Lisa Jacobs

and oxaliplatin). Continue until disease progression or unacceptable toxicity.

Dose Modification

Infusion Reactions

Mild to moderate reactions: Reduce infusion rate by 50% for remainder of infusion. **Severe reactions:** Discontinue infusion. Depending on severity, consider permanent discontinuation.

Skin Toxicity

For all CTCAE grade 3 skin toxicities, withhold treatment for 1–2 doses until improved to better than grade 3. Then, reduce dose as follows: **First occurrence of CTCAE grade 3:** Resume at same dose. **Second occurrence of CTCAE grade 3:** Reduce dose to 80% of initial dose. **Third occurrence of CTCAE grade 3:** Reduce dose to 60% of initial dose. **Fourth occurrence of CTCAE grade 3:** Permanently discontinue.

Dosage in Renal/Hepatic Impairment

No dose adjustment.

SIDE EFFECTS

Common (65%–57%): Erythema, acneiform dermatitis, pruritus. **Frequent** (26%–20%): Fatigue, abdominal pain, skin exfoliation, paronychia (soft tissue infection around nailbed), nausea, rash, diarrhea, constipation, skin fissures. **Occasional** (19%–10%): Vomiting, acne, cough, peripheral edema, dry skin. **Rare** (7%–2%): Stomatitis, mucosal inflammation, eyelash growth, conjunctivitis, increased lacrimation.

ADVERSE EFFECTS/TOXIC REACTIONS

Pulmonary fibrosis, severe dermatologic toxicity (complicated by infectious sequelae) occur

manifested as ...otension oc... urs in 39% ...tal bullous ...rted. Severe ...ease risk of ...nlight may ... cause ocular toxicities including keratitis, ulcerative keratitis, corneal ulceration.

NURSING CONSIDERATIONS

BASELINE ASSESSMENT

Assess serum magnesium, calcium prior to therapy, periodically during therapy, and for 8 wks after completion of therapy. Assess *KRAS* mutational status in colorectal tumors and confirm the absence of a *RAS* mutation.

INTERVENTION/EVALUATION

Assess for skin, ocular, mucosal, pulmonary toxicity; report effects. Median time to development of skin/ocular toxicity is 14–15 days; resolution after last dosing is 84 days. Monitor serum electrolytes for hypomagnesemia, hypocalcemia. Offer antiemetic if nausea/vomiting occurs. Monitor daily pattern of bowel activity, stool consistency.

PATIENT/FAMILY TEACHING

• Do not have immunizations without physician's approval (drug lowers resistance). • Avoid contact with those who have recently received a live virus vaccine. • Avoid crowds, those with infection. • There is a potential risk for development of fetal abnormalities if pregnancy occurs; take measures to prevent pregnancy. • Report skin reactions, including rash, sloughing, blisters, erosions. • Report difficulty breathing, fever with cough, lung pain; may indicate life-threatening lung inflammation. • Limit sun, UV exposure. Wear protective sunscreen, hats, and clothing while outdoors.

P

Side Effects section in each drug monograph specifies the frequency of particular side effects.

Adverse Reactions highlight the particularly dangerous side effects.

High Alert drugs are shaded in blue for easy identification.

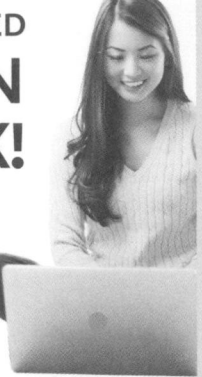

Saunders

NURSING DRUG HANDBOOK 2022

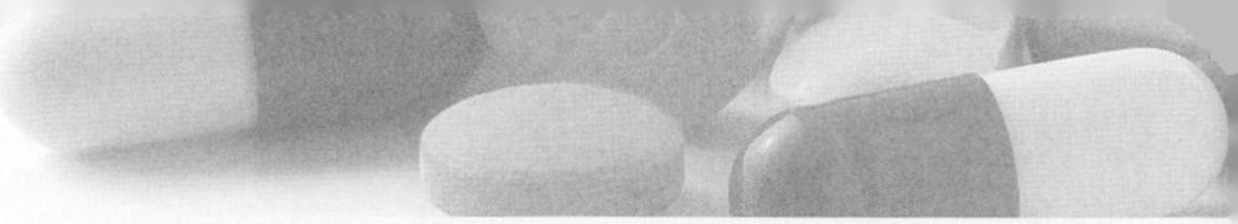

Saunders

NURSING DRUG HANDBOOK 2022

ROBERT J. KIZIOR, BS, RPH
Department of Pharmacy
Alexian Brothers Medical Center
Elk Grove Village, Illinois

KEITH J. HODGSON, RN, BSN, CCRN
Staff Nurse, Intensive Care Unit
Former Staff Nurse, Emergency Department
St. Joseph's Hospital
Tampa, Florida

ELSEVIER

Elsevier
3251 Riverport Lane
St. Louis, Missouri 63043

SAUNDERS NURSING DRUG HANDBOOK 2022 ISBN: 978-0-323-79890-7
ISSN: 1098-8661

Notice

Practitioners and researchers must always rely on their own experience and knowledge in evaluating and using any information, methods, compounds, or experiments described herein. Because of rapid advances in the medical sciences, in particular, independent verification of diagnoses and drug dosages should be made. To the fullest extent of the law, no responsibility is assumed by Elsevier, authors, editors, or contributors for any injury and/or damage to persons or property as a matter of products liability, negligence, or otherwise, or from any use or operation of any methods, products, instructions, or ideas contained in the material herein.

International Standard Book Number: 978-0-323-79890-7

Executive Content Strategist: Sonya Seigafuse
Senior Content Development Manager: Lisa Newton
Senior Content Development Specialist: Tina Kaemmerer
Publishing Services Manager: Catherine Jackson
Senior Project Manager/Specialist: Carrie Stetz
Design Direction: Bridget Hoette

Printed in China

Last digit is the print number: 9 8 7 6 5 4 3 2

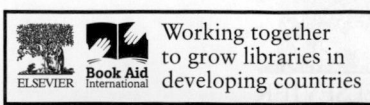

CONTENTS

AUTHOR BIOGRAPHIES

Robert (Bob) J. Kizior, BS, RPh

Bob graduated from the University of Illinois School of Pharmacy and is licensed to practice in the state of Illinois. He has worked as a hospital pharmacist for more than 40 years at Alexian Brothers Medical Center in Elk Grove Village, Illinois—a suburb of Chicago. Bob is the Pharmacy Surgery Coordinator for the Department of Pharmacy, where he participates in educational programs for pharmacists, nurses, physicians, and patients. He plays a major role in coordinating pharmacy services in the OR satellite. Bob is a former adjunct faculty member at William Rainey Harper Community College in Palatine, Illinois.

An avid sports fan, Bob also has eclectic tastes in music that range from classical, big band, rock 'n' roll, and jazz to country and western. Bob spends much of his free time reviewing the professional literature to stay current on new drug information.

Keith J. Hodgson, RN, BSN, CCRN

Keith was born into a loving family in Chicago, Illinois. His mother, Barbara B. Hodgson, was an author and publisher of several medication products, and her work has been a part of his life since he was a child. By the time he was 4 years old, Keith was already helping his mother with the drug cards by stacking the draft pages that were piled up throughout their home.

Because of his mother's influence, Keith contemplated becoming a nurse in college, but his mind was fully made up after he shadowed his sister in the Emergency Department. Keith received his Associates Degree in Nursing from Hillsborough Community College and his Bachelor of Science in Nursing from the University of South Florida in Tampa, Florida. Keith started his career in the Emergency Department and now works in the Trauma/Neurological/Surgical Intensive Care Unit at St. Joseph's Hospital in Tampa, Florida.

Keith's favorite interests include music, reading, Kentucky basketball, and, if he gets the chance, watching every minute of the Olympic Games.

REVIEWERS

James Graves, PharmD
Clinical Pharmacist
University of Missouri Hospital
Columbia, Missouri

Joshua J. Neumiller, PharmD, CDCES, FADCES, FASCP
Vice-Chair & Allen I. White Distinguished Associate Professor
Department of Pharmacotherapy
College of Pharmacy and Pharmaceutical Sciences
Washington State University
Spokane, Washington

CONSULTANTS*

Katherine B. Barbee, MSN, ANP, F-NP-C
Kaiser Permanente
Washington, District of Columbia

Marla J. DeJong, RN, MS, CCRN, CEN, Capt
Wilford Hall Medical Center
Lackland Air Force Base, Texas

Diane M. Ford, RN, MS, CCRN
Andrews University
Berrien Springs, Michigan

Denise D. Hopkins, PharmD
College of Pharmacy
University of Arkansas
Little Rock, Arkansas

Barbara D. Horton, RN, MS
Arnot Ogden Medical Center School of Nursing
Elmira, New York

Mary Beth Jenkins, RN, CCRN, CAPA
Elliott One Day Surgery Center
Manchester, New Hampshire

Kelly W. Jones, PharmD, BCPS
McLeod Family Medicine Center
McLeod Regional Medical Center
Florence, South Carolina

Linda Laskowski-Jones, RN, MS, CS, CCRN, CEN
Christiana Care Health System
Newark, Delaware

Jessica K. Leet, RN, BSN
Cardinal Glennon Children's Hospital
St. Louis, Missouri

Denise Macklin, BSN, RNC, CRNI
President, Professional Learning Systems, Inc.
Marietta, Georgia

Judith L. Myers, MSN, RN
Health Sciences Center
St. Louis University School of Nursing
St. Louis, Missouri

Kimberly R. Pugh, MSEd, RN, BS
Nurse Consultant
Baltimore, Maryland

Regina T. Schiavello, BSN, RNC
Wills Eye Hospital
Philadelphia, Pennsylvania

Gregory M. Susla, PharmD, FCCM
National Institutes of Health
Bethesda, Maryland

*The authors acknowledge the work of the consultants in previous editions.

ACKNOWLEDGMENTS

I would like to thank my co-author Bob Kizior for his knowledge, experience, support, and friendship. We would like to give special thanks to Sonya Seigafuse, Charlene Ketchum, Carrie Stetz, Tina Kaemmerer, and the entire Elsevier team for their superior dedication, hard work, and belief in us. Without this wonderful team, none of this would be possible.

Keith J. Hodgson, RN, BSN, CCRN

DEDICATION

I dedicate my work to the practicing nurse, those aspiring to become nurses, and to all health care professionals who are dedicated to the art and science of healing.

Bob Kizior, BS, RPh

I dedicate this work to my wife, Jen Hodgson, the love of my life; my sister, Lauren, a foundation for our family; my sister, Kathryn, for her love and support; my father, David Hodgson, the best father a son could have; my brothers-in-law, Andy and Nick, great additions to the family; the grandchildren, Paige Olivia, Logan James, Ryan James, and Dylan Boyd; and to my band of brothers, Peter, Jamie, Miguel, Ritch, George, Jon, Domingo, Ben, Craig, Pat, and Shay.

We also make a special dedication to Barbara B. Hodgson, RN, OCN. She truly was a piece of something wonderful. Barbara often gave her love and support without needing any in return and would do anything for a smile. Not only was she a colleague and a friend, she was also a small business owner, an artist, a dreamer, and an innovator. We hope the pride we offer in her honor comes close to what she always gave us. Her dedication and perseverance lives on.

Keith J. Hodgson, RN, BSN, CCRN

BIBLIOGRAPHY

Lexi-Comp's Drug Information Handbook, ed 29, Hudson, OH, 2020–2021, Lexi-Comp.

Medical Letter on Drugs and Therapeutics: 2019–2020, *Pharmacists Letter*: 2020.

Takemoto CK, Hodding JH, Kraus DM: *Lexi-Comp's Pediatric Dosage Handbook*, ed 26, Hudson, OH, 2019–2020, Lexi-Comp.

Trissel LA: *Handbook of Injectable Drugs*, ed 19, Bethesda, MD, 2016, American Society of Health-System Pharmacists.

ILLUSTRATION CREDITS

Kee JL, Hayes ER, McCuiston LE, editors: *Pharmacology: A Nursing Process Approach*, ed 7, Philadelphia, 2012, Saunders.

NEWLY APPROVED MEDICATIONS

Alpelisib (Piqray)	A kinase inhibitor for advanced or metastatic breast cancer
Avapritinib (Ayvakit)	A kinase inhibitor for advanced gastrointestinal stromal tumor (GIST)
Bempedoic acid (Nexletol)	An adenosine triphosphate–citrate lyase inhibitor for hypercholesterolemia
Capmatinib (Tabrecta)	A kinase inhibitor for metastatic non–small-cell lung cancer
Cenobamate (Xcopri)	An anticonvulsant for partial-onset seizures
Daratumumab/hyaluronidase-fihj) (Darzalex Faspro)	Combination antibody and hyaluronidase for multiple myeloma
Darolutamide (Nubeqa)	An oral androgen receptor inhibitor for nonmetastatic castration-resistant prostate cancer
Diroximel fumarate (Vumerity)	An oral capsule for treatment of multiple sclerosis
Elexacaftor/tezacaftor/ivacaftor (Trikafta)	Combination product for cystic fibrosis
Enfortumab vedotin-ejfv (Padcev)	A monoclonal antibody for advanced urothelial cancer
Entrectinib (Rozlytrek)	A kinase inhibitor for metastatic non–small-cell lung cancer and certain solid tumors
Eptinezumab-jjmr (Vyepti)	A calcitonin gene–related peptide receptor antagonist prevention of migraine
Esketamine (Spravato)	An NMDA receptor antagonist nasal spray for treatment-resistant depression
Fam-trastuzumab deruxtecan-nxki (Enhertu)	A monoclonal antibody/topoisomerase inhibitor for HER2-positive breast cancer
Isatuximab-irfc (Sarclisa)	A monoclonal antibody for multiple myeloma
Lumateperone (Caplyta)	An atypical antipsychotic for schizophrenia
Ozanimod (Zeposia)	An oral sphingosine 1-phosphate receptor modulator for relapsing forms of multiple sclerosis
Polatuzumab vedotin-piiq (Polivy)	A monoclonal antibody for relapsed or refractory diffuse large B-cell lymphoma
Rimegepant (Nurtec ODT)	A calcitonin gene–related peptide receptor antagonist for acute treatment of migraine
Ripretinib (Qinlock)	A kinase inhibitor for advanced gastrointestinal stromal tumor (GIST)
Sacituzumab govitecan-hziy (Trodelvy)	A monoclonal antibody for advanced breast cancer
Selinexor (Xpovio)	A nuclear export inhibitor of relapsed or refractory multiple myeloma

Selpercatinib (Retevmo)	A kinase inhibitor for metastatic non–small-cell lung cancer
Trastuzumab/hyaluronidase (Herceptin Hylecta)	A subcutaneous injection formulation for HER2-overexpressing breast cancer
Tucatinib (Tukysa)	A kinase inhibitor for advanced breast cancer
Ubrogepant (Ubrelvy)	A calcitonin gene–related peptide receptor antagonist for acute treatment of migraine
Upadacitinib (Rinvoq)	A Janus kinase inhibitor for moderate to severe rheumatoid arthritis
Zanubrutinib (Brukinsa)	A kinase inhibitor for mantle cell lymphoma

PREFACE

Nurses are faced with the ever-challenging responsibility of ensuring safe and effective drug therapy for their patients. Not surprisingly, the greatest challenge for nurses is keeping up with the overwhelming amount of new drug information, including the latest FDA-approved drugs and changes to already approved drugs, such as new uses, dosage forms, warnings, and much more. Nurses must integrate this information into their patient care quickly and in an informed manner.

Saunders Nursing Drug Handbook 2022 is designed as an easy-to-use source of current drug information to help the busy nurse meet these challenges. What separates this book from others is that it guides the nurse through patient care to better practice and better care. This handbook contains the following:

1. **An IV compatibility chart.** This handy chart is bound into the handbook to prevent accidental loss.
2. **The Drug Classifications section.** The action and uses for some of the most common clinical and pharmacotherapeutic classes are presented. Unique to this handbook, each class provides an at-a-glance table that compares all the generic drugs within the classification according to product availability, dosages, side effects, and other characteristics. Its half-page color tab ensures you can't miss it!
3. **An alphabetical listing of drug entries by generic name.** Blue letter thumb tabs help you page through this section quickly. Information on medications that contain a Black Box Alert is an added feature of the drug entries. This alert identifies those medications for which the FDA has issued a warning that the drugs may cause serious adverse effects. Tall Man lettering, with emphasis on certain syllables to avoid confusing similar sounding/looking medications, is shown in capitalized letters (e.g., oxy**CODONE**). High Alert drugs with a color icon HIGH ALERT are considered dangerous by The Joint Commission and the Institute for Safe Medication Practices (ISMP) because if they are administered incorrectly, they may cause life-threatening or permanent harm to the patient. The entire High Alert generic drug entry sits on a shaded background so that it's easy to spot! To make scanning pages easier, each new entry begins with a shaded box containing the generic name, pronunciation, trade name(s), fixed combination(s), and classification(s).
4. **A comprehensive reference section.** Appendixes include vital information on calculation of doses; controlled drugs; chronic wound care; drugs of abuse; equianalgesic dosing; herbals: common natural medicines; lifespan, cultural aspects, and pharmacogenomics of drug therapy; normal laboratory values; drug interactions; antidotes or reversal agents; preventing medication errors; parenteral fluid administration; and Common Terminology Criteria for Adverse Events (CTCAE).
5. **Drugs by Disorder.** You'll find Drugs by Disorder in the front of the book for easy reference. It lists common disorders and the drugs most often used for treatment.
6. **The index.** The comprehensive index is located at the back of the book on light blue pages. Undoubtedly the best tool to help you navigate the handbook, the comprehensive index is organized by showing generic drug names in **bold,** trade names in regular type, classifications in *italics,* and the page number of the main drug entry listed first and in **bold.**

A DETAILED GUIDE TO THE SAUNDERS NURSING DRUG HANDBOOK

An intensive review by consultants and reviewers helped us to revise the **Saunders Nursing Drug Handbook** so that it is most useful in both educational and clinical practice. The main objective of the handbook is to provide essential drug information in a user-friendly format. The bulk of the handbook contains an alphabetical listing of drug entries by generic name.

To maintain the portability of this handbook and meet the challenge of keeping content current, we have also included additional information for some medications on the Evolve® Internet site. Users can also choose from 100 monographs for the most commonly used medications and customize and print drug cards. Evolve® also includes drug alerts (e.g., medications removed from the market) and drug updates (e.g., new drugs, updates on existing entries). Information is periodically added, allowing the nurse to keep abreast of current drug information.

We have incorporated the IV Incompatibilities/Compatibilities heading. The drugs listed in this section are compatible or incompatible with the generic drug when administered directly by IV push, via a Y-site, or via IV piggyback. We have highlighted the intravenous drug administration and handling information with a special heading icon and have broken it down by Reconstitution, Rate of Administration, and Storage.

We present entries in an order that follows the logical thought process the nurse undergoes whenever a drug is ordered for a patient:

- What is the drug?
- How is the drug classified?
- What does the drug do?
- What is the drug used for?
- Under what conditions should you **not** use the drug?
- How do you administer the drug?
- How do you store the drug?
- What is the dose of the drug?
- What should you monitor the patient for once he or she has received the drug?
- What do you assess the patient for?
- What interventions should you perform?
- What should you teach the patient?

The following are included within the drug entries:

Generic Name, Pronunciation, Trade Names. Each entry begins with the generic name and pronunciation, followed by the U.S. and Canadian trade names. Exclusively Canadian trade names are followed by a maple leaf ✱. Trade names that were most prescribed in the year 2019 are underlined in this section.
Black Box Alert. This feature highlights drugs that carry a significant risk of serious or life-threatening adverse effects. Black Box Alerts are ordered by the FDA.
Do Not Confuse With. Drug names that sound similar to the generic and/or trade names are listed under this heading to help you avoid potential medication errors.
Fixed-Combination Drugs. Where appropriate, fixed-combinations, or drugs made up of two or more generic medications, are listed with the generic drug.
Pharmacotherapeutic and **Clinical Classification Names.** Each entry includes both the pharmacotherapeutic and clinical classifications for the generic drug.
Action/Therapeutic Effect. This section describes how the drug is predicted to behave, with the expected therapeutic effect(s) under a separate heading.
Pharmacokinetics. This section includes the absorption, distribution, metabolism, excretion, and half-life of the medication. The half-life is bolded in blue for easy access.

Uses/Off-Label. The listing of uses for each drug includes both the FDA uses and the off-label uses. The off-label heading is shown in bold blue for emphasis.
Precautions. This heading incorporates a discussion about when the generic drug is contraindicated or should be used with caution. The cautions warn the nurse of specific situations in which a drug should be closely monitored.
Lifespan Considerations ⌛. This section includes pregnancy/lactation data and age-specific information concerning children and elderly people.
Interactions. This heading enumerates drug, food, and herbal interactions with the generic drug. As the number of medications a patient receives increases, awareness of drug interactions becomes more important. Also included is information about therapeutic and toxic blood levels in addition to effects the drug may have on lab results.
Product Availability. Each drug monograph gives the form and availability of the drug. The icon identifies noncrushable drug forms.
Administration/Handling. Instructions for administration are given for each route of administration (e.g., IV, IM, PO, rectal). Special handling, such as refrigeration, is also included where applicable. The routes in this section are always presented in the order IV, IM, SQ, and PO, with subsequent routes in alphabetical order (e.g., Ophthalmic, Otic, Topical). **IV administration** is broken down by reconstitution, rate of administration (how fast the IV should be given), and storage (including how long the medication is stable once reconstituted).
IV Incompatibilities/IV Compatibilities. These sections give the nurse the most comprehensive compatibility information possible when administering medications by direct IV push, via a Y-site, or via IV piggyback.
Indications/Routes/Dosage. Each entry provides specific dosing guidelines for adults, elderly, children, and patients with renal and/or hepatic impairment. Dose modification for toxicity has been added where applicable. Dosages are clearly indicated for each approved indication and route.
Side Effects. Side effects are defined as those responses that are usually predictable with the drug, are **not** life-threatening, and may or may not require discontinuation of the drug. Unique to this handbook, side effects are grouped by frequency listed from highest occurrence percentage to lowest so that the nurse can focus on patient care without wading through myriad signs and symptoms of side effects.
Adverse Effects/Toxic Reactions. Adverse effects and toxic reactions are very serious and often life-threatening undesirable responses that require prompt intervention from a health care provider.
Nursing Considerations. Nursing considerations are organized as care is organized:

- What needs to be assessed or done before the first dose is administered? (Baseline Assessment)
- What interventions and evaluations are needed during drug therapy? (Intervention/Evaluation)
- What teaching is needed for the patient and family? (Patient/Family Teaching)

Saunders Nursing Drug Handbook is an easy-to-use source of current drug information for nurses, students, and other health care providers. It is our hope that this handbook will help you provide quality care to your patients.

We welcome any comments to improve future editions of the handbook. Please contact us via the publisher at *http://evolve.elsevier.com/SaundersNDH*.

Robert J. Kizior, BS, RPh
Keith J. Hodgson, RN, BSN, CCRN

DRUGS BY DISORDER

Note: Not all medications appropriate for a given condition are listed, nor are those not listed inappropriate.

Generic names appear first, followed by brand names in parentheses.

Alcohol dependence
Acamprosate (Campral)
Disulfiram (Antabuse)
Naltrexone (Depade, ReVia, Vivitrol)

Allergic conjunctivitis
Alcaftadine (Lastacaft)
Azelastine – generic
Bepotastine (Bepreve)
Cetirizine (Zerviate)
Cromolyn – generic
Emedastine (Emadine)
Epinastine (Elestat)
Ketorolac (Acular)
Ketotifen (Alaway, Zaditor)
Lodoxamide (Alomide)
Loteprednol (Alrex, Lotemax)
Nedocromil (Alocril)
Olopatadine (Pataday, Patanol, Pazeo)
Prednisone (Pred Mild)

Allergic rhinitis
Nasal spray
Azelastine (Astelin, Astepro)
Azelastine/fluticasone (Dymista)
Beclomethasone (Beconase AQ, Qnasl)
Budesonide (Rhinocort Allergy Spray)
Ciclesonide (Omnaris, Zetonna)
Flunisolide
Fluticasone (Flonase Sensimist Allergy Relief)
Mometasone (Nasonex)
Nasal spray
Olopatadine (Patanase)
Triamcinolone (Nasacort Allergy 24 HR)
Oral form
Cetirizine (Zyrtec Allergy)
Cetirizine/pseudoephedrine (Zyrtec-D 12 hour)
Desloratadine (Clarinex)
Desloratadine/pseudoephedrine (Clarinex-D 12 hour)
Fexofenadine (Allegra)
Fexofenadine/pseudoephedrine (Allegra-D 12 hour, Allegra-D 24 hour)
Levocetirizine (Xyzal Allergy 24 hour)
Loratadine (Alavert, Claritin)
Loratadine/pseudoephedrine (Alavert-D 12 hour, Claritin-D 12 hour, Claritin-D 24 hour)
Montelukast (Singulair)

Alzheimer's disease
Acetylcholinesterase inhibitors
Donepezil (Aricept)
Galantamine (Razadyne)
Rivastigmine (Exelon Patch)
NMDA receptor antagonist
Memantine (Namenda)
NMDA receptor antagonist/ acetylcholinesterase inhibitor
Namzaric

Angina
Amlodipine (Norvasc)
Atenolol (Tenormin)
Diltiazem (Cardizem, Dilacor)
Isosorbide (Imdur, Isordil)
Metoprolol (Lopressor)
Nadolol (Corgard)
Nicardipine (Cardene)
Nifedipine (Adalat, Procardia)
Nitroglycerin
Propranolol (Inderal)
Verapamil (Calan, Isoptin)

Anxiety
Alprazolam (Xanax)
Buspirone (BuSpar)
Diazepam (Valium)

Hydroxyzine (Atarax, Vistaril)
Lorazepam (Ativan)
Oxazepam (Serax)
Paroxetine (Paxil)
Trazodone (Desyrel)
Venlafaxine (Effexor)

Arrhythmias
Adenosine (Adenocard)
Amiodarone (Cordarone, Pacerone)
Digoxin (Lanoxin)
Diltiazem (Cardizem, Dilacor)
Disopyramide (Norpace)
Dofetilide (Tikosyn)
Dronedarone (Multaq)
Esmolol (Brevibloc)
Flecainide (Tambocor)
Ibutilide (Corvert)
Lidocaine
Metoprolol (Lopressor)
Mexiletine (Mexitil)
Propafenone (Rythmol)
Propranolol (Inderal)
Sotalol (Betapace)
Verapamil (Calan, Isoptin)

Arthritis, rheumatoid
Conventional DMARDs
Hydroxychloroquine (Plaquenil)
Leflunomide (Arava)
Methotrexate (Otrexup, Rasuvo, Trexall)
Sulfasalazine (Azulfidine)
Biologic agents
TNF inhibitors
Adalimumab (Humira)
Certolizumab pegol (Cimzia)
Etanercept (Enbrel)
Golimumab (Simponi, Simponi Aria)
Infliximab (Remicade, Inflectra, Renflexis)
IL-6 inhibitors
Sarilumab (Kevzara)
Tocilizumab (Actemra)
Other biologic agents
Abatacept (Orencia)
Anakinra (Kineret)
Rituximab (Rituxan)
JAK inhibitors
Baricitinib (Olumiant)
Tofacitinib (Xeljanz, Xeljanz XR)
Upadacitinib (Rincoq)

Asthma
Short-acting beta-2 agonists (SABA)
Albuterol (ProAir HFA, Proventil HFA, Ventolin HFA, ProAir RespiClick)
Levalbuterol (Xopenex HFA)
Short-acting muscarinic antagonists (SAMA)
Ipratropium (Atrovent HFA)
Inhaled corticosteroids
Beclomethasone (QVAR)
Budesonide (Pulmicort)
Ciclesonide (Alvesco)
Flunisolide (Aerospan)
Fluticasone (Arnuity Ellipta, Flovent Diskus)
Mometasone (Asmanex)
Long-acting beta-2 agonists (LABA)
Formoterol (Perforomist)
Salmeterol (Serevent)
Inhaled corticosteroid/LABA combinations
Budesonide/formoterol (Symbicort)
Fluticasone/vilanterol (Breo Ellipta)
Fluticasone/Salmeterol (Advair, AirDuo RespiClick)
Mometasone, formoterol (Dulera)
Inhaled long-acting muscarinic antagonist (LAMA)
Tiotropium (Spiriva)

Atrial fibrillation
Oral anticoagulants
Vitamin K antagonist
Warfarin (Coumadin)
Direct thrombin inhibitor
Dabigatran (Pradaxa)
Direct factor Xa inhibitors
Apixaban (Eliquis)
Edoxaban (Savaysa)
Rivaroxaban (Xarelto)
Rate control
Beta adrenergic blockers
Atenolol (Tenormin)
Bisoprolol
Carvedilol (Coreg, Coreg CR)
Metoprolol (Lopressor, Toprol XL)
Nadolol (Corgard)
Propranolol (Inderal LA, InnoPran XL)
Calcium channel blockers

Diltiazem (Cardizem CD, Cartia XT, Taztia XT, Tiazac)
Verapamil (Calan, Verelan)
Other
Amiodarone (Pacerone)
Digoxin (Digitek, Lanoxin)
Rhythm control
Amiodarone (Pacerone)
Dronedarone (Multaq)
Dofetilide (Tikosyn)
Flecainide
Propafenone (Rythmol SR)
Sotalol (Betapace, Sotalol AF)

Attention-deficit hyperactivity disorder (ADHD)
Amphetamine (Adzenys XR-ODT, Dyanavel XR)
Atomoxetine (Strattera)
Clonidine (Catapres, Kapvay)
Desipramine (Norpramin)
Dexmethylphenidate (Focalin, Focalin XR)
Dextroamphetamine (Dexedrine, ProCentra, Zenzedi)
Guanfacine (Intuniv)
Lisdexamfetamine (Vyvanse)
Methylphenidate (Aptensio XR, Concerta, Cotempla XR-ODT, Daytrana, Focalin, Focalin XR, Jornay PM, Metadate CD, Methylin, QuilliChew ER, Quillivant XR, Ritalin)
Mixed amphetamine (dextroamphetamine and amphetamine salts) (Adderall, Adderall XR, Mydayis)

Benign prostatic hypertrophy (BPH)
Alfuzosin (Uroxatral)
Doxazosin (Cardura)
Dutasteride (Avodart)
Fesoterodine (Toviaz)
Finasteride (Proscar)
Mirabegron (Myrbetriq)
Silodosin (Rapaflo)
Tadalafil (Cialis)
Tamsulosin (Flomax)
Terazosin (Hytrin)
Tolterodine (Detrol)

Bipolar disorder
Aripiprazole (Abilify)
Asenapine (Saphris)
Carbamazepine (Tegretol)
Lamotrigine (Lamictal)
Lithium (Lithobid)
Lurasidone (Latuda)
Olanzapine (Zyprexa)
Olanzapine/fluoxetine (Symbyax)
Oxcarbazepine (Trileptal)
Paliperidone (Invega)
Quetiapine (Seroquel)
Risperidone (Risperdal)
Valproic acid (Depakene, Depakote)
Ziprasidone (Geodon)

Bladder hyperactivity
Darifenacin (Enablex)
Oxybutynin (Ditropan, Gelnique)
Solifenacin (VESIcare)
Tolterodine (Detrol)
Trospium (Sanctura)

Bronchospasm
Albuterol (Proventil, Ventolin)
Bitolterol (Tornalate)
Levalbuterol (Xopenex)
Metaproterenol (Alupent)
Salmeterol (Serevent)
Terbutaline (Brethine)

Cancer
Abarelix (Plenaxis)
Abemaciclib (Verzenio)
Abiraterone (Zytiga)
Acalabrutinib (Calquence)
Ado-trastuzumab (Kadcyla)
Afatinib (Gilotrif)
Aldesleukin (Proleukin)
Alemtuzumab (Campath)
Alitretinoin (Panretin)
Altretamine (Hexalen)
Anastrozole (Arimidex)
Apalutamide (Erleada)
Alpelisib (Piqray)
Arsenic trioxide (Trisenox)
Asparaginase (Elspar)
Atezolizumab (Tecentriq)
Avapritinib (Ayvakit)
Avelumab (Bavencio)
Axitinib (Inlyta)
Azacitidine (Vidaza)
BCG (TheraCys, Tice BCG)
Belinostat (Beleodaq)

Bendamustine (Treanda)
Bevacizumab (Avastin)
Bexarotene (Targretin)
Bicalutamide (Casodex)
Binimetinib (Mektovi)
Bleomycin (Blenoxane)
Blinatumomab (Blincyto)
Bortezomib (Velcade)
Bosutinib (Bosulif)
Brentuximab (Adcetris)
Brigatinib (Alunbrig)
Busulfan (Myleran)
Cabazitaxel (Jevtana)
Capmatinib (Tabrecta)
Cabozantinib (Cabometyx)
Capecitabine (Xeloda)
Carboplatin (Paraplatin)
Carfilzomib (Kyprolis)
Carmustine (BiCNU)
Ceritinib (Zykadia)
Cetuximab (Erbitux)
Chlorambucil (Leukeran)
Cisplatin (Platinol)
Cladribine (Leustatin)
Clofarabine (Clolar)
Cobimetinib (Cotellic)
Copanlisib (Aliqopa)
Crizotinib (Xalkori)
Cyclophosphamide (Cytoxan)
Cytarabine (Ara-C, Cytosar)
Dabrafenib (Tafinlar)
Dacarbazine (DTIC)
Dacomitinib (Vizimpro)
Dactinomycin (Cosmegen)
Daratumumab (Darzalex)
Daratumumab/hyaluronidase (Darzalex Faspro)
Darolutamide (Nubeqa)
Dasatinib (Sprycel)
Daunorubicin (Cerubidine, DaunoXome)
Degarelix (Firmagon)
Denileukin (Ontak)
Dinutuximab (Unituxin)
Docetaxel (Taxotere)
Doxorubicin (Adriamycin, Doxil)
Durvalumab (Imfinzi)
Duvelisib (Copiktra)
Elotuzumab (Empliciti)
Enasidenib (IDHIFA)
Encorafenib (Braftovi)
Enfortumab vedotin (Padcev)
Entrectinib (Rozlytrek)
Enzalutamide (Xtandi)
Epirubicin (Ellence)
Erdafitinib (Balversa)
Eribulin (Halaven)
Erlotinib (Tarceva)
Estramustine (Emcyt)
Etoposide (VePesid)
Everolimus (Afinitor)
Fam-trastuzumab (Enhertu)
Fludarabine (Fludara)
Fluorouracil
Flutamide (Eulexin)
Fulvestrant (Faslodex)
Gefitinib (Iressa)
Gemcitabine (Gemzar)
Gilteritinib (Xospata)
Glasdegib (Daurismo)
Goserelin (Zoladex)
Hydroxyurea (Hydrea)
Ibritumomab (Zevalin)
Ibrutinib (Imbruvica)
Idarubicin (Idamycin)
Idelalisib (Zydelig)
Ifosfamide (Ifex)
Imatinib (Gleevec)
Inotuzumab ozogamicin (Besponsa)
Interferon alfa-2b (Intron A)
Ipilimumab (Yervoy)
Irinotecan (Camptosar)
Isatuximab (Sarclisa)
Ivosidenib (Tibsovo)
Ixabepilone (Ixempra)
Ixazomib (Ninlaro)
Lapatinib (Tykerb)
Larotrectinib (Vitrakvi)
Letrozole (Femara)
Leuprolide (Lupron)
Lenvatinib (Lenvima)
Lomustine (CeeNU)
Lorlatinib (Lorbrena)
Mechlorethamine (Mustargen)
Megestrol (Megace)
Melphalan (Alkeran)
Mercaptopurine (Purinethol)
Methotrexate
Midostaurin (Rydapt)
Mitomycin (Mutamycin)
Mitotane (Lysodren)
Mitoxantrone (Novantrone)
Moxetumomab (Lumoxiti)

Necitumumab (Portrazza)
Nelarabine (Arranon)
Neratinib (Nerlynx)
Nilotinib (Tasigna)
Nilutamide (Nilandron)
Niraparib (Zejula)
Nivolumab (Opdivo)
Obinutuzumab (Gazyva)
Ofatumumab (Arzerra)
Olaparib (Lynparza)
Olaratumab (Lartruvo)
Omacetaxine (Synribo)
Osimertinib (Tagrisso)
Oxaliplatin (Eloxatin)
Paclitaxel (Taxol)
Palbociclib (Ibrance)
Panitumumab (Vectibix)
Panobinostat (Farydak)
Pazopanib (Votrient)
Pegaspargase (Oncaspar)
Pembrolizumab (Keytruda)
Pemetrexed (Alimta)
Pentostatin (Nipent)
Pertuzumab (Perjeta)
Plicamycin (Mithracin)
Polatuzumab (Polivy)
Pomalidomide (Pomalyst)
Ponatinib (Iclusig)
Pralatrexate (Folotyn)
Procarbazine (Matulane)
Ramucirumab (Cyramza)
Rasburicase (Elitek)
Regorafenib (Stivarga)
Ribociclib (Kisqali)
Ripretinib (Qinlock)
Rituximab (Rituxan)
Rituximab/hyaluronidase (Rituxan Hycela)
Romidepsin (Istodax)
Rucaparib (Rubraca)
Sacitumumab (Trodelvy)
Selinexor (Xpovio)
Selpercatinib (Retevmo)
Sipuleucel-T (Provenge)
Sonidegib (Odomzo)
Sorafenib (Nexavar)
Streptozocin (Zanosar)
Sunitinib (Sutent)
Talazoparib (Talzenna)
Tamoxifen (Nolvadex)
Temozolomide (Temodar)
Temsirolimus (Torisel)
Teniposide (Vumon)
Thioguanine
Thiotepa (Thioplex)
Tipifarnib (Zarnestra)
Tipiracil/trifluridine (Lonsurf)
Tisagenlecleucel (Kymriah)
Topotecan (Hycamtin)
Toremifene (Fareston)
Tositumomab (Bexxar)
Trabectedin (Yondelis)
Trametinib (Mekinist)
Trastuzumab (Herceptin)
Trastuzumab/hyaluronidase (Herceptin Hylecta)
Tretinoin (ATRA, Vesanoid)
Tucatinib (Tukysa)
Valrubicin (Valstar)
Vandetanib (Caprelsa)
Vemurafenib (Zelboraf)
Venetoclax (Venclexta)
Vinblastine (Velban)
Vincristine (Oncovin)
Vinorelbine (Navelbine)
Vismodegib (Erivedge)
Vorinostat (Zolinza)
Zanubrutinib (Brukinsa)
Ziv-aflibercept (Zaltrap)

Cerebrovascular accident (CVA)

Aspirin
Clopidogrel (Plavix)
Heparin
Nimodipine (Nimotop)
Prasugrel (Effient)
Warfarin (Coumadin)

Chronic obstructive pulmonary disease (COPD)

Inhaled short-acting antimuscarinic

Ipratropium (Atrovent HFA)

Inhaled short-acting Beta-2 agonists (SABA)

Albuterol (ProAir HFA, Proventil HFA, Ventolin HFA)
Levalbuterol (Xopenex HFA)

Inhaled short-acting Beta-2 agonist (SABA)/short-acting antimuscarinic (SAMA)

Albuterol/Ipratropium (Combivent Respimat)

Inhaled long-acting Beta-2 agonists (LABA)
Arformoterol (Brovana)
Indacaterol (Arcapta Neohaler)
Olodaterol (Striverdi Respimat)
Salmeterol (Serevent Diskus)
Formoterol (Perforomist)
Inhaled long-acting antimuscarinic agents (LAMA)
Aclidinium (Tudorza Pressair)
Glycopyrrolate (Seebri Neohaler)
Revefenacin (Yupelri)
Tiotropium (Spiriva Respimat)
Umeclidinium (Incruse Ellipta)
Inhaled long-acting Beta-2 agonists (LABA)/long-acting antimuscarinic agents (LAMA)
Glycopyrrolate/formoterol (Bevespi)
Glycopyrrolate/indacaterol (Utibron Neohaler)
Tiotropium/olodaterol (Stiolto Respimat)
Umeclidinium/vilanterol (Anoro Ellipta)
Inhaled corticosteroids
Beclomethasone (QVAR)
Budesonide (Pulmicort)
Ciclesonide (Alvesco)
Flunisolide (Aerospan HFA)
Fluticasone (Flovent Diskus, Flovent HFA)
Mometasone (Asmanex HFA, Asmanex Twisthaler)
Inhaled corticosteroids/long-acting Beta-2 agonists (LABA)
Fluticasone/salmeterol (Advair Diskus)
Fluticasone/vilanterol (Breo Ellipta)
Budesonide/formoterol (Symbicort)
Inhaled corticosteroids/long-acting Beta-2 agonists (LABA)/long-acting antimuscarinic agents (LAMA)
Fluticasone/vilanterol/umeclidinium (Trelegy Ellipta)

Constipation
Bisacodyl (Dulcolax)
Docusate (Colace)
Lactulose (Kristalose)
Lubiprostone (Amitiza)
Methylcellulose (Citrucel)
Milk of magnesia (MOM)
Polyethylene glycol (MiraLAX)
Psyllium (Metamucil)
Senna (Senokot)

Crohn's disease
Azathioprine
Adalimumab (Humira)
Certolizumab (Cimzia)
Corticosteroids
Infliximab (Inflectra, Remicade)
6-Mercaptopurine
Ustekinumab (Stelara)
Vedolizumab (Entyvio)

Deep vein thrombosis (DVT)
Dalteparin (Fragmin)
Edoxaban (Savaysa)
Enoxaparin (Lovenox)
Heparin
Tinzaparin (Innohep)
Warfarin (Coumadin)

Depression
SSRIs
Citalopram (Celexa)
Escitalopram (Lexapro)
Fluoxetine (Prozac, Prozac Weekly)
Paroxetine (Paxil, Paxil CR)
Sertraline (Zoloft)
SNRIs
Desvenlafaxine (Pristiq, Khedezla)
Duloxetine (Cymbalta)
Venlafaxine (Effexor XR)
Levomilnacipran (Fetzima)
TCAs
Amitriptyline (Elavil)
Nortriptyline (Pamelor)
MAOIs
Phenelzine (Nardil)
Selegiline (Emsam)
Other
Bupropion (Wellbutrin SR, Aplenzin, Forfivo XL)
Esketamine (Spravato)
Mirtazapine (Remeron, Remeron SolTab)
Trazodone (Oleptro)
Vilazodone (Viibryd)
Vortioxetine (Trintellix)

Diabetes
Biguanides
Metformin (Glucophage, Glucophage XR, Glumetza, Fortamet, Riomet)
Sulfonylureas
Glimepiride (Amaryl, Glipizide, Glucotrol, Glucotrol XL)

Glyburide (Glynase)
GLP-1 receptor agonists
Albiglutide (Tanzeum)
Dulaglutide (Trulicity)
Exenatide (Byetta, Bydureon)
Liraglutide (Victoza)
Lixisenatide (Adlyxin)
Semaglutide (Ozempic)
DDP-4 inhibitors
Alogliptin (Nesina)
Linagliptin (Tradjenta)
Saxagliptin (Onglyza)
Sitagliptin (Januvia)
SGLT2 inhibitors
Canagliflozin (Invokana)
Dapagliflozin (Farxiga)
Empagliflozin (Jardiance)
Ertugliflozin (Steglatro)
Meglitinides
Nateglinide (Starlix)
Repaglinide (Prandin)
Thiazolidinediones
Pioglitazone (Actos)
Rosiglitazone (Avandia)
Alpha-glucosidase inhibitors
Acarbose (Precose)
Miglitol (Glyset)
Other
Colesevelam (Welchol)
Bromocriptine (Cycloset)
Pramlintide (Symlin)
Insulin
Rapid-acting
Insulin aspart (Fiasp, Novolog)
Insulin glulisine (Apidra)
Insulin lispro (Admelog, Humalog)
Insulin inhalation powder (Afrezza)
Regular insulin
Humulin R
Novolin R
Intermediate insulin
NPH (Humulin N, Novolin N)
Long-acting insulin
Insulin detemir (Levemir)
Insulin glargine (Lantus, Toujeo, Basaglar)
Insulin degludec (Tresiba)

Diabetic peripheral neuropathy
Amitriptyline (Elavil)
Bupropion (Wellbutrin)
Capsaicin (Trixaicin)
Carbamazepine (Tegretol)
Citalopram (Celexa)
Desipramine (Norpramin)
Duloxetine (Cymbalta)
Gabapentin (Neurontin)
Lamotrigine (Lamictal)
Lidocaine patch (Lidoderm)
Nortriptyline (Pamelor)
Oxcarbazepine (Trileptal)
Oxycodone (OxyContin)
Paroxetine (Paxil)
Pregabalin (Lyrica)
Tramadol (Ultram)
Valproic acid (Depakote)
Venlafaxine, extended-release (Effexor XR)

Diarrhea
Bismuth subsalicylate (Pepto-Bismol)
Diphenoxylate and atropine (Lomotil)
Fidaxomicin (Dificid)
Kaolin-pectin (Kaopectate)
Loperamide (Imodium)
Octreotide (Sandostatin)
Rifaximin (Xifaxan)

Edema
Amiloride (Midamor)
Bumetanide (Bumex)
Chlorthalidone (Hygroton)
Ethacrynic acid (Edecrin)
Furosemide (Lasix)
Hydrochlorothiazide (Hydrodiuril)
Indapamide (Lozol)
Metolazone (Zaroxolyn)
Spironolactone (Aldactone)
Torsemide (Demadex)
Triamterene (Dyrenium)

Epilepsy
Brivaracetam (Briviact)
Carbamazepine (Tegretol)
Cenobamate (Xcopri)
Clobazam (Onfi)
Clonazepam (Klonopin)
Clorazepate (Tranxene)
Diazepam (Valium)
Eslicarbazepine (Aptiom)
Ethosuximide (Zarontin)
Ezogabine (Potiga)

Fosphenytoin (Cerebyx)
Gabapentin (Neurontin)
Lacosamide (Vimpat)
Lamotrigine (Lamictal, Lamictal ODT, Lamictal XR)
Levetiracetam (Keppra)
Lorazepam (Ativan)
Midazolam (Versed)
Oxcarbazepine (Trileptal)
Perampanel (Fycompa)
Phenobarbital
Phenytoin (Dilantin)
Pregabalin (Lyrica)
Primidone (Mysoline)
Rufinamide (Banzel)
Tiagabine (Gabitril)
Topiramate (Qudexy XR, Topamax, Trokendi XR)
Valproic acid (Depakene, Depakote)
Vigabatrin (Sabril)
Zonisamide (Zonegran)

Esophageal reflux, esophagitis
Cimetidine (Tagamet)
Dexlansoprazole (Dexilant)
Esomeprazole (Nexium)
Famotidine (Pepcid)
Lansoprazole (Prevacid)
Nizatidine (Axid)
Omeprazole (Prilosec)
Pantoprazole (Protonix)
Rabeprazole (AcipHex)
Ranitidine (Zantac)

Fever
Acetaminophen (Tylenol)
Aspirin
Ibuprofen (Advil, Caldolor, Motrin)
Naproxen (Aleve, Anaprox, Naprosyn)

Fibromyalgia
Acetaminophen (Tylenol)
Amitriptyline (Elavil)
Carisoprodol (Soma)
Citalopram (Celexa)
Cyclobenzaprine (Flexeril)
Duloxetine (Cymbalta)
Fluoxetine (Prozac)
Gabapentin (Neurontin)
Milnacipran (Savella)
Paroxetine (Paxil)
Pregabalin (Lyrica)
Tramadol (Ultram)
Venlafaxine (Effexor)

Gastric/duodenal ulcer
Cimetidine (Tagamet)
Esomeprazole (Nexium)
Famotidine (Pepcid)
Lansoprazole (Prevacid)
Nizatidine (Axid)
Omeprazole (Prilosec)
Pantoprazole (Protonix)
Rabeprazole (AcipHex)
Ranitidine (Zantac)
Sucralfate (Carafate)

Gastritis
Cimetidine (Tagamet)
Famotidine (Pepcid)
Nizatidine (Axid)
Ranitidine (Zantac)

Gastroesophageal reflux disease (GERD)
H_2 receptor antagonists
Cimetidine (Tagamet HB)
Famotidine (Pepcid)
Nizatidine
Ranitidine (Zantac)
Proton pump inhibitors (PPIs)
Dexlansoprazole (Dexilant)
Esomeprazole (Nexium)
Lansoprazole (Prevacid)
Omeprazole (Prilosec)
Rabeprazole (AcipHex)

Glaucoma
Acetazolamide (Diamox)
Apraclonidine (Iopidine)
Betaxolol (Betoptic)
Bimatoprost (Lumigan)
Brimonidine (Alphagan)
Brinzolamide (Azopt)
Carbachol
Dorzolamide (Trusopt)
Echothiophate iodide (Phospholine)
Latanoprost (Xalatan)
Levobunolol (Betagan)
Pilocarpine (Isopto Carpine)
Tafluprost (Zioptan)

Timolol (Timoptic)
Travoprost (Travatan)
Unoprostone (Rescula)

Gout
Anti-inflammatory agents
Anakinra (Kineret)
Canakinumab (Ilaris)
Colchicine (Colcrys, Mitigare)
Ibuprofen (Motrin)
Naproxen (Naprosyn)
Prednisone
Urate-lowering agents
Allopurinol (Zyloprim)
Febuxostat (Uloric)
Probenecid
Pegloticase (Krystexxa)

Heart failure
Angiotensin-converting enzyme (ACE) inhibitors
Captopril
Enalapril (Vasotec)
Fosinopril
Lisinopril (Prinivil, Zestril)
Quinapril (Accupril)
Ramipril (Altace)
Angiotensin receptor blockers (ARBs)
Candesartan (Atacand)
Losartan (Cozaar)
Valsartan (Diovan)
Angiotensin receptor-neprilysin inhibitor
Sacubitril/valsartan (Entresto)
Beta adrenergic blockers
Bisoprolol
Carvedilol (Coreg)
Metoprolol succinate (Toprol XL)
Cardiac glycoside
Digoxin (Digitek, Lanoxin)
Diuretics (loop)
Bumetanide (Bumex)
Furosemide (Lasix)
Torsemide (Demadex)
HCN channel blocker
Ivabradine (Corlanor)
Mineralocorticoid receptor antagonists
Eplerenone (Inspra)
Spironolactone (Aldactone)
Vasodilators
Isosorbide/hydralazine (BiDil)

Hepatitis B
Adefovir (Hepsera)
Entecavir (Baraclude)
Lamivudine (Epivir)
Peginterferon alpha-2a (Pegasys)
Telbivudine (Tyzeka)
Tenofovir (Viread)

Hepatitis C
Daclatasvir (Daklinza)
Elbasvir/grazoprevir (Zepatier)
Glecaprevir/pibrentasvir (Mavyret)
Ledipasvir/sofosbuvir (Harvoni)
Ombitasvir/paritaprevir/ritonavir (Technivie)
Ombitasvir/paritaprevir/ritonavir/dasabuvir (Viekira Pak)
Peginterferon alfa-2a (Pegasys)
Peginterferon alfa-2b (Pegintron)
Ribavirin (Copegus, Rebetol, Ribasphere)
Simeprevir (Olysio)
Sofosbuvir (Sovaldi)
Sofosbuvir/velpatasvir (Epclusa)
Sofosbuvir/velpatasvir/voxilaprevir (Vosevi)

Human immunodeficiency virus (HIV)
Abacavir/dolutegravir/lamivudine (Triumeq)
Abacavir (Ziagen)
Atazanavir (Reyataz)
Bictegravir/emtricitabine/tenofovir alafenamide (Biktarvy)
Cobicistat (Tybost)
Darunavir (Prezista)
Delavirdine (Rescriptor)
Didanosine (Videx)
Dolutegravir (Tivicay)
Dolutegravir/lamivudine (Dovato)
Doravirine (Pifeltro)
Doravirine/lamivudine/tenofovir (Delstrigo)
Efavirenz (Sustiva)
Efavirenz/lamivudine/tenofovir disoproxil (Symfi)
Elvitegravir (Vitekta)
Elvitegravir/cobicistat/emtricitabine, tenofovir (Genova/Stribild)

Emtricitabine (Emtriva)
Emtricitabine/tenofovir (Truvada)
Enfuvirtide (Fuzeon)
Etravirine (Intelence)
Fosamprenavir (Lexiva)
Ibalizumab-uiyk (Trogarzo)
Indinavir (Crixivan)
Lamivudine (Epivir)
Lamivudine/tenofovir (Cimduo)
Lopinavir/ritonavir (Kaletra)
Maraviroc (Selzentry)
Nelfinavir (Viracept)
Nevirapine (Viramune)
Raltegravir (Isentress)
Rilpivirine (Edurant)
Ritonavir (Norvir)
Saquinavir (Invirase)
Stavudine (Zerit)
Tenofovir (Viread)
Tesamorelin (Egrifta)
Tipranavir (Aptivus)
Zidovudine (AZT, Retrovir)

Hyperphosphatemia
Aluminum salts
Calcium salts
Ferric citrate (Auryxia)
Lanthanum (Fosrenol)
Sevelamer (Renagel)

Hypertension
Thiazide diuretics
Hydrochlorothiazide
Loop diuretics
Bumetanide (Bumex)
Furosemide (Lasix)
Aldosterone antagonists
Eplerenone (Inspra)
Spironolactone (Aldactone)
ACE inhibitors
Benazepril (Lotensin)
Enalapril (Vasotec)
Lisinopril (Zestril, Prinivil)
Quinapril (Accupril)
Ramipril (Altace)
ARBs
Azilsartan (Edarbi)
Candesartan (Atacand)
Irbesartan (Avapro)
Losartan (Cozaar)
Valsartan (Diovan)
Calcium channel blockers dihydropyridines
Amlodipine (Norvasc)
Nifedipine (Adalat CC, Procardia XL)
Nondihydropyridines
Diltiazem (Cardizem LA, Taztia XT)
Verapamil (Calan)
Beta blockers
Atenolol (Tenormin)
Carvedilol (Coreg, Coreg CR)
Labetalol
Metoprolol (Lopressor, Toprol XL)
Nebivolol (Bystolic)
Central alpha-adrenergic agonists
Clonidine (Catapres)
Direct vasodilators
Hydralazine (Apresoline)

Hypertriglyceridemia
Atorvastatin (Lipitor)
Colesevelam (Welchol)
Fenofibrate (Tricor)
Fluvastatin (Lescol)
Gemfibrozil (Lopid)
Icosapent (Vascepa)
Lovastatin (Mevacor)
Niacin (Niaspan)
Omega-3 acid ethyl esters (Lovaza)
Pravastatin (Pravachol)
Rosuvastatin (Crestor)
Simvastatin (Zocor)

Hyperuricemia
Allopurinol (Zyloprim)
Febuxostat (Uloric)
Pegloticase (Krystexxa)
Probenecid (Benemid)

Hypotension
Dobutamine (Dobutrex)
Dopamine (Intropin)
Ephedrine
Epinephrine
Norepinephrine (Levophed)
Phenylephrine (Neo-Synephrine)

Hypothyroidism
Levothyroxine (Levoxyl, Synthroid)
Liothyronine (Cytomel)
Thyroid

Idiopathic thrombocytopenic purpura (ITP)
Cyclophosphamide (Cytoxan)
Dexamethasone (Decadron)
Hydrocortisone (Solu-Cortef)
Immune globulin intravenous
Methylprednisolone (Solu-Medrol)
Prednisone
Rh_0(D) immune globulin (RhoGAM)
Rituximab (Rituxan)

Inflammatory bowel disease (Crohn's disease, ulcerative colitis)
Aminosalicylates
Mesalamine: Oral: (Apriso, Asacol HD, Delzicol, Lialda, Pentasa); Rectal: (Rowasa, Canasa)
5-ASA pro-drugs
Balsalazide (Colazal, Giazo)
Olsalazine (Dipentum)
Sulfasalazine (Azulfidine)
Corticosteroids
Budesonide (Entocort EC, Uceris)
Hydrocortisone (Colocort, Cortenema)
Prednisone (Rayos)
Immunosuppressants
Azathioprine (Azasan, Imuran)
Cyclosporine (Sandimmune)
Mercaptopurine (Purixan)
Methotrexate (Otrexup, Rasuvo)
TNF inhibitors
Adalimumab (Humira)
Certolizumab pegol (Cimzia)
Golimumab (Simponi, Simponi Aria)
Infliximab (Remicade, Inflectra, Renflexis)
Integrin receptor antagonists
Natalizumab (Tysabri)
Vedolizumab (Entyvio)
Interleukin antagonist
Ustekinumab (Stelara)
JAK inhibitor
Tofacitinib (Xeljanz)

Insomnia
Benzodiazepine receptor agonists
Eszopiclone (Lunesta)
Zaleplon (Sonata)
Zolpidem (Ambien, Zolpimist, Edluar, Intermezzo)
Benzodiazepines
Estazolam
Flurazepam (Dalmane)
Lorazepam (Ativan)
Temazepam (Restoril)
Melatonin receptor agonist
Ramelteon (Rozerem)
Orexin receptor antagonist
Suvorexant (Belsomra)

Irritable bowel syndrome with constipation
Chloride channel activator
lubiprostone (Amitiza)
Guanylate cyclase-C receptor agonist
Linaclotide (Linzess)

Irritable bowel syndrome with diarrhea
Antibiotic
Rifaximin (Xifaxan)
Mu-opioid receptor agonist/ delta-opioid receptor antagonist
Eluxadoline (Viberzi)
5-HT modulators
Alosetron (Lotronex)
Ondansetron (Zofran)

Lipid disorders
Statins
Atorvastatin (Lipitor)
Fluvastatin (Lescol)
Lovastatin (Altoprev)
Pitavastatin (Livalo)
Pravastatin (Pravachol)
Rosuvastatin (Crestor)
Simvastatin (Zocor)
Cholesterol absorption inhibitor
Ezetimibe (Zetia)
PCSK9 inhibitors
Alirocumab (Praluent)
Evolocumab (Repatha)
Bile acid sequestrants
Colesevelam (Welchol)
Colestipol (Colestid)
Cholestyramine (Questran)
Fibrates
Gemfibrozil (Lopid)

Fenofibrate (Lipofen, Lofibra, Tricor, Antara, Fibricor, Trilipix)

Fish oil

Icosapent ethyl (Vascepa)
Omega-3 acid ethyl esters (Lovaza)

Migraine prevention

Eptinezumab (Vyepti)
Erenumab-aooe (Aimovig)
Fremanezumab (Ajovy)
Galcanezumab-gnlm (Emgality)

Migraine treatment

Almotriptan (Axert)
Dihydroergotamine (DHE 45, Migranal)
Eletriptan (Relpax)
Ergotamine/caffeine (Cafergot)
Frovatriptan (Frova)
Naratriptan (Amerge)
Rimegepant (Nurtec)
Rizatriptan (Maxalt)
Sumatriptan (Imitrex)
Ubrogepant (Ubrelvy)
Zolmitriptan (Zomig, Zomig-ZMT)

Multiple sclerosis (MS)

Alemtuzumab (Lemtrada)
Daclizumab (Zinbryta)
Dalfampridine (Ampyra)
Dimethyl fumarate (Tecfidera)
Diroximel (Vumerity)
Fingolimod (Gilenya)
Glatiramer (Copaxone)
Interferon beta-1a (Avonex, Rebif)
Interferon beta-1b (Betaseron, Extavia)
Mitoxantrone (Novantrone)
Natalizumab (Tysabri)
Ocrelizumab (Ocrevus)
Peginterferon beta-la (Plegridy)
Siponimod (Mayzent)
Teriflunomide (Aubagio)

Myelodysplastic syndrome

Azacitidine (Vidaza)
Clofarabine (Clolar)
Decitabine (Dacogen)
Lenalidomide (Revlimid)

Myocardial infarction (MI)

Alteplase (Activase)
Aspirin
Atenolol (Tenormin)
Captopril (Capoten)
Clopidogrel (Plavix)
Dalteparin (Fragmin)
Diltiazem (Cardizem, Dilacor)
Enalapril (Vasotec)
Enoxaparin (Lovenox)
Heparin
Lidocaine
Lisinopril (Prinivil, Zestril)
Metoprolol (Lopressor)
Morphine
Nitroglycerin
Propranolol (Inderal)
Quinapril (Accupril)
Ramipril (Altace)
Reteplase (Retavase)
Warfarin (Coumadin)

Nausea

Aprepitant (Emend)
Chlorpromazine (Thorazine)
Dexamethasone (Decadron)
Dimenhydrinate (Dramamine)
Dronabinol (Marinol)
Droperidol (Inapsine)
Fosaprepitant (Emend)
Fosnetupitant/palonosetron (Akynzeo)
Granisetron (Kytril)
Hydroxyzine (Vistaril)
Lorazepam (Ativan)
Meclizine (Antivert)
Metoclopramide (Reglan)
Nabilone (Cesamet)
Ondansetron (Zofran)
Ozanimod (Zeposia)
Palonosetron (Aloxi)
Prochlorperazine (Compazine)
Promethazine (Phenergan)
Rolapitant (Varubi)

Obsessive-compulsive disorder (OCD)

Citalopram (Celexa)
Clomipramine (Anafranil)
Escitalopram (Lexapro)
Fluoxetine (Prozac)
Fluvoxamine (Luvox)
Paroxetine (Paxil)
Sertraline (Zoloft)

Organ transplant, rejection prophylaxis
Azathioprine (Imuran)
Basiliximab (Simulect)
Belatacept (Nulojix)
Cyclophosphamide (Cytoxan, Neosar)
Cyclosporine (Sandimmune)
Daclizumab (Zenapax)
Everolimus (Zortress)
Mycophenolate (CellCept)
Sirolimus (Rapamune)
Tacrolimus (Prograf)

Osteoarthritis
Acetaminophen (Tylenol)
Celecoxib (Celebrex)
Diclofenac (Cataflam, Pennsaid, Voltaren)
Duloxetine (Cymbalta)
Etodolac (Lodine)
Flurbiprofen (Ansaid)
Ibuprofen (Motrin)
Ketoprofen (Orudis)
Meloxicam (Mobic)
Nabumetone (Relafen)
Naproxen (Naprosyn)
Sulindac (Clinoril)
Tramadol (Ultram)

Osteoporosis
Bisphosphonates
Alendronate (Binosto, Fosamax)
Ibandronate (Boniva)
Risedronate (Actonel, Atelvia)
Zoledronic acid (Reclast)
Anti-RANK ligand antibody
Denosumab (Prolia)
Parathyroid hormone receptor agonists
Abaloparatide (Tymlos)
Teriparatide (Forteo)
Sclerostin inhibitor
Romosozumab (Evenity)
Selective estrogen receptor modulator (SERM)
Raloxifene
Conjugated estrogens/bazedoxifene (Duavee)
Calcitonin
Miacalcin injection
Nasal spray (generic)

Paget's disease
Alendronate (Fosamax)
Calcitonin (Miacalcin)
Etidronate (Didronel)
Pamidronate (Aredia)
Risedronate (Actonel)
Tiludronate (Skelid)
Zoledronic acid (Reclast)

Pain, mild to moderate
Acetaminophen (Tylenol)
Aspirin
Celecoxib (Celebrex)
Codeine
Diclofenac (Cataflam, Voltaren, Zipsor)
Diflunisal (Dolobid)
Etodolac (Lodine)
Flurbiprofen (Ansaid)
Ibuprofen (Advil, Caldolor, Motrin)
Ketorolac (Toradol)
Naproxen (Anaprox, Naprosyn)
Salsalate (Disalcid)
Tramadol (Ultram)

Pain, moderate to severe
Butorphanol (Stadol)
Fentanyl (Onsolis, Sublimaze)
Hydromorphone (Dilaudid)
Methadone (Dolophine)
Morphine (MS Contin)
Morphine/naltrexone (Embeda)
Nalbuphine (Nubain)
Oxycodone (OxyFast, Roxicodone)
Oxymorphone (Opana)
Ziconotide (Prialt)

Panic attack disorder
Alprazolam (Xanax)
Clonazepam (Klonopin)
Paroxetine (Paxil)
Sertraline (Zoloft)
Venlafaxine (Effexor)

Parkinson's disease
Carbidopa/levodopa
Immediate-release (Sinemet)
Orally disintegrating
Sustained-release (Sinemet CR)
Extended-release (Rytary)
Intrajejunal infusion (Duopa)
Dopamine agonists

Apomorphine (Apokyn)
Pramipexole (Mirapex)
Ropinirole (Requip)
Rotigotine (Neupro)
COMT inhibitors
Entacapone (Comtan)
Tolcapone (Tasmar)
MAO-B inhibitors
Rasagiline (Azilect)
Safinamide (Xadago)
Selegiline (Eldepryl, Zelapar)

Peptic ulcer disease
H_2 receptor antagonists
Cimetidine (Tagamet HB)
Famotidine (Pepcid)
Nizatidine
Ranitidine (Zantac)
Proton pump inhibitors (PPIs)
Dexlansoprazole (Dexilant)
Esomeprazole (Nexium)
Lansoprazole (Prevacid)
Omeprazole (Prilosec)
Rabeprazole (AcipHex)

Pneumonia
Amoxicillin (Amoxil)
Amoxicillin/clavulanate (Augmentin)
Ampicillin (Polycillin)
Azithromycin (Zithromax)
Cefaclor (Ceclor)
Cefpodoxime (Vantin)
Ceftriaxone (Rocephin)
Cefuroxime (Kefurox, Zinacef)
Clarithromycin (Biaxin)
Co-trimoxazole (Bactrim, Septra)
Erythromycin
Gentamicin (Garamycin)
Levofloxacin (Levaquin)
Linezolid (Zyvox)
Moxifloxacin (Avelox)
Piperacillin/tazobactam (Zosyn)
Tobramycin (Nebcin)
Vancomycin (Vancocin)

Pneumonia, *pneumocystis jirovecii*
Atovaquone (Mepron)
Clindamycin (Cleocin)
Co-trimoxazole (Bactrim, Septra)
Pentamidine (Pentam)
Trimethoprim (Proloprim)

Post-traumatic stress disorder (PTSD)
Amitriptyline (Elavil)
Aripiprazole (Abilify)
Citalopram (Celexa)
Escitalopram (Lexapro)
Fluoxetine (Prozac)
Imipramine (Tofranil)
Lamotrigine (Lamictal)
Olanzapine (Zyprexa)
Paroxetine (Paxil)
Phenelzine (Nardil)
Prazosin (Minipress)
Propranolol (Inderal)
Quetiapine (Seroquel)
Risperidone (Risperdal)
Sertraline (Zoloft)
Topiramate (Topamax)
Valproic acid (Depakote)
Venlafaxine (Effexor)
Ziprasidone (Geodon)

Pruritus
Amcinonide (Cyclocort)
Cetirizine (Zyrtec)
Clemastine (Tavist)
Clobetasol (Temovate)
Cyproheptadine (Periactin)
Desloratadine (Clarinex)
Desonide (Tridesilon)
Desoximetasone (Topicort)
Diphenhydramine (Benadryl)
Fluocinolone (Synalar)
Fluocinonide (Lidex)
Halobetasol (Ultravate)
Hydrocortisone (Cort-Dome, Hytone)
Hydroxyzine (Atarax, Vistaril)
Prednisolone (Prelone)
Prednisone (Deltasone)
Promethazine (Phenergan)

Psoriasis
Vitamin D analogs
Calcipotriene (Dovonex, Sorilux)
Calcitriol (Vectical)
Retinoids
Acitretin (Soriatane)
Tazarotene (Tazorac)
Phosphodiesterase 4 (PDE4) inhibitor
Apremilast (Otezla)
Immunosuppressants

Cyclosporine (Neoral)
Methotrexate (Otrexup, Rasuvo)
TNF inhibitors
Adalimumab (Humira)
Certolizumab pegol (Cimzia)
Etanercept (Enbrel)
Infliximab (Remicade, Inflectra, Renflexis)
IL 12-23 antagonist
Ustekinumab (Stelara)
IL 17A antagonists
Brodalumab (Siliq)
Ixekizumab (Taltz)
Secukinumab (Cosentyx)
IL 23 antagonists
Guselkumab (Tremfya)
Risankizumab (Skyrizi)
Tildrakizumab (Ilumya)

Psychotic disorders
Aripiprazole (Abilify)
Asenapine (Saphris)
Brexpiprazole (Rexulti)
Cariprazine (Vraylar)
Chlorpromazine (Thorazine)
Clozapine (Clozaril)
Fluphenazine (Prolixin)
Haloperidol (Haldol)
Iloperidone (Fanapt)
Loxapine (Adasuve)
Lumateperone (Caplyta)
Lurasidone (Latuda)
Olanzapine (Zyprexa, Zyprexa Zydis)
Paliperidone (Invega)
Pimavanserin (Nuplazid)
Quetiapine (Seroquel, Seroquel XR)
Risperidone (Risperdal)
Thioridazine (Mellaril)
Thiothixene (Navane)
Ziprasidone (Geodon)

Pulmonary arterial hypertension
Ambrisentan (Letairis)
Bosentan (Tracleer)
Epoprostenol (Flolan)
Iloprost (Ventavis)
Macitentan (Opsumit)
Riociguat (Adempas)
Selexipag (Uptravi)
Sildenafil (Revatio)
Tadalafil (Adcirca)
Treprostinil (Remodulin, Tyvaso)

Respiratory distress syndrome (RDS)
Beractant (Survanta)
Calfactant (Infasurf)
Poractant alfa (Curosurf)

Restless legs syndrome
Cabergoline (Dostinex)
Carbamazepine (Tegretol)
Carbidopa/levodopa (Sinemet)
Clonazepam (Klonopin)
Gabapentin (Horizant, Neurontin)
Levodopa
Pramipexole (Mirapex)
Pregabalin (Lyrica)
Ropinirole (Requip)
Rotigotine (Neupro)

Schizophrenia
Aripiprazole (Abilify)
Asenapine (Saphris)
Brexpiprazole (Rexulti)
Cariprazine (Vraylar)
Chlorpromazine (Thorazine)
Clozapine (Clozaril)
Fluphenazine (Prolixin)
Haloperidol (Haldol)
Iloperidone (Fanapt)
Lumateperone (Caplyta)
Lurasidone (Latuda)
Olanzapine (Zyprexa, Zyprexa Zydis)
Paliperidone (Invega, Invega Sustenna)
Quetiapine (Seroquel, Seroquel XR)
Risperidone (Risperdal)
Thioridazine (Mellaril)
Thiothixene (Navane)
Ziprasidone (Geodon)

Smoking cessation
Bupropion (Zyban)
Nicotine (NicoDerm, Nicotrol)
Varenicline (Chantix)

Thrombosis
Apixaban (Eliquis)
Dalteparin (Fragmin)
Edoxaban (Savaysa)
Enoxaparin (Lovenox)
Fondaparinux (Arixtra)
Heparin

Tinzaparin (Innohep)
Warfarin (Coumadin)

Thyroid disorders
Levothyroxine (Levoxyl, Synthroid)
Liothyronine (Cytomel)
Thyroid

Transient ischemic attack (TIA)
Aspirin
Clopidogrel (Plavix)
Prasugrel (Effient)
Warfarin (Coumadin)

Tremor
Atenolol (Tenormin)
Chlordiazepoxide (Librium)
Diazepam (Valium)
Lorazepam (Ativan)
Metoprolol (Lopressor)
Nadolol (Corgard)
Propranolol (Inderal)

Tuberculosis (TB)
Bedaquiline (Sirturo)
Cycloserine (Seromycin)
Ethambutol (Myambutol)
Isoniazid (INH)
Pyrazinamide
Rifabutin (Mycobutin)
Rifampin (Rifadin)
Rifapentine (Priftin)

Urticaria
Cetirizine (Zyrtec)
Cimetidine (Tagamet)
Clemastine (Tavist)
Cyproheptadine (Periactin)
Diphenhydramine (Benadryl)
Hydroxyzine (Atarax, Vistaril)
Loratadine (Claritin)
Promethazine (Phenergan)
Ranitidine (Zantac)

Vertigo
Dimenhydrinate (Dramamine)
Diphenhydramine (Benadryl)
Meclizine (Antivert)
Scopolamine (Trans-Derm Scop)

Vomiting
Aprepitant (Emend)
Chlorpromazine (Thorazine)
Dexamethasone (Decadron)
Dimenhydrinate (Dramamine)
Dronabinol (Marinol)
Droperidol (Inapsine)
Fosaprepitant (Emend)
Granisetron (Kytril)
Hydroxyzine (Vistaril)
Lorazepam (Ativan)
Meclizine (Antivert)
Metoclopramide (Reglan)
Nabilone (Cesamet)
Ondansetron (Zofran)
Palonosetron (Aloxi)
Prochlorperazine (Compazine)
Promethazine (Phenergan)
Rolapitant (Varubi)
Scopolamine (Trans-Derm Scop)
Trimethobenzamide (Tigan)

Weight management
Sympathomimetic amines
Benzphetamine
Diethylpropion
Phendimetrazine
Phentermine (Adipex, Lomaira)
Phentermine/topiramate (Qsymia)
Lipase inhibitor
Orlistat (Alli, Xenical)
Serotonin receptor agonist
Lorcaserin (Belviq)
Opioid antagonist/antidepressant
Naltrexone/bupropion (Contrave)
GLP-1 receptor agonist
Liraglutide (Saxenda)

Zollinger-Ellison syndrome
Aluminum salts
Cimetidine (Tagamet)
Esomeprazole (Nexium)
Famotidine (Pepcid)
Lansoprazole (Prevacid)
Omeprazole (Prilosec)
Pantoprazole (Protonix)
Rabeprazole (AcipHex)
Ranitidine (Zantac)

DRUG CLASSIFICATION CONTENTS

Beta-Adrenergic Blockers

USES

Management of hypertension, angina pectoris, arrhythmias, hypertrophic subaortic stenosis, migraine headaches, MI (prevention), glaucoma.

ACTION

Beta-adrenergic blockers competitively block beta adrenergic receptors, located primarily in myocardium, and $beta_2$-adrenergic receptors, located primarily in bronchial and vascular smooth muscle. By occupying beta-receptor sites, these agents prevent naturally occurring or administered epinephrine/norepinephrine from exerting their effects. The results are basically opposite to those of sympathetic stimulation.

Effects of $beta_1$ blockade include slowing heart rate, decreasing cardiac output and contractility; effects of $beta_2$ blockade include bronchoconstriction, increased airway resistance in pts with asthma or COPD. Beta blockers can affect cardiac rhythm/automaticity (decrease sinus rate, SA/AV conduction; increase refractory period in AV node); decrease systolic and diastolic B/P; exact mechanism unknown but may block peripheral receptors, decrease sympathetic outflow from CNS, or decrease renin release from kidney. All beta blockers mask tachycardia that occurs with hypoglycemia. When applied to the eye, reduce intraocular pressure and aqueous production.

BETA-ADRENERGIC BLOCKERS

Name	Availability	Indication	Dosage Range	Frequent or Severe Side Effects
Acebutolol (Sectral)	**C:** 200 mg, 400 mg	HTN, ventricular arrhythmia	**HTN:** Initially, 400 mg once daily or 2 divided doses. Usual dose: 200–1200 mg once/d or divided bid **Arrhythmia:** Initially, 200 mg 2 times/day. Gradually increase to 300–600 mg 2 times/day	**Class:** Fatigue, depression, bradycardia, decreased exercise tolerance, erectile dysfunction, heart failure, may aggravate hypoglycemia, increase incidence of diabetes, insomnia, increase triglycerides, decrease cholesterol. Sudden withdrawal may exacerbate angina and myocardial infarction.

Atenolol (Tenormin)	**T:** 25 mg, 50 mg, 100 mg	HTN, angina, MI	**Angina:** Initially, 50 mg once daily. May increase to 100 mg once daily after one wk **HTN:** Initially, 50 mg once daily. May increase to 100 mg once daily after 2 wks **MI:** 50 mg bid or 100 mg once daily	
Bisoprolol (Zebeta)	**T:** 5 mg, 10 mg	HTN	Initially, 5 mg once daily. May increase to 10 mg/day, then 20 mg/day. Usual dose: 5–10 mg/day	
Carvedilol (Coreg)	**T:** 3.125 mg, 6.25 mg, 12.5 mg, 25 mg **C (SR):** 10 mg, 20 mg, 40 mg, 80 mg	HF, LVD after MI, HTN	**Immediate-Release HF:** Initially, 3.25 mg 2 times/day. May increase at 2-wk intervals to 6.25 mg 2 times/day, then 12.5 mg 2 times/day, then 25 mg 2 times/day **LVD after MI:** Initially, 6.25 mg 2 times/day. May increase q3–10 days to 12.5 mg 2 times/day, then 25 mg 2 times/day **HTN:** Initially, 6.25 mg 2 times/day. May increase q7–14 days to 12.5 mg 2 times/day, then 25 mg 2 times/day **Extended-Release HF:** 10–80 mg once daily **LVD after MI:** 10–80 mg once daily **HTN:** 20–80 mg once daily	
Labetalol (Trandate)	**T:** 100 mg, 200 mg, 300 mg	HTN	Initially, 100 mg 2 times/day. May increase q2–3 days in 100 mg 2 times/day increments Usual dose: 200–1,200 mg 2 times/day	

Continued

BETA-ADRENERGIC BLOCKERS—cont'd

Metoprolol (Lopressor [IR], Toprol XL [SR])	**T (IR)**: 50 mg, 100 mg **T (SR)**: 25 mg, 50 mg	HTN, angina, HF, MI	**IR:** **Angina**: Initially, 50 mg 2 times/day. May increase up to 400 mg/day **HTN**: Initially, 100 mg once daily. May increase at weekly intervals up to 450 mg/divided bid or tid **Post-MI**: 100 mg bid **SR:** **Angina**: 100–400 mg once daily **HF**: 12.5–200 mg once daily **HTN**: 25–400 mg once daily	
Nadolol (Corgard)	**T**: 20 mg, 40 mg, 80 mg	HTN, angina	**Angina, HTN**: Initially, 40 mg once/day. Usual dose: 40–320 mg once daily	
Nebivolol (Bystolic)	**T**: 2.5 mg, 5 mg, 10 mg, 20 mg	HTN	Initially, 5 mg once daily. May increase at 2-wk intervals up to 40 mg once daily	
Pindolol (Visken)	**T**: 5 mg, 10 mg	HTN	Initially, 5 mg 2 times/day. May increase to 10–40 mg/day. **Maximum:** 60 mg/day divided bid	

Name	Availability	Indication	Dosage Range	Frequent or Severe Side Effects
Propranolol (Inderal)	**T (IR)**: 10 mg, 20 mg, 40 mg, 60 mg, 80 mg **C (SR)**: 60 mg, 80 mg, 120 mg, 160 mg **S**: 4 mg/mL, 8 mg/mL **I**: 1 mg/mL	HTN, angina, MI, arrhythmias, migraine, essential tremor, hypertrophic subaortic stenosis	**IR:** **Angina**: 80–320 mg/day in 2–4 divided doses **Arrhythmias**: 10–30 mg 3–4 times/day **HTN**: 40 mg bid up to 240 mg/day in 2–3 divided doses **Hypertrophic subaortic stenosis:** 20–40 mg 3–4 times/day **Post-MI**: 180–240 mg/day in 2–4 divided doses **Migraine:** Initially, 80 mg/day. May increase gradually up to 240 mg/day in divided doses **Tremor:** Initially, 40 mg 2 times/day. Usual dose: 120–320 mg/day **SR:** **Angina**: Initially, 80 mg once daily. May increase q3–7days up to 320 mg/day **HTN**: 80–120 mg once daily at bedtime **Migraine:** Initially, 80 mg once daily Gradually increase up to 240 mg once daily **Hypertrophic subaortic stenosis:** 80–160 mg once daily	

C, Capsules; ***HF,*** heart failure; ***HTN,*** hypertension; ***I,*** injection; ***LVD,*** left ventricular dysfunction; ***MI,*** acute myocardial infarction; ***S,*** solution; ***SR,*** sustained-release; ***T,*** tablets.

Asthma/COPD

USES

Asthma: Chronic lung disorder marked by recurring episodes of airway obstruction (e.g., labored breathing with wheezing and coughing) and feeling of chest constriction. Asthma is triggered by hyper-reactivity to various stimuli (e.g., allergens, rapid change in air temperature). The obstruction is usually reversible with air flow good between attacks of asthma. Medication treatment includes inhaled corticosteroid (ICS), short-acting beta$_2$-agonist (SABA) as a reliever agent, inhaled anti-muscarinic agent as a reliever agent, leukotriene-receptor antagonist (LTRA), inhaled long-acting beta$_2$-agonist (LABA), anti–immunoglobulin E (IgE) agent, anti–interleukin-5 (IL-5) agent, oral corticosteroids, theophylline (rarely used).

COPD: Disorder that persistently obstructs bronchial airflow. COPD is frequently related to cigarette smoking and mainly involves two related diseases: chronic bronchitis and emphysema. The obstruction is usually permanent with progression over time. Medication treatment includes inhaled corticosteroid (ICS), inhaled antimuscarinic agent (LAMA), and inhaled long-acting beta$_2$-agonist (LABA).

ACTION

Inhaled corticosteroids: Exact mechanism unknown. May act as anti-inflammatories, decrease mucus secretion.

Beta$_2$-adrenergic agonists: Stimulate beta receptors in lung, relax bronchial smooth muscle, increase vital capacity, decrease airway resistance.

Antimuscarinics: Inhibit cholinergic receptors on bronchial smooth muscle (block acetylcholine action).

Leukotriene modifiers: Decrease effect of leukotrienes, which increase migration of eosinophils, producing mucus/edema of airway wall, causing bronchoconstriction.

IgE: Inhibits the binding of IgE to high-affinity receptors on surface of mast cells and basophils.

IL-5: Binds to IL-5, reducing the production and survival of eosinophils.

Methylxanthines: Directly relax smooth muscle of bronchial airway, pulmonary blood vessels (relieve bronchospasm, increase vital capacity). Increase cyclic 3,5-adenosine monophosphate.

ASTHMA/COPD

Name	Availability	Dosage Range	Side Effects
Antimuscarinics			
Aclidinium (Tudorza)	**Inhalation powder:** 400 mcg/actuation	**A:** 400 mcg 2 times/day	Headache, nasopharyngitis, cough
Glycopyrrolate (Seebri Neohaler)	**Inhalation capsule:** 15.6 mcg/cap	**A:** One inhalation 2 times/day	Fatigue, diarrhea, nausea, arthralgia, nasopharyngitis, upper respiratory tract infection, wheezing
Ipratropium (Atrovent)	**NEB:** 0.02% (500 mcg) **MDI:** 17 mcg/actuation	**A (NEB):** 500 mcg q6–8h **A (MDI):** 2 puffs 4 times/day	Upper respiratory tract infection, bronchitis, sinusitis, headache, dyspnea
Revefenacin (Yupelri)	Inhalation solution for nebulization. Each vial contains 175 mcg/3 mL solution	One 175-mcg vial (3 mL) once daily	Cough, nasopharyngitis, upper respiratory tract infection, headache, back pain
Tiotropium (Spiriva, Spiriva Respimat)	**Inhalation powder:** 18 mcg/capsule **Aerosol solution:** 1.25 mcg/inhalation	**A:** Once/day (inhaled twice) **Aerosol solution:** 2 inhalations once daily	Xerostomia, upper respiratory tract infection, sinusitis, pharyngitis
Umeclidinium (Incruse Ellipta)	**Inhalation powder:** 62.5 mcg/blister	**A:** One inhalation once daily	Nasopharyngitis, upper respiratory tract infection, cough, arthralgia
Bronchodilators			
Arformoterol (Brovanna)	**NEB:** 15 mcg/2 mL	**NEB:** 15 mcg 2 times/day	Pain, diarrhea, sinusitis, leg cramps, dyspnea, rash, flu syndrome, peripheral edema

Continued

Asthma/COPD—cont'd

Albuterol (ProAir HFA, ProAir Respiclick Proventil HFA, Ventolin HFA)	**DPI**: 90 mcg/actuation **MDI**: 90 mcg/actuation **NEB**: 2.5 mg/3 mL, 2.5 mg/0.5 mL, 0.63–1.25 mg/3 mL	**DPI**: 1–2 inhalations q4–6h as needed **MDI**: 2 inhalations q4–6h as needed **NEB**: 1.25–5 mg q4–6h as needed	Tachycardia, skeletal muscle tremors, muscle cramping, palpitations, insomnia, hypokalemia, increased serum glucose
Albuterol/ipratropium (Combivent Respimat, DuoNeb)	**MDI**: 90 mcg albuterol/18 mcg ipratropium/actuation **NEB**: 2.5 mg albuterol/0.5 mg ipratropium/3 mL	**MDI**: 1 inhalation 4 times/day as needed **NEB**: 2.5 mg/0.5 mg 4 times/day as needed	Same as individual listing for albuterol and ipratropium
Formoterol (Foradil, Perforomist)	**NEB**: 20 mcg/2 mL	**NEB**: 20 mcg q12h	Diarrhea, nausea, asthma exacerbation, bronchitis, infection
Indacaterol (Arcapta)	**DPI**: 75 mcg/capsule	**DPI**: 75 mcg once daily	Cough, oropharyngeal pain, nasopharyngitis, headache, nausea
Levalbuterol (Xopenex)	**MDI**: 45 mcg/actuation **NEB**: 0.31, 0.63, 1.25 mg/3 mL, 1.25 mg/0.5 mL	**MDI**: 2 inhalations q4–6h as needed **NEB**: 0.31–1.25 mg q6–8h	Tremor, rhinitis, viral infection, headache, nervousness, asthma, pharyngitis, rash
Olodaterol (Striverdi Respimat)	**MDI**: 2.5 mcg/actuation	**MDI**: 2 inhalations once daily	Nasopharyngitis, rash, dizziness, cough, bronchitis, upper respiratory tract infections
Salmeterol (Serevent Diskus)	**DPI**: 50 mcg/blister	**DPI**: 50 mcg q12h	Headache, pain, throat irritation, nasal congestion, bronchitis, pharyngitis
Inhaled Corticosteroids			
Beclomethasone (Qvar)	**MDI**: 40, 80 mcg/inhalation	**MDI**: 40–320 mcg 2 times/day	Cough, hoarseness, headache, pharyngitis
Budesonide (Pulmicort Flexhaler, Pulmicort Respules)	**DPI: (Flexhaler)**: 90,180 mcg/inhalation **DPI: (Turbuhaler)**: 200 mcg/inhalation **NEB: (Respules)**: 0.25, 0.5 mg/2 mL	**DPI: (Flexhaler)**: 180–720 mcg 2 times/day **DPI: (Turbuhaler)**: 400–2,400 mcg/day in 2–4 divided doses **NEB: (Respules)**: 250–500 mcg 1–2 times/day or 1 mg once daily	Headache, nausea, respiratory infection, rhinitis

Name	Availability	Dosage Range	Side Effects
Ciclesonide (Alvesco HFA)	**HFA:** 80, 160 mcg/inhalation	**HFA:** 80–320 mcg 2 times/day	Headache, nasopharyngitis, upper respiratory infection, epistaxis, nasal congestion, sinusitis
Fluticasone (Arnuity Ellipta, Flovent Diskus, Flovent HFA)	**DPI: (Flovent Diskus):** 50, 100, 250 mcg/blister **(Arnuity Ellipta):** 100 mcg, 200 mcg/activation **MDI: (Flovent HFA):** 44, 110, 220 mcg/inhalation	**DPI: (Flovent Diskus):** 100–1,000 mcg 2 times/day **(Arnuity Ellipta):** 100–200 mcg once daily **MDI: (Flovent HFA):** 88–880 mcg 2 times/day	Headache, nasal congestion, pharyngitis, sinusitis, respiratory infections
Mometasone (Asmanex Twisthaler)	**DPI:** 110–220 mcg/inhalation	**DPI:** 220–880 mcg once daily in evening or 220 mcg bid	Same as beclomethasone
Long Acting Antimuscarinic Agent/Long-Acting Beta$_2$-Agonist (LAMA/LABA)			
Aclidinium/formoterol (Duaklir Pressair)	400 mcg/12 mcg/inhalation	1 inhalation bid	Headache, upper respiratory tract infections
Glycopyrrolate/formoterol (Bevespi Aerosphere)	9 mcg/4.8 mcg/inhalation	2 inhalation bid	Urinary tract infection, cough
Glycopyrrolate/indacaterol (Utibron Neohaler)	15.6 mcg/27.5 mcg/cap	1 inhalation bid	Nasopharyngitis, hypertension
Tiotropium/olodaterol (Stiolto Respimat)	2.5 mcg/2.5 mcg/inhalation	2 inhalation once daily	Nasopharyngitis, cough, back pain
Umeclidinium/vilanterol (Anoro Ellipta)	62.5 mcg/25 mcg/inhalation	1 inhalation once/day	Pharyngitis, sinusitis, lower respiratory tract infections, constipation, diarrhea, muscle spasms, neck/chest pain

Continued

Asthma/COPD—cont'd

Leukotriene Modifiers			
Montelukast (Singulair)	**T:** 4 mg, 5 mg, 10 mg	**A:** 10 mg/day **C (6–14 yrs):** 5 mg/day **C (2–5 yrs):** 4 mg/day	Dyspepsia, increased LFTs, cough, nasal congestion, headache, dizziness, fatigue
Zafirlukast (Accolate)	**T:** 10 mg, 20 mg	**A, C (12 yrs and older):** 20 mg 2 times/day **C (5–11 yrs):** 10 mg 2 times/day	Headache, nausea, diarrhea, infection
PDE-4 Inhibitor			
Roflumilast (Daliresp)	**T:** 500 mcg	**A:** 500 mcg once daily	Headache, dizziness, insomnia
Inhaled Corticosteroid/Long-Acting Beta$_2$-Agonist (ICS/LABA)			
Fluticasone propionate/salmeterol (Advair Diskus)	100, 250, 500 mcg/50 mcg blister	100–500 mcg bid	Same as individual listing for fluticasone and salmeterol
Fluticasone propionate/salmeterol (Advair HFA)	45, 115, 230 mcg/21 mcg/inhalation	2 inhalations bid	Same as individual listing for fluticasone and salmeterol
Fluticasone propionate/salmeterol (AirDuo Respiclick)	55, 113, 232 mcg/14 mcg/inhalation	1 inhalation bid	Same as individual listing for fluticasone and salmeterol
Fluticasone furoate/vilanterol (Breo Ellipta)	100, 200 mcg/25 mcg/inhalation	1 inhalation once/day	Nasopharyngitis, upper respiratory tract infection, headache, oral candidiasis
Budesonide/formoterol (Symbicort)	80, 160 mcg/4.5 mcg/inhalation	80–160 mcg/25 mcg bid	Same as individual listing for budesonide and formoterol
Mometasone/formoterol (Dulera)	100, 200 mcg/5 mcg/inhalation	2 inhalations bid	Same as individual listing for mometasone and formoterol

Name	Availability	Dosage Range	Side Effects
Inhaled Corticosteroid/ Long Acting Antimuscarinic Agent /Long-Acting Beta$_2$-Agonist (ICS/LAMA/LABA)			
Fluticasone furoate/umeclidinium/ vilanterol (Trelegy Ellipta)	100 mcg/62.5 mcg/25 mcg/ inhalation	1 inhalation once/day	Same as individual listing for fluticasone, umeclidinium, and vilanterol
Anti-IgE Antibody			
Omalizumab (Xolair)	**I:** 150 mg	**SQ:** 75–300 mcg q4wks	Arthralgia, pain, fatigue, dizziness, fracture, pruritus, earache
Anti-Interleukin-5 Antibodies (Eosinophilia Asthma)			
Benralizumab (Fasenra)	**I:** 30 mg/mL	**SQ:** 30 mg q4wks times 3 doses, then q8wks	Injection site reactions, urticaria, angioedema, rash
Dupilumab (Dupixent)	**I:** 200 mg/1.14 mL, 300 mg/2 mL prefilled syringes	**SQ:** Initially, 400 mg, then 200 mg q2wks or 600 mg, then 300 mg q2wks	Injection-site reactions, transient eosinophilia, eosinophilic pneumonia, vasculitis, conjunctivitis
Mepolizumab (Nucala)	**I:** 100 mg	100 mg **SQ** q4wks	Headache, injection site reaction, fatigue, back pain
Resilizumab (Cinqair)	**I:** 100 mg/10-mL vial	3 mg/kg **IV** q4wks	Antibody development, increased CPK, myalgia, oropharyngeal pain

A, Adults; ***C** (dosage),* children; ***DPI,*** dry powder inhaler; ***HFA,*** hydrofluoroalkane; ***MDI,*** metered dose inhaler; ***NEB,*** nebulizatlon; ***T,*** tablets.

Calcium Channel Blockers

USES

Treatment of essential hypertension, treatment of and prophylaxis of angina pectoris (including vasospastic, chronic stable, unstable), prevention/control of supraventricular tachyarrhythmias, prevention of neurologic damage due to subarachnoid hemorrhage.

ACTION

Calcium channel blockers inhibit the flow of extracellular Ca^{2+} ions across cell membranes of cardiac cells, vascular tissue. They relax arterial smooth muscle, depress the rate of sinus node pacemaker, slow AV conduction, decrease heart rate, produce negative inotropic effect (rarely seen clinically due to reflex response). Calcium channel blockers decrease coronary vascular resistance, increase coronary blood flow, reduce myocardial oxygen demand. Degree of action varies with individual agent.

CALCIUM CHANNEL BLOCKERS

Name	Availability	Indications	Dosage Range	Side Effects
Amlodipine (Norvasc)	**T:** 2.5 mg, 5 mg, 10 mg	HTN, angina	**HTN:** Initially, 2.5–5 mg once daily. May titrate q7–14 days up to 10 mg/day **Angina:** 5–10 mg once daily	Headache, peripheral edema, dizziness, flushing, rash, gingival hyperplasia, tachycardia
Diltiazem (Cardizem)	**T:** 30 mg, 60 mg, 90 mg, 120 mg **(ER):** 120 mg, 180 mg, 240 mg, 300 mg, 360 mg, 420 mg **C (SR-12HR):** 60 mg, 90 mg, 120 mg, **(ER-24HR):** 120 mg, 180 mg, 240 mg, 300 mg, 360 mg, 420 mg **I:** 5 mg/mL	**PO:** HTN, angina **IV:** Arrhythmias	**See monograph** **HTN:** 120–540 mg/day **Angina:** 120–480 mg/day **I:** 20–25 mg IV bolus, then 5–15 mg/hr infusion	Constipation, flushing, hypotension, dizziness, AV block, bradycardia, headache, edema, HF
Felodipine (Plendil)	**T:** 2.5 mg, 5 mg, 10 mg	HTN	Initially, 5 mg/day. May increase q2wks Usual dose: 5–10 mg/day	Headache, peripheral edema, dizziness, flushing, rash, gingival hyperplasia, tachycardia

Isradipine	**C**: 2.5 mg, 5 mg	HTN	Initially, 2.5 mg 2 times/day. May increase at 2–4 wk intervals at 2.5–5 mg increments. Usual dose: 5–10 mg 2 times/day	Headache, peripheral edema, dizziness, flushing, rash, gingival hyperplasia, tachycardia
Nicardipine (Cardene)	**C (IR)**: 20 mg, 30 mg **C (ER)**: 30 mg, 45 mg,60 mg **I**: 2.5 mg/mL	HTN, angina	**Angina/HTN**: Initially, 20–30 mg 3 times/day. May increase q3days. Usual dose: 20–40 mg 3 times/day	Headache, peripheral edema, dizziness, flushing, rash, gingival hyperplasia, tachycardia
Nifedipine (Adalat, Procardia)	**C (IR)**: 10 mg, 20 mg **T (ER)**: 30 mg, 60 mg, 90 mg	HTN, angina	**HTN (ER)**: Initially, 30–60 mg once daily Usual dose: 90–120 mg once daily **Angina (IR)**: 10–20 mg tid or **(ER)**: Initially, 30–60 mg once daily. Titrate up to 90 mg daily. **Maximum**: 120 mg	Headache, peripheral edema, dizziness, flushing, rash, gingival hyperplasia, tachycardia
Nimodipine (Nimotop, Nymalize)	**C**: 30 mg **S**: 60 mg/20 mL	Prevent neurologic damage following subarachnoid hemorrhage	60 mg q4h for 21 days	Nausea, reduced B/P, headache, rash, diarrhea
Verapamil (Calan, Isoptin)	**T (IR)**: 40 mg, 80 mg, 120 mg **T (SR)**: 120 mg, 180 mg, 240 mg	HTN, angina	**Angina (IR)**: Initially, 40–120 mg 3 times/day. Usual dose: 80–160 mg tid or **(SR)**: Initially, 180 mg at HS. May increase at weekly intervals up to 480 mg/day **HTN (IR)**: Initially, 80 mg 3 times/day Usual dose: 240–480 mg/day in divided doses **(SR)**: Initially, 120–180 mg/day. May increase at wkly intervals to 240 mg/day, then 180 mg 2 times/day **Maximum**: 240 mg 2 times/day	Constipation, dizziness, tachycardia, AV block, bradycardia, headache, edema, HF

C, Capsules; ***CR,*** controlled-release; ***ER,*** extended-release; ***HTN,*** hypertension; ***I,*** injection; ***IR,*** immediate-release; ***S,*** solution; ***SR,*** sustained-release; ***T,*** tablets.

Chemotherapeutic Agents

USES

Treatment of a variety of cancers; may be palliative or curative. Treatment of choice in hematologic cancers. Often used as adjunctive therapy (e.g., with surgery or irradiation); most effective when tumor mass has been removed or reduced by radiation. Often used in combinations to increase therapeutic results, decrease toxic effects. Certain agents may be used in nonmalignant conditions: polycythemia vera, psoriasis, rheumatoid arthritis, or immunosuppression in organ transplantation (used only in select cases that are severe and unresponsive to other forms of therapy). Refer to individual monographs.

ACTION

Most antineoplastics can be divided into alkylating agents, antimetabolites, anthracyclines, plant alkaloids, and topoisomerase inhibitors. These agents affect cell division or DNA synthesis. Newer agents (monoclonal antibodies and tyrosine kinase inhibitors) directly target a molecular abnormality in certain types of cancer. Hormones modulate tumor cell behavior without directly attacking those cells. Some agents are classified as miscellaneous.

CHEMOTHERAPEUTIC AGENTS

Name	Uses	Category	Side Effects
Abemaciclib (Verzenio)	Breast cancer, advanced or metastatic	Cyclin-dependent kinase inhibitor	Fatigue, diarrhea, nausea, anemia, decreased absolute lymphocyte count, neutropenia, thrombocytopenia, leukopenia, increased ALT, AST, serum creatinine
Abiraterone (Zytiga)	Prostate cancer	Antiandrogen	Joint swelling, hypokalemia, edema, muscle discomfort, hot flashes, diarrhea, UTI, cough, hypertension, arrhythmia, dyspepsia, upper respiratory tract infection
Acalabrutinib (Calquence)	Mantle cell lymphoma (previously treated)	Tyrosine kinase inhibitor	Headache, fatigue, skin rash, diarrhea, nausea, neutropenia, bruising, anemia, myalgia

Aldesleukin (Proleukin)	Melanoma (metastatic), renal cell (metastatic)	Biologic response modifier	Hypotension, sinus tachycardia, nausea, vomiting, diarrhea, renal impairment, anemia, rash, fatigue, agitation, pulmonary congestion, dyspnea, fever, chills, oliguria, weight gain, dizziness
Alectinib (Alecensa)	Non–small-cell lung cancer (NSCLC), metastatic	Kinase inhibitor	Constipation, fatigue, edema, myalgia
Anastrozole (Arimidex)	Breast cancer	Aromatase inhibitor	Peripheral edema, chest pain, nausea, vomiting, diarrhea, constipation, abdominal pain, anorexia, pharyngitis, vaginal hemorrhage, anemia, leukopenia, rash, weight gain, diaphoresis, increased appetite, pain, headaches, dizziness, depression, paresthesia, hot flashes, increased cough, dry mouth, asthenia, dyspnea, phlebitis
Apalutamide (Erleada)	Prostate cancer, non-metastatic, castration-resistant	Antiandrogen	Hypertension, fatigue, skin rash, hypercholesterolemia, hyperglycemia, hypertriglyceridemia, hyperkalemia, diarrhea, anemia, leukopenia, lymphocytopenia
Alpelisib (Piqray)	Breast cancer, advanced or metastatic	Phosphatidylinositol 3-kinase inhibitor	Skin rash, fatigue, hyperglycemia, diarrhea, nausea, lymphocytopenia, increased alanine aminotransferase, creatinine
Arsenic trioxide (Trisenox)	Acute promyelocytic leukemia (APL)	Miscellaneous	AV block, GI hemorrhage, hypertension, hypoglycemia, hypokalemia, hypomagnesemia, neutropenia, oliguria, prolonged QT interval, seizures, sepsis, thrombocytopenia
Asparaginase (Elspar)	Acute lymphoblastic leukemia (ALL)	Miscellaneous	Anorexia, nausea, vomiting, hepatic toxicity, pancreatitis, nephrotoxicity, clotting factor abnormalities, malaise, confusion, lethargy, EEG changes, respiratory distress, fever, hyperglycemia, depression, stomatitis, allergic reactions, drowsiness
Atezolizumab (Tecentriq)	NSCLC, metastatic, urothelial carcinoma, locally advanced or metastatic	Miscellaneous	Fatigue, decreased appetite, nausea, UTI, constipation, pyrexia
Avapritinib (Ayvakit)	Gastrointestinal stromal tumor, unresectable or metastatic	PDGFR-alpha blocker, tyrosine kinase inhibitor	Fatigue, cognitive dysfunction, nausea, leukopenia; decreased phosphate, potassium, albumin, sodium; increased bilirubin, aspartate aminotransferase
Avelumab (Bavencio)	Merkel cell carcinoma	PD-L1 blocking antibody	Fatigue, musculoskeletal pain, diarrhea, nausea, infusion-related reactions, rash, decreased appetite, peripheral edema

Continued

CHEMOTHERAPEUTIC AGENTS—cont'd

Name	Uses	Category	Side Effects
Axitinib (Inlyta)	Renal cell carcinoma, advanced	Kinase inhibitor	Diarrhea, hypertension, fatigue, decreased appetite, nausea, dysphoria, vomiting, asthenia, constipation
Azacitidine (Vidaza)	Myelodysplastic (MDS) syndrome	DNA methylation inhibitor	Edema, hypokalemia, weight loss, myalgia, cough, dyspnea, upper respiratory tract infection, back pain, pyrexia, weakness
BCG (TheraCys, Tice BCG)	Bladder cancer	Biologic response modulator	Nausea, vomiting, anorexia, diarrhea, dysuria, hematuria, cystitis, urinary urgency, anemia, malaise, fever, chills
Belinostat (Beleodaq)	Peripheral T-cell lymphoma	Miscellaneous	Nausea, fatigue, pyrexia, anemia, vomiting
Bendamustine (Treanda)	Chronic lymphocytic leukemia (CLL), non-Hodgkin lymphoma (NHL)	Alkylating agent	Neutropenia, pyrexia, thrombocytopenia, nausea, anemia, leukopenia, vomiting
Bevacizumab (Avastin)	Cervical cancer, persistent/recurrent/metastatic, colorectal cancer, metastatic, glioblastoma, NSCLC, nonsquamous	Monoclonal antibody	Increased B/P, fatigue, blood clots, diarrhea, decreased WBCs, headaches, decreased appetite, stomatitis
Bexarotene (Targretin)	Cutaneous T-cell lymphoma	Miscellaneous	Anemia, dermatitis, fever, hypercholesterolemia, infection, leukopenia, peripheral edema
Bicalutamide (Casodex)	Prostate cancer, metastatic	Antiandrogen	Gynecomastia, hot flashes, breast pain, nausea, diarrhea, constipation, nocturia, impotence, pain, muscle pain, asthenia, abdominal pain
Binimetinib (Mektovi)	Melanoma (unresectable or metastatic)	Kinase inhibitor	Fatigue, nausea, diarrhea, vomiting, anemia, hemorrhage; increased CPK, serum creatinine
Bleomycin (Blenoxane)	Head/neck cancers, Hodgkin lymphoma, malignant pleural effusion, testicular cancer	Antibiotic	Nausea, vomiting, anorexia, stomatitis, hyperpigmentation, alopecia, pruritus, hyperkeratosis, urticaria, pneumonitis progression to fibrosis, weight loss, rash

Blinatumomab (Blincyto)	ALL	Miscellaneous	Pyrexia, headache, peripheral edema, febrile neutropenia, nausea, hypokalemia, tremor, rash, constipation
Bortezomib (Velcade)	Mantle cell lymphoma, multiple myeloma	Proteasome inhibitor	Anxiety, dizziness, headaches, insomnia, peripheral neuropathy, pruritus, rash, abdominal pain, decreased appetite, constipation, diarrhea, dyspepsia, nausea, vomiting, arthralgia, dyspnea, asthenia, edema, pain
Bosutinib (Bosulif)	Chronic myelogenous leukemia (CML)	Kinase inhibitor	Nausea, diarrhea, thrombocytopenia, vomiting, abdominal pain, anemia, fever, fatigue
Brentuximab (Adcetris)	Anaplastic large cell lymphoma, Hodgkin lymphoma (relapsed, refractory, post-autologous hematopoietic stem cell transplant)	Miscellaneous	Neutropenia, peripheral sensory neuropathy, fatigue, nausea, anemia, upper respiratory tract infection, diarrhea, pyrexia, thrombocytopenia, cough, vomiting
Brigatinib (Alunbrig)	NSCLC, metastatic	Kinase inhibitor	Nausea, diarrhea, fatigue, cough, headache
Busulfan (Myleran)	CML	Alkylating agent	Nausea, vomiting, hyperuricemia, myelosuppression, skin hyperpigmentation, alopecia, anorexia, weight loss, diarrhea, stomatitis
Cabazitaxel (Jevtana)	Prostate cancer, metastatic	Microtubule inhibitor	Neutropenia, anemia, leukopenia, thrombocytopenia, diarrhea, fatigue, nausea, vomiting, constipation, asthenia, abdominal pain, hematuria, anorexia, peripheral neuropathy, dyspnea, alopecia
Capmatinib (Tabrecta)	NSCLC, metastatic	MET inhibitor, tyrosine kinase inhibitor	Peripheral edema, nausea, vomiting, lymphocytopenia, fatigue; decreased albumin, glucose, phosphate, sodium; increased alanine aminotransferase, creatinine
Capecitabine (Xeloda)	Breast cancer, metastatic, colorectal cancer	Antimetabolite	Nausea, vomiting, diarrhea, stomatitis, myelosuppression, palmar-plantar erythrodysesthesia syndrome, dermatitis, fatigue, anorexia
Carboplatin (Paraplatin)	Ovarian cancer, advanced	Alkylating agent	Nausea, vomiting, nephrotoxicity, myelosuppression, alopecia, peripheral neuropathy, hypersensitivity, ototoxicity, asthenia, diarrhea, constipation

Continued

CHEMOTHERAPEUTIC AGENTS—cont'd

Name	Uses	Category	Side Effects
Carfilzomib (Kyprolis)	Multiple myeloma, relapsed/refractory	Proteasome inhibitor	Anemia, fatigue, nausea, thrombocytopenia, dyspnea, diarrhea, pyrexia
Carmustine (BiCNU)	Brain tumors, multiple myeloma, Hodgkin lymphoma, relapsed/refractory, NHL, relapsed/refractory	Alkylating agent	Anorexia, nausea, vomiting, myelosuppression, pulmonary fibrosis, pain at injection site, diarrhea, skin discoloration
Ceritinib (Zykadia)	NSCLC, metastatic	Kinase inhibitor	Diarrhea, nausea, increased LFTs, vomiting, abdominal pain, fatigue, decreased appetite, constipation
Cetuximab (Erbitux)	Colorectal cancer, metastatic, head/neck cancer, squamous cell	Monoclonal antibody	Dyspnea, hypotension, acne-like rash, dry skin, weakness, fatigue, fever, constipation, abdominal pain
Chlorambucil (Leukeran)	CLL	Alkylating agent	Myelosuppression, dermatitis, nausea, vomiting, hepatic toxicity, anorexia, diarrhea, abdominal discomfort, rash
Cisplatin (Platinol-AQ)	Bladder cancer, advanced, ovarian cancer, metastatic, testicular cancer, metastatic	Alkylating agent	Nausea, vomiting, nephrotoxicity, myelosuppression, neuropathies, ototoxicity, anaphylactic-like reactions, hyperuricemia, hypomagnesemia, hypophosphatemia, hypokalemia, hypocalcemia, pain at injection site
Cladribine (Leustatin)	Hairy cell leukemia	Antimetabolite	Nausea, vomiting, diarrhea, myelosuppression, chills, fatigue, rash, fever, headaches, anorexia, diaphoresis
Cobimetinib (Cotellic)	Melanoma, unresectable or metastatic	Kinase inhibitor	Diarrhea, photosensitivity reaction, nausea, vomiting, pyrexia, increased ALT, AST, alkaline phosphatase
Copanlisib (Alqopa)	Follicular lymphoma (relapsed)	Phosphatidylinositol 3-kinase inhibitor	Hypertension, decreased energy, hyperglycemia, hypertriglyceridemia, hypophosphatemia, hyperuricemia, diarrhea, nausea, decreased Hgb, leukopenia, decreased absolute lymphocyte count, neutropenia, thrombocytopenia, serious infection
Crizotinib (Xalkori)	NSCLC, metastatic	Tyrosine kinase inhibitor	Vision disorders, nausea, vomiting, diarrhea, edema, constipation

Cyclophosphamide (Cytoxan)	ALL, AML, breast cancer, CML, Hodgkin lymphoma, multiple myeloma, NHL, ovarian carcinoma	Alkylating agent	Nausea, vomiting, hemorrhagic cystitis, myelosuppression, alopecia, interstitial pulmonary fibrosis, amenorrhea, azoospermia, diarrhea, darkening skin/fingernails, headaches, diaphoresis
Cytarabine (Ara-C, Cytosar)	AML, ALL, CML, meningeal leukemia	Antimetabolite	Anorexia, nausea, vomiting, stomatitis, esophagitis, diarrhea, myelosuppression, alopecia, rash, fever, neuropathies, abdominal pain
Dabrafenib (Tafinlar)	Melanoma, metastatic or unresectable	Kinase inhibitor	Hyperkeratosis, headache, pyrexia, arthralgia, constipation, alopecia, rash, cough, palmar-plantar erythrodysesthesia syndrome, papilloma
Dacarbazine (DTIC)	Hodgkin lymphoma, metastatic malignant melanoma	Alkylating agent	Nausea, vomiting, anorexia, hepatic necrosis, myelosuppression, alopecia, rash, facial flushing, photosensitivity, flu-like symptoms, confusion, blurred vision
Dacomitinib (Vizimpro)	NSCLC	Tyrosine kinase inhibitor	Skin rash, paronychia, xeroderma, alopecia, pruritus, hypoalbuminemia, hyperglycemia, hypocalcemia, hypokalemia, hyponatremia, weight loss, diarrhea, stomatitis, anemia, lymphocytopenia
Daratumumab (Darzalex)	Multiple myeloma, relapsed/refractory	Monoclonal antibody	Fatigue, nausea, infusion reactions, back pain, pyrexia, nausea, upper respiratory tract infections
Daratumumab/ hyaluronidase (Darzalex Faspro)	Multiple myeloma, newly diagnosed, relapsed/refractory	Anti-CD38, monoclonal antibody	Decreased hemoglobin, neutrophils, platelet count; leukopenia, lymphocytopenia
Darolutamide (Nubeqa)	Prostate cancer, nonmetastatic, castration-resistant	Antiandrogen	Fatigue, neutropenia; increased bilirubin, aspartate aminotransferase
Dasatinib (Sprycel)	ALL, CML	Tyrosine kinase inhibitor	Pyrexia, pleural effusion, febrile neutropenia, GI bleeding, pneumonia, thrombocytopenia, dyspnea, anemia, cardiac failure, diarrhea
Daunorubicin (Cerubidine)	ALL, AML	Anthracycline	HF, nausea, vomiting, stomatitis, mucositis, diarrhea, hematuria, myelosuppression, alopecia, fever, chills, abdominal pain

Continued

CHEMOTHERAPEUTIC AGENTS—cont'd

Name	Uses	Category	Side Effects
Daunorubicin liposomal (DaunoXome)	Kaposi sarcoma	Anthracycline	Nausea, diarrhea, abdominal pain, anorexia, vomiting, stomatitis, myelosuppression, rigors, back pain, headaches, neuropathy, depression, dyspnea, fatigue, fever, cough, allergic reactions, diaphoresis
Dinutuximab (Unituxin)	Neuroblastoma	Monoclonal antibody	Pain, arthralgia, myalgia, neuralgia, pyrexia, hypotension, vomiting, diarrhea, urticaria, hypoxia
Docetaxel (Taxotere)	Breast cancer, NSCLC, prostate, gastric, head/neck cancers	Antimicrotubular	Hypotension, nausea, vomiting, diarrhea, mucositis, myelosuppression, rash, paresthesia, hypersensitivity, fluid retention, alopecia, asthenia, stomatitis, fever
Doxorubicin (Adriamycin)	Breast cancer, metastatic cancers	Anthracycline	Cardiotoxicity, including HF; arrhythmias, nausea, vomiting, stomatitis, esophagitis, GI ulceration, diarrhea, anorexia, hematuria, myelosuppression, alopecia, hyperpigmentation of nail beds and skin, local inflammation at injection site, rash, fever, chills, urticaria, lacrimation, conjunctivitis
Doxorubicin liposomal (Doxil)	AIDS-related Kaposi sarcoma, multiple myeloma, ovarian cancer, advanced	Anthracycline	Neutropenia, palmar-plantar erythrodysesthesia syndrome, cardiomyopathy, HF
Durvalumab (Imfinzi)	Urothelial carcinoma, advanced or metastatic	PD-L1 blocking antibody	Fatigue, musculoskeletal pain, constipation, decreased appetite, nausea, peripheral edema, UTI
Duvelisib (Copiktra)	Chronic lymphocytic leukemia/small lymphocytic lymphoma (relapsed or refractory), follicular lymphoma (relapsed or refractory)	Kinase inhibitor	Edema, fatigue, headache, skin rash, hypophosphatemia, hyponatremia, diarrhea, nausea, neutropenia; increased serum lipase/amylase
Elotuzumab (Empliciti)	Multiple myeloma, relapsed/refractory	Immunostimulatory antibody	Fatigue, diarrhea, pyrexia, constipation, cough, peripheral neuropathy, nasopharyngitis, decreased appetite, upper respiratory tract infections, pneumonia
Enasidenib (Idhifa)	AML, refractory	Isocitrate dehydrogenase-2 inhibitor	Nausea, vomiting, diarrhea, elevated bilirubin, decreased appetite

Enasidenib (IDHIFA)	Acute myeloid leukemia (relapsed/refractory)	IDH2 inhibitor	Decreased calcium, potassium, nausea, diarrhea, decreased appetite, vomiting, leukocytosis, increased bilirubin
Encorafenib (Braftovi)	Melanoma (unresectable or metastatic)	Kinase inhibitor	Fatigue, hyperkeratosis, alopecia, skin rash, hyperglycemia, nausea, anemia; increased serum creatinine
Enfortumab vedotin (Padcev)	Urothelial cancer, locally advanced or metastatic	Anti-nectin-4 antibody drug conjugate, monoclonal antibody	Fatigue, peripheral neuropathy, skin rash, alopecia, nausea, diarrhea, dysgeusia, lymphocytopenia, ocular toxicity, dry eye syndrome; decreased phosphate, potassium, appetite, hemoglobin
Entrectinib (Rozlytrek)	NSCLC, metastatic; solid tumors	Tropomyosin receptor kinase (TRK) inhibitor, tyrosine kinase inhibitor	Edema, fatigue, dizziness, dysesthesia, hyperuricemia, hypernatremia, hypocalcemia, constipation, dysgeusia, diarrhea, nausea, anemia, lymphocytopenia; increased aspartate aminotransferase, alanine aminotransferase, creatinine
Enzalutamide (Xtandi)	Prostate cancer, metastatic	Antiandrogen	Fatigue, weakness, back pain, diarrhea, tissue swelling, musculoskeletal pain, headache, upper respiratory tract infections, blood in urine, spinal cord compression
Epirubicin (Ellence)	Breast cancer, adjuvant	Anthracycline	Anemia, leukopenia, neutropenia, infection, mucositis
Erdafitinib (Balversa)	Urothelial carcinoma (locally advanced or metastatic)	Kinase inhibitor	Fatigue, onycholysis, hyperphosphatemia, stomatitis, diarrhea, decreased Hgb, increased serum creatinine
Erlotinib (Tarceva)	NSCLC, pancreatic cancer	Tyrosine kinase inhibitor	Diarrhea, rash, nausea, vomiting
Etoposide (VePesid)	Small-cell lung cancer, testicular cancer	Podophyllotoxin derivative	Nausea, vomiting, anorexia, myelosuppression, alopecia, diarrhea, drowsiness, peripheral neuropathies

Continued

CHEMOTHERAPEUTIC AGENTS—cont'd

Name	Uses	Category	Side Effects
Everolimus (Afinitor)	Breast cancer, advanced, neuroendocrine tumors, renal cell carcinoma, advanced, subependymal giant cell astrocytoma	mTOR kinase inhibitor	Stomatitis, infections, asthenia, fatigue, cough, diarrhea
Exemestane (Aromasin)	Breast cancer	Aromatase inactivator	Dyspnea, edema, hypertension, mental depression
Fam-trastuzumab deruxtecan-nxki (Enhertu)	Breast cancer, unresectable or metastatic	Anti-HER2, antibody drug conjugate, monoclonal antibody, topoisomerase I inhibitor	Fatigue, alopecia, nausea, vomiting, constipation, diarrhea, anemia
Fludarabine (Fludara)	CLL	Antimetabolite	Nausea, diarrhea, stomatitis, bleeding, anemia, myelosuppression, skin rash, weakness, confusion, visual disturbances, peripheral neuropathy, coma, pneumonia, peripheral edema, anorexia
Fluorouracil (Adrucil, Efudex)	Breast, colon, gastric, pancreatic, rectal cancers, basal cell carcinoma	Antimetabolite	Nausea, vomiting, stomatitis, GI ulceration, diarrhea, anorexia, myelosuppression, alopecia, skin hyperpigmentation, nail changes, headaches, drowsiness, blurred vision, fever
Flutamide (Eulexin)	Prostate cancer	Antiandrogen	Hot flashes, nausea, vomiting, diarrhea, hepatitis, impotence, decreased libido, rash, anorexia
Fulvestrant (Faslodex)	Breast cancer, metastatic or advanced	Estrogen receptor antagonist	Asthenia, pain, headaches, injection site pain, flu-like symptoms, fever, nausea, vomiting, constipation, anorexia, diarrhea, peripheral edema, dizziness, depression, anxiety, rash, increased cough, UTI
Gefitinib (Iressa)	NSCLC	Tyrosine kinase inhibitor	Diarrhea, rash, acne, nausea, dry skin, vomiting, pruritus, anorexia
Gemcitabine (Gemzar)	Breast, NSCLC, ovarian, pancreatic cancers	Antimetabolite	Increased LFT, nausea, vomiting, diarrhea, stomatitis, hematuria, myelosuppression, rash, mild paresthesia, dyspnea, fever, edema, flu-like symptoms, constipation

Gilteritinib (Xospata)	AML, relapsed or refractory	Kinase inhibitor	Edema, fatigue, malaise, hyperglycemia, hypertriglyceridemia, hypocalcemia, hypoalbuminemia, arthralgia, myalgia, increased serum creatinine
Glasdegib (Daurismo)	AML	Hedgehog pathway inhibitor	Edema, fatigue, hyponatremia, hypomagnesemia, nausea, anemia, hemorrhage, febrile neutropenia, increased serum creatinine
Goserelin (Zoladex)	Breast cancer, prostate cancer	Hormone agonist	Hot flashes, sexual dysfunction, erectile dysfunction, gynecomastia, lethargy, pain, lower urinary tract symptoms, headaches, nausea, depression, diaphoresis
Hydroxyurea (Hydrea)	CML, head/neck cancers	Antimetabolite	Anorexia, nausea, vomiting, stomatitis, diarrhea, constipation, myelosuppression, fever, chills, malaise
Ibrutinib (Imbruvica)	CLL, small lymphocytic lymphoma, mantle cell lymphoma, Waldenstrom macroglobulinemia	Kinase inhibitor	Neutropenia, thrombocytopenia, diarrhea, anemia, musculoskeletal pain, rash, nausea, bruising, fatigue, hemorrhage, pyrexia
Idarubicin (Idamycin PFS)	AML	Anthracycline	HF, arrhythmias, nausea, vomiting, stomatitis, myelosuppression, alopecia, rash, urticaria, hyperuricemia, abdominal pain, diarrhea, esophagitis, anorexia
Idelalisib (Zydelig)	CLL, follicular B-cell NHL, small lymphocytic lymphoma	Kinase inhibitor	Diarrhea, pyrexia, fatigue, nausea, cough, abdominal pain, pneumonia, increased ALT/AST
lenalidomide (Revlimid)	Mantle cell lymphoma, multiple myeloma, myelodysplastic syndromes	Immunomodulator	Diarrhea, pruritus, rash, fatigue, DVT, pulmonary embolism, thrombocytopenia, neutropenia, upper respiratory tract infection, cellulitis, hypertension, peripheral neuropathy
Ifosfamide (Ifex)	Testicular cancer	Alkylating agent	Nausea, vomiting, hemorrhagic cystitis, myelosuppression, alopecia, lethargy, drowsiness, confusion, hallucinations, hematuria
Imatinib (Gleevec)	ALL, CML, dermatofibrosarcoma protuberans, gastrointestinal stromal tumors (GIST), chronic eosinophilic leukemias, myelodysplastic/myeloproliferative disease	Tyrosine kinase inhibitor	Nausea, fluid retention, hemorrhage, musculoskeletal pain, arthralgia, weight gain, pyrexia, abdominal pain, dyspnea, pneumonia

Continued

CHEMOTHERAPEUTIC AGENTS—cont'd

Name	Uses	Category	Side Effects
Inotuzumab ozogamicin (Besponsa)	Acute lymphoblastic leukemia (relapsed/refractory)	Monoclonal antibody	Fatigue, headache, increased GGT, lipase, nausea, abdominal pain, thrombocytopenia, neutropenia, anemia, leukopenia, lymphocytopenia, increased ALT, AST, alkaline phosphatase, infection, fever
Interferon alfa-2b (Intron-A)	AIDS-related Kaposi sarcoma, follicular lymphoma, hairy cell leukemia, malignant melanoma	Miscellaneous	Mild hypotension, hypertension, tachycardia with high fever, nausea, diarrhea, altered taste, weight loss, thrombocytopenia, myelosuppression, rash, pruritus, myalgia, arthralgia associated with flu-like symptoms
Ipilimumab (Yervoy)	Melanoma, unresectable or metastatic, melanoma, adjuvant	Miscellaneous	Fatigue, diarrhea, pruritus, rash, colitis
Irinotecan (Camptosar)	Colorectal cancer, metastatic, pancreatic adenocarcinoma, metastatic	Camptothecin	Diarrhea, nausea, vomiting, abdominal cramps, anorexia, stomatitis, increased AST, severe myelosuppression, alopecia, diaphoresis, rash, weight loss, dehydration, increased serum alkaline phosphatase, headaches, insomnia, dizziness, dyspnea, cough, asthenia, rhinitis, fever, back pain, chills
Isatuximab-irfc (Sarclisa)	Multiple myeloma, relapsed or refractory	Anti-CD38, monoclonal antibody	Diarrhea, anemia, lymphocytopenia, neutropenia, thrombocytopenia, infusion-related reaction
Ivosidenib (Tibsovo)	AML newly diagnosed (relapsed/refractory)	IDH1 Inhibitor	Edema, fatigue, diarrhea, nausea, decreased Hgb, leukocytosis, hypomagnesemia, hypokalemia, hyponatremia
Ixabepilone (Ixempra)	Breast cancer	Antimicrotubular	Peripheral sensory neuropathy, fatigue, myalgia, alopecia, nausea, vomiting, stomatitis, diarrhea, anorexia, abdominal pain
Ixazomib (Ninlaro)	Multiple myeloma	Proteasome inhibitor	Diarrhea, constipation, thrombocytopenia, peripheral neuropathy, nausea, peripheral edema, back pain, vomiting
Lapatinib (Tykerb)	Breast cancer	Tyrosine kinase inhibitor	Diarrhea, palmar-plantar erythrodysesthesia, nausea, rash, vomiting, fatigue
Larotrectinib (Vitrakvi)	Solid tumors	Tyrosine kinase inhibitor	Neurotoxicity, fatigue, dizziness, hypoalbuminemia, nausea, vomiting, anemia, cough

Lenvatinib (Lenvima)	Renal cell carcinoma, advanced, thyroid cancer, differentiated	Kinase inhibitor	Hypertension, fatigue, diarrhea, arthralgia, decreased weight, nausea, stomatitis, headache, vomiting, proteinuria, abdominal pain
Letrozole (Femara)	Breast cancer in post-menopausal women	Aromatase inhibitor	Hypertension, nausea, vomiting, constipation, diarrhea, abdominal pain, anorexia, rash, pruritus, musculoskeletal pain, arthralgia, fatigue, headaches, dyspnea, coughing, hot flashes
Leuprolide (Lupron)	Prostate cancer, advanced	Hormone agonist	Hot flashes, gynecomastia, nausea, vomiting, constipation, anorexia, dizziness, headaches, insomnia, paresthesia, bone pain
Lomustine (CeeNU)	Brain tumors, Hodgkin lymphoma	Alkylating agent	Anorexia, nausea, vomiting, stomatitis, hepatotoxicity, nephrotoxicity, myelosuppression, alopecia, confusion, slurred speech
Lorlatinib (Lorbrena)	NSCLC, metastatic	Tyrosine kinase inhibitor	Edema, peripheral neuropathy, hypercholesterolemia, hypertriglyceridemia, anemia, dyspnea
Megestrol (Megace)	Breast cancer, endometrial cancer	Hormone	Deep vein thrombosis, Cushing-like syndrome, alopecia, carpal tunnel syndrome, weight gain, nausea
Melphalan (Alkeran)	Multiple myeloma, ovarian cancer	Alkylating agent	Anorexia, nausea, vomiting, myelosuppression, diarrhea, stomatitis
Mercaptopurine (Purinethol)	ALL	Antimetabolite	Anorexia, nausea, vomiting, stomatitis, hepatic toxicity, myelosuppression, hyperuricemia, diarrhea, rash
Methotrexate (Rheumatrex)	ALL, trophoblastic neoplasms, breast cancer, head and neck cancer, cutaneous T-cell lymphoma, lung cancer, advanced NHL, osteosarcoma	Antimetabolite	Nausea, vomiting, stomatitis, GI ulceration, diarrhea, hepatic toxicity, renal failure, cystitis, myelosuppression, alopecia, urticaria, acne, photosensitivity, interstitial pneumonitis, fever, malaise, chills, anorexia
Midostaurin (Rhydapt)	AML, aggressive systemic mastocytosis (ASM)	Kinase inhibitor	Febrile neutropenia, nausea, mucositis, vomiting, headache, petechiae, musculoskeletal pain, epistaxis, hyperglycemia, upper respiratory tract infections

Continued

CHEMOTHERAPEUTIC AGENTS—cont'd

Name	Uses	Category	Side Effects
Mitomycin (Mutamycin)	Gastric cancer, pancreatic cancer	Antibiotic	Anorexia, nausea, vomiting, stomatitis, diarrhea, renal toxicity, myelosuppression, alopecia, pruritus, fever, hemolytic uremic syndrome, weakness
Mitotane (Lysodren)	Adrenocortical carcinoma	Miscellaneous	Anorexia, nausea, vomiting, diarrhea, skin rashes, depression, lethargy, drowsiness, dizziness, adrenal insufficiency, blurred vision, impaired hearing
Mitoxantrone (Novantrone)	Acute nonlymphocytic leukemias, prostate cancer, advanced hormone refractory	Anthracenedione	HF, tachycardia, EKG changes, chest pain, nausea, vomiting, stomatitis, mucositis, myelosuppression, rash, alopecia, urine discoloration (bluish green), phlebitis, diarrhea, cough, headaches, fever
Moxetumomab (Lumoxiti)	Hairy cell leukemia (relapsed or refractory)	Anti-CD22	Peripheral edema, capillary leak syndrome, fatigue, headache, hypoalbuminemia, nausea, decreased Hgb, neutropenia; increased serum ALT, AST, creatinine
Necitumumab (Portrazza)	NSCLC (squamous) metastatic	Epidermal growth factor receptor (EGFR) antagonist	Rash, hypomagnesemia
Nelarabine (Arranon)	T-cell acute lymphoblastic leukemia/lymphoma	Antimetabolite	Anemia, neutropenia, thrombocytopenia, nausea, vomiting, diarrhea, fatigue, fever, dyspnea, severe neurologic events (convulsions, peripheral neuropathy)
Neratinib (Nerlynx)	Breast cancer	Kinase inhibitor	Diarrhea, nausea, abdominal pain, fatigue, vomiting, stomatitis, muscle spasms increase AST/ALT, UTI
Nilotinib (Tasigna)	CML	Tyrosine kinase inhibitor	Rash, pruritus, nausea, fatigue, headache, constipation, diarrhea, vomiting, thrombocytopenia, neutropenia
Nilutamide (Nilandron)	Prostate cancer, metastatic	Antiandrogen	Hypertension, angina, hot flashes, nausea, anorexia, increased hepatic enzymes, dizziness, dyspnea, visual disturbances, impaired adaptation to dark, constipation, decreased libido
Niraparib (Zejula)	Epithelial carcinoma, fallopian tube or peritoneal cancer	PARP inhibitor	Thrombocytopenia, anemia, neutropenia, leukopenia, palpitations, nausea, vomiting, stomatitis, UTI, elevated AST/ALT, dyspnea, hypertension

Nivolumab (Opdivo)	Melanoma, unresectable or metastatic, head and neck cancer, squamous cell (recurrent or metastatic), Hodgkin lymphoma, NSCLC, metastatic, renal cell cancer, advanced	Miscellaneous	Fatigue, dyspnea, musculoskeletal pain, decreased appetite, cough, nausea, constipation
Obinutuzumab (Gazyva)	CLL, follicular lymphoma	Monoclonal antibody	Infusion reactions, thrombocytopenia, febrile neutropenia, lymphopenia, bone marrow failure, tumor lysis syndrome
Ofatumumab (Arzerra)	CLL	Monoclonal antibody	Fever, cough, diarrhea, fatigue, rash, infections, septic shock, neutropenia, thrombocytopenia, infusion reactions
Olaparib (Lynparza)	Ovarian cancer, advanced	Miscellaneous	Anemia, fatigue, nausea, vomiting, diarrhea, dysgeusia, dyspepsia, headache, decreased appetite
Olaratumab (Lartruvo)	Soft tissue sarcoma	PDGFR-alpha blocking antibody	Nausea, fatigue, musculoskeletal pain, mucositis, alopecia, vomiting, neuropathy, headache
Omacetaxine (Synribo)	CML	Protein synthesis inhibitor	Diarrhea, nausea, fatigue, pyrexia, asthenia, vomiting, anorexia, headache, thrombocytopenia, neutropenia, leukopenia, lymphopenia
Osimertinib (Tagrisso)	NSCLC, metastatic	Kinase inhibitor	Diarrhea, rash, dry skin, nail toxicity
Oxaliplatin (Eloxatin)	Colon cancer	Alkylating agent	Fatigue, neuropathy, abdominal pain, dyspnea, diarrhea, nausea, vomiting, anorexia, fever, edema, chest pain, anemia, thrombocytopenia, thromboembolism, altered hepatic function tests
Paclitaxel (Taxol)	Breast cancer, Kaposi sarcoma, NSCLC, ovarian cancer	Antimicrotubular	Hypertension, bradycardia, ECG changes, nausea, vomiting, diarrhea, mucositis, myelosuppression, alopecia, peripheral neuropathies, hypersensitivity reaction, arthralgia, myalgia

Continued

CHEMOTHERAPEUTIC AGENTS—cont'd

Name	Uses	Category	Side Effects
Palbociclib (Ibrance)	Breast cancer, advanced	Kinase inhibitor	Neutropenia, leukopenia, fatigue, anemia, upper respiratory tract infection, nausea, stomatitis, alopecia, diarrhea, thrombocytopenia, decreased appetite, vomiting, asthenia, peripheral neuropathy, epistaxis
Panitumumab (Vectibix)	Colorectal cancer metastatic	Monoclonal antibody	Pulmonary fibrosis, severe dermatologic toxicity, infusion reactions, abdominal pain, nausea, vomiting, constipation, skin rash, fatigue
Panobinostat (Farydak)	Multiple myeloma	Miscellaneous	Diarrhea, fatigue, nausea, peripheral edema, decreased appetite, pyrexia, vomiting
Pazopanib (Votrient)	Renal cell carcinoma, soft tissue sarcoma	Kinase inhibitor	Diarrhea, hypertension, nausea, fatigue, vomiting, hepatotoxicity, hemorrhagic events
Pegaspargase (Oncaspar)	ALL	Miscellaneous	Hypotension, anorexia, nausea, vomiting, hepatotoxicity, pancreatitis, depression of clotting factors, malaise, confusion, lethargy, EEG changes, respiratory distress, hypersensitivity reaction, fever, hyperglycemia, stomatitis
Pemetrexed (Alimta)	NSCLC, nonsquamous, mesothelioma	Antimetabolite	Anorexia, constipation, diarrhea, neuropathy, anemia, chest pain, dyspnea, rash, fatigue
Pentostatin (Nipent)	Hairy cell leukemia	Antibiotic	Nausea, vomiting, hepatic disorders, elevated hepatic function tests, leukopenia, anemia, thrombocytopenia, rash, fever, upper respiratory infection, fatigue, hematuria, headaches, myalgia, arthralgia, diarrhea, anorexia
Pertuzumab (Perjeta)	Breast cancer, metastatic	HER2/neu receptor antagonist	Alopecia, diarrhea, nausea, neutropenia, rash, fatigue, peripheral neuropathy
Polatuzumab vedotin-piiq (Polivy)	Diffuse large B-cell lymphoma, relapsed or refractory	Anti-CD79B antibody drug conjugate, monoclonal antibody	Peripheral neuropathy, neutropenia, diarrhea, thrombocytopenia, anemia; decreased calcium; increased creatinine
Pomalidomide (Pomalyst)	Multiple myeloma, relapsed/refractory	Immunomodulator	Dyspnea, fatigue, peripheral edema, anorexia, rash, neutropenia, leukopenia, thrombocytopenia
Ponatinib (Iclusig)	ALL, CML	Kinase inhibitor	Abdominal pain, rash, fatigue, hypertension, pyrexia, myelosuppression, arthralgia, vomiting

Procarbazine (Matulane)	Hodgkin lymphoma, NHLs, CNS tumors	Alkylating agent	Nausea, vomiting, stomatitis, diarrhea, constipation, myelosuppression, pruritus, hyperpigmentation, alopecia, myalgia, paresthesia, confusion, lethargy, mental depression, fever, hepatic toxicity, arthralgia, respiratory disorders
Ramucirumab (Cyramza)	Colorectal cancer, metastatic, gastric cancer, advanced or metastatic, NSCLC, metastatic	Miscellaneous	Diarrhea, hypertension
Regorafenib (Stivarga)	Colorectal cancer, GIST	VEGF inhibitor	Asthenia, fatigue, mucositis, weight loss, fever, GI perforation, hemorrhage, infections, palmer-planter erythrodysesthesia syndrome (PPES)
Ribociclib (Kisqali)	Breast cancer, metastatic or advanced	Kinase inhibitor	Neutropenia, nausea, fatigue, diarrhea, leukopenia, alopecia, vomiting, headache
Ripretinib (Qinlock)	Gastrointestinal stromal tumor, advanced	KIT inhibitor, PDGFR-alpha blocker, tyrosine kinase inhibitor	Alopecia, abdominal pain, constipation, decreased appetite, diarrhea, fatigue; increased INR, prolonged partial thromboplastin time
Rituximab (Rituxan)	CLL, NHL	Monoclonal antibody	Hypotension, arrhythmias, peripheral edema, nausea, vomiting, abdominal pain, leukopenia, thrombocytopenia, neutropenia, rash, pruritus, urticaria, angioedema, myalgia, headaches, dizziness, throat irritation, rhinitis, bronchospasm, hypersensitivity reaction
Rucaparib (Rubraca)	Ovarian cancer, advanced	PARP inhibitor	Nausea, fatigue, vomiting, anemia, decreased appetite, diarrhea, thrombocytopenia, dyspnea, increased AST/ALT, decreased Hgb, platelets, ANC
Sacituzumab govitecan-hziy (Trodelvy)	Breast cancer (triple negative, metastatic, refractory)	Anti-Trop-2 antibody, drug conjugate, monoclonal antibody, topoisomerase I inhibitor	Alopecia, hyperglycemia, hypermagnesemia, constipation, diarrhea, vomiting, anemia, leukopenia, neutropenia, fatigue; decreased albumin, calcium, sodium; prolonged prothrombin time

Continued

CHEMOTHERAPEUTIC AGENTS—cont'd

Name	Uses	Category	Side Effects
Selinexor (Xpovio)	Diffuse large B-cell lymphoma (relapsed or refractory), multiple myeloma (relapsed or refractory)	Nuclear export inhibitor	Fatigue, weight loss, hyponatremia, nausea, decreased appetite, diarrhea, vomiting, thrombocytopenia, anemia, neutropenia, infection
Sipuleucel-T (Provenge)	Prostate cancer, metastatic	Miscellaneous	Chills, fatigue, fever, back pain, nausea, headache, joint ache
Sonidegib (Odomzo)	Basal cell carcinoma, locally advanced	Hedgehog pathway inhibitor	Muscle spasms, alopecia, dysgeusia, fatigue, nausea, diarrhea, decreased weight, musculoskeletal pain, myalgia, headache, abdominal pain, vomiting, pruritus
Sorafenib (Nexavar)	Hepatocellular cancer, renal cell cancer, advanced, thyroid cancer	Tyrosine kinase inhibitor	Fatigue, alopecia, nausea, vomiting, anorexia, constipation, diarrhea, neuropathy, dyspnea, cough, asthenia, pain
Selpercatinib (Retevmo)	NSCLC (metastatic, RET fusion positive), thyroid, medullary cancer (RET mutant), thyroid cancer (RET fusion positive)	RET kinase inhibitor, tyrosine kinase inhibitor	Edema, hypertension, fatigue, leukopenia, thrombocytopenia; decreased albumin, calcium; increased alkaline phosphatase, ALT, AST, creatinine
Sunitinib (Sutent)	GIST, pancreatic neuroendocrine tumors, advanced, renal cell carcinoma, advanced	Tyrosine kinase inhibitor	Hypotension, edema, fatigue, headache, fever, dizziness, rash, hyperpigmentation, diarrhea, nausea, dyspepsia, altered taste, vomiting, neutropenia, thrombocytopenia, increased ALT/AST
Tamoxifen (Nolvadex-D)	Breast cancer	Estrogen receptor antagonist	Skin rash, nausea, vomiting, anorexia, menstrual irregularities, hot flashes, pruritus, vaginal discharge or bleeding, myelosuppression, headaches, tumor or bone pain, ophthalmic changes, weight gain, confusion
Talazoparib (Talzenna)	Breast cancer	PARP inhibitor	Fatigue, hyperglycemia, nausea, decreased Hgb, anemia, neutropenia, increased serum AST, ALT, alkaline phosphatase

Temozolomide (Temodar)	Anaplastic astrocytoma, glioblastoma multiforme	Alkylating agent	Amnesia, fever, infection, leukopenia, neutropenia, peripheral edema, seizures, thrombocytopenia
Temsirolimus (Torisel)	Renal cell carcinoma, advanced	mTOR kinase inhibitor	Rash, asthenia, mucositis, nausea, edema, anorexia, thrombocytopenia, leukopenia
Thioguanine (Tabloid)	AML	Antimetabolite	Anorexia, stomatitis, myelosuppression, hyperuricemia, nausea, vomiting, diarrhea
Thiotepa (Thioplex)	Bladder cancer, papillary, breast cancer	Alkylating agent	Anorexia, nausea, vomiting, mucositis, myelosuppression, amenorrhea, reduced spermatogenesis, fever, hypersensitivity reactions, pain at injection site, headaches, dizziness, alopecia
Tipiracil/trifluridine (Lonsurf)	Colorectal cancer, metastatic	Miscellaneous	Asthenia, fatigue, nausea, diarrhea, vomiting, decreased appetite, pyrexia, abdominal pain
Tisagenlecleucel (Kymriah)	Acute lymphoblastic leukemia (relapsed/refractory); diffuse large B-cell lymphoma (relapsed/refractory)	Chimeric antigen receptor T-cell immunotherapy	Hypotension, tachycardia, hypertension, hypokalemia, hypophosphatemia, decreased appetite, vomiting, diarrhea, nausea, anemia, neutropenia, thrombocytopenia, lymphocytopenia, leukopenia, infection, acute renal failure, fever
Topotecan (Hycamtin)	Cervical cancer, recurrent or resistant, ovarian cancer, metastatic, SCLC, relapsed	Camptothecin	Nausea, vomiting, diarrhea, constipation, abdominal pain, stomatitis, anorexia, neutropenia, leukopenia, thrombocytopenia, anemia, alopecia, headaches, dyspnea, paresthesia
Toremifene (Fareston)	Breast cancer	Estrogen receptor antagonist	Elevated hepatic function tests, nausea, vomiting, constipation, skin discoloration, dermatitis, dizziness, hot flashes, diaphoresis, vaginal discharge or bleeding, ocular changes, cataracts, anxiety
Trabectedin (Yondelis)	Soft tissue sarcoma	Alkylating agent	Nausea, vomiting, fatigue, diarrhea, decreased appetite, peripheral edema, dyspnea, headache, increased ALT, AST, alkaline phosphatase, neutropenia, thrombocytopenia, anemia

Continued

CHEMOTHERAPEUTIC AGENTS—cont'd

Name	Uses	Category	Side Effects
Trametinib (Mekinist)	Melanoma, metastatic or unresectable	MEK inhibitor	Rash, peripheral edema, pyrexia, malignancies, fatigue, hemorrhagic events, HF
Trastuzumab (Herceptin)	Gastric cancer, metastatic, breast cancer, metastatic	Monoclonal antibody	HF, heart murmur (S_3 gallop), nausea, vomiting, diarrhea, abdominal pain, anorexia, rash, peripheral edema, back or bone pain, asthenia (loss of strength, energy), headaches, insomnia, dizziness, cough, dyspnea, rhinitis, pharyngitis
Trastuzumab/hyaluronidase (Herceptin Hylecta)	Breast cancer, adjuvant treatment, metastatic	Anti-HER2 tyrosine kinase inhibitor	Fatigue, alopecia, nausea, diarrhea, neutropenia
Tretinoin (Vesanoid)	Acute promyelocytic leukemia	Miscellaneous	Flushing, nausea, vomiting, diarrhea, constipation, dyspepsia, mucositis, leukocytosis, dry skin/mucous membranes, rash, pruritus, alopecia, dizziness, anxiety, insomnia, headaches, depression, confusion, intracranial hypertension, agitation, dyspnea, shivering, fever, visual changes, earaches, hearing loss, bone pain, myalgia, arthralgia
Tucatinib (Tukysa)	Breast cancer, human epidermal growth factor receptor 2 positive, advanced, unresectable or metastatic	Anti-HER2 tyrosine kinase inhibitor	Palmar-plantar erythrodysesthesia, abdominal pain, diarrhea, nausea, hepatotoxicity, fatigue, headache; decreased magnesium, phosphate, potassium; increased ALT
Valrubicin (Valstar)	Bladder cancer	Anthracycline	Dysuria, hematuria, urinary frequency/incontinence/urgency
Vandetanib (Caprelsa)	Thyroid cancer, medullary	Tyrosine kinase inhibitor	Diarrhea, rash, acne, nausea, hypertension, headache, fatigue, decreased appetite, abdominal pain
Vemurafenib (Zelboraf)	Melanoma, metastatic or unresectable	Kinase inhibitor	Arthralgia, alopecia, fatigue, malignancies, dermatological reactions
Venetoclax (Vencelexta)	CLL	BCL-2 inhibitor	Diarrhea, neutropenia, anemia, nausea, upper respiratory tract infections, thrombocytopenia, fatigue

Vinblastine (Velban)	Mycosis fungoides, Hodgkin lymphoma, lymphocytic lymphoma, testicular cancer, Kaposi sarcoma	Vinca alkaloid	Nausea, vomiting, stomatitis, constipation, myelosuppression, alopecia, peripheral neuropathy, loss of deep tendon reflexes, paresthesia, diarrhea
Vincristine (Oncovin)	ALL, Hodgkin lymphoma, non-Hodgkin lymphomas, Wilm's tumor, neuroblastoma, rhabdomyosarcoma	Vinca alkaloid	Nausea, vomiting, stomatitis, constipation, pharyngitis, polyuria, myelosuppression, alopecia, numbness, paresthesia, peripheral neuropathy, loss of deep tendon reflexes, headaches, abdominal pain
Vincristine liposomal (Marqibo)	ALL	Vinca alkaloid	Constipation, nausea, pyrexia, fatigue, peripheral neuropathy, febrile neutropenia, diarrhea, anemia, reduced appetite, insomnia
Vinorelbine (Navelbine)	NSCLC	Vinca alkaloid	Elevated LFT, nausea, vomiting, constipation, ileus, anorexia, stomatitis, myelosuppression, alopecia, vein discoloration, venous pain, phlebitis, interstitial pulmonary changes, asthenia, fatigue, diarrhea, peripheral neuropathy, loss of deep tendon reflexes
Vismodegib (Erivedge)	Basal cell carcinoma, metastatic or locally advanced	Hedgehog pathway inhibitor	Alopecia, muscle spasms, dysgenesia, weight loss, fatigue, nausea, diarrhea, reduced appetite, vomiting, arthralgia
Vorinostat (Zolinza)	Cutaneous T-cell lymphoma	Histone deacetylase inhibitor	Diarrhea, fatigue, nausea, thrombocytopenia, anorexia, dysgeusia
Zanubrutinib (Brukinsa)	Mantle cell lymphoma, relapsed or refractory	Bruton tyrosine kinase inhibitor	Skin rash, diarrhea, petechiae, lymphocytosis, neutropenia, thrombocytopenia, leukopenia, upper respiratory tract infection; increased ALT, bilirubin, uric acid
Ziv-aflibercept (Zaltrap)	Colorectal cancer, metastatic	Miscellaneous	Leukopenia, neutropenia, diarrhea, proteinuria, increased ALT/AST, stomatitis, thrombocytopenia, hypertension, epistaxis, headache, abdominal pain

AV, Atrioventricular; ***C,*** capsules; ***EEG,*** electroencephalogram; ***ECG,*** electrocardiogram; ***GI,*** gastrointestinal; ***HF,*** heart failure; ***I,*** injection; ***LFT,*** liver function test; ***T,*** tablets; ***UTI,*** urinary tract infection.

Contraception

ACTION	CLASSIFICATION	
Combination oral contraceptives decrease fertility primarily by inhibition of ovulation. In addition, they can promote thickening of the cervical mucus, thereby creating a physical barrier for the passage of sperm. Also, they can modify the endometrium, making it less favorable for nidation.	Oral contraceptives either contain both an estrogen and a progestin (combination oral contraceptives) or contain only a progestin (progestin-only oral contraceptives). The combination oral contraceptives have four subgroups: *Monophasic:* Daily estrogen and progestin dosage remains constant.	*Biphasic:* Estrogen remains constant, but the progestin dosage increases during the second half of the cycle. *Triphasic:* Progestin changes for each phase of the cycle. *Four-phasic:* Contains four progestin/estrogen dosing combinations during the 20-day cycle.

COMMON COMPLAINTS WITH ORAL CONTRACEPTIVES

Too much estrogen	Nausea, bloating, breast tenderness, increased B/P, melasma, headache
Too little estrogen	Early or midcycle breakthrough bleeding, increased spotting, hypomenorrhea
Too much progestin	Breast tenderness, headache, fatigue, changes in mood
Too little progestin	Late breakthrough bleeding
Too much androgen	Increased appetite, weight gain, acne, oily skin, hirsutism, decreased libido, increased breast size, breast tenderness, increased LDL cholesterol, decreased HDL cholesterol

B/P, Blood pressure; ***HDL,*** high-density lipoprotein; ***LDL,*** low-density lipoprotein.

CONTRACEPTIVES

Name	Estrogen Content	Progestin Content
Low-Dose Monophasic Pills		
Aubra Aviane Falmina Lessina Lutera Orsythia Sronyx	EE 20 mcg	Levonorgestrel 0.1 mg
Junel 1/20 Junel Fe 1/20 Loestrin Fe 1/20 Microgestin Fe 1/20 Tarina Fe 1/20 EQ	EE 20 mcg	Norethindrone 1 mg
Altavera Levora Marlissa Portia-28	EE 30 mcg	Levonorgestrel 0.15 mg
Cryselle-28 Elinest Low-Ogestrel-28	EE 30 mcg	Norgestrel 0.3 mg
Junel 1.5/30 Junel Fe 1.5/30 Larin 1.5/30 Loestrin Fe 1.5/30 Microgestin 1.5/30 Microgestin Fe 1.5/30	EE 30 mcg	Norethindrone acetate 1.5 mg

Continued

CONTRACEPTIVES—cont'd

Name	Estrogen Content	Progestin Content
Apri Juleber Reclipsen	EE 30 mcg	Desogestrel 0.15 mg
Ocella Syeda	EE 30 mcg	Drospirenone 3 mg
Yasmin Kelnor 1/35 Zovia 1/35	EE 35 mcg	Ethynodiol diacetate 1 mg
Estarylla Mononessa Previfem Sprintec	EE 35 mcg	Norgestimate 0.25 mg
Balziva Femcon Fe	EE 35 mcg	Norethindrone 0.4 mg
Nortrel 1/35 Ortho-Novum 1/35	EE 35 mcg	Norethindrone 1 mg (total of 21 mg/cycle)
High-Dose Monophasic Pills		
Kelnor 1/50–28	EE 50 mcg	Ethynodiol diacetate 1 mg
Ogestrel 0.5/50	EE 50 mcg	Norgestrel 0.5 mg

Biphasic Pills		
Azurette Kariva Mircette	EE 20 mcg × 21 days, placebo × 2 days, 10 mcg × 5 days	Desogestrel 0.15 mg × 21 days
Triphasic Pills		
Tilia Fe Tri-Legest Fe	EE 20 mcg × 5 days, 30 mcg × 7 days, 35 mcg × 9 days	Norethindrone 1 mg × 21 days
Ortho Tri-Cyclen Lo	EE 25 mcg × 21 days	Norgestimate 0.18 mg × 7 days, 0.215 mg × 7 days, 0.25 mg × 7 days
Caziant Cyclessa Velivet	EE 25 mcg × 21 days	Desogestrel 0.1 mg × 7 days, 0.125 mg × 7 days, 0.15 mg × 7 days
Enpresse Trivora	EE 30 mcg × 6 days, 40 mcg × 5 days. 30 mcg × 10 days	Levonorgestrel 0.05 mg × 6 days, 0.075 mg × 5 days, 0.125 mg × 10 days
Ortho Tri-Cyclen Tri-Previfem Tri-Sprintec	EE 35 mcg × 21 days	Norgestimate 0.18 mg × 7 days, 0.215 mg × 7 days, 0.25 mg × 7 days
Aranelle Leena	EE 35 mcg × 21 days	Norethindrone 0.5 mg × 7 days, 1 mg × 9 days, 0.5 mg × 5 days
Nortrel 7/7/7 Ortho-Novum 7/7/7	EE 35 mcg × 21 days	Norethindrone 0.5 mg × 7 days, 0.75 mg × 7 days, 1 mg × 7 days
Four Phasic		
Natazia	Estradiol 3 mg × 2 days, then 2 mg × 22 days, then 1 mg × 2 days, then 2-day pill-free interval	Dienogest none × 2 days, then 2 mg × 5 days, then 3 mg × 17 days, then none for 4 days

Continued

CONTRACEPTIVES—cont'd

Name	Estrogen Content	Progestin Content
Extended-Cycle Pills		
Loestrin FE	EE 20 mcg × 24 days	Norethindrone 1 mg × 24 days
Jolessa	EE 30 mcg × 84 days	Levonorgestrel 0.15 mg × 84 days
Quartette	EE 20 mcg × 42 days, 25 mcg × 21 days, 30 mcg × 21 days, then 10 mcg × 7 days	Levonorgestrel 0.15 mg × 84 days
Seasonique	EE 30 mcg × 84 days, 10 mcg × 7 days	Levonorgestrel 0.15 mg × 84 days
Yaz Gianvi	EE 20 mcg × 24 days	Drospirenone 3 mg × 24 days
Continuous Cycle Pill		
Amethyst	EE 20 mcg	Levonorgestrel 90 mcg
Progestin-Only Pills		
Camilla Errin Nora-BE Slynd	N/A	Norethindrone 0.35 mg Norethindrone 0.35 mg Norethindrone 0.35 mg Drospirenone 4 mg x 24 days
Emergency Contraception		
Plan B	N/A	Levonorgestrel 0.75-mg tablets taken 12 hrs apart
Ella	N/A	Ulipristal 30 mg one time within 5 days after unprotected intercourse

Hormonal Alternative to Oral Contraception

Annovera Depo-Provera CI Medroxyprogesterone Acetate	EE 13 mcg/day None	Segesterone acetate 150 mcg/day Medroxyprogesterone 150 mg
Depo-SubQ Provera 104	None	Medroxyprogesterone 104 mg
Kyleena	None	19.5 mg for 5 yrs
Liletta	None	52 mg for 3 yrs
Mirena	None	Levonorgestrel 20 mcg/day for up to 5 yrs
NuvaRing	EE 15 mcg/day	Etonogestrel 0.12 mg/day
Skyla	None	13.5 mg for 3 yrs

EE, Ethinyl estradiol.

Corticosteroids

USES	ACTION
Replacement therapy in adrenal insufficiency, including Addison's disease. Symptomatic treatment of multiorgan disease/conditions. Rheumatoid arthritis (RA), osteoarthritis, severe psoriasis, ulcerative colitis, lupus erythematosus, anaphylactic shock, acute exacerbation of asthma, status asthmaticus, organ transplant.	Suppress migration of polymorphonuclear leukocytes (PML) and reverse increased capillary permeability by their anti-inflammatory effect. Suppress immune system by decreasing activity of lymphatic system.

Continued

CORTICOSTEROIDS

Name	Availability	Route of Administration	Side Effects
Beclomethasone (Beconase, Qnasl, QVAR)	**Aerosol (oral inhalation), QVAR:** 40 mcg/ inhalation, 80 mcg/inhalation **Aerosol (spray, intranasal), Qnasl:** 80 mcg/ inhalation **Suspension (intranasal), Beconase:** 42 mcg/ inhalation	Inhalation, intranasal	**I:** Cough, dry mouth/throat, headaches, throat irritation, increased blood glucose **Nasal:** Headaches, sore throat, intranasal ulceration, increased blood glucose
Betamethasone (Celestone)	**I:** 6 mg/ml	IV, intralesional, intra-articular	Nausea, vomiting, increased appetite, weight gain, insomnia, increased blood glucose
Budesonide (Pulmicort, Rhinocort)	**Nasal:** 32 mcg/spray **Suspension for nebulization:** 250 mcg, 500 mcg	Intranasal	Headaches, sore throat, intranasal ulceration, increased blood glucose
Cortisone (Cortone)	**T:** 5 mg, 10 mg, 25 mg	PO	Insomnia, nervousness, increased appetite, indigestion, increased blood glucose
Dexamethasone (Decadron)	**T:** 0.5 mg, 1 mg, 4 mg, 6 mg **OS:** 0.5 mg/5 ml **I:** 4 mg/ml, 10 mg/ml	PO, parenteral	Insomnia, weight gain, increased appetite, increased blood glucose
Fludrocortisone (Florinef)	**T:** 0.1 mg	PO	Edema, headache, peptic ulcer, increased blood glucose
Flunisolide (Nasalide)	**Nasal:** 25 mcg/spray	Inhalation, intranasal	Headache, nasal congestion, pharyngitis, upper respiratory infections, altered taste/ smell, increased blood glucose
Fluticasone (Flonase, Flovent)	**Inhalation:** 44 mcg, 110 mg, 220 mcg **Nasal:** 50 mg, 100 mcg	Inhalation, intranasal	Headache, burning/stinging, nasal congestion, upper respiratory infections, increased blood glucose
Hydrocortisone (Solu-Cortef)	**T:** 5 mg, 10 mg, 25 mg **I:**100 mg, 250 mg, 500 mg, 1 g	PO, parenteral	Insomnia, headache, nausea, vomiting, increased blood glucose

Methylprednisolone (Solu-Medrol)	**T:** 4 mg **I:** 40 mg, 125 mg, 500 mg, 1 g, 2 g	PO, parenteral	Headache, insomnia, nervousness, increased appetite, nausea, vomiting, increased blood glucose
Prednisolone (Prelone)	**T:** 5 mg **OS:** 5 mg/5 ml, 15 mg/5 ml	PO	Headache, insomnia, weight gain, nausea, vomiting, increased blood glucose
Prednisone	**T:** 1 mg, 2.5 mg, 5 mg, 10 mg, 20 mg, 50 mg	PO	Headache, insomnia, weight gain, nausea, vomiting, increased blood glucose
Triamcinolone (Kenalog, Nasacort AQ)	**Injection, suspension:** 10 mg/ml, 40 mg/ml **Intranasal, suspension:** 55 mcg/ inhalation	IM, inhalation (nasal)	**PO:** Insomnia, increased appetite, nausea, vomiting, increased blood glucose **I:** Cough, dry mouth/throat, headaches, throat irritation, increased blood glucose

I, Injection; ***OS,*** oral suspension; ***T,*** tablets.

Diuretics

USES

Thiazides: Management of edema resulting from a number of causes (e.g., HF, hepatic cirrhosis); hypertension either alone or in combination with other antihypertensives.

Loop: Management of edema associated with HF, cirrhosis of the liver, and renal disease. Furosemide used in treatment of hypertension alone or in combination with other antihypertensives.

Potassium-sparing: Adjunctive treatment with thiazides, loop diuretics in treatment of HF and hypertension.

ACTION

Increase the excretion of water/sodium and other electrolytes via the kidneys. Exact mechanism of antihypertensive effect unknown; may be due to reduced plasma volume or decreased peripheral vascular resistance. Subclassifications of diuretics are based on their mechanism and site of action.

Thiazides: Act at cortical diluting segment of nephron, block reabsorption of Na, CI, and water; promote excretion of Na, CI, K, and water.

Loop: Act primarily at the thick ascending limb of Henle's loop to inhibit Na, CI, and water absorption.

Potassium-sparing: Spironolactone blocks aldosterone action on distal nephron (causes K retention, Na excretion). Triamterene, amiloride act on distal nephron, decreasing Na reuptake, reducing K secretion.

DIURETICS

Name	Availability	Dosage Range	Side Effects
Thiazide, Thiazide-related			
Chlorothiazide (Diuril)	**T:** 250 mg, 500 mg **S:** 250 mg/5 mL **I:** 500 mg	**Edema:** 500–1,000 mg 1–2 times/day **HTN:** 500–2,000 mg/day in 1–2 divided doses	**CLASS** Hyperuricemia, hypokalemia, hypomagnesemia, hyperglycemia, hyponatremia, hypercalcemia, hypercholesterolemia, hypertriglyceridemia, pancreatitis, rash, photosensitivity
Chlorthalidone	**Hygroton:** 25 mg, 50 mg, 100 mg	**Edema:** Initially, 50–100 mg once daily or 100 mg every other day **Maximum:** 200 mg/day	
Hydrochlorothiazide	**T:** 12.5 mg, 25 mg, 50 mg **C:** 12.5 mg	**Edema:** 25–100 mg/day in 1–2 divided doses **HTN:** Initially, 12.5–25 mg once daily. May increase up to 50 mg/day in 1 or 2 divided doses	
Indapamide (Lozol)	**T:** 1.25 mg, 2.5 mg	**Edema:** Initially, 2.5 mg/day. May increase after 1 wk to 5 mg/day **HTN:** Initially, 2.5 mg/day. May increase q4wks to 2.5 mg, then to 5 mg/day	
Metolazone (Zaroxolyn)	**T:** 2.5 mg, 5 mg, 10 mg	**Edema:** 2.5–20 mg once daily **HTN:** 2.5–5 mg once daily	
Loop			
Bumetanide (Bumex)	**T:** 0.5 mg, 1 mg, 2 mg **I:** 0.25 mg/mL	**Edema:** Initially, 0.5–2 mg/dose 1–2 times/day **Maximum:** 10 mg/day	**CLASS** Dehydration, hypokalemia, hyponatremia, hypomagnesemia, hyperglycemia, metabolic alkalosis, hyperuricemia, blood dyscrasias, rash, hypercholesterolemia, hypertriglyceridemia
Furosemide (Lasix)	**T:** 20 mg, 40 mg, 80 mg **OS:** 10 mg/mL, 40 mg/5 mL **I:** 10 mg/mL	**HTN:** 20–80 mg/day in 2 divided doses **Edema: PO:** 20–80 mg/dose. May increase by 20–40 mg/dose up to 600 mg/day. **IV:** 20–40 mg/dose. May increase by 20 mg/dose. **Maximum:** 200 mg/dose	
Torsemide (Demadex)	**T:** 5 mg, 10 mg, 20 mg, 100 mg **I:** 10 mg/mL	**Edema:** 10–200 mg/day **HTN:** Initially, 5 mg/day. May increase after 4–6 wks to 10 mg/day	

Continued

DIURETICS—cont'd

Name	Availability	Dosage Range	Side Effects
Potassium-sparing			
Amiloride (Midamor)	**T:** 5 mg	**HF/Edema:** Initially, 5 mg/day. May increase to 10 mg/day	Hyperkalemia, nausea, abdominal pain, diarrhea, rash, headache
Eplerenone (Inspra)	**T:** 25 mg, 50 mg	**HF:** Initially, 25 mg/day, titrate to 50 mg once daily **HTN:** Initially, 50 mg/day. May increase to 50 mg 2 times/day	Hyperkalemia, hyponatremia
Spironolactone (Aldactone)	**T:** 25 mg, 50 mg, 100 mg	**Edema:** 25–200 mg/day in 1 or 2 divided doses **HTN:** 50–100 mg/day in 1 or 2 divided doses **Hypokalemia:** 25–100 mg/day **HF:** Initially, 12.5–25 mg once daily **Maximum:** 50 mg/day	Hyperkalemia, nausea, vomiting, abdominal cramps, diarrhea, hyponatremia, gynecomastia, menstrual abnormalities, rash
Triamterene (Dyrenium)	**C:** 50 mg, 100 mg	**Edema, HTN:** 100–300 mg/day in 1–2 divided doses	Hyperkalemia, nausea, abdominal pain, nephrolithiasis

C, Capsules; ***HF,*** heart failure; ***HTN,*** hypertension; ***I,*** injection; ***OS,*** oral solution; ***S,*** suspension; ***T,*** tablets.

H_2 Antagonists

USES	ACTION
Short-term treatment of duodenal ulcer (DU), active benign gastric ulcer (GU), maintenance therapy of DU, pathologic hypersecretory conditions (e.g., Zollinger-Ellison syndrome), gastroesophageal reflux disease (GERD), and prevention of upper GI bleeding in critically ill pts.	Inhibits gastric acid secretion by interfering with histamine at the histamine H_2 receptors in parietal cells. Decreases basal acid secretion and food-stimulated acid secretion.

H_2 ANTAGONISTS

Name	Availability	Usual Adult Dose	Class Side Effects
Cimetidine (Tagamet)	**T**: 200 mg, 300 mg, 400 mg, 800 mg **L**: 300 mg/5 mL	200–400 mg bid	Severe effects uncommon. Hepatitis, hematologic toxicity, CNS effects (e.g., headache, fatigue, cognitive impairment)
Famotidine (Pepcid)	**T**: 10 mg, 20 mg, 40 mg **OS**: 40 mg/5 mL **I**: 10 mg/mL	20–40 mg bid	
Nizatidine (Axid)	**OS**: 15 mg/mL **C**: 75 mg, 150 mg, 300 mg	150 mg bid	

C, Capsules; ***CNS,*** central nervous system; ***I,*** injection; ***L,*** liquid; ***OS,*** oral suspension; ***T,*** tablets.

Hepatitis C Virus Infection

Hepatitis C virus (HCV) infection is the leading blood-borne infection in the US. HCV is transmitted by exposure to infected blood products. Risk factors for acquiring HCV include injection drug use, receiving contaminated blood products, needle sticks, and vertical transmission. If untreated, HCV may progress to chronic HCV and long-term sequelae including cirrhosis and hepatocellular carcinoma. There are seven known genotypes of HCV (genotypes 1–7) which impact the selection of initial therapy and treatment response. Genotype 1 is the most common and is further subtyped into genotypes 1a and 1b.

Currently, there are two indirect-acting antivirals and seven direct-acting antivirals approved for the treatment of chronic HCV

ACTION

Indirect Acting Antivirals (IAA)

Alpha Interferons (peginterferons): Induces immune response against HCV, inhibiting viral replication

Ribavirin: Exact mechanism unknown but has activity against several RNA and DNA viruses

Direct Acting Antivirals (DAA)

NS3/4A Protease Inhibitors (PIs): Targets the serine protease NS3/NS4 that is responsible for processing HCV polyprotein and producing new viruses.

Nonstructural Protein 5A (NS5A) Inhibitors: Suppress the NS5A protein, which is essential for viral assembly and replication.

Nonstructural Protein 5B (NS5B) Inhibitors: Suppress the NS5B RNA-dependent RNA polymerase that is responsible for HCV replication.

ANTI-HEPATITIS C VIRUS PREPARATIONS

Name	Type	Genotype	Dosage	Side Effects
Elbasvir, grazoprevir (Zepatier)	DAA NS5A/NS3/4A protease inhibitor	1, 4	**Genotype 1a:** One tablet daily for 12 wks (16 wks with baseline NS5A polymorphins) **Genotype 1b:** One tablet daily for 12 wks **Genotype 4:** One tablet daily for 12 wks (16 wks peginterferon/ribavirin experienced)	Fatigue, headache, nausea
Glecaprevir, pibrentasvir (Mavyret)	DAA NS5A/NS3/4A protease inhibitor	1, 2, 3, 4, 5, 6	**Genotypes 1, 2, 3, 4, 5, 6:** Three tablets once daily. Treatment duration 8–16 wks based on patients that are mono-infected, and coinfected with compensated liver disease (with or without cirrhosis) and with or without renal impairment	Headache, fatigue, nausea, diarrhea, increased serum bilirubin
Simeprevir (Olysio)	DAA (NS3/4A-PI)	1, 4	150 mg once daily plus peginterferon and ribavirin for 12 wks, then additional 12–36 wks of peginterferon and ribavirin 150 mg once daily plus sofosbuvir for 12 wks without cirrhosis or 24 wks with cirrhosis	(With peginterferon, ribavirin): Rash, itching, nausea, photosensitivity (With sofosbuvir): Fatigue, headache, nausea, insomnia, pruritus, rash, dizziness, diarrhea
Sofosbuvir (Sovaldi)	DAA (NS5B)	1, 2, 3, 4	**Genotypes 1, 4:** 400 mg once daily plus peginterferon and ribavirin for 12 wks 400 mg once daily plus simeprevir for 12 wks without cirrhosis or 24 wks with cirrhosis **Genotypes 2, 3:** 400 mg once daily plus ribavirin for 12 wks for genotype 2 or 24 wks for genotype 3	(With peginterferon, ribavirin): Fatigue, headache, nausea, insomnia, anemia (With simeprevir): Fatigue, headache, nausea, insomnia, pruritus, rash, dizziness, diarrhea
Ledipasvir, Sofosbuvir (Harvoni)	DAA (NS5A/NS5B)	1, 4, 5, 6	**Genotype 1:** One tablet (90 mg/400 mg) for 12 wks in treatment-naïve pt with or without cirrhosis and treatment-experienced pt without cirrhosis; for 24 wks for treatment-experienced pts with cirrhosis **Genotypes 4, 5, 6:** One tablet daily for 12 wks	Fatigue, headache, nausea, diarrhea, insomnia; elevations in bilirubin, lipase, and creatinine kinase

Continued

ANTI-HEPATITIS C VIRUS PREPARATIONS—cont'd

Name	Type	Genotype	Dosage	Side Effects
Ombitasvir, paritaprevir, ritonavir, dasabuvir (Viekira Pak)	DAA (NS5A/protease inhibitor/CYP3A inhibitor/polymerase inhibitor)	1	Two ombitasvir, paritaprevir, ritonavir tablets (12.5 mg, 75 mg, 50 mg) once daily in the morning plus one dasabuvir 250 mg tablet 2 times/day Patients with **genotype 1a or 1b with cirrhosis** will also receive ribavirin for 12 wks (genotype 1a with cirrhosis: 12–24 wks based on treatment history; liver transplant pts: 24 wks)	(With ribavirin): Fatigue, nausea, itching, insomnia (Without ribavirin): Nausea, itching, insomnia
Peginterferon alfa 2a (Pegasys)	IAA (Interferon)	1, 2, 3, 4	180 mcg SQ wkly for 12–48 wks based on antiviral regimen, pt history, response	(With ribavirin): Fatigue, weakness, fever, myalgia, headache
Peginterferon alfa 2b (PegIntron)	IAA (Interferon)	1, 2, 3, 4	1.5 mcg/kg SQ wkly for 12–48 wks based on antiviral regimen, pt history, response	(With ribavirin): Injection site reaction, fatigue, weakness, headache, rigors, fever, nausea, myalgia, insomnia, mood instability, hair loss
Ribavirin (Copegus, Ribasphere)	IAA (Nucleoside analogue)	1, 2, 3, 4	**Genotypes 2, 3** 400 mg 2 times/day (with peginterferon) **Genotypes 1, 4** <75 kg: 400 mg qam; and 600 mg qpm; 75 kg or greater: 600 mg 2 times/day	(With peginterferon): Fatigue, weakness, headache, rigors, fever, nausea, myalgia, insomnia, mood instability, hair loss
Daclatasvir (Daklinza)	DAA (NS5A)	3	60 mg once daily with sofosbuvir for 12 wks	Headache, fatigue
Ombitasvir, paritaprevir, ritonavir (Technivie)	DAA (NS5A/protease inhibitor/CYP3A inhibitor)	4	Two tablets once daily with ribavirin for 12 wks	Asthenia, fatigue, nausea, insomnia
Sofosbuvir/velpatasvir (Epclusa)	DAA (NS5B/NS5A)	1, 2, 3, 4, 5, 6	One tablet daily for 12 wks	Insomnia, anemia, headache, fatigue, nausea, diarrhea
Sofosbuvir/velpatasvir/voxilaprevir (VOSEVI)	DAA (NS5B/NS5A/protease inhibitor)	1, 2, 3, 4, 5, 6	One tablet daily for 12 wks	Headache, fatigue, diarrhea, nausea

Hormones

USES

Functions of the body are regulated by two major control systems: the nervous system and the endocrine (hormone) system. Together they maintain homeostasis and control different metabolic functions in the body.

Hormones are concerned with control of different metabolic functions in the body (e.g., rates of chemical reactions in cells, transporting substances through cell membranes, cellular metabolism [growth/secretions]). By definition, a hormone is a chemical substance secreted into body fluids by cells and has control over other cells in the body.

Hormones can be local or general:

- *Local hormones* have specific local effects (e.g., acetylcholine, which is secreted at parasympathetic and skeletal nerve endings).
- *General hormones* are mostly secreted by specific endocrine glands (e.g., epinephrine/norepinephrine are secreted by the adrenal medulla in response to sympathetic stimulation), transported in the blood to all parts of the body, causing many different reactions.

Some general hormones affect all or almost all cells of the body (e.g., thyroid hormone from the thyroid gland increases the rate of most chemical reactions in almost all cells of the body); other general hormones affect only specific tissue (e.g., ovarian hormones are specific to female sex organs and secondary sexual characteristics of the female).

ACTION

Endocrine hormones almost never directly act intracellularly affecting chemical reactions. They first combine with hormone receptors either on the cell surface or inside the cell (cell cytoplasm or nucleus). The combination of hormone and receptors alters the function of the receptor, and the receptor is the direct cause of the hormone effects. Altered receptor function may include the following:

Altered cell permeability, which causes a change in protein structure of the receptor, usually opening or closing a channel for one or more ions. The movement of these ions causes the effect of the hormone.

Activation of intracellular enzymes immediately inside the cell membrane (e.g., hormone combines with receptor that then becomes the activated enzyme adenyl cyclase, which causes formation of cAMP).

◀ALERT▶ cAMP has effects inside the cell. It is not the hormone but cAMP that causes these effects.

Regulation of hormone secretion is controlled by an internal control system, the negative feedback system:

- Endocrine gland oversecretes.
- Hormone exerts more and more of its effect.

Continued

Hormones—cont'd

ACTION—cont'd

- Target organ performs its function.
- Too much function in turn feeds back to endocrine gland to decrease secretory rate.

The endocrine system contains many glands and hormones. A summary of the important glands and their hormones secreted are as follows:

The pituitary gland (hypophysis) is a small gland found in the sella turcica at the base of the brain. The pituitary is divided into two portions physiologically: the anterior pituitary (adenohypophysis) and the posterior pituitary (neurohypophysis). Six important hormones are secreted from the anterior pituitary and two from the posterior pituitary.

Anterior pituitary hormones:
- Growth hormone (GH)
- Adrenocorticotropin (corticotropin)
- Thyroid-stimulating hormone (thyrotropin) (TSH)
- Follicle-stimulating hormone (FSH)
- Luteinizing hormone (LH)
- Prolactin

Posterior pituitary hormones:
- Antidiuretic hormone (vasopressin)
- Oxytocin

Almost all secretions of the pituitary hormones are controlled by hormonal or nervous signals from the hypothalamus. The hypothalamus is a center of information concerned with the well-being of the body, which in turn is used to control secretions of the important pituitary hormones just listed. Secretions from the posterior pituitary are controlled by nerve signals originating in the hypothalamus; anterior pituitary hormones are controlled by hormones secreted within the hypothalamus. These hormones are as follows:
- Thyrotropin-releasing hormone (TRH) releasing thyroid-stimulating hormone
- Corticotropin-releasing hormone (CRH) releasing adrenocorticotropin
- Growth hormone–releasing hormone (GHRH) releasing growth hormone and growth hormone inhibitory hormone (GHIH) (same as somatostatin)
- Gonadotropin-releasing hormone (GnRH) releasing the two gonadotropic hormones, LH and FSH
- Prolactin inhibitory factor (PIF) causing inhibition of prolactin and prolactin-releasing factor

Anterior Pituitary Hormones

All anterior pituitary hormones (except growth hormone) have as their principal effect stimulating target glands.

Growth Hormone (GH)

Growth hormone affects almost all tissues of the body. GH (somatotropin) causes growth in almost all tissues of the body (increases cell size, increases mitosis with increased number of cells, and differentiates certain types of cells). Metabolic effects include increased rate of protein synthesis, mobilization of fatty acids from adipose tissue, decreased rate of glucose utilization.

Thyroid-Stimulating Hormone (TSH)

Thyroid-stimulating hormone controls secretion of the thyroid hormones. The thyroid gland is located immediately below the larynx on either side of and anterior to the trachea and secretes two significant hormones, thyroxine (T_4) and triiodothyronine (T_3), which have a profound effect on increasing the metabolic rate of the body. The thyroid gland also secretes calcitonin, an important hormone for calcium metabolism. Calcitonin promotes deposition of calcium in the bones, which decreases calcium concentration in the extracellular fluid.

Adrenocorticotropin

Adrenocorticotropin causes the adrenal cortex to secrete adrenocortical hormones. The adrenal glands lie at the superior poles of the two kidneys. Each gland is composed of two distinct parts: the adrenal medulla and the cortex. The adrenal medulla, related to the sympathetic nervous system, secretes the hormones epinephrine and norepinephrine. When stimulated, they cause constriction of blood vessels, increased activity of the heart inhibitory effects on the GI tract, and dilation of the pupils. The adrenal cortex secretes corticosteroids, of which there are two major types: mineralocorticoids and glucocorticoids. Aldosterone, the principal mineralocorticoid, primarily affects electrolytes of the extracellular fluids. Cortisol, the principal glucocorticoid, affects glucose, protein, and fat metabolism.

Luteinizing Hormone

Luteinizing hormone plays an important role in ovulation and causes secretion of female sex hormones by the ovaries and testosterone by the testes.

Follicle-Stimulating Hormone

Follicle-stimulating hormone causes growth of follicles in the ovaries before ovulation and promotes formation of sperm in the testes.

Ovarian sex hormones are estrogens and progestins. Estradiol is the most important estrogen; progesterone is the most important progestin.

Estrogens mainly promote proliferation and growth of specific cells in the body and are responsible for development of most of the secondary sex characteristics. Primarily cause cellular proliferation and growth of tissues of sex organs/other tissue related to reproduction. Ovaries, fallopian tubes, uterus, vagina increase in size. Estrogen initiates growth of breast and milk-producing apparatus, external appearance.

Progesterone stimulates secretion of the uterine endometrium during the latter half of the female sexual cycle, preparing the uterus for implantation of the fertilized ovum. Decreases the frequency of uterine contractions (helps prevent expulsion of the implanted ovum). Progesterone promotes development of breasts, causing alveolar cells to proliferate, enlarge, and become secretory in nature.

Testosterone is secreted by the testes and formed by the interstitial cells of Leydig. Testosterone production increases under the stimulus of the anterior pituitary gonadotropic hormones. It is responsible for distinguishing characteristics of the masculine body (stimulates the growth of male sex organs and promotes the development of male secondary sex characteristics, e.g., distribution of body hair; effect on voice, protein formation, and muscular development).

Prolactin

Prolactin promotes the development of breasts and secretion of milk.

POSTERIOR PITUITARY HORMONES

Antidiuretic Hormone (ADH) (Vasopressin)

ADH can cause antidiuresis (decreased excretion of water by the kidneys). In the presence of ADH, the permeability of the renal-collecting ducts and tubules to water increases, which allows water to be absorbed, conserving water in the body. ADH in higher concentrations is a very potent vasoconstrictor, constricting arterioles everywhere in the body, increasing B/P.

Oxytocin

Oxytocin contracts the uterus during the birthing process, esp. toward the end of the pregnancy, helping expel the baby. Oxytocin also contracts myoepithelial cells in the breasts, causing milk to be expressed from the alveoli into the ducts so that the baby can obtain it by suckling.

Continued

Hormones—cont'd

ACTION—cont'd

PANCREAS

The pancreas is composed of two tissue types: *acini* (secrete digestive juices in the duodenum) and *islets of Langerhans* (secrete insulin/glucagons directly into the blood). The islets of Langerhans contain three cells: alpha, beta, and delta. Alpha cells secrete glucagon, beta cells secrete insulin, and delta cells secrete somatostatin.

Insulin promotes glucose entry into most cells, thus controlling the rate of metabolism of most carbohydrates. Insulin also affects fat metabolism.

Glucagon effects are opposite those of insulin, the most important of which is increasing blood glucose concentration by releasing it from the liver into the circulating body fluids.

Somatostatin (same chemical as secreted by the hypothalamus) has multiple inhibitory effects: depresses secretion of insulin and glucagon, decreases GI motility, decreases secretions/absorption of the GI tract.

Human Immunodeficiency Virus (HIV) Infection

USES

Antiretroviral (ARV) agents are used in the treatment of HIV infection.

An ARV regimen for treatment-naive patients generally consists of two nucleoside reverse transcriptase inhibitors (NRTIs) in combination with a third ARV medication from one of three drug classes: an integrase inhibitor (INSTI), non-nucleoside reverse transcriptase inhibitor, or a protease inhibitor (PI) with either cobicistat or ritonavir.

ACTION

Nucleoside reverse transcriptase inhibitors compete with natural substrates for formation of proviral DNA by reverse transcriptase inhibiting viral replication.

Nucleotide reverse transcriptase inhibitors (NtRTIs) inhibit reverse transcriptase by competing with the natural substrate deoxyadenosine triphosphate and by DNA chain termination.

Non-nucleoside reverse transcriptase inhibitors directly bind to reverse transcriptase and block RNA-dependent and DNA-dependent DNA polymerase activities by disrupting the enzyme's catalytic site.

Protease inhibitors (PIs) bind to the active site of HIV-1 protease and prevent the processing of viral gag and gag-pol polyprotein precursors resulting in immature, noninfectious mal particles.

Fusion inhibitors interfere with the entry of HIV-1 into cells by inhibiting fusion of viral and cellular membranes. *CCR5 coreceptor antagonist* selectively binds to human chemokine receptor CCR5 present on cell membrane preventing HIV-1 from entering cells.

Integrase inhibitor inhibits catalytic activity of HIV-1 integrase, an HIV-1 encoded enzyme required for viral replication.

ANTIRETROVIRAL AGENTS FOR TREATMENT OF HIV INFECTION

Name	Availability	Dosage Range	Side Effects
Nucleoside Analogues			
Abacavir (Ziagen)	**T:** 300 mg **OS:** 20 mg/mL	**A:** 300 mg 2 times/day or 600 mg once daily	Nausea, vomiting, malaise, rash, fever, headaches, asthenia, fatigue, hypersensitivity reactions
Didanosine (Videx EC)	**DR:** 125 mg, 200 mg, 250 mg, 400 mg **OS:** 2 g/bottle, 4 g/bottle	**DR (weighing 60 kg or more):** 400 mg once daily; **(weighing 25–59 kg):** 250 mg once daily; **(weighing 20–24 kg):** 200 mg once daily **OS (weighing more than 60 kg):** 200 mg q12h or 400 mg once daily; **(weighing less than 60 kg):** 125 mg q12h or 250 mg once daily	Peripheral neuropathy, pancreatitis, diarrhea, nausea, vomiting, headaches, insomnia, rash, hepatitis, seizures
Emtricitabine (Emtriva)	**C:** 200 mg **OS:** 10 mg/mL	**A:** 200 mg/day **(C)** 240 mg/day **(OS)**	Headaches, insomnia, depression, diarrhea, nausea, vomiting, rhinitis, asthenia, rash
Lamivudine (Epivir)	**T:** 100 mg, 150 mg, 300 mg **OS:** 5 mg/mL, 10 mg/mL	**A:** 150 mg 2 times/day or 300 mg once daily **C:** 4 mg/kg 2 times/day	Diarrhea, malaise, fatigue, headaches, nausea, vomiting, abdominal pain, peripheral neuropathy, arthralgia, myalgia, skin rash
Stavudine (Zerit)	**C:** 15 mg, 20 mg, 30 mg, 40 mg **OS:** 1 mg/mL	**A (weighing more than 60 kg):** 40 mg 2 times/day (20 mg 2 times/day if peripheral neuropathy occurs); **(weighing 60 kg or less):** 30 mg 2 times/day (15 mg 2 times/day if peripheral neuropathy occurs)	Peripheral neuropathy, anemia, leukopenia, neutropenia
Zidovudine (Retrovir)	**C:** 100 mg **T:** 300 mg **Syrup:** 50 mg/5 mL, 10 mg/mL	**A:** 300 mg 2 times/day	Anemia, granulocytopenia, myopathy, nausea, malaise, fatigue, insomnia

Continued

ANTIRETROVIRAL AGENTS FOR TREATMENT OF HIV INFECTION—cont'd

Nucleotide Analogues			
Tenofovir TAF (Vemlidy)	**T**: 25 mg	**A**: 25 mg once daily	Headache, abdominal pain, fatigue, cough, nausea, back pain
Tenofovir TDF (Viread)	**T**: 300 mg	**A**: 300 mg once daily	Nausea, vomiting, diarrhea, headache, fatigue
Non-nucleoside Analogues			
Delavirdine (Rescriptor)	**T**: 100 mg, 200 mg	**A**: 200 mg 3 times/day for 14 days, then 400 mg 3 times/day	Rash, nausea, headaches, elevated hepatic function tests
Efavirenz (Sustiva)	**C**: 50 mg, 200 mg **T**: 600 mg	**A**: 600 mg/day **C**: 200–600 mg/day based on weight	Headaches, dizziness, insomnia, fatigue, rash, nightmares
Etravirine (Intelence)	**T**: 100 mg, 200 mg	**A**: 200 mg 2 times/day	Skin reactions (e.g., Stevens-Johnson syndrome, erythema multiforme), nausea, abdominal pain, vomiting
Nevirapine (Viramune, Viramune XR)	**T**: 200 mg **T (ER)**: 400 mg **S**: 50 mg/mL	**A**: 200 mg/day for 14 days, then (if no rash) 200 mg 2 times/day	Rash, nausea, fatigue, fever, headaches, abnormal hepatic function tests
Rilpivirine (Edurant)	**T**: 25 mg	**A**: 25 mg once daily with a meal	Depression, insomnia, headache, rash
Protease Inhibitors			
Atazanavir (Reyataz)	**C**: 100 mg, 150 mg, 200 mg, 300 mg	**A**: 400 mg/day or 300 mg (with 100 mg ritonavir) once daily	Headaches, diarrhea, abdominal pain, nausea, rash
Darunavir (Prezista)	**T**: 400 mg, 600 mg	**A**: 600 mg 2 times/day (with ritonavir 100 mg) or 800 mg once daily with ritonavir 100 mg	Diarrhea, nausea, vomiting, headaches, skin rash, constipation
Fosamprenavir (Lexiva)	**T**: 700 mg **OS**: 50 mg/mL	**A**: 1,400–2,800 mg/day with 100 mg ritonavir	Headaches, fatigue, rash, nausea, diarrhea, vomiting, abdominal pain

Indinavir (Crixivan)	**C:** 200 mg, 400 mg	**A:** 800 mg q8h or 800 mg 2 times/day with ritonavir 100 mg	Nephrolithiasis, hyperbilirubinemia, abdominal pain, asthenia, fatigue, flank pain, nausea, vomiting, diarrhea, headaches, insomnia, dizziness, altered taste
Lopinavir/ritonavir (Kaletra)	**C:** 133/33 mg **OS:** 80/20 mg	**A:** 400 mg/100 mg 2 times/day or 800 mg/200 mg once daily **C (4–12 yrs):** 10–13 mg/kg 2 times/day	Diarrhea, nausea, vomiting, abdominal pain, headaches, rash
Nelfinavir (Viracept)	**T:** 250 mg **Oral Powder:** 50 mg/g	**A:** 750 mg q8h or 1,250 mg 2 times/day **C:** 20–25 mg/kg q8h	Diarrhea, fatigue, asthenia, headaches, hypertension, impaired concentration
Ritonavir (Norvir)	**C:** 100 mg **OS:** 80 mg/mL	**A:** Titrate up to 800 mg/day based on protease inhibitor	Nausea, vomiting, diarrhea, altered taste, fatigue, elevated LFTs and triglyceride levels
Saquinavir (Invirase)	**C:** 200 mg **T:** 500 mg	**A:** 1,000 mg 2 times/day with ritonavir 100 mg	Diarrhea, elevated LFTs, hypertriglycerides, cholesterol, abnormal fat accumulation, hyperglycemia
Tipranavir (Aptivus)	**C:** 250 mg **OS:** 100 mg/mL	**A:** 500 mg (with 200 mg ritonavir) 2 times/day	Diarrhea, nausea, fatigue, headaches, vomiting
Fusion Inhibitors			
Enfuvirtide (Fuzeon)	**I:** 108 mg (90 mg when reconstituted)	**Subcutaneous:** 90 mg 2 times/day	Insomnia, depression, peripheral neuropathy, decreased appetite, constipation, asthenia, cough

Continued

ANTIRETROVIRAL AGENTS FOR TREATMENT OF HIV INFECTION—cont'd

CCR5 Antagonists			
Maraviroc (Selzentry)	**T**: 150 mg, 300 mg	**A**: 300 mg 2 times/day **CYP3A4 inducers:** 600 mg 2 times/day **CYP3A4 inhibitors:** 150 mg 2 times/day	Cough, pyrexia, upper respiratory tract infections, rash, musculoskeletal symptoms, abdominal pain, dizziness
Integrase Inhibitor			
Raltegravir (Isentress)	**T**: 400 mg	**A**: 400 mg 2 times/day	Nausea, headache, diarrhea, pyrexia
Dolutegravir (Tivicay)	**T**: 50 mg	**A**: 50 mg once daily or 50 mg bid (with CYP3A inducers or resistance)	Insomnia, headache
Monoclonal Antibody			
Ibalizumab-uiyk (Trogarzo)	**I**: 200 mg	**IV**: Initially, 2000 mg as a single dose, then 800 mg q14days	Dizziness, diarrhea; decreased Hgb, leukocytes, neutrophils, platelets; increased serum bilirubin, creatinine

A, Adults; ***C,*** capsules; ***C*** *(dosage)*, children; ***DR,*** delayed-release; ***ER,*** extended-release; ***I,*** injection; ***IV,*** intravenous; ***OS,*** oral solution; ***S,*** suspension; ***T,*** tablets; ***TAF,*** tenofovir alafenamide; ***TDF,*** tenofovir disoproxil fumarate.

FIXED-COMBINATION THERAPIES

Brand Name	Generic Name	Dosage
Atripla	Efavirenz 600 mg Emtricitabine 200 mg Tenofovir (TDF) 300 mg	1 tablet once daily
Biktarvy	Bictegravir 50 mg Emtricitabine 200 mg Tenofovir (TAF) 25 mg	1 tablet once daily
Cimduo	Lamivudine 300 mg Tenofovir (TDF) 300 mg	1 tablet once daily
Combivir	Lamivudine 150 mg Zidovudine 300 mg	1 tablet twice daily
Complera	Emtricitabine 200 mg Rilpivirine 27.5 mg Tenofovir (TDF) 300 mg	1 tablet once daily
Delstrigo	Doravirine 100 mg Lamivudine 300 mg Tenofovir 300 mg	1 tablet once daily
Descovy	Emtricitabine 200 mg Tenofovir (TAF) 25 mg	1 tablet once daily
Dovato	Dolutegravir 50 mg Lamivudine 300 mg	1 tablet once daily
Epzicom	Abacavir 600 mg Lamivudine 300 mg	1 tablet once daily

Continued

FIXED-COMBINATION THERAPIES—cont'd

Brand Name	Generic Name	Dosage
Evotaz	Atazanavir 300 mg Cobicistat 150 mg	1 tablet once daily
Genvoya	Cobicistat 150 mg Elvitegravir 150 mg Emtricitabine 200 mg Tenofovir (TAF) 10 mg	1 tablet once daily
Juluca	Dolutegravir 50 mg Rilpivirine 25 mg	1 tablet once daily
Odefsey	Emtricitabine 200 mg Rilpivirine 25 mg Tenofovir (TAF) 25 mg	1 tablet once daily
Prezcobix	Cobicistat 150 mg Darunavir 800 mg	1 tablet once daily
Stribild	Cobicistat 150 mg Elvitegravir 150 mg Emtricitabine 200 mg Tenofovir (TDF) 300 mg	1 tablet once daily
Symfi	Efavirenz 400 mg Lamivudine 300 mg Tenofovir (TDF) 300 mg	1 tablet once daily
Symtuza	Cobicistat 150 mg Darunavir 800 mg Emtricitabine 200 mg Tenofovir 10 mg	1 tablet once daily

Triumeq	Abacavir 600 mg Dolutegravir 50 mg Lamivudine 300 mg	1 tablet once daily
Trizivir	Abacavir 300 mg Lamivudine 150 mg Zidovudine 300 mg	1 tablet twice daily
Truvada	Emtricitabine 200 mg Tenofovir (TDF) 300 mg	1 tablet once daily

TAF, Tenofovir alafenamide; ***TDF,*** tenofovir disoproxil fumarate.

Immunosuppressive Agents

USES	ACTION
Improvement of both short- and long-term allograft survivals.	*Basiliximab:* An interleukin-2 (IL-2) receptor antagonist inhibiting IL-2 binding. This prevents activation of lymphocytes, and the response of the immune system to antigens is impaired. *Cyclosporine:* Inhibits production and release of IL-2. *Daclizumab:* An IL-2 receptor antagonist inhibiting IL-2 binding. *Mycophenolate:* A prodrug that reversibly binds and inhibits inosine monophosphate dehydrogenase (IMPD), resulting in inhibition of purine nucleotide synthesis, inhibiting DNA and RNA synthesis and subsequent synthesis of T and B cells. *Sirolimus:* Inhibits IL-2–stimulated T-lymphocyte activation and proliferation, which may occur through formation of a complex. *Tacrolimus:* Inhibits IL-2–stimulated T-lymphocyte activation and proliferation, which may occur through formation of a complex.

IMMUNOSUPPRESSIVE AGENTS

Name	Availability	Dosage	Side Effects
Basiliximab (Simulect)	**I:** 10 mg, 20 mg	20 mg for 2 doses (on day of transplant, then 4 days after transplantation)	Abdominal pain, asthenia, cough, dizziness, dyspnea, dysuria, edema, hypertension, infection, tremors
Cyclosporine (Neoral, Sandimmune)	**C:** 25 mg, 50 mg, 100 mg **S:** 100 mg/mL **I:** 50 mg/mL	Dose dependent on type of transplant and formulation	Hypertension, hyperkalemia, nephrotoxicity, coarsening of facial features, hirsutism, gingival hyperplasia, nausea, vomiting, diarrhea, hepatotoxicity, hyperuricemia, hypertriglyceridemia, hypercholesterolemia, tremors, paresthesia, seizures, risk of infection/malignancy
Mycophenolate (CellCept, Myfortic)	**Cellcept:** **C:** 250 mg **I:** 500 mg **S:** 200 mg/mL **T:** 500 mg **Myfortic:** **T(DR):** 180 mg, 320 mg	**Cellcept:** 1–1.5 g 2 times/day based on type of transplant **Myfortic:** **Renal:** 720 mg 2 times/day	Diarrhea, vomiting, leukopenia, neutropenia, infections
Sirolimus (Rapamune)	**S:** 1 mg/mL **T:** 0.5 mg, 1 mg, 2 mg	2–6 mg/day	Dyspnea, leukopenia, thrombocytopenia, hyperlipidemia, abdominal pain, acne, arthralgia, fever, diarrhea, constipation, headaches, vomiting, weight gain
Tacrolimus (Prograf)	**C:** 0.5 mg, 1 mg, 5 mg **I:** 5 mg/mL **C(ER):** 0.5 mg, 1 mg, 5 mg **T(ER):** 0.75 mg, 1 mg, 4 mg	**Heart:** 0.075 mg/kg/day in 2 divided doses q12h **Kidney:** 0.1–0.2 mg/kg/day in 2 divided doses q12h **Liver:** 0.1–0.15 mg/kg/day in 2 divided doses q12h	Nephrotoxicity, neurotoxicity, hyperglycemia, nausea, vomiting, photophobia, infections, hypertension, hyperlipidemia

C, Capsules; ***DR***, delayed release; ***ER***, extended release; ***I***, injection; ***S***, oral solution or suspension; ***T***, tablets.

Laxatives

USES

Short-term treatment of constipation; colon evacuation before rectal/bowel examination; prevention of straining (e.g., after anorectal surgery, MI); to reduce painful elimination (e.g., episiotomy, hemorrhoids, anorectal lesions); modification of effluent from ileostomy, colostomy; prevention of fecal impaction; removal of ingested poisons.

ACTION

Laxatives ease or stimulate defecation. Mechanisms by which this is accomplished include (1) attracting, retaining fluid in colonic contents due to hydrophilic or osmotic properties; (2) acting directly or indirectly on mucosa to decrease absorption of water and NaCl; or (3) increasing intestinal motility, decreasing absorption of water and NaCl by virtue of decreased transit time.

Bulk-forming: Act primarily in small/large intestine. Retain water in stool, may bind water, ions in colonic lumen (soften feces, increase bulk); may increase colonic bacteria growth (increases fecal mass). Produce soft stool in 1–3 days.

Osmotic agents: Act in colon. Similar to saline laxatives. Osmotic action may be enhanced in distal ileum/colon by bacterial metabolism to lactate, other organic acids. This decrease in pH increases motility, secretion. Produce soft stool in 1–3 days.

Saline: Acts in small/large intestine, colon (sodium phosphate). Poorly, slowly absorbed; causes hormone cholecystokinin release from duodenum (stimulates fluid secretion, motility); possesses osmotic properties; produces watery stool in 2–6 hrs (small doses produce semifluid stool in 6–12 hrs).

Stimulant: Acts in colon. Enhances accumulation of water/electrolytes in colonic lumen, enhances intestinal motility. May act directly on intestinal mucosa. Produces semifluid stool in 6–12 hrs.

◄**ALERT**► Bisacodyl suppository acts in 15–60 min.

Stool softener: Acts in small/large intestine. Hydrates and softens stools by its surfactant action, facilitating penetration of fat and water into stool. Produces soft stool in 1–3 days.

LAXATIVES

Name	Onset of Action	Uses	Side Effects/Precautions
Bulk-forming			
Methylcellulose (Citrucel)	12–24 hrs up to 3 days	Treatment of constipation for postpartum women, elderly, pts with diverticulosis, irritable bowel syndrome, hemorrhoids	Gas, bloating, esophageal obstruction, colonic obstruction, calcium and iron malabsorption
Psyllium (Metamucil)	Same as methylcellulose	Treatment of chronic constipation and constipation associated with rectal disorders; management of irritable bowel syndrome	Diarrhea, constipation, abdominal cramps, esophageal/colon obstruction, bronchospasm
Stool Softener			
Docusate (Colace, Surfak)	1–3 days	Treatment of constipation due to hard stools, in painful anorectal conditions, and for those who need to avoid straining during bowel movements	Stomachache, mild nausea, cramping, diarrhea, irritated throat (with liquid and syrup dose forms)
Saline			
Magnesium citrate (Citrate of Magnesia, Citro-Mag)	30 min–3 hrs	Bowel evacuation prior to certain surgical and diagnostic procedures	Hypotension, abdominal cramping, diarrhea, gas formation, electrolyte abnormalities
Magnesium hydroxide	30 min–3 hrs	Short-term treatment of occasional constipation	Electrolyte abnormalities can occur; use caution in pts with renal or cardiac impairment; diarrhea, abdominal cramps, hypotension
Sodium phosphate (Fleet Phospho-Soda)	2–15 min	Relief of occasional constipation; bowel evacuation prior to certain surgical and diagnostic procedures	Electrolyte abnormalities; do not use for pts with HF, severe renal impairment, ascites, GI obstruction, active inflammatory bowel disease

Continued

LAXATIVES—cont'd

Osmotic			
Lactulose (Kristalose)	24–48 hrs	Short-term relief of constipation, treatment of hyperammonemia-induced encephalopathy	Nausea, vomiting, diarrhea, abdominal cramping, bloating, gas
Polyethylene glycol (MiraLax)	24–48 hrs	Short-term relief of constipation	Bitter taste, diarrhea
Stimulant			
Bisacodyl (Dulcolax)	**PO:** 6–12 hrs **Rectal:** 15–60 min	Short-term relief of constipation	Electrolyte imbalance, abdominal discomfort, gas, potential for overuse/abuse
Senna (Senokot)	6–12 hrs	Short-term relief of constipation	Abdominal discomfort, cramps

GI, Gastrointestinal; ***HF***, heart failure.

Multiple Sclerosis

Multiple sclerosis (MS) is the most common autoimmune disorder affecting the central nervous system. MS is a demyelinating disease where insulating covers of nerve cells in the brain and spinal cord are damaged, which disrupts the ability of parts of the nervous system to communicate. Symptoms may include double vision, blindness in one eye, muscle weakness, trouble with sensation or coordination.

Presently, there is no cure for MS. Treatment attempts to improve function and prevent new attacks.

MEDICATIONS FOR MULTIPLE SCLEROSIS

Name	Dosage	Side Effects
Alemtuzumab (Lemtrada)	12 mg IV once daily for 5 days followed 1 year later by 12 mg IV once daily for 3 days	Rigors, tremors nausea, vomiting, rash, fatigue, hypotension, urticaria, pruritus, skeletal pain, headache, diarrhea, neutropenia, anemia, thrombocytopenia, respiratory toxicity (dyspnea, cough, pneumonitis, infections)
Cladribine (Mavenclad)	Recommended cumulative dosage: 3.5 mg/kg body weight administered orally and divided into 2 yearly treatment courses (1.75 mg/kg/treatment course)	Upper respiratory tract infection, headache, lymphopenia
Daclizumab (Zinbryta)	150 mg SQ once monthly	Autoimmune disorders (hepatitis, lymphadenopathy, noninfectious colitis), depression, severe hypersensitivity reactions, infections
Dimethyl fumarate (Tecfidera)	240 mg PO bid	Flushing, abdominal pain, diarrhea, nausea, vomiting, dyspepsia, lymphopenia, hepatotoxicity, progressive multifocal leukoencephalopathy (PML)
Diroximel fumarate (Vumerity)	**PO:** Initially, 231 mg twice daily; after 7 days, increase to maintenance dose of 462 mg twice daily	Flushing, abdominal pain, diarrhea, nausea, infection, pruritus, skin rash, erythema, albuminuria, vomiting, dyspepsia, lymphocytopenia; increased serum AST

MEDICATIONS FOR MULTIPLE SCLEROSIS—cont'd

Name	Dosage	Side Effects
Fingolimod (Gilenya)	0.5 mg PO once daily	Headache, back pain, cough, infections, hypersensitivity reactions, elevated LFTs, bradycardia, AV block, macular edema, decreased pulmonary function
Glatiramer (Copaxone, Glatopa)	**Copaxone:** 20 mg SQ once daily or 40 mg 3 times/wk **Glatopa:** 20 mg SQ once daily	Pain, erythema, inflammation, pruritus at injection site, arthralgia, transient chest pain, post-injection reactions (chest pain, palpitations, dyspnea)
Interferon beta 1a (Avonex, Rebif)	**Avonex:** 30 mcg IM wkly **Rebif:** 44 mcg 3 times/wk	Headache, flu-like symptoms, myalgia, depression with suicidal ideation, generalized pain, asthenia, chills, injection site reaction, hypersensitivity reactions, anemia, hepatotoxicity
Interferon beta 1b (Betaseron, Extavia)	250 mcg SQ every other day	Headache, flu-like symptoms, myalgia, upper respiratory tract infection, depression with suicidal ideation, generalized pain, asthenia, chills, fever, injection site reaction, hypersensitivity reactions, anemia, hepatotoxicity, seizures
Mitoxantrone	12 mg/m2 IV q3mos	Nausea, vomiting, diarrhea, cough, headache, stomatitis, abdominal discomfort, fever, alopecia, cardiotoxicity, myelosuppression, acute/chronic myeloid leukemia
Natalizumab (Tysabri)	300 mg IV q4wks	Headache, fatigue, depression, arthralgia, infections, hypersensitivity reactions, hepatotoxicity, PML
Ocrelizumab (Ocrevus)	600 mg IV q6mos	Infusion reactions (pruritus, rash, urticaria, erythema), respiratory tract infections, skin infections, malignancies, PML
Ozanimod (Zeposia)	**PO**: Initially, 0.23 mg once daily on days 1–4; then 0.46 mg once daily on days 5–7. **Maintenance:** 0.92 mg once daily starting on day 8	Infection, upper respiratory tract infection, hypertension, orthostatic hypotension, UTI; increased serum ALT, AST

Name	Dosage	Side Effects
Pegylated interferon beta 1a (Plegridy)	125 mcg SQ q2wks	Headache, flu-like symptoms, myalgia, depression with suicidal ideation, generalized pain, asthenia, chills, injection site reaction, hypersensitivity reactions, anemia, hepatotoxicity, elevated LFTs, seizures
Siponimod (Mayzent)	Titration required for treatment initiation Recommended maintenance dosage: 2 mg	Headache, hypertension, increased serum ALT, AST
Teriflunomide (Aubagio)	7 or 14 mg PO once daily	Headache, diarrhea, nausea, alopecia, paresthesia, abdominal pain, elevated LFTs, neutropenia, leukopenia, hepatic failure, acute renal failure, toxic epidermal necrolysis

ALT, Alanine aminotransferase; ***AST,*** aspartate aminotransferase; ***bid,*** twice daily; ***IM,*** intramuscular; ***IV,*** intravenous; ***LFT,*** liver function test; ***PML,*** progressive multifocal leukoencephalopathy; ***PO,*** oral; ***SQ,*** subcutaneous; ***UTI,*** urinary tract infection.

Nonsteroidal Anti-Inflammatory Drugs (NSAIDs)

USES

Provide symptomatic relief from *pain/inflammation* in the treatment of musculoskeletal disorders (e.g., rheumatoid arthritis [RA], osteoarthritis, ankylosing spondylitis), *analgesic* for low to moderate pain, *reduction in fever* (many agents not suited for routine/prolonged therapy due to toxicity). By virtue of its action on platelet function, aspirin is used in treatment or prophylaxis of diseases associated with hypercoagulability (reduces risk of stroke/heart attack).

ACTION

Exact mechanism for anti-inflammatory, analgesic, antipyretic effects unknown. Inhibition of enzyme cyclooxygenase, the enzyme responsible for prostaglandin synthesis, appears to be a major mechanism of action. May inhibit other mediators of inflammation (e.g., leukotrienes). Direct action on hypothalamus heat-regulating center may contribute to antipyretic effect.

Continued

NSAIDs

Name	Availability	Dosage Range	Side Effects
Aspirin	**Caplet:** 500 mg **Suppository:** 300 mg, 600 mg **T:** 325 mg **T (EC):** 81 mg, 325 mg **T (Chew):** 81 mg	**Analgesic/antipyretic:** 325–650 mg q4–6h prn or 975 mg q6h prn or 500–1000 mg q4–6h prn	GI discomfort, dizziness, headaches, increased risk of bleeding
Celecoxib (Celebrex)	**C:** 50 mg, 100 mg, 200 mg, 400 mg	200 mg q12h (**Maximum:** 600 mg day 1, then 400 mg/day)	Diarrhea, back pain, dizziness, heartburn, headaches, nausea, abdominal pain
Diclofenac (Voltaren, Zipsor, Zorvolex)	**T:** 25 mg, 50 mg, 75 mg **C (Zipsor):** 25 mg **C (Zorvolex):** 18 mg, 35 mg	50 mg tid **(Zipsor):** 25 mg 4 times/day **(Zorvolex):** 18–35 mg 3 times/day	Indigestion, constipation, diarrhea, nausea, headaches, fluid retention, abdominal cramps
Diflunisal (Dolobid)	**T:** 500 mg	**Arthritis:** 0.5–1 g/day in 2 divided doses **Maximum:** 1.5 g/day **P:** 500 mg once, then 250 mg q8–12h	Headaches, abdominal cramps, indigestion, diarrhea, nausea
Etodolac (Lodine)	**T:** 400 mg, 500 mg **T (ER):** 400 mg, 500 mg, 600 mg **C:** 200 mg, 300 mg	**Arthritis:** 400 mg 2 times/day or 300 mg 2–3 times/day or 500 mg 2 times/day. **(ER):** 400 mg up to 1,000 mg once daily **P:** 200–400 mg q6–8h as needed	Indigestion, dizziness, headaches, bloated feeling, diarrhea, nausea, weakness, abdominal cramps
Fenoprofen (Nalfon)	**C:** 200 mg, 400 mg **T:** 600 mg	**Arthritis:** 400–600 mg 3–4 times/day **P:** 200 mg q4–6h as needed	Nausea, indigestion, anxiety, constipation, shortness of breath, heartburn
Ibuprofen (Advil, Caldolor, Motrin)	**I:** 100 mg/mL **T:** 100 mg, 200 mg, 400 mg, 600 mg, 800 mg **T (Chew):** 50 mg, 100 mg **C:** 200 mg **S:** 100 mg/5 mL	**Inflammatory disease:** 400–800 mg/dose 3–4 times/day **P:** 200–400 mg/dose q4–6h as needed	Dizziness, abdominal cramps, abdominal pain, heartburn, nausea

Indomethacin (Indocin, Tivorbex)	**(Tivorbex):** 20 mg, 40 mg **C:** 25 mg, 50 mg **C (SR):** 75 mg **S:** 25 mg/5 mL	**Arthritis:** 25–50 mg/dose 2–3 times/day **Maximum:** 200 mg/day **P: (Tivorbex only):** 20 mg 3 times/day or 40 mg 2–3 times/day	Fluid retention, dizziness, headaches, abdominal pain, indigestion, nausea
Ketoprofen (Orudis KT)	**C:** 25 mg, 50 mg **C (ER):** 200 mg	**Arthritis:** 50 mg 4 times/day or 75 mg 3 times/day **ER:** 200 mg once daily **P:** 25–50 mg q6–8h as needed	Headaches, anxiety, abdominal pain, bloated feeling, constipation, diarrhea, nausea
Ketorolac (Toradol)	**T:** 10 mg **I:** 15 mg/mL, 30 mg/mL	**P: (PO):** 10 mg q4–6h as needed; **(IM/IV):** 60–120 mg/day in divided doses	Fluid retention, abdominal pain, diarrhea, dizziness, headaches, nausea
Meloxicam (Mobic, Vivlodex)	**C: (Vivlodex):** 5 mg, 10 mg **T: (Mobic):** 7.5 mg, 15 mg **S:** 7.5 mg/5 mL	**Arthritis: (Mobic):** 7.5–15 mg once daily **(Vivlodex):** 5–10 mg once daily	Heartburn, indigestion, nausea, diarrhea, headaches
Nabumetone (Relafen)	**T:** 500 mg, 750 mg	**Arthritis:** 1–2 g/day in 1–2 divided doses	Fluid retention, dizziness, headaches, abdominal pain, constipation, diarrhea, nausea
Naproxen (Anaprox, Naprosyn)	**T:** 250 mg, 375 mg, 500 mg **T (CR):** 375 mg, 500 mg **S:** 125 mg/5 mL	**Arthritis:** 500–1,000 mg/day in 2 divided doses **Maximum:** 1,500 mg/day **P:** 500 mg once, then 500 mg q12h or 250 mg q6–8h as needed	Tinnitus, fluid retention, shortness of breath, dizziness, drowsiness, headaches, abdominal pain, constipation, heartburn, nausea
Oxaprozin (Daypro)	**C:** 600 mg **T:** 600 mg	**Arthritis:** 600–1,200 mg once daily	Constipation, diarrhea, nausea, indigestion
Piroxicam (Feldene)	**C:** 10 mg, 20 mg	**Arthritis:** 10–20 mg/day in 1–2 divided doses	Abdominal pain, stomach pain, nausea
Sulindac (Clinoril)	**T:** 150 mg, 200 mg	**Arthritis:** 150 mg bid	Dizziness, abdominal pain, constipation, diarrhea, nausea

A, Adults; ***C,*** capsules; ***CR,*** controlled-release; ***ER,*** extended-release; ***GI,*** gastrointestinal; ***I,*** injection; ***P,*** pain; ***S,*** suspension; ***SR,*** sustained-release; ***T,*** tablets.

Nutrition: Enteral

	INDICATIONS	ROUTES OF ENTERAL NUTRITION DELIVERY
Enteral nutrition (EN), also known as *tube feedings,* provides food/nutrients via the GI tract using special formulas, delivery techniques, and equipment. All routes of EN consist of a tube through which liquid formula is infused.	Tube feedings are used in pts with major trauma, burns; those undergoing radiation and/or chemotherapy; pts with hepatic failure, severe renal impairment, physical or neurologic impairment; preop and postop to promote anabolism; prevention of cachexia, malnutrition; dysphagia, pts requiring mechanical ventilation.	**Nasogastric (NG):** **INDICATIONS:** Most common for short-term feeding in pts unable or unwilling to consume adequate nutrition by mouth. Requires at least a partially functioning GI tract. **ADVANTAGES:** Does not require surgical intervention and is fairly easily inserted. Allows full use of digestive tract. Decreases abdominal distention, nausea, vomiting that may be caused by hyperosmolar solutions. **DISADVANTAGES:** Temporary. May be easily pulled out during routine nursing care. Has potential for pulmonary aspiration of gastric contents, risk of reflux esophagitis, regurgitation. **Nasoduodenal (ND), Nasojejunal (NJ):** **INDICATIONS:** Pts unable or unwilling to consume adequate nutrition by mouth. Requires at least a partially functioning GI tract. **ADVANTAGES:** Does not require surgical intervention and is fairly easily inserted. Preferred for pts at risk for aspiration. Valuable for pts with gastroparesis.

DISADVANTAGES: Temporary. May be pulled out during routine nursing care. May be dislodged by coughing, vomiting. Small lumen size increases risk of clogging when medication is administered via tube, more susceptible to rupturing when using infusion device. Must be radiographed for placement, frequently extubated.

GASTROSTOMY:

INDICATIONS: Pts with esophageal obstruction or impaired swallowing; pts in whom NG, ND, or NJ not feasible; when long-term feeding indicated.

ADVANTAGES: Permanent feeding access. Tubing has larger bore, allowing noncontinuous (bolus) feeding (300–400 ml over 30–60 min q3–6h). May be inserted endoscopically using local anesthetic (procedure called *percutaneous endoscopic gastrostomy* [PEG]).

DISADVANTAGES: Requires surgery; may be inserted in conjunction with other surgery or endoscopically (see **ADVANTAGES**). Stoma care required. Tube may be inadvertently dislodged. Risk of aspiration, peritonitis, cellulitis, leakage of gastric contents.

JEJUNOSTOMY:

INDICATIONS: Pts with stomach or duodenal obstruction, impaired gastric motility; pts in whom NG, ND, or NJ not feasible; when long-term feeding indicated.

ADVANTAGES: Allows early postop feeding (small bowel function is least affected by surgery). Risk of aspiration reduced. Rarely pulled out inadvertently.

DISADVANTAGES: Requires surgery (laparotomy). Stoma care required. Risk of intraperitoneal leakage. Can be dislodged easily.

INITIATING ENTERAL NUTRITION

With continuous feeding, initiation of isotonic (about 300 mOsm/L) or moderately hypertonic feeding (up to 495 mOsm/L) can be given full strength, usually at a slow rate (30–50 ml/hr) and gradually increased (25 ml/hr q6–24h). Formulas with osmolality greater than 500 mOsm/L are generally started at half strength and gradually increased in rate, then concentration. Tolerance is increased if the rate and concentration are not increased simultaneously.

Continued

Nutrition: Enteral—cont'd

SELECTION OF FORMULAS

Protein: Has many important physiologic roles and is the primary source of nitrogen in the body. Provides 4 kcal/g protein. Sources of protein in enteral feedings: sodium caseinate, calcium caseinate, soy protein, dipeptides.

Carbohydrate (CHO): Provides energy for the body and heat to maintain body temperature. Provides 3.4 kcal/g carbohydrate. Sources of CHO in enteral feedings: corn syrup, cornstarch, maltodextrin, lactose, sucrose, glucose.

Fat: Provides concentrated source of energy. Referred to as *kilocalorie dense* or *protein sparing.* Provides 9 kcal/g fat. Sources of fat in enteral feedings: corn oil, safflower oil, medium-chain triglycerides.

Electrolytes, vitamins, trace elements: Contained in formulas (not found in specialized products for renal/hepatic insufficiency).

All products containing protein, fat, carbohydrate, vitamin, electrolytes, trace elements are nutritionally complete and designed to be used by pts for long periods.

COMPLICATIONS

MECHANICAL: Usually associated with some aspect of the feeding tube.

Aspiration pneumonia: Caused by delayed gastric emptying, gastroparesis, gastroesophageal reflux, or decreased gag reflex. May be prevented or treated by reducing infusion rate, using lower-fat formula, feeding beyond pylorus, checking residuals, using small-bore feeding tubes, elevating head of bed 30–45 degrees during and for 30–60 min after intermittent feeding, and regularly checking tube placement.

Esophageal, mucosal, pharyngeal irritation, otitis: Caused by using large-bore NG tube. Prevented by use of small bore whenever possible.

Irritation, leakage at ostomy site: Caused by drainage of digestive juices from site. Prevented by close attention to skin/stoma care.

Tube, lumen obstruction: Caused by thickened formula residue, formation of formula-medication complexes. Prevented by frequently irrigating tube with clear water (also before and after giving formulas/medication), avoiding instilling medication if possible.

GASTROINTESTINAL: Usually associated with formula, rate of delivery, unsanitary handling of solutions or delivery system.

Diarrhea: Caused by low-residue formulas, rapid delivery, use of hyperosmolar formula, hypoalbuminemia, malabsorption, microbial contamination, or rapid GI transit time. Prevented by using fiber supplemented formulas, decreasing rate of delivery, using dilute formula, and gradually increasing strength.

Cramps, gas, abdominal distention: Caused by nutrient malabsorption, rapid delivery of refrigerated formula. Prevented by delivering formula by continuous methods, giving formulas at room temperature, decreasing rate of delivery.

Nausea, vomiting: Caused by rapid delivery of formula, gastric retention. Prevented by reducing rate of delivery, using dilute formulas, selecting low-fat formulas.

Constipation: Caused by inadequate fluid intake, reduced bulk, inactivity. Prevented by supplementing fluid intake, using fiber-supplemented formula, encouraging ambulation.

MONITORING

METABOLIC: Fluid/serum electrolyte status should be monitored. Refer to monitoring section. In addition, the very young and very old are at greater risk of developing complications such as dehydration or overhydration.

Daily: Estimate nutrient intake, fluid intake/output, weight of pt, clinical observations.

Weekly: Serum electrolytes (potassium, sodium, magnesium, calcium, phosphorus), blood glucose, BUN, creatinine, hepatic function tests (e.g., AST, ALT, alkaline phosphatase), 24-hr urea and creatinine excretion, total iron-binding capacity (TIBC) or serum transferrin, triglycerides, cholesterol.

Monthly: Serum albumin.

Other: Urine glucose, acetone (when blood glucose is greater than 250), vital signs (temperature, respirations, pulse, B/P) q8h.

DRUG THERAPY: DOSAGE FOR SELECTION/ ADMINISTRATION:
Drug therapy should not have to be compromised in pts receiving enteral nutrition:
- Temporarily discontinue medications not immediately necessary.
- Consider an alternate route for administering medications (e.g., transdermal, rectal, intravenous).
- Consider alternate medications when current medication is not available in alternate dosage forms.

ENTERAL ADMINISTRATION OF MEDICATIONS:
Medications may be given via feeding tube with several considerations:
- Tube type
- Tube location in the GI tract.
- Site of drug action.
- Site of drug absorption.
- Effects of food on drug absorption.
- Use of liquid dosage forms is preferred whenever possible; many tablets may be crushed; contents of many capsules may be emptied and given through large-bore feeding tubes.
- Many oral products should not be crushed (e.g., sustained-release, enteric coated, capsule granules).
- Some medications should not be given with enteral formulas because they form precipitates that may clog the feeding tube and reduce drug absorption.
- Feeding tube should be flushed with water before and after administration of medications to clear any residual medication.

Continued

Nutrition: Enteral—cont'd

	INDICATIONS	COMPONENTS OF PN
Parenteral nutrition (PN), also known as *total parenteral nutrition* (TPN) or *hyperalimentation* (HAL), provides required nutrients to pts by IV route of administration. The goal of PN is to maintain or restore nutritional status caused by disease, injury, or inability to consume nutrients by other means.	Conditions when pt is unable to use alimentary tract via oral, gastrostomy, or jejunostomy route. Impaired absorption of protein caused by obstruction, inflammation, or antineoplastic therapy. Bowel rest necessary because of GI surgery or ileus, fistulas, or anastomotic leaks. Conditions with increased metabolic requirements (e.g., burns, infection, trauma). Preserve tissue reserves (e.g., acute renal failure). Inadequate nutrition from tube feeding methods.	To meet IV nutritional requirements, six essential categories in PN are needed for tissue synthesis and energy balance. *Protein:* In the form of crystalline amino acids (CAA), primarily used for protein synthesis. Several products are designed to meet specific needs for pts with renal failure (e.g., NephrAmine), hepatic disease (e.g., Hepat Amine), stress/trauma (e.g., Aminosyn HBC), use in neonates and pediatrics (e.g., Aminosyn PF, TrophAmine). Calories: 4 kcal/g protein. *Energy:* In the form of dextrose, available in concentrations of 5%–70%. Dextrose less than 10% may be given peripherally; concentrations greater than 10% must be given centrally. Calories: 3.4 kcal/g dextrose. *IV fat emulsion:* Available in 10% and 20% concentrations. Provides a concentrated source of energy/calories (9 kcal/g fat) and is a source of essential fatty acids. May be administered peripherally or centrally.

ROUTE OF ADMINISTRATION

Electrolytes: Major electrolytes (calcium, magnesium, potassium, sodium; also acetate, chloride, phosphate). Doses of electrolytes are individualized, based on many factors (e.g., renal/hepatic function, fluid status).

Vitamins: Essential components in maintaining metabolism and cellular function; widely used in PN.

Trace elements: Necessary in long-term PN administration. Trace elements include zinc, copper, chromium, manganese, selenium, molybdenum, iodine.

Miscellaneous: Additives include insulin, albumin, heparin, and H_2 blockers (e.g., cimetidine, ranitidine, famotidine). Other medication may be included, but compatibility for admixture should be checked on an individual basis.

PN is administered via either peripheral or central vein.

Peripheral: Usually involves 2–3 L/day of 5%–10% dextrose with 3%–5% amino acid solution along with IV fat emulsion. Electrolytes, vitamins, trace elements are added according to pt needs. Peripheral solutions provide about 2,000 kcal/day and 60–90 g protein/day.

ADVANTAGES: Lower risks vs. central mode of administration.

DISADVANTAGES: Peripheral veins may not be suitable (esp. in pts with illness of long duration); more susceptible to phlebitis (due to osmolalities greater than 600 mOsm/L); veins may be viable only 1–2 wks; large volumes of fluid are needed to meet nutritional requirements, which may be contraindicated in many pts.

Central: Usually utilizes hypertonic dextrose (concentration range of 15%–35%) and amino acid solution of 3%–7% with IV fat emulsion. Electrolytes, vitamins, trace elements are added according to pt needs. Central solutions provide 2,000–4,000 kcal/day. Must be given through large central vein with high blood flow, allowing rapid dilution, avoiding phlebitis/thrombosis (usually through percutaneous insertion of catheter into subclavian vein, then advancement of catheter to superior vena cava).

ADVANTAGES: Allows more alternatives/flexibility in establishing regimens; allows ability to provide full nutritional requirements without need of daily fat emulsion; useful in pts who are fluid restricted (increased concentration), those needing large nutritional requirements (e.g., trauma, malignancy), or those for whom PN indicated more than 7–10 days.

DISADVANTAGES: Risk with insertion, use, maintenance of central line; increased risk of infection, catheter-induced trauma, and metabolic changes.

Continued

Nutrition: Enteral—cont'd

MONITORING

May vary slightly from institution to institution.

Baseline: CBC, platelet count, prothrombin time (PT), weight, body length/head circumference (in infants), serum electrolytes, glucose, BUN, creatinine, uric acid, total protein, cholesterol, triglycerides, bilirubin, alkaline phosphatase, lactate dehydrogenase (LDH), AST, albumin, prealbumin, other tests as needed.

Daily: Weight, vital signs (temperature, pulse, respirations [TPR]), nutritional intake (kcal, protein, fat), serum electrolytes (potassium, sodium chloride), glucose (serum, urine), acetone, BUN, osmolarity, other tests as needed.

2–3 times/wk: CBC, coagulation studies (PT, partial thromboplastin time [PTT]), serum creatinine, calcium, magnesium, phosphorus, acid-base status, other tests as needed.

Weekly: Nitrogen balance, total protein, albumin, prealbumin, transferrin, hepatic function tests (AST, ALT), serum alkaline phosphatase, LDH, bilirubin, Hgb, uric acid, cholesterol, triglycerides, other tests as needed.

COMPLICATIONS

Mechanical: Malfunction in system for IV delivery (e.g., pump failure; problems with lines, tubing, administration sets, catheter). Pneumothorax, catheter misdirection, arterial puncture, bleeding, hematoma formation may occur with catheter placement.

Infectious: Infections (pts often more susceptible to infections), catheter sepsis (e.g., fever, shaking, chills, glucose intolerance where no other site of infection is identified).

Metabolic: Includes hyperglycemia, elevated serum cholesterol and triglycerides, abnormal serum hepatic function tests.

Fluid, electrolyte, acid-base disturbances: May alter serum potassium, sodium, phosphate, magnesium levels.

Nutritional: Clinical effects seen may be due to lack of adequate vitamins, trace elements, essential fatty acids.

DRUG THERAPY/ADMINISTRATION METHODS: Compatibility of other intravenous medications pts may be administered while receiving parenteral nutrition is an important concern.

Intravenous medications usually are given as a separate admixture via piggyback to the parenteral nutrition line, but in some instances may be added directly to the parenteral nutrition solution. Because of the possibility of incompatibility when adding medication directly to the parenteral nutrition solution, specific criteria should be considered:

- Stability of the medication in the parenteral nutrition solution
- Properties of the medication, including pharmacokinetics that determine if the medication is appropriate for continuous infusion
- Documented chemical and physical compatibility with the parenteral nutrition solution

In addition, when medication is given via piggyback using the parenteral nutrition line, important criteria should include the following:

- Stability of the medication in the parenteral nutrition solution
- Documented chemical and physical compatibility with the parenteral nutrition solution

Obesity Management

USES	ACTIONS
Adjunct to diet and physical activity in the treatment of chronic, relapsing obesity.	Two categories of medications are used for weight control. *Appetite suppressants:* Block neuronal uptake of norepinephrine, serotonin, dopamine, causing a feeling of fullness or satiety. *Digestion inhibitors:* Reversible lipase inhibitors that block the breakdown and absorption of fats, decreasing appetite and reducing calorie intake.

ANOREXIANTS

Name	Availability	Dosage	Side Effects
Diethylpropion (Tenuate, Tenuate Dospan)	**T:** 25 mg, **T (CR):** 75 mg	25 mg 3–4 times/day or 75 mg once daily in midmorning	Headaches, euphoria, palpitations, hypertension, pulmonary hypertension, valvular heart disease, seizures, bone marrow depression, dependence, withdrawal psychosis
Liraglutide (Victoza)	**I:** 18 mg/3 mL	**SQ:** Initially, 0.6 mg/day. May increase by 0.6 mg/day wkly up to 3 mg/day	Diarrhea, constipation, dyspepsia, fatigue, vomiting, increased heart rate, renal impairment
Lorcaserin (BelViq, Belviq XR)	**C:** 10 mg **T:** 20 mg	**(Belviq):** 10 mg 2 times/day **(Belviq XR):** 20 mg once daily	Nausea, headache, dizziness, fatigue, dry mouth, diarrhea, constipation, hypoglycemia, hallucinations, decreased white/red blood cells, euphoria, cognitive impairment
Naltrexone/ bupropion (Contrave)	**T:** 8 mg/90 mg	Titrate wkly up to 2 tablets 2 times/day (1 tablet once daily, then 1 tablet 2 times/day, then 2 tablets in AM and 1 in PM, then 2 tablets 2 times/day)	Suicidal ideation, mood changes, seizures, increased HR with or without B/P, allergic reactions, hepatic toxicity, nausea, vomiting, headache, dizziness, dry mouth, angle-closure glaucoma

Continued

ANOREXIANTS—cont'd

Name	Availability	Dosage	Side Effects
Orlistat (Alli, Xenical)	**C**: 60 mg, 120 mg	**Alli:** 60 mg up to tid with meals **Xenical:** 120 mg tid with each meal containing fat	Flatulence, rectal incontinence, oily stools, cholelithiasis, abdominal/rectal pain, hepatitis, pancreatitis, nausea
Phentermine (Apidex-P, Suprenza)	**C**: 15 mg, 30 mg, 37.5 mg **T**: 37.5 mg **T (ODT)**: 15 mg, 30 mg, 37.5 mg	15–37.5 mg/day in 1 or 2 divided doses **ODT**: 15–37.5 mg once daily in morning	Headaches, euphoria, palpitations, hypertension, pulmonary hypertension, valvular heart disease, tremor, dependence, withdrawal psychosis, CNS stimulation, GI complaints
Phentermine/ topiramate (Qsymia)	**C**: 13.75 mg/23 mg	3.75 mg/23 mg to 15 mg/92 mg once daily in the morning	Paresthesia, dizziness, insomnia, depression, tachycardia, cognitive impairment, angle-closure glaucoma, hypokalemia, metabolic acidosis, constipation, dry mouth, suicidal ideation, kidney stones

AS, Appetite suppressant; ***B/P,*** blood pressure; ***C,*** capsules; ***CNS,*** central nervous system; ***CR,*** controlled-release; ***DI,*** digestion inhibitor; ***GI,*** gastrointestinal; ***HR,*** heart rate; ***I,*** injection; ***ODT,*** orally disintegrating tablets; ***SQ,*** subcutaneous; ***T,*** tablets.

Osteoporosis

HISTORY

Osteoporosis is a bone disease that can lead to fractures. Bone mineral density (BMD) is reduced, bone microarchitecture is disrupted, and the amount and variety of proteins in bone are altered. Osteoporosis primarily affects women after menopause (postmenopausal osteoporosis) but may develop in men, in anyone in the presence of particular hormonal disorders (e.g., parathyroid glands), after overconsumption of dietary proteins, or as a result of medications (e.g., glucocorticoids). Several pharmacologic options, along with lifestyle changes, that can be used to prevent and/or treat osteoporotic fractures include calcium and vitamin D supplements in patients having inadequate dietary intake of calcium, bisphosphonates, selective estrogen receptor modulator (SERM), parathyroid hormone (PTH), calcitonin, and monoclonal antibodies.

ACTION

Bisphosphonates: Inhibit bone resorption via actions on osteoclasts or osteoclast precursors, decrease rate of bone resorption, leading to an indirect increase in BMD.

Selective estrogen receptor modulator (SERM): Decreases bone resorption increasing BMD and decreasing the incidence of fractures.

Parathyroid hormone: Stimulates osteoblast function, increasing gastrointestinal calcium absorption and increasing renal tubular reabsorption of calcium. This increases BMD, bone mass, and strength, resulting in a decrease in osteoporosis-related fractures.

Calcitonin: Inhibitor of bone resorption. Efficacy not observed in early postmenopausal women and is used only in women with osteoporosis who are at least 5 yrs beyond menopause.

Monoclonal antibody: Inhibits the RANK ligand (RANKL), a cytokine member of the tumor necrosis factor family. This inhibits osteoclast formation, function, and survival, which decreases bone resorption and increases bone mass and strength in cortical and trabecular bone.

Sclerostin inhibitor: Sclerostin is an osteocyte-derived glycoprotein that inhibits bone formation. Inhibition of sclerostin induces osteoblast activity and bone formation, decreasing bone resorption and increasing bone mineral density.

Continued

BISPHOSPHONATES

Name	Availability	Dosage	Class Side Effects
Alendronate (Binosto, Fosamax)	**T:** 5 mg, 10 mg, 35 mg, 40 mg, 70 mg **S:** 70 mg/75 mL	**Prevention:** 5 mg/day or 35 mg/wk **Treatment:** 10 mg/day or 70 mg/wk	Hypocalcemia, may cause jaw osteonecrosis (rarely); GI (e.g., heartburn, esophageal irritation, esophagitis, abdominal pain, diarrhea); severe bone, joint, or muscle pain. IV: acute-phase reaction (e.g., low-grade fever, myalgia, arthralgia) within 1–3 days of the infusion
Ibandronate (Boniva)	**T:** 150 mg **I:** 1 mg/mL	**Prevention and treatment:** 150 mg/mo **IV Injection: Treatment:** 3 mg/3 mos	
Risedronate (Actonel)	**T:** 5 mg, 30 mg, 35 mg, 150 mg **T (DR):** 35 mg	**Prevention and treatment:** 5 mg/day, 35 mg/wk, or 150 mg/mo	
Zoledronic acid (Reclast)	**I:** 5 mg	**Prevention: IV:** 5 mg every 2 yrs **Treatment: IV:** 5 mg every yr	

SERM

Name	Availability	Dosage	Side Effects
Raloxifene (Evista)	**T:** 60 mg	**Prevention and treatment:** 60 mg/day	Leg cramps, hot flashes, increased risk of thromboembolic events and stroke

PARATHYROID HORMONE

Name	Availability	Dosage	Class Side Effects
Abaloparatide (Tymos)	**I**: 2,000 mcg/mL prefilled pen delivers 80 mcg/dose	**Treatment:** 80 mcg subcutaneously once daily	Muscle cramps, injection site reactions, tachycardia, hypotension, increased serum uric acid concentration, hypercalciuria, dizziness, nausea, headache, hypercalcemia
Teriparatide (Forteo)	**I**: 250 mcg/mL syringe delivers 20 mcg/dose	**Treatment**: 20 mcg subcutaneously once daily	

CALCITONIN

Name	Availability	Dosage	Side Effects
Calcitonin (Fortical, Miacalcin)	**I (Miacalcin):** 200 units/mL **Nasal (Fortical, Miacalcin):** 200 units/activation	**Treatment: IM/SQ (Miacalcin)**: 100 units every other day **Nasal:** 200 units in 1 nostril daily	Rhinitis, local nasal irritation. **Injection:** nausea, local inflammation, flushing of face, hands

MONOCLONAL ANTIBODY RANKL INHIBITOR

Name	Availability	Dosage	Side Effects
Denosumab (Prolia)	**I**: 60 mg/mL	**SQ**: 60 mg once every 6 mos	Dermatitis, rash, eczema, hypocalcemia. May cause jaw osteonecrosis (rarely)

DR, Delayed-release; ***I,*** injection; ***S,*** solution (oral); ***T,*** tablet.

SCLEROSTIN INHIBITOR

Name	Availability	Dosage	Side Effects
Romosozumab (Evenity)	**I:** 105 mg/1.17 mL syringe	**SQ:** 210 mg (2 injections) once every mo for up to 12 doses	Arthralgia, headache

SQ, subcutaneous.

Parkinson's Disease Treatment

USES	ACTION
To slow or stop clinical progression of Parkinson's disease and to improve function and quality of life in pts with Parkinson's disease, a progressive neurodegenerative disorder.	Normal motor function is dependent on the synthesis and release of dopamine by neurons projecting from the substantia nigra to the corpus striatum. In Parkinson's disease, disruption of this pathway results in diminished levels of the neurotransmitter dopamine. Medication is aimed at providing improved function using the lowest effective dose.

TYPES OF MEDICATIONS FOR PARKINSON'S DISEASE DOPAMINE PRECURSOR

Levodopa/carbidopa:

Levodopa: Dopamine precursor supplementation to enhance dopaminergic neurotransmission. A small amount of levodopa crosses the blood-brain barrier and is decarboxylated to dopamine, which is then available to stimulate dopaminergic receptors.
Carbidopa: Inhibits peripheral decarboxylation of levodopa, decreasing its conversion to dopamine in peripheral tissues, which results in an increased availability of levodopa for transport across the blood-brain barrier.

COMT INHIBITORS

Entacapone, tolcapone: Reversible inhibitor of catechol-*O*-methyltransferase (COMT). COMT is responsible for catalyzing levodopa. In the presence of a decarboxylase inhibitor (carbidopa), COMT becomes the major metabolizing enzyme for levodopa in the brain and periphery. By inhibiting COMT, higher plasma levels of levodopa are attained, resulting in more dopaminergic stimulation in the brain and lessening the symptoms of Parkinson's disease.

DOPAMINE RECEPTOR AGONISTS

Bromocriptine: Stimulates postsynaptic dopamine type 2 receptors in the neostriatum of the CNS.
Pramipexole: Stimulates dopamine receptors in the striatum of the CNS.
Ropinirole: Stimulates postsynaptic dopamine D2 type receptors within the caudate putamen in the brain.

MONOAMINE OXIDASE B INHIBITORS

Rasagiline, Safinamide, Selegiline: Increase dopaminergic activity due to inhibition of monoamine oxidase type B (MAO B). MAO B is involved in the oxidative deamination of dopamine in the brain.

ADENOSINE A2A RECEPTOR ANTAGONIST

Istradefylline: Attenuates excessive activity of the striato-pallidal neurons in pts with Parkinson's Disease. Possibly increases dopaminergic activity in the brain.

Parkinson's Disease Treatment

MEDICATIONS FOR TREATMENT OF PARKINSON'S DISEASE

Name	Type	Availability	Dosage	Side Effects
Amantadine **Gocovri** **Osmolex ER**	Dopamine agonist	**C:** 100 mg **Syrup:** 10 mg/mL **T:** 100 mg **ER Caps (Gocovri):** 68.5 mg, 137 mg **ER Tabs (Osmolex ER):** 129 mg, 193 mg, 258 mg	100 mg 2 times/day. May increase up to 400 mg/day in divided doses **ER Caps:** 274 mg once at bedtime **ER Tabs:** 129–322 mg once daily in the morning	Cognitive impairment, confusion, insomnia, hallucinations, livido reticularis
Carbidopa/ levodopa (Rytary, Sinemet, Sinemet CR)	Dopamine precursor	**OD:** 10/100 mg, 25/100 mg, 25/250 mg **Immediate-release (Sinemet):** 10/100 mg, 25/100 mg, 25/250 mg **ER (Sinemet CR):** 25/100 mg, 50/200 mg **(Rytary):** 23.75 mg/95 mg, 36.25 mg/145 mg, 48.75 mg/ 195 mg, 61.25 mg/245 mg	300–1,500 mg levodopa in divided doses **Sinemet:** 300–1,500 mg levodopa in divided doses **Sinemet CR:** Initially, 400 mg/day in 2 divided doses. May increase up to 1,600 mg levodopa in divided doses **Rytary:** Initially, 23.75 mg/95 mg 3 times/ day May increase up to 612.5 mg/2,450 mg per day in divided doses	Anorexia, nausea, orthostatic hypotension initially; hallucinations, confusion, sleep disturbances with chronic use, constipation, dry mouth, headache, dyskinesia
Entacapone (Comtan)	COMT inhibitor	**T:** 200 mg	200 mg 3–4 times/day up to **maximum** of 8 times/day (1,600 mg)	Dyskinesias, nausea, diarrhea, urine discoloration
Istradefylline (Nourianz)	Adenosine A2a Receptor Antagonist	**T:** 20 mg, 40 mg	20–40 mg once daily	Dyskinesia, hallucinations, psychotic behavior, impulse control disorders
Pramipexole (Mirapex, Mirapex ER)	Dopamine agonist	**T:** 0.125 mg, 0.25 mg, 0.5 mg, 0.75 mg, 1 mg, 1.5 mg **ER:** 0.375 mg, 0.75 mg, 1.5 mg, 2.25 mg, 3 mg, 3.75 mg, 4.5 mg	**T:** Initially, 0.125 mg 3 times/day May increase q5–7 days. Usual dose: 0.5–1.5 mg 3 times/day **ER:** Initially, 0.375 mg once daily May increase q5–7 days by 0.75 mg/dose up to 4.5 mg once daily	Side effects similar to carbidopa/ levodopa. Lower risk of dyskinesias, higher risk of hallucinations, sleepiness, edema. May cause excessive daytime sleepiness, impair impulse control (e.g., gambling)

Continued

MEDICATIONS FOR TREATMENT OF PARKINSON'S DISEASE—cont'd

Name	Type	Availability	Dosage	Side Effects
Rasagiline (Azilect)	MAO B inhibitor	**T:** 0.5 mg, 1 mg	0.5–1 mg once daily	Nausea, orthostatic hypotension, hallucinations, insomnia, dry mouth, constipation, vivid dreams. Many potential drug interactions.
Ropinirole (Requip, Requip XL)	Dopamine agonist	**T:** 0.25 mg, 0.5 mg, 1 mg, 2 mg, 3 mg, 4 mg, 5 mg **XL:** 2 mg, 4 mg, 6 mg, 8 mg, 12 mg	**T:** Initially, 0.25 mg 3 times/day. May increase at wkly intervals to 0.5 mg 3 times/day, then 0.75 mg 3 times/day, then 1 mg 3 times/day May then increase by 1.5 mg/day up to 9 mg/day, then by 3 mg/day up to total dose of 24 mg/day in divided doses **XL:** Initially, 2 mg/day for 1–2 wks, then increase by 2 mg/day at wkly intervals	Side effects similar to carbidopa/levodopa. Lower risk of dyskinesias, higher risk of hallucinations, sleepiness, edema. May cause excessive daytime sleepiness, impair impulse control (e.g., gambling)
Rotigotine (Neupro)	Dopamine agonist	**Transdermal patch:** 1 mg/24 hrs, 2 mg/24 hrs, 3 mg/24 hrs, 4 mg/24 hrs, 6 mg/24 hrs, 8 mg/24 hrs	Early stage: Initially, 2 mg/24 hrs up to 6 mg/24 hrs Advanced stage: Initially, 4 mg/24 hrs up to 8 mg/24 hrs	Side effects similar to carbidopa/levodopa. Lower risk of dyskinesias, higher risk of hallucinations, sleepiness, edema. May cause excessive daytime sleepiness, impair impulse control (e.g., gambling)
Safinamide (Xadago)	MAO B inhibitor	**T:** 50 mg, 100 mg	Initially, 50 mg once daily. May increase after 2 wks to 100 mg once daily	Dyskinesia, falls, hallucinations, nausea, insomnia. Many potential drug interactions
Selegiline (Eldepryl, Zelapar)	MAO B inhibitor	**C (Eldepryl):** 5 mg **OD (Zelapar):** 1.25 mg	**C:** 5 mg with breakfast and lunch **OD:** 1.25–2.5 mg daily in the morning	Nausea, orthostatic hypotension, hallucinations, insomnia, dry mouth, constipation, vivid dreams. Many potential drug interactions
Tolcapone (Tasmar)	COMT inhibitor	**T:** 100 mg	Initially, 100 mg 3 times/day. May increase to 200 mg 3 times/day	Dyskinesias, nausea, diarrhea, urine discoloration

C, Capsules; ***COMT,*** catechol-*O*-methyltransferase; ***CR,*** controlled-release; ***ER,*** extended-release; ***I,*** Injection; ***MAO B,*** monoamine oxidase B; ***OD,*** orally disintegrating; ***T,*** tablets; ***XL,*** extended-release.

Proton Pump Inhibitors

USES

Treatment of various gastric disorders, including gastric and duodenal ulcers, gastroesophageal reflex disease (GERD), pathologic hypersecretory conditions.

ACTION

Binds to the activated proton pump on the apical membrane of parietal cells. Inhibits acid secretion into the gastric lumen.

PROTON PUMP INHIBITORS

Name	Availability	Indications	Usual Adult Dosage	Class Side Effects
Dexlansoprazole (Dexilant)	**C:** 30 mg, 60 mg	Erosive esophagitis, heartburn associated with nonerosive GERD	30–60 mg/day	Generally well tolerated. Most common: headache, nausea, constipation, diarrhea, flatulence, abdominal pain. Long-term use associated with *C. difficile* infection, risk of fractures, hypomagnesemia.
Esomeprazole (Nexium)	**C:** 20 mg, 40 mg **I:** 20 mg, 40 mg	*Helicobacter pylori* eradication, GERD, erosive esophagitis	20–40 mg/day	
Lansoprazole (Prevacid)	**C:** 15 mg, 30 mg **T (ODT):** 15 mg, 30 mg	Duodenal ulcer, gastric ulcer, NSAID-associated gastric ulcer, hypersecretory conditions, *H. pylori* eradication, GERD, erosive esophagitis	15–30 mg/day	
Omeprazole (Prilosec)	**C:** 10 mg, 20 mg, 40 mg	Duodenal ulcer, gastric ulcer, hypersecretory conditions, *H. pylori* eradication, GERD, erosive esophagitis	20–40 mg/day	
Omeprazole and Sodium Bicarbonate (Zegerid)	**P:** 20 mg, 40 mg	Duodenal ulcer, benign gastric ulcer, GERD, erosive esophagitis	20–40 mg/day	
Pantoprazole (Protonix)	**T:** 20 mg, 40 mg **I:** 40 mg	Erosive esophagitis, hypersecretory conditions	40 mg/day	
Rabeprazole (Aciphex)	**T:** 20 mg **S:** 5 mg, 10 mg	Duodenal ulcer, hypersecretory conditions, *H. pylori* eradication, GERD, erosive esophagitis	20 mg/day	

C, Capsules; ***GERD,*** gastroesophageal reflux disease; ***I,*** Injection; ***NSAID,*** nonsteroidal anti-inflammatory drug; ***ODT,*** orally disintegrating tablets; ***P,*** powder for suspension; ***S,*** sprinkles; ***T,*** tablets.

Rheumatoid Arthritis

Rheumatoid arthritis (RA) is an autoimmune disease associated with progressive disability, systemic complications, early death, and socioeconomic costs. RA affects most joints and their surrounding tissues. RA is characterized by synovial inflammation and hyperplasia, autoantibody production (e.g., rheumatoid factor), cartilage and bone destruction, and systemic features (e.g., cardiovascular, pulmonary, psychological, skeletal disorders). The clinical hallmark of RA is polyarticular synovial inflammation of peripheral joints (typically in the hands, resulting in pain, stiffness, and some degree of irreversible joint damage; deformity; and disability).

Medications used in RA include disease-modifying antirheumatic drugs (DMARDs) and biologic agents, including tumor necrosis factor (TNT) inhibitors.

Combination treatment useful in pts with a long duration of disease or clinical features indicating a poor prognosis.

DMARDS

Name	Dosage	Side Effects/Comments
Hydroxychloroquine (Plaquenil)	Induction: 400–600 mg/day for 4–12 wks Maintenance: 200–400 mg/day	**Side Effects:** Nausea, epigastric pain, hemolysis may occur in pts with G6PD deficiency, retinal toxicity with long-term use
Leflunomide (Arava)	Induction: 100 mg/day for 3 days Maintenance: 10–20 mg/day	**Side Effects:** Diarrhea, respiratory tract infection, hypertension, headache, reversible alopecia, rash, myelosuppression, and/or elevated hepatic enzymes **Comments:** Contraindicated for use during pregnancy
Methotrexate (oral) (Rheumatrex, Trexall) Methotrexate (injectable) (Otrexup, Rasuvo)	Induction: 7.5–10 mg PO once wkly Maintenance: 7.5–25 mg PO once wkly Induction: 7.5 PO once wkly Maintenance: 10–25 mg IM or SQ once wkly	**Side Effects:** Stomatitis, anorexia, nausea, vomiting, diarrhea, abdominal cramps, hepatic enzyme elevations, thrombocytopenia **Comments:** Not recommended in pts with CrCl <30 mL/min; should not be prescribed for women who are or may become pregnant
Sulfasalazine (Azulfidine)	Induction: 3–4 g/day in divided doses Maintenance: 2 g/day in divided doses	**Side Effects:** Headache, nausea, anorexia, rash, hemolysis may occur in pts with G6PD deficiency

BIOLOGIC AGENTS

TNF Inhibitors

Name	Dosage	Side Effects/Comments
Adalimumab (Humira)	40 mg SQ once wkly or q2wks	**Side Effects:** Headache, skin rash, positive ANA titer, antibody development, injection site reaction (erythema, itching, pain, swelling), upper respiratory tract infection **Comments:** Increased risk for serious infections (e.g., tuberculosis, invasive fungal infections), avoid use in pts with recent history of malignancy or preexisting demyelinating disorders
Certolizumab (Cimzia)	Induction: 400 mg SQ at 0, 2, 4 wks Maintenance: 200 mg SQ every other wk or 400 mg q4wks	**Side Effects:** Nausea, infection, upper respiratory tract infection, skin rash **Comments:** See adalimumab
Etanercept (Enbrel)	25 mg SQ 2 times/wk or 50 mg SQ once wkly	**Side Effects:** Headache, skin rash, diarrhea, injection site reactions (e.g., erythema, swelling), upper respiratory tract infection, rhinitis **Comments:** See adalimumab
Golimumab (Simponi, Simponi Aria)	**Simponi:** 50 mg SQ once monthly **Simponi Aria:** Induction: 2 mg/kg IV at 0 and 4 wks Maintenance: 2 mg/kg IV q8wks	**Side Effects:** Positive ANA titer, upper respiratory tract infection (e.g., nasopharyngitis, rhinitis) **Comments:** See adalimumab
Infliximab (Remicade) Biosimilars: Inflectra, Renflexis	Induction: 3 mg/kg IV at 0, 2, and 6 wks Maintenance: 3 mg/kg IV q8wks	**Side Effects:** Nausea, diarrhea, abdominal pain, increased ANA titer, upper respiratory tract infection, sinusitis, cough, pharyngitis **Comments:** See adalimumab

Continued

OTHER BIOLOGIC AGENTS

Name	Dosage	Side Effects/Comments
Abatacept (Orencia)	**IV**: 500 mg, 750 mg, or 1,000 mg IV at 0, 2, and 4 wks, then q4wks **SQ**: 125 mg SQ once wkly	**Side Effects:** Nausea, UTIs, acute exacerbation of COPD, hypertension, headache, dizziness **Comments:** May increase risk of serious infections (e.g., pneumonia, pyelonephritis, cellulitis, diverticulitis)
Baricitinib (Olumiant)	2 mg PO once daily	**Side Effects:** Upper respiratory tract infection, nausea. Thrombotic events, malignancy, GI perforation, cytopenias, dyslipidemia, increased hepatic transaminases reported **Comments:** Screening for tuberculosis recommended
Rituximab (Rituxan)	1,000 mg IV twice, 2 wks apart	**Side Effects:** Hypotension, peripheral edema, abdominal pair anemia, arthralgia, infusion site reactions **Comments:** Pts at high risk for hepatitis B virus infection should be screened before beginning therapy
Sarilumab (Kevzara)	**SQ**: 200 mg q2wks	**Side Effects:** Neutropenia, increased ALT, injection site reactions (e.g., erythema), upper respiratory tract infections, UTI **Comments:** Screening for tuberculosis recommended
Tocilizumab (Actemra)	**IV**: Induction: 4 mg/kg IV q4wks Maintenance: 8 mg/kg q4 wks **SQ**: Induction: 162 mg SQ every other wk Maintenance: 162 mg once wkly	**Side Effects:** Hypertension, upper abdominal pain, increased ALT/ AST, injection site reactions, neutropenia, dyslipidemia **Comments:** Severe complications including GI perforation and hypersensitivity with anaphylaxis have been reported
Tofacitinib (Xeljanz), Xeljanz XR)	5 mg PO bid **XR**: 11 mg PO once daily	**Side Effects:** Diarrhea, nasopharyngitis, upper respiratory infections, headache hypertension, increased LFTs, dyslipidemia, cytopenias have been reported **Comments:** Screening for tuberculosis recommended, increased incidence of solid cancers detected
Upadacitinbi (Rinvoq)	15 mg PO once daily	**Side Effects:** Upper respiratory tract infections, nausea, cough, pyrexia **Comments:** Screening for tuberculosis recommended

ALT, Alanine transaminase; ***ANA,*** antinuclear antibodies; ***CNS,*** central nervous system; ***COPD,*** chronic obstructive pulmonary disease; ***GI,*** gastrointestinal; ***IM,*** intramuscular; ***IV,*** intravenous; ***LFT,*** liver function test; ***PO,*** oral; ***SQ,*** subcutaneous; ***UTI,*** urinary tract Infection.

Rhinitis Preparations

USES

Relieve symptoms associated with allergic rhinitis. These symptoms include rhinorrhea, nasal congestion, pruritus, sneezing, postnasal drip, nasal pain.

Allergic rhinitis or hay fever is an inflammation of the nasal airways occurring when an allergen (e.g., pollen) is inhaled. This triggers antibody production. The antibodies bind to mast cells, which contain histamine. Histamine is released, causing symptoms of allergic rhinitis.

ACTION

Intranasal corticosteroids: Depress migration of polymorphonuclear leucocytes and fibroblasts, reverse capillary permeability, and stabilize nasal membranes to prevent/control inflammation. First-line therapy for moderate to severe symptoms or where nasal congestion is the dominant complaint.

Intranasal antihistamines: Reduce histamine-mediated symptoms of allergic rhinitis, including pruritus, sneezing, rhinorrhea, watery eyes. Second-line therapy for intermittent nasal symptoms where congestion is not dominant.

Intranasal mast cell stabilizers: Inhibit the mast cell release of histamine and other inflammatory mediators.

Intranasal anticholinergics: Block acetylcholine in the nasal mucosa. Effective in treating rhinorrhea associated with allergic rhinitis.

Intranasal decongestants: Vasoconstrict the respiratory mucosa, provide short-term relief of nasal congestion. Used only as adjuvant therapy for 3–5 days.

Oral antihistamines (second generation): First-line therapy for mild symptoms or where sneezing/itching is primary complaint (see antihistamine classification).

Oral decongestants: For primary complaint of nasal congestion.

CORTICOSTEROIDS—INTRANASAL

Generic (Brand)	Adult Dose	Pediatric Dose	Side Effects
Beclomethasone (Beconase AQ) (Qnasl)	Beconase AQ: 1–2 sprays in each nostril 2 times/day Qnasl: 80 mcg/spray: 2 sprays in each nostril once daily	Beconase AQ: 6–11 yrs: 1–2 sprays in each nostril 2 times/day Qnasl: 4–11 yrs: 40 mcg/spray: 1 spray in each nostril once daily	Mild dryness, irritation, burning, stinging, bleeding of nasal mucosa, throat irritation, epistaxis, headache
Budesonide (Rhinocort Allergy Spray, Rhinocort Aqua)	Rhinocort Aqua: 1–4 sprays in each nostril daily Rhinocort Allergy Spray: 1–2 sprays in each nostril once daily	Rhinocort Allergy Spray, Rhinocort Aqua: 6–11 yrs: 1–2 sprays in each nostril daily	

Continued

CORTICOSTEROIDS—INTRANASAL—cont'd

Generic (Brand)	Adult Dose	Pediatric Dose	Side Effects
Ciclesonide (Omnaris, Zetonna)	Omnaris: 2 sprays in each nostril daily Zetonna: 1 spray in each nostril daily	Omnaris: 6–11 yrs: 2 sprays in each nostril daily (seasonal allergic rhinitis only)	
Flunisolide (Nasalide)	2 sprays in each nostril 2 or 3 times/day (**maximum:** 8 sprays in each nostril daily)	6–14 yrs: 2 sprays in each nostril 2 times/day or 1 spray in each nostril 3 times/day (**maximum:** 4 sprays in each nostril daily)	
Fluticasone (Flonase Sensimist, Flonase Allergy Relief)	Flonase, Flonase Allergy Relief, Flonase Sensimist: 1–2 sprays in each nostril once daily	Flonase Sensimist: 2–11 yrs: 1 spray in each nostril daily Flonase Allergy Relief: 4–11 yrs: 1 spray in each nostril once daily	
Fluticasone/Azelastine (Dymista)	1 spray in each nostril 2 times/day	Not indicated in children younger than 6 yrs	
Mometasone (Nasonex)	2 sprays in each nostril daily	2–11 yrs: 1 spray in each nostril daily	
Triamcinolone (Nasacort Allergy 24 HR, Nasacort AQ)	1–2 sprays in each nostril daily	2–5 yrs: 1 spray in each nostril once daily 6–11 yrs: 1–2 sprays in each nostril daily	

ANTIHISTAMINES—INTRANASAL

Generic (Brand)	Adult Dose	Pediatric Dose	Side Effects
Azelastine Astepro 0.1%, 0.15%	Azelastine: 1–2 sprays in each nostril 2 times/day Astepro 0.1%, 0.15%: 1–2 sprays in each nostril two times/day or 2 sprays each nostril once daily (for seasonal allergic rhinitis)	Azelastine: 5–11 yrs: 1 spray in each nostril 2 times/day Astepro 0.1%: 2–5 yrs: 1 spray 2 times/day Astepro 0.1% or 0.15%: 6–11 yrs: 1 spray 2 times/day	Nasal discomfort, epistaxis, somnolence, headache
Azelastine/Fluticasone (Dymista)	1 spray in each nostril 2 times/day	Not approved for children younger than 6 yrs	
Olopatadine (Patanase)	2 sprays in each nostril 2 times/day	6–11 yrs: 1 spray in each nostril 2 times/day	

MAST CELL STABILIZERS

Generic (Brand)	Adult Dose	Pediatric Dose	Side Effects
Cromolyn (NasalCrom)	1 spray in each nostril 3–4 times/day	2–11 yrs: 1 spray in each nostril 3–4 times/day	Nasal irritation, unpleasant taste

ANTICHOLINERGICS

Generic (Brand)	Adult Dose	Pediatric Dose	Side Effects
Ipratropium (Atrovent) 0.03%	2 sprays in each nostril 2–3 times/day	6–12 yrs: 2 sprays in each nostril 2–3 times/day	Nasal irritation, dizziness, headache
Ipratropium (Atrovent) 0.06%	2 sprays in each nostril 3–4 times/day	5–12 yrs: 2 sprays in each nostril 3–4 times/day	

DECONGESTANTS

Generic (Brand)	Adult Dose	Pediatric Dose	Side Effects
Oxymetazoline (Afrin, Neo-Synephrine 12 HR)	2–3 sprays 2 times/day	6–11 yrs: 2–3 sprays 2 times/day	Insomnia, tachycardia, nervousness, nausea, vomiting, transient burning, headache, rebound congestion if used longer than 72 hrs
Phenylephrine (Neo-Synephrine Cold and Sinus, Vicks Sinus)	2–3 drops/sprays q4h as needed (0.25% or 0.5%)	6–11 yrs: 2–3 drops/sprays (0.25%) q4h as needed 1–5 yrs: 2–3 drops/sprays (0.125%) q4h as needed	Restlessness, nervousness, headache, rebound nasal congestion, burning, stinging, dryness

Continued

Alzheimer's Disease

Dementia is a general term used describing a decline in mental ability that is severe enough to interfere with the function of daily living. Alzheimer's disease (AD) is the most common cause of dementia. Cognitive loss in AD is associated with depletion of acetylcholine (involved with learning and memory). AD is confirmed only at autopsy and is characterized by the presence of beta-amyloid plaques on the outer portions of neurons.

Currently, two classes of medications are used as therapies for AD, ***acetylcholinesterase inhibitors (AChEIs)*** and an ***N-methyl-D-aspartate (NMDA) receptor antagonist.***

AChEIs increase the concentration of acetylcholine and may have beneficial effects on dementia. NMDA receptor antagonist mechanism of action is unclear, but may reduce glutamatergic overstimulation at the NMDA receptor, which may have symptomatic benefits on dementia.

ACETYLCHOLINESTERASE INHIBITORS

Name	Uses	Availability	Dose/Titration	Adverse Effects
Donepezil (Aricept, Aricept ODT)	Mild, moderate, severe AD	**T**: 5 mg, 10 mg, 23 mg **ODT**: 5 mg, 10 mg	Initially, 5 mg once daily, may increase to 10 mg once daily after 4–6 wks. After 3 months, if suboptimal response, may increase to 23 mg once daily	Nausea, vomiting, abdominal cramping, diarrhea, bradycardia, syncope
Galantamine (Razadyne, Razadyne ER)	Mild, moderate AD	**T**: 4 mg, 8 mg, 12 mg **OS**: 4 mg/mL **ER**: 8 mg, 16 mg, 24 mg	**T, OS**: Initially, 4 mg bid; may increase to 8 mg bid after 4 wks, then to 12 mg bid after additional 4 wks **ER**: Initially, 8 mg once daily, may increase to 16 mg once daily after 4 wks, then to 24 mg once daily after additional 4 wks	Nausea, vomiting, diarrhea, weight loss, decreased appetite, syncope

Name	Uses	Availability	Dose/Titration	Adverse Effects
Rivastigmine (Exelon, Exelon Patch)	Mild, moderate AD Patch also approved for severe AD	**C:** 1.5 mg, 3 mg, 4.5 mg, 6 mg **OS:** 2 mg/mL **PATCH:** 4.6 mg/24 hrs, 9.5 mg/24 hrs, 13.3 mg/24 hrs	**C, OS:** Initially, 1.5 mg bid, may increase in increments of 1.5 mg bid every 2 wks up to 6 mg bid	Nausea, vomiting, abdominal cramping, diarrhea, bradycardia, syncope, loss of appetite, weight loss
NMDA Receptor Antagonist				
Memantine (Namenda, Namenda XR)	Moderate, severe AD	**T:** 5 mg, 10 mg **OS:** 2 mg/mL **XR:** 7 mg, 14 mg, 21 mg, 28 mg	**T, OS:** Initially, 5 mg once daily, may increase in increments of 5 mg/wk up to 10 mg bid	Dizziness, headache, diarrhea, constipation, confusion
NMDA Receptor Antagonist/ Acetylcholinesterase Inhibitor				
Memantine/donepezil (Namzaric)	Moderate, severe AD	**ER:** 14/10 mg, 28/10 mg	**14/10 mg:** Once/d in evening in patients previously stabilized on memantine 5 mg bid or 14 mg once daily and donepezil 10 mg once/d **28/10 mg:** Once daily in evening in patients previously stabilized on memantine 10 mg bid or 28 mg once daily and donepezil 10 mg once daily	Refer to individual agents for adverse effects

C: Capsule, ***ER:*** extended-release, ***OS:*** oral solution, ***T:*** tablet, ***XR:*** extended-release

Angiotensin-Converting Enzyme (ACE) Inhibitors

USES	ACTION	
Treatment of hypertension (HTN), adjunctive therapy for heart failure (HF).	*Antihypertensive:* Inhibits angiotensin-converting enzyme (ACE). ACE catalyzes conversion of angiotensin I to angiotensin II, a potent vasoconstrictor that also stimulates aldosterone secretion by adrenal cortex. Beneficial effects in HTN/HF appear to be suppression of the renin-angiotensin-aldosterone system. Reduces peripheral arterial resistance.	*HF:* Decreases peripheral vascular resistance (afterload), pulmonary capillary wedge pressure (preload); improves cardiac output, exercise tolerance.

ACE INHIBITORS

Name	Availability	Uses	Dosage Range (per day)	Frequent or Severe Side Effects
Benazepril (Lotensin)	**T:** 5 mg, 10 mg, 20 mg, 40 mg	HTN	**HTN**: Initially, 10 mg/day. Usual dose: 20–80 mg once daily or divided bid	**Class Effects** Cough, hypotension, rash, acute renal failure (in pts with renal artery stenosis), angioedema, hyperkalemia, mild-moderate loss of taste, hepatotoxicity, pancreatitis, blood dyscrasias, renal damage
Captopril (Capoten)	**T:** 12.5 mg, 25 mg, 50 mg, 100 mg	HTN HF	**HTN**: Initially, 12.5–25 mg 2–3 times/day. Usual dose: 50–100 mg 2 times/day **HF**: Initially, 6.25 mg 3 times/day. Target: 50 mg 3 times/day	
Enalapril (Vasotec)	**T:** 2.5 mg, 5 mg, 10 mg, 20 mg **IV:** 1.25 mg/mL	HTN HF	**HTN**: Initially, 2.5–5 mg/day; may increase at 1–2 wk intervals. Usual dose: 5–40 mg once/d or divided bid **HF**: Initially, 2.5 mg 2 times/day, may increase at 1–2 wk intervals. Target: 20 mg/day in 1–2 divided doses	
Fosinopril (Monopril)	**T:** 10 mg, 20 mg, 40 mg	HTN HF	**HTN**: Initially, 10 mg/day Usual dose: 10–80 mg once daily **HF**: Initially, 5–10 mg/day Target: 10–40 mg/day	

Name	Availability	Uses	Dosage Range (per day)	Frequent or Severe Side Effects
Lisinopril (Prinivil, Zestril)	**T:** 2.5 mg, 5 mg, 10 mg, 20 mg, 40 mg	HTN HF	**HTN**: Initially, 5–10 mg/day. Usual dose: 10–40 mg once daily **HF**: Initially, 2.5–5 mg/day. Target: 20–40 mg/day	
Moexipril (Univasc)	**T:** 7.5 mg, 15 mg	HTN	**HTN**: Initially, 3.75–7.5 mg/day. Usual dose: 7.5–30 mg/day in 1–2 divided doses	
Perindopril (Aceon)	**T:** 2 mg, 4 mg, 6 mg	HTN	**HTN**: Initially, 4 mg/day. May increase at 1–2 wk intervals. Usual dose: 4–8 mg once daily or divided bid	
Quinapril (Accupril)	**T:** 5 mg, 10 mg, 20 mg, 40 mg	HTN HF	**HTN**: Initially, 10–20 mg once daily. Usual dose: 10–40 mg once daily or divided bid **HF**: Initially, 5 mg 2 times/day. Titrate to 20–40 mg/day in 2 divided doses	
Ramipril (Altace)	**C:** 1.25 mg, 2.5 mg, 5 mg, 10 mg	HTN HF	**HTN**: Initially, 2.5 mg once daily. Usual dose: 2.5–20 mg once daily or divided bid **HF**: Initially, 1.25–2.5 mg once daily. Target: 10 mg once daily	
Trandolapril (Mavik)	**T:** 1 mg, 2 mg, 4 mg	HTN HF	**HTN**: Initially, 1–2 mg once daily. Usual dose: 2–8 mg once daily or divided bid **HF**: Initially, 1 mg once daily. Target: 4 mg once daily	

C, Capsules; ***HF,*** heart failure; ***HTN,*** hypertension; ***T,*** tablets.

Angiotensin II Receptor Antagonists

USES

Treatment of hypertension (HTN) alone or in combination with other antihypertensives. Treatment of heart failure (HF).

ACTION

Angiotensin II receptor antagonists (AIIRA) block vasoconstrictor and aldosterone-secreting effects on angiotensin II by selectively blocking the binding of angiotensin II to AT_1 receptors in vascular smooth muscle and the adrenal gland, causing vasodilation and a decrease in aldosterone effects.

ANGIOTENSIN II RECEPTOR ANTAGONISTS

Name	Availability	Uses	Dosage Range (per day)	Frequent or Severe Side Effects
Azilsartan (Edarbi)	**T:** 40 mg, 80 mg	HTN	40–80 mg once daily	**Class Effects** Hypotension, rash, acute renal failure (in pts with renal artery stenosis), hyperkalemia, mild-moderate loss of taste, hepatotoxicity, pancreatitis, blood dyscrasias, renal damage
Candesartan (Atacand)	**T:** 4 mg, 8 mg, 16 mg, 32 mg	HTN, HF	Initially, 16 mg once daily. Usual dose: 8–32 mg in 1–2 divided doses. Initially, 4–8 mg once daily. Double dose at 2 wk intervals. Target: 32 mg once daily	
Eprosartan (Teveten)	**T:** 400 mg, 600 mg	HTN	Initially, 600 mg/day. Usual dose: 600 mg once daily	
Irbesartan (Avapro)	**T:** 75 mg, 150 mg, 300 mg	HTN Nephropathy	150–300 mg once daily 300 mg once daily	
Losartan (Cozaar)	**T:** 25 mg, 50 mg, 100 mg	HTN Nephropathy	Initially, 50 mg once daily. Usual dose: 25–100 mg/once daily or divided bid Initially, 50 mg/day; may increase to 100 mg/day	
Olmesartan (Benicar)	**T:** 5 mg, 20 mg, 40 mg	HTN	Initially, 20 mg once daily. May increase to 40 mg once daily after 2 wks	

Name	Availability	Uses	Dosage Range (per day)	Frequent or Severe Side Effects
Telmisartan (Micardis)	**T:** 40 mg, 80 mg	HTN CV risk reduction	Initially, 40 mg once daily. Usual dose: 40–80 mg once daily. 80 mg once daily	
Valsartan (Diovan)	**T:** 80 mg, 160 mg	HTN HF Post MI	Initially, 80 or 160 mg once daily. Usual dose: 80–320 mg once daily Initially, 20–40 mg 2 times/day. Titrate to 80–160 mg 2 times/day Initially, 20 mg 2 times/day. Titrate to target of 160 mg 2 times/day	

CV, Cardiovascular; ***HF,*** heart failure; ***HTN,*** hypertension; ***MI,*** myocardial infarction; ***T,*** tablets.

Antianxiety Agents

USES

Anxiety disorders are the most common form of psychiatric illness and include generalized anxiety disorder (GAD), panic disorder, obsessive-compulsive disorder (OCD), social anxiety disorder (SAD), posttraumatic stress disorder (PTSD), and acute stress disorder. Treatment options for anxiety disorders include pharmacotherapy and psychological therapy (e.g., behavioral therapy). A selective serotonin reuptake inhibitor (SSRI) or a serotonin norepinephrine reuptake inhibitor (SNRI) is generally used for initial treatment. Benzodiazepines can provide immediate relief of anxiety symptoms and are often used as adjuncts to SSRIs and SNRIs (see classification Antidepressants for SSRI and SNRI charts).

ACTION

Benzodiazepines: The exact mechanism is unknown, but they may increase the inhibiting effect of gamma-aminobutyric acid (GABA), which inhibits nerve impulse transmission by binding to specific benzodiazepine receptors in various areas of the central nervous system (CNS).

Continued

ANTIANXIETY AGENTS

Name	Availability	Uses	Dosage	Side Effects
Benzodiazepine				
Alprazolam (Xanax)	**T:** 0.25 mg, 0.5 mg, 1 mg, 2 mg **S:** 1 mg/ml **ER:** 0.5 mg, 1 mg, 2 mg, 3 mg **ODT:** 0.25 mg, 0.5 mg, 1 mg, 2 mg	Anxiety, panic disorder	Initially, 0.25–0.5 mg 3 times/day. May increase every 3–4 days. **Maximum:** 4 mg/day	Drowsiness, weakness, fatigue, ataxia, slurred speech, confusion, lack of coordination, impaired memory, paradoxical agitation, dizziness, nausea
Clonazepam (Klonopin)	**T:** 0.5 mg, 1 mg, 2 mg **ODT:** 0.125, 0.25, 0.5, 1, 2 mg	Anxiety, panic disorder	Anxiety: 1–4 mg divided bid	Drowsiness, ataxia, behavioral disturbances
Clorazepate (Tranxene)	**T:** 3.75 mg, 7.5 mg, 15 mg **SD:** 11.25 mg, 22.5 mg	Anxiety, alcohol withdrawal, anticonvulsant	7.5–15 mg 2–4 times/day	Hypotension, drowsiness, fatigue, ataxia, memory impairment, headache, nausea
Diazepam (Valium)	**T:** 2 mg, 5 mg, 10 mg **S:** 5 mg/5 mL **I:** 5 mg/mL	Anxiety, alcohol withdrawal, anticonvulsant, muscle relaxant	2–10 mg, 2–4 times/day	Hypotension, ataxia, drowsiness, fatigue, vertigo
Lorazepam (Ativan)	**T:** 0.5 mg, 1 mg, 2 mg **S:** 2 mg/mL **I:** 2 mg/mL, 4 mg/mL	Anxiety, alcohol withdrawal	Initially, 2–3 mg/day in 2–3 divided doses. Usual dose: 2–6 mg/day in divided doses	Sedation, respiratory depression, ataxia, dizziness, headache

Nonbenzodiazepine				
Buspirone (BuSpar)	**T:** 5 mg, 7.5 mg, 10 mg, 15 mg, 30 mg	Anxiety	Initially, 7.5 mg 2 times/day. May increase every 2–3 days by 2.5 mg bid. **Maximum:** 30 mg 2 times/day	Dizziness, light-headedness, headaches, nausea, restlessness
Hydroxyzine (Atarax, Vistaril)	**T:** 10 mg, 25 mg, 50 mg **C:** 25 mg, 50 mg, 100 mg **S:** 10 mg/5 mL	Anxiety	50–100 mg 4 times/day	Drowsiness; dry mouth, nose, and throat

C, Capsules; ***CR,*** controlled-release; ***ER,*** extended-release; ***I,*** injection; ***ODT,*** orally disintegrating tablet; ***S,*** solution; ***SD,*** single dose; ***T,*** tablets.

Antiarrhythmics

USES

Prevention and treatment of cardiac arrhythmias, such as premature ventricular contractions, ventricular tachycardia, premature atrial contractions, paroxysmal atrial tachycardia, atrial fibrillation, and flutter.

ACTION

The antiarrhythmics are divided into four classes based on their effects on certain ion channels and/or receptors located on the myocardial cell membrane. Class I is further divided into three subclasses (IA, IB, IC) based on electrophysiologic effects.

Class I: Blocks cardiac sodium channels and slows conduction velocity, prolonging refractory period, and decreasing automaticity of sodium-dependent tissue.

Class IA: Blocks sodium and potassium channels.

Class IB: Shortens the repolarization phase.

Class IC: Slows conduction velocity; no effect on repolarization phase.

Class II: Slows sinus and atrioventricular (AV) nodal conduction.

Class III: Blocks cardiac potassium channels, prolonging the repolarization phase of electrical cells.

Class IV: Inhibits the influx of calcium through its channels, causing slower conduction through the sinus and AV nodes; decreases contractility.

ANTIARRHYTHMICS

Name	Availability	Uses	Dosage Range	Side Effects
Class IA				
Disopyramide (Norpace, Norpace CR)	**C:** 100 mg, 150 mg **C (ER):** 100 mg, 150 mg	AF, WPW, PSVT, PVCs, VT	**C:** 100–200 mg q6h **ER:** 200–400 mg q12h	Dry mouth, blurred vision, urinary retention, HF, proarrhythmia, heart block, nausea, vomiting, diarrhea, hypoglycemia, nervousness
Procainamide (Procan-SR, Pronestyl)	**I:** 100 mg/mL, 500 mg/mL	AF, WPW, PVCs, VT	Loading dose: 15–18 mg/kg over 20–30 min. Maintenance dose: 1–4 mg/min as a continuous infusion	Hypotension, fever, agranulocytosis, SLE, headaches, proarrhythmia, confusion, disorientation, GI symptoms, hypotension

Quinidine (Quinaglute, Quinidex)	**T:** 200 mg, 300 mg **T (ER):** 300 mg, 324 mg **I:** 80 mg/mL	AF, WPW, PVCs, VT	**A (PO):** 400 mg q6h. **(ER):** 300 mg q8–12h or 648 mg q8h	Diarrhea, hypotension, nausea, vomiting, cinchonism, fever, bitter taste, heart block, thrombocytopenia, proarrhythmia
Class IB				
Lidocaine (Xylocaine)	**I:** 300 mg for IM **IV Infusion:** 2 mg/mL, 4 mg/mL	PVCs, VT, VF	**IV:** Initially, 1–1.5 mg/kg. May repeat 0.5–0.75 mg/kg q5–10 min. **Maximum cumulative dose:** 3 mg/kg, then 1–4 mg/min infusion	Drowsiness, agitation, muscle twitching, seizures, paresthesia, proarrhythmia, slurred speech, tinnitus, cardiac depression, bradycardia, asystole
Mexiletine (Mexitil)	**C:** 150 mg, 200 mg, 250 mg	PVCs, VT, VF	**A:** Initially, 200 mg q8h. Adjust every 2–3 days in 50–100 mg increments. **Maximum:** 1,200 mg/day	Drowsiness, agitation, muscle twitching, seizures, paresthesia, proarrhythmia, nausea, vomiting, blood dyscrasias, hepatitis, fever
Class IC				
Flecainide (Tambocor)	**T:** 50 mg, 100 mg, 150 mg	AF, PSVT, life-threatening ventricular arrhythmias	**A:** Initially, 100 mg q12h. May increase by 50 mg q12h at 4 day intervals. **Maximum:** 400 mg/day	Dizziness, tremors, bradycardia, heart block, HF, GI upset, neutropenia, flushing, blurred vision, metallic taste, proarrhythmia
Propafenone (Rythmol)	**T:** 150 mg, 225 mg, 300 mg **ER:** 225 mg, 325 mg, 425 mg	PAF, WPW, life-threatening ventricular arrhythmias	**A: T:** Initially, 150 mg q8h. May increase at 3–4 day intervals up to 300 mg q8h **ER:** Initially, 225 mg q12h. May increase at a minimum of 5 days up to 425 mg q12h	Dizziness, blurred vision, altered taste, nausea, exacerbation of asthma, proarrhythmia, bradycardia, heart block, HF, GI upset, bronchospasm, hepatotoxicity

Continued

ANTIARRHYTHMICS—cont'd

Name	Availability	Uses	Dosage Range	Side Effects
Class II (Beta-Blockers)				
Acebutolol (Sectral)	**C:** 100 mg, 200 mg, 400 mg	Ventricular arrhythmias	**A:** Initially, 200 mg 2 times/day Maintenance: 600–1200 mg/day in divided doses	Bradycardia, hypotension, depression, nightmares, fatigue, sexual dysfunction, SLE, arthritis, myalgia
Esmolol (Brevibloc)	**I:** 10 mg/mL	Supraventricular tachycardia	**A:** 50–200 mcg/kg/min	Hypotension, heart block, HF, bronchospasm
Propranolol (Inderal)	**T:** 10 mg, 20 mg, 40 mg	Tachyarrhythmias	**A:** Initially, 10–30 mg 3–4 times/day Maintenance: 10–40 mg 3–4 times/day	Bradycardia, hypotension, depression, nightmares, fatigue, sexual dysfunction, heart block, bronchospasm
Class III				
Amiodarone (Cordarone, Pacerone)	**T:** 100 mg, 200 mg, 400 mg **I:** 50 mg/mL	AF, PAF, PSVT, life-threatening ventricular arrhythmias	**A (PO):** 800–1,600 mg/day in divided doses for 1–3 wks, then 600–800 mg/day in divided doses **(IV):** 150 mg bolus, then 900 mg over 18 hrs	Blurred vision, photophobia, constipation, ataxia, proarrhythmia, pulmonary fibrosis, bradycardia, heart block, hyperthyroidism or hypothyroidism, peripheral neuropathy, GI upset, blue-gray skin, optic neuritis, hypotension
Dofetilide (Tikosyn)	**C:** 125 mcg, 250 mcg, 500 mcg	AF, A flutter	**A:** Individualized	Torsades de pointes, hypotension
Dronedarone (Multaq)	**T:** 400 mg	AF, A flutter	**A (PO):** 400 mg 2 times/day	Diarrhea, nausea, abdominal pain, vomiting, asthenia
Ibutilide (Corvert)	**I:** 0.1 mg/mL	AF, A flutter	**A (greater than 60 kg):** 1 mg over 10 min; **(less than 60 kg):** 0.01 mg/kg over 10 min	Torsades de pointes

Sotalol (Betapace)	**T:** 80 mg, 120 mg, 160 mg	AF, PAF, PSVT, life-threatening ventricular arrhythmias	**A:** Initially, 80 mg 2 times/day May increase at 3 day intervals up to 160 mg 2 times/day	Fatigue, dizziness, dyspnea, bradycardia, proarrhythmia, heart block, hypotension, bronchospasm
Class IV (Calcium Channel Blockers)				
Diltiazem (Cardizem)	**I:** 25 mg/mL vials **Infusion:** 1 mg/mL	AF, A flutter, PSVT	**A (IV):** 20–25 mg bolus, then infusion of 5–15 mg/hr	Hypotension, bradycardia, dizziness, headaches, heart block, asystole, HF
Verapamil (Calan, Isoptin)	**I:** 5 mg/2 mL	AF, A flutter, PSVT	**A (IV):** 5–10 mg	Hypotension, bradycardia, dizziness, headaches, constipation, heart block, HF, asystole, fatigue, edema, nausea

A, Adults; ***AF,*** atrial fibrillation; ***A flutter,*** atrial flutter; ***C,*** capsules; ***HF,*** heart failure; ***ER,*** extended-release; ***I,*** injection; ***PAF,*** paroxysmal atrial fibrillation; ***PSVT,*** paroxysmal supraventricular tachycardia; ***PVCs,*** premature ventricular contractions; ***SLE,*** systemic lupus erythematosus; ***SR,*** sustained-release; ***T,*** tablets; ***VT,*** ventricular tachycardia; ***WPW,*** Wolff-Parklnson-White syndrome.

Antibiotics

USES

Treatment of wide range of gram-positive or gram-negative bacterial infections, suppression of intestinal flora before surgery, control of acne, prophylactically to prevent rheumatic fever, prophylactically in high-risk situations (e.g., some surgical procedures or medical conditions) to prevent bacterial infection.

ACTION

Antibiotics are natural or synthetic compounds that have the ability to kill or suppress the growth of microorganisms.

One means of classifying antibiotics is by their antimicrobial spectrum. Narrow-spectrum agents are effective against few microorganisms (e.g., aminoglycosides are effective against gram-negative aerobes), whereas broad-spectrum agents are effective against a wide variety of microorganisms (e.g., fluoroquinolones are effective against gram-positive cocci and gram-negative bacilli).

Antimicrobial agents may also be classified based on their mechanism of action.

- Agents that inhibit cell wall synthesis or activate enzymes that disrupt the cell wall, causing a weakening in the cell, cell lysis, and death. Include penicillins, cephalosporins, vancomycin, imidazole antifungal agents.
- Agents that act directly on the cell wall, affecting permeability of cell membranes, causing leakage of intracellular substances. Include antifungal agents amphotericin and nystatin, polymyxin, colistin.
- Agents that bind to ribosomal subunits, altering protein synthesis and eventually causing cell death. Include aminoglycosides.
- Agents that affect bacterial ribosome function, altering protein synthesis and causing slow microbial growth. Do not cause cell death. Include chloramphenicol, clindamycin, erythromycin, tetracyclines.
- Agents that inhibit nucleic acid metabolism by binding to nucleic acid or interacting with enzymes necessary for nucleic acid synthesis. Inhibit DNA or RNA synthesis. Include rifampin, metronidazole, fluoroquinolones (e.g., ciprofloxacin).
- Agents that inhibit specific metabolic steps necessary for microbial growth, causing a decrease in essential cell components or synthesis of nonfunctional analogues of normal metabolites. Include trimethoprim, sulfonamides.
- Agents that inhibit viral DNA synthesis by binding to viral enzymes necessary for DNA synthesis, preventing viral replication. Include acyclovir, vidarabine.

SELECTION OF ANTIMICROBIAL AGENTS

The goal of therapy is to achieve antimicrobial action at the site of infection sufficient to inhibit the growth of the microorganism. The agent selected should be the most active against the most likely infecting organism, least likely to cause toxicity or allergic reaction. Factors to consider in selection of an antimicrobial agent include the following:

- Sensitivity pattern of the infecting microorganism
- Location and severity of infection (may determine route of administration)
- Pt's ability to eliminate the drug (status of renal and hepatic function)
- Pt's defense mechanisms (includes both cellular and humoral immunity)
- Pt's age, pregnancy status, genetic factors, allergies, CNS disorder, preexisting medical problems

CATEGORIZATION OF ORGANISMS BY GRAM STAINING

Gram-Positive Cocci	Gram-Negative Cocci	Gram-Positive Bacilli	Gram-Negative Bacilli
Aerobic *Staphylococcus aureus* *Staphylococcus epidermidis* *Streptococcus pneumoniae* *Streptococcus pyogenes* *Viridans streptococci* *Enterococcus faecalis* *Enterococcus faecium* **Anaerobic** *Peptostreptococcus spp.* *Peptococcus spp.*	**Aerobic** *Neisseria gonorrhoeae* *Neisseria meningitidis* *Moraxella catarrhalis*	**Aerobic** *Listeria monocytogenes* *Bacillus anthracis* *Corynebacterium diphtheriae* **Anaerobic** *Clostridium difficile* *Clostridium perfringens* *Clostridium tetani* *Actinomyces spp.*	**Aerobic** *Escherichia coli* *Klebsiella pneumoniae* *Proteus mirabilis* *Serratia marcescens* *Acinetobacter spp.* *Pseudomonas aeruginosa* *Enterobacter spp.* *Haemophilus influenzae* *Legionella pneumophila* **Anaerobic** *Bacteroides fragilis* *Fusobacterium spp.*

Antibiotic: Aminoglycosides

USES

Treatment of serious infections when other less-toxic agents are not effective, are contraindicated, or require adjunctive therapy (e.g., with penicillins or cephalosporins). Used primarily in the treatment of infections caused by gram-negative microorganisms, such as those caused by *Proteus, Klebsiella, Pseudomonas, Escherichia coli, Serratia,* and *Enterobacter.* Inactive against most gram-positive microorganisms. Not well absorbed systemically from GI tract (must be administered parenterally for systemic infections). Oral agents are given to suppress intestinal bacteria.

ACTION

Bactericidal. Transported across bacterial cell membrane; irreversibly bind to specific receptor proteins of bacterial ribosomes. Interfere with protein synthesis, preventing cell reproduction and eventually causing cell death.

ANTIBIOTIC: AMINOGLYCOSIDES

Name	Availability	Dosage Range	Class Side Effects
Amikacin	**I:** 50 mg/mL, 250 mg/mL	**A:** 5–7.5 mg/kg q8h or 15–20 mg/kg once daily **C:** 5–7.5 mg/kg q8h	Nephrotoxicity, neurotoxicity, ototoxicity (both auditory and vestibular), hypersensitivity (skin itching, redness, rash, swelling)
Gentamicin	**I:** 10 mg/mL, 40 mg/mL	**A:** 4–7 mg/kg once daily or 1–2.5 mg/kg q8–12h **C:** 2–2.5 mg/kg q8h	
Plazomicin (Zemdri)	**I:** 50 mg/mL	**A:** 15 mg/kg q24h	Decreased renal function, diarrhea, hypertension, headache, nausea, vomiting, hypotension
Tobramycin	**I:** 10 mg/mL, 40 mg/mL	**A:** 5–7 mg/kg once daily or 1–2.5 mg/kg q8h **C:** 2–2.5 mg/kg q8h	

A, Adults; ***C** (dosage),* children; ***I,*** injection; ***T,*** tablets.

Antibiotic: Carbapenems

Carbapenems are a class of beta-lactam antibiotics that are used to treat severe or high-risk bacterial infections. They may be used in the treatment of intra-abdominal infections, complicated urinary tract infections, pneumonia, and sepsis.

SPECTRUM OF ACTIVITY

Doripenem, imipenem, and meropenem exhibit broad spectrum activity against gram-negative bacteria including most *Enterobacteriaceae* (e.g., *Escherichia coli, Klebsiella pneumoniae, Enterobacter, Citrobacter, Proteus mirabilis,* and *Serratia marcescens*) and good activity against *Pseudomonas aeruginosa* and *Acinetobacter* species.

Meropenem/vaborbactam exhibits activity against *Enterobacter cloacae* species complex, *E. coli*, and *K. pneumoniae.*

Carbapenems exhibit narrower activity against gram-positive bacteria including methicillin-sensitive strains of *Staphylococcus* and *Streptococcus* species.

Carbapenems exhibit good activity against anaerobes (e.g., *Bacteroides fragilis*).

ACTION

Inhibit bacterial cell wall synthesis by binding to one or more of the penicillin-binding proteins, causing cell lysis and death.

ANTIBIOTIC: CARBAPENEMS

Name	Indications	Dosage Range	Side Effects
Doripenem (Dorbax)	Intra-abdominal infection Complicated urinary tract infection (including pyelonephritis)	500 mg q8h	Headache, diarrhea, nausea, skin rash, anemia
Ertapenem (Invanz)	Acute pelvic infections Community-acquired pneumonia Complicated intra-abdominal infections, skin and skin structure, and UTI	1 g once daily	Diarrhea, vomiting, nausea, abdominal pain, increased AST, ALT

Continued

ANTIBIOTIC: CARBAPENEMS

Name	Indications	Dosage Range	Side Effects
Imipenem (Primaxin)	Lower respiratory tract infections Urinary tract infections. Intra-abdominal infections. Gynecologic infections Bacterial septicemia Bone and joint infections Skin and skin structure infections Endocarditis	500–1,000 mg q6h or 1,000 mg q8h	Decreased hematocrit, hemoglobin, eosinophilia, thrombocythemia, increased ALT, AST
Meropenem (Merrem)	Meningitis Intra-abdominal infection Pneumonia Sepsis	1.5-6 g daily divided q8h	Headache, pain, skin rash, nausea, diarrhea, constipation, vomiting, anemia
Meropenem/vaborbactam (Vabomere)	Complicated urinary tract infection (including pyelonephritis)	4 g (2 g meropenem/2 g vabor-bactam) q8h	Headache, diarrhea, phlebitis/infusion site reactions

Antibiotic: Cephalosporins

USES

Broad-spectrum antibiotics, which, like penicillins, may be used in a number of diseases, including respiratory diseases, skin and soft tissue infection, bone/joint infections, and genitourinary infections and prophylactically in some surgical procedures.

First-generation cephalosporins have activity against gram-positive organisms (e.g., streptococci and most staphylococci) and activity against some gram-negative organisms, including *Escherichia coli, Klebsiella pneumoniae,* and *Proteus mirabilis.*

ACTION

Second-generation cephalosporins have same effectiveness as first-generation and increased activity against gram-negative organisms, including *Haemophilus influenzae, Neisseria gonorrhoeae, E. coli,* and *Klebsiella*. Cefoxitin has activity against gram-negative bacilli *Bacteroides fragilis* and certain *Enterobacteriaceae.*

Third-generation cephalosporins are less active against gram-positive organisms but active against gram-negative bacteria including *Haemophilus influenzae,* and *Proteus, Citrobacter, Serratia,* Enterobacteriaceae (*E. coli*), *and Klebsiella* species. Ceftazidime has activity against *Pseudomonas aeruginosa.*

Fourth-generation cephalosporins have good activity against gram-positive organisms (e.g., *Staphylococcus aureus*) and gram-negative organisms (e.g., *Pseudomonas aeruginosa, E. coli, Klebsiella,* and *Proteus*). Cefepime penetrates the CNS and can be used in treating meningitis.

Fifth-generation cephalosporins have good activity against gram-positive organisms (e.g., *Staphylococcus aureus, Streptococcus* spp.) and gram-negative organisms (e.g., *E. coli, Klebsiella* spp.). Ceftaroline has activity against multidrug-resistant *Staphylococcus aureus*, including MRSA, VRSA, and VISA.

Cephalosporins inhibit cell wall synthesis or activate enzymes that disrupt the cell wall, causing cell lysis and cell death. May be bacteriostatic or bactericidal. Most effective against rapidly dividing cells.

ANTIBIOTIC: CEPHALOSPORINS

Name	Availability	Dosage Range	Side Effects
First-Generation			
Cefadroxil (Duricef)	**C:** 500 mg **T:** 1 g **S:** 125 mg/5 mL, 250 mg/5 mL, 500 mg/5 mL	**A:** 500 mg–1 g **C:** 15 mg/kg ql2h	Abdominal cramps/pain, fever, nausea, vomiting, diarrhea, headaches, oral/vaginal candidiasis

Continued

ANTIBIOTIC: CEPHALOSPORINS—cont'd

Name	Availability	Dosage Range	Side Effects
Cefazolin (Ancef)	**I:** 500 mg, 1 g, 2 g	**A:** 500 mg–2 g q6–8h **C:** 25–100 mg/kg/day divided q6–8h	Fever, rash, diarrhea, nausea, pain at injection site
Cephalexin (Keflex, Keftab)	**C:** 250 mg, 500 mg **T:** 250 mg, 500 mg, 1 g	**A:** 250 mg–1 g q6–12h **C:** 25–100 mg/kg/day divided q6–8h	Headache, abdominal pain, diarrhea, nausea, dyspepsia
Second-Generation			
Cefaclor (Ceclor)	**C:** 250 mg, 500 mg **T (ER):** 500 mg **S:** 125 mg/5 mL, 187 mg/5 mL, 250 mg/5 mL, 375 mg/5 mL	**A:** 250–500 mg q8h **ER:** 500 mg q12h **C:** 20–40 mg/kg/day q8–12h	Rash, diarrhea, increased transaminases May have serum sickness-like reaction
Cefotetan	**I:**1g, 2 g	**A:** 500 mg–3 g q12h **C:** 20–40 mg/kg q12h	Diarrhea, increased AST, ALT, hypersensitivity reactions
Cefoxitin (Mefoxin)	**I:**1g, 2 g	**A:** 1–2 g q6–8h **C:** 80–160 mg/kg/day divided q6h	Diarrhea
Cefprozil (Cefzil)	**T:** 250 mg, 500 mg **S:** 125 mg/5 mL, 250 mg/5 mL	**A:** 500 mg q12–24h **C:** 7.5–15 mg/kg q12h	Dizziness, abdominal pain, diarrhea, nausea, increased AST, ALT
Cefuroxime (Ceftin, Kefurox, Zinacef)	**T:** 125 mg, 250 mg, 500 mg **S:** 125 mg/5 mL, 250 mg/5 mL **I:** 750 mg, 1.5 g	**A (PO):** 125–500 mg q12h **(IM/IV):** 750 mg–1.5 g q8–12h **C (PO):** 10–15 mg/kg q12h **(IM/IV):** 75–150 mg/kg/day divided q8h	Diarrhea, nausea, vomiting, thrombophlebitis, increased AST, ALT
Third-Generation			
Cefdinir (Omnicef)	**C:** 300 mg **S:** 125 mg/5 mL	**A:** 300 mg q12h or 600 mg once daily **C:** 7 mg/kg q12h or 14 mg/kg once daily	Headache, hyperglycemia, abdominal pain, diarrhea, nausea
Cefditoren (Spectracef)	**T:** 200 mg, 400 mg	**A:** 200–400 mg q12h **C: (>11 yrs):** 200–400 mg q12h	Diarrhea, nausea
Cefotaxime (Claforan)	**I:** 500 mg, 1 g, 2 g	**A:** 1–2 g q4–12h **C:** 50–300 mg/kg/day divided q4–6h	Rash, diarrhea, nausea, pain at injection site

Cefpodoxime (Vantin)	**T:** 100 mg, 200 mg **S:** 50 mg/5 mL, 100 mg/5 mL	**A:** 100–400 mg q12h **C:** 5 mg/kg q12h	Rash, diarrhea, nausea
Ceftazidime (Fortaz, Tazicef, Tazidime)	**I:** 500 mg, 1 g, 2 g	**A:** 500 mg–2 g q8—12h **C:** 30–50 mg/kg q8h	Diarrhea, pain at injection site
Ceftibuten (Cedax)	**C:** 400 mg **S:** 90 mg/5 mL, 180 mg/5 mL	**A:** 400 mg once daily **C:** 4.5 mg/kg bid or 9 mg/kg once daily	Headache, nausea, diarrhea
Ceftriaxone (Rocephin)	**I:** 250 mg, 500 mg, 1 g, 2 g	**A:** 1–2 g q12–24h **C:** 50–100 mg/kg/day divided q12–24h	Rash, diarrhea, eosinophilia, increased AST, ALT
Fourth-Generation			
Cefepime (Maxipime)	**I:** 1g, 2g	**A:** 1–2 g q8–12h **C:** 50 mg/kg q8–12h	Rash, diarrhea, nausea, increased AST, ALT
Fifth-Generation			
Ceftaroline (Teflaro)	**I:** 400 mg, 600 mg	**A:** 600 mg q12h	Headache, insomnia, rash, pruritus, diarrhea, nausea
Fixed-Combinations			
Ceftazidime/avibactam (Avycaz)	**I:** 2 g ceftazidime/0.5 g avibactam	**A:** 2.5 g q8h	Nausea, vomiting, constipation, anxiety
Ceftolozane/tazobactam (Zerbaxa)	**I:** 1 g ceftolozane/0.5 g tazobactam	**A:** 1.5 g q8h	Nausea, diarrhea, headache, pyrexia

A, Adults; ***C,*** capsules; ***C*** *(dosage),* children; ***ER,*** extended-release; ***I,*** injection; ***S,*** suspension; ***T,*** tablets.

Antibiotic: Fluoroquinolones

USES

Fluoroquinolones act against a wide range of gram-negative and gram-positive organisms. They are used primarily in the treatment of lower respiratory infections, skin/skin structure infections, urinary tract infections, and sexually transmitted diseases.

ACTION

Bactericidal. Inhibit DNA gyrase in susceptible microorganisms, interfering with bacterial DNA replication and repair.

ANTIBIOTIC: FLUOROQUINOLONES

Name	Availability	Dosage Range	Side Effects, Comments
Ciprofloxacin (Cipro)	**T:** 100 mg, 250 mg, 500 mg, 750 mg **S:** 250 mg/5 mL, 500 mg/5 mL **I:** 200 mg, 400 mg	**A (PO):** 250–750 mg q12h **(IV):** 200–400 mg q12h	Dizziness, headaches, anxiety, drowsiness, insomnia, abdominal pain, nausea, diarrhea, vomiting, phlebitis (parenteral) Good aerobic gram-negative activity. Considered most active against *Pseudomonas aeruginosa (PsAg)*
Delafloxacin (Baxdela)	**T:** 450 mg **I:** 300 mg	**A (PO):** 450 mg q12h **(IV):** 300 mg q12h	Nausea, diarrhea, headache, elevation of transaminases, vomiting Best aerobic gram-positive activity, good aerobic gram-negative activity including fluoroquinolone susceptible *PsAg*
Levofloxacin (Levaquin)	**T:** 250 mg, 500 mg, 750 mg **I:** 250 mg, 500 mg, 750 mg **OS:** 250 mg/10 mL	**A (PO/IV):** 250–750 mg/day as single dose	Headache, insomnia, dizziness, rash, nausea, diarrhea, constipation Good aerobic gram-positive activity, good aerobic gram-negative activity including fluoroquinolone susceptible *PsAg*
Moxifloxacin (Avelox)	**T:** 400 mg **I:** 400 mg	**A:** 400 mg/day	Headache, dizziness, insomnia, nausea, diarrhea Good aerobic gram-positive activity, less aerobic gram-negative activity including fluoroquinolone susceptible *PsAg* Has anaerobic coverage

A, Adults; ***I,*** injection; ***OS,*** oral solution; ***PO,*** oral; ***S,*** suspension; ***T,*** tablets.

Antibiotic: Macrolides

USES

Macrolides act primarily against most gram-positive microorganisms and some gram-negative cocci. Azithromycin and clarithromycin appear to be more potent than erythromycin. Macrolides are used in the treatment of pharyngitis/tonsillitis, sinusitis, chronic bronchitis, pneumonia, uncomplicated skin/skin structure infections.

ACTION

Bacteriostatic or bactericidal. Reversibly binds to the P site of the 50S ribosomal subunit of susceptible organisms, inhibiting RNA-dependent protein synthesis.

ANTIBIOTIC: MACROLIDES

Name	Availability	Dosage Range	Side Effects
Azithromycin (Zithromax)	**T**: 250 mg, 600 mg **S**: 100 mg/5 mL, 200 mg/5 mL, 1-g packet **I**: 500 mg	**A (PO)**: 500 mg once, then 250 mg once daily **(IV)**: 500 mg/day **C (PO/IV)**: 5–10 mg/kg once daily	**PO**: Nausea, diarrhea, vomiting, abdominal pain **IV**: Pain, redness, swelling at injection site
Clarithromycin (Biaxin)	**T**: 250 mg, 500 mg **T (XL)**: 500 mg **S**: 125 mg/5 mL	**A**: 250–500 mg q12h (or XL 1,000 mg once daily) **C**: 7.5 mg/kg q12h	Headaches, loss of taste, nausea, vomiting, diarrhea, abdominal pain/discomfort
Erythromycin (EES, Eryc, EryPed, Ery-Tab, Erythrocin, PCE)	**T**: 200 mg, 250 mg, 333 mg, 400 mg, 500 mg **C**: 250 mg **S**: 100 mg/2.5 mL, 125 mg/5 mL, 200 mg/5 mL, 250 mg/5 mL, 400 mg/5 mL	**A (PO)**: 250–500 mg q6h **(IV)**: 500 mg–1 g q6h **C (PO)**: 7.5 mg/kg q6h **(IV)**: 15–20 mg/kg/day in divided doses q6h	**PO**: Nausea, vomiting, diarrhea, abdominal pain **IV**: Inflammation, phlebitis at injection site

A, Adults; ***C,*** capsules; ***C (dosage),*** children; ***I,*** injection; ***S,*** suspension; ***T,*** tablets; ***XL,*** long-acting.

Antibiotic: Penicillins

USES

Penicillins (also referred to as beta-lactam antibiotics) may be used to treat a large number of infections, including pneumonia and other respiratory diseases, urinary tract infections, septicemia, meningitis, intra-abdominal infections, gonorrhea and syphilis, and bone/joint infection.

Penicillins are classified based on an antimicrobial spectrum:
Natural penicillins are very active against gram-positive cocci but ineffective against most strains of *Staphylococcus aureus* (inactivated by enzyme penicillinase).
Penicillinase-resistant penicillins are effective against penicillinase-producing *Staphylococcus aureus* but are less effective against gram-positive cocci than the natural penicillins.
Broad-spectrum penicillins are effective against gram-positive cocci and some gram-negative bacteria (e.g., *Haemophilus influenzae, Escherichia coli, Proteus mirabilis, Salmonella,* and *Shigella*).
Extended-spectrum penicillins are effective against gram-negative organisms, including *Pseudomonas aeruginosa, Enterobacter, Proteus* spp., *Klebsiella, Serratia* spp., and *Acinetobacter* spp.

ACTION

Penicillins inhibit cell wall synthesis or activate enzymes, which disrupt the bacterial cell wall, causing cell lysis and cell death. May be bacteriostatic or bactericidal. Most effective against bacteria undergoing active growth and division.

ANTIBIOTIC: PENICILLINS

Name	Availability	Dosage Range	Side Effects
Natural			
Penicillin G benzathine (Bicillin, Bicillin LA)	**I:** 600,000 units, 1.2 million units, 2.4 million units	**A:** 1.2–2.4 million units as single dose **C:** 25,000–50,000 units/kg as single dose	Mild diarrhea, nausea, vomiting, headaches, sore mouth/tongue, vaginal itching/discharge, allergic reaction (including anaphylaxis, skin rash, urticaria, pruritus)

Penicillin G potassium (Pfizerpen)	**I:** 1, 2, 3, 5 million-unit vials	**A:** 2–4 million units q4h **C:** 100,000–400,000 units/kg/day divided q4–6h	Rash, injection site reaction, phlebitis
Penicillin V potassium (Apo-Pen-VK)	**T:** 250 mg, 500 mg **S:** 125 mg/5 mL, 250 mg/5 mL	**A:** 250–500 mg q6–8h **C:** 25–50 mg/kg/day in divided doses q6–8h	Diarrhea, nausea, vomiting
Penicillinase-Resistant			
Dicloxacillin (Dynapen, Pathocil)	**C:** 125 mg, 250 mg, 500 mg **S:** 62.5 mg/5 mL	**A:** 125–500 mg q6h **C:** 25–50 mg/kg/day divided q6h	Abdominal pain, diarrhea, nausea
Nafcillin (Unipen)	**I:** 500 mg, 1 g, 2 g	**A (IV):** 500 mg–2 g q4–6h **C (IV):** 50–200 mg/kg/day in divided doses q4–6h	Inflammation, pain, phlebitis, increased risk of interstitial nephritis
Oxacillin (Bactocill)	**C:** 250 mg, 500 mg **S:** 250 mg/5 mL **I:** 250 mg, 500 mg, 1 g, 2 g	**A (IV):** 1–2 g q4–6h **C (IV):** 25–50 mg/kg q6h	Diarrhea, nausea, vomiting, increased risk of hepatotoxicity, interstitial nephritis
Broad-Spectrum			
Amoxicillin (Amoxil, Trimox)	**T:** 125 mg, 250 mg, 500 mg, 875 mg **C:** 250 mg, 500 mg **S:** 200 mg/5 mL, 400 mg/5 mL, 125 mg/5 mL, 250 mg/5 mL	**A:** 250–500 mg q8h or 500–875 g q12h **C:** 20–90 mg/kg/day divided q8–12h	Diarrhea, colitis, nausea

Continued

ANTIBIOTIC: PENICILLINS—cont'd

Name	Availability	Dosage Range	Side Effects
Amoxicillin/ clavulanate (Augmentin)	**T**: 250 mg, 500 mg, 875 mg **T (chewable)**: 125 mg, 200 mg, 250 mg, 400 mg **S**: 125 mg/5 mL, 200 mg/5 mL, 250 mg/5 mL, 400 mg/5 mL	**A**: 875 mg q12h or 250–500 mg q8h **C**: 25–90 mg/kg/day divided q12h	Diarrhea, rash, nausea, vomiting
Ampicillin (Principen)	**C**: 250 mg, 500 mg **S**: 125 mg/5 mL, 250 mg/5 mL **I**: 125 mg, 250 mg, 500 mg, 1 g, 2 g	**A (PO)**: 250–500 mg q6h **(IV)**: 500 mg–2 g q6h **C (PO)**: 12.5–50 mg/kg q6h **(IV)**: 25–50 mg/kg q6h	Nausea, vomiting, diarrhea
Ampicillin/sulbactam (Unasyn)	**I**: 1.5 g, 3 g	**A**: 1.5–3 g q6h **C**: 25–50 mg/kg q6h	Local pain at injection site, rash, diarrhea
Extended-Spectrum			
Piperacillin/tazobactam (Zosyn)	**I**: 2.25 g, 3.375 g, 4.5 g	**A**: 3.375 g q6h or 4.5 g q6–8h **C**: 240–300 mg/kg/day divided q8h	Diarrhea, insomnia, headache, fever, rash

A, Adults; ***C,*** capsules; ***C (dosage),*** children; ***I,*** injection; ***PO,*** oral; ***S,*** suspension; ***T,*** tablets.

Anticoagulants/Antiplatelets/Thrombolytics

USES

Treatment and prevention of venous thromboembolism, acute MI, acute cerebral embolism; reduce risk of acute MI; reduction of total mortality in pts with unstable angina; prevent occlusion of saphenous grafts following open heart surgery; prevent embolism in select pts with atrial fibrillation, prosthetic heart valves, valvular heart disease, cardiomyopathy. Heparin also used for acute/chronic consumption coagulopathies (disseminated intravascular coagulation).

ACTION

Anticoagulants: Inhibit blood coagulation by preventing the formation of new clots and extension of existing ones *but do not dissolve formed clots.* Anticoagulants are subdivided. *Heparin* (including low molecular weight heparin): Indirectly interferes with blood coagulation by blocking the conversion of prothrombin to thrombin and fibrinogen to fibrin. *Coumarin:* Acts indirectly to prevent synthesis in the liver of vitamin K–dependent clotting factors. *Direct Thrombin Inhibitors:* Inhibit thrombin from converting fibrinogen to fibrin. *Factor Xa Inhibitors:* Inhibit platelet activation and fibrin clot formation.

Antiplatelets: Interfere with platelet aggregation. Effects are irreversible for life of platelet. Medications in this group act by different mechanisms. Aspirin irreversibly inhibits cyclo-oxygenase and formation of thromboxane A_2. Clopidogrel, dipyridamole, prasugrel, and ticlopidine have similar effects as aspirin and are known as adenosine diphosphate (ADP) inhibitors. Abciximab, eptifibatide, and tirofiban block binding of fibrinogen to the glycoprotein IIb/IIIa receptor on platelet surface (known as platelet glycoprotein IIb/IIIa receptor antagonists).

Thrombolytics: Act directly or indirectly on fibrinolytic system to dissolve clots (converting plasminogen to plasmin, an enzyme that digests fibrin clot).

ANTICOAGULANTS/ANTIPLATELETS/THROMBOLYTICS

Name	Availability	Uses	Side Effects
Anticoagulants			
Direct Thrombin Inhibitors			
Argatroban	**I:** 100 mg/mL	Prevent/treat VTE in pts with HIT or at risk for HIT undergoing PCI	Bleeding, hypotension, hematuria

Continued

ANTICOAGULANTS/ANTIPLATELETS/THROMBOLYTICS—cont'd

Name	Availability	Uses	Side Effects
Bivalirudin (Angiomax)	**I:** 250-mg vials	Pts with unstable angina undergoing PTCA	Bleeding, hypotension, pain, headache, nausea, back pain
Dabigatran (Pradaxa)	**C:** 75 mg, 110 mg, 150 mg	Reduce risk for stroke/embolism with nonvalvular atrial fibrillation, prevent/treat DVT/PE, postoperative prophylaxis of DVT/ PE following hip replacement	Bleeding, gastritis, dyspepsia
Desirudin (Iprivask)	**I:** 15 mg	Prophylaxis of DVT following hip surgery	Bleeding, drainage from a wound, nausea, anemia, DVT, serious allergic reactions
Heparin, Low Molecular Weight Heparins			
Dalteparin (Fragmin)	**I:** 2,500 units, 5,000 units, 7,500 units, 10,000 units	Prevent DVT following hip surgery, abdominal surgery, unstable angina or non–Q-wave MI	Bleeding, hematoma, increased ALT, AST, pain at injection site, bruising, pruritus, fever, thrombocytopenia
Enoxaparin (Lovenox)	**I:** 30 mg, 40 mg, 60 mg, 80 mg, 100 mg, 120 mg, 150 mg	Prevent DVT following hip surgery, knee surgery, abdominal surgery, unstable angina or non–Q-wave MI, acute illness	Bleeding, thrombocytopenia, hematoma, increased ALT, AST, nausea, bruising Injection site reactions, anemia, diarrhea, fever
Heparin	**I:** 1,000 units/mL, 2,500 units/mL, 5,000 units/mL, 7,500 units/mL, 10,000 units/mL, 20,000 units/mL	Prevent/treat VTE	Bleeding, thrombocytopenia, skin rash, itching, burning Increased hepatic transaminase
Factor Xa Inhibitor			
Apixaban (Eliquis)	**T:** 2.5 mg, 5 mg	Reduce risk of stroke/embolism in nonvalvular atrial fibrillation. Prevent VTE post hip/knee replacement surgery, prevent/treat recurrence	Bleeding, nausea, anemia Confusion, increased AST, ALT

Betrixaban (Bevyxxa)	**C:** 40 mg, 80 mg	Prophylaxis of VTE in adults with acute medical illness at risk for thromboembolic complications due to restricted mobility, other VTE risk factors	Bleeding, nausea, diarrhea, UTI, hypokalemia, hypertension, headache
Edoxaban (Savaysa)	**T:** 15 mg, 30 mg, 60 mg	Prevent thromboembolism in nonvalvular atrial fibrillation, treat DVT/PT	Bleeding, anemia, rash, abnormal liver function tests
Fondaparinux (Arixtra)	**I:** 2.5 mg, 5 mg, 7.5 mg, 10 mg	Prophylaxis of DVT following hip fracture, abdominal surgery, hip surgery, knee surgery, treat DVT/PE	Bleeding, thrombocytopenia, hematoma, fever, nausea, anemia Increased AST, ALT; insomnia, dizziness, hypokalemia
Rivaroxaban (Xarelto)	**T:** 10 mg	Prevent DVT post knee, hip replacement Prevent thromboembolism in atrial fibrillation Prevent/treat DVT/PE	Bleeding, abdominal pain, fatigue, muscle spasms, anxiety, depression, UTI, increased AST, ALT
Coumarin			
Warfarin (Coumadin)	**PO:** 1 mg, 2 mg, 2.5 mg, 3 mg, 4 mg, 5 mg, 6 mg, 7.5 mg, 10 mg **I:** 5 mg	Prevent/treat VTE in pts, prevent systemic embolism in pts with heart valve replacement, valve heart disease, MI, atrial fibrillation	Bleeding, skin necrosis, anorexia, nausea, vomiting, diarrhea, rash, abdominal cramps, purple toe syndrome, drug interactions (see individual monograph)
Antiplatelets			
Abciximab (ReoPro)	**I:** 2 mg/mL	Adjunct to PCI to prevent acute cardiac ischemic complications (with heparin and aspirin)	Bleeding, hypotension, nausea, vomiting, back pain, allergic reactions, thrombocytopenia
Aspirin	**PO:** 81 mg, 165 mg, 325 mg, 500 mg, 650 mg	TIA, acute MI, chronic stable/unstable angina, revascularization procedures, prevent reinfarction and thromboembolism post MI	Tinnitus, dizziness, hypersensitivity, dyspepsia, minor bleeding, GI ulceration

Continued

ANTICOAGULANTS/ANTIPLATELETS/THROMBOLYTICS—cont'd

Name	Availability	Uses	Side Effects
Clopidogrel (Plavix)	**PO:** 75 mg	Reduce risk of stroke, MI, or vascular death in pts with recent MI, noncardioembolic stroke, peripheral artery disease, reduce CV death, MI, stroke, reinfarction in pts with non-STEMI/STEMI	Bleeding, rash, pruritus, bruising, epistaxis
Cangrelor (Kengreal)	**I:** 50 mg	Adjunct to PCI to reduce risk of MI, repeat coronary revascularization, stent thrombosis	Bleeding
Eptifibatide (Integrilin)	**I:** 0.75 mg/mL, 2 mg/mL	Treat acute coronary syndrome	Bleeding, hypotension
Prasugrel (Effient)	**PO:** 5 mg, 10 mg	Reduce thrombotic cardiovascular events in pts with ACS to be managed with PCI (including stenting)	Bleeding, hypotension
Ticagrelor (Brilinta)	**PO:** 60 mg, 90 mg	Reduce thrombotic cardiovascular events in pts with ACS	Bleeding, dyspnea
Tirofiban (Aggrastat)	**I:** 50 mcg/mL, 250 mcg/mL	Treat acute coronary syndrome	Bleeding, thrombocytopenia, bradycardia, pelvic pain
Vorapaxar (Zontivity)	**T:** 2.08 mg	Reduce thrombotic cardiovascular events (e.g., MI, stroke) in pts with history of MI or peripheral arterial disease	Bleeding
Thrombolytics			
Alteplase (Activase)	**I:** 50 mg, 100 mg	Acute MI, acute ischemic stroke, pulmonary embolism	Bleeding, epistaxis
Tenecteplase (TNKase)	**I:** 50 mg	Acute MI	Bleeding, hematuria

ACS, Acute coronary syndrome; ***DVT,*** deep vein thrombosis; ***HIT,*** heparin-induced thrombocytopenia; ***I,*** injection; ***MI,*** myocardial infarction; ***PCI,*** percutaneous coronary intervention; ***PO,*** oral; ***PTCA,*** percutaneous transluminal coronary angioplasty; ***STEMI,*** ST segment elevation MI; ***T,*** tablet; ***TIA,*** transient ischemic attack; ***VTE,*** venous thromboembolism.

Anticonvulsants

USES

Anticonvulsants are used to treat seizures. Seizures can be divided into two broad categories: partial seizures and generalized seizures. *Partial seizures* begin locally in the cerebral cortex, undergoing limited spread. Simple partial seizures do not involve loss of consciousness but may evolve secondarily into generalized seizures. Complex partial seizures involve impairment of consciousness.

Generalized seizures may be convulsive or nonconvulsive and usually produce immediate loss of consciousness.

ACTION

Anticonvulsants can prevent or reduce excessive discharge of neurons with seizure foci or decrease the spread of excitation from seizure foci to normal neurons. The exact mechanism is unknown but may be due to (1) suppressing sodium influx, (2) suppressing calcium influx, or (3) increasing the action of gamma-aminobutyric acid (GABA), which inhibits neurotransmitters throughout the brain.

ANTICONVULSANTS

Name	Availability	Uses	Dosage Range	Side Effects
Brivaracetam (Briviact)	**I**: 10 mg/mL **S**: 10 mg/mL **T**: 10 mg, 25 mg, 50 mg, 75 mg, 100 mg	Partial-onset seizure	**A**: Initially, 50 mg bid. (May decrease to 25 mg bid or increase to 100 mg bid)	Nausea, vomiting, dizziness, fatigue, angioedema, psychiatric symptoms
Carbamazepine (Carbatrol, Carnexiv, Epitol, Tegretol, Tegretol XR)	**S**: 100 mg/5 mL **T (chewable)**: 100 mg **T**: 200 mg **T (ER)**: 100 mg, 200 mg, 400 mg **C (ER)**: 100 mg, 200 mg, 300 mg **I**:10 mg/mL	Complex partial, tonic-clonic, mixed seizures; trigeminal neuralgia	**Note:** Refer to monograph for IV dosage **A**: Initially, 400 mg/day in 2 divided doses. May increase up to 200 mg/day at wkly intervals up to 800–1,600 mg/day in 2–3 doses **C**: Initially, 200 mg/day in 2 divided doses. May increase by 100 mg/day at wkly intervals up to 400–800 mg/day in 3–4 doses	Dizziness, diplopia, leukopenia, drowsiness, blurred vision, headache, ataxia, nausea, vomiting, hyponatremia, rash, pruritus

Continued

ANTICONVULSANTS—cont'd

Name	Availability	Uses	Dosage Range	Side Effects
Cenobamate (Xcopri)	**T:** 12.5 mg, 25 mg, 50 mg, 100 mg, 150 mg, 200 mg	Partial-onset seizures in adults	Initially, 12.5 mg once daily; titrate to the recommended maintenance dose of 200 mg once daily. **Maximum:** 400 mg once daily	Somnolence, dizziness, fatigue, diplopia, headache
Clonazepam (Klonopin)	**T:** 0.5 mg, 1 mg, 2 mg	Petit mal, akinetic, myoclonic, absence seizures	**A:** Initially, not to exceed 1.5 mg in 3 divided doses. May increase q3days up to 2–8 mg/day in 1–2 divided doses	CNS depression, sedation, ataxia, confusion, depression, behavior disorders, respiratory depression
Ezogabine (Potiga)	**T:** 50 mg, 200 mg, 300 mg, 400 mg	Partial onset seizures	**A:** Initially, 100 mg 3 times/day. May increase at weekly intervals up to 150 mg/day. Usual dose: 200–400 mg 3 times/day	Dizziness, somnolence, fatigue, confusion, vertigo, tremor, balance disorder, urinary retention
Fosphenytoin (Cerebyx)	**I:** 50 mg PE/mL	Status epilepticus, seizures occurring during neurosurgery	**A:** 15–20 mg PE/kg bolus, then 4–6 mg PE/kg/day maintenance	Burning, itching, paresthesia, nystagmus, ataxia
Gabapentin (Neurontin)	**C:** 100 mg, 300 mg, 400 mg **S:** 250 mg/5 mL	Partial and generalized seizures	**A:** 300 mg 3 times/day. Usual dose: 900–1,800 mg/day in 3 doses	CNS depression, fatigue, drowsiness, dizziness, ataxia, nystagmus, blurred vision, confusion; may cause weight gain
Lacosamide (Vimpat)	**T:** 50 mg, 100 mg, 150 mg, 200 mg **S:** 10 mg/mL **I:** 10 mg/mL	Adjunctive therapy, partial seizures	**A:** Monotherapy: Initially, 100 mg 2 times/day. May increase at wkly intervals by 50 mg 2 times/day. Maintenance: 150–200 mg 2 times/day Adjunctive: Initially, 50 mg 2 times/day. May increase by 50 mg 2 times/day. Maintenance: 100–200 mg 2 times/day	Diplopia, headache, dizziness, nausea

Lamotrigine (Lamictal)	**T:** 25 mg, 100 mg, 150 mg, 200 mg **T (ER):** 25 mg, 50 mg, 100 mg, 200 mg, 250 mg, 300 mg **T (ODT):** 25 mg, 50 mg, 100 mg, 200 mg **T (Chew):** 5 mg, 25 mg	Partial seizures, primary generalized tonic-clonic seizures, generalized seizures of Lennox-Gastaut syndrome	**A:** Refer to individual monograph	Dizziness, ataxia, drowsiness, diplopia, nausea, rash, headache, vomiting, insomnia, incoordination
Levetiracetam (Keppra)	**T:** 250 mg, 500 mg, 750 mg, 1,000 mg **S:** 100 mg/ml **T (ER):** 500 mg, 750 mg	Adjunctive therapy, partial seizures, primary tonic-clonic seizures, myoclonic seizures	**A: T:** Initially, 500 mg 2 times/day. May increase q2wks by 500mg/dose. Usual dose: 1,500 mg 2 times/day **ER:** Initially, 1,000 mg once daily. May increase q2wks by 1,000 mg/day up to 3,000 mg once daily	Dizziness, drowsiness, weakness, irritability, hallucinations, psychosis
Oxcarbazepine (Trileptal)	**T:** 150 mg, 300 mg, 600 mg **T (ER):** 150 mg, 300 mg, 600 mg	Partial seizures	**A: T:** 600 mg/day in 2 divided doses. May increase by 600 mg/day at wkly intervals up to 1,200 mg/day in 2 divided doses **ER:** 600 mg once daily. May increase by 600 mg/day at wkly intervals up to 1,200–2,400 mg/day	Drowsiness, dizziness, headaches, diplopia, ataxia, nausea, vomiting, hyponatremia, skin reactions
Perampanel (Fycompa)	**S:** 0.5 mg/ml **T:** 2 mg, 4 mg, 6 mg, 8 mg, 10 mg, 12 mg	Partial onset seizure, primary generalized tonic-clonic seizure	**A, C (12 yrs or older):** Initially, 2 mg daily at hs May increase by 2 mg/d at wkly intervals **Usual dose:** 8–12 mg qhs	Weight gain, abnormal gait, dizziness, headache, somnolence, serious psychiatric reactions
Phenobarbital	**T:** 30 mg, 60 mg, 100 mg **I:** 65 mg, 130 mg	Tonic-clonic, partial seizures; status epilepticus	**A (PO):** 100–300 mg/day **(IM/IV):** 200–600 mg **C (PO):** 3–5 mg/kg/day **(IM/IV):** 100–400 mg	CNS depression, sedation, paradoxical excitement and hyperactivity, rash, hypotension

Continued

ANTICONVULSANTS—cont'd

Name	Availability	Uses	Dosage Range	Side Effects
Phenytoin (Dilantin)	**C:** 30 mg, 100 mg **T (Chewable):** 50 mg **S:** 125 mg/5 mL **I:** 50 mg/mL	Tonic-clonic, psychomotor seizures	**A:** Initially, 100 mg 3 times/day. May increase at 7–10 day intervals. Usual dose: 400 mg/day **C:** Initially, 5 mg/kg/day in 2–3 divided doses May increase at 7–10 day intervals. Usual dose: 4–8 mg/kg/day in 1–3 doses	Nystagmus, ataxia, hypertrichosis, gingival hyperplasia, rash, osteomalacia, lymphadenopathy
Pregabalin (Lyrica)	**C:** 25 mg, 50 mg, 75 mg, 100 mg, 150 mg, 200 mg, 225 mg, 300 mg	Adjunctive therapy, partial seizures	**A:** Initially, 150 mg/day (75 mg 2 times/day or 50 mg 3 times/day) up to 600 mg/day in 2 or 3 doses	Confusion, drowsiness, dizziness, ataxia, weight gain, dry mouth, blurred vision, peripheral edema, myopathy, angioedema, decreased platelet count
Primidone (Mysoline)	**T:** 50 mg, 250 mg	Complex partial, akinetic, tonic-clonic seizures	**A:** 750–1250 mg/day in 3–4 doses **C:** 10–25 mg/kg/day	CNS depression, sedation, paradoxical excitement and hyperactivity, rash, dizziness, ataxia
Rufinamide (Banzel)	**S:** 40 mg/mL **T:** 200 mg, 400 mg	Lennox-Gastaut syndrome (adjunct)	**A:** Initially, 400–800 mg/day in 2 divided doses May increase by 400–800 mg/day every other day **C:** Initially, 10 mg/kg/day in 2 divided doses May increase by 10 mg/kg/day every other day up to 45 mg/kg/day **Maximum:** 3,200 mg/day	Fatigue, dizziness, headache, nausea, drowsiness
Tiagabine (Gabitril)	**T:** 4 mg, 12 mg, 16 mg, 20 mg	Partial seizures	**A:** Initially, 4 mg up to 56 mg/day in 2–4 doses May increase by 4–8 mg/day at wkly intervals **C:** Initially, 4 mg up to 32 mg/day in 2–4 doses May increase by 4–8 mg/day at wkly intervals	Dizziness, asthenia, nervousness, anxiety, tremors, abdominal pain

Topiramate (Topamax)	**T**: 25 mg, 100 mg, 200 mg **C (Sprinkle)**: 15 mg, 25 mg **C (ER 24HR Sprinkle): (Qudexy XR)**: 25 mg, 50 mg, 100 mg, 150 mg **C XR (Trokendi XR)**: 25 mg, 50 mg, 100 mg, 200 mg	Partial seizures, Lennox-Gastaut syndrome	See individual monograph	Drowsiness, dizziness, headache, ataxia, confusion, weight loss, diplopia
Valproic acid (Depakene, Depakote)	**C**: 250 mg **S**: 250 mg/5 mL **Sprinkles:** 125 mg **T**: 125 mg, 250 mg, 500 mg **T (ER)**: 500 mg **I**: 100 mg/mL	Complex partial, absence seizures	**A, C**: Initially, 15 mg/kg/day. May increase by 5–10 mg/kg/day at wkly intervals up to 60 mg/kg/day	Nausea, vomiting, tremors, thrombocytopenia, hair loss, hepatic dysfunction, weight gain, decreased platelet function
Vigabatrin (Sabril)	**T**: 500 mg **PS**: 500 mg	Infantile spasms, refractory complex partial seizures	**A**: Initially, 500 mg 2 times/day. May increase by 500 mg increments at wkly intervals up to 1,500 mg 2 times/day **C**: Initially, 250 mg 2 times/day. May increase by 500 mg/day at wkly intervals up to 1,000 mg 2 times/day	Vision changes, eye pain, abdominal pain, agitation, confusion, mood/mental changes, abnormal coordination, weight gain
Zonisamide (Zonegran)	**C**: 100 mg	Partial seizures	**A**: Initially, 100 mg/day. May increase to 200 mg/day after 2 wks, then 300 mg/day up to 400 mg/day at 2 wk intervals	Drowsiness, dizziness, anorexia, diarrhea, weight loss, agitation, irritability, rash, nausea, cognitive side effects, kidney stones

A, Adults; ***C,*** capsules; ***C*** *(dosage),* children; ***ER,*** extended-release; ***I,*** injection; ***ODT,*** orally disintegrating tablets; ***PE,*** phenytoin equivalent; ***PO,*** oral; ***PS,*** powder sachet; ***qhs,*** every night at bedtime; ***S,*** suspension; ***T,*** tablets.

Antidepressants

USES

Used primarily for the treatment of depression. Depression can be a chronic or recurrent mental disorder presenting with symptoms such as depressed mood, loss of interest or pleasure, guilt feelings, disturbed sleep/appetite, low energy, and difficulty in thinking. Depression can also lead to suicide.

ACTION

Antidepressants include tricyclics, monoamine oxidase inhibitors (MAOIs), selective serotonin reuptake inhibitors (SSRIs), serotonin-norepinephrine reuptake inhibitors (SNRIs), and other antidepressants. Depression may be due to reduced functioning of monoamine neurotransmitters (e.g., norepinephrine, serotonin [5-HT], dopamine) in the CNS (decreased amount and/or decreased effects at the receptor sites). Antidepressants block metabolism, increase amount/effects of monoamine neurotransmitters, and act at receptor sites (change responsiveness/sensitivities of both presynaptic and postsynaptic receptor sites).

ANTIDEPRESSANTS

Name	Availability	Uses	Dosage Range (per day)	Side Effects
Tricyclics				
Amitriptyline (Elavil)	**T:** 10 mg, 25 mg, 50 mg, 75 mg, 100 mg, 150 mg	Depression, neuropathic pain	Initially, 25–100 mg at bedtime or in divided doses. Usual dose: 100–300 mg/day	Drowsiness, blurred vision, constipation, confusion, postural hypotension, cardiac conduction defects, weight gain, seizures, dry mouth
Desipramine (Norpramin)	**T:** 10 mg, 25 mg, 50 mg, 75 mg, 100 mg, 150 mg	Depression, neuropathic pain	Initially, 25–100 mg at bedtime or in divided doses. Usual dose: 100–300 mg/day	Dizziness, drowsiness, fatigue, headache, anorexia, diarrhea, nausea

Imipramine (Tofranil)	**T:** 10 mg, 25 mg, 50 mg **C:** 75 mg, 100 mg, 125 mg, 150 mg	Depression, enuresis, neuropathic pain, panic disorder, ADHD	Initially, 25–100 mg at bedtime or in divided doses. Usual dose: 100–300 mg/day	Dizziness, fatigue, headache, vomiting, xerostomia
Nortriptyline (Aventyl, Pamelor)	**C:** 10 mg, 25 mg, 50 mg, 75 mg **S:** 10 mg/5 mL	Depression, neuropathic pain, smoking cessation	Initially, 50–100 mg once daily. Usual dose: 50–150 mg once daily	Dizziness, fatigue, headache, anorexia, xerostomia
Selective Serotonin Reuptake Inhibitors				
Citalopram (Celexa)	**T:** 10 mg, 20 mg, 40 mg **ODT:** 40 mg **S:** 10 mg/5 mL	Depression, OCD, panic discrder	20–40 mg	**Class Side Effects:** Restlessness, sleep disturbances, nausea, diarrhea, headache, fatigue, sexual dysfunction, weight gain; increased risk of bleeding; may prolong QT interval
Escitalopram (Lexapro)	**T:** 5 mg, 10 mg, 20 mg **S:** 5 mg/5 mL	Depression, GAD	10–20 mg	
Fluoxetine (Prozac)	**C:** 10 mg, 20 mg, 40 mg **C (DR):** 90 mg **T:** 10 mg, 20 mg **S:** 20 mg/5 mL	Depression, OCD, bulimia, panic disorder, anorexia, bipolar disorder, premenstrual syndrome	Initially, 10–20 mg once daily. Usual dose: 20 mg once daily **DR:** 90 mg once wkly	
Paroxetine (Paxil)	**T:** 10 mg, 20 mg, 30 mg, 40 mg **S:** 10 mg/5 mL **ER:** 12.5 mg, 25 mg, 37.5 mg	Depression, OCD, panic attack, SAD	Initially/usual dose: 20 mg once daily **ER:** Initially, 12.5–25 mg once daily. Usual dose: 25 mg once daily	

Continued

ANTIDEPRESSANTS—cont'd

Name	Availability	Uses	Dosage Range (per day)	Side Effects
Sertraline (Zoloft)	**T:** 25 mg, 50 mg, 100 mg **S:** 20 mg/ml	Depression, OCD, panic attack	50–200 mg	
Vortioxetine (Trintellix)	**T:** 5 mg, 10 mg, 15 mg, 20 mg	Depression	Initially, 10 mg once daily. Usual dose: 10–20 mg once daily	
Serotonin-Norepinephrine Reuptake Inhibitors				
Desvenlafaxine (Pristiq)	**T:** 25 mg, 50 mg, 100 mg	Depression	50–100 mg	**Class Side Effects:** Similar to SSRIs. Additionally, sweating, tachycardia, urinary retention, increase in blood pressure
Duloxetine (Cymbalta)	**C:** 20 mg, 30 mg, 60 mg	Depression, fibromyalgia, neuropathic pain	Initially, 30–60 mg once daily. Usual dose: 60 mg once daily or 2 divided doses	
Venlafaxine (Effexor)	**T:** 25 mg, 37.5 mg, 50 mg, 75 mg, 100 mg, 150 mg, 225 mg **T (ER):** 37.5 mg, 75 mg, 150 mg	Depression, anxiety	Initially, 25 mg 3 times or **(ER):** 37.5 mg once daily. Usual dose: 75 mg 3 times/day or **(ER):** 75–225 mg once daily	
Other				
Brexpiprazole (Rexulti)	**T:** 0.25 mg, 0.5 mg, 1 mg, 2 mg, 3 mg, 4 mg	Depression	Initially, 0.5–1 mg/day. May increase at wkly intervals to 1 mg/day **Maximum:** 3 mg/day	Weight gain, akathisia
Bupropion (Wellbutrin)	**T:** 75 mg, 100 mg **SR:** 100 mg, 150 mg, 200 mg	Depression, smoking cessation, ADHD, bipolar disorder	Initially, 100 mg 2 times/day. Usual dose: 100 mg 3 times/day **SR:** Initially, 150 mg once daily. Usual dose: 150 mg 2 times/day	Insomnia, irritability, seizures

Esketamine (Spravato)	**Nasal Spray:** delivers 2 sprays containing a total of 28 mg of esketamine	Depression	Induction Phase Wks 1–4: Administer twice per wk day 1 (starting dose): 56 mg. Subsequent doses: 56 mg or 84 mg. Maintenance Phase Wks 5–8: Give once wkly as 56 mg or 84 mg. Wk 9 and thereafter: Administer q2wks or once wkly as 56 mg or 84 mg	Anxiety, dissociation, dizziness, hypertension, hypoesthesia, lethargy, nausea, sedation, vertigo, vomiting
Mirtazapine (Remeron)	**T:** 7.5 mg, 15 mg, 30 mg, 45 mg	Depression	Initially, 15 mg once at bedtime. Usual dose: 30–45 mg once daily	Sedation, dry mouth, weight gain, agranulocytosis, hepatic toxicity
Trazodone (Desyrel)	**T:** 50 mg, 100 mg, 150 mg, 300 mg **ER:** 150 mg, 300 mg	Depression	Initially, 75 mg 2 times/day or **(ER):** 150 mg once daily. Usual dose: 150 mg bid or **(ER):** 150–375 mg once daily	Sedation, orthostatic hypotension, priapism
Vilazodone (Viibryd)	**T:** 10 mg, 20 mg, 40 mg	Depression	Initially, 10 mg once daily. Usual dose: 40 mg once daily	Diarrhea, nausea, dizziness, dry mouth, insomnia, vomiting, decreased libido

ADHD, Attention-deficit hyperactivity disorder; ***C,*** capsules; ***DR,*** delayed-release; ***ER,*** extended-release; ***GAD,*** generalized anxiety disorder; ***OC,*** oral concentrate; ***OCD,*** obsessive-compulsive disorder; ***ODT,*** orally disintegrating tablets; ***S,*** suspension; ***SAD,*** social anxiety disorder; ***SR,*** sustained-release; ***T,*** tablets.

Antidiabetics

USES

Insulin: Treatment of insulin-dependent diabetes (type 1) and non–insulin-dependent diabetes (type 2). Also used in acute situations such as ketoacidosis, severe infections, major surgery in otherwise non–insulin-dependent diabetics. Administered to pts receiving parenteral nutrition. Drug of choice during pregnancy. All insulins, including long-acting insulins, can cause hypoglycemia and weight gain.

Alpha-glucosidase inhibitors: Adjunct to diet and exercise for management of type 2 diabetes mellitus.

Biguanides: Adjunct to diet and exercise for management of type 2 diabetes mellitus.

ACTION

Dipeptidyl peptidase 4 inhibitors (DPP-4): Adjunct to diet and exercise for management of type 2 diabetes mellitus.

Meglitinide: Adjunct to diet and exercise for management of type 2 diabetes mellitus.

Sulfonylureas: Adjunct to diet and exercise for management of type 2 diabetes mellitus.

Thiazolidinediones: Adjunct to diet and exercise for management of type 2 diabetes mellitus.

Sodium-glucose co-transporter 2 (SGLT2): Adjunct to diet and exercise for management of type 2 diabetes mellitus.

Insulin: A hormone synthesized and secreted by beta cells of Langerhans' islet in the pancreas. Controls storage and utilization of glucose, amino acids, and fatty acids by activated transport systems/enzymes. Inhibits breakdown of glycogen, fat, protein. Insulin lowers blood glucose by inhibiting glycogenolysis and gluconeogenesis in liver; stimulates glucose uptake by muscle, adipose tissue. Activity of insulin is initiated by binding to cell surface receptors.

Alpha-glucosidase inhibitors: Work locally in small intestine, slowing carbohydrate breakdown and glucose absorption.

Biguanides: Inhibit hepatic gluconeogenesis, glycogenolysis; enhance insulin sensitivity in muscle and fat.

DPP-4: Inhibit degradation of endogenous incretins, which increases insulin secretion, decreases glucagon secretion.

Meglitinide: Stimulates pancreatic insulin secretion.

Sulfonylureas: Stimulate release of insulin from beta cells of the pancreas.

Thiazolidinediones: Enhance insulin sensitivity in muscle and fat.

SGLT2: Blocks glucose reabsorption in proximal tubule in the kidney, increases urinary glucose excretion.

ANTIDIABETICS

INSULIN

Type	Onset	Peak	Duration	Comments
Rapid-Acting				
Apidra, glulisine	10–15 min	1–1.5 hrs	3–5 hrs	Refrigerate unopened vial. Do not freeze. Stable at room temperature for 28 days after opening Can mix with NPH
Admelog, lispro	15–30 min	2 hrs	6–7 hrs	Refrigerate unopened vial. Do not freeze. Stable at room temperature for 28 days after opening
Humalog, lispro	15–30 min	0.5–2.5 hrs	6–8 hrs	Refrigerate unopened vial. Do not freeze. Stable at room temperature for 28 days after opening Can mix with NPH

Novolog, aspart	10–20 min	1–3 hrs	3–5 hrs	Refrigerate unopened vial. Do not freeze. Stable at room temperature for 28 days after opening Can mix with NPH
Fiasp, aspart	15–20 min	1.5–2.5 hrs	5–7 hrs	Refrigerate unopened vial. Do not freeze. Stable at room temperature for 28 days after opening
Short-Acting				
Humulin R, Novolin R, regular	30–60 min	1–5 hrs	6–10 hrs	Refrigerate unopened vial. Do not freeze. Stable at room temperature for 28 days after opening Can mix with NPH
Intermediate-Acting				
Humulin N, Novolin N, NPH	1–2 hrs	6–14 hrs	16–24 hrs	Refrigerate unopened vial. Do not freeze. Stable at room temperature for 31 days after opening (Pen 14 days) Can mix with aspart, lispro, glulisine
Long-Acting				
Basaglar, glargine	1–4 hrs	No significant peak	24 hrs	Do NOT mix with other insulins Refrigerate unopened vial. Do not freeze. Stable at room temperature for 28 days after opening
Lantus, glargine	1–4 hrs	No significant peak	24 hrs	Do NOT mix with other insulins Refrigerate unopened vial. Do not freeze. Stable at room temperature for 28 days after opening
Semglee, glargine	Not available	12 hrs	24 hrs	Do NOT mix with other insulins. Refrigerate unused vial; do not refrigerate prefilled pen. Do not freeze. Vial: stable at room temperature for 28 days after opening vial. Pre-filled pen: stable at room temperature per expiration date until used; then stable for 28 days

Continued

ANTIDIABETICS—cont'd

Type	Onset	Peak	Duration	Comments
Levemir, detemir	0.8–2 hrs	No significant peak	12–24 hrs (dose dependent)	Do NOT mix with other insulins Refrigerate unopened vial. Do not freeze. Stable at room temperature for 42 days after opening
Toujeo, glargine	1–6 hrs	No significant peak	Longer than 24 hrs	Do NOT mix with other insulins Refrigerate unopened vial. Do not freeze. Stable at room temperature for 42 days after opening
Tresiba, degludec	0.5–1.5 hrs	12 hrs	42 hrs	Do NOT mix with other insulins Refrigerate unopened vial. Do not freeze. Stable at room temperature for 56 days after opening

Oral Agents

Name	Availability	Dosage Range	Side Effects
Sulfonylureas			
Glimepiride (Amaryl)	**T:** 1 mg, 2 mg, 4 mg	Initially, 1–2 mg/day. May increase by 1–2 mg q1–2 wks. **Maximum:** 8 mg/day	Hypoglycemia, dizziness, headache, nausea, flu-like syndrome
Glipizide (Glucotrol)	**T:** 5 mg, 10 mg **T (XL):** 5 mg	**T:** Initially, 5 mg/day. May increase by 2.5–5 mg q3–4 days. **(XL):** Initially, 5 mg/day. **Maximum:** 20 mg/day	Dizziness, nervousness, anxiety, diarrhea, tremor
Glyburide (DiaBeta, Micronase)	**T:** 1.25 mg, 2.5 mg, 5 mg **PT:** 1.5 mg, 3 mg	**T:** Initially, 2.5–5 mg/day. May increase by 2.5 mg/day at wkly intervals up to 20 mg/day **PT:** Initially, 1.5–3 mg/day. May increase by 1.5 mg at wkly intervals up to 12 mg/day	Dizziness, headache, nausea

Alpha-Glucosidase Inhibitors			
Acarbose (Precose)	**T:** 25 mg, 50 mg, 100 mg	Initially, 25 mg 3 times/day. May increase at 4–8 wk intervals. Usual dose: 50–100 mg 3 times/day	Flatulence, diarrhea, abdominal pain, increased risk of hypoglycemia when used with insulin or sulfonylureas
Miglitol (Glyset)	**T:** 25 mg, 50 mg, 100 mg	Initially, 25 mg 3 times/day. May increase at 4–8 wk intervals to 50 mg 3 times/day, then 100 mg 3 times/day	Flatulence, diarrhea, abdominal pain, rash
Dipeptidyl Peptidase Inhibitors			
Alogliptin (Nesina)	**T:** 6.25 mg, 12.5 mg, 25 mg	6.25–25 mg/day	Nasopharyngitis, cough, headache, upper respiratory tract infections
Linagliptin (Tradjenta)	**T:** 5 mg	5 mg/day	Arthralgia, back pain, headache
Saxagliptin (Onglyza)	**T:** 2.5 mg, 5 mg	2.5–5 mg/day	Upper respiratory tract infection, urinary tract infection, headache
Sitagliptin (Januvia)	**T:** 25 mg, 50 mg, 100 mg	25–100 mg/day	Nasopharyngitis, upper respiratory infection, headaches, modest weight gain, increased incidence of hypoglycemia when added to a sulfonylurea
Biguanides			
Metformin (Glucophage)	**T:** 500 mg, 850 mg, 1,000 mg **XR:** 500 mg, 750 mg, 1,000 mg	**T:** Initially, 500 mg 2 times/day or 850 mg once daily. May increase by 500 mg/day at wkly intervals up to 2,550 mg/day **XR:** Initially, 500–1,000 mg/day. May increase by 500 mg/day at wkly intervals up to 2,500 mg/day	Nausea, vomiting, diarrhea, loss of appetite, metallic taste, lactic acidosis (rare but potentially fatal complication)

Continued

ANTIDIABETICS—cont'd

Name	Availability	Dosage Range	Side Effects
Glucagon-Like Peptide-1 (GLP-1)			
Albiglutide (Tanzeum)	**I:** 30 mg, 50 mg	30–50 mg once wkly	Diarrhea, nausea, upper respiratory tract infection, injection site reaction
Exenatide (Byetta)	**I:** 5 mcg, 10 mcg	5–10 mcg 2 times/day	Diarrhea, dizziness, dyspnea, headaches, nausea, vomiting
Exenatide extended-release (Bydureon)	**I:** 2 mg	2 mg once wkly	Diarrhea, nausea, headache
Liraglutide (Victoza)	**I:** 0.6 mg, 1.2 mg, 1.8 mg (6 mg/mL)	Initially, 0.6 mg/day. May increase at weekly intervals up to 1.2 mg/day, then 1.8 mg/day	Headache, nausea, diarrhea
Lixisenatide (Adlyxin)	**I:** 50 mcg/mL, 100 mcg/mL	20 mcg SC once daily	Nausea, vomiting, headache, dizziness
Semaglutide (Ozempic, Rybelsus)	**I:** 2 mg/1.5 mL delivers 0.25 mg, 0.5 mg or 1 mg per injection **T:** 3 mg, 7 mg, 14 mg	**SQ:** Initially, 0.25 mg once wkly for 4 wks, then 0.5 mg for at least 4 wks up to maximum of 1 mg once wkly. **PO:** Initially, 3 mg once daily for 30 days, then 7 mg once daily for 30 days, then 14 mg once daily thereafter	**SQ:** Increased amylase, lipase, nausea, diarrhea, vomiting, abdominal pain, constipation, dyspepsia **PO:** Nausea, vomiting, abdominal pain, diarrhea, constipation
Meglitinides			
Nateglinide (Starlix)	**T:** 60 mg, 120 mg	60–120 mg 3 times/day	Hypoglycemia, upper respiratory infection, dizziness, back pain, flu-like syndrome

Repaglinide (Prandin)	**T:** 0.5 mg, 1 mg, 2 mg	0.5–1 mg with each meal. Usual dose: 0.5–4 mg/day (**Maximum:** 16 mg/day)	Headache, hypoglycemia, upper respiratory infection
SGLT2			
Canagliflozin (Invokana)	**T:** 100 mg, 300 mg	100–300 mg/day before first meal of day	Genital mycotic infections, recurrent urinary tract infections, increased urinary frequency, hypotension, increased serum creatinine, LDL, Hgb, Hct. Hyperkalemia, hypermagnesemia, hyperphosphatemia, fractures
Dapagliflozin (Farxiga)	**T:** 5 mg, 10 mg	5–10 mg/day in morning	Genital mycotic infections, recurrent urinary tract infections, increased urinary frequency, hypotension, increased serum creatinine, LDL, Hgb, Hct. Hyperphosphatemia, fractures
Empagliflozin (Jardiance)	**T:** 10 mg, 25 mg	10–25 mg/day in morning	Genital mycotic infections, recurrent urinary tract infections, increased urinary frequency, hypotension, increased serum creatinine, LDL, Hgb, Hct
Ertugliflozin (Steglatro)	**T:** 5 mg, 15 mg	Initially, 5 mg once daily in morning. **Maximum:** 15 mg once daily	Genital candidiasis, headache, back pain, urinary frequency, vulvovaginal pruritus, nasopharyngitis

Continued

ANTIDIABETICS—cont'd

Name	Availability	Dosage Range	Side Effects
Thiazolidinediones			
Pioglitazone (Actos)	**T:** 15 mg, 30 mg, 45 mg	15–30 mg/day	Mild to moderate peripheral edema, weight gain, increased risk of HF, associated with reduced bone mineral density and increased incidence of fractures
Rosiglitazone (Avandia)	**T:** 2 mg, 4 mg, 8 mg	Initially, 4 mg/day. May increase at 8–12 wks to 8 mg/day as a single or 2 divided doses	Increased cholesterol, weight gain, back pain, upper respiratory tract infection
Miscellaneous			
Bromocriptine (Cycloset)	**T:** 0.8 mg	1.6–4.8 mg/day	Nausea, fatigue, dizziness, vomiting
Colesevelam (Welchol)	**T:** 625 mg **S:** 1.875 g, 3.75 g packet	3.75 g/day	Constipation, dyspepsia, nausea
Pramlintide (Symlin)	**I:** 1,500 mcg/1.5 mL, 2,700 mcg/2.7 mL	Type 1: 15–60 mcg immediately prior to meals Type 2: 60–120 mcg immediately prior to meals	Abdominal pain, anorexia, headaches, nausea, vomiting, severe hypoglycemia may occur when used in combination with insulin (reduction in dosages of short-acting, including premixed, insulins recommended)

HF, Heart failure; ***I,*** injection; ***PT,*** prestab; ***S,*** suspension; ***T,*** tablets; ***XL,*** extended-release; ***XR,*** extended-release.

Antidiarrheals

USES	ACTION	
Acute diarrhea, chronic diarrhea of inflammatory bowel disease, reduction of fluid from ileostomies.	*Systemic agents:* Act as smooth muscle receptors (enteric) disrupting peristaltic movements, decreasing GI motility, increasing transit time of intestinal contents.	*Local agents:* Adsorb toxic substances and fluids to large surface areas of particles in the preparation. Some of these agents coat and protect irritated intestinal walls. May have local anti-inflammatory action.

ANTIDIARRHEALS

Name	Availability	Type	Dosage Range
Bismuth (Pepto-Bismol)	**T**: 262 mg **C**: 262 mg **L**: 130 mg/15 mL, 262 mg/15 mL, 524 mg/15 mL	Local	**A**: 2 **T** or 30 mL **C (9–12 yrs)**: 1 **T** or 15 mL **C (6–8 yrs)**: 2/3 **T** or 10 mL **C (3–5 yrs)**: 1/3 **T** or 5 mL
Diphenoxylate with atropine (Lomotil)	**T**: 2.5 mg **L**: 2.5 mg/5 mL	Systemic	**A**: 5 mg 4 times/day **C**: 0.3–0.4 mg/kg/day in 4 divided doses **(L)**
Loperamide (Imodium)	**C**: 2 mg **T**: 2 mg **L**: 1 mg/5 mL, 1 mg/mL	Systemic	**A**: Initially, 4 mg (**Maximum:** 16 mg/day) **C (9–12 yrs)**: 2 mg 3 times/day **C (6–8 yrs)**: 2 mg 2 times/day **C (2–5 yrs)**: 1 mg 3 times/day **(L)**

A, Adults; ***C,*** capsules; ***C (dosage),*** children; ***L,*** liquid; ***S,*** suspension; ***T,*** tablets.

Antifungals: Systemic Mycoses

Systemic mycoses are subdivided into opportunistic infections (candidiasis, aspergillosis, cryptococcosis, and mucormycosis) that are seen primarily in debilitated or immunocompromised hosts and nonopportunistic infections (blastomycosis, histoplasmosis, and coccidioidomycosis) that occur in any host. Treatment can be difficult because these infections often resist treatment and may require prolonged therapy.

ANTIFUNGALS: SYSTEMIC MYCOSES

Name	Indications	Side Effects
Amphotericin B	Potentially life-threatening fungal infections, including aspergillosis, blastomycosis, coccidioidomycosis, cryptococcosis, histoplasmosis, systemic candidiasis	Fever, chills, headache, nausea, vomiting, nephrotoxicity, hypokalemia, hypomagnesemia, hypotension, dyspnea, arrhythmias, abdominal pain, diarrhea, increased hepatic function tests
Amphotericin B lipid complex (Abelcet)	Invasive fungal infections	Chills, fever, hypotension, headache, nausea, vomiting
Amphotericin B liposomal (AmBisome)	Empiric therapy for presumed fungal infections in febrile neutropenic pts, treatment of cryptococcal meningitis in HIV-infected pts, treatment of *Aspergillus, Candida, Cryptococcus* infections, treatment of visceral leishmaniasis	Peripheral edema, tachycardia, hypotension, chills, insomnia, headache
Amphotericin colloidal dispersion (Amphotec)	Invasive *Aspergillus*	Hypotension, tachycardia, chills, fever, vomiting
Anidulafungin (Eraxis)	Candidemia, esophageal candidiasis	Diarrhea, hypokalemia, increased hepatic function tests, headache

Caspofungin (Cancidas)	Candidemia, invasive aspergillosis, empiric therapy for presumed fungal infections in febrile neutropenic pts	Headache, nausea, vomiting, diarrhea, increased hepatic function tests
Fluconazole (Diflucan)	Treatment of vaginal candidiasis; oropharyngeal, esophageal candidiasis; and cryptococcal meningitis. Prophylaxis to decrease incidence of candidiasis in pts undergoing bone marrow transplant receiving cytotoxic chemotherapy and/or radiation	Nausea, vomiting, abdominal pain, diarrhea, dysgeusia, increased hepatic function tests, liver necrosis, hepatitis, cholestasis, headache, rash, pruritus, eosinophilia, alopecia
Isavuconazonium (Cresemba)	Treatment of invasive aspergillosis, invasive mucormycosis	Nausea, vomiting, diarrhea, increased hepatic enzymes, hypokalemia, constipation, dyspnea, cough, peripheral edema, back pain
Itraconazole (Sporanox)	Blastomycosis, histoplasmosis, aspergillosis, onychomycosis, empiric therapy of febrile neutropenic pts with suspected fungal infections, treatment of oropharyngeal and esophageal candidiasis	Congestive heart failure, peripheral edema, nausea, vomiting, abdominal pain, diarrhea, increased hepatic function tests, liver necrosis, hepatitis, cholestasis, headache, rash, pruritus, eosinophilia
Ketoconazole (Nizoral)	Candidiasis, chronic mucocutaneous candidiasis, oral thrush, candiduria, blastomycosis, coccidioidomycosis	Nausea, vomiting, abdominal pain, diarrhea, gynecomastia, increased LFTs, liver necrosis, hepatitis, cholestasis, headache, rash, pruritus, eosinophilia
Micafungin (Mycamine)	Esophageal candidiasis, *Candida* infections, prophylaxis in pts undergoing hematopoietin stem cell transplantation	Fever, chills, hypokalemia, hypomagnesemia, hypocalcemia, myelosuppression, thrombocytopenia, nausea, vomiting, abdominal pain, diarrhea, increased LFTs, dizziness, headache, rash, pruritus, pain or inflammation at injection site, fever
Posaconazole (Noxafil)	Prevent invasive aspergillosis and *Candida* infections in pts 13 yrs and older who are immunocompromised, treatment of oropharyngeal candidiasis	Fever, headaches, nausea, vomiting, diarrhea, abdominal pain, hypokalemia, cough, dyspnea
Voriconazole (Vfend)	Invasive aspergillosis, candidemia, esophageal candidiasis, serious fungal infections	Visual disturbances, nausea, vomiting, abdominal pain, diarrhea, increased LFTs, liver necrosis, hepatitis, cholestasis, headache, rash, pruritus, eosinophilia

Antiglaucoma Agents

USES

Reduction of elevated intraocular pressure (IOP) in pts with open-angle glaucoma and ocular hypertension.

ACTION

Medications decrease IOP by two primary mechanisms: decreasing aqueous humor (AH) production or increasing AH outflow.

- *Alpha$_2$ agonists:* Activate receptors in ciliary body, inhibiting aqueous secretion and increasing uveoscleral aqueous outflow.
- *Beta blockers:* Reduce production of aqueous humor.
- *Carbonic anhydrase inhibitors:* Decrease production of AH by inhibiting enzyme carbonic anhydrase.
- *Prostaglandins:* Increase outflow of aqueous fluid through uveoscleral route.
- *Rho kinase inhibitors:* Inhibits the norepinephrine transporter. Decreases resistance in the trabecular meshwork outflow pathway, decreases aqueous humor production, and increases outflow of aqueous humor.

ANTIGLAUCOMA AGENTS

Name	Availability	Dosage Range	Side Effects
Alpha$_2$ Agonists			
Apraclonidine (Iopidine)	**S:** 0.5%, 1%	1 drop bid or tid	Fatigue, somnolence, local allergic reaction, dry eyes, stinging
Brimonidine (Alphagan HP)	**S:** 0.1%, 0.15%, 0.2%	1 drop bid or tid	Same as apraclonidine

Prostaglandins			
Bimatoprost (Lumigan)	**S**: 0.01%	1 drop daily in evening	Conjunctival hyperemia; darkening of iris, eyelids; increase in length, thickness, and number of eyelashes; local irritation; itching; dryness; blurred vision
Latanoprost (Xalatan)	**S**: 0.005%	1 drop daily in evening	See bimatoprost
Latanoprostene bunod (Vyzulta)	**S**: 0.0024%	1 drop every evening	Conjunctival hyperemia, eye irritation, eye pain, iris pigmentation
Tafluprost (Zioptan)	**S**: 0.0015%	1 drop daily in evening	See bimatoprost
Travoprost (Travatan)	**S**: 0.004%	1 drop daily in evening	See bimatoprost
Beta Blockers			
Betaxolol (Betoptic, Betoptic-S)	**Suspension (Betoptic-S)**: 0.25% **S (Betoptic)**: 0.5%	Betoptic-S: 1 drop 2 times/day Betoptic: 1–2 drops 2 times/day	Fatigue, dizziness, bradycardia, respiratory depression, mask symptoms of hypoglycemia, block effects of beta agonists in treatment of asthma
Carteolol (Ocupress)	**S**: 1%	1 drop 2 times/day	Same as betaxolol
Levobunolol (Betagan)	**S**: 0.25%, 0.5%	1 drop 1–2 times/day	Same as betaxolol
Metipranolol (OptiPranolol)	**S**: 0.3%	1 drop 2 times/day	Same as betaxolol
Timolol (Betimol, Istalol, Timoptic, Timoptic XE)	**S**: 0.25%, 0.5% **G, Timoptic XE**: 0.25%, 0.5%	**S**: 1 drop 2 times/day (Istalol): 1 drop daily **G**: 1 drop daily	Same as betaxolol
Carbonic Anhydrase Inhibitors			
Brinzolamide (Azopt)	**Suspension**: 1%	1 drop 3 times/day	Bitter taste, stinging, redness, burning, conjunctivitis, dry eyes, blurred vision
Dorzolamide (Trusopt)	**S**: 2%	1 drop 3 times/day	Same as brinzolamide

Continued

ANTIGLAUCOMA AGENTS—cont'd

Name	Availability	Dosage Range	Side Effects
Rho Kinase Inhibitors			
Netarsudil (Rhopressa)	**S**: 0.02%	1 drop every evening	Conjunctival hyperemia, corneal verticillata, instillation site pain, conjunctival hemorrhage, blurred vision, increased lacrimation, reduced visual acuity
Combinations			
Brimonidine/timolol (Combigan)	0.2%/0.5%	1 drop bid	See individual agents
Brinzolamide/brimonidine (Simbrinza)	1%/0.2%	1 drop tid	See individual agents
Timolol/dorzolamide (Cosopt)	0.5%/2%	1 drop bid	See individual agents

C, Capsules; ***G,*** gel; ***O,*** ointment; ***S,*** solution; ***T,*** tablets.

Antihistamines

USES

Symptomatic relief of upper respiratory allergic disorders. Allergic reactions associated with other drugs respond to antihistamines, as do blood transfusion reactions. Used as a second-choice drug in treatment of angioneurotic edema. Effective in treatment of acute urticaria and other dermatologic conditions. May also be used for preop sedation, Parkinson's disease, and motion sickness.

ACTION

Antihistamines (H_1 antagonists) inhibit vasoconstrictor effects and vasodilator effects on endothelial cells of histamine. They block increased capillary permeability, formation of edema/wheal caused by histamine. Many antihistamines can bind to receptors in CNS, causing primarily depression (decreased alertness, slowed reaction times, drowsiness) but also stimulation (restlessness, nervousness, inability to sleep). Some may counter motion sickness.

ANTIHISTAMINES

Name	Availability	Dosage Range	Side Effects
Cetirizine (Zyrtec)	**T**: 5 mg, 10 mg **C**: 5 mg, 10 mg **T (Chew)**: 5 mg/10 mg **S**: 5 mg/5 mL	**A**: 5–10 mg/day **C (6–12 yrs)**: 5–10 mg/day **C (2–5 yrs)**: 2.5–5 mg/day	Headache, somnolence, fatigue, abdominal pain, dry mouth
Desloratadine (Clarinex)	**T**: 5 mg **ODT**: 2.5 mg, 5 mg **S**: 0.5 mg/mL	**A, C (12 yrs and older)**: 5 mg/day **C (6–11 yrs)**: 2.5 mg/day **C (1–5 yrs)**: 1.25 mg/day **C (6–11 mos)**: 1 mg/day	Dizziness, fatigue, headache, nausea
Dimenhydrinate (Dramamine)	**T**: 50 mg **T (Chew)**: 25 mg, 50 mg	**A**: 50–100 mg q4–6h **C**: 12.5–50 mg q6–8h	Dizziness, drowsiness, headache, nausea
Diphenhydramine (Benadryl)	**T**: 25 mg, 50 mg **C**: 25 mg, 50 mg **L**: 12.5 mg/5 mL	**A**: 25–50 mg q6–8h **C (6–11 yrs)**: 12.5–25 mg q4–6h **C (2–5 yrs)**: 6.25 mg q4–6h	Chills, confusion, dizziness, fatigue, headache, sedation, nausea
Fexofenadine (Allegra)	**T**: 30 mg, 60 mg, 180 mg **ODT**: 30 mg **S**: 30 mg/5 mL	**A**: 60 mg q12h or 180 mg/day **C (2–11 yrs)**: 30 mg q12h **(6–23 mos)**: 15 mg bid	Headache, vomiting, fatigue, diarrhea
Hydroxyzine (Atarax)	**T**: 10 mg, 25 mg, 50 mg **C**: 25 mg, 50 mg, 100 mg **S**: 10 mg/5 mL	**A**: 25 mg q6–8h **C**: 2 mg/kg/day in divided doses q6–8h	Dizziness, drowsiness, fatigue, headache
Levocetirizine (Xyzal)	**T**: 5 mg **S**: 2.5 mg/mL	**A, C (12 yrs and older)**: 5 mg once daily in evening **C (6–11 yrs)**: 2.5 mg once daily in evening **(6 mos–5 yrs)**: 1.25 mg once daily	Fatigue, fever, somnolence, vomiting

Continued

ANTIHISTAMINES—cont'd

Name	Availability	Dosage Range	Side Effects
Loratadine (Claritin)	**ODT**: 10 mg **T (Chew)**: 5 mg **T**: 10 mg **S**: 1 mg/mL	**A**: 10 mg/day **C (6–12 yrs)**: 10 mg/day **(2–5 yrs)**: 5 mg/day	Fatigue, headache, malaise, somnolence, abdominal pain
Promethazine (Phenergan)	**T**: 12.5 mg, 25 mg, 50 mg **S**: 6.25 mg/5 mL	**A**: 25 mg at bedtime or 12.5 mg q8h **C**: 0.5 mg/kg at bedtime or 0.1 mg/kg q6–8h	Confusion, dizziness, drowsiness, fatigue, constipation, nausea, vomiting

A, Adults; ***C,*** capsules; ***C** (dosage),* children; ***L,*** liquid; ***ODT,*** orally disintegrating tablet; ***S,*** syrup; ***SR,*** sustained-release; ***T,*** tablets.

Antihyperlipidemics

USES

Cholesterol management.

ACTION

Bile acid sequestrants: Bind bile acids in the intestine; prevent active transport and reabsorption and enhance bile acid excretion. Depletion of hepatic bile acid results in the increased conversion of cholesterol to bile acids.

HMG-CoA reductase inhibitors (statins): Inhibit HMG-CoA reductase, the last regulated step in the synthesis of cholesterol. Cholesterol synthesis in the liver is reduced.

Niacin (nicotinic acid): Reduces hepatic synthesis of triglycerides and secretion of very low density lipoprotein (VLDL) by inhibiting the mobilization of free fatty acids from peripheral tissues.

Fibric acid: Increases the oxidation of fatty acids in the liver, resulting in reduced secretion of triglyceride-rich lipoproteins, and increases lipoprotein lipase activity and fatty acid uptake.

Cholesterol absorption inhibitor: Acts in the gut wall to prevent cholesterol absorption through the intestinal villi.

Omega fatty acids: Exact mechanism unknown. Mechanisms may include inhibition of acyl-CoA, decreased lipogenesis in liver, increased lipoprotein lipase activity.

PCSK9 inhibitors: Binds with high-affinity and specificity to LDL cholesterol receptors, promoting their degradation.

Adenosine triphosphate–citrate lyase (ACL) inhibitor: ACL is an enzyme involved in hepatic cholesterol synthesis. Increases LDL from blood.

ANTIHYPERLIPIDEMICS

Name	Primary Effect	Dosage	Comments/Side Effects
Bile Acid Sequestrants			
Cholestyramine (Prevalite, Questran)	Decreases LDL Increases HDL, TG	4 g 1–2 times/day. May increase over 1 mo interval. Usual dose: 8–16 g/day in 2 divided doses	**Class Side Effects:** Constipation, heartburn, nausea, eructation, and bloating May increase triglyceride levels. Avoid use with triglyceride levels greater than 300 mg/dL
Colesevelam (Welchol)	Decreases LDL Increases HDL, TG	3.75 g once daily or 1.875 g 2 times/day	
Colestipol (Colestid)	Decreases LDL Increases TG	**G:** Initially, 5 g once or twice daily. May increase by 5 g/day q1–2 mos. Maintenance: 5–30 g/day. **T:** Initially, 2 g once or twice daily. May increase by 2 g 2 times/day at 1–2 mo intervals. Maintenance: 2–16 g/day	
Cholesterol Absorption Inhibitor			
Ezetimibe (Zetia)	Decreases LDL Increases HDL Decreases TG	10 mg once daily	Administer at least 2 hrs before or 4 hrs after bile acid sequestrants **Side Effects:** Dizziness, headache, fatigue, diarrhea, abdominal pain, arthralgia, sinusitis, pharyngitis
Fibric Acid Derivatives			
Fenofibrate (Antara, Lofibra, Tricor, Triglide)	Decreases TG Decreases LDL Increases HDL	**Antara:** 43–130 mg/day **Lofibra:** 67–200 mg/day **Tricor:** 48–145 mg/day **Triglide:** 50–160 mg/day **Fenoglide:** 40–120 mg/day **Lipofen:** 50–150 mg/day	May increase levels of ezetimibe. Concomitant use of statins may increase rhabdomyolysis, elevate CPK levels, and cause myoglobinuria **Side Effects:** Abdominal pain, constipation, diarrhea, respiratory complaints, headache, fever, flu-like syndrome, asthenia

Continued

ANTIHYPERLIPIDEMICS—cont'd

Name	Primary Effect	Dosage	Comments/Side Effects
Fenofibric acid (Fibricor, Trilipix)	Decreases TG, LDL Increases HDL	**Trilipix:** 45–135 mg/day **Fibricor:** 35–105 mg/day	May give without regard to meals. Concomitant use of statins may increase rhabdomyolysis **Side Effects:** Headache, upper respiratory tract infection, pain, nausea, dizziness, nasopharyngitis
Gemfibrozil (Lopid)	Decreases TG Increases HDL	600 mg 2 times/day	Give 30 min before breakfast and dinner. Concomitant use of statins may increase rhabdomyolysis, elevate CPK levels, and cause myoglobinuria **Side Effects:** Fatigue, vertigo, headache, rash, eczema, diarrhea, abdominal pain, nausea, vomiting, constipation
Niacin			
Niacin, nicotinic acid (Niacor, Niaspan)	Decreases LDL,TG Increases HDL	**Regular-release (Niacor):** 1 g tid **Extended-release (Niaspan):** 1 g at bedtime	Diabetics may experience a dose-related elevation in glucose **Side Effects:** Increased LFT, hyperglycemia, dyspepsia, itching, flushing, dizziness, insomnia
Statins			
Atorvastatin (Lipitor)	Decreases LDL,TG Increases HDL	Initially, 10–20 mg/day Range: 10–80 mg/day	May interact with CYP3A4 inhibitors (e.g., amiodarone, diltiazem, cyclosporine, grapefruit juice) increasing risk of myopathy **Side Effects:** Myalgia, myopathy, rhabdomyolysis, headache, chest pain, peripheral edema, dizziness, rash, abdominal pain, constipation, diarrhea, dyspepsia, nausea, flatulence, increased LFT, back pain, sinusitis
Fluvastatin (Lescol)	Decreases LDL,TG Increases HDL	40–80 mg/day	Primarily metabolized by CYP2C9 enzyme system. May increase levels of phenytoin, rifampin. May lower fluvastatin levels **Side Effects:** Headache, fatigue, dyspepsia, diarrhea, nausea, abdominal pain, myalgia, myopathy, rhabdomyolysis

Lovastatin (Mevacor)	Decreases LDL, TG Increases HDL	Initially, 20 mg/day. Adjust at 4 wk intervals **Maximum:** 80 mg/day	May interact with CYP3A4 inhibitors (e.g., amiodarone, diltiazem, cyclosporine, grapefruit products) increasing risk of myopathy **Side Effects:** Increased CPK levels, headache, dizziness, rash, constipation, diarrhea, abdominal pain, dyspepsia, nausea, flatulence, myalgia, myopathy, rhabdomyolysis
Pitavastatin (Livalo)	Decreases LDL, TG Increases HDL	Initially, 2 mg/day. May increase at 4 wk intervals to 4 mg/day	Erythromycin, rifampin may increase concentration **Side Effects:** Myalgia, back pain, diarrhea, constipation, pain in extremities
Pravastatin (Pravachol)	Decreases LDL, TG Increases HDL	Initially, 40 mg/day. Titrate to response Range: 10–80 mg/day	May be less likely to be involved in drug interactions Cyclosporine may increase pravastatin levels **Side Effects:** Chest pain, headache, dizziness, rash, nausea, vomiting, diarrhea, increased LFTs, cough, flu-like symptoms, myalgia, myopathy, rhabdomyolysis
Rosuvastatin (Crestor)	Decreases LDL, TG Increases HDL	Initially, 10–20 mg/day Titrate to response Range: 5–40 mg/day	May be less likely to be involved in drug interactions Cyclosporine may increase rosuvastatin levels **Side Effects:** Chest pain, peripheral edema, headache, rash, dizziness, vertigo, pharyngitis, diarrhea, nausea, constipation, abdominal pain, dyspepsia, sinusitis, flu-like symptoms, myalgia, myopathy, rhabdomyolysis
ACL Inhibitor			
Bempedoic acid (Nexletol)	Decreases LDL	180 mg once daily	Back pain, extremity pain, elevated liver enzymes, hyperuricemia, gout, tendonitis

Continued

ANTIHYPERLIPIDEMICS—cont'd

Name	Primary Effect	Dosage	Comments/Side Effects
Simvastatin (Zocor)	Decreases LDL,TG Increases HDL	5–40 mg/day	May interact with CYP3A4 inhibitors (e.g., amiodarone, diltiazem, cyclosporine, grapefruit products) increasing risk of myopathy **Side Effects:** Constipation, flatulence, dyspepsia, increased LFTs, increased CPK, upper respiratory tract infection
Omega Fatty Acids			
Icosapent (Vascepa)	Decreases TG	2 g 2 times/day	**Side Effects:** Arthralgia
Lovaza	Decreases TG Increases LDL, HDL	2 g 2 times/day or 4 g once daily	Use with caution with fish or shellfish allergy **Side Effects:** Eructation, dyspepsia, taste perversion
PCSK9 Inhibitors			
Alirocumab (Praluent)	Decreases LDL	**SQ:** 75 mg q2wks	**Side Effects:** Hypersensitivity reactions (e.g., rash), nasopharyngitis, injection site reactions, influenza
Evolcumab (Repatha)	Decreases LDL	**SQ:** 140 mg q2wks or 420 mg qmo	**Side Effects:** Nasopharyngitis, upper respiratory tract infection, influenza, back pain, injection site reactions

CPK, Creatine phosphokinase; ***G,*** granules; ***HDL,*** high-density lipoprotein; ***LDL,*** low-density lipoprotein; ***SQ,*** subcutaneous; ***T,*** tablets; ***TG,*** triglycerides.

Antihypertensives

USES	ACTION
Treatment of mild to severe hypertension.	Many groups of medications are used in the treatment of hypertension. *ACE inhibitors:* Decrease conversion of angiotensin I to angiotensin II, a potent vasoconstrictor, reducing peripheral vascular resistance and B/P. *Alpha agonists (central action):* Stimulate $alpha_2$-adrenergic receptors in the cardiovascular centers of the CNS, reducing sympathetic outflow and producing an antihypertensive effect. *Alpha antagonists (peripheral action):* Block $alpha_1$-adrenergic receptors in arterioles and veins, inhibiting vasoconstriction and decreasing peripheral vascular resistance, causing a fall in B/P. *Angiotensin receptor blockers:* Block vasoconstrictor effects of angiotensin II by blocking the binding of angiotensin II to AT1 receptors in vascular smooth muscle, helping blood vessels to relax and reduce B/P. *Beta blockers:* Decrease B/P by inhibiting $beta_1$ adrenergic receptors, which lowers heart rate, heart workload, and the heart's output of blood. *Calcium channel blockers:* Reduce B/P by inhibiting flow of extracellular calcium across cell membranes of vascular tissue, relaxing arterial smooth muscle. *Diuretics:* Inhibit sodium (Na) reabsorption, increasing excretion of Na and water. Reduce plasma, extracellular fluid volume, and peripheral vascular resistance. *Renin inhibitors:* Directly inhibit renin, decreasing plasma renin activity (PRA), inhibiting conversion of angiotensinogen to angiotensin, producing antihypertensive effect. *Vasodilators:* Directly relax arteriolar smooth muscle, decreasing vascular resistance. Exact mechanism unknown.

ANTIHYPERTENSIVES

Name	Availability	Dosage Range	Side Effects
ACE Inhibitors			
Benazepril (Lotensin)	**T:** 5 mg, 10 mg, 20 mg, 40 mg	20–80 mg/day as single or 2 divided doses	Postural dizziness, headache, cough
Captopril	**T:** 12.5 mg, 25 mg, 50 mg, 100 mg	50–100 mg 2 times/day	Rash, cough, hyperkalemia
Enalapril (Vasotec)	**T:** 2.5 mg, 5 mg, 10 mg, 20 mg	5–40 mg/day in 1–2 divided doses	Hypotension, chest pain, syncope, headache, dizziness, fatigue
Fosinopril	**T:** 10 mg, 20 mg, 40 mg	10–80 mg once daily or divided bid	Dizziness, cough, hyperkalemia
Lisinopril (Prinivil, Zestril)	**T:** 2.5 mg, 5 mg, 10 mg, 20 mg, 30 mg, 40 mg	10–40 mg once daily	Hypotension, headache, fatigue, dizziness, hyperkalemia, cough
Quinapril	**T:** 5 mg, 10 mg, 20 mg, 40 mg	10–80 mg once daily or divided bid	Hypotension, dizziness, fatigue, headache, myalgia, hyperkalemia
Ramipril (Altace)	**T or C:** 1.25 mg, 2.5 mg, 5 mg, 10 mg	2.5–20 mg once daily or divided bid	Cough, hypotension, angina, headache, dizziness, hyperkalemia
Alpha Agonists: Central Action			
Clonidine (Catapres)	**T:** 0.1 mg, 0.2 mg, 0.3 mg **P:** 0.1 mg/hr, 0.2 mg/hr, 0.3 mg/hr	**PO:** 0.1–0.8 mg divided bid or tid **Topical:** 0.1–0.6 mg/wk	Sedation, dry mouth, heart block, rebound hypertension, contact dermatitis with patch, bradycardia, drowsiness
Alpha Agonists: Peripheral Action			
Doxazosin (Cardura)	**T:** 1 mg, 2 mg, 4 mg, 8 mg	**PO:** 2–16 mg/day	Dizziness, vertigo, headaches
Prazosin (Minipress)	**C:** 1 mg, 2 mg, 5 mg	**PO:** 6–20 mg/day	Dizziness, light-headedness, headaches, drowsiness, palpitations, fluid retention
Terazosin (Hytrin)	**C:** 1 mg, 2 mg, 5 mg, 10 mg	**PO:** 1–20 mg/day	Dizziness, headaches, asthenia (loss of strength, energy)

Angiotensin Receptor Blockers			
Azilsartan (Edarbi)	**T:** 40 mg, 80 mg	40–80 mg once daily	Diarrhea, hypotension, nausea, cough
Candesartan (Atacand)	**T:** 4 mg, 8 mg, 16 mg, 32 mg	8–32 mg once daily or divided bid	Hypotension, dizziness, headache, hyperkalemia
Eprosartan (Teveten)	**T:** 400 mg, 600 mg	600 mg once daily	Headache, cough, dizziness
Irbesartan (Avapro)	**T:** 75 mg, 150 mg, 300 mg	150–300 mg once daily	Fatigue, diarrhea, cough
Losartan (Cozaar)	**T:** 25 mg, 50 mg, 100 mg	25–100 mg once daily or divided bid	Chest pain, fatigue, hypoglycemia, weakness, cough, hypotension
Olmesartan (Benicar)	**T:** 5 mg, 20 mg, 40 mg	20–40 mg once daily	Dizziness, headache, diarrhea, flu-like symptoms
Valsartan (Diovan)	**T:** 80 mg, 160 mg, 320 mg	80–320 mg once daily	Dizziness, fatigue, increased BUN
Beta Blockers			
Atenolol (Tenormin)	**T:** 25 mg, 50 mg, 100 mg	50–100 mg once daily	Fatigue, bradycardia, reduced exercise tolerance, increased triglycerides, bronchospasm, sexual dysfunction, masked hypoglycemia
Bisoprolol (Zebeta)	**T:** 5 mg, 10 mg	5–20 mg once daily	Fatigue, insomnia, diarrhea, arthralgia, upper respiratory infections
Carvedilol (Coreg, Coreg CR)	**T:** 3.125 mg, 6.25 mg, 12.5 mg, 25 mg **CR:** 10 mg, 20 mg, 40 mg, 80 mg	**T:** 12.5–50 mg divided bid **CR:** 20–80 mg once daily	Orthostatic hypotension, fatigue, dizziness
Metoprolol (Lopressor)	**T:** 25 mg, 37.5 mg, 50 mg, 75 mg, 100 mg	100–450 mg bid or tid	Hypotension, bradycardia, fatigue, 1st degree heart block, dizziness
Metoprolol XL (Toprol XL)	**T:** 25 mg, 50 mg, 100 mg, 200 mg	25–400 mg once daily	Same as metoprolol
Nebivolol (Bystolic)	**T:** 2.5 mg, 5 mg, 10 mg, 20 mg	5–40 mg once daily	Upper respiratory tract infection, dizziness, fatigue

Continued

ANTIHYPERTENSIVES—cont'd

Name	Availability	Dosage Range	Side Effects
Calcium Channel Blockers			
Amlodipine (Norvasc)	**T:** 2.5 mg, 5 mg, 10 mg	2.5–10 mg once daily	Headache, fatigue, peripheral edema, flushing, worsening heart failure, rash, gingival hyperplasia, tachycardia
Diltiazem CD (Cardizem CD)	**C:** 120 mg, 180 mg, 240 mg, 300 mg	240–360 mg once daily	Dizziness, headache, bradycardia, heart block, worsening heart failure, edema, constipation
Felodipine (Plendil)	**T:** 2.5 mg, 5 mg, 10 mg	2.5–10 mg once daily	Headache, flushing, peripheral edema, rash, gingival hyperplasia, tachycardia
Nifedipine XL (Adalat CC, Procardia XL)	**T:** 30 mg, 60 mg, 90 mg	30–90 mg once daily	Flushing, peripheral edema, headache, dizziness, nausea
Verapamil SR (Calan SR)	**T:** 120 mg, 180 mg, 240 mg **T (Sustained-Release):** 120 mg, 180 mg	**T (Immediate-Release):** 80–160 mg tid **T (Sustained-Release):** 240–480 mg once daily or divided bid	Headache, gingival hyperplasia, constipation
Diuretics			
Chlorthalidone (Hygroton)	**T:** 25 mg, 50 mg	12.5–25 mg/day	Same as hydrochlorothiazide
Hydrochlorothiazide (Hydrodiuril)	**T:** 25 mg, 50 mg	12.5–50 mg/day	Hypokalemia, hyperuricemia, hypomagnesemia, hyperglycemia Pancreatitis, rash, photosensitivity, hyponatremia, hypercalcemia, hypercholesterolemia, hypertriglyceridemia

Renin Inhibitor			
Aliskiren (Tekturna)	**T:** 150 mg, 300 mg	**PO:** 150–300 mg/day	Diarrhea, dyspepsia, headache, dizziness, fatigue, upper respiratory tract infection
Vasodilators			
Hydralazine (Apresoline)	**T:** 10 mg, 25 mg, 50 mg, 100 mg	**PO:** 40–300 mg/day	Headaches, palpitations, aggravation of angina, dizziness, fluid retention, nasal congestion
Minoxidil (Loniten)	**T:** 2.5 mg, 10 mg	**PO:** 10–40 mg/day	Rapid/irregular heartbeat, hypertrichosis, peripheral edema, aggravation of angina, fluid retention

C, Capsules; ***P,*** patch; ***PO,*** oral; ***T,*** tablets.

Antimigraine (Triptans)

USES	ACTION
Treatment of migraine headaches with or without aura in adults 18 yrs and older.	Triptans are selective agonists of the serotonin (5-HT) receptor in cranial arteries, which cause vasoconstriction and reduce inflammation associated with antidromic neuronal transmission correlating with relief of migraine headache.

TRIPTANS

Name	Availability	Dosage Range	Contraindications	Common Side Effects
Almotriptan (Axert)	**T:** 6.25 mg, 12.5 mg	6.25–12.5 mg; may repeat after 2 hrs (**Maximum:** 25 mg/day)	Ischemic heart disease, angina pectoris, arrhythmias, previous MI, uncontrolled hypertension, hemiplegic or basilar migraine, peripheral vascular disease	Drowsiness, dizziness, paresthesia, nausea, vomiting, headache, xerostomia
Eletriptan (Relpax)	**T:** 20 mg, 40 mg	**A:** 20–40 mg; may repeat after 2 hrs (**Maximum:** 80 mg/day)	Same as almotriptan	Chest pain, dizziness, drowsiness, headache, paresthesia, nausea, xerostomia, weakness
Frovatriptan (Frova)	**T:** 2.5 mg	2.5 mg; may repeat after 2 hrs; no more than 3 **T**/day (**Maximum:** 7.5 mg/day)	Same as almotriptan	Hot/cold sensations, dizziness, fatigue, headaches, skeletal pain, dyspepsia, flushing, paresthesia, drowsiness, xerostomia, nausea
Naratriptan (Amerge)	**T:** 1 mg, 2.5 mg	1–2.5 mg; may repeat once after 4 hrs (**Maximum:** 5 mg/day)	Same as almotriptan plus severe renal/hepatic disease	Neck pain, pain, nausea, fatigue
Rizatriptan (Maxalt, Maxalt-MLT)	**T:** 5 mg, 10 mg **DT:** 5 mg, 10 mg	5 or 10 mg; may repeat after 2 hrs (**Maximum:** 30 mg/day)	Same as almotriptan	Chest pain, drowsiness, xerostomia, weakness, paresthesia, nausea, dizziness, drowsiness, fatigue

Sumatriptan (Imitrex, Sumavel DosePro, Onzetra, Xsail, Zecuity)	**T**: 25 mg, 50 mg, 100 mg **NS**: 5 mg, 10 mg, 20 mg **I**: 4 mg, 6 mg **NP**: 8 pouches of 2 nose pieces each 11 mg/piece	**PO**: 25–100 mg; may repeat after 2 hrs (**Maximum:** 200 mg/day) **NS**: 5–20 mg; may repeat after 2 hrs (**Maximum:** 40 mg/day) **SQ**: 3–6 mg; may repeat after 1 hr (**Maximum:** 12 mg/day) **NP**: 22 mg; may repeat after 2 hrs (**Maximum:** 44 mg/day)	Same as almotriptan plus severe hepatic dysfunction	*Oral:* Hot/cold flashes, paresthesia, malaise, fatigue *Injection:* Atypical sensations, flushing, chest pain/discomfort, injection site reaction, dizziness, vertigo, paresthesia, bleeding, bruising, swelling, erythema at injection site *Nasal:* Discomfort, nausea, vomiting, altered taste *Transdermal:* Localized pain, skin discoloration, allergic contact dermatitis, pruritus, local irritation
Zolmitriptan (Zomig, Zomig-ZMT)	**T**: 2.5 mg, 5 mg **DT**: 2.5 mg, 5 mg **NS**: 2.5 mg/0.1 mL, 5 mg/0.1 mL	**PO**: 2.5–5 mg; may repeat after 2 hrs (**Maximum:** 10 mg/day) **NS**: 1 spray (2.5 or 5 mg) at onset of migraine headache; may repeat after 2 hrs (**Maximum:** 10 mg/day)	Same as almotriptan plus symptomatic Wolff-Parkinson-White syndrome	Atypical sensations, pain, nausea, dizziness, asthenia, drowsiness

A, Adults; ***DT,*** disintegrating tablets; ***I,*** injection; ***NP,*** nasal powder; ***NS,*** nasal spray; ***SQ,*** subcutaneous; ***T,*** tablets.

Antipsychotics

USES	ACTION	SIDE EFFECTS (Please refer to individual monographs)
Antipsychotics are primarily used in managing schizophrenia. They may also be used in treatment of bipolar disorder, schizoaffective disorder, and irritability associated with autism. The goals in treating schizophrenia include targeting symptoms, preventing relapse, and increasing adaptive functioning. Use of antipsychotic medications is the mainstay of schizophrenia management.	The precise mechanism of action of antipsychotic medications is unknown, but they have been categorized into two groups: *Typical (traditional):* Associated with high dopamine antagonism and low serotonin antagonism. *Atypical:* Those having moderate to high dopamine antagonism and high serotonin antagonism and those having low dopamine antagonism and high serotonin antagonism.	*Typical versus atypical:* Typical antipsychotics are associated with a greater risk of extrapyramidal side effects, and atypicals are associated with a greater risk of weight gain. *Endocrine:* Hyperprolactinemia, weight gain, increased risk of diabetes. *Cardiovascular:* Orthostatic hypotension, electrocardiographic changes. *Lipids:* Increased triglycerides, cholesterol. *Central nervous system:* Dystonic reactions, akathisia, pseudo-parkinsonism, tardive dyskinesia, sedation, risk of seizures.

TYPICAL ANTIPSYCHOTICS

Name	Uses	Dosage (Oral)
Fluphenazine	Adult psychosis	1–5 mg/day
Haloperidol (Haldol)	Adult and child psychosis	1–15 mg/day
Thioridazine	Adult, adolescent, child schizophrenia and psychosis	200–800 mg/day
Thiothixene (Navane)	Adult and adolescent schizophrenia	Moderate: 15 mg/day Severe: 20–30 mg/day

ATYPICAL ANTIPSYCHOTICS

Name	Uses	Dosage
Aripiprazole (Abilify)	Adult and adolescent schizophrenia; adult and child bipolar I disorder; adult major depressive disorder; irritability with adolescent autism	10–15 mg/day
Brexpiprazole (Rexulti)	Adult schizophrenia; adult major depressive disorder	2–4 mg/day
Cariprazine (Vraylar)	Adult schizophrenia, bipolar I discrder (manic or mixed episodes)	1.5–6 mg/day
Clozapine (Clozaril)	Schizophrenia; suicidal behavior in adult schizophrenia and schizoaffective disorder	300–450 mg/day
Iloperidone (Fanapt)	Adult schizophrenia	12–24 mg/day
Lumateperone (Caplyta)	Adult schizophrenia	40–160 mg/day
Lurasidone (Latuda)	Adult schizophrenia, bipolar I disorder (manic or mixed episodes)	40–160 mg/day
Olanzapine (Zyprexa)	Adult, adolescent, and child schizophrenia; adult, adolescent mania in bipolar I disorder	10–20 mg/day
Paliperidone (Invega)	Adult and adolescent schizophrenia; adult schizoaffective disorder	3–12 mg/day
Quetiapine (Seroquel)	Adult and adolescent schizophrenia; adult, adolescent, and child bipolar I disorder	400–800 mg/day
Risperidone (Risperdal)	Adult and adolescent schizophrenia; adult, adolescent, and child bipolar I disorder; irritability with adolescent and child autism	4–8 mg/day
Ziprasidone (Geodon)	Adult schizophrenia; manic or mixed episodes associated with adult bipolar I disorder	40–160 mg/day

Antivirals

USES

Treatment of HIV infection. Treatment of cytomegalovirus (CMV) retinitis in pts with AIDS, acute herpes zoster (shingles), genital herpes (recurrent), mucosal and cutaneous herpes simplex virus (HSV), chickenpox, and influenza A viral illness.

ACTION

Effective antivirals must inhibit virus-specific nucleic acid/protein synthesis. Possible mechanisms of action of antivirals used for non-HIV infection may include interference with viral DNA synthesis and viral replication, inactivation of viral DNA polymerases, incorporation and termination of the growing viral DNA chain, prevention of release of viral nucleic acid into the host cell, or interference with viral penetration into cells.

ANTIVIRALS

Name	Availability	Uses	Side Effects
Abacavir (Ziagen)	**T:** 300 mg **OS:** 20 mg/mL	HIV infection	Nausea, vomiting, loss of appetite, diarrhea, headaches, fatigue, hypersensitivity reactions
Acyclovir (Zovirax)	**T:** 400 mg, 800 mg **C:** 200 mg **I:** 50 mg/mL	Mucosal/cutaneous HSV-1 and HSV-2, varicella-zoster (shingles), genital herpes, herpes simplex, encephalitis, chickenpox	Malaise, anorexia, nausea, vomiting, light-headedness
Adefovir (Hepsera)	**T:** 10 mg	Chronic hepatitis B	Asthenia, headaches, abdominal pain, nausea, diarrhea, flatulence, dyspepsia
Amantadine (Symmetrel)	**T:** 100 mg **C:** 100 mg **S:** 50 mg/5 mL	Influenza A	Anxiety, dizziness, headaches, nausea, loss of appetite
Cidofovir (Vistide)	**I:** 75 mg/mL	CMV retinitis	Decreased urination, fever, chills, diarrhea, nausea, vomiting, headaches, loss of appetite

Darunavir (Prezista)	**T:** 75 mg, 150 mg, 400 mg, 600 mg, 800 mg	HIV infection	Diarrhea, nausea, vomiting, headaches, skin rash, constipation
Delavirdine (Rescriptor)	**T:** 100 mg, 200 mg	HIV infection	Diarrhea, fatigue, rash, headaches, nausea
Didanosine (Videx)	**C:** 125 mg, 200 mg, 250 mg, 400 mg **Powder for suspension:** 2 g, 4 g	HIV infection	Peripheral neuropathy, anxiety, headaches, rash, nausea, diarrhea, dry mouth
Efavirenz (Sustiva)	**C:** 50 mg, 200 mg **T:** 600 mg	HIV infection	Diarrhea, dizziness, headaches, insomnia, nausea, vomiting, drowsiness
Etravirine (Intelence)	**T:** 25 mg, 100 mg, 200 mg	HIV infection	Rash, nausea, abdominal pain, vomiting
Famciclovir (Famvir)	**T:** 125 mg, 250 mg, 500 mg	Herpes zoster, genital herpes, herpes labialis, mucosal/cutaneous herpes simplex	Headaches, nausea
Foscarnet (Foscavir)	**I:** 24 mg/mL	CMV retinitis, HSV infections	Decreased urination, abdominal pain, nausea, vomiting, dizziness, fatigue, headaches
Ganciclovir (Cytovene)	**I:** 500 mg	CMV retinitis, CMV disease	Sore throat, fever, unusual bleeding/bruising
Indinavir (Crixivan)	**C:** 200 mg, 400 mg	HIV infection	Blood in urine, weakness, nausea, vomiting, diarrhea, headaches, insomnia, altered taste
Lamivudine (Epivir)	**T:** 100 mg, 150 mg, 300 mg **OS:** 5 mg/mL, 10 mg/mL	HIV infection, chronic hepatitis B	Nausea, vomiting, abdominal pain, paresthesia
Lopinavir/ritonavir (Kaletra)	**T:** 100 mg/25 mg, 200 mg/50 mg **OS:** 80 mg/20 mg per mL	HIV infection	Diarrhea, nausea

Continued

ANTIVIRALS—cont'd

Name	Availability	Uses	Side Effects
Maraviroc (Selzentry)	**T**: 150 mg, 300 mg	HIV infection	Cough, pyrexia, upper respiratory tract infection, rash, musculoskeletal symptoms, abdominal pain, dizziness
Nelfinavir (Viracept)	**T**: 250 mg, 625 mg	HIV infection	Diarrhea
Oseltamivir (Tamiflu)	**C**: 30 mg, 45 mg, 75 mg **S**: 6 mg/mL	Influenza A or B	Diarrhea, nausea, vomiting
Raltegravir (Isentress)	**T**: 400 mg **T (chew)**: 25 mg, 100 mg	HIV infection	Nausea, headache, diarrhea, pyrexia
Ribavirin (Virazole)	**Aerosol**: 6 g **OS**: 40 mg/mL **T**: 200 mg, 400 mg, 600 mg	Lowers respiratory infections in infants, children due to respiratory syncytial virus (RSV), chronic hepatitis C	Anemia
Ritonavir (Norvir)	**C**: 100 mg **T**: 100 mg **OS**: 80 mg/mL	HIV infection	Weakness, diarrhea, nausea, decreased appetite, vomiting, altered taste
Saquinavir (Invirase)	**C**: 200 mg **T**: 500 mg	HIV infection	Weakness, diarrhea, nausea, oral ulcers, abdominal pain
Stavudine (Zerit)	**C**: 15 mg, 20 mg, 30 mg, 40 mg **OS**: 1 mg/mL	HIV infection	Paresthesia, decreased appetite, chills, fever, rash

Tenofovir (Viread)	**T:** 150 mg, 200 mg, 250 mg, 300 mg **Powder (oral):** 40 mg/g	HIV infection	Diarrhea, nausea, pharyngitis, headaches
Valacyclovir (Valtrex)	**T:** 500 mg, 1 g	Herpes zoster, genital herpes, herpes labialis, chickenpox	Headaches, nausea
Valganciclovir (Valcyte)	**T:** 450 mg **OS:** 50 mg/mL	CMV retinitis	Anemia, abdominal pain, diarrhea, headaches, nausea, vomiting, paresthesia
Zanamivir (Relenza)	**Inhalation:** 5 mg	Influenza A and B	Cough, diarrhea, dizziness, headaches, nausea, vomiting
Zidovudine (Retrovir)	**C:** 100 mg **S:** 50 mg/5 mL **I:** 10 mg/mL	HIV infection	Fatigue, fever, chills, headaches, nausea, muscle pain

C, Capsules; ***I,*** injection; ***OS,*** oral solution; ***S,*** syrup; ***T,*** tablets.

Sedative-Hypnotics

USES

Treatment of insomnia (i.e., difficulty falling asleep initially, frequent awakening, awakening too early).

ACTION

Benzodiazepines are the most widely used agents and largely replace barbiturates due to greater safety, lower incidence of drug dependence. Benzodiazepines nonselectively bind to at least three receptor subtypes accounting for sedative, anxiolytic, relaxant, and anticonvulsant properties. Benzodiazepines enhance the effect of the inhibitory neurotransmitter gamma-aminobutyric acid (GABA), which inhibits impulse transmission in the CNS reticular formation in brain. Benzodiazepines decrease sleep latency, number of nocturnal awakenings, and time spent in awake stage of sleep; increase total sleep time. The *nonbenzodiazepines* zaleplon and zolpidem preferentially bind with one receptor subtype, reducing sleep latency and nocturnal awakenings and increasing total sleep time. Ramelteon is a selective agonist of melatonin receptors (responsible for determining circadian rhythms and synchronizing sleep-wake cycles).

SEDATIVE-HYPNOTICS

Name	Availability	Dosage Range	Side Effects
Benzodiazepines			
Estazolam	**T:** 1 mg, 2 mg	**A:** 1–2 mg **E:** 0.5–1 mg	Daytime sedation, memory and psychomotor impairment, tolerance, withdrawal reactions, rebound insomnia, dependence
Flurazepam	**C:** 15 mg, 30 mg	**A/E:** 15–30 mg **E:** 15 mg	Headaches, unpleasant taste, dry mouth, dizziness, anxiety, nausea
Temazepam (Restoril)	**C:** 7.5 mg, 15 mg, 30 mg	**A:** 15–30 mg **E:** 7.5–15 mg	Same as flurazepam

Continued

SEDATIVE-HYPNOTICS—cont'd

Name	Availability	Dosage Range	Side Effects
Nonbenzodiazepines			
Doxepin (Silenor)	**T:** 3 mg, 6 mg	**A, E:** 3–6 mg	Somnolence, dizziness, nausea, upper respiratory tract infections, nasopharyngitis, hypertension, headache
Eszopiclone (Lunesta)	**T:** 1 mg, 2 mg, 3 mg	**A:** 1–3 mg **E:** 1–2 mg	Headaches, unpleasant taste, dry mouth, dizziness, anxiety, nausea
Ramelteon (Rozerem)	**T:** 8 mg	**A, E:** 8 mg	Headaches, dizziness, fatigue, nausea
Suvorexant (Belsomra)	**T:** 5 mg, 10 mg, 15 mg, 20 mg	**A, E:** 10–20 mg	Next day somnolence, leg weakness
Zaleplon (Sonata)	**C:** 5 mg, 10 mg	**A:** 10–20 mg **E:** 5 mg	Headaches, dizziness, myalgia, drowsiness, asthenia, abdominal pain
Zolpidem (Ambien, Ambien CR, Edluar, Intermezzo, Zolpimist)	**T:** 5 mg, 10 mg **CR:** 6.25 mg, 12.5 mg **SL (Edluar):** 5 mg, 10 mg **(Intermezzo):** 1.75 mg, 3.5 mg **OS:** 5 mg/actuation	**OS, T, SL (Edluar):** 5 mg (females, elderly); 5–10 mg (males) (Intermezzo): 1.75 mg (females, elderly); 3.5 mg (males) **CR:** 6.25 mg (females, elderly); 6.25–12.5 mg (males)	Dizziness, daytime drowsiness, headaches, confusion, depression, hangover, asthenia

A, Adults; ***C,*** capsules; ***CR,*** controlled-release; ***E,*** elderly; ***OS,*** oral solution; ***SL,*** sublingual; ***T,*** tablets.

Skeletal Muscle Relaxants

USES

Central acting muscle relaxants: Adjunct to rest, physical therapy for relief of discomfort associated with acute, painful musculoskeletal disorders (i.e., local spasms from muscle injury).

Baclofen, dantrolene, diazepam: Treatment of spasticity characterized by heightened muscle tone, spasm, loss of dexterity caused by multiple sclerosis, cerebral palsy, spinal cord lesions, CVA.

ACTION

Central acting muscle relaxants: Exact mechanism unknown. May act in CNS at various levels to depress polysynaptic reflexes; sedative effect may be responsible for relaxation of muscle spasm.

Baclofen, diazepam: May mimic actions of gamma-aminobutyric acid on spinal neurons; do not directly affect skeletal muscles.

Dantrolene: Acts directly on skeletal muscle, relieving spasticity.

SKELETAL MUSCLE RELAXANTS

Name	Indication	Dosage Range	Side Effects/Comments
Baclofen (Lioresal)	Spasticity associated with multiple sclerosis, spinal cord injury	Initially 5 mg 3 times/day Increase by 5 mg 3 times/day q3days **Maximum:** 20 mg 4 times/day	Drowsiness, dizziness, GI effects Caution with renal impairment, seizure disorders Withdrawal syndrome (e.g., hallucinations, psychosis, seizures)
Carisoprodol (Rela)	Discomfort due to acute, painful, musculoskeletal conditions	250–350 mg 4 times/day	Drowsiness, dizziness, GI effects Hypomania at higher than recommended doses Withdrawal syndrome Hypersensitivity reaction (skin reaction, bronchospasm, weakness, burning eyes, fever) or idiosyncratic reaction (weakness, visual or motor disturbances, confusion) usually occurring within first 4 doses

Continued

SKELETAL MUSCLE RELAXANTS—cont'd

Chlorzoxazone (Lorzone)	Discomfort due to acute, painful, musculoskeletal conditions	Initially 250–500 mg 3–4 times/day **Maximum:** 750 mg 3–4 times/day	Drowsiness, dizziness, GI effects, rare hepatotoxicity Hypersensitivity reaction (urticaria, itching) Urine discoloration to orange, red, or purple
Cyclobenzaprine (Flexeril)	Muscle spasm, pain, tenderness, restricted movement due to acute, painful, musculoskeletal conditions	Initially 5–10 mg 3 times/day	Drowsiness, dizziness, GI effects Anticholinergic effects (dry mouth, urinary retention) Quinidine-like effects on heart (QT prolongation) Long half-life
Dantrolene (Dantrium)	Spasticity associated with multiple sclerosis, cerebral palsy, spinal cord injury	Initially 25 mg/day for 1 wk, then 25 mg 3 times/day for 1 wk, then 50 mg 3 times/day for 1 wk, then 100 mg 3 times/day **Maximum:** 100 mg 4 times/day	Drowsiness, dizziness, GI effects Contraindicated with hepatic disease Dose-dependent hepatotoxicity Diarrhea that is dose dependent and may be severe, requiring discontinuation
Diazepam (Valium)	Spasticity associated with cerebral palsy, spinal cord injury; reflex spasm due to muscle, joint trauma or inflammation	2–10 mg 3–4 times/day	Drowsiness, dizziness, GI effects Abuse potential
Metaxalone (Skelaxin)	Discomfort due to acute, painful, musculoskeletal conditions	800 mg 3–4 times/day	Drowsiness (low risk), dizziness, GI effects Paradoxical muscle cramps Mild withdrawal syndrome Contraindicated in serious hepatic or renal disease
Methocarbamol (Robaxin)	Discomfort due to acute, painful, musculoskeletal conditions	Initially 1,500 mg 4 times/day Maintenance: 1,000 mg 4 times/day	Drowsiness, dizziness, GI effects Urine discoloration to brown, brown-black, or green

Name	Indication	Dosage Range	Side Effects/Comments
Orphenadrine (Norflex)	Discomfort due to acute, painful, musculoskeletal conditions	100 mg 2 times/day	Drowsiness, dizziness, GI effects Long half-life Anticholinergic effects (dry mouth, urinary retention) Rare aplastic anemia Some products may contain sulfites
Tizanidine (Zanaflex)	Spasticity	Initially 4 mg q6–8h (**maximum** 3 times/day), may increase by 2–4 mg as needed/tolerated **Maximum:** 36 mg (limited information on doses greater than 24 mg)	Drowsiness, dizziness, GI effects Hypotension (20% decrease in B/P) Hepatotoxicity (usually reversible) Withdrawal syndrome (hypertension, tachycardia, hypertonia) Effect is short lived (3–6 hrs) Dose cautiously with creatinine clearance less than 25 mL/min

B/P, Blood pressure; ***GI,*** gastrointestinal.

Smoking Cessation Agents

Tobacco smoking is associated with the development of lung cancer and chronic obstructive pulmonary disease. Smoking is harmful not just to the smoker but also to family members, coworkers, and others breathing cigarette smoke.

Quitting smoking decreases the risk of developing lung cancer, other cancers, heart disease, stroke, and respiratory illnesses. Several medications have proved useful as smoking cessation aids. Nausea and lightheadedness are possible signs of overdose of nicotine warranting a reduction in dosage.

SMOKING CESSATION AGENTS

Name	Availability	Dose Duration	Cautions/Side Effects	Comments
Bupropion (Zyban)	**T:** 150 mg	150 mg every morning for 3 days, then 150 mg 2 times/day Start 1–2 wks before quit date **Duration:** 7–12 wks up to 6 mos for maintenance	History of seizure, eating disorder, use of MAOI within previous 14 days, bipolar disorder **Side Effects:** Insomnia, dry mouth, tremor, rash	Stop smoking during second wk of treatment and use counseling support services along with medication

Nicotine gum (Nicorette)	**Squares:** 2 mg, 4 mg	1 gum q1–2h for 6 wks, then q2–4h for 3 wks then q4–8h for 3 wks **Maximum:** 24 pieces/day **Duration:** up to 12 wks	Recent MI (within 2 wks), serious arrhythmias, serious or worsening angina pectoris **Side Effects:** Dyspepsia, mouth soreness, hiccups	2 mg recommended for pts smoking less than 25 cigarettes/day, 4 mg for pts smoking 25 or more cigarettes/day Chew until a peppery or minty taste emerges and then "park" between cheek and gums to facilitate nicotine absorption through oral mucosa Chew slowly and intermittently to avoid jaw ache and achieve maximum benefit Only water should be taken 15 min before and during chewing
Nicotine inhaler (Nicotrol)	**Cartridge:** 10 mg (delivers 4 mg nicotine)	4–16 cartridges daily; taper frequency of use over the last 6–12 wks **Duration:** up to 6 mos	Recent MI (within 2 wks), serious arrhythmias, serious or worsening angina pectoris **Side Effects:** Local irritation of mouth and throat, coughing, rhinitis	Use at or above room temperature (cold temperatures decrease amount of nicotine inhaled)
Nicotine lozenge (Nicorette Lozenges)	**Lozenges:** 2 mg, 4 mg	One lozenge q1–2h for 6 wks, then q2–4h for 3 wks, then q4–8h for 3 wks **Duration:** 12 wks **Maximum:** 5 lozenges in 6 hrs; 20 lozenges in 1 day	Recent MI (within 2 wks), serious arrhythmias, serious or worsening angina pectoris **Side Effects:** Local skin reaction, insomnia, nausea, sore throat	First cigarette smoked within 30 min of waking, use 4 mg; after 30 min of waking, use 2 mg Use at least 9 lozenges/day first 6 wks Only 1 lozenge at a time, 5 per 6 hrs and 20 per 24 hrs Do not chew or swallow
Nicotine nasal spray (Nicotrol NS)	10 mg/ml (delivers 0.5 mg/spray)	8–40 doses/day A dose consists of one 0.5 mg delivery to each nostril; initial dose is 1–2 sprays/hr, increasing as needed **Duration:** 3–6 mos	Recent MI (within 2 wks), serious arrhythmias, serious or worsening angina pectoris **Side Effects:** Nasal irritation	Do not sniff, swallow, or inhale through nose while administering nicotine doses (may increase irritation) Tilt head back slightly for best results

SMOKING CESSATION AGENTS—cont'd

Nicotine patch (NicoDerm CQ)	**Nicoderm CQ:** 7 mg/24 hrs, 14 mg/24 hrs, 21 mg/24 hrs **Nicotrol:** 5 mg/16 hrs, 10 mg/16 hrs, 15 mg/16 hrs	Apply upon waking on quit date: **Nicoderm CQ (greater than 10 cigarettes/day):** 21 mg/24 hrs for 4 wks, then 14 mg/24 hrs for 2 wks, then 7 mg/24 hrs for 2 wks **(10 or fewer cigarettes/day):** 14 mg/24 hrs for 6 wks, then 7 mg/24 hrs for 2 wks	Recent MI (within 2 wks), serious arrhythmias, serious or worsening angina pectoris **Side Effects:** Local skin reaction, insomnia	The 16- and 24-hr patches are of comparable efficacy Begin with a lower-dose patch in pts smoking 10 or fewer cigarettes/day Place new patch on relatively hair-free location, usually between neck and waist, in the morning If insomnia occurs, remove the 24-hr patch prior to bedtime or use the 16-hr patch Rotate patch site to diminish skin irritation
Varenicline (Chantix)	**T:** 0.5 mg, 1 mg	**Days 1–3:** 0.5 mg daily; **days 4–7:** 0.5 mg 2 times/day; **day 8 to end of treatment:** 1 mg 2 times/day **Duration:** begin 1 wk before set quit date, continue for 12 wks. May use additional 12 wks if failed to quit after first 12 wks	**Side Effects:** Nausea; sleep disturbances; headaches; may impair ability to drive, operate machinery; depressed mood; altered behavior; suicidal ideation reported	Use lower dosage if not able to tolerate nausea and vomiting Use counseling support services along with medication

B/P, Blood pressure; ***MAOI,*** monoamine oxidase inhibitor; ***MI,*** myocardial infarction; ***T,*** tablets.

Vitamins

INTRODUCTION

Vitamins are organic substances required for growth, reproduction, and maintenance of health and are obtained from food or supplementation in small quantities (vitamins cannot be synthesized by the body or the rate of synthesis is too slow/inadequate to meet metabolic needs). Vitamins are essential for energy transformation and regulation of metabolic processes. They are catalysts for all reactions using proteins, fats, carbohydrates for energy, growth, and cell maintenance.

WATER SOLUBLE

Water-soluble vitamins include vitamin C (ascorbic acid), B_1 (thiamine), B_2 (riboflavin), B_3 (niacin), B_5 (pantothenic acid), B_6 (pyridoxine), folic acid, B_{12} (cyanocobalamin). Water-soluble vitamins act as coenzymes for almost every cellular reaction in the body. B-complex vitamins differ from one another in both structure and function but are grouped together because they first were isolated from the same source (yeast and liver).

FAT SOLUBLE

Fat-soluble vitamins include vitamins A, D, E, and K. They are soluble in lipids and are usually absorbed into the lymphatic system of the small intestine and then into the general circulation. Absorption is facilitated by bile. These vitamins are stored in the body tissue when excessive quantities are consumed. May be toxic when taken in large doses (see sections on individual vitamins).

VITAMINS

Name	Uses	Deficiency	Side Effects
Vitamin A (Aquasol A)	Required for normal growth, bone development, vision, reproduction, maintenance of epithelial tissue	Dry skin, poor tooth development, night blindness	**High dosages:** Hepatotoxicity, cheilitis, facial dermatitis, photosensitivity, mucosal dryness
Vitamin B_1 (thiamine)	Important in red blood cell formation, carbohydrate metabolism, neurologic function, myocardial contractility, growth, energy production	Fatigue, anorexia, growth retardation	**Large parenteral doses:** May cause pain on injection
Vitamin B_2 (riboflavin)	Necessary for function of coenzymes in oxidation-reduction reactions, essential for normal cellular growth, assists in absorption of iron and pyridoxine	Numbness in extremities, blurred vision, photophobia, cheilosis	Orange-yellow discoloration in urine

Continued

VITAMINS—cont'd

Name	Uses	Deficiency	Side Effects
Vitamin B_3 (niacin)	Coenzyme for many oxidation-reduction reactions	Pellagra, headache, anorexia, memory loss, insomnia	**High dosages (more than 500 mg):** Nausea, vomiting, diarrhea, gastritis, hepatotoxicity, skin rash, facial flushing, headaches
Vitamin B_5 (pantothenic acid)	Precursor to coenzyme A, important in synthesis of cholesterol, hormones, fatty acids	Natural deficiency unknown	Occasional GI disturbances (e.g., diarrhea)
Vitamin B_6 (pyridoxine)	Enzyme cofactor for amino acid metabolism, essential for erythrocyte production, Hgb synthesis	Neuritis, anemia, lymphopenia	**High dosages:** May cause sensory neuropathy
Vitamin B_{12} (cyanocobalamin)	Coenzyme in cells, including bone marrow, CNS, and GI tract, necessary for lipid metabolism, formation of myelin	Gastrointestinal disorders, anemias, poor growth	Skin rash, diarrhea, pain at injection site
Vitamin C (ascorbic acid)	Cofactor in various physiologic reactions, necessary for collagen formation, acts as antioxidant	Poor wound healing, bleeding gums, scurvy	**High dosages:** May cause calcium oxalate crystalluria, esophagitis, diarrhea
Vitamin D (Calciferol)	Necessary for proper formation of bone, calcium, mineral homeostasis, regulation of parathyroid hormone, calcitonin, phosphate	Rickets, osteomalacia	Hypercalcemia, kidney stones, renal failure, hypertension, psychosis, diarrhea, nausea, vomiting, anorexia, fatigue, headaches, altered mental status
Vitamin E (Aquasol E)	Antioxidant, promotes formation, functioning of red blood cells, muscle, other tissues	Red blood cell breakdown	**High dosages:** GI disturbances, malaise, headaches

CNS, Central nervous system; ***GI,*** gastrointestinal.

abacavir/ dolutegravir/ lamivudine

a-**bak**-a-veer/**doe**-loo-**teg**-ra-vir/la-**miv**-yoo-deen
(Triumeq)

■ BLACK BOX ALERT ■ Serious, sometimes fatal hypersensitivity reactions, lactic acidosis, severe hepatomegaly with steatosis (fatty liver) have occurred with abacavir-containing products, esp. in pts who carry the HLA-B*5701 allele. Restarting abacavir following a hypersensitivity reaction may be life-threatening. May cause hepatitis B virus reactivation.

Do not confuse abacavir with entecavir, or dolutegravir with elvitegravir or raltegravir, or lamivudine with telbivudine or lamotrigine.

FIXED-COMBINATION(S)

abacavir/dolutegravir/lamivudine (antiretrovirals): 600 mg/50 mg/300 mg.

◆CLASSIFICATION

PHARMACOTHERAPEUTIC: Integrase inhibitor (INSTI), reverse transcriptase inhibitor, nucleoside. **CLINICAL:** Antiretroviral.

USES

Treatment of HIV-1 infection, in adults and children weighing at least 40 kg.

PRECAUTIONS

Contraindications: Hypersensitivity to abacavir, dolutegravir, lamivudine. Pts who test positive for the HLA-B*5701 allele. Concomitant use of dofetilide. Pts with moderate to severe hepatic impairment. **Cautions:** Diabetes, hepatic/renal impairment, coronary artery disease, history of hepatitis or tuberculosis, prior hypersensitivity reaction to INSTIs. Use in children with history of pancreatitis or risk factors for developing pancreatitis. Not recommended in pts with resistance-associated integrase substitutions or clinically suspected integrase strand transfer inhibitor resistance; creatinine clearance less than 50 mL/min; mild hepatic impairment; children weighing less than 40 kg.

ACTION

Abacavir interferes with HIV viral RNA-dependent DNA polymerase. Dolutegravir inhibits HIV integrase by blocking strand transfer step of retroviral DNA integration (essential for HIV replication cycle). Lamivudine inhibits reverse transcriptase by viral DNA chain termination. **Therapeutic Effect:** Interferes with HIV replication, slowing progression of HIV infection.

PHARMACOKINETICS

Abacavir, lamivudine rapidly absorbed and widely distributed. Abacavir distributes into cerebrospinal fluid (CSF) and erythrocytes. Abacavir metabolized by alcohol dehydrogenase and glucuronyl transferase. Dolutegravir metabolized in liver. Protein binding: abacavir: 50%; dolutegravir: 98.9%; lamivudine: less than 36%. Peak plasma concentration: dolutegravir: 2–3 hrs. Excretion: abacavir: urine (primary); dolutegravir: feces (53%), urine (31%); lamivudine: urine (70%). **Half-life:** abacavir: 1.5 hrs; dolutegravir: 14 hrs; lamivudine: 5–7 hrs.

⌛ LIFESPAN CONSIDERATIONS

Pregnancy/Lactation: Breastfeeding not recommended due to risk of postnatal HIV transmission. Unknown if distributed in breast milk. **Children:** Safety and efficacy not established in pts weighing less than 40 kg. **Elderly:** May have increased risk of adverse effects; worsening of hepatic, renal, cardiac function.

INTERACTIONS

DRUG: Dolutegravir may increase concentration/effect of **dofetilide** (contraindicated). **Fosphenytoin, phenytoin, nevirapine, oxcarbazepine, phenobarbital, primidone** may decrease concentration of dolutegravir. **Lamivudine** may increase adverse/toxic effects of **emtricitabine.** **HERBAL:** **St. John's wort** may decrease effect of dolutegravir. **FOOD:** None known. **LAB VALUES:** May increase serum amylase, ALT, AST, bilirubin, cholesterol, creatine kinase (CK), creatinine, glucose, lipase, triglycerides. May decrease Hgb, Hct, neutrophils.

AVAILABILITY (Rx)

Fixed-Dose Combination Tablet: abacavir 600 mg/dolutegravir 50 mg/lamivudine 300 mg.

ADMINISTRATION/HANDLING

PO

• Give without regard to food. • Administer at least 2 hrs before or at least 6 hrs after giving medications containing aluminum, calcium, iron, magnesium (supplements, antacids, laxatives).

INDICATIONS/ROUTES/DOSAGE

HIV Infection

PO: ADULTS, ELDERLY, CHILDREN WEIGHING 40 KG OR MORE: 1 tablet once daily.

Dosage in Renal Impairment

Creatinine clearance less than 50 mL/min: Not recommended.

Dosage in Hepatic Impairment

Mild impairment: Consider use of individual components. **Moderate to severe impairment:** Contraindicated.

SIDE EFFECTS

Rare (3%–1%): Insomnia, fatigue, headache, abdominal pain/distension, dyspepsia, flatulence, gastroesophageal reflux disease, fever, lethargy, anorexia, arthralgia, myositis, somnolence, pruritus, depression, abnormal dreams, dizziness, nausea, diarrhea, rash.

ADVERSE EFFECTS/ TOXIC REACTIONS

Serious and sometimes fatal hypersensitivity reactions including anaphylaxis, severe diarrhea, dyspnea, hypotension, intractable nausea/vomiting, multi-organ failure, pharyngitis may occur within the first 6 wks of treatment with abacavir (8% of pts). If therapy is discontinued, pts co-infected with hepatitis B or C virus have an increased risk for viral replication, worsening of hepatic function, and may experience hepatic decompensation and/or failure. May induce immune recovery syndrome (inflammatory response to dormant opportunistic infections such as *Mycobacterium avium*, cytomegalovirus, PCP, tuberculosis, or acceleration of autoimmune disorders such as Graves' disease, polymyositis, Guillain-Barré). Fatal cases of lactic acidosis, severe hepatomegaly with steatosis have been reported. Hepatic failure occurred in 1% of pts taking dolutegravir-containing products. Abacavir-containing products may increase risk of myocardial infarction, erythema multiform, Stevens-Johnson Syndrome, toxic epidermal necrolysis. May increase risk of pancreatitis.

NURSING CONSIDERATIONS

BASELINE ASSESSMENT

Obtain CBC, BMP, LFT, CD4+ count, viral load, HIV-1 RNA level. Obtain weight in kilograms. Screen for HLA-B* 5701 allele, hepatitis B or C virus infection before initiating therapy. Question for prior hypersensitivity reactions (especially to abacavir-containing products); history of diabetes, coronary artery disease, hepatic/renal impairment. Receive full medication history, including herbal products. Offer emotional support.

INTERVENTION/EVALUATION

Monitor CBC, BMP, LFT periodically. Immediately discontinue if hypersensitivity reaction is suspected, even when other diagnoses are possible (e.g., pneumonia, bronchitis, pharyngitis, influenza, gastroenteritis, reactions to other medications). Stop treatment if 3 or more of the following symptoms occur: rash, fever, GI disturbances (diarrhea, nausea, vomiting), flu-like symptoms, respiratory distress. If hypersensitivity reaction is related to abacavir, do not restart treatment (may cause more severe reactions and/or death within hours). Assess for hepatic impairment (bruising, hematuria, jaundice, right upper abdominal pain, nausea, vomiting, weight loss). Screen for immune recovery syndrome, rhabdomyolysis (muscle weakness, myalgia, decreased urinary output). Pediatric pts should be closely monitored for symptoms of pancreatitis (severe, steady abdominal pain often radiating to the back; clammy skin, reduced B/P; nausea and vomiting accompanied by abdominal pain). Monitor daily stool pattern, consistency; I&Os. Assess dietary pattern; monitor for weight loss. Screen for toxic skin reactions. Monitor for symptoms of MI (jaw/chest/left arm pain or pressure, dyspnea, diaphoresis, vomiting).

PATIENT/FAMILY TEACHING

• Blood levels will be monitored periodically. • Treatment does not cure HIV infection nor reduce risk of transmission. Practice safe sex with barrier methods or abstinence. • As immune system strengthens, it may respond to dormant infections hidden within the body. Report any new fever, chills, body aches, cough, night sweats, shortness of breath. • Antiretrovirals may cause excess body fat in upper back, neck, breast, trunk; may cause decreased body fat in legs, arms, face. • Drug resistance can form if therapy is interrupted for even a short time; do not run out of supply. • Report signs of abdominal pain, darkened urine, decreased urine output, yellowing of skin or eyes, clay colored stools, weight loss. • Do not breastfeed. • Small, frequent meals may offset anorexia, nausea. • Take dose at least 2 hrs before or at least 6 hrs after other medications containing aluminum, calcium, iron, magnesium (supplements, antacids, laxatives). • Do not take newly prescribed medications, including OTC drugs, unless approved by doctor who originally started treatment.

abaloparatide

a-**bal**-oh-**par**-a-tide
(Tymlos)

BLACK BOX ALERT May cause a dose-dependent increase in the incidence of osteosarcoma. It is unknown whether abaloparatide will cause osteosarcoma in humans. Avoid use in pts at risk for osteosarcoma (e.g., pts with Paget's disease of bone or unexplained elevations of alkaline phosphatase, pediatric and young adults with open epiphyses, pts with bone metastasis or skeletal malignancies, hereditary disorders predisposing to osteosarcoma, or prior history of external beam or implant radiation involving the skeleton. Cumulative use of parathyroid analogs (e.g., teriparatide) for more than 2 yrs during a pt's lifetime is not recommended.

Do not confuse abaloparatide with teriparatide.

◆CLASSIFICATION

PHARMACOTHERAPEUTIC: Parathyroid hormone receptor analog. **CLINICAL:** Osteoporosis agent.

USES

Treatment of postmenopausal women with osteoporosis at high risk for fracture, defined as history of osteoporotic fracture, multiple risk factors for fracture, or pts who have failed or are intolerant to other osteoporosis therapy.

PRECAUTIONS

Contraindications: Hypersensitivity to abaloparatide. **Cautions:** Pts at risk for hypercalcemia (e.g., hyperparathyroidism, renal impairment, severe dehydration; history of hypercalciuria, urolithiasis). Avoid use in pts at increased risk for osteosarcoma (e.g., pts with Paget's disease of bone or unexplained elevations of alkaline phosphatase, open epiphyses, bone or skeletal malignancies, hereditary disorders predisposing to osteosarcoma, prior radiation therapy involving the skeleton). Not recommended in pts with cumulative use of parathyroid analogs greater than 2 yrs during lifetime.

ACTION

Acts as an agonist at the PTH1 receptor. **Therapeutic Effect:** Stimulates osteoblast function and increases bone mass, decreasing risk of fractures.

PHARMACOKINETICS

Widely distributed. Metabolism not specified. Degraded into small peptides via proteolytic enzymes. Protein binding: 70%. Peak plasma concentration: 0.51 hrs. Excreted primarily in urine. Not expected to be removed by dialysis. **Half-life:** 1.7 hrs.

⌛ LIFESPAN CONSIDERATIONS

Pregnancy/Lactation: Not indicated in females of reproductive potential. Unknown if distributed in breast milk or crosses the placenta. **Children:** Safety and efficacy not established. **Elderly:** No age-related precautions noted.

INTERACTIONS

DRUG: None known. **HERBAL:** None significant. **FOOD:** None known. **LAB VALUES:** May increase serum calcium, uric acid; urine calcium.

AVAILABILITY (Rx)

Prefilled Injector Pens: 3120 mcg/1.56 mL (2000 mcg/mL). Delivers 30 doses of 80 mcg.

ADMINISTRATION/HANDLING

SQ

• Visually inspect for particulate matter or discoloration. Solution should appear clear, colorless. • Do not use if solution is cloudy, discolored, or if visible particles are observed. • Insert needle subcutaneously into the periumbilical region of the abdomen (avoid a 2-inch area around the navel) and inject solution. • Do not inject into areas of active skin disease or injury such as sunburns, skin rashes, inflammation, skin infections, or active psoriasis. • Do not administer IV or intramuscularly. • Rotate injection sites. **Storage** • Refrigerate unused injector pens. • After first use, store at room temperature for up to 30 days. • Do not freeze or expose to heating sources.

INDICATIONS/ROUTES/DOSAGE

Postmenopausal Osteoporosis

SQ: ADULTS, ELDERLY: 80 mcg once daily. Give with supplemental calcium and vitamin D if dietary intake is inadequate.

Dosage in Renal Impairment

No dose adjustment.

Dosage in Hepatic Impairment

Not specified; use caution.

SIDE EFFECTS

Frequent (58%): Injection site reactions (edema, pain, redness). **Occasional (10%–5%):** Dizziness, nausea, headache, palpitations. **Rare (3%–2%):** Fatigue, upper abdominal pain, vertigo.

ADVERSE EFFECTS/TOXIC REACTIONS

May increase risk of osteosarcoma. Hypercalcemia reported in 3% of pts. Tachycardia occurred in 2% of pts (usually within 15 min after injection). Orthostatic hypotension reported in 4% of pts (usually within 4 hrs after injection). Hypercalciuria and urolithiasis reported in 20% and 2% of pts, respectively. Immunogenicity (auto-abaloparatide antibodies) occurred in 49% of pts.

NURSING CONSIDERATIONS

BASELINE ASSESSMENT

Obtain baseline parathyroid hormone level. Screen for risk of osteosarcoma, hypercalcemia (as listed in Precautions); prior use of parathyroid analogs. Assess pt's willingness to self-inject medication.

INTERVENTION/EVALUATION

Monitor bone mineral density, parathyroid hormone level; serum calcium. Monitor urinary calcium levels, esp. in pts with preexisting hypercalciuria or active urolithiasis. Due to risk of orthostatic hypotension, administer the first several doses with the pt in the lying or sitting position. Monitor for orthostatic hypotension (dizziness, palpitations, tachycardia, nausea, syncope). If orthostatic hypotension occurs, place pt in supine position. Assess need for calcium, vitamin D supplementation.

PATIENT/FAMILY TEACHING

• Receive the first several injections while lying or sitting down. Slowly go from lying to standing to avoid an unusual drop in blood pressure. Immediately sit or lie down if dizziness, near-fainting, palpitations occur. • Report symptoms of high calcium levels (e.g., constipation, lethargy, nausea, vomiting, weakness); severe bone pain. • An increased heart rate may occur after injection and will usually subside within 6 hrs. • A healthcare provider will show you how to properly prepare and inject your medication. You must demonstrate correct preparation and injection techniques before using medication at home. • Vitamin D and calcium supplementation may be required if dietary intake is inadequate.

abatacept

TOP 100

a-**bay**-ta-sept
(Orencia)
Do not confuse Orencia, Orencia ClickJect

◆CLASSIFICATION

PHARMACOTHERAPEUTIC: Selective T-cell co-stimulation modulator.
CLINICAL: Antirheumatic: disease modifying.

USES

Reduction of signs and symptoms, progression of structural damage in adults with moderate to severe rheumatoid arthritis (RA) alone or in combination with methotrexate. Treatment of active adult psoriatic arthritis. Treatment of moderate to severe active polyarticular juvenile idiopathic arthritis in pts 2 yrs and older. May use alone or in combination with methotrexate. **Note:** Do not use with anakinra or tumor necrosis factor [TNF] antagonists.

PRECAUTIONS

Contraindications: Hypersensitivity to abatacept. **Cautions:** Chronic, latent, or localized infection; conditions predisposing to infections (diabetes, indwelling catheters, renal failure, open wounds); COPD (higher incidence of adverse effects); elderly, hx recurrent infections.

ACTION

Inhibits T-cell (T-lymphocyte) activation (binds to CD80 and CD86 on antigen-presenting cells (APCs); blocks CD28 interaction between APCs and T-cells). Activated T-cells are found in synovium of rheumatoid arthritic patients. **Therapeutic Effect:** Induces positive clinical response in adult pts with moderate to severely active RA or juvenile idiopathic arthritis.

PHARMACOKINETICS

Higher clearance with increasing body weight. Age, gender do not affect clearance. **Half-life:** 8–25 days.

⌛ LIFESPAN CONSIDERATIONS

Pregnancy/Lactation: Crosses placenta; unknown if distributed in breast milk. **Children:** Safety and efficacy not established in pts younger than 6 yrs. **Elderly:** Cautious use due to increased risk of serious infection and malignancy.

INTERACTIONS

DRUG: **Anakinra, anti-TNF agents, baricitinib, pimecrolimus, rituximab, tacrolimus (topical), tocilizumab** may increase adverse effects. May decrease therapeutic effects of **BCG (intravesical), vaccines (live).** May increase concentration/effects of **belimumab, natalizumab, tofacitinib, vaccines (live).** **HERBAL:** **Echinacea** may decrease concentration/effect. **FOOD:** None known. **LAB VALUES:** None significant.

AVAILABILITY (Rx)

IV Injection, Powder for Reconstitution: 250 mg. **SQ Injection, Solution:** 50 mg/0.4 mL, 87.5 mg/0.7 mL, 125 mg/mL single-dose prefilled syringe.

ADMINISTRATION/HANDLING

IV

Reconstitution • Reconstitute each vial with 10 mL Sterile Water for Injection using the silicone-free syringe provided with each vial and an 18- to 21-gauge needle. • Rotate solution gently to prevent foaming until powder is completely dissolved. • From a 100-mL 0.9% NaCl infusion bag, withdraw and discard an amount equal to the volume of the reconstituted vials (for 2 vials remove 20 mL, for 3 vials remove 30 mL, for 4 vials remove 40 mL), resulting in final volume of 100 mL. • Slowly add the reconstituted solution from each vial into the infusion bag using the same syringe provided with each vial. • Concentration in the infusion bag will be 10 mg/mL or less abatacept.

Rate of administration • Infuse over 30 min using a 0.2 to 1.2 micron low protein-binding filter.

Storage • Store vials, prefilled syringes in refrigerator. • Any reconstitution that has been prepared by using siliconized syringes will develop translucent particles and must be discarded. • Solution should appear clear and colorless to pale yellow. Discard if solution is discolored or contains precipitate. • Solution is stable for up to 24 hrs after reconstitution. • Reconstituted solution may be stored at room temperature or refrigerated.

SQ

• Allow syringe to warm to room temperature (30–60 min). • Inject in front of thigh, outer areas of upper arms, or abdomen. • Avoid areas that are tender, bruised, red, scaly, or hard. • Do not rub injection site. • Rotate injection sites.

IV INCOMPATIBILITIES

Do not infuse concurrently in same IV line as other agents.

INDICATIONS/ROUTES/DOSAGE

Note: Discontinue in pts developing serious infection.

Rheumatoid Arthritis (RA), Psoriatic Arthritis (PsA)

IV: ADULTS, ELDERLY WEIGHING 101 KG OR MORE: 1 g (4 vials) given as a 30-min infusion. Following initial therapy, give at 2 wks and 4 wks after first infusion, then q4wks thereafter. **WEIGHING 60–100 KG:** 750 mg (3 vials) given as a 30-min infusion. Following initial therapy, give at 2 wks and 4 wks after first infusion, then q4wks thereafter. **WEIGHING 59 KG OR LESS:** 500 mg (2 vials) given as a 30-min infusion. Following initial therapy, give at 2 wks and 4 wks after first infusion, then q4wks thereafter.

SQ: (RA): Following a single IV infusion, 125 mg given within 24 hrs of infusion, then 125 mg once a week (SQ administration may be initiated without an IV loading dose). **(PsA):** Give without an IV loading dose. 125 mg once weekly.

Transitioning from IV to SQ: Give 1st SQ dose instead of next scheduled IV dose.

Juvenile Idiopathic Arthritis

Note: Dose based on body weight at each administration.

IV: CHILDREN 6 YRS AND OLDER, WEIGHING LESS THAN 75 KG: 10 mg/kg. **CHILDREN WEIGHING 75–100 KG:** 750 mg. **WEIGHING MORE THAN 100 KG:** 1,000 mg. Following initial therapy, give 2 wks and 4 wks after first infusion, then q4wks thereafter.

SQ: CHILDREN 2 YRS AND OLDER, ADOLESCENTS WEIGHING 50 KG OR MORE: 125 mg once weekly. **WEIGHING 25–49 KG:** 87.5 mg once weekly. **WEIGHING 10–24 KG:** 50 mg once weekly.

Dosage Adjustment for Toxicity
Discontinue in pts developing a serious infection.

Dosage in Renal/Hepatic Impairment
No dose adjustment.

SIDE EFFECTS

Frequent (18%): Headache. **Occasional (9%–6%):** Dizziness, cough, back pain, hypertension, nausea.

ADVERSE EFFECTS/TOXIC REACTIONS

Upper respiratory tract infection, nasopharyngitis, sinusitis, UTI, influenza, bronchitis occur in 5% of pts. Serious infections, including pneumonia, cellulitis, diverticulitis, acute pyelonephritis, occur in 3% of pts. Hypersensitivity reaction (rash, urticaria, hypotension, dyspnea) occurs rarely. May increase risk of malignancies.

NURSING CONSIDERATIONS

BASELINE ASSESSMENT

Assess onset, type, location, duration of pain/inflammation. Inspect appearance of affected joint for immobility, deformities, skin condition. Screen for latent TB infection prior to initiating therapy.

INTERVENTION/EVALUATION

Assess for therapeutic response: relief of pain, stiffness, swelling; increased joint mobility; reduced joint tenderness; improved grip strength. Monitor for hypersensitivity reaction. Diligently screen for infection.

PATIENT/FAMILY TEACHING

• Notify physician if infection, hypersensitivity reaction, infusion-related reaction occurs. • Do not receive live vaccines during treatment or within 3 mos of its discontinuation. • COPD pts must report worsening of respiratory symptoms.

abemaciclib

a-**bem**-a-**sye**-klib
(Verzenio)
Do not confuse abemaciclib with palbociclib or ribociclib.

◆CLASSIFICATION

PHARMACOTHERAPEUTIC: Cyclin-dependent kinase inhibitor. **CLINICAL:** Antineoplastic.

USES

Used in combination with an aromatase inhibitor as initial endocrine-based therapy for treatment of postmenopausal women with hormone receptor (HR)-positive, human epidermal growth factor receptor 2 (HER2)-negative advanced or metastatic breast cancer. Used in combination with fulvestrant for treatment of women with HR-positive, HER2-negative advanced or metastatic breast cancer with disease progression following endocrine therapy. Used as monotherapy for treatment of adults with HR-positive, HER2-negative advanced or metastatic breast cancer with disease progression following endocrine therapy and prior chemotherapy in the metastatic setting.

PRECAUTIONS

Contraindications: Hypersensitivity to abemaciclib. **Cautions:** Baseline anemia, leukopenia, neutropenia, thrombocytopenia; hepatic/renal impairment, conditions predisposing to infection (e.g., diabetes, immunocompromised pts, open wounds), history of venous thromboembolism. Avoid concomitant use of strong CYP3A inhibitors, strong CYP3A inducers.

ACTION

Blocks retinoblastoma tumor suppressor protein phosphorylation and prevents progression through cell cycle, resulting in arrest of G1 phase. **Therapeutic Effect:** Inhibits tumor cell growth and survival.

PHARMACOKINETICS

Widely distributed. Metabolized in liver. Protein binding: 96.3%. Peak plasma concentration: 8 hrs. Steady-state reached in 5 days. Excreted in feces (81%), urine (3%). **Half-life:** 18.3 hrs.

LIFESPAN CONSIDERATIONS

Pregnancy/Lactation: Avoid pregnancy; may cause fetal harm/malformations. Females of reproductive potential should use effective contraception during treatment and up to 3 wks after discontinuation. Unknown if distributed in breast milk. Breastfeeding not recommended during treatment and up to 3 wks after discontinuation. May impair fertility in males. **Children:** Safety and efficacy not established. **Elderly:** No age-related precautions noted.

INTERACTIONS

DRUG: **Strong CYP3A inhibitors (e.g., clarithromycin, ketoconazole, ritonavir), moderate CYP3A inhibitors (e.g., erythromycin, diltiazem, dronedarone, fluconazole)** may increase concentration/effect. **Strong CYP3A inducers (e.g., carbamazepine, phenytoin, rifampin)** may decrease concentration/effect. May decrease effect of **BCG (intravesical), vaccines (live).** May enhance adverse/toxic effects of **natalizumab, vaccines (live). Pimecrolimus, tacrolimus** may enhance adverse/toxic effects. **HERBAL:** **Echinacea** may decrease therapeutic effect. **FOOD:** **Grapefruit products** may increase concentration/effect. **LAB VALUES:** May increase serum ALT, AST, bilirubin, creatinine. May decrease ANC, Hgb, Hct, lymphocytes, leukocytes, neutrophils, platelets.

AVAILABILITY (Rx)

Tablets: 50 mg, 100 mg, 150 mg, 200 mg.

ADMINISTRATION/HANDLING

PO

• Give without regard to food. • Administer whole; do not crush, cut, or divide tablets. Do not give broken or cracked tablets. • If a dose is missed or vomiting occurs, do not give extra dose. Administer next dose at regularly scheduled time.

INDICATIONS/ROUTES/DOSAGE

Breast Cancer

PO: ADULTS, ELDERLY: Monotherapy: 200 mg twice daily. **In combination with fulvestrant (and a gonadotropin-releasing hormone agonist if pre- or perimenopausal) or an aromatase inhibitor:** 150 mg twice daily. Continue until disease progression or unacceptable toxicity. Recommended dose of fulvestrant is 500 mg once on days 1, 15, 29, then monthly thereafter.

Dose Reduction for Adverse Events

Monotherapy: Starting dose: 200 mg twice daily. **FIRST DOSE REDUCTION:** 150 mg twice daily. **SECOND DOSE REDUCTION:** 100 mg twice daily. **THIRD DOSE REDUCTION:** 50 mg twice daily. **In combination with fulvestrant or an aromatase inhibitor: STARTING DOSE:** 150 mg twice daily. **FIRST DOSE REDUCTION:** 100 mg twice daily. **SECOND DOSE REDUCTION:** 50 mg twice daily.

Dose Modification

Based on Common Terminology Criteria for Adverse Events (CTCAE).

Diarrhea

Note: At first sign of loose stools, recommend treatment with antidiarrheal agents and hydration.
Grade 1 diarrhea: No dose adjustment. **Grade 2 diarrhea:** If toxicity does not resolve to Grade 1 or less within 24 hrs, withhold treatment until resolved. Then resume at same dose level. **Recurrent or persistent Grade 2 diarrhea at same dose level despite supportive measures:** Withhold treatment until recovery to Grade 1 or less, then resume at reduced dose level. **Grade 3 or 4 diarrhea or required hospitalization:** Withhold treatment until recovery to Grade 1 or less, then resume at reduced dose level.

Hematologic Toxicity

Grade 1 or 2 hematologic toxicity: No dose adjustment. **Grade 3 hematologic toxicity:** Withhold treatment until recovery to Grade 2 or less, then resume at same dose level. **Grade 3 (recurrent) or Grade 4 hematologic toxicity:** Withhold treatment until recovery to Grade 2 or less, then resume at reduced dose level.

Hepatotoxicity

Grade 1 or 2 hepatotoxicity without serum bilirubin elevation greater than 2 times ULN: No dose adjustment. **Recurrent or persistent Grade 2 hepatotoxicity; Grade 3 hepatotoxicity without serum bilirubin elevation greater than 2 times ULN:** Withhold treatment until recovery to Grade 1 or less, then resume at reduced dose level. **Serum ALT, AST elevation greater than 3 times ULN with serum bilirubin elevation greater than 2 times ULN (in the absence of cholestasis); Grade 4 hepatotoxicity:** Permanently discontinue.

Other Toxicities

Any other Grade 1 or 2 toxicities: No dose adjustment. **Recurrent or persistent Grade 2 toxicity that does not resolve to Grade 1 (or baseline) within 7 days despite supportive measures:** Withhold treatment until recovery to Grade 1 or less, then resume at reduced dose level. **Any other Grade 3 or 4 toxicities:** Withhold treatment until resolved to Grade 1 or less, then resume at reduced dose level.

Concomitant Use of Strong CYP3A Inhibitors

If strong CYP3A inhibitor cannot be discontinued, reduce initial dose to 100 mg twice daily if pt taking 200 mg or 150 mg twice daily regimen. If dose was already reduced to 100 mg twice daily due to adverse effects, reduce dose to 50 mg twice daily. If CYP3A inhibitor is discontinued, increase dose (after 3–5 half-lives of CYP3A inhibitor have elapsed) to the dose used prior to initiating strong CYP3A inhibitor.

Dosage in Renal Impairment

Mild to moderate impairment: No dose adjustment. **Severe impairment, ESRD:** Not specified.

Dosage in Hepatic Impairment

Mild to moderate impairment: No dose adjustment. **Severe impairment:** Reduce dose frequency to once daily.

SIDE EFFECTS

Note: Side effects may vary if pt treated concomitantly with an aromatase inhibitor. **Frequent (90%–35%):** Diarrhea, fatigue, asthenia, nausea, decreased appetite, abdominal pain, vomiting. **Occasional (20%–10%):** Headache, cough, constipation, arthralgia, dry mouth, decreased weight, stomatitis, dysgeusia, alopecia, dizziness, pyrexia, dehydration.

ADVERSE EFFECTS/TOXIC REACTIONS

Anemia, leukopenia, neutropenia, thrombocytopenia is an expected response to therapy. Diarrhea occurred in 81–90% of pts. Grade 3 diarrhea occurred in 9–20% of pts. Diarrhea may increase risk of dehydration and infection. Neutropenia reported in 37–41% of pts. Grade 3 or 4 hepatotoxicity occurred in up to 4% of pts. Venous thromboembolism including cerebral venous thrombosis, subclavian and axillary vein thrombosis, inferior vena cava thrombosis, DVT, PE, pelvic venous thrombosis reported in 5% of pts taking concomitant aromatase inhibitor therapy. Infections including upper respiratory infection, UTI, pulmonary infection occurred in 39% of pts taking concomitant aromatase inhibitor therapy.

NURSING CONSIDERATIONS

BASELINE ASSESSMENT

Obtain ANC, CBC, BMP, LFT. Confirm HR-positive, HER2-negative status. Obtain pregnancy test prior to initiation. Question current breastfeeding status. Stress importance of antidiarrheal if diarrhea occurs. Question history of hepatic impairment, venous thromboembolism. Question usual bowel movement patterns, stool characteristics. Receive full medication history and screen for interactions. Screen for active infection. Assess hydration status. Offer emotional support.

INTERVENTION/EVALUATION

Monitor CBC for myelosuppression; LFT for hepatotoxicity q2wks for first 2 mos, then monthly for 2 mos, then as clinically indicated. Monitor for hepatotoxicity (abdominal pain, ascites, confusion, dark-colored urine, jaundice). Monitor daily pattern of bowel activity, stool consistency. Ensure compliance of antidiarrheal therapy if diarrhea occurs. If treatment-related toxicities occur, consider referral to specialist. Be alert for serious infection, opportunistic infection, sepsis. Monitor for venous thromboembolism (arm/leg pain, swelling; chest pain, dyspnea, hypoxia, tachycardia). Ensure adequate hydration, nutrition. Monitor weight, I&Os.

PATIENT/FAMILY TEACHING

• Treatment may depress your immune system and reduce your ability to fight infection. Report symptoms of infection such as body aches, burning with urination, chills, cough, fatigue, fever. Avoid those with active infection. • Report symptoms of bone marrow depression such as bruising, fatigue, fever, shortness of breath, weight loss; bleeding easily, bloody urine or stool. • Therapy may cause severe diarrhea, which may lead to dehydration and infection. Drink plenty of fluids. Take antidiarrheal medication as prescribed at the first sign of loose stools. • Treatment may cause fetal harm; avoid pregnancy. • Females of child-bearing potential should use effective contraception during treatment and for at least 3 wks after last dose. Do not breastfeed. • Report symptoms of DVT (swelling, pain, hot feeling in the arms or legs), lung embolism (difficulty breathing, chest pain, rapid heart rate); liver problems (bruising, contusion; amber, dark, orange-colored urine; right upper abdominal pain, yellowing of the skin or eyes). • Do not take newly prescribed medications unless approved by the prescriber who originally started treatment. • Do not ingest grapefruit products.

abiraterone

TOP 100

a-bir-**a**-ter-one
(Yonsa, Zytiga)
Do not confuse Zytiga with Zetia or ZyrTEC.

◆CLASSIFICATION

PHARMACOTHERAPEUTIC: Antiandrogen. **CLINICAL:** Antineoplastic.

USES

Treatment of metastatic castration-resistant prostate cancer in combination with prednisone or methylprednisolone. Treatment of metastatic, high-risk castration-sensitive prostate cancer (in combination with prednisone).

PRECAUTIONS

Contraindications: Hypersensitivity to abiraterone. Use in women who are pregnant or may become pregnant. **Cautions:** History of cardiovascular disease (especially HF, recent MI, or ventricular arrhythmia) due to potential for hypertension, hypokalemia, fluid retention; moderate hepatic impairment; adrenal insufficiency. Avoid use with strong CYP3A4 inducers.

ACTION

Selectively and irreversibly inhibits CYP17, an enzyme needed for androgen biosynthesis (expressed in testicular, adrenal, or prostatic tumor tissue). Inhibits formation of testosterone precursors DHEA and androstenedione. **Therapeutic Effect:** Lowers serum testosterone to castrate levels.

PHARMACOKINETICS

Protein binding: 99%. Primarily excreted in feces. Peak plasma concentration: 2 hrs. **Half-life:** 12 hrs (up to 19 hrs with hepatic impairment).

LIFESPAN CONSIDERATIONS

Pregnancy/Lactation: Contraindicated in women who are or may become pregnant. **Children:** Safety and efficacy not established. **Elderly:** No age-related precautions noted.

INTERACTIONS

DRUG: May increase concentration/effects of **doxorubicin (conventional), thioridazine.** May decrease concentration/effect of **tamoxifen. CYP3A4 inducers (e.g., carbamazepine, ketoconazole, ritonavir), dabrafenib, enzalutamide, lorlatinib** may decrease concentration/effect. **HERBAL:** **St. John's wort** may decrease concentration/effect. **FOOD:** Do not give with **food** (no **food** should be consumed for at least 2 hrs before or 1 hr after dose). **LAB VALUES:** May increase serum ALT, AST, bilirubin, triglycerides. May decrease serum potassium, phosphate.

AVAILABILITY (Rx)

Tablets: *(Yonsa):* 125 mg. *(Zytiga):* 250 mg, 500 mg.

ADMINISTRATION/HANDLING

PO

• *(Yonsa):* May give without regard to food. • Do not break, crush, dissolve, or divide tablets. Give whole with water. • *(Zytiga):* Give on empty stomach only (at least 1 hr before or 2 hrs after food). • Give with water. • Administer whole. Do not break, crush, dissolve, or divide tablets. Women who are or may become pregnant should wear gloves if handling the tablets.

INDICATIONS/ROUTES/DOSAGE

ALERT Consider increased dosage of predniSONE during unusual stress or infection. Interrupting predniSONE therapy may induce adrenocorticoid insufficiency.

Metastatic Castration-Resistant Prostate Cancer

PO: ADULTS, ELDERLY: *(Yonsa):* 500 mg once daily (with methylPREDNISolone 4 mg 2 times/day). *(Zytiga):* 1,000 mg once daily (with predniSONE 5 mg 2 times/day).

Dosage Modification

Hepatic Enzymes Greater Than Upper Limit of Normal (ULN) (During Treatment)

Lab Values	Recommendation
ALT, AST elevations greater than 5 × ULN or bilirubin greater than 3 × ULN with 1,000 mg	Interrupt treatment and restart at 750 mg once ALT, AST less than 2.5 × ULN or bilirubin less than 1.5 × ULN.
ALT, AST elevations greater than 5 × ULN or bilirubin greater than 3 × ULN with 750 mg	Interrupt treatment and restart at 500 mg once ALT, AST less than 2.5 × ULN or bilirubin less than 1.5 × ULN.

If hepatotoxicity occurs at reduced dose of 500 mg daily, discontinue treatment.

Dosage Adjustment for Concomitant Strong CYP3A4 Inducers

Increase abiraterone dose to 1,000 mg twice daily.

Dosage in Renal Impairment

No dose adjustment.

Dosage in Hepatic Impairment

Mild impairment: No dosage adjustment necessary. **Moderate impairment:** Reduce dose to 250 mg daily. Discontinue if serum ALT, AST greater than 5 times ULN or serum bilirubin greater than 3 times ULN. **Severe impairment:** Avoid use.

SIDE EFFECTS

Frequent (30%–26%): Joint swelling/discomfort, peripheral edema, muscle spasm, musculoskeletal pain, hypokalemia. **Occasional (19%–6%):** Hot flashes, diarrhea, UTI, cough, hypertension, urinary frequency, nocturia. **Rare (less than 6%):** Heartburn, upper respiratory tract infection.

ADVERSE EFFECTS/ TOXIC REACTIONS

Mineralocorticoid excess (severe fluid retention, hypokalemia, hypertension) may compromise pts with prior cardiovascular history. Safety not established in pts with left ventricular ejection fraction less than 50%. Tachycardia, atrial fibrillation, supraventricular tachycardia, atrial flutter, complete AV block, bradyarrhythmia reported in 7% of pts. Chest pain, unstable angina, HF reported in less than 4% of pts. Stress, infection, or interruption of daily steroids may cause adrenocortical insufficiency. Hepatotoxicity (serum ALT, AST greater than 5 times ULN) reported in 2% of pts. Pts with hepatic impairment are more likely to develop hepatotoxicity.

NURSING CONSIDERATIONS

BASELINE ASSESSMENT

Obtain baseline BMP, LFT. Evaluate history of HF, myocardial infarction, arrhythmias, angina pectoris, peripheral edema, hepatic impairment, adrenal or pituitary abnormalities, left ventricular ejection fraction (if applicable). Question possibility of pregnancy before treatment. Question history of corticosteroid intolerance if applicable.

INTERVENTION/EVALUATION

Monitor BMP, LFT. Monitor for mineralocorticoid excess (hypokalemia, hypertension, fluid retention) at least once monthly. Assess for cardiac arrhythmia if hypokalemia occurs. Obtain ECG for palpitations, dyspnea, dizziness. Monitor for signs and symptoms of adrenocortical insufficiency during predniSONE interruption, periods of stress, infection. Measure serum ALT, AST, alkaline phosphatase, bilirubin every 2 wks for 3 mos, then monthly. If hepatotoxicity occurs, dosage modification will be necessary. Pts with moderate hepatic impairment must have LFT every wk for first month, then every 2 wks for 2 mos, then monthly. If serum ALT, AST above 5 times ULN or serum bilirubin above 3 times ULN, treatment should be discontinued.

PATIENT/FAMILY TEACHING

• Must be taken on empty stomach (no food 2 hrs before and 1 hr after dose). • If taken with food, toxic levels may result. • Sexually active men must wear condoms during treatment and for 1 wk after treatment. • Women who are pregnant or are planning pregnancy may not touch medication without gloves. • Dizziness, palpitations, headache, confusion, muscle weakness, leg swelling/discomfort may become more apparent during periods of unusual stress, infection, or interruption of predniSONE therapy. • Blood tests will be performed routinely. • Report signs of liver problems (yellowing of skin, bruising, light-colored stool, right upper quadrant pain), chest pain, palpitations. • An increase in urinary frequency or nocturia is expected as treatment becomes therapeutic. • Do not chew, crush, dissolve, or divide tablets.

acalabrutinib

a-**kal**-a-**broo**-ti-nib
(Calquence)
Do not confuse acalabrutinib with afatinib, cabozantinib, ibrutinib, or lenvatinib.

◆CLASSIFICATION

PHARMACOTHERAPEUTIC: Bruton tyrosine kinase inhibitor. **CLINICAL:** Antineoplastic.

USES

Treatment of adults with mantle cell lymphoma (MCL) who have received at least one prior therapy. Treatment of adults with chronic lymphocytic leukemia or small lymphocytic lymphoma.

PRECAUTIONS

Contraindications: Hypersensitivity to acalabrutinib. **Cautions:** Baseline anemia, neutropenia, thrombocytopenia; active infection, conditions predisposing to infection (e.g., diabetes, renal failure, immunocompromised pts, open wounds); history of atrial fibrillation, atrial flutter; pts at risk for hemorrhage (e.g., history of intracranial/GI bleeding, coagulation disorders, recent trauma; concomitant use of anticoagulants, antiplatelets, NSAIDS).

ACTION

Inhibits enzymatic activity of Bruton tyrosine kinase (BTK); a signaling molecule that promotes malignant B-cell proliferation and survival. **Therapeutic Effect:** Decreases malignant B-cell proliferation and survival.

PHARMACOKINETICS

Rapidly absorbed and widely distributed. Metabolized in liver. Protein binding: 97.5%. Peak plasma concentration: 0.75 hrs. Steady-state maintained over 12 hrs. Excreted in feces (84%), urine (12%). **Half-life:** 0.9 hrs (metabolite: 6.9 hrs).

LIFESPAN CONSIDERATIONS

Pregnancy/Lactation: Avoid pregnancy; may cause fetal harm. Unknown if distributed in breast milk. Breastfeeding not recommended during treatment and for at least 2 wks after discontinuation. **Children:** Safety and efficacy not established. **Elderly:** No age-related precautions noted.

INTERACTIONS

DRUG: **Strong CYP3A4 inhibitors (e.g., clarithromycin, ketoconazole, ritonavir), moderate CYP3A inhibitors (e.g., erythromycin, diltiazem, fluconazole, verapamil)** may increase concentration/effect. **Strong CYP3A4 inducers (e.g., carbamazepine, phenytoin, rifampin)** may decrease concentration/effect. May decrease effect of **BCG (intravesical), vaccines (live).** May enhance adverse/toxic effects of **natalizumab, vaccines (live). Pimecrolimus, tacrolimus** may enhance adverse/toxic effects. **HERBAL:** **Echinacea, St. John's wort** may decrease concentration/effect. **FOOD:** None known. **LAB VALUES:** May decrease Hgb, platelets, neutrophils.

AVAILABILITY (Rx)

Capsules: 100 mg.

ADMINISTRATION/HANDLING

PO

• Give without regard to food. • Administer whole with a glass of water; do not break, cut, or open capsule. • If a dose is missed, may administer dose up to 3 hrs after regularly scheduled time. If more than 3 hrs have elapsed, do not give dose. Administer next dose at regularly scheduled time. • Give at least 2 hrs before aluminum-, magnesium-, or calcium-containing antacids, H2-receptor antagonists.

INDICATIONS/ROUTES/DOSAGE

Mantle Cell Lymphoma

PO: ADULTS, ELDERLY: 100 mg approximately q12h. Continue until disease progression or unacceptable toxicity.

Chronic Lymphocytic Leukemia or Small Lymphocytic Lymphoma

PO: ADULTS, ELDERLY: (Single-agent therapy): 100 mg q12h. Continue until disease progression or unacceptable toxicity. **(Combination therapy with obinutuzumab):** 100 mg q12h. Continue until disease progression or unacceptable toxicity. Begin acalabrutinib at cycle 1 (28-day cycle); obinutuzumab given for 6 cycles beginning at cycle 2.

Dose Modification

Based on Common Terminology Criteria for Adverse Events (CTCAE).

Grade 3 or 4 nonhematologic toxicities; Grade 3 thrombocytopenia with bleeding; Grade 4 thrombocytopenia; Grade 4 neutropenia lasting longer than 7 days: First and second occurrence: Withhold treatment until recovery to Grade 1 or baseline, then resume at 100 mg twice daily. **Third occurrence:** Withhold treatment until recovery to Grade 1 or baseline, then resume at 100 mg once daily. **Fourth occurrence:** Permanently discontinue.

Chronic Lymphocytic Leukemia or Small Lymphocytic Lymphoma

PO: ADULTS, ELDERLY: (Single-agent therapy): 100 mg q12h. Continue until disease progression or unacceptable toxicity. **(Combination therapy with obinutuzumab):** 100 mg q12h. Continue until disease progression or unacceptable toxicity. Begin acalabrutinib at cycle 1 (28-day cycle); obinutuzumab given for 6 cycles beginning at cycle 2.

Concomitant Use of Strong CYP3A Inhibitors

Avoid use. If short-term treatment with CYP3A inhibitor is unavoidable (e.g., anti-infectives for up to 7 days), withhold acalabrutinib until strong CYP3A inhibitor is discontinued.

Concomitant Use of Moderate CYP3A Inhibitors
Decrease frequency to 100 mg once daily.

Concomitant Use of Strong CYP3A Inducers
If strong CYP3A inducer cannot be discontinued, increase acalabrutinib dose to 200 mg twice daily.

Dosage in Renal Impairment
Mild to moderate impairment: No dose adjustment. **Severe impairment:** Not specified; use caution.

Dosage in Hepatic Impairment
Mild to moderate impairment: No dose adjustment. **Severe impairment:** Not specified; use caution.

SIDE EFFECTS

Frequent (39%–18%): Headache, diarrhea, fatigue, myalgia, bruising, nausea, rash. **Occasional (15%–13%):** Abdominal pain, constipation, vomiting.

ADVERSE EFFECTS/TOXIC REACTIONS

Anemia, neutropenia, thrombocytopenia is an expected response to therapy. Serious and sometimes fatal hemorrhagic events including intracranial hemorrhage, GI bleeding, epistaxis occurred in 2% of pts. Petechiae, bruising reported in 50% of pts. Serious bacterial, viral, fungal infections occurred in 18% of pts. Infections due to hepatitis B virus reactivation was reported. New primary malignancies including skin cancer (7% of pts), nonskin carcinomas (11% of pts) have occurred. Progressive Multifocal Leukoencephalopathy (PML), an opportunistic viral infection of the brain caused by the JC virus, may result in progressive permanent disability and death. Atrial fibrillation/atrial flutter reported in 3% of pts.

NURSING CONSIDERATIONS

BASELINE ASSESSMENT

Obtain ANC, CBC; PT/INR if on anticoagulation; pregnancy test in females of reproductive potential. Screen for active infection. Question history of atrial fibrillation, atrial flutter; intracranial/GI bleeding, coagulation disorders, recent trauma; previous skin cancers. Conduct baseline dermatological exam and assess skin for open/unhealed wounds, lesions, moles. Question current breastfeeding status. Receive full medication history and screen for interactions. Offer emotional support.

INTERVENTION/EVALUATION

Monitor CBC periodically for cytopenias. Closely monitor for HBV reactivation; symptoms of PML (altered mental status, seizures, visual disturbances, generalized or unilateral weakness). Obtain ECG if chest pain, dyspnea, palpitations occur. Be alert for serious infection, opportunistic infection, sepsis; nonskin carcinomas. Monitor for hemorrhagic events including intracranial hemorrhage (altered mental status, aphasia, blindness, hemiparesis, unequal pupils, seizures), GI bleeding (hematemesis, melena, rectal bleeding), epistaxis. Assess skin for new lesions, moles. Ensure adequate hydration.

PATIENT/FAMILY TEACHING

• Treatment may depress your immune system and reduce your ability to fight infection. Report symptoms of infection such as body aches, burning with urination, chills, cough, fatigue, fever. Avoid those with active infection. • Report symptoms of bone marrow depression such as bruising, fatigue, fever, shortness of breath, weight loss; bleeding easily, bloody urine or stool. • Avoid pregnancy. Breastfeeding not recommended during treatment and for at least 2 wks after last dose. • PML, an opportunistic viral infection of the brain, may cause progressive, permanent disabilities and death. Report symptoms of PML, brain hemorrhage such as confusion, memory loss, paralysis, trouble speaking, vision loss, seizures, weakness • Treatment may cause new cancers, heart arrhythmias (chest pain, dizziness, fainting, palpitations, slow or rapid heart rate, irregular heart rate), reactivation of HBV. • Immediately report bleeding of any kind. • Do not take newly prescribed medications unless approved by the prescriber who originally started treatment. • Do not ingest grapefruit products.

acetaminophen

TOP 100

a-**seet**-a-**min**-oh-fen
(Abenol ✦, Acephen, Apo-Acetaminophen ✦, Atasol ✦, Feverall, Mapap, Ofirmev, Tempra ✦, Tylenol, Tylenol 8HR Arthritis Pain, Tylenol Children's, Tylenol Infants, Tylenol Extra Strength)

■ **BLACK BOX ALERT** ■ Potential for severe liver injury. Acetaminophen injection associated with acute liver failure.

Do not confuse Acephen with Aciphex, Feverall with Fiberall, Fioricet with Fiorinal, Percocet with Percodan, Tylenol with atenolol, timolol, Tylenol PM, or Tylox, or Vicodin with Hycodan.

FIXED-COMBINATION(S)

Tylenol with Codeine: acetaminophen/codeine: 120 mg/12 mg per 5 mL. **Endocet:** acetaminophen/oxyCODONE: 325 mg/5 mg, 325 mg/7.5 mg, 325 mg/10 mg. **Fioricet:** acetaminophen/caffeine/butalbital: 325 mg/40 mg/50 mg. **Hycet:** acetaminophen/HYDROcodone: 325 mg/7.5 mg per 15 mL. **Norco:** acetaminophen/HYDROcodone: 325 mg/5 mg, 325 mg/7.5 mg, 325 mg/10 mg. **Percocet:** acetaminophen/oxyCODONE: 325 mg/5 mg. **Tylenol with Codeine:** acetaminophen/codeine: 300 mg/15 mg, 300 mg/30 mg, 300 mg/60 mg. **Ultracet:** acetaminophen/traMADol: 325 mg/37.5 mg. **Vicodin:** acetaminophen/HYDROcodone: 300 mg/5 mg. **Vicodin ES:** acetaminophen/HYDROcodone: 300 mg/7.5 mg. **Vicodin HP:** acetaminophen/HYDROcodone: 300 mg/10 mg. **Xartemis XR:** acetaminophen/oxyCODONE: 325 mg/7.5 mg. **Xodol:** acetaminophen/HYDROcodone: 300 mg/5 mg, 300 mg/7.5 mg, 300 mg/10 mg.

◆CLASSIFICATION

PHARMACOTHERAPEUTIC: Central analgesic. **CLINICAL:** Nonnarcotic analgesic, antipyretic.

USES

PO, rectal: Temporary relief of mild to moderate pain, headache, fever.
IV: (Additional) Management of moderate to severe pain when combined with opioid analgesia.

PRECAUTIONS

Contraindications: Hypersensitivity to acetaminophen, severe hepatic impairment or severe active liver disease. **Cautions:** Sensitivity to acetaminophen; severe renal impairment; alcohol dependency, hepatic impairment, or active hepatic disease; chronic malnutrition and hypovolemia (Ofirmev); G6PD deficiency (hemolysis may occur). Limit dose to less than 4 g/day.

ACTION

Analgesic: Activates descending serotonergic inhibitory pathways in CNS. Antipyretic: Inhibits hypothalamic heat-regulating center. **Therapeutic Effect:** Results in antipyresis. Produces analgesic effect.

PHARMACOKINETICS

Route	Onset	Peak	Duration
PO	Less than 60 min	1–3 hrs	4–6 hrs

Rapidly, completely absorbed from GI tract; rectal absorption variable. Protein binding: 20%–50%. Widely distributed to most body tissues. Metabolized in liver. Excreted in urine. Removed by hemodialysis. **Half-life:** 1–4 hrs (increased in pts with hepatic disease, elderly, neonates; decreased in children).

⌛ LIFESPAN CONSIDERATIONS

Pregnancy/Lactation: Crosses placenta; distributed in breast milk. Routinely used in all stages of pregnancy; appears safe for short-term use. **Children/Elderly:** No age-related precautions noted.

INTERACTIONS

DRUG: **Alcohol** (chronic use), **hepatotoxic medications (e.g., phenytoin), strong CYP3A4 inducers (e.g., carbamazepine, phenytoin, rifampin)** may increase risk of hepatotoxicity with prolonged high dose or single toxic dose. **Dasatinib, probenecid** may increase concentration/effect. **HERBAL:** None significant. **FOOD:** **Food** may decrease rate of absorption. **LAB VALUES:** May increase serum ALT, AST, bilirubin; prothrombin levels (may indicate hepatotoxicity).

AVAILABILITY (OTC)

Caplets: 325 mg, 500 mg, 650 mg. **Capsules:** 325 mg, 500 mg. **Elixir:** 160 mg/5 mL. **Injection, Solution (Ofirmev):** 1,000 mg/100 mL glass vial. **Liquid (Oral):** 160 mg/5 mL. **Solution (Oral Drops):** 80 mg/0.8 mL. **Suppository:** 80 mg, 120 mg, 325 mg, 650 mg. **Suspension:** 160 mg/5 mL. **Syrup:** 160 mg/5 mL. **Tablets:** 325 mg, 500 mg. **Tablets (Chewable):** 80 mg. **Tablets (Orally Disintegrating):** 80 mg, 160 mg.

Caplets: (Extended-Release [Tylenol Arthritis Pain]): 650 mg.

ADMINISTRATION/HANDLING

IV

Reconstitution • Does not require further dilution. • Store at room temperature. • Withdraw doses less than 1,000 mg. • Place in separate empty, sterile container.

Rate of administration • Infuse over 15 min.

Stability • Once opened or transferred, stable for 6 hrs at room temperature.

PO

• Give without regard to food. • Tablets may be crushed. • Do not crush extended-release caplets. • Suspension: Shake well before use. • Take with full glass of water.

Rectal

• Moisten suppository with cold water before inserting well up into rectum. • Do not freeze suppositories.

INDICATIONS/ROUTES/DOSAGE

Note: Over-the-counter (OTC) use of acetaminophen should be limited to 3,000 mg/day.

Analgesia and Antipyresis

IV: ADULTS, ELDERLY, ADOLESCENTS WEIGHING 50 KG OR MORE: 1,000 mg q6h or 650 mg q4h. **Maximum single dose:** 1,000 mg; **maximum total daily dose:** 4,000 mg. **ADULTS, ADOLESCENTS WEIGHING LESS THAN 50 KG:** 15 mg/kg q6h or 12.5 mg/kg q4h. **Maximum single dose:** 750 mg; **maximum total daily dose:** 75 mg/kg/day (3,750 mg). **CHILDREN 2–12 YRS:** 15 mg/kg q6h or 12.5 mg/kg q4h. **Maximum single dose:** 750 mg. **Maximum:** 75 mg/kg/day, not to exceed 3,750 mg/day. **INFANTS AND CHILDREN LESS THAN 2 YRS (FEVER ONLY):** 7.5–15 mg/kg q6h. **Maximum:** 60 mg/kg/day. **NEONATES (FEVER ONLY):** (Limited data available) Loading dose: 20 mg/kg. **PMA 37 or greater than 37 wks:** 10 mg/kg/dose q6h. **Maximum:** 40 mg/kg/day. **PMA 33–36 wks:** 10 mg/kg/dose q8h. **Maximum:** 40 mg/kg/day. **PMA 28–32 wks:** 10 mg/kg/dose q12h. **Maximum:** 22.5 mg/kg/day.

PO: ADULTS, ELDERLY, CHILDREN 13 YRS AND OLDER: (Regular Strength) 325–650 mg q4–6h. **Maximum:** 3,250 mg/day unless directed by health care provider. **Extra Strength:** 1000 mg q6h. **Maximum:** 3,000 mg/day unless directed by health care provider. **Extended-Release:** 1300 mg q8h. **Maximum:** 3,900 mg/day. **CHILDREN 12 YRS AND YOUNGER:** (Weight dosing preferred; if not available, use age. Doses may be repeated q4h. **Maximum:** 5 doses/day.)

Age	Weight (Kg)	Dose
11–12 yrs	32.7–43.2	480 mg
9–10 yrs	27.3–32.6	400 mg
6–8 yrs	21.8–27.2	320 mg
4–5 yrs	16.4–21.7	240 mg
2–3 yrs	10.9–16.3	160 mg
1–<2 yrs	8.2–10.8	120 mg
4–11 mos	5.4–8.1	80 mg
0–3 mos	2.7–5.3	40 mg

NEONATES: Term: 10–15 mg/kg/dose q4–6h. **Maximum:** 75 mg/kg/day. **GA 33–37 wks or term less than 10 days:** 10–15 mg/kg/dose q6h. **Maximum:** 60 mg/kg/day. **GA 28–32 wks:** 10–12 mg/kg/dose q6–8h. **Maximum:** 40 mg/kg/day.

Rectal: ADULTS, ELDERLY, CHILDREN 12 YRS AND OLDER: 325–650 mg q4–6h. **Maximum:** 4 g/24 hrs. **CHILDREN: (7–11 YRS):** 325 mg q4–6h. **Maximum:** 1,625 mg/day. **(4–6 YRS):** 120 mg q4–6h. **Maximum:** 600 mg/day. **(1–3 YRS):** 80 mg q4–6h. **Maximum:** 400 mg/day. **(6–11 mos):** 80 mg q6h. **Maximum:** 320 mg/day. **NEONATES:** Term: Initially, 30 mg/kg/once, then 20 mg/kg/dose q6–8h. **Maximum:** 75 mg/kg/day. **GA 33–37 wks or term less than 10 days:** Initially, 30 mg/kg once, then 15 mg/kg/dose q8h. **Maximum:** 60 mg/kg/day. **GA 28–32 wks:** 20 mg/kg/dose q12h. **Maximum:** 40 mg/kg/day.

Dosage in Renal Impairment

Creatinine Clearance	Frequency
Oral	
10–50 mL/min	q6h
Less than 10 mL/min	q8h
Continuous renal replacement therapy	q6h
IV	
30 mL/min or less (use caution, decrease daily dose, extend dosing interval)	

Dosage in Hepatic Impairment

Use with caution. IV contraindicated in pts with severe impairment.

SIDE EFFECTS

Rare: Hypersensitivity reaction.

ADVERSE EFFECTS/TOXIC REACTIONS

Early Signs of Acetaminophen Toxicity: Anorexia, nausea, diaphoresis, fatigue within first 12–24 hrs. **Later Signs of Toxicity:** Vomiting, right upper quadrant tenderness, elevated LFTs within 48–72 hrs after ingestion. **Antidote:** Acetylcysteine (see Appendix J for dosage).

NURSING CONSIDERATIONS

BASELINE ASSESSMENT

If given for analgesia, assess onset, type, location, duration of pain. Effect of medication is reduced if full pain response recurs prior to next dose. Assess for fever. Assess LFT in pts with chronic usage or history of hepatic impairment, alcohol abuse.

INTERVENTION/EVALUATION

Assess for clinical improvement and relief of pain, fever. **Therapeutic serum level:** 10–30 mcg/mL; **toxic serum level:** greater than 200 mcg/mL. Do not exceed maximum daily recommended dose: 4 g/day.

PATIENT/FAMILY TEACHING

• Consult physician for use in children younger than 2 yrs, oral use longer than 5 days (children) or longer than 10 days (adults), or fever lasting longer than 3 days. • Severe/recurrent pain or high/continuous fever may indicate serious illness. • Do not take more than 4 g/day (3 g/day if using OTC [over-the-counter]). Actual OTC dosing recommendations may vary by product and/or manufacturer. Many nonprescription combination products contain acetaminophen. Avoid alcohol.

acetylcysteine

a-**seet**-il-**sis**-teen
(Acetadote, Mucomyst ✱, Parvolex ✱)

Do not confuse acetylcysteine with acetylcholine, or Mucomyst with Mucinex.

◆CLASSIFICATION

PHARMACOTHERAPEUTIC: Respiratory inhalant, intratracheal. **CLINICAL:** Mucolytic, antidote acetylcysteine with acetylcholine, or Mucomyst with Mucinex.

USES

Inhalation: Adjunctive treatment for abnormally viscid mucous secretions present in acute and chronic bronchopulmonary disease and in pulmonary complications of cystic fibrosis and surgery, diagnostic bronchial studies. **Injection, PO:** Antidote in acute acetaminophen toxicity.

PRECAUTIONS

Contraindications: Hypersensitivity to acetylcysteine. **Cautions:** Pts with bronchial asthma; debilitated pts with severe respiratory insufficiency (increases risk of anaphylactoid reaction).

ACTION

Mucolytic splits linkage of mucoproteins, reducing viscosity of pulmonary secretions. Acetaminophen toxicity: Hepatoprotective by restoring hepatic glutathione and enhancing nontoxic sulfate conjugation of acetaminophen. **Therapeutic Effect:** Facilitates removal of pulmonary secretions by coughing, postural drainage, mechanical means. Protects against acetaminophen overdose-induced hepatotoxicity.

LIFESPAN CONSIDERATIONS

Pregnancy/Lactation: Unknown if distributed in breast milk. **Children/Elderly:** No age-related precautions noted.

INTERACTIONS

DRUG: None significant. **HERBAL:** None significant. **FOOD:** None known. **LAB VALUES:** None significant.

AVAILABILITY (Rx)

Inhalation Solution: ***(Mucomyst):*** 10% (100 mg/mL), 20% (200 mg/mL). **Injection Solution:** ***(Acetadote):*** 20% (200 mg/mL).

ADMINISTRATION/HANDLING

IV

The total dose is 300 mg/kg administered over 21 hrs. Dose preparation is based on pt weight. Total volume administered should be adjusted for pts less than 40 kg and for pts requiring fluid restriction. Store unopened vials at room temperature. Following dilution in D_5W, solution is stable for 24 hrs at room temperature. Color change of opened vials may occur (does not affect potency).

Three-Bag Method (as Antidote): Loading, Second, and Third Doses, Pts Weighing 40 kg or More

Loading dose: 150 mg/kg in 200 mL of diluent administered over 60 min.
Second dose: 50 mg/kg in 500 mL of diluent administered over 4 hrs.
Third dose: 100 mg/kg in 1,000 mL of diluent administered over 16 hrs.

Pts Weighing More Than 20 kg but Less Than 40 kg

Loading dose: 150 mg/kg in 100 mL of diluent administered over 60 min.
Second dose: 50 mg/kg in 250 mL of diluent administered over 4 hrs.
Third dose: 100 mg/kg in 500 mL of diluent administered over 16 hrs.

Pts Weighing Less Than or Equal to 20 kg

Loading dose: 150 mg/kg in 3 mL/kg of body weight of diluent administered over 60 min.
Second dose: 50 mg/kg in 7 mL/kg of body weight of diluent administered over 4 hrs.
Third dose: 100 mg/kg in 14 mL/kg of body weight of diluent administered over 16 hrs.

PO

• For treatment of acetaminophen overdose. • Give as 5% solution. • Dilute 20% solution 1:3 with cola, orange juice, other soft drink. • Give within 1 hr of preparation.

Inhalation, Nebulization

• 20% solution may be diluted with 0.9% NaCl or sterile water; 10% solution may be used undiluted.

IV COMPATIBILITIES

Cefepime (Maxipime), cefTAZidime (Fortaz).

INDICATIONS/ROUTES/DOSAGE

Bronchopulmonary Disease

Inhalation, Nebulization

◀ALERT▶ Bronchodilators should be given 10–15 min before acetylcysteine.

ADULTS, ELDERLY, CHILDREN: 3–5 mL (20% solution) 3–4 times/day or 6–10 mL (10% solution) 3–4 times/day. Range: 1–10 mL (20% solution) q2–6h or 2–20 mL (10% solution) q2–6h. **INFANTS:** 1–2 mL (20%) or 2–4 mL (10%) 3–4 times/day.

Intratracheal: ADULTS, CHILDREN: 1–2 mL of 10% or 20% solution instilled into tracheostomy q1–4h.

Acetaminophen Overdose

◀ALERT▶ It is essential to initiate treatment as soon as possible after overdose and, in any case, within 24 hrs of ingestion.

PO: ***(Oral Solution 5%):*** **ADULTS, ELDERLY, CHILDREN:** Loading dose of 140 mg/kg, followed in 4 hrs by maintenance dose of 70 mg/kg q4h for 17 additional doses (or until acetaminophen assay reveals nontoxic level). Repeat dose if emesis occurs within 1 hr of administration.

IV: ADULTS, ELDERLY, CHILDREN: (Consists of 3 doses. Total Dose: 300 mg/kg.) 150 mg/kg infused over 60 min, then 50 mg/kg infused over 4 hrs, then 100 mg/kg infused over 16 hrs (see Administration/Handling for dilution). **WEIGHING MORE THAN 100 KG:** (Consists of 3 doses. Total Dose: 30 g.) 15 g over 60 min; 5 g over 4 hrs; 10 g over 16 hrs. Duration of administration may vary depending on acetaminophen levels and LFTs obtained during treatment. Pts who still have detectable levels of acetaminophen or elevated LFT results continue to benefit from additional acetylcysteine administration beyond 24 hrs.

Diagnostic Bronchial Studies

Inhalation, Nebulization: ADULTS: 1–2 mL of 20% solution or 2–4 mL of 10% solution 2–3 times before the procedure.

SIDE EFFECTS

IV: (10%): Nausea, vomiting. **(7%–6%):** Acute flushing, erythema. **(4%):** Pruritus. **Frequent: Inhalation:** Stickiness on face, transient unpleasant odor. **Occasional: Inhalation:** Increased bronchial secretions, throat irritation, nausea, vomiting, rhinorrhea. **Rare: Inhalation:** Rash. **PO:** Facial edema, bronchospasm, wheezing, nausea, vomiting.

ADVERSE EFFECTS/TOXIC REACTIONS

Large doses may produce severe nausea/vomiting. **(Less than 2%):** Serious anaphylactoid reactions including cough, wheezing, stridor, respiratory distress, bronchospasm, hypotension, and death have been known to occur with IV administration.

NURSING CONSIDERATIONS

BASELINE ASSESSMENT

Mucolytic: Assess pretreatment respirations for rate, depth, rhythm. **IV antidote:** Obtain baseline LFT, PT/INR, and drug screen. For use as antidote, obtain acetaminophen level to determine need for treatment with acetylcysteine.

INTERVENTION/EVALUATION

If bronchospasm occurs, discontinue treatment, notify physician; bronchodilator may be added to therapy. Monitor rate, depth, rhythm, type of respiration (abdominal, thoracic). Observe sputum for color, consistency, amount. **IV antidote:** Administer within 8 hrs of acetaminophen ingestion for maximal hepatic protection; ideally, within 4 hrs after immediate-release and 2 hrs after liquid acetaminophen formulations.

PATIENT/FAMILY TEACHING

• Slight, disagreeable sulfuric odor from solution may be noticed during initial administration but disappears quickly. • Adequate hydration is important part of therapy. • Follow guidelines for proper coughing and deep breathing techniques. • Auscultate lung sounds.

acyclovir

a-**sye**-klo-veer
(Apo-Acyclovir 🍁, Zovirax)

Do not confuse acyclovir with ganciclovir, Retrovir, or valACYclovir, or Zovirax with Doribax, Valtrex, Zithromax, Zostrix, Zyloprim, or Zyvox.

FIXED-COMBINATION(S)

Lipsovir: acyclovir/hydrocortisone (a steroid): 5%/1%.

◆CLASSIFICATION

PHARMACOTHERAPEUTIC: Synthetic nucleoside. **CLINICAL:** Antiviral. Acyclovir with ganciclovir, Retrovir, or valACYclovir, or Zovirax with Doribax, Valtrex, Zithromax, Zostrix, Zyloprim, or Zyvox.

USES

Parenteral
Treatment of initial and prophylaxis of recurrent mucosal and cutaneous herpes simplex virus (HSV-1 and HSV-2) in immunocompromised pts. Treatment of severe initial episodes of herpes genitalis in immunocompetent pts. Treatment of herpes simplex encephalitis including neonatal herpes simplex virus. Treatment of herpes zoster (shingles) in immunocompromised pts.

Oral
Treatment of initial episodes and prophylaxis of recurrent herpes simplex (HSV-2 genital herpes). Treatment of chickenpox (varicella). Acute treatment of herpes zoster (shingles).

OFF-LABEL: (Parenteral/Oral): Prevention of HSV reactivation in HIV-positive pts; hematopoietic stem cell transplant (HSCT); during periods of neutropenia in pts with cancer; prevention of VZV reactivation in allogenic HSCT; treatment of disseminated HSC or VZV in immunocompromised pts with cancer; empiric treatment of suspected encephalitis in immunocompromised pts with cancer; treatment of initial and prophylaxis of recurrent mucosal and cutaneous herpes simplex infections in immunocompromised pts.

Topical
Cream: Treatment of recurrent herpes labialis (cold sores) in immunocompetent pts. **Ointment:** Management of initial genital herpes. Treatment of mucocutaneous HSV in immunocompromised pts.

PRECAUTIONS

Contraindications: Use in neonates when acyclovir is reconstituted with Bacteriostatic Water for Injection containing benzyl alcohol. Hypersensitivity to acyclovir, valACYclovir. **Cautions:** Immunocompromised pts (thrombocytopenic purpura/hemolytic uremic syndrome reported); elderly, renal impairment, use of other nephrotoxic medications. **IV Use:** Pts with underlying neurologic abnormalities, serious hepatic/electrolyte abnormalities, substantial hypoxia.

ACTION

Acyclovir is converted to acyclovir triphosphate, which competes for viral DNA polymerase, becoming part of DNA chain. **Therapeutic Effect:** Inhibits DNA synthesis and viral replication. Virustatic.

PHARMACOKINETICS

15%–30% absorbed from GI tract. Bioavailability: 10%–20%; minimal absorption following topical application. Protein binding: 9%–36%. Widely distributed. Partially metabolized in liver. Excreted primarily in urine. Removed by hemodialysis. **Half-life:** 2.5 hrs (increased in renal impairment).

⌛ LIFESPAN CONSIDERATIONS

Pregnancy/Lactation: Crosses placenta; distributed in breast milk. **Children:** Safety and efficacy not established in pts younger than 2 yrs (younger than 1 yr for IV use). **Elderly:** Age-related renal impairment may require decreased dosage. May experience more neurologic effects (e.g., agitation, confusion, hallucinations).

INTERACTIONS

DRUG: **Foscarnet** may increase nephrotoxic effect. May increase adverse effects of **tizanidine.** May decrease therapeutic effect of **Varicella virus vaccine, zoster vaccine.** **HERBAL:** None significant. **FOOD:** None known. **LAB VALUES:** May increase serum ALT, AST, BUN, creatinine.

AVAILABILITY (Rx)

Cream: 5%. **Injection, Powder for Reconstitution:** 500 mg. **Injection, Solution:** 50 mg/mL. **Ointment:** 5%. **Oral Suspension:** 200 mg/5 mL. **Tablets:** 400 mg, 800 mg.

Capsules: 200 mg.

ADMINISTRATION/HANDLING

IV

Reconstitution • Dilute with at least 100 mL D_5W or 0.9 NaCl. Final concentration should be 7 mg/mL or less. (Concentrations greater than 10 mg/mL increase risk of phlebitis.)

Rate of administration • Infuse over at least 1 hr (nephrotoxicity due to crystalluria and renal tubular damage may occur with too-rapid rate). • Maintain adequate hydration during infusion and for 2 hrs following IV administration.

Storage • Store vials at room temperature. • IV infusion (piggyback) stable for 24 hrs at room temperature.

PO

• May give without regard to food. • Do not crush/break capsules. • Store capsules at room temperature.

Topical

Ointment • Avoid contact with eye. • Use finger cot/rubber glove to prevent autoinoculation.

Cream • Apply to cover only cold sores or area with symptoms. • Rub until it disappears.

IV INCOMPATIBILITIES

Aztreonam (Azactam), diltiaZEM (Cardizem), DOBUTamine (Dobutrex), DOPamine (Intropin), levoFLOXacin (Levaquin), meropenem (Merrem IV), ondansetron (Zofran), piperacillin and tazobactam (Zosyn).

IV COMPATIBILITIES

Allopurinol (Alloprim), amikacin (Amikin), ampicillin, ceFAZolin (Ancef), cefotaxime (Claforan), cefTAZidime (Fortaz), cefTRIAXone (Rocephin), cimetidine (Tagamet), clindamycin (Cleocin), diphenhydrAMINE (Benadryl), famotidine (Pepcid), fluconazole (Diflucan), gentamicin, heparin, HYDROmorphone (Dilaudid), imipenem (Primaxin), LORazepam (Ativan), magnesium sulfate, methylPREDNISolone (SOLU), metoclopramide (Reglan), metroNIDAZOLE (Flagyl), morphine, multivitamins, potassium chloride, propofol (Diprivan), raNITIdine (Zantac), vancomycin.

INDICATIONS/ROUTES/DOSAGE

Genital Herpes (Initial Episode)

IV: ADULTS, ELDERLY: 5–10 mg/kg q8h for 2–7 days. Followed with oral therapy to complete at least 10 days of therapy.

PO: ADULTS, ELDERLY, CHILDREN 12 YRS AND OLDER: 200 mg q4h 5 times/day for 10 days or 400 mg 3 times/day for 7–10 days. **CHILDREN YOUNGER THAN 12 YRS:** 40–80 mg/kg/day in 3–4 divided doses for 5–10 days. **Maximum:** 1,200 mg/day.

Topical: ADULTS: (Ointment): 0.5 inch for 4-inch square surface q3h (6 times/day) for 7 days.

Genital Herpes (Recurrent)

Intermittent Therapy

PO: ADULTS, ELDERLY, CHILDREN 12 YRS AND OLDER: 400 mg 3 times/day for 5 days or 800 mg 2 times/day for 5 days or 800 mg 3 times/day for 2 days. **CHILDREN YOUNGER THAN 12 YRS:** 20 mg/kg 3 times/day for 5 days. **Maximum:** 400 mg/dose.

Chronic Suppressive Therapy

PO: ADULTS, ELDERLY, CHILDREN 12 YRS AND OLDER: 400 mg 2 times/day for up to 12 mos. **CHILDREN YOUNGER THAN 12 YRS:** 20 mg/kg twice daily. **Maximum:** 400 mg/dose.

Herpes Simplex Mucocutaneous
PO: ADULTS, ELDERLY: 400 mg 3 times/day or 200 mg 5 times/day for 7–10 days. **CHILDREN:** 20 mg/kg 4 times/day for 5–7 days. **Maximum:** 800 mg/dose.
IV: ADULTS, ELDERLY, CHILDREN: 5 mg/kg/dose q8h for 7–14 days.
Topical: ADULTS: ***(Ointment):*** 0.5 inch for 4-inch square surface q3h (6 times/day) for 7 days.

Herpes Simplex Encephalitis
IV: ADULTS, ELDERLY, CHILDREN 12 YRS AND OLDER: 10 mg/kg q8h for 14–21 days. **CHILDREN 3 MOS–YOUNGER THAN 12 YRS:** 10–15 mg/kg q8h for 14–21 days.

Herpes Zoster (Shingles)
IV: ADULTS, CHILDREN 12 YRS AND OLDER: (immunocompromised) 10–15 mg/kg/dose q8h for 10–14 days. **CHILDREN YOUNGER THAN 12 YRS:** (immunocompromised) 10 mg/kg/dose q8h for 7–10 days.
PO: ADULTS, ELDERLY, CHILDREN 12 YRS AND OLDER: 800 mg q4h 5 times/day for 7–10 days.

Herpes Labialis (Cold Sores)
Topical: ADULTS, ELDERLY, CHILDREN 12 YRS AND OLDER: Apply to affected area 5 times/day for 4 days. **Buccal Tablet:** 50 mg as a single dose to upper gum region.

Varicella-Zoster (Chickenpox)
◀ALERT▶ Begin treatment within 24 hrs of onset of rash.
PO: ADULTS, ELDERLY, CHILDREN OLDER THAN 12 YRS AND CHILDREN 2–12 YRS, WEIGHING 40 KG OR MORE: 800 mg 5 times/day for 5–7 days. **CHILDREN 2–12 YRS, WEIGHING LESS THAN 40 KG:** 20 mg/kg 4 times/day for 5 days. **Maximum:** 800 mg/dose.

Usual Neonatal Dosage
HSV (treatment) (IV): 20 mg/kg/dose q8–12h for 14–21 days.
HSV (chronic suppression) (PO): 300 mg/m^2/dose q8h –(after completing a 14–21 day course of IV therapy) for 6 mos.
Varicella-Zoster (IV): 10–15 mg/kg/dose q8h for 5–10 days.

Dosage in Renal Impairment
Dosage and frequency are modified based on severity of infection and degree of renal impairment.
PO: Normal dose 200 mg q4h, 200 mg q8h, or 400 mg q12h. **Creatinine clearance 10 mL/min and less:** 200 mg q12h.
PO: Normal dose 800 mg q4h. **Creatinine clearance greater than 25 mL/min:** Give usual dose and at normal interval, 800 mg q4h. **Creatinine clearance 10–25 mL/min:** 800 mg q8h. **Creatinine clearance less than 10 mL/min:** 800 mg q12h.
IV:

Creatinine Clearance	Dosage
Greater than 50 mL/min	100% of normal q8h
25–50 mL/min	100% of normal q12h
10–24 mL/min	100% of normal q24h
Less than 10 mL/min	50% of normal q24h
Hemodialysis (HD)	2.5–5 mg/kg q24h (give after HD)
Peritoneal dialysis (PD)	50% normal dose q24h
Continuous renal replacement therapy (CRRT)	5–10 mg/kg q12–24h (q12h for viral meningoencephalitis/VZV infection)

Dosage in Hepatic Impairment
Mild to moderate impairment: No dose adjustment. **Severe impairment:** Use caution.

SIDE EFFECTS

Frequent: Parenteral (9%–7%): Phlebitis or inflammation at IV site, nausea, vomiting. **Topical (28%):** Burning, stinging. **Occasional: Parenteral (3%):** Pruritus, rash, urticaria. **PO (12%–6%):** Malaise, nausea. **Topical (4%):** Pruritus. **Rare: PO (3%–1%):** Vomiting, rash, diarrhea, headache. **Parenteral (2%–1%):** Confusion, hallucinations, seizures, tremors. **Topical (less than 1%):** Rash.

ADVERSE EFFECTS/TOXIC REACTIONS

Rapid parenteral administration, excessively high doses, or fluid and electrolyte imbalance may produce renal failure. Toxicity not reported with oral or topical use.

NURSING CONSIDERATIONS

BASELINE ASSESSMENT

Question for history of allergies, esp. to acyclovir. Assess herpes simplex lesions before treatment to compare baseline with treatment effect.

INTERVENTION/EVALUATION

Assess IV site for phlebitis (heat, pain, red streaking over vein). Evaluate cutaneous lesions. Ensure adequate ventilation. Manage chickenpox and disseminated herpes zoster with strict isolation. Encourage fluid intake.

PATIENT/FAMILY TEACHING

• Drink adequate fluids. • Do not touch lesions with bare fingers to prevent spreading infection to new site. • Continue therapy for full length of treatment. • Space doses evenly. • Use finger cot/rubber glove to apply topical ointment. • Avoid sexual intercourse during duration of lesions to prevent infecting partner. • Acyclovir does not cure herpes infections. • Pap smear should be done at least annually due to increased risk of cervical cancer in women with genital herpes.

adalimumab

TOP 100

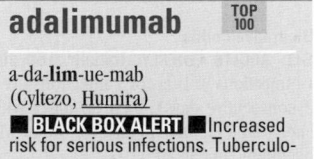

a-da-**lim**-ue-mab
(Cyltezo, Humira)

BLACK BOX ALERT Increased risk for serious infections. Tuberculosis, invasive fungal infections, bacterial and viral opportunistic infections have occurred. Test for tuberculosis prior to and during treatment. Lymphoma, other malignancies reported in children/adolescents. Hepatosplenic T-cell lymphoma reported primarily in pts with Crohn's disease or ulcerative colitis and concomitant azaTHIOprine or mercaptopurine.

Do not confuse Humira with HumaLOG or HumuLIN, or adalimumab with belimumab or ipilimumab.

◆CLASSIFICATION

PHARMACOTHERAPEUTIC: Monoclonal antibody. **CLINICAL:** Antirheumatic, disease modifying; GI agent; TNF blocking agent.

USES

Reduces signs/symptoms, progression of structural damage and improves physical function in adults with moderate to severe RA. May be used alone or in combination with other disease-modifying antirheumatic drugs. First-line treatment of moderate to severe RA, treatment of psoriatic arthritis, treatment of ankylosing spondylitis, to induce/maintain remission of moderate to severe active Crohn's disease, moderate to severe plaque psoriasis in pts 6 yrs of age and older. Reduces signs and symptoms of moderate to severe active polyarticular juvenile rheumatoid arthritis in pts 2 yrs and older. Treatment of active ulcerative colitis in pts unresponsive to immunosuppressants. Treatment of moderate to severe hidradenitis suppurativa. Treatment of uveitis (noninfectious intermediate, posterior and panuveitis) in adults.

PRECAUTIONS

Contraindications: Hypersensitivity to adalimumab. Severe infections (e.g., sepsis, TB). **Cautions:** Pts with chronic infections or pts at risk for infections (e.g., diabetes, indwelling catheters, renal failure, open wounds), elderly, decreased left ventricular function, HF, demyelinating disorders, invasive fungal infections, history of malignancies.

ACTION

Binds specifically to tumor necrosis factor (TNF) alpha cell, blocking its interaction with cell surface TNF receptors and cytokine-driven inflammatory processes. **Therapeutic Effect:** Decreases signs/symptoms of RA, psoriatic arthritis, ankylosing spondylitis, Crohn's disease, ulcerative colitis. Inhibits progression of rheumatoid and psoriatic arthritis. Reduces epidermal thickness, inflammation of plaque psoriasis.

PHARMACOKINETICS

Metabolism not specified. Elimination not specified. **Half-life:** 10–20 days.

⌛ LIFESPAN CONSIDERATIONS

Pregnancy/Lactation: Unknown if distributed in breast milk. **Children:** Safety and efficacy not established. **Elderly:** Cautious use due to increased risk of serious infection and malignancy.

INTERACTIONS

DRUG: May increase the adverse effects of **abatacept, anakinra, belimumab, canakinumab, natalizumab, tofacitinib, vaccines (live), vedolizumab.** May decrease the therapeutic effect of **BCG (intravesical), vaccines (live).** May increase the immunosuppressive effects of **certolizumab, infliximab. Tocilizumab** may increase immunosuppressive effect. **HERBAL: Echinacea** may decrease effects. **FOOD:** None known. **LAB VALUES:** May increase serum cholesterol, other lipids, alkaline phosphatase.

AVAILABILITY (Rx)

Injection Solution: 10 mg/0.2 mL, 20 mg/0.4 mL, 40 mg/0.8 mL, 40 mg/0.4 mL, 80 mg/0.8 mL in prefilled syringes.

ADMINISTRATION/HANDLING

SQ

• Refrigerate; do not freeze. • Discard unused portion. • Rotate injection sites. Give new injection at least 1 inch from an old site and never into area where skin is tender, bruised, red, or hard. • Give in thigh or lower abdomen. • Avoid areas within 2 inches of navel.

INDICATIONS/ROUTES/DOSAGE

Rheumatoid Arthritis (RA)

SQ: ADULTS, ELDERLY: 40 mg every other wk. Dose may be increased to 40 mg/wk in pts not taking methotrexate.

Ankylosing Spondylitis, Psoriatic Arthritis

SQ: ADULTS, ELDERLY: 40 mg every other wk.

Crohn's Disease

SQ: ADULTS, ELDERLY, CHILDREN 6 YRS AND OLDER WEIGHING 40 KG OR MORE: Initially, 160 mg given as 4 injections on day 1 or 2 injections/day over 2 days, then 80 mg 2 wks later (day 15). **Maintenance:** 40 mg every other wk beginning at day 29. **CHILDREN 6 YRS AND OLDER WEIGHING 17–39 KG:** 80 mg (2 40-mg injections on day 1), then 40 mg 2 wks later. **Maintenance:** 20 mg every other wk beginning at day 29.

Plaque Psoriasis, Uveitis

SQ: ADULTS, ELDERLY: Initially, 80 mg as a single dose, then 40 mg every other wk starting 1 wk after initial dose.

Juvenile Rheumatoid Arthritis

SQ: CHILDREN 2 YRS AND OLDER, WEIGHING 10–14 KG: 10 mg every other wk. **WEIGHING 15–29 KG:** 20 mg every other wk. **WEIGHING 30 KG OR MORE:** 40 mg every other wk.

Ulcerative Colitis

SQ: ADULTS, ELDERLY: Initially, 160 mg (4 injections in 1 day or 2 injections over 2 consecutive days), then 80 mg 2 wks later (day 15), then 40 mg every other wk beginning on day 29.

Hidradenitis Suppurativa

SQ: ADULTS, ELDERLY: Initially, 160 mg (4 injections day 1) or 80 mg (2 injections on days 1 and 2), then 80 mg 2 wks later (day 15), then 40 mg weekly beginning day 29.

Dosage in Renal/Hepatic Impairment

No dose adjustment.

SIDE EFFECTS

Frequent (20%): Injection site erythema, pruritus, pain, swelling. **Occasional (12%–9%):** Headache, rash, sinusitis, nausea. **Rare (7%–5%):** Abdominal or back pain, hypertension.

ADVERSE EFFECTS/TOXIC REACTIONS

Hypersensitivity reactions (rash, urticaria, hypotension, dyspnea), infections (primarily upper respiratory tract, bronchitis, urinary tract) occur rarely. May increase risk of serious infections (pneumonia, tuberculosis, cellulitis, pyelonephritis, septic arthritis). May increase risk of reactivation of hepatitis B virus in pts who are chronic carriers. May cause new-onset or exacerbation of central nervous demyelinating disease; worsening and new-onset HF. May increase risk of malignancies. Immunogenicity (anti-adalimumab autoantibodies) occurred in 12% of pts.

NURSING CONSIDERATIONS

BASELINE ASSESSMENT

Assess onset, type, location, duration of pain or inflammation. Inspect appearance of affected joints for immobility, deformities, skin condition. Review immunization status/screening for TB. If pt is to self-administer, instruct on SQ injection technique, including areas of the body acceptable for injection sites.

INTERVENTION/EVALUATION

Monitor lab values, particularly CBC. Assess for therapeutic response: relief of pain, stiffness, swelling; increased joint mobility; reduced joint tenderness; improved grip strength.

PATIENT/FAMILY TEACHING

• Injection site reaction generally occurs in first month of treatment and decreases in frequency during continued therapy. • Do not receive live vaccines during treatment. • Report rash, nausea. • A healthcare provider will show you how to properly prepare and inject your medication. You must demonstrate correct preparation and injection techniques before using medication.

ado-trastuzumab emtansine

ado-tras-**tooz**-oo-mab
(Kadcyla)

■ **BLACK BOX ALERT** ■ Do not substitute ado-trastuzumab for trastuzumab. Hepatotoxicity, hepatic failure may lead to death. Monitor hepatic function prior to each dose. May decrease left ventricular ejection fraction (LVEF). Embryo-fetal toxicity may result in birth defects and/or fetal demise.

Do not confuse ado-trastuzumab with trastuzumab.

◆CLASSIFICATION

PHARMACOTHERAPEUTIC: Anti-HER2. Antibody drug conjugate. Antimicrotubular. Monoclonal antibody. **CLINICAL:** Antineoplastic.

USES

Treatment of HER2-positive, metastatic breast cancer in pts who have previously received trastuzumab and a taxane agent separately or in combination, or pts who have developed recurrence within 6 mos of completing adjuvant therapy. Treatment (single agent) of human epidermal growth factor receptor 2 (HER2)–positive early breast cancer in pts with residual invasive disease after taxane and trastuzumab-based treatment.

PRECAUTIONS

Contraindications: Hypersensitivity to trastuzumab. **Cautions:** History of cardiomyopathy, HF, MI, arrhythmias, hepatic disease, thrombocytopenia, pulmonary disease, peripheral neuropathy, pregnancy.

ACTION

Binds to HER2 receptor and undergoes receptor-mediated lysosomal degradation, resulting in intracellular release of DM1-containing cytotoxic catabolites. Binding of DM1 to tubulin disrupts microtubule networks in the cell. **Therapeutic Effect:** Inhibits tumor cell survival in HER2-positive breast cancer.

PHARMACOKINETICS

Metabolized in liver. Protein binding: 93%. Peak plasma concentration: 30–90 min. **Half-life:** 4 days.

LIFESPAN CONSIDERATIONS

Pregnancy/Lactation: May cause fetal harm. Use contraception during treatment and up to 6 mos after discontinuation. Unknown if distributed in breast milk. Do not breastfeed. **Children:** Safety and efficacy not established. **Elderly:** No age-related precautions noted.

INTERACTIONS

DRUG: May decrease the therapeutic effect of **BCG (intravesical), vaccines (live).** May increase adverse effects of **belimumab, natalizumab, vaccines (live). Strong CYP3A4 inhibitors (e.g., clarithromycin, ketoconazole, ritonavir)** may increase concentration/effect. **HERBAL:** **Echinacea** may decrease therapeutic effect. **FOOD:** None known. **LAB VALUES:** May increase serum ALT, AST, bilirubin. May decrease platelets, serum potassium.

AVAILABILITY (Rx)

Lyophilized Powder for Injection: 100-mg vial, 160-mg vial.

ADMINISTRATION/HANDLING

◀ALERT▶ Use 0.22-micron in-line filter. Do not administer IV push or bolus.

IV

Reconstitution • Use proper chemotherapy precautions. • Slowly inject 5 mL of Sterile Water for Injection into 100-mg vial or 8 mL Sterile Water for Injection for 160-mg vial. • Final concentration: 20 mg/mL. • Gently swirl until completely dissolved. • Do not shake. • Inspect for particulate matter/discoloration. • Calculate dose from 20 mg/mL vial. • Further dilute in 250 mL of 0.9% NaCl only. • Invert bag to mix (do not shake).

Rate of administration • Infuse using 0.22-micron in-line filter. • Infuse initial dose over 90 min. • Infuse subsequent doses over 30 min. • Slow or interrupt infusion rate if hypersensitivity reaction occurs.

Storage • Refrigerate unused vials. • Reconstituted vials, diluted solutions should be used immediately (may be refrigerated for up to 24 hrs).

IV INCOMPATIBILITIES

Do not use dextrose-containing solutions.

INDICATIONS/ROUTES/DOSAGE

Note: Do not substitute with conventional trastuzumab (Herceptin).

Metastatic Breast Cancer

IV infusion: ADULTS/ELDERLY: 3.6 mg/kg every 3 wks until disease progression or unacceptable toxicity. **Maximum:** 3.6 mg/kg.

Breast Cancer, Early, HER2 Positive, Adjuvant Therapy

IV infusion: ADULTS/ELDERLY: 3.6 mg/kg q3wks for 14 cycles (in the absence of disease recurrence or unacceptable toxicity).
Maximum: 3.6 mg/kg.

Dose Modification

Reduction Schedule for Adverse Effects

Initial dose: 3.6 mg/kg. First reduction: 3 mg/kg. Second reduction: 2.4 mg/kg.

Hepatotoxicity

Elevated serum ALT, AST: If less than 5 times upper limit of normal (ULN), continue same dose. If 5–20 times ULN, hold until less than 5 times ULN and reduce by one dose level. If greater than 20 times ULN, discontinue. **Elevated serum bilirubin:** Hold until less than 1.5 times ULN, then continue same dose. If 3–10 times ULN, hold until less than 1.5 times ULN, then reduce by one dose level. If greater than 10 times ULN, discontinue.

Cardiotoxicity

Left ventricular dysfunction: If LVEF greater than 45%, continue same dose. If LVEF 40%–45% with a decrease less than 10% from baseline, continue dose (or reduce) and repeat LVEF in 3 wks. If LVEF 40%–45% with decrease greater than 10% from baseline, hold and repeat assessment in 3 wks. Discontinue therapy if no recovery within 10% of baseline, LVEF less than 40%, or symptomatic HF.

Thrombocytopenia

Platelet count 25,000–50,000 cells/mm³: Withhold treatment until improved to 75,000 cells/mm³, then continue same dose. **Platelet count less than 25,000 cells/mm³:** Withhold treatment until improved to 75,000 cells/mm³, then reduce dose level.

Dosage in Renal/Hepatic Impairment

No dose adjustment.

SIDE EFFECTS

Frequent (40%–21%): Nausea, fatigue, musculoskeletal pain, headache, constipation, diarrhea. **Occasional (19%–7%):** Abdominal pain, vomiting, pyrexia, arthralgia, asthenia, cough, dry mouth, stomatitis, myalgia, insomnia, rash, dizziness, dyspepsia, chills, dysgeusia, peripheral edema. **Rare (6%–3%):** Pruritus, blurry vision, dry eye, conjunctivitis, lacrimation.

ADVERSE EFFECTS/TOXIC REACTIONS

Hepatotoxicity may include elevated transaminase, nodular regenerative hyperplasia, portal hypertension. Left ventricular dysfunction reported in 1.8% of pts. Interstitial lung disease (ILD), including pneumonitis, may lead to ARDS. Hypersensitivity reactions reported in 1.4% of pts. Thrombocytopenia (34% of pts) may increase risk of bleeding. Peripheral neuropathy observed rarely. Approx. 5.3% of pts tested positive for anti–ado-trastuzumab antibodies (immunogenicity).

NURSING CONSIDERATIONS

BASELINE ASSESSMENT

Obtain baseline CBC, BMP; PT/INR if on anticoagulants. Confirm HER2-positive titer. Screen for baseline HF, hepatic impairment, peripheral edema, pulmonary disease, thrombocytopenia. Obtain negative pregnancy test before initiating treatment. Question current breastfeeding status. Obtain baseline echocardiogram for LVEF status.

INTERVENTION/EVALUATION

Observe for hypersensitivity reactions during infusion. Monitor LFT, potassium levels before and during treatment. Obtain LVEF q3mos or with any dose reduction regarding LVEF status. Assess for bruising, jaundice, right upper quadrant (RUQ) abdominal pain. Obtain anti–ado-trastuzumab antibody titer if immunogenicity suspected. Obtain stat ECG for palpitations or irregular pulse, chest X-ray for difficulty breathing, cough, fever. Monitor for neurotoxicity (peripheral neuropathy).

PATIENT/FAMILY TEACHING

• Blood levels will be monitored routinely. • Avoid pregnancy. • Contraception should be used during treatment and up to 6 mos after discontinuation. • Report black/tarry stools, RUQ abdominal pain, nausea, bruising, yellowing of skin or eyes, difficulty breathing, palpitations, bleeding. • Avoid alcohol. • Treatment may reduce the heart's ability to pump; expect routine echocardiograms. • Report bleeding of any kind or extremity numbness, tingling, weakness, pain.

afatinib

a-fa-ti-nib
(Gilotrif)
Do not confuse afatinib with ibrutinib, dasatinib, gefitinib, or SUNItinib.

◆CLASSIFICATION

PHARMACOTHERAPEUTIC: Epidermal growth factor receptor (EGFR) inhibitor. Tyrosine kinase inhibitor. **CLINICAL:** Antineoplastic.

USES

First-line treatment of metastatic non–small-cell lung cancer (NSCLC) in pts with epidermal growth factor (EDGF) exon 19 deletions or exon 21 (L858R) substitution mutations. Treatment of metastatic, squamous NSCLC progressing after platinum-based chemotherapy.

PRECAUTIONS

Contraindications: Hypersensitivity to afatinib. **Cautions:** Hepatic impairment; severe renal impairment; pts with hx of keratitis, severe dry eye, ulcerative keratitis, or use of contact lenses; hypovolemia; pulmonary disease; ulcerative lesions. Patients with GI disorders associated with diarrhea (e.g., Crohn's disease), cardiac risk factors, and/or decreased left ventricular ejection fraction.

ACTION

Highly selective blocker of ErbB family (e.g., EGFR, HER2); irreversibly binds to intracellular tyrosine kinase domain. **Therapeutic Effect:** Inhibits tumor growth, causes tumor regression.

PHARMACOKINETICS

Readily absorbed following PO administration. Enzymatic metabolism is minimal. Protein binding: 95%. Peak plasma concentration: 2–5 hrs. Excreted in feces (85%), urine (4%). **Half-life:** 37 hrs.

⌛ LIFESPAN CONSIDERATIONS

Pregnancy/Lactation: May cause fetal harm. Unknown if distributed in breast milk. Must either discontinue drug or discontinue breastfeeding. Contraception recommended during treatment and up to 2 wks after discontinuation. **Children:** Safety and efficacy not established. **Elderly:** No age-related precautions noted.

INTERACTIONS

DRUG: **P-glycoprotein inhibitors (e.g., amiodarone, cycloSPORINE, ketoconazole)** may increase concentration/effect. **P-glycoprotein inducers (e.g., carBAMazepine, rifAMPin)** may decrease concentration/effect. **HERBAL:** None significant. **FOOD:** **High-fat meals** may decrease absorption. **LAB VALUES:** May increase serum ALT, AST. May decrease serum potassium.

AVAILABILITY (Rx)

Tablets: 20 mg, 30 mg, 40 mg.

ADMINISTRATION/HANDLING

PO

• Give at least 1 hr before or 2 hrs after meal. Do not take missed dose within 12 hrs of next dose.

INDICATIONS/ROUTES/DOSAGE

Metastatic NSCLC, Metastatic Squamous NSCLC

PO: ADULTS/ELDERLY: Initially, 40 mg once daily until disease progression or no longer tolerated. Do not take missed dose within 12 hrs of next dose.

Dose Modification

Chronic use of P-glycoprotein (P-gp) inhibitors: Reduce daily dose by 10 mg. Resume previous dose after discontinuation of inhibitor if tolerated. **Chronic use of P-glycoprotein inducers:** Increase daily dose by 10 mg if tolerated. May resume initial dose 2–3 days after discontinuation of P-gp inducer. **Moderate to severe diarrhea (more than 48 hrs):** Withhold dose until resolution to mild diarrhea. **Moderate cutaneous skin reaction (more than**

7 days): Withhold dose until reaction resolves, then reduce dose appropriately. **Suspected keratitis:** Withhold until appropriately ruled out. If keratitis confirmed, continue only if benefits outweigh risks.

Permanent Discontinuation

Discontinue if persistent severe diarrhea, respiratory distress, severe dry eye, or life-threatening bullous, blistering, exfoliating lesions, persistent ulcerative keratitis, interstitial lung disease, symptomatic left ventricular dysfunction occurs.

Dosage in Renal/Hepatic Impairment

eGFR 15–29 mL/min: Decrease dose to 30 mg. **Severe impairment:** Avoid use.

SIDE EFFECTS

Frequent (96%–58%): Diarrhea, rash, dermatitis, stomatitis, paronychia (nail infection). **Occasional (31%–11%):** Dry skin, decreased appetite, pruritus, epistaxis, weight loss, cystitis, pyrexia, cheilitis (lip inflammation), rhinorrhea, conjunctivitis.

ADVERSE EFFECTS/TOXIC REACTIONS

Diarrhea may lead to severe, sometimes fatal, dehydration or renal impairment. Bullous and exfoliative skin lesions occur rarely. Rash, erythema, acneiform lesions occur in 90% of pts. Palmar-plantar erythrodysesthesia syndrome (PPES), a chemotherapy-induced skin condition that presents with redness, swelling, numbness, skin sloughing of the hands and feet, has been reported. Interstitial lung disease (ILD), including pulmonary infiltration, pneumonitis, ARDS, allergic alveolitis, reported in 2% of pts. Hepatotoxicity reported in 10% of pts. Keratitis symptoms, such as eye inflammation, lacrimation, light sensitivity, blurred vision, red eye, occurred in 1% of pts.

NURSING CONSIDERATIONS

BASELINE ASSESSMENT

Obtain baseline CBC, BMP, visual acuity. Obtain negative pregnancy test before initiating therapy. Question current breastfeeding status. Screen for history/comorbidities, contact lens use. Receive full medication history, including herbal products. Assess skin for lesions, ulcers, open wounds.

INTERVENTION/EVALUATION

Monitor renal/hepatic function tests, urine output. Encourage PO intake. Assess for hydration status. Offer antidiarrheal medication for loose stool. Report oliguria, dark or concentrated urine. Immediately report skin lesions, vision changes, dry eye, severe diarrhea. Obtain chest X-ray if ILD suspected. Assess skin for dermal changes, toxicities.

PATIENT/FAMILY TEACHING

• Most pts experience diarrhea, and severe cases may lead to dehydration or kidney failure; maintain adequate hydration. • Avoid pregnancy; contraception should be used during treatment and up to 2 wks after discontinuation. • Report any yellowing of skin or eyes, abdominal pain, bruising, black/tarry stools, dark urine, decreased urine output. • Minimize exposure to sunlight. • Immediately report eye problems (pain, swelling, blurred vision, vision changes) or skin blistering/redness. • Do not eat 1 hr before or 2 hrs after dose. • Do not wear contact lenses (may increase risk of keratitis).

albumin

al-**bue**-min
(Albuked-5, Albuked-25, AlbuRx, Albutein, Flexbumin, Kedbumin, Plasbumin-5, Plasbumin-25)
Do not confuse albumin with albuterol, or Buminate with bumetanide.

◆CLASSIFICATION

PHARMACOTHERAPEUTIC: Plasma protein fraction. **CLINICAL:** Blood derivative.

USES

Hypovolemia plasma volume expansion, maintenance of cardiac output in treatment of shock or impending shock. May be useful in treatment of ovarian hyperstimulation syndrome, acute/severe nephrosis, cirrhotic ascites, adult respiratory distress syndrome (ARDS), cardiopulmonary bypass, hemodialysis. **OFF-LABEL:** Large-volume paracentesis. In cirrhotics, with diuretics to help facilitate diuresis.

PRECAUTIONS

Contraindications: Hypersensitivity to albumin. Pts at risk for volume overload (e.g., severe anemia, HF, renal insufficiency). Dilution with Sterile Water for Injection may cause hemolysis or acute renal failure. **Cautions:** Pts for whom sodium restriction is necessary, hepatic/renal failure (added protein load). Avoid 25% concentration in preterm infants (risk of intraventricular hemorrhage).

ACTION

Blood volume expander. **Therapeutic Effect:** Provides increase in intravascular oncotic pressure, mobilizes fluids into intravascular space.

PHARMACOKINETICS

Route	Onset	Peak	Duration
IV	15 min (in well-hydrated pt)	N/A	Dependent on initial blood volume

Distributed throughout extracellular fluid. **Half-life:** 15–20 days.

LIFESPAN CONSIDERATIONS

Pregnancy/Lactation: Unknown if drug crosses placenta or is distributed in breast milk. **Children/Elderly:** No age-related precautions noted.

INTERACTIONS

DRUG: None significant. **HERBAL:** None significant. **FOOD:** None known. **LAB VALUES:** May increase serum alkaline phosphatase.

AVAILABILITY (Rx)

Injection Solution: (5%): 50 mL, 250 mL, 500 mL. **(25%):** 20 mL, 50 mL, 100 mL.

ADMINISTRATION/HANDLING

IV

Reconstitution • A 5% solution may be made from 25% solution by adding 1 volume 25% to 4 volumes 0.9% NaCl (NaCl preferred). Do not use Sterile Water for Injection (life-threatening hemolysis, acute renal failure can result).

Rate of administration • Give by IV infusion. Rate is variable, depending on use, blood volume, concentration of solute. 5%: Do not exceed 2–4 mL/min in pts with normal plasma volume, 5–10 mL/min in pts with hypoproteinemia. 25%: Do not exceed 1 mL/min in pts with normal plasma volume, 2–3 mL/min in pts with hypoproteinemia. 5% is administered undiluted; 25% may be administered undiluted or diluted in 0.9% NaCl. • May give without regard to pt blood group or Rh factor.

Storage • Store at room temperature. Appears as clear brownish, odorless, moderately viscous fluid. • Do not use if solution has been frozen, appears turbid, contains sediment, or if not used within 4 hrs of opening vial.

IV INCOMPATIBILITIES

Lipids, micafungin (Mycamine), midazolam (Versed), vancomycin (Vancocin), verapamil (Isoptin).

IV COMPATIBILITIES

DiltiaZEM (Cardizem), LORazepam (Ativan).

INDICATIONS/ROUTES/DOSAGE

◀ALERT▶ 5% should be used in hypovolemic or intravascularly depleted pts. 25% should be used in pts in whom fluid and sodium intake must be minimized.

Usual Dosage

IV: ADULTS, ELDERLY: Initially, 25 g; may repeat in 15–30 min if response is inadequate.

Hypovolemia
IV: ADULTS, ELDERLY, ADOLESCENTS: 5% albumin: 12.5–25 g (250–500 mL), repeat after 15–30 min, as needed. **CHILDREN:** 0.5–1 g/kg/dose (10–20 mL/kg/dose of 5% albumin). Repeat in 30-min intervals as needed.

Hemodialysis
IV: ADULTS, ELDERLY: 50–100 mL (12.5–25 g) of 25% albumin as needed.

Dosage in Renal/Hepatic Impairment
No dose adjustment.

SIDE EFFECTS

Occasional: Hypotension. **Rare:** High dose in repeated therapy: altered vital signs, chills, fever, increased salivation, nausea, vomiting, urticaria, tachycardia.

ADVERSE EFFECTS/TOXIC REACTIONS

Fluid overload may occur, marked by increased B/P, distended neck veins. Pulmonary edema may occur, evidenced by labored respirations, dyspnea, rales, wheezing, coughing. Neurologic changes, including headache, weakness, blurred vision, behavioral changes, incoordination, isolated muscle twitching, may occur.

NURSING CONSIDERATIONS

BASELINE ASSESSMENT

Obtain B/P, pulse, respirations immediately before administration. Adequate hydration required before albumin is administered.

INTERVENTION/EVALUATION

Monitor B/P for hypotension/hypertension. Assess frequently for evidence of fluid overload, pulmonary edema (see **Adverse Effects/Toxic Reactions**). Check skin for flushing, urticaria. Monitor I&O ratio (watch for decreased output). Assess for therapeutic response (increased B/P, decreased edema).

albuterol

TOP 100

al-**bue**-ter-ol
(Airomir ✱, ProAir HFA, ProAir RespiClick, Proventil HFA, Ventolin HFA)
Do not confuse albuterol with albumin or atenolol, Proventil with Bentyl, PriLOSEC, or Prinivil, or Ventolin with Benylin or Vantin.

FIXED-COMBINATION(S)

Combivent Respimat: albuterol/ipratropium (a bronchodilator): 100 mcg/20 mcg per actuation. **DuoNeb:** albuterol/ipratropium 3 mg/0.5 mg.

◆CLASSIFICATION

PHARMACOTHERAPEUTIC: Sympathomimetic (adrenergic $beta_2$-agonist). **CLINICAL:** Bronchodilator.

USES

Treatment or prevention of bronchospasm due to reversible obstructive airway disease, prevention of exercise-induced bronchospasm. **OFF-LABEL:** Treatment of asthma in children under 4 yrs of age.

PRECAUTIONS

Contraindications: Hypersensitivity to albuterol. Severe hypersensitivity to milk protein (dry powder inhalation). **Cautions:** Hypertension, cardiovascular disease, hyperthyroidism, diabetes, HF, convulsive disorders, glaucoma, hypokalemia, arrhythmias.

ACTION

Stimulates $beta_2$-adrenergic receptors in lungs, resulting in relaxation of bronchial smooth muscle (little effect on HR). **Therapeutic Effect:** Relieves bronchospasm and reduces airway resistance.

PHARMACOKINETICS

Route	Onset	Peak	Duration
PO	15–30 min	2–3 hrs	4–6 hrs
PO (extended-release)	30 min	2–4 hrs	12 hrs
Inhalation	5–15 min	0.5–2 hrs	2–5 hrs

Rapidly, well absorbed from GI tract; rapidly absorbed from bronchi after inhalation. Metabolized in liver. Primarily excreted in urine. **Half-life:** 3.8–6 hrs.

⌛ LIFESPAN CONSIDERATIONS

Pregnancy/Lactation: Appears to cross placenta; unknown if distributed in breast milk. May inhibit uterine contractility. **Children:** Safety and efficacy not established in pts younger than 2 yrs (syrup) or younger than 6 yrs (tablets). **Elderly:** May be more sensitive to tremor or tachycardia due to age-related increased sympathetic sensitivity.

INTERACTIONS

DRUG: Beta-blockers (e.g., carvedilol, labetalol, metoprolol) may decrease bronchodilation. **MAOIs (e.g., phenelzine, selegiline), linezolid, sympathomimetics (e.g., dopamine, norepinephrine)** may increase hypertensive effect. **HERBAL:** None significant. **FOOD:** None known. **LAB VALUES:** May increase blood glucose. May decrease serum potassium.

AVAILABILITY (Rx)

Powder Breath Activated Inhalation Aerosol: ***(ProAir RespiClick):*** 90 mcg/actuation. **Inhalation Aerosol Solution:** ***(ProAir HFA, Proventil HFA, Ventolin HFA):*** 90 mcg/spray. **Solution for Nebulization:** 0.63 mg/3 mL (0.021%), 1.25 mg/3 mL (0.042%), 2.5 mg/3 mL (0.084%), 5 mg/mL (0.5%). **Syrup:** 2 mg/5 mL. **Tablets:** 2 mg, 4 mg.

Tablets (Extended-Release): 4 mg, 8 mg.

ADMINISTRATION/HANDLING

Inhalation Aerosol

• Shake container well before inhalation. • Prime prior to first use. A spacer is recommended for use with MDI. • Wait 2 min before inhaling second dose (allows for deeper bronchial penetration). • Rinse mouth with water immediately after inhalation (prevents mouth/throat dryness).

Inhalation Powder

• Device is breath activated. • Do not use with spacer. • Do not wash or put any part of inhaler to water.

Nebulization

• Administer over 5–15 min.

INDICATIONS/ROUTES/DOSAGE

Acute Bronchospasm, Exacerbation of Asthma

Inhalation: **ADULTS, ELDERLY, CHILDREN OLDER THAN 12 YRS:** **(Acute, Severe):** 4–8 puffs q20min for 3 doses, then taper as tolerated. **CHILDREN 12 YRS AND YOUNGER:** **Acute, Severe:** 4–8 puffs q20min for 3 doses, then q1–4h as needed. **Nebulization:** **ADULTS, ELDERLY, CHILDREN OLDER THAN 12 YRS:** **Acute, Severe:** 2.5–5 mg q20min for 3 doses, then 2.5–10 mg q1–4h or 10–15 mg/hr continuously. **CHILDREN 12 YRS AND YOUNGER:** 0.15 mg/kg q20min for 3 doses (minimum: 2.5 mg), then 0.15–0.3 mg/kg q1–4h as needed. **Maximum:** 10 mg q1–4h as needed or 0.5 mg/kg/hr by continuous inhalation.

Bronchospasm

Nebulization: **ADULTS, ELDERLY, CHILDREN 12 YRS AND OLDER:** 2.5 mg 3–4 times/day as needed. **CHILDREN 2–11 YRS:** (Greater than 15 kg): 0.63–2.5 mg 3 to 4 times/day. **Maximum:** 10 mg/day. (10–15 kg): 0.63–1.25 mg 3–4 times/day as needed. **Maximum:** 10 mg/day. **Inhalation:** **ADULTS, ELDERLY, CHILDREN:** 2 puffs q4–6h as needed.

Exercise-Induced Bronchospasm
Inhalation: ADULTS, ELDERLY, CHILDREN 5 YRS AND OLDER: 2 puffs 5–20 min before exercise. **CHILDREN 4 YRS AND YOUNGER:** 1–2 puffs 5–20 min before exercise.

Dosage in Renal/Hepatic Impairment
No dose adjustment.

SIDE EFFECTS

Frequent (27%–4%): Headache, restlessness, nervousness, tremors, nausea, dizziness, throat dryness and irritation, pharyngitis, B/P changes including hypertension, heartburn, transient wheezing. **Occasional (3%–2%):** Insomnia, asthenia, altered taste. **Inhalation:** Dry, irritated mouth or throat; cough, bronchial irritation. **Rare:** Drowsiness, diarrhea, dry mouth, flushing, diaphoresis, anorexia.

ADVERSE EFFECTS/TOXIC REACTIONS

Excessive sympathomimetic stimulation may produce palpitations, ectopy, tachycardia, chest pain, slight increase in B/P followed by substantial decrease, chills, diaphoresis, blanching of skin. Too-frequent or excessive use may lead to decreased bronchodilating effectiveness and severe, paradoxical bronchoconstriction.

NURSING CONSIDERATIONS

BASELINE ASSESSMENT

Assess lung sounds, pulse, B/P, color, characteristics of sputum noted. Offer emotional support (high incidence of anxiety due to difficulty in breathing and sympathomimetic response to drug).

INTERVENTION/EVALUATION

Monitor rate, depth, rhythm, type of respiration; quality and rate of pulse; ECG; serum potassium, glucose; ABG determinations. Assess lung sounds for wheezing (bronchoconstriction), rales.

PATIENT/FAMILY TEACHING

• Follow guidelines for proper use of inhaler. • Increase fluid intake (decreases lung secretion viscosity). • Do not take more than 2 inhalations at any one time (excessive use may produce paradoxical bronchoconstriction or decreased bronchodilating effect). • Rinsing mouth with water immediately after inhalation may prevent mouth/throat dryness. • Avoid excessive use of caffeine derivatives (chocolate, coffee, tea, cola, cocoa).

alectinib

al-**ek**-ti-nib
(Alecensa, Alecensaro ✤)
Do not confuse alectinib with afatinib, ibrutinib, imatinib, or gefitinib.

◆CLASSIFICATION

PHARMACOTHERAPEUTIC: Tyrosine kinase inhibitor. Anaplastic lymphoma kinase (ALK) inhibitor. **CLINICAL:** Antineoplastic.

USES

Treatment of pts with anaplastic lymphoma kinase (ALK)–positive metastatic non–small-cell lung cancer (NSCLC).

PRECAUTIONS

Contraindications: Hypersensitivity to alectinib. **Cautions:** Baseline anemia, leukopenia; bradycardia, bradyarrhythmias, chronic edema, diabetes, dehydration, electrolyte imbalance, hepatic/renal impairment, HF, ocular disease, pulmonary disease, history of thromboembolism.

ACTION

Inhibits ALK. ALK gene abnormalities may result in expression of oncogenic fusion proteins, which alter signaling and result in increased cellular proliferation/survival in tumors. **Therapeutic Effect:** Inhibition of ALK decreases tumor cell viability.

PHARMACOKINETICS

Metabolized in liver. Protein binding: Greater than 99%. Peak plasma concentration: 4 hrs. Steady state reached in 7 days. Excreted in feces (98%), urine (less than 0.5%). **Half-life:** 33 hrs.

LIFESPAN CONSIDERATIONS

Pregnancy/Lactation: Avoid pregnancy; may cause fetal harm. Females of reproductive potential should use effective contraception during treatment and for at least 1 wk after discontinuation. Unknown if distributed in breast milk. Breastfeeding not recommended during treatment and for at least 1 wk after discontinuation. **Males:** Males with female partners of reproductive potential must use barrier methods during treatment and up to 3 mos after discontinuation. **Children/Elderly:** Safety and efficacy not established.

INTERACTIONS

DRUG: **Beta blockers (e.g., atenolol, carvedilol, metoprolol), calcium channel blockers (e.g., diltiazem, verapamil), digoxin** may increase risk of bradycardia. **HERBAL:** None significant. **FOOD:** **High-fat, high-calorie meals** increase absorption/exposure. **LAB VALUES:** May increase serum alkaline phosphatase, ALT, AST, bilirubin, CPK, creatinine, glucose. May decrease serum calcium, potassium, phosphate, sodium; Hgb, Hct, lymphocytes, RBCs.

AVAILABILITY (Rx)

Capsules: 150 mg.

ADMINISTRATION/HANDLING

PO

• Give with food. • Administer whole; do not break, crush, cut, or open capsules. • If a dose is missed or vomiting occurs during administration, give next dose at regularly scheduled time.

INDICATIONS/ROUTES/DOSAGE

Non–Small-Cell Lung Cancer

PO: ADULTS, ELDERLY: 600 mg twice daily until disease progression or unacceptable toxicity.

Dose Reduction Schedule

First dose reduction: 450 mg twice daily. **Second dose reduction:** 300 mg twice daily. Permanently discontinue if unable to tolerate 300 mg twice daily.

Dose Modification

Bradycardia

Symptomatic bradycardia: Withhold treatment until recovery to asymptomatic bradycardia or to a heart rate of 60 bpm or greater, then resume at reduced dose level (if pt not taking concomitant medications known to cause bradycardia). **Symptomatic bradycardia in pts taking concomitant medications known to cause bradycardia:** Withhold treatment until recovery to asymptomatic bradycardia or heart rate of 60 bpm or greater. If concomitant medication can be adjusted or discontinued, then resume at same dose. If concomitant medication cannot be adjusted or discontinued, then resume at reduced dose level. **Life-threatening bradycardia in pts who are not taking concomitant medications known to cause bradycardia:** Permanently discontinue. **Life-threatening bradycardia in pts who are taking concomitant medications known to cause bradycardia:** Withhold treatment until recovery to asymptomatic bradycardia or heart rate of 60 bpm or greater. If concomitant medication can be adjusted or discontinued, then resume at reduced dose level with frequent monitoring. Permanently discontinue if bradycardia recurs despite dose reduction.

CPK Elevation

CPK elevation greater than 5 times upper limit of normal (ULN): Withhold treatment until recovery to baseline or less than or equal to 2.5 times ULN, then resume at same dose. **CPK elevation greater than 10 times ULN or second occurrence of CPK elevation**

greater than 5 times ULN: Withhold treatment until recovery to baseline or less than or equal to 2.5 times ULN, then resume at reduced dose level.

Hepatotoxicity

Serum ALT or AST elevation greater than 5 times ULN with total bilirubin less than or equal to 2 times ULN: Withhold treatment until serum ALT or AST recovers to baseline or less than or equal to 3 times ULN, then resume at reduced dose level. **Serum ALT or AST elevation greater than 3 times ULN with total serum bilirubin greater than 2 times ULN in the absence of cholestasis or hemolysis:** Permanently discontinue. **Total bilirubin elevation greater than 3 times ULN:** Withhold treatment until recovery to baseline or less than or equal to 1.5 times ULN, then resume at reduced dose level.

Pulmonary

Any grade treatment-related interstitial lung disease/pneumonitis: Permanently discontinue.

Dosage in Renal Impairment

Mild to moderate impairment: No dose adjustment. **Severe impairment:** Not specified; use caution.

Dosage in Hepatic Impairment

Mild impairment: No dose adjustment. **Moderate to severe impairment:** Not specified; use caution.

SIDE EFFECTS

Frequent (41%–19%): Fatigue, asthenia, constipation, edema (peripheral, generalized, eyelid, periorbital), myalgia, musculoskeletal pain, cough, generalized rash, papular rash, pruritus, macular rash, maculopapular rash, acneiform dermatitis, erythema, nausea. **Occasional (18%–10%):** Headache, diarrhea, dyspnea, back pain, vomiting, increased weight, blurred vision, vitreous floaters, visual impairment, reduced visual acuity, asthenopia, diplopia, photosensitivity.

ADVERSE EFFECTS/TOXIC REACTIONS

Approx. 23% of pts required at least one dose reduction. Median time to first dose reduction was 48 days. Decreased Hgb levels were reported in 56% of pts. Drug-induced hepatotoxicity with elevations of serum ALT/AST greater than 5 times ULN reported in 4%–5% of pts. Most reported cases of hepatotoxicity occurred during first 2 mos of therapy. Grade 3 interstitial lung disease occurred in less than 1% of pts. Symptomatic bradycardia reported in 7.5% of pts. Severe myalgia, musculoskeletal pain occurred in 29% of pts. CPK elevation occurred in 43% of pts. Other serious adverse effects may include endocarditis, hemorrhage (unspecified), intestinal perforation, pulmonary embolism.

NURSING CONSIDERATIONS

BASELINE ASSESSMENT

Obtain baseline CBC, BMP, LFT; pregnancy test in females of reproductive potential. Obtain baseline ECG in pts with history of arrhythmias, HF, concurrent use of medications known to cause bradycardia. Question history of hepatic/renal impairment, pulmonary embolism, diabetes, cardiac/pulmonary disease. Screen for medication known to cause bradycardia. Assess visual acuity. Verify ALK-positive NSCLC test prior to initiation.

INTERVENTION/EVALUATION

Monitor CBC routinely; LFTs q2wks during first 2 mos of treatment, then periodically thereafter (or more frequently in pts with hepatic impairment). Obtain BMP, serum ionized calcium, magnesium if arrhythmia or severe dehydration occurs. Monitor vital signs (esp. heart rate). Obtain ECG for bradycardia, chest pain, dyspnea. Worsening cough, fever, dyspnea may indicate interstitial lung disease/pneumonitis. Monitor for hepatotoxicity, hyperglycemia, vision changes, myalgia, musculoskeletal pain.

PATIENT/FAMILY TEACHING

• Report history of heart problems including extremity swelling, HF, slow heart rate. Therapy may decrease your heart rate; report dizziness, chest pain, palpitations, or fainting. • Worsening cough, fever, or shortness of breath may indicate severe lung inflammation. • Avoid pregnancy; contraception recommended during treatment and for up to 7 days after final dose. Do not breastfeed. Males with female partners of reproductive potential should use condoms during sexual activity during treatment and up to 3 mos after final dose. • Blurry vision, confusion, frequent urination, increased thirst, fruity breath may indicate high blood sugar levels. • Report any yellowing of skin or eyes, upper abdominal pain, bruising, black/tarry stools, dark urine. • Do not take newly prescribed medication unless approved by doctor who originally started treatment. • Avoid prolonged sun exposure/tanning beds. Use high SPF sunscreen and lip balm to protect against sunburn. • Take with food. • Avoid alcohol.

alendronate

a-**len**-dro-nate
(Binosto, Fosamax)
Do not confuse alendronate with risedronate, or Fosamax with Flomax.

FIXED-COMBINATION(S)

Fosamax Plus D: alendronate/cholecalciferol (vitamin D analogue): 70 mg/2,800 international units, 70 mg/5,600 international units.

◆CLASSIFICATION

PHARMACOTHERAPEUTIC: Bisphosphonate. **CLINICAL:** Bone resorption inhibitor, calcium regulator.

USES

Fosamax: Treatment of glucocorticoid-induced osteoporosis in men and women with low bone mineral density who are receiving at least 7.5 mg predniSONE (or equivalent). Treatment and prevention of osteoporosis in males and postmenopausal women. Treatment of Paget's disease of the bone in pts who are symptomatic, at risk for future complications, or with alkaline phosphatase equal to or greater than 2 times ULN. **Binosto:** Treatment of osteoporosis in males and postmenopausal women.

PRECAUTIONS

Contraindications: Hypocalcemia, abnormalities of the esophagus, inability to stand or sit upright for at least 30 min, sensitivity to alendronate or other bisphosphonates; oral solution or effervescent tablet should not be used in pts at risk for aspiration. **Cautions:** Renal impairment, dysphagia, esophageal disease, gastritis, ulcers, or duodenitis.

ACTION

Inhibits bone resorption via actions on osteoclasts or osteoclast precursors. **Therapeutic Effect:** Leads to indirect increase in bone mineral density. **Paget's Disease:** Inhibits bone resorption, leading to an indirect decrease in bone formation, but bone has a more normal architecture.

PHARMACOKINETICS

Poorly absorbed after PO administration. Protein binding: 78%. After PO administration, rapidly taken into bone, with uptake greatest at sites of active bone turnover. Excreted in urine, feces (as unabsorbed drug). **Terminal half-life:** Greater than 10 yrs (reflects release from skeleton as bone is resorbed).

⌛ LIFESPAN CONSIDERATIONS

Pregnancy/Lactation: Possible incomplete fetal ossification, decreased maternal weight gain, delay in delivery. Unknown if distributed in breast milk. Breastfeeding not recommended. **Children:** Safety and efficacy not established. **Elderly:** No age-related precautions noted.

INTERACTIONS

DRUG: **Antacids, calcium, iron, magnesium salts** may decrease the concentration/effect. **Aspirin, NSAIDs (e.g., ibuprofen, ketorolac, naproxen)** may increase adverse effects (e.g., increased risk of ulcer). **HERBAL:** None significant. **FOOD:** Concurrent **beverages, dietary supplements, food** may interfere with absorption. **Caffeine** may reduce efficacy. **LAB VALUES:** Reduces serum calcium, phosphate. Significant decrease in serum alkaline phosphatase noted in pts with Paget's disease.

AVAILABILITY (Rx)

Oral Solution: 70 mg/75 mL. **Tablets:** 5 mg, 10 mg, 35 mg, 40 mg, 70 mg. **Effervescent Tablets: (Binosto):** 70 mg.

ADMINISTRATION/HANDLING

PO

• Give at least 30 min before first food, beverage, or medication of the day. **Tablets, effervescent:** Dissolve in 4 oz water. Wait at least 5 min after effervescence stops. Stir for 10 sec and drink. **Oral solution:** Follow with at least 2 oz of water.

INDICATIONS/ROUTES/DOSAGE

Note: Consider discontinuing after 3–5 yrs for osteoporosis in pts at low risk for fractures.

Osteoporosis (in Men)

PO: ADULTS, ELDERLY: 10 mg once daily in the morning or 70 mg weekly.

Glucocorticoid-Induced Osteoporosis

PO: ADULTS, ELDERLY: 70 mg once weekly or 10 mg once daily.

Postmenopausal Osteoporosis

PO: ADULTS, ELDERLY: **Treatment:** 10 mg once daily in the morning or 70 mg weekly. **ADULTS, ELDERLY:** **Prevention:** 5 mg once daily in the morning or 35 mg weekly.

Paget's Disease

PO: ADULTS, ELDERLY: 40 mg once daily in the morning for 6 mos.

Dosage in Renal Impairment

Not recommended in pts with creatinine clearance less than 35 mL/min.

Dosage in Hepatic Impairment

No dose adjustment.

SIDE EFFECTS

Frequent (8%–7%): Back pain, abdominal pain. **Occasional (3%–2%):** Nausea, abdominal distention, constipation, diarrhea, flatulence. **Rare (less than 2%):** Rash; severe bone, joint, muscle pain.

ADVERSE EFFECTS/TOXIC REACTIONS

Overdose produces hypocalcemia, hypophosphatemia, significant GI disturbances. Esophageal irritation occurs if not given with 6–8 oz of plain water or if pt lies down within 30 min of administration. May increase risk of osteonecrosis of the jaw.

NURSING CONSIDERATIONS

BASELINE ASSESSMENT

Obtain baseline serum calcium, phosphate, alkaline phosphatase. Hypocalcemia, vitamin D deficiency must be corrected before beginning therapy. Assess pt's ability to remain upright for at least 30 minutes.

INTERVENTION/EVALUATION

Monitor chemistries (esp. serum calcium, phosphorus, alkaline phosphatase levels).

PATIENT/FAMILY TEACHING

• Expected benefits occur only when medication is taken with full glass (6–8 oz) of plain water, first thing in the morning and at least 30 min before first food, beverage, or medication of the day is taken. Any other beverage (mineral water, orange juice, coffee) significantly reduces absorption of medication.

• Do not lie down for at least 30 min after taking medication (potentiates delivery to stomach, reducing risk of esophageal irritation). • Report new swallowing difficulties, pain when swallowing, chest pain, new/worsening heartburn. • Consider weight-bearing exercises, modify behavioral factors (e.g., cigarette smoking, alcohol consumption). • Supplemental calcium and vitamin D should be taken if dietary intake inadequate.

alirocumab

al-i-**rok**-ue-mab
(Praluent)
Do not confuse alirocumab with adalimumab or raxibacumab.

◆CLASSIFICATION

PHARMACOTHERAPEUTIC: Proprotein convertase subtilisin kexin 9 (PCSK9) inhibitor, monoclonal antibody. **CLINICAL:** Antihyperlipidemic.

USES

Adjunct to diet, alone or in combination with other lipid-lowering therapies (e.g., statins, ezetimibe) for treatment of primary hyperlipidemia (including heterozygous familial hypercholesterolemia [HeFH]) to reduce low-density lipoprotein cholesterol (LDL-C). To reduce risk of MI, stroke, and unstable angina requiring hospitalization in adults with established cardiovascular disease.

PRECAUTIONS

Contraindications: Severe hypersensitivity to alirocumab. **Cautions:** Hepatic impairment.

ACTION

Prevents binding of PCSK9 to LDL receptors on hepatocytes. Increases hepatic uptake of LDL. **Therapeutic Effect:** Lowers LDL levels.

PHARMACOKINETICS

Distributed primarily in circulatory system. Metabolized by protein degradation into small peptides, amino acids. Peak plasma concentration: 3–7 days. Steady state reached by 2–3 doses. **Half-life:** 17–20 days.

⌛ LIFESPAN CONSIDERATIONS

Pregnancy/Lactation: May cross placental barrier, esp. during second and third trimesters. Unknown if distributed in breast milk. Human immunoglobulin G is present in breast milk. **Children:** Safety and efficacy not established. **Elderly:** No age-related precautions noted.

INTERACTIONS

DRUG: May enhance adverse effects/toxicity of **belimumab**. **HERBAL:** None significant. **FOOD:** None known. **LAB VALUES:** Expected to decrease serum LDL-C levels. May increase serum ALT, AST.

AVAILABILITY (Rx)

Injection Solution: 75 mg/mL, 150 mg/mL in single-dose, prefilled syringe or pen.

ADMINISTRATION/HANDLING

SQ

• Visually inspect for particulate matter or discoloration. Solution should appear clear, colorless to pale yellow. • Allow pen/syringe to warm to room temperature for 30–40 min prior to use. • Subcutaneously insert needle into abdomen, thigh, or upper arm region and inject solution. It may take up to 20 sec to fully inject dose. • Do not inject into areas of active skin disease or injury such as sunburns, skin rashes, inflammation, or skin infections. • Rotate injection sites.

Storage • Refrigerate unused pens/syringes in outer carton. • Do not freeze. • Discard if pen/syringe has been at room temperature more than 24 hrs or longer. • Protect from light.

INDICATIONS/ROUTES/DOSAGE

Hyperlipidemia, Secondary Prevention of Cardiovascular Events

SQ: ADULTS, ELDERLY: 75 mg once every 2 wks or 300 mg every 4 wks. May increase to maximum dose of 150 mg once every 2 wks if response inadequate. If a dose is missed, administer within 7 days of scheduled dose, then resume normal schedule. If missed dose is not within 7 days, wait until next scheduled dose. Less frequent dosing: 300 mg q4wks.

Dosage in Renal Impairment

No dose adjustment.

Dosage in Hepatic Impairment

Mild to moderate impairment: No dose adjustment. **Severe impairment:** Use caution.

SIDE EFFECTS

Occasional (11%–7%): Nasopharyngitis, injection site reactions (e.g., erythema, itching, swelling, pain/tenderness, bruising/contusion). **Rare (5%–2%):** Diarrhea, bronchitis, myalgia, muscle spasm, sinusitis, cough, musculoskeletal pain.

ADVERSE EFFECTS/TOXIC REACTIONS

Serious hypersensitivity reactions (e.g., pruritus, rash, urticaria), including some serious events (e.g., hypersensitivity vasculitis, hypersensitivity reactions requiring hospitalization), have been reported. Infections such as UTI (5% of pts) and influenza (6% of pts) have occurred. Neurologic events such as confusion, memory impairment reported in less than 1% of pts. Immunogenicity (anti-alirocumab antibodies) reported in 5% of pts. Pts who developed neutralizing antibodies had a higher incidence of injection site reactions.

NURSING CONSIDERATIONS

BASELINE ASSESSMENT

Obtain baseline LDL-C level, LFT. Question history of hypersensitivity reaction, hepatic impairment. Assess skin for sunburns, skin rashes, inflammation, or skin infections.

INTERVENTION/EVALUATION

Obtain LDL-C level within 4–8 wks after treatment initiation or with any dose titration. Monitor for hypersensitivity reactions. If hypersensitivity reaction occurs, discontinue therapy and treat symptoms accordingly; monitor until symptoms resolve. Monitor for infections including UTI, influenza.

PATIENT/FAMILY TEACHING

• A healthcare provider will show you how to properly prepare and inject your medication. You must demonstrate correct preparation and injection techniques before using medication. • Treatment may cause serious allergic reactions such as itching, hives, rash, or more serious reactions requiring hospitalization. If allergic reaction occurs, immediately seek medical attention. • Do not reuse prefilled pens/syringes.

allopurinol

al-oh-**pure**-i-nol
(Aloprim, Zyloprim)

Do not confuse allopurinol with Apresoline or haloperidol, or Zyloprim with Zorprin or Zovirax.

FIXED-COMBINATION(S)

Duzallo: allopurinol/lesinurad (uric acid transporter-1 inhibitor): 200 mg/200 mg, 300 mg/200 mg.

◆CLASSIFICATION

PHARMACOTHERAPEUTIC: Xanthine oxidase inhibitor. **CLINICAL:** Antigout agent.

USES

PO: Management of primary or secondary gout (e.g., acute attack, nephropathy). Treatment of secondary hyperuricemia that may occur during cancer treatment. Management of recurrent uric acid and calcium oxalate calculi. **Injection:** Management of elevated uric acid in cancer treatment for leukemia, lymphoma, or solid tumor malignancies.

PRECAUTIONS

Contraindications: Severe hypersensitivity to allopurinol. **Cautions:** Renal/hepatic impairment; pts taking diuretics, mercaptopurine or azaTHIOprine, other drugs causing myelosuppression. Do not use in asymptomatic hyperuricemia.

ACTION

Decreases uric acid production by inhibiting xanthine oxidase, an enzyme responsible for converting xanthine to uric acid. **Therapeutic Effect:** Reduces uric acid concentrations in serum and urine.

PHARMACOKINETICS

Route	Onset	Peak	Duration
PO, IV	2–3 days	1–3 wks	1–2 wks

Well absorbed from GI tract. Widely distributed. Protein binding: less than 1%. Metabolized in liver. Excreted primarily in urine. Removed by hemodialysis. **Half-life:** 1–3 hrs; metabolite, 12–30 hrs.

LIFESPAN CONSIDERATIONS

Pregnancy/Lactation: Unknown if drug crosses placenta or is distributed in breast milk. **Children/Elderly:** No age-related precautions noted.

INTERACTIONS

DRUG: **Angiotensin-converting enzyme (ACE) inhibitors (e.g., enalapril, lisinopril)** may increase potential for hypersensitivity reactions. **Antacids** may decrease absorption. May increase concentration/effects of **azaTHIOprine, didanosine, mercaptopurine.** May increase adverse effects of **pegloticase.** May increase anticoagulant effect of **vitamin K antagonists (e.g., warfarin).** May decrease concentration/effect of **capecitabine.** **HERBAL:** None significant. **FOOD:** None known. **LAB VALUES:** May increase serum BUN, alkaline phosphatase, ALT, AST, creatinine.

AVAILABILITY (Rx)

Injection, Powder for Reconstitution: *(Aloprim):* 500 mg. **Tablets:** *(Zyloprim):* 100 mg, 300 mg.

ADMINISTRATION/HANDLING

IV

Reconstitution • Reconstitute 500-mg vial with 25 mL Sterile Water for Injection (concentration of 20 mg/mL). • Further dilute with 0.9% NaCl or D_5W (50–100 mL) to a concentration of 6 mg/mL or less.

Rate of administration • Infuse over 15–60 min. Daily doses can be given as a single infusion or in equally divided doses at 6-, 8-, or 12-hr intervals.

Storage • Solution should appear clear and colorless. • Store unreconstituted vials at room temperature. • Do not refrigerate reconstituted and/or diluted solution. Must administer within 10 hrs of preparation. • Do not use if precipitate forms or solution is discolored.

PO

• Give after meals with plenty of fluid. • Fluid intake should yield slightly alkaline urine and output of approximately 2 L in adults. • Dosages greater than 300 mg/day to be administered in divided doses.

IV INCOMPATIBILITIES

Amikacin (Amikin), carmustine (BiCNU), cefotaxime (Claforan), clindamycin (Cleocin), cytarabine (Ara-C), dacarbazine (DTIC), diphenhydrAMINE (Benadryl), DOXOrubicin (Adriamycin), doxycycline (Vibramycin), gentamicin, haloperidol (Haldol), hydrOXYzine (Vistaril), IDArubicin (Idamycin), imipenem-cilastatin (Primaxin), methylPREDNISolone (SOLU-

Medrol), metoclopramide (Reglan), ondansetron (Zofran), streptozocin (Zanosar), tobramycin, vinorelbine (Navelbine).

IV COMPATIBILITIES

Bumetanide (Bumex), calcium gluconate, furosemide (Lasix), heparin, HYDROmorphone (Dilaudid), LORazepam (Ativan), morphine, potassium chloride.

INDICATIONS/ROUTES/DOSAGE

◀ALERT▶ Doses greater than 300 mg should be given in divided doses.

Gout

PO: ADULTS, ELDERLY: Initially, 100 mg/day. Increase at 2–4 wk intervals needed to achieve desired serum uric acid level. **Mild:** 200–300 mg/day. **Moderate to severe:** 400–600 mg/day in 2–3 divided doses. **Maximum:** 800 mg/day.

Secondary Hyperuricemia Associated With Chemotherapy

Note: Begin 1–2 days before initiating induction of chemotherapy. May continue for 3–7 days after chemotherapy. **PO: ADULTS, CHILDREN OLDER THAN 10 YRS:** 600–800 mg/day in 2–3 divided doses. **CHILDREN 6–10 YRS:** 300 mg/day in 2–3 divided doses. **CHILDREN YOUNGER THAN 6 YRS:** 150 mg/day in 3 divided doses.

◀ALERT▶ IV: Daily dose can be given as single infusion or at 6-, 8-, or 12-hr intervals.

IV: ADULTS, ELDERLY, CHILDREN 10 YRS OR OLDER: 200–400 mg/m²/day. **CHILDREN YOUNGER THAN 10 YRS:** 200 mg/m²/day. **Maximum:** 600 mg/day.

Recurrent Uric Acid Calcium Oxalate Calculi

PO: ADULTS: 200–300 mg/day in single or 2–3 divided doses.

Dosage in Renal Impairment

Dosage is modified based on creatinine clearance. **PO:** Removed by hemodialysis. Administer dose following hemodialysis or administer 50% supplemental dose.

IV/PO

Creatinine Clearance	Dosage
10–20 mL/min	200 mg/day
3–9 mL/min	100 mg/day
Less than 3 mL/min	100 mg at extended intervals
HD	100 mg q48h (increase cautiously to 300 mg)

Dosage in Hepatic Impairment

No dose adjustment.

SIDE EFFECTS

Occasional: PO: Drowsiness, unusual hair loss. **IV:** Rash, nausea, vomiting. **Rare:** Diarrhea, headache.

ADVERSE EFFECTS/TOXIC REACTIONS

Pruritic maculopapular rash, possibly accompanied by malaise, fever, chills, joint pain, nausea, vomiting should be considered a toxic reaction. Severe hypersensitivity reaction may follow appearance of rash. Bone marrow depression, hepatotoxicity, peripheral neuritis, acute renal failure occur rarely.

NURSING CONSIDERATIONS

BASELINE ASSESSMENT

Obtain baseline BMP, LFT. Instruct pt to drink minimum of 2,500–3,000 mL of fluid daily while taking medication.

INTERVENTION/EVALUATION

Discontinue medication immediately if rash or other evidence of allergic reaction occurs. Monitor I&O (output should be at least 2,000 mL/day). Assess serum chemistries, uric acid, hepatic function. Assess urine for cloudiness, unusual color, odor. **Gout:** Assess for therapeutic response: relief of pain, stiffness, swelling; increased joint mobility; reduced joint tenderness; improved grip strength.

PATIENT/FAMILY TEACHING

• May take 1 wk or longer for full therapeutic effect. • Maintain adequate hydration; drink 2,500–3,000 mL of fluid daily while taking medication. • Avoid tasks that require alertness, motor skills until response to drug is established. • Avoid alcohol (may increase uric acid).

almotriptan

al-moe-**trip**-tan

Do not confuse almotriptan with alvimopan, or Axert with Antivert.

◆CLASSIFICATION

PHARMACOTHERAPEUTIC: Serotonin receptor agonist (5-HT_{1B}). **CLINICAL:** Antimigraine.

USES

Acute treatment of migraine headache with or without aura in adults. Acute treatment of migraine headache in adolescents 12–17 yrs with history of migraine with or without aura and having attacks usually lasting 4 or more hrs when left untreated.

PRECAUTIONS

Contraindications: Hypersensitivity to almotriptan. Cerebrovascular disease (e.g., recent stroke, transient ischemic attacks), peripheral vascular disease (e.g., ischemic bowel disease), hemiplegic or basilar migraine, ischemic heart disease (including angina pectoris, history of MI, silent ischemia, and Prinzmetal's angina), uncontrolled hypertension, use within 24 hrs of ergotamine-containing preparations or another 5-HT_{1B} agonist. **Cautions:** Mild to moderate renal or hepatic impairment, pt profile suggesting cardiovascular risks, controlled hypertension; history of CVA, sulfonamide allergy.

ACTION

Binds selectively to serotonin receptors in cranial arteries producing a vasoconstrictive effect. Decreases inflammation associated with relief of migraine. **Therapeutic Effect:** Produces relief of migraine headache.

PHARMACOKINETICS

Well absorbed after PO administration. Protein binding: 35%. Metabolized by liver. Primarily excreted in urine. **Half-life:** 3–4 hrs.

⌛ LIFESPAN CONSIDERATIONS

Pregnancy/Lactation: Unknown if distributed in breast milk. **Children:** Safety and efficacy not established in pts younger than 12 yrs. **Elderly:** No age-related precautions noted.

INTERACTIONS

DRUG: **Ergot derivatives (e.g., dihydroergotamine, ergotamine)** may increase vasoconstrictive effect. **Strong CYP3A4 inhibitors (e.g., clarithromycin, ketoconazole, ritonavir)** may increase concentration/effect. **MAOIs (e.g., phenelzine, selegiline)** may increase concentration/effect. **HERBAL:** None significant. **FOOD:** None known. **LAB VALUES:** None significant.

AVAILABILITY (Rx)

Tablets: 6.5 mg, 12.5 mg.

ADMINISTRATION/HANDLING

PO

• Swallow whole; do not break, crush, dissolve, or divide tablets. • Take with full glass of water. • May give without regard to food.

INDICATIONS/ROUTES/DOSAGE

Migraine Headache

PO: ADULTS, ELDERLY, ADOLESCENTS 12–17 YRS: Initially, 6.25–12.5 mg as a single dose. If headache returns, dose may be repeated after 2 hrs. **Maximum:** 2 doses/24 hrs (25 mg).

Concurrent Use of CYP3A4 Inhibitors

ADULTS, ELDERLY: Recommended initial dose is 6.25 mg, maximum daily dose is 12.5 mg. Avoid use in pts with renal or hepatic impairment AND use of CYP3A4 inhibitors.

Dosage in Renal Impairment
Creatinine clearance 30 mL/min or less: Initially, 6.25 mg in a single dose. **Maximum:** 12.5 mg/day.

Dosage in Hepatic Impairment
Initially, 6.25 mg in a single dose. **Maximum:** 12.5 mg/day.

SIDE EFFECTS

Rare (2%–1%): Nausea, dry mouth, headache, dizziness, somnolence, paresthesia, flushing.

ADVERSE EFFECTS/TOXIC REACTIONS

Excessive dosage may produce tremor, redness of extremities, decreased respirations, cyanosis, seizures, chest pain. Serious arrhythmias occur rarely but particularly in pts with hypertension, diabetes, obesity, smokers, and those with strong family history of coronary artery disease.

NURSING CONSIDERATIONS

BASELINE ASSESSMENT

Question for history of peripheral vascular disease, cardiac conduction disorders, CVA. Question pt regarding onset, location, duration of migraine, and possible precipitating factors.

INTERVENTION/EVALUATION

Evaluate for relief of migraine headache and associated photophobia, phonophobia (sound sensitivity), nausea, vomiting.

PATIENT/FAMILY TEACHING

• Take a single dose as soon as symptoms of an actual migraine attack appear. • Medication is intended to relieve migraine, not to prevent or reduce number of attacks. • Lie down in quiet, dark room for additional benefit after taking medication. • Avoid tasks that require alertness, motor skills until response to drug is established. • Report immediately if palpitations, pain or tightness in chest or throat, or pain or weakness of extremities occurs. • Swallow whole; do not chew, crush, dissolve, or divide tablets.

alpelisib

al-pe-lis-ib
(Piqray)
Do not confuse alpelisib with duvelisib, copanlisib, or idelalisib.

◆CLASSIFICATION

PHARMACOTHERAPEUTIC: Phosphatidylinositol 3-kinase (P13K) inhibitor. **CLINICAL:** Antineoplastic.

USES

Used (in combination with fulvestrant) for the treatment of men and postmenopausal women and with hormone receptor (HR)–positive, human epidermal growth factor receptor 2 (HER2)–negative, PIK3CA-mutated, advanced or metastatic breast cancer following progression on or after an endocrine-based regimen.

PRECAUTIONS

Contraindications: Hypersensitivity to alpelisib. **Cautions:** Baseline anemia, lymphopenia, thrombocytopenia. History of diabetes, dermatologic disease, pulmonary disease; pts at risk for hyperglycemia (e.g., diabetes, chronic use of corticosteroids); concomitant use of strong CYP3A inducers, BCRP inhibitors, CYP2C9 substrates. Not recommended in pts with history of Stevens-Johnson syndrome, erythema multiforme, toxic epidermal necrolysis.

ACTION

Alpelisib has selective activity against P13Ka. Mutations in the catalytic a-subunit of P13K (P13KCA) leads to P13Ka and Akt signaling, cellular transformation and tumor generation. By inhibiting phosphorylation of P13K downstream, alpelisib shows activity in cell lines with PIK3CA mutation. **Therapeutic Effect:** Inhibits tumor cell activity.

A

PHARMACOKINETICS

Widely distributed. Metabolized by enzymatic hydrolysis. Protein binding: 89%. Peak plasma concentration: 2–4 hrs. Steady state reached in 3 days. Excreted in feces (81%), urine (14%). **Half-life:** 8–9 hrs.

⌛ LIFESPAN CONSIDERATIONS

Pregnancy/Lactation: Avoid pregnancy; may cause fetal harm. Females of reproductive potential must use effective contraception during treatment and for at least 7 days after discontinuation. Unknown if distributed in breast milk. Breastfeeding not recommended during treatment and for at least 7 days after discontinuation. May impair fertility in both females and males. **Males:** Males with female partners of reproductive potential must use barrier methods during treatment and for at least 7 days after discontinuation. **Children:** Safety and efficacy not established. **Elderly:** No age-related precautions noted.

INTERACTIONS

DRUG: **BCRP inhibitors (e.g., methotrexate, imatinib, rosuvastatin, topotecan)** may increase concentration/effect. **Strong CYP3A4 inducers (e.g., carbamazepine, phenytoin, rifampin)** may decrease concentration/effect. May decrease concentration/effect of **CYP2C9 substrates (e.g., warfarin).** **HERBAL:** **St. John's wort** may decrease concentration/effect. **FOOD:** None known. **LAB VALUES:** May increase serum ALT, creatinine, GGT, lipase. May decrease lymphocytes, Hgb, platelets; serum albumin, calcium, magnesium, potassium. May increase or decrease serum glucose. May prolong aPTT.

AVAILABILITY (Rx)

Tablets: 50 mg, 150 mg, 200 mg.

ADMINISTRATION/HANDLING

PO

• Give with food. • Administer tablets whole; do not break, crush, or divide. Tablets cannot be chewed. Do not give if tablet is broken, cracked, or not intact. • If vomiting occurs after administration, give next dose at regularly scheduled time (do not give additional dose). • If a dose is missed, may give within 9 hrs of regularly scheduled time. After more than 9 hrs, skip dose and give next regularly scheduled time.

INDICATIONS/ROUTES/DOSAGE

Breast Cancer

PO: ADULTS, ELDERLY: 300 mg once daily (in combination with 500 mg of fulvestrant on days 1, 15, 29, then monthly). Continue until disease progression or unacceptable toxicity.

Dose Reduction Schedule for Adverse Events

First Dose Reduction: 250 mg once daily. **Second Dose Reduction:** 200 mg once daily.

Dose Modification

Based on Common Terminology Criteria for Adverse Events (CTCAE).

Diarrhea

Grade 1 diarrhea: No dose adjustment. **Grade 2 diarrhea:** Withhold treatment until improved to Grade 1 or 0, then resume at same dose level. **Grade 3 or 4 diarrhea:** Withhold treatment until improved to Grade 1 or 0, then resume at reduced dose level.

Dermatologic Toxicity

Grade 1 or 2 rash: No dose adjustment. **Grade 3 rash:** Withhold treatment until improved to Grade 1 or 0, then resume at same dose level for first occurrence or reduced dose level for second occurrence. **Grade 4 rash (severe bullous, blistering, or exfoliating skin):** Permanently discontinue.

Hyperglycemia

Grade 1 hyperglycemia: No dose adjustment. **Grade 2 hyperglycemia:** No dose adjustment. If fasting plasma glucose (FPG) does not decrease to less than or equal to 160 mg/dL or 8.9 mmol/L within

21 days, reduce dose level. **Grade 3 hyperglycemia:** Withhold treatment. If FPG decreases to less than or equal to 160 mg/dL or 8.9 mmol/L within 3–5 days, resume at reduced dose level. If FPG does not decrease within 3–5 days, consider referral to specialist to manage hyperglycemia. If FPG does not decrease within 21 days with specialized therapy, permanently discontinue. **Grade 4 hyperglycemia:** Withhold treatment. Recheck FPG after 24 hrs of hyperglycemic treatment. If FPG decreases to less than 500 mg/dL or 27.8 mmol/L, follow guidelines for Grade 3 hyperglycemia. If FPG is remains greater than 500 mg/dL or 27.8 mmol/L, permanently discontinue.

Other Toxicities

Any other Grade 1 or 2 toxicities: No dose adjustment. **Any other Grade 3 toxicities:** Withhold treatment until improved to Grade 1 or 0, then resume at reduced dose level. **Any other Grade 4 toxicities:** Permanently discontinue.

Dosage in Renal Impairment

Mild to moderate impairment: No dose adjustment. **Severe impairment:** Not specified; use caution.

Dosage in Hepatic Impairment

Mild to severe impairment: Not specified; use caution.

SIDE EFFECTS

Frequent (52%–19%): Diarrhea, rash, nausea, fatigue, asthenia, decreased appetite, stomatitis, mouth ulceration, vomiting, decreased weight, alopecia, mucosal inflammation. **Occasional** (18%–11%): Dry skin, xerosis, xeroderma, pruritus, dysgeusia, headache, abdominal pain, peripheral edema, pyrexia, mucosal dryness, dyspepsia.

ADVERSE EFFECTS/TOXIC REACTIONS

Anemia, lymphopenia, thrombocytopenia are expected responses to therapy. Severe hypersensitivity reactions, including anaphylaxis, may occur. Grade 3 or 4 hypersensitivity reactions reported in less than 1% of pts. Severe cutaneous reactions, including Stevens-Johnson syndrome and erythema multiforme, reported in 0.4% and 1% of pts, respectively. Hyperglycemia reported in 65% of pts. Grade 3 hyperglycemia and Grade 4 hyperglycemia reported in 33% and 4% of pts, respectively. Ketoacidosis reported in less than 1% of pts. Pneumonitis, interstitial lung disease reported in 2% of pts. Diarrhea reported in 58% of pts. Severe diarrhea may cause dehydration, acute kidney injury. UTI reported in 10% of pts.

NURSING CONSIDERATIONS

BASELINE ASSESSMENT

Obtain CBC, fasting plasma glucose; pregnancy test in female pts of reproductive potential. Confirm compliance of effective contraception. Question history of diabetes, pulmonary disease, dermatologic diseases. Recommend adequate glycemic control before initiation. Assess usual bowel movement patterns, stool characteristics. Assess hydration status. Receive full medication history and screen for interactions. Offer emotional support.

INTERVENTION/EVALUATION

Monitor plasma blood glucose levels as clinically indicated. Consider ABG, radiologic test if ILD/pneumonitis (excessive cough, dyspnea, fever, hypoxia) is suspected. Monitor for hyperglycemia (blurred vision, confusion, excessive thirst, Kussmaul respirations, polyuria). Monitor for skin toxicities, cutaneous reactions; hypersensitivity reactions, anaphylaxis (dyspnea, fever, hypotension, rash, tachycardia). If treatment-related toxicities occur, consider referral to specialist. Monitor daily pattern of bowel activity, stool consistency; I&Os, hydration status. If dermatologic toxicities occur, consider topical corticosteroid; addition of oral antihistamine. If hyperglycemia occurs, start or adjust antidiabetic/hyperglycemic treatment as appropriate.

PATIENT/FAMILY TEACHING

• Severe allergic reactions such as dizziness, hives, palpitations, rash, shortness of breath, tongue swelling may occur. • Treatment may cause severe rashes, peeling, or blistering of the skin. • Severe diarrhea may cause dehydration, kidney injuries. Drink plenty of fluids. • Report symptoms of high blood sugar levels (blurred vision, excessive thirst/hunger, headache, frequent urination); lung inflammation (excessive coughing, difficulty breathing, chest pain); toxic skin reactions (itching, peeling, rash, redness, swelling); UTI (fever, urinary frequency, burning during urination, foul-smelling urine). • Females and males of childbearing potential must use reliable contraception during treatment and for at least 7 days after last dose. Do not breastfeed. • Do not take newly prescribed medications unless approved by the prescriber who originally started treatment.

ALPRAZolam

al-**praz**-oh-lam
(ALPRAZolam Intensol, ALPRAZolam XR, Apo-Alpraz ✱, Xanax, Xanax XR)

■ **BLACK BOX ALERT** ■ Concomitant use of benzodiazepines and opioids may result in profound sedation, respiratory depression, coma, and death. Reserve concomitant of these drugs for use in pts for whom alternative treatment options are inadequate. Limit dosages and durations to the minimum required. Follow pts for signs and symptoms of respiratory depression and sedation.

Do not confuse ALPRAZolam with LORazepam, or Xanax with Tenex, Tylox, Xopenex, Zantac, or ZyrTEC.

◆CLASSIFICATION

PHARMACOTHERAPEUTIC: Benzodiazepine (Schedule IV). **CLINICAL:** Antianxiety.

USES

Management of generalized anxiety disorders (GAD). Short-term relief of symptoms of anxiety, panic disorder, with or without agoraphobia. Anxiety associated with depression. **OFF-LABEL:** Anxiety in children. Preoperative anxiety.

PRECAUTIONS

Contraindications: Hypersensitivity to ALPRAZolam. Acute narrow angle-closure glaucoma, concurrent use with ketoconazole or itraconazole or other strong CYP3A4 inhibitors. **Cautions:** Renal/hepatic impairment, predisposition to urate nephropathy, obese pts. Concurrent use of CYP3A4 inhibitors/inducers and major CYP3A4 substrates; debilitated pts, respiratory disease, depression (esp. suicidal risk), elderly (increased risk of severe toxicity). History of substance abuse.

ACTION

Enhances the inhibitory effects of the neurotransmitter gamma-aminobutyric acid in the brain. **Therapeutic Effect:** Produces anxiolytic effect due to CNS depressant action.

PHARMACOKINETICS

Well absorbed from GI tract. Protein binding: 80%. Metabolized in liver. Primarily excreted in urine. Minimal removal by hemodialysis. **Half-life:** 6–27 hrs.

⌛ LIFESPAN CONSIDERATIONS

Pregnancy/Lactation: Crosses placenta; distributed in breast milk. Chronic ingestion during pregnancy may produce withdrawal symptoms, CNS depression in neonates. **Children:** Safety and efficacy not established. **Elderly:** Use small initial doses with gradual increase to avoid ataxia (muscular incoordination) or excessive sedation. May have increased risk of falls, delirium.

INTERACTIONS

DRUG: **CNS depressants (e.g., alcohol, morphine, zolpidem)** may increase CNS depression. **Strong CYP3A4**

inhibitors (e.g., clarithromycin, ketoconazole, ritonavir) may increase concentration/effect. **Strong CYP3A4 inducers (e.g., carbamazepine, phenytoin, rifampin)** may decrease concentration/effect. HERBAL: **Herbals with sedative properties (e.g., chamomile, kava kava, valerian)** may increase CNS depression. **St. John's wort** may decrease effects. FOOD: **Grapefruit products** may increase level, effects. LAB VALUES: None significant.

AVAILABILITY (Rx)

Oral Solution: ***(Alprazolam Intensol):*** 1 mg/mL. **Tables (Orally Disintegrating):** 0.25 mg, 0.5 mg, 1 mg, 2 mg. **Tablets (Immediate-Release):** ***(Xanax)*:** 0.25 mg, 0.5 mg, 1 mg, 2 mg.

Tablets (Extended-Release): ***(Xanax XR):*** 0.5 mg, 1 mg, 2 mg, 3 mg.

ADMINISTRATION/HANDLING

PO, Immediate-Release

• May give without regard to food. • Tablets may be crushed. • If oral intake is not possible, may be given sublingually.

PO, Extended-Release

• Administer once daily. • Do not break, crush, dissolve, or divide extended-release tablets. Swallow whole.

PO, Orally Disintegrating

• Place tablet on tongue, allow to dissolve. • Swallow with saliva. • Administration with water not necessary. • If using ½ tab, discard remaining ½ tab.

INDICATIONS/ROUTES/DOSAGE

Anxiety Disorders

PO: ***(Immediate-Release, Oral Concentrate, ODT)*:** ADULTS: Initially, 0.25–0.5 mg 3 times/day. May titrate q3–4days. **Maximum:** 4 mg/day in divided doses. CHILDREN, YOUNGER THAN 18 YRS: 0.125 mg 3 times/day. May increase by 0.125–0.25 mg/dose. **Maximum:** 0.06 mg/kg/day or 0.02 mg/kg/dose. Range: 0.375–3 mg/day. ELDERLY, DEBILITATED PTS, PTS WITH HEPATIC DISEASE OR LOW SERUM ALBUMIN: Initially, 0.25 mg 2–3 times/day. Gradually increase to optimum therapeutic response.

Panic Disorder

PO: ***(Immediate-Release, Oral Concentrate, ODT)*:** ADULTS: Initially, 0.5 mg 3 times/day. May increase at 3- to 4-day intervals in increments of 1 mg or less a day. Range: 5–6 mg/day. **Maximum:** 10 mg/day. ELDERLY: Initially, 0.125–0.25 mg twice daily. May increase in 0.125-mg increments until desired effect attained.

PO: ***(Extended-Release)*:**

◀ALERT▶ To switch from immediate-release to extended-release form, give total daily dose (immediate-release) as a single daily dose of extended-release form.

ADULTS: Initially, 0.5–1 mg once daily. May titrate at 3- to 4-day intervals. Range: 3–6 mg/day. ELDERLY: Initially, 0.5 mg once daily.

Dosage in Renal Impairment

No dose adjustment.

Dosage in Hepatic Impairment

Severe disease: ***(Immediate-Release):*** 0.25 mg 2–3 mg times/day. ***(Extended-Release):*** 0.5 mg once daily.

SIDE EFFECTS

Frequent (41%–20%): Ataxia, light-headedness, drowsiness, slurred speech (particularly in elderly or debilitated pts). **Occasional (15%–5%):** Confusion, depression, blurred vision, constipation, diarrhea, dry mouth, headache, nausea. **Rare (4% or less):** Behavioral problems such as anger, impaired memory; paradoxical reactions (insomnia, nervousness, irritability).

ADVERSE EFFECTS/TOXIC REACTIONS

Concomitant use with opioids may result in profound sedation, respiratory depression, coma, and death. Abrupt or too-rapid withdrawal may result in restlessness, irritability, insomnia, hand tremors, abdominal/muscle cramps, diaphoresis, vomiting, seizures. Overdose results in drowsiness, confusion, diminished reflexes, coma. Blood dyscrasias noted rarely. **Antidote:** Flumazenil (see Appendix J for dosage).

NURSING CONSIDERATIONS

BASELINE ASSESSMENT

Assess degree of anxiety; assess for drowsiness, dizziness, light-headedness. Assess motor responses (agitation, trembling, tension), autonomic responses (cold/clammy hands, diaphoresis). Initiate fall precautions.

INTERVENTION/EVALUATION

For pts on long-term therapy, perform hepatic/renal function tests, CBC periodically. Assess for paradoxical reaction, particularly during early therapy. Evaluate for therapeutic response: calm facial expression, decreased restlessness, insomnia. Monitor respiratory and cardiovascular status.

PATIENT/FAMILY TEACHING

• Drowsiness usually disappears during continued therapy. • If dizziness occurs, change positions slowly from recumbent to sitting position before standing. • Avoid tasks that require alertness, motor skills until response to drug is established. • Smoking reduces drug effectiveness. • Sour hard candy, gum, sips of water may relieve dry mouth. • Do not abruptly withdraw medication after long-term therapy. • Avoid alcohol. • Do not take other medications without consulting physician.

alteplase

HIGH ALERT

al-te-plase
(Activase, Cathflo Activase)
Do not confuse alteplase or Activase with Altace, or Activase with Cathflo Activase.

◆CLASSIFICATION

PHARMACOTHERAPEUTIC: Tissue plasminogen activator (tPA). **CLINICAL:** Thrombolytic.

USES

Treatment of ST-elevation MI (STEMI) for lysis of thrombi in coronary arteries, acute ischemic stroke (AIS), acute massive pulmonary embolism (PE). Treatment of occluded central venous catheters. **OFF-LABEL:** Acute peripheral occlusive disease, prosthetic valve thrombosis. Acute ischemic stroke presenting 3–4½ hrs after onset of symptoms.

PRECAUTIONS

Contraindications: Hypersensitivity to alteplase. Active internal bleeding, AV malformation or aneurysm, bleeding diathesis CVA, intracranial neoplasm, intracranial or intraspinal surgery or trauma, recent (within past 2 mos), severe uncontrolled hypertension, suspected aortic dissection. **Cautions:** Recent (within 10 days) major surgery or GI bleeding, OB delivery, organ biopsy, recent trauma or CPR, left heart thrombus, endocarditis, severe hepatic disease, pregnancy, elderly, cerebrovascular disease, diabetic retinopathy, thrombophlebitis, occluded AV cannula at infected site.

ACTION

Binds to fibrin in a thrombus and converts entrapped plasminogen to plasmin, initiating local fibrinolysis. **Therapeutic Effect:** Degrades fibrin clots, fibrinogen, other plasma proteins.

PHARMACOKINETICS

Rapidly metabolized in liver. Primarily excreted in urine. **Half-life:** 35 min.

LIFESPAN CONSIDERATIONS

Pregnancy/Lactation: Use only when benefit outweighs potential risk to fetus. Unknown if drug crosses placenta or is distributed in breast milk. **Children:** Safety and efficacy not established. **Elderly:** May have increased risk of bleeding; monitor closely.

INTERACTIONS

DRUG: **Heparin, low molecular weight heparins, medications altering platelet function (e.g., clopidogrel, NSAIDs), oral anticoagulants (e.g., warfarin)** increase risk of bleeding. May increase anticoagulant effect of **desirudin.** **HERBAL:** **Herbals with anticoagulant/antiplatelet properties (e.g., garlic, ginger, ginkgo biloba)** may increase adverse effects. **FOOD:** None known. **LAB VALUES:** Decreases plasminogen, fibrinogen levels during infusion, decreases clotting time (confirms the presence of lysis). May decrease Hgb, Hct.

AVAILABILITY (Rx)

Injection, Powder for Reconstitution: ***(Cathflo Activase):*** 2 mg, ***(Activase):*** 50 mg, 100 mg.

ADMINISTRATION/HANDLING

IV

Reconstitution • ***(Activase):*** Reconstitute immediately before use with Sterile Water for Injection. • Reconstitute 100-mg vial with 100 mL Sterile Water for Injection (50-mg vial with 50 mL sterile water) without preservative to provide a concentration of 1 mg/mL. • ***(Activase Cathflo):*** Add 2.2 mL Sterile Water for Injection to provide concentration of 1 mg/mL. • Avoid excessive agitation; gently swirl or slowly invert vial to reconstitute.

Rate of administration • ***(Activase):*** Give by IV infusion via infusion pump (see Indications/Routes/Dosage). • If minor bleeding occurs at puncture sites, apply pressure for 30 sec; if unrelieved, apply pressure dressing. • If uncontrolled hemorrhage occurs, discontinue infusion immediately (slowing rate of infusion may produce worsening hemorrhage). • Avoid undue pressure when drug is injected into catheter (can rupture catheter or expel clot into circulation). • Instill dose into occluded catheter. • After 30 min, assess catheter function by attempting to aspirate blood. • If still occluded, let dose dwell an additional 90 min. • If function not restored, a second dose may be instilled.

Storage • ***(Activase):*** Store vials at room temperature. • After reconstitution, solution appears colorless to pale yellow. • Solution is stable for 8 hrs after reconstitution. Discard unused portions.

IV INCOMPATIBILITIES

DOBUTamine (Dobutrex), DOPamine (Intropin), heparin.

IV COMPATIBILITIES

Lidocaine, metoprolol (Lopressor), morphine, nitroglycerin, propranolol (Inderal).

INDICATIONS/ROUTES/DOSAGE

Acute MI

IV infusion: ADULTS WEIGHING MORE THAN 67 KG: **Total dose:** 100 mg over 90 min, starting with 15-mg bolus over 1–2 min, then 50 mg over 30 min, then 35 mg over 60 min. **ADULTS WEIGHING 67 KG OR LESS:** **Total dose:** Start with 15-mg bolus over 1–2 min, then 0.75 mg/kg over 30 min (**maximum:** 50 mg), then 0.5 mg/kg over 60 min (**maximum:** 35 mg). **Maximum total dose:** 100 mg.

Acute Pulmonary Emboli

IV infusion: ADULTS: 100 mg over 2 hrs. Institute or reinstitute heparin near end or immediately after infusion when activated partial thromboplastin time (aPTT) or thrombin time (TT) returns to twice normal or less.

Acute Ischemic Stroke

◄ **ALERT** ► Dose should be given within the first 3 hrs of the onset of symptoms. Recommended total dose: 0.9 mg/kg. **Maximum:** 90 mg.

IV infusion: ADULTS WEIGHING 100 KG OR LESS: 0.09 mg/kg as IV bolus over 1 min, then 0.81 mg/kg as continuous infusion over 60 min. WEIGHING MORE THAN 100 KG: 9 mg bolus over 1 min, then 81 mg as continuous infusion over 60 min.

Central Venous Catheter Clearance

IV: ADULTS, ELDERLY: Up to 2 mg; may repeat after 2 hrs. If catheter functional, withdraw 4–5 mL blood to remove drug and residual clot.

Usual Neonatal Dosage

Occluded IV catheter: Use 1 mg/mL conc (**maximum:** 2 mg/2 mL) leave in lumen up to 2 hrs, then aspirate.
Systemic thrombosis: 0.1–0.6 mg/kg/hr for 6 hrs. Usual dose: 0.5 mg/kg/hr.

Dosage in Renal/Hepatic Impairment

No dose adjustment.

SIDE EFFECTS

Frequent: Superficial bleeding at puncture sites, decreased B/P. **Occasional:** Allergic reaction (rash, wheezing, bruising).

ADVERSE EFFECTS/TOXIC REACTIONS

Severe internal hemorrhage, intracranial hemorrhage may occur. Lysis of coronary thrombi may produce atrial or ventricular arrhythmias or stroke.

NURSING CONSIDERATIONS

BASELINE ASSESSMENT

Assess for contraindications to therapy. Obtain baseline B/P, apical pulse. Record weight. Evaluate 12-lead ECG, cardiac enzymes, serum electrolytes. Assess Hct, platelet count, prothrombin time (PT), activated partial thromboplastin time (aPTT), fibrinogen level before therapy is instituted. Type and screen blood.

INTERVENTION/EVALUATION

Perform continuous cardiac monitoring for arrhythmias. Check B/P, pulse, respirations q15min until stable, then hourly. Check peripheral pulses, heart and lung sounds. Monitor for chest pain relief and notify physician of continuation or recurrence (note location, type, intensity). Assess for bleeding: overt blood, occult blood in any body substance. Monitor aPTT per protocol. Maintain B/P; avoid any trauma that might increase risk of bleeding (e.g., injections, shaving). Assess neurologic status frequently.

amikacin

am-i-**kay**-sin

BLACK BOX ALERT May cause neurotoxicity, nephrotoxicity, and/or neuromuscular blockade and respiratory paralysis. Ototoxicity usually is irreversible; nephrotoxicity usually is reversible.

Do not confuse amikacin or Amikin with Amicar, or amikacin with anakinra.

◆CLASSIFICATION

PHARMACOTHERAPEUTIC: Aminoglycoside. **CLINICAL:** Antibiotic.

USES

Treatment of serious infections (e.g., bone infections, respiratory tract infections, septicemia) due to *Pseudomonas,* other gram-negative organisms (*Proteus, Serratia, E. coli, Enterobacter, Klebsiella*). **OFF-LABEL:** *Mycobacterium avium* complex (MAC).

PRECAUTIONS

Contraindications: Hypersensitivity to amikacin, other aminoglycosides. **Cautions:** Preexisting renal impairment, auditory or vestibular impairment, hypocalcemia, elderly, neuromuscular disorder, dehydration, concomitant use of neurotoxic or nephrotoxic medications.

ACTION

Inhibits protein synthesis in susceptible bacteria by binding to 30S ribosomal unit. **Therapeutic Effect:** Interferes with protein synthesis of susceptible microorganisms.

PHARMACOKINETICS

Rapid, complete absorption after IM administration. Protein binding: 0%–10%. Widely distributed (penetrates blood-brain barrier when meninges are inflamed). Excreted unchanged in urine. Removed by hemodialysis. **Half-life:** 2–4 hrs (increased in renal impairment, neonates; decreased in cystic fibrosis, burn pts, febrile pts).

LIFESPAN CONSIDERATIONS

Pregnancy/Lactation: Readily crosses placenta; small amounts distributed in breast milk. May produce fetal nephrotoxicity. **Children:** Neonates, premature infants may be more susceptible to toxicity due to immature renal function. **Elderly:** Higher risk of toxicity due to age-related renal impairment, increased risk of hearing loss.

INTERACTIONS

DRUG: **Foscarnet, mannitol** may increase nephrotoxic effect. **Penicillin** may decrease concentration/effect. **HERBAL:** None significant. **FOOD:** None known. **LAB VALUES:** May increase serum creatinine, BUN, ALT, AST, bilirubin, LDH. May decrease serum calcium, magnesium, potassium, sodium. **Therapeutic levels:** Peak: life-threatening infections: 25–40 mcg/mL; serious infections: 20–25 mcg/mL; urinary tract infections: 15–20 mcg/mL. **Trough:** Less than 8 mcg/mL. **Toxic levels:** Peak: greater than 40 mcg/mL; **trough:** greater than 10 mcg/mL.

AVAILABILITY (Rx)

Injection Solution: 250 mg/mL.

ADMINISTRATION/HANDLING

IV

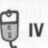

Reconstitution • Dilute to concentration of 0.25–5 mg/mL in 0.9% NaCl or D_5W.
Rate of administration • Infuse over 30–60 min.
Storage • Store vials at room temperature. • Solution appears clear but may become pale yellow (does not affect potency). • Intermittent IV infusion (piggyback) is stable for 24 hrs at room temperature, 2 days if refrigerated. • Discard if precipitate forms or dark discoloration occurs.

IM

• To minimize discomfort, give deep IM slowly. • Less painful if injected into gluteus maximus rather than in lateral aspect of thigh.

IV INCOMPATIBILITIES

Amphotericin, azithromycin (Zithromax), propofol (Diprivan).

IV COMPATIBILITIES

Amiodarone (Cordarone), aztreonam (Azactam), calcium gluconate, cefepime (Maxipime), cimetidine (Tagamet), ciprofloxacin (Cipro), clindamycin (Cleocin), dexmedetomidine (Precedex), dilTIAZem (Cardizem), diphenhydrAMINE (Benadryl), enalapril (Vasotec), esmolol (BreviBloc), fluconazole (Diflucan), furosemide (Lasix), levoFLOXacin (Levaquin), LORazepam (Ativan), magnesium sulfate, midazolam (Versed), morphine, ondansetron (Zofran), potassium chloride, raNITIdine (Zantac), vancomycin.

INDICATIONS/ROUTES/DOSAGE

Usual Parenteral Dosage

Note: Individualization of dose is critical due to low therapeutic index. Initial and periodic peak and trough levels should be determined.

IV, IM: ADULTS, ELDERLY, CHILDREN, INFANTS: 5–7.5 mg/kg/dose q8h. **NEONATES:** 15 mg/kg/dose (interval based on disease, age, weight).

Dosage in Renal Impairment

Dosage and frequency are modified based on degree of renal impairment and serum drug concentration. After a loading dose of 5–7.5 mg/kg, maintenance dose and frequency are based on serum creatinine levels and creatinine clearance.

Adults

Creatinine Clearance	Dosing Interval
50 mL/min or greater	No dose adjustment
10–50 mL/min	q24–72h
Less than 10 mL/min	q48–72h
Hemodialysis	q48–72h (give after HD on dialysis days)
Continuous renal replacement therapy (CRRT)	Initially, 10 mg/kg, then 7.5 mg/kg q24–48h

Dosage in Hepatic Impairment

No dose adjustment.

SIDE EFFECTS

Frequent: Phlebitis, thrombophlebitis. **Occasional:** Rash, fever, urticaria, pruritus. **Rare:** Neuromuscular blockade (difficulty breathing, drowsiness, weakness).

ADVERSE EFFECTS/TOXIC REACTIONS

Serious reactions include nephrotoxicity (increased thirst, decreased appetite, nausea, vomiting, increased BUN and serum creatinine levels, decreased creatinine clearance); neurotoxicity (muscle twitching, visual disturbances, seizures, paresthesia); ototoxicity (tinnitus, dizziness, loss of hearing).

NURSING CONSIDERATIONS

BASELINE ASSESSMENT

Obtain BUN, serum creatinine. Dehydration must be treated prior to aminoglycoside therapy. Establish baseline hearing acuity before beginning therapy. Question for history of allergies, esp. to aminoglycosides and sulfite. Obtain specimen for culture, sensitivity before giving first dose (therapy may begin before results are known).

INTERVENTION/EVALUATION

Monitor I&O (maintain hydration), urinalysis. Monitor results of serum peak/trough levels. Be alert to ototoxic, neurotoxic, nephrotoxic symptoms (see Adverse Effects/Toxic Reactions). Check IM injection site for pain, induration. Evaluate IV site for phlebitis. Assess for skin rash, diarrhea, superinfection (particularly genital/anal pruritus), changes of oral mucosa. When treating pts with neuromuscular disorders, assess respiratory response carefully. **Therapeutic levels:** Peak: life-threatening infections: 25–40 mcg/mL; serious infections: 20–25 mcg/mL; urinary tract infections: 15–20 mcg/mL. **Trough:** Less than 8 mcg/mL. **Toxic levels:** Peak: greater than 40 mcg/mL; **trough:** greater than 10 mcg/mL.

PATIENT/FAMILY TEACHING

• Continue antibiotic for full length of treatment. • Space doses evenly. • IM injection may cause discomfort. • Report any hearing, visual, balance, urinary problems, even after therapy is completed. • Do not take other medications without consulting physician.

amiodarone HIGH ALERT

a-mi-**oh**-da-rone
(Nexterone, Pacerone)

BLACK BOX ALERT Pts should be hospitalized when amiodarone is initiated. Alternative therapies should be tried first before using amiodarone. Only indicated for pts with life-threatening arrhythmias due to risk of toxicity. Pulmonary toxicity may occur without symptoms. Hepatotoxicity is common, usually mild (rarely possible). Can exacerbate arrhythmias.

Do not confuse amiodarone with aMILoride, dronedarone, or Cordarone with Cardura.

CLASSIFICATION

PHARMACOTHERAPEUTIC: Cardiac agent. **CLINICAL:** Antiarrhythmic. Class III.

USES

Management of life-threatening recurrent ventricular fibrillation (VF) or recurrent hemodynamically unstable ventricular tachycardia (VT) unresponsive to other therapy. **OFF-LABEL:** Treatment of atrial fibrillation, paroxysmal supraventricular tachycardia (SVT); ventricular tachyarrhythmias.

PRECAUTIONS

Contraindications: Hypersensitivity to amiodarone, iodine. Bradycardia-induced syncope (except in the presence of a pacemaker), second- and third-degree AV block (except in presence of a pacemaker); severe sinus node dysfunction, causing marked sinus bradycardia; cardiogenic shock. **Cautions:** May prolong QT interval. Thyroid disease, electrolyte imbalance, hepatic disease, hypotension, left ventricular dysfunction, pulmonary disease. Pts taking warfarin, surgical pts.

ACTION

Inhibits adrenergic stimulation; affects Na, K, Ca channels; prolongs action potential and refractory period in myocardial tissue. Decreases AV conduction and sinus node function. **Therapeutic Effect:** Suppresses arrhythmias.

PHARMACOKINETICS

Route	Onset	Peak	Duration
PO	3 days–3 wks	1 wk–5 mos	7–50 days after discontinuation

Slowly, variably absorbed from GI tract. Protein binding: 96%. Extensively metabolized in liver. Excreted via bile; not removed by hemodialysis. **Half-life:** 26–107 days; metabolite: 61 days.

LIFESPAN CONSIDERATIONS

Pregnancy/Lactation: Crosses placenta; distributed in breast milk. May adversely affect fetal development. **Children:** Safety and efficacy not established. **Elderly:** May be more sensitive to effects on thyroid function. May experience increased incidence of ataxia, other neurotoxic effects.

INTERACTIONS

DRUG: May increase QT interval–prolonging effect of **citalopram, clarithromycin, erythromycin, nilotinib, quetiapine, ribociclib, thioridazine, voriconazole. Fingolimod, levofloxacin** may enhance QT interval-prolonging effect. **Beta blockers (e.g., atenolol, carvedilol, metoprolol), calcium channel blockers (e.g., diltiaZEM, verapamil), digoxin, sofosbuvir** may increase the bradycardic effect. **HERBAL: Herbals with hypotensive properties (e.g., garlic, ginger, ginkgo biloba)** may increase concentration/effects. **St. John's wort** may decrease concentration/effect. May increase concentration/effect of **red yeast rice. FOOD: Grapefruit products** may alter effect. Avoid use during therapy. **LAB VALUES:** May increase serum ALT, AST, alkaline phosphatase, ANA titer. May cause changes in ECG, thyroid function test results. **Therapeutic serum level:** 0.5–2.5 mcg/mL; toxic serum level not established.

AVAILABILITY (Rx)

Infusion (Pre-Mix): Nexterone: 150 mg/100 mL; 360 mg/200 mL. **Injection, Solution:** 150 mg/3 mL, 450 mg/9 mL, 900 mg/18 mL. **Tablets:** ***(Pacerone):*** 100 mg, 200 mg, 400 mg.

ADMINISTRATION/HANDLING

IV

Reconstitution • Infusions longer than 2 hrs must be administered/diluted in glass or polyolefin bottles. • Dilute loading dose (150 mg) in 100 mL D_5W (1.5 mg/mL). • Dilute maintenance dose (900 mg) in 500 mL D_5W (1.8 mg/mL). Concentrations greater than 3 mg/mL cause peripheral vein phlebitis.

Rate of administration • Does not need protection from light during administration. • Administer through central venous catheter (CVC) if possible, using in-line filter. • Bolus over 10 min (15 mg/min) not to exceed 30 mg/min; then 1 mg/min over 6 hrs; then 0.5 mg/min over 18 hrs. • Infusions longer than 1 hr, concentration not to exceed 2 mg/mL unless CVC used.

Storage • Store at room temperature. • Stable for 24 hrs when diluted in glass or polyolefin containers; stable for 2 hrs when diluted in PVC containers.

PO

• Give consistently with regard to meals to reduce GI distress. • Tablets may be crushed. • Do not give with grapefruit products.

IV INCOMPATIBILITIES

CeFAZolin (Ancef), heparin, sodium bicarbonate.

IV COMPATIBILITIES

Dexmedetomidine (Precedex), DOBUTamine (Dobutrex), DOPamine (Intropin), furosemide (Lasix), insulin (regular), labetalol (Normodyne), lidocaine, LORazepam (Ativan), midazolam (Versed), morphine, nitroglycerin, norepinephrine (Levophed), phenylephrine (Neo-Synephrine), potassium chloride, vancomycin.

INDICATIONS/ROUTES/DOSAGE

Ventricular Arrhythmias

PO: ADULTS, ELDERLY: Initially, 400 mg q8–12h for 1–2 wks, then decrease to 200–400 mg once daily. **Maintenance:** 200–400 mg/day.

IV infusion: ADULTS, ELDERLY: Initially, 150 mg over 10 min, then 1 mg/min over 6 hrs; then 0.5 mg/min. Continue this rate over at least 18 hrs or until complete transition or oral. Breakthrough stable VT: 150 mg in 100 mL D_5W or NS over 10 min. 1–6 mg/mL.

Dosage in Renal Impairment

No dose adjustment.

Dosage in Hepatic Impairment

Use caution.

SIDE EFFECTS

Expected: Corneal microdeposits noted in almost all pts treated for more than 6 mos (can lead to blurry vision). **Occasional (greater than 3%): PO:** Constipation, headache, decreased appetite, nausea, vomiting, paresthesia, photosensitivity, muscular incoordination. **Parenteral:** Hypotension, nausea, fever, bradycardia. **Rare (less than 3%): PO:** Bitter or metallic taste, decreased libido, dizziness, facial flushing, blue-gray coloring of skin (face, arms, and neck), blurred vision, bradycardia, asymptomatic corneal deposits, rash, visual disturbances, halo vision.

ADVERSE EFFECTS/TOXIC REACTIONS

Serious, potentially fatal pulmonary toxicity (alveolitis, pulmonary fibrosis, pneumonitis, acute respiratory distress syndrome) may begin with progressive dyspnea and cough with crackles, decreased breath sounds, pleurisy, HF, or hepatotoxicity. May worsen existing arrhythmias or produce new arrhythmias.

NURSING CONSIDERATIONS

BASELINE ASSESSMENT

Obtain baseline serum ALT, AST, alkaline phosphatase, ECG; pulmonary function tests, CXR in pts with pulmonary disease. Assess B/P, apical pulse immediately before drug is administered (if pulse is 60/min or less or systolic B/P is less than 90 mm Hg, withhold medication, contact physician).

INTERVENTION/EVALUATION

Monitor for symptoms of pulmonary toxicity (progressively worsening dyspnea, cough). Dosage should be discontinued or reduced if toxicity occurs. Assess pulse for quality, rhythm, bradycardia. Monitor ECG for cardiac changes (e.g., widening of QRS, prolongation of PR and QT intervals). Notify physician of any significant interval changes. Assess for nausea, fatigue, paresthesia, tremor. Monitor for signs of hypothyroidism (periorbital edema, lethargy, pudgy hands/feet, cool/pale skin, vertigo, night cramps) and hyperthyroidism (hot/dry skin, bulging eyes [exophthalmos], frequent urination, eyelid edema, weight loss, difficulty breathing). Monitor serum ALT, AST, alkaline phosphatase for evidence of hepatic toxicity. Assess skin, cornea for bluish discoloration in pts who have been on drug therapy longer than 2 mos. Monitor thyroid function test results. If elevated hepatic enzymes occur, dosage reduction or discontinuation is necessary. Monitor for therapeutic serum level (0.5–2.5 mcg/mL). Toxic serum level not established.

PATIENT/FAMILY TEACHING

• Protect against photosensitivity reaction on skin exposed to sunlight. • Bluish skin discoloration gradually disappears when drug is discontinued. • Report shortness of breath, cough. • Outpatients should monitor pulse before taking medication. • Do not abruptly discontinue medication. • Compliance with therapy regimen is essential to control arrhythmias. • Restrict salt, alcohol intake. • Avoid grapefruit products. • Recommend ophthalmic exams q6mos. • Report any vision changes, signs/symptoms of cardiac arrhythmias.

amitriptyline

a-mi-**trip**-ti-leen
(Levate ✱)

■ BLACK BOX ALERT ■ Increased risk of suicidal thinking and behavior in children, adolescents, young adults 18–24 yrs with major depressive disorder, other psychiatric disorders.

Do not confuse amitriptyline with aminophylline, imipramine, or nortriptyline, or Elavil with Eldepryl, enalapril, Equanil, or Mellaril.

FIXED-COMBINATION(S)

Limbitrol: amitriptyline/chlordiazePOXIDE (an antianxiety): 12.5 mg/5 mg, 25 mg/10 mg.

◆CLASSIFICATION

PHARMACOTHERAPEUTIC: Tricyclic. **CLINICAL:** Antidepressant.

USES

Treatment of unipolar, major depression. **OFF-LABEL:** Neuropathic pain, related to diabetic neuropathy or postherpetic neuralgia; treatment of migraine. Treatment of depression in children, posttraumatic stress disorder (PTSD).

PRECAUTIONS

Contraindications: Hypersensitivity to amitriptyline. Acute recovery period after MI, coadministered with or within 14 days of MAOIs. **Cautions:** Prostatic hypertrophy, history of urinary retention or obstruction, narrow-angle glaucoma, diabetes, seizures, hyperthyroidism, cardiac/hepatic/renal disease, schizophrenia, xerostomia, visual problems, constipation or bowel obstruction, elderly, increased intraocular pressure (IOP), hiatal hernia, suicidal ideation.

ACTION

Blocks reuptake of neurotransmitters (norepinephrine, serotonin) at presynaptic membranes, increasing synaptic concentration in the CNS. **Therapeutic Effect:** Antidepressant effect.

PHARMACOKINETICS

Rapidly and well absorbed from GI tract. Protein binding: 90%. Metabolized in liver. Primarily excreted in urine. Minimal removal by hemodialysis. **Half-life:** 10–26 hrs.

⌛ LIFESPAN CONSIDERATIONS

Pregnancy/Lactation: Crosses placenta; minimally distributed in breast milk. **Children:** More sensitive to increased dosage, toxicity, increased risk of suicidal ideation, worsening of depression. **Elderly:** Increased risk of toxicity. Increased sensitivity to anticholinergic effects. Caution in pts with cardiovascular disease.

INTERACTIONS

DRUG: **CNS depressants (e.g., alcohol, morphine, zolpidem)** may increase CNS depression. May increase CNS depressant effect of **azelastine. Aclidinium, ipratropium, tiotropium, umeclidinium** may increase anticholinergic effect. May increase arrhythmogenic effect of **dronedarone. MAOIs (e.g., phenelzine, selegiline)** may increase the serotonergic effect. HERBAL: **Herbals with sedative properties (e.g., chamomile, kava kava, valerian)** may increase CNS depression. **St. John's wort** may decrease concentration/effects. FOOD: None known. LAB VALUES: May alter ECG readings (flattened T wave), serum glucose (increase or decrease). **Therapeutic serum level:** Peak: 120–250 ng/mL; **toxic serum level:** greater than 500 ng/mL.

AVAILABILITY (Rx)

Tablets: 10 mg, 25 mg, 50 mg, 75 mg, 100 mg, 150 mg.

ADMINISTRATION/HANDLING

PO

• Give with food or milk if GI distress occurs.

INDICATIONS/ROUTES/DOSAGE

Depression

PO: ADULTS: Initially, 25–50 mg/day as a single dose at bedtime, or in divided doses. May gradually increase in increments of 25–50 mg at 1-wk (or greater) intervals up to 100–300 mg/day. Titrate to lowest effective dosage. **ELDERLY:** Initially, 10–25 mg once daily at bedtime. **ADOLESCENTS:** Initially, 10 mg 3 times/day and 20 mg at bedtime. **Maximum:** 200 mg/day.

Pain Management

PO: ADULTS, ELDERLY: Initially, 10–25 mg once daily at bedtime. May increase gradually in 10–25 mg increments over at least 1 wk up to 150 mg/day. **CHILDREN:** Initially, 0.1 mg/kg. May increase over 2 wks to 0.5–2 mg/kg at bedtime.

Dosage in Renal/Hepatic Impairment

Use with caution.

SIDE EFFECTS

Frequent: Dizziness, drowsiness, dry mouth, orthostatic hypotension, headache, increased appetite, weight gain, nausea, unusual fatigue, unpleasant taste. **Occasional:** Blurred vision, confusion, constipation, hallucinations, delayed micturition, eye pain, arrhythmias, fine muscle tremors, parkinsonian syndrome, anxiety, diarrhea, diaphoresis, heartburn, insomnia. **Rare:** Hypersensitivity, alopecia, tinnitus, breast enlargement, photosensitivity.

ADVERSE EFFECTS/TOXIC REACTIONS

Overdose may produce confusion, seizures, severe drowsiness, changes in cardiac conduction, fever, hallucinations, agitation, dyspnea, vomiting, unusual fatigue, weakness. Abrupt withdrawal after prolonged therapy may produce headache, malaise, nausea, vomiting, vivid dreams. Blood dyscrasias, cholestatic jaundice occur rarely.

NURSING CONSIDERATIONS

BASELINE ASSESSMENT

Observe and record behavior. Assess psychological status, thought content, suicidal ideation, sleep patterns, appearance, interest in environment. For pts on long-term therapy, hepatic/renal function tests, blood counts should be performed periodically.

INTERVENTION/EVALUATION

Supervise suicidal-risk pt closely during early therapy (as depression lessens, energy level improves, increasing suicide potential). Assess appearance, behavior, speech pattern, level of interest, mood. Monitor B/P for hypotension, pulse, arrhythmias. **Therapeutic serum level:** Peak: 120–250 ng/mL; **toxic serum level:** greater than 500 ng/mL. **Maximum:** 200 mg/day.

PATIENT/FAMILY TEACHING

• Go slowly from lying to standing. • Tolerance to postural hypotension, sedative and anticholinergic effects usually develops during early therapy. • Maximum therapeutic effect may be noted in 2–4 wks. • Sensitivity to sun may occur. • Report visual disturbances. • Do not abruptly discontinue medication. • Avoid tasks that require alertness, motor skills until response to drug is established. • Avoid alcohol. • Sips of water may relieve dry mouth.

amLODIPine

TOP 100

am-**loe**-di-peen
(Katerzia, Norvasc)
Do not confuse amLODIPine with aMILoride, or Norvasc with Navane or Vascor.

FIXED-COMBINATION(S)

Amturnide: amLODIPine/aliskiren (a renin inhibitor)/hydroCHLOROthiazide (a diuretic): 5 mg/150 mg/12.5 mg, 5 mg/300 mg/12.5 mg, 5 mg/300 mg/25 mg, 10 mg/300 mg/12.5 mg, 10 mg/300 mg/25 mg. **Azor:** amLODIPine/olmesartan (an angiotensin II receptor antagonist): 5 mg/20 mg, 10 mg/20 mg, 5 mg/40 mg, 10 mg/40 mg. **Caduet:** amLODIPine/atorvastatin (hydroxymethylglutaryl-CoA [HMG-CoA] reductase inhibitor): 2.5 mg/10 mg, 2.5 mg/20 mg, 2.5 mg/40 mg, 5 mg/10 mg, 10 mg/10 mg, 5 mg/20 mg, 10 mg/20 mg, 5 mg/40 mg, 10 mg/40 mg, 5 mg/80 mg, 10 mg/80 mg. **Exforge:** amLODIPine/valsartan (an angiotensin II receptor antagonist): 5 mg/160 mg, 10 mg/160 mg, 5 mg/320 mg, 10 mg/320 mg. **Exforge HCT:** amLODIPine/valsartan/hydroCHLOROthiazide (a diuretic): 5 mg/160 mg/12.5 mg, 5 mg/160 mg/25 mg, 10 mg/160 mg/12.5 mg, 10 mg/160 mg/25 mg, 10 mg/320 mg/25 mg. **Lotrel:** amLODIPine/benazepril (an angiotensin-converting enzyme [ACE] inhibitor): 2.5 mg/10 mg, 5 mg/10 mg, 5 mg/20 mg, 5 mg/40 mg, 10 mg/20 mg, 10 mg/40 mg. **Prestalia:** amLODIPine/perindopril (an ACE inhibitor): 2.5 mg/3.5 mg; 5 mg/7 mg; 10 mg/14 mg. **Tekamlo:** amLODIPine/aliskiren (a renin inhibitor): 5 mg/150 mg, 5 mg/300 mg, 10 mg/150 mg, 10 mg/300 mg. **Tribenzor:** amLODIPine/olmesartan/hydroCHLOROthiazide: 5 mg/20 mg/12.5 mg, 5 mg/40 mg/12.5 mg, 5 mg/40 mg/25 mg, 10 mg/40 mg/12.5 mg, 10 mg/40 mg/25 mg. **Twynsta:** amLODIPine/telmisartan (an angiotensin II receptor antagonist): 5 mg/40 mg, 5 mg/80 mg, 10 mg/40 mg, 10 mg/80 mg.

◆CLASSIFICATION

PHARMACOTHERAPEUTIC: Calcium channel blocker (dihydropyridine). **CLINICAL:** Antihypertensive, antianginal.

USES

Management of hypertension, coronary artery disease (chronic stable angina, vasospastic [Prinzmetal's or variant] angina).

PRECAUTIONS

Contraindications: Hypersensitivity to amLODIPine. **Cautions:** Hepatic impairment, severe aortic stenosis, hypertrophic cardiomyopathy with outflow tract obstruction.

ACTION

Inhibits calcium movement across cardiac and vascular smooth muscle cell membranes during depolarization. **Therapeutic Effect:** Dilates coronary arteries, peripheral arteries/arterioles. Decreases total peripheral vascular resistance and B/P by vasodilation.

PHARMACOKINETICS

Route	Onset	Peak	Duration
PO	0.5–1 hr	N/A	24 hrs

Slowly absorbed from GI tract. Protein binding: 95%–98%. Metabolized in liver. Excreted primarily in urine. Not removed by hemodialysis. **Half-life:** 30–50 hrs (increased in elderly, pts with hepatic cirrhosis).

LIFESPAN CONSIDERATIONS

Pregnancy/Lactation: Unknown if drug crosses placenta or is distributed in breast milk. **Children:** Safety and efficacy not established. **Elderly:** Half-life may be increased, more sensitive to hypotensive effects.

INTERACTIONS

DRUG: **Strong CYP3A4 inducers (e.g., carbamazepine, phenytoin, rifampin)** may decrease concentration/effect. **Antihepaciviral combination products** may increase concentration/effect. May increase concentration/effect of **fosphenytoin, lomitapide, phenytoin, simvastatin.** **HERBAL:** **St. John's wort** may decrease concentration/effect. **Herbals with hypotensive properties (e.g., garlic, ginger, gingko biloba)** may increase risk of hypotension. **FOOD:** **Grapefruit products** may increase concentration, hypotensive effects. **LAB VALUES:** May increase hepatic enzyme levels.

AVAILABILITY (Rx)

Oral Suspension: 1 mg/mL. **Tablets:** 2.5 mg, 5 mg, 10 mg.

ADMINISTRATION/HANDLING

PO

- May give without regard to food.

INDICATIONS/ROUTES/DOSAGE

Hypertension

PO: ADULTS: Initially, 2.5–5 mg/day as a single dose. May titrate every 7–14 days. **Maximum:** 10 mg/day. **SMALL-FRAME, FRAGILE, ELDERLY, ADDITION TO OTHER ANTIHYPERTENSIVES:** 2.5 mg/day as a single dose. May titrate q7–14 days. **Maximum:** 10 mg/day. **CHILDREN 6–17 YRS:** 2.5–5 mg/day.

CAD (Angina)

PO: ADULTS: 5–10 mg/day as a single dose. **ELDERLY, PTS WITH HEPATIC INSUFFICIENCY:** 5 mg/day as a single dose.

Dosage in Renal Impairment

No dose adjustment.

Dosage in Hepatic Impairment

ADULTS, ELDERLY: **Hypertension:** Initially, 2.5 mg/day. **Angina:** Initially, 5 mg/day. Titrate slowly in pts with severe impairment.

SIDE EFFECTS

Frequent (greater than 5%): Peripheral edema, headache, flushing. **Occasional (5%–1%):** Dizziness, palpitations, nausea, unusual fatigue or weakness (asthenia). **Rare (less than 1%):** Chest pain, bradycardia, orthostatic hypotension.

ADVERSE EFFECTS/ TOXIC REACTIONS

Overdose may produce excessive peripheral vasodilation, marked hypotension with reflex tachycardia, syncope.

NURSING CONSIDERATIONS

BASELINE ASSESSMENT

Assess baseline renal/hepatic function tests, B/P, apical pulse.

INTERVENTION/EVALUATION

Assess B/P (if systolic B/P is less than 90 mm Hg, withhold medication, contact physician). Assess skin for flushing. Question for headache, asthenia.

PATIENT/FAMILY TEACHING

- Do not abruptly discontinue medication. • Compliance with therapy regimen is essential to control hypertension. • Avoid tasks that require alertness, motor skills until response to drug is established. • Do not ingest grapefruit products.

amoxicillin

a-**mox**-i-sil-in
(Novamoxin 🍁)
Do not confuse amoxicillin with amoxapine or Atarax.

CLASSIFICATION

PHARMACOTHERAPEUTIC: Penicillin. **CLINICAL:** Antibiotic.

USES

Treatment of susceptible infections due to streptococci, *E. coli, E. faecalis, P. mirabilis, H. influenzae, N. gonorrhoeae*, including ear, nose, and throat; lower respiratory tract; skin and skin structure; UTIs; acute uncomplicated gonorrhea; *H. pylori*. **OFF-LABEL:** Treatment of Lyme disease and typhoid fever. Postexposure prophylaxis for anthrax exposure.

PRECAUTIONS

Contraindications: Serious hypersensitivity to amoxicillin, other beta-lactams. **Cautions:** History of allergies (esp. cephalosporins), infectious mononucleosis, renal impairment, asthma.

ACTION

Inhibits bacterial cell wall synthesis by binding to PCN-binding proteins. **Therapeutic Effect:** Bactericidal in susceptible microorganisms.

PHARMACOKINETICS

Well absorbed from GI tract. Protein binding: 20%. Partially metabolized in liver. Primarily excreted in urine. Removed by hemodialysis. **Half-life:** 1–1.3 hrs (increased in renal impairment).

LIFESPAN CONSIDERATIONS

Pregnancy/Lactation: Crosses placenta, appears in cord blood, amniotic fluid. Distributed in breast milk in low concentrations. May lead to allergic sensitization, diarrhea, candidiasis, skin rash in infant. **Children:** Immature renal function in neonate/young infant may delay renal excretion. **Elderly:** Age-related renal impairment may require dosage adjustment.

INTERACTIONS

DRUG: **Allopurinol** may increase incidence of rash. **Probenecid** may increase concentration, toxicity risk. **Tetracyclines** may decrease therapeutic effect. **HERBAL:** None significant. **FOOD:** None known. **LAB VALUES:** May increase serum ALT, AST, bilirubin, BUN, creatinine, LDH. May cause positive Coombs' test.

AVAILABILITY (Rx)

Capsules: 250 mg, 500 mg. **Powder for Oral Suspension:** 125 mg/5 mL, 200 mg/5 mL, 250 mg/5 mL, 400 mg/5 mL. **Tablets:** 500 mg, 875 mg. **Tablets (Chewable):** 125 mg, 250 mg.

ADMINISTRATION/HANDLING

PO

• Give without regard to food. • Instruct pt to chew/crush chewable tablets thoroughly before swallowing. • Oral suspension dose may be mixed with formula, milk, fruit juice, water, cold drink. • Give immediately after mixing. • After reconstitution, oral suspension is stable for 14 days at either room temperature or refrigerated.

INDICATIONS/ROUTES/DOSAGE

Usual Dosage

PO: ADULTS, ELDERLY: 500–1000 mg q8–12h. **INFANTS OLDER THAN 3 MOS, CHILDREN, ADOLESCENTS:** 25–50 mg/kg/day in divided doses q8h. **Maximum Dose:** 500 mg. **INFANTS 3 MOS AND YOUNGER:** 25–50 mg/kg/day in divided doses. **NEONATE:** 20–30 mg/kg/day in divided doses q12h.

Dosage in Renal Impairment

◀ALERT▶ Immediate-release 875-mg tablet should not be used in pts with creatinine clearance less than 30 mL/min. Dosage interval is modified based on creatinine clearance. **Creatinine clearance 10–30 mL/min: ADULTS:** 250–500 mg q12h. **CHILDREN:** 8–20 mg/kg/dose q12h. **Creatinine clearance less than 10 mL/min: ADULTS:** 250–500 mg q24h. **CHILDREN:** 8–20 mg/kg/dose q24h.

Dosage in Hepatic Impairment

No dose adjustment.

SIDE EFFECTS

Frequent: GI disturbances (mild diarrhea, nausea, vomiting), headache, oral/

vaginal candidiasis. **Occasional:** Generalized rash, urticaria.

ADVERSE EFFECTS/TOXIC REACTIONS

Antibiotic-associated colitis, other superinfections (abdominal cramps, severe watery diarrhea, fever) may result from altered bacterial balance in GI tract. Severe hypersensitivity reactions, including anaphylaxis, acute interstitial nephritis, occur rarely.

NURSING CONSIDERATIONS

BASELINE ASSESSMENT

Question for history of allergies (esp. penicillins, cephalosporins), renal impairment.

INTERVENTION/EVALUATION

Promptly report rash, diarrhea (fever, abdominal pain, mucus and blood in stool may indicate antibiotic-associated colitis). Be alert for superinfection: fever, vomiting, diarrhea, anal/genital pruritus, black "hairy" tongue, oral mucosal changes (ulceration, pain, erythema). Monitor renal/hepatic function tests.

PATIENT/FAMILY TEACHING

• Continue antibiotic for full length of treatment. • Space doses evenly. • Take with meals if GI upset occurs. • Thoroughly crush or chew the chewable tablets before swallowing. • Report rash, diarrhea, other new symptoms.

amoxicillin/ clavulanate

a-**mox**-i-sil-in/**klav**-yoo-la-nate
(Augmentin, Augmentin ES 600, Clavulin ✱)
Do not confuse Augmentin with amoxicillin or Azulfidine.

◆CLASSIFICATION

PHARMACOTHERAPEUTIC: Penicillin. **CLINICAL:** Antibiotic.

USES

Treatment of susceptible infections due to *streptococci, E. coli, E. faecalis, P. mirabilis,* beta-lactamase producing *H. influenzae, Klebsiella* spp., *M. catarrhalis*, and *S. aureus* (not methicillin-resistant *Staphylococcus aureus* [MRSA]), including lower respiratory, skin and skin structure, UTIs, otitis media, sinusitis. **OFF-LABEL:** Chronic antimicrobial suppression of prosthetic joint infection.

PRECAUTIONS

Contraindications: Hypersensitivity to amoxicillin, clavulanate, any penicillins; history of cholestatic jaundice or hepatic impairment with amoxicillin/clavulanate therapy. Augmentin XR (additional): Severe renal impairment (creatinine clearance less than 30 mL/min), hemodialysis pt. **Cautions:** History of allergies, esp. cephalosporins; renal impairment, infectious mononucleosis.

ACTION

Amoxicillin inhibits bacterial cell wall synthesis by binding to PCN-binding proteins. Clavulanate inhibits bacterial beta-lactamase protecting amoxicillin from degradation. **Therapeutic Effect:** Amoxicillin is bactericidal in susceptible microorganisms. Clavulanate protects amoxicillin from enzymatic degradation.

PHARMACOKINETICS

Well absorbed from GI tract. Protein binding: 20%. Partially metabolized in liver. Primarily excreted in urine. Removed by hemodialysis. **Half-life:** 1–1.3 hrs (increased in renal impairment).

⌛ LIFESPAN CONSIDERATIONS

Pregnancy/Lactation: Crosses placenta, appears in cord blood, amniotic fluid. Distributed in breast milk in low concentrations. May lead to allergic sensitization, diarrhea, candidiasis, skin rash in infant. **Children:** Immature renal function in neonate/young infant may delay renal excretion. **Elderly:** Age-related renal impairment may require dosage adjustment.

INTERACTIONS

DRUG: **Allopurinol** may increase incidence of rash. **Probenecid** may increase concentration, toxicity risk. **Tetracyclines** may decrease therapeutic effect. **HERBAL:** None significant. **FOOD:** None known. **LAB VALUES:** May increase serum ALT, AST. May cause positive Coombs' test.

AVAILABILITY (Rx)

Powder for Oral Suspension: ***(Amoclan, Augmentin):*** 125 mg–31.25 mg/5 mL, 200 mg–28.5 mg/5 mL, 250 mg–62.5 mg/5 mL, 400 mg–57 mg/5 mL, 600 mg–42.9 mg/5 mL. **Tablets:** ***(Augmentin):*** 250 mg–125 mg, 500 mg–125 mg, 875 mg–125 mg. **Tablets (Chewable):** ***(Augmentin):*** 200 mg–28.5 mg, 400 mg–57 mg.

(Non-Crushable) **Tablets (Extended-Release):** 1,000 mg–62.5 mg.

ADMINISTRATION/HANDLING

PO

• Store tablets at room temperature. • After reconstitution, oral suspension is stable for 10 days but should be refrigerated. • May mix dose of suspension with milk, formula, or juice and give immediately. • Give without regard to meals. • Give with food to increase absorption, decrease stomach upset. • Instruct pt to chew/crush chewable tablets thoroughly before swallowing. • Do not break, crush, dissolve, or divide extended-release tablets.

INDICATIONS/ROUTES/DOSAGE

Note: Dosage based on amoxicillin component.

Usual Adult Dosage

PO: ADULTS, ELDERLY: 250 mg q8h or 500 mg q8–12h or 875 mg q12h or ***(Extended-Release)*** 2,000 mg q12h.

Usual Pediatric Dosage

PO: CHILDREN OLDER THAN 3 MOS, WEIGHING 40 KG OR MORE: (Mild-Moderate): 500 mg q12h or 250 mg q8h. **(Severe):** 875 mg q12h or 500 mg q8h. ***(Extended-Release):*** 2,000 mg q12h. **WEIGHING LESS THAN 40 KG: (Mild-Moderate):** 25 mg/kg/day in 2 divided doses or 20 mg/kg/day in 3 divided doses. **(Severe):** 45 mg/kg/day in 2 divided doses or 40 mg/kg/day in 3 divided doses. **Maximum single dose:** 500 mg. **YOUNGER THAN 3 MOS:** Amoxicillin 30 mg/kg/day divided q12h using 125 mg/5mL suspension only. **NEONATES:** 30 mg/kg/day (using 125 mg/5 mL suspension) in divided doses q12h.

Dosage in Renal Impairment

◀ALERT▶ Do not use 875-mg tablet or extended-release tablets for creatinine clearance less than 30 mL/min. Dosage and frequency are modified based on creatinine clearance. **Creatinine clearance 10–30 mL/min:** 250–500 mg q12h. **Creatinine clearance less than 10 mL/min:** 250–500 mg q24h. **HD:** 250–500 mg q24h, give dose during and after dialysis. **PD:** 250 mg q12h.

Dosage in Hepatic Impairment

No dose adjustment (see Contraindications).

SIDE EFFECTS

Occasional (9%–4%): Diarrhea, loose stools, nausea, skin rashes, urticaria. **Rare (less than 3%):** Vomiting, vaginitis, abdominal discomfort, flatulence, headache.

ADVERSE EFFECTS/TOXIC REACTIONS

Antibiotic-associated colitis, other superinfections (abdominal cramps, severe watery diarrhea, fever) may result from altered bacterial balance in GI tract. Severe hypersensitivity reactions, including anaphylaxis, acute interstitial nephritis, occur rarely.

NURSING CONSIDERATIONS

BASELINE ASSESSMENT

Question for history of allergies, esp. penicillins, cephalosporins, renal impairment.

INTERVENTION/EVALUATION

Promptly report rash, diarrhea (fever, abdominal pain, mucus and blood in stool may indicate antibiotic-associated colitis). Be alert for signs of superinfection, including fever, vomiting, diarrhea, black "hairy" tongue, ulceration or changes of oral mucosa, anal/genital pruritus. Monitor renal/hepatic tests with prolonged therapy.

PATIENT/FAMILY TEACHING

• Continue antibiotic for full length of treatment. • Space doses evenly. • Take with meals if GI upset occurs. • Thoroughly crush or chew the chewable tablets before swallowing. • Notify physician if rash, diarrhea, other new symptoms occur.

amphotericin B HIGH ALERT

am-foe-**ter**-i-sin

(Abelcet, AmBisome, Fungizone ✱)

■ BLACK BOX ALERT ■ (Nonliposomal) To be used primarily for pts with progressive, potentially fatal fungal infection. Not to be used for noninvasive forms of fungal disease (oral thrush, vaginal candidiasis).

◆CLASSIFICATION

PHARMACOTHERAPEUTIC: Polyene antifungal. **CLINICAL:** Antifungal, antiprotozoal.

USES

Abelcet: Treatment of invasive fungal infections refractory or intolerant to Fungizone. **AmBisome:** Empiric treatment of fungal infection in febrile neutropenic pts. *Aspergillus, Candida* species, *Cryptococcus* infections refractory to Fungizone or pt with renal impairment or toxicity with Fungizone. Treatment of cryptococcal meningitis in HIV-infected pts. Treatment of visceral leishmaniasis. **Fungizone:** Treatment of life-threatening fungal infections caused by susceptible fungi, including *Candida* spp., *Histoplasma, Cryptococcus, Aspergillus, Blastomyces.* **OFF-LABEL: Abelcet:** Serious *Candida* infections. **AmBisome:** Treatment of systemic histoplasmosis infection.

PRECAUTIONS

Contraindications: Hypersensitivity to amphotericin B. **Cautions:** Concomitant use with other nephrotoxic drugs; renal impairment.

ACTION

Generally fungistatic but may become fungicidal with high dosages or very susceptible microorganisms. Binds to sterols in fungal cell membrane. **Therapeutic Effect:** Alters fungal cell membrane permeability, allowing loss of potassium, other cellular components, resulting in cell death.

PHARMACOKINETICS

Protein binding: 90%. Widely distributed. Metabolism not specified. Cleared by nonrenal pathways. Minimal removal by hemodialysis. Amphotec and Abelcet are not dialyzable. **Half-life:** Fungizone, 24 hrs (increased in neonates and children); Abelcet, 7.2 days; AmBisome, 100–153 hrs; Amphotec, 26–28 hrs.

⌛ LIFESPAN CONSIDERATIONS

Pregnancy/Lactation: Crosses placenta; unknown if distributed in breast milk. **Children:** Safety and efficacy not established, but use the least amount for therapeutic regimen. **Elderly:** No age-related precautions noted.

INTERACTIONS

DRUG: **Foscarnet** may increase nephrotoxic effect. May decrease therapeutic effect of *Saccharomyces boulardii.* **HERBAL:** None significant. **FOOD:** None known. **LAB VALUES:** May increase serum ALT, AST, alkaline phosphatase, BUN, creatinine. May decrease serum calcium, magnesium, potassium.

AVAILABILITY (Rx)

Injection, Powder for Reconstitution: ***(AmBisome, Fungizone):*** 50 mg. **Injection, Suspension:** ***(Abelcet):*** 5 mg/mL (20 mL).

ADMINISTRATION/HANDLING

IV

• Use strict aseptic technique; no bacteriostatic agent or preservative is present in diluent.

Reconstitution • ***(Abelcet):*** Shake 20-mL (100-mg) vial gently until contents are dissolved. Withdraw required dose using 5-micron filter needle (supplied by manufacturer). • Dilute with D_5W to 1–2 mg/mL. • ***(AmBisome):*** Reconstitute each 50-mg vial with 12 mL Sterile Water for Injection to provide concentration of 4 mg/mL. • Shake vial vigorously for 30 sec. Withdraw required dose and inject syringe contents through a 5-micron filter into an infusion of D_5W to provide final concentration of 1–2 mg/mL (0.2–0.5 mg/mL for infants and small children). • ***(Fungizone):*** Add 10 mL Sterile Water for Injection to each 50-mg vial. • Further dilute with 250–500 mL D_5W. • Final concentration should not exceed 0.1 mg/mL (0.25 mg/mL for central infusion).

Rate of administration • Give by slow IV infusion. Infuse conventional amphotericin over 4–6 hrs; Abelcet over 2 hrs (shake contents if infusion longer than 2 hrs); AmBisome over 1–2 hrs.

Storage • ***(Abelcet):*** Refrigerate unreconstituted solution. Reconstituted solution is stable for 48 hrs if refrigerated, 6 hrs at room temperature. • ***(AmBisome):*** Refrigerate unreconstituted solution. Reconstituted vials are stable for 24 hrs when refrigerated. Concentration of 1–2 mg/mL is stable for 6 hrs. • ***(Fungizone):*** Refrigerate unused vials. • Once reconstituted, vials stable for 24 hrs at room temperature, 7 days if refrigerated. • Diluted solutions stable for 24 hrs at room temperature, 2 days if refrigerated.

IV INCOMPATIBILITIES

Note: Abelcet, AmBisome, Amphotec: Do not mix with any other drug, diluent, or solution. Fungizone: Allopurinol (Aloprim), aztreonam (Azactam), calcium gluconate, cefepime (Maxipime), cimetidine (Tagamet), ciprofloxacin (Cipro), dexmedetomidine (Precedex), diphenhydrAMINE (Benadryl), DOPamine (Intropin), enalapril (Vasotec), filgrastim (Neupogen), fluconazole (Diflucan), foscarnet (Foscavir), magnesium sulfate, meropenem (Merrem IV), ondansetron (Zofran), piperacillin and tazobactam (Zosyn), potassium chloride, propofol (Diprivan).

IV COMPATIBILITIES

LORazepam (Ativan).

INDICATIONS/ROUTES/DOSAGE

Usual Abelcet Dose

IV infusion: ADULTS, CHILDREN: 5 mg/kg once daily.

Usual AmBisome Dose

IV infusion: ADULTS: 3–6 mg/kg/day. **CHILDREN:** 3–5 mg/kg/day.

Fungizone, Usual Dose

IV infusion: ADULTS, ELDERLY: Dosage based on pt tolerance and severity of infection. Initially, 1-mg test dose is given over 20–30 min. If tolerated, usual dose is 0.3–1.5 mg/kg/day. Once therapy established, may give q48h at 1–1.5 mg/kg q48h. **Maximum:** 1.5 mg/kg/day.

CHILDREN: Test dose of 0.1 mg/kg/dose (**maximum:** 1 mg) is infused over 30–60 min. If test dose is tolerated, usual initial dose is 0.25–0.5 mg/kg/day. Gradually increase dose until desired dose achieved. **Maximum:** 1.5 mg/kg/day. Once therapy is established, may give 1–1.5 mg/kg q48h. **NEONATES:** Initially, 1 mg/kg/dose once daily up to 1.5 mg/kg/day for short term. Once therapy established, may give 1–1.5 mg/kg q48h.

Dosage in Renal/Hepatic Impairment

No dose adjustment.

SIDE EFFECTS

Frequent (greater than 10%): Abelcet: Chills, fever, increased serum creatinine, multiple organ failure. **AmBisome:** Hypokalemia, hypomagnesemia, hyperglycemia, hypocalcemia, edema, abdominal pain, back pain, chills, chest pain, hypotension, diarrhea, nausea, vomiting, headache, fever, rigors, insomnia, dyspnea, epistaxis, increased hepatic/renal function test results. **Amphotec:** Chills, fever, hypotension, tachycardia, increased serum creatinine, hypokalemia, bilirubinemia. **Amphocin:** Fever, chills, headache, anemia, hypokalemia, hypomagnesemia, anorexia, malaise, generalized pain, nephrotoxicity.

ADVERSE EFFECTS/TOXIC REACTIONS

Cardiovascular toxicity (hypotension, ventricular fibrillation), anaphylaxis occur rarely. Altered vision/hearing, seizures, hepatic failure, coagulation defects, multiple organ failure, sepsis may occur. Each alternative formulation is less nephrotoxic than conventional amphotericin (Amphocin).

NURSING CONSIDERATIONS

BASELINE ASSESSMENT

Obtain baseline BMP, LFT, serum magnesium, ionized calcium. Question for history of allergies, esp. to amphotericin B, sulfite. Avoid, if possible, other nephrotoxic medications. Obtain premedication orders (antipyretics, antihistamines, antiemetics, corticosteroids) to reduce adverse reactions during IV therapy.

INTERVENTION/EVALUATION

Monitor B/P, temperature, pulse, respirations; assess for adverse reactions (fever, tremors, chills, anorexia, nausea, vomiting, abdominal pain) q15min twice, then q30min for 4 hrs of initial infusion. If symptoms occur, slow infusion, administer medication for symptomatic relief. For severe reaction, stop infusion and notify physician. Evaluate IV site for phlebitis. Monitor I&O, renal function tests for nephrotoxicity. Monitor CBC, BMP (esp. potassium), LFT, serum magnesium.

PATIENT/FAMILY TEACHING

• Prolonged therapy (wks or mos) is usually necessary. • Fever reaction may decrease with continued therapy. • Muscle weakness may be noted during therapy (due to hypokalemia).

ampicillin

am-pi-**sil**-in

Do not confuse ampicillin with aminophylline.

◆CLASSIFICATION

PHARMACOTHERAPEUTIC: Penicillin. **CLINICAL:** Antibiotic.

USES

Treatment of susceptible infections due to streptococci, *S. pneumoniae*, staphylococci (non–penicillinase-producing), meningococci, *Listeria*, some *Klebsiella*, *E. coli*, *H. influenzae*, *Salmonella*, *Shigella*, including GI, GU, respiratory infections, meningitis, endocarditis prophylaxis. **OFF-LABEL:** Surgical prophylaxis for liver transplantation.

PRECAUTIONS

Contraindications: Hypersensitivity to ampicillin or any penicillin. Infections caused by penicillinase-producing organisms. **Cautions:** History of allergies, esp. cephalosporins, renal impairment, asthmatic pts, infectious mononucleosis.

ACTION

Inhibits cell wall synthesis in susceptible microorganisms by binding to PCN binding protein. **Therapeutic Effect:** Bactericidal in susceptible microorganisms.

PHARMACOKINETICS

Moderately absorbed from GI tract. Protein binding: 15%–25%. Widely distributed. Partially metabolized in liver. Primarily excreted in urine. Removed by hemodialysis. **Half-life:** 1–1.5 hrs (increased in renal impairment).

LIFESPAN CONSIDERATIONS

Pregnancy/Lactation: Crosses placenta; appears in cord blood, amniotic fluid. Distributed in breast milk in low concentrations. May lead to allergic sensitization, diarrhea, candidiasis, skin rash in infant. **Children:** Immature renal function in neonates/young infants may delay renal excretion. **Elderly:** Age-related renal impairment may require dosage adjustment.

INTERACTIONS

DRUG: **Allopurinol** may increase incidence of rash. **Probenecid** may increase concentration, toxicity risk. **Tetracyclines** may decrease therapeutic effect. **HERBAL:** None significant. **FOOD:** None known. **LAB VALUES:** May increase serum ALT, AST. May cause positive Coombs' test.

AVAILABILITY (Rx)

Capsules: 500 mg. **Injection, Powder for Reconstitution:** 125 mg, 250 mg, 500 mg, 1 g, 2 g. **Powder for Oral Suspension:** 125 mg/5 mL, 250 mg/5 mL.

ADMINISTRATION/HANDLING

IV

Reconstitution • For IV injection, dilute each vial with 5 mL Sterile Water for Injection or 0.9% NaCl (10 mL for 1- and 2-g vials). **Maximum concentration:** 100 mg/mL for IV push. • For intermittent IV infusion (piggyback), further dilute with 50–100 mL 0.9% NaCl. **Maximum concentration:** 30 mg/mL.

Rate of administration • For IV injection, give over 3–5 min (125–500 mg) or over 10–15 min (1–2 g). For intermittent IV infusion (piggyback), infuse over 15–30 min. • Due to potential for hypersensitivity/anaphylaxis, start initial dose at few drops per min, increase slowly to ordered rate; stay with pt first 10–15 min, then check q10min.

Storage • IV solution, diluted with 0.9% NaCl, is stable for 8 hrs at room temperature or 2 days if refrigerated. • If diluted with D_5W, is stable for 2 hrs at room temperature or 3 hrs if refrigerated. • Discard if precipitate forms.

IM

• Reconstitute each vial with Sterile Water for Injection or Bacteriostatic Water for Injection (consult individual vial for specific volume of diluent). • Stable for 1 hr. • Give deeply in large muscle mass.

PO

• Oral suspension, after reconstitution, is stable for 7 days at room temperature, 14 days if refrigerated. • Shake oral suspension well before using. • Give orally 1–2 hrs before meals for maximum absorption.

IV INCOMPATIBILITIES

DiltiaZEM (Cardizem), midazolam (Versed), ondansetron (Zofran).

IV COMPATIBILITIES

Calcium gluconate, cefepime (Maxipime), dexmedetomidine (Precedex), DOPamine (Intropin), famotidine (Pepcid), furosemide (Lasix), heparin, HYDROmorphone

(Dilaudid), insulin (regular), levoFLOXacin (Levaquin), lipids, magnesium sulfate, morphine, multivitamins, potassium chloride, propofol (Diprivan).

INDICATIONS/ROUTES/DOSAGE

Usual Dosage

PO: ADULTS, ELDERLY: 250–500 mg q6h. **CHILDREN:** 50–100 mg/kg/day in divided doses q6h. **Maximum:** 2 g/day. **IV, IM: ADULTS, ELDERLY:** 1–2 g q4–6h or 50–250 mg/kg/day in divided doses. **Maximum:** 12 g/day. **CHILDREN:** 50–200 mg/kg/day in divided doses q6h. **Maximum:** 8–12 g/day. **NEONATES:** 50 mg/kg/dose q6–12h.

Dosage in Renal Impairment

Creatinine Clearance	Dosage
10–50 mL/min	Administer q6–12h
Less than 10 mL/min	Administer q12–24h
Hemodialysis	1–2 g q12–24h
Peritoneal dialysis	250 mg q12h
Continuous renal replacement therapy (CRRT)	2g, then 1–2 g q6–8h

Dosage in Hepatic Impairment

No dose adjustment.

SIDE EFFECTS

Frequent: Pain at IM injection site, GI disturbances (mild diarrhea, nausea, vomiting), oral or vaginal candidiasis. **Occasional:** Generalized rash, urticaria, phlebitis, thrombophlebitis (with IV administration), headache. **Rare:** Dizziness, seizures (esp. with IV therapy).

ADVERSE EFFECTS/TOXIC REACTIONS

Antibiotic-associated colitis, other superinfections (abdominal cramps, severe watery diarrhea, fever) may result from altered bacterial balance in GI tract. Severe hypersensitivity reactions, including anaphylaxis, acute interstitial nephritis, occur rarely.

NURSING CONSIDERATIONS

BASELINE ASSESSMENT

Question for history of allergies, esp. penicillins, cephalosporins; renal impairment.

INTERVENTION/EVALUATION

Promptly report rash (although common with ampicillin, may indicate hypersensitivity) or diarrhea (fever, abdominal pain, mucus and blood in stool may indicate antibiotic-associated colitis). Evaluate IV site for phlebitis. Check IM injection site for pain, induration. Monitor I&O, urinalysis, renal function tests. Be alert for superinfection: fever, vomiting, diarrhea, anal/genital pruritus, oral mucosal changes (ulceration, pain, erythema).

PATIENT/FAMILY TEACHING

• Continue antibiotic for full length of treatment. • Space doses evenly. • More effective if taken 1 hr before or 2 hrs after food/beverages. • Discomfort may occur with IM injection. • Report rash, diarrhea, or other new symptoms.

ampicillin/sulbactam

amp-i-**sil**-in/sul-**bak**-tam
(Unasyn)

◆CLASSIFICATION

PHARMACOTHERAPEUTIC: Penicillin. **CLINICAL:** Antibiotic.

USES

Treatment of susceptible infections, including intra-abdominal, skin/skin structure, gynecologic infections, due to beta-lactamase–producing organisms, including *H. influenzae, E. coli, Klebsiella, Acinetobacter, Enterobacter, S. aureus,* and *Bacteroides* spp. **OFF-LABEL:** Endocarditis, community-acquired pneumonia, surgical prophylaxis, pelvic inflammatory disease.

PRECAUTIONS

Contraindications: Hypersensitivity to ampicillin, any penicillins, or sulbactam. Hx of cholestatic jaundice, hepatic impairment associated with ampicillin/sulbactam. **Cautions:** History of allergies, esp. cephalosporins; renal impairment; infectious mononucleosis; asthmatic pts.

ACTION

Ampicillin inhibits bacterial cell wall synthesis by binding to PCN-binding proteins. Sulbactam inhibits bacterial beta-lactamase, protecting ampicillin from degradation. **Therapeutic Effect:** Bactericidal in susceptible microorganisms.

PHARMACOKINETICS

Protein binding: 28%–38%. Widely distributed. Partially metabolized in liver. Primarily excreted in urine. Removed by hemodialysis. **Half-life:** 1–1.3 hrs (increased in renal impairment).

LIFESPAN CONSIDERATIONS

Pregnancy/Lactation: Crosses placenta; appears in cord blood, amniotic fluid. Distributed in breast milk in low concentrations. May lead to allergic sensitization, diarrhea, candidiasis, skin rash in infant. **Children:** Safety and efficacy not established in pts younger than 1 yr. **Elderly:** Age-related renal impairment may require dosage adjustment.

INTERACTIONS

DRUG: Allopurinol may increase incidence of rash. **Probenecid** may increase concentration, toxicity risk. **Tetracyclines** may decrease therapeutic effect. **HERBAL:** None significant. **FOOD:** None known. **LAB VALUES:** May increase serum ALT, AST, alkaline phosphatase, LDH, creatinine. May cause positive Coombs' test.

AVAILABILITY (Rx)

Injection, Powder for Reconstitution: 1.5 g (ampicillin 1 g/sulbactam 0.5 g), 3 g (ampicillin 2 g/sulbactam 1 g).

ADMINISTRATION/HANDLING

IV

Reconstitution • For IV injection, dilute with Sterile Water for Injection to provide concentration of 375 mg/mL. • For intermittent IV infusion (piggyback), further dilute with 50–100 mL 0.9% NaCl.

Rate of administration • For IV injection, give slowly over minimum of 10–15 min. • For intermittent IV infusion (piggyback), infuse over 15–30 min. • Due to potential for hypersensitivity/anaphylaxis, start initial dose at few drops per min, increase slowly to ordered rate; stay with pt first 10–15 min, then check q10min.

Storage • IV solution, diluted with 0.9% NaCl, is stable for up to 72 hrs if refrigerated (4 hrs if diluted with D_5W). • Discard if precipitate forms.

IM

• Reconstitute each 1.5-g vial with 3.2 mL Sterile Water for Injection or lidocaine to provide concentration of 250 mg ampicillin/125 mg sulbactam/mL. • Give deeply into large muscle mass within 1 hr after preparation.

IV INCOMPATIBILITIES

Amiodarone (Cordarone), diltiaZEM (Cardizem), IDArubicin (Idamycin), ondansetron (Zofran).

IV COMPATIBILITIES

Famotidine (Pepcid), heparin, insulin (regular), morphine.

INDICATIONS/ROUTES/DOSAGE

Usual Dosage Range

IV, IM: ADULTS, ELDERLY, CHILDREN 13 YRS AND OLDER: 1.5–3 g q6h. **Maximum:** 12 g/day. **IV: CHILDREN 12 YRS AND YOUNGER:** 100–200 mg ampicillin/kg/day in divided doses q6h. **Maximum:** 12 g/day (Unasyn), 8 g/day (ampicillin). **NEONATES:** 100 mg (ampicillin)/kg/day in divided doses q8–12h.

Dosage in Renal Impairment

Dosage and frequency are modified based on creatinine clearance and severity of infection.

Creatinine Clearance	Dosage
Greater than 30 mL/min	No dose adjustment
15–30 mL/min	1.5–3 g q12h
5–14 mL/min	1.5–3 g q24h
Hemodialysis	1.5–3 g q12–24h (after HD on dialysis days)
Peritoneal dialysis	1.5–3 g q12–24h
Continuous renal replacement therapy (CRRT)	3 g, then 1.5–3 g q6–12h

Dosage in Hepatic Impairment

No dose adjustment.

SIDE EFFECTS

Frequent: Diarrhea, rash (most common), urticaria, pain at IM injection site, thrombophlebitis with IV administration, oral or vaginal candidiasis. **Occasional:** Nausea, vomiting, headache, malaise, urinary retention.

ADVERSE EFFECTS/TOXIC REACTIONS

Antibiotic-associated colitis, other superinfections (abdominal cramps; severe, watery diarrhea; fever) may result from altered bacterial balance in GI tract. Severe hypersensitivity reactions, including anaphylaxis, acute interstitial nephritis, blood dyscrasias may occur. High dosage may produce seizures.

NURSING CONSIDERATIONS

BASELINE ASSESSMENT

Question for history of allergies, esp. penicillins, cephalosporins; renal impairment.

INTERVENTION/EVALUATION

Promptly report rash (although common with ampicillin, may indicate hypersensitivity) or diarrhea (fever, abdominal pain, mucus and blood in stool may indicate antibiotic-associated colitis). Evaluate IV site for phlebitis. Check IM injection site for pain, induration. Monitor I&O, urinalysis, renal function tests. Be alert for superinfection: fever, vomiting, diarrhea, anal/genital pruritus, oral mucosal changes (ulceration, pain, erythema).

PATIENT/FAMILY TEACHING

• Take antibiotic for full length of treatment. • Space doses evenly. • Discomfort may occur with IM injection. • Report rash, diarrhea, or other new symptoms.

anastrozole

HIGH ALERT

an-**as**-troe-zole

(Arimidex)

Do not confuse anastrozole with letrozole, or Arimidex with Imitrex.

◆CLASSIFICATION

PHARMACOTHERAPEUTIC: Aromatase inhibitor. **CLINICAL:** Antineoplastic hormone.

USES

Treatment of advanced breast cancer in postmenopausal women who have developed progressive disease while receiving tamoxifen therapy. First-line therapy in advanced or metastatic breast cancer in postmenopausal women. Adjuvant treatment in early hormone receptor–positive breast cancer in postmenopausal women. **OFF-LABEL:** Treatment of recurrent or metastatic endometrial or uterine cancers; treatment of ovarian cancer.

PRECAUTIONS

Contraindications: Hypersensitivity to anastrozole. Pregnancy, women who may become pregnant. **Cautions:** Preexisting ischemic cardiac disease, osteopenia (higher risk of developing osteoporosis), hyperlipidemia. May increase fall risk with fractures during therapy in pts with history of osteoporosis.

ACTION

Inhibits aromatase, preventing conversion of androstenedione to estrone, and testosterone to estradiol. **Therapeutic Effect:** Decreases tumor mass or delays tumor progression.

PHARMACOKINETICS

Well absorbed into systemic circulation (absorption not affected by food). Protein binding: 40%. Metabolized in liver. Eliminated by biliary system and, to a lesser extent, kidneys. **Mean half-life:** 50 hrs in postmenopausal women. Steady-state plasma levels reached in approximately 7 days.

LIFESPAN CONSIDERATIONS

Pregnancy/Lactation: Crosses placenta; may cause fetal harm. Unknown if distributed in breast milk. **Children:** Safety and efficacy not established. **Elderly:** No age-related precautions noted.

INTERACTIONS

DRUG: **Estrogen therapies** may reduce concentration/effects. **Tamoxifen** may reduce plasma concentration. **HERBAL:** None significant. **FOOD:** None known. **LAB VALUES:** May elevate serum GGT level in pts with liver metastases. May increase serum ALT, AST, alkaline phosphatase, total cholesterol, LDL.

AVAILABILITY (Rx)

Tablets: 1 mg.

ADMINISTRATION/HANDLING

PO

- Give without regard to food.

INDICATIONS/ROUTES/DOSAGE

Breast Cancer (Advanced)

PO: ADULTS, ELDERLY: 1 mg once daily (continue until tumor progresses).

Breast Cancer (Early, Adjuvant)

PO: ADULTS, ELDERLY: 1 mg once daily.

Dosage in Renal/Hepatic Impairment

No dose adjustment.

SIDE EFFECTS

Frequent (16%–8%): Asthenia, nausea, headache, hot flashes, back pain, vomiting, cough, diarrhea. **Occasional (6%–4%):** Constipation, abdominal pain, anorexia, bone pain, pharyngitis, dizziness, rash, dry mouth, peripheral edema, pelvic pain, depression, chest pain, paresthesia. **Rare (2%–1%):** Weight gain, diaphoresis.

ADVERSE EFFECTS/TOXIC REACTIONS

Thrombophlebitis, anemia, leukopenia occur rarely. Vaginal hemorrhage occurs rarely (2%).

NURSING CONSIDERATIONS

BASELINE ASSESSMENT

Obtain baseline bone mineral density, total cholesterol, LDL, mammogram, clinical breast exam.

INTERVENTION/EVALUATION

Monitor for asthenia, dizziness; assist with ambulation if needed. Assess for headache, pain. Offer antiemetic for nausea, vomiting. Monitor for onset of diarrhea; offer antidiarrheal medication.

PATIENT/FAMILY TEACHING

- Notify physician if nausea, asthenia, hot flashes become unmanageable.

anidulafungin

a-**nid**-ue-la-**fun**-jin
(Eraxis)

CLASSIFICATION

PHARMACOTHERAPEUTIC: Echinocandin. **CLINICAL:** Antifungal.

USES

Treatment of candidemia, other forms of *Candida* infections (e.g., intra-abdominal abscess, peritonitis), esophageal candidiasis.

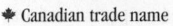

PRECAUTIONS

Contraindications: Hypersensitivity to anidulafungin, other echinocandins. **Cautions:** Hepatic impairment.

ACTION

Inhibits synthesis of the enzyme glucan (vital component of fungal cell formation), preventing fungal cell wall formation. **Therapeutic Effect:** Fungistatic.

PHARMACOKINETICS

Distributed in tissue. Moderately bound to albumin. Protein binding: 84%–99%. Slow chemical degradation; 30% excreted in feces over 9 days. Not removed by hemodialysis. **Half-life:** 40–50 hrs.

LIFESPAN CONSIDERATIONS

Pregnancy/Lactation: May be embryotoxic. Crosses placental barrier. Unknown if distributed in breast milk. **Children:** Safety and efficacy not established. **Elderly:** No age-related precautions noted.

INTERACTIONS

DRUG: May decrease effect of *Saccharomyces boulardii*. **HERBAL:** None significant. **FOOD:** None known. **LAB VALUES:** May increase serum alkaline phosphatase, amylase, ALT, AST, bilirubin, calcium, creatinine, CPK, LDH, lipase. May decrease serum albumin, bicarbonate, magnesium, protein, potassium; Hgb, Hct, WBCs, neutrophils, platelet count. May prolong prothrombin time (PT).

AVAILABILITY (Rx)

Injection, Powder for Reconstitution: 50-mg vial, 100-mg vial.

ADMINISTRATION/HANDLING

IV

Reconstitution • Reconstitute each 50-mg vial with 15 mL Sterile Water for Injection (100 mg with 30 mL). Swirl, do not shake. • Further dilute 50 mg with 50 mL D_5W or 0.9% NaCl (100 mg with 100 mL, 200 mg with 200 mL).

Rate of administration • Do not exceed infusion rate of 1.1 mg/min. Not for IV bolus injection.

Storage • Refrigerate unreconstituted vials. Reconstituted vials are stable for 24 hrs at room temperature. Infusion solution is stable for 48 hrs at room temperature.

IV INCOMPATIBILITIES

Amphotericin B (Abelcet, AmBisome), ertapenem (INVanz), sodium bicarbonate.

IV COMPATIBILITIES

Dexamethasone (Decadron), famotidine (Pepcid), furosemide (Lasix), HYDROmorphone (Dilaudid), LORazepam (Ativan), methylPREDNISolone (SOLU), morphine. Refer to IV Compatibility Chart in front of book.

INDICATIONS/ROUTES/DOSAGE

◀ALERT▶ Duration of treatment based on pt's clinical response. In general, treatment is continued for at least 14 days after last positive culture.

Candidemia, Other *Candida* Infections

IV: ADULTS, ELDERLY: Give single 200-mg loading dose on day 1, followed by 100 mg/day thereafter for at least 14 days after last positive culture.

Esophageal Candidiasis

IV: ADULTS, ELDERLY: 200 mg daily for 14–21 days. May transition to fluconazole (oral).

Dosage in Renal/Hepatic Impairment

No dose adjustment.

SIDE EFFECTS

Rare (3%–1%): Diarrhea, nausea, headache, rigors, peripheral edema.

ADVERSE EFFECTS/TOXIC REACTIONS

Hypokalemia occurs in 4% of pts. Hypersensitivity reaction characterized by facial flushing, hypotension, pruritus, urticaria, rash occurs rarely. Hepatitis, elevated LFT, hepatic failure was reported.

NURSING CONSIDERATIONS

BASELINE ASSESSMENT

Obtain baseline CBC, BMP, LFT. Obtain specimens for fungal culture prior to therapy. Treatment may be instituted before results are known.

INTERVENTION/EVALUATION

Monitor for evidence of hepatic dysfunction, hypokalemia. Monitor daily pattern of bowel activity, stool consistency. Assess for rash, urticaria.

PATIENT/FAMILY TEACHING

- For esophageal candidiasis, maintain diligent oral hygiene.

apalutamide

ap-a-**loot**-a-mide
(Erleada)

Do not confuse apalutamide with bicalutamide, enzalutamide, or niltamide.

◆CLASSIFICATION

PHARMACOTHERAPEUTIC: Antiandrogen. **CLINICAL:** Antineoplastic.

USES

Treatment of nonmetastatic castration-resistant prostate cancer (NM-CRPC), metastatic, castration-sensitive prostate cancer.

PRECAUTIONS

Contraindications: Hypersensitivity to apalutamide. Use in women who are pregnant or may become pregnant. **Cautions:** History of cardiovascular disease (HF, ischemic heart disease), hypothyroidism, conditions predisposing to seizure activity (traumatic brain injury, brain tumor, prior CVA, seizure disorder). Pts at risk for fractures (frequent falls, osteoporosis, chronic corticosteroid therapy), hyperglycemia (e.g., diabetes, recent surgery, chronic use of corticosteroids).

ACTION

Binds directly to ligands of androgen receptor, preventing androgen-receptor translocation, DNA binding, and receptor-mediated transcription. **Therapeutic Effect:** Decreases proliferation of tumor cells, increases apoptosis, resulting in decreased tumor volume.

PHARMACOKINETICS

Rapidly absorbed and widely distributed. Metabolized in liver. Protein binding: 96%. Peak plasma concentration: 2 hrs. Steady-state reached in 4 wks. Excreted in urine (65%), feces (24%). **Half-life:** 3 days.

⌛ LIFESPAN CONSIDERATIONS

Pregnancy/Lactation: Not indicated in female population. Males with female partners of reproductive potential must use effective contraception during treatment and up to 3 mos after discontinuation. May cause fetal harm if administered in pregnant females. May cause decreased fertility in males. **Children:** Safety and efficacy not established. **Elderly:** No age-related precautions noted.

INTERACTIONS

DRUG: **Strong CYP3A4 inhibitors (e.g., clarithromycin, ketoconazole, ritonavir), strong CYP2C8 inhibitors (e.g., gemfibrozil, trimethoprim), P-gp inhibitors (e.g., amiodarone, azithromycin, captopril, carvedilol, cyclosporine, felodipine, ticagrelor)** may increase concentration/effect. **Strong CYP3A4 inducers (e.g., carbamazepine, phenytoin, rifampin)** may decrease concentration/effect. **HERBAL:** None significant. **FOOD:** None known. **LAB VALUES:** May decrease Hgb, Hct, leukocytes, lymphocytes, RBCs. May increase serum cholesterol, glucose, potassium, triglycerides.

AVAILABILITY (Rx)

Tablets: 60 mg.

ADMINISTRATION/HANDLING

PO

• Give without regard to food. • Swallow tablets whole; do not break, cut, crush, or divide.

INDICATIONS/ROUTES/DOSAGE

Non-Metastatic Castration-Resistant Prostate Cancer, Metastatic Castration-Sensitive Prostate Cancer

PO: ADULTS, ELDERLY: 240 mg once daily (in combination with a gonadotropin-releasing hormone analog agonist or antagonist [if not received orchiectomy]). Continue until disease progression or unacceptable toxicity.

Dose Modification

Based on Common Terminology Criteria for Adverse Effects (CTCAE).

Toxicities or Intolerable Side Effects

Any Grade 3 toxicity or intolerable side effect: Withhold treatment until resolved to Grade 1 or less, then resume at same dose. If applicable, may decrease dose to 180 mg or 120 mg once daily. **Seizures:** Permanently discontinue.

Dosage in Renal/Hepatic Impairment

Mild to moderate impairment: No dose adjustment. **Severe impairment:** ESRD: Not specified; use caution.

SIDE EFFECTS

Frequent (39%–16%): Fatigue, asthenia, hypertension, rash, urticaria, conjunctivitis, stomatitis, diarrhea, nausea, arthralgia, decreased weight. **Occasional (14%–6%):** Hot flush, decreased appetite, early satiety, hypophagia, peripheral edema, penile/scrotal edema, pruritus.

ADVERSE EFFECTS/TOXIC REACTIONS

Anemia, leukopenia, lymphopenia are expected responses to therapy. Increased incidence of falls (16% of pts) and fractures (12% of pts) was reported. Seizures reported in less than 1% of pts. Hypothyroidism reported in 8% of pts. Higher incidence of ischemic heart disease (4% of pts), HF (2% of pts) has occurred.

NURSING CONSIDERATIONS

BASELINE ASSESSMENT

Obtain baseline CBC, BMP, TSH; B/P. Question history of cardiovascular disease (HF, ischemic heart disease), hypothyroidism, seizure disorder. Assess risk for falls and fractures. Receive full medication history and screen for interactions. Offer emotional support.

INTERVENTION/EVALUATION

Monitor CBC, BMP, TSH; B/P periodically. Monitor for symptoms of hypothyroidism (bradycardia, constipation, depression, fatigue, muscle weakness, weight gain), hyperglycemia, seizure activity. Assess skin for rash. Question for any incidence of falls, suspected fractures.

PATIENT/FAMILY TEACHING

• Sexually active men must wear condoms with sexual activity during treatment and for at least 3 mos after last dose. • Women who are pregnant or who plan on becoming pregnant should not handle medication. • Treatment may increase risk of falls and fractures. Go slowly from lying to standing. Use caution during strenuous activity. • Slow heart rate, constipation, depression, fatigue may indicate low thyroid levels. • Immediately report symptoms of seizure activity (confusion, convulsions, loss of consciousness). • Report symptoms of elevated blood sugar levels (blurred vision, headache, increased thirst, frequent urination). • Do not take newly prescribed medications unless approved by the prescriber who originally started treatment.

apixaban

a-**pix**-a-ban
(Eliquis)

■ BLACK BOX ALERT ■ Discontinuation in absence of alternative anticoagulation increases risk for thrombotic events. Spinal or epidural hematoma resulting in paralysis may occur with neuraxial anesthesia or spinal/epidural puncture.

Do not confuse apixaban with rivaroxaban, argatroban, or dabigatran.

◆CLASSIFICATION

PHARMACOTHERAPEUTIC: Factor Xa inhibitor. **CLINICAL:** Anticoagulant.

USES

Reduces risk for stroke, systemic embolism in pts with nonvalvular atrial fibrillation. Prophylaxis of DVT following hip or knee replacement surgery. Treatment of DVT and PE. Reduces risk of recurrent DVT/PE following initial therapy. **OFF-LABEL:** Prevention of recurrent stroke or TIA.

PRECAUTIONS

Contraindications: Severe hypersensitivity to apixaban. Active pathologic bleeding. **Cautions:** Mild to moderate hepatic impairment, severe renal impairment (may increase bleeding risk). Avoid use in pts with severe hepatic impairment, prosthetic heart valve, significant rheumatic heart disease.

ACTION

Selectively, directly, and reversibly inhibits free and clot-bound factor Xa, a key factor in the intrinsic and extrinsic pathway of blood coagulation cascade. **Therapeutic Effect:** Inhibits clot-induced platelet aggregation, fibrin clot formation.

PHARMACOKINETICS

Readily absorbed after PO administration. Peak plasma concentration: 3–4 hrs. Protein binding: 87%. Metabolized in liver. Excreted primarily in urine, feces. **Half-life:** 12 hrs.

⌛ LIFESPAN CONSIDERATIONS

Pregnancy/Lactation: Unknown if distributed in breast milk. **Children:** Safety and efficacy not established. **Elderly:** No age-related precautions noted.

INTERACTIONS

DRUG: **Strong CYP3A4 inducers (e.g., carBAMazepine, rifAMPin)** may decrease level/effect. **Anticoagulants (e.g., dabigatran, heparin, warfarin), antiplatelets (e.g., aspirin, clopidogrel), NSAIDs (e.g., diclofenac, ibuprofen, naproxen), strong CYP3A4 inhibitors (e.g., ketoconazole, clarithromycin)** may increase concentration, bleeding risk. **HERBAL:** **St. John's wort** may decrease concentration/effect. **Herbals with anticoagulant/antiplatelet properties (e.g., garlic, ginger, ginkgo biloba)** may increase risk of bleeding. **FOOD:** **Grapefruit products** may increase concentration/effect. **LAB VALUES:** May decrease platelet count, Hgb, LFT.

AVAILABILITY (Rx)

Tablets: 2.5 mg, 5 mg.

ADMINISTRATION/HANDLING

◀ALERT▶ Discontinuation in absence of alternative anticoagulation increases risk for thrombotic events.

PO

• Give without regard to food. • If elective surgery or invasive procedures with moderate or high risk for bleeding, discontinue apixaban at least 24–48 hrs prior to procedure.

INDICATIONS/ROUTES/DOSAGE

Nonvalvular Atrial Fibrillation

PO: **ADULTS, ELDERLY:** 5 mg twice daily. In pts with at least 2 of the following characteristics: age 80 yrs or older, body weight 60 kg or less, serum creatinine 1.5 mg/dL or greater, concurrent use with CYP3A4, or P-gp inhibitors (e.g., ketoconazole, ritonavir), reduce dose to 2.5 mg twice daily.

DVT/PE Treatment
PO: ADULTS, ELDERLY: 10 mg twice daily for 7 days, then 5 mg twice daily.

DVT Prophylaxis (Hip/Knee Replacement)
Note: Begin 12–24 hrs postoperatively.
ADULTS, ELDERLY: 2.5 mg twice daily (approx. 30 days for hip; 10–14 days for knee).

DVT Prophylaxis, Reduce Risk Recurrent DVT/PE
PO: ADULTS, ELDERLY: 2.5 mg twice daily (after at least 6 mos of treatment).

Dosage in Renal Impairment
DVT/PE/Reduce risk recurrent DVT, postoperative: No adjustment. **Nonvalvular A-fib, HD: SCR LESS THAN 1.5:** No adjustment. **SCR 1.5 OR GREATER, OLDER THAN 80 YRS, WEIGHING 60 KG OR LESS:** 2.5 mg 2 times/day.

Dosage in Hepatic Impairment
Mild impairment: No dose adjustment. **Moderate impairment:** Use caution. **Severe impairment:** Not recommended.

SIDE EFFECTS

Rare (3%–1%): Nausea, ecchymosis.

ADVERSE EFFECTS/TOXIC REACTIONS

Increased risk for bleeding/hemorrhagic events. May cause serious, potentially fatal bleeding, accompanied by one or more of the following: a decrease in Hgb of 2 g/dL or more; a need for 2 or more units of packed RBCs; bleeding occurring at one of the following sites: intracranial, intraspinal, intraocular, pericardial, intra-articular, intramuscular with compartment syndrome, retroperitoneal. Serious reactions include jaundice, cholestasis, cytolytic hepatitis, Stevens-Johnson syndrome, hypersensitivity reaction, anaphylaxis.

NURSING CONSIDERATIONS

BASELINE ASSESSMENT

Obtain CBC. Question history of bleeding disorders, recent surgery, spinal punctures, intracranial hemorrhage, bleeding ulcers, open wounds, anemia, hepatic impairment. Obtain full medication history including herbal products.

INTERVENTION/EVALUATION

Periodically monitor CBC, stool for occult blood. Be alert for complaints of abdominal/back pain, headache, confusion, weakness, vision change (may indicate hemorrhage). Question for increased menstrual bleeding/discharge. Assess for any sign of bleeding: bleeding at surgical site, hematuria, blood in stool, bleeding from gums, petechiae, ecchymosis.

PATIENT/FAMILY TEACHING

• Do not take/discontinue any medication except on advice from physician. • Avoid alcohol, aspirin, NSAIDs, herbal supplements, grapefruit products. • Consult physician before surgery, dental work. • Use electric razor, soft toothbrush to prevent bleeding. • Report blood-tinged mucus from coughing, heavy menstrual bleeding, headache, vision problems, weakness, abdominal pain, frequent bruising, bloody urine or stool, joint pain or swelling.

apremilast

a-**pre**-mi-last
(Otezla)
Do not confuse apremilast with roflumilast.

◆CLASSIFICATION

PHARMACOTHERAPEUTIC: Phosphodiesterase 4 (PDE4) enzyme inhibitor. **CLINICAL:** Antipsoriatic arthritis agent.

USES

Treatment of adult pts with active psoriatic arthritis, moderate to severe plaque psoriasis who are candidates for phototherapy or systemic therapy. Treatment of oral ulcers associated with Behcet's disease.

PRECAUTIONS

Contraindications: Hypersensitivity to apremilast. **Cautions:** History of depression, severe renal impairment, suicidal ideation. Pts with latent infections (e.g., TB, viral hepatitis).

ACTION

Selectively inhibits PDE4, increasing cyclic AMP (cAMP) and regulation of inflammatory mediators. **Therapeutic Effect:** Reduces psoriatic arthritis exacerbations.

PHARMACOKINETICS

Readily absorbed after PO administration. Protein binding: 68%. Peak plasma concentration: 2.5 hrs. Metabolized in liver. Excreted in urine (58%), feces (39%). **Half-life:** 6–9 hrs.

⌛ LIFESPAN CONSIDERATIONS

Pregnancy/Lactation: Unknown if distributed in breast milk. Not recommended for nursing mothers. **Children:** Safety and efficacy not established. **Elderly:** No age-related precautions noted.

INTERACTIONS

DRUG: **Strong CYP3A4 inducers (e.g., carbamazepine, phenytoin, rifampin)** may decrease concentration/effect. **HERBAL:** **St. John's wort** may decrease concentration/effect. **FOOD:** None significant. **LAB VALUES:** None known.

AVAILABILITY (Rx)

Tablets: 10 mg, 20 mg, 30 mg.

ADMINISTRATION/HANDLING

PO

- Give without regard to food. Administer whole; do not crush, cut, dissolve, or divide.

INDICATIONS/ROUTES/DOSAGE

Behcet's Disease, Psoriatic Arthritis, Plaque Psoriasis

PO: ADULTS/ELDERLY: Initially, titrate dose from day 1–day 5. **Day 1:** 10 mg in AM only. **Day 2:** 10 mg in AM; 10 mg in PM. **Day 3:** 10 mg in AM; 20 mg in PM. **Day 4:** 20 mg in AM; 20 mg in PM. **Day 5:** 20 mg in AM; 30 mg in PM. **Day 6/maintenance:** 30 mg twice daily.

Dosage in Renal Impairment (Creatinine Clearance less than 30 mL/min)

Days 1–3: 10 mg in AM. **Days 4–5:** 20 mg in AM, using only am schedule. **Day 6/maintenance:** 30 mg once daily.

Dosage in Hepatic Impairment

No dose adjustment.

SIDE EFFECTS

Occasional (9%–4%): Nausea, diarrhea, headache, upper respiratory tract infection. **Rare (3% or less):** Vomiting, nasopharyngitis, upper abdominal pain.

ADVERSE EFFECTS/TOXIC REACTIONS

Increased risk of depression reported in less than 1% of pts. Weight decrease of 5%–10% of body weight occurred in 10% of pts.

NURSING CONSIDERATIONS

BASELINE ASSESSMENT

Obtain baseline weight, vital signs. Question history of depression, severe renal impairment, suicidal ideations. Screen for prior allergic reactions to drug class. Receive full medication history including herbal products. Assess degree of joint pain, range of motion, mobility.

INTERVENTION/EVALUATION

Be alert for worsening depression, suicidal ideation. Monitor for weight loss. Assess for dehydration if diarrhea occurs. Assess improvement of joint pain, range of motion, mobility.

PATIENT/FAMILY TEACHING

- Report changes in mood or behavior, thoughts of suicide, self-destructive behavior. Report weight loss of any kind. • Increase fluid intake if dehydration suspected. • Immediately notify physician if pregnancy suspected. • Do not chew, crush, dissolve, or divide tablets.

aprepitant/ fosaprepitant

a-**prep**-i-tant/fos-a-**prep**-i-tant
(Cinvanti, Emend)
Do not confuse fosaprepitant with aprepitant, fosamprenavir, or fospropofol.

◆CLASSIFICATION

PHARMACOTHERAPEUTIC: Neurokinin receptor antagonist. **CLINICAL:** Antinausea, antiemetic.

USES

PO/IV: Prevention of nausea, vomiting associated with repeat courses of moderately to highly emetogenic cancer chemotherapy. **PO:** Prevention of postop nausea, vomiting.

PRECAUTIONS

Contraindications: Hypersensitivity to aprepitant or fosaprepitant. Concurrent use with pimozide. **Cautions:** Severe hepatic impairment. Concurrent use of medications metabolized through CYP3A4 (e.g., docetaxel, etoposide, ifosfamide, imatinib, irinotecan, PACLitaxel, vinblastine, vinCRIStine, vinorelbine).

ACTION

Inhibits substance P receptor, augments antiemetic activity of 5-HT_3 receptor antagonists. **Therapeutic Effect:** Prevents acute and delayed phases of chemotherapy-induced emesis.

PHARMACOKINETICS

Moderately absorbed from GI tract. Crosses blood-brain barrier. Extensively metabolized in liver. Protein binding: greater than 95%. Eliminated primarily by liver metabolism (not excreted renally). **Half-life:** 9–13 hrs.

⌛ LIFESPAN CONSIDERATIONS

Pregnancy/Lactation: Unknown if drug crosses placenta or is distributed in breast milk. **Children:** Safety and efficacy not established. **Elderly:** No age-related precautions noted.

INTERACTIONS

DRUG: **Strong CYP3A4 inhibitors (e.g., ketoconazole, clarithromycin)** may increase concentration/effect. **Strong CYP3A4 inducers (e.g., carBAMazepine, rifAMPin)** may decrease concentration/effect. May decrease effectiveness of **hormonal contraceptives, warfarin.** May increase concentration/effects of **bosutinib, budesonide, cobimetinib, neratinib, simeprevir.** **HERBAL:** **St. John's wort** may decrease concentration/effect. **FOOD:** **Grapefruit products** may increase concentration/effect. **LAB VALUES:** May increase serum ALT, AST, alkaline phosphatase, BUN, creatinine, glucose. May produce proteinuria.

AVAILABILITY (Rx)

Capsules: ***(Emend):*** 40 mg, 80 mg, 125 mg. **Injection, Emulsion:** ***(Cinvanti):*** 130 mg/18 mL. **Injection, Powder for Reconstitution:** ***(Fosaprepitant):*** 150 mg. **Oral Suspension:** 125 mg.

ADMINISTRATION/HANDLING

PO

• Give without regard to food. • Administer whole; do not cut, crush, or open capsules. • Suspension (prepared by healthcare provider in oral dispenser). Dispense in pt's mouth along inner cheek. Suspension is stable for 72 hrs if refrigerated or up to 3 hrs at room temperature.

IV (Emend)

Reconstitution • Reconstitute each vial with 5 mL 0.9% NaCl. • Add to 145 mL 0.9% NaCl to provide a final concentration of 1 mg/mL.

Rate of administration • Infuse over 20–30 min 30 min prior to chemotherapy. **Storage** • Refrigerate unreconstituted vials. • After reconstitution, solution is stable at room temperature for 24 hrs.

IV Emulsion (Cinvanti)

Reconstitution • For 130-mg dose, dilute 18 mL of Cinvanti into 100 mL 0.9% NaCl or D_5W infusion bag. • For 100-mg dose, dilute 14 mL of Cinvanti into 100 mL 0.9% NaCl or D_5W infusion bag. • Mix by gentle inversion (4–5 times). • Do not shake.

Rate of administration • Infuse over 30 minutes. Use only non-DEHP tubing for administration. For IV injection, no further dilution is necessary. Inject over 2 min.

IV INCOMPATIBILITIES

Do not infuse with any solutions containing calcium or magnesium.

INDICATIONS/ROUTES/DOSAGE

Prevention of Chemotherapy-Induced Nausea, Vomiting

Note: Administer in combination with a 5-HT_3 antagonist on day 1 and dexamethasone on days 1 through 4.

PO: ADULTS, ELDERLY, CHILDREN 12 YRS OR YOUNGER WEIGHING 30 KG OR MORE: 125 mg 1 hr before chemotherapy on day 1 and 80 mg once daily in the morning on days 2 and 3.

IV: ADULTS, ELDERLY (SINGLE-DOSE REGIMEN): *(Emend):* 150 mg over 20–30 min 30 min before chemotherapy. *(Cinvanti):* 100–130 mg over 30 min or IV injection over 2 min approx. 30 min before chemotherapy.

Prevention of Postop Nausea, Vomiting

PO: ADULTS, ELDERLY: 40 mg once within 3 hrs prior to induction of anesthesia.

Dosage in Renal/Hepatic Impairment

No dose adjustment. Caution in severe hepatic impairment.

SIDE EFFECTS

Frequent (17%–10%): Fatigue, nausea, hiccups, diarrhea, constipation, anorexia. **Occasional (8%–4%):** Headache, vomiting, dizziness, dehydration, heartburn. **Rare (3% or less):** Abdominal pain, epigastric discomfort, gastritis, tinnitus, insomnia.

ADVERSE EFFECTS/TOXIC REACTIONS

Neutropenia, mucous membrane disorders occur rarely.

NURSING CONSIDERATIONS

BASELINE ASSESSMENT

Assess for dehydration (poor skin turgor, dry mucous membranes, longitudinal furrows in tongue).

INTERVENTION/EVALUATION

Monitor hydration, nutritional status, I&O. Assess bowel sounds for peristalsis. Assist with ambulation if dizziness occurs. Provide supportive measures. Monitor daily pattern of bowel activity, stool consistency.

PATIENT/FAMILY TEACHING

• Relief from nausea/vomiting generally occurs shortly after drug administration. • Report persistent vomiting, headache. • May decrease effectiveness of oral contraceptives.

argatroban

HIGH ALERT

ar-**gat**-roe-ban

Do not confuse argatroban with Aggrastat.

◆CLASSIFICATION

PHARMACOTHERAPEUTIC: Direct thrombin inhibitor. **CLINICAL:** Anticoagulant.

USES

Prophylaxis or treatment of thrombosis in heparin-induced thrombocytopenia (HIT) in pts with HIT or at risk of developing HIT undergoing percutaneous coronary procedures. **OFF-LABEL:** Maintain extracorporeal circuit patency of continuous renal replacement therapy (CRRT) in pts with HIT.

PRECAUTIONS

Contraindications: Hypersensitivity to argatroban, active major bleeding. **Cautions:** Severe hypertension, immediately following lumbar puncture, spinal anesthesia, major surgery, pts with congenital or acquired bleeding disorders, gastrointestinal ulcerations, hepatic impairment, critically ill pts.

ACTION

Direct thrombin inhibitor that reversibly binds to thrombin-active sites of free and clot-associated thrombin. Inhibits thrombin-catalyzed or thrombin-induced reactions, including fibrin formation, activation of coagulant factors V, VIII, and XIII; inhibits protein C formation, platelet aggregation. **Therapeutic Effect:** Produces anticoagulation.

PHARMACOKINETICS

Distributed primarily in extracellular fluid. Protein binding: 54%. Metabolized in liver. Primarily excreted in the feces, presumably through biliary secretion. **Half-life:** 39–51 min (prolonged in hepatic failure).

LIFESPAN CONSIDERATIONS

Pregnancy/Lactation: Unknown if excreted in breast milk. **Children:** Safety and efficacy not established. **Elderly:** No age-related precautions noted.

INTERACTIONS

DRUG: **Anticoagulants (e.g., dabigatran, heparin, rivaroxaban, warfarin), antiplatelets (e.g., aspirin, clopidogrel), NSAIDs (e.g., diclofenac, ibuprofen, naproxen)** may increase anticoagulant effect. **HERBAL:** **Herbals with anticoagulant/antiplatelet properties (e.g., garlic, ginger, ginkgo biloba)** may increase risk of bleeding. **FOOD:** None known. **LAB VALUES:** Prolongs prothrombin time (PT), activated partial thromboplastin time (aPTT), international normalized ratio (INR). May decrease Hgb, Hct.

AVAILABILITY (Rx)

Infusion (Pre-Mix): 125 mg/125 mL, 250 mg/250 mL. **Injection Solution:** 250 mg/2.5 mL vial.

ADMINISTRATION/HANDLING

IV

Reconstitution • Dilute each 250-mg vial with 250 mL 0.9% NaCl, D_5W to provide a final concentration of 1 mg/mL.

Rate of administration • Initial rate of administration is based on body weight at 2 mcg/kg/min (e.g., 50-kg pt infuse at 6 mL/hr). Dosage should not exceed 10 mcg/kg/min.

Storage • Discard if solution appears cloudy or an insoluble precipitate is noted. • Following reconstitution, stable for 96 hrs at room temperature or refrigerated. • Avoid direct sunlight.

IV INCOMPATIBILITIES

Amiodarone (Cordarone).

IV COMPATIBILITIES

DiphenhydrAMINE (Benadryl), DOBUTamine (Dobutrex), DOPamine (Intropin), furosemide (Lasix), midazolam (Versed), morphine, vasopressin (Pitressin). Refer to IV Compatibility Chart in front of book.

INDICATIONS/ROUTES/DOSAGE

Heparin-Induced Thrombocytopenia (HIT)

IV infusion: **ADULTS, ELDERLY:** Initially, 2 mcg/kg/min administered as a continuous infusion. After initial infusion, dose may be adjusted until steady-state aPTT is 1.5–3 times initial baseline value, not to exceed 100 sec. Dosage should not exceed 10 mcg/kg/min.

Percutaneous Coronary Intervention

IV infusion: **ADULTS, ELDERLY:** Initially, administer bolus of 350 mcg/kg over 3–5 min, then infuse at 25 mcg/kg/min. Check ACT (activated clotting time) 5–10 min following bolus. If ACT is less than

300 sec, give additional bolus 150 mcg/kg, increase infusion to 30 mcg/kg/min. If ACT is greater than 450 sec, decrease infusion to 15 mcg/kg/min. Recheck ACT in 5–10 min. Once ACT of 300–450 sec achieved, continue dose through duration of procedure.

Dosage in Renal Impairment
No dose adjustment.

Dosage in Hepatic Impairment
Moderate to severe impairment: ADULTS, ELDERLY: Initially, 0.5 mcg/kg/min. CHILDREN: Initially, 0.2 mcg/kg/min. Adjust dose in increments of 0.05 mcg/kg/min or less.

SIDE EFFECTS

Frequent (8%–3%): Dyspnea, hypotension, fever, diarrhea, nausea, pain, vomiting, infection, cough.

ADVERSE EFFECTS/TOXIC REACTIONS

Ventricular tachycardia, atrial fibrillation occur occasionally. Major bleeding, sepsis occur rarely.

NURSING CONSIDERATIONS

BASELINE ASSESSMENT

Obtain CBC, PT, aPTT. Determine initial B/P. Minimize need for multiple injection sites, blood draws, catheters.

INTERVENTION/EVALUATION

Assess for any sign of bleeding: bleeding at surgical site, hematuria, melena, bleeding from gums, petechiae, ecchymoses, bleeding from injection sites. Handle pt carefully and infrequently to prevent bleeding. Assess for decreased B/P, increased pulse rate, complaint of abdominal/back pain, severe headache (may indicate hemorrhage). Monitor ACT, PT, aPTT, platelet count, Hgb, Hct. Question for increase in discharge during menses. Assess for hematuria. Observe skin for any occurring ecchymoses, petechiae, hematoma. Use care in removing any dressing, tape.

PATIENT/FAMILY TEACHING

• Use electric razor, soft toothbrush to prevent cuts, gingival trauma. • Report any sign of bleeding, including red/dark urine, black/red stool, coffee-ground vomitus, blood-tinged mucus from cough.

ARIPiprazole TOP 100

ar-i-**pip**-ra-zole
(Abilify, Abilify Maintena, Aristada Initio)

BLACK BOX ALERT Increased risk of mortality in elderly pts with dementia-related psychosis, mainly due to pneumonia, HF. Increased risk of suicidal thinking and behavior in children, adolescents, young adults 18–24 yrs with major depressive disorder, other psychiatric disorders.

Do not confuse Abilify with Ambien, or ARIPiprazole with esomeprazole, omeprazole, pantoprazole, or RABEprazole (proton pump inhibitors).

CLASSIFICATION

PHARMACOTHERAPEUTIC: Quinolinone antipsychotic. CLINICAL: Second-generation (atypical) antipsychotic agent.

USES

PO: Treatment of schizophrenia. Treatment of bipolar disorder. Adjunct treatment in major depressive disorder. Treatment of irritability associated with autism in children 6–17 yrs of age. Treatment of Tourette disorder. **IM: (Extended-Release): Abilify Maintena:** Treatment of schizophrenia in adults. Maintenance monotherapy treatment of bipolar 1 disorder in adults. **Aristada Initio:** In combination with oral aripiprazole for initiation of Aristada when used for treatment of schizophrenia. OFF-LABEL: Schizoaffective disorder, depression with psychotic features, aggression, bipolar disorder (children), conduct disorder (children), psychosis/agitation related to Alzheimer's dementia.

PRECAUTIONS

Contraindications: Hypersensitivity to ARIPiprazole. **Cautions:** Concurrent use of CNS depressants (including alcohol), disorders in which CNS depression is a feature, cardiovascular or cerebrovascular diseases (may induce hypotension), Parkinson's disease (potential for exacerbation), history of seizures or conditions that may lower seizure threshold (Alzheimer's disease), diabetes mellitus. Pts at risk for pneumonia. Elderly with dementia.

ACTION

Provides partial agonist activity at DOPamine (D2, D3) and serotonin (5-HT_{1A}) receptors and antagonist activity at serotonin (5-HT_{2A}) receptors. **Therapeutic Effect:** Improves symptoms associated with schizophrenia, bipolar disorder, autism, depression.

PHARMACOKINETICS

Well absorbed through GI tract. Protein binding: 99% (primarily albumin). Reaches steady levels in 2 wks. Metabolized in liver. Excreted in feces (55%), urine (25%). Not removed by hemodialysis. **Half-life:** 75 hrs.

LIFESPAN CONSIDERATIONS

Pregnancy/Lactation: Unknown if drug crosses placenta. May be distributed in breast milk. Breastfeeding not recommended. **Children:** Safety and efficacy not established. **Elderly:** May increase risk of mortality in pts with dementia-related psychosis.

INTERACTIONS

DRUG: **CYP3A4 inducers (e.g., carBAMazepine, rifampin)** may decrease concentration/effect. **CYP3A4 inhibitors (e.g., erythromycin, ketoconazole, ritonavir)** may increase concentration/effect. **CNS depressants (e.g., alcohol, morphine, oxycodone, zolpidem)** may increase CNS depression. **Strong CYP2D6 inhibitors (e.g., fluoxetine, paroxetine)** may increase concentration/effect. **HERBAL:** **Herbals with sedative properties (e.g., chamomile, kava kava, valerian)** may increase CNS depression. **St. John's wort** may decrease concentration/effect. **FOOD:** None known. **LAB VALUES:** May increase serum glucose. May decrease neutrophils, leukocytes.

AVAILABILITY (Rx)

Injection, Prefilled Syringe: ***(Abilify Maintena):*** 300 mg, 400 mg. **Injection, Suspension (Extended-Release *[Aristada Initio]*):** 675 mg. **Oral Solution:** 1 mg/mL. **Tablets:** 2 mg, 5 mg, 10 mg, 15 mg, 20 mg, 30 mg. **Orally Disintegrating Tablets:** 10 mg, 15 mg.

ADMINISTRATION/HANDLING

IM (Abilify Maintena)

Vial • Reconstitute 400-mg vial with 1.9 mL Sterile Water for Injection (300-mg vial with 1.5 mL) to provide a concentration of 100 mg/0.5 mL. Once reconstituted, administer in gluteal muscle. Do not administer via IV or subcutaneously.

Prefilled syringe • Reconstitute at room temperature by rotating syringe plunger to release diluent. Shake until suspension is uniform. • Inject full syringe content immediately following reconstitution.

PO

• Give without regard to food.

Orally Disintegrating Tablet

• Remove tablet, place entire tablet on tongue. • Do not break, split tablet. • May give without liquid.

INDICATIONS/ROUTES/DOSAGE

Note: May substitute oral solution/tablet mg per mg up to 25 mg. For 30-mg tablets, give 25 mg oral solution.

Strong CYP3A4 inducers: ARIPiprazole dose should be doubled. **Strong CYP3A4 inhibitors:** ARIPiprazole dose should be reduced by 50%.

Schizophrenia

PO: ADULTS, ELDERLY: Initially, 10–15 mg once daily. May increase up to 30 mg/day. Titrate dose by 5 mg/day at minimum of 2-wk intervals. **CHILDREN 13–17 YRS:** Initially, 2 mg/day for 2 days, then 5 mg/day for 2 days. May further increase to target dose of 10 mg/day. May then increase in increments of 5 mg up to maximum of 30 mg/day. **IM: ADULTS, ELDERLY:** ***(Abilify Maintena):*** Initially, 400 mg monthly (separate doses by at least 26 days). ***(Aristada Initio):*** 675 mg once (single dose) with 30 mg aripiprazole with first IM dose of Aristada.

Bipolar Disorder

PO: ADULTS, ELDERLY: Monotherapy: Initially, 10–15 mg once daily. May increase in increments of 5–10 mg/day of at least 1-wk intervals to 30 mg/day. **Adjunct to lithium or valproic acid:** Initially, 10–15 mg. May increase to 30 mg/day based on pt tolerance. **CHILDREN 10–17 YRS:** Initially, 2 mg/day for 2 days, then 5 mg/day for 2 days. May further increase to a target of 10 mg/day. Give subsequent dose increases of 5 mg/day. **Maximum:** 30 mg/day. **IM: ADULTS, ELDERLY:** ***(Abilify Maintena):*** Initially, 400 mg monthly (separate doses by at least 26 days). Tolerability should be established using oral therapy before initiation of parenteral therapy. Continue oral therapy for 14 days during initiation of parenteral therapy.

Major Depressive Disorder (Adjunct to Antidepressants)

PO: ADULTS, ELDERLY: ***(Abilify):*** Initially, 2–5 mg/day. May increase up to maximum of 15 mg/day. Titrate dose in 5-mg increments of at least 1-wk intervals.

Irritability With Autism

PO: CHILDREN 6–17 YRS: Initially, 2 mg/day for 7 days followed by increase to 5 mg/day. Subsequent increases made in 5-mg increments at intervals of at least 1 wk. **Maximum:** 15 mg/day.

Tourette Disorder

PO: CHILDREN 6–17 YRS WEIGHING 50 KG OR MORE: 2 mg/day for 2 days; then 5 mg/day for 5 days with target dose of 10 mg on day 8. **Maximum:** 20 mg/day. **LESS THAN 50 KG:** 2 mg/day for 2 days, then 5 mg/day. **Maximum:** 10 mg/day.

Dosage in Renal/Hepatic Impairment

No dose adjustment.

SIDE EFFECTS

Frequent (11%–5%): Weight gain, headache, insomnia, vomiting. **Occasional (4%–3%):** Light-headedness, nausea, akathisia, drowsiness. **Rare (2% or less):** Blurred vision, constipation, asthenia (loss of strength, energy), anxiety, fever, rash, cough, rhinitis, orthostatic hypotension.

ADVERSE EFFECTS/TOXIC REACTIONS

Extrapyramidal symptoms, neuroleptic malignant syndrome, tardive dyskinesia, hyperglycemia, ketoacidosis, hyperosmolar coma, CVA, TIA occur rarely. Prolonged QT interval occurs rarely. May cause leukopenia, neutropenia, agranulocytosis.

NURSING CONSIDERATIONS

BASELINE ASSESSMENT

Assess behavior, appearance, emotional status, response to environment, speech pattern, thought content. Correct dehydration, hypovolemia. Assess for suicidal tendencies. Question history (or family history) of diabetes. Obtain serum blood glucose level.

INTERVENTION/EVALUATION

Periodically monitor weight. Monitor for extrapyramidal symptoms (abnormal movement), tardive dyskinesia (protrusion of tongue, puffing of cheeks, chewing/puckering of the mouth). Periodically monitor B/P, pulse (particularly in pts with preexisting cardiovascular disease). Monitor serum blood glucose levels during therapy. Assess for therapeutic response (greater interest in surroundings, improved self-care, increased ability to concentrate, relaxed facial expression).

PATIENT/FAMILY TEACHING

• Avoid alcohol. • Avoid tasks that require alertness, motor skills until response to drug is established. • Report worsening depression, suicidal ideation, unusual changes in behavior, extrapyramidal effects.

aspirin

TOP 100 HIGH ALERT

as-pir-in
(Asaphen E.C. ✱, Ascriptin, Bayer, Bufferin, Durlaza, Ecotrin, Entrophen ✱, Novasen ✱)
Do not confuse aspirin or Ascriptin with Afrin, Aricept, or Ecotrin with Epogen.

FIXED-COMBINATION(S)

Aggrenox: aspirin/dipyridamole (an antiplatelet agent): 25 mg/200 mg. **Fiorinal:** aspirin/butalbital/caffeine (a barbiturate): 325 mg/50 mg/40 mg. **Lortab/ASA:** aspirin/HYDROcodone (an analgesic): 325 mg/5 mg. **Percodan:** aspirin/oxyCODONE (an analgesic): 325 mg/2.25 mg, 325 mg/4.5 mg. **Pravigard:** aspirin/pravastatin (a cholesterol-lowering agent): 81 mg/20 mg, 81 mg/40 mg, 81 mg/80 mg, 325 mg/20 mg, 325 mg/40 mg, 325 mg/80 mg. **Yosprala:** aspirin/omeprazole (a proton pump inhibitor [PPI]) 325 mg/40 mg, 81 mg/40 mg.

◆CLASSIFICATION

PHARMACOTHERAPEUTIC: Nonsteroidal anti-inflammatory drug (NSAID). **CLINICAL:** Anti-inflammatory, antipyretic, analgesic, anti-platelet.

USES

Treatment of mild to moderate pain, fever. Reduces inflammation related to rheumatoid arthritis (RA), juvenile arthritis, osteoarthritis, rheumatic fever. Used as platelet aggregation inhibitor in the prevention of transient ischemic attacks (TIAs), cerebral thromboembolism, MI or reinfarction. **Durlaza:** Reduce risk of MI in pts with CAD or stroke in pts who have had TIA or ischemic stroke. **OFF-LABEL:** Prevention of preeclampsia; alternative therapy for preventing thromboembolism associated with atrial fibrillation when warfarin cannot be used; pericarditis associated with MI; prosthetic valve thromboprophylaxis. Adjunctive treatment of Kawasaki's disease. Complications associated with autoimmune disorders, colorectal cancer.

PRECAUTIONS

Contraindications: Hypersensitivity to NSAIDs. Pts with asthma rhinitis, nasal polyps; inherited or acquired bleeding disorders; use in children (younger than 16 yrs) for viral infections with or without fever. **Cautions:** Platelet/bleeding disorders, severe renal/hepatic impairment, dehydration, erosive gastritis, peptic ulcer disease, sensitivity to tartrazine dyes, elderly (chronic use of doses 325 mg or greater). Avoid use in pregnancy, especially third trimester.

ACTION

Irreversibly inhibits cyclo-oxygenase enzyme, resulting in a decreased formation of prostaglandin precursors. Irreversibly inhibits formation of thromboxane, resulting in inhibiting platelet aggregation. **Therapeutic Effect:** Reduces inflammatory response, intensity of pain; decreases fever; inhibits platelet aggregation.

PHARMACOKINETICS

Route	Onset	Peak	Duration
PO	1 hr	2–4 hrs	4–6 hrs

Rapidly and completely absorbed from GI tract; enteric-coated absorption delayed; rectal absorption delayed and incomplete. Protein binding: High. Widely distributed. Rapidly hydrolyzed to salicylate. **Half-life:** 15–20 min (aspirin); 2–3 hrs (salicylate at low dose); more than 20 hrs (salicylate at high dose).

LIFESPAN CONSIDERATIONS

Pregnancy/Lactation: Readily crosses placenta; distributed in breast milk. May prolong gestation and labor, decrease fetal birth weight, increase incidence of stillbirths, neonatal mortality, hemorrhage. Avoid use during last trimester (may adversely affect fetal cardiovascular system: premature closure of ductus arteriosus). **Children:** Caution in pts with acute febrile illness (Reye's syndrome). **Elderly:** May be more susceptible to toxicity; lower dosages recommended.

INTERACTIONS

DRUG: **Alcohol, NSAIDs (e.g., ibuprofen, ketorolac, naproxen)** may increase risk of GI effects (e.g., ulceration). **Antacids, urinary alkalinizers** increase excretion. **Anticoagulants, (e.g. enoxaparin, warfarin), heparin, thrombolytics, ticagrelor** increase risk of bleeding. **Apixaban, dabigatran, edoxaban, rivaroxaban** may increase anticoagulant effect. **HERBAL:** **Herbals with anticoagulant/antiplatelet properties (e.g., garlic, ginger, ginkgo biloba)** may increase risk of bleeding. **FOOD:** None known. **LAB VALUES:** May alter serum ALT, AST, alkaline phosphatase, uric acid; prolongs prothrombin time (PT) platelet function assay. May decrease serum cholesterol, potassium, T_3, T_4.

AVAILABILITY (OTC)

Caplets: 325 mg, 500 mg. **Suppositories:** 300 mg, 600 mg. **Tablets:** 325 mg. **Tablets (Chewable):** 81 mg.

Extended-Release Capsule: (Durlaza) 162.5 mg. **Tablets (Enteric-Coated):** 81 mg, 325 mg, 500 mg, 650 mg.

ADMINISTRATION/HANDLING

PO

• Do not break, crush, dissolve, or divide enteric-coated tablets or extended-release capsule. • May give with water, milk, meals if GI distress occurs.

Rectal

• Refrigerate suppositories; do not freeze. • If suppository is too soft, chill for 30 min in refrigerator or run cold water over foil wrapper. • Moisten suppository with cold water before inserting well into rectum.

INDICATIONS/ROUTES/DOSAGE

Analgesia, Fever

PO: ADULTS, ELDERLY, CHILDREN 12 YRS AND OLDER AND WEIGHING 50 KG OR MORE: 325–1,000 mg q4–6h prn. **Maximum:** 4 g/day. **RECTAL:** 300–600 mg q4h prn. **INFANTS, CHILDREN WEIGHING LESS THAN 50 KG:** 10–15 mg/kg/dose q4–6h. **Maximum:** 4 g/day or 90 mg/kg/day.

Revascularization

PO: ADULTS, ELDERLY: 80–325 mg/day.

Kawasaki's Disease

PO: CHILDREN: 80–100 mg/kg/day in divided doses q6h up to 14 days (until fever resolves for at least 48 hrs). After fever resolves, 1–5 mg/kg once daily for at least 6–8 wks.

MI, Stroke (Risk Reduction)

PO: ADULTS, ELDERLY: *(Durlaza):* 162.5 mg once daily.

Dosage in Renal/Hepatic Impairment

Avoid use in severe impairment.

SIDE EFFECTS

Occasional: GI distress (including abdominal distention, cramping, heartburn, mild nausea); allergic reaction (including bronchospasm, pruritus, urticaria).

ADVERSE EFFECTS/TOXIC REACTIONS

High doses of aspirin may produce GI bleeding and/or gastric mucosal lesions. Dehydrated, febrile children may experience aspirin toxicity quickly. Reye's syndrome, characterized by persistent vomiting, signs of brain dysfunction, may occur in children taking aspirin with recent viral infection (chickenpox, common cold, or flu). Low-grade aspirin toxicity characterized by tinnitus, generalized pruritus (may be severe), headache, dizziness, flushing, tachycardia, hyperventilation, diaphoresis, thirst. Marked toxicity characterized by hyperthermia, restlessness, seizures, abnormal breathing patterns, respiratory failure, coma.

NURSING CONSIDERATIONS

BASELINE ASSESSMENT

Do not give to children or teenagers who have or have recently had viral infections (increases risk of Reye's syndrome). Do not use if vinegar-like odor is noted (indicates chemical breakdown). Assess history of GI bleed, peptic ulcer disease, OTC use of products that may contain aspirin. Assess type, location, duration of pain, inflammation. Inspect appearance of affected joints for immobility, deformities, skin condition. **Therapeutic serum level for antiarthritic effect:** 20–30 mg/dL (toxicity occurs if level is greater than 30 mg/dL).

INTERVENTION/EVALUATION

Monitor urinary pH (sudden acidification, pH from 6.5 to 5.5, may result in toxicity). Assess skin for evidence of ecchymosis. If given as antipyretic, assess temperature directly before and 1 hr after giving medication. Evaluate for therapeutic response: relief of pain, stiffness, swelling; increased joint mobility; reduced joint tenderness; improved grip strength.

PATIENT/FAMILY TEACHING

• Do not, chew, crush, dissolve, or divide enteric-coated tablets. • Avoid alcohol, OTC pain/cold products that may contain aspirin. • Report ringing of the ears or persistent abdominal GI pain, bleeding. • Therapeutic anti-inflammatory effect noted in 1–3 wks. • Behavioral changes, persistent vomiting may be early signs of Reye's syndrome; contact physician.

atenolol HIGH ALERT

a-**ten**-oh-lol
(Tenormin)

■ BLACK BOX ALERT ■ Do not abruptly discontinue; taper gradually to avoid acute tachycardia, hypertension, ischemia.

Do not confuse atenolol with albuterol, timolol, or Tylenol, or Tenormin with Imuran, Norpramin, or thiamine.

◆CLASSIFICATION

PHARMACOTHERAPEUTIC: Beta$_1$-adrenergic blocker. **CLINICAL:** Antihypertensive, antianginal, antiarrhythmic.

USES

Treatment of hypertension, alone or in combination with other agents; management of angina pectoris; management of pts with definite/suspected MI to reduce CV mortality. **OFF-LABEL:** Arrhythmia (esp. supraventricular and ventricular tachycardia), thyrotoxicosis.

PRECAUTIONS

Contraindications: Hypersensitivity to atenolol. Cardiogenic shock, uncompensated HF, second- or third-degree heart block (except with functioning pacemaker), sinus bradycardia, sinus node dysfunction. **Cautions:** Elderly, renal impairment, peripheral vascular disease, diabetes, thyroid disease, bronchospastic disease, compensated HF, myasthenia gravis, psychiatric disease, history of anaphylaxis to allergens, concurrent use with digoxin, verapamil, or diltiaZEM.

ACTION

Blocks beta$_1$-adrenergic receptors in cardiac tissue. **Therapeutic Effect:** Slows sinus node heart rate, decreasing cardiac output, B/P. Decreases myocardial oxygen demand.

PHARMACOKINETICS

Route	Onset	Peak	Duration
PO	1 hr	2–4 hrs	24 hrs

Incompletely absorbed from GI tract. Protein binding: 6%–16%. Minimal liver metabolism. Primarily excreted unchanged in urine. Removed by hemodialysis. **Half-life:** 6–9 hrs (increased in renal impairment).

LIFESPAN CONSIDERATIONS

Pregnancy/Lactation: Readily crosses placenta; distributed in breast milk. Avoid use during first trimester. May produce bradycardia, apnea, hypoglycemia, hypothermia during delivery; low birth-weight infants. **Children:** No age-related precautions noted. **Elderly:** Age-related peripheral vascular disease, renal impairment require caution.

INTERACTIONS

DRUG: **Alpha$_2$ agonists (e.g., clonidine)** may increase AV-blocking effect. **Strong CYP3A4 inducers (e.g., carbamazepine, rifampin)** may decrease concentration/effect. **Dronedarone, fingolimod, rivastigmine** may increase bradycardic effect. May increase vasoconstriction of **ergot derivatives (e.g., dihydroergotamine, ergotamine).** **HERBAL:** **Herbals with hypertensive properties (e.g., licorice, yohimbe)** or **hypotensive properties (e.g., garlic, ginger, ginkgo biloba)** may alter effects. **St. John's wort** may decrease concentration/effect. **FOOD:** None known. **LAB VALUES:** May increase serum ANA titer, serum BUN, creatinine, potassium, uric acid, lipoprotein, triglycerides.

AVAILABILITY (Rx)

Tablets: 25 mg, 50 mg, 100 mg.

ADMINISTRATION/HANDLING

PO

• Give without regard to food. • Tablets may be crushed.

INDICATIONS/ROUTES/DOSAGE

Hypertension

PO: **ADULTS:** Initially, 25–50 mg once daily. After 1–2 wks, may increase dose up to 100 mg once daily. **ELDERLY:** Usual initial dose, 25 mg/day. **CHILDREN:** Initially, 0.5–1 mg/kg/dose given once daily. Range: 0.5–1.5 mg/kg/day. **Maximum:** 2 mg/kg/day up to 100 mg/day.

Angina Pectoris

PO: **ADULTS:** Initially, 50 mg once daily. May increase dose up to 200 mg once daily. **ELDERLY:** Usual initial dose, 25 mg/day.

Post-MI

PO: **ADULTS:** 100 mg once daily or 50 mg twice daily. Begin within first 24 hrs post-MI, then continue indefinitely.

Dosage in Renal Impairment

Dosage interval is modified based on creatinine clearance.

Creatinine Clearance	Maximum Dosage
15–35 mL/min	50 mg/day
Less than 15 mL/min	25 mg/day
Hemodialysis (HD)	Give dose post-HD or give 25–50 mg supplemental dose

Dosage in Hepatic Impairment

No dose adjustment.

SIDE EFFECTS

Atenolol is generally well tolerated, with mild and transient side effects. **Frequent:** Hypotension manifested as cold extremities, constipation or diarrhea, diaphoresis, dizziness, fatigue, headache, nausea. **Occasional:** Insomnia, flatulence, urinary frequency, impotence or decreased libido, depression. **Rare:** Rash, arthralgia, myalgia, confusion (esp. in the elderly), altered taste.

ADVERSE EFFECTS/TOXIC REACTIONS

Overdose may produce profound bradycardia, hypotension. Abrupt withdrawal may result in diaphoresis, palpitations, headache, tremors. May precipitate HF, MI in pts with cardiac disease; thyroid storm in pts with thyrotoxicosis; peripheral ischemia in pts with existing peripheral vascular disease. Hypoglycemia may occur in previously controlled diabetes. Thrombocytopenia (unusual bruising, bleeding) occurs rarely. **Antidote:** Glucagon (see Appendix J for dosage).

NURSING CONSIDERATIONS

BASELINE ASSESSMENT

Assess B/P, apical pulse immediately before drug is administered (if pulse is 60/min or less, or systolic B/P is less than 90 mm Hg, withhold medication, contact physician). **Antianginal:** Record onset, quality (sharp, dull, squeezing), radiation, location, intensity, duration of anginal pain, precipitating factors (exertion, emotional stress). Assess baseline renal/hepatic function tests.

INTERVENTION/EVALUATION

Monitor B/P for hypotension, pulse for bradycardia, respiration for difficulty in breathing, ECG. Monitor daily pattern of bowel activity, stool consistency. Assess for evidence of HF: dyspnea (particularly on exertion or lying down), nocturnal cough, peripheral edema, distended neck veins. Monitor I&O (increased weight, decreased urinary output may indicate HF). Assess extremities for pulse quality, changes in temperature (may indicate worsening peripheral vascular disease). Assist with ambulation if dizziness occurs.

PATIENT/FAMILY TEACHING

• Do not abruptly discontinue medication. • Compliance with therapy essential to control hypertension, angina. • To reduce hypotensive effect, go from lying to standing slowly. • Avoid tasks that require alertness, motor skills until response to drug is established. • Advise diabetic pts to monitor blood glucose carefully (may mask signs of hypoglycemia). • Report dizziness, depression, confusion, rash, unusual bruising/bleeding. • Outpatients should monitor B/P, pulse before taking medication, following correct technique. • Restrict salt, alcohol intake. • Therapeutic antihypertensive effect noted in 1–2 wks.

atezolizumab

a-te-zoe-**liz**-ue-mab
(Tecentriq)
Do not confuse atezolizumab with daclizumab, certolizumab, eculizumab, omalizumab, or tocilizumab.

◆CLASSIFICATION

PHARMACOTHERAPEUTIC: Programmed death-ligand 1 (PD-L1) blocking antibody. Monoclonal antibody. **CLINICAL:** Antineoplastic.

USES

Treatment of pts with locally advanced or metastatic urothelial carcinoma who have disease progression during or following platinum-containing chemotherapy or have disease progression within 12 mos of neoadjuvant or adjuvant treatment with platinum-containing chemotherapy. First-line treatment of metastatic non–small-cell lung cancer (NSCLC) as first-line monotherapy for certain pts, in combination with bevacizumab, paclitaxel, and carboplatin; or in combination with paclitaxel (protein bound) and carboplatin in pts with no EGFR or ALK genome tumor aberrations. Treatment of metastatic NSCLC in pts with disease progression during or following platinum-containing chemotherapy. Pts should have disease progression on approved therapy for EGFR or ALK genomic tumor mutation before receiving atezolizumab. Treatment of unresectable locally advanced or metastatic triple-negative breast cancer (in combination with paclitaxel [protein bound]) in pts whose tumors express PD-L1. First-line treatment of extensive-stage small-cell lung cancer (in combination with carboplatin and etoposide). Treatment of hepatocellular carcinoma (in combination with bevacizumab).

PRECAUTIONS

Contraindications: Hypersensitivity to atezolizumab. **Cautions:** Active infection;

baseline anemia, lymphopenia; pts at risk for hyperglycemia (e.g., diabetes, chronic use of corticosteroids); conditions predisposing to infection (e.g., diabetes, renal failure, immunocompromised pts, open wounds); pts at risk for dehydration, electrolyte imbalance; hepatic impairment, peripheral or generalized edema, neuropathy, optic disorders, interstitial lung disease; history of venous thromboembolism, intestinal obstruction, pancreatitis.

ACTION

Binds to PD-L1 to selectively prevent the interaction between PD-L1 and B7.1 receptors. PD-L1 is an immune checkpoint protein expressed on tumor cells. **Therapeutic Effect:** Restores antitumor T-cell function.

PHARMACOKINETICS

Metabolism not specified. Steady state reached in 6–9 wks. Elimination not specified. **Half-life:** 27 days.

LIFESPAN CONSIDERATIONS

Pregnancy/Lactation: Avoid pregnancy; may cause fetal harm. Unknown if distributed in breast milk; however, human immunoglobulin G is present in breast milk. Breastfeeding not recommended during treatment and for at least 5 mos after discontinuation. Females of reproductive potential should use effective contraception during treatment and up to 5 mos after discontinuation. May impair fertility in females. **Children:** Safety and efficacy not established. **Elderly:** No age-related precautions noted.

INTERACTIONS

DRUG: None known. **HERBAL:** None significant. **FOOD:** None known. **LAB VALUES:** May increase serum alkaline phosphatase, ALT, AST, creatinine, glucose. May decrease serum albumin, sodium; lymphocytes, Hgb, Hct, RBCs.

AVAILABILITY (Rx)

Injection Solution: 840 mg/14 mL, 1,200 mg/20 mL (60 mg/mL).

ADMINISTRATION/HANDLING

IV

Reconstitution • Visually inspect solution for particulate matter or discoloration. Solution should appear clear to slightly yellow. Discard if solution is cloudy or discolored or if visible particles are present. • Do not shake vial. • Withdraw 20 mL of solution from vial and dilute into a 250-mL polyvinyl chloride, polyethylene, or polyolefin infusion bag containing 0.9% NaCl. Dilute with 0.9% NaCl only. • Mix by gentle inversion. • Do not shake. • Discard partially used or empty vials.

Rate of administration • Infuse over 60 min using sterile, nonpyrogenic, low protein-binding, 0.2- to 0.22-micron in-line filter. • If first infusion is tolerated, all subsequent infusions may be delivered over 30 mins. • Do not administer as IV bolus.

Storage • Refrigerate diluted solution up to 24 hrs or store at room temperature for no more than 6 hrs (includes time of preparation and infusion). • Do not freeze. • Do not shake.

IV INCOMPATIBILITIES

Do not administer with other medications. Infuse via dedicated line.

INDICATIONS/ROUTES/DOSAGE

NSCLC

IV: ADULTS, ELDERLY: 1,200 mg on day 1 q3wks (in combination with bevacizumab, paclitaxel [protein bound], or carboplatin) for 4–6 cycles, then 1,200 mg on day 1 (followed by bevacizumab) q3wks. Following combination chemotherapy, may continue atezolizumab as single agent at 800 mg q2wks or 1,200 mg q3wks or 1,680 mg q4wks. Continue until disease progression or unacceptable toxicity.

Urothelial Carcinoma

IV: ADULTS, ELDERLY: 840 mg q2wks or 1,200 mg q3wks or 1,680 mg q4wks until disease progression or unacceptable toxicity. No dose reductions are recommended.

Breast Cancer (Triple-Negative), Locally Advanced or Metastatic
IV: ADULTS, ELDERLY: 840 mg on days 1 and 15 q4wks (in combination with paclitaxel [protein bound]) until disease progression or unacceptable toxicity.

Small-Cell Lung Cancer (Extensive-Stage), First-Line Treatment
IV: ADULTS, ELDERLY: Induction: 1,200 mg on day 1 q3wks (in combination with carboplatin and etoposide) for 4 cycles, followed by single-agent maintenance therapy of 840 mg once q2wks; or 1,200 mg once q3wks; or 1,680 mg once q4wks. Continue until disease progression or unacceptable toxicity.

Hepatocellular Carcinoma
IV: ADULTS, ELDERLY: 1,200 mg (followed by bevacizumab 15 mg/kg on same day) q3wks. If bevacizumab is discontinued, continue atezolizumab as single agent at 800 mg q2wks or 1,200 mg q3wks or 1,680 mg q4wks.

Dose Modification
Based on Common Terminology Criteria for Adverse Events (CTCAE). **Withhold treatment for any of the following toxic reactions:** Grade 2 or 3 diarrhea or colitis; Grade 2 pneumonitis; serum AST or ALT elevation 3–5 times upper limit of normal (ULN) or serum bilirubin elevation 1.5–3 times ULN; symptomatic hypophysitis, adrenal insufficiency, hypothyroidism, hyperthyroidism; Grade 3 or 4 hyperglycemia; Grade 3 rash; Grade 2 ocular inflammatory toxicity, Grade 2 or 3 pancreatitis, Grade 3 or 4 infection, Grade 2 infusion-related reactions. **Restarting treatment after interruption of therapy:** Resume treatment when adverse effects return to Grade 0 or 1. **Permanently discontinue for any of the following toxic reactions:** Grade 3 or 4 diarrhea or colitis; Grade 3 or 4 pneumonitis; serum AST or ALT elevation greater than 5 times ULN or serum bilirubin elevation 3 times ULN; Grade 4 hypophysitis; Grade 4 rash; Grade 3 or 4 ocular inflammatory toxicity; Grade 4 or any grade recurrent pancreatitis; Grade 3 or 4 infusion-related reactions; any occurrence of encephalitis, Guillain-Barré, meningitis, meningoencephalitis, myasthenic syndrome/myasthenia gravis.

Dosage in Renal Impairment
No dose adjustment.

Dosage in Hepatic Impairment
Mild impairment: No dose adjustment. **Moderate to severe impairment:** Not specified; use caution.

SIDE EFFECTS

Frequent (52%–18%): Fatigue, decreased appetite, nausea, pyrexia, constipation, diarrhea, peripheral edema. **Occasional (17%–13%):** Abdominal pain, vomiting, dyspnea, back/neck pain, rash, arthralgia, cough, pruritus.

ADVERSE EFFECTS/TOXIC REACTIONS

May cause severe immune-mediated events including adrenal insufficiency (0.4% of pts), interstitial lung disease or pneumonitis (3% of pts), colitis or diarrhea (20% of pts), hepatitis (2%–3% of pts), hypophysitis (0.2% of pts), hyperthyroidism (1% of pts), hypothyroidism (4% of pts), rash (up to 37% of pts), new-onset diabetes with ketoacidosis (0.2% of pts), pancreatitis (0.1% of pts); meningoencephalitis, myasthenic syndrome/myasthenia gravis, Guillain-Barré, ocular inflammatory toxicity (less than 1% of pts). Severe, sometimes fatal infections, including sepsis, herpes encephalitis, mycobacterial infection, occurred in 38% of pts. Urinary tract infections were the most common cause of Grade 3 or higher infection, occurring in 7% of pts. Severe infusion-related reactions reported in less than 1% of pts. Other adverse events, including acute kidney injury, dehydration, dyspnea, encephalitis, hematuria, intestinal obstruction, meningitis, neuropathy, pneumonia, urinary obstruction, venous thromboembolism, were reported. Immunogenicity (auto-atezolizumab antibodies) occurred in 42% of pts.

NURSING CONSIDERATIONS

BASELINE ASSESSMENT

Obtain baseline CBC, BMP, LFT, thyroid panel, urine pregnancy, urinalysis; vital signs. Screen for history of pituitary/pulmonary/thyroid disease, autoimmune disorders, diabetes, hepatic impairment, venous thromboembolism. Conduct full dermatologic/neurologic/ophthalmologic exam. Verify use of effective contraception in females of reproductive potential. Screen for active infection. Assess hydration status.

INTERVENTION/EVALUATION

Monitor CBC, BMP, LFT, thyroid panel, vital signs. Diligently monitor for immune-mediated adverse events as listed in Adverse Effects/Toxic Reactions. Notify physician if any CTCAE toxicities occur and initiate proper treatment. Obtain chest X-ray if interstitial lung disease, pneumonitis suspected. Due to high risk for dehydration/diarrhea, strictly monitor I&O. Encourage PO intake. If corticosteroid therapy is initiated for immune-mediated events, monitor capillary blood glucose and screen for corticosteroid side effects. Report any changes in neurologic status, including nuchal rigidity with fever, positive Kernig's sign, positive Brudzinski's sign, altered mental status, seizures. Diligently monitor for infection.

PATIENT/FAMILY TEACHING

• Blood levels will be routinely monitored. • Avoid pregnancy; treatment may cause birth defects. Do not breastfeed. Females of childbearing potential should use effective contraception during treatment and for at least 5 mos after final dose. • Treatment may cause serious or life-threatening inflammatory reactions. Report signs and symptoms of treatment-related inflammatory events in the following body systems: colon (severe abdominal pain or diarrhea); eye (blurry vision, double vision, unequal pupil size, sensitivity to light, eyelid drooping); lung (chest pain, cough, shortness of breath); liver (bruising easily, amber-colored urine, clay-colored/tarry stools, yellowing of skin or eyes); pituitary (persistent or unusual headache, dizziness, extreme weakness, fainting, vision changes); thyroid (trouble sleeping, high blood pressure, fast heart rate [overactive thyroid]), (fatigue, goiter, weight gain [underactive thyroid]), neurologic (confusion, headache, seizures, neck rigidity with fever, severe nerve pain or loss of motor function). • Immediately report allergic reactions, bleeding of any kind, signs of infection. • Treatment may cause severe diarrhea. Drink plenty of fluids.

atoMOXetine

at-oh-**mox**-e-teen
(Apo-Atomoxetine ♣, Strattera)

■ BLACK BOX ALERT ■ Increased risk of suicidal thinking and behavior in children and adolescents with attention-deficit hyperactivity disorder (ADHD).

Do not confuse atomoxetine with atorvastatin.

◆CLASSIFICATION

PHARMACOTHERAPEUTIC: Norepinephrine reuptake inhibitor. **CLINICAL:** Psychotherapeutic agent.

USES

Treatment of ADHD.

PRECAUTIONS

Contraindications: Hypersensitivity to atomoxetine. Narrow-angle glaucoma, use with or within 14 days of MAOIs. Pheochromocytoma or history of pheochromocytoma. Severe cardiovascular or vascular disease. **Cautions:** Hypertension, tachycardia, cardiovascular disease (e.g., structural abnormalities, cardiomyopathy), urinary retention, moderate or severe hepatic impairment, suicidal ideation, emergent psychotic or manic symptoms, comorbid bipolar disorder, renal impairment, poor metabolizers of CYP2D6 metabolized drugs (e.g., FLUoxetine, PARoxetine). Pts predisposed to hypotension.

ACTION

Selectively inhibits reuptake of norepinephrine. **Therapeutic Effect:** Improves symptoms of ADHD.

PHARMACOKINETICS

Rapidly absorbed after PO administration. Protein binding: 98% (primarily to albumin). Excreted in urine (80%), feces (17%). Not removed by hemodialysis. **Half-life:** 4–5 hrs (increased in moderate to severe hepatic insufficiency).

LIFESPAN CONSIDERATIONS

Pregnancy/Lactation: Unknown if distributed in breast milk. **Children:** Safety and efficacy not established in pts younger than 6 yrs. May produce suicidal thoughts in children and adolescents. **Elderly:** Age-related hepatic/renal impairment, cardiovascular or cerebrovascular disease may increase risk of adverse effects.

INTERACTIONS

DRUG: **MAOIs** may increase concentration/effect. **Strong CYP2D6 inhibitors (e.g., FLUoxetine, paroxetine)** may increase concentration/effect. **HERBAL:** None significant. **FOOD:** None known. **LAB VALUES:** May increase hepatic enzymes, serum bilirubin.

AVAILABILITY (Rx)

Capsules: 10 mg, 18 mg, 25 mg, 40 mg, 60 mg, 80 mg, 100 mg.

ADMINISTRATION/HANDLING

PO

• Give without regard to food. • Swallow capsules whole, do not break or open (powder in capsule is ocular irritant). Give as single daily dose in the morning or 2 evenly divided doses in morning and late afternoon/early evening.

INDICATIONS/ROUTES/DOSAGE

Note: May discontinue without tapering dose.

Attention-Deficit Hyperactivity Disorder (ADHD)

PO: ADULTS, CHILDREN 6 YRS AND OLDER WEIGHING 70 KG OR MORE: Initially, 40 mg once daily. May increase after at least 3 days to 80 mg daily. May further increase to 100 mg/day after 2–4 additional wks to achieve optimal response. **Maximum:** 100 mg. **CHILDREN 6 YRS AND OLDER WEIGHING LESS THAN 70 KG:** Initially, 0.5 mg/kg/day. May increase after at least 3 days to 1.2 mg/kg/day. **Maximum:** 1.4 mg/kg/day or 100 mg, whichever is less.

Dosage in Hepatic Impairment

Expect to administer 50% of normal atomoxetine dosage to pts with moderate hepatic impairment and 25% of normal dosage to pts with severe hepatic impairment.

Dosage in Renal Impairment

No dose adjustment.

Dosage With Strong CYP2D6 Inhibitors

ADULTS: Initially, 40 mg/day. May increase to 80 mg/day after minimum of 4 wks. **CHILDREN:** Initially, 0.5 mg/kg/day. May increase to 1.2 mg/kg/day only after minimum 4-wk interval.

SIDE EFFECTS

Frequent: Headache, dyspepsia, nausea, vomiting, fatigue, decreased appetite, dizziness, altered mood. **Occasional:** Tachycardia, hypertension, weight loss, delayed growth in children, irritability. **Rare:** Insomnia, sexual dysfunction in adults, fever.

ADVERSE EFFECTS/TOXIC REACTIONS

Urinary retention, urinary hesitancy may occur. In overdose, gastric lavage, activated charcoal may prevent systemic absorption. Severe hepatic injury occurs rarely.

NURSING CONSIDERATIONS

BASELINE ASSESSMENT

Assess pulse, B/P before therapy, following dose increases, and periodically during therapy. Assess attention span, interactions with others.

INTERVENTION/EVALUATION

Monitor urinary output; complaints of urinary retention/hesitancy may be a related adverse reaction. Monitor B/P, pulse periodically and following dose increases. Monitor for growth, attention span, hyperactivity, unusual changes in behavior, suicidal ideation. Assist with ambulation if dizziness occurs. Be alert to mood changes. Monitor fluid and electrolyte status in pts with significant vomiting.

PATIENT/FAMILY TEACHING

• Take last dose early in evening to avoid insomnia. • Report palpitations, fever, vomiting, irritability. • Monitor growth rate, weight. • Report changes in behavior, suicidal ideation, chest pain, palpitations, dyspnea.

atorvaSTATin TOP 100

a-**tor**-va-sta-tin
(Lipitor)

Do not confuse atorvastatin with atomoxetine, lovastatin, nystatin, pitavastatin, pravastatin, or simvastatin, or Lipitor with Levatol, lisinopril, or Zocor.

FIXED-COMBINATION(S)

Caduet: atorvastatin/amLODIPine (calcium channel blocker): 10 mg/2.5 mg, 10 mg/5 mg, 10 mg/10 mg, 20 mg/2.5 mg, 20 mg/5 mg, 20 mg/10 mg, 40 mg/2.5 mg, 40 mg/5 mg, 40 mg/10 mg, 80 mg/5 mg, 80 mg/10 mg.

◆CLASSIFICATION

PHARMACOTHERAPEUTIC: Hydroxymethylglutaryl CoA (HMG-CoA) reductase inhibitor. **CLINICAL:** Antihyperlipidemic.

USES

Dyslipidemias: Primary prevention of cardiovascular disease in high-risk pts. Reduces risk of stroke and heart attack in pts with type 2 diabetes with or without evidence of heart disease. Reduces risk of stroke in pts with or without evidence of heart disease with multiple risk factors other than diabetes. Adjunct to diet therapy in management of hyperlipidemias (reduces elevations in total cholesterol, LDL-C, apolipoprotein B, triglycerides in pts with primary hypercholesterolemia), homozygous familial hypercholesterolemia, heterozygous familial hypercholesterolemia in pts 10–17 yrs of age, females more than 1 yr postmenarche. **OFF-LABEL:** Secondary prevention in pts who have experienced a noncardioembolic stroke/TIA or following an acute coronary syndrome (ACS) event.

PRECAUTIONS

Contraindications: Hypersensitivity to atorvastatin. Active hepatic disease, breastfeeding, pregnancy or women who may become pregnant, unexplained elevated LFT results. **Cautions:** Anticoagulant therapy; history of hepatic disease; substantial alcohol consumption; pts with prior stroke/TIA; concomitant use of potent CYP3A4 inhibitors; elderly (predisposed to myopathy).

ACTION

Inhibits HMG-CoA reductase, the enzyme that catalyzes the early step in cholesterol synthesis. Results in an increase of expression in LDL receptors on hepatocyte membranes and a stimulation of LDL catabolism. **Therapeutic Effect:** Decreases LDL and VLDL, plasma triglyceride levels; increases HDL concentration.

PHARMACOKINETICS

Poorly absorbed from GI tract. Protein binding: greater than 98%. Metabolized in liver. Primarily excreted in feces (biliary). **Half-life:** 14 hrs.

LIFESPAN CONSIDERATIONS

Pregnancy/Lactation: Distributed in breast milk. Contraindicated during pregnancy. May produce fetal skeletal malformation. **Children:** Safety and efficacy not established. **Elderly:** No age-related precautions noted.

INTERACTIONS

DRUG: **Strong CYP3A4 inhibitors (e.g., clarithromycin, ketoconazole, ritonavir)** may increase concentration, risk of rhabdomyolysis. **CycloSPORINE** may increase concentration. **Gemfibrozil, fibrates, niacin, colchicine** may increase risk of myopathy, rhabdomyolysis. **Strong CYP3A4 inducers (e.g., carbamazepine, phenytoin, rifampin)** may decrease concentration/effect. **HERBAL:** **St. John's wort** may decrease concentration/effect. **FOOD:** **Grapefruit products** may increase concentration/effect. **Red yeast rice** may increase concentration/effect. (2.4 mg lovastatin per 600 mg rice). **LAB VALUES:** May increase serum transaminase, creatinine kinase concentrations.

AVAILABILITY (Rx)

Tablets: 10 mg, 20 mg, 40 mg, 80 mg.

ADMINISTRATION/HANDLING

PO

• Give without regard to food or time of day. • Do not break, crush, dissolve, or divide film-coated tablets.

INDICATIONS/ROUTES/DOSAGE

Do not use in pts with active hepatic disease. **Note:** Individualize dosage based on baseline LDL/cholesterol, goal of therapy, pt response. **Maximum dose with strong CYP3A4 inhibitors:** 20 mg/day.

Dyslipidemias

PO: ADULTS, ELDERLY: Initially, 10–20 mg/day (40 mg in pts requiring greater than 45% reduction in LDL-C). Range: 10–80 mg/day.

Heterozygous Hypercholesterolemia

PO: ADULTS: Initially, 40–80 mg once daily. **Maximum:** 80 mg/day. **CHILDREN 10–17 YRS:** Initially, 10 mg/day. May increase incrementally by doubling dose at monthly intervals. **Maximum:** 80 mg/day.

Dosage in Renal Impairment

No dose adjustment.

Dosage in Hepatic Impairment

See contraindications.

SIDE EFFECTS

Common: Atorvastatin is generally well tolerated. Side effects are usually mild and transient. **Frequent (16%):** Headache. **Occasional (5%–2%):** Myalgia, rash, pruritus, allergy. **Rare (less than 2%–1%):** Flatulence, dyspepsia, depression.

ADVERSE EFFECTS/TOXIC REACTIONS

Potential for cataracts, photosensitivity, myalgia, rhabdomyolysis.

NURSING CONSIDERATIONS

BASELINE ASSESSMENT

Obtain cholesterol, triglycerides, LFT. Question for possibility of pregnancy before initiating therapy. Obtain dietary history.

INTERVENTION/EVALUATION

Monitor for headache. Assess for rash, pruritus, malaise. Monitor cholesterol, triglyceride lab values for therapeutic response. Monitor LFTs, CPK.

PATIENT/FAMILY TEACHING

• Follow special diet (important part of treatment). • Periodic lab tests are essential part of therapy. • Do not take other medications without consulting physician. • Do not chew, crush, dissolve, or divide tablets. • Report dark urine, muscle fatigue, bone pain. • Avoid excessive alcohol intake, large quantities of grapefruit products.

avapritinib

a-va-**pri**-ti-nib
(Ayvakit)
Do not confuse avapritinib with acalabrutinib, afatinib, alectinib, axitinib, enasidenib, ibrutinib, or imatinib.

◆Classification

PHARMACOTHERAPEUTIC: PDGFR-alpha blocker. Tyrosine kinase inhibitor.
CLINICAL: Antineoplastic.

USES

Treatment of adults with unresectable or metastatic GI stromal tumor (GIST) harboring a platelet derived growth factor receptor alpha (PDGFRA) exon 18 mutation, including PDGFRA D842V mutations.

PRECAUTIONS

Contraindications: Hypersensitivity to avapritinib. **Cautions:** Baseline anemia, leukopenia, neutropenia, thrombocytopenia. Severe hepatic/renal impairment; conditions predisposing to infection (e.g., diabetes, immunocompromised, open wounds). History of intracranial/GI bleeding; anxiety, depression, suicidal ideation/behavior. Avoid concomitant use of strong or moderate CYP3A inhibitors, strong or moderate CYP3A inducers.

ACTION

Blocks PDGFRA targeting PDGFRA, PDGFR, and KIT mutants, which may result in autophosphorylation/activation of these receptors and lead to tumor cell proliferation. Avapritinib inhibits autophosphorylation of PDGFRA, KIT exon mutations. **Therapeutic Effect:** Inhibits tumor growth and survival associated with bowel, esophagus, stomach cancer.

PHARMACOKINETICS

Widely distributed. Metabolized in liver. Protein binding: 99%. Peak plasma concentration: 2–4 hrs. Steady state reached in 15 days. Excreted in feces (70%), urine (18%). **Half-life:** 32–57 hrs.

⌛ LIFESPAN CONSIDERATIONS

Pregnancy/Lactation: Avoid pregnancy; may cause fetal harm. Females and males of reproductive potential must use effective contraception during treatment and for at least 6 wks after discontinuation. Unknown if distributed in breast milk. Breastfeeding not recommended during treatment and for at least 2 wks after discontinuation. May impair fertility in both females and males. **Children:** Safety and efficacy not established. **Elderly:** No age-related precautions noted.

INTERACTIONS

DRUG: Alcohol, hydroxyzine, lorazepam, opioids (e.g., oxycodone), zolpidem may increase CNS depression. **Strong CYP3A4 inhibitors (e.g., clarithromycin, ketoconazole, ritonavir)** may increase concentration/effect. **Strong CYP3A4 inducers (e.g., carbamazepine, phenytoin, rifampin), moderate CYP3A inducers (e.g., bosentan, nafcillin)** may decrease concentration/effect. **HERBAL: St. John's wort** may decrease concentration/effect. **Herbals with sedative properties (e.g., chamomile, kava kava, valerian)** may increase CNS depression. **FOOD: Grapefruit products** may increase concentration/effect. **LAB VALUES:** May increase serum alkaline phosphatase, ALT, AST, bilirubin, creatinine. May decrease Hgb, leukocytes, neutrophils, platelets; serum albumin, magnesium, phosphate, potassium, sodium. May increase or decrease serum glucose. May prolong aPTT, PT; increase INR.

AVAILABILITY (Rx)

Tablets: 100 mg, 200 mg, 300 mg.

ADMINISTRATION/HANDLING

PO

• Give on empty stomach, at least 1 hr before or 2 hrs after meal. • Administer tablets whole; do not break, crush, or divide. Tablet cannot be chewed. • If vomiting occurs after administration, give next dose at regularly scheduled time (do not give additional dose). • If a dose is missed, do not give within 8 hrs of next scheduled dose.

INDICATIONS/ROUTES/DOSAGE

GI Stromal Tumor

PO: ADULTS, ELDERLY: 300 mg once daily. Continue until disease progression or unacceptable toxicity. If unable to discontinue moderate CYP3A inhibitor, reduce starting dose to 100 mg once daily.

Dose Reduction Schedule for Adverse Events

First dose reduction: 200 mg once daily. **Second dose reduction:** 100 mg once daily. **Unable to tolerate 100 mg dose:** Permanently discontinue.

Dose Modification

Based on Common Terminology Criteria for Adverse Events (CTCAE).

Central Nervous System (CNS) Effects

Grade 1 effects: Continue at same dose or withhold treatment until resolved or improved to baseline, then resume at same dose or reduced dose level. **Grade 2 or 3 effects:** Withhold treatment until resolved, or improved to Grade 1 or baseline, then resume at same dose or reduced dose level. **Grade 4 effects:** Permanently discontinue.

Intracranial Hemorrhage

Grade 1 or 2 intracranial hemorrhage: For first occurrence, withhold treatment until resolved, then resume at reduced dose level. For second occurrence, permanently discontinue. **Grade 3 or 4 intracranial hemorrhage:** Permanently discontinue.

Other Toxicities

Any other Grade 3 or 4 toxicities: Withhold treatment until improved to Grade 2 or less, then resume at same dose or reduced dose level.

Dosage in Renal Impairment

Mild to moderate impairment (CrCl 30–89 mL/min): No dose adjustment.
Severe impairment (CrCl 15–29 mL/min), ESRD: Not specified; use caution.

Dosage in Hepatic Impairment

Mild to moderate impairment: No dose adjustment.
Severe impairment: Not specified; use caution.

SIDE EFFECTS

Frequent (72%–22%): Edema (conjunctival, face, eye, eyelid, generalized, periorbital, peripheral, localized, orbital, testicular), nausea, fatigue, asthenia, cognitive impairment, vomiting, decreased appetite, diarrhea, increased lacrimation, abdominal pain, constipation, rash, dizziness. **Occasional (17%–8%):** Headache, dyspepsia, sleep disorders, insomnia, somnolence, dysgeusia, ageusia, hair color changes, dyspnea, pyrexia, alopecia, decreased weight, hypertension.

ADVERSE EFFECTS/TOXIC REACTIONS

Anemia, leukopenia, neutropenia, thrombocytopenia is an expected response to therapy. Intracranial hemorrhage, subdural hematoma reported in 1%–3% of pts. CNS effects including dizziness, hallucinations, cognitive impairment (e.g., amnesia confusion, dementia, encephalopathy, memory/mental impairment), mood disorders (e.g., agitation, anxiety, depression, dysphoria, personality change, suicidal ideation) reported in 58% of pts. Median onset of CNS effects was 6 wks. Grade 1 or 2 nausea and vomiting has occurred. Other serious reactions including pleural effusion, sepsis (3% of pts); GI hemorrhage, acute kidney injury (2% of pts); pneumonia, tumor hemorrhage (1% of pts) has occurred. Palmar-plantar erythrodysesthesia syndrome (PPES), a chemotherapy-induced skin condition that presents with redness, swelling, numbness, skin sloughing of the hands and feet reported in 1% of pts. Hyperthyroidism, hypothyroidism reported in 3% of pts.

NURSING CONSIDERATIONS

BASELINE ASSESSMENT

Obtain CBC, BMP, LFT; pregnancy test in female pts of reproductive potential. Confirm compliance of effective contraception. Question history of anxiety, depression, mood disorder, suicidal ideation and behavior; hepatic/renal impairment, intracranial/GI hemorrhage. Assess usual bowel movement patterns, stool characteristics. Assess hydration status. Screen for active infection. Receive full medication history and screen for interactions. Conduct baseline neurologic exam. Offer emotional support.

INTERVENTION/EVALUATION

Obtain CBC, BMP, LFT as clinically appropriate. Conduct regular neurologic exams to assess CNS effects, symptoms of intracranial bleeding (aphasia, blindness, confusion, facial droop, hemiplegia, seizures). Assess skin for dermal toxicities, PPES. Diligently screen for suicidal ideation and behavior; new-onset or worsening of anxiety, depression, mood disorder. Consult mental health professional if mood disorder suspected. Monitor daily pattern of bowel activity, stool consistency; I&Os, hydration status. Monitor for GI bleeding, infections (cough, fatigue, fever); drug toxicities if discontinuation of CYP3A inhibitor is unavoidable.

PATIENT/FAMILY TEACHING

• Treatment may depress your immune system response and reduce your ability to fight infection. Report symptoms of infection such as body aches, chills, cough, fatigue, fever. Avoid those with active infection. • Seek immediate medical attention if thoughts of suicide, new-onset or worsening of anxiety, depression, or changes in mood occur. • Nervous system changes including altered memory, confusion, delirium, difficulty speaking, gait disturbance, numbness, tremors may occur. Avoid tasks that require alertness, motor skills if neurologic effects are occurring. • Report symptoms of liver problems (abdominal pain, bruising, clay-colored stool, amber- or dark-colored urine, yellowing of the skin or eyes); hemorrhagic stroke (confusion, difficulty speaking, one-sided weakness, loss of vision). • Females and males of childbearing potential must use reliable contraception during treatment and for at least 6 wks after last dose. Do not breastfeed. • Treatment may cause diarrhea, dehydration. Drink plenty of fluids. • There is a high risk of interactions with other medications. Do not take newly prescribed medications unless approved by the prescriber who originally started treatment. • Avoid grapefruit products, herbal supplements (esp. St. John's wort).

avelumab

a-**vel**-ue-mab
(Bavencio)
Do not confuse avelumab with durvalumab, nivolumab, or olaratumab.

◆CLASSIFICATION

PHARMACOTHERAPEUTIC: Programmed death ligand-1 (PD-L1) blocking antibody. Monoclonal antibody.
CLINICAL: Antineoplastic.

USES

Treatment of adults and pediatric pts 12 yrs and older with metastatic Merkel cell carcinoma. Treatment of pts with locally advanced or metastatic urothelial carcinoma as first-line maintenance treatment or who have disease progression during or following platinum-containing chemotherapy or have disease progression within 12 mos of neoadjuvant or adjuvant treatment with platinum-containing chemotherapy. First-line treatment of advanced renal cell carcinoma (in combination with axitinib).

PRECAUTIONS

Contraindications: Hypersensitivity to avelumab. **Cautions:** Acute infection, conditions predisposing to infection (e.g., diabetes, immunocompromised pts, renal failure, open wounds); corticosteroid intolerance, hematologic cytopenias, hepatic impairment, interstitial lung disease, renal insufficiency; history of autoimmune disorders (Crohn's disease, demyelinating polyneuropathy, Guillain-Barré syndrome, Hashimoto's thyroiditis, hyperthyroidism, myasthenia gravis, rheumatoid arthritis, Type I diabetes, vasculitis); CVA, diabetes, intestinal obstruction, pancreatitis.

ACTION

Binds to PD-L1 and blocks interaction with both PD-L1 and B7.1 receptors while still allowing interaction between PD-L2 and PD-L1. PD-L1 is an immune check point protein expressed on tumor cells, down regulating anti-tumor T-cell function. **Therapeutic Effect:** Restores immune responses, including T-cell anti-tumor function.

PHARMACOKINETICS

Widely distributed. Degraded into small peptides and amino acids via proteolytic enzymes. Steady state reached in 4–6 wks. Excretion not specified. **Half-life:** 6.1 days.

LIFESPAN CONSIDERATIONS

Pregnancy/Lactation: Avoid pregnancy; may cause fetal harm. Females of reproductive potential should use effective contraception during treatment and for at least 1 mo after discontinuation. Unknown if distributed in breast milk. However, human immunoglobulin G (IgG) is present in breast milk and is known to cross the placenta. Breastfeeding not recommended during treatment and for at least 1 mo after discontinuation. **Children:** Safety and efficacy not established in pts younger than 12 yrs. **Elderly:** No age-related precautions noted.

INTERACTIONS

DRUG: May enhance adverse effects/toxicity of **belimumab**. **HERBAL:** None significant. **FOOD:** None known. **LAB VALUES:** May decrease Hgb, Hct, lymphocytes, neutrophils, platelets, RBCs. May increase serum alkaline phosphatase, ALT, AST, amylase, bilirubin, glucose, GGT, lipase.

AVAILABILITY (Rx)

Injection: 200 mg/10 mL (20 mg/mL).

ADMINISTRATION/HANDLING

IV

Preparation • Visually inspect for particulate matter or discoloration. Solution should appear clear and colorless to slightly yellow in color. • Do not use if solution is cloudy, discolored, or if visible particles are observed. • Withdraw proper volume from vial and inject into a 250-mL bag of 0.9% NaCl or 0.45% NaCl. • Gently invert to mix; avoid foaming. • Do not shake. • Diluted solution should be clear, colorless, and free of particles.

Rate of administration • Infuse over 60 min via dedicated IV line using a sterile, nonpyrogenic, low protein-binding in-line filter.

Storage • Refrigerate unused vials. • May refrigerate diluted solution for no more than 24 hrs or store at room temperature for no more than 4 hrs. If refrigerated, allow diluted solution to warm to room temperature before infusing. • Do not freeze or shake. • Protect from light.

IV INCOMPATIBILITIES

Do not mix or infuse with other medications.

INDICATIONS/ROUTES/DOSAGE

Note: Premedicate with acetaminophen and an antihistamine prior to the first 4 infusions. Consider premedication for subsequent infusions based on prior infusion reactions.

Urothelial Carcinoma, Merkel Cell Carcinoma

IV: ADULTS, ELDERLY, CHILDREN: 800 mg once q2wks or 10 mg/kg every 2 wks. Continue until disease progression or unacceptable toxicity.

Renal Cell Carcinoma (Advanced)

IV: ADULTS, ELDERLY: 800 mg once q2wks or 10 mg/kg q2wks (in combination with axitinib) until disease progression or unacceptable toxicity.

Dose Modification

Infusion-Related Reactions

CTCAE Grade 1 or 2: Interrupt or decrease rate of infusion. **CTCAE Grade 3 or 4:** Permanently discontinue.

Endocrinopathies (e.g., Adrenal Insufficiency, Hyperglycemia, Hyperthyroidism, Hypothyroidism) (Treatment-Induced)

CTCAE Grade 3 or 4 endocrinopathies: Withhold treatment until resolved to Grade 1 or 0, then resume therapy after corticosteroid taper. Consider hormone replacement therapy if hypothyroidism occurs.

Colitis (Treatment-Induced)

CTCAE Grade 2 or 3 diarrhea or colitis: Withhold treatment until resolved to Grade 1 or 0, then resume therapy after corticosteroid taper. **CTCAE Grade 4 diarrhea or colitis; recurrent Grade 3 diarrhea or colitis:** Permanently discontinue.

Hepatitis (Treatment-Induced)

Serum ALT/AST greater than 3 and up to 5 times upper limit normal (ULN) or serum bilirubin greater than 1.5 and up to 3 times ULN): Withhold treatment until resolved to Grade 1 or 0, then resume therapy. **Serum ALT/AST greater than 5 times upper limit normal (ULN) or serum bilirubin greater than 3 times ULN):** Permanently discontinue.

Nephritis and Renal Dysfunction (Treatment-Induced)

Serum creatinine greater than 1.5 and up to 6 times ULN: Withhold treatment until resolved to Grade 1 or 0, then resume therapy after corticosteroid taper. **Serum creatinine greater than 6 times ULN:** Permanently discontinue. **Other moderate or severe symptoms of treatment-induced reactions (e.g., arthritis, bullous dermatitis, encephalitis, erythema multiform, exfoliative dermatitis, demyelination, Guillain-Barré syndrome, hemolytic anemia, histiocytic necrotizing lymphadenitis, hypophysitis, hypopituitarism, iritis, myasthenia gravis, myocarditis, myositis, pancreatitis, pemphigoid, psoriasis, Stevens Johnson Syndrome/toxic epidermal necrolysis, rhabdomyolysis, uveitis, vasculitis):** Withhold treatment until resolved to Grade 1 or 0, then resume therapy after corticosteroid taper. **Life-threatening adverse effects, recurrent severe immune-mediated reactions; requirement of predniSONE 10 mg/day or greater (or equivalent) for more than 2 wks; persistent Grade 2 or 3 immune-mediated reaction lasting 12 wks or longer:** Permanently discontinue.

Pneumonitis (Treatment-Induced)

CTCAE Grade 2 pneumonitis: Withhold treatment until resolved to Grade 1 or 0, then resume therapy after corticosteroid taper. **CTCAE Grade 3 or 4 or recurrent Grade 2 pneumonitis:** Permanently discontinue.

Dosage in Renal/Hepatic Impairment

Not specified; use caution.

SIDE EFFECTS

Note: Percentage of side effects may vary depending on indication of treatment.

Frequent (50%–18%): Fatigue, musculoskeletal pain, diarrhea, rash, infusion reactions (back pain, chills, pyrexia, hypotension), nausea, decreased appetite, peripheral edema, cough. **Occasional (17%–10%):** Constipation, arthralgia, abdominal pain, decreased weight, dizziness, vomiting, hypertension, dyspnea, pruritus, headache.

ADVERSE EFFECTS/TOXIC REACTIONS

Anemia, neutropenia, thrombocytopenia is an expected response to therapy. May cause severe, sometimes fatal cases of immune-mediated reactions such as pneumonitis (1% of pts), hepatitis (1% of pts), colitis (2% of pts), adrenal insufficiency (1% of pts), hypothyroidism, hyperthyroidism (6% of pts), type 1 diabetes mellitus including ketoacidosis (less than 1% of pts), nephritis (less than 1% of pts), other immune-mediated effects (less than 1%). Cellulitis, CVA, dyspnea, ileus, pericardial effusion, small bowel/intestinal obstruction, renal failure, respiratory failure, septic shock, transaminitis, urosepsis may occur. Immunogenicity (auto-avelumab antibodies) reported in 4% of pts.

NURSING CONSIDERATIONS

BASELINE ASSESSMENT

Obtain ANC, CBC, BMP (esp. serum creatinine, creatinine clearance; BUN), TSH, vital signs; urine pregnancy. Question current breastfeeding status. Verify use of contraception in female pts of reproductive potential. Question history of prior hypersensitivity reaction, infusion-related reactions, allergy to corticosteroids/prednisone. Screen for history of autoimmune disorders, diabetes, pituitary/pulmonary/thyroid disease, renal insufficiency. Obtain nutrition consult. Offer emotional support.

INTERVENTION/EVALUATION

Monitor ANC, CBC, BMP, creatinine clearance, thyroid panel (if applicable); vital signs. Diligently monitor for infusion-related reactions, treatment-related toxicities, esp. during initial infusions. If immune-mediated reactions occur, consider referral to specialist; pt may require treatment with corticosteroids. Screen for allergic reactions, acute infections (cellulitis, sepsis, UTI), hepatitis, pulmonary events (dyspnea, pneumonitis, pneumonia). Monitor strict I&O, hydration status, stool frequency and consistency. Encourage proper calorie intake and nutrition. Assess skin for rash, lesions, dermal toxicities.

PATIENT/FAMILY TEACHING

• Treatment may depress your immune system and reduce your ability to fight infection. Report symptoms of infection such as body aches, burning with urination, chills, cough, fatigue, fever. Avoid those with active infection. • Avoid pregnancy; treatment may cause birth defects. Do not breastfeed. Females of childbearing potential should use effective contraception during treatment and for at least 1 mo after discontinuation. • Serious adverse reactions may affect lungs, liver, intestines, kidneys, hormonal glands, nervous system, which may require anti-inflammatory medication. • Immediately report any serious or life-threatening inflammatory symptoms in the following body systems: colon (severe abdominal pain/swelling, diarrhea); kidneys (decreased or dark-colored urine, flank pain); lung (chest pain, severe cough, shortness of breath); liver (bruising, dark-colored urine, clay-colored/tarry stools, nausea, yellowing of the skin or eyes); nervous system (paralysis, weakness); pituitary (persistent or unusual headaches, dizziness, extreme weakness, fainting, vision changes); skin (blisters, bubbling, inflammation, rash); thyroid (trouble sleeping, high blood pressure, fast heart rate [overactive thyroid]; fatigue, goiter, weight gain [underactive thyroid]); vascular (low blood pressure, vein/artery pain or irritation). • Do not take any over-the-counter anti-inflammatory medications unless approved by your doctor.

axitinib

ax-**i**-ti-nib
(Inlyta)
Do not confuse axitinib with afatinib, ibrutinib, or imatinib.

◆CLASSIFICATION

PHARMACOTHERAPEUTIC: Vascular endothelial growth factor (VEGF) inhibitor. Tyrosine kinase inhibitor. **CLINICAL:** Antineoplastic.

USES

Treatment of advanced renal cell carcinoma after failure of one prior systemic chemotherapy.

PRECAUTIONS

Contraindications: Hypersensitivity to axitinib. **Cautions:** Pts with increased risk or history of thrombotic events (CVA, MI), GI perforation or fistula formation, renal/hepatic impairment, hypertension, HF. Do not use in pts with untreated brain metastasis or recent active GI bleeding.

ACTION

Inhibits vascular endothelial growth factor receptors. **Therapeutic Effect:** Blocks tumor growth, inhibits angiogenesis.

PHARMACOKINETICS

Metabolized in liver. Protein binding: greater than 99%. Excreted primarily in feces with a lesser amount excreted in urine. **Half-life:** 2.5–6 hrs.

⧗ LIFESPAN CONSIDERATIONS

Pregnancy/Lactation: May cause fetal harm. Unknown whether distributed in breast milk. **Children:** Safety and efficacy not established. **Elderly:** No age-related precautions noted.

INTERACTIONS

DRUG: Strong CYP3A4 inhibitors (e.g., erythromycin, ketoconazole, ritonavir) may significantly increase concentration; do not use concurrently. If used, reduce dose by 50%. Coadministration with **strong CYP3A4 inducers (e.g., rifAMPin, phenytoin, carBAMazepine, PHENobarbital)** may significantly decrease concentration/effect, do not use concurrently. **HERBAL: St. John's wort** may decrease concentration/effect. **FOOD: Grapefruit products** may increase concentration/effect. **LAB VALUES:** May decrease Hgb, WBC count, platelets, lymphocytes; serum calcium, alkaline phosphatase, albumin, sodium, phosphate, bicarbonate. May increase serum ALT, AST, bilirubin, BUN, creatinine, serum potassium, lipase, amylase; urine protein. May alter serum glucose.

AVAILABILITY (Rx)

Film-Coated Tablets: 1 mg, 5 mg.

ADMINISTRATION/HANDLING

PO

• Give without regard to food. • Swallow tablets whole with full glass of water.

INDICATIONS/ROUTES/DOSAGE

Renal Cell Carcinoma

PO: ADULTS, ELDERLY: Initially, 5 mg twice daily, given approximately 12 hrs apart. If tolerated (no adverse events above Grade 2, B/P normal, and no antihypertension use for at least 2 consecutive wks), may increase to 7 mg twice daily, then 10 mg twice daily. For adverse effects, may decrease to 3 mg twice daily, then 2 mg twice daily if adverse effects persist.

Dose Modification

Dosage with concomitant strong CYP3A4 inhibitors: Reduce dose by 50%. (Avoid concomitant use if possible.)

Dosage in Renal Impairment

No dose adjustment. Use caution in ESRD.

Dosage in Hepatic Impairment

Mild impairment: No dose adjustment. **Moderate impairment:** Reduce initial dose by 50%. **Severe impairment:** Not recommended.

SIDE EFFECTS

Frequent (55%–20%): Diarrhea, hypertension, fatigue, decreased appetite, nausea, dysphonia, palmar-plantar erythrodysesthesia (hand-foot) syndrome, weight loss, vomiting, asthenia, constipation. **Occasional (19%–11%):** Hypothyroidism, cough, stomatitis, arthralgia, dyspnea, abdominal pain, headache, peripheral pain, rash, proteinuria, dysgeusia. **Rare (10%–2%):** Dry skin, dyspepsia, dizziness, myalgia, pruritus, epistaxis, alopecia, hemorrhoids, tinnitus, erythema.

ADVERSE EFFECTS/TOXIC REACTIONS

Arterial and venous thrombotic events (MI, CVA), GI perforation, fistula, hemorrhagic events (including cerebral hemorrhage, hematuria, hemoptysis, GI bleeding), hypertensive crisis, cardiac failure have been observed and can be fatal. Hypothyroidism requiring thyroid hormone replacement has been noted. Reversible posterior leukoencephalopathy syndrome (RPLS) has been observed.

NURSING CONSIDERATIONS

BASELINE ASSESSMENT

Obtain baseline BMP, LFT, renal function test, urine protein, serum amylase, lipase, phosphate before initiation of, and periodically throughout, treatment. Offer emotional support. Assess medical history, esp. hepatic function abnormalities. B/P should be well controlled prior to initiating treatment. Stop medication at least 24 hrs prior to scheduled surgery. Monitor thyroid function before and periodically throughout treatment.

INTERVENTION/EVALUATION

Monitor CBC, BMP, LFT, renal function test, urine protein, serum amylase, lipase, phosphate, thyroid tests. Monitor daily pattern of bowel activity, stool consistency. Assess for evidence of bleeding or hemorrhage. Assess for hypertension. For persistent hypertension despite use of antihypertensive medications, dose should be reduced. Permanently discontinue if signs or symptoms of RPLS occur (extreme lethargy, increased B/P from pt baseline, pyuria). Contact physician if changes in voice, redness of skin, or rash is noted.

PATIENT/FAMILY TEACHING

• Avoid crowds, those with known infection. • Avoid contact with anyone who recently received live virus vaccine; do not receive vaccinations. • Swallow tablet whole; do not chew, crush, dissolve, or divide. • Avoid grapefruit products. • Report persistent diarrhea, extreme fatigue, abdominal pain, yellowing of skin or eyes, bruising easily; bleeding of any kind, esp. bloody stool or urine; confusion, seizure activity, vision loss, trouble speaking, chest pain; difficulty breathing, leg pain or swelling.

azilsartan

a-zil-**sar**-tan
(Edarbi)

■ **BLACK BOX ALERT** ■ May cause fetal injury, mortality. Discontinue as soon as possible once pregnancy is detected.
Do not confuse azilsartan with losartan, irbesartan, or valsartan.

FIXED-COMBINATION(S)

Edarbyclor: azilsartan/chlorthalidone, a diuretic: 40 mg/12.5 mg, 40 mg/25 mg.

◆CLASSIFICATION

PHARMACOTHERAPEUTIC: Angiotensin II receptor blocker (ARB). **CLINICAL:** Antihypertensive.

USES

Treatment of hypertension alone or in combination with other antihypertensives.

PRECAUTIONS

Contraindications: Hypersensitivity to azilsartan. Concomitant use with aliskiren in pts with diabetes. **Cautions:** Renal/hepatic impairment, unstented renal artery stenosis, significant aortic/mitral stenosis, severe HF, volume depletion/salt-depleted pts, history of angioedema.

ACTION

Inhibits vasoconstriction, aldosterone-secreting effects of angiotensin II, blocking the binding of angiotensin II to AT_1 receptors in vascular smooth muscle and adrenal gland tissue. **Therapeutic Effect:** Produces vasodilation, decreases peripheral resistance, decreases B/P.

PHARMACOKINETICS

Hydrolyzed to active metabolite in GI tract. Moderately absorbed (60%). Peak plasma concentration: 1.5–3 hrs. Metabolized in liver. Protein binding: greater than 99%. Excreted in feces (55%), urine (42%). **Half-life:** 11 hrs.

LIFESPAN CONSIDERATIONS

Pregnancy/Lactation: May cause fetal harm when administered during third trimester. Unknown if distributed in breast milk. Breastfeeding not recommended. **Children:** Safety and efficacy not established. **Elderly:** Elevated creatinine levels may occur in pts older than 75 yrs.

INTERACTIONS

DRUG: **ACE inhibitors (e.g., enalapril, lisinopril), potassium-sparing diuretics (e.g., spironolactone, triamterene), potassium supplements** may increase risk of hyperkalemia. **NSAIDs, COX-2 inhibitors (e.g., celecoxib)** may decrease effect. **Hypotensive agents** may increase hypotensive effects. May increase concentration/effect of **lithium**. **HERBAL:** **Herbals with hypertensive properties (e.g., licorice, yohimbe)** or **hypotensive properties (e.g., garlic, ginger, ginkgo biloba)** may alter effects. **FOOD:** None known.

LAB VALUES: May increase serum creatinine. May decrease Hgb, Hct.

AVAILABILITY (Rx)

Tablets: 40 mg, 80 mg.

ADMINISTRATION/HANDLING

PO

- May give without regard to food.

INDICATIONS/ROUTES/DOSAGE

Hypertension

PO: ADULTS, ELDERLY: Initially, 40 mg once daily. May increase up to 80 mg once daily.

Dosage in Renal/Hepatic Impairment

No dose adjustment.

SIDE EFFECTS

Occasional (2%–0.4%): Diarrhea, orthostatic hypotension. **Rare (0.3%):** Nausea, fatigue, muscle spasm, cough.

ADVERSE EFFECTS/TOXIC REACTIONS

Oliguria, acute renal failure may occur in pts with history of renal artery stenosis, severe HF, volume depletion.

NURSING CONSIDERATIONS

BASELINE ASSESSMENT

Obtain baseline Hgb, Hct, BMP, LFT. Obtain B/P, apical pulse immediately before each dose, in addition to regular monitoring (be alert to fluctuations). Question for possibility of pregnancy. Assess medication history (esp. diuretics). Question history of hepatic/renal impairment, renal artery stenosis, severe HF.

INTERVENTION/EVALUATION

Maintain hydration (offer fluids frequently). Monitor serum electrolytes, B/P, pulse, hepatic/renal function. Observe for symptoms of hypotension. If excessive reduction in B/P occurs, place pt in supine position, feet slightly elevated. Correct volume or salt depletion prior to treatment.

PATIENT/FAMILY TEACHING

• Take measures to avoid pregnancy. If pregnancy occurs, inform physician immediately. • Low blood pressure is more likely to occur if pt takes diuretics or other medications to control hypertension, consumes low-salt diet, experiences vomiting or diarrhea, or becomes dehydrated. • Change positions slowly, particularly from lying to standing position. • Report light-headedness or dizziness; lie down immediately. • Report swollen extremities or decreased urine output despite fluid intake.

azithromycin

a-**zith**-roe-**mye**-sin
(AzaSite, Zithromax)
Do not confuse azithromycin with azaTHIOprine or erythromycin, or Zithromax with Fosamax or Zovirax.

◆CLASSIFICATION

PHARMACOTHERAPEUTIC: Macrolide. **CLINICAL:** Antibiotic.

USES

IV/PO: Treatment of susceptible infections due to *Chlamydia pneumoniae, C. trachomatis, H. influenzae, Legionella, M. catarrhalis, Mycoplasma pneumoniae, N. gonorrhoeae, S. aureus., S. pneumoniae, S. pyogenes,* including mild to moderate infections of upper respiratory tract (pharyngitis, tonsillitis), lower respiratory tract (acute bacterial exacerbations, COPD, pneumonia), uncomplicated skin and skin-structure infections, sexually transmitted diseases (nongonococcal urethritis, cervicitis due to *C. trachomatis*), chancroid. Prevents disseminated *Mycobacterium avium* complex (MAC). Treatment of mycoplasma pneumonia, community-acquired pneumonia, pelvic inflammatory disease (PID). Prevention/treatment of MAC in pts with advanced HIV infection. **OFF-LABEL:** Prophylaxis of endocarditis. Prevention of pulmonary exacerbations in pts with cystic fibrosis. **Ophthalmic:** Treatment of bacterial conjunctivitis caused by susceptible infections due to *H. influenzae, S. aureus, S. mitis, S. pneumoniae.* Prevention of pulmonary exacerbations in pts with cystic fibrosis.

PRECAUTIONS

Contraindications: Hypersensitivity to azithromycin, erythromycin, or other macrolide antibiotics. History of cholestatic jaundice/hepatic impairment associated with prior azithromycin therapy. **Cautions:** Hepatic/renal impairment, myasthenia gravis, hepatocellular and/or cholestatic hepatitis (with or without jaundice), hepatic necrosis. May prolong QT interval.

ACTION

Binds to ribosomal receptor sites of susceptible organisms, inhibiting RNA-dependent protein synthesis. **Therapeutic Effect:** Bacteriostatic or bactericidal, depending on drug dosage.

PHARMACOKINETICS

Rapidly absorbed from GI tract. Protein binding: 7%–50%. Widely distributed. Metabolized in liver. Excreted primarily by biliary excretion. **Half-life:** 68 hrs.

LIFESPAN CONSIDERATIONS

Pregnancy/Lactation: Unknown if distributed in breast milk. **Children:** Safety and efficacy not established in pts younger than 16 yrs for IV use and younger than 6 mos for oral use. **Elderly:** No age-related precautions in those with normal renal function.

INTERACTIONS

DRUG: **Aluminum/magnesium-containing antacids** may decrease concentration (give 1 hr before or 2 hrs after antacid). May increase concentration/effect of **amiodarone, colchicine, cycloSPORINE, dabigatran, dronedarone, edoxaban, pazopanib, QT-pro-**

longing medications, thioridazine, topotecan, toremifene, ziprasidone. QUEtiapine may increase concentration. **HERBAL**: None significant. **FOOD**: None known. **LAB VALUES**: May increase serum creatine phosphokinase (CPK), ALT, AST, bilirubin, LDH, potassium.

AVAILABILITY (Rx)

Injection, Powder for Reconstitution: ***(Zithromax):*** 500 mg. **Ophthalmic Solution:** ***(AzaSite)***: 1%. **Oral Packet:** 1g. **Oral Suspension:** ***(Zithromax):*** 100 mg/5 mL, 200 mg/5 mL. **Tablets:** 250 mg, 600 mg.

ADMINISTRATION/HANDLING

IV

Reconstitution • Reconstitute each 500-mg vial with 4.8 mL Sterile Water for Injection to provide concentration of 100 mg/mL. • Shake well to ensure dissolution. • Further dilute with 250 or 500 mL 0.9% NaCl or D_5W to provide final concentration of 2 mg/mL with 250 mL diluent or 1 mg/mL with 500 mL diluent.

Rate of administration • Infuse over 60 min (2 mg/mL). Infuse over 3 hrs (1 mg/mL).

Storage • Store vials at room temperature. • Following reconstitution, diluted solution is stable for 24 hrs at room temperature or 7 days if refrigerated.

PO

• Give without regard to food. • May store suspension at room temperature. Stable for 10 days after reconstitution.

Ophthalmic

• Place gloved finger on lower eyelid and pull out until a pocket is formed between eye and lower lid. • Place prescribed number of drops into pocket. • Instruct pt to close eye gently for 1 to 2 min (so that medication will not be squeezed out of sac) and to apply digital pressure to lacrimal sac at inner canthus for 1 min to minimize systemic absorption.

IV INCOMPATIBILITIES

CefTRIAXone (Rocephin), ciprofloxacin (Cipro), famotidine (Pepcid), furosemide (Lasix), ketorolac (Toradol), levoFLOXacin (Levaquin), morphine, piperacillin/tazobactam (Zosyn), potassium chloride.

IV COMPATIBILITIES

Ceftaroline (Teflaro), doripenem (Doribax), ondansetron (Zofran), tigecycline (Tygacil), diphenhydrAMINE (Benadryl).

INDICATIONS/ROUTES/DOSAGE

Usual Dosage Range

PO: ADULTS, ELDERLY: 250–600 mg once daily or 1–2 g as single dose. **ADOLESCENTS, CHILDREN, INFANTS**: 5–12 mg/kg/dose (usually 10–12 mg/kg on day 1, then 5–6 mg/kg thereafter). **Usual maximum total course:** 1,500–2,000 mg. **NEONATES**: 10–20 mg/kg once daily.

IV: ADULTS, ELDERLY: 250–500 mg once daily **ADOLESCENTS, CHILDREN, INFANTS, NEONATES**: 10 mg/kg once daily.

Mild to Moderate Respiratory Tract, Skin, Soft Tissue Infections

PO: ADULTS, ELDERLY: 500 mg day 1, then 250 mg days 2–5.

MAC Prevention

PO: ADULTS, ELDERLY, ADOLESCENTS: 1,200 mg once weekly or 600 mg twice weekly. **CHILDREN**: 20 mg/kg once weekly. **Maximum:** 1,200 mg/dose or 5 mg/kg once daily. **Maximum:** 250 mg/dose.

MAC Treatment

PO: ADULTS, ELDERLY: 500–600 mg/day. **CHILDREN**: 10–12 mg/kg/day (**maximum:** 500 mg).

Otitis Media

PO: CHILDREN 6 MOS AND OLDER: 30 mg/kg as single dose (**maximum:** 1,500 mg) or 10 mg/kg/day for 3 days (**maximum:** 500 mg) or 10 mg/kg on day 1 (**maximum:** 500 mg), then 5 mg/kg on days 2–5 (**maximum:** 250 mg).

Pharyngitis, Tonsillitis
PO: ADULTS, ELDERLY, CHILDREN: 12 mg/kg (**maximum:** 500 mg) on day 1, then 6 mg/kg (**maximum:** 250 mg) on days 2–5.

Pneumonia, Community-Acquired
PO: *(Zmax):* **ADULTS, ELDERLY:** 2 g as single dose.
PO: ADULTS, ELDERLY, CHILDREN 16 YRS AND OLDER: 500 mg on day 1, then 250 mg on days 2–5 or 500 mg/day IV for 2 days, then 500 mg/day PO to complete course of therapy. **CHILDREN 6 MOS–15 YRS:** 10 mg/kg on day 1 (**maximum:** 500 mg), then 5 mg/kg (**maximum:** 250 mg) on days 2–5.

Bacterial Conjunctivitis
Ophthalmic: ADULTS, ELDERLY: 1 drop in affected eye twice daily for 2 days, then 1 drop once daily for 5 days.

Dosage in Renal/Hepatic Impairment
Use caution.

SIDE EFFECTS

Occasional: Systemic: Nausea, vomiting, diarrhea, abdominal pain. **Ophthalmic:** Eye irritation. **Rare: Systemic:** Headache, dizziness, allergic reaction.

ADVERSE EFFECTS/TOXIC REACTIONS

Antibiotic-associated colitis, other superinfections may result from altered bacterial balance in GI tract. Acute interstitial nephritis, hepatotoxicity occur rarely.

NURSING CONSIDERATIONS

BASELINE ASSESSMENT

Question for history of hepatitis, allergies to azithromycin, erythromycins. Assess for infection (WBC count, appearance of wound, evidence of fever).

INTERVENTION/EVALUATION

Check for GI discomfort, nausea, vomiting. Monitor daily pattern of bowel activity and stool consistency. Monitor LFT, CBC. Assess for hepatotoxicity: malaise, fever, abdominal pain, GI disturbances. Be alert for superinfection: fever, vomiting, diarrhea, anal/genital pruritus, oral mucosal changes (ulceration, pain, erythema).

PATIENT/FAMILY TEACHING

• Continue therapy for full length of treatment. • Avoid concurrent administration of aluminum- or magnesium-containing antacids. • Bacterial conjunctivitis: Do not wear contact lenses.

aztreonam

az-**tree**-o-nam
(Azactam, Cayston)

◆CLASSIFICATION

PHARMACOTHERAPEUTIC: Monobactam. **CLINICAL:** Antibiotic.

USES

Injection: Treatment of infections caused by susceptible gram-negative microorganisms *P. aeruginosa, E. coli, S. marcescens, K. pneumoniae, P. mirabilis, H. influenzae, Enterobacter, Citrobacter* spp., including lower respiratory tract, skin/skin structure, intra-abdominal, gynecologic, complicated/uncomplicated UTIs; septicemia; cystic fibrosis. **Oral inhalation: (Cayston):** Improve respiratory symptoms in cystic fibrosis pts with *P. aeruginosa.* **OFF-LABEL:** Surgical prophylaxis.

PRECAUTIONS

Contraindications: Hypersensitivity to aztreonam. **Cautions:** History of allergy, esp. cephalosporins, penicillins; renal impairment; bone marrow transplant pts with risk factors for toxic epidermal necrolysis (TEN).

ACTION

Binds to penicillin-binding proteins, which inhibits bacterial cell wall synthesis. **Therapeutic Effect:** Bactericidal.

PHARMACOKINETICS

Completely absorbed after IM administration. Protein binding: 56%–60%. Partially metabolized by hydrolysis. Primarily excreted unchanged in urine. Removed by hemodialysis. **Half-life:** 1.4–2.2 hrs (increased in renal/hepatic impairment).

LIFESPAN CONSIDERATIONS

Pregnancy/Lactation: Crosses placenta, distributed in amniotic fluid; low concentration in breast milk. **Children:** Safety and efficacy not established in pts younger than 9 mos. **Elderly:** Age-related renal impairment may require dosage adjustment.

INTERACTIONS

DRUG: None significant. **HERBAL:** None significant. **FOOD:** None known. **LAB VALUES:** May increase serum alkaline phosphatase, creatinine, LDH, ALT, AST levels. Produces a positive Coombs' test. May prolong partial thromboplastin time (PTT), prothrombin time (PT).

AVAILABILITY (Rx)

Injection, Infusion Solution: ***(Azactam):*** Premix 1 g/50 mL, 2 g/50 mL. **Injection, Powder for Reconstitution:** ***(Azactam):*** 1 g, 2 g. **Oral Inhalation, Powder for Reconstitution:** ***(Cayston):*** 75 mg.

ADMINISTRATION/HANDLING

IV

Reconstitution • For IV push, dilute each gram with 6–10 mL Sterile Water for Injection. • For intermittent IV infusion, further dilute with 50–100 mL D_5W or 0.9% NaCl. Final concentration not to exceed 20 mg/mL.

Rate of administration • For IV push, give over 3–5 min. • For IV infusion, administer over 20–60 min.

Storage • Store vials at room temperature. • Solution appears colorless to light yellow. • Following reconstitution, solution is stable for 48 hrs at room temperature or 7 days if refrigerated. • Discard if precipitate forms. Discard unused portions.

IM

• Reconstitute with at least 3 mL diluent per gram of aztreonam. • Shake immediately, vigorously after adding diluent. • Inject deeply into large muscle mass. • Following reconstitution, solution is stable for 48 hrs at room temperature or 7 days if refrigerated.

Inhalation

• Administer only with an Altera nebulizer system. • Nebulize over 2–3 min. • Give bronchodilator 15 min–4 hrs (short-acting) or 30 min–12 hrs (long-acting) before administration. • Reconstituted solution must be used immediately.

IV INCOMPATIBILITIES

Acyclovir (Zovirax), amphotericin (Fungizone), LORazepam (Ativan), metroNIDAZOLE (Flagyl), vancomycin (Vancocin).

IV COMPATIBILITIES

Bumetanide (Bumex), calcium gluconate, cimetidine (Tagamet), diltiaZEM (Cardizem), diphenhydrAMINE (Benadryl), DOBUTamine (Dobutrex), DOPamine (Intropin), famotidine (Pepcid), furosemide (Lasix), heparin, HYDROmorphone (Dilaudid), insulin (regular), magnesium sulfate, morphine, potassium chloride, propofol (Diprivan).

INDICATIONS/ROUTES/DOSAGE

Severe Infections

IV: ADULTS, ELDERLY: 2 g q6–8h. **Maximum:** 8 g/day. **CHILDREN:** 30 mg/kg q6–8h. **Maximum:** 8 g/day (120 mg/kg/day).

Mild to Moderate Infections

IV: ADULTS, ELDERLY: 1–2 g q8–12h. **Maximum:** 8 g/day. **CHILDREN:** 30 mg/kg q8h. **Maximum:** 3,000 mg/day.

UTI

IM/IV: ADULTS, ELDERLY: 0.5–1 g q8–12h.

Usual Neonatal Dosage

IV: 30 mg/kg/dose q6–12h.

Cystic Fibrosis

Note: Pretreatment with a bronchodilator is recommended.

IV: CHILDREN: 50 mg/kg/dose q6–8h up to 200 mg/kg/day. **Maximum:** 8 g/day.

Inhalation (nebulizer): ADULTS, CHILDREN 7 YRS OR OLDER: 75 mg 3 times/day (at least 4 hrs apart) for 28 days, then off for 28-day cycle.

Dosage in Renal Impairment

Dosage and frequency are modified based on creatinine clearance and severity of infection:

Creatinine Clearance	Dosage
10–30 mL/min	50% usual dose at usual intervals
Less than 10 mL/min	25% usual dose at usual intervals
Hemodialysis	500 mg–2 g, then 25% of initial dose at usual interval
Continuous renal replacement therapy (CRRT)	2 g, then 1 g q8–12h or 2g q12h

Dosage in Hepatic Impairment

Use with caution.

SIDE EFFECTS

Frequent (greater than 5%): Cayston: Cough, nasal congestion, wheezing, pharyngolaryngeal pain, pyrexia, chest discomfort, abdominal pain, vomiting. **Occasional (less than 3%):** Discomfort and swelling at IM injection site, nausea, vomiting, diarrhea, rash. **Rare (less than 1%):** Phlebitis or thrombophlebitis at IV injection site, abdominal cramps, headache, hypotension.

ADVERSE EFFECTS/TOXIC REACTIONS

Antibiotic-associated colitis, other superinfections may result from altered bacterial balance in GI tract. Severe hypersensitivity reactions, including anaphylaxis, occur rarely.

NURSING CONSIDERATIONS

BASELINE ASSESSMENT

Question for history of allergies, esp. to aztreonam, other antibiotics.

INTERVENTION/EVALUATION

Evaluate for phlebitis, pain at IM injection site. Assess for GI discomfort, nausea, vomiting. Monitor daily pattern of bowel activity, stool consistency. Assess skin for rash. Be alert for superinfection: fever, vomiting, diarrhea, anal/genital pruritus, oral mucosal changes (ulceration, pain, erythema). Monitor renal/hepatic function.

PATIENT/FAMILY TEACHING

- Report nausea, vomiting, diarrhea, rash.

B

baclofen

bak-loe-fen
(Gablofen, Lioresal, Ozobax)

■ **BLACK BOX ALERT** ■ Abrupt withdrawal of intrathecal form has resulted in severe hyperpyrexia, obtundation, rebound or exaggerated spasticity, muscle rigidity, leading to organ failure, death.

Do not confuse baclofen with Bactroban or Beclovent, or Lioresal with lisinopril or Lotensin.

◆CLASSIFICATION

PHARMACOTHERAPEUTIC: Skeletal muscle relaxant. **CLINICAL:** Antispastic, analgesic in trigeminal neuralgia.

USES

Oral: Management of reversible spasticity associated with multiple sclerosis, spinal cord lesions. **Intrathecal:** Management of severe spasticity of spinal cord or cerebral origin in pts 4 yrs of age and older. **OFF-LABEL:** Treatment of bladder spasms, spasticity in cerebral palsy, intractable hiccups or pain, Huntington's chorea, trigeminal neuralgia.

PRECAUTIONS

Contraindications: Hypersensitivity to baclofen. **Intrathecal:** IV, IM, SQ, or epidural administration in addition to intrathecal use. **Cautions:** Renal impairment, seizure disorder, elderly, autonomic dysreflexia, reduced GI motility, GI or urinary obstruction; respiratory, pulmonary, peptic ulcer disease.

ACTION

Inhibits transmission of monosynaptic or polysynaptic reflexes at spinal cord level possibly by hyperpolarization of primary afferent fiber terminals. **Therapeutic Effect:** Relieves muscle spasticity.

PHARMACOKINETICS

Well absorbed from GI tract. Protein binding: 30%. Partially metabolized in liver. Primarily excreted in urine. **Half-life:** 2.5–4 hrs.

LIFESPAN CONSIDERATIONS

Pregnancy/Lactation: Unknown if crosses placenta or distributed in breast milk. **Children:** Safety and efficacy not established in pts younger than 12 yrs. Limited published data in children. **Elderly:** Increased risk of CNS toxicity (hallucinations, sedation, confusion, mental depression); age-related renal impairment may require decreased dosage.

INTERACTIONS

DRUG: **CNS depressants (e.g., alcohol, morphine, oxyCODONE, zolpidem)** may increase CNS depressant effect. **HERBAL:** **Herbals with sedative properties (e.g., chamomile, kava kava, valerian)** may increase CNS depression. **FOOD:** None known. **LAB VALUES:** May increase serum ALT, AST, alkaline phosphatase, glucose.

AVAILABILITY (Rx)

Intrathecal Injection Solution: 500 mcg/mL, 1,000 mcg/mL, 2,000 mcg/mL. **Oral Solution:** 5 mg/5 mL. **Tablets:** 5 mg, 10 mg, 20 mg.

ADMINISTRATION/HANDLING

PO

• Give with food or milk. • Tablets may be crushed.

Intrathecal

• For screening, a 50 mcg/mL concentration should be used for injection. • For maintenance therapy, solution should be diluted for pts who require concentrations other than 500 mcg/mL or 2,000 mcg/mL.

INDICATIONS/ROUTES/DOSAGE

◀ALERT▶ Avoid abrupt withdrawal.

B

Spasticity

PO: ADULTS, CHILDREN 12 YRS AND OLDER: Initially, 5 mg 3 times daily. May increase by 15 mg/day (5 mg/dose) at 3-day intervals until optimal response achieved. Range: 40–80 mg/day. **Maximum:** 80 mg/day. **ELDERLY:** Initially, 5 mg 2–3 times daily. May gradually increase dosage.

Intrathecal Dose

ADULTS, ELDERLY, CHILDREN 4 YRS AND OLDER: Initially, 50 mcg as screening dose (25 mcg in very small pediatric pts) for 1 dose; observe pt for 4–8 hrs for positive response (decrease in muscle tone and/or frequency and/or severity of spasm). If response is inadequate, give 75 mcg 24h after 1st dose. If response is still inadequate, give 100 mcg 24h after 2nd dose. Initial pump dose: give double screening dose (unless efficacy of bolus maintained greater than 8 hrs, then screening dose). After 24h, dose may be increased/decreased only once q24h until satisfactory response.

Dosage in Renal Impairment
Use caution.

Dosage in Hepatic Impairment
No dose adjustment.

SIDE EFFECTS

Frequent (greater than 10%): Transient drowsiness, asthenia, dizziness, nausea, vomiting. **Occasional (10%–2%):** Headache, paresthesia, constipation, anorexia, hypotension, confusion, nasal congestion. **Rare (less than 1%):** Paradoxical CNS excitement or restlessness, slurred speech, tremor, dry mouth, diarrhea, nocturia, impotence.

ADVERSE EFFECTS/TOXIC REACTIONS

Abrupt discontinuation may produce hallucinations, seizures. Overdose results in blurred vision, seizures, myosis, mydriasis, severe muscle weakness, strabismus, respiratory depression, vomiting.

NURSING CONSIDERATIONS

BASELINE ASSESSMENT

Record onset, type, location, duration of muscular spasm, pain. Check for immobility, stiffness, swelling.

INTERVENTION/EVALUATION

For pts on long-term therapy, BMP, LFT, CBC should be performed periodically. Assess for paradoxical reaction. Observe for drowsiness, dizziness, ataxia. Assist with ambulation at all times. Evaluate for therapeutic response: decreased intensity of skeletal muscle spasm, pain.

PATIENT/FAMILY TEACHING

• Drowsiness usually diminishes with continued therapy. • Avoid tasks that require alertness, motor skills until response to drug is established. • Do not abruptly withdraw medication after long-term therapy (may result in muscle rigidity, rebound spasticity, high fever, altered mental status). • Avoid alcohol, CNS depressants.

baricitinib

bar-i-**sye**-ti-nib
(Olumiant)

BLACK BOX ALERT Increased risk for developing bacterial, viral, invasive fungal infections including tuberculosis, cryptococcosis, pneumocystosis, that may lead to hospitalization or death. Infections often occurred in combination with immunosuppressants (methotrexate, other disease-modifying antirheumatic drugs). Closely monitor for development of infection. Test for latent tuberculosis prior to treatment and during treatment, regardless of initial result. Treatment of latent TB should be initiated before initiation. Lymphomas, other malignancies were reported. Thromboembolic events including DVT, pulmonary embolism, arterial thrombosis have occurred.

B

Do not confuse baricitinib with ceritinib, gefitinib, pacritinib, tofacitinib, or sunitinib.

◆CLASSIFICATION

PHARMACOTHERAPEUTIC: Janus-associated kinase inhibitor. **CLINICAL:** Antirheumatic agent. Disease modifying.

USES

Treatment of adults with moderately to severely active rheumatoid arthritis who have had an inadequate response to one or more TNF antagonist therapies. May be used alone or in combination with methotrexate or other nonbiologic disease-modifying antirheumatic drugs (DMARDs).

PRECAUTIONS

Hypersensitivity to baricitinib. **Cautions:** Baseline anemia, lymphopenia, neutropenia; hepatic/renal impairment, elderly, hypercholesterolemia; history of arterial or venous thromboembolic events (CVA, DVT, MI, PE), pts at risk for thrombosis (immobility, indwelling venous catheter/access device, morbid obesity, underlying atherosclerosis, genetic hypercoagulable conditions); recent travel or residence in TB or mycosis endemic areas; history of chronic opportunistic infections (esp. bacterial, invasive fungal, mycobacterial, protozoal, viral, TB); history of HIV, herpes zoster, hepatitis B or C virus infection; conditions predisposing to infection (e.g., diabetes, renal failure, immunocompromised pts, open wounds), pts at risk for GI perforation (e.g., Crohn's disease, diverticulitis, GI tract malignancies, peptic ulcers, peritoneal malignancies), pts who reside or travel to where TB is endemic. Concomitant use of strong organic anion transporter 2 (OAT3) inhibitors (e.g., probenecid), JAK inhibitors, biologic DMARDs, potent immunosuppressants (e.g., azathioprine or cyclosporine) not recommended.

ACTION

Inhibits JAK enzymes, which are intracellular enzymes involved in stimulating hematopoiesis and immune cell function via a signaling pathway. **Therapeutic Effect:** Reduces inflammation, tenderness, swelling of joints; slows or prevents progressive joint destruction in rheumatoid arthritis (RA).

PHARMACOKINETICS

Rapidly absorbed and widely distributed. Metabolized in liver. Protein binding: 50%. Peak plasma concentration: 1 hr. Excreted in urine (75%), feces (20%). **Half-life:** 12 hrs.

⧖ LIFESPAN CONSIDERATIONS

Pregnancy/Lactation: Unknown if distributed in breast milk. Breastfeeding not recommended. **Children:** Safety and efficacy not established. **Elderly:** Increased risk for serious infections, malignancy.

INTERACTIONS

DRUG: May diminish therapeutic effects of **live vaccines, BCG (intravesical). Immunosuppressants (e.g., azathioprine, cyclosporine)** may increase risk for added immunosuppression, infection. May enhance adverse/toxic effects of **biologic disease-modifying drugs (DMARDs), natalizumab, tacrolimus, tofacitinib, vaccines (live). Probenecid** may increase concentration/effect. **HERBAL: St. John's wort** may decrease concentration/effect. **FOOD:** None known. **LAB VALUES:** May increase serum ALT, AST, CPK, cholesterol (HDL, LDL, total), triglycerides; platelets. May decrease ANC, Hgb, absolute lymphocyte count.

AVAILABILITY (Rx)

Tablets: 1 mg, 2 mg.

ADMINISTRATION/HANDLING

PO

- Give without regard to food.

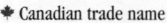

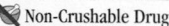

B

INDICATIONS/ROUTES/DOSAGE

◀ ALERT ▶ Do not initiate in pts with severe, active infection (systemic/localized), absolute lymphocyte count less than 500 cells/mm^3, ANC less than 1000 cells/mm^3, Hgb less than 8 g/dL. Do not use in combination with biologic DMARDs or with strong immunosuppressants (e.g., azathioprine or cyclosporine).

Rheumatoid Arthritis

PO: ADULTS, ELDERLY: 2 mg once daily.

Dose Modification

Anemia

Hgb less than 8 g/dL: Withhold treatment until Hgb is greater than or equal to 8 gm/dL.

Lymphopenia

Absolute lymphocyte count (ALC) less than 500 cells/mm^3: Withhold treatment until ALC is greater than or equal to 500 cells/mm^3.

Neutropenia

ANC less than 1000 cells/mm^3: Withhold treatment until ANC is greater than or equal to 1000 cells/mm^3.

Serious Infection

Withhold treatment until serious infection is resolved, then resume as clinically indicated.

Dosage in Renal Impairment

eGFR less than 60 mL/min: Not recommended.

Dosage in Hepatic Impairment

Mild to moderate impairment: No dose adjustment. **Severe impairment:** Not recommended.

SIDE EFFECTS

Rare (2%–1%): Nausea, acne.

ADVERSE EFFECTS/TOXIC REACTIONS

Neutropenia, lymphopenia may increase risk of infection. Serious and sometimes fatal infections (bacterial, mycobacterial, viral, invasive fungal, other opportunistic infection) may occur. Serious infections may include aspergillosis, BK virus, cellulitis, cryptococcosis, cytomegalovirus, esophageal candidiasis, herpes zoster histoplasmosis, listeriosis, pneumocystosis, pneumonia, tuberculosis, UTI, sepsis. Upper respiratory tract infections including epiglottitis, laryngitis, nasopharyngitis, pharyngitis, pharyngotonsillitis, sinusitis, tracheitis, tonsillitis reported in 16% of pts. May increase risk of new malignancies. May induce viral reactivation of hepatitis B or C virus infection, herpes zoster, HIV. Thrombosis including DVT, pulmonary embolism, arterial thrombosis have occurred. May increase risk of GI perforation. Platelet count greater than 600,000 cells/mm^3 occurred in 1% of pts.

NURSING CONSIDERATIONS

BASELINE ASSESSMENT

Obtain CBC, BMP, LFT, lipid panel; pregnancy test in females of reproductive potential. Assess onset, location, duration of pain, inflammation. Inspect appearance of affected joints for immobility, deformities. Evaluate for active TB and test for latent infection prior to and during treatment. Induration of 5 mm or greater with purified protein derivative (PPD) is considered a positive result when assessing for latent TB. Consider treatment with antimycobacterial therapy in pts with latent TB. Question history of arterial/venous thrombosis, hepatic/renal impairment, HIV infection, hepatitis B or C virus infection, diverticulitis, malignancies. Screen for active infection. Assess skin for open wounds. Receive full medication history and screen for interactions.

INTERVENTION/EVALUATION

Assess for therapeutic response: relief of pain, stiffness, swelling; increased joint mobility; reduced joint tenderness; improved grip strength. Monitor

CBC, LFT periodically. Monitor for TB regardless of baseline PPD. Consider discontinuation if acute infection, opportunistic infection, sepsis occurs; initiate appropriate antimicrobial therapy. Immediately report any hemorrhaging, melena, abdominal pain, hemoptysis (may indicate GI perforation). Monitor for symptoms of DVT (leg or arm pain/swelling), CVA (aphasia, altered mental status, headache, hemiplegia, vision loss), MI (chest pain, dyspnea, syncope, diaphoresis, arm/jaw pain), PE (chest pain, dyspnea, tachycardia).

PATIENT/FAMILY TEACHING

• Treatment may depress your immune system response and reduce your ability to fight infection. Report symptoms of infection such as body aches, chills, cough, fatigue, fever. Avoid those with active infection. • Expect routine tuberculosis screening. Report any travel plans to possible endemic areas. • Do not receive live vaccines. • Report symptoms of DVT (swelling, pain, hot feeling in the arms or legs; discoloration of extremity), lung embolism (difficulty breathing, chest pain, rapid heart rate), stroke (confusion, one-sided weakness or paralysis, difficulty speaking). • Treatment may cause life-threatening arterial blood clots; report symptoms of heart attack (chest pain, difficulty breathing, jaw pain, nausea, pain that radiates to the arm or jaw, sweating), stroke (blindness, confusion, one-sided weakness, loss of consciousness, trouble speaking, seizures). • Report symptoms of liver problems such as bruising, confusion, dark or amber-colored urine, right upper abdominal pain, or yellowing of the skin or eyes. • Immediately report severe or persistent abdominal pain, bloody stool, fever; may indicate tear in GI tract. • Treatment may cause reactivation of chronic viral infections, new cancers.

basiliximab

ba-si-**lik**-si-mab
(Simulect)

■ BLACK BOX ALERT ■ Must be prescribed by a physician experienced in immunosuppression therapy and organ transplant management.

Do not confuse basiliximab with daclizumab or brentuximab.

CLASSIFICATION

PHARMACOTHERAPEUTIC: Monoclonal antibody. **CLINICAL:** Immunosuppressive.

USES

Adjunct with cycloSPORINE, corticosteroids in prevention of acute organ rejection in pts receiving renal transplant. **OFF-LABEL:** Treatment of refractory graft-vs-host disease, prevention of liver or cardiac transplant rejection.

PRECAUTIONS

Contraindications: Hypersensitivity to basiliximab. **Cautions:** Re-exposure to subsequent courses of basiliximab.

ACTION

Binds to and blocks receptor of interleukin-2, a protein that stimulates proliferation of T lymphocytes, which play a major role in organ transplant rejection. **Therapeutic Effect:** Impairs response of immune system to antigens, prevents acute renal transplant rejection.

PHARMACOKINETICS

Half-life: 4–10 days (adults); 5–17 days (children).

LIFESPAN CONSIDERATIONS

Pregnancy/Lactation: Unknown if crosses placenta or distributed in breast milk. Breastfeeding not recommended. **Children/Elderly:** No age-related precautions noted.

B

INTERACTIONS

DRUG: May decrease therapeutic effect of **BCG (intravesical), vaccines (live).** May increase adverse effects of **belimumab, natalizumab, vaccines (live). HERBAL: Echinacea** may decrease therapeutic effect. **FOOD:** None known. **LAB VALUES:** May alter serum calcium, glucose, potassium; Hgb, Hct. May increase serum cholesterol, BUN, creatinine, uric acid. May decrease serum magnesium, phosphate; platelet count.

AVAILABILITY (Rx)

Injection, Powder for Reconstitution: 10 mg, 20 mg.

ADMINISTRATION/HANDLING

IV

Reconstitution • Reconstitute 10-mg vial with 2.5 mL or 20-mg vial with 5 mL Sterile Water for Injection. • Shake gently to dissolve. • May further dilute with 25–50 mL 0.9% NaCl or D_5W to a final concentration of 0.4 mg/mL. • Gently invert to avoid foaming. • Do not shake.

Rate of administration • Give as IV bolus over 10 min or as IV infusion over 20–30 min.

Storage • Refrigerate unused vials. • After reconstitution, use within 4 hrs (24 hrs if refrigerated). • Discard if precipitate forms.

IV INCOMPATIBILITIES

Specific information not available. Do not add other medications simultaneously through same IV line.

INDICATIONS/ROUTES/DOSAGE

Prophylaxis of Organ Rejection

IV: ADULTS, ELDERLY, CHILDREN WEIGHING 35 KG OR MORE: 20 mg within 2 hrs before transplant surgery and 20 mg 4 days after transplant. **CHILDREN WEIGHING LESS THAN 35 KG:** 10 mg within 2 hrs before transplant surgery and 10 mg 4 days after transplant.

Dosage in Renal/Hepatic Impairment

No dose adjustment.

SIDE EFFECTS

Frequent (greater than 10%): GI disturbances (constipation, diarrhea, dyspepsia), CNS effects (dizziness, headache, insomnia, tremor), respiratory tract infection, dysuria, acne, leg or back pain, peripheral edema, hypertension. **Occasional (10%–3%):** Angina, neuropathy, abdominal distention, tachycardia, rash, hypotension, urinary disturbances (urinary frequency, genital edema, hematuria), arthralgia, hirsutism, myalgia.

ADVERSE EFFECTS/TOXIC REACTIONS

Severe, acute hypersensitivity reactions including anaphylaxis characterized by bronchospasm, capillary leak syndrome, cytokine release syndrome, dyspnea, HF, hypotension, pulmonary edema, pruritus, respiratory failure, tachycardia, rash, urticaria, wheezing have been reported. May increase risk of cytomegalovirus infection.

NURSING CONSIDERATIONS

BASELINE ASSESSMENT

Obtain CBC, BMP, serum ionized calcium, phosphate, uric acid; vital signs, particularly B/P, pulse rate. Question current breastfeeding status.

INTERVENTION/EVALUATION

Diligently monitor CBC, electrolytes, renal function. Assess B/P for hypertension/hypotension, pulse for evidence of tachycardia. Question for GI disturbances, CNS effects, urinary changes. Monitor for presence of wound infection, signs of infection (fever, sore throat, unusual bleeding/bruising), hypersensitivity reaction.

PATIENT/FAMILY TEACHING

• Report difficulty in breathing or swallowing, palpitations, bruising/bleeding, rash, itching, swelling of lower extremities, weakness. • Female pts should take measures to avoid pregnancy; avoid breastfeeding.

B

beclomethasone

be-kloe-**meth**-a-sone
(Beconase AQ, QNASL, QVAR RediHaler)
Do not confuse beclomethasone with betamethasone or dexamethasone, or Beconase with baclofen.

◆CLASSIFICATION

PHARMACOTHERAPEUTIC: Adrenocorticosteroid. **CLINICAL:** Anti-inflammatory, immunosuppressant.

USES

Inhalation: Maintenance and prophylactic treatment of asthma in pts 5 yrs and older. **Intranasal: Beconase AQ:** Relief of seasonal/perennial rhinitis; prevention of nasal polyp recurrence after surgical removal; treatment of nonallergic rhinitis. **QNASL:** Treatment of seasonal and perennial allergic rhinitis in pts 4 yrs and older. **OFF-LABEL:** Prevention of seasonal rhinitis (nasal form).

PRECAUTIONS

Contraindications: Hypersensitivity to beclomethasone. **Oral Inhalation:** Acute exacerbation of asthma, status asthmaticus. **Cautions:** Cardiovascular disease, cataracts, diabetes, elderly, glaucoma, hepatic/renal impairment, myasthenia gravis, risk for osteoporosis, peptic ulcer disease, seizure disorder, thyroid disease, ulcerative colitis; following acute MI. Avoid use in pts with untreated viral, fungal, or bacterial systemic infections.

ACTION

Controls or prevents inflammation by altering rate of protein synthesis; depresses migration of polymorphonuclear leukocytes, fibroblasts; reverses capillary permeability. **Therapeutic Effect: Inhalation:** Inhibits bronchoconstriction, produces smooth muscle relaxation, decreases mucus secretion. **Intranasal:** Decreases response to seasonal, perennial rhinitis.

PHARMACOKINETICS

Rapidly absorbed from pulmonary, nasal, GI tissue. Metabolized in liver. Protein binding: 87%. Excreted in feces (60%), urine (12%). **Half-life:** 2–4.5 hrs.

⌛ LIFESPAN CONSIDERATIONS

Pregnancy/Lactation: Unknown if crosses placenta or distributed in breast milk. **Children:** Prolonged treatment/high dosages may decrease short-term growth rate, cortisol secretion. **Elderly:** No age-related precautions noted.

INTERACTIONS

DRUG: May enhance hyponatremic effect of **desmopressin.** May decrease effect of **aldesleukin, BCG (intravesical).** May increase adverse effects of **loxapine, natalizumab. HERBAL: Echinacea** may decrease effects. **FOOD:** None known. **LAB VALUES:** None significant.

AVAILABILITY (Rx)

Oral Inhalation: 40 mcg/inhalation, 80 mcg/inhalation. **Nasal Inhalation:** ***(Beconase AQ):*** 42 mcg/inhalation. ***(QNASL):*** 40 mcg/actuation, 80 mcg/actuation.

ADMINISTRATION/HANDLING

Inhalation

• Shake container well. • Instruct pt to exhale completely, place mouthpiece between lips, inhale, hold breath as long as possible before exhaling. • Allow at least 1 min between inhalations. • Rinse mouth after each use (decreases dry mouth, hoarseness, thrush).

Intranasal

• Instruct pt to clear nasal passages as much as possible before use. • Tilt pt's head slightly forward. • Insert spray tip into nostril, pointing toward nasal passages, away from nasal septum. • Spray into one nostril while pt

B

holds the other nostril closed, concurrently inhaling through nose to permit medication as high into nasal passages as possible.

INDICATIONS/ROUTES/DOSAGE

Asthma

Oral inhalation: *(QVAR):* **ADULTS, ELDERLY, CHILDREN 12 YRS AND OLDER:** (Pts not on inhaled corticosteroids): Initially 40–80 mcg twice daily. (Previously on inhaled corticosteroids): Initially, 40–320 mcg twice daily. **Maximum:** 320 mcg twice daily. **CHILDREN 5–11 YRS:** Initially, 40 mcg twice daily. **Maximum:** 80 mcg twice daily.

Rhinitis, Prevention of Recurrence of Nasal Polyps

Nasal inhalation: *(Beconase AQ):* **ADULTS, ELDERLY, CHILDREN 12 YRS AND OLDER:** 1–2 sprays (42 or 84 mcg) in each nostril twice daily. **Maximum:** 336 mcg/day. **CHILDREN 6–11 YRS:** 1 spray (42 mcg) in each nostril twice daily (total dose: 168 mcg daily). May increase to 2 sprays (84 mcg) 2 times/day (total dose 336 mcg daily). Once adequate control achieved, decrease to 1 spray (42 mcg) in each nostril twice daily (total dose: 168 mcg daily).

Allergic Rhinitis

Nasal inhalation: *(QNASL):* **ADULTS, ELDERLY, CHILDREN 12 YRS AND OLDER:** 80 mcg/spray: 2 sprays in each nostril daily. **Maximum:** 320 mcg (4 sprays/day). **CHILDREN 4–11 YRS:** 40 mcg/spray: 1 spray each nostril once daily. **Maximum:** 80 mcg/day.

Dosage in Renal/Hepatic Impairment

No dose adjustment.

SIDE EFFECTS

Frequent: Inhalation (14%–4%): Throat irritation, dry mouth, hoarseness, cough. **Intranasal:** Nasal burning, mucosal dryness. **Occasional: Inhalation** (3%–2%): Localized fungal infection (thrush). **Intranasal:** Nasal-crusting epistaxis, sore throat, ulceration of nasal mucosa. **Rare: Inhalation:** Transient bronchospasm, esophageal candidiasis. **Intranasal:** Nasal and pharyngeal candidiasis, eye pain.

ADVERSE EFFECTS/TOXIC REACTIONS

Acute hypersensitivity reaction (urticaria, angioedema, severe bronchospasm) occurs rarely. Change from systemic to local steroid therapy may unmask previously suppressed bronchial asthma condition.

NURSING CONSIDERATIONS

BASELINE ASSESSMENT

Establish baseline history for asthma, rhinitis. Question for hypersensitivity to corticosteroids.

INTERVENTION/EVALUATION

Monitor respiratory status. Auscultate lung sounds. Observe for signs of oral candidiasis. In pts receiving bronchodilators by inhalation concomitantly with inhaled steroid therapy, advise use of bronchodilator several minutes before corticosteroid aerosol (enhances penetration of steroid into bronchial tree).

PATIENT/FAMILY TEACHING

• Do not change dose schedule or stop taking drug; must taper off gradually under medical supervision. • **Inhalation:** Maintain diligent oral hygiene. • Rinse mouth with water immediately after inhalation (prevents mouth/throat dryness, fungal infection of mouth). • Report sore throat or mouth. • **Intranasal:** Report symptoms that do not improve; or if sneezing, nasal irritation occurs. • Clear nasal passages prior to use. • Improvement may take days to several weeks.

belatacept

bel-**at**-a-sept
(Nulojix)

■ BLACK BOX ALERT ■ Must be administered by personnel trained in administration/handling of immunosuppression therapy. Increased risk of malignancies, infection. Increased risk of posttransplant lymphoproliferative disorder (PTLD), mainly in central nervous system. Not recommended for hepatic transplants due to increased risk of graft loss, death.

◆CLASSIFICATION

PHARMACOTHERAPEUTIC: Selective T-cell costimulation blocker. **CLINICAL:** Immunosuppressive agent.

USES

Prevention of acute organ rejection in pts receiving kidney transplants (in combination with basiliximab induction, mycophenolate mofetil, corticosteroids). For use in Epstein-Barr virus (EBV) seropositive kidney transplant recipients.

PRECAUTIONS

Contraindications: Hypersensitivity to belatacept. Transplant pts who are Epstein-Barr virus (EBV) seronegative or unknown sero-status. **Cautions:** History of opportunistic infections: bacterial, mycobacterial, invasive fungal, viral, protozoal (e.g., histoplasmosis, aspergillosis, candidiasis, coccidioidomycosis, listeriosis, HIV, tuberculosis, pneumocystosis). Recent open wounds, ulcerations. Not recommended in liver transplants. Avoid use of live vaccines.

ACTION

Fusion protein acting as a selective T-cell (lymphocyte) costimulation blocker (binds to CD80 and CD86 receptors on antigen presenting cells [APC]). **Therapeutic Effect:** Blocks reaction between APC and T cells needed to activate T lymphocytes. Prevents renal transplant rejection.

PHARMACOKINETICS

Half-life: 8–10 days.

LIFESPAN CONSIDERATIONS

Pregnancy/Lactation: Unknown if crosses placenta or distributed in breast milk. Must either discontinue breastfeeding or discontinue drug. **Children:** Safety and efficacy not established. **Elderly:** No age-related precautions noted.

INTERACTIONS

DRUG: May decrease therapeutic effect of **BCG (intravesical), vaccines (live).** May increase adverse effects of **belimumab, natalizumab, vaccines (live). HERBAL: Echinacea** may reduce therapeutic effect. **FOOD:** None known. **LAB VALUES:** May increase serum potassium, cholesterol, uric acid, glucose; urine protein. May decrease serum calcium, magnesium, phosphate, potassium; Hgb, Hct, WBC.

AVAILABILITY (Rx)

Lyophilized Powder for Injection: 250 mg per vial.

ADMINISTRATION/HANDLING

◀ALERT▶ Use only silicone-free disposable syringe provided. Using different syringe may produce translucent particles. Administer via dedicated line only.

IV

Reconstitution • Reconstitute vial with 10.5 mL of suitable diluent (0.9% NaCl, D_5W or Sterile Water for Injection) using provided syringe, 18- to 20-gauge needle. • Direct stream to glass wall (avoids foaming). • Swirl gently (do not shake). • Discard if opaque particles, discoloration, or foreign particles are present. • Infusion bag must match diluent (0.9% NaCl with 0.9% NaCl, D_5W with D_5W; may use Sterile Water for Injection with NaCl or D_5W). • To mix infusion bag, withdraw and discard volume equal to the volume of reconstituted solution. • Using same silicone-free disposable syringe, gently inject reconstituted solution into 100- to 250-mL bag (based on concentration). • Final concentration of infusion bag should range from 2 mg/mL to 10 mg/mL. • IV infusion stable for 24 hrs at room temperature.

Rate of administration • Infuse over 30 min using infusion set with a 0.2- to 1.2-micron low-protein-binding filter.

Storage • Refrigerate vials. • Solution should be clear to slightly opalescent and colorless to slightly yellow. • May refrigerate solution up to 24 hrs. • Discard if reconstituted solution remains at room temperature longer than 24 hrs.

INDICATIONS/ROUTES/DOSAGE

Note: Dosage based on actual body weight at time of transplantation. Do not modify dose unless a change in body weight is greater than 10%.

Prophylaxis of Acute Kidney Transplant Rejection (in Combination With an Immunosuppressant)

IV: ADULTS, ELDERLY: Initial phase: 10 mg/kg on day 1 (day of transplantation, prior to implantation), day 5, end of wks 2, 4, 8, and 12 after transplantation. **Maintenance:** 5 mg/kg end of wk 16 following transplantation, then q4wks thereafter (plus or minus 3 days).

Dosage Modification

Infusion is based on actual body weight at the time of transplantation; modify dose for weight changes greater than 10% during treatment. Prescribed dose must be evenly divisible by 12.5 to match closest increment (0, 12.5, 25, 37.5, 50, 62.5, 75, 87.5, 100) in mg. For example, the actual dose for a 64-kg pt is 637.5 mg or 650 mg, not 640 mg.

Dosage in Renal/Hepatic Impairment

No dose adjustment.

SIDE EFFECTS

Frequent (45%–20%): Anemia, diarrhea, UTI, peripheral edema, constipation, hypertension, pyrexia, nausea, cough, vomiting, headache. **Occasional (19%–5%):** Abdominal pain, hypotension, arthralgia, hematuria, upper respiratory infection, insomnia, nasopharyngitis, back pain, dyspnea, influenza, dysuria, bronchitis, stomatitis, anxiety, dizziness, abdominal pain, muscle tremor, acne, alopecia, hyperhidrosis.

ADVERSE EFFECTS/TOXIC REACTIONS

Serious conditions, including malignancies (esp. skin cancer), progressive multifocal leukoencephalopathy (caused by JC virus), cytomegalovirus, polyoma virus nephropathy, viral reactivation (herpes zoster, hepatitis), may occur. Other opportunistic infections (bacterial, fungal, viral, protozoal) may cause tuberculosis, cryptococcal meningitis, Chagas' disease, West Nile encephalitis, Guillain-Barré syndrome, cerebral aspergillosis. Additional complications, including chronic allograft nephropathy, renal tubular necrosis, renal artery necrosis, atrial fibrillation, hematoma at incision site, wound dehiscence, lymphocele, arteriovenous fistula thrombosis, hydronephrosis, urinary incontinence, anti-belatacept antibody formation, were reported.

NURSING CONSIDERATIONS

BASELINE ASSESSMENT

Obtain baseline CBC, serum chemistries, renal function, glomerular filtration rate (GFR). Evaluate pt for active tuberculosis or latent infection prior to initiating treatment and periodically during therapy. Induration of 5 mm or greater with tuberculin skin test should be considered a positive result when assessing whether treatment for latent tuberculosis is necessary. Assess baseline mental status to compare any worsening cognitive symptoms. Obtain Epstein-Barr virus (EBV) serology prior to treatment (contraindicated in pts who are EBV seronegative). Note any skin

B

discoloration, ulcers, excoriation, lesions. Question history of hypertension/hypotension, arrhythmia, diabetes, HIV. Receive full medication history. Question possibility of pregnancy.

INTERVENTION/EVALUATION

Monitor B/P, vital signs, I&O, weight. Monitor CBC, renal function, serum electrolytes (hypokalemia may result in changes in muscle strength, muscle cramps, altered mental status, cardiac arrhythmias). Routinely monitor serum glucose levels for new-onset diabetes after transplantation, corticosteroid use. Monitor for fever, tenderness over transplantation site, skin lesions, changing characteristics of moles, neurologic deterioration related to PTLD or PML.

PATIENT/FAMILY TEACHING

• Therapy may increase risk of malignancies and life-threatening infections. • Treatment is given with immunosuppressive therapy with basiliximab induction, corticosteroids. • Report history of HIV, opportunistic infections, hepatitis, coughing of blood, or close relatives with active tuberculosis. • Avoid sunlight, sunlamps. • Seek immediate attention if toxic reactions occur. • Do not receive live vaccines. • Report pregnancy or plans of becoming pregnant. • Adhere to strict dosing schedule. • Report chest pain, palpitations, edema, fever, night sweats, weight loss, swollen glands, flu-like symptoms, stomach pain, vomiting, diarrhea, weakness, or urinary changes (color, frequency, odor, concentration, burning, blood).

belinostat

beh-**lih**-noh-**stat**
(Beleodaq)

◆CLASSIFICATION

PHARMACOTHERAPEUTIC: Histone deacetylase (HDAC) inhibitor. **CLINICAL:** Antineoplastic.

USES

Treatment of relapsed or refractory peripheral T-cell lymphoma (PTCL).

PRECAUTIONS

Contraindications: Hypersensitivity to belinostat. **Cautions:** Pts with high tumor burden, hx of hepatic impairment, thrombocytopenia. Avoid use in pts with active infection.

ACTION

Inhibits enzymatic activity of histone deacetylases by catalyzing removal of acetyl groups from lysine residues of histones and nonhistone proteins. **Therapeutic Effect:** Inhibits tumor cell growth and metastasis; causes tumor cellular death (apoptosis).

PHARMACOKINETICS

Limited tissue distribution. Metabolized in liver. Protein binding: 93%–95%. Excreted primarily in urine. **Half-life:** 1.1 hrs.

LIFESPAN CONSIDERATIONS

Pregnancy/Lactation: Avoid pregnancy; may cause fetal harm. Females of reproductive potential must use effective contraception during treatment and for at least 6 mos after discontinuation. Unknown if distributed in breast milk. Breastfeeding not recommended during treatment and for at least 2 wks after discontinuation. May impair fertility. **Males:** Males with female partners of reproductive potential must use effective contraception during treatment and for at least 3 mos after discontinuation. **Children:** Safety and efficacy not established. **Elderly:** No age-related precautions noted.

INTERACTIONS

DRUG: **Strong UGT1A1 inhibitors (e.g., atazanavir)** may increase concentration/effect. May decrease therapeutic effect of **BCG (intravesical)**. **HERBAL:** None known. **FOOD:** None significant. **LAB VALUES:** May decrease ANC, Hgb/Hct, lymphocytes, platelets, WBC; serum potassium. May increase blood lactic dehydrogenase, serum creatinine.

B

AVAILABILITY (Rx)

Lyophilized Powder for Injection: 500 mg vial.

ADMINISTRATION/HANDLING

IV

Reconstitution • Maintain standard chemotherapy preparation and handling precautions. • Reconstitute each vial with 9 mL of Sterile Water for Injection, using suitable syringe for final concentration of 50 mg/mL. • Gently swirl contents until completely dissolved. • Visually inspect for particulate matter. • Do not use if cloudiness or particulate matter observed. • Withdraw required dosage and mix into infusion bag containing 250 mL of 0.9% NaCl.

Rate of administration • Infuse over 30 min using 0.22-micron in-line filter. • May extend infusion time to 45 min if infusion site pain or other infusion-related symptoms occur.

Storage • Reconstituted vial may be stored at room temperature (max 77°F/25°C) for up to 12 hrs. • Infusion bag may be stored at room temperature (max 77°F/25°C) for up to 36 hrs.

INDICATIONS/ROUTES/DOSAGE

Peripheral T-Cell Lymphoma

IV infusion: ADULTS/ELDERLY: 1,000 mg/m^2 once daily on days 1–5 of a 21-day cycle. Cycles may be repeated every 21 days until disease progression or unacceptable toxicity.

Dose Modification

ANC should be greater than or equal to 1,000 cells/mm^3 and platelet count greater than or equal to 50,000 cells/mm^3 prior to start of each cycle or prior to resuming treatment following toxicity. Discontinue treatment if ANC nadir less than 500 cells/mm^3 or recurrent platelet count nadir less than 25,000 cells/mm^3 after two dose reductions. Other toxicities must be Grade 2 or less prior to resuming treatment.

Hematologic Toxicities

Platelet count greater than 25,000 cells/mm^3 or ANC greater than 500 cells/mm^3: No change. **Platelet count less than 25,000 cells/mm^3 or ANC less than 500 cells/mm^3:** Decrease dose by 25% (750 mg/m^2).

Nonhematologic Toxicities

Any Grade 3 or 4: Decrease dose by 25% (750 mg/m^2). **Recurrence of Grade 3 or 4 adverse reaction after two dosage reductions:** Discontinue treatment. **Nausea, vomiting, diarrhea:** Only modify dose if duration is greater than 7 days with supportive management. **Pts with reduced UGT1A1 activity:** Reduce starting dose to 750 mg/m^2 in pts known to be homozygous for UGT1A1*28 allele.

Dosage in Renal/Hepatic Impairment

No dose adjustment.

SIDE EFFECTS

Frequent (47%–29%): Nausea, fatigue, pyrexia, vomiting, anemia. **Occasional (23%–10%):** Constipation, diarrhea, dyspepsia, rash, peripheral edema, cough, pruritus, chills, decreased appetite, headache, infusion site pain, abdominal pain, hypotension, phlebitis, dizziness.

ADVERSE EFFECTS/TOXIC REACTIONS

Anemia, lymphopenia, neutropenia, thrombocytopenia are expected responses to therapy. Serious and sometimes fatal infections including pneumonia, sepsis have occurred. May cause hepatotoxicity, LFT abnormalities, tumor lysis syndrome. GI toxicities including severe diarrhea, nausea, vomiting may require use of antiemetic and antidiarrheal medication or result in dosage reduction. Nineteen percent of pts required treatment discontinuation related to toxic anemia, febrile neutropenia, multiorgan failure, ventricular fibrillation (rare).

B

NURSING CONSIDERATIONS

BASELINE ASSESSMENT

Obtain ANC, CBC, BMP, LFT, vital signs; pregnancy test in females of reproductive potential. Question history of anemia, arrhythmias, hepatic impairment, peripheral edema, or if pt homozygous for UGT1A1 allele (may require reduced starting dose). Screen for active infection. Receive full medication history including herbal products.

INTERVENTION/EVALUATION

Monitor blood counts (esp. ANC, Hgb/Hct, WBC, platelet count) weekly; hepatic/renal function prior to start of first dose of each cycle, vital signs. Monitor for symptoms of hypokalemia. Screen for tumor lysis syndrome (electrolyte imbalance, uric acid nephropathy, acute renal failure). Obtain ECG if arrhythmia, palpitations occur. Monitor for infections (cough, fatigue, fever). If serious infection or sepsis occurs, initiate appropriate antimicrobial therapy. Offer antiemetics if nausea, vomiting occurs.

PATIENT/FAMILY TEACHING

• Blood levels will be routinely monitored. • Avoid pregnancy; treatment may cause birth defects or miscarriage. Do not breastfeed. • Report any abdominal pain, black/tarry stools, bruising, yellowing of skin or eyes, dark urine, decreased urine output. • Severe diarrhea may lead to dehydration. • Body aches, burning with urination, chills, cough, difficulty breathing, fever may indicate an acute infection.

bempedoic acid (Nexletol)

bem-pe-**doe**-ik-**as**-id
(Nexletol)
Do not confuse Nexletol with Tegretol or nadolol.

◆CLASSIFICATION

PHARMACOTHERAPEUTIC: Adenosine triphosphate–citrate lyase (ACL) inhibitor. **CLINICAL:** Antihyperlipidemic agent.

USES

Adjunct to diet and maximally tolerated statin therapy for the treatment of adults with heterozygous familial hypercholesterolemia (HeFH) or established atherosclerotic cardiovascular disease who require additional lowering of LDL-C.

PRECAUTIONS

Contraindications: Hypersensitivity to bempedoic acid. **Cautions:** History of hyperuricemia, gout; pts at risk for tendon rupture (e.g., renal failure, previous tendon rupture, concomitant use of corticosteroids or fluoroquinolone drugs; pts older than 60 yrs of age). Avoid concomitant use of simvastatin dose greater than 20 mg; pravastatin dose greater than 40 mg.

ACTION

Inhibits cholesterol synthesis in the liver. Interferes with hepatic cholesterol biosynthesis by inhibiting adenosine triphosphate–citrate lyase and HMG-COA reductase. **Therapeutic Effect:** Lowers LDL-C.

PHARMACOKINETICS

Widely distributed. Metabolized in liver. Protein binding: 99%. Peak plasma concentration: 3.5 hrs. Steady state reached in 7 days. Excreted in urine (70%), feces (30%). **Half-life:** 21 ± 11 hrs.

⌛ LIFESPAN CONSIDERATIONS

Pregnancy/Lactation: Avoid pregnancy; may cause fetal harm. May possibly effect the synthesis of biologically active substances in breast milk that are derived from cholesterol, which may cause fetal harm. Breastfeeding not recommended. **Children:** Safety and efficacy not established. **Elderly:** May have increased risk of tendon rupture.

B

INTERACTIONS

DRUG: May increase concentration/risk of myopathy of pravastatin, simvastatin. May increase concentration/effects of elagolix, eluxadoline, grazoprevir, revefenacin, voxilaprevir. **HERBAL:** **Red yeast** may increase risk of myopathy. **FOOD:** None known. **LAB VALUES:** May increase serum ALT, AST, BUN, creatine kinase, creatinine, uric acid; platelets. May decrease Hgb, leukocytes.

AVAILABILITY (Rx)

Tablets: 180 mg.

ADMINISTRATION/HANDLING

PO

- Give without regard to food.

INDICATIONS/ROUTES/DOSAGE

HeFH, Hyperlipidemia

PO: ADULTS, ELDERLY: 180 mg once daily.

Dosage in Renal Impairment

Mild to moderate impairment: No dose adjustment. **Severe impairment, ESRD:** Not specified; use caution.

Dosage in Hepatic Impairment

Mild to moderate impairment: No dose adjustment. **Severe impairment:** Not specified; use caution.

SIDE EFFECTS

Rare (3%): Muscle spasm, back pain, abdominal pain, extremity pain.

ADVERSE EFFECTS/TOXIC REACTIONS

Hyperuricemia reported in 26% of pts. Tendon rupture (e.g., Achilles tendon, biceps tendon, rotator cuff), tendonitis reported in less than 1% of pts. Tendon rupture may occur more frequently in pts with renal failure, previous tendon rupture; pts taking concomitant corticosteroids or fluoroquinolone drugs; pts older than 60 yrs of age. Upper respiratory tract infection reported in 5% of pts. Bronchitis reported in 3% of pts. Atrial fibrillation, gout reported in 2% of pts. Benign prostatic hyperplasia reported in 1% of pts.

NURSING CONSIDERATIONS

BASELINE ASSESSMENT

Obtain baseline lipid levels; pregnancy test in female pts of reproductive potential. Obtain dietary history, esp. fat consumption. Question history of gout, tendon rupture, tendonitis. Question use of concomitant corticosteroids or fluoroquinolones (due to increased risk of tendon rupture).

INTERVENTION/EVALUATION

Obtain lipid levels within 8–12 wks after initiation. Monitor for tendon rupture, tendonitis (joint pain, swelling, inflammation, popping). Obtain CK level if myopathy (muscle atrophy/pain/weakness, dyspnea, gait disturbance) is suspected. Monitor for hyperuricemia (joint pain/inflammation/redness).

PATIENT/FAMILY TEACHING

• Maintain proper diet and exercise. • Tendon inflammation/swelling, tendon rupture may occur; report bruising, pain, swelling, snapping, or popping of joints/tendons. Certain antibiotics/steroids may increase risk of tendon rupture. • Report signs of myopathy (e.g., muscle pain/weakness, shortness of breath, difficulty rising from chair or walking upstairs), gout (e.g., joint pain/swelling/redness/warmth). • Treatment may cause fetal harm; avoid pregnancy. Do not breastfeed.

benazepril

ben-**ay**-ze-pril

(Lotensin)

■ BLACK BOX ALERT ■ May cause fetal injury, mortality. Discontinue as soon as possible once pregnancy is detected.

Do not confuse benazepril with enalapril, lisinopril, or Benadryl, or Lotensin with Lioresal.

B

FIXED-COMBINATION(S)

Lotensin HCT: benazepril/hydrochlorothiazide (a diuretic): 5 mg/6.25 mg, 10 mg/12.5 mg, 20 mg/12.5 mg, 20 mg/25 mg. **Lotrel:** benazepril/amLODIPine (a calcium blocker): 2.5 mg/10 mg, 5 mg/10 mg, 5 mg/20 mg, 5 mg/40 mg, 10 mg/20 mg, 10 mg/40 mg.

◆CLASSIFICATION

PHARMACOTHERAPEUTIC: Angiotensin-converting enzyme (ACE) inhibitor. **CLINICAL:** Antihypertensive.

USES

Treatment of hypertension. Used alone or in combination with other antihypertensives.

PRECAUTIONS

Contraindications: Hypersensitivity to benazepril. History of angioedema with or without previous treatment with ACE inhibitors. Use with aliskiren in pts with diabetes. Coadministration with or within 36 hrs of switching to or from a neprilysin inhibitor (e.g., sacubitril). **Cautions:** Renal impairment; hypertrophic cardiomyopathy without flow tract obstruction; severe aortic stenosis; before, during, or immediately following major surgery; unstented renal artery stenosis; diabetes mellitus, pregnancy, breastfeeding. Concomitant use of potassium-sparing diuretics, potassium supplements.

ACTION

Decreases rate of conversion of angiotensin I to angiotensin II, a potent vasoconstrictor. Results in lower levels of angiotensin II, causing an increase in plasma renin activity and decreased aldosterone secretion. **Therapeutic Effect:** Lowers B/P.

PHARMACOKINETICS

Route	Onset	Peak	Duration
PO	1 hr	2–4 hrs	24 hrs

Partially absorbed from GI tract. Protein binding: 97%. Metabolized in liver. Primarily excreted in urine. Minimal removal by hemodialysis. **Half-life:** 35 min; metabolite, 10–11 hrs.

⌛ LIFESPAN CONSIDERATIONS

Pregnancy/Lactation: Crosses placenta. Unknown if distributed in breast milk. May cause fetal, neonatal mortality or morbidity. **Children:** Safety and efficacy not established. **Elderly:** May be more sensitive to hypotensive effects.

INTERACTIONS

DRUG: **Aliskiren** may increase hyperkalemic effect. May increase potential for allergic reactions to **allopurinol. Angiotensin II receptor blockers (ARB) (e.g., losartan, valsartan)** may increase adverse effects. May increase adverse effects of **lithium, sacubitril.** **HERBAL:** **Herbals with hypertensive properties (e.g., licorice, yohimbe)** or **hypotensive properties (e.g., garlic, ginger, ginkgo biloba)** may alter effects. **FOOD:** None known. **LAB VALUES:** May increase serum potassium, ALT, AST, alkaline phosphatase, bilirubin, BUN, creatinine, glucose. May decrease serum sodium; Hgb, Hct. May cause positive ANA titer.

AVAILABILITY (Rx)

Tablets: 5 mg, 10 mg, 20 mg, 40 mg.

ADMINISTRATION/HANDLING

- Give without regard to food.

INDICATIONS/ROUTES/DOSAGE

Hypertension (Monotherapy)

PO: ADULTS, ELDERLY: Initially, 5–10 mg/day. Titrate based on pt response up to 40 mg daily in 1 or 2 divided doses. **CHILDREN 6 YRS AND OLDER:** Initially, 0.2 mg/kg/day (up to 10 mg/day). Maintenance: 0.1–0.6 mg/kg/day. **Maximum:** 0.6 mg/kg or 40 mg/day.

Hypertension (Combination Therapy)

PO: ADULTS: Discontinue diuretic 2–3 days before initiating benazepril, then dose

B

as noted above. If unable to discontinue diuretic, begin benazepril at 5 mg/day.

Dosage in Renal Impairment

CrCl less than 30 mL/min: ADULTS: Initially, 5 mg/day titrated up to maximum of 40 mg/day. **CHILDREN:** Not recommended. **HD, PD:** 25%–50% of usual dose; supplement dose not necessary.

Dosage in Hepatic Impairment

Use caution.

SIDE EFFECTS

Frequent (6%–3%): Cough, headache, dizziness. **Occasional (2%):** Fatigue, drowsiness, nausea. **Rare (less than 1%):** Rash, fever, myalgia, diarrhea, loss of taste.

ADVERSE EFFECTS/TOXIC REACTIONS

Excessive hypotension ("first-dose syncope") may occur in pts with HF, severe salt or volume depletion. Angioedema, hyperkalemia occur rarely. Agranulocytosis, neutropenia may be noted in pts with renal impairment, collagen vascular disease (scleroderma, systemic lupus erythematosus). Nephrotic syndrome may occur in pts with history of renal disease.

NURSING CONSIDERATIONS

BASELINE ASSESSMENT

Obtain CBC before therapy begins and q2wks for 3 mos, then periodically thereafter. Obtain B/P immediately before each dose, in addition to regular monitoring (be alert to fluctuations).

INTERVENTION/EVALUATION

Assist with ambulation if dizziness occurs. Monitor B/P, renal function, urinary protein, serum potassium. Monitor CBC with differential if pt has collagen vascular disease or renal impairment. If excessive reduction in B/P occurs, place pt in supine position with legs elevated. Monitor pt with renal impairment, autoimmune disease, or taking drugs that affect leukocytes or immune response.

PATIENT/FAMILY TEACHING

• To reduce hypotensive effect, go from lying to standing slowly. • Full therapeutic effect may take 2–4 wks. • Skipping doses or noncompliance with drug therapy may produce severe rebound hypertension. • Report dizziness, persistent cough.

bendamustine

ben-da-**mus**-teen
(Belrapzo, Bendeka, Treanda)
Do not confuse bendamustine with carmustine or lomustine.

◆CLASSIFICATION

PHARMACOTHERAPEUTIC: Alkylating agent. **CLINICAL:** Antineoplastic.

USES

Treatment of chronic lymphocytic leukemia (CLL). Treatment of indolent B-cell non-Hodgkin's lymphoma (NHL) that has progressed during or within 6 mos of treatment with riTUXimab or a riTUXimab-containing regimen. **OFF-LABEL:** Treatment of mantle cell lymphoma, relapsed multiple myeloma. First-line treatment for follicular lymphoma. Treatment of Waldenström's macroglobulinemia.

PRECAUTIONS

Contraindications: Hypersensitivity to bendamustine. (Bendeka only): polyethylene glycol 400, or propylene glycol mono-thioglycerol. **Cautions:** Baseline cytopenias, hepatic/renal impairment, conditions predisposing to infection (e.g., diabetes, renal failure, immunocompromised pts, open wounds); dermatologic disease, HF, dehydration; pts at high risk for tumor lysis syndrome (high tumor burden); history of hepatitis B virus infection, herpes zoster infection.

ACTION

Alkylates and cross-links double-stranded DNA. **Therapeutic Effect:** Inhibits tumor cell growth, causes cell death.

PHARMACOKINETICS

Metabolized in liver and via hydrolysis to metabolites. Protein binding: 94%–96%. Excreted in urine (50%), feces (25%). **Half-life:** 40 min.

LIFESPAN CONSIDERATIONS

Pregnancy/Lactation: May cause fetal harm. Unknown if distributed in breast milk. Impaired spermatogenesis, azoospermia have been reported in male pts. **Children:** Safety and efficacy not established. **Elderly:** No age-related precautions noted.

INTERACTIONS

DRUG: **CYP1A2 inducers (e.g., carbamazepine, rifampicin)** may decrease concentration/effect. **CYP1A2 inhibitors (e.g., ciprofloxacin, fluvoxamine)** may increase concentration/effect. **Allopurinol** may increase risk of severe skin toxicities. May decrease therapeutic effect of **BCG (intravesical). HERBAL:** None significant. **FOOD:** None known. **LAB VALUES:** May increase serum AST, bilirubin, creatinine, glucose, uric acid. May decrease WBCs, neutrophils, Hgb, platelets; serum potassium, sodium, calcium.

AVAILABILITY (Rx)

Injection Powder for Reconstitution: ***(Treanda):*** 25 mg, 100 mg. **Injection:** ***(Belrapzo, Bendeka):*** 100 mg/4 mL.

ADMINISTRATION/HANDLING

IV

Reconstitution • Reconstitute each 100-mg vial with 20 mL Sterile Water for Injection (25-mg vial with 5 mL) for final concentration of 5 mg/mL. • Powder should completely dissolve in 5 min. • Discard if particulate matter is observed. • Withdraw volume needed for required dose (based on 5 mg/mL concentration) and immediately transfer to 500-mL infusion bag of 0.9% NaCl for final concentration of 0.2–0.6 mg/mL. • Reconstituted solution must be transferred to infusion bag within 30 min of reconstitution. • After transferring, thoroughly mix contents of infusion bag.

Rate of administration • Infuse over 30 min for CLL or 60 min for NHL.

Storage • Reconstituted solution should appear clear and colorless to pale yellow. • Final solution is stable for 24 hrs if refrigerated or 3 hrs at room temperature. • Administration must be completed within these stability time frames.

INDICATIONS/ROUTES/DOSAGE

◀ALERT▶ Antiemetics are recommended to prevent nausea and vomiting.

Chronic Lymphocytic Leukemia

IV infusion: ADULTS/ELDERLY: 100 mg/m^2 given over 30 min daily on days 1 and 2 of a 28-day cycle as a single agent, up to 6 cycles.

Non-Hodgkin's Lymphoma

IV infusion: ADULTS/ELDERLY: 120 mg/m^2 on days 1 and 2 of a 21-day cycle as a single agent, up to 8 cycles.

Dose Modification

Hematologic toxicity Grade 4 or greater: Withhold until ANC 1,000 cells/mm^3 or greater, platelet 75,000 cells/mm^3 or greater. **CLL: toxicity Grade 3 or greater:** Reduce dose to 50 mg/m^2 on days 1 and 2 of each treatment cycle. **Recurrence:** Reduce dose to 25 mg/^{2} on days 1 and 2 of each cycle. **NHL: hematologic toxicity Grade 4 or nonhematologic toxicity Grade 3 or greater:** Reduce dose to 90 mg/m^2 on days 1 and 2 of each cycle. **Recurrence:** Reduce dose to 60 mg/m^2 on days 1 and 2 of each treatment cycle.

Dosage in Renal Impairment

Not recommended in pts with CrCl less than 30 mL/min.

Dosage in Hepatic Impairment

Not recommended in pts with serum ALT/AST 2.5–10 times ULN and total bilirubin

B

1.5–3 times ULN, or total bilirubin greater than 3 times ULN.

SIDE EFFECTS

Note: Frequency and occurrence of side effects may vary depending on indication of treatment.

Frequent (75%–21%): Nausea, fatigue, vomiting, anorexia, diarrhea, pyrexia, constipation, decreased appetite, cough, headache. **Occasional (18%–6%):** Decreased weight, rash, dyspnea, stomatitis, dehydration, back pain, dizziness, chills, peripheral edema, abdominal pain, insomnia, dyspepsia, asthenia, pharyngeal pain, anxiety, dysgeusia, tachycardia, depression, chest pain, infusion site pain, catheter site pain, arthralgia, pruritus, hypotension. **Rare (5%):** Extremity pain, bone pain, abdominal distension, wheezing, nasal congestion, dry skin, night sweats, hyperhidrosis.

ADVERSE EFFECTS/TOXIC REACTIONS

Grade 3–4 myelosuppression reported in 98% of pts. Infections including sepsis, septic shock, herpes zoster, upper respiratory tract infection, UTI, sinusitis, pneumonia, febrile neutropenia, oral candidiasis, nasopharyngitis were reported. Reactivation of cytomegalovirus, hepatitis B virus, mycobacterium tuberculosis, herpes zoster was reported. Tumor lysis syndrome may present as acute renal failure, hypocalcemia, hyperuricemia, hyperphosphatemia. Infusion reactions (e.g., chills, fever, pruritus, rash), anaphylaxis were reported. Fatal skin reactions including Stevens-Johnson syndrome, toxic epidermal necrolysis, DRESS syndrome (drug reaction with eosinophilia and systemic symptoms, also known as multiorgan hypersensitivity) have been reported. DRESS may present with facial swelling, eosinophilia, fever, lymphadenopathy, rash, which may be associated with other organ systems, such as hepatitis, hematologic abnormalities, myocarditis, nephritis. Serious, sometimes fatal, hepatotoxicity may occur. Premalignant and malignant disease including myelodysplastic syndrome, myeloproliferative disorders, acute myeloid leukemia, bronchial carcinoma were reported. Skin and soft tissue infusion site extravasation with secondary cellulitis, exfoliation may occur. Other reactions may include acute renal failure, cardiac failure, pulmonary fibrosis, hemolysis, dermatitis, skin necrosis, atrial fibrillation, myocardial infarction, pneumonitis.

NURSING CONSIDERATIONS

BASELINE ASSESSMENT

Obtain CBC, BMP, LFT; pregnancy test in females of reproductive potential. Screen for active infection. Assess usual bowel movement patterns, stool characteristics. Ensure adequate hydration in pts at risk for tumor lysis syndrome. Question history of hepatic/renal impairment; history of hepatitis B virus infection, herpes zoster infection. Verify use of effective contraception in female pts of reproductive potential. Conduct baseline dermatologic exam. Receive full medication history and screen for interactions. Ensure patency of IV access. Offer emotional support.

INTERVENTION/EVALUATION

Monitor CBC for myelosuppression; BMP; LFT for hepatotoxicity; renal function (CrCl, GFR). Hematologic nadirs usually occur in 3rd wk of therapy. An increase of serum creatinine greater than 0.4 mg/dL from baseline may indicate renal injury. Obtain serum calcium, phosphate, uric acid if tumor lysis syndrome is suspected (presents as acute renal failure, electrolyte imbalance, cardiac arrhythmias, seizures). Monitor for infusion-related reactions, hypersensitivity reactions (anaphylaxis, chills, fever, rash), renal toxicity (anuria, hypertension, generalized edema, flank pain), extravasation injuries (redness, swelling, pain, necrosis of injection site), secondary malignancies, HBV reactivation (amber- to orange-colored urine, fatigue, jaundice, nausea, vomiting). Assess skin for dermal toxicities, DRESS. Monitor daily pattern of bowel activity, stool consistency; I&Os. Ensure adequate hydration, nutrition. Monitor for infections (cough, fatigue, fever). If serious infection, sepsis occurs, initiate appropriate antimicrobial therapy.

PATIENT/FAMILY TEACHING

• Treatment may depress your immune system response and reduce your ability to fight infection. Report symptoms of infection such as body aches, chills, cough, fatigue, fever. Avoid those with active infection. • Report symptoms of bone marrow depression such as bruising, fatigue, fever, shortness of breath, weight loss; bleeding easily, bloody urine or stool. • Therapy may cause life-threatening tumor lysis syndrome (a condition caused by the rapid breakdown of cancer cells), which can cause kidney failure. Report decreased urination, amber-colored urine; confusion, difficulty breathing, fatigue, fever, muscle or joint pain, palpitations, seizures, vomiting. • Treatment may cause diarrhea, dehydration. Drink plenty of fluids. • Use effective contraception. Do not breastfeed. • Report symptoms of liver problems (abdominal pain, bruising, clay-colored stool, amber- or dark-colored urine, yellowing of the skin or eyes), kidney problems (decreased urine output, flank pain, darkened urine), skin reactions (rash, skin eruptions); UTI (fever, urinary frequency, burning during urination, foul-smelling urine), skin problems (rash, sloughing, necrotic tissue, dermal toxicity).•Report symptoms of drug-induced hypersensitivity syndrome (fever, swollen face/lymph nodes, skin rash/peeling/inflammation). • Allergic reactions such as chills, fever, rash may occur during infusion. Anaphylaxis (difficulty breathing, low blood pressure, severe rash, swelling of lips and tongue, rapid heart rate, can be life threatening. If allergic reaction occurs, seek immediate medical attention. • Treatment may cause reactivation of chronic viral infections, new cancers.

benralizumab

ben-ra-**liz**-ue-mab
(Fasenra)
Do not confuse benralizumab with certolizumab, daclizumab, eculizumab, efalizumab, mepolizumab, natalizumab, omalizumab, pembrolizumab, reslizumab, tocilizumab, or vedolizumab.

◆CLASSIFICATION

PHARMACOTHERAPEUTIC: Interleukin-5 receptor alpha-directed cytolytic. Monoclonal antibody. **CLINICAL:** Antiasthmatic.

USES

Add-on maintenance treatment of pts with severe asthma, aged 12 yrs and older, and with an eosinophilic phenotype.

PRECAUTIONS

Contraindications: Hypersensitivity to benralizumab. **Cautions:** History of helminth (parasite) infection; long-term use of corticosteroids. Not indicated for treatment of other eosinophilic conditions; relief of acute bronchospasm or status asthmaticus.

ACTION

Exact mechanism unknown. Inhibits signaling of interleukin-5 cytokine, reducing production and survival of eosinophils responsible for asthmatic inflammation and pathogenesis. **Therapeutic Effect:** Prevents inflammatory process; relieves signs/symptoms of asthma.

B

PHARMACOKINETICS

Widely distributed. Degraded into small peptides and amino acids via proteolytic enzymes. **Half-life:** 15 days.

LIFESPAN CONSIDERATIONS

Pregnancy/Lactation: Unknown if distributed in breast milk. However, human immunoglobulin G is present in breast milk and is known to cross placenta. **Children:** Safety and efficacy not established in pts younger than 12 yrs. **Elderly:** No age-related precautions noted.

INTERACTIONS

DRUG: May increase adverse effects of **belimumab. HERBAL:** None significant. **FOOD:** None known. **LAB VALUES:** None known.

AVAILABILITY (Rx)

Injection Solution (Prefilled Syringe, Auto-Injector): 30 mg/mL.

ADMINISTRATION/HANDLING

SQ

Preparation • Remove prefilled syringe from refrigerator and allow solution to warm to room temperature (approx. 30 min) with needle cap intact. • Visually inspect for particulate matter or discoloration. Solution should appear clear, colorless to slightly yellow in color. Do not use if solution is cloudy, discolored, or visible particles are observed.

Administration • Follow manufacturer guidelines regarding use of plunger. • Insert needle subcutaneously into upper arm, outer thigh, or abdomen and inject solution. • Do not inject into areas of active skin disease or injury such as sunburns, skin rashes, inflammation, skin infections, or active psoriasis. • Do not administer IV or intramuscularly. • Rotate injection sites.

Storage • Refrigerate prefilled syringes in original carton until time of use. Once warmed to room temperature, do not place back into refrigerator. • Do not freeze or expose to heating sources. • Do not shake. • Protect from light.

INDICATIONS/ROUTES/DOSAGE

Asthma (Severe)

SQ: ADULTS, ELDERLY, CHILDREN: 30 mg once q4wks for the first 3 doses, then once q8wks thereafter.

Dosage in Renal/Hepatic Impairment

Not specified; use caution.

SIDE EFFECTS

Occasional (8%–3%): Headache, pyrexia.

ADVERSE EFFECTS/TOXIC REACTIONS

Hypersensitivity reactions including anaphylaxis, angioedema, bronchospasm, hypotension, urticaria, rash were reported. Hypersensitivity reactions typically occurred hrs to days after administration. Infections including bacterial/viral pharyngitis may occur. Unknown if treatment will influence the immunological response to helminth (parasite) infection. Immunogenicity (auto-benralizumab antibodies) reported in 13% of pts.

NURSING CONSIDERATIONS

BASELINE ASSESSMENT

Obtain apical pulse, oxygen saturation. Auscultate lung fields. Question history of parasitic infection, hypersensitivity reaction. Pts with preexisting helminth (parasite) infection should be treated prior to initiation. Inhaled or systemic corticosteroids should not be suddenly discontinued upon initiation. Corticosteroids that are not gradually reduced may cause withdraw symptoms or unmask conditions that were originally suppressed with corticosteroid therapy.

INTERVENTION/EVALUATION

Monitor rate, depth, rhythm of respirations. Assess lungs for wheezing, rales. Monitor oxygen saturation. Interrupt or discontinue treatment if hypersensitivity reaction, opportunistic infection (esp. parasite infection, herpes zoster infection); worsening of asthma-related symptoms (esp. in pts tapering off corticosteroids) occurs. Obtain pulmonary function test to assess disease improvement.

Monitor for increased use of rescue inhalers; may indicate deterioration of asthma.

PATIENT/FAMILY TEACHING

• Treatment not indicated for relief of acute asthmatic episodes. • Have a rescue inhaler readily available. • Increased use of rescue inhaler may indicate worsening of asthma. • Seek medical attention if asthma symptoms worsen or remain uncontrolled after starting therapy. • Immediately report allergic reactions such as difficulty breathing, itching, hives, rash, swelling of the face or tongue. • Report infections of any kind. • Do not stop corticosteroid therapy unless directed by prescriber.

bethanechol

be-**than**-e-kole
(Duvoid ✱, Urecholine)
Do not confuse bethanechol with betaxolol.

◆CLASSIFICATION

PHARMACOTHERAPEUTIC: Parasympathomimetic choline ester. **CLINICAL**: Cholinergic.

USES

Treatment of acute postoperative and postpartum nonobstructive urinary retention, neurogenic atony of urinary bladder with retention. **OFF-LABEL**: Treatment of gastroesophageal reflux.

PRECAUTIONS

Contraindications: Hypersensitivity to bethanechol. Mechanical obstruction of GI/GU tract, GI or bladder wall instability, hyperthyroidism, asthma, peptic ulcer disease, epilepsy, pronounced bradycardia or hypotension, parkinsonism, CAD, vasomotor instability, bladder neck obstruction, spastic GI disturbances, acute inflammatory lesions of the GI tract, peritonitis, marked vagotonia. **Cautions**: Bladder reflux infection.

ACTION

Stimulates parasympathetic nervous system, increasing bladder muscle tone and causing contractions, which initiates urination. Also stimulates gastric motility, increasing gastric tone, and may restore peristalsis. **Therapeutic Effect:** May initiate urination, bladder emptying. Stimulates gastric, intestinal motility.

PHARMACOKINETICS

Route	Onset	Peak	Duration
PO	30–90 min	60 min	6 hrs

Poorly absorbed following PO administration. Does not cross blood-brain barrier. **Half-life:** Unknown.

⌛ LIFESPAN CONSIDERATIONS

Pregnancy/Lactation: Unknown if crosses placenta or distributed in breast milk. **Children/Elderly**: No age-related precautions noted.

INTERACTIONS

DRUG: **Beta blockers (e.g., labetalol, metoprolol), anticholinesterase inhibitors (e.g., donepezil, rivastigmine)** may increase effect/toxicity. **HERBAL**: None significant. **FOOD**: None known. **LAB VALUES**: May increase serum amylase, lipase, ALT, AST.

AVAILABILITY (Rx)

Tablets: 5 mg, 10 mg, 25 mg, 50 mg.

ADMINISTRATION/HANDLING

PO

• Administer 1 hr before or 2 hrs after meals.

INDICATIONS/ROUTES/DOSAGE

Nonobstructive Urinary Retention, Neurogenic Bladder

PO: ADULTS, ELDERLY: Usual dose: 10–50 mg 3–4 times/day. Minimum effective dose determined by giving 5–10 mg initially, repeating same amount at 1-hr intervals until desired response is achieved or a maximum of 50 mg is reached.

B

Dosage in Renal/Hepatic Impairment
No dose adjustment.

SIDE EFFECTS

Occasional: Belching, changes in vision, blurred vision, diarrhea, urinary urgency or frequency. **Rare:** Dyspnea, chest tightness, bronchospasm.

ADVERSE EFFECTS/TOXIC REACTIONS

Overdose produces CNS stimulation (insomnia, anxiety, orthostatic hypotension), cholinergic stimulation (headache, increased salivation/diaphoresis, nausea, vomiting, flushed skin, abdominal pain, seizures).

NURSING CONSIDERATIONS

BASELINE ASSESSMENT

Ensure pt has emptied bladder prior to procedure.

INTERVENTION/EVALUATION

Monitor urine output. Palpate bladder for evidence of urinary retention.

PATIENT/FAMILY TEACHING.

- Report nausea, vomiting, diarrhea, diaphoresis, increased salivary secretions, irregular heartbeat, muscle weakness, severe abdominal pain, difficulty breathing.

bevacizumab

TOP 100 HIGH ALERT

be-va-**siz**-ue-mab
(Avastin, Mvasi, Zirabev)

■ BLACK BOX ALERT ■ May result in development of GI perforation, presented as intra-abdominal abscess, fistula, wound dehiscence, wound healing complications. Severe, sometimes fatal, hemorrhagic events including central nervous system/GI/vaginal bleeding, epistaxis, hemoptysis, pulmonary hemorrhage have occurred.

Do not confuse Avastin with Astelin, or bevacizumab with cetuximab or riTUXimab.

◆CLASSIFICATION

PHARMACOTHERAPEUTIC: Vascular endothelial growth factor (VEGF) inhibitor. Monoclonal antibody. **CLINICAL:** Antineoplastic.

USES

First- or second-line combination chemotherapy with 5-fluorouracil (5-FU) for treatment of pts with colorectal cancer. Second-line treatment of colorectal cancer after progression of first-line treatment with bevacizumab. Treatment with CARBOplatin and PACLitaxel for nonsquamous, non–small-cell lung cancer (NSCLC). Treatment of renal cell carcinoma (metastatic) with interferon alfa, brain cancer (glioblastoma) that has progressed following prior therapy. Treatment of platinum-resistant recurrent epithelial ovarian, fallopian tube, or primary peritoneal cancer (in combination with PACLitaxel, DOXOrubicin [liposomal] or topotecan). Treatment of stage III or IV epithelial ovarian, fallopian tube, or primary peritoneal cancer following initial surgical resection (in combination with carboplatin and paclitaxel), then single-agent bevacizumab. Treatment of platinum-sensitive ovarian cancer. Treatment of persistent, recurrent, or metastatic cervical cancer (in combination with PACLitaxel and either CISplatin or topotecan). **OFF-LABEL:** Adjunctive therapy in malignant mesothelioma, ovarian cancer, prostate cancer, age-related macular degeneration. Treatment of metastatic breast cancer.

PRECAUTIONS

Contraindications: Hypersensitivity to bevacizumab. **Cautions:** Cardiovascular disease, acquired coagulopathy, preexisting hypertension, pts at risk of thrombocytopenia. Pts with CNS metastasis. Do not administer within 28 days of major surgery or active bleeding. Pts at risk for hemorrhage (e.g., history of GI bleeding, fistulas, coagulation disorders, recent trauma; concomitant use of anticoagulants, NSAIDS, antiplatelets), History of thromboembolism (CVA, DVT,

MI], transient ischemic attack [TIA]), GI perforation or hemorrhage; pts at risk for thrombosis (immobility, indwelling venous catheter/access device, morbid obesity, genetic hypercoagulable conditions).

ACTION

Binds to and neutralizes vascular endothelial growth factor, preventing association with endothelial receptors. **Therapeutic Effect:** Inhibition of microvascular growth retards growth of all tissue, including metastatic tissue.

PHARMACOKINETICS

Clearance varies by body weight, gender, tumor burden. **Half-life:** 20 days (range: 11–50 days).

LIFESPAN CONSIDERATIONS

Pregnancy/Lactation: May possess teratogenic effects. Potential for fertility impairment. May decrease maternal and fetal body weight, increase risk of skeletal fetal abnormalities. Breastfeeding not recommended. **Children:** Safety and efficacy not established. **Elderly:** Higher incidence of severe adverse reactions in pts older than 65 yrs.

INTERACTIONS

DRUG: May increase cardiotoxic effect of **anthracyclines.** May decrease therapeutic effect of **BCG (intravesical).** May increase adverse effects of **belimumab. Sunitinib** may increase adverse effects. **HERBAL:** None significant. **FOOD:** None known. **LAB VALUES:** May decrease Hgb, Hct, platelet count, WBC; serum potassium, sodium. May increase urine protein.

AVAILABILITY (Rx)

Injection Solution: 100 mg/4 mL, 400 mg/16 mL vials.

ADMINISTRATION/HANDLING

IV

◀ALERT▶ Do not give by IV push or bolus.

Reconstitution • Dilute prescribed dose in 100 mL 0.9% NaCl. • Avoid dextrose-containing solutions. • Discard any unused portion.

Rate of administration • Usually given following other chemotherapy. Infuse initial dose over 90 min. • If first infusion is well tolerated, second infusion may be administered over 60 min. • If 60-min infusion is well tolerated, all subsequent infusions may be administered over 30 min.

Storage • Diluted solution may be stored for up to 8 hrs if refrigerated.

IV INCOMPATIBILITIES

Do not mix with dextrose solutions.

INDICATIONS/ROUTES/DOSAGE

Colorectal Cancer (With Fluorouracil-Based Chemotherapy)

IV: ADULTS, ELDERLY: 5 mg/kg q2wks (in combination with bolus-IFL) or 10 mg/kg q2wks in combination with FOLFOX4).

Colorectal Cancer Progression (Following Initial Bevacizumab/Fluorouracil-Based Chemotherapy)

IV: ADULTS, ELDERLY: 5 mg/kg q2wks or 7.5 mg/kg q3wks (in combination with fluoropyrimidine-irinotecan– or fluoropyrimidine-oxaliplatin–based regimen).

Non–Small-Cell Lung Cancer (NSCLC)

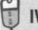

IV: ADULTS, ELDERLY: 15 mg/kg q3wks (in combination with CARBOplatin and PACLitaxel) for 6 cycles.

Metastatic Renal Cell Carcinoma

IV: ADULTS, ELDERLY: 10 mg/kg once q2wks (with interferon alfa).

Brain Cancer

IV: ADULTS, ELDERLY: 10 mg/kg q2wks (as monotherapy).

Ovarian Cancer (Platinum-Resistant)

IV: ADULTS, ELDERLY: 10 mg/kg q2wks with PACLitaxel, DOXOrubicin (liposomal), or wkly topotecan or 15 mg/kg q3wks (with topotecan q3wks).

B

Ovarian Cancer (Platinum-Sensitive)
IV: ADULTS, ELDERLY: 15 mg/kg q3wks with CARBOplatin/PACLitaxel for 6–8 cycles, then 15 mg/kg q3wks as a single agent or 15 mg/kg with CARBOplatin/gemcitabine for 6–10 cycles, then 15 mg/kg q3wks as a single agent. Continue until disease progression or unacceptable toxicity.

Ovarian Cancer (Following Initial Surgery)
IV: ADULTS, ELDERLY: 15 mg/kg q3wks with CARBOplatin/PACLitaxel for 6 cycles, then 15 mg/kg q3wks as a single agent for total of up to 22 cycles. Continue until disease progression.

Cervical Cancer
IV: ADULTS, ELDERLY: 15 mg/kg q3wks (in combination with PACLitaxel and either CISplatin or topotecan). Continue until disease progression or unacceptable toxicity.

Dose Adjustment for Toxicity
Temporary suspension: Mild to moderate proteinuria, severe hypertension not controlled with medical management. **Permanent discontinuation:** Wound dehiscence requiring intervention, GI perforation, tracheoesophageal fistula, Grade 4 fistula, fistula formation involving any internal organ, hypertensive crisis, serious bleeding, nephrotic syndrome, arterial or venous thromboembolism, hypertensive encephalopathy, posterior reversible encephalopathy syndrome, severe infusion reaction, HF.

Dosage in Renal/Hepatic Impairment
No dose adjustment.

SIDE EFFECTS

Frequent (73%–25%): Asthenia, vomiting, anorexia, hypertension, epistaxis, stomatitis, constipation, headache, dyspnea. **Occasional (21%–15%):** Altered taste, dry skin, exfoliative dermatitis, dizziness, flatulence, excessive lacrimation, skin discoloration, weight loss, myalgia. **Rare (8%–6%):** Nail disorder, skin ulcer, alopecia, confusion, abnormal gait, dry mouth.

ADVERSE EFFECTS/TOXIC REACTIONS

Fatal GI perforations reported in up to 3% of pts. Serious fistula formations in bladder, biliary, bronchopleural, tracheoesophageal, renal, vaginal sites may occur. Necrotizing fasciitis due to poor wound healing complications, GI perforation may occur. Severe bleeding events including CNS hemorrhage, GI bleeding, epistaxis, hemoptysis, hematemesis, pulmonary hemorrhage, vaginal bleeding were reported. Thromboembolic events including CVA, DVT, MI, TIA. Posterior reversible encephalopathy syndrome (PRES) reported in less than 1% of pts. Renal injury, proteinuria, nephrotic syndrome may occur. Infusion-related reactions including altered mental status, chest pain, diaphoresis, hypertension crisis, hypoxia, rigors, wheezing may occur. Palmar-plantar erythrodysesthesia (redness, swelling, numbness, skin sloughing of the hands and feet) reported in 5% of pts. Other reactions may include ovarian failure, HF.

NURSING CONSIDERATIONS

BASELINE ASSESSMENT

Obtain baseline CBC, serum potassium, sodium levels at regular intervals during therapy. Assess for proteinuria with urinalysis. For pts with 2+ or greater urine dipstick reading, a 24-hr urine collection is advised. Question history as listed in PRECAUTIONS. Screen for active infection.

INTERVENTION/EVALUATION

Monitor CBC for myelosuppression; renal function (CrCl, GFR). Monitor for GI perforation, GI bleeding, bloody stool; symptoms of intracranial bleeding (aphasia, blindness, confusion, facial droop, hemiplegia, seizures); symptoms of MI (chest pain, diaphoresis, left arm/jaw pain, increased serum troponin, ST segment elevation), CVA (aphasia, altered mental status, facial droop, hemiplegia, vision loss), DVT (leg or arm pain/swelling), PE (chest pain, dyspnea, tachycardia), HF (dyspnea, peripheral edema, palpitations, exercise intolerance). Monitor B/P for hypertension. Persistent hypertension despite medical management may indicate hypertensive crisis. Reversible posterior leukoencephalopathy syndrome should be considered in pts with seizure, headache, visual disturbances, confusion, altered mental status. An increase of serum creatinine greater than 0.4 mg/dL from baseline may indicate renal injury. Monitor for infusion-related reactions. Assess proteinuria with urinalysis. Monitor daily pattern of bowel activity, stool consistency.

PATIENT/FAMILY TEACHING

• Treatment may depress your immune system and reduce your ability to fight infection. Report symptoms of infection such as body aches, burning with urination, chills, cough, fatigue, fever. Avoid those with active infection. • Treatment may worsen high blood pressure. • Therapy may cause life-threatening blood clots or bleeding; report symptoms of heart attack (chest pain, difficulty breathing, jaw pain, nausea, pain that radiates to the left arm, sweating), DVT (swelling, pain, hot feeling in the arms or legs; discoloration of extremity), stroke (confusion, difficulty speaking, one-sided weakness or paralysis, loss of vision). • Stomach/pelvic pain, vomiting, fever may indicate GI perforation (tear). • Neurologic changes including altered mental status, seizures, headache, blurry vision, trouble speaking, one-sided weakness may indicate stroke, high blood pressure crisis, or life-threatening brain swelling. • Report abdominal pain, vomiting, constipation, headache. • Do not receive immunizations without physician's approval (lowers body's resistance). • Avoid pregnancy.

bictegravir/emtricitabine/tenofovir

bik-**teg**-ra-vir/**em**-trye-**sye**-ta-been/ten-**oh**-foe-veer
(Biktarvy)

BLACK BOX ALERT Serious, sometimes fatal lactic acidosis and severe hepatomegaly with steatosis (fatty liver) have been reported. Severe exacerbations of hepatitis B virus (HBV) reported in pts co-infected with HIV-1 and HBV following discontinuation. If discontinuation occurs, monitor hepatic function for at least several months. Initiate anti-HBV therapy if warranted.

Do not confuse bictegravir/emtricitabine/tenofovir (Biktarvy) with elvitegravir/cobicistat/emtricitabine/tenofovir (Stribild), emtricitabine/rilpivirine/tenofovir (Complera), efavirenz/emtricitabine/tenofovir (Atripla), or emtricitabine/tenofovir (Truvada).

FIXED-COMBINATION(S)

Biktarvy: bictegravir/emtricitabine/tenofovir: 50 mg/200 mg/25 mg.

CLASSIFICATION

PHARMACOTHERAPEUTIC: Integrase inhibitor, nucleoside reverse transcriptase inhibitor, nucleotide reverse transcriptase inhibitor. **CLINICAL:** Antiretroviral.

USES

Indicated as complete regimen for treatment of HIV-1 infection in adults who are antiretroviral naïve or to replace the current antiretroviral regimen in pts who are virologically suppressed (HIV-1 RNA less than 50 copies/mL) on a stable antiretroviral regimen for at least 3 mos with no history of treatment failure and no known substitutions associated with resistance to the individual components of bictegravir/emtricitabine/tenofovir.

B

PRECAUTIONS

Contraindications: Hypersensitivity to bictegravir/emtricitabine/tenofovir. Concomitant use of dofetilide, rifampin. **Cautions:** Mild to moderate hepatic/renal impairment. History of depression, suicidal ideation; hepatitis B or C virus infection. Concomitant use of nephrotoxic medications. Not recommended in pts with creatinine clearance less than 30 mL/min; severe hepatic impairment.

ACTION

Bictegravir inhibits strand transfer activity of HIV-1 integrase, essential for viral replication. Emtricitabine inhibits HIV-1 reverse transcriptase by competing with natural substrates, resulting in chain termination. Tenofovir inhibits HIV reverse transcriptase by interfering with HIV viral RNA-dependent DNA polymerase. **Therapeutic Effect:** Interferes with HIV replication, slowing progression of HIV infection.

PHARMACOKINETICS

Widely distributed. Bictegravir metabolized in liver. Emtricitabine phosphorylated by cellular enzymes. Tenofovir metabolized by enzymatic hydrolysis, mediated by macrophages and hepatocytes. Protein binding: (bictegravir): greater than 99%; (emtricitabine): less than 4%; (tenofovir): 80%. Peak plasma concentration: (bictegravir): 2–4 hrs; (emtricitabine): 1.5–2 hrs; (tenofovir): 0.5–2 hrs. Bictegravir excreted in feces (60%), urine (35%). Emtricitabine excreted in urine (70%), feces (14%). Tenofovir excreted in urine, feces (32%), (less than 1%). **Half-life:** (bictegravir): 17 hrs; (emtricitabine): 10 hrs; (tenofovir): 0.5 hrs.

⌛ LIFESPAN CONSIDERATIONS

Pregnancy/Lactation: Breastfeeding not recommended due to risk of postnatal HIV transmission. Distributed in breast milk. **Children:** Safety and efficacy not established. **Elderly:** Not specified; use caution.

INTERACTIONS

DRUG: May significantly increase concentration/effect of **dofetilide** (contraindicated). **Rifampin** may significantly decrease concentration/effect (contraindicated). **Carbamazepine, oxcarbazepine, phenobarbital, primidone** may decrease concentration of tenofovir. **Adefovir, fosphenytoin, phenytoin** may decrease therapeutic effect of tenofovir. **HERBAL:** **St. John's wort** may decrease concentration/effect of bictegravir, tenofovir. **FOOD:** None known. **LAB VALUES:** May increase serum amylase, ALT, AST, cholesterol, creatine kinase, creatinine. May decrease neutrophils.

AVAILABILITY (Rx)

Fixed-Dose Combination Tablets: bictegravir 50 mg/emtricitabine 200 mg/tenofovir 25 mg.

ADMINISTRATION/HANDLING

PO

• Give without regard to food. • Administer at least 2 hrs before medications containing aluminum, calcium, iron, magnesium (supplements, antacids, laxatives).

INDICATIONS/ROUTES/DOSAGE

HIV Infection

PO: ADULTS, ELDERLY: 1 tablet once daily.

Dosage in Renal Impairment

CrCl greater than or equal to 30 mL/min: No dose adjustment. **CrCl less than or equal to 30 mL/min:** Not recommended.

Dosage in Hepatic Impairment

Mild to moderate impairment: No dose adjustment. **Severe impairment:** Not recommended.

SIDE EFFECTS

Occasional (6%–2%): Diarrhea, nausea, headache, fatigue, abnormal dreams, dizziness, insomnia, vomiting, flatulence, dyspepsia, abdominal pain, rash.

ADVERSE EFFECTS/TOXIC REACTIONS

If therapy is discontinued, pts coinfected with hepatitis B virus have an increased risk for viral replication, worsening of hepatic function, and may experience hepatic decompensation and/or failure. May induce immune reconstitution syndrome (inflammatory response to dormant opportunistic infections, such as *Mycobacterium avium*, cytomegalovirus, PCP, tuberculosis, or acceleration of autoimmune disorders such as Graves' disease, polymyositis, Guillain-Barré). Acute renal failure, Fanconi syndrome (renal tubular injury with severe hypophosphatemia) were reported. Fatal cases of lactic acidosis, severe hepatomegaly with steatosis have occurred. Suicidal ideation, depression, suicide attempt reported in less than 1% of pts (primarily occurred in pts with prior psychiatric illness).

NURSING CONSIDERATIONS

BASELINE ASSESSMENT

Obtain BUN, serum creatinine, creatinine clearance, GFR; CD4+ count, viral load, HIV-1 RNA level; urine glucose, urine protein. Obtain serum phosphate level in pts with chronic kidney disease. Test all pts for hepatitis B virus infection. Question history of depression, suicidal ideation. Receive full medication history (including herbal products); screen for contraindications/interactions. Offer emotional support.

INTERVENTION/EVALUATION

Monitor CD4+ count, viral load, HIV-1 RNA level for treatment effectiveness. Monitor renal function as clinically indicated. An increase in serum creatinine greater than 0.4 mg/dL from baseline may indicate renal impairment. If discontinuation of drug regimen occurs, monitor hepatic function for at least several months. Initiate anti-HBV therapy if warranted. Cough, dyspnea, fever, excess of band cells on CBC may indicate acute infection (WBC count may be unreliable in pts with uncontrolled HIV infection). Screen for immune reconstitution syndrome. Monitor daily pattern of bowel activity, stool consistency; I&Os.

PATIENT/FAMILY TEACHING

• Drug resistance can form if therapy is interrupted; do not run out of supply. • As immune system strengthens, it may respond to dormant infections hidden within the body. Report body aches, chills, cough, fever, night sweats, shortness of breath. • Treatment may cause kidney failure. Report flank pain, darkened urine, decreased urine output. • Practice safe sex with barrier methods or abstinence. • Lactating females should not breastfeed.

binimetinib

bin-i-**me**-ti-nib
(Mektovi)
Do not confuse binimetinib with alectinib, bosutinib, brigatinib, cobimetinib, encorafenib, neratinib or trametinib, or Mektovi with Mekinist.

◆CLASSIFICATION

PHARMACOTHERAPEUTIC: Mitogen-activated extracellular (MEK) kinase inhibitor. **CLINICAL:** Antineoplastic.

USES

Treatment of pts with unresectable or metastatic melanoma with a BRAF V600E or V600K mutation (in combination with encorafenib).

PRECAUTIONS

Contraindications: Hypersensitivity to binimetinib. **Cautions:** Baseline anemia, leukopenia, lymphopenia, neutropenia; pts at risk for hemorrhage (e.g., history

B

of GI bleeding, coagulation disorders, recent trauma; concomitant use of anticoagulants, NSAIDs, antiplatelets), hepatic/renal impairment, pulmonary disease, cardiovascular disease, HF. History of thromboembolism (deep vein thrombosis [DVT], pulmonary embolism [PE]); pts at risk for thrombosis (immobility, indwelling venous catheter/access device, morbid obesity, genetic hypercoagulable conditions).

ACTION

Potent and selective inhibitor of mitogen-activated extracellular kinase (MEK) pathway. Inhibits MEK1 and MEK2, which are upstream regulators of the ERK pathway. The ERK pathway promotes cellular proliferation. MEK1 and MEK2 are part of the BRAF pathway. **Therapeutic Effect:** Increases apoptosis and reduces tumor growth.

PHARMACOKINETICS

Widely distributed. Metabolized in liver. Protein binding: 97%. Peak plasma concentration: 1.6 hrs. Excreted in feces (62%), urine (31%). **Half-life:** 3.5 hrs.

LIFESPAN CONSIDERATIONS

Pregnancy/Lactation: Avoid pregnancy; may cause fetal harm. Females of reproductive potential should use effective contraception during treatment and for up to 4 wks after discontinuation. Unknown if distributed in breast milk. Breastfeeding not recommended during treatment and up to 3 days after discontinuation. **Children:** Safety and efficacy not established. **Elderly:** No age-related precautions noted.

INTERACTIONS

DRUG: None significant. **HERBAL:** None significant. **FOOD:** None known. **LAB VALUES:** May increase serum alkaline phosphatase, ALT, AST, creatine phosphokinase, creatinine, GGT. May decrease Hct, Hgb, leukocytes, lymphocytes, neutrophils, RBCs; serum sodium.

AVAILABILITY (Rx)

Tablets: 15 mg.

ADMINISTRATION/HANDLING

PO

• Give without regard to food. • If a dose is missed or vomiting occurs after administration, give next dose at regularly scheduled time. • Do not give a missed dose within 6 hrs of next dose.

INDICATIONS/ROUTES/DOSAGE

Metastatic Melanoma

PO: ADULTS, ELDERLY: 45 mg twice daily (in combination with encorafenib). Continue until disease progression or unacceptable toxicity.

Dose Reduction for Adverse Reactions

First dose reduction: 30 mg twice daily. **Unable to tolerate 30 mg dose:** Permanently discontinue.

Dose Modification

Based on Common Terminology Criteria for Adverse Events (CTCAE). See prescribing information for encorafenib for recommended dose modification. If encorafenib is discontinued, binimetinib must also be discontinued.

Cardiomyopathy

Asymptomatic, absolute decrease in left ventricular ejection fraction (LVEF) greater than 10% from baseline and below lower limit of normal (LLN): Withhold treatment for up to 4 wks. If LVEF is at or above LLN, and the decrease from baseline is 10% or less, and pt is asymptomatic, then resume at reduced dose. If LVEF does not recover within 4 wks, permanently discontinue. **Symptomatic HF or absolute decrease in LVEF of greater than 20% from baseline that is also below LLN:** Permanently discontinue.

Dermatologic Reactions

Grade 2 skin reaction: If not improved within 2 wks, withhold treatment until improved to Grade 1 or 0. Resume at same dose for first occurrence or reduce dose if reaction is recurrent. **Grade 3 skin reaction:** Withhold treatment until improved to Grade 1 or 0. Resume at same dose for first occurrence or reduce dose if reaction is recurrent. **Grade 4 skin reaction:** Permanently discontinue.

Hepatotoxicity

Grade 2 serum ALT, AST elevation: Maintain dose. If not improved within 2 wks, withhold treatment until improved to Grade 1 or 0 (or to pretreatment baseline), then resume at same dose. **Grade 3 or 4 serum ALT, AST elevation:** See Other Adverse Reactions.

Ocular Toxicities

Symptomatic serious retinopathy; retinal pigment epithelial detachment: Withhold treatment for up to 10 days. If symptoms improve and become asymptomatic, resume at same dose. If not improved, resume at reduced dose or permanently discontinue. **Retinal vein occlusion:** Permanently discontinue.

Pulmonary Toxicity

Grade 2 interstitial lung disease: Withhold treatment for up to 4 wks. If improved to Grade 1 or 0, resume at reduced dose. If not resolved within 4 wks, permanently discontinue. **Grade 3 or 4 interstitial lung disease:** Permanently discontinue.

Rhabdomyolysis, Elevated Serum CPK

Grade 4 asymptomatic CPK elevation; any CPK elevation with symptoms or with renal impairment: Withhold treatment for up to 4 wks. If improved to Grade 1 or 0, resume at reduced dose. If not resolved within 4 wks, permanently discontinue.

Uveitis

Grade 1–3 uveitis: Withhold treatment for up to 6 wks if Grade 1 or 2 uveitis does not respond to medical therapy or if Grade 3 uveitis occurs. If improved, resume at same dose or reduced dose. If not improved, permanently discontinue. **Grade 4 uveitis:** Permanently discontinue.

Other Adverse Reactions (Including Hemorrhage)

Any recurrent Grade 2 reaction; first occurrence of any Grade 3 reaction: Withhold treatment for up to 4 wks. If improved to Grade 1 or 0 (or to pretreatment baseline), resume at reduced dose. If not improved, permanently discontinue. **First occurrence of any Grade 4 reaction:** Permanently discontinue or withhold treatment for up to 4 wks. If improved to Grade 1 or 0 (or to pretreatment baseline), resume at reduced dose. If not improved, permanently discontinue. **Recurrent Grade 3 reaction:** Consider permanent discontinuation. **Recurrent Grade 4 reaction:** Permanently discontinue.

Thromboembolism

Uncomplicated deep vein thrombosis (DVT); pulmonary embolism (PE): Withhold treatment until improved to Grade 1 or 0, then resume at reduced dose. **Life-threatening PE:** Permanently discontinue.

Dosage in Renal Impairment

Mild to severe impairment: Not specified; use caution.

Dosage in Hepatic Impairment

Mild impairment: No dose adjustment. **Moderate to severe impairment:** 30 mg twice daily.

SIDE EFFECTS

Frequent (43%–20%): Fatigue, nausea, diarrhea, vomiting, abdominal pain, constipation, rash, visual impairment. **Occasional (18%–13%):** Pyrexia, dizziness, peripheral edema.

ADVERSE EFFECTS/TOXIC REACTIONS

Anemia, leukopenia, lymphopenia, neutropenia is an expected response to

B

therapy. Cardiomyopathy reported in 7% of pts. DVT reported in 6% of pts. PE reported in 3% of pts. Ocular toxicities including serious retinopathy, retinal detachment, macular edema, retinal vein occlusion may occur. Uveitis, including iritis and iridocyclitis, occurred in 4% of pts. Interstitial lung disease, pneumonitis reported in less than 1% of pts. Grade 3 or 4 hepatotoxicity reported in 3%–6% of pts. Rhabdomyolysis occurs rarely. Serious hemorrhagic events including GI bleeding, rectal bleeding (4% of pts), hematochezia (3% of pts) may occur. Fatal intracranial hemorrhage reported in 2% of pts in the setting of new or progressive brain metastases. Colitis, panniculitis reported in less than 10% of pts.

NURSING CONSIDERATIONS

BASELINE ASSESSMENT

Confirm presence of BRAF V600E or V600K mutation in tumor specimen before initiation. Obtain baseline CBC, BMP, LFT, CPK; pregnancy test in females of reproductive potential. Question history of cardiovascular disease, genetic hypercoagulable conditions, hypersensitivity reactions, HF, pulmonary disease, thrombosis. Obtain echocardiogram for LVEF. Screen for active infection. Verify use of effective contraception in females of reproductive potential. Offer emotional support.

INTERVENTION/EVALUATION

Monitor CBC for anemia, leukopenia, lymphopenia, neutropenia; LFT for hepatotoxicity (bruising, hematuria, jaundice, right upper abdominal pain, nausea, vomiting, weight loss); CPK for rhabdomyolysis (amber-colored urine, flank pain, decreased urine output, muscle aches). Assess skin for dermal toxicities. Assess for eye pain/redness, visual changes at each office visit. Assess LVEF by echocardiogram 1 mo after initiation, then q2–3mos thereafter during treatment. If treatment withheld due to change in LVEF, monitor LVEF q2wks. Monitor for symptoms of DVT (leg or arm pain/swelling), PE (chest pain, dyspnea, tachycardia), HF (dyspnea, peripheral edema, palpitations, exercise intolerance). Monitor for GI bleeding, bloody stool; symptoms of intracranial bleeding (aphasia, blindness, confusion, facial droop, hemiplegia, seizures). Obtain ABG, radiologic test if interstitial lung disease or pneumonitis suspected. Diligently screen for infections.

PATIENT/FAMILY TEACHING

• Treatment may depress your immune system and reduce your ability to fight infection. Report symptoms of infection such as body aches, chills, cough, fatigue, fever. Avoid those with active infection. • Expect frequent cardiac function tests, eye exams, skin exams. • Therapy may cause toxic skin reactions, vision changes, or decrease the heart's ability to pump blood. • Report GI bleeding such as bloody stools or rectal bleeding. • Report symptoms of liver problems (bruising, confusion; amber, dark, orange-colored urine; right upper abdominal pain, yellowing of the skin or eyes); lung problems (severe cough, difficulty breathing, lung pain, shortness of breath), DVT (swelling, pain, hot feeling in the arms or legs; discoloration of extremity), lung embolism (difficulty breathing, chest pain, rapid heart rate), hemorrhagic stroke (confusion, difficulty speaking, one-sided weakness or paralysis, loss of vision), HF (shortness of breath, palpitations; swelling of legs, ankle, feet); rhabdomyolysis (dark-colored urine, decreased urinary output, fatigue, muscle aches). • Report any vision changes, eye redness. • Use effective contraception to avoid pregnancy. Do not breastfeed.

B

bisoprolol

HIGH ALERT

bi-**soe**-proe-lol
(Apo-Bisoprolol ✱)
Do not confuse bisoprolol with metoprolol.

FIXED-COMBINATION(S)

Ziac: bisoprolol/hydroCHLOROthiazide (a diuretic): 2.5 mg/6.25 mg, 5 mg/6.25 mg, 10 mg/6.25 mg.

◆CLASSIFICATION

PHARMACOTHERAPEUTIC: Beta$_1$ selective adrenergic blocker. **CLINICAL:** Antihypertensive.

USES

Management of hypertension, alone or in combination with other medications. **OFF-LABEL:** Chronic stable angina pectoris, premature ventricular contractions, supraventricular arrhythmias, HF.

PRECAUTIONS

Contraindications: Hypersensitivity to bisoprolol. Cardiogenic shock, marked sinus bradycardia, overt HF, second- or third-degree heart block (except in pts with pacemaker). **Cautions:** Concurrent use of digoxin, verapamil, diltiaZEM, HF, history of severe anaphylaxis to allergens, renal/hepatic impairment, hyperthyroidism, diabetes, bronchospastic disease, myasthenia gravis, psychiatric disease, peripheral vascular disease, Raynaud's disease.

ACTION

Selectively blocks beta$_1$-adrenergic receptors. **Therapeutic Effect:** Slows sinus heart rate, decreases B/P.

PHARMACOKINETICS

Well absorbed from GI tract. Protein binding: 26%–33%. Metabolized in liver. Primarily excreted in urine. Not removed by hemodialysis. **Half-life:** 9–12 hrs (increased in renal impairment).

LIFESPAN CONSIDERATIONS

Pregnancy/Lactation: Readily crosses placenta; distributed in breast milk. Avoid use during first trimester. May produce bradycardia, apnea, hypoglycemia, hypothermia during delivery, low-birth-weight infants. **Children:** Safety and efficacy not established. **Elderly:** Age-related peripheral vascular disease may increase risk of decreased peripheral circulation.

INTERACTIONS

DRUG: **Alpha$_2$ agonists (e.g., cloNIDine)** may increase AV-blocking effect. **Strong CYP3A4 inducers (e.g., carBAMazepine, phenytoin, rifAMPin)** may decrease concentration/effect. **Dronedarone, fingolimod, rivastigmine** may increase bradycardic effect. May increase vasoconstriction of **ergot derivatives (e.g., dihydroergotamine, ergotamine).** **HERBAL:** **Herbals with hypertensive properties (e.g., licorice, yohimbe)** or **hypotensive properties (e.g., garlic, ginger, ginkgo biloba)** may alter effects. **St John's wort** may decrease concentration/effect. **FOOD:** None known. **LAB VALUES:** May increase ANA titer, serum BUN, creatinine, potassium, uric acid, lipoproteins, triglycerides.

AVAILABILITY (Rx)

Tablets: 5 mg, 10 mg.

ADMINISTRATION/HANDLING

PO

- Give without regard to food.

INDICATIONS/ROUTES/DOSAGE

Hypertension

PO: ADULTS, ELDERLY: Initially, 2.5–5 mg once daily. May increase to 10 mg, then to 20 mg once daily. Usual dose: 2.5–10 mg once daily.

Dosage in Renal Impairment

CrCl less than 40 mL/min: ADULTS, ELDERLY: Initially, give 2.5 mg.

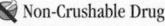

B

Dosage in Hepatic Impairment
Cirrhosis, hepatitis: Initially, 2.5 mg.

SIDE EFFECTS

Frequent (11%–8%): Fatigue, headache. **Occasional (4%–2%):** Dizziness, arthralgia, peripheral edema, URI, rhinitis, pharyngitis, diarrhea, nausea, insomnia. **Rare (less than 2%):** Chest pain, asthenia, dyspnea, vomiting, bradycardia, dry mouth, diaphoresis, decreased libido, impotence.

ADVERSE EFFECTS/ TOXIC REACTIONS

Overdose may produce profound bradycardia, hypotension. Abrupt withdrawal may result in diaphoresis, palpitations, headache, tremors. May precipitate HF, MI in pts with cardiac disease, thyroid storm in pts with thyrotoxicosis, peripheral ischemia in those with existing peripheral vascular disease. Hypoglycemia may occur in previously controlled diabetes. Thrombocytopenia, unusual bruising/bleeding occur rarely.

NURSING CONSIDERATIONS

BASELINE ASSESSMENT

Assess baseline renal/hepatic function tests. Assess B/P, apical pulse immediately before drug is administered (if pulse is 60/min or less or systolic B/P is less than 90 mm Hg, withhold medication, contact physician).

INTERVENTION/EVALUATION

Monitor B/P, pulse for quality, irregular rate, bradycardia. Assist with ambulation if dizziness occurs. Assess for peripheral edema. Monitor daily pattern of bowel activity, stool consistency. Assess neurologic status.

PATIENT/FAMILY TEACHING

• Do not abruptly discontinue medication. • Compliance with therapy regimen is essential to control hypertension. • If dizziness occurs, sit or lie down immediately. • Avoid tasks that require alertness, motor skills until response to drug is established. • Take pulse properly before each dose and report excessively slow pulse rate (less than 60 beats/min). Report numbness of extremities, dizziness. • Do not use nasal decongestants, OTC cold preparations (stimulants) without physician's approval. • Restrict salt, alcohol intake.

blinatumomab

blin-a-**toom**-oh-mab
(Blincyto)

■ BLACK BOX ALERT ■ Cytokine release syndrome (CRS) or neurologic toxicities, which may be life threatening or fatal, have occurred. Interrupt or discontinue treatment as recommended.

Do not confuse blinatumomab with ibritumomab or tositumomab.

◆CLASSIFICATION

PHARMACOTHERAPEUTIC: Anti-CD19/CD3 bispecific T-cell engager. Monoclonal antibody. **CLINICAL:** Antineoplastic.

USES

Treatment of Philadelphia chromosome-negative relapsed or refractory B-cell precursor acute lymphoblastic leukemia (ALL) in adults and children. Treatment of B-cell precursor ALL in first or second complete remission with minimal residual disease.

PRECAUTIONS

Contraindications: Hypersensitivity to blinatumomab. **Cautions:** Baseline anemia, leukopenia, neutropenia, thrombocytopenia; active infection or pts at increased risk of infection (diabetes, indwelling catheters), hepatic/renal impairment, high tumor burden, history of cognitive or seizure disorders, syncope, elderly.

ACTION

Binds to CD19 expressed on B cells and CD3 expressed on T cells. Activates endogenous T cells, forming a cytolytic synapse between a cytotoxic T cell and the cancer target B cell. **Therapeutic Effect:** Inhibits tumor cell growth and metastasis in ALL.

PHARMACOKINETICS

Widely distributed. Metabolism not specified; degrades into small peptides and amino acids via catabolic pathway. Protein binding: Not specified. Steady state reached within 24 hrs. Excretion not specified; negligible amounts excreted in urine. **Half-life:** 2.1 hrs.

LIFESPAN CONSIDERATIONS

Pregnancy/Lactation: May cause fetal harm. Avoid pregnancy. Unknown if distributed in breast milk. Must either discontinue drug or discontinue breastfeeding. **Children:** Safety and efficacy not established. **Elderly:** May have increased risk of neurologic toxicities, including cognitive disorder, encephalopathy, confusion, seizure; serious infections, hepatic impairment.

INTERACTIONS

DRUG: May decrease therapeutic effect of **BCG (intravesical), vaccines (live).** May increase adverse effects of **natalizumab, vaccines (live). HERBAL: Echinacea** may decrease therapeutic effect. **FOOD:** None known. **LAB VALUES:** May decrease immunoglobulins, Hgb, Hct, neutrophils, leukocytes, platelets; serum albumin, magnesium, phosphate, potassium. May increase serum ALT, AST, bilirubin, GGT, glucose; body weight.

AVAILABILITY (Rx)

Injection, Lyophilized Powder for Reconstitution: 35 mcg/vial.

ADMINISTRATION/HANDLING

IV

• Hospitalization is recommended for the first 9 days of the first cycle and the first 2 days of the second cycle. For all subsequent cycle starts and reinitiation (e.g., if treatment is interrupted for 4 or more hrs), supervision by a healthcare professional or hospitalization is recommended. • Do not flush infusion line after administration, esp. when changing infusion bags. Flushing of infusion line can result in excess dosage and complications. • At end of infusion, any used solution in IV bag and IV lines should be disposed of in accordance with local requirements.

Premedication • Premedicate with dexamethasone 20 mg IV 1 hr prior to the first dose of each cycle, prior to step dose (such as cycle 1 on day 8), or when restarting an infusion after an interruption of 4 or more hrs.

Reconstitution • Reconstitution guidelines are highly specific. Infusion bags must be prepared by personnel trained in aseptic preparations and admixing of oncologic drugs following strict environmental specifications at a USP 797 compliant facility using ISO Class 5 laminar flow hood or better. • See manufacturer guidelines for details.

Rate of administration • Administer as continuous IV infusion at a constant flow rate using an infusion pump. The pump should be programmable, lockable, nonelastomeric, and have an alarm. • Infusion bags should be infused over 24–48 hrs. Infuse the total 240-mL solution according to the instructions on the pharmacy label of the bag at one of the following constant rates: 10 mL/hr over 24 hrs, or 5 mL/hr over 48 hrs. • Infuse via dedicated line. • Use sterile, nonpyrogenic, low protein-binding, 0.2-micron in-line filter.

Storage • Refrigerate unused vials and IV solution stabilizer until time of use. • Protect from light. • Do not freeze. • Reconstituted vials may be stored at room temperature up to 4 hrs or refrigerated up to 24 hrs. • Prepared IV bag solutions may be stored at room temperature up to 48 hrs or refrigerated up to 8 days. • If prepared IV bag solution is not administered with the infusion time frame and temperature

B

indicated, it must be discarded; do not refrigerate again.

INDICATIONS/ROUTES/DOSAGE

Note: See Administration/Handling.

Acute Lymphoblastic Leukemia (ALL)

IV: ADULTS, ELDERLY, CHILDREN: A treatment course consists of up to 2 cycles for induction followed by 3 additional cycles for consolidation and up to 4 additional cycles of continued therapy. Cycles 1–5 consist of 4 wks of continuous IV infusion followed by a 2-wk treatment-free interval. Cycles 6–9 consist of 4 wks of continuous IV infusion followed by an 8-wk treatment-free interval. **PTS WEIGHING 45 KG OR MORE:** (Induction cycle 1): Administer 9 mcg/day on days 1–7, then at 28 mcg/day on days 8–28 as continuous infusion. (Induction cycle 2, consolidation cycles 3–5, continued therapy cycles 6–9): Administer 28 mcg/day on days 1–28. **PTS WEIGHING LESS THAN 45 KG:** (Cycle 1): 5 mcg/m^2/day (not to exceed 9 mcg/day) on days 1–7 and 15 mcg/m^2/day (**Maximum:** 28 mcg/day) on days 8–28 as continuous infusion. (Induction cycle 2, consolidation cycles 3–5, continued therapy cycles 6–9): Administer 15 mcg/m^2/day (**Maximum:** 28 mcg/day) on days 1–28.

Acute Lymphoblastic Leukemia, Minimal Residual Disease (MRD)–Positive

IV: ADULTS, ELDERLY, CHILDREN: A treatment course consists of 1 induction cycle followed by up to 3 additional cycles for consolidation. Each cycle consists of 4 wks of continuous infusion followed by a 2-wk treatment-free interval. **PTS WEIGHING 45 KG OR MORE:** Administer 28 mcg/day on days 1–28. **PTS WEIGHING LESS THAN 45 KG:** Administer 15 mcg/m^2/day (**Maximum:** 28 mcg/day) on days 1–28.

Dose Modification

Based on Common Terminology Criteria for Adverse Events (CTCAE). **Note:** If interruption after an adverse event is no longer than 7 days, continue the same cycle to a total of 28 days of infusion inclusive of the days before and after the interruption in that cycle. If interruption due to an adverse event is longer than 7 days, start new cycle.

Cytokine Release Syndrome

CTCAE Grade 3: Withhold until resolved, then restart at 9 mcg/day. Increase dose to 28 mcg/day after 7 days if toxicity does not occur. **CTCAE Grade 4:** Permanently discontinue.

Neurological Toxicity

CTCAE Grade 3: Withhold until no more than Grade 1 for at least 3 days, then restart at 9 mcg/day. Increase dose to 28 mcg/day after 7 days if toxicity does not recur. If toxicity occurred at 9 mcg/day, or if toxicity takes more than 7 days to resolve, permanently discontinue. **CTCAE Grade 4:** Permanently discontinue.

Seizure

Permanently discontinue if more than one seizure occurs.

Other Clinically Relevant Adverse Reactions

CTCAE Grade 3: Withhold until no more than Grade 1, then restart at 9 mcg/day. Increase dose to 28 mcg/day after 7 days if toxicity does not recur. If toxicity takes more than 14 days to resolve, permanently discontinue. **CTCAE Grade 4:** Consider permanent discontinuation.

Elevated Hepatic Enzymes

Interrupt treatment if ALT/AST rise to greater than 5 times upper limit of normal (ULN) or bilirubin rises to more than 3 times ULN. Consider dose recommendation as listed in other clinically relevant adverse reactions or as ordered by prescriber.

Dosage in Renal Impairment

CrCl equal to or greater than 30 mL/min: No dose adjustment. **CrCl less than 30 mL/min or hemodialysis:** Not specified; use caution.

Dosage in Hepatic Impairment

Not specified; use caution. Hepatic toxicity during treatment: see dose modification.

SIDE EFFECTS

Frequent (62%–36%): Pyrexia, headache. **Occasional (25%–5%):** Peripheral edema, nausea, tremor, constipation, diarrhea, cough, fatigue, dyspnea, insomnia, chills, abdominal pain, dizziness, back pain, extremity pain, vomiting, bone pain, chest pain, decreased appetite, arthralgia, hypotension, hypertension, tachycardia, confusion, paresthesia. **Rare (4%–2%):** Aphasia, memory impairment.

ADVERSE EFFECTS/TOXIC REACTIONS

Myelosuppression (principally, anemia, leukopenia, neutropenia, thrombocytopenia) is an expected outcome of treatment. Cytokine release syndrome (CRS) may be life threatening or fatal. Symptoms of CRS may include asthenia, hypotension, nausea, pyrexia; elevated ALT/AST, bilirubin; disseminated intravascular coagulation (DIC), capillary leak syndrome, hemophagocytic lymphohistiocytosis/macrophage activation syndrome (HLH/MAS). Infusion reactions have occurred and may be clinically indistinguishable from CRS. Neurologic toxicities such as altered level of consciousness, balance disorders, confusion, disorientation encephalopathy, seizures, speech disorders, syncope occurred in approx. 50% of pts and may affect ability to drive or operate machinery. Median time to onset of neurologic toxicity was 7 days. CTCAE Grade 3 toxicities or higher occurred in 15% of pts. Serious infections such as opportunistic infections, bacterial/viral/fungal infections, sepsis, pneumonia, catheter-site infections occurred in 25% of pts. Other life-threatening or fatal events may include tumor lysis syndrome, neutropenia/febrile neutropenia, leukoencephalopathy. Medication preparation and administration errors have occurred, resulting in underdose or overdose. Immunogenicity (anti-blinatumomab antibodies) occurred in less than 1% of pts.

NURSING CONSIDERATIONS

BASELINE ASSESSMENT

Obtain CBC, BMP, LFT, serum magnesium, phosphate, ionized calcium, vital signs. Consider electrolyte correction before starting treatment. Screen for home medications requiring narrow therapeutic index. Screen for active infection, history of seizures, hepatic/renal impairment, cognitive disorders. Verify pregnancy status in women of childbearing potential. Assess plans of breastfeeding. Conduct full neurologic assessment.

INTERVENTION/EVALUATION

Monitor CBC, LFT, serum electrolytes (correct as indicated), vital signs. Monitor closely for cytokine release syndrome, neurologic toxicities, serious infection, tumor lysis syndrome, hepatic impairment. Keep area around IV site clean to reduce risk of infection. Do not adjust setting of infusion pump. Pump changes may result in dosing errors. Do not flush IV line after infusion completion. Initiate fall precautions. Monitor I&O.

PATIENT/FAMILY TEACHING

• Treatment may cause life-threatening side effects that must be immediately treated by medical personnel. • Report symptoms of cytokine release syndrome, such as chills, facial swelling, fever, low blood pressure, nausea, vomiting, weakness; any infusion-related reactions, such as difficulty breathing or skin rash. • Report any neurologic problems, such as confusion, difficulty speaking or slurred speech, loss of consciousness, loss of balance, or seizures. • Treatment may lower your white blood cell count and increase your risk of infection. Report any signs of infection, such as fever, cough, fatigue, or burning with urination. Keep area around IV catheter clean at all times to reduce risk of infection. • Do not change or alter settings on infusion pump, even if the pump alarm sounds. Any changes made to the infusion pump by anyone other than trained medical personnel can result in a dose that is too high or too low and may be life threatening. • Report symptoms of liver problems, such as bruising, confusion, dark or amber-colored urine, right upper abdominal pain, or yellowing of the skin or eyes. • Avoid tasks that require alertness, motor skills until response to drug is established. Do not drive or operate machinery. • Hospitalization is required when starting therapy.

bortezomib

HIGH ALERT

bor-**tez**-oh-mib
(Velcade)

CLASSIFICATION

PHARMACOTHERAPEUTIC: Proteasome inhibitor. **CLINICAL:** Antineoplastic.

USES

Treatment of relapsed or refractory mantle cell lymphoma. Treatment of multiple myeloma. **OFF-LABEL:** Treatment of Waldenström's macroglobulinemia; peripheral or cutaneous T-cell lymphoma; systemic light-chain amyloidosis.

PRECAUTIONS

Contraindications: Hypersensitivity to bortezomib, boron, or mannitol; intrathecal administration. **Cautions:** Concomitant use of CYP3A4 inhibitors, history of syncope, concomitant use of antihypertensives; dehydration, diabetes, hepatic impairment, preexisting cardiac disease, neuropathy.

ACTION

Inhibits proteasomes (enzyme complexes regulating protein homeostasis within the cell). **Therapeutic Effect:** Produces cell-cycle arrest, apoptosis.

PHARMACOKINETICS

Widely distributed. Protein binding: 83%. Primarily metabolized by enzymatic action. Significant biliary excretion, with lesser amount excreted in urine. **Half-life:** 9–15 hrs.

LIFESPAN CONSIDERATIONS

Pregnancy/Lactation: May induce degenerative effects in ovary, degenerative changes in testes. May affect male/female fertility. Breastfeeding not recommended. **Children:** Safety and efficacy not established. **Elderly:** Increased incidence of Grade 3 or 4 thrombocytopenia.

INTERACTIONS

DRUG: **CYP3A4 inhibitors (e.g., itraconazole, ketoconazole)** may increase concentration/toxicity. **CYP3A4 inducers (e.g., rifAMPin)** may decrease concentration/effect (avoid use). **HERBAL:** **Green tea, green tea extracts** may diminish effect. **St. John's wort** may decrease level/effect. **FOOD:** **Grapefruit products** may increase concentration. **LAB VALUES:** May significantly decrease WBC, Hgb, Hct, platelet count, neutrophils.

AVAILABILITY (Rx)

Injection, Powder for Reconstitution: 3.5 mg.

ADMINISTRATION/HANDLING

IV

Reconstitution • Reconstitute vial with 3.5 mL 0.9% NaCl to provide a concentration of 1 mg/mL.
Rate of administration • Give as bolus IV injection over 3–5 sec.
Storage • Store unopened vials at room temperature. • Once reconstituted, solution may be stored at room temperature for up to 3 days or for 5 days if refrigerated.

SQ

Reconstitution • Reconstitute vial with 1.4 mL 0.9% NaCl to provide a concentration of 2.5 mg/mL.

INDICATIONS/ROUTES/DOSAGE

Mantle Cell Lymphoma (Initial Treatment)
IV: ADULTS, ELDERLY: 1.3 mg/m^2 days 1, 4, 8, 11 of a 21-day cycle for 6 cycles (in combination with riTUXimab, cyclophosphamide,

DOXOrubicin, and predniSONE). If response is seen at cycle 6, may continue for 2 additional cycles.

Mantle Cell Lymphoma (Relapsed)

IV, SQ: ADULTS, ELDERLY: Treatment cycle consists of 1.3 mg/m^2 twice wkly on days 1, 4, 8, and 11 for 2 wks of a 21-day treatment for 8 cycles. Therapy extending beyond 8 cycles may be given by standard schedule.

Multiple Myeloma (Initial Treatment)

IV, SQ: ADULTS, ELDERLY: (with melphalan and predniSONE) 1.3 mg/m^2 on days 1, 4, 8, 11, 22, 25, 29, 32 of a 42-day cycle for 4 cycles, then 1.3 mg/m^2 on days 1, 8, 22, 29 of a 42-day cycle for 5 cycles.

Multiple Myeloma (Relapsed)

IV, SQ: ADULTS, ELDERLY: 1.3 mg/m^2 twice wkly for 2 wks on days 1, 4, 8, 11 of a 21-day treatment cycle for 8 cycles. Therapy extending beyond 8 cycles may be given once wkly for 4 wks followed by a 13-day rest period.

Dosage Adjustment Guidelines

Withhold therapy at onset of CTCAE Grade 3 nonhematologic or Grade 4 hematologic toxicities, excluding neuropathy. When symptoms resolve, resume therapy at a 25% reduced dosage.

Dosage Adjustment Guidelines With Neuropathic Pain, Peripheral Sensory Neuropathy

For CTCAE Grade 1 toxicity with pain or Grade 2 (interfering with function but not activities of daily living [ADL]), 1 mg/m^2. For Grade 2 toxicity with pain or Grade 3 (interfering with ADL), withhold drug until toxicity is resolved, then reinitiate with 0.7 mg/m^2. For Grade 4 toxicity (permanent sensory loss that interferes with function), discontinue bortezomib.

Dosage in Renal Impairment

No dose adjustment.

Dosage in Hepatic Impairment

Mild impairment: No initial adjustment. **Moderate (bilirubin greater than 1.5–3 times upper limit of normal [ULN]) to severe (bilirubin greater than 3 times ULN) impairment:** Decrease initial dose to 0.7 mg/m^2 (based on tolerance may increase to 1 mg/m^2 or decrease to 0.5 mg/m^2).

SIDE EFFECTS

Expected (65%–36%): Fatigue, malaise, asthenia, nausea, diarrhea, anorexia, constipation, fever, vomiting. **Frequent (28%–21%):** Headache, insomnia, arthralgia, limb pain, edema, paresthesia, dizziness, rash. **Occasional (18%–11%):** Dehydration, cough, anxiety, bone pain, muscle cramps, myalgia, back pain, abdominal pain, taste alteration, dyspepsia, pruritus, hypotension (including orthostatic hypotension), rigors, blurred vision.

ADVERSE EFFECTS/TOXIC REACTIONS

Thrombocytopenia occurs in 40% of pts. GI, intracerebral hemorrhage are associated with drug-induced thrombocytopenia. Anemia occurs in 32% of pts. New onset or worsening of existing neuropathy occurs in 37% of pts. Symptoms may improve in some pts upon drug discontinuation. Pneumonia occurs occasionally.

NURSING CONSIDERATIONS

BASELINE ASSESSMENT

Obtain baseline CBC. Ensure adequate hydration prior to initiation of therapy. Antiemetics, antidiarrheals may be effective in preventing, treating nausea, vomiting, diarrhea.

INTERVENTION/EVALUATION

Routinely assess B/P; monitor pt for orthostatic hypotension. Maintain strict I&O. Monitor CBC, esp. platelet count, throughout treatment. Monitor renal, hepatic, pulmonary function throughout therapy. Encourage adequate fluid intake to prevent dehydration. Monitor temperature and be alert to high potential for fever. Monitor for peripheral neuropathy (burning sensation, neuropathic pain, paresthesia, hyperesthesia). Avoid IM injections, rectal temperatures, other traumas that may induce bleeding.

B

PATIENT/FAMILY TEACHING

• Report new/worsening vomiting, bruising/bleeding, breathing difficulties. • Discuss importance of pregnancy testing, avoidance of pregnancy, measures to prevent pregnancy. • Increase fluid intake. • Avoid tasks that require mental alertness, motor skills until response to drug is established.

bosutinib

boe-**sue**-ti-nib
(Bosulif)

◆CLASSIFICATION

PHARMACOTHERAPEUTIC: BCR-ABL tyrosine kinase inhibitor. **CLINICAL:** Antineoplastic.

USES

Treatment of chronic, accelerated, or blast phase Philadelphia chromosome–positive chronic myelogenous leukemia (Ph+CML) with resistance or intolerance to prior therapy. Treatment of newly diagnosed chronic phase Ph+CML.

PRECAUTIONS

Contraindications: Hypersensitivity to bosutinib. **Cautions:** Baseline anemia, thrombocytopenia, neutropenia; hepatic impairment, recent diarrhea, pulmonary edema, HF, fluid retention. Pts with history of pancreatitis, moderate to severe renal impairment. Avoid concurrent use of CYP3A4 inducers/inhibitors.

ACTION

Inhibits Bcr-Abl tyrosine kinase, a translocation-created enzyme, created by the Philadelphia chromosome abnormality noted in chronic myelogenous leukemia (CML). Inhibits Src-family kinase, including Src, Lyn, and Hck. **Therapeutic Effect:** Inhibits tumor cell growth and proliferation in chronic, accelerated, or blast phase CML.

PHARMACOKINETICS

Well absorbed following oral administration. Protein binding: 94%. Metabolized in liver. Excreted in feces (91%), urine (3%). **Half-life:** 22.5 hrs.

⧖ LIFESPAN CONSIDERATIONS

Pregnancy/Lactation: Potential for embryo/fetal toxicity. Avoid pregnancy. Must use effective contraception during treatment and for at least 30 days after treatment. Unknown if distributed in breast milk. Avoid breastfeeding. **Children:** Safety and efficacy not established. **Elderly:** No age-related precautions noted.

INTERACTIONS

DRUG: **Strong CYP3A inhibitors and/or P-glycoprotein (P-gp) inhibitors (e.g., clarithromycin, ketoconazole, ritonavir, miSOPROStol, nafcillin, salmeterol), moderate CYP3A4 inhibitors (e.g., ciprofloxacin, diltiaZEM, erythromycin, verapamil)** may increase concentration/effect. **Strong CYP3A4 inducers (e.g., rifAMPin, phenytoin, PHENobarbital), moderate CYP3A4 inducers (e.g., bosentan, nafcillin, modafinil)** may decrease concentration/effect. **Proton pump inhibitors (e.g., omeprazole, pantoprazole)** may reduce absorption, concentration. **HERBAL:** **St. John's wort** may decrease effectiveness. **Bitter orange, pomegranate, star fruit** may increase concentration/effect. **FOOD:** **Grapefruit products** may decrease bosutinib concentration. **LAB VALUES:** May decrease Hgb, platelets, WBCs, serum phosphorous. May increase serum ALT, AST, bilirubin, lipase.

AVAILABILITY (Rx)

Tablets: 100 mg, 400 mg, 500 mg.

ADMINISTRATION/HANDLING

PO

• Give with food. Do not break, crush, dissolve, or divide tablets.

B

INDICATIONS/ROUTES/DOSAGE

Ph+CML (Resistant or Intolerant to Prior Therapy)

PO: ADULTS, ELDERLY: 500 mg once daily. Continue until disease progression or unacceptable toxicity. If complete hematologic response not achieved by wk 8 or complete cytogenetic response not achieved by wk 12, in absence of Grade 3 or higher adverse reactions, may increase to 600 mg once daily.

Ph+CML (Newly Diagnosed Chronic Phase)

PO: ADULTS, ELDERLY: 400 mg once daily. Continue until disease progression or unacceptable toxicity.

CML With Baseline Renal Impairment

Ph+CML (intolerant): CrCl less than 30 mL/min: 300 mg once daily. **CrCl 30–50 mL/min:** 400 mg once daily. **Ph+CML (newly diagnosed): CrCl less than 30 mL/min:** 200 mg once daily. **CrCl 30–50 mL/min:** 300 mg once daily.

CML With Baseline Hepatic Impairment

PO: ADULTS: 200 mg once daily with food.

Dosage Modification

Hepatotoxicity: Withhold treatment until serum ALT, AST less than or equal to 2.5 times ULN. Then, resume at 400 mg once daily with food. Discontinue if recovery lasts longer than 4 wks or hepatotoxicity, including elevated serum bilirubin levels greater than 2 times ULN. **Severe diarrhea:** Withhold until recovery to low-grade diarrhea. Then, resume at 400 mg once daily with food. **Myelosuppression:** Withhold until absolute neutrophil count greater than 1,000 cells/mm^3 and platelet count greater than 50,000 cells/mm^3. Then, resume at same dose if recovery occurs within 2 wks. May reduce dose to 400 mg for recovery lasting greater than 2 wks.

SIDE EFFECTS

Frequent (82%–35%): Diarrhea, nausea, vomiting, abdominal pain, rash. **Occasional (26%–10%):** Pyrexia, fatigue, headache, cough, peripheral edema, arthralgia, anorexia, upper respiratory infection, asthenia, back pain, nasopharyngitis, dizziness, pruritus.

ADVERSE EFFECTS/TOXIC REACTIONS

Severe fluid retention may result in pleural effusion, pericardial effusion, pulmonary edema, ascites. Neutropenia, thrombocytopenia, anemia is an expected response of drug therapy. Severe diarrhea may result in fluid loss, electrolyte imbalance, hypotension. Hepatotoxicity occurred in 7%–9% of pts.

NURSING CONSIDERATIONS

BASELINE ASSESSMENT

Offer emotional support. Assess baseline weight, BMP, LFT. Confirm negative pregnancy test before initiating treatment. Obtain full medication history, including vitamins, herbal products. Screen for peripheral edema, signs/symptoms of HF, anemia.

INTERVENTION/EVALUATION

Weigh daily and monitor for unexpected rapid weight gain, edema. Monitor for changes in serum electrolytes, LFT during treatment. Offer antiemetics for nausea, vomiting. Monitor daily pattern of bowel activity, stool consistency. Monitor CBC for neutropenia, thrombocytopenia, anemia. Assess for bruising, hematuria, jaundice, right upper abdominal pain, weight loss, or acute infection (fever, diaphoresis, lethargy, productive cough).

PATIENT/FAMILY TEACHING

• Blood levels will be drawn routinely. • Take with meals. • Drink plenty of fluids (diarrhea may result in dehydration). • Swallow whole; do not break, chew, crush, dissolve, or divide tablets. • Use effective contraception. Do not breastfeed. • Report urine changes, bloody or clay-colored stools, upper abdominal pain, nausea, vomiting, bruising, persistent diarrhea, fever, cough, difficulty breathing, chest pain. • Immediately report any newly prescribed medications. • Avoid alcohol, grapefruit products. • Discuss using antacids for indigestion, heartburn, upset stomach (omeprazole, lansoprazole, pantoprazole may reduce absorption, concentration of bosutinib). • Separate antacid dosing by more than 2 hrs before and after medication.

brentuximab vedotin

bren-**tux**-i-mab ve-**doe**-tin
(Adcetris)

BLACK BOX ALERT JC virus infection resulting in progressive multifocal leukoencephalopathy and death can occur.

◆CLASSIFICATION

PHARMACOTHERAPEUTIC: Monoclonal antibody, anti-CD30. **CLINICAL:** Antineoplastic.

USES

Treatment of relapsed or refractory classical Hodgkin's lymphoma after failure of autologous hematopoietic stem cell transplant (HSCT) or after failure of at least two prior multiagent chemotherapy regimens or in pts who are not transplant candidates. Treatment of classical Hodgkin's lymphoma, previously untreated stage III or IV. Treatment of classical Hodgkin's lymphoma in pts at high risk of relapse or progression as post autologous HSCT consolidation. Treatment of systemic anaplastic large-cell lymphoma (ALCL) after failure of at least one prior multiagent chemotherapy regimen. Treatment of previously untreated systemic ALCL, peripheral T-cell lymphoma (CD30-expressing) in combination with cyclophosphamide, DOXOrubicin, and predniSONE. Treatment of primary cutaneous ALCL in pts receiving prior systemic therapy. Treatment of CD30-expressing mycosis fungoides.

PRECAUTIONS

Contraindications: Hypersensitivity to brentuximab. Avoid use with bleomycin (increased risk for pulmonary toxicity). **Cautions:** Renal/hepatic impairment, peripheral neuropathy, infusion reactions, neutropenia, tumor lysis syndrome, Stevens-Johnson syndrome, pregnancy.

ACTION

Binds to CD30-expressing cells, allowing the antibody to direct the drug to a target on lymphoma cells, disrupting the microtubule network within the cell. **Therapeutic Effect:** Induces cell cycle arrest, cell death.

PHARMACOKINETICS

Minimally metabolized. Protein binding: 68%–82%. Excreted primarily in feces (72%). **Half-life:** 4–6 days.

⌛ LIFESPAN CONSIDERATIONS

Pregnancy/Lactation: May cause fetal harm (embryo-fetal toxicities). Unknown if distributed in breast milk. **Children/Elderly:** Safety and efficacy not established.

INTERACTIONS

DRUG: **Strong CYP3A4 inhibitors (e.g., atazanavir, clarithromycin, ketoconazole)** increase concentration/effect. **CYP3A4 inducers (e.g., rifAMPin)** may reduce concentration/effect. May decrease therapeutic effect of **BCG (intravesical), vaccines (live).** May increase adverse effects of **belimumab, bleomycin, natalizumab, vaccines (live).** **HERBAL:** **Echinacea** may decrease effect. **FOOD:** None known. **LAB VALUES:** May decrease Hgb, Hct, WBC, RBC, platelets. May increase serum bicarbonate, lactate dehydrogenase, glucose, albumin, magnesium, sodium.

AVAILABILITY (Rx)

Injection, Powder for Reconstitution: 50-mg single-use vial.

ADMINISTRATION/HANDLING

IV

Reconstitution • Reconstitute each 50-mg vial with 10.5 mL Sterile Water for Injection, directing the stream toward wall of vial and not at powder. • Gently swirl (do not shake). • This will yield a concentration of 5 mg/mL. • The dose for pts weighing over 100 kg should be calculated for 100 kg. • Reconstituted solution must be transferred to infusion bag with a minimum 100 mL diluent, yielding a final concentration of 0.4–1.8 mg/mL brentuximab. • Gently invert bag to mix solution.

Rate of administration • Infuse over 30 min.

Storage • Discard if solution contains particulate or is discolored; solution should appear clear to slightly opalescent, colorless. • May store solution at 36°–46°F. • Use within 24 hrs after reconstitution.

IV COMPATIBILITIES

0.9% NaCl, D_5W, lactated Ringer's.

INDICATIONS/ROUTES/DOSAGE

◀ALERT▶ Do not give by IV bolus or IV push.

Hodgkin's Lymphoma (Relapsed or Refractory)

IV infusion: ADULTS, ELDERLY: 1.8 mg/kg (**Maximum:** 180 mg) infused over 30 min q3wks. Continue treatment until disease progression or unacceptable toxicity.

Hodgkin's Lymphoma (After HSCT)

IV infusion: ADULTS/ELDERLY: 1.8 mg/kg (**Maximum:** 180 mg) infused over 30 min every 3 wks. Continue treatment until a maximum of 16 cycles, disease progression, or unacceptable toxicity occurs. Begin within 4–6 wks post HSCT or upon recovery from HSCT.

Hodgkin's Lymphoma (Previously Untreated)

IV infusion: ADULTS, ELDERLY: 1.2 mg/kg (**Maximum:** 120 mg) q2wks (in combination with doxorubicin, vinblastine, and dacarbazine [AVD]). Begin within 1 hr after completion of AVD until a maximum of 12 doses, disease progression, or unacceptable toxicity occurs.

Mycosis Fungoides

IV infusion: ADULTS, ELDERLY: 1.8 mg/kg (**Maximum:** 180 mg) q3wks. Continue until a maximum of 16 cycles, disease progression, or unacceptable toxicity.

Systemic Anaplastic Large-Cell Lymphoma (ALCL) (Relapsed)

IV infusion: ADULTS/ELDERLY: 1.8 mg/kg (**Maximum:** 180 mg) infused over 30 min q3wks. Continue treatment until disease progression or unacceptable toxicity occurs.

Systemic ALCL, Peripheral T-Cell Lymphoma (CD30-Expressing) (Previously Untreated)

IV infusion: ADULTS/ELDERLY: 1.8 mg/kg (**Maximum:** 180 mg) q3wks for 6–8 doses (in combination with cyclophosphamide, DOXOrubicin, and predniSONE).

Primary Cutaneous ALCL (Relapsed)

IV infusion: ADULTS/ELDERLY: 1.8 mg/kg (**Maximum:** 180 mg) q3wks for up to 16 cycles.

Dosage in Renal Impairment

CrCl less than 30 mL/min: Avoid use.

Dosage in Hepatic Impairment

Mild impairment: Initial dose 1.2 mg/kg (**Maximum:** 120 mg) q3wks. **Moderate to severe impairment:** Avoid use.

SIDE EFFECTS

◀ALERT▶ Effects present as mild, manageable.

Frequent (52%–22%): Peripheral neuropathy, fatigue, respiratory tract infection,

B

nausea, diarrhea, fever, rash, abdominal pain, cough, vomiting. **Occasional (19%–11%):** Headache, dizziness, constipation, chills, bone/muscle pain, insomnia, peripheral edema, alopecia. **Rare (10%–5%):** Anxiety, muscle spasm, decreased appetite, dry skin.

ADVERSE EFFECTS/TOXIC REACTIONS

Myelosuppression characterized as neutropenia (54% of pts), peripheral neuropathy (52% of pts), thrombocytopenia (28% of pts), anemia (19% of pts) have occurred. Infusion reactions (including anaphylaxis), Stevens-Johnson syndrome have been reported. Tumor lysis syndrome may lead to acute renal failure. Progressive multifocal leukoencephalopathy (changes in mood, confusion, loss of memory, decreased strength or weakness on one side of body, changes in speech, walking, and vision) has been reported.

NURSING CONSIDERATIONS

BASELINE ASSESSMENT

Obtain baseline CBC before treatment begins and as needed to monitor response and toxicity but particularly prior to each dosing cycle. Question for evidence of peripheral neuropathy (hypoesthesia, hyperesthesia, paresthesia, burning sensation, neuropathic pain or weakness). Pts experiencing new or worsening neuropathy may require a delay, dose change, or discontinuation of treatment.

INTERVENTION/EVALUATION

Offer antiemetics to control nausea, vomiting. Monitor for hematologic toxicity (fever, sore throat, signs of local infection, bruising, unusual bleeding), symptoms of anemia (excessive fatigue, weakness). Assess response to medication. Monitor and report nausea, vomiting, diarrhea. Monitor daily pattern of bowel activity, stool consistency. Assess skin for evidence of rash.

PATIENT/FAMILY TEACHING

• Avoid crowds, persons with known infections. • Report signs of infection at once (fever, flu-like symptoms). • Avoid contact with those who recently received live virus vaccine. • Do not receive immunizations without physician's approval (drug lowers body resistance). • Promptly report fever, easy bruising, or unusual bleeding from any site. • Male pts should be warned of potential risk to their reproductive capacities.

brexpiprazole

brex-**pip**-ra-zole
(Rexulti)

■ **BLACK BOX ALERT** ■ Elderly pts with dementia-related psychosis are at increased risk of death, mainly due to HF, pneumonia. Increased risk of suicidal thoughts and behaviors in patients aged 24 yrs and younger with major depression, other psychiatric disorders.

Do not confuse brexpiprazole with ARIPiprazole, esomeprazole, omeprazole, or pantoprazole, or RABEprazole.

◆CLASSIFICATION

PHARMACOTHERAPEUTIC: DOPamine agonist. **CLINICAL:** Second-generation (atypical) antipsychotic agent.

USES

Adjunctive therapy to antidepressants for the treatment of major depressive disorder. Treatment of schizophrenia. **OFF-LABEL:** Psychosis/agitation associated with dementia.

PRECAUTIONS

Contraindications: Hypersensitivity to brexpiprazole. **Cautions:** Concurrent use of CNS depressants (including alcohol) antihypertensives, disorders in which

CNS depression is a feature, cardiovascular or cerebrovascular disease (may induce hypotension), Parkinson's disease, Parkinson's disease dementia, Lewy body dementia, history of seizures or conditions that may lower seizure threshold (Alzheimer's disease). Pts at risk for aspiration pneumonia, elderly, HF, diabetes. Pts at high risk for suicide. Preexisting low WBC/ANC, history of drug-induced leukopenia/neutropenia, dehydration.

ACTION

Exact mechanism of action unknown. Provides partial agonist activity at DOPamine and serotonin ($5\text{-}HT_1A$) receptors and antagonist activity at serotonin ($5\text{-}HT_2A$) receptors. **Therapeutic Effect:** Diminishes schizophrenic, depressive behavior.

PHARMACOKINETICS

Widely distributed. Metabolized in liver. Protein binding: greater than 99%. Peak plasma concentration: 4 hrs. Steady state reached in 10–12 days. Excreted in urine (25%), feces (46%). **Half-life:** 86–91 hrs.

⌛ LIFESPAN CONSIDERATIONS

Pregnancy/Lactation: Unknown if distributed in breast milk. May cause extrapyramidal and/or withdrawal symptoms in neonates if given in third trimester. **Children:** Safety and efficacy not established. **Elderly:** May have increased risk for adverse effects due to age-related hepatic, renal, cardiac disease. May increase risk of death in elderly pts with dementia-related psychosis.

INTERACTIONS

DRUG: **Alcohol** may potentiate cognitive and motor effects. **Strong CYP3A4 inducers (e.g., carBAMazepine, rifAMPin)** may decrease concentration/effect. **Strong CYP3A4 inhibitors (e.g., itraconazole, ketoconazole), strong CYP2D6 inhibitors (e.g., FLUoxetine, PARoxetine)** may increase concentration/effect. **Metoclopramide** may increase adverse effects. **HERBAL:** **St John's wort** may decrease concentration. **Gotu kola, kava kava, valerian** may increase CNS depression. **FOOD:** None known. **LAB VALUES:** May decrease leukocytes, neutrophils. May increase serum blood glucose, lipid levels.

AVAILABILITY (Rx)

Tablets: 0.25 mg, 0.5 mg, 1 mg, 2 mg, 3 mg, 4 mg.

ADMINISTRATION/HANDLING

PO

- Give without regard to food.

INDICATIONS/ROUTES/DOSAGE

Major Depressive Disorder (MDD)

PO: ADULTS, ELDERLY: Initially, 0.5–1 mg once daily. May increase at weekly intervals up to 1 mg (if initial dose is 0.5 mg) once daily, then up to target dose of 2 mg once daily. **Maximum:** 3 mg once daily.

Schizophrenia

PO: ADULTS, ELDERLY: Initially, 1 mg once daily on days 1–4. May increase to 2 mg once daily on days 5–7, then to 4 mg once daily on day 8 based on clinical response and tolerability. **Maximum:** 4 mg once daily.

Dosage in Renal Impairment

CrCl less than 60 mL/min: Maximum: 2 mg once daily for MDD, or 3 mg once daily for schizophrenia.

Dosage in Hepatic Impairment

Maximum: 2 mg once daily for MDD, or 3 mg once daily for schizophrenia.

CYP2D6 poor metabolizers or pts taking strong CYP2D6 inhibitors or strong CYP3A4 inhibitors: Administer half of the usual dose. **CYP2D6 poor metabolizers taking strong/moderate CYP3A4 inhibitors or pts taking strong/moderate CYP2D6 inhibitors with strong/moderate CYP3A4 inhibitors:** Administer a quarter of the usual dose. **Pts taking strong CYP3A4 inducers:** Double the usual dose over 1–2 wks.

B

SIDE EFFECTS

Occasional (9%–4%): Headache, nasopharyngitis, dyspepsia, akathisia, somnolence, tremor. **Rare (3%–1%):** Constipation, fatigue, increased appetite, weight gain, anxiety, restlessness, dizziness, diarrhea, blurry vision, dry mouth, salivary hypersecretion, abdominal pain, flatulence, myalgia, abnormal dreams, insomnia, hyperhidrosis.

ADVERSE EFFECTS/TOXIC REACTIONS

May increase risk of death in elderly pts with dementia-related psychosis. Most deaths appeared to be cardiovascular (e.g., HF, sudden death) or infectious (e.g., pneumonia) in nature. Increased incidence of suicidal thoughts and behaviors in pts 24 yrs and younger was reported. May increase risk of neuroleptic malignant syndrome (NMS). Symptoms of NMS may include hyperpyrexia, muscle rigidity, altered mental status, autonomic instability (irregular pulse or blood pressure, tachycardia, diaphoresis, and cardiac dysrhythmia), elevated creatinine, phosphokinase, myoglobinuria (rhabdomyolysis), acute renal failure. Metabolic changes such as hyperglycemia, ketoacidosis, hyperosmolar coma, diabetes, dyslipidemia, dystonia, and weight gain may occur. Other adverse effects may include leukopenia, neutropenia, agranulocytosis, orthostatic hypotension, syncope, cerebrovascular events (e.g., CVA, transient ischemic attack), seizures, hyperthermia, dysphagia, cognitive or motor impairment, tardive dyskinesia.

NURSING CONSIDERATIONS

BASELINE ASSESSMENT

Obtain baseline BMP, capillary blood glucose, vital signs; CBC in pts with preexisting low WBC or history of leukopenia or neutropenia. Receive full medication history and screen for drug interactions. Assess behavior, appearance, emotional state, response to environment, speech pattern, thought content. Correct dehydration, hypovolemia. Assess for suicidal tendencies, history of dementia-related psychosis, HF, CVA, NMS, diabetes.

INTERVENTION/EVALUATION

Monitor weight, BMP, capillary blood glucose, vital signs. Diligently monitor for extrapyramidal symptoms, tardive dyskinesia, hypotension, syncope, cerebrovascular or cardiovascular dysfunction, NMS. Assess for therapeutic response (greater interest in surroundings, improved self-care, increased ability to concentrate, relaxed facial expression).

PATIENT/FAMILY TEACHING

• Avoid alcohol. • Avoid tasks that require alertness, motor skills until response to drug is established. • Report worsening depression, suicidal ideation, abnormal changes in behavior. • Treatment may cause life-threatening conditions such as involuntary, uncontrollable movements, elevated body temperature, altered mental status, high or low blood pressure, seizures. • Pts with HF or active pneumonia are at increased risk of sudden death. • Immediately report fever, cough, increased sputum production, palpitations, fainting, or signs of HF.

brigatinib

bri-**ga**-ti-nib
(Alunbrig)
Do not confuse brigatinib with axitinib, cabozantinib, ceritinib, crizotinib, erlotinib, imatinib.

◆CLASSIFICATION

PHARMACOTHERAPEUTIC: Anaplastic lymphoma tyrosine kinase inhibitor. **CLINICAL:** Antineoplastic.

USES

First-line treatment of pts with anaplastic lymphoma kinase (ALK)–positive metastatic non–small-cell lung cancer (NSCLC).

B

PRECAUTIONS

Contraindications: Hypersensitivity to brigatinib. **Cautions:** Baseline anemia, leukopenia. History of symptomatic bradycardia, bradyarrhythmias, diabetes, hepatic/renal impairment, hypertension, ocular disease, pancreatitis, pulmonary disease. Concomitant use of strong CYP3A inhibitors, beta blockers, calcium channel blockers (see Interactions).

ACTION

A broad-spectrum kinase inhibitor (activity against EGFR, ALK, ROSI, IGF-1R and FLT-3). Inhibits ALK downstream signaling proteins. Has activity against cells expressing EML4-ALK. **Therapeutic Effect:** Expresses anti-tumor activity against EML-ALK mutant forms shown in NSCLC in pts progressed with crizotinib.

PHARMACOKINETICS

Widely distributed. Metabolized in liver. Protein binding: 66%. Peak plasma concentration: 1–4 hrs. Excreted in feces (65%), urine (25%). **Half-life:** 25 hrs.

LIFESPAN CONSIDERATIONS

Pregnancy/Lactation: Avoid pregnancy; may cause fetal harm. Females of reproductive potential should use effective nonhormonal contraception during treatment and for at least 4 mos after discontinuation. Unknown if distributed in breast milk. Breastfeeding not recommended during treatment and for at least 1 wk after discontinuation. **Males:** Males with female partners of reproductive potential should use barrier methods during sexual activity during treatment for at least 3 mos after discontinuation. **Children:** Safety and efficacy not established. **Elderly:** No age-related precautions noted.

INTERACTIONS

DRUG: **Strong CYP3A4 inhibitors (e.g., clarithromycin, itraconazole, ritonavir)** may increase concentration/effect. **Strong CYP3A4 inducers (e.g., carbamazepine, phenytoin, rifampin)** may decrease concentration/effect. May decrease effectiveness of hormonal contraceptives. Concomitant use of **beta blockers (e.g., atenolol, carvedilol, metoprolol), calcium channel blockers (e.g., diltiazem, verapamil), digoxin** may increase risk of symptomatic bradycardia. **HERBAL:** **St. John's wort** may decrease concentration/effect. **FOOD:** **Grapefruit products** may increase concentration/effect. **LAB VALUES:** May increase serum alkaline phosphatase, ALT, AST, amylase, bilirubin, CPK, glucose, lipase. May decrease Hct, Hgb, lymphocytes, RBCs; serum phosphate. May prolong aPTT.

AVAILABILITY (Rx)

Tablets: 30 mg, 90 mg, 180 mg.

ADMINISTRATION/HANDLING

PO

• Give with or without food. • Administer tablets whole; do not break, crush, cut, or divide. • If a dose is missed or vomiting occurs after administration, do not give extra dose. Administer next dose at regularly scheduled time.

INDICATIONS/ROUTES/DOSAGE

Non–Small-Cell Lung Cancer (Metastatic, ALK-Positive)

PO: ADULTS, ELDERLY: 90 mg once daily for 7 days. If 90-mg dose is tolerated, then increase to 180 mg once daily. Continue until disease progression or unacceptable toxicity. **Note:** If treatment is interrupted for 14 days (or more) for reasons other than toxic reactions, restart at 90 mg once daily for 7 days before increasing to the dose that was previously tolerated.

Dose Reduction Schedule

First dose reduction: 90 MG ONCE DAILY: Reduce to 60 mg once daily. **180 MG ONCE DAILY:** Reduce to 120 mg once daily. **Second dose reduction: 90 MG ONCE DAILY:** Permanently discontinue. **180**

MG ONCE DAILY: Reduce to 90 mg once daily. **Third dose reduction: 90 MG ONCE DAILY:** N/A. **180 MG ONCE DAILY:** Reduce to 60 mg once daily. **Note:** Once dose has been reduced, do not subsequently increase dose. If pt is unable to tolerate 60-mg dose, permanently discontinue.

Dose Modification

Based on Common Terminology Criteria for Adverse Events (CTCAE).

Symptomatic Bradycardia

Withhold treatment until recovery to asymptomatic bradycardia or to a heart rate of 60 bpm or greater, then resume at reduced dose level (if pt not taking concomitant medications known to cause bradycardia). **Symptomatic bradycardia in pts taking concomitant medications known to cause bradycardia:** Withhold treatment until recovery to asymptomatic bradycardia or heart rate of 60 bpm or greater. If concomitant medication can be adjusted or discontinued, then resume at same dose. If concomitant medication cannot be adjusted or discontinued, then resume at reduced dose level. **Life-threatening bradycardia in pts who are not taking concomitant medications known to cause bradycardia:** Permanently discontinue. **Life-threatening bradycardia in pts who are taking concomitant medications known to cause bradycardia:** Withhold treatment until recovery to asymptomatic bradycardia or heart rate of 60 bpm or greater. If concomitant medication can be adjusted or discontinued, then resume at reduced dose level with frequent monitoring. Permanently discontinue if symptomatic bradycardia recurs despite dose reduction.

CPK Elevation

Grade 3 CPK elevation (greater than 5 times upper limit of normal [ULN]): Withhold treatment until recovery to baseline or less than or equal to 2.5 times ULN, then resume at same dose. **Grade 4 CPK elevation (greater than 10 times ULN) or recurrence of Grade 3 CPK elevation:** Withhold treatment until recovery to baseline or less than or equal to 2.5 times ULN, then resume at reduced dose level.

Hyperglycemia

Grade 3 serum glucose elevation (greater than 250 mg/dL or 13.9 mmol/L): If adequate medical management of hyperglycemia cannot be achieved, withhold treatment until adequately controlled. Consider dose reduction or permanent discontinuation.

Hypertension

Grade 3 hypertension (systolic B/P greater than or equal to 160 mm Hg or diastolic B/P greater than or equal to 100 mm Hg); concomitant use of more than one antihypertensive drug; required medical intervention; requirement of aggressive hypertensive therapy: Withhold treatment until recovery to Grade 1 or 0, then resume at reduced dose level. **Grade 4 hypertension (first occurrence) or recurrence of Grade 3 hypertension:** Withhold treatment until recovery to Grade 1 or 0, then either resume at reduced dose level or permanently discontinue. **Recurrence of Grade 4 hypertension:** Permanently discontinue.

Lipase/Amylase Elevation

Grade 3 serum amylase or lipase elevation (greater than 2 times upper limit of normal [ULN]): Withhold treatment until recovery to Grade 1 or 0 (or baseline), then resume at same dose. **Grade 4 serum amylase or lipase elevation (greater than 5 times ULN) or recurrence of Grade 3 serum lipase or amylase elevation:** Withhold treatment until recovery to Grade 1 or 0, then resume at reduced dose level.

Pulmonary

Grade 1 pulmonary symptoms during the first 7 days of therapy: Withhold treatment until recovery to baseline, then resume at same dose level. Do not increase dose if interstitial lung disease (ILD)/pneumonitis suspected. **Grade 1 pulmonary symptoms after the first 7 days of therapy:** Withhold treatment until recovery to baseline, then resume at same dose level. **Grade 2 pulmonary symptoms during the first 7 days of therapy:** Withhold treatment until recovery to baseline, then resume at reduced dose level. Do not increase dose if ILD/ pneumonitis suspected. **Grade 2 pulmonary symptoms after the first 7 days of therapy:** Withhold treatment until recovery to baseline, then resume at same dose level. If ILD/pneumonitis is suspected, resume at reduced dose level. With any recurrence of ILD/pneumonitis or any Grade 3 or 4 pulmonary symptoms, permanently discontinue.

Visual Disturbance

Grade 2 or 3 visual disturbance: Withhold treatment until recovery to baseline, then resume at reduced dose level. **Grade 4 visual disturbance:** Permanently discontinue.

Other Toxicities

Any other Grade 3 toxicity: Withhold treatment until recovery to baseline, then resume at same dose level. **Recurrence of any other Grade 3 toxicity:** Withhold treatment until recovery to baseline, then either resume at reduced dose level or permanently discontinue. **First occurrence of any other Grade 4 toxicity:** Withhold treatment until recovery to baseline, then either resume at reduced dose level or permanently discontinue. **Recurrence of any other Grade 4 toxicity:** Permanently discontinue. **Concomitant use of strong CYP3A inhibitors:** Reduce daily dose by 50% if strong CYP3A inhibitor cannot be discontinued. If strong CYP3A inhibitor is discontinued, then resume the dose that was previously tolerated before starting CYP3A inhibitor.

Dosage in Renal Impairment

Mild to moderate impairment: No dose adjustment. **Severe impairment:** Not specified; use caution.

Dosage in Hepatic Impairment

Mild impairment: No dose adjustment. **Moderate to severe impairment:** Not specified; use caution.

SIDE EFFECTS

Frequent (33%–19%): Nausea, fatigue, headache, dyspnea, vomiting, decreased appetite, diarrhea, constipation. **Occasional (18%–9%):** Cough, abdominal pain, rash (acneiform dermatitis, exfoliative rash, pruritic rash, pustular rash), pyrexia, arthralgia, peripheral neuropathy, muscle spasm, extremity pain, hypertension, back pain, myalgia.

ADVERSE EFFECTS/TOXIC REACTIONS

Anemia, leukopenia are expected responses to therapy. Serious events, such as ILD/pneumonitis (3%–9% of pts), hypertension (6%–21% of pts), symptomatic bradycardia (6%–7% of pts), visual disturbance (blurred vision, diplopia, reduced visual acuity, macular edema, vitreous floaters, visual field defect, vitreous detachment, cataract [7%–10% of pts]), CPK elevation (27%–48% of pts), pancreatic enzyme elevation (27%–39%), hyperglycemia (43% of pts), may occur.

NURSING CONSIDERATIONS

BASELINE ASSESSMENT

Obtain baseline CBC, CPK, BMP, LFT; pregnancy test in females of reproductive potential. Obtain baseline ECG in pts with history of arrhythmia, HF. Question plans for breastfeeding. Question history of hepatic/renal impairment, diabetes, cardiac/ pulmonary disease, hypertension, pancreatitis. Receive full medication history and screen for interactions. Assess visual acuity. Verify ALK-positive NSCLC test prior to initiation. Obtain nutritional consult. Offer emotional support.

INTERVENTION/EVALUATION

Monitor CBC, CPK, BMP, LFT; vital signs (esp. heart rate) periodically. Obtain serum amylase, lipase in pts with severe abdominal pain, nausea, periumbilical ecchymosis (Cullen's sign), flank ecchymosis (Grey Turner's sign). Monitor for hepatotoxicity, hyperglycemia, vision changes, myalgia, musculoskeletal pain, interstitial lung disease/pneumonitis. If treatment-related toxicities occur, consider referral to specialist; pt may require treatment with corticosteroids. Screen for acute infections. Monitor I&O, hydration status, stool frequency and consistency. Encourage proper calorie intake and nutrition. Assess skin for rash, lesions.

PATIENT/FAMILY TEACHING

• Treatment may depress your immune system and reduce your ability to fight infection. Report symptoms of infection, such as body aches, burning with urination, chills, cough, fatigue, fever. Avoid those with active infection. • Therapy may decrease your heart rate, which may be life threatening; report dizziness, chest pain, palpitations, or fainting. • Worsening cough, fever, or shortness of breath may indicate severe lung inflammation. • Use effective contraception. Do not breastfeed. • Blurry vision, confusion, frequent urination, increased thirst, fruity breath may indicate high blood sugar levels. • Report abdominal pain, bruising around belly button or flank bruising, black/tarry stools, dark-colored urine, decreased urine output, severe muscle aches, yellowing of the skin or eyes. • Do not take newly prescribed medication unless approved by the doctor who originally started treatment. • Do not ingest grapefruit products.

brivaracetam

briv-a-ra-se-tam
(Briviact, Brivlera ✱)
Do not confuse brivaracetam with levETIRAcetam.

◆CLASSIFICATION

PHARMACOTHERAPEUTIC: Synaptic vesicle protein 2A ligand. **CLINICAL:** Anticonvulsant, miscellaneous.

USES

PO: Monotherapy or adjunctive therapy in the treatment of partial-onset seizures in pts 4 years and older with epilepsy. **IV:** Treatment in pts 16 yrs and older.

PRECAUTIONS

Contraindications: Hypersensitivity to brivaracetam. **Cautions:** Baseline neutropenia, hepatic impairment; pts at high risk for suicide; history of depression, mood disorder, psychiatric disorder; history of drug abuse.

ACTION

Exact mechanism unknown. Has high affinity for synaptic vesicle protein 2A in the brain. **Therapeutic Effect:** Prevents seizure activity.

PHARMACOKINETICS

Rapidly, completely absorbed following PO administration. Metabolized primarily by enzymatic hydrolysis, mediated by hepatic and extrahepatic amidase. Protein binding: less than or equal to 20%. Peak plasma concentration: 1 hr. Primarily excreted in urine (95%). **Half-life:** 9 hrs.

⌛ LIFESPAN CONSIDERATIONS

Pregnancy/Lactation: Unknown if distributed in breast milk. Must either discontinue drug or discontinue breastfeeding. **Children:** Safety and efficacy not established in pts younger than 16 yrs. **Elderly:** Not specified; use caution.

INTERACTIONS

DRUG: **RifAMPin** may decrease concentration/effect. May increase concentration/effect of **carBAMazepine. CNS depressants (e.g., alcohol, morphine, oxyCODONE, zolpidem)** may increase CNS depressant effect. **HERBAL:** **Herbals with sedative properties (e.g., chamomile, kava kava, valerian)** may increase CNS depression. **FOOD:** None known. **LAB VALUES:** May decrease neutrophils, WBCs. May increase serum phenytoin (free and total) levels.

AVAILABILITY (Rx)

Tablets: 10 mg, 25 mg, 50 mg, 75 mg, 100 mg. **Oral Solution:** 10 mg/mL. **Injection Solution:** 50 mg/5 mL.

ADMINISTRATION/HANDLING

IV

Reconstitution • Visually inspect for particulate matter or discoloration. Do not use if particulate matter or discoloration observed. • May be given without further dilution or may be mixed with 0.9% NaCl, 5% dextrose injection.

Rate of administration • Give over 2–15 min.

Storage • Injection solution should appear clear and colorless. • Diluted solution should not be stored more than 4 hrs at room temperature. Do not freeze.

PO

• Give without regard to food. • Administer tablets whole; do not crush, cut, dissolve, or divide. • Oral solution should appear slightly viscous, clear, colorless to yellowish in color, and have a raspberry flavor. • Store oral solution at room temperature. • Discard unused oral solution remaining after 5 mos of first opening bottle. • Do not freeze oral solution. Oral solution should be delivered using calibrated measuring device (does not require dilution). May give oral solution via nasogastric tube or gastrostomy tube.

INDICATIONS/ROUTES/DOSAGE

Partial-Onset Seizures (Monotherapy or Adjunctive Therapy)

PO/IV: ADULTS, ADOLESCENTS 16 YRS AND OLDER: Initially, 50 mg twice daily. May either decrease to 25 mg twice daily or increase to 100 mg twice daily. **Maintenance:** 25–100 mg twice daily. **Maximum:** 200 mg/day. When initiating treatment, gradual dose escalation is not required. Injection solution should be administered at same dose and same frequency as tablets and oral solution. Gradually taper dose to discontinue treatment (50 mg/day on a weekly basis with final week of treatment at dose of 20 mg/day). **ELDERLY:** Consider initiating at lower end of the dosage range. **PO: CHILDREN 4–15 YRS WEIGHING 50 KG OR MORE:** Initially, 25–50 mg twice daily. May increase up to maximum of 100 mg twice daily. **WEIGHING 20–49 KG:** Initially, 0.5–1 mg/kg twice daily. May increase up to maximum of 2 mg/kg twice daily. **WEIGHING 11–19 KG:** Initially, 0.5–1.25 mg/kg twice daily. May increase up to maximum of 2.5 mg/kg twice daily.

Dose Modification

Concomitant use with rifAMPin: May need to increase brivaracetam dosage by 100% (double dose).

Dosage in Renal Impairment

No dosage adjustment. Not recommended in pts with ESRD undergoing dialysis (not studied).

Dosage in Hepatic Impairment

Mild to severe impairment: Initially, 25 mg twice daily. **Maintenance:** 25–75 mg twice daily. **Maximum:** 75 mg twice daily.

SIDE EFFECTS

Occasional (16%–9%): Somnolence, sedation, dizziness, fatigue. **Rare (5%–2%):** Nausea, vomiting, ataxia, balance disorder,

B

abnormal coordination, nystagmus, irritability, constipation.

ADVERSE EFFECTS/TOXIC REACTIONS

Sudden discontinuance may increase risk of seizure frequency and status epilepticus. May increase risk of suicidal thoughts or behavior. Psychiatric events including nonpsychotic behavior (anger, agitation, aggression, anxiety, apathy, depression, hyperactivity, irritability, mood swings, nervousness, restlessness, tearfulness) and psychotic symptoms (psychotic behavior with acute psychosis, delirium, hallucinations, paranoia) occurred in 13% of pts. Hypersensitivity reactions including bronchospasm, angioedema were reported. Clinically significant decreased WBC count (less than 3,000 cells/mm^3) and decreased neutrophil count (less than 1,000 cells/mm^3) occurred in 1.8% and 0.3% of pts, respectively.

NURSING CONSIDERATIONS

BASELINE ASSESSMENT

Obtain CBC in pts with baseline neutropenia. Review history of seizure disorder (intensity, frequency, duration, LOC). Initiate seizure precautions, fall precautions. Question history of hypersensitivity reaction, hepatic impairment, psychiatric disorder; history of suicidal thoughts or behavior. Obtain urine pregnancy in female pts of reproductive potential.

INTERVENTION/EVALUATION

Periodically monitor CBC in pts with neutropenia. Monitor phenytoin levels in pts taking concomitant phenytoin (treatment may increase phenytoin levels). Observe for recurrence of seizure activity. Assess for clinical improvement (decrease in intensity/frequency of seizures). Diligently monitor for depression, changes in behavior, psychosis, suicidal ideation. Assist with ambulation if dizziness occurs.

PATIENT/FAMILY TEACHING

• Drowsiness usually diminishes with continued therapy. • Avoid tasks that require alertness, motor skills until response to drug is established. • Do not abruptly discontinue medication (may precipitate seizures). • Strict maintenance of drug therapy is essential for seizure control. • Report anxiety, anger, depression, mood swings, hostile behavior, thoughts of suicide, unusual changes in behavior. • Difficulty breathing, swelling of tongue or throat may indicate emergent allergic reaction. • Avoid alcohol.

brodalumab

broe-dal-ue-mab
(Siliq)

■ BLACK BOX ALERT ■ Suicidal ideation and behavior, including completed suicides, were reported with brodalumab. Screen for history of depression, suicidal ideation. Recommend mental health consultation for pts with suicidal ideation and behavior. Pts must seek immediate medical attention if new-onset suicidal ideation, anxiety, depression, mood change occur.

Do not confuse brodalumab with avelumab, dupilumab, durvalumab, nivolumab, or sarilumab.

◆CLASSIFICATION

PHARMACOTHERAPEUTIC: Anti-interleukin 17-receptor antibody. Monoclonal antibody. **CLINICAL:** Anti-psoriasis agent.

USES

Treatment of moderate to severe plaque psoriasis in adults who are candidates for systemic therapy or phototherapy and have failed to respond or have lost response to other systemic therapies.

PRECAUTIONS

Contraindications: Hypersensitivity to brodalumab. Crohn's disease. **Cautions:**

Baseline neutropenia; history of anxiety, depression, suicidal ideation and behavior, mood disorder; concomitant immunosuppressant therapy, conditions predisposing to infection (e.g., diabetes, immunocompromised pts, renal failure, open wounds), prior exposure to tuberculosis. Concomitant use of live vaccines not recommended. Not recommended in pts with active TB.

ACTION

Selectively binds to the IL-17A receptor, inhibiting the release of pro-inflammatory cytokines (involved in the pathogenesis of immune-mediated diseases, including plaque psoriasis). **Therapeutic Effect:** Blocks cytokine-induced responses.

PHARMACOKINETICS

Widely distributed. Metabolism: not specified. Degraded into small peptides and amino acids via catabolic pathway. Peak plasma concentration: 3 days. Steady state reached in 4 wks. Excretion not specified. **Half-life:** Not specified.

LIFESPAN CONSIDERATIONS

Pregnancy/Lactation: Unknown if distributed in breast milk. However, human immunoglobulin G (IgG) is present in breast milk and is known to cross the placenta. **Children:** Safety and efficacy not established. **Elderly:** No age-related precautions noted.

INTERACTIONS

DRUG: May decrease therapeutic effect of **BCG (intravesical), vaccines (live).** May increase adverse effects of **belimumab, natalizumab, vaccines (live). HERBAL: Echinacea** may decrease therapeutic effect. **FOOD:** None known. **LAB VALUES:** May decrease neutrophils.

AVAILABILITY (Rx)

Injection Solution: 210 mg/1.5 mL in prefilled single-dose syringe.

ADMINISTRATION/HANDLING

SQ

Preparation • Remove prefilled syringe from refrigerator and allow solution to warm to room temperature (approx. 30 min) with needle cap intact. • Visually inspect for particulate matter or discoloration. Solution should appear clear, colorless to slightly yellow in color. Do not use if solution is cloudy, discolored, or if visible particles are observed.

Administration • Insert needle subcutaneously into upper arms, outer thigh, or abdomen, and inject solution. • Do not inject into areas of active skin disease or injury such as sunburns, skin rashes, inflammation, skin infections, or active psoriasis. • Do not administer IV or intramuscularly. • Rotate injection sites.

Storage • Refrigerate prefilled syringes in original carton until time of use. • May store at room temperature for up to 14 days. Once warmed to room temperature, do not place back into refrigerator. • Do not freeze or expose to heating sources. • Do not shake. • Protect from light.

INDICATIONS/ROUTES/DOSAGE

Plaque Psoriasis

SQ: ADULTS, ELDERLY: Initially, 210 mg once at wks 0, 1, 2, followed by 210 mg once q2wks thereafter. **Permanent discontinuation:** Consider discontinuation in pts who have not achieved an adequate response after 12–16 wks.

Dosage in Renal/Hepatic Impairment

Not specified; use caution.

SIDE EFFECTS

Occasional (5%–4%): Arthralgia, headache. **Rare (3%–1%):** Fatigue, diarrhea, oropharyngeal pain, nausea, myalgia, injection site reactions (bruising, erythema, hemorrhage, pain, pruritus), conjunctivitis.

B

ADVERSE EFFECTS/TOXIC REACTIONS

Suicidal ideation and behavior, including completed suicides, were reported. May increase risk of tuberculosis. Infections such as bronchitis, influenza, nasopharyngitis, pharyngitis, upper respiratory tract infection, tinea infections, UTI may occur. May cause exacerbation of Crohn's disease and ulcerative colitis. Immunogenicity (auto-brodalumab antibodies) occurred in 3% of pts.

NURSING CONSIDERATIONS

BASELINE ASSESSMENT

Obtain CBC in pts with known history of neutropenia. Screen for active infection. Pts should be evaluated for active tuberculosis and tested for latent infection prior to initiating treatment and periodically during therapy. Induration of 5 mm or greater with tuberculin skin test should be considered a positive test result when assessing if treatment for latent tuberculosis is necessary. Verify pt has not received live vaccines prior to initiation. Question history of Crohn's disease, ulcerative colitis, hypersensitivity reaction; anxiety, depression, mood disorder, suicidal ideation and behavior. Conduct dermatological exam; record characteristics of psoriatic lesions. Assess pt's willingness to self-inject medication.

INTERVENTION/EVALUATION

Diligently monitor for suicidal ideation and behavior, new onset or worsening of anxiety, depression, mood disorder. Consult mental health professional if mood disorder suspected. Monitor for symptoms of tuberculosis, including those who tested negative for latent tuberculosis infection prior to initiation. Interrupt or discontinue treatment if serious infection, opportunistic infection, or sepsis occurs, and initiate appropriate antimicrobial therapy. Monitor for hypersensitivity reaction, symptoms of inflammatory bowel disease. Assess skin for improvement of lesions.

PATIENT/FAMILY TEACHING

• Seek immediate medical attention if thoughts of suicide, new onset or worsening of anxiety, depression, or changes in mood occurs. • A healthcare provider will show you how to properly prepare and inject your medication. You must demonstrate correct preparation and injection techniques before using medication at home. • Treatment may depress your immune system response and reduce your ability to fight infection. Report symptoms of infection, such as body aches, chills, cough, fatigue, fever. Avoid those with active infection. • Do not receive live vaccines. • Expect frequent tuberculosis screening. • Report travel plans to possible endemic areas. • Treatment may cause worsening of Crohn's disease or cause inflammatory bowel disease. Report abdominal pain, diarrhea, weight loss.

budesonide

TOP 100

bue-**des**-oh-nide
(Entocort EC, Pulmicort Flexhaler, Pulmicort, Rhinocort Allergy, Uceris)
Do not confuse budesonide with Budeprion.

FIXED-COMBINATION(S)

Symbicort: budesonide/formoterol (bronchodilator): 80 mcg/4.5 mcg, 160 mcg/4.5 mcg.

CLASSIFICATION

PHARMACOTHERAPEUTIC: Glucocorticosteroid. **CLINICAL:** Anti-inflammatory, antiallergy.

USES

Nasal: (Rx): Management of seasonal or perennial allergic rhinitis in adults and children 6 yrs and older. **(OTC):** Relief of hay fever, other upper respiratory allergies in adults and children 6 yrs and older. **Nebulization, oral inhalation:** Maintenance or prophylaxis therapy for asthma in pts 6 yrs and older (dry powder inhaler) or 12 mos to 8 yrs (nebulization). **PO:** Treatment of mild to moderate active Crohn's disease. Maintenance of clinical remission of mild to moderate Crohn's disease. Induction of remission in active, mild to moderate ulcerative colitis. **OFF-LABEL: PO:** Treatment of eosinophilic esophagitis. **Nebulization/inhalation:** Acute exacerbation of COPD.

PRECAUTIONS

Contraindications: Hypersensitivity to budesonide (nebulization/inhalation), primary treatment of status asthmaticus, acute episodes of asthma. Not for relief of acute bronchospasms. **Nasal:** Use in children younger than 6 yrs of age. **Cautions:** Thyroid disease, hepatic impairment, renal impairment, cardiovascular disease, diabetes, glaucoma, cataracts, myasthenia gravis, pts at risk for osteoporosis, seizures, GI disease, post acute MI, elderly.

ACTION

Inhibits accumulation of inflammatory cells; controls rate of protein synthesis; decreases migration of polymorphonuclear leukocytes (reverses capillary permeability and lysosomal stabilization at cellular level). **Therapeutic Effect:** Relieves symptoms of allergic rhinitis, asthma, Crohn's disease.

PHARMACOKINETICS

Form	Onset	Peak	Duration
Pulmicort Respules	2–8 days	4–6 wks	—
Rhinocort Aqua	10 hrs	2 wks	—

Minimally absorbed from nasal tissue; moderately absorbed from inhalation. Protein binding: 88%. Primarily metabolized in liver. **Half-life:** 2–3 hrs.

⌛ LIFESPAN CONSIDERATIONS

Pregnancy/Lactation: Unknown if drug crosses placenta or is distributed in breast milk. **Children:** Prolonged treatment or high dosages may decrease short-term growth rate, cortisol secretion. **Elderly:** No age-related precautions noted.

INTERACTIONS

DRUG: CYP3A4 inhibitors (e.g., clarithromycin, ketoconazole, ritonavir) may increase concentration. May decrease effect of **aldesleukin, BCG (intravesical).** May increase adverse effects of **natalizumab. HERBAL: Echinacea** may decrease effects. **FOOD: Grapefruit products** may increase systemic exposure. **LAB VALUES:** May decrease serum potassium.

AVAILABILITY (Rx)

Oral Inhalation Powder: ***(Pulmicort Flexhaler):*** 90 mcg per inhalation; 180 mcg per inhalation. **Inhalation Suspension for Nebulization:** ***(Pulmicort):*** 0.25 mg/2 mL; 0.5 mg/2 mL; 1 mg/2 mL. **Nasal Spray:** ***(Rhinocort Allergy, Rhinocort Aqua):*** 32 mcg/spray.

Delayed-Release Capsules: ***(Entocort EC):*** 3 mg. **Extended-Release Capsules:** ***(Uceris):*** 9 mg.

ADMINISTRATION/HANDLING

Inhalation

• Hold inhaler in upright position to load dose. Do not shake prior to use. Prime prior to first use only. • Place mouthpiece between lips and inhale forcefully and deeply. Do not exhale through inhaler; do not use a spacer. • Rinsing mouth after each use decreases incidence of candidiasis.

Intranasal

• Instruct pt to clear nasal passages before use. • Tilt pt's head slightly forward. • Insert spray tip into nostril, pointing toward nasal passages, away from nasal septum. • Spray into one nostril while pt holds other nostril closed and concurrently inspires through nostril to allow medication as high into nasal passages as possible.

Nebulization

• Shake well before use. • Administer with mouthpiece or face mask. • Rinse mouth following treatment.

B

PO

• May take with or without food. Swallow whole. Do not break, crush, dissolve, or divide capsule or tablet.

INDICATIONS/ROUTES/DOSAGE

Rhinitis

Intranasal: (Rx): ADULTS, ELDERLY, CHILDREN 6 YRS AND OLDER: 1 spray (32 mcg) in each nostril once daily. **Maximum:** 4 sprays in each nostril once daily for adults and children 12 yrs and older; 2 sprays in each nostril once daily for children 6–11 yrs.

Intranasal: (OTC): ADULTS, ELDERLY, CHILDREN 6 YRS AND OLDER: 2 sprays in each nostril once daily. May decrease to 1 spray in each nostril once daily.

Bronchial Asthma

Nebulization: CHILDREN 12 MOS–8 YRS: (Previous therapy with bronchodilators alone): 0.5 mg/day as single dose or 2 divided doses. **Maximum:** 0.5 mg/day. **(Previous therapy with inhaled corticosteroids):** 0.5 mg/day as single dose or 2 divided doses. **Maximum:** 1 mg/day. **(Previous therapy of oral corticosteroids):** 1 mg/day as single dose in 2 divided doses. **Maximum:** 1 mg/day.

Oral inhalation: (Pulmicort Flexhaler): **ADULTS, ELDERLY:** Initially, 360 mcg 2 times/day. **Maximum:** 720 mcg 2 times/day. **CHILDREN 6 YRS AND OLDER:** 180 mcg 2 times/day. **Maximum:** 360 mcg 2 times/day.

Crohn's Disease

PO (capsule): ADULTS, ELDERLY: 9 mg once daily for up to 8 wks. Recurring episodes may be treated with a repeat 8-wk course of treatment. **Maintenance of remission:** 6 mg once daily for up to 3 mos.

Ulcerative Colitis

PO (tablet): ADULTS, ELDERLY: 9 mg once daily in morning for up to 8 wks.

Dosage in Renal/Hepatic Impairment

No dose adjustment.

SIDE EFFECTS

Frequent (greater than 3%): Nasal: Mild nasopharyngeal irritation, burning, stinging, dryness; headache, cough. **Inhalation:** Flu-like symptoms, headache, pharyngitis. **Occasional (3%–1%): Nasal:** Dry mouth, dyspepsia, rebound congestion, rhinorrhea, loss of taste. **Inhalation:** Back pain, vomiting, altered taste, voice changes, abdominal pain, nausea, dyspepsia.

ADVERSE EFFECTS/TOXIC REACTIONS

Acute hypersensitivity reaction (urticaria, angioedema, severe bronchospasm) occurs rarely.

NURSING CONSIDERATIONS

BASELINE ASSESSMENT

Question for hypersensitivity to any corticosteroids, components. Auscultate lung sounds.

INTERVENTION/EVALUATION

Monitor for relief of symptoms. Auscultate lung sounds. Observe proper use of medication delivery device to ensure correct technique.

PATIENT/FAMILY TEACHING

• Improvement noted in 24 hrs, but full effect may take 3–7 days. • Report if no improvement in symptoms or if sneezing, nasal irritation occurs.

bumetanide

bue-**met**-a-nide

(Bumex, Burinex ✱)

BLACK BOX ALERT Excess dosage can lead to profound diuresis with fluid and electrolyte loss.

Do not confuse bumetanide with Buminate.

◆CLASSIFICATION

PHARMACOTHERAPEUTIC: Loop diuretic. **CLINICAL:** Diuretic.

USES

Management of edema associated with HF, renal disease, or hepatic disease.

PRECAUTIONS

Contraindications: Hypersensitivity to bumetanide. Anuria, hepatic coma, severe electrolyte depletion (until condition improves or is corrected). **Cautions:** Severe hypersensitivity to sulfonamides; hypotension.

ACTION

Enhances excretion of sodium, chloride, and, to lesser degree, potassium by direct action at ascending limb of loop of Henle and in proximal tubule. **Therapeutic Effect:** Produces diuresis.

PHARMACOKINETICS

Route	Onset	Peak	Duration
PO	30–60 min	60–120 min	4–6 hrs
IV	Rapid	15–30 min	2–3 hrs

Completely absorbed from GI tract (absorption decreased in HF, nephrotic syndrome). Protein binding: 94%–96%. Partially metabolized in liver. Primarily excreted in urine. Not removed by hemodialysis. **Half-life:** 1–1.5 hrs.

LIFESPAN CONSIDERATIONS

Pregnancy/Lactation: Unknown if drug is distributed in breast milk. **Children:** Safety and efficacy not established. **Elderly:** May be more sensitive to hypotension/electrolyte effects. Increased risk for circulatory collapse or thrombolytic episode. Age-related renal impairment may require reduced or extended dosage interval.

INTERACTIONS

DRUG: **Agents inducing hypokalemia (e.g., metOLazone, hydroCHLOROthiazide)** may increase risk of hypokalemia. **NSAIDs (e.g., diclofenac, naproxen)** may increase effect. May increase hyponatremic effect of **desmopressin.** **HERBAL:** **Herbals with hypertensive properties (e.g., licorice, yohimbe)** or **hypotensive properties (e.g., garlic, ginger, ginkgo biloba)** may alter effects. **FOOD:** None known. **LAB VALUES:** May increase serum glucose, BUN, uric acid; urinary phosphate. May decrease serum calcium, chloride, magnesium, potassium, sodium.

AVAILABILITY (Rx)

Injection Solution: 0.25 mg/mL. **Tablets:** 0.5 mg, 1 mg, 2 mg.

ADMINISTRATION/HANDLING

IV

Rate of administration • May give undiluted but is compatible with D_5W, 0.9% NaCl, or lactated Ringer's solution. • Administer IV push over 1–2 min. • May give through Y tube or 3-way stopcock. • May give as continuous infusion. **Storage** • Store at room temperature. • Stable for 24 hrs if diluted.

PO

• Give with food to avoid GI upset, preferably with breakfast (may prevent nocturia).

IV INCOMPATIBILITIES

Midazolam (Versed).

IV COMPATIBILITIES

Aztreonam (Azactam), cefepime (Maxipime), dexmedetomidine (Precedex), dilTIAZem (Cardizem), DOBUTamine (Dobutrex), furosemide (Lasix), LORazepam (Ativan), milrinone (Primacor), morphine, piperacillin and tazobactam (Zosyn), propofol (Diprivan).

INDICATIONS/ROUTES/DOSAGE

Edema, HF

PO: ADULTS, ELDERLY: 0.5–2 mg 1–2 times/day. May repeat in 4–5 hrs for up to 2 doses. **Maximum:** 10 mg/day.
IV, IM: ADULTS, ELDERLY: 0.5–1 mg/dose; may repeat in 2–3 hrs for up to 2 doses (**Maximum:** 10 mg/day) or 0.5–2 mg/hr by continuous IV infusion. Repeat loading dose before increasing infusion rate.

B

Usual Pediatric Dosage

IV, IM, PO: CHILDREN: 0.015–0.1 mg/kg/dose q6–24h. **Maximum:** 10 mg/day. **NEONATES:** 0.01–0.05 mg/kg/dose q12–48h.

Dosage in Renal/Hepatic Impairment

Use caution; contraindicated in anuria, hepatic coma.

SIDE EFFECTS

Expected: Increased urinary frequency and urine volume. **Frequent (5%):** Muscle cramps, dizziness, hypotension, headache, nausea. **Occasional (3%–1%):** Impaired hearing, pruritus, ECG changes, weakness, hives, abdominal pain, dyspepsia, musculoskeletal pain, rash, nausea, vomiting. **Rare (less than 1%):** Chest pain, ear pain, fatigue, dry mouth, premature ejaculation, impotence, nipple tenderness.

ADVERSE EFFECTS/TOXIC REACTIONS

Vigorous diuresis may lead to profound water and electrolyte depletion, resulting in hypokalemia, hyponatremia, dehydration, coma, circulatory collapse. Ototoxicity manifested as deafness, vertigo, tinnitus may occur, esp. in pts with severe renal impairment or those taking other ototoxic drugs. Blood dyscrasias, acute hypotensive episodes have been reported.

NURSING CONSIDERATIONS

BASELINE ASSESSMENT

Obtain baseline vital signs, esp. B/P for hypotension, before administration. Assess baseline electrolytes, particularly for hypokalemia, hyponatremia. Assess for edema. Observe skin turgor, mucous membranes for hydration status. Initiate I&O, obtain baseline weight.

INTERVENTION/EVALUATION

Continue to monitor B/P, vital signs, electrolytes, I&O, weight. Note extent of diuresis. Watch for changes from initial assessment (hypokalemia may result in muscle weakness, tremor, muscle cramps, altered mental status, cardiac arrhythmias; hyponatremia may result in confusion, thirst, cold/clammy skin).

PATIENT/FAMILY TEACHING

• Expect increased urinary frequency/volume. • Report auditory abnormalities (e.g., sense of fullness in ears, tinnitus). • Eat foods high in potassium such as whole grains (cereals), legumes, meat, bananas, apricots, orange juice, potatoes (white, sweet), raisins. • Rise slowly from sitting/lying position.

buprenorphine

TOP 100

bue-pre-**nor**-feen
(Belbuca, Buprenex, Butrans, Probuphine)

BLACK BOX ALERT **Transdermal, Immediate-Release, Injection:** Prolonged use during pregnancy may result in neonatal abstinence syndrome. Potential for abuse, misuse, and diversion. Do not exceed dose of one 20 mcg/hr patch due to risk of QT interval prolongation. May cause potentially life-threatening respiratory depression. **Implant:** Potential for implant migration, protrusion, expulsion, and nerve damage associated with insertion and removal.

Do not confuse Buprenex with Bumex, or buprenorphine with buPROPion.

FIXED-COMBINATION(S)

Bunavail: buprenorphine/naloxone (narcotic antagonist): 2.1 mg/0.3 mg; 4.2 mg/0.7 mg; 6.3 mg/1 mg. **Suboxone:** buprenorphine/naloxone: 2 mg/0.5 mg, 4 mg/1 mg, 8 mg/2 mg, 12 mg/3 mg. **Zubsolv:** buprenorphine/naloxone: 1.4 mg/0.36 mg; 5.7 mg/1.4 mg.

◆CLASSIFICATION

PHARMACOTHERAPEUTIC: Opioid agonist, partial agonist (Schedule V). **CLINICAL:** Opioid dependence adjunct, analgesic.

USES

Sublingual tablet: Treatment of opioid dependence. **Implant:** Maintenance treatment of opioid dependence in pts who achieved/sustained prolonged clinical stability on low to moderate doses of a transmucosal buprenorphine product for 3 months or longer with no need for supplemental dosing or adjustments. **Injection:** Relief of moderate to severe pain. **Transdermal, buccal film:** Moderate to severe chronic pain requiring continuous around-the-clock opioid analgesic for extended period. **OFF-LABEL:** Injection: Heroin/opioid withdrawal in hospitalized pts.

PRECAUTIONS

Contraindications: Hypersensitivity to buprenorphine. **Additional: Transdermal patch, buccal film, immediate-release injection:** Significant respiratory depression, severe asthma in an unmonitored setting or in absence of resuscitative equipment, known or suspected GI obstruction, including paralytic ileus. **Cautions:** Hepatic/renal impairment, elderly, debilitated, pediatric pts, head injury/increased intracranial pressure, pts at risk for respiratory depression, hyperthyroidism, myxedema, adrenal cortical insufficiency (e.g., Addison's disease), urethral stricture, CNS depression, morbid obesity, toxic psychosis, prostatic hypertrophy, delirium tremens, kyphoscoliosis, biliary tract dysfunction, acute pancreatitis, acute abdominal conditions, acute alcoholism, pts with prolonged QT syndrome, concurrent use of antiarrhythmics, hypovolemia, cardiovascular disease, ileus, bowel obstruction, hx of seizure disorder.

ACTION

Binds to mu opioid receptors within CNS. **Therapeutic Effect:** Suppresses opioid withdrawal symptoms, cravings. Alters pain perception, emotional response to pain.

PHARMACOKINETICS

Route	Onset	Peak	Duration
Sublingual	15 min	1 hr	6 hrs
IV	Less than 15 min	Less than 1 hr	6 hrs
IM	15 min	1 hr	6 hrs

Excreted primarily in feces, with lesser amount eliminated in urine. Protein binding: High. **Half-life: Parenteral:** 2–3 hrs; **Sublingual:** 37 hrs (increased in hepatic impairment).

LIFESPAN CONSIDERATIONS

Pregnancy/Lactation: Crosses placenta. Distributed in breast milk. Breastfeeding not recommended. Neonatal withdrawal noted in infant if mother was treated with buprenorphine during pregnancy, with onset of withdrawal symptoms generally noted on day 1, manifested as hypertonia, tremor, agitation, myoclonus. Apnea, bradycardia, seizures occur rarely. **Children:** Safety and efficacy of injection form not established in those 2–12 yrs. Safety and efficacy of tablet, fixed-combination form not established in pts 16 yrs or younger. **Elderly:** Age-related hepatic impairment may require dosage adjustment.

INTERACTIONS

DRUG: **CNS depressants (e.g., lorazepam, morphine, zolpidem), MAOIs (e.g., phenelzine, selegiline)** may increase CNS or respiratory depression, hypotension. **CYP3A4 inhibitors (e.g., clarithromycin, ketoconazole, ritonavir)** may increase plasma concentration. **CYP3A4 inducers (e.g., carBAMazepine, phenytoin, rifAMPin)** may cause increased clearance of buprenorphine. **HERBAL:** **Herbals with sedative properties (e.g., chamomile, kava kava, valerian)** may increase CNS depression. **St. John's wort** may decrease concentration/effect. **FOOD:** None known. **LAB VALUES:** May increase serum amylase, lipase.

AVAILABILITY (Rx)

Buccal Film: 75 mcg, 150 mcg, 300 mcg, 450 mcg, 600 mcg, 750 mcg, 900 mcg. **Implant: *(Probuphine)*:** Set of 4 implants, each containing 74.2 mg of buprenorphine (equivalent to 80 mg of buprenorphine hydrochloride). **Injection Solution: *(Buprenex)*:** 0.3 mg/1 mL. **Sublingual Tablets:** 2 mg, 8 mg. **Transdermal Weekly Patch: *(Butrans)*:** 5 mcg/hr, 7.5 mcg/hr, 10 mcg/hr, 15 mcg/hr, 20 mcg/hr.

ADMINISTRATION/HANDLING

IV

Reconstitution • May be diluted with lactated Ringer's solution, D_5W, 0.9% NaCl.

Rate of administration • If given as IV push, administer over at least 2 min.

IM

• Give deep IM into large muscle mass.

Buccal Film

Moisten inside cheek. Apply with dry finger. Press and hold in place for 5 sec. Keep film in place until dissolved (approx 30 min). Do not chew, swallow, touch, or move film. Do not cut/tear. Avoid areas with open sores/lesions.

Sublingual

• Instruct pt to dissolve tablet(s) under tongue; avoid swallowing (reduces drug bioavailability). • For doses greater than 2 tablets, either place all tablets at once or 2 tablets at a time under the tongue.

Storage • Store parenteral form at room temperature. • Protect from prolonged exposure to light. • Store tablets at room temperature.

Transdermal

• Apply to clean, dry, intact, nonirritated, hairless skin of upper outer arm, upper chest, upper back, or side of chest. Hair at application site should be clipped; do not shave. • Clean site with clear water and allow to dry. Do not use soaps, alcohol, oils (may increase absorption). Press patch in place and hold for 15 seconds. • Wait minimum of 21 days before reapplying to same site. • Avoid exposing patch to external heat sources. Incidental exposure to water is acceptable. Patch may be taped in place with first-aid tape. • If patch falls off during 7-day dosing interval, apply new patch to a different skin site.

IV INCOMPATIBILITIES

DiazePAM (Valium), furosemide (Lasix), LORazepam (Ativan).

IV COMPATIBILITIES

Allopurinol (Aloprim, Zyloprim), aztreonam (Azactam), cefepime (Maxipime), diphenhydrAMINE (Benadryl), granisetron (Kytril), haloperidol (Haldol), heparin, linezolid (Zyvox), midazolam (Versed), piperacillin/tazobactam (Zosyn), promethazine (Phenergan), propofol (Diprivan).

INDICATIONS/ROUTES/DOSAGE

Opioid Dependence

Sublingual: ADULTS, CHILDREN 13 YRS AND OLDER: 8 mg on day 1, then 16 mg on day 2 and subsequent induction days. Range: 12–16 mg/day (usually over 3–4 days). **Maintenance:** Target dose 12–16 mg/day. Pts should be switched to buprenorphine/naloxone combination for maintenance and unsupervised therapy. **Implant:** Four implants inserted subdermally in upper arm for 6 mos of treatment.

Moderate to Severe Acute Pain

IM/IV: ADULTS, ELDERLY, CHILDREN 13 YRS AND OLDER: 0.3 mg (1 mL) q6–8h prn; may repeat once 30–60 min after initial dose. **CHILDREN 2–12 YRS:** 2–6 mcg/kg q4–6h prn.

Moderate to Severe Chronic Pain

Transdermal: ADULTS, ELDERLY: (OPIOID NAÏVE): Initial dose 5 mcg/hr once q7days. **(OPIOID EXPERIENCED):** Discontinue all other around-the-clock opioid medications. Initial dose based on morphine equivalent dose: (Less than 30 mg): Initially 5 mcg/hr q7days. (30–80 mg): 10 mcg/hr q7days. (Greater than 80 mg): 20 mcg/hr q7days.

B

Buccal: ADULTS, ELDERLY: (OPIOID NAIVE): Initially, 75 mcg once or q12h for 4 days, then 150 mcg q12h. (OPIOID EXPERIENCED): Taper current opioid to no more than 30 mg oral morphine equivalent. **Based on opioid dose before tapering:** 75 mcg once daily or q12h for less than 30 mg; 150 mcg q12h for 30–89 mg; 300 mcg q12h for 90–160 mg.

Dosage in Renal Impairment
Use caution.

Dosage in Hepatic Impairment
Injection: Use caution.
Transdermal: No adjustment.

SIDE EFFECTS

Frequent (67%–10%): Sedation, dizziness, nausea. **Butrans (more than 5%):** Nausea, headache, pruritus at application site, dizziness, rash, vomiting, constipation, dry mouth. **Implant (more than 5%):** Headache, nausea, vomiting, constipation. **Occasional (5%–1%):** Headache, hypotension, vomiting, miosis, diaphoresis. **Rare (less than 1%):** Dry mouth, pallor, visual abnormalities, injection site reaction.

ADVERSE EFFECTS/TOXIC REACTIONS

Overdosage results in cold, clammy skin, weakness, confusion, severe respiratory depression, cyanosis, pinpoint pupils, seizures, extreme drowsiness progressing to stupor, coma.

NURSING CONSIDERATIONS

BASELINE ASSESSMENT

Obtain baseline B/P, pulse rate. Assess mental status, alertness. Assess type, location, intensity of pain. Obtain history of pt's last opioid use. Assess for early signs of withdrawal symptoms before initiating therapy.

INTERVENTION/EVALUATION

Monitor for change in respirations, B/P, rate/quality of pulse, mental status. Assess lab results. Initiate deep breathing, coughing exercises, particularly in pts with pulmonary impairment. Assess for clinical improvement; record onset of relief of pain. Monitor strictly for compliance, signs of abuse or misuse.

PATIENT/FAMILY TEACHING

• Change positions slowly to avoid dizziness, orthostatic hypotension. • Avoid tasks that require alertness, motor skills until response to drug is established. • Avoid alcohol, sedatives, antidepressants, tranquilizers.

buPROPion

bue-**proe**-pee-on
(Aplenzin, Forfivo XL, Wellbutrin SR, Wellbutrin XL)

■ BLACK BOX ALERT ■
Increased risk of suicidal thinking and behavior in children, adolescents, young adults 18–24 yrs with major depressive disorder, other psychiatric disorders. Agitation, hostility, depressed mood also reported. Use in smoking cessation may cause serious neuropsychiatric events.

Do not confuse Aplenzin with Relenza, buPROPion with busPIRone, Wellbutrin SR with Wellbutrin XL, or Zyban with Diovan or Zagam.

◆CLASSIFICATION

PHARMACOTHERAPEUTIC: Dopamine/norepinephrine reuptake inhibitor. **CLINICAL:** Antidepressant, smoking cessation aid.

USES

Treatment of major depressive disorder (MDD), seasonal affective disorder (SAD). Zyban assists in smoking cessation. **OFF-LABEL:** Treatment of ADHD in adults, children. Depression associated with bipolar disorder.

PRECAUTIONS

Contraindications: Hypersensitivity to buPROPion. Current or prior diagnosis

B

of anorexia nervosa or bulimia, seizure disorder, use of MAO inhibitors (concurrently or within 14 days of discontinuing either bupropion or the MAOI); pts undergoing abrupt discontinuation of alcohol or sedatives. Initiation of buPROPion in pts receiving linezolid or IV methylene blue. **Aplenzin, Forfivo XL, Wellbutrin XL (additional):** Conditions increasing seizure risk, severe head injury, stroke, CNS tumor/infection. **Forfivo XL (additional):** Pts receiving other dosage forms of bupropion. **Cautions:** History of seizure, cranial or head trauma, cardiovascular disease, history of hypertension or coronary artery disease, elderly, pts at high risk for suicide, renal/hepatic impairment. Concurrent use of antipsychotics, antidepressants, theophylline, steroids, stimulants, hypoglycemic agents, excessive use of alcohol, sedatives/hypnotics, opioids.

ACTION

Blocks reuptake of neurotransmitters, (DOPamine, norepinephrine) at CNS presynaptic membranes. **Therapeutic Effect:** Relieves depression. Eliminates nicotine withdrawal symptoms.

PHARMACOKINETICS

Rapidly absorbed from GI tract. Protein binding: 84%. Crosses the blood-brain barrier. Metabolized in liver. Primarily excreted in urine. **Half-life:** 14 hrs.

LIFESPAN CONSIDERATIONS

Pregnancy/Lactation: Unknown if drug crosses placenta or is distributed in breast milk. **Children:** More sensitive to increased dosage, toxicity; increased risk of suicidal ideation, worsening of depression. Safety and efficacy not established. **Elderly:** More sensitive to anticholinergic, sedative, cardiovascular effects. Age-related renal impairment may require dosage adjustment.

INTERACTIONS

DRUG: **CNS depressants (e.g., alcohol, morphine, oxyCODONE, zolpidem)** may increase CNS depressant effect. **MAOIs (e.g., phenelzine, selegiline)** may increase hypertensive effect. May decrease concentration of **tamoxifen.** May increase concentration of **aripiprazole, brexpiprazole, iloperidone, metoclopramide, thioridazine.** May increase adverse effects of **citalopram, vortioxetine.** **HERBAL:** **Herbals with sedative properties (e.g., chamomile, kava kava, valerian)** may increase CNS depression. **FOOD:** None known. **LAB VALUES:** May decrease WBC.

AVAILABILITY (Rx)

Tablets: 75 mg, 100 mg.

Extended-Release Tablets: (24 hr): ***(Aplenzin):*** 174 mg, 348 mg, 522 mg ***(Forfivo XL):*** 450 mg ***(Wellbutrin XL):*** 150 mg, 300 mg. **Sustained-Release Tablets: (12 hr):** ***(Wellbutrin SR):*** 100 mg, 150 mg, 200 mg; ***(Zyban):*** 150 mg.

ADMINISTRATION/HANDLING

PO

• Give without regard to food (give with food if GI irritation occurs). • Give at least 4-hr interval for immediate onset and 8-hr interval for sustained-release tablet to avoid seizures. • Give Aplenzin once daily in the morning. • Avoid bedtime dosage (decreases risk of insomnia). • Do not break, crush, dissolve, or divide sustained-, extended-release preparations.

INDICATIONS/ROUTES/DOSAGE

Depression

PO: ***(Immediate-Release):*** **ADULTS, ELDERLY:** Initially, 100 mg twice daily. May increase to 100 mg 3 times/day no sooner than 3 days after beginning therapy. **Maximum:** 150 mg 3 times/day.

PO: ***(Sustained-Release):*** **ADULTS, ELDERLY:** Initially, 150 mg/day as a single dose in the morning. May increase to 150 mg twice daily as early as day 4 after beginning therapy. **Maximum:** 400 mg/day in 2 divided doses.

PO: ***(Extended-Release):*** **ADULTS, ELDERLY:** 150 mg once daily. May increase to 300 mg once daily as early as day 4.

If no clinical improvement after 2 wks, may increase to 450 mg once daily. **Maximum:** 450 mg/day. ***(Aplenzin):*** Initially, 174 mg once daily in morning; may increase as soon as 4 days to 348 mg/day.

Smoking Cessation
PO: ADULTS, ELDERLY: ***(Zyban):*** Initially, 150 mg/day for 3 days, then 150 mg twice daily for 7–12 wks.

SAD
PO: ADULTS, ELDERLY: ***(Wellbutrin XL):*** 150 mg/day for 1 wk, then 300 mg/day. Begin in autumn (Sept–Nov). End of treatment begins in spring (Mar–Apr) by decreasing dose to 150 mg/day for 2 wks before discontinuation. ***(Aplenzin):*** 174 mg once daily. May increase after 1 wk to 348 mg once daily.

Dosage in Renal Impairment
Use caution.

Dosage in Hepatic Impairment
Mild to moderate impairment: Use caution, reduce dosage. **Severe impairment:** Use extreme caution. **Maximum:** ***(Aplenzin):*** 174 mg every other day. ***(Wellbutrin):*** 75 mg/day. ***(Wellbutrin SR):*** 100 mg/day or 150 mg every other day. ***(Wellbutrin XL):*** 150 mg every other day. ***(Zyban):*** 150 mg every other day.

SIDE EFFECTS

Frequent (32%–18%): Constipation, weight gain or loss, nausea, vomiting, anorexia, dry mouth, headache, diaphoresis, tremor, sedation, insomnia, dizziness, agitation. **Occasional (10%–5%):** Diarrhea, akinesia, blurred vision, tachycardia, confusion, hostility, fatigue.

ADVERSE EFFECTS/TOXIC REACTIONS

Risk of seizures increases in pts taking more than 150 mg/dose; in pts with history of bulimia, seizure disorders, discontinuing drugs that may lower seizure threshold.

NURSING CONSIDERATIONS

BASELINE ASSESSMENT

Assess psychological status, thought content, suicidal tendencies, appearance. For pts on long-term therapy, hepatic/renal function tests should be performed periodically.

INTERVENTION/EVALUATION

Supervise suicidal-risk pt closely during early therapy and dose changes (as depression lessens, energy level improves, increasing suicide potential). Assess appearance, behavior, speech pattern, level of interest, mood changes.

PATIENT/FAMILY TEACHING

• Full therapeutic effect may be noted in 4 wks. • Avoid tasks that require alertness, motor skills until response to drug is established. • Report signs/symptoms of seizure, worsening depression, suicidal ideation, unusual behavioral changes. • Avoid alcohol. • Do not chew, crush, dissolve, or divide sustained-, extended-release tablets.

busPIRone

bue-**spye**-rone
Do not confuse busPIRone with buPROPion.

◆CLASSIFICATION

PHARMACOTHERAPEUTIC: Nonbarbiturate. **CLINICAL:** Antianxiety.

USES

Management of anxiety disorders. Short-term relief of symptoms of anxiety. **OFF-LABEL:** Augmenting medication for antidepressants.

PRECAUTIONS

Contraindications: Hypersensitivity to busPIRone. Concomitant use of MAOIs intended to treat depression or within 14 days of discontinuing MAOIs intended

B

to treat depression. Concomitant use of MAOIs within 14 days of discontinuing buspirone. Initiation of buspirone in pts receiving IV methylene blue or linezolid. **Cautions:** Concurrent use of MAOIs, severe hepatic/renal impairment (not recommended).

ACTION

Exact mechanism of action unknown. Binds to serotonin, DOPamine at presynaptic neurotransmitter receptors in CNS. **Therapeutic Effect:** Produces anxiolytic effect.

PHARMACOKINETICS

Rapidly and completely absorbed from GI tract. Protein binding: 95%. Metabolized in liver. Primarily excreted in urine. Not removed by hemodialysis. **Half-life:** 2–3 hrs.

LIFESPAN CONSIDERATIONS

Pregnancy/Lactation: Unknown if drug crosses placenta or is distributed in breast milk. **Children:** Safety and efficacy not established. **Elderly:** No age-related precautions noted.

INTERACTIONS

DRUG: **CNS depressants (e.g., alcohol, morphine, oxyCODONE, zolpidem)** may increase CNS depressant effect. May increase adverse effects of **MAOIs (e.g., phenelzine, selegiline).** May increase serotonergic effects of **SSRIs (e.g., citalopram, FLUoxetine, sertraline). CYP3A4 inhibitors (e.g., erythromycin, ketoconazole)** may increase concentration/effect. **CYP3A4 inducers (e.g., rifAMPin)** may decrease concentration/effect. **HERBAL:** **Herbals with sedative properties (e.g., chamomile, kava kava, valerian)** may increase CNS depression. **St. John's wort** may decrease concentration/effect. **FOOD:** **Grapefruit products** may increase concentration, risk of toxicity. **LAB VALUES:** May produce false-positive urine metanephrine/catecholamine assay test.

AVAILABILITY (Rx)

Tablets: 5 mg, 7.5 mg, 10 mg, 15 mg, 30 mg.

ADMINISTRATION/HANDLING

PO

- Give without regard to food. Must be consistent.

INDICATIONS/ROUTES/DOSAGE

Anxiety Disorders

PO: ADULTS, ELDERLY: Initially, 10–15 mg/day in 2–3 divided doses. May increase every 2–3 days in increments of 2.5 mg twice daily. **Maintenance:** 10–15 mg twice daily. **Maximum:** 30 mg twice daily.

Dosage in Renal/Hepatic Impairment

Not recommended in severe impairment.

SIDE EFFECTS

Frequent (12%–6%): Dizziness, drowsiness, nausea, headache. **Occasional (5%–2%):** Nervousness, fatigue, insomnia, dry mouth, light-headedness, mood swings, blurred vision, poor concentration, diarrhea, paresthesia. **Rare:** Muscle pain/stiffness, nightmares, chest pain, involuntary movements.

ADVERSE EFFECTS/TOXIC REACTIONS

No evidence of drug tolerance, psychological or physical dependence, withdrawal syndrome. Overdose may produce severe nausea, vomiting, dizziness, drowsiness, abdominal distention, excessive pupil constriction.

NURSING CONSIDERATIONS

BASELINE ASSESSMENT

Assess degree/manifestations of anxiety. Offer emotional support. Assess motor responses (agitation, trembling, tension), autonomic responses (cold, clammy hands; diaphoresis).

INTERVENTION/EVALUATION

For pts on long-term therapy, CBC, LFT, renal function tests should be performed periodically. Assist with ambulation if drowsiness, dizziness occur. Evaluate for therapeutic response: calm facial expression, decreased restlessness, lessened insomnia, mental status.

PATIENT/FAMILY TEACHING

• Improvement may be noted in 7–10 days, but optimum therapeutic effect generally takes 3–4 wks. • Drowsiness usually disappears during continued therapy. • If dizziness occurs, slowly go from lying to standing. • Avoid tasks that require alertness, motor skills until response to drug is established. • Avoid alcohol, grapefruit products. • Be consistent in taking with regard to food.

C

cabazitaxel

ka-**baz**-i-**tax**-el
(Jevtana)

■ BLACK BOX ALERT ■ All pts should be premedicated with a corticosteroid, an antihistamine, and an H_2 serum antagonist prior to infusion. Severe hypersensitivity reactions have occurred. Immediately discontinue infusion and give appropriate treatment if hypersensitivity reaction occurs. Neutropenic deaths reported. CBC, particularly ANC, should be obtained prior to and during treatment. Do not administer with neutrophil count 1,500 cells/mm^3 or less.

Do not confuse cabazitaxel with PACLitaxel or Paxil, or Jevtana with Januvia, Levitra, or Sentra.

◆CLASSIFICATION

PHARMACOTHERAPEUTIC: Microtubule inhibitor. **CLINICAL:** Antineoplastic.

USES

Used in combination with predniSONE for treatment of castration-resistant metastatic prostate cancer previously treated with a DOCEtaxel-containing regimen.

PRECAUTIONS

Contraindications: Hypersensitivity to cabazitaxel. Severe hepatic impairment (total serum bilirubin greater than 3 times upper limit of normal [ULN]). Neutrophil count of 1,500 cells/mm^3 or less, history of hypersensitivity to polysorbate 80. **Cautions:** Mild to moderate hepatic impairment (bilirubin equal to or less than 3 times ULN), elderly, pregnancy, renal impairment (CrCl less than 30 mL/min). Pts at risk for developing GI complications (e.g., GI ulceration, concomitant use of NSAIDs).

ACTION

Binds to tubulin to promote assembly into microtubules and inhibits disassembly, which stabilizes microtubules. Inhibits microtubule depolymerization/cell division. **Therapeutic Effect:** Arrests the cell cycle, inhibiting tumor proliferation.

PHARMACOKINETICS

Widely distributed. Metabolized in liver. Protein binding: 89%–92%. Excreted in feces (76%), urine (3.7%). **Half-life:** 95 hrs.

⌛ LIFESPAN CONSIDERATIONS

Pregnancy/Lactation: May cause fetal harm. Crosses placental barrier. Breastfeeding not recommended. **Children:** Safety and efficacy not established. **Elderly:** Pts 65 yrs and older have 5% greater risk of developing neutropenia, fatigue, dizziness, fever, urinary tract infection, dehydration.

INTERACTIONS

DRUG: **Strong CYP3A4 inhibitors (e.g., atazanavir, clarithromycin, ketoconazole, ritonavir)** may increase concentration/effect; avoid use. **Strong CYP3A4 inducers (e.g., carBAMazepine, PHENobarbital, phenytoin, rifAMPin)** may decrease cabazitaxel concentration effects. **Live virus vaccine** may potentiate virus replication, increase vaccine's side effects, decrease response to vaccine. **HERBAL:** **Echinacea** may decrease therapeutic effect. **St. John's wort** may decrease concentration/effect. **FOOD:** **Grapefruit products** may increase concentration/effects. **LAB VALUES:** May increase serum bilirubin. May decrease Hgb, Hct, neutrophils, platelets.

AVAILABILITY (Rx)

Injection: 60 mg/1.5 mL

ADMINISTRATION/HANDLING

◀ALERT▶ Wear gloves during preparation, handling. Two-step dilution process must be performed under aseptic conditions to prepare second (final) infusion solution. Medication undergoes two dilutions. After second dilution, administration should be initiated within 30 min.

Reconstitution

Step 1, first dilution • Each vial of cabazitaxel contains 60 mg/1.5 mL; must first be mixed with entire contents of supplied diluent. • Once reconstituted, solution contains 10 mg/mL of cabazitaxel. • When transferring diluent, direct needle onto inside vial wall and inject slowly to limit foaming. • Remove syringe and needle, then gently mix initial diluted solution by repeated inversions for at least 45 sec to ensure full mixing of drug and diluent. • Do not shake. • Allow any foam to dissipate.

Step 2, final dilution • Withdraw recommended dose and further dilute with 250 mL 0.9% NaCl or D_5W. • If dose greater than 65 mg is required, use larger volume of 0.9% NaCl or D_5W so that concentration of 0.26 mg/mL is not exceeded. • Concentration of final diluted solution should be between 0.10 and 0.26 mg/mL.

Rate of administration • Infuse over 1 hr using in-line 0.22-micron filter.

Storage • Store vials at room temperature. • First dilution solution stable for 30 min. • Final diluted solution stable for 8 hrs at room temperature or 24 hrs if refrigerated.

INDICATIONS/ROUTES/DOSAGE

◀ALERT▶ Antihistamine (dexchlorpheniramine 5 mg, diphenhydrAMINE 25 mg, or equivalent antihistamine), corticosteroid (dexamethasone 8 mg or equivalent), and H_2 antagonist (raNITIdine 50 mg or equivalent H_2 antagonist) should be given at least 30 min prior to each dose to reduce risk/severity of hypersensitivity.

Metastatic Prostate Cancer

◀ALERT▶ Monitoring of CBC is essential on wkly basis during cycle 1 and before each treatment cycle thereafter so that the dose can be adjusted.

IV infusion: ADULTS, ELDERLY: 20–25 mg/m² given as 1-hr infusion q3wks in combination with predniSONE.

Dose Modification

Grade 3 neutropenia, febrile neutropenia, Grade 3 or persistent diarrhea, neuropathy: Reduce dosage to 20 mg/m² after treatment interruption.

Dosage With Strong CYP3A Inhibitors

Consider dose reduction by 25%.

Dosage in Renal Impairment

CrCl less than 15 mL/min: Use caution.

Dosage in Hepatic Impairment

Mild impairment: 20 mg/m². **Moderate impairment:** 15 mg/m². **Severe impairment:** Contraindicated.

SIDE EFFECTS

Frequent (47%–16%): Diarrhea, fatigue, nausea, vomiting, constipation, esthesia, abdominal pain, anorexia, back pain. **Occasional (13%–5%):** Peripheral neuropathy, fever, dyspnea, cough, arthralgia, dysgeusia, dyspepsia, alopecia, peripheral edema, weight decrease, urinary tract infection, dizziness, headache, muscle spasm, dysuria, hematuria, mucosal inflammation, dehydration.

ADVERSE EFFECTS/TOXIC REACTIONS

Myelosuppression is an expected response to therapy, but more severe reactions including severe neutropenia, febrile neutropenia may be life threatening. Hypersensitivity reaction may include generalized rash, erythema, hypotension, bronchospasm. 94% of pts develop Grade 1–4 neutropenia and associated complications including anemia, thrombocytopenia, sepsis. GI abnormalities, hypertension, arrhythmias, renal failure may occur.

NURSING CONSIDERATIONS

BASELINE ASSESSMENT

Obtain ANC, CBC, BMP, LFT, serum testosterone. Assess ANC, CBC prior to each infusion. Question history of hypersensitivity reaction; renal/hepatic impairment; intolerance to corticosteroids. Receive full medication history and screen for interactions.

INTERVENTION/EVALUATION

Monitor CBC, ANC on wkly basis during cycle 1 and before each treatment cycle thereafter; do not administer if ANC less than 1,500 cells/mm^3. Monitor serum ALT, AST, renal function. Monitor for hypersensitivity reaction (rash, erythema, dyspnea). Encourage adequate fluid intake. Monitor daily pattern of bowel activity, stool consistency. Offer antiemetics if nausea, vomiting occur. Closely monitor for signs/symptoms of neutropenia.

PATIENT/FAMILY TEACHING

• Treatment may depress your immune system and reduce your ability to fight infection. Report symptoms of infection such as body aches, burning with urination, chills, cough, fatigue, fever. Avoid those with active infection. • Report symptoms of bone marrow depression (e.g., bruising, fatigue, fever, shortness of breath, weight loss; bleeding easily, bloody urine or stool). • Report fever, chills, persistent sore throat, unusual bruising/bleeding, pale skin, fatigue. • Avoid tasks that require alertness, motor skills until response to drug is established. • Maintain strict oral hygiene. • Do not have immunizations without physician approval (drug lowers body's resistance). • Avoid those who have received a live virus vaccine. • Avoid grapefruit products. • Diarrhea may cause dehydration; drink plenty of fluids.

calcitonin

kal-si-**toe**-nin
(Calcimar 🍁, Miacalcin)
Do not confuse calcitonin with calcitriol, or Miacalcin with Micatin.

◆CLASSIFICATION

PHARMACOTHERAPEUTIC: Synthetic hormone. **CLINICAL:** Calcium regulator, bone resorption inhibitor.

USES

Parenteral: Treatment of Paget's disease of bone, hypercalcemia, postmenopausal osteoporosis in women greater than 5 yrs postmenopause. **Intranasal:** Postmenopausal osteoporosis in women more than 5 yrs postmenopause.

PRECAUTIONS

Contraindications: Hypersensitivity to calcitonin, salmon. **Cautions:** None known.

ACTION

Antagonizes effects of parathyroid hormone. Increases jejunal secretion of water, sodium, potassium, chloride. Inhibits osteoclast bone resorption. Promotes renal excretion of calcium, phosphate, sodium, magnesium, potassium by decreasing tubular reabsorption. **Therapeutic Effect:** Regulates serum calcium concentrations.

PHARMACOKINETICS

Nasal form rapidly absorbed. Injection form rapidly metabolized primarily in kidneys. Primarily excreted in urine. **Half-life: Nasal:** 43 min; **Injection:** 70–90 min.

⌛ LIFESPAN CONSIDERATIONS

Pregnancy/Lactation: Does not cross placenta; unknown if distributed in breast milk. Safe usage during lactation not established (inhibits lactation in animals). **Children:** Safety and efficacy not established. **Elderly:** No age-related precautions noted.

INTERACTIONS

DRUG: May decrease concentration/effect of **lithium.** May increase concentration/effect of **zoledronic acid**. **HERBAL:** None significant. **FOOD:** None known. **LAB VALUES:** None significant.

AVAILABILITY (Rx)

Injection Solution: ***(Miacalcin):*** 200 units/mL. **Nasal Spray:** ***(Miacalcin Nasal):*** 200 units/activation.

ADMINISTRATION/HANDLING

IM, SQ

• IM route preferred if injection volume greater than 2 mL. Subcutaneous injection for outpatient self-administration unless volume greater than 2 mL. • Skin test should be performed before therapy in pts suspected of sensitivity to calcitonin. • Bedtime administration may reduce nausea, flushing.

Intranasal

• Refrigerate unopened nasal spray. Store at room temperature after initial use. • Instruct pt to clear nasal passages. • Tilt head slightly forward. • Insert spray tip into nostril, pointing toward nasal passages, away from nasal septum. • Spray into one nostril while pt holds other nostril closed and concurrently inspires through nose to deliver medication as high into nasal passage as possible. Spray into one nostril daily. • Discard after 30 doses.

INDICATIONS/ROUTES/DOSAGE

Skin Testing Before Treatment in Pts With Suspected Sensitivity to Calcitonin-Salmon

Note: A detailed skin testing protocol is available from the manufacturer.

Paget's Disease

IM, SQ: ADULTS, ELDERLY: 100 units/day.

Postmenopausal Osteoporosis

IM, SQ: ADULTS, ELDERLY: 100 units daily with adequate calcium and vitamin D intake. **Intranasal: ADULTS, ELDERLY:** 200 units/day as a single spray in one nostril, alternating nostrils daily.

Hypercalcemia

IM, SQ: ADULTS, ELDERLY: Initially, 4 units/kg q12h; may increase to 8 units/kg q12h if no response in 2 days; may further increase to 8 units/kg q6–12h.

Dosage in Renal/Hepatic Impairment

No dose adjustment.

SIDE EFFECTS

Frequent: IM, SQ (10%): Nausea (may occur soon after injection; usually diminishes with continued therapy), inflammation at injection site. **Nasal (12%–10%):** Rhinitis, nasal irritation, redness, mucosal lesions. **Occasional: IM, SQ (5%–2%):** Flushing of face, hands. **Nasal (5%–3%):** Back pain, arthralgia, epistaxis, headache. **Rare: IM, SQ:** Epigastric discomfort, dry mouth, diarrhea, flatulence. **Nasal:** Itching of earlobes, pedal edema, rash, diaphoresis.

ADVERSE EFFECTS/TOXIC REACTIONS

Pts with a protein allergy may develop a hypersensitivity reaction (rash, dyspnea, hypotension, tachycardia).

NURSING CONSIDERATIONS

BASELINE ASSESSMENT

Obtain serum calcium, phosphate level.

INTERVENTION/EVALUATION

Ensure rotation of injection sites; check for inflammation. Assess vertebral bone mass (document stabilization/improvement). Assess for allergic response: rash, urticaria, swelling, dyspnea, tachycardia, hypotension. Monitor serum electrolytes, calcium, alkaline phosphatase.

PATIENT/FAMILY TEACHING

• Instruct pt/family on aseptic technique, proper injection method of subcutaneous medication, including rotation of sites, proper administration of nasal medication. • Nausea is transient and usually decreases over time. • Immediately report rash, itching, shortness of breath, significant nasal irritation. • Improvement in biochemical abnormalities and bone pain usually occurs in the first few months of treatment. • Improvement of neurologic lesions may take more than a year.

calcium acetate

(Eliphos, PhosLo)

calcium carbonate

(Apo-Cal ♣, Caltrate 600 ♣, OsCal ♣, Titralac, Tums)

calcium chloride

(Cal-Citrate, Citracal, Osteocit ♣)

C

calcium glubionate

calcium gluconate

kal-si-um

Do not confuse Citracal with Citrucel, OsCal with Asacol, or PhosLo with Prosom.

CLASSIFICATION

PHARMACOTHERAPEUTIC: Electrolyte replenisher. **CLINICAL**: Antacid, antihypocalcemic, antihyperkalemic, antihypermagnesemic, antihyperphosphatemic.

USES

Parenteral (calcium chloride): Treatment of hypocalcemia and conditions secondary to hypocalcemia (e.g., seizures, arrhythmias), emergency treatment of severe hypermagnesemia; **(calcium gluconate):** Treatment of hypocalcemia and conditions secondary to hypocalcemia (e.g., seizures, arrhythmias). **Calcium carbonate:** Antacid, dietary supplement. **Calcium acetate:** Controls hyperphosphatemia in end-stage renal disease. **OFF-LABEL (Calcium chloride):** Calcium channel blocker overdose, severe hyperkalemia, malignant arrhythmias associated with hypermagnesemia.

PRECAUTIONS

Contraindications: Hypersensitivity to calcium formulation. **All preparations:** Calcium-based renal calculi, hypercalcemia, ventricular fibrillation. **Calcium chloride:** Digoxin toxicity. **Calcium gluconate: Neonates:** Concurrent IV use with cefTRIAXone. **Cautions**: Chronic renal impairment, hypokalemia, concurrent use with digoxin.

ACTION

Essential for function, integrity of nervous, muscular, skeletal systems. Plays an important role in normal cardiac/renal function, respiration, blood coagulation, cell membrane and capillary permeability. Assists in regulating release/storage of hormones/neurotransmitters. Neutralizes/reduces gastric acid (increases pH). **Calcium acetate:** Binds with dietary phosphate, forming insoluble calcium phosphate. **Calcium chloride, calcium gluconate:** Moderates nerve and muscle performance by regulating action potential excitation threshold. **Therapeutic Effect:** Replaces calcium in deficiency states; controls hyperphosphatemia in end-stage renal disease; relieves heartburn, indigestion.

PHARMACOKINETICS

Moderately absorbed from small intestine (absorption depends on presence of vitamin D metabolites, pH). Primarily eliminated in feces.

LIFESPAN CONSIDERATIONS

Pregnancy/Lactation: Distributed in breast milk. Unknown whether calcium chloride or calcium gluconate is distributed in breast milk. **Children**: Risk of extreme irritation, possible tissue necrosis or sloughing with IV calcium preparations. Restrict IV use due to small vasculature. **Elderly**: Oral absorption may be decreased.

INTERACTIONS

DRUG: Hypercalcemia may increase **digoxin** toxicity. Oral form may decrease absorption of **bisphosphonates (e.g., risedronate), calcium channel blockers (e.g., amLODIPine, dilTIAZem, verapamil), tetracycline derivatives, thyroid products.** **HERBAL**: None significant. **FOOD**: **Food** may increase calcium absorption. **LAB VALUES**: May increase serum pH, calcium, gastrin. May decrease serum phosphate, potassium.

AVAILABILITY (Rx)

Calcium Acetate (667 mg = 169 mg calcium)

Capsules: 667 mg. **Tablets**: ***(Eliphos):*** 667 mg.

Calcium Carbonate (1 g = 400 mg calcium)
Tablets: 500 mg, 600 mg, 1,250 mg, 1,500 mg. **Tablets (Chewable):** 500 mg, 750 mg, 1,000 mg.

Calcium Chloride
Injection Solution: 10% (100 mg/mL) equivalent to 27.2 mg elemental calcium per mL.

Calcium Gluconate (1 g = 93 mg calcium)
Injection Solution: 10%.

ADMINISTRATION/HANDLING

IV

Dilution: ***(Calcium Chloride):*** May give undiluted or may dilute with 0.9% NaCl or Sterile Water for Injection. ***(Calcium Gluconate):*** May give undiluted or may dilute with 100 mL 0.9% NaCl or D5W.

Rate of administration: ***(Calcium Chloride):*** **Note:** Rapid administration may produce bradycardia, metallic/chalky taste, hypotension, sensation of heart, peripheral vasodilation. • **IV push:** Infuse slowly at maximum rate of 50–100 mg/min (in cardiac arrest, may administer over 10–20 sec). • **IV infusion:** Dilute to maximum final concentration of 20 mg/mL and infuse over 1 hr or no faster than 45–90 mg/kg/hr. Give via a central line. Do **NOT** use scalp, small hand or foot veins. Stop infusion if pt complains of pain or discomfort. ***(Calcium Gluconate):*** **Note:** Rapid administration may produce vasodilation, hypotension, arrhythmias, syncope, cardiac arrest. • **IV push:** Infuse slowly over 3–5 min or at maximum rate of 50–100 mg/min (in cardiac arrest, may administer over 10–20 sec). • **IV infusion:** Dilute 1–2 g in 100 mL 0.9% NaCl or D_5W and infuse over 1 hr.

Storage • Store at room temperature. • Once diluted, stable for 24 hrs at room temperature.

PO

(Calcium Acetate): Administer with plenty of fluids during meals to optimize effectiveness. ***(Calcium Carbonate):*** Administer with or immediately following meals with plenty of water (give with meals if used for phosphate binding). Instruct pt to thoroughly chew chewable tablets before swallowing.

IV INCOMPATIBILITIES

Calcium chloride: Amphotericin B complex (Abelcet, AmBisome, Amphotec), pantoprazole (Protonix), phosphate-containing solutions, propofol (Diprivan), sodium bicarbonate. **Calcium gluconate:** Amphotericin B complex (Abelcet, AmBisome, Amphotec), fluconazole (Diflucan).

IV COMPATIBILITIES

Calcium chloride: Amikacin (Amikin), DOBUTamine (Dobutrex), lidocaine, milrinone (Primacor), morphine, norepinephrine (Levophed). **Calcium gluconate:** Ampicillin, aztreonam (Azactam), ceFAZolin (Ancef), cefepime (Maxipime), ciprofloxacin (Cipro), DOBUTamine (Dobutrex), enalapril (Vasotec), famotidine (Pepcid), furosemide (Lasix), heparin, lidocaine, lipids, magnesium sulfate, meropenem (Merrem IV), midazolam (Versed), milrinone (Primacor), norepinephrine (Levophed), piperacillin and tazobactam (Zosyn), potassium chloride, propofol (Diprivan).

INDICATIONS/ROUTES/DOSAGE

Hyperphosphatemia

PO: ***(Calcium Acetate):*** **ADULTS, ELDERLY:** Initially, 1334 mg 3 times/day with meals. May increase gradually (q2–3wks) to decrease serum phosphate level to less than 6 mg/dL as long as hypercalcemia does not develop. Usual dose: 2,001–2,668 mg with each meal.

Hypocalcemia

IV: ***(Calcium Chloride):*** **ADULTS, ELDERLY:** (Acute, symptomatic): 200–1,000 mg at intervals of q1–3days. (Severe, symptomatic): 1 g over 10 min; may repeat q60min until symptoms resolve. **CHILDREN, NEONATES:** 2.7–5 mg/kg q4–6h as needed (**Maximum:** 1,000 mg).

IV: ***(Calcium Gluconate):*** **ADULTS, ELDERLY:** (Mild): 1–2 g over 2 hrs; (Moderate to severe, asymptomatic): 4 g over 4 hrs; (Severe, symptomatic): 1–2 g over 10 min; may repeat q60min until symptoms resolve. **CHILDREN:** 200–500 mg/kg/day as a continuous infusion or in 4 divided doses. (**Maximum:** 1,000 mg). **NEONATES:** 200 mg/kg q6–12h or 400 mg/kg/day as a continuous infusion.

Antacid

PO: ***(Calcium Carbonate):*** **ADULTS, ELDERLY:** 1–4 tabs as needed. **Maximum:** 8,000 mg/day. **CHILDREN 12 YRS AND OLDER:** 500–3,000 mg for up to 2 wks. **Maximum:** 7,500 mg/day. **CHILDREN 6–11 YRS:** 750–800 mg/day for up to 2 wks. **Maximum:** 3,000 mg/day. **CHILDREN 2–5 YRS:** 375–400 mg/day for up to 2 wks. **Maximum:** 1,500 mg/day.

Cardiac Arrest

IV: ***(Calcium Chloride):*** **ADULTS, ELDERLY:** 500–1,000 mg over 2–5 min. May repeat as necessary. **CHILDREN, NEONATES:** 20 mg/kg. May repeat in 10 min if necessary. If effective, consider IV infusion of 20–50 mg/kg/hr. **Maximum:** 2,000 mg/dose.

Supplement

PO: ***(Calcium Carbonate):*** **ADULTS, ELDERLY:** 500 mg–4 g/day in 1–3 divided doses. **CHILDREN OLDER THAN 4 YRS:** 750 mg 3 times/day. **CHILDREN 2–4 YRS:** 750 mg 2 times/day. ***(Calcium Citrate):*** **ADULTS, ELDERLY:** 0.5–2 g 2–4 times/day. **CHILDREN:** 45–65 mg/kg/day in 4 divided doses.

Dosage in Renal/Hepatic Impairment

No dose adjustment.

SIDE EFFECTS

Frequent: **PO:** Chalky taste. **Parenteral:** Pain, rash, redness, burning at injection site; flushing, nausea, vomiting, diaphoresis, hypotension. **Occasional:** **PO:** Mild constipation, fecal impaction, peripheral edema, metabolic alkalosis (muscle pain, restlessness, slow respirations, altered taste). **Calcium carbonate:** Milk-alkali syndrome (headache, decreased appetite, nausea, vomiting, unusual fatigue). **Rare:** Urinary urgency, painful urination.

ADVERSE EFFECTS/TOXIC REACTIONS

Hypercalcemia: Early signs: Constipation, headache, dry mouth, increased thirst, irritability, decreased appetite, metallic taste, fatigue, weakness, depression. **Later signs:** Confusion, drowsiness, hypertension, photosensitivity, arrhythmias, nausea, vomiting, painful urination.

NURSING CONSIDERATIONS

BASELINE ASSESSMENT

Assess B/P, ECG and cardiac rhythm, renal function, serum magnesium, phosphate, calcium, ionized calcium.

INTERVENTION/EVALUATION

Monitor serum BMP, calcium, ionized calcium, magnesium, phosphate; B/P, cardiac rhythm, renal function. Monitor for signs of hypercalcemia.

PATIENT/FAMILY TEACHING

• Do not take within 1–2 hrs of other oral medications, fiber-containing foods. • Avoid excessive use of alcohol, tobacco, caffeine.

canagliflozin

kan-a-gli-**floe**-zin
(Invokana)

Do not confuse canagliflozin with dapagliflozin, empagliflozin, or ertugliflozin.

FIXED-COMBINATION(S)

Invokamet: canagliflozin/metFORMIN (an antidiabetic): 50 mg/500 mg, 50 mg/1,000 mg, 150 mg/500 mg, 150 mg/1,000 mg.

◆CLASSIFICATION

PHARMACOTHERAPEUTIC: Sodium-glucose cotransporter 2 (SGLT2) inhibitor. **CLINICAL:** Antidiabetic.

USES

Adjunctive treatment to diet and exercise to improve glycemic control in pts with type 2 diabetes mellitus; risk reduction of major cardiovascular events (cardiovascular death, nonfatal MI, and nonfatal stroke) in adults with type 2 diabetes and established CV disease; reduce risk of end-stage kidney disease, doubling of serum creatinine, cardiovascular death, and hospitalization for HF in pts with type 2 diabetes mellitus and diabetic nephropathy with albuminuria.

PRECAUTIONS

Contraindications: Hypersensitivity to canagliflozin; pts who are being treated for glycemic control without established cardiovascular disease or multiple cardiovascular risk factors with severe renal impairment (eGFR less than 30 mL/min). **Cautions:** Concomitant use of loop diuretics, other hypoglycemic agents (e.g., insulin, insulin secretagogues), baseline systolic hypotension, renal impairment, hypovolemia/dehydration, recent genital mycotic infection; pts at risk for diabetic ketoacidosis (insulin dose reduction, acute febrile illness, reduced calorie intake, surgery, alcohol abuse, history of pancreatitis). Not recommended in pts with active bladder cancer, diabetic ketoacidosis, type 1 diabetes mellitus, severe renal impairment (eGFR less than 30 mL/min) when used for glycemic control.

ACTION

Inhibits SGLT2 in proximal renal tubule, reducing reabsorption of filtered glucose from tubular lumen and lowering renal threshold for glucose. Reduces reabsorption of sodium and increases delivery of sodium to the distal tubule. **Therapeutic Effect:** Increases urinary excretion of glucose; lowers serum glucose levels. Reduces cardiac preload and afterload; downregulates sympathetic activity.

PHARMACOKINETICS

Rapidly absorbed and widely distributed. Metabolized in liver. Peak plasma concentration: 1–2 hrs. Protein binding: 99%. Excreted in feces (42%), urine (33%). **Half-life:** 11–13 hrs.

⌛ LIFESPAN CONSIDERATIONS

Pregnancy/Lactation: Not recommended during second or third trimester. Unknown if distributed in breast milk. Breastfeeding not recommended. **Children:** Safety and efficacy not established. **Elderly:** May have increased risk for adverse reactions (e.g., hypotension, syncope, dehydration).

INTERACTIONS

DRUG: **CarBAMazepine, fosphenytoin, PHENobarbital, phenytoin** may decrease concentration/effect. May increase hypotensive effect of **loop diuretics (e.g., bumetanide, furosemide). Insulin, insulin secretagogues (e.g., glyBURIDE)** may increase risk of hypoglycemia. May increase concentration/effects of **digoxin.** **HERBAL:** **Fenugreek, garlic, ginkgo, ginger, ginseng** may increase hypoglycemic effect. **FOOD:** None known. **LAB VALUES:** May increase serum low-density lipoprotein-cholesterol (LDL-C), Hgb, creatinine, magnesium, phosphate, potassium. May decrease glomerular filtration rate. Expected to result in positive urine glucose test. May interfere with 1,5-anhydrogluitol (1,5-AG) assay.

AVAILABILITY (Rx)

Tablets: 100 mg, 300 mg.

ADMINISTRATION/HANDLING

PO

- Give before first meal of the day.

INDICATIONS/ROUTES/DOSAGE

Type 2 Diabetes Mellitus

PO: ADULTS/ELDERLY: 100 mg daily before first meal. May increase to 300 mg daily if glomerular filtration rate (GFR) greater than 60 mL/min.

C

Dose Modification

Concomitant use of insulin, insulin secretagogue: Consider lowering dose of insulin or insulin secretagogue to reduce hypoglycemic events.

Concomitant Use of UGT Inducers (e.g., rifampin, phenytoin, ritonavir)

eGFR 60 mL/min or greater: Increase dose to 200 mg once daily in pts taking concurrent 100-mg dose. May increase dose to 300 mg once daily in pts tolerating 200-mg dose who require additional glycemic control. **eGFR less than 60 mL/min:** Increase dose to 200 mg once daily in pts taking concurrent 100 mg dose. Consider additional antihyperglycemic agents who require additional glycemic control.

Dosage in Renal Impairment

GFR 30–59 mL/min: 100 mg daily (maximum). **GFR less than 30 mL/min:** Permanently discontinue.

Dosage in Hepatic Impairment

No dose adjustment.

SIDE EFFECTS

Occasional (5%): Increased urination. **Rare (3%–2%):** Thirst, nausea, constipation.

ADVERSE EFFECTS/TOXIC REACTIONS

May increase risk of lower limb amputations. Symptomatic hypotension (orthostatic hypotension, postural dizziness, syncope) may occur, esp. in pts who are elderly, use concomitant loop diuretics, or have baseline systolic hypotension. Intravascular volume depletion/contraction may cause acute kidney injury requiring dialysis. Fatal cases of ketoacidosis were reported. Hypoglycemic events were reported in pts using concomitant insulin, insulin secretagogues. Infections including influenza, nasopharyngitis, pyelonephritis, urosepsis, UTI, genital mycotic infections (male and female), upper respiratory tract infection may occur. Necrotizing fasciitis of the perineum (Fournier's gangrene), a life-threatening necrotizing infection of the genital and perineum region that requires urgent surgical intervention, has been reported. An increased risk of bone fracture was reported. Hypersensitivity reactions including anaphylaxis, angioedema, urticaria have occurred.

NURSING CONSIDERATIONS

BASELINE ASSESSMENT

Obtain BUN, serum creatinine, eGFR, CrCl, blood glucose level, Hgb A1c; B/P. Assess hydration status. Correct volume depletion before initiation. Assess pt's understanding of diabetes management, routine home glucose monitoring. Obtain dietary consult for nutritional education. Question history of renal impairment, type 1 diabetes, ketoacidosis. In pts requiring surgery, consider suspending treatment at least 3 days before surgery.

INTERVENTION/EVALUATION

Monitor BUN, serum creatinine, eGFR, CrCl, blood glucose level, Hgb A1c; B/P periodically. Monitor for ketoacidosis (e.g., dehydration, confusion, extreme thirst, sweet-smelling breath, Kussmaul respirations, nausea), hypoglycemia (anxiety, confusion, diaphoresis, diplopia, dizziness, headache, hunger, perioral numbness, tachycardia, tremors), hyperglycemia (fatigue, Kussmaul respirations, polyphagia, polyuria, polydipsia, nausea, vomiting). Pts presenting with metabolic acidosis should be screened for ketoacidosis, regardless of serum glucose levels. Concomitant use of beta blockers (e.g., carvedilol, metoprolol) may mask symptoms of hypoglycemia. Monitor for acute kidney injury (dark-colored urine, flank pain, decreased urine output, muscle aches), infections (cough, fatigue, fever), urinary tract infections (dysuria, fever, flank pain, malaise), mycotic infections, Fournier's gangrene (perineal necrosis). Screen for glucose-altering conditions (fever, increased activity or stress, surgical procedures). Monitor weight, I&Os. Monitor for hypersensitivity reactions (anaphylaxis, angioedema, urticaria). Diligently monitor for new leg ulcers, sores, pain; wound may lead to amputation.

PATIENT/FAMILY TEACHING

• Diabetes mellitus requires lifelong control. Diet and exercise are principal parts of treatment; do not skip or delay meals. Test blood sugar regularly. Monitor daily calorie intake. • When taking combination drug therapy or when glucose conditions are altered (excessive alcohol ingestion, insufficient carbohydrate intake, hormone deficiencies, critical illness), have a low blood sugar treatment available (e.g., glucagon, oral dextrose). • Genital itching or discharge may indicate yeast infection. • Report symptoms of perineal necrosis (e.g., discoloration, pain, swelling of the scrotum, penis, or perineum). • Therapy may increase risk for dehydration, low blood pressure, which may cause kidney failure. Report decreased urination, amber-colored urine, flank pain, fatigue, swelling of the hands or feet. Drink enough fluids to maintain adequate hydration. Pts with HF should be cautious of overhydration. • Report symptoms of UTI, kidney infection (back pain, pelvic pain, burning while urinating, cloudy or foul-smelling urine), allergic reactions (difficulty breathing, rash, wheezing; swelling of the face or tongue). • Go slowly from lying to standing. • Do not breastfeed. • Treatment may cause loss of limbs; immediately report new leg ulcers, pain, tenderness.

candesartan

kan-de-**sar**-tan
(Atacand)

BLACK BOX ALERT May cause fetal injury, mortality. Discontinue as soon as possible once pregnancy is detected.

FIXED-COMBINATION(S)

Atacand HCT: candesartan/hydroCHLOROthiazide (a diuretic): 16 mg/12.5 mg, 32 mg/12.5 mg.

◆CLASSIFICATION

PHARMACOTHERAPEUTIC: Angiotensin II receptor blocker. **CLINICAL:** Antihypertensive.

USES

Treatment of hypertension alone or in combination with other antihypertensives, HF: NYHA class II–IV.

PRECAUTIONS

Contraindications: Hypersensitivity to candesartan. Concomitant use with aliskiren in pts with diabetes mellitus. **Cautions:** Significant aortic/mitral stenosis, renal/hepatic impairment, unstented (unilateral/bilateral) renal artery stenosis, HF (may induce hypotension when treatment initiated).

ACTION

Blocks vasoconstriction, aldosterone-secreting effects of angiotensin II, inhibiting binding of angiotensin II to AT_1 receptors. **Therapeutic Effect:** Produces vasodilation; decreases peripheral resistance, B/P.

PHARMACOKINETICS

Route	Onset	Peak	Duration
PO	2–3 hrs	6–8 hrs	Greater than 24 hrs

Rapidly, completely absorbed. Protein binding: greater than 99%. Undergoes minor hepatic metabolism to inactive metabolite. Excreted unchanged in urine and in feces through biliary system. Not removed by hemodialysis. **Half-life:** 9 hrs.

⌛ LIFESPAN CONSIDERATIONS

Pregnancy/Lactation: Unknown if distributed in breast milk. May cause fetal/neonatal morbidity/mortality. **Children:** Safety and efficacy not established in pts younger than 1 yr. **Elderly:** No age-related precautions noted.

C

INTERACTIONS

DRUG: May increase risk of **lithium** toxicity. **NSAIDs (e.g., ibuprofen, ketorolac, naproxen)** may decrease antihypertensive effect. **Aliskiren** may increase hyperkalemic effect. May increase adverse/toxicity of **ACE inhibitors (e.g., benazepril, lisinopril). HERBAL: Herbals with hypertensive properties (e.g., licorice, yohimbe)** or **hypotensive properties (e.g., garlic, ginger, ginkgo biloba)** may alter effects. **FOOD:** None known. **LAB VALUES:** May increase serum BUN, alkaline phosphatase, bilirubin, creatinine, ALT, AST. May decrease Hgb, Hct.

AVAILABILITY (Rx)

Tablets: 4 mg, 8 mg, 16 mg, 32 mg.

ADMINISTRATION/HANDLING

PO

- Give without regard to food.

INDICATIONS/ROUTES/DOSAGE

Hypertension

Note: Antihypertensive effect usually seen in 2 wks. Maximum effect within 4–6 wks.

PO: ADULTS, ELDERLY: Initially, 8 mg once daily. Evaluate response q4–6wks Range: 8–32 mg once daily. **CHILDREN 6–16 YRS WEIGHING MORE THAN 50 KG:** Initially, 8–16 mg/day in 1–2 divided doses. Range: 4–32 mg. **Maximum:** 32 mg/day. **50 KG OR LESS:** Initially, 4–8 mg in 1–2 divided doses. Range: 2–16 mg/day. **Maximum:** 32 mg/day. **CHILDREN 1–5 YRS:** Initially, 0.2 mg/kg/day in 1–2 divided doses. Range: 0.05–0.4 mg/kg/day. **Maximum:** 0.4 mg/kg/day.

HF

PO: ADULTS, ELDERLY: Initially, 4–8 mg once daily. May double dose at approximately 2-wk intervals up to a target dose of 32 mg/day.

Dosage in Renal/Hepatic Impairment

Mild to moderate impairment: No dose adjustment. **Severe impairment:** Use caution.

SIDE EFFECTS

Occasional (6%–3%): Upper respiratory tract infection, dizziness, back/leg pain. **Rare (2%–1%):** Pharyngitis, rhinitis, headache, fatigue, diarrhea, nausea, dry cough, peripheral edema.

ADVERSE EFFECTS/TOXIC REACTIONS

Overdosage may cause hypotension, tachycardia. Bradycardia occurs less often. May increase risk of renal failure, hyperkalemia.

NURSING CONSIDERATIONS

BASELINE ASSESSMENT

Obtain B/P immediately before each dose in addition to regular monitoring (be alert to fluctuations). Obtain pregnancy test in females of reproductive potential. Assess medication history (esp. diuretic). Question for history of hepatic/renal impairment, renal artery stenosis. Obtain serum BUN, creatinine, LFT.

INTERVENTION/EVALUATION

Maintain hydration (offer fluids frequently). Assess for evidence of upper respiratory infection. Assist with ambulation if dizziness occurs. Monitor electrolytes, renal function, urinalysis. Assess B/P for hypertension/hypotension. If excessive reduction in B/P occurs, place pt in supine position, feet slightly elevated.

PATIENT/FAMILY TEACHING

• Hypertension requires lifelong control. • Inform female pts regarding potential for fetal injury, mortality with second- and third-trimester exposure to candesartan. • Report suspected pregnancy. • Avoid tasks that require alertness, motor skills until response to drug is established. • Report any sign of infection (sore throat, fever). • Caution against exercising during hot weather (risk of dehydration, hypotension).

capecitabine

TOP 100 HIGH ALERT

kap-e-**sye**-ta-bine
(Xeloda)

■ BLACK BOX ALERT ■ May increase anticoagulant effect of warfarin. Fatal hemorrhagic events have occurred.

Do not confuse capecitabine with decitabine or emtricitabine, or Xeloda with Xenical.

◆ CLASSIFICATION

PHARMACOTHERAPEUTIC: Antimetabolite. **CLINICAL:** Antineoplastic.

USES

Treatment of metastatic breast cancer as monotherapy or in combination with docetaxel after failure of prior anthracycline-containing regimen. Treatment of metastatic colorectal cancer. Adjuvant (postsurgical) treatment of Dukes C colon cancer. **OFF-LABEL:** Gastric cancer, pancreatic cancer, esophageal cancer, ovarian cancer, neuroendocrine tumors, hepatobiliary cancer.

PRECAUTIONS

Contraindications: Severe renal impairment (CrCl less than 30 mL/min), dihydropyrimidine dehydrogenase (DPD) deficiency, hypersensitivity to capecitabine, 5-fluorouracil (5-FU). **Cautions:** Existing bone marrow depression, hepatic impairment, mild to moderate renal impairment, previous cytotoxic therapy/radiation therapy, elderly (60 yrs of age or older).

ACTION

Enzymatically converted to 5-fluorouracil (5-FU). Inhibits enzymes necessary for synthesis of essential cellular components. **Therapeutic Effect:** Interferes with DNA synthesis, RNA processing, protein synthesis.

PHARMACOKINETICS

Readily absorbed from GI tract. Protein binding: less than 60%. Metabolized in liver. Primarily excreted in urine. **Half-life:** 45 min.

⌛ LIFESPAN CONSIDERATIONS

Pregnancy/Lactation: May cause fetal harm. Unknown if distributed in breast milk. **Children:** Safety and efficacy not established. **Elderly:** May be more sensitive to GI side effects.

INTERACTIONS

DRUG: May increase concentration, toxicity of **warfarin, phenytoin.** Myelosuppression may be enhanced when given concurrently with **bone marrow depressants. Live virus vaccines** may potentiate virus replication, increase vaccine side effects, decrease pt's antibody response to vaccine. May decrease therapeutic effect of **BCG (intravesical). Allopurinol** may decrease concentration/effect. **HERBAL: Echinacea** may decrease therapeutic effect. **FOOD:** None known. **LAB VALUES:** May increase serum alkaline phosphatase, bilirubin, ALT, AST. May decrease Hgb, Hct, WBC. May increase PT/INR.

AVAILABILITY (Rx)

Tablets: 150 mg, 500 mg.

ADMINISTRATION/HANDLING

- Give within 30 min after meals with water.
- Administer whole; do not cut, crush.

INDICATIONS/ROUTES/DOSAGE

Metastatic Breast Cancer (as Monotherapy or in Combination With Docetaxel), Metastatic Colorectal Cancer, Adjuvant (Postsurgery) Treatment of Dukes C Colon Cancer

PO: ADULTS, ELDERLY: Initially, 2,500 mg/m^2/day in 2 equally divided doses approximately q12h apart for 2 wks. Follow with a 1-wk rest period; given in 3-wk cycles.

Dosage in Renal Impairment

CrCl 51–80 mL/min: No adjustment. **CrCl 30–50 mL/min:** 75% of normal dose. **CrCl less than 30 mL/min:** Contraindicated.

Dosage in Hepatic Impairment

No dose adjustment at start of therapy; interrupt therapy for Grade 3 or 4 hyperbilirubinemia until bilirubin is 3 times ULN or less.

C

SIDE EFFECTS

Frequent (55%–25%): Diarrhea, nausea, vomiting, stomatitis, fatigue, anorexia, dermatitis. **Occasional (24%–10%):** Constipation, dyspepsia, headache, dizziness, insomnia, edema, myalgia, pyrexia, dehydration, dyspnea, back pain. **Rare (less than 10%):** Mood changes, depression, sore throat, epistaxis, cough, visual abnormalities.

ADVERSE EFFECTS/TOXIC REACTIONS

Serious reactions include myelosuppression (neutropenia, thrombocytopenia, anemia), cardiovascular toxicity (angina, cardiomyopathy, DVT), respiratory toxicity (dyspnea, epistaxis, pneumonia), lymphedema. Palmar-plantar erythrodysesthesia syndrome (PPES), presenting as redness, swelling, numbness, skin sloughing of hands and feet, may occur.

NURSING CONSIDERATIONS

BASELINE ASSESSMENT

Assess sensitivity to capecitabine or 5-fluorouracil. Obtain baseline Hgb, Hct, serum chemistries, renal function.

INTERVENTION/EVALUATION

Monitor for severe diarrhea, nausea, vomiting; if dehydration occurs, fluid and electrolyte replacement therapy should be initiated. Assess hands/feet for PPES. Monitor CBC for evidence of bone marrow depression. Monitor renal/hepatic function. Monitor for blood dyscrasias (fever, sore throat, signs of local infection, unusual bruising/bleeding from any site), symptoms of anemia (excessive fatigue, weakness).

PATIENT/FAMILY TEACHING

- Report nausea, vomiting, diarrhea, hand-and-foot syndrome, stomatitis.
- Do not have immunizations without physician's approval (drug lowers body's resistance).
- Avoid contact with those who have recently received live virus vaccine.
- Promptly report fever higher than 100.5°F, sore throat, signs of local infection, unusual bruising/bleeding from any site.

capmatinib

kap-**ma**-ti-nib
(Tabrecta)

Do not confuse capmatinib with cabozantinib, capecitabine, ceritinib, cobimetinib, crizotinib, or imatinib.

◆CLASSIFICATION

PHARMACOTHERAPEUTIC: Mesenchymal-epithelial transition (MET) tyrosine kinase inhibitor. **CLINICAL:** Antineoplastic.

USES

Treatment of adults with metastatic non–small-cell lung cancer (NSCLC) whose tumors have a mutation that leads to MET exon 14 skipping.

PRECAUTIONS

Contraindications: Hypersensitivity to capmatinib. **Cautions:** Baseline anemia, leukopenia, lymphopenia; hepatic impairment, pulmonary disease; concomitant use of CYP3A inhibitors, CYP1A2 substrates, P-glycoprotein substrates, breast cancer resistance protein (BCRP) substrates. Avoid concomitant use of strong or moderate CYP3A inducers.

ACTION

Inhibits MET phosphorylation (including the mutant variant produced by exon 14 skipping), which increases downstream MET signaling. **Therapeutic Effect:** Decreases tumor cell growth.

PHARMACOKINETICS

Widely distributed. Metabolized in liver and by aldehyde oxidase. Protein binding: 96%. Peak plasma concentration: 1–2 hrs. Steady state reached in 3 days. Excreted in feces (78%), urine (22%). **Half-life:** 6.5 hrs.

LIFESPAN CONSIDERATIONS

Pregnancy/Lactation: Avoid pregnancy; may cause fetal harm. Female and male pts of reproductive potential must use effective contraception during treatment and for at least 7 days after discontinuation. Unknown if distributed in breast milk. Breastfeeding not recommended during treatment and for at least 7 days after discontinuation. **Children:** Safety and efficacy not established. **Elderly:** No age-related precautions noted.

INTERACTIONS

DRUG: **Strong CYP3A4 inducers (e.g., carBAMazepine, phenytoin, rifAMPin), moderate CYP3A inducers (e.g., bosentan, efavirenz, nafcillin)** may decrease concentration/effect. May increase concentration/effect of **alpelisib, cladribine, ozanimod, pazopanib, topotecan, vinCRIStine.** HERBAL: None significant. FOOD: None known. LAB VALUES: May increase serum alkaline phosphatase, ALT, AST, amylase, creatinine, GGT, lipase, potassium. May decrease serum albumin, glucose, phosphate, sodium, magnesium; Hgb, leukocytes, lymphocytes.

AVAILABILITY (Rx)

Tablets: 150 mg, 200 mg.

ADMINISTRATION/HANDLING

PO

- Give with or without regard to food.
- Administer tablets whole; do not break, crush, or divide. Tablet cannot be chewed.
- If vomiting occurs after administration, give next dose at regularly scheduled time (do not give additional dose).

INDICATIONS/ROUTES/DOSAGE

Non–Small-Cell Lung Cancer

PO: ADULTS, ELDERLY: 400 mg twice daily.

Dose Reduction Schedule for Adverse Events

First dose reduction: 300 mg twice daily. **Second dose reduction:** 200 mg twice daily. **Unable to tolerate 200 mg dose:** Permanently discontinue.

Dose Modification

Based on Common Terminology Criteria for Adverse Events (CTCAE).

Serum ALT/AST elevation

Grade 3 serum ALT/AST elevation (without total bilirubin elevation): Withhold treatment until improved to baseline. If improved within 7 days, resume at same dose. If not improved within 7 days, resume at reduced dose level. **Grade 4 serum ALT/AST elevation (without total bilirubin elevation):** Permanently discontinue. **Serum ALT/AST elevation greater than 3 times ULN (with total bilirubin elevation greater than 2 times ULN):** Permanently discontinue.

Hyperbilirubinemia

Grade 2 increased total bilirubin (without ALT/AST elevation): Withhold treatment until improved to baseline. If improved within 7 days, resume at same dose. If not improved within 7 days, resume at reduced dose level. **Grade 3 increased total bilirubin (without ALT/AST elevation):** Withhold treatment until improved to baseline. If improved within 7 days, resume at reduced dose level. If not improved within 7 days, permanently discontinue. **Grade 4 increased total bilirubin (without ALT/AST elevation):** Permanently discontinue.

Interstitial Lung Disease (ILD)

Any grade treatment-related ILD: Permanently discontinue.

Other Toxicities

Any Grade 2 toxicities: No dose adjustment. If intolerable, consider withholding treatment until resolved, then resume at reduced dose level. **Any Grade 3 toxicity:** Withhold treatment until resolved, then resume at reduced dose level. **Any Grade 4 toxicities:** Permanently discontinue.

C

Dosage in Renal Impairment

Mild to moderate impairment: No dose adjustment. **Severe impairment:** Not specified; use caution.

Dosage in Hepatic Impairment

Mild to severe impairment: Not specified; use caution.

SIDE EFFECTS

Frequent (52%–18%): Peripheral edema, fatigue, asthenia, nausea, vomiting, dyspnea, decreased appetite, constipation, diarrhea, cough. **Occasional (15%–less than 10%):** Noncardiac chest pain, back pain, pyrexia, decreased weight, pruritus, urticaria.

ADVERSE EFFECTS/TOXIC REACTIONS

Anemia, leukopenia, lymphopenia is an expected response to therapy. Pneumonitis, ILD reported in 5% of pts. Hepatotoxicity reported in 13% of pts. Photosensitivity reactions from UV exposure may increase risk of sunburn, skin erythema. Acute kidney injury, cellulitis reported in less than 10% of pts.

NURSING CONSIDERATIONS

BASELINE ASSESSMENT

Obtain CBC, BMP, LFTs; pregnancy test in females of reproductive potential. Confirm compliance of effective contraception. Confirm presence of mutation that leads to MET exon 14 skipping in tumor expression. Question history of hepatic impairment, pulmonary disease. Screen for active infection. Receive full medication history and screen for interactions. Offer emotional support.

INTERVENTION/EVALUATION

Monitor LFTs q2wks for 3 mos, then monthly thereafter (or more frequently in pts with hepatotoxicity). Monitor BUN, CrCl, serum creatinine periodically for acute kidney injury. An increase of serum creatinine greater than 0.4 mg/dL from baseline may indicate renal impairment. Consider ABG, radiologic test if ILD/pneumonitis (excessive cough, dyspnea, fever, hypoxia) is suspected. Monitor for drug toxicities if discontinuation or dose reduction of concomitant CYP3A inhibitor, P-glycoprotein inhibitor, CYP1A2 inhibitor is unavoidable.

PATIENT/FAMILY TEACHING

• Treatment may depress your immune system response and reduce your ability to fight infection. Report symptoms of infection such as body aches, chills, cough, fatigue, fever. Avoid those with active infection. • Report symptoms of lung inflammation (excessive coughing, difficulty breathing, chest pain); toxic skin reactions (itching, peeling, rash, redness, swelling); liver problems (abdominal pain, bruising, clay-colored stool, amber- or dark-colored urine, yellowing of the skin or eyes), kidney problems (decreased urine output, flank pain, darkened urine). • Females and males of childbearing potential must use reliable contraception during treatment and for at least 7 days after last dose. Do not breastfeed. • Avoid prolonged sun exposure/tanning beds. Use high SPF sunscreen, lip balm, clothing to protect against sunburn. • There is a high risk of interactions with other medications. Do not take newly prescribed medications unless approved by prescriber who originally started therapy. • Avoid grapefruit products, herbal supplements (esp. St. John's wort).

captopril

kap-toe-pril

■ BLACK BOX ALERT ■ May cause injury/death to developing fetus. Discontinue as soon as possible once pregnancy is detected.

Do not confuse captopril with calcitriol, Capitrol, carvedilol, enalapril, fosinopril, lisinopril, Monopril, or quinapril.

FIXED-COMBINATION(S)

Capozide: captopril/hydroCHLOROthiazide (a diuretic): 25 mg/15 mg, 25 mg/25 mg, 50 mg/15 mg, 50 mg/25 mg.

C

◆CLASSIFICATION

PHARMACOTHERAPEUTIC: Angiotensin-converting enzyme (ACE) inhibitor. **CLINICAL:** Antihypertensive, vasodilator.

USES

Treatment of hypertension, HF, diabetic nephropathy, post-MI to improve survival in pts with left ventricular dysfunction.

PRECAUTIONS

Contraindications: Hypersensitivity to captopril. History of angioedema from previous treatment with ACE inhibitors, concomitant use with aliskiren in pts with diabetes mellitus. Coadministration with or within 36 hrs of switching to or from a neprilysin inhibitor (e.g., sacubitril). **Cautions:** Renal impairment; hypertrophic cardiomyopathy with outflow obstruction before, during, or immediately after major surgery. Unstented unilateral/bilateral renal artery stenosis. Concomitant use of potassium-sparing diuretics, potassium supplements.

ACTION

Suppresses renin-angiotensin-aldosterone system (prevents conversion of angiotensin I to angiotensin II, a potent vasoconstrictor; may inhibit angiotensin II at local vascular and renal sites). Decreases plasma angiotensin II, increases plasma renin activity, decreases aldosterone secretion. **Therapeutic Effect:** Lowers BP. Improves HF, diabetic neuropathy.

PHARMACOKINETICS

Route	Onset	Peak	Duration
PO	0.25 hr	0.5–1.5 hrs	Dose-related

Rapidly, well absorbed from GI tract (absorption decreased in presence of food). Protein binding: 25%–30%. Metabolized in liver. Primarily excreted in urine. Removed by hemodialysis. **Half-life:** Less than 3 hrs (increased in renal impairment).

LIFESPAN CONSIDERATIONS

Pregnancy/Lactation: Crosses placenta; distributed in breast milk. May cause fetal/neonatal mortality/morbidity. **Children:** Safety and efficacy not established. **Elderly:** May be more sensitive to hypotensive effects.

INTERACTIONS

DRUG: **Aliskiren** may increase hyperkalemic effect. May increase potential for allergic reactions to **allopurinol. Angiotensin II receptor blockers (ARBs) (e.g., losartan, valsartan)** may increase adverse effects. May increase adverse effects of **lithium, sacubitril. HERBAL: Herbals with hypertensive properties (e.g., licorice, yohimbe)** or **hypotensive properties (e.g., garlic, ginger, ginkgo biloba)** may alter effects. **FOOD: Licorice** may cause sodium and water retention, hypokalemia. **LAB VALUES:** May increase serum BUN, alkaline phosphatase, bilirubin, creatinine, potassium, ALT, AST. May decrease serum sodium. May cause positive ANA titer.

AVAILABILITY (Rx)

Tablets: 12.5 mg, 25 mg, 50 mg, 100 mg.

ADMINISTRATION/HANDLING

PO

• Administer 1 hr before or 2 hrs after meals for maximum absorption (food may decrease drug absorption). • Tablets may be crushed.

INDICATIONS/ROUTES/DOSAGE

Hypertension

PO: ADULTS, ELDERLY: Initially, 12.5–25 mg 2–3 times/day. May increase by 12.5–25 mg/dose at 1–2-wk intervals up to 50 mg 3 times/day. Add diuretic before further increase in dose. **CHILDREN, ADOLESCENTS:** 0.3–0.5 mg 3 times/day. **Maximum:** 6 mg/kg/day in 3 divided doses. **INFANTS:** 0.1–0.3 mg/kg/dose. May titrate up to maximum of 6 mg/kg/day in 3 divided doses. Usual range: 2.5–6 mg/kg/day in 3 divided doses. **NEONATES:** 0.01–0.1 mg/kg/dose q8–24h. **Maximum:** 0.5 mg/kg/dose q6–24h.

HF

PO: ADULTS, ELDERLY: Initially, 6.25 mg 3 times/day. **Target dose:** 50 mg 3 times/day.

Post-MI

PO: ADULTS, ELDERLY: Initially, 6.25 mg. If tolerated, then 12.5 mg 3 times/day. Increase to 25 mg 3 times/day over several days, up to target dose of 50 mg 3 times/day over several wks.

Diabetic Nephropathy

PO: ADULTS, ELDERLY: 25 mg 3 times/day.

Dosage in Renal Impairment

CrCl 10–50 mL/min: 75% of normal dosage. **CrCl less than 10 mL/min:** 50% of normal dosage.

Dosage in Hepatic Impairment

No dose adjustment.

SIDE EFFECTS

Frequent (7%–4%): Rash. **Occasional (4%–2%):** Pruritus, dysgeusia. **Rare (less than 2%):** Headache, cough, insomnia, dizziness, fatigue, paresthesia, malaise, nausea, diarrhea or constipation, dry mouth, tachycardia.

ADVERSE EFFECTS/TOXIC REACTIONS

Hypotension ("first-dose syncope") may occur in pts with HF and in those who are severely sodium/volume depleted. Angioedema, hyperkalemia occur rarely. Agranulocytosis, neutropenia noted in those with collagen vascular disease (scleroderma, systemic lupus erythematosus), renal impairment. Nephrotic syndrome noted in those with history of renal disease.

NURSING CONSIDERATIONS

BASELINE ASSESSMENT

Obtain B/P immediately before each dose in addition to regular monitoring (be alert to fluctuations). In pts with prior renal disease or receiving dosages greater than 150 mg/day, test urine for protein by dipstick method with first urine of day before therapy begins and periodically thereafter. In pts with renal impairment, autoimmune disease, or taking drugs that affect leukocytes or immune response, obtain CBC before beginning therapy, q2wks for 3 mos, then periodically thereafter.

INTERVENTION/EVALUATION

Assess skin for rash, pruritus. Assist with ambulation if dizziness occurs. Monitor urinalysis for proteinuria. Monitor serum potassium levels in pts on concurrent diuretic therapy. Monitor B/P, serum BUN, creatinine, CBC. Discontinue medication, contact physician if angioedema occurs.

PATIENT/FAMILY TEACHING

• Full therapeutic effect of B/P reduction may take several wks. • Skipping doses or voluntarily discontinuing drug may produce severe rebound hypertension. • Limit alcohol intake. • Immediately report if swelling of face, lips, or tongue, difficulty breathing, vomiting, diarrhea, excessive perspiration, dehydration, persistent cough, sore throat, fever occur. • Inform physician if pregnant or planning to become pregnant. • Rise slowly from sitting/lying position.

carBAMazepine

kar-ba-**maz**-e-peen
(Carbatrol, Epitol, Equetro, TEGretol, TEGretol XR)

■ **BLACK BOX ALERT** ■ Potentially fatal aplastic anemia, agranulocytosis reported. Potentially fatal, severe dermatologic reactions (e.g., Stevens-Johnson syndrome, toxic epidermal necrolysis) may occur. Risk increased in pts with the variant HLA-β* 1502 allele, almost exclusively in pts of Asian ancestry.

Do not confuse carBAMazepine with OXcarbazepine, eslicarbazepine, or TEGretol with Mebaral, Toprol XL, Toradol, or TRENtal.

◆CLASSIFICATION

PHARMACOTHERAPEUTIC: Iminostilbene derivative. **CLINICAL:** Anticonvulsant.

USES

Carbatrol, Epitol, TEGretol, TEGretol XR: Treatment of partial seizures with complex symptomatology, generalized tonic-clonic seizures, mixed seizure patterns, pain relief of trigeminal, glossopharyngeal neuralgia. **Equetro:** Acute manic and mixed episodes associated with bipolar disorder. **OFF-LABEL:** Neuropathic pain in critically ill pts.

PRECAUTIONS

Contraindications: Concomitant use or within 14 days of use of MAOIs, myelosuppression. Concomitant use of delavirdine or other NNRT inhibitors that are substrates of CYP3A4. Hypersensitivity to carBAMazepine, tricyclic antidepressants. **Cautions:** High risk of suicide, increased IOP, hepatic or renal impairment, history of cardiac impairment, ECG abnormalities, elderly.

ACTION

Decreases sodium ion influx into neuronal membranes (may depress activity in thalamus, decreasing synaptic transmission or decreasing temporal stimulation, leading to neural discharge). **Therapeutic Effect:** Produces anticonvulsant effect.

PHARMACOKINETICS

Slowly, completely absorbed from GI tract. Protein binding: 75%–90%. Metabolized in liver. Primarily excreted in urine. Not removed by hemodialysis. **Half-life:** 25–65 hrs (decreased with chronic use).

⌛ LIFESPAN CONSIDERATIONS

Pregnancy/Lactation: Crosses placenta; distributed in breast milk. Accumulates in fetal tissue. **Children:** Behavioral changes more likely to occur. **Elderly:** More susceptible to confusion, agitation, AV block, bradycardia, syndrome of inappropriate antidiuretic hormone (SIADH).

INTERACTIONS

DRUG: CYP3A4 inhibitors (e.g., cimetidine, clarithromycin, azole antifungals, protease inhibitors) may increase concentration. **CYP3A4 inducers (e.g., rifAMPin, phenytoin)** may decrease concentration/effects. May decrease concentration/effects of **hormonal contraceptives, warfarin, traZODone.** May decrease concentration/effects of **abemaciclib, apixaban, axitinib, bosutinib, brigatinib, dronedarone, nifedipine, ranolazine, regorafenib, vorapaxar, voriconazole.** May decrease therapeutic effect of **BCG (intravesical). HERBAL: Gotu kola, kava kava, valerian** may increase CNS depression. **St. John's wort** may decrease concentration/effect. **FOOD: Grapefruit products** may increase concentration/effect. **LAB VALUES:** May increase serum BUN, glucose, alkaline phosphatase, bilirubin, ALT, AST, cholesterol, HDL, triglycerides. May decrease serum calcium, thyroid hormone (T_3, T_4 index) levels. **Therapeutic serum level:** 4–12 mcg/mL; **toxic serum level:** greater than 12 mcg/mL.

AVAILABILITY (Rx)

Oral Suspension: 100 mg/5 mL. **Tablets:** 200 mg. **Tablets:** ***(Chewable):*** 100 mg.

Capsules: ***(Extended-Release):*** 100 mg, 200 mg, 300 mg. **Tablets:** ***(Extended-Release):*** 100 mg, 200 mg, 400 mg.

ADMINISTRATION/HANDLING

PO

• Store oral suspension, tablets at room temperature. • To reduce GI distress, give tablets or extended-release tablets with food. May give extended-release capsules without regard to food. Give extended-release capsules whole; do not cut or crush. Capsules may be opened and beads sprinkled on food (e.g., applesauce). • Give extended-release tablets whole; do not break, cut, or crush. Extended-release formulations cannot be chewed. • Shake oral suspension well. Do not administer simultaneously with other liquid medicine.

INDICATIONS/ROUTES/DOSAGE

◀ALERT▶ Suspension must be given on a 3–4 times/day schedule; tablets on a 2–4 times/day schedule; extended-release capsules 2 times/day. ***(Carnexiv):*** 70% of total oral dose given as four 30-min infusions separated by 6 hrs.

Seizure Control

PO: ADULTS, ELDERLY, CHILDREN OLDER THAN 12 YRS: Initially, 2–3 mg/kg/day (100–200 mg/day). May increase dose by 200 mg or less per day in time increments of at least q5days. Usual dose: 800–1,200 mg/day in 2–4 divided doses. **Maximum: ADULTS, ELDERLY:** 1,600 mg/day; **CHILDREN OLDER THAN 15 YRS:** 1,200 mg/day; **CHILDREN 13–15 YRS:** 1,000 mg/day. **CHILDREN 6–12 YRS:** Initially, 100 mg twice daily (tablets) or 4 times/day (oral suspension). May increase by 100 mg/day at wkly intervals. **Usual dose:** 400–800 mg/day. **Maximum:** 1,000 mg/day. **CHILDREN YOUNGER THAN 6 YRS:** Initially, 10–20 mg/kg/day 2–3 times/day (tablets) or 4 times/day (suspension). May increase at wkly intervals until optimal response and therapeutic levels are achieved. **Maximum:** 35 mg/kg/day.

Trigeminal, Glossopharyngeal Neuralgia, Diabetic Neuropathy

PO: ADULTS, ELDERLY: Initially, 200 mg/day as single dose (extended-release), or 100 mg in 2 divided doses (immediate-release), or 50 mg 4 times/day (oral suspension). May increase by 200 mg/day as needed. Give extended release in 2 divided doses if total daily dose exceeds 200 mg. **Usual dose:** 600–800 mg daily. **Maximum:** 1,200 mg/day.

Bipolar Disorder

PO: ADULTS, ELDERLY: Initially, 100–400 mg/day in 2 divided doses. May adjust dose in 200-mg increments q1–4 days. **Usual range:** 600–1,200 mg/day. **Maximum:** 1,600 mg/day in divided doses.

Dosage in Renal Impairment

CrCl less than 10 mL/min: 75% of normal dose. **HD:** 75% of normal dose. **CRRT:** 75% of normal dose.

Dosage in Hepatic Impairment

Use caution.

SIDE EFFECTS

Frequent (greater than 10%): Vertigo, somnolence, ataxia, fatigue, leukopenia, rash, urticaria, nausea, vomiting. **Occasional (10%–1%):** Headache, diplopia, blurred vision, thrombocytopenia, dry mouth, edema, fluid retention, increased weight. **Rare (less than 1%):** Tremors, visual disturbances, lymphadenopathy, jaundice, involuntary muscle movements, nystagmus, dermatitis.

ADVERSE EFFECTS/TOXIC REACTIONS

Toxic reactions appear as blood dyscrasias (aplastic anemia, agranulocytosis, thrombocytopenia, leukopenia, leukocytosis, eosinophilia), cardiovascular disturbances (HF, hypotension/hypertension, thrombophlebitis, arrhythmias), dermatologic effects (rash, urticaria, pruritus, photosensitivity). Abrupt withdrawal may precipitate status epilepticus.

NURSING CONSIDERATIONS

BASELINE ASSESSMENT

CBC, serum iron determination, urinalysis, BUN should be performed before therapy begins and periodically during therapy. **Seizures:** Review history of seizure disorder (intensity, frequency, duration, level of consciousness [LOC]). Initiate seizure precautions. **Neuralgia:** Assess facial pain, stimuli that may cause facial pain. **Bipolar:** Assess mental status, cognitive abilities.

INTERVENTION/EVALUATION

Seizures: Observe frequently for recurrence of seizure activity. Monitor therapeutic levels. Assess for clinical improvement (decrease in intensity, frequency of seizures). Assess for clinical evidence of early toxicity (fever, sore throat, mouth ulcerations, unusual bruising/bleeding, joint pain). **Neuralgia:** Avoid triggering tic douloureux (draft, talking, washing face, jarring bed, hot/warm/cold food or liquids). **Bipolar:** Monitor for suicidal ideation, behavioral changes. Observe for excessive sedation. **Therapeutic serum level:** 4–12 mcg/mL; **toxic serum level:** greater than 12 mcg/mL.

PATIENT/FAMILY TEACHING

• Do not abruptly discontinue medication after long-term use (may precipitate seizures). • Strict maintenance of therapy is essential for seizure control. • Avoid tasks that require alertness, motor skills until response to drug is established. • Report visual disturbances. • Blood tests should be repeated frequently during first 3 mos of therapy and at monthly intervals thereafter for 2–3 yrs. • Do not take oral suspension simultaneously with other liquid medicine. • Do not ingest grapefruit products. • Report serious skin reactions.

carbidopa/levodopa

kar-bi-doe-pa/**lee**-voe-doe-pa
(Apo-Levocarb ✦, Duopa, Rytary, Sinemet, Sinemet CR)
Do not confuse Sinemet with Serevent.

FIXED-COMBINATION(S)

Stalevo: carbidopa/levodopa/entacapone (antiparkinson agent): 12.5 mg/50 mg/200 mg, 18.75 mg/75 mg/200 mg, 25 mg/100 mg/200 mg, 31.25 mg/125 mg/200 mg, 37.5 mg/150 mg/200 mg, 50 mg/200 mg/200 mg.

◆CLASSIFICATION

PHARMACOTHERAPEUTIC: DOPamine precursor. Decarboxylase inhibitor. **CLINICAL:** Antiparkinson agent.

USES

Treatment of Parkinson's disease, postencephalitic parkinsonism, symptomatic parkinsonism following CNS injury by carbon monoxide poisoning, manganese intoxication. **Duopa:** Treatment of motor fluctuations in advanced Parkinson's disease. **OFF-LABEL:** Restless legs syndrome.

PRECAUTIONS

Contraindications: Hypersensitivity to carbidopa/levodopa. Concurrent use with MAOIs or use within 14 days. (Tablets only): Narrow-angle glaucoma. **Cautions:** History of MI, arrhythmias, bronchial asthma, emphysema, severe cardiac, pulmonary, renal/hepatic impairment; active peptic ulcer, treated open-angle glaucoma, seizure disorder, pts at risk for hypotension; elderly.

ACTION

Levodopa is converted to DOPamine in basal ganglia, increasing DOPamine concentration in brain, inhibiting hyperactive cholinergic activity. Carbidopa prevents peripheral breakdown of levodopa, making more levodopa available for transport into brain. **Therapeutic Effect:** Treats symptoms associated with Parkinson's disease.

PHARMACOKINETICS

Rapidly and completely absorbed from GI tract. Widely distributed. Excreted primarily in urine. Levodopa is converted to DOPamine. Excreted primarily in urine. **Half-life:** 1–2 hrs (carbidopa); 1–3 hrs (levodopa).

⌛ LIFESPAN CONSIDERATIONS

Pregnancy/Lactation: Unknown if drug crosses placenta or is distributed in breast milk. May inhibit lactation. Breastfeeding not recommended. **Children:** Safety and efficacy not established. **Elderly:** More sensitive to effects of levodopa. Anxiety, confusion, nervousness more common when receiving anticholinergics.

INTERACTIONS

DRUG: **Antipsychotics, pyridoxine** may decrease therapeutic effect. May increase adverse effects of **MAOIs (e.g., phenelzine, selegiline).** **HERBAL:** None significant. **FOOD:** **High-protein** diets may cause decreased or erratic response to levodopa. **LAB VALUES:** May increase serum BUN, LDH, alkaline phosphatase, bilirubin, ALT, AST. May decrease Hgb, Hct, WBC.

AVAILABILITY (Rx)

Enteral Suspension: ***(Duopa):*** 100-mL cassette containing 4.63 mg carbidopa and 20 mg levodopa per mL. **Tablets:** ***(Immediate-Release [Sinemet]):*** 10 mg carbidopa/100 mg levodopa, 25 mg carbidopa/100 mg levodopa, 25 mg carbidopa/250 mg levodopa. **Tablets:** ***(Orally Disintegrating Immediate-Release):*** 10 mg carbidopa/100 mg levodopa, 25 mg carbidopa/100 mg levodopa, 25 mg carbidopa/250 mg levodopa.

Capsules: ***(Extended-Release [Rytary]):*** carbidopa/levodopa: 23.75 mg/95 mg, 36.25 mg/145 mg, 48.75 mg/195 mg, 61.25 mg/245 mg. **Tablets:** ***(Extended-Release [Sinemet CR]):*** 25 mg carbidopa/100 mg levodopa, 50 mg carbidopa/200 mg levodopa.

ADMINISTRATION/HANDLING

Note: Space doses evenly over waking hours.

Enteral Suspension

• Refrigerate. Remove 20 min prior to administration.

PO

• Scored tablets may be crushed. • Give with meals to decrease GI upset. • Do not crush or chew extended-release tablets.

PO

• ***(Parcopa):*** Place orally disintegrating tablet on top of tongue. Tablet will dissolve in seconds; pt to swallow with saliva. Not necessary to administer with liquid.

INDICATIONS/ROUTES/DOSAGE

Parkinsonism

PO: ADULTS, ELDERLY: ***(Immediate-Release Orally Disintegrating Tablet):*** Initially, 25/100 mg 3 times/day. May increase daily or every other day by 1 tablet up to 200/2,000 mg daily. ***(Extended-Release): (Sinemet CR)*** 50/200 mg 2 times/day at least 6 hrs apart. Intervals between doses of Sinemet CR should be 4–8 hrs while awake, with smaller doses at end of day if doses are not equal. May adjust q3days. **Maximum:** 8 tablets/day. ***(Rytary):*** Initially, 23.75/95 mg 3 times/day for 3 days, then to 36.25/145 mg 3 times/day. Frequency may be increased to maximum of 5 times/day if needed and tolerated. **Maximum daily dose:** 612.5/2450 mg/day. ***(Enteral Suspension):*** **Maximum:** 2000 mg (1 container) over 16 hrs through NJ or PEG tube via infusion pump. Also take oral immediate-release in evening after disconnecting pump. Refer to manufacturer's guidelines for morning dose, continuous dose escalation, titration instructions.

Dosage in Renal/Hepatic Impairment

Use caution.

SIDE EFFECTS

Frequent (80%–50%): Involuntary movements of face, tongue, arms, upper body; nausea/vomiting; anorexia. **Occasional:** Depression, anxiety, confusion, nervousness, urinary retention, palpitations, dizziness, light-headedness, decreased appetite, blurred vision, constipation, dry mouth, flushed skin, headache, insomnia, diarrhea, unusual fatigue, darkening of urine and sweat. **Rare:** Hypertension, ulcer, hemolytic anemia (marked by fatigue).

ADVERSE EFFECTS/TOXIC REACTIONS

High incidence of involuntary choreiform, dystonic, dyskinetic movements may occur in pts on long-term therapy. Numerous mild to severe CNS and psychiatric disturbances may occur (reduced attention span, anxiety, nightmares, daytime drowsiness, euphoria, fatigue, paranoia, psychotic episodes, depression, hallucinations).

NURSING CONSIDERATIONS

BASELINE ASSESSMENT

Assess symptoms of Parkinson's disease (e.g., muscular rigidity, pen rolling motion, gait disturbance, tremors), emotional state. Receive full medication history and screen for interactions.

INTERVENTION/EVALUATION

Be alert to neurologic effects (headache, lethargy, mental confusion, agitation). Monitor for evidence of dyskinesia (difficulty with movement). Assess for clinical reversal of symptoms (improvement of tremor of head and hands at rest, mask-like facial expression, shuffling gait, muscular rigidity). Monitor B/P (standing, sitting, supine).

PATIENT/FAMILY TEACHING

• Avoid tasks that require alertness, motor skills until response to drug is established. • Take with food to minimize GI upset. • Effects may be delayed from several wks to mos. • May cause darkening of urine or sweat (not harmful). • Report any uncontrolled movement of face, eyelids, mouth, tongue, arms, hands, legs; mental changes; palpitations; severe or persistent nausea/vomiting; difficulty urinating. • Report exacerbations of asthma, underlying depression, psychosis.

CARBOplatin HIGH ALERT

kar-boe-**plat-in**

BLACK BOX ALERT Must be administered by personnel trained in administration/handling of chemotherapeutic agents (high potential for severe reactions, including anaphylaxis [may occur within minutes of administration] and sudden death). Profound myelosuppression (anemia, thrombocytopenia) has occurred. Vomiting may occur.

Do not confuse CARBOplatin with CISplatin or oxaliplatin, or with Platinol.

◆CLASSIFICATION

PHARMACOTHERAPEUTIC: Alkylating agent. Platinum analog. **CLINICAL:** Antineoplastic.

USES

Treatment of advanced ovarian carcinoma. Palliative treatment of recurrent ovarian cancer. **OFF-LABEL:** Brain tumors, Hodgkin's and non-Hodgkin's lymphomas, malignant melanoma, retinoblastoma; treatment of breast, bladder, cervical, endometrial, esophageal, small-cell lung, non–small-cell lung, head and neck, testicular carcinomas; germ cell tumors, osteogenic sarcoma.

PRECAUTIONS

Contraindications: Hypersensitivity to CARBOplatin. History of severe allergic reaction to CISplatin, platinum compounds, mannitol; severe bleeding, severe myelosuppression. **Cautions:** Moderate bone marrow depression, renal impairment, elderly.

ACTION

Inhibits DNA synthesis by cross-linking with DNA strands, preventing cell division. **Therapeutic Effect:** Interferes with DNA function.

PHARMACOKINETICS

Protein binding: Low. Hydrolyzed in solution to active form. Primarily excreted in urine. **Half-life:** 2.6–5.9 hrs.

LIFESPAN CONSIDERATIONS

Pregnancy/Lactation: If possible, avoid use during pregnancy, esp. first trimester. May cause fetal harm. Unknown if distributed in breast milk. Breastfeeding not recommended. **Children:** Safety and efficacy not established. **Elderly:** Pe-

C

ripheral neurotoxicity increased, myelotoxicity may be more severe. Age-related renal impairment may require decreased dosage, careful monitoring of blood counts.

INTERACTIONS

DRUG: **Bone marrow depressants (e.g., cladribine)** may increase myelosuppression. May increase adverse effects of **cloZAPine, natalizumab, leflunomide.** May increase immunosuppressive effect of **baricitinib, fingolimod.** May increase concentration/effect of **bexarotene.** May decrease therapeutic effect of **BCG (intravesical), vaccines (live).** May increase adverse effects of **vaccines (live).** **HERBAL:** None significant. **Echinacea** may decrease therapeutic effect. **FOOD:** None known. **LAB VALUES:** May decrease serum calcium, magnesium, potassium, sodium. May increase serum BUN, alkaline phosphatase, bilirubin, creatinine, AST.

AVAILABILITY (Rx)

Injection Solution: 10 mg/mL (5 mL, 15 mL, 45 mL, 60 mL).

ADMINISTRATION/HANDLING

◀ALERT▶ May be carcinogenic, mutagenic, teratogenic. Handle with extreme care during preparation/administration.

IV

Reconstitution • Dilute with D_5W or 0.9% NaCl to a final concentration as low as 0.5 mg/mL.

Rate of administration • Infuse over 15–60 min. • Rarely, anaphylactic reaction occurs minutes after administration. Use of epinephrine, corticosteroids alleviates symptoms.

Storage • Store vials at room temperature. • After dilution, solution is stable for 8 hrs.

IV INCOMPATIBILITIES

Amphotericin B complex (Abelcet, AmBisome, Amphotec).

IV COMPATIBILITIES

Etoposide (VePesid), granisetron (Kytril), ondansetron (Zofran), PACLitaxel (Taxol), palonosetron (Aloxi).

INDICATIONS/ROUTES/DOSAGE

Note: Doses commonly calculated by target AUC.

Ovarian Carcinoma

IV: ADULTS: Target AUC 5–6 over 1 hr on day 1; repeat q3 wks for 3–6 cycles (in combination with paclitaxel). Do not repeat dose until neutrophil and platelet counts are within acceptable levels.

Dose Modification

Platelets less than 50,000 cells/mm³ or ANC less than 500 cells/mm³: Give 75% of dose.

Dosage in Renal Impairment

Initial dosage is based on creatinine clearance; subsequent dosages are based on pt's tolerance, degree of myelosuppression.

Creatinine Clearance	Dosage Day 1
60 mL/min or greater	360 mg/m²
41–59 mL/min	250 mg/m²
16–40 mL/min	200 mg/m²

Dosage in Hepatic Impairment

No dose adjustment.

SIDE EFFECTS

Frequent (80%–65%): Nausea, vomiting. **Occasional (17%–4%):** Generalized pain, diarrhea/constipation, peripheral neuropathy. **Rare (3%–2%):** Alopecia, asthenia, hypersensitivity reaction (erythema, pruritus, rash, urticaria).

ADVERSE EFFECTS/TOXIC REACTIONS

Myelosuppression may be severe, resulting in anemia, infection (sepsis, pneumonia), major bleeding. Prolonged treatment may result in peripheral neurotoxicity.

NURSING CONSIDERATIONS

BASELINE ASSESSMENT

Obtain ECG, CBC, serum chemistries, renal function test. Offer emotional support. Do not repeat treatment until WBC recovers from previous therapy. Transfusions may be needed in pts receiving prolonged therapy (myelosuppression increased in those with previous therapy, renal impairment).

INTERVENTION/EVALUATION

Monitor pulmonary function studies, hepatic/renal function tests, CBC, serum electrolytes. Monitor for fever, sore throat, signs of local infection, unusual bruising/bleeding from any site, symptoms of anemia (excessive fatigue, weakness).

PATIENT/FAMILY TEACHING

• Nausea, vomiting generally abate within 24 hrs. • Do not have immunizations without physician's approval (drug lowers body's resistance). • Avoid contact with those who have recently received live virus vaccine.

carfilzomib

kar-**fil**-zoh-mib
(Kyprolis)
Do not confuse carfilzomib with crizotinib, ixazomib, PAZOpanib.

◆CLASSIFICATION

PHARMACOTHERAPEUTIC: Proteasome inhibitor. **CLINICAL:** Antineoplastic.

USES

Treatment of pts with multiple myeloma who have received at least 2 prior therapies including bortezomib and an immunomodulatory agent and have demonstrated disease progression on or within 60 days of completion of last therapy. In combination with dexamethasone, lenalidomide, and dexamethasone; or daratumumab and dexamethasone for treatment of relapsed multiple myeloma who have received 1 to 3 prior therapies.

PRECAUTIONS

Contraindications: Hypersensitivity to carfilzomib. **Cautions:** Preexisting HF, decreased left ventricular ejection fraction, myocardial abnormalities, complications of pulmonary hypertension (e.g., dyspnea), hepatic impairment, thrombocytopenia.

ACTION

Blocks action of proteasomes (responsible for intracellular protein homeostasis). **Therapeutic Effect:** Produces cell cycle arrest and apoptosis.

PHARMACOKINETICS

Protein binding: 97%. Rapidly, extensively metabolized. Excreted primarily extrahepatically. Minimal removal by hemodialysis. **Half-life:** Equal to or less than 1 hr on day 1 of cycle 1. Proteasome inhibition was maintained for 48 hrs or longer following first dose of carfilzomib for each week of dosing.

⌛ LIFESPAN CONSIDERATIONS

Pregnancy/Lactation: Avoid pregnancy. May cause fetal harm. Unknown if excreted in breast milk. **Children:** Safety and efficacy not established. **Elderly:** No age-related precautions noted.

INTERACTIONS

DRUG: May decrease levels/effect of **BCG (intravesical)**. May increase myelosuppressive effect of **myelosuppressants (e.g., cladribine). Oral contraceptives** may increase risk of thrombosis. **HERBAL:** None significant. **FOOD:** None known. **LAB VALUES:** May increase serum creatinine, glucose, creatinine, ALT, AST, bilirubin, calcium. May decrease RBC, Hgb, Hct, absolute neutrophil count (ANC), platelet count; serum magnesium, phosphate, potassium, sodium.

C

AVAILABILITY (Rx)

Injection Powder for Reconstitution (Single-Use Vial): 10 mg, 30 mg, 60 mg.

ADMINISTRATION/HANDLING

IV

Reconstitution • Reconstitute 60-mg vial with 29 mL Sterile Water for Injection (30-mg vial with 15 mL, 10 mg with 5 mL), directing solution to inside wall of vial (minimizes foaming). • Swirl and invert vial slowly for 1 min or until completely dissolved. • Do not shake. • If foaming occurs, rest vial for 2–5 min until subsided. • Withdraw calculated dose from vial and dilute into 50–100 mL D_5W (depending on dose and infusion duration). • Final concentration of reconstituted solution: 2 mg/mL.

Rate of administration • Infuse over 10–30 min (depending on the dose regimen) via dedicated IV line. Flush line before and after with NaCl or D_5W. • Do not administer as a bolus.

Storage • Refrigerate unused vials. • Reconstituted solution may be refrigerated up to 24 hrs. • At room temperature, use diluted solution within 4 hrs.

IV INCOMPATIBILITIES

Do not mix with other IV medications or additives. Flush IV administration line with NaCl or D_5W immediately before and after carfilzomib administration.

INDICATIONS/ROUTES/DOSAGE

◀ALERT▶ Dose is calculated using pt's actual body surface area at baseline. Pts with a body surface area greater than 2.2 m^2 should receive dose based on a body surface area of 2.2 m^2. No dose adjustment needed for weight changes of less than or equal to 20%.

◀ALERT▶ Prior to each dose in cycle 1, give 250 mL to 500 mL NaCl bolus. Give an additional 250 mL to 500 mL IV fluid following administration. Continue IV hydration in subsequent cycles (reduces risk of renal toxicity, tumor lysis syndrome). Premedicate with dexamethasone 4 mg PO or IV prior to all doses during cycle 1 and prior to all doses during first cycle of dose escalation to 27 mg/m^2 (reduces incidence, severity of infusion reactions). Reinstate dexamethasone premedication (4 mg PO or IV) if symptoms develop or reappear during subsequent cycles.

Multiple Myeloma, Relapsed/Refractory (Single-Agent 20/27 mg/m^2 Regimen)

IV infusion: ADULTS, ELDERLY: Cycle 1: 20 mg/m^2 over 10 min on days 1 and 2. If tolerated, increase to 27 mg/m^2 over 10 min on days 8, 9, 15, and 16 of a 28-day cycle. Cycles 2–12: 27 mg/m^2 over 10 min on days 1, 2, 8, 9, 15, and 16 of a 28-day cycle. Cycles 13 and beyond: 27 mg/m^2 over 10 min on days 1, 2, 15, and 16 of a 28-day cycle. Continue until disease progression or unacceptable toxicity.

Multiple Myeloma, Relapsed/Refractory (Single-Agent 20/56 mg/m^2 Regimen)

IV infusion: ADULTS, ELDERLY: Cycle 1: 20 mg/m^2 over 30 min on days 1 and 2. If tolerated, increase to 56 mg/m^2 over 30 min on days 8, 9, 15, and 16 of a 28-day cycle. Cycles 2–12: 56 mg/m^2 over 30 min on days 1, 2, 8, 9, 15, and 16 of a 28-day cycle. Cycles 13 and beyond: 56 mg/m^2 over 30 min on days 1, 2, 15, and 16 of a 28-day cycle. Continue until disease progression or unacceptable toxicity.

Multiple Myeloma, Relapsed/Refractory (In Combination With Lenalidomide and Dexamethasone)

IV infusion: ADULTS, ELDERLY: Cycle 1: 20 mg/m^2 over 10 min on days 1 and 2. If tolerated, increase to 27 mg/m^2 over 10 min on days 8, 9, 15, and 16 of a 28-day cycle. Cycles 2–12: 27 mg/m^2 over 10 min on days 1, 2, 8, 9, 15, and 16 of a 28-day cycle. Cycles 13–18: 27 mg/m^2 over 10 min on days 1, 2, 15, and 16 of a 28-day cycle. Beginning with cycle 19, lenalidomide and dexamethasone may be continued (until disease progression or unacceptable toxicity) without carfilzomib.

Multiple Myeloma, Relapsed/Refractory (in Combination With Dexamethasone)
IV infusion: ADULTS, ELDERLY: Cycle 1: 20 mg/m² over 30 min on days 1 and 2. If tolerated, increase to 56 mg/m² over 30 min on days 8, 9, 15, and 16 of a 28-day cycle. Cycle 2 and beyond: 56 mg/m² over 30 min on days 1, 2, 8, 9, 15, and 16 of a 28-day cycle. Continue until disease progression or unacceptable toxicity.

Multiple Myeloma, Relapsed/Refractory (in Combination With Dexamethasone; 20/70 mg/m² Regimen [once-wkly dosing])
IV infusion: ADULTS, ELDERLY: Cycle 1: 20 mg/m² over 30 min on day 1. Increase dose to 70 mg/m² over 30 min on days 8 and 15 of a 28-day treatment cycle. Cycle 2 and beyond: 70 mg/m² over 30 min on days 1, 8, and 15 of a 28-day treatment cycle. Continue until disease progression or unacceptable toxicity.

Multiple Myeloma, Relapsed/Refractory (in combination with daratumumab and dexamethasone; 20/56 mg/m² regimen [twice-weekly dosing])
IV infusion: ADULTS, ELDERLY: Cycle 1: 20 mg/m² on days 1 and 2; if tolerated, increase to 56 mg/m² on days 8, 9, 15, and 16 of a 28-day cycle. **Cycles 2 and thereafter:** 56 mg/m² on days 1, 2, 8, 9, 15, and 16 of a 28-day cycle; continue until disease progression or unacceptable toxicity.

Multiple Myeloma, Relapsed/Refractory (in combination with daratumumab and dexamethasone; 20/70 mg/m² regimen [once-weekly dosing])
IV infusion: Cycle 1: 20 mg/m² on day 1; if tolerated, increase dose to 70 mg/m² on days 8 and 15 of a 28-day cycle. **Cycles 2 and thereafter:** 70 mg/m² over on days 1, 8, and 15 of a 28-day cycle; continue until disease progression or unacceptable toxicity.

Dose Modification
Hematologic Toxicity
Grade 3 or 4 neutropenia: Withhold dose. Continue at same dose if fully recovered prior to next scheduled dose. If recovered to Grade 2, reduce dose by one dose level. If dose tolerated, may escalate to previous dose. **Grade 4 thrombocytopenia:** Withhold dose. Continue at same dose if fully recovered prior to next scheduled dose. If recovered to Grade 3, reduce dose by one dose level. If dose tolerated, may escalate to previous dose.
Cardiotoxicity
Grade 3 or 4, new onset or worsening of HF, decreased LVF, myocardial ischemia: Withhold dose until resolved or at baseline. After resolution, restart at reduced dose level. If dose tolerated, may escalate to previous dose.
Hepatotoxicity
Grade 3 or 4 elevation of bilirubin, transaminases: Withhold dose until resolved or at baseline. After resolution, restart at reduced dose level. If dose tolerated, may escalate to previous dose.
Peripheral Neuropathy
Grade 3 or 4: Withhold dose until resolved or at baseline. After resolution, restart at reduced dose level. If dose tolerated, may escalate to previous dose.
Pulmonary Toxicity
Pulmonary hypertension: Withhold dose until resolved or at baseline. After resolution, restart at reduced dose level. If dose tolerated, may escalate to previous dose. **Grade 3 or 4 pulmonary complications:** Withhold dose until resolved or at baseline. After resolution, restart at reduced dose level. If dose tolerated, may escalate to previous dose.
Renal Toxicity
Serum creatinine 2 times or greater from baseline: Withhold dose until renal function improves to Grade 1 or baseline. After resolution, restart at reduced dose level. If dose tolerated, may escalate to previous dose.

Dosage in Renal/Hepatic Impairment
No dose adjustment.

SIDE EFFECTS

Frequent (56%–20%): Fatigue, anemia, nausea, exertional dyspnea, diarrhea, fever, headache, cough, peripheral edema, vom-

C

iting, constipation, back pain. **Occasional (18%–14%):** Insomnia, chills, arthralgia, muscle spasms, hypertension, asthenia, extremity pain, dizziness, hypoesthesia (decreased sensitivity to touch), anorexia.

ADVERSE EFFECTS/TOXIC REACTIONS

Pneumonia (10% of pts), acute renal failure (4% of pts), pyrexia (3% of pts), and HF (3% of pts) were reported. Adverse reactions leading to discontinuation occurred in 15% of pts. Upper respiratory tract infection reported in 28% of pts. HF, pulmonary edema, decrease in ejection fraction were reported in 7% of pts. Infusion reaction characterized by chills, fever, wheezing, facial flushing, dyspnea, vomiting, chest tightness can occur immediately following or up to 24 hrs after administration. Tumor lysis syndrome occurs rarely.

NURSING CONSIDERATIONS

BASELINE ASSESSMENT

Obtain accurate height and weight. Obtain full history of home medications including vitamins, herbal products. Ensure hydration status and maintain throughout treatment. Obtain CBC, BMP, LFT. Assess vital signs, O_2 saturation. Platelet nadirs occur around day 8 of each 28-day cycle and recover to baseline by start of the next 28-day cycle.

INTERVENTION/EVALUATION

Monitor for fluid overload. Monitor platelet count frequently; adjust dose according to grade of thrombocytopenia. Obtain serum ALT, AST, bilirubin for evidence of hepatotoxicity. Monitor vital signs, O_2 saturation routinely. Monitor cardiac function and manage as needed. Assess for palpitations, tachycardia. Assess for anemia-related dizziness, exertional dyspnea, fatigue, weakness, syncope. Monitor for acute infection (fever, diaphoresis, lethargy, oral mucosal changes, productive cough), bloody stools, bruising, hematuria, DVT, pulmonary embolism. Encourage nutritional intake and assess anorexia, weight loss. Reinforce birth control compliance. Monitor daily pattern of bowel activity, stool consistency. Offer antiemetics if nausea, vomiting occur. Monitor for symptoms of neutropenia.

PATIENT/FAMILY TEACHING

• Immediately report any newly prescribed medications. • May alter taste of food or decrease appetite. • Report bloody stool/urine, increased bruising, difficulty breathing, weakness, dizziness, palpitations, weight loss. • Maintain strict oral hygiene. • Do not have immunizations without physician approval (drug lowers body's resistance). • Avoid those who have recently taken live virus vaccine. • Avoid crowds, those with symptoms of viral illness.

cariprazine

kar-**ip**-ra-zeen
(Vraylar)

■ **BLACK BOX ALERT** ■ Elderly pts treated with antipsychotic drugs are at an increased risk of death. Treatment not approved in pts with dementia-related psychosis.

Do not confuse cariprazine with Compazine or mirtazapine.

◆CLASSIFICATION

PHARMACOTHERAPEUTIC: Serotonin receptor antagonist. **CLINICAL:** Second-generation (atypical) antipsychotic.

USES

Treatment of schizophrenia. Acute treatment of manic or mixed episodes and major depression associated with bipolar I disorder.

PRECAUTIONS

Contraindications: Hypersensitivity to cariprazine. **Cautions:** Baseline leukopenia, neutropenia; hx of drug-induced leukopenia, neutropenia; debilitated, diabetes mellitus, dyslipidemia, elderly, hepatic impairment, Parkinson's disease, pts at risk for hypotension (dehydration, hypovolemia, concomitant use of antihypertensives), pts at risk for aspiration, dysphagia; history of cardiovascular disease (e.g., ischemic heart disease, HF, cardiac arrhythmias); pts at risk for CVA, TIA; hx of seizures. Concomitant use of medications that lower seizure threshold. Avoid concomitant use of CYP3A inducers.

ACTION

Exact mechanism unknown. Partial agonist of central DOPamine D_2 and serotonin 5-HT_{1A} receptors and antagonist of serotonin 5-HT_{2A} receptors. **Therapeutic Effect:** Diminishes symptoms of psychotic behavior.

PHARMACOKINETICS

Widely distributed. Metabolized in liver. Protein binding: 91%–97%. Peak plasma concentration: 3–6 hrs. Mean plasma concentrations decrease approx. 50% after 1 wk from last dose. Excreted primarily in urine (21%). **Half-life:** 2–4 days.

LIFESPAN CONSIDERATIONS

Pregnancy/Lactation: Avoid pregnancy; may cause fetal harm. May increase risk of extrapyramidal symptoms and/or withdrawal syndrome in neonates. Unknown if distributed in breast milk. Must either discontinue drug or discontinue breastfeeding. **Children:** Safety and efficacy not established. **Elderly:** May increase risk of adverse effects due to age-related cardiac/hepatic/renal impairment.

INTERACTIONS

DRUG: **Strong CYP3A inhibitors (e.g., clarithromycin, ketoconazole, ritonavir)** may increase concentration/effect. **Strong CYP3A inducers (e.g., carBAMazepine, rifampin), moderate CYP3A inducers (e.g., nafcillin)** may decrease concentration/effect; avoid use. **Alcohol, antidepressants (e.g., sertraline, nortriptyline), benzodiazepines (e.g., diazePAM, LORazepam), opioids (e.g., morphine), phenothiazines (e.g., thioridazine), sedative/hypnotics (e.g., zolpidem)** may increase CNS depression. **Metoclopramide** may increase adverse effects. HERBAL: **St. John's wort** may decrease concentration/effect. **Herbs with sedative properties (e.g., chamomile, kava kava, valerian)** may increase CNS depression. FOOD: **Grapefruit products** may increase concentration/effect. LAB VALUES: May increase serum ALT, AST; CPK. May decrease serum sodium.

AVAILABILITY (Rx)

Capsules: 1.5 mg, 3 mg, 4.5 mg, 6 mg.

ADMINISTRATION/HANDLING

PO

Give without regard to food. Administer whole; do not break, crush, cut, or open capsule.

INDICATIONS/ROUTES/DOSAGE

Schizophrenia

PO: ADULTS, ELDERLY: Initially, 1.5 mg once daily. May increase to 3 mg on day 2 if tolerated. May further increase in increments of 1.5–3 mg based on clinical response and tolerability. **Note:** Due to long half-life, changes in dosage will not be reflected in plasma for several wks. Range: 1.5–6 mg once daily.

Bipolar I Disorder (Manic or Mixed Episodes)

PO: ADULTS, ELDERLY: 1.5 mg once on day 1, then increase to 3 mg once daily on day 2. May further increase in increments of 1.5–3 mg based on clinical response and tolerability. Range: 3–6 mg once daily.

Concomitant Use of Strong CYP3A Inhibitors

Pts starting strong CYP3A inhibitor while on stable dose of cariprazine: Reduce maintenance cariprazine dose by 50%. Pts taking cariprazine 4.5 mg/day should reduce dosage to 1.5 mg/

day or 3 mg/day. Pts taking 1.5 mg/day, adjust dosing to every other day. If the strong CYP3A inhibitor is discontinued, cariprazine may need to be increased. **Pts starting cariprazine while on CYP3A inhibitor:** 1.5 mg once on day 1; no dose on day 2; 1.5 mg once on day 3. After day 3, increase dose to 3 mg once daily as tolerated. If strong CYP3A inhibitor is discontinued, cariprazine may need to be increased.

Bipolar I (Major Depression)

PO: ADULTS, ELDERLY: Initially: 0.5–1.5 mg once daily; increase based on response and tolerability to 3 mg on day 15. **Maximum:** 3 mg/day.

Dosage in Renal Impairment

Mild to moderate impairment: No dose adjustment. **Severe impairment:** Treatment not recommended.

Dosage in Hepatic Impairment

Mild to moderate impairment: No dose adjustment. **Severe impairment:** Treatment not recommended.

SIDE EFFECTS

Frequent (26%–11%): Bradykinesia, cogwheel rigidity, drooling, dyskinesia, masked faces, muscle rigidity, dystonia, tremor, salivary hypersecretion, torticollis, trismus, insomnia, akathisia, headache. **Occasional (5%–3%):** Nausea, constipation, restlessness, vomiting, dizziness, agitation, anxiety, dyspepsia, abdominal pain, diarrhea, fatigue, asthenia, back pain, toothache, hypertension, decreased appetite. **Rare (2%–1%):** Dry mouth, weight gain, extremity pain, somnolence, sedation, cough, tachycardia, arthralgia.

ADVERSE EFFECTS/TOXIC REACTIONS

May increase risk of hypotension, orthostatic hypotension, syncope; diabetes mellitus, DKA, hyperglycemia, hyperglycemic hyperosmolar nonketotic coma; leukopenia, neutropenia, febrile neutropenia; aspiration, dysphagia, gastritis, gastric reflux; extrapyramidal symptoms including akathisia, dystonia, parkinsonism, tardive dyskinesia; suicidal ideation. May cause neuroleptic malignant syndrome (NMS), manifested by altered mental status, cardiac arrhythmias, diaphoresis, labile blood pressure, malignant hyperthermia, muscle rigidity, rhabdomyolysis, renal failure. May increase risk of death in pts with dementia-related psychosis. Cognitive and motor impairment reported in 7% of pts. May increase seizure-like activity related to decrease in seizure threshold. Infectious processes including nasopharyngitis, urinary tract infection reported in 1% of pts. Hypersensitivity reactions including angioedema, rash, pruritus have occurred.

NURSING CONSIDERATIONS

BASELINE ASSESSMENT

Obtain baseline fasting lipid profile, fasting plasma glucose level, vital signs; Hgb A1c in pts with diabetes; ANC, CBC in pts with baseline leukopenia, neutropenia. Receive full medication history, including herbal products, and screen for interactions. Assess appearance, behavior, speech pattern, levels of interest. Verify pregnancy status. Question history of diabetes, cardiovascular disease, CVA, dysphagia, hepatic impairment, hypersensitivity reaction, TIA, seizures.

INTERVENTION/EVALUATION

Monitor ANC, CBC, fasting lipid profile, fasting plasma glucose levels periodically. Assess mental status for anxiety, depression, suicidal ideation (esp. at initiation and with change in dosage), social function. Due to long half-life, any change in dosage will not be fully reflected for several wks; monitor closely for adverse effects during the following wks. Monitor for hypersensitivity reaction, dysphagia, tardive dyskinesia, extrapyramidal symptoms, metabolic changes including hyperglycemia. Screen for infection. Monitor for neuroleptic malignant syndrome.

PATIENT/FAMILY TEACHING

• Immediately report thoughts of suicide or plans to commit suicide. • Avoid tasks that require alertness until response to drug is established. • Therapy may increase blood sugar levels. Monitor for blurry vision, confusion, frequent urination, fruity-smelling breath, thirst, weakness. • Treatment may cause fetal harm. Avoid pregnancy. Do not breastfeed. • Treatment may lower ability to fight infection. • Swallow capsules whole; do not chew, crush, cut, or open capsules. • Do not ingest grapefruit products or herbal products. Report drooling, muscle rigidity, lockjaw, tremors, or inability to control muscle movements. • Treatment may increase risk of seizures. • Report confusion, palpitations, profuse sweating, fluctuating blood pressure, unusually high core body temperature, muscle rigidity, dark-colored urine or decreased urine output; may indicate life-threatening neurologic event called neuroleptic malignant syndrome (NMS).

carvedilol

TOP 100 HIGH ALERT

kar-**ve**-dil-ole
(Apo-Carvedilol ✦, Coreg, Coreg CR)
Do not confuse carvedilol with atenolol or carteolol, or Coreg with Corgard, Cortef, or Cozaar.

◆CLASSIFICATION

PHARMACOTHERAPEUTIC: Beta-adrenergic blocker. **CLINICAL:** Antihypertensive.

USES

Treatment of mild to severe HF, left ventricular dysfunction following MI, hypertension. **OFF-LABEL:** Treatment of angina pectoris, idiopathic cardiomyopathy.

PRECAUTIONS

Contraindications: Hypersensitivity to carvedilol. Bronchial asthma or related bronchospastic conditions, cardiogenic shock, decompensated HF requiring intravenous inotropic therapy, severe hepatic impairment, second- or third-degree AV block, severe bradycardia, or sick sinus syndrome (except in pts with pacemaker). **Cautions:** Diabetes, myasthenia gravis, mild to moderate hepatic impairment. Withdraw gradually to avoid acute tachycardia, hypertension, and/or ischemia. Pts suspected of having Prinzmetal's angina, pheochromocytoma, hx of severe anaphylaxis to allergens.

ACTION

Possesses nonselective beta-blocking and alpha-adrenergic blocking activity. Causes vasodilation. **Therapeutic Effect: Hypertension:** Reduces cardiac output, exercise-induced tachycardia, reflex orthostatic tachycardia; reduces peripheral vascular resistance. **HF:** Decreases pulmonary capillary wedge pressure, heart rate, systemic vascular resistance; increases stroke volume index.

PHARMACOKINETICS

Route	Onset	Peak	Duration
PO	30 min	1–2 hrs	24 hrs

Rapidly, extensively absorbed from GI tract. Protein binding: 98%. Metabolized in liver. Excreted primarily via bile into feces. Minimally removed by hemodialysis. **Half-life:** 7–10 hrs. Food delays rate of absorption.

⌛ LIFESPAN CONSIDERATIONS

Pregnancy/Lactation: Unknown if drug crosses placenta or is distributed in breast milk. May produce bradycardia, apnea, hypoglycemia, hypothermia during delivery; may contribute to low birth-weight infants. **Children:** Safety and efficacy not established. **Elderly:** Incidence of dizziness may be increased.

INTERACTIONS

DRUG: **Calcium channel blockers (e.g., diltiaZEM, verapamil), digoxin, CYP2C9 inhibitors (e.g., amiodarone, fluconazole)** increase risk of cardiac conduction disturbances. **CYP2D6 inhib-**

itors (e.g., **FLUoxetine, PARoxetine**) may increase concentration/side effects; may enhance slowing of HR or cardiac conduction. May decrease bronchodilation effect of **beta$_2$ agonists (e.g., albuterol, salmeterol).** May increase concentration/effects of **pazopanib, topotecan. Rivastigmine** may increase risk of bradycardia. HERBAL: **Herbals with hypertensive properties (e.g., licorice, yohimbe)** or **hypotensive properties (e.g., garlic, ginger, ginkgo biloba)** may alter effects. FOOD: None known. LAB VALUES: May increase serum creatinine, bilirubin, ALT, AST, PT.

AVAILABILITY (Rx)

Tablets ***(Immediate-Release):*** 3.125 mg, 6.25 mg, 12.5 mg, 25 mg.

Capsules: ***(Extended-Release [Coreg CR]):*** 10 mg, 20 mg, 40 mg, 80 mg.

ADMINISTRATION/HANDLING

PO

• Give with food (slows rate of absorption, reduces risk of orthostatic effects). • Do not crush or cut extended-release capsules. • Capsules may be opened and sprinkled on applesauce for immediate use.

INDICATIONS/ROUTES/DOSAGE

Hypertension

PO: ***(Immediate-Release):*** **ADULTS, ELDERLY:** Initially, 6.25 mg twice daily. May double at intervals of 1–2 wks to 12.5 mg twice daily, then to 25 mg twice daily. **Maximum:** 25 mg twice daily. ***(Extended-Release):*** Initially, 20 mg once daily. May increase to 40 mg once daily after 1–2 wks, then to 80 mg once daily. **Maximum:** 80 mg once daily.

HF

PO: ***(Immediate-Release):*** **ADULTS, ELDERLY:** Initially, 3.125 mg twice daily. May double at 2-wk intervals to highest tolerated dosage. **Maximum: WEIGHING MORE THAN 85 KG:** 50 mg twice daily; **LESS THAN 85 KG:** 25 mg twice daily. ***(Extended-Release):*** Initially, 10 mg once daily for 2 wks. May increase to 20 mg, 40 mg, and 80 mg over successive intervals of at least 2 wks. **Maximum:** 80 mg/day.

Left Ventricular Dysfunction Following MI

PO: ***(Immediate-Release):*** **ADULTS, ELDERLY:** Initially, 3.125 mg twice daily for 2 wks. May increase at intervals of 3–10 days up to 25 mg twice daily (85 kg or less) or 50 mg twice daily (greater than 85 kg). ***(Extended-Release):*** Initially, 10–20 mg once daily. May increase incrementally in intervals of 3–10 days. Target dose: 80 mg once daily.

Dosage in Renal Impairment

No dose adjustment.

Dosage in Hepatic Impairment

Contraindicated in severe impairment.

SIDE EFFECTS

Frequent (6%–4%): Fatigue, dizziness. **Occasional (2%):** Diarrhea, bradycardia, rhinitis, back pain. **Rare (less than 2%):** Orthostatic hypotension, drowsiness, UTI, viral infection.

ADVERSE EFFECTS/TOXIC REACTIONS

Overdose may produce profound bradycardia, hypotension, bronchospasm, cardiac insufficiency, cardiogenic shock, cardiac arrest. Abrupt withdrawal may result in diaphoresis, palpitations, headache, tremors. May precipitate HF, MI in pts with cardiac disease; thyroid storm in pts with thyrotoxicosis; peripheral ischemia in pts with existing peripheral vascular disease. Hypoglycemia may occur in pts with previously controlled diabetes. May mask symptoms of hypoglycemia.

NURSING CONSIDERATIONS

BASELINE ASSESSMENT

Assess B/P, apical pulse immediately before drug is administered (if pulse is 60 beats/min or less or systolic B/P is less than 90 mm Hg, withhold medication, contact physician). Receive full medication history and screen for interactions.

INTERVENTION/EVALUATION

Monitor B/P for hypotension, respirations for dyspnea. Take standing systolic B/P 1 hr after dosing as guide for tolerance. Assess pulse for quality, regularity, rate; monitor for bradycardia. Monitor ECG for cardiac arrhythmias. Assist with ambulation if dizziness occurs. Assess for evidence of HF: dyspnea (particularly on exertion or lying down), night cough, peripheral edema, distended neck veins. Monitor I&O (increase in weight, decrease in urine output may indicate HF).

PATIENT/FAMILY TEACHING

• Full therapeutic effect of B/P may take 1–2 wks. • Take with food. • Abruptly stopping treatment or missing multiple doses may cause beta-blocker withdrawal symptoms (fast heart rate, high blood pressure, palpitations, sweating, tremors). • Compliance with therapy regimen is essential to control hypertension. • Report excessive fatigue, prolonged dizziness. • Do not use nasal decongestants, OTC cold preparations (stimulants) without physician's approval. • Monitor B/P, pulse before taking medication. • Restrict salt, alcohol intake.

caspofungin

kas-poe-**fun**-jin
(Cancidas)

◆CLASSIFICATION

PHARMACOTHERAPEUTIC: Echinocandin antifungal. **CLINICAL:** Antifungal.

USES

Treatment of invasive aspergillosis, candidemia, *Candida* infection (intra-abdominal abscess, peritonitis, esophageal, pleural space) in pts aged 3 months and older. Empiric therapy for presumed fungal infections in febrile neutropenia.

PRECAUTIONS

Contraindications: Hypersensitivity to caspofungin. **Cautions:** Concurrent use of cycloSPORINE, hepatic impairment.

ACTION

Inhibits synthesis of glucan, a vital component of fungal cell wall formation, damaging fungal cell membrane. **Therapeutic Effect:** Fungistatic.

PHARMACOKINETICS

Distributed in tissue. Protein binding: 97%. Metabolized in liver. Excreted in urine (50%), feces (30%). Not removed by hemodialysis. **Half-life:** 40–50 hrs.

LIFESPAN CONSIDERATIONS

Pregnancy/Lactation: May be embryotoxic. Crosses placental barrier. Distributed in breast milk. **Children:** Safety and efficacy not established. **Elderly:** Age-related moderate renal impairment may require dosage adjustment.

INTERACTIONS

DRUG: **CycloSPORINE** may increase concentration. **RifAMPin** may decrease concentration. May decrease concentration/effect of **tacrolimus.** May decrease therapeutic effect of ***saccharomyces boulardii.*** **HERBAL:** None significant. **FOOD:** None known. **LAB VALUES:** May increase serum alkaline phosphatase, bilirubin, creatinine, ALT, AST, urine protein. May decrease serum albumin, bicarbonate, potassium, magnesium; Hgb, Hct.

AVAILABILITY (Rx)

Injection Powder for Reconstitution: 50-mg, 70-mg vials.

ADMINISTRATION/HANDLING

IV

Reconstitution • Reconstitute 50-mg or 70-mg vial with 0.9% NaCl, Sterile Water for Injection, or Bacteriostatic Water for Injection. Further dilute in 0.9% NaCl or D_5W to maximum concentration of 0.5 mg/mL.

C

Rate of administration • Infuse over 60 min.
Storage • Refrigerate vials but warm to room temperature before preparing with diluent. • Reconstituted solution, diluted solution, may be stored at room temperature for 1 hr before infusion. • Final infusion solution can be stored at room temperature for 24 hrs or 48 hrs if refrigerated. • Discard if solution contains particulate or is discolored.

IV INCOMPATIBILITIES

Cefepime (Maxipime), ceftaroline (Teflaro), cefTAZidime (Fortaz), cefTRIAXone (Rocephin), furosemide (Lasix).

IV COMPATIBILITIES

Aztreonam (Azactam), DAPTOmycin (Cubicin), fluconazole (Diflucan), linezolid (Zyvox), meropenem (Merrem IV), piperacillin/tazobactam (Zosyn), vancomycin.

INDICATIONS/ROUTES/DOSAGE

Aspergillosis

Note: Continue for minimum of 6–12 wks.
IV: ADULTS, ELDERLY: Give single 70-mg loading dose on day 1, followed by 50 mg/day thereafter. **CHILDREN 3 MOS–17 YRS:** 70 mg/m^2 on day 1, then 50 mg/m^2 daily. **Maximum:** 70 mg loading dose or daily dose.

Candidemia

Note: Continue for at least 14 days after last positive culture.
IV: ADULTS, ELDERLY: Initially, 70 mg on day 1, followed by 50 mg daily. **CHILDREN 3 MOS–17 YRS:** 70 mg/m^2 on day 1, then 50 mg/m^2 daily. **Maximum:** 70-mg loading dose, 50-mg daily dose.

Esophageal Candidiasis

Note: Continue for 14–21 days after symptom resolution.
IV: ADULTS, ELDERLY: 50 mg/day. **CHILDREN 3 MOS–17 YRS:** 50 mg/m^2 daily. **Maximum:** 50 mg.

Empiric Therapy

Note: Continue for minimum 14 days if fungal infection confirmed (continue for 7 days after resolution of neutropenia/clinical symptoms).
IV: ADULTS, ELDERLY: Initially 70 mg, then 50 mg/day. May increase to 70 mg/day. **CHILDREN 3 MOS–17 YRS:** 70 mg/m^2 on day 1, then 50 mg/m^2 daily. **Maximum:** 70 mg loading dose or daily dose.

Dosage in Renal Impairment

No dose adjustment.

Dosage in Hepatic Impairment

Mild: No adjustment. **Moderate: CHILD-PUGH SCORE 7–9:** Decrease dose to 35 mg/day. **Severe:** No clinical experience.

SIDE EFFECTS

Frequent (26%): Fever. **Occasional (11%–4%):** Headache, nausea, phlebitis. **Rare (3% or less):** Paresthesia, vomiting, diarrhea, abdominal pain, myalgia, chills, tremor, insomnia.

ADVERSE EFFECTS/TOXIC REACTIONS

Hypersensitivity reaction (rash, facial edema, pruritus, sensation of warmth), including anaphylaxis, may occur. May cause hepatic dysfunction, hepatitis (drug-induced), or hepatic failure.

NURSING CONSIDERATIONS

BASELINE ASSESSMENT

Obtain baseline CBC, BMP, LFT, serum magnesium. Determine baseline temperature. Question history of prior hypersensitivity reaction.

INTERVENTION/EVALUATION

Assess for signs/symptoms of hepatic dysfunction. Monitor LFT in pts with preexisting hepatic impairment. Monitor CBC, serum potassium. Monitor for fever, hypersensitivity reaction.

PATIENT/FAMILY TEACHING

• Report rash, facial swelling, itching, difficulty breathing, abdominal pain, yellowing of skin or eyes, dark-colored urine, nausea.

cefaclor

sef-a-klor
(Novo-Cefaclor ♣)
Do not confuse cefaclor with cephalexin.

◆CLASSIFICATION

PHARMACOTHERAPEUTIC: Second-generation cephalosporin. **CLINICAL:** Antibiotic.

USES

Treatment of susceptible infections due to *S. pneumoniae, S. pyogenes, S. aureus, H. influenzae, E. coli, M. catarrhalis, Klebsiella* spp., *P. mirabilis*, including acute otitis media, bronchitis, pharyngitis/tonsillitis, respiratory tract, skin/skin structure, UTIs.

PRECAUTIONS

Contraindications: History of hypersensitivity/anaphylactic reaction to cefaclor, cephalosporins. **Cautions:** Severe renal impairment, history of penicillin allergy. Extended release not approved in children younger than 16 yrs.

ACTION

Binds to bacterial cell membranes, inhibits cell wall synthesis. **Therapeutic Effect:** Bactericidal.

PHARMACOKINETICS

Well absorbed from GI tract. Protein binding: 25%. Widely distributed. Partially metabolized in liver. Primarily excreted in urine. Moderately removed by hemodialysis. **Half-life:** 0.6–0.9 hr (increased in renal impairment).

LIFESPAN CONSIDERATIONS

Pregnancy/Lactation: Readily crosses placenta. Distributed in breast milk. **Children:** No age-related precautions noted in pts older than 1 mo. **Elderly:** Age-related renal impairment may require dosage adjustment.

INTERACTIONS

DRUG: **Probenecid** may increase concentration/effect. **HERBAL:** None significant. **FOOD:** None known. **LAB VALUES:** May increase serum BUN, alkaline phosphatase, bilirubin, creatinine, LDH, ALT, AST. May cause positive direct/indirect Coombs' test.

AVAILABILITY (Rx)

Capsules: 250 mg, 500 mg. **Powder for Oral Suspension:** 125 mg/5 mL, 250 mg/5 mL, 375 mg/5 mL. **Tablets (Extended-Release):** 500 mg.

ADMINISTRATION/HANDLING

PO

• After reconstitution, oral solution is stable for 14 days if refrigerated. • Shake oral suspension well before using. • Give without regard to food; if GI upset occurs, give with food, milk.

INDICATIONS/ROUTES/DOSAGE

Usual Dosage

PO: ADULTS, ELDERLY: 250–500 mg q8h or 500 mg q12h (extended-release). **CHILDREN:** 20–40 mg/kg/day divided q8–12h. **Maximum:** 1 g/day.

Otitis Media

PO: CHILDREN: 40 mg/kg/day divided q12h. **Maximum:** 1 g/day.

Pharyngitis

CHILDREN: 20 mg/kg/day divided q12h. **Maximum:** 1 g/day.

Dosage in Renal Impairment

Use caution.

Dosage in Hepatic Impairment

No dose adjustment.

SIDE EFFECTS

Frequent: Oral candidiasis, mild diarrhea, mild abdominal cramping, vaginal candidiasis. **Occasional:** Nausea, serum sickness–like reaction (fever, joint pain; usually occurs after second course of therapy and resolves after drug is discontinued). **Rare:** Allergic reaction (pruritus, rash, urticaria).

ADVERSE EFFECTS/TOXIC REACTIONS

Antibiotic-associated colitis (abdominal cramps, severe watery diarrhea, fever), other superinfections may result from altered bacterial balance in GI tract. Nephrotoxicity may occur, esp. in pts with preexisting renal disease. Pts with history of penicillin allergy are at increased risk for developing a severe hypersensitivity reaction (severe pruritus, angioedema, bronchospasm, anaphylaxis).

NURSING CONSIDERATIONS

BASELINE ASSESSMENT

Obtain baseline CBC, renal function tests. Question for history of allergies, particularly cephalosporins, penicillins.

INTERVENTION/EVALUATION

Assess oral cavity for white patches on mucous membranes, tongue (thrush). Monitor daily pattern of bowel activity, stool consistency. Mild GI effects may be tolerable (increasing severity may indicate onset of antibiotic-associated colitis). Monitor I&O, renal function tests for nephrotoxicity. Be alert for superinfection: fever, vomiting, diarrhea, anal/genital pruritus, oral mucosal changes (ulceration, pain, erythema).

PATIENT/FAMILY TEACHING

• Continue therapy for full length of treatment. • Doses should be evenly spaced. • May cause GI upset (may take with food, milk). • Chewable tablets must be chewed; do not swallow whole. • Refrigerate oral suspension. • Report persistent diarrhea.

cefadroxil

sef-a-**drox**-il
(Apo-Cefadroxil ✱)

◆CLASSIFICATION

PHARMACOTHERAPEUTIC: First-generation cephalosporin. **CLINICAL:** Antibiotic.

USES

Treatment of susceptible infections due to group A streptococci, staphylococci, *S. pneumoniae, H. influenzae, Klebsiella* spp., *E. coli, P. mirabilis*, including impetigo, pharyngitis/tonsillitis, skin/skin structure, UTIs. **OFF-LABEL:** Chronic suppression of prosthetic joint infection.

PRECAUTIONS

Contraindications: History of hypersensitivity/anaphylactic reaction to cefadroxil, cephalosporins. **Cautions:** Severe renal impairment, history of penicillin allergy. History of GI disease (colitis).

ACTION

Binds to bacterial cell membranes, inhibits cell wall synthesis. **Therapeutic Effect:** Bactericidal.

PHARMACOKINETICS

Well absorbed from GI tract. Protein binding: 15%–20%. Widely distributed. Primarily excreted in urine. Removed by hemodialysis. **Half-life:** 1.2–1.5 hrs (increased in renal impairment).

⌛ LIFESPAN CONSIDERATIONS

Pregnancy/Lactation: Readily crosses placenta. Distributed in breast milk. **Children:** No age-related precautions noted. **Elderly:** Age-related renal impairment may require dosage adjustment.

INTERACTIONS

DRUG: **Probenecid** may increase concentration/effect. **HERBAL:** None significant. **FOOD:** None known. **LAB VALUES:** May increase serum BUN, alkaline phosphatase, bilirubin, creatinine, LDH, ALT, AST. May cause positive direct/indirect Coombs' test.

AVAILABILITY (Rx)

Capsules: 500 mg. **Powder for Oral Suspension:** 250 mg/5 mL, 500 mg/5 mL. **Tablets:** 1 g.

ADMINISTRATION/HANDLING

PO

• After reconstitution, oral solution is stable for 14 days if refrigerated. • Shake oral suspension well before using. • Give without regard to food; if GI upset occurs, give with food, milk.

INDICATIONS/ROUTES/DOSAGE

Usual Dosage

PO: ADULTS, ELDERLY: 1–2 g/day as single dose or in 2 divided doses. **CHILDREN:** 30 mg/kg/day as a single dose or in 2 divided doses. **Maximum:** 2 g/day.

Dosage in Renal Impairment

After initial 1-g dose, dosage and frequency are modified based on creatinine clearance and severity of infection.

Creatinine Clearance	Dosage
26–50 mL/min	q12h
10–25 mL/min	q24h
Less than 10 mL/min	q36h

Dosage in Hepatic Impairment

No dose adjustment.

SIDE EFFECTS

Frequent: Oral candidiasis, mild diarrhea, mild abdominal cramping, vaginal candidiasis. **Occasional:** Nausea, unusual bruising/bleeding, serum sickness–like reaction (fever, joint pain; usually occurs after second course of therapy and resolves after drug is discontinued). **Rare:** Allergic reaction (rash, pruritus, urticaria), thrombophlebitis (pain, redness, swelling at injection site).

ADVERSE EFFECTS/TOXIC REACTIONS

Antibiotic-associated colitis, other superinfections (abdominal cramps, severe watery diarrhea, fever) may result from altered bacterial balance in GI tract. Nephrotoxicity may occur, esp. in pts with preexisting renal disease. Pts with history of penicillin allergy are at increased risk for developing a severe hypersensitivity reaction (severe pruritus, angioedema, bronchospasm, anaphylaxis).

NURSING CONSIDERATIONS

BASELINE ASSESSMENT

Obtain CBC, renal function tests. Question for history of allergies, particularly cephalosporins, penicillins.

INTERVENTION/EVALUATION

Assess oral cavity for white patches on mucous membranes, tongue (thrush). Monitor daily pattern of bowel activity, stool consistency. Mild GI effects may be tolerable (increasing severity may indicate onset of antibiotic-associated colitis). Monitor I&O, renal function tests for nephrotoxicity. Be alert for superinfection: fever, vomiting, diarrhea, anal/genital pruritus, oral mucosal changes (ulceration, pain, erythema).

PATIENT/FAMILY TEACHING

• Continue therapy for full length of treatment. • Doses should be evenly spaced. • May cause GI upset (may take with food, milk). • Refrigerate oral suspension. • Report persistent diarrhea.

ceFAZolin

sef-a-**zoe**-lin

Do not confuse ceFAZolin with cefOXitin, cefprozil, cefTRIAXone, or cephalexin.

◆CLASSIFICATION

PHARMACOTHERAPEUTIC: First-generation cephalosporin. **CLINICAL:** Antibiotic.

USES

Treatment of susceptible infections due to *S. aureus, S. epidermidis,* group A beta-hemolytic streptococci, *S. pneumoniae, E. coli, P. mirabilis, Klebsiella* spp., *H. influenzae,* including biliary tract, bone and joint, genital, respiratory tract, skin/skin structure infections; UTIs, endocarditis, perioperative prophylaxis, septicemia. **OFF-LABEL:** Prophylaxis against infective endocarditis.

PRECAUTIONS

Contraindications: History of hypersensitivity/anaphylactic reaction to ceFAZolin, cephalosporins. **Cautions:** Severe renal impairment, history of penicillin allergy, history of seizures.

ACTION

Binds to bacterial cell membranes, inhibits cell wall synthesis. **Therapeutic Effect:** Bactericidal.

PHARMACOKINETICS

Widely distributed. Protein binding: 85%. Primarily excreted unchanged in urine. Moderately removed by hemodialysis. **Half-life:** 1.4–1.8 hrs (increased in renal impairment).

LIFESPAN CONSIDERATIONS

Pregnancy/Lactation: Readily crosses placenta; distributed in breast milk. **Children:** No age-related precautions noted. **Elderly:** Age-related renal impairment may require reduced dosage.

INTERACTIONS

DRUG: **Probenecid** may increase concentration/effect. **HERBAL:** None significant. **FOOD:** None known. **LAB VALUES:** May increase serum BUN, alkaline phosphatase, bilirubin, creatinine, LDH, ALT, AST. May cause positive direct/indirect Coombs' test.

AVAILABILITY (Rx)

Injection, Powder for Reconstitution: 500 mg, 1 g. **Ready-to-Hang Infusion:** 1 g/50 mL, 2 g/100 mL.

ADMINISTRATION/HANDLING

IV

Reconstitution • Reconstitute each 1 g with at least 10 mL Sterile Water for Injection or 0.9% NaCl. • May further dilute in 50–100 mL D_5W or 0.9% NaCl (decreases incidence of thrombophlebitis).

Rate of administration • For IV push, administer over 3–5 min (**maximum concentration:** 100 mg/mL). • For intermittent IV infusion (piggyback), infuse over 30–60 min (**maximum concentration:** 20 mg/mL).

Storage • Solution appears light yellow to yellow in color. • Reconstituted solution stable for 24 hrs at room temperature or for 10 days if refrigerated. • IV infusion (piggyback) stable for 48 hrs at room temperature or for 14 days if refrigerated.

IM

• To minimize discomfort, inject deep IM slowly. • Less painful if injected into gluteus maximus rather than lateral aspect of thigh.

IV INCOMPATIBILITIES

Amikacin (Amikin), amiodarone (Cordarone), HYDROmorphone (Dilaudid).

IV COMPATIBILITIES

Calcium gluconate, dexamethasone (Decadron), dilTIAZem (Cardizem), famotidine (Pepcid), heparin, insulin (regular), lidocaine, LORazepam (Ativan), magnesium sulfate, meperidine (Demerol), metoclopramide (Reglan), midazolam (Versed), morphine, multivitamins, ondansetron (Zofran), potassium chloride, propofol (Diprivan).

INDICATIONS/ROUTES/DOSAGE

Usual Dosage Range

IV, IM: **ADULTS:** 1–1.5 g q6–12h (usually q8h). **Maximum:** 12 g/day. **CHILDREN OLDER THAN 1 MO:** 25–100 mg/kg/day divided q6–8h. **Maximum:** 6 g/day. **NEONATES:** 50–150 mg/kg/day in 2–4 divided doses.

Dosage in Renal Impairment

Dosing frequency is modified based on creatinine clearance.

Creatinine Clearance	Dosage
11–34 mL/min	50% usual dose q12h

Creatinine Clearance	Dosage
10 mL/min or less	50% usual dose q18–24h
HD	500 mg–1 g q24h
PD	500 mg q12h
CRRT	
CVVH	Loading dose 2 g, then 1–2 g q12h
CVVHD/CVVHDF	Loading dose 2 g, then 1 g q8h or 2 g q12h

Dosage in Hepatic Impairment

No dose adjustment.

SIDE EFFECTS

Frequent: Discomfort with IM administration, oral candidiasis (thrush), mild diarrhea, mild abdominal cramping, vaginal candidiasis. **Occasional:** Nausea, serum sickness–like reaction (fever, joint pain; usually occurs after second course of therapy and resolves after drug is discontinued). **Rare:** Allergic reaction (rash, pruritus, urticaria), thrombophlebitis (pain, redness, swelling at injection site).

ADVERSE EFFECTS/TOXIC REACTIONS

Antibiotic-associated colitis, other superinfections (abdominal cramps, severe watery diarrhea, fever) may result from altered bacterial balance in GI tract. Nephrotoxicity may occur, esp. in pts with preexisting renal disease. Pts with history of penicillin allergy are at increased risk for developing severe hypersensitivity reaction (severe pruritus, angioedema, bronchospasm, anaphylaxis).

NURSING CONSIDERATIONS

BASELINE ASSESSMENT

Obtain CBC, renal function tests. Question for history of allergies, particularly cephalosporins, penicillins.

INTERVENTION/EVALUATION

Evaluate IM site for induration and tenderness. Assess oral cavity for white patches on mucous membranes, tongue (thrush). Monitor daily pattern of bowel activity, stool consistency. Mild GI effects may be tolerable (increasing severity may indicate onset of antibiotic-associated colitis). Monitor I&O, renal function tests for nephrotoxicity. Be alert for superinfection: fever, vomiting, diarrhea, anal/genital pruritus, oral mucosal changes (ulceration, pain, erythema).

PATIENT/FAMILY TEACHING

• Discomfort may occur with IM injection.

cefdinir

sef-di-neer

(Omnicef ✱)

◆CLASSIFICATION

PHARMACOTHERAPEUTIC: Third-generation cephalosporin. **CLINICAL:** Antibiotic.

USES

Treatment of susceptible infections due to *S. pyogenes, S. pneumoniae, H. influenzae, H. parainfluenzae, M. catarrhalis,* including community-acquired pneumonia, acute exacerbation of chronic bronchitis, acute maxillary sinusitis, pharyngitis, tonsillitis, uncomplicated skin/skin structure infections, otitis media.

PRECAUTIONS

Contraindications: Hypersensitivity to cefdinir. History of anaphylactic reaction to cephalosporins. **Cautions:** Hypersensitivity to penicillins; renal impairment.

ACTION

Binds to bacterial cell membranes, inhibits cell wall synthesis. **Therapeutic Effect:** Bactericidal.

PHARMACOKINETICS

Moderately absorbed from GI tract. Protein binding: 60%–70%. Widely distributed. Not appreciably metabolized. Primarily excreted in urine. Minimally removed by hemodialysis. **Half-life:** 1–2 hrs (increased in renal impairment).

C

LIFESPAN CONSIDERATIONS

Pregnancy/Lactation: Crosses placenta. Not detected in breast milk. **Children:** Newborns, infants may have lower renal clearance. **Elderly:** Age-related renal impairment may require decreased dosage or increased dosing interval.

INTERACTIONS

DRUG: Antacids, iron preparations may interfere with absorption. **Probenecid** increases concentration/effect. **HERBAL:** None significant. **FOOD:** None known. **LAB VALUES:** May produce false-positive reaction for urine ketones. May increase serum alkaline phosphatase, bilirubin, LDH, ALT, AST.

AVAILABILITY (Rx)

Capsules: 300 mg. **Powder for Oral Suspension:** 125 mg/5 mL, 250 mg/5 mL.

ADMINISTRATION/HANDLING

PO

• Give without regard to food. Give at least 2 hrs before or after antacids or iron supplements. • Twice-daily doses should be given 12 hrs apart. • Shake oral suspension well before administering. • Store mixed suspension at room temperature for 10 days.

INDICATIONS/ROUTES/DOSAGE

Usual Dosage Range

PO: ADULTS, ELDERLY: 300 mg q12h or 600 mg once daily. **CHILDREN 6 MOS–12 YRS:** 7 mg/kg q12h or 14 mg/kg once daily. **Maximum:** 600 mg/day.

Dosage in Renal Impairment

CrCl less than 30 mL/min: 300 mg/day or 7 mg/kg as single daily dose. **Maximum:** 300 mg. **Hemodialysis pts:** 300 mg or 7 mg/kg/dose every other day. **Maximum:** 300 mg.

Dosage in Hepatic Impairment

No dose adjustment.

SIDE EFFECTS

Frequent: Oral candidiasis, mild diarrhea, mild abdominal cramping, vaginal candidiasis. **Occasional:** Nausea, serum sickness–like reaction (fever, joint pain; usually occurs after second course of therapy and resolves after drug is discontinued). **Rare:** Allergic reaction (rash, pruritus, urticaria).

ADVERSE EFFECTS/TOXIC REACTIONS

Antibiotic-associated colitis, other superinfections (abdominal cramps, severe watery diarrhea, fever) may result from altered bacterial balance in GI tract. Nephrotoxicity may occur, esp. in pts with preexisting renal disease. Pts with history of penicillin allergy are at increased risk for developing a severe hypersensitivity reaction (severe pruritus, angioedema, bronchospasm, anaphylaxis).

NURSING CONSIDERATIONS

BASELINE ASSESSMENT

Obtain CBC, renal function tests. Question for hypersensitivity to cefdinir or other cephalosporins, penicillins.

INTERVENTION/EVALUATION

Observe for rash. Monitor daily pattern of bowel activity, stool consistency. Mild GI effects may be tolerable (increasing severity may indicate onset of antibiotic-associated colitis). Be alert for superinfection: fever, vomiting, diarrhea, anal/genital pruritus, oral mucosal changes (ulceration, pain, erythema). Monitor hematology reports.

PATIENT/FAMILY TEACHING

• Take antacids 2 hrs before or following medication. • Continue medication for full length of treatment; do not skip doses. • Doses should be evenly spaced. • Report persistent severe diarrhea, rash, muscle aches, fever, enlarged lymph nodes, joint pain.

cefepime

sef-e-**peem**
(Maxipime)
Do not confuse cefepime with cefixime or cefTAZidime.

◆CLASSIFICATION

PHARMACOTHERAPEUTIC: Fourth-generation cephalosporin. **CLINICAL:** Antibiotic.

USES

Susceptible infections due to aerobic gram-negative organisms including *P. aeruginosa,* gram-positive organisms including *S. aureus.* Treatment of empiric febrile neutropenia, intra-abdominal infections, skin/skin structure infections, UTIs, pneumonia. **OFF-LABEL:** Brain abscess, malignant otitis externa, septic lateral/cavernous sinus thrombus.

PRECAUTIONS

Contraindications: History of anaphylactic reaction to penicillins, hypersensitivity to cefepime, cephalosporins. **Cautions:** Renal impairment, history of seizure disorder, GI disease (colitis), elderly.

ACTION

Binds to bacterial cell wall membranes, inhibits cell wall synthesis. **Therapeutic Effect:** Bactericidal.

PHARMACOKINETICS

Well absorbed after IM administration. Protein binding: 20%. Widely distributed. Primarily excreted in urine. Removed by hemodialysis. **Half-life:** 2–2.3 hrs (increased in renal impairment, elderly pts).

LIFESPAN CONSIDERATIONS

Pregnancy/Lactation: Unknown if distributed in breast milk. **Children:** No age-related precautions noted in pts older than 2 mos. **Elderly:** Age-related renal impairment may require reduced dosage or increased dosing interval. Elderly pts with renal insufficiency may have an increased risk of encephalopathy, seizures.

INTERACTIONS

DRUG: **Probenecid** may increase concentration/effect. May increase **aminoglycoside** concentration. **HERBAL:** None significant. **FOOD:** None known. **LAB VALUES:** May increase serum BUN, alkaline phosphatase, bilirubin, LDH, ALT, AST. May cause positive direct/indirect Coombs' test.

AVAILABILITY (Rx)

Injection, Powder for Reconstitution: 1 g, 2 g. **Injection, Premix:** 1 g (50 mL), 2 g (100 mL).

ADMINISTRATION/HANDLING

IV

Reconstitution • Add 10 mL of diluent for 1-g and 2-g vials. • Further dilute with 50–100 mL 0.9% NaCl or D_5W.
Rate of administration • For intermittent IV infusion (piggyback), infuse over 30 min. For direct IV, administer over 5 min.
Storage • Solution is stable for 24 hrs at room temperature, 7 days if refrigerated.

IM

• Add 2.4 mL Sterile Water for Injection, 0.9% NaCl, or D_5W to 1-g and 2-g vials. • Inject into a large muscle mass (e.g., upper gluteus maximus).

IV INCOMPATIBILITIES

Acyclovir (Zovirax), amphotericin (Fungizone), cimetidine (Tagamet), ciprofloxacin (Cipro), CISplatin (Platinol), dacarbazine (DTIC), DAUNOrubicin (Cerubidine), diazePAM (Valium), diphenhydrAMINE (Benadryl), DOBUTamine (Dobutrex), DOPamine (Intropin), DOXOrubicin (Adriamycin), droperidol (Inapsine), famotidine (Pepcid), ganciclovir (Cytovene), haloperidol (Haldol), magnesium, magnesium sulfate, manni-

C

tol, metoclopramide (Reglan), morphine, ofloxacin (Floxin), ondansetron (Zofran), vancomycin (Vancocin).

IV COMPATIBILITIES

Bumetanide (Bumex), calcium gluconate, furosemide (Lasix), HYDROmorphone (Dilaudid), LORazepam (Ativan), propofol (Diprivan).

INDICATIONS/ROUTES/DOSAGE

Usual Dosage Range

IV: ADULTS, ELDERLY: 1–2 g q8–12h. **CHILDREN:** 50 mg/kg q8–12h. **Maximum:** 2,000 mg/dose. **NEONATES:** 30 mg/kg q12h up to 50 mg/kg q8–12h.

Dosage in Renal Impairment

Dosage and frequency are modified based on creatinine clearance and severity of infection.

Creatinine Clearance	Dosage
30–60 mL/min	500 mg q24h–2 g q12h
11–29 mL/min	500 mg–2 g q24h
10 mL/min or less	250 mg–1 g q24h
Hemodialysis	Initially, 1 g, then 0.5–1 g q24h or 1–2 g q48–72h
Peritoneal dialysis	Normal dose q48h
Continuous renal replacement therapy	Initially, 2 g, then 1 g q8h or 2 g q12h

Dosage in Hepatic Impairment

No dose adjustment.

SIDE EFFECTS

Frequent: Discomfort with IM administration, oral candidiasis (thrush), mild diarrhea, mild abdominal cramping, vaginal candidiasis. **Occasional:** Nausea, serum sickness–like reaction (fever, joint pain; usually occurs after second course of therapy and resolves after drug is discontinued). **Rare:** Allergic reaction (rash, pruritus, urticaria), thrombophlebitis (pain, redness, swelling at injection site).

ADVERSE EFFECTS/TOXIC REACTIONS

Antibiotic-associated colitis, other superinfections (abdominal cramps, severe watery diarrhea, fever) may result from altered bacterial balance in GI tract. Nephrotoxicity may occur, esp. in pts with preexisting renal disease. Pts with history of penicillin allergy are at increased risk for developing a severe hypersensitivity reaction (severe pruritus, angioedema, bronchospasm, anaphylaxis).

NURSING CONSIDERATIONS

BASELINE ASSESSMENT

Obtain CBC, renal function tests. Question for history of allergies, particularly cephalosporins, penicillins.

INTERVENTION/EVALUATION

Evaluate IM site for induration and tenderness. Assess oral cavity for white patches on mucous membranes, tongue (thrush). Monitor daily pattern of bowel activity, stool consistency. Mild GI effects may be tolerable (increasing severity may indicate onset of antibiotic-associated colitis). Monitor I&O, CBC, renal function tests for nephrotoxicity. Be alert for superinfection: fever, vomiting, diarrhea, anal/genital pruritus, oral mucosal changes (ulceration, pain, erythema).

PATIENT/FAMILY TEACHING

• Discomfort may occur with IM injection. • Continue therapy for full length of treatment. • Doses should be evenly spaced. • Report persistent diarrhea.

cefixime

sef-**ix**-eem
(Suprax)
Do not confuse cefixime with cefepime, or Suprax with Sporanox or Surbex.

CLASSIFICATION

PHARMACOTHERAPEUTIC: Third-generation cephalosporin. **CLINICAL:** Antibiotic.

USES

Treatment of susceptible infections due to *S. pneumoniae, S. pyogenes, M. catarrhalis, H. influenzae, E. coli, P. mirabilis,* including otitis media, acute bronchitis, acute exacerbations of chronic bronchitis, pharyngitis, tonsillitis, uncomplicated UTI.

PRECAUTIONS

Contraindications: History of hypersensitivity/anaphylactic reaction to cefixime, cephalosporins. **Cautions:** History of penicillin allergy, renal impairment.

ACTION

Binds to bacterial cell membranes, inhibits cell wall synthesis. **Therapeutic Effect:** Bactericidal.

PHARMACOKINETICS

Moderately absorbed from GI tract. Protein binding: 65%–70%. Widely distributed. Primarily excreted in urine. Minimally removed by hemodialysis. **Half-life:** 3–4 hrs (increased in renal impairment).

LIFESPAN CONSIDERATIONS

Pregnancy/Lactation: Not recommended during labor and delivery. Unknown if distributed in breast milk. **Children:** Safety and efficacy not established in pts younger than 6 mos. **Elderly:** Age-related renal impairment may require dosage adjustment.

INTERACTIONS

DRUG: **Probenecid** may increase concentration/effect. **HERBAL:** None significant. **FOOD:** None known. **LAB VALUES:** May increase serum BUN, alkaline phosphatase, bilirubin, creatinine, LDH, ALT, AST. May cause a positive direct/indirect Coombs' test.

AVAILABILITY (Rx)

Oral Suspension: 100 mg/5 mL, 200 mg/5 mL, 500 mg/5 mL. **Capsules:** 400 mg. **Tablets (Chewable):** 100 mg, 200 mg.

ADMINISTRATION/HANDLING

PO

• Give without regard to food. • After reconstitution, oral suspension is stable for 14 days at room temperature or refrigerated. • Shake oral suspension well before administering. Chewable tablets must be chewed or crushed before swallowing.

INDICATIONS/ROUTES/DOSAGE

Usual Dosage

PO: ADULTS: 400 mg/day as a single dose or in 2 divided doses. **INFANTS, CHILDREN, ADOLESCENTS:** 8 mg/kg/day as a single dose or in 2 divided doses. **Maximum:** 400 mg/day.

Dosage in Renal Impairment

Dosage is modified based on creatinine clearance.

Creatinine Clearance	Dosage
21–60 mL/min	260 mg/day
20 mL/min or less	200 mg/day
Hemodialysis	260 mg/day

Dosage in Hepatic Impairment

No dose adjustment.

SIDE EFFECTS

Frequent: Oral candidiasis (thrush), mild diarrhea, mild abdominal cramping, vaginal candidiasis. **Occasional:** Nausea, serum sickness–like reaction (arthralgia, fever; usually occurs after second course of therapy and resolves after drug is discontinued). **Rare:** Allergic reaction (rash, pruritus, urticaria).

ADVERSE EFFECTS/TOXIC REACTIONS

Antibiotic-associated colitis, other superinfections (abdominal cramps, severe watery diarrhea, fever) may result from altered bacterial balance in GI tract. Nephrotoxicity may occur, esp. in pts with preexisting renal disease. Pts with history of penicillin allergy are at increased risk for developing a severe hypersensitivity reaction (severe pruritus, angioedema, bronchospasm, anaphylaxis).

NURSING CONSIDERATIONS

BASELINE ASSESSMENT

Obtain CBC, renal function tests. Question for hypersensitivity to cefixime or other cephalosporins, penicillins.

INTERVENTION/EVALUATION

Assess oral cavity for white patches on mucous membranes, tongue (thrush). Monitor daily pattern of bowel activity, stool consistency. Mild GI effects may be tolerable (increasing severity may indicate onset of antibiotic-associated colitis). Monitor renal function tests for evidence of nephrotoxicity. Be alert for superinfection: fever, vomiting, diarrhea, anal/genital pruritus, oral mucosal changes (ulceration, pain, erythema).

PATIENT/FAMILY TEACHING

• Continue medication for full length of treatment; do not skip doses. • Doses should be evenly spaced. • May cause GI upset (may take with food or milk). • Report persistent diarrhea.

cefotaxime

sef-oh-**tax**-eem

Do not confuse cefotaxime with cefOXitin, ceftizoxime, or cefuroxime, or Claforan with Claritin.

◆CLASSIFICATION

PHARMACOTHERAPEUTIC: Third-generation cephalosporin. **CLINICAL:** Antibiotic.

USES

Treatment of susceptible infections (active vs. most gram-negative [not *Pseudomonas*] and gram-positive cocci [not *Enterococcus*]), including bone, joint, GU, gynecologic, intra-abdominal, lower respiratory tract, skin/skin structure infections; septicemia, meningitis, perioperative prophylaxis. **OFF-LABEL:** Surgical prophylaxis.

PRECAUTIONS

Contraindications: History of hypersensitivity/anaphylactic reaction to cefotaxime, cephalosporins. **Cautions:** History of penicillin allergy, colitis, renal impairment with CrCl less than 30 mL/min.

ACTION

Binds to bacterial cell membranes, inhibits cell wall synthesis. **Therapeutic Effect:** Bactericidal.

PHARMACOKINETICS

Widely distributed to CSF. Protein binding: 30%–50%. Partially metabolized in liver. Primarily excreted in urine. Moderately removed by hemodialysis. **Half-life:** 1 hr (increased in renal impairment).

LIFESPAN CONSIDERATIONS

Pregnancy/Lactation: Readily crosses placenta. Distributed in breast milk. **Children:** No age-related precautions noted. **Elderly:** Age-related renal impairment may require dosage adjustment.

INTERACTIONS

DRUG: **Probenecid** may increase concentration/effect. **HERBAL:** None significant. **FOOD:** None known. **LAB VALUES:** May cause positive direct/indirect Coombs' test. May increase serum BUN, creatinine, ALT, AST, alkaline phosphatase.

AVAILABILITY (Rx)

Injection, Powder for Reconstitution: 500 mg, 1 g.

ADMINISTRATION/HANDLING

IV

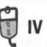

Reconstitution • Reconstitute with 10 mL Sterile Water for Injection or 0.9% NaCl to provide a maximum concentration of 100 mg/mL. • May further dilute with 50–100 mL 0.9% NaCl or D_5W.

Rate of administration • For IV push, administer over 3–5 min. • For intermittent IV infusion (piggyback), infuse over 15–30 min.

Storage • Solution appears light yellow to amber. • IV infusion (piggyback) is stable for 24 hrs at room temperature, 5 days if refrigerated. • Discard if precipitate forms.

IM

• Reconstitute with Sterile Water for Injection or Bacteriostatic Water for Injection to provide a concentration of 230–330 mg/mL. • To minimize discomfort, inject deep IM slowly. Less painful if injected into gluteus maximus than lateral aspect of thigh. For 2-g IM dose, give at 2 separate sites.

IV INCOMPATIBILITIES

Allopurinol (Aloprim), filgrastim (Neupogen), fluconazole (Diflucan), vancomycin (Vancocin).

IV COMPATIBILITIES

dilTIAZem (Cardizem), famotidine (Pepcid), HYDROmorphone (Dilaudid), LORazepam (Ativan), magnesium sulfate, midazolam (Versed), morphine, propofol (Diprivan).

INDICATIONS/ROUTES/DOSAGE

Usual Dosage Range

IV, IM: ADULTS, ELDERLY: Uncomplicated infection: 1 g q12h. **Moderate to severe infection:** 1–2 g q8h. **Life-threatening infection:** 2 g q4h. **INFANTS, CHILDREN, ADOLESCENTS:** 150–180 mg/kg/day in divided doses q8h. **Maximum:** 8 g/day. **NEONATES:** 50 mg/kg/dose q8–12h.

Dosage in Renal Impairment

Creatinine Clearance	Dosage Interval
10–50 mL/min	6–12 hrs
Less than 10 mL/min	24 hrs
Hemodialysis	1–2g q24h
Peritoneal dialysis	1g q24h
CVVH	1–2 g q8–12h
CVVHD	1–2g q8h
CVVHDF	1–2g q6–8h

Dosage in Hepatic Impairment

No dose adjustment.

SIDE EFFECTS

Frequent: Discomfort with IM administration, oral candidiasis (thrush), mild diarrhea, mild abdominal cramping, vaginal candidiasis. **Occasional:** Nausea, serum sickness–like reaction (fever, joint pain; usually occurs after second course of therapy and resolves after drug is discontinued). **Rare:** Allergic reaction (rash, pruritus, urticaria), thrombophlebitis (pain, redness, swelling at injection site).

ADVERSE EFFECTS/TOXIC REACTIONS

Antibiotic-associated colitis, other superinfections (abdominal cramps, severe watery diarrhea, fever) may result from altered bacterial balance in GI tract. Nephrotoxicity may occur, esp. in pts with preexisting renal disease. Pts with history of penicillin allergy are at increased risk for developing a severe hypersensitivity reaction (severe pruritus, angioedema, bronchospasm, anaphylaxis).

NURSING CONSIDERATIONS

BASELINE ASSESSMENT

Question for history of allergies, particularly cephalosporins, penicillins.

INTERVENTION/EVALUATION

Check IM injection sites for induration, tenderness. Assess oral cavity for white patches on mucous membranes, tongue (thrush). Monitor daily pattern of bowel activity, stool consistency. Mild GI effects may be tolerable (increasing severity may indicate onset of antibiotic-associated colitis). Monitor I&O, renal function tests for nephrotoxicity. Be alert for superinfection: fever, vomiting, diarrhea, anal/genital pruritus, oral mucosal changes (ulceration, pain, erythema).

PATIENT/FAMILY TEACHING

• Discomfort may occur with IM injection. • Doses should be evenly spaced. • Continue antibiotic therapy for full length of treatment.

C

cefpodoxime

sef-poe-**dox**-eem

◆CLASSIFICATION

PHARMACOTHERAPEUTIC: Third-generation cephalosporin. **CLINICAL:** Antibiotic.

USES

Treatment of susceptible infections due to *S. pneumoniae, S. pyogenes, S. aureus, H. influenzae, M. catarrhalis, E. coli, Proteus, Klebsiella* spp., including acute maxillary sinusitis, chronic bronchitis, community-acquired pneumonia, otitis media, pharyngitis, tonsillitis, skin/skin structure infections, UTIs.

PRECAUTIONS

Contraindications: History of hypersensitivity/anaphylactic reaction to cefpodoxime, cephalosporins. **Cautions:** Renal impairment, history of penicillin allergy.

ACTION

Binds to bacterial cell membranes, inhibits cell wall synthesis. **Therapeutic Effect:** Bactericidal.

PHARMACOKINETICS

Well absorbed from GI tract (food increases absorption). Protein binding: 18%–23%. Widely distributed. Primarily excreted unchanged in urine. Partially removed by hemodialysis. **Half-life:** 2.3 hrs (increased in renal impairment, elderly pts).

⌛ LIFESPAN CONSIDERATIONS

Pregnancy/Lactation: Readily crosses placenta. Distributed in breast milk. **Children:** Safety and efficacy not established in pts younger than 6 mos. **Elderly:** Age-related renal impairment may require dosage adjustment.

INTERACTIONS

DRUG: High doses of **antacids containing aluminum, H_2 antagonists (e.g., famotidine, ranitidine)** may decrease absorption. **Probenecid** may increase concentration/effect. **HERBAL:** None significant. **FOOD:** **Food** enhances absorption. **LAB VALUES:** May increase serum BUN, alkaline phosphatase, bilirubin, creatinine, LDH, ALT, AST. May cause positive direct/indirect Coombs' test.

AVAILABILITY (Rx)

Oral Suspension: 50 mg/5 mL, 100 mg/5 mL. **Tablets:** 100 mg, 200 mg.

ADMINISTRATION/HANDLING

PO

• Administer tablet with food (enhances absorption). • Administer suspension without regard to food. • After reconstitution, oral suspension is stable for 14 days if refrigerated.

INDICATIONS/ROUTES/DOSAGE

Usual Dosage Range

PO: ADULTS, ELDERLY: 100–400 mg q12h. **CHILDREN:** 10 mg/kg/day in 2 divided doses. **Maximum:** 200 mg/dose.

Dosage in Renal Impairment

For pts with CrCl less than 30 mL/min, usual dose is given q24h. For pts on hemodialysis, usual dose is given 3 times/wk after dialysis.

Dosage in Hepatic Impairment

No dose adjustment.

SIDE EFFECTS

Frequent: Oral candidiasis (thrush), mild diarrhea, mild abdominal cramping, vaginal candidiasis. **Occasional:** Nausea, serum sickness–like reaction (fever, joint pain; usually occurs after second course of therapy and resolves after drug is discontinued). **Rare:** Allergic reaction (pruritus, rash, urticaria).

ADVERSE EFFECTS/TOXIC REACTIONS

Antibiotic-associated colitis, other superinfections (abdominal cramps, severe watery diarrhea, fever) may result from altered bacterial balance in GI tract. Nephrotoxicity may occur, esp. in pts with preexisting renal disease. Pts with history of penicillin allergy are at increased risk for developing a severe hypersensitivity reaction (severe pruritus, angioedema, bronchospasm, anaphylaxis).

NURSING CONSIDERATIONS

BASELINE ASSESSMENT

Obtain CBC, renal function tests. Question for history of allergies, particularly cephalosporins, penicillins.

INTERVENTION/EVALUATION

Assess oral cavity for white patches on mucous membranes, tongue (thrush). Monitor daily pattern of bowel activity, stool consistency. Mild GI effects may be tolerable (increasing severity may indicate onset of antibiotic-associated colitis). Monitor I&O, renal function tests for nephrotoxicity. Be alert for superinfection: fever, vomiting, diarrhea, anal/genital pruritus, oral mucosal changes (ulceration, pain, erythema).

PATIENT/FAMILY TEACHING

• Doses should be evenly spaced. • Shake oral suspension well before using. • Take tablets with food (enhances absorption). • Continue antibiotic therapy for full length of treatment. • Refrigerate oral suspension. • Report persistent diarrhea.

cefprozil

sef-proe-zil
(Apo-Cefprozil ✱)

Do not confuse cefprozil with ceFAZolin, or Cefzil with Cefol, Ceftin, or Kefzol.

◆CLASSIFICATION

PHARMACOTHERAPEUTIC: Second-generation cephalosporin. **CLINICAL:** Antibiotic.

USES

Treatment of susceptible infections due to *S. pneumoniae, S. pyogenes, S. aureus, H. influenzae, M. catarrhalis,* including pharyngitis, tonsillitis, otitis media, secondary bacterial infection of acute bronchitis, acute bacterial exacerbation of chronic bronchitis, uncomplicated skin/skin structure infections, acute sinusitis.

PRECAUTIONS

Contraindications: History of hypersensitivity/anaphylactic reaction to cefprozil, cephalosporins. **Cautions:** Severe renal impairment, history of penicillin allergy.

ACTION

Binds to bacterial cell membranes, inhibits cell wall synthesis. **Therapeutic Effect:** Bactericidal.

PHARMACOKINETICS

Well absorbed from GI tract. Protein binding: 36%–45%. Widely distributed. Primarily excreted in urine. Moderately removed by hemodialysis. **Half-life:** 1.3 hrs (increased in renal impairment).

⌛ LIFESPAN CONSIDERATIONS

Pregnancy/Lactation: Readily crosses placenta. Distributed in breast milk. **Children:** Safety and efficacy not established in pts younger than 6 mos. **Elderly:** Age-related renal impairment may require dosage adjustment.

INTERACTIONS

DRUG: **Probenecid** may increase concentration/effect. **HERBAL:** None significant. **FOOD:** None known. **LAB VALUES:** May cause positive direct/indirect Coombs' test. May increase serum BUN, creatinine, alkaline phosphatase, ALT, AST.

AVAILABILITY (Rx)

Oral Suspension: 125 mg/5 mL, 250 mg/5 mL. **Tablets:** 250 mg, 500 mg.

C

ADMINISTRATION/HANDLING

PO

• Give without regard to food; if GI upset occurs, give with food, milk. • After reconstitution, oral suspension is stable for 14 days if refrigerated. • Shake oral suspension well before using.

INDICATIONS/ROUTES/DOSAGE

Usual Dosage Range

PO: ADULTS, ELDERLY: 250–500 mg q12h or 500 mg q24h. **CHILDREN, ADOLESCENTS:** 7.5–15 mg/kg/day in 2 divided doses. **Maximum:** 500 mg/dose. Do not exceed adult dose.

Dosage in Renal Impairment

CrCl less than 30 mL/min: 50% of usual dose at usual interval. **Hemodialysis:** Administer dose after completion of dialysis.

Dosage in Hepatic Impairment

No dose adjustment.

SIDE EFFECTS

Frequent: Oral candidiasis (thrush), mild diarrhea, mild abdominal cramping, vaginal candidiasis. **Occasional:** Nausea, serum sickness–like reaction (fever, joint pain; usually occurs after second course of therapy and resolves after drug is discontinued). **Rare:** Allergic reaction (pruritus, rash, urticaria).

ADVERSE EFFECTS/TOXIC REACTIONS

Antibiotic-associated colitis, other superinfections (abdominal cramps, severe watery diarrhea, fever) may result from altered bacterial balance in GI tract. Nephrotoxicity may occur, esp. in pts with preexisting renal disease. Pts with history of penicillin allergy are at increased risk for developing a severe hypersensitivity reaction (severe pruritus, angioedema, bronchospasm, anaphylaxis).

NURSING CONSIDERATIONS

BASELINE ASSESSMENT

Obtain CBC, renal function tests. Question for history of allergies, particularly cephalosporins, penicillins.

INTERVENTION/EVALUATION

Assess oral cavity for evidence of stomatitis. Monitor daily pattern of bowel activity, stool consistency. Mild GI effects may be tolerable (but increasing severity may indicate onset of antibiotic-associated colitis). Monitor I&O, renal function tests for nephrotoxicity. Be alert for superinfection: fever, vomiting, diarrhea, anal/genital pruritus, oral mucosal changes (ulceration, pain, erythema).

PATIENT/FAMILY TEACHING

• Doses should be evenly spaced. • Continue antibiotic therapy for full length of treatment. • May cause GI upset (may take with food or milk). • Report persistent diarrhea.

ceftaroline

sef-**tar**-o-leen
(Teflaro)

◆CLASSIFICATION

PHARMACOTHERAPEUTIC: Fifth-generation cephalosporin. **CLINICAL:** Antibiotic.

USES

Treatment of susceptible infections due to gram-positive and gram-negative organisms, including *S. pneumoniae, S. aureus* (methicillin-susceptible only), *H. influenzae, Klebsiella pneumoniae, E. coli,* including acute bacterial skin and skin structure infections, community-acquired bacterial pneumonia.

PRECAUTIONS

Contraindications: History of hypersensitivity/anaphylactic reaction to ceftaroline, cephalosporins. **Cautions:** History of allergy to penicillin, severe renal impairment with CrCl less than 50 mL/min, elderly.

ACTION

Binds to bacterial cell membranes, inhibits cell wall synthesis. **Therapeutic Effect:** Bactericidal.

PHARMACOKINETICS

Protein binding: 20%. Widely distributed in plasma. Not metabolized. Primarily excreted in urine. Hemodialyzable. **Half-life:** 1.6 hrs (increased in renal impairment).

LIFESPAN CONSIDERATIONS

Pregnancy/Lactation: Unknown if distributed in breast milk. **Children:** Safety and efficacy not established. **Elderly:** Age-related renal impairment may require dose adjustment.

INTERACTIONS

DRUG: **Probenecid** may increase concentration/effect. **HERBAL:** None significant. **FOOD:** None known. **LAB VALUES:** May cause positive direct/indirect Coombs' test. May increase serum BUN, creatinine. May decrease serum potassium.

AVAILABILITY (Rx)

Injection, Powder for Reconstitution: 400-mg, 600-mg single-use vial.

ADMINISTRATION/HANDLING

◀ALERT▶ Give by intermittent IV infusion (piggyback). Do not give IV push.

Reconstitution • Reconstitute either 400-mg or 600-mg vial with 20 mL Sterile Water for Injection. • Mix gently to dissolve powder. • Further dilute with 50–250 mL D_5W, 0.9% NaCl.

Rate of administration • Infuse over 5–60 min.

Storage • Discard if particulate is present. • Following reconstitution, solution should appear clear, light to dark yellow. • Solution is stable for 6 hrs at room temperature or 24 hrs if refrigerated.

IV INCOMPATIBILITIES

Fluconazole (Diflucan), vancomycin (Vancocin).

IV COMPATIBILITIES

Famotidine (Pepcid), HYDROmorphone (Dilaudid), LORazepam (Ativan), magnesium sulfate, midazolam (Versed), morphine, propofol (Diprivan).

INDICATIONS/ROUTES/DOSAGE

Usual Dosage

IV: ADULTS, ELDERLY: 600 mg q12h. **CHILDREN 2–18 YRS (WEIGHING MORE THAN 33 KG):** 400 mg q8h or 600 mg q12h. **(WEIGHING 33 KG OR LESS):** 12 mg/kg q8h. **CHILDREN 2 MOS TO LESS THAN 2 YRS:** 8 mg/kg q8h.

Dosage in Renal Impairment

Creatinine Clearance	Dosage
30–50 mL/min	400 mg q12h
15–29 mL/min	300 mg q12h
End-stage renal disease, hemodialysis	200 mg every 12 hrs (give after dialysis)

Dosage in Hepatic Impairment

No dose adjustment.

SIDE EFFECTS

Occasional (5%–4%): Diarrhea, nausea. **Rare (3%–2%):** Allergic reaction (rash, pruritus, urticaria), phlebitis.

ADVERSE EFFECTS/TOXIC REACTIONS

Antibiotic-associated colitis, other superinfections (abdominal cramps, severe watery diarrhea, fever) may result from altered bacterial balance in GI tract. Nephrotoxicity may occur, esp. with preexisting renal disease. Pts with history of penicillin allergy are at increased risk for developing a severe hypersensitivity reaction (severe pruritus, angioedema, bronchospasm, anaphylaxis).

NURSING CONSIDERATIONS

BASELINE ASSESSMENT

Obtain CBC, renal function tests. Question for hypersensitivity to other cephalosporins, penicillins. For pts on hemodialysis, administer medication after dialysis.

C

INTERVENTION/EVALUATION

Assess oral cavity for white patches on mucous membranes, tongue (thrush). Monitor daily pattern of bowel activity, stool consistency. Mild GI effects may be tolerable, but increasing severity may indicate onset of antibiotic-associated colitis. Monitor I&O, renal function tests for evidence of nephrotoxicity. Be alert for superinfection: fever, vomiting, severe genital/anal pruritus, moderate to severe diarrhea, oral mucosal changes (ulceration, pain, erythema).

PATIENT/FAMILY TEACHING

• Continue medication for full length of treatment. • Doses should be evenly spaced.

cefTAZidime

sef-**taz**-i-deem
(Fortaz, Tazicef)
Do not confuse cefTAZidime with ceFAZolin, cefepime, or cefTRIAXone.

◆CLASSIFICATION

PHARMACOTHERAPEUTIC: Third-generation cephalosporin. **CLINICAL:** Antibiotic.

USES

Treatment of susceptible infections due to gram-negative organisms (including *Pseudomonas* and *Enterobacteriaceae*), including bone, joint, CNS (including meningitis), gynecologic, intra-abdominal, lower respiratory tract, skin/skin structure infections; UTI, septicemia. Treatment of CNS infections due to *H. influenzae, N. meningitidis,* including meningitis. **OFF-LABEL:** Bacterial endophthalmitis.

PRECAUTIONS

Contraindications: History of hypersensitivity/anaphylactic reaction to cefTAZidime, cephalosporins. **Cautions:** Severe renal impairment, history of penicillin allergy, seizure disorder.

ACTION

Binds to bacterial cell membranes, inhibits cell wall synthesis. **Therapeutic Effect:** Bactericidal.

PHARMACOKINETICS

Widely distributed, including to CSF. Protein binding: 5%–17%. Primarily excreted in urine. Removed by hemodialysis. **Half-life:** 2 hrs (increased in renal impairment).

⌛ LIFESPAN CONSIDERATIONS

Pregnancy/Lactation: Readily crosses placenta. Distributed in breast milk. **Children:** No age-related precautions noted. **Elderly:** Age-related renal impairment may require dosage adjustment.

INTERACTIONS

DRUG: **Probenecid** may increase concentration/effect. **HERBAL:** None significant. **FOOD:** None known. **LAB VALUES:** May increase serum BUN, alkaline phosphatase, creatinine, LDH, ALT, AST. May cause positive direct/indirect Coombs' test.

AVAILABILITY (Rx)

Injection Powder for Reconstitution: ***(Fortaz, Tazicef):*** 500 mg, 1 g, 2 g. **Injection Premix:** 1 g/50 mL.

ADMINISTRATION/HANDLING

◀ALERT▶ Give by IM injection, direct IV injection (IV push), or intermittent IV infusion (piggyback).

IV

Reconstitution • Add 10 mL Sterile Water for Injection to each 1 g to provide concentration of 90 mg/mL. • May further dilute with 50–100 mL 0.9% NaCl, D_5W, or other compatible diluent.
Rate of administration • For IV push, administer over 3–5 min (**maximum concentration:** 180 mg/mL). • For in-

termittent IV infusion (piggyback), infuse over 15–30 min.

Storage • Solution appears light yellow to amber, tends to darken (color change does not indicate loss of potency). • IV infusion (piggyback) stable for 12 hrs at room temperature or 3 days if refrigerated. • Discard if precipitate forms.

IM

Reconstitution • Add 1.5 mL Sterile Water for Injection or lidocaine 1% to 500-mg vial or 3 mL to 1-g vial to provide a concentration of 280 mg/mL. • To minimize discomfort, inject deep IM slowly. Less painful if injected into gluteus maximus than lateral aspect of thigh.

IV INCOMPATIBILITIES

Amphotericin B complex (Abelcet, AmBisome, Amphotec), fluconazole (Diflucan), IDArubicin, midazolam (Versed), vancomycin (Vancocin).

IV COMPATIBILITIES

DiltiaZEM (Cardizem), famotidine (Pepcid), heparin, HYDROmorphone (Dilaudid), lipids, morphine, propofol (Diprivan).

INDICATIONS/ROUTES/DOSAGE

Usual Dosage Range

IV, IM: ADULTS, ELDERLY: 500 mg–2 g q8–12h.

IV: CHILDREN 1 MO–12 YRS: Mild to moderate infection: 90–150 mg/kg/day in divided doses q8h. **Maximum:** 3 g/day. **Severe infection:** 200 mg/kg/day in divided doses q8h. **Maximum:** 6 g/day. **NEONATES 0–4 WKS:** 50 mg/kg/dose q8–12h.

Dosage in Renal Impairment

Dosage and frequency are modified based on creatinine clearance and severity of infection.

Creatinine Clearance	Dosage
31–50 mL/min	1g q12h
16–30 mL/min	1g q24h
6–15 mL/min	500 mg q24h
Less than 6 mL/min	500 mg q48h
Hemodialysis	0.5–1 g q24h or 1–2 g q48–72h (give post hemodialysis on dialysis days)
Peritoneal dialysis	Initially, 1 g, then 0.5 g q24h
Continuous renal replacement therapy	Initially, 2 g, then 1 g q8h or 2 g q12h

Dosage in Hepatic Impairment

No dose adjustment.

SIDE EFFECTS

Frequent: Discomfort with IM administration, oral candidiasis (thrush), mild diarrhea, mild abdominal cramping, vaginal candidiasis. **Occasional:** Nausea, serum sickness–like reaction (fever, joint pain; usually occurs after second course of therapy and resolves after drug is discontinued). **Rare:** Allergic reaction (pruritus, rash, urticaria), thrombophlebitis (pain, redness, swelling at injection site).

ADVERSE EFFECTS/TOXIC REACTIONS

Antibiotic-associated colitis, other superinfections (abdominal cramps, severe watery diarrhea, fever) may result from altered bacterial balance in GI tract. Nephrotoxicity may occur, esp. in pts with preexisting renal disease. Pts with history of penicillin allergy are at increased risk for developing a severe hypersensitivity reaction (severe pruritus, angioedema, bronchospasm, anaphylaxis).

NURSING CONSIDERATIONS

BASELINE ASSESSMENT

Obtain CBC, renal function tests. Question for history of allergies, particularly cephalosporins, penicillins.

INTERVENTION/EVALUATION

Evaluate IV site for phlebitis (heat, pain, red streaking over vein). Assess IM in-

C

jection sites for induration, tenderness. Check oral cavity for white patches on mucous membranes, tongue (thrush). Monitor daily pattern of bowel activity, stool consistency. Mild GI effects may be tolerable (increasing severity may indicate onset of antibiotic-associated colitis). Monitor I&O, renal function tests for nephrotoxicity. Be alert for superinfection: fever, vomiting, diarrhea, anal/genital pruritus, oral mucosal changes (ulceration, pain, erythema).

PATIENT/FAMILY TEACHING

• Discomfort may occur with IM injection. • Doses should be evenly spaced. • Continue antibiotic therapy for full length of treatment.

cefTAZidime/avibactam

sef-**taz**-i-deem/**a**-vi-**bak**-tam
(Avycaz)
Do not confuse cefTAZidime with ceFAZolin or cefepime, or avibactam with sulbactam or tazobactam.

◆CLASSIFICATION

PHARMACOTHERAPEUTIC: Cephalosporin/beta-lactamase inhibitor. **CLINICAL:** Antibacterial.

USES

Used in combination with metroNIDAZOLE for treatment of complicated intra-abdominal infections caused by the following susceptible microorganisms: *E. cloacae, E. coli, K. pneumoniae, K. oxytoca, P. mirabilis, P. stuartii,* and *P. aeruginosa* in adults and pediatric pts 3 mos and older. Treatment of complicated urinary tract infections, including pyelonephritis, caused by the following susceptible microorganisms: *C. freundii, C. koseri, E. aerogenes, E. cloacae, E. coli, K. pneumoniae, Proteus* spp., and *P. aeruginosa* in adults and pediatric pts 3 mos and older. Treatment of hospital-acquired bacterial pneumonia and ventilator-associated bacterial pneumonia (HAP/VAP) caused by the following susceptible microorganisms: *K. pneumoniae, E. cloacae, E. coli, Serratia marcescens, P. mirabilis, P. aeruginosa,* and *Haemophilus influenzae.*

PRECAUTIONS

Contraindications: Hypersensitivity to avibactam-containing products, cefTAZidime, cephalosporins. **Cautions:** History of renal impairment, seizure disorder, encephalopathy, recent *C. difficile* (C-diff) infection or antibiotic-associated colitis. Hypersensitivity to penicillins, other beta-lactams.

ACTION

Inhibits cell wall synthesis by binding to bacterial cell membrane. Bacterial action of cefTAZidime is mediated through binding to essential penicillin-binding proteins. Avibactam inactivates some beta-lactamases and protects cefTAZidime from degradation by certain beta-lactamases. **Therapeutic Effect:** Bactericidal.

PHARMACOKINETICS

Widely distributed. Excreted unchanged as parent drug; not significantly metabolized in liver. Protein binding: less than 10%. Removed extensively by hemodialysis (55% of dose). Eliminated in urine (80%–90% unchanged). **Half-life:** 2.7 hrs (dependent on dose and severity of renal impairment).

⌛ LIFESPAN CONSIDERATIONS

Pregnancy/Lactation: CefTAZidime is excreted in breast milk in low concentrations. Unknown if avibactam is excreted in breast milk. **Children:** Safety and efficacy not established. **Elderly:** May have increased risk of adverse effects (due to renal impairment).

INTERACTIONS

DRUG: May decrease therapeutic effect of **BCG (intravesical). HERBAL:** None significant. **FOOD:** None known. **LAB VALUES:** May increase serum alkaline phosphatase, ALT, GGT, LDH. May decrease platelets, eosinophils, leukocytes, lymphocytes, serum potassium. May result in positive Coombs' test or false-positive elevated urine glucose.

AVAILABILITY (Rx)

◀ALERT▶ CefTAZidime/avibactam is a combination product.

Injection, Powder for Reconstitution: 2 gm cefTAZidime/0.5 gm avibactam.

ADMINISTRATION/HANDLING

IV

Reconstitution • Reconstitute vial with 10 mL of one of the following solutions: 0.9% NaCl, Sterile Water for Injection or 5% Dextrose Injection. • Shake gently until powder is completely dissolved. • Visually inspect for particulate matter or discoloration. Solution should appear clear to slightly yellow in color. • Final concentration of vial will equal approx. 0.167 g/mL of cefTAZidime and 0.042 g/mL of avibactam. • Further dilute with 50 mL to 250 mL 0.9% NaCl or 5% Dextrose Injection.

Rate of administration • Infuse over 2 hrs.

Storage • Diluted solution may be stored at room temperature up to 12 hrs or refrigerated up to 24 hrs. • Infuse within 12 hrs once removed from refrigerator. • Do not freeze.

INDICATIONS/ROUTES/DOSAGE

Complicated Intra-Abdominal Infections

IV: ADULTS, ELDERLY: 2.5 g (cefTAZidime 2 g/avibactam 0.5 g) q8h for 5–14 days (in combination with metroNIDAZOLE). **INFANTS 6 MOS AND OLDER, CHILDREN, ADOLESCENTS YOUNGER THAN 18 YRS:** 50 mg cefTAZidime/kg/dose q8h; **Maximum:** 2g cefTAZidime/dose. **INFANTS 3 MOS TO LESS THAN 6 MOS:** 40 mg cefTAZidime/kg/dose q8h.

Complicated Urinary Tract Infections Including Pyelonephritis

IV: ADULTS, ELDERLY: 2.5 g (2 g cefTAZidime/0.5 g avibactam) q8h for 7–14 days. **INFANTS 6 MOS AND OLDER, CHILDREN, ADOLESCENTS YOUNGER THAN 18 YRS:** 50 mg cefTAZidime/kg/dose q8h. **Maximum:** 2 g cefTAZidime/dose. **INFANTS 3 MOS TO LESS THAN 6 MOS:** 40 mg cefTAZidime/kg/dose q8h.

HAP/VAP

IV: ADULTS, ELDERLY: 2.5 g (2 g cefTAZidime/0.5 g avibactam) q8h for 7–14 days.

Dosage in Renal Impairment

Note: Infuse after hemodialysis on hemodialysis days. Dosage is modified based on creatinine clearance.

Creatinine Clearance	Dosage
Greater than 50 mL/min	2.5 g (2 g/0.5 g) q8h
31–50 mL/min	1.25 g (1 g/0.25 g) q8h
16–30 mL/min	0.94 g (0.75 g/0.19 g) q12h
6–15 mL/min	0.94 g (0.75 g/0.19 g) q24h
Less than or equal to 5 mL/min	0.94 g (0.75 g/0.19 g) q48h

Dosage in Hepatic Impairment

No dose adjustment.

SIDE EFFECTS

Occasional (14%–5%): Vomiting, nausea, abdominal pain, anxiety, rash. **Rare (4%–2%):** Constipation, dizziness.

ADVERSE EFFECTS/TOXIC REACTIONS

May cause worsening of renal function or acute renal failure in pts with renal impairment. Clinical cure rates were lower in pts with CrCl 30–50 mL/min compared with those with CrCl greater than 50 mL/min, and in pts receiving metroNIDAZOLE combination therapy. Blood and lymphatic disorders such as agranulocytosis, hemolytic anemia, leukopenia, lymphocytosis, neutropenia, thrombocytopenia were reported. Hypersensitivity reactions, including anaphylaxis or severe skin reactions, have been reported in pts treated with beta-lactam antibacterial drugs. *C. difficile* (C-diff)–associated diarrhea, with severity ranging from mild diarrhea to fatal colitis, was reported. C-diff infection may occur more than 2 mos after treat-

C

ment completion. Central nervous system reactions including asterixis, coma, encephalopathy, neuromuscular excitability, myoclonus, nonconvulsive status epilepticus, seizures have been reported in pts receiving cefTAZidime, esp. in pts with renal impairment. May increase risk of development of drug-resistant bacteria when used in the absence of a proven or strongly suspected bacterial infection. Skin and subcutaneous tissue disorders such as angioedema, erythema multiforme, pruritus, Stevens-Johnson syndrome, toxic epidermal necrolysis were reported in pts receiving cefTAZidime. Other reported adverse effects, including infusion site inflammation/hematoma/thrombosis, jaundice, candidiasis, dysgeusia, paresthesia, tubulointerstitial nephritis, vaginal inflammation, occur rarely.

NURSING CONSIDERATIONS

BASELINE ASSESSMENT

Obtain baseline CBC, BUN, serum creatinine, potassium; CrCl, GFR, LFT; bacterial culture and sensitivity; vital signs. Question history of recent *C. difficile* infection, renal impairment, seizure disorder; hypersensitivity reaction to beta-lactams, carbapenem, cephalosporins, PCN. Assess skin for wounds; assess hydration status. Question pt's usual stool characteristics (color, frequency, consistency).

INTERVENTION/EVALUATION

Monitor CBC, BMP, renal function periodically. For pts with changing renal function, monitor renal function test daily and adjust dose accordingly. Diligently monitor I&Os. Observe daily pattern of bowel activity, stool consistency (increased severity may indicate antibiotic-associated colitis). If frequent diarrhea occurs, obtain *C. difficile* toxin screen and initiate isolation precautions until test result confirmed; manage proper fluids levels/PO intake, electrolyte levels, protein intake. Antibacterial drugs that are not directed against *C. difficile* infection may need to be discontinued. Report any sign of hypersensitivity reaction.

PATIENT/FAMILY TEACHING

• It is essential to complete drug therapy despite symptom improvement. Early discontinuation may result in antibacterial resistance or increased risk of recurrent infection. • Report any episodes of diarrhea, esp. in the mos following treatment completion. Frequent diarrhea, fever, abdominal pain, blood-streaked stool may indicate infectious diarrhea and may be contagious to others. • Report abdominal pain, black/tarry stools, bruising, yellowing of skin or eyes; dark urine, decreased urine output; skin problems such as development of sores, rash, skin bubbling/necrosis. • Drink plenty of fluids. • Report any nervous system changes such as anxiety, confusion, hallucinations, muscle jerking, or seizure-like activity. • Severe allergic reactions such as hives, palpitations, shortness of breath, rash, tongue-swelling may occur.

ceftolozane/ tazobactam

cef-**tol**-oh-zane/tay-zoe-**bak**-tam
(Zerbaxa)

Do not confuse ceftolozane with cefTAZidime, or tazobactam with avibactam or sulbactam.

◆CLASSIFICATION

PHARMACOTHERAPEUTIC: Cephalosporin/beta-lactamase inhibitor. **CLINICAL:** Antibacterial.

USES

Used in combination with metroNIDAZOLE for treatment of complicated intra-abdominal infections caused by the following susceptible gram-negative and gram-positive microorganisms: *B. fragilis, E. cloacae, E. coli, K. oxytoca, K. pneumoniae, P. mirabilis, P. aeruginosa, S. anginosus, S. constellatus,* and *S. salivarius* in pts 18 yrs or older. Treatment of complicated urinary tract infections, including pyelonephritis, caused by the following susceptible gram-negative microorganisms: *E. coli, K. pneumoniae, P. mirabilis,* and *P. aeruginosa* in pts 18 yrs or older. Treatment of hospital-acquired pneumonia and ventilator-associated bacterial pneumonia in pts 18 yrs and older caused by *E. cloacae, E. coli, Haemophilus influenzae, K. oxytoca, K. pneumoniae, P. mirabilis, P. aeruginosa,* and *Serratia marcescens*.

PRECAUTIONS

Contraindications: Hypersensitivity to ceftolozane/tazobactam, piperacillin/tazobactam, or other beta-lactams. **Cautions:** History of atrial fibrillation, electrolyte imbalance–associated arrhythmias, recent *C. difficile* (C-diff) infection or antibiotic-associated colitis, renal/hepatic impairment, seizure disorder; prior hypersensitivity to penicillins, other cephalosporins.

ACTION

Inhibits cell wall synthesis by binding to bacterial cell membrane. Bacterial action of ceftolozane is mediated through binding to essential penicillin-binding proteins. Tazobactam inactivates certain beta-lactamases and binds to certain chromosomal and plasmid-mediated bacterial beta-lactamases. **Therapeutic Effect:** Bactericidal.

PHARMACOKINETICS

Widely distributed. Excreted unchanged as parent drug; not significantly metabolized in liver. Protein binding: 16%–30%. Eliminated in urine (95% unchanged). Removed extensively by hemodialysis. **Half-life:** 2.7 hrs (dependent on dose and severity of renal impairment).

LIFESPAN CONSIDERATIONS

Pregnancy/Lactation: Unknown if distributed in breast milk. **Children:** Safety and efficacy not established. **Elderly:** May have increased risk of adverse effects (due to renal impairment).

INTERACTIONS

DRUG: **Probenecid** may increase concentration/effect. **HERBAL:** None significant. **FOOD:** None known. **LAB VALUES:** May increase serum alkaline phosphatase, ALT, AST, GGT. May decrease Hgb, Hct, platelets; serum potassium, magnesium, phosphate. May result in positive Coombs' test.

AVAILABILITY (Rx)

◀ALERT▶ Ceftolozane/tazobactam is a combination product.

Injection Powder for Reconstitution: 1 g ceftolozane/0.5 g tazobactam.

ADMINISTRATION/HANDLING

IV

Reconstitution • Reconstitute vial with 10 mL of Sterile Water for Injection or 0.9% NaCl. • Shake gently until powder is completely dissolved. • Final volume of vial will equal approx. 11.4 mL. • Visually inspect for particulate matter or discoloration. Solution should appear clear, colorless to slightly yellow in color. • Withdraw required volume from reconstituted vial and inject into diluent bag containing 100 mL 0.9% NaCl or 5% dextrose injection as follows:

Ceftolozane/ Tazobactam	Volume to Withdraw From Reconstituted Vial
1.5 g (1 g/0.5 g)	11.4 mL
750 mg (500 mg/250 mg)	5.7 mL
375 mg (250 mg/125 mg)	2.9 mL
150 mg (100 mg/50 mg)	1.2 mL

Rate of administration • Infuse over 60 min.

Storage • Refrigerate intact vials. • Reconstituted vial may be held for 1 hr prior to transfer to diluent bag. • May refrigerate diluted solution up to 7 days or store at room temperature up to 24 hrs. • Do not freeze.

INDICATIONS/ROUTES/DOSAGE

Complicated Intra-Abdominal Infections

IV: ADULTS, ELDERLY: 1.5 g (ceftolozane 1 g/tazobactam 0.5 g) q8h for 4–14 days (in combination with metroNIDAZOLE).

C

Complicated Urinary Tract Infections Including Pyelonephritis
IV: ADULTS, ELDERLY: 1.5 g (ceftolozane 1 g/tazobactam 0.5 g) q8h for 7 days.

Pneumonia, Hospital-Acquired or Ventilator-Associated
IV: ADULTS, ELDERLY: 3 g (ceftolozane) q8h for 7 days (longer course may be required).

Dosage in Renal Impairment
CrCl 30–50 mL/min: 750 mg (500 mg/250 mg) q8h. **CrCl 15–29 mL/min:** 375 mg (250 mg/125 mg) q8h. **End-stage renal disease or on hemodialysis:** 750 mg (500 mg/250 mg) loading dose, then 150 mg (100 mg/50 mg) maintenance dose q8h for the remainder of the treatment period. **Note:** Administer after hemodialysis on hemodialysis days.

Dosage in Hepatic Impairment
No dose adjustment.

SIDE EFFECTS

Occasional (6%–3%): Nausea, diarrhea, pyrexia, insomnia, headache, vomiting. **Rare (2%–1%):** Constipation, anxiety, hypotension, rash, abdominal pain, dizziness, tachycardia, dyspnea, urticaria, gastritis, abdominal distention, dyspepsia, flatulence.

ADVERSE EFFECTS/TOXIC REACTIONS

Clinical cure rates were lower in pts with CrCl 30–50 mL/min compared with those with CrCl greater than 50 mL/min, and in pts receiving metroNIDAZOLE combination therapy. Hypersensitivity reactions including anaphylaxis or severe skin reactions have been reported with use of beta-lactam antibacterial drugs. *Clostridium difficile* (C-diff)–associated diarrhea, with severity ranging from mild diarrhea to fatal colitis, was reported. C-diff infection may occur more than 2 mos after treatment completion. May increase risk of development of drug-resistant bacteria when used in the absence of a proven or strongly suspected bacterial infection. Atrial fibrillation reported in 1.2% of pts. Other reported adverse events such as angina pectoris, infections (candidiasis, oropharyngeal infection, fungal urinary tract infection), paralytic ileus, venous thrombosis occur rarely.

NURSING CONSIDERATIONS

BASELINE ASSESSMENT

Obtain baseline CBC, serum BUN, creatinine; CrCl, GFR, LFT; bacterial culture and sensitivity; vital signs. Question history of atrial fibrillation, recent *C. difficile* infection, hepatic/renal impairment, hypersensitivity reaction to beta-lactams, cephalosporins, penicillins, carbapenem. Assess skin for wounds; assess hydration status. Question pt's usual stool characteristics (color, frequency, consistency).

INTERVENTION/EVALUATION

Monitor CBC, BMP, renal function test periodically; serum magnesium, ionized calcium in pts at risk for arrhythmias. For pts with changing renal function, monitor renal function test daily and adjust dose accordingly. Diligently monitor I&Os. Observe daily pattern of bowel activity, stool consistency (increased severity may indicate antibiotic-associated colitis). If frequent diarrhea occurs, obtain *C. difficile* toxin screen and initiate isolation precautions until test result confirmed; manage proper fluids levels/PO intake, electrolyte levels, protein intake. Antibacterial drugs that are not directed against C-diff infection may need to be discontinued. Report any signs of hypersensitivity reaction.

PATIENT/FAMILY TEACHING

• It is essential to complete drug therapy despite symptom improvement. Early discontinuation may result in antibacterial resistance or increased risk of recurrent infection. • Report any episodes of diarrhea, esp. the following mos after treatment completion. Frequent diarrhea, fever, abdominal pain, blood-streaked stool may indicate infectious diarrhea and may be contagious to others. • Report abdominal pain, black/tarry stools, bruising, yellowing of skin or eyes; dark urine, decreased urine output. • Drink plenty of fluids. • Severe allergic reactions such as hives, palpitations, rash, shortness of breath, tongue swelling may occur.

cefTRIAXone

sef-trye-**ax**-own

Do not confuse cefTRIAXone with ceFAZolin, cefOXitin, or ceftazidime.

◆CLASSIFICATION

PHARMACOTHERAPEUTIC: Third-generation cephalosporin. **CLINICAL:** Antibiotic.

USES

Treatment of susceptible infections due to gram-negative aerobic organisms, some gram-positive organisms, including respiratory tract, GU tract, skin and skin structure, bone and joint, intra-abdominal, pelvic inflammatory disease (PID), biliary tract/urinary tract infections; bacterial septicemia, meningitis, perioperative prophylaxis, acute bacterial otitis media. **OFF-LABEL:** Complicated gonococcal infections, STDs, Lyme disease, salmonellosis, shigellosis, atypical community-acquired pneumonia.

PRECAUTIONS

Contraindications: History of hypersensitivity/anaphylactic reaction to cefTRIAXone, cephalosporins. Hyperbilirubinemic neonates, esp. premature infants, should not be treated with cefTRIAXone (can displace bilirubin from its binding to serum albumin, causing bilirubin encephalopathy). Do not administer with calcium-containing IV solutions, including continuous calcium-containing infusion such as parenteral nutrition (in neonates) due to the risk of precipitation of cefTRIAXone-calcium salt. **Cautions:** Hepatic impairment, history of GI disease (esp. ulcerative colitis, antibiotic-associated colitis). History of penicillin allergy.

ACTION

Binds to bacterial cell membranes, inhibits cell wall synthesis. **Therapeutic Effect:** Bactericidal.

PHARMACOKINETICS

Widely distributed, including to CSF. Protein binding: 83%–96%. Primarily excreted in urine. Not removed by hemodialysis. **Half-life: IV:** 4.3–4.6 hrs; **IM:** 5.8–8.7 hrs (increased in renal impairment).

LIFESPAN CONSIDERATIONS

Pregnancy/Lactation: Readily crosses placenta. Distributed in breast milk. **Children:** May displace bilirubin from serum albumin. Contraindicated in hyperbilirubinemic neonates. **Elderly:** Age-related renal impairment may require dosage adjustment.

INTERACTIONS

DRUG: **Probenecid** may increase excretion/effect. **Calcium salts** may increase adverse/toxic effects. **HERBAL:** None significant. **FOOD:** None known. **LAB VALUES:** May increase serum BUN, alkaline phosphatase, bilirubin, creatinine, LDH, ALT, AST. May cause positive direct/indirect Coombs' test.

AVAILABILITY (Rx)

Injection, Powder for Reconstitution: 250 mg, 500 mg, 1 g, 2 g. **Intravenous Solution:** 1 g/50 mL, 2 g/50 mL.

ADMINISTRATION/HANDLING

IV

Reconstitution • Add 2.4 mL Sterile Water for Injection to each 250 mg to provide concentration of 100 mg/mL. • May further dilute with 50–100 mL 0.9% NaCl, D_5W.

Rate of administration • For IV push, administer over 1–4 min (**maximum concentration:** 40 mg/mL). • For intermittent IV infusion (piggyback), infuse over 30 min.

Storage • Solution appears light yellow to amber. • IV infusion (piggyback) is stable for 2 days at room temperature, 10 days if refrigerated. • Discard if precipitate forms.

IM

• Add 0.9 mL Sterile Water for Injection, 0.9% NaCl, D_5W, or lidocaine to each 250 mg to provide concentration of 250 mg/mL. • To minimize discomfort, inject deep IM slowly. Less painful if injected into gluteus maximus than lateral aspect of thigh.

IV INCOMPATIBILITIES

Amphotericin B complex (Abelcet, AmBisome, Amphotec), famotidine (Pepcid), fluconazole (Diflucan), labetalol (Normodyne), Lactated Ringer's injection, vancomycin (Vancocin).

IV COMPATIBILITIES

DiltiaZEM (Cardizem), heparin, lidocaine, metroNIDAZOLE (Flagyl), morphine, propofol (Diprivan).

INDICATIONS/ROUTES/DOSAGE

Usual Dosage Range

IM/IV: ADULTS, ELDERLY: 1–2 g q12–24h. **CHILDREN: Mild to moderate infection:** 50–75 mg/kg/day in 1–2 divided doses. **Maximum:** 1 g/day. **Severe infection:** 100 mg/kg/day divided q12–24h. **Maximum:** 4 g/day. **NEONATES:** 50 mg/kg/dose given once daily.

Dosage in Renal/Hepatic Impairment

Dosage modification is usually unnecessary, but hepatic/renal function test results should be monitored in pts with renal and hepatic impairment or severe renal impairment.

SIDE EFFECTS

Frequent: Discomfort with IM administration, oral candidiasis (thrush), mild diarrhea, mild abdominal cramping, vaginal candidiasis. **Occasional:** Nausea, serum sickness–like reaction (fever, joint pain; usually occurs after second course of therapy and resolves after drug is discontinued). **Rare:** Allergic reaction (rash, pruritus, urticaria), thrombophlebitis (pain, redness, swelling at injection site).

ADVERSE EFFECTS/TOXIC REACTIONS

Antibiotic-associated colitis, other superinfections (abdominal cramps, severe watery diarrhea, fever) may result from altered bacterial balance in GI tract. Nephrotoxicity may occur, esp. in pts with preexisting renal disease. Pts with history of penicillin allergy are at increased risk for developing a severe hypersensitivity reaction (severe pruritus, angioedema, bronchospasm, anaphylaxis).

NURSING CONSIDERATIONS

BASELINE ASSESSMENT

Obtain CBC, renal function tests. Question for history of allergies, particularly cephalosporins, penicillins.

INTERVENTION/EVALUATION

Assess oral cavity for white patches on mucous membranes, tongue (thrush). Monitor daily pattern of bowel activity, stool consistency. Mild GI effects may be tolerable (increasing severity may indicate onset of antibiotic-associated colitis). Monitor I&O, renal function tests for nephrotoxicity, CBC. Be alert for superinfection: fever, vomiting, diarrhea, anal/genital pruritus, oral mucosal changes (ulceration, pain, erythema).

PATIENT/FAMILY TEACHING

• Discomfort may occur with IM injection. • Doses should be evenly spaced. • Continue antibiotic therapy for full length of treatment.

cefuroxime

sef-ue-**rox**-eem

Do not confuse Ceftin with Cefzil or Cipro, cefuroxime with cefotaxime, cefprozil, or deferoxamine, or Zinacef with Zithromax.

C

◆CLASSIFICATION

PHARMACOTHERAPEUTIC: Second-generation cephalosporin. **CLINICAL:** Antibiotic.

USES

Treatment of susceptible infections due to group B streptococci, pneumococci, staphylococci, *H. influenzae, E. coli, Enterobacter, Klebsiella,* including acute/chronic bronchitis, gonorrhea, impetigo, early Lyme disease, otitis media, pharyngitis/tonsillitis, sinusitis, skin/skin structure, UTI, perioperative prophylaxis.

PRECAUTIONS

Contraindications: History of hypersensitivity/anaphylactic reaction to cefuroxime, cephalosporins. **Cautions:** Severe renal impairment, history of penicillin allergy. Pts with hx of colitis, GI malabsorption, seizures.

ACTION

Binds to bacterial cell membranes, inhibits cell wall synthesis. **Therapeutic Effect:** Bactericidal.

PHARMACOKINETICS

Rapidly absorbed from GI tract. Protein binding: 33%–50%. Widely distributed, including to CSF. Primarily excreted unchanged in urine. Moderately removed by hemodialysis. **Half-life:** 1.3 hrs (increased in renal impairment).

LIFESPAN CONSIDERATIONS

Pregnancy/Lactation: Readily crosses placenta. Distributed in breast milk. **Children:** No age-related precautions noted. **Elderly:** Age-related renal impairment may require dosage adjustment.

INTERACTIONS

DRUG: **Probenecid** may increase concentration/effect. **Antacids, H_2-receptor antagonists (e.g., cimetidine, famotidine), proton pump inhibitors (e.g., pantoprazole)** may decrease absorption. May decrease therapeutic effect of **BCG (intravesical).** **HERBAL:** None significant. **FOOD:** None known. **LAB VALUES:** May increase serum BUN, creatinine, alkaline phosphatase, bilirubin, LDH, ALT, AST. May cause positive direct/indirect Coombs' test.

AVAILABILITY (Rx)

Injection Powder for Reconstitution: 750 mg, 1.5 g. **Tablets:** 250 mg, 500 mg.

ADMINISTRATION/HANDLING

IV

Reconstitution • Reconstitute 750 mg in 8 mL (1.5 g in 14 mL) Sterile Water for Injection to provide a concentration of 100 mg/mL. • For intermittent IV infusion (piggyback), further dilute with 50–100 mL 0.9% NaCl or D_5W.

Rate of administration • For IV push, administer over 3–5 min. • For intermittent IV infusion (piggyback), infuse over 15–30 min.

Storage • Solution appears light yellow to amber (may darken, but color change does not indicate loss of potency). • IV infusion (piggyback) is stable for 24 hrs at room temperature, 7 days if refrigerated. • Discard if precipitate forms.

IM

• To minimize discomfort, inject deep IM slowly in large muscle mass.

PO

• Give tablets without regard to food (give 400-mg dose with food). • If GI upset occurs, give with food, milk. • Avoid crushing tablets due to bitter taste.

IV INCOMPATIBILITIES

Fluconazole (Diflucan), midazolam (Versed), vancomycin (Vancocin).

IV COMPATIBILITIES

DiltiaZEM (Cardizem), HYDROmorphone (Dilaudid), morphine, propofol (Diprivan).

C

INDICATIONS/ROUTES/DOSAGE

Usual Dosage

IV, IM: ADULTS, ELDERLY: 750 mg–1.5 g q8h up to 1.5 g q6h for severe infections. **INFANTS, CHILDREN, ADOLESCENTS: Mild to moderate infection:** 75–100 mg/kg/day divided q8h. **Maximum:** 1,500 mg/dose. **Severe infection:** 100–200 mg/kg/day divided into 3–4 doses. **Maximum:** 1,500 mg/dose. **NEONATES:** 50 mg/kg/dose q8–12h.

PO: ADULTS, ELDERLY: 250–500 mg twice daily **INFANTS, CHILDREN, ADOLESCENTS:** 20–30 mg/kg/day in 2 divided doses. **Maximum:** 1 g/day (500 mg/dose).

Dosage in Renal Impairment

Adult dosage frequency is modified based on creatinine clearance and severity of infection.

Creatinine Clearance	Dosage
IV	
Greater than 20 mL/min	q8h
10–20 mL/min	q12h
Less than 10 mL/min	q24h
Peritoneal dialysis	Dose q24h
Continuous renal replacement therapy	1 g q12h
PO	
Greater than 30 mL/min	No adjustment
10–29 mL/min	q24h
Less than 10 mL/min	q48h

Dosage in Hepatic Impairment

No dose adjustment.

SIDE EFFECTS

Frequent: Discomfort with IM administration, oral candidiasis (thrush), mild diarrhea, mild abdominal cramping, vaginal candidiasis. **Occasional:** Nausea, serum sickness–like reaction (fever, joint pain; usually occurs after second course of therapy and resolves after drug is discontinued). **Rare:** Allergic reaction (rash, pruritus, urticaria), thrombophlebitis (pain, redness, swelling at injection site).

ADVERSE EFFECTS/TOXIC REACTIONS

Antibiotic-associated colitis, other superinfections (abdominal cramps, severe watery diarrhea, fever) may result from altered bacterial balance in GI tract. Nephrotoxicity may occur, esp. in pts with preexisting renal disease. Pts with history of penicillin allergy are at increased risk for developing a severe hypersensitivity reaction (severe pruritus, angioedema, bronchospasm anaphylaxis).

NURSING CONSIDERATIONS

BASELINE ASSESSMENT

Obtain CBC, renal function tests. Question for history of allergies, particularly cephalosporins, penicillins.

INTERVENTION/EVALUATION

Assess oral cavity for white patches on mucous membranes, tongue (thrush). Monitor daily pattern of bowel activity, stool consistency. Mild GI effects may be tolerable (increasing severity may indicate onset of antibiotic-associated colitis). Monitor I&O, renal function tests for nephrotoxicity. Be alert for superinfection: fever, vomiting, diarrhea, anal/genital pruritus, oral mucosal changes (ulceration, pain, erythema).

PATIENT/FAMILY TEACHING

• Discomfort may occur with IM injection. • Doses should be evenly spaced. • Continue antibiotic therapy for full length of treatment. • May cause GI upset (may take with food, milk).

celecoxib

TOP 100

sel-e-**kox**-ib

(CeleBREX)

BLACK BOX ALERT Increased risk of serious cardiovascular thrombotic events, including MI, CVA. Increased risk of severe GI reactions, including ulceration, bleeding, perforation of stomach, intestines.

Do not confuse CeleBREX with CeleXA, Cerebyx, or Clarinex.

◆CLASSIFICATION

PHARMACOTHERAPEUTIC: NSAID, COX-2 selective. **CLINICAL:** Anti-inflammatory.

USES

Relief of signs/symptoms of osteoarthritis, rheumatoid arthritis (RA) in adults. Treatment of acute pain, primary dysmenorrhea. Relief of signs/symptoms associated with ankylosing spondylitis. Treatment of juvenile rheumatoid arthritis (JRA) in pts 2 yrs and older and weighing 10 kg or more.

PRECAUTIONS

◀ALERT▶ May increase cardiovascular risk when high doses are given to prevent colon cancer.

Contraindications: Hypersensitivity to celecoxib, sulfonamides, aspirin, other NSAIDs. Active GI bleeding. Pts experiencing asthma, urticaria, or allergic reactions to aspirin, other NSAIDs. Treatment of perioperative pain in coronary artery bypass graft (CABG) surgery. **Cautions:** History of GI disease (bleeding/ulcers); concurrent use with aspirin, anticoagulants, smoking; alcohol, elderly, debilitated pts, hypertension, asthma, renal/hepatic impairment. Pts with edema, cerebrovascular disease, ischemic heart disease, HF, known or suspected deficiency of cytochrome P450 isoenzyme 2C9. Pediatric pts with systemic-onset juvenile idiopathic arthritis.

ACTION

Inhibits cyclooxygenase-2, the enzyme responsible for prostaglandin synthesis. **Therapeutic Effect:** Reduces inflammation, relieves pain.

PHARMACOKINETICS

Rapidly absorbed from GI tract. Widely distributed. Protein binding: 97%. Metabolized in liver. Primarily eliminated in feces. **Half-life:** 11.2 hrs.

⌛ LIFESPAN CONSIDERATIONS

Pregnancy/Lactation: Unknown if drug crosses placenta or is distributed in breast milk. Avoid use during third trimester (may adversely affect fetal cardiovascular system: premature closure of ductus arteriosus). **Children:** Safety and efficacy not established. **Elderly:** No age-related precautions noted.

INTERACTIONS

DRUG: May increase concentration/effect of **lithium, methotrexate. Aspirin** may increase adverse effects. May increase nephrotoxic effects of **cycloSPORINE, tenofovir. HERBAL: Herbals with anticoagulant/antiplatelet properties (e.g., garlic, ginger, ginkgo biloba)** may increase adverse effects. **FOOD:** None known. **LAB VALUES:** May increase serum ALT, AST, alkaline phosphatase, creatinine, BUN. May decrease serum phosphate.

AVAILABILITY (Rx)

Capsules: 50 mg, 100 mg, 200 mg, 400 mg.

ADMINISTRATION/HANDLING

PO

- May give without regard to food.
- Capsules may be swallowed whole or opened and mixed with applesauce.

INDICATIONS/ROUTES/DOSAGE

Note: Consider reduced initial dose of 50% in poor CYP2C9 metabolizers.

Osteoarthritis

PO: ADULTS, ELDERLY: 200 mg/day as a single dose or 100 mg twice daily.

Rheumatoid Arthritis (RA)

PO: ADULTS, ELDERLY: 100–200 mg twice daily.

Juvenile Rheumatoid Arthritis (JRA)

PO: CHILDREN 2 YRS AND OLDER, WEIGHING MORE THAN 25 KG: 100 mg twice daily. **WEIGHING 10–25 KG:** 50 mg twice daily.

Acute Pain, Primary Dysmenorrhea

PO: ADULTS, ELDERLY: Initially, 400 mg with additional 200 mg on day 1, if needed. **Maintenance:** 200 mg twice daily as needed.

C

Ankylosing Spondylitis

PO: ADULTS, ELDERLY: 200 mg/day as a single dose or in 2 divided doses. May increase to 400 mg/day if no effect is seen after 6 wks.

Dosage in Renal Impairment

Not recommended in severe renal impairment.

Dosage in Hepatic Impairment

Decrease dose by 50% in pts with moderate hepatic impairment. Not recommended in severe hepatic impairment.

SIDE EFFECTS

Frequent (16%–5%): Diarrhea, dyspepsia, headache, upper respiratory tract infection. **Occasional (less than 5%):** Abdominal pain, flatulence, nausea, back pain, peripheral edema, dizziness, insomnia, rash.

ADVERSE EFFECTS/TOXIC REACTIONS

Increased risk of cardiovascular events (MI, CVA), serious, potentially life-threatening GI bleeding.

NURSING CONSIDERATIONS

BASELINE ASSESSMENT

Assess onset, type, location, duration of pain/inflammation. Inspect appearance of affected joints for immobility, deformity, skin condition. Assess for allergy to sulfa, aspirin, or NSAIDs (contraindicated).

INTERVENTION/EVALUATION

Assess for therapeutic response: pain relief; decreased stiffness, swelling; increased joint mobility; reduced joint tenderness; improved grip strength. Observe for bleeding, bruising, weight gain.

PATIENT/FAMILY TEACHING

• If GI upset occurs, take with food. • Avoid aspirin, alcohol (increases risk of GI bleeding). • Immediately report chest pain, jaw pain, sweating, confusion, difficulty speaking, one-sided weakness (may indicate heart attack or stroke).

cenobamate

sen-oh-**bam**-ate

(Xcopri)

Do not confuse cenobamate with carisbamate, felbamate, or meprobamate.

◆Classification

PHARMACOTHERAPEUTIC: Voltage-gated sodium channel inhibitor, gamma-aminobutyric acid ($GABA_A$) modulator. **CLINICAL:** Anticonvulsant.

USES

Treatment of partial-onset (focal) seizures in adults.

PRECAUTIONS

Contraindications: Hypersensitivity to cenobamate. Familial short-QT syndrome. **Cautions:** Hepatic/renal impairment; pts at high risk for suicide ideation and behavior, substance abuse (e.g., history of depression, mood disorder, psychiatric disorder; history of drug abuse). Concomitant use of QT interval–shortening drugs.

ACTION

Inhibits voltage-gated sodium channels, reducing repetitive neuronal firing. Acts as a positive allosteric modulator of the gamma-aminobutyric acid ($GABA_A$) ion channel. **Therapeutic Effect:** Prevents seizure activity.

PHARMACOKINETICS

Widely distributed. Extensively metabolized in liver. Protein binding: 60% (primarily to albumin). Peak plasma concentration: 1-4 hrs. Excreted in urine (88%), feces (5%). **Half-life:** 50-60 hrs.

⌛ LIFESPAN CONSIDERATIONS

Pregnancy/Lactation: Oral contraceptives may become ineffective with therapy. Females of reproductive potential should use additional or alternative nonhormonal contraception during treatment. Unknown if distributed in breast milk. **Children:** Safety and efficacy not established. **Elderly:** Not specified; use caution.

INTERACTIONS

DRUG: **CNS depressants (e.g., alcohol, lorazepam, morphine, zolpidem)** may increase CNS effects. May decrease concentration/effect of **antihepaciviral combination products, avapritinib, axitinib, bosutinib, capmatinib, cobimetinib, neratinib, olaparib, oral contraceptives, ranolazine.** **HERBAL:** **Herbals with sedative properties (e.g., chamomile, kava kava, valerian)** may increase CNS depression. **FOOD:** None known. **LAB VALUES:** May increase serum ALT, AST, potassium.

AVAILABILITY (Rx)

Tablets: 12.5 mg, 25 mg, 50 mg, 100 mg, 150 mg, 200 mg.

ADMINISTRATION/HANDLING

PO

• Give without regard to food. • Tablets cannot be chewed or crushed.

INDICATIONS/ROUTES/DOSAGE

Partial-Onset Seizures

PO: ADULTS: Initially, 12.5 mg once daily on wks 1 and 2, then increase based on clinical response and tolerability. **Titration: Weeks 3 and 4:** 25 mg once daily. **Weeks 5 and 6:** 50 mg once daily. **Weeks 7 and 8:** 100 mg once daily. **Weeks 9 and 10:** 150 mg once daily. **Maintenance dose (week 11 and thereafter):** 200 mg once daily. **Maximum:** May increase dose above 200 mg by increments of 50 mg once daily q2wks up to 400 mg based on clinical response and tolerability. **Discontinuation:** Gradually reduce over a period of 2 wks.

Concomitant Use of Other Medications

Carbamazepine, lamotrigine, CYP2B6 substrates, CYP3A substrates: Because of potential of reduced efficacy, consider increasing dose of carBAMazepine, lamotrigine, CYP2B6 substrates, CYP3A substrates as needed. **Clobazam, phenobarbital, phenytoin, CYP2C19 substrates:** Because of potential of increased concentration/effect, consider reducing dose of clobazam, phenobarbital, phenytoin, CYP2C19 substrates as needed.

Dosage in Renal Impairment

Mild to severe impairment: Use caution. Consider dose reduction. **ESRD, HD:** Not recommended.

Dosage in Hepatic Impairment

Mild to moderate impairment: Maximum dose is 200 mg once daily. **Severe impairment:** Not recommended.

SIDE EFFECTS

Note: Frequency of side effects is dose dependent. **Frequent (22%-14%):** Somnolence, dizziness, fatigue. **Occasional (12%-5%):** Headache, nystagmus, diplopia, nausea, balance disorder. **Rare (4%-1%):** Constipation, vomiting, gait disturbance, tremor, diarrhea, ataxia, dysgeusia, abdominal pain, palpitations, blurry vision, decreased weight, back pain, dyspepsia, dysmenorrhea, memory impairment, decreased appetite, musculoskeletal chest pain, sedation, aphasia, asthenia, dry mouth, pollakiuria, dysarthria, vertigo, hiccups, vertigo, rash.

ADVERSE EFFECTS/TOXIC REACTIONS

Sudden discontinuance may increase risk of seizure frequency, status epilepticus; physical withdrawal symptoms (decreased appetite, depressed mood, insomnia, muscle aches, tremor). Drug reaction with eosinophilia and systemic symptoms (DRESS), also known as multiorgan hypersensitivity, has been reported. DRESS may present with facial swelling, eosinophilia, fever, lymphadenopathy, rash, which may be associated with other organ systems, such as hepatitis, hematologic abnormalities, myocarditis, nephritis. Shortening of QT interval of greater than 20 msec reported in 6%-17% of pts. Pts with familial short QT syndrome have an increased risk of sudden death, ventricular fibrillation. May increase risk of suicidal behavior and ideation. Other psychological disorders may include confusion, euphoria, irritability. Increased incidence of appendicitis was reported. Infections including nasopharyngitis (4% of pts), pharyngitis, (2% of pts), UTI (5% of pts) have occurred.

C

NURSING CONSIDERATIONS

BASELINE ASSESSMENT

Review history of seizure disorder (intensity, frequency, duration). Initiate seizure precautions, fall precautions. Question history of familial short-QT syndrome, hepatic/renal impairment. Question history of anxiety, depression, mood disorder, suicidal ideation and behavior. Obtain pregnancy test in females of reproductive potential. Assess for potential of abuse/misuse (e.g., drug seeking behavior, mental health conditions, history of substance abuse). Receive full medication history and screen for interactions.

INTERVENTION/EVALUATION

Observe for recurrence of seizure activity. Assess for clinical improvement (decrease in intensity, frequency of seizures). Monitor for CNS effects during titration or discontinuation. Monitor for symptoms of DRESS; cardiac effects (palpitations, syncope), esp. during titration. Diligently assess for suicidal ideation and behavior; new onset or worsening of anxiety, depression, mood disorder. Consult mental health professional if mood disorder suspected.

PATIENT/FAMILY TEACHING

• Strict maintenance of drug therapy is essential for seizure control. • Avoid tasks that require alertness, motor skills until response to drug is established. • Do not abruptly discontinue medication (may cause seizures; symptoms of withdrawal syndrome). • Treatment may affect the electrical properties of the heart; report palpitations, loss of consciousness. • Seek immediate medical attention if thoughts of suicide or new onset or worsening of anxiety, depression, or changes in mood occur. • Avoid alcohol, nervous system depressants. • Report symptoms of drug-induced hypersensitivity syndrome (e.g., fever, swollen face/lymph nodes, skin rash/peeling/inflammation). • There is a high risk of interactions with other medications. Do not take newly prescribed medications unless approved by prescriber who originally started therapy. • Oral contraceptives may become ineffective. Additional or alternative contraceptive measures are recommended.

cephalexin

sef-a-**lex**-in
(Keflex)
Do not confuse cephalexin with cefaclor, ceFAZolin, or ciprofloxacin.

◆CLASSIFICATION

PHARMACOTHERAPEUTIC: First-generation cephalosporin. **CLINICAL:** Antibiotic.

USES

Treatment of susceptible infections due to staphylococci, group A *streptococcus, K. pneumoniae, E. coli, P. mirabilis, H. influenzae, M. catarrhalis,* including respiratory tract, genitourinary tract, skin, soft tissue, bone infections; otitis media; follow-up to parenteral therapy. **OFF-LABEL:** Suppression of prosthetic joint infection.

PRECAUTIONS

Contraindications: History of hypersensitivity/anaphylactic reaction to cephalexin, cephalosporins. **Cautions:** Renal impairment, history of GI disease (esp. ulcerative colitis, antibiotic-associated colitis), history of penicillin allergy.

ACTION

Binds to bacterial cell membranes, inhibits cell wall synthesis. **Therapeutic Effect:** Bactericidal.

PHARMACOKINETICS

Rapidly absorbed from GI tract (delayed in young children). Protein binding: 10%–15%. Widely distributed. Primarily excreted unchanged in urine. Moderately removed by hemodialysis. **Half-life:** 0.9–1.2 hrs (increased in renal impairment).

LIFESPAN CONSIDERATIONS

Pregnancy/Lactation: Readily crosses placenta. Distributed in breast milk. **Children:** No age-related precautions noted. **Elderly:** Age-related renal impairment may require dosage adjustment.

INTERACTIONS

DRUG: **Probenecid** may increase concentration/effect. **HERBAL:** None significant. **FOOD:** None known. **LAB VALUES:** May increase serum BUN, creatinine, alkaline phosphatase, bilirubin, LDH, ALT, AST. May cause positive direct/indirect Coombs' test.

AVAILABILITY (Rx)

Capsules: 250 mg, 500 mg, 750 mg. **Powder for Oral Suspension:** 125 mg/5 mL, 250 mg/5 mL. **Tablets:** 250 mg, 500 mg.

ADMINISTRATION/HANDLING

PO

• After reconstitution, oral suspension is stable for 14 days if refrigerated. • Shake oral suspension well before using. • Give without regard to food. If GI upset occurs, give with food, milk.

INDICATIONS/ROUTES/DOSAGE

Usual Dosage Range

PO: ADULTS, ELDERLY: 250–1,000 mg q6h or 500 mg q12h. **Maximum:** 4 g/day. **INFANTS, CHILDREN, ADOLESCENTS: (Mild to moderate infections):** 25–50 mg/kg/day divided q6–12h. **Maximum:** 2 g/day. **(Severe infections):** 75–100 mg/kg/day. **Maximum:** 4 g/day.

Dosage in Renal Impairment

After usual initial dose, dosing frequency is modified based on creatinine clearance and severity of infection.

Creatinine Clearance	Dosage
60 mL/min or greater	No adjustment
30–59 mL/min	Maximum: 1,000 mg/day
15–29 mL/min	250 mg q8-12h
5–14 mL/min	250 mg q24h
1–4 mL/min	250 mg q48-60h
Hemodialysis	250–500 mg q12–24h (administer after dialysis session)

Dosage in Hepatic Impairment

No dose adjustment.

SIDE EFFECTS

Frequent: Oral candidiasis, mild diarrhea, mild abdominal cramping, vaginal candidiasis. **Occasional:** Nausea, serum sickness–like reaction (fever, joint pain; usually occurs after second course of therapy and resolves after drug is discontinued). **Rare:** Allergic reaction (rash, pruritus, urticaria).

ADVERSE EFFECTS/TOXIC REACTIONS

Antibiotic-associated colitis, other superinfections (abdominal cramps, severe watery diarrhea, fever) may result from altered bacterial balance in GI tract. Nephrotoxicity may occur, esp. in pts with preexisting renal disease. Pts with history of penicillin allergy are at increased risk for developing a severe hypersensitivity reaction (severe pruritus, angioedema, bronchospasm, anaphylaxis).

NURSING CONSIDERATIONS

BASELINE ASSESSMENT

Obtain CBC, renal function tests. Question for history of allergies, particularly cephalosporins, penicillins.

INTERVENTION/EVALUATION

Assess oral cavity for white patches on mucous membranes, tongue (thrush). Monitor daily pattern of bowel activity, stool consistency. Mild GI effects may be tolerable (increasing severity may indicate onset of antibiotic-associated colitis). Monitor I&O, renal function tests for nephrotoxicity. Be alert for superinfection: fever, vomiting, diarrhea, anal/genital pruritus, oral mucosal changes (ulceration, pain, erythema). With prolonged therapy, monitor renal/hepatic function tests.

PATIENT/FAMILY TEACHING

• Doses should be evenly spaced. • Continue therapy for full length of treatment. • May cause GI upset (may take with food, milk). • Refrigerate oral suspension. • Report persistent diarrhea.

ceritinib

se-**ri**-ti-nib
(Zykadia)
Do not confuse ceritinib with crizotinib, gefitinib, imatinib, or lapatinib.

◆CLASSIFICATION

PHARMACOTHERAPEUTIC: Anaplastic lymphoma kinase inhibitor. **CLINICAL:** Antineoplastic.

USES

Treatment of pts with anaplastic lymphoma kinase (ALK)–positive metastatic non–small-cell lung cancer (NSCLC).

PRECAUTIONS

Contraindications: Hypersensitivity to ceritinib. **Cautions:** Bradyarrhythmias/ventricular arrhythmias, diabetes, dehydration, electrolyte imbalance (e.g., hypomagnesemia, hypokalemia), hepatic impairment, HF, ocular disease, pulmonary disease. Medications that prolong QT interval. Not recommended in pts with congenital long QT syndrome. Avoid use of medications that cause bradycardia.

ACTION

Potent inhibitor of ALK involved in the pathogenesis of NSCLC. ALK gene abnormalities may result in expression of oncogenic fusion proteins, resulting in increased cell proliferation/survival in tumor cells. **Therapeutic Effect:** Reduces proliferation of tumor cells expressing the genetic abnormality.

PHARMACOKINETICS

Well absorbed after PO administration. Metabolized in liver. Peak plasma concentration: 4–6 hrs. Protein binding: 97%. Eliminated in feces (92%), urine (1.3%). **Half-life:** 41 hrs.

⌛ LIFESPAN CONSIDERATIONS

Pregnancy/Lactation: Avoid pregnancy; may cause fetal harm. Contraception recommended during treatment and for at least 2 wks after discontinuation. Unknown if distributed in breast milk. **Children:** Safety and efficacy not established. **Elderly:** No age-related precautions noted.

INTERACTIONS

DRUG: Strong CYP3A4 inhibitors (e.g., clarithromycin, ketoconazole, ritonavir) may increase concentration/effect; avoid use. **Strong CYP3A4 inducers (e.g., carBAMazepine, phenytoin, rifAMPin)** may decrease concentration/effect; avoid use. **QT interval-prolonging medications (e.g., amiodarone, azithromycin, haloperidol, moxifloxacin)** may increase risk of QT interval prolongation, cardiac arrhythmias. **Amiodarone, dronedarone** may increase risk of bradycardia. May increase concentration/effects of **aprepitant, bosutinib, budesonide, cobimetinib, colchicine, eletriptan, ivabradine. HERBAL: St. John's wort** may decrease effectiveness. **FOOD: All food** may increase absorption/effect. **Grapefruit products** may increase concentration/effect; avoid use. **LAB VALUES:** May decrease Hgb, phosphate. May increase serum ALT, AST, bilirubin, creatinine, glucose, lipase.

AVAILABILITY (Rx)

Tablets: 150 mg.

ADMINISTRATION/HANDLING

PO

• Give with food. • Administer whole; do not break, cut, or open. • If a dose is missed, take dose unless next dose due within 12 hrs. If vomiting occurs, do not administer an additional dose.

INDICATIONS/ROUTES/DOSAGE

Non–Small-Cell Lung Cancer

PO: ADULTS/ELDERLY: 450 mg once daily until disease progression or unacceptable toxicity.

Dosage in Renal Impairment

Mild to moderate impairment: CrCl 30–90 mL/min: No dose adjustment. **Severe impairment:** Not specified; use caution.

Dosage in Hepatic Impairment

Mild to moderate impairment: No dose adjustment. **Severe impairment:** Decrease dose by 1/3 (round to nearest 150 mg).

Dose Modification

Cardiotoxicity

QTc interval greater than 500 msec on at least 2 separate ECGs: Withhold until QTc interval is less than 481 msec, or recovery to baseline (if baseline QTc interval is greater than or equal to 481 msec), then resume with a 150-mg dose reduction.

QTc prolongation in combination with torsades de pointes or polymorphic ventricular tachycardia or serious arrhythmia: Permanently discontinue.

Symptomatic, non–life-threatening bradycardia: Withhold until recovery to asymptomatic bradycardia or heart rate of 60 beats/min or greater. Evaluate concomitant medications known to cause bradycardia and adjust dose as tolerated (reduction not specified).

Clinically significant, life-threatening bradycardia requiring intervention or life-threatening bradycardia in pts taking concomitant medications known to cause bradycardia or hypotension: Withhold until recovery to asymptomatic bradycardia or heart rate of 60 beats/min or greater. If concomitant medication can be adjusted or discontinued, then resume with a 150-mg dose reduction.

Life-threatening bradycardia in pts who are not taking concomitant medications known to cause bradycardia or hypotension: Permanently discontinue.

Concomitant use of strong CYP3A inhibitors: If concomitant use unavoidable, reduce ceritinib dose by one third, rounded to the nearest 150-mg dose strength. After discontinuation of a strong CYP3A inhibitor, resume ceritinib dose that was taken prior to initiating strong CYP3A inhibitor.

Gastrointestinal Toxicity

Severe or intolerable diarrhea, nausea, vomiting despite optimal antiemetic or antidiarrheal therapy: Withhold until improved, then resume with a 150-mg dose reduction.

Hepatotoxicity

ALT, AST greater than 5 times upper limit of normal (ULN) with total bilirubin elevation less than or equal to 2 times ULN: Withhold until recovery to baseline or less than or equal to 2 times ULN, then resume with a 150-mg dose reduction.

ALT, AST greater than 3 times ULN with total bilirubin elevation greater than or equal to 2 times ULN in the absence of cholestasis or hemolysis: Permanently discontinue.

Hyperglycemia

Persistent hyperglycemia greater than 250 mL/dL despite optimal antihyperglycemic therapy: Withhold until hyperglycemia is adequately controlled, then resume with a 150-mg dose reduction. If adequate control cannot be achieved with optimal medical management, then permanently discontinue.

Pulmonary Toxicity

Any grade treatment related to interstitial lung disease/pneumonitis: Permanently discontinue.

Intolerability/Toxicity

If unable to tolerate 300-mg dose: Permanently discontinue.

SIDE EFFECTS

Frequent (86%–52%): Diarrhea, nausea, vomiting, abdominal pain, fatigue, asthenia. **Occasional (34%–9%):** Decreased appetite, constipation, paresthesia, muscular weakness, gait disturbance, peripheral motor/sensory neuropathy, hypotonia, polyneuropathy, dyspepsia, gastric reflux disease, dysphagia, rash, maculopapular rash, acneiform dermatitis, vision impairment, blurred vision, photopsia, presbyopia, reduced visual acuity.

ADVERSE EFFECTS/TOXIC REACTIONS

Approximately 60% of pts required at least one dose reduction. Median time to first dose reduction was approximately 7 wks. Decreased Hgb levels reported in 84% of pts. Severe or persistent GI toxicity including nausea, vomiting, diarrhea occurred in 96% of pts; severe cases reported in 14% of pts. Drug-induced hepatotoxicity with elevation of serum ALT 5 times ULN occurred in 27% of pts. Bradycardia, severe interstitial lung disease (ILD), QT interval prolongation, ILD reported in 3% of pts. Grade 3–4 hyperglycemia reported in 13% of pts; diabetics have a sixfold increase in risk; pts receiving corticosteroids have twofold increase in risk. Fatal adverse reactions including pneumonia, respiratory failure, ILD/pneumonitis, pneumothorax, gastric hemorrhage, general physical health deterioration, tuberculosis, cardiac tamponade, sepsis occurred in 5% of pts.

NURSING CONSIDERATIONS

BASELINE ASSESSMENT

Obtain baseline CBC, BMP, LFT; capillary blood glucose, O_2 saturation, urine pregnancy, vital signs. Obtain baseline ECG in pts with history of arrhythmias, HF, electrolyte imbalance, or concurrent use of medications known to prolong QTc interval. Question possibility of pregnancy or plans of breastfeeding. Assess hydration status. Screen for history/comorbidities. Receive full medication history including herbal products, esp. CYP3A inhibitors or inducers, medications that prolong QT interval. Assess visual acuity. Verify ALK-positive NSCLC test prior to initiation.

INTERVENTION/EVALUATION

Monitor CBC routinely; LFT monthly (or more frequently in pts with elevated hepatic enzymes). Obtain BMP, serum ionized calcium, magnesium if arrhythmia or dehydration occurs. Monitor vital signs (esp. heart rate). Obtain ECG for bradycardia, chest pain, dyspnea; chest X-ray if ILD, pneumonitis, pneumothorax suspected. Worsening cough, fever, or shortness of breath may indicate pneumonitis. Monitor for hepatic dysfunction, hyperglycemia, sepsis, vision changes. Assess hydration status. Encourage PO intake. Offer antidiarrheal medication for loose stool, antiemetic for nausea, vomiting.

PATIENT/FAMILY TEACHING

• Most pts experience diarrhea, nausea, vomiting, which may lead to dehydration; drink plenty of fluids. • Report history of heart problems, including extremity swelling, HF, congenital long QT syndrome, palpitations, syncope. Therapy may decrease your heart rate; report dizziness, chest pain, palpitations, or fainting. • Worsening cough, fever, or shortness of breath may indicate severe lung inflammation. • Avoid pregnancy; contraception recommended during treatment and up to 2 wks after final dose. Do not breastfeed. • Blurry vision, confusion, frequent urination, increased thirst, fruity breath may indicate high blood sugar levels. • Report any yellowing of skin or eyes, upper abdominal pain, bruising, black/tarry stools, dark urine. • Immediately report any newly prescribed medications. • Take on empty stomach only; do not eat 2 hrs before or 2 hrs after any dose. • Avoid alcohol. Do not consume grapefruit products.

C

certolizumab pegol

ser-toe-**liz**-ue-mab
(Cimzia)

BLACK BOX ALERT Serious, sometimes fatal cases of tuberculosis, invasive fungal infections, or other opportunistic infections, including viral and bacterial infection, have been reported. Lymphoma reported in children/adolescents receiving other TNF-blocking medications.

◆CLASSIFICATION

PHARMACOTHERAPEUTIC: Antirheumatic, disease modifying. GI agent. Tumor necrosis factor (TNF) blocker. **CLINICAL:** Anti-inflammatory agent.

USES

Treatment of moderate to severe active rheumatoid arthritis, moderate to severe active Crohn's disease, active ankylosing spondylitis, active psoriatic arthritis, moderate to severe plaque psoriasis, axial spondyloarthritis, nonradiographic.

PRECAUTIONS

Contraindications: Hypersensitivity to certolizumab. **Cautions:** Chronic, latent, or localized infection; preexisting or recent-onset CNS demyelinating disorders, moderate to severe HF, underlying hematologic disorders, elderly. Pts who have resided in regions where TB is endemic, pts who are hepatitis B virus carriers. Use of live vaccines.

ACTION

Binds to and neutralizes human TNF-alpha activity. Elevated levels of TNF-alpha play a role in inflammation (Crohn's disease) and joint destruction (RA). **Therapeutic Effect:** Reduces signs and symptoms of Crohn's disease and joint destruction associated with rheumatoid arthritis.

PHARMACOKINETICS

Higher clearance with increasing body weight. Peak plasma concentrations: 54–171 hrs. **Half-life:** 14 days.

⌛ LIFESPAN CONSIDERATIONS

Pregnancy/Lactation: Unknown if distributed in breast milk. **Children:** Safety and efficacy not established. **Elderly:** Use cautiously due to higher risk of infection.

INTERACTIONS

DRUG: May increase adverse effects of **abatacept, anakinra, canakinumab, natalizumab, vaccines (live), vedolizumab.** May decrease therapeutic effects of **BCG (intravesical), vaccines (live). HERBAL: Echinacea** may decrease therapeutic effect. **FOOD:** None known. **LAB VALUES:** May increase serum alkaline phosphatase, ALT, AST, bilirubin; aPTT.

AVAILABILITY (Rx)

Injection, Powder for Reconstitution: 200 mg. **Injection, Solution:** 200 mg/mL in a single-use prefilled syringe.

ADMINISTRATION/HANDLING

SQ

Reconstitution • Bring to room temperature before reconstitution. • Reconstitute with 1 mL Sterile Water for Injection. • Gently swirl without shaking, using syringe with 20-gauge needle. • Leave undisturbed to fully reconstitute (may take as long as 30 min). • Using a new 20-gauge needle, withdraw reconstituted solution into syringe for final concentration of 1 mL (200 mg). Use separate syringes for multiple vials. • Switch each 20-gauge needle to a 23-gauge needle and inject full contents of each syringe subcutaneously into separate sites on the abdomen or thigh.

Storage • Store vial in refrigerator. • Once powder reconstituted, solution should appear clear to opalescent, colorless to pale yellow. • Discard if solution is discolored or contains precipitate. • Reconstituted solution is stable for up to 2 hrs at room temperature or 24 hrs if refrigerated.

C

INDICATIONS/ROUTES/DOSAGE

Note: Each 400-mg dose is given as two injections of 200 mg each.

Crohn's Disease

SQ: Initially, 400 mg (given as two subcutaneous injections of 200 mg) and at weeks 2 and 4. **Maintenance:** In pts who obtain a therapeutic response, 400 mg q4wks.

Rheumatoid Arthritis, Ankylosing Spondylitis, Psoriatic Arthritis

SQ: ADULTS, ELDERLY: Initially, 400 mg and at weeks 2 and 4. **Maintenance:** 200 mg q2wks or 400 mg q4wks.

Plaque Psoriasis

SQ: ADULTS, ELDERLY: 400 mg every other week. **PTS WEIGHING 90 KG OR LESS:** 400 mg at wks 0, 2, and 4, then 200 mg q every other wk may be used.

Axial Spondyloarthritis, Nonradiographic

SQ: ADULTS, ELDERLY: Initially, 400 mg, repeat dose 2 and 4 wks after initial dose. **Maintenance:** 200 mg q2wks or 400 mg q4wks.

Dosage Modification

Discontinue for hypersensitivity reaction, lupus-like syndrome, serious infection, sepsis, hepatitis B virus reactivation.

Dosage in Renal/Hepatic Impairment

No dose adjustment.

SIDE EFFECTS

Occasional (6%): Arthralgia. **Rare (less than 1%):** Abdominal pain, diarrhea.

ADVERSE EFFECTS/TOXIC REACTIONS

Upper respiratory tract infection occurs in 20% of pts. UTI occurs in 7% of pts. Serious infections such as pneumonia, pyelonephritis occur in 3% of pts. Hypersensitivity reaction (rash, urticaria, hypotension, dyspnea) occurs rarely. May increase risk of malignancies (e.g., lymphoma).

NURSING CONSIDERATIONS

BASELINE ASSESSMENT

Obtain baseline CBC, urinalysis, C-reactive protein. Do not initiate treatment in pts with active infections, including chronic or localized infection. TB test should be obtained before initiation.

INTERVENTION/EVALUATION

Monitor pts for infection during and after treatment. If pt develops an infection, treatment should be discontinued. Monitor lab results, especially WBC count, urinalysis, C-reactive protein for evidence of infection.

PATIENT/FAMILY TEACHING

• Report cough, fever, flu-like symptoms. • Do not receive live virus vaccine during treatment or within 3 mos after last dose.

cetirizine

se-**teer**-i-zeen
(Apo-Cetirizine 🍁, Quzyttir, Reactine 🍁, Zerviate, ZyrTEC ALLERGY)
Do not confuse cetirizine with levocetirizine, or ZyrTEC with Xanax, Zantac, Zocor, or ZyPREXA.

FIXED-COMBINATION(S)

ZyrTEC D 12 Hour Tablets: cetirizine/pseudoephedrine: 5 mg/120 mg.

◆CLASSIFICATION

PHARMACOTHERAPEUTIC: Histamine H_1 antagonist (second generation). **CLINICAL:** Antihistamine.

USES

Relief of symptoms (sneezing, rhinorrhea, postnasal discharge, nasal pruritus, ocular pruritus, tearing) of upper respiratory allergies; relieves itching due to urticaria. **Quzyttir:** Treatment of acute urticaria. **Zerviate:** Treatment of ocular itching associated with allergic conjunctivitis.

PRECAUTIONS

Contraindications: Hypersensitivity to cetirizine, hydrOXYzine. **Cautions:** Elderly, hepatic/renal impairment.

ACTION

Competes with histamine for H_1-receptor sites on effector cells in GI tract, blood vessels, respiratory tract. **Therapeutic Effect:** Prevents allergic response, produces mild bronchodilation, blocks histamine-induced bronchitis.

PHARMACOKINETICS

Route	Onset	Peak	Duration
PO	Less than 1 hr	4–8 hrs	Less than 24 hrs

Well absorbed from GI tract. Protein binding: 93%. Undergoes low first-pass metabolism; not extensively metabolized. Primarily excreted in urine. **Half-life:** 6.5–10 hrs.

LIFESPAN CONSIDERATIONS

Pregnancy/Lactation: Not recommended during first trimester of pregnancy. Distributed in breast milk. Breastfeeding not recommended. **Children:** Less likely to cause anticholinergic effects. **Elderly:** More sensitive to anticholinergic effects (e.g., dry mouth, urinary retention). Dizziness, sedation, confusion may occur.

INTERACTIONS

DRUG: **Alcohol, CNS depressants (e.g., LORazepam, morphine, zolpidem)** may increase CNS depression. **Anticholinergics (e.g., aclidinium, ipratropium, umeclidinium)** may increase anticholinergic effect. **HERBAL:** **Herbs with sedative properties (e.g., chamomile, kava kava, valerian)** may increase CNS depression. **FOOD:** None known. **LAB VALUES:** May suppress wheal and flare reactions to antigen skin testing unless drug is discontinued 4 days before testing.

AVAILABILITY (Rx)

Capsules: 10 mg. **Injection:** 10 mg/mL. **Ophthalmic:** 0.24%. **Oral Solution:** 5 mg/5 mL. **Tablets:** 5 mg, 10 mg. **Tablets (Chewable):** 5 mg, 10 mg. **Tablets (Dispersible):** 10 mg.

ADMINISTRATION/HANDLING

PO

- Give without regard to food.

IV

- Administer IV push over 1–2 min.

Ophthalmic

- Remove contact lenses before administration (wait at least 10 min before inserting contact lenses). • Use immediately after opening. Wash hands; do not touch dropper tip to eyelids.

INDICATIONS/ROUTES/DOSAGE

◀ALERT▶ May cause drowsiness at dosage greater than 10 mg/day.

Upper Respiratory Allergies, Urticaria

PO: ADULTS, CHILDREN OLDER THAN 5 YRS: Initially, 5–10 mg/day as single dose. **Maximum:** 10 mg/day. **ELDERLY:** 5 mg once daily. **Maximum:** 5 mg/day. **CHILDREN 2–5 YRS:** 2.5 mg/day. May increase up to 5 mg/day as a single dose or in 2 divided doses. **CHILDREN 12–23 MOS:** Initially, 2.5 mg/day. May increase up to 5 mg/day in 2 divided doses. **CHILDREN 6–11 MOS:** 2.5 mg once daily.

Acute Urticaria

IV: ADULTS, ELDERLY: Initially, 10 mg once daily. May increase to 10 mg twice daily. **CHILDREN 12 YRS AND OLDER, ADOLESCENTS:** 10 mg q24h. **CHILDREN 6–11 YRS:** 5–10 mg q24h. **CHILDREN 6 MOS TO 5 YRS:** 2.5 mg q24h.

Allergic Conjunctivitis

OPHTH: ADULTS, ELDERLY, ADOLESCENTS, CHILDREN 2 YRS AND OLDER: Instill 1 drop in affected eye twice daily (about 8 hrs apart).

Dosage in Renal Impairment

ADULTS: GFR 50 mL/min or less: 5 mg once daily. **CHILDREN:** GFR 10–29 mL/min: reduce dose by 50 %. GFR <10 mL/min: Not recommended.

C

Dosage in Hepatic Impairment
No dose adjustment.

SIDE EFFECTS

Occasional (10%–2%): Pharyngitis, dry mucous membranes, nausea, vomiting, abdominal pain, headache, dizziness, fatigue, thickening of mucus, drowsiness, photosensitivity, urinary retention.

ADVERSE EFFECTS/TOXIC REACTIONS

Children may experience paradoxical reaction (restlessness, insomnia, euphoria, nervousness, tremor). Dizziness, sedation, confusion more likely to occur in elderly.

NURSING CONSIDERATIONS

BASELINE ASSESSMENT

Assess lung sounds. Assess severity of rhinitis, urticaria, other symptoms.

INTERVENTION/EVALUATION

For upper respiratory allergies, increase fluids to maintain thin secretions and offset thirst. Monitor symptoms for therapeutic response.

PATIENT/FAMILY TEACHING

• Avoid tasks that require alertness, motor skills until response to drug is established. • Avoid alcohol.

cetuximab

HIGH ALERT

se-**tux**-i-mab
(Erbitux)

■ BLACK BOX ALERT ■ Severe infusion reactions (bronchospasm, stridor, urticaria, hypotension, cardiac arrest) have occurred, especially with first infusion in pts with head and neck cancer. Cardiopulmonary arrest reported in pts receiving radiation in combination with cetuximab.

Do not confuse cetuximab with bevacizumab.

◆CLASSIFICATION

PHARMACOTHERAPEUTIC: Epidermal growth factor receptor (EGFR) inhibitor, monoclonal antibody. **CLINICAL:** Antineoplastic.

USES

Colorectal cancer, metastatic: Treatment of KRAS wild type, EGFR-expressing, metastatic colorectal cancer as first-line treatment (in combination with FOLFIRI [irinotecan, fluorouracil, and leucovorin]); in combination with irinotecan in pts refractory or intolerant to irinotecan-based chemotherapy; or as a single agent in pts who failed irinotecan- and oxaliplatin-based chemotherapy or who are intolerant to irinotecan. **Head and neck cancer, squamous cell:** Treatment of advanced squamous cell cancer of head/neck (with radiation). Treatment of recurrent or metastasized squamous cell carcinoma of head/neck progressing after platinum-based therapy. First-line treatment of squamous cell carcinoma of head and neck in combination with platinum-based therapy with 5-FU. **OFF-LABEL:** EGFR-expressing advanced non–small-cell lung cancer (NSCLC). Treatment of unresectable squamous cell skin cancer.

PRECAUTIONS

Contraindications: Hypersensitivity to cetuximab. **Cautions:** Preexisting IgE antibodies to cetuximab, coronary artery disease, HF, arrhythmias, pulmonary disease.

ACTION

Specifically binds to and inhibits epidermal growth factor receptor (EGFR), blocking phosphorylation/activation of receptor-associated kinases. **Therapeutic Effect:** Inhibits tumor cell growth, inducing apoptosis (cell death).

PHARMACOKINETICS

Reaches steady-state levels by the third wkly infusion. Clearance decreases as dose increases. **Half-life:** 114 hrs (range: 75–188 hrs).

⌛ LIFESPAN CONSIDERATIONS

Pregnancy/Lactation: Crosses placental barrier; may cause fetal harm;

abortifacient. Breastfeeding not recommended. **Children:** Safety and efficacy not established. **Elderly:** No age-related precautions noted.

INTERACTIONS

DRUG: None significant. **HERBAL:** None significant. **FOOD:** None known. **LAB VALUES:** May decrease WBCs; serum calcium, magnesium, potassium.

AVAILABILITY (Rx)

Injection Solution: 2 mg/mL (50 mL, 100 mL).

ADMINISTRATION/HANDLING

IV

◀ALERT▶ Do not give by IV push or bolus.

Reconstitution • Does not require reconstitution. • Solution should appear clear, colorless; may contain a small amount of visible, white particulates. • Do not shake or dilute. • Infuse with a low protein-binding 0.22-micron in-line filter.

Rate of administration • First dose should be given as a 120-min infusion. • Maintenance infusion should be infused over 60 min. • Maximum infusion rate should not exceed 5 mL/min.

Storage • Refrigerate vials. • Infusion containers are stable for up to 12 hrs if refrigerated, up to 8 hrs at room temperature. • Discard unused portions.

IV COMPATIBILITIES

Irinotecan (Camptosar).

INDICATIONS/ROUTES/DOSAGE

Head/Neck Cancer, Metastatic Colorectal Cancer

IV: ADULTS, ELDERLY: Initially, 400 mg/m^2 as a loading dose. **Maintenance:** 250 mg/m^2 infused over 60 min wkly. Continue until disease progression or unacceptable toxicity.

Dosage in Renal/Hepatic Impairment

No dose adjustment.

SIDE EFFECTS

Frequent (90%–25%): Acneiform rash, malaise, fever, nausea, diarrhea, constipation, headache, abdominal pain, anorexia, vomiting. **Occasional (16%–10%):** Nail disorder, back pain, stomatitis, peripheral edema, pruritus, cough, insomnia. **Rare (9%–5%):** Weight loss, depression, dyspepsia, conjunctivitis, alopecia.

ADVERSE EFFECTS/TOXIC REACTIONS

Anemia occurs in 10% of pts. Severe infusion reaction (rapid onset of airway obstruction, hypotension, severe urticaria) occurs rarely. Dermatologic toxicity, pulmonary embolus, leukopenia, renal failure occur rarely.

NURSING CONSIDERATIONS

BASELINE ASSESSMENT

Monitor Hgb, Hct, serum potassium, magnesium. Assess for evidence of anemia. Question possibility of pregnancy. Question history of hypersensitivity reaction.

INTERVENTION/EVALUATION

Monitor for evidence of infusion reaction (rapid onset of bronchospasm, stridor, hoarseness, urticaria, hypotension) during infusion and for at least 1 hr postinfusion. Pts may experience first severe infusion reaction during later infusions. Assess skin for evidence of dermatologic toxicity (development of inflammatory sequelae, dry skin, exfoliative dermatitis, rash). Monitor CBC, serum electrolytes, acute onset or worsening pulmonary symptoms.

PATIENT/FAMILY TEACHING

• Do not have immunizations without physician's approval (drug lowers resistance). • Avoid contact with anyone who recently received a live virus vaccine. • Avoid crowds, those with infection. • Wear sunscreen, limit sun exposure (sunlight can exacerbate skin reactions). • Avoid pregnancy. • Report cardiac or lung symptoms, severe rash.

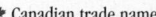

C

chlorambucil

HIGH ALERT

klor-**am**-bue-sil
(Leukeran)

■ BLACK BOX ALERT ■ May cause myelosuppression. Affects fertility; potential for carcinogenic, mutagenic, teratogenic effects. May cause azoospermia.

Do not confuse Leukeran with Alkeran, Leukine, or Myleran.

◆CLASSIFICATION

PHARMACOTHERAPEUTIC: Alkylating agent, nitrogen mustard. **CLINICAL:** Antineoplastic.

USES

Treatment of chronic lymphocytic leukemia (CLL), Hodgkin's and non-Hodgkin's lymphomas (NHL). **OFF-LABEL:** Nephrotic syndrome in children, Waldenström's macroglobulinemia.

PRECAUTIONS

Contraindications: Hypersensitivity to chlorambucil. Previous allergic reaction to other alkylating agents, prior resistance to chlorambucil, pregnancy. **Extreme Cautions:** Treatment within 4 wks after full-course radiation therapy or myelosuppressive drug regimen. **Cautions:** History of bone marrow suppression, head trauma, hepatic impairment, nephrotic syndrome, seizure disorder; administration of live vaccines to immunocompromised pts.

ACTION

Inhibits DNA, RNA synthesis by cross-linking with DNA strands. **Therapeutic Effect:** Interferes with DNA replication and RNA transcription.

PHARMACOKINETICS

Rapidly, completely absorbed from GI tract. Protein binding: 99%. Metabolized in liver to active metabolite. Not removed by hemodialysis. **Half-life:** 1.5 hrs; metabolite, 2.5 hrs.

LIFESPAN CONSIDERATIONS

Pregnancy/Lactation: If possible, avoid use during pregnancy, esp. first trimester. Breastfeeding not recommended. **Children:** No age-related precautions noted. When taken for nephrotic syndrome, may increase risk of seizures. **Elderly:** No age-related precautions noted.

INTERACTIONS

DRUG: May decrease therapeutic effect of **BCG (intravesical), vaccines (live).** May increase adverse effects of **vaccines (live).** May increase myelosuppressive effect of **myelosuppressants (e.g., cladribine). HERBAL: Echinacea** may decrease therapeutic effect. **FOOD: Acidic foods, spicy foods** may delay absorption. **LAB VALUES:** May increase serum alkaline phosphatase, AST, uric acid.

AVAILABILITY (Rx)

Tablets: 2 mg.

ADMINISTRATION/HANDLING

PO

- Give 30–60 min before food.

INDICATIONS/ROUTES/DOSAGE

Chronic Lymphocytic Leukemia (CLL)

PO: ADULTS, ELDERLY: 0.1 mg/kg/day for 3–6 wks or 0.4 mg/kg pulsed doses administered intermittently, biweekly or monthly (increased by 0.1 mg/kg/dose until response/toxicity observed).

Hodgkin's Lymphoma (HL)

PO: ADULTS, ELDERLY, ADOLESCENTS, CHILDREN, INFANTS 7 MOS OR OLDER: 6 mg/m^2 once daily (maximum: 10 mg) on days 1–14 of 28-day cycle for 6–10 cycles.

Non-Hodgkin's Lymphoma (NHL)

PO: ADULTS, ELDERLY: 0.1 mg/kg/day for 3–6 wks.

Dosage in Renal Impairment

CrCl 10–50 mL/min: 75% of dose. **CrCl less than 10 mL/min:** 50% of dose.

C

Dosage in Hepatic Impairment
Use caution.

SIDE EFFECTS

Expected: GI effects (nausea, vomiting, anorexia, diarrhea, abdominal distress), generally mild, last less than 24 hrs, occur only if single dose exceeds 20 mg. **Occasional:** Rash, dermatitis, pruritus, oral ulcerations. **Rare:** Alopecia, urticaria, erythema, hyperuricemia.

ADVERSE EFFECTS/TOXIC REACTIONS

Hematologic toxicity due to severe myelosuppression occurs frequently, manifested as neutropenia, anemia, thrombocytopenia. After discontinuation of therapy, thrombocytopenia, neutropenia usually last for 1–2 wks, but may persist for 3–4 wks. Neutrophil count may continue to decrease for up to 10 days after last dose. Toxicity appears to be less severe with intermittent drug administration. Overdosage may produce seizures in children. Excessive serum uric acid level, hepatotoxicity occur rarely.

NURSING CONSIDERATIONS

BASELINE ASSESSMENT

Obtain CBC before therapy and wkly during therapy, WBC count 3–4 days following each wkly, CBC during first 3–6 wks of therapy (4–6 wks if pt on intermittent dosing schedule).

INTERVENTION/EVALUATION

Monitor CBC, serum uric acid, LFT. Monitor for hematologic toxicity (fever, sore throat, signs of local infection, unusual bruising/bleeding from any site), symptoms of anemia (excessive fatigue, weakness). Assess skin for rash, pruritus, urticaria.

PATIENT/FAMILY TEACHING

• Treatment may depress your immune system and reduce your ability to fight infection. Report symptoms of infection such as body aches, burning with urination, chills, cough, fatigue, fever. Avoid those with active infection. • Report symptoms of bone marrow depression (e.g., bruising, fatigue, fever, shortness of breath, weight loss; bleeding easily, bloody urine or stool). • Increase fluid intake (may protect against hyperuricemia). • Avoid acidic or spicy foods; may delay absorption of medication. • Do not have immunizations without physician's approval (drug lowers resistance). • Avoid contact with those who have recently received live virus vaccine.

cinacalcet

sin-a-**kal**-set
(Sensipar)

◆CLASSIFICATION

PHARMACOTHERAPEUTIC: Calcium receptor agonist. **CLINICAL:** Calcimimetic.

USES

Treatment of severe hypercalcemia in pts with primary parathyroid carcinoma. Treatment of secondary hyperparathyroidism in pts with chronic renal disease on dialysis. Treatment of severe hypercalcemia in pts with primary hyperparathyroidism unable to undergo parathyroidectomy.

PRECAUTIONS

Contraindications: Hypersensitivity to cinacalcet. Serum calcium lower than the lower limit of normal range. **Cautions:** Cardiovascular disease, moderate to severe hepatic impairment, seizure disorder.

ACTION

Increases sensitivity of calcium-sensing receptor on parathyroid gland to activation by extracellular calcium, thus lowering parathyroid hormone (PTH), calcium, and phosphorus levels. **Therapeutic Effect:** Prevents progressive bone disease and adverse effects associated with disorders of mineral metabolism.

PHARMACOKINETICS

Extensively distributed after PO administration. Protein binding: 93%–97%. Metabolized in liver. Excreted in urine (80%), feces (15%). **Half-life:** 30–40 hrs.

LIFESPAN CONSIDERATIONS

Pregnancy/Lactation: May cross placental barrier; unknown if distributed in breast milk. Safe usage during lactation not established (potential adverse reaction in infants). **Children:** Safety and efficacy not established. **Elderly:** No age-related precautions noted.

INTERACTIONS

DRUG: **Strong CYP3A4 inhibitors (e.g., erythromycin, ketoconazole, ritonavir)** increase concentration/effect. May increase concentration/effect of **thioridazine.** May decrease concentration/effect of **tamoxifen. HERBAL:** None significant. **FOOD:** **High-fat meals** increase plasma concentration. **LAB VALUES:** May decrease serum calcium, phosphorus.

AVAILABILITY (Rx)

Tablets: 30 mg, 60 mg, 90 mg.

ADMINISTRATION/HANDLING

PO

• Store at room temperature. • Do not break, crush, dissolve, or divide film-coated tablets. • Administer with food or shortly after a meal.

INDICATIONS/ROUTES/DOSAGE

Hypercalcemia in Parathyroid Carcinoma; Primary Hyperparathyroidism

PO: ADULTS, ELDERLY: Initially, 30 mg twice daily. Titrate dosage sequentially (60 mg twice daily, 90 mg twice daily, and 90 mg 3–4 times/day) every 2–4 wks as needed to normalize serum calcium level. **Maximum:** 360 mg/day (as 90 mg 4 times/day).

Secondary Hyperparathyroidism

PO: ADULTS, ELDERLY: Initially, 30 mg once daily. Titrate dosage sequentially (60, 90, 120, and 180 mg once daily) every 2–4 wks to maintain iPTH level between 150 and 300 pg/mL. **Maximum:** 180 mg/day.

Dosage in Renal Impairment

No dose adjustment.

Dosage in Hepatic Impairment

Moderate to severe impairment: Use caution.

SIDE EFFECTS

Frequent (31%–21%): Nausea, vomiting, diarrhea. **Occasional (15%–10%):** Myalgia, dizziness. **Rare (7%–5%):** Asthenia, hypertension, anorexia, noncardiac chest pain.

ADVERSE EFFECTS/TOXIC REACTIONS

Overdose may lead to hypocalcemia, seizures, worsening of HF.

NURSING CONSIDERATIONS

BASELINE ASSESSMENT

Establish baseline serum electrolyte levels (esp. serum calcium, phosphate, ionized calcium).

INTERVENTION/EVALUATION

Monitor serum calcium, phosphate, ionized calcium for hyperparathyroidism. Monitor daily pattern of bowel activity, stool consistency. Obtain order for antidiarrhea, antiemetic medication to prevent serum electrolyte imbalance. Assess for evidence of dizziness; institute fall risk precautions.

PATIENT/FAMILY TEACHING

• Take with food or shortly after a meal. • Do not chew, crush, dissolve, or divide film-coated tablets. • Notify physician if vomiting, diarrhea, cramping, muscle pain, numbness occurs.

C

ciprofloxacin

sip-roe-**flox**-a-sin
(Cetraxal, Ciloxan, Cipro)

BLACK BOX ALERT May increase risk of tendonitis, tendon rupture. May exacerbate myasthenia gravis.

Do not confuse Ciloxan with Cytoxan, or Cipro with Ceftin, or ciprofloxacin with cephalexin.

FIXED-COMBINATION(S)

Cipro HC Otic: ciprofloxacin/hydrocortisone (a steroid): 0.2%/1%. **CiproDex Otic:** ciprofloxacin/dexamethasone (a corticosteroid): 0.3%/0.1%.

◆CLASSIFICATION

PHARMACOTHERAPEUTIC: Fluoroquinolone. **CLINICAL:** Antibiotic.

USES

Treatment of susceptible infections due to *E. coli, K. pneumoniae, E. cloacae, P. mirabilis, P. vulgaris, P. aeruginosa, H. influenzae, M. catarrhalis, S. pneumoniae, S. aureus* (methicillin susceptible), *S. epidermidis, S. pyogenes, C. jejuni, Shigella* spp., *S. typhi* including intra-abdominal, bone, joint, lower respiratory tract, skin/skin structure infections; UTIs, infectious diarrhea, prostatitis, sinusitis, typhoid fever, febrile neutropenia. **Ophthalmic:** Treatment of superficial ocular infections. **Otic:** Treatment of acute otitis externa due to susceptible strains of *P. aeruginosa* or *S. aureus*. **OFF-LABEL:** Treatment of chancroid. Acute pulmonary exacerbations in cystic fibrosis, disseminated gonococcal infections, prophylaxis to *Neisseria meningitidis* following close contact with infected person. Infectious diarrhea (children); periodontitis.

PRECAUTIONS

Contraindications: Hypersensitivity to ciprofloxacin, other quinolones. Concurrent use of tiZANidine. **Cautions:** Renal impairment, CNS disorders, seizures, rheumatoid arthritis, history of QT prolongation, uncorrected hypokalemia, hypomagnesemia, myasthenia gravis. Suspension not used through feeding or gastric tubes. Use in children (due to adverse events to joints/surrounding tissue).

ACTION

Inhibits enzyme, DNA gyrase, in susceptible bacteria, interfering with bacterial cell replication. **Therapeutic Effect:** Bactericidal.

PHARMACOKINETICS

Well absorbed from GI tract. Protein binding: 20%–40%. Widely distributed including to CSF. Metabolized in liver. Primarily excreted in urine. Minimal removal by hemodialysis. **Half-life:** 3–5 hrs (increased in renal impairment, elderly).

⌛ LIFESPAN CONSIDERATIONS

Pregnancy/Lactation: Unknown if distributed in breast milk. If possible, do not use during pregnancy/lactation (risk of arthropathy to fetus/infant). **Children:** Arthropathy may occur. **Elderly:** Age-related renal impairment may require dosage adjustment.

INTERACTIONS

DRUG: Antacids, calcium, magnesium, zinc, iron preparations, sucralfate may decrease absorption. May increase effects of **caffeine, oral anticoagulants (e.g., warfarin).** May increase concentration/effect of **pimozide, tizanidine**. May increase concentration, toxicity of **theophylline. HERBAL: Dong quai, St. John's wort** may increase photosensitization. **FOOD:** None known. **LAB VALUES:** May increase serum alkaline phosphatase, creatine kinase (CK), LDH, ALT, AST.

AVAILABILITY (Rx)

Infusion Solution: 200 mg/100 mL, 400 mg/200 mL. **Ophthalmic Ointment:** ***(Ciloxan):*** 0.3%. **Ophthalmic Solution:** ***(Ciloxan):*** 0.3%. **Otic Solution: *(Cetraxal):*** 0.2% (single-dose container: 0.25 mL).

Suspension, Oral: 250 mg/5 mL, 500 mg/5 mL. **Tablets:** 100 mg, 250 mg, 500 mg, 750 mg.

C

ADMINISTRATION/HANDLING

IV

Reconstitution • Available prediluted in infusion container ready for use. Final concentration not to exceed 2 mg/mL.

Rate of administration • Infuse over 60 min (reduces risk of venous irritation).

Storage • Store at room temperature. • Solution appears clear, colorless to slightly yellow.

PO

• May be given with food to minimize GI upset. • Give at least 2 hrs before or 6 hrs after antacids, calcium, iron, zinc-containing products. • Do not administer suspension through feeding or gastric tubes. • **NG tube:** Crush immediate-release tablet and mix with water. Flush tube before/after administration.

Ophthalmic

• Place gloved finger on lower eyelid and pull out until a pocket is formed between eye and lower lid. • Place ointment or drops into pocket. • Instruct pt to close eye gently for 1–2 min (so that medication will not be squeezed out of the sac). • Instruct pt using ointment to roll eyeball to increase contact area of drug to eye. • Instruct pt using solution to apply digital pressure to lacrimal sac at inner canthus for 1 min to minimize systemic absorption. • Do not use ophthalmic solution for injection.

IV INCOMPATIBILITIES

Ampicillin and sulbactam (Unasyn), cefepime (Maxipime), dexamethasone (Decadron), furosemide (Lasix), heparin, hydrocortisone (Solu-Cortef), methylPREDNISolone (Solu-Medrol), phenytoin (Dilantin), sodium bicarbonate.

IV COMPATIBILITIES

Calcium gluconate, diltiaZEM (Cardizem), DOBUTamine (Dobutrex), DOPamine (Intropin), lidocaine, LORazepam (Ativan), magnesium, midazolam (Versed), potassium chloride.

INDICATIONS/ROUTES/DOSAGE

Note: Not recommended as first choice in pregnancy/lactation or in children younger than 18 yrs due to adverse events related to joints/surrounding tissue.

Usual Dosage Range

PO: ADULTS, ELDERLY: 250–750 mg q12h. **CHILDREN: Mild to moderate infections:** 10 mg/kg twice daily. **Maximum:** 500 mg/dose. **Severe infections:** 15–20 mg/kg twice daily. **Maximum:** 750 mg/dose.

IV: ADULTS, ELDERLY: 200–400 mg q12h. **CHILDREN:** 10 mg/kg q8–12h. **Maximum:** 400 mg/dose.

Usual Ophthalmic Dosage

ADULTS, ELDERLY, CHILDREN: ***(Solution):*** 1–2 drops q2h while awake for 2 days, then 1–2 drops q4h while awake for 5 days. ***(Ointment):*** Apply 3 times/day for 2 days, then 2 times/day for 5 days.

Usual Otic Dosage

ADULTS, ELDERLY, CHILDREN: Otic solution 0.2%. Instill 0.25 mL (0.5 mg) 2 times/day for 7 days.

Dosage in Renal Impairment

Dosage and frequency are modified based on creatinine clearance and the severity of the infection.

Creatinine Clearance	Dosage
Immediate-Release	
30–50 mL/min	PO: 250–500 mg q12h
5–29 mL/min	250–500 mg q18h
ESRD, HD, PD	250–500 mg q24h
Extended-Release	
< 30 mL/min	500 mg q24h
ESRD, HD, PD	500 mg q24h
IV 5–29 mL/min	200–400 mg q18–24h

Dosage in Hepatic Impairment

No dose adjustment.

C

SIDE EFFECTS

Frequent (5%–2%): Nausea, diarrhea, dyspepsia, vomiting, constipation, flatulence, confusion, crystalluria. **Ophthalmic:** Burning, crusting in corner of eye. **Occasional (less than 2%):** Abdominal pain/discomfort, headache, rash. **Ophthalmic:** Altered taste, sensation of foreign body in eye, eyelid redness, itching. **Rare (less than 1%):** Dizziness, confusion, tremors, hallucinations, hypersensitivity reaction, insomnia, dry mouth, paresthesia.

ADVERSE EFFECTS/TOXIC REACTIONS

Superinfection (esp. enterococcal, fungal), nephropathy, cardiopulmonary arrest, cerebral thrombosis may occur. Hypersensitivity reaction (rash, pruritus, blisters, edema, burning skin), photosensitivity have occurred. Sensitization to ophthalmic form may contraindicate later systemic use of ciprofloxacin. May exacerbate muscle weakness in pts with myasthenia gravis. Dermatologic conditions such as toxic epidermal necrolysis, Stevens-Johnson syndrome have been reported. Cases of severe hepatotoxicity have occurred. May increase risk of tendonitis, tendon rupture.

NURSING CONSIDERATIONS

BASELINE ASSESSMENT

Question for history of hypersensitivity to ciprofloxacin, quinolones; myasthenia gravis, renal/hepatic impairment.

INTERVENTION/EVALUATION

Obtain urinalysis for microscopic analysis for crystalluria prior to and during treatment. Evaluate food tolerance. Monitor daily pattern of bowel activity, stool consistency. Encourage hydration (reduces risk of crystalluria). Monitor for dizziness, headache, visual changes, tremors. Assess for chest, joint pain. **Ophthalmic:** Observe therapeutic response.

PATIENT/FAMILY TEACHING

• It is essential to complete drug therapy despite improvement of symptoms. Early discontinuation may result in antibacterial resistance or increase the risk of recurrent infection. • Frequent diarrhea, fever, abdominal pain, blood-streaked stool may indicate infectious diarrhea and may be contagious to others. • Maintain adequate hydration. • Do not take antacids within 2 hrs of ciprofloxacin (reduces/destroys effectiveness). • Shake suspension well before using; do not chew microcapsules in suspension. • Report tendon pain or swelling. • Avoid exposure to sunlight/artificial light (may cause photosensitivity reaction).

CISplatin

HIGH ALERT

sis-**pla**-tin

BLACK BOX ALERT Cumulative renal toxicity may be severe. Dose-related toxicities include myelosuppression, nausea, vomiting. Ototoxicity, especially pronounced in children, noted by tinnitus, loss of high-frequency hearing, deafness. Must be administered by personnel trained in administration/handling of chemotherapeutic agents. Anaphylactic reaction can occur within minutes of administration. Avoid confusion between CISplatin and CARBOplatin.

Do not confuse CISplatin with CARBOplatin or oxaliplatin.

CLASSIFICATION

PHARMACOTHERAPEUTIC: Alkylating agent. **CLINICAL:** Antineoplastic.

USES

Treatment of metastatic testicular cancers, metastatic ovarian cancers, advanced bladder cancer. **OFF-LABEL:** Breast, cervical, endometrial, esophageal, gastric, head and neck, lung (small-cell, non–small-cell) carcinomas; Hodgkin's and non-Hodgkin's lymphomas;

malignant melanoma, neuroblastoma, osteosarcoma, soft tissue sarcoma, Wilms' tumor.

PRECAUTIONS

Contraindications: Hypersensitivity to CISplatin. Hearing impairment, myelosuppression, preexisting renal impairment. **Cautions:** Elderly, renal impairment.

ACTION

Inhibits DNA synthesis by cross-linking with DNA strands. Cell cycle–phase nonspecific. **Therapeutic Effect:** Prevents cellular division.

PHARMACOKINETICS

Widely distributed. Protein binding: greater than 90%. Undergoes rapid nonenzymatic conversion to inactive metabolite. Excreted in urine. Removed by hemodialysis. **Half-life:** 58–73 hrs (increased in renal impairment).

LIFESPAN CONSIDERATIONS

Pregnancy/Lactation: If possible, avoid use during pregnancy, esp. first trimester. Breastfeeding not recommended. **Children:** Ototoxic effects may be more severe. **Elderly:** Age-related renal impairment may require dosage adjustment.

INTERACTIONS

DRUG: **Bone marrow depressants (e.g., PACLitaxel)** may increase myelosuppression. **Live virus vaccines** may potentiate virus replication, increase vaccine side effects, decrease pt's antibody response to vaccine. **HERBAL:** **Echinacea** may decrease therapeutic effect. **FOOD:** None known. **LAB VALUES:** May increase serum BUN, creatinine, uric acid, AST. May decrease CrCl, serum calcium, magnesium, phosphate, potassium, sodium. May cause positive Coombs' test.

AVAILABILITY (Rx)

Injection Solution: 1 mg/mL (50 mL, 100 mL, 200 mL).

ADMINISTRATION/HANDLING

◀ALERT▶ Wear protective gloves during handling. May be carcinogenic, mutagenic, teratogenic. Handle with extreme care during preparation/administration.

IV

Dilution • Dilute desired dose in 250–1,000 mL 0.9% NaCl, D_5/0.45% NaCl, or D_5/0.9% NaCl to concentration of 0.05–2 mg/mL. Solution should have final NaCl concentration of 0.2% or greater.

Rate of administration • Infuse over 6–8 hrs (per protocol). • Avoid rapid infusion (increases risk of nephrotoxicity, ototoxicity). • Monitor for anaphylactic reaction during first few minutes of infusion.

Storage • Protect from sunlight. • Do not refrigerate (may precipitate). Discard if precipitate forms. IV infusion: Stable for 72 hrs at 39°F–77°F.

IV INCOMPATIBILITIES

Amphotericin B complex (Abelcet, AmBisome, Amphotec), cefepime (Maxipime), piperacillin and tazobactam (Zosyn), sodium bicarbonate.

IV COMPATIBILITIES

Etoposide (VePesid), granisetron (Kytril), heparin, HYDROmorphone (Dilaudid), lipids, LORazepam (Ativan), magnesium sulfate, mannitol, morphine, ondansetron (Zofran), palonosetron (Aloxi).

INDICATIONS/ROUTES/DOSAGE

Note: Pretreatment hydration with 1–2 liters of fluid recommended. Adequate hydration, urine output greater than 100 mL/hr should be maintained for 24 hrs after administration. Verify any cisplatin dose exceeding 100 mg/m^2/course.

Bladder Cancer

IV: ADULTS, ELDERLY: (Single agent): 50–70 mg/m^2 q3–4wks.

Ovarian Cancer

IV: ADULTS, ELDERLY: 75–100 mg/m² q3–4wks.

Testicular Cancer

IV: ADULTS, ELDERLY: 20 mg/m² daily for 5 days repeated q3wks (in combination with bleomycin and etoposide).

Dosage in Renal Impairment

Dosage is modified based on CrCl, BUN.

◀ALERT▶ Repeated courses of CISplatin should not be given until serum creatinine is less than 1.5 mg/100 mL and/or BUN is less than 25 mg/100 mL.

Creatinine Clearance	Dosage
10–50 mL/min	75% of normal dose
Less than 10 mL/min	50% of normal dose
Hemodialysis	50% of dose post dialysis
Peritoneal dialysis	50% of dose
Continuous renal replacement therapy	75% of dose

Dosage in Hepatic Impairment

No dose adjustment.

SIDE EFFECTS

Frequent: Nausea, vomiting (occurs in more than 90% of pts, generally beginning 1–4 hrs after administration and lasting up to 24 hrs); myelosuppression (affecting 25%–30% of pts, with recovery generally occurring in 18–23 days). **Occasional:** Peripheral neuropathy (with prolonged therapy [4–7 mos]). Pain/redness at injection site, loss of taste, appetite. **Rare:** Hemolytic anemia, blurred vision, stomatitis.

ADVERSE EFFECTS/TOXIC REACTIONS

Anaphylactic reaction (angioedema, wheezing, tachycardia, hypotension) may occur in first few minutes of administration in pt previously exposed to CISplatin. Nephrotoxicity occurs in 28%–36% of pts treated with a single dose, usually during second wk of therapy. Ototoxicity (tinnitus, hearing loss) occurs in 31% of pts treated with a single dose (more severe in children). Symptoms may become more frequent, severe with repeated doses.

NURSING CONSIDERATIONS

BASELINE ASSESSMENT

Obtain baseline CBC, BMP, LFT. Pts should be well hydrated before and 24 hrs after medication to ensure adequate urinary output (100 mL/hr), decrease risk of nephrotoxicity.

INTERVENTION/EVALUATION

Measure all emesis, urine output (general guideline requiring immediate notification of physician: 750 mL/8 hrs, urinary output less than 100 mL/hr). Monitor I&O q1–2h beginning with pretreatment hydration, continue for 48 hrs after dose. Assess vital signs q1–2h during infusion. Monitor urinalysis, serum electrolytes, LFT, renal function tests, CBC, platelet count for changes from baseline.

PATIENT/FAMILY TEACHING

• Report signs of ototoxicity (tinnitus, hearing loss). • Do not have immunizations without physician's approval (lowers body's resistance). • Avoid contact with those who have recently taken oral polio vaccine. • Report if nausea/vomiting continues at home. • Report signs of peripheral neuropathy.

citalopram

sye-**tal**-o-pram
(CeleXA)

BLACK BOX ALERT Increased risk of suicidal thinking and behavior in children, adolescents, young adults 18–24 yrs with major depressive disorder, other psychiatric disorders.

Do not confuse CeleXA with CeleBREX, Cerebyx, Ranexa, or ZyPREXA.

◆CLASSIFICATION

PHARMACOTHERAPEUTIC: Selective serotonin reuptake inhibitor. **CLINICAL:** Antidepressant.

C

USES

Treatment of unipolar major depression. **OFF-LABEL:** Treatment of alcohol abuse, diabetic neuropathy, obsessive-compulsive disorder, smoking cessation, GAD, panic disorder.

PRECAUTIONS

Contraindications: Hypersensitivity to citalopram, use of MAOIs intended to treat psychiatric disorders (concurrently or within 14 days of discontinuing either citalopram or MAOI), initiation in pts receiving linezolid or methylene blue. Concurrent use with pimozide. **Cautions:** Elderly, hepatic/renal impairment, seizure disorder. Not recommended in pts with congenital long QT syndrome, bradycardia, recent MI, uncompensated HF, hypokalemia, or hypomagnesemia; pts at high risk of suicide.

ACTION

Blocks uptake of the neurotransmitter serotonin at CNS presynaptic neuronal membranes, increasing its availability at postsynaptic receptor sites. **Therapeutic Effect:** Relieves symptoms of depression.

PHARMACOKINETICS

Well absorbed after PO administration. Protein binding: 80%. Extensively metabolized in liver. Excreted in urine. **Half-life:** 35 hrs.

⌛ LIFESPAN CONSIDERATIONS

Pregnancy/Lactation: Distributed in breast milk. **Children:** May cause increased anticholinergic effects, hyperexcitability. **Elderly:** More sensitive to anticholinergic effects (e.g., dry mouth), more likely to experience dizziness, sedation, confusion, hypotension, hyperexcitability.

INTERACTIONS

DRUG: **CYP2C19 inhibitors (e.g., fluconazole), other medications prolonging QT interval (e.g., amiodarone, azithromycin, ciprofloxacin, haloperidol)** may increase risk of QT prolongation. **Linezolid, MAOIs (e.g., phenelzine, selegiline), triptans** may cause serotonin syndrome (excitement, diaphoresis, rigidity, hyperthermia, autonomic hyperactivity, coma). **Strong CYP3A4 inducers (e.g., carBAMazepine, phenytoin, rifAMPin)** may decrease concentration/effect. **HERBAL:** **St. John's wort** may decrease concentration/effect. **FOOD:** None known. **LAB VALUES:** May decrease serum sodium.

AVAILABILITY (Rx)

Oral Solution: 10 mg/5 mL. **Tablets:** 10 mg, 20 mg, 40 mg.

ADMINISTRATION/HANDLING

PO

- Give without regard to food.

INDICATIONS/ROUTES/DOSAGE

Note: Doses greater than 40 mg not recommended.

Depression

PO: **ADULTS YOUNGER THAN 60 YRS:** Initially, 20 mg once daily in the morning or evening. May increase in 20-mg increments at intervals of no less than 1 wk. **Maximum:** 40 mg/day. **ELDERLY 60 YRS OR OLDER:** 20 mg once daily. **Maximum:** 20 mg/day.

Dose Modification

Hepatic impairment; poor metabolizers of CYP2C19; concomitant use of CYP2C19 inhibitors: 20 mg once daily. **Maximum:** 20 mg/day.

Dosage in Renal Impairment

Mild to moderate impairment: No dose adjustment. **Severe impairment:** Use caution.

SIDE EFFECTS

Frequent (21%–11%): Nausea, dry mouth, drowsiness, insomnia, diaphoresis. **Occasional (8%–4%):** Tremor, diarrhea, abnormal ejaculation, dyspepsia, fatigue, anxiety, vomiting, anorexia. **Rare (3%–2%):** Sinusitis, sexual dysfunction, menstrual disorder, abdominal pain, agitation, decreased libido.

ADVERSE EFFECTS/TOXIC REACTIONS

Overdose manifested as dizziness, drowsiness, tachycardia, confusion, seizures, torsades de pointes, ventricular tachycardia, sudden death. Serotonin syndrome or neuroleptic malignant syndrome (NMS)–like reactions have been reported.

NURSING CONSIDERATIONS

BASELINE ASSESSMENT

CBC, LFT should be performed periodically for pts on long-term therapy. Observe, record behavior. Assess psychological status, thought content, sleep pattern, appearance, interest in environment. Screen for bipolar disorder.

INTERVENTION/EVALUATION

Supervise suicidal-risk pt closely during early therapy (as depression lessens, energy level improves, increasing suicide potential). Assess appearance, behavior, speech pattern, level of interest, mood.

PATIENT/FAMILY TEACHING

• Do not stop taking medication or increase dosage. • Avoid alcohol. • Avoid tasks that require alertness, motor skills until response to drug is established. • Report worsening depression, suicidal ideation, unusual changes in behavior.

clarithromycin

HIGH ALERT

kla-**rith**-roe-**mye**-sin
(Apo-Clarithromycin ✦, PMS-Clarithromycin ✦)

Do not confuse clarithromycin with Claritin, clindamycin, or erythromycin.

◆CLASSIFICATION

PHARMACOTHERAPEUTIC: Macrolide. **CLINICAL:** Antibiotic.

USES

Treatment of susceptible infections due to *C. pneumoniae, H. influenzae, H. parainfluenzae, H. pylori, M. catarrhalis, M. avium, M. pneumoniae, S. aureus, S. pneumoniae, S. pyogenes*, including bacterial exacerbation of bronchitis, otitis media, acute maxillary sinusitis, *Mycobacterium avium* complex (MAC), pharyngitis, tonsillitis, *H. pylori* duodenal ulcer, community-acquired pneumonia, skin and soft tissue infections. Prevention of MAC disease. **OFF-LABEL:** Prophylaxis of infective endocarditis, pertussis, Lyme disease.

PRECAUTIONS

Contraindications: Hypersensitivity to clarithromycin, other macrolide antibiotics. History of QT prolongation or ventricular arrhythmias, including torsades de pointes. History of cholestatic jaundice or hepatic impairment with prior use of clarithromycin. Concomitant use with colchicine (in pts with renal/hepatic impairment), statins, pimozide, ergotamine, dihydroergotamine. **Cautions:** Hepatic/renal impairment, elderly with severe renal impairment, myasthenia gravis, coronary artery disease. Pts at risk of prolonged cardiac repolarization. Avoid use with uncorrected electrolytes (e.g., hypokalemia, hypomagnesemia), clinically significant bradycardia, class IA or III antiarrhythmics (see Classification).

ACTION

Binds to ribosomal receptor sites of susceptible organisms, inhibiting protein synthesis of bacterial cell wall. **Therapeutic Effect:** Bacteriostatic; may be bactericidal with high dosages or very susceptible microorganisms.

PHARMACOKINETICS

Well absorbed from GI tract. Protein binding: 65%–75%. Widely distributed (except CNS). Metabolized in liver. Primarily excreted in urine. Not removed by hemodialysis. **Half-life:** 3–7 hrs; metabolite, 5–9 hrs (increased in renal impairment).

C

LIFESPAN CONSIDERATIONS

Pregnancy/Lactation: Unknown if distributed in breast milk. **Children:** Safety and efficacy not established in pts younger than 6 mos. **Elderly:** Age-related renal impairment may require dosage adjustment.

INTERACTIONS

DRUG: May increase concentration/effects of **acalabrutinib, ado-trastuzumab, axitinib, bosutinib, budesonide, eletriptan, lovastatin.** May increase QT-prolonging effects of **dronedarone.** **HERBAL:** **St. John's wort** may decrease concentration/effect. **FOOD:** None known. **LAB VALUES:** May increase serum BUN, ALT, AST, alkaline phosphatase, LDH, creatinine, PT. May decrease WBC.

AVAILABILITY (Rx)

Oral Suspension: 125 mg/5 mL, 250 mg/5 mL. **Tablets:** 250 mg, 500 mg.

Tablets (Extended-Release): 500 mg.

ADMINISTRATION/HANDLING

PO

• Give immediate-release tablets, oral suspension without regard to food. • Give q12h (rather than twice daily). • Shake suspension well before each use. • Extended-release tablets should be given with food. • Do not break, crush, dissolve, or divide extended-release tablets.

INDICATIONS/ROUTES/DOSAGE

Usual Dosage Range

PO: ADULTS, ELDERLY: 250–500 mg q12h or 1,000 mg once daily (2 × 500-mg extended-release tablets). **CHILDREN 6 MOS AND OLDER:** *(Immediate-Release):* 7.5 mg/kg q12h. **Maximum:** 500 mg/dose.

Dosage in Renal Impairment

CrCl less than 30 mL/min: Reduce dose by 50% and administer once or twice daily. **HD:** Administer dose after dialysis complete.

Combination With Atazanavir or Ritonavir	
CrCl 30–60 mL/min	Decrease dose by 50%
CrCl less than 30 mL/min	Decrease dose by 75%

Dosage in Hepatic Impairment

No dose adjustment.

SIDE EFFECTS

Occasional (6%–3%): Diarrhea, nausea, altered taste, abdominal pain. **Rare (2%–1%):** Headache, dyspepsia.

ADVERSE EFFECTS/TOXIC REACTIONS

Antibiotic-associated colitis, other superinfections (abdominal cramps, severe watery diarrhea, fever) may result from altered bacterial balance in GI tract. Hepatotoxicity, thrombocytopenia occur rarely.

NURSING CONSIDERATIONS

BASELINE ASSESSMENT

Question pt for allergies to clarithromycin, erythromycins.

INTERVENTION/EVALUATION

Monitor daily pattern of bowel activity, stool consistency. Mild GI effects may be tolerable, but increasing severity may indicate onset of antibiotic-associated colitis. Be alert for superinfection: fever, vomiting, diarrhea, anal/genital pruritus, oral mucosal changes (ulceration, pain, erythema).

PATIENT/FAMILY TEACHING

• It is essential to complete drug therapy despite improvement of symptoms. Early discontinuation may result in antibacterial resistance or increase the risk of recurrent infection. • Frequent diarrhea, fever, abdominal pain, blood-streaked stool may indicate infectious diarrhea and may be contagious to others. • Biaxin may be taken without regard to food. Take Biaxin XL with food.

clevidipine

clev-eye-di-peen
(Cleviprex)
Do not confuse clevidipine with amlodipine, cladribine, clofarabine, clozapine, or Cleviprex with Claravis.

◆CLASSIFICATION

PHARMACOTHERAPEUTIC: Dihydropyridine calcium channel blocker. **CLINICAL:** Antihypertensive.

USES

Management of hypertension when oral therapy is not feasible or not desirable.

PRECAUTIONS

Contraindications: Hypersensitivity to clevidipine. Allergy to soy or egg products; abnormal lipid metabolism (e.g., acute pancreatitis, lipoid nephrosis, pathologic hyperlipidemia if accompanied by hyperlipidemia), severe aortic stenosis. **Cautions:** HF; pt with disorders of lipid metabolism.

ACTION

Causes potent arterial vasodilation by inhibiting the influx of calcium during depolarization in arterial smooth muscle. **Therapeutic Effect:** Decreases mean arterial pressure (MAP) by reducing systemic vascular resistance.

PHARMACOKINETICS

Widely and rapidly distributed. Full recovery of therapeutic B/P occurs 5–15 min. after discontinuation. Onset of effects: 2–4 min. Metabolized via hydrolysis by esterases in blood and extravascular tissue. Protein binding: 99.5%. Excreted in urine (74%), feces (22%). **Half-life:** 15 min.

⌛ LIFESPAN CONSIDERATIONS

Pregnancy/Lactation: Unknown if distributed in breast milk. May depress uterine contractions during labor and delivery. **Children:** Safety and efficacy not established. **Elderly:** Start at low end of dosing range. May experience greater hypotensive effect.

INTERACTIONS

DRUG: None significant. **HERBAL:** **Herbals with hypotensive properties (e.g., garlic, ginger, hawthorn)** may enhance effect. **Yohimbe** may decrease effect. **FOOD:** None known. **LAB VALUES:** May increase serum BUN, potassium, triglycerides, uric acid.

AVAILABILITY (Rx)

Injection, Emulsion: 50 mL (0.5 mg/mL), 100 mL (0.5 mg/mL).

ADMINISTRATION/HANDLING

IV

Preparation • Do not dilute. • To ensure uniformity of emulsion, gently invert vial several times before use. • Visually inspect for particulate matter or discoloration. Emulsion should appear milky white. Discard if discoloration or particulate matter is observed.

Rate of administration • Titrate to desired effect using infusion pump via peripheral or central line.

Storage • Refrigerate unused vial in original carton. • May store at controlled room temperature (77°F) for up to 2 mos. • Do not freeze. • Do not return to refrigerator once warmed to room temperature. Once the stopper is punctured, use within 12 hrs. • Discard unused portions.

IV INCOMPATIBILITIES

May be administered with, but not diluted in, solutions including Sterile Water for Injection, 0.9% NaCl, dextrose-containing solutions, lactated Ringer's, 10% amino acid. Do not administer with other medications.

C

INDICATIONS/ROUTES/DOSAGE

Note: Individualize dosage depending on desired B/P and pt response. See manufacturer guidelines for dose conversion.

Hypertension

IV: ADULTS, ELDERLY: Initiate infusion at 1–2 mg/hr. **Titration:** Initially, dosage may be doubled at short (90-sec) intervals. As B/P approaches goal, an increase in dosage should be less than double, and time intervals between dose adjustments should be lengthened to q5–10 min. **Maintenance:** Desired therapeutic effect generally occurs at a rate of 4–6 mg/hr (pts with severe hypertension may require limited doses up to 32 mg/hr). **Maximum:** 16 mg/hr (no more than 21 mg/hr or 1000 mL is recommended per 24 hrs due to lipid load).

Dosage in Renal Impairment

No dose adjustment.

Dosage in Hepatic Impairment

Not specified; use caution.

SIDE EFFECTS

Occasional (6%–3%): Headache, insomnia, nausea, vomiting. **Rare (less than 1%):** Syncope, dyspnea.

ADVERSE EFFECTS/TOXIC REACTIONS

May cause atrial fibrillation, hypotension, reflex tachycardia. Rebound hypertension may occur in pts who are not transitioned to oral antihypertensives after discontinuation. Dihydropyridine calcium channel blockers are known to have negative inotropic effects, which may exacerbate HF. Rebound hypertension may cause emergent hypertensive crisis, which may cause CVA, myocardial infarction, renal failure, HF, seizures.

NURSING CONSIDERATIONS

BASELINE ASSESSMENT

Screen for history of defective lipid metabolism, pancreatitis, hypertriglyceridemia, severe aortic stenosis; allergy to soy products, eggs products. Assess B/P, apical pulse immediately before initiation.

INTERVENTION/EVALUATION

Monitor B/P, pulse rate. Generally, an increase of 1–2 mg/hour will produce an additional 2–4 mm Hg decrease in systolic B/P. If an oral antihypertensive is required to wean off infusion, consider the delay of onset of oral medication's effect. Pts who receive prolonged IV infusions and are not changed to other antihypertensives should be monitored for rebound hypertension for at least 8 hrs after discontinuation. Obtain serum triglyceride level in pts receiving prolonged infusions. Monitor for atrial fibrillation, hypotension, reflex tachycardia; exacerbation of HF in pts with history of HF. Beta blockers should be discontinued only after a gradual reduction in dose.

PATIENT/FAMILY TEACHING

• In some pts, an oral blood pressure medication may need to be started; compliance is essential to control high blood pressure. • Life-threatening high blood pressure crisis may occur up to 8 hrs after stopping infusion; report severe anxiety, chest pain, difficulty breathing, headache, stroke-like symptoms (confusion, difficulty speaking, paralysis, one-sided weakness, vision loss).

clindamycin

klin-da-**mye**-sin
(Cleocin, Cleocin T, Clindagel, Clindesse)

■ BLACK BOX ALERT ■ May cause severe, potentially fatal colitis characterized by severe, persistent diarrhea, severe abdominal cramps, passage of blood and mucus.

Do not confuse Cleocin with Clinoril or Cubicin, or clindamycin with clarithromycin, Claritin, or vancomycin.

◆CLASSIFICATION

PHARMACOTHERAPEUTIC: Lincosamide. **CLINICAL:** Antibiotic.

C

USES

Systemic: Treatment of aerobic gram-positive staphylococci and streptococci (not enterococci), *Fusobacterium, Bacteroides* spp., and *Actinomyces* for treatment of respiratory tract infections, skin/soft tissue infections, sepsis, intra-abdominal infections, infections of female pelvis and genital tract, bacterial endocarditis prophylaxis for dental and upper respiratory procedures in penicillin-allergic pts, perioperative prophylaxis. **Topical:** Treatment of acne vulgaris. **Intravaginal:** Treatment of bacterial vaginosis. **OFF-LABEL:** Treatment of actinomycosis, babesiosis, erysipelas, malaria, otitis media, *Pneumocystis jiroveci* pneumonia (PCP), sinusitis, toxoplasmosis. **PO:** Bacterial vaginosis.

PRECAUTIONS

Contraindications: Hypersensitivity to clindamycin. **Cautions:** Severe hepatic dysfunction; history of GI disease (especially colitis).

ACTION

Inhibits protein synthesis of bacterial cell wall by binding to bacterial ribosomal receptor sites. Topically, decreases fatty acid concentration on skin. **Therapeutic Effect:** Bacteriostatic or bacteriocidal.

PHARMACOKINETICS

Rapidly absorbed from GI tract. Protein binding: 92%–94%. Widely distributed. Metabolized in liver. Primarily excreted in urine. Not removed by hemodialysis. **Half-life:** 1.6–5.3 hrs (increased in renal/hepatic impairment, premature infants).

LIFESPAN CONSIDERATIONS

Pregnancy/Lactation: Readily crosses placenta. Distributed in breast milk. **Topical/Vaginal:** Unknown if distributed in breast milk. **Children:** Caution in pts younger than 1 mo. **Elderly:** No age-related precautions noted.

INTERACTIONS

DRUG: None significant. **HERBAL: St. John's wort** may decrease concentration/effect. **FOOD:** None known. **LAB VALUES:** May increase serum alkaline phosphatase, ALT, AST.

AVAILABILITY (Rx)

Capsules: 75 mg, 150 mg, 300 mg. **Vaginal Cream:** 2%. **Topical Gel:** 1%. **Infusion, Premix:** 300 mg/50 mL, 600 mg/50 mL, 900 mg/50 mL. **Injection Solution:** 150 mg/mL. **Lotion:** 1%. **Oral Solution:** 75 mg/5 mL. **Vaginal Suppositories:** 100 mg. **Topical Swabs:** 1%.

ADMINISTRATION/HANDLING

IV

Reconstitution • Dilute 300–600 mg with 50 mL D_5W or 0.9% NaCl (900–1,200 mg with 100 mL).

Rate of administration • Infuse over at least 10–60 min at rate not exceeding 30 mg/min. Severe hypotension, cardiac arrest can occur with rapid administration. • No more than 1.2 g should be given in a single infusion.

Storage • Reconstituted IV infusion (piggyback) is stable for 16 days at room temperature, 32 days if refrigerated.

IM

• Do not exceed 600 mg/dose. • Administer deep IM.

PO

• Store capsules at room temperature. • After reconstitution, oral solution is stable for 2 wks at room temperature. • Do not refrigerate oral solution (avoids thickening). • Give with at least 8 oz water (minimizes esophageal ulceration). • Give without regard to food.

Topical

• Wash skin; allow to dry completely before application. • Shake topical lotion

C

well before each use. • Apply liquid, solution, or gel in thin film to affected area. • Avoid contact with eyes or abraded areas.

Vaginal, Cream or Suppository
• Use one applicatorful or suppository at bedtime. • Fill applicator that comes with cream or suppository to indicated level. • Instruct pt to lie on back with knees drawn upward and spread apart. • Insert applicator into vagina and push plunger to release medication. • Withdraw, wash applicator with soap and warm water. • Wash hands promptly to avoid spreading infection.

IV INCOMPATIBILITIES

Allopurinol (Aloprim), fluconazole (Diflucan).

IV COMPATIBILITIES

Amiodarone (Cordarone), diltiaZEM (Cardizem), heparin, HYDROmorphone (Dilaudid), magnesium sulfate, midazolam (Versed), morphine, multivitamins, propofol (Diprivan).

INDICATIONS/ROUTES/DOSAGE

Usual Dosage
IV, IM: ADULTS, ELDERLY: 600–2,700 mg/day in 2–4 divided doses. **Maximum IM dose:** 600 mg. **CHILDREN:** 20–40 mg/kg/day in 3–4 divided doses. **Maximum:** 2,700 mg/day. **CHILDREN YOUNGER THAN 1 MO:** 5 mg/kg/dose q6–12h. **NEONATES:** 15–20 mg/kg/day divided q6–8h.

PO: ADULTS, ELDERLY: 150–450 mg q6h. **Maximum:** 1,800 mg/day. **INFANTS, CHILDREN, ADOLESCENTS:** 8–40 mg/kg/day in divided doses q6–8h. **Maximum:** 1,800 mg/day. **NEONATES:** 5 mg/kg/dose q6–12 hrs.

Bacterial Vaginosis
Intravaginal: ***(Cream):*** **ADULTS:** One applicatorful at bedtime for 3 days in nonpregnant pts or for 7 days in pregnant pts. ***(Clindesse):*** **ADULTS:** One applicatorful once daily as single dose in nonpregnant pts. **Suppository: ADULTS:** Once daily into vagina at bedtime for 3 days.

Acne Vulgaris
Topical: ADULTS: Apply thin layer to affected area twice daily (pledget, lotion, solution); once daily (gel, foam).

Dosage in Renal/Hepatic Impairment
No dose adjustment.

SIDE EFFECTS

Frequent: Systemic: Abdominal pain, nausea, vomiting, diarrhea. **Topical:** Dry, scaly skin. **Vaginal:** Vaginitis, pruritus. **Occasional: Systemic:** Phlebitis; pain, induration at IM injection site; allergic reaction, urticaria, pruritus. **Topical:** Contact dermatitis, abdominal pain, mild diarrhea, burning, stinging. **Vaginal:** Headache, dizziness, nausea, vomiting, abdominal pain. **Rare: Vaginal:** Hypersensitivity reaction.

ADVERSE EFFECTS/TOXIC REACTIONS

Antibiotic-associated colitis, other superinfections (abdominal cramps, severe watery diarrhea, fever) may occur during and several wks after clindamycin therapy (including topical form). Blood dyscrasias (leukopenia, thrombocytopenia), nephrotoxicity (proteinuria, azotemia, oliguria) occur rarely. Thrombophlebitis with IV administration.

NURSING CONSIDERATIONS

BASELINE ASSESSMENT

Obtain baseline WBC. Question pt for history of allergies. Avoid, if possible, concurrent use of neuromuscular blocking agents.

INTERVENTION/EVALUATION

Monitor daily pattern of bowel activity, stool consistency. Report diarrhea promptly due to potential for serious colitis (even with topical or vaginal administration). Assess skin for rash (dryness, irritation) with topical application. With all routes of administration, be alert for superinfection: fever, vomiting, diarrhea, anal/genital pruritus, oral mucosal changes (ulceration, pain, erythema).

PATIENT/FAMILY TEACHING

• It is essential to complete drug therapy despite improvement of symptoms. Early discontinuation may result in antibacterial resistance or increase the risk of recurrent infection. • Frequent diarrhea, fever, abdominal pain, blood-streaked stool may indicate infectious diarrhea and may be contagious to others. • Take oral doses with at least 8 oz water. • Use caution when applying topical clindamycin concurrently with peeling or abrasive acne agents, soaps, alcohol-containing cosmetics to avoid cumulative effect. • Do not apply topical preparations near eyes, abraded areas. • **Vaginal:** In event of accidental contact with eyes, rinse with large amounts of cool tap water. • Do not engage in sexual intercourse during treatment. • Wear sanitary pad to protect clothes against stains. Tampons should not be used.

cloBAZam

kloe-**ba**-zam
(Onfi, Sympazan)
Do not confuse cloBAZam with clonazePAM or cloZAPine.

◆CLASSIFICATION

PHARMACOTHERAPEUTIC: Benzodiazepine (Schedule IV). **CLINICAL:** Anticonvulsant.

USES

Adjunctive treatment of seizures associated with Lennox-Gastaut syndrome in pts 2 yrs of age and older. **OFF-LABEL:** Catamenial epilepsy; epilepsy (monotherapy).

PRECAUTIONS

Contraindications: Hypersensitivity to cloBAZam. **Cautions:** Elderly, debilitated, mild to moderate hepatic impairment, preexisting muscle weakness or ataxia, concomitant CNS depressants, impaired gag reflex, respiratory disease, sleep apnea, concomitant poor CYP2C19 metabolizers, pts at risk for falls, myasthenia gravis, narrow-angle glaucoma.

ACTION

Potentiates neurotransmission of gamma-aminobutyric acid (GABA) by binding to GABA receptor. Depresses nerve impulse transmission in motor cortex. **Therapeutic Effect:** Decreases seizure activity.

PHARMACOKINETICS

Rapidly absorbed after PO administration. Metabolized in liver. Peak plasma concentration: 0.5–4 hrs. Protein binding: 80–90%. Primarily excreted in urine. Unknown if removed by dialysis. **Half-life:** 36–42 hrs.

⌛ LIFESPAN CONSIDERATIONS

Pregnancy/Lactation: Excreted in breast milk. Hormonal contraceptives may have decreased effectiveness. Nonhormonal contraception recommended. **Children:** Safety and efficacy not established in pts younger than 2 yrs. **Elderly:** May have decreased clearance levels (initial dose 5 mg/day).

INTERACTIONS

DRUG: **CYP2C19 inhibitors (e.g., fluconazole, fluvoxaMINE, omeprazole, ticlopidine)** may increase concentration/effect. **Alcohol, other CNS depressants (e.g., LORazepam, morphine, zolpidem)** may increase CNS depression. May decrease effects of **hormonal contraceptives. CYP2C19 inducers (e.g., prednisone, rifAMPin)** may decrease concentration/effect. **OLANZapine** may increase adverse effects. **HERBAL:** **Herbs with sedative properties (e.g., chamomile, kava kava, valerian)** may increase CNS depression. **St. John's wort** may decrease concentration/effect. **FOOD:** None known. **LAB VALUES:** None significant.

C

AVAILABILITY (Rx)

Oral Suspension: 2.5 mg/mL. **Tablets:** 10 mg, 20 mg. **Oral Film:** 5 mg, 10 mg, 20 mg.

ADMINISTRATION/HANDLING

• May give without regard to food. • Tablets may be crushed and mixed with applesauce. • Shake suspension well. Use oral syringe supplied with suspension.

Oral Film

• Apply on top of tongue where it can dissolve. Apply only one at a time. • Do not give with liquids; ensure swallowing of a normal manner. • Pt should not chew, spit, or talk as film dissolves.

INDICATIONS/ROUTES/DOSAGE

Seizure Control (Lennox-Gastaut Syndrome)

PO: CHILDREN WEIGHING 30 KG OR LESS: Initially, 5 mg once daily for at least 7 days, then increase to 5 mg twice for at least 7 days, then increase to 10 mg twice daily. **Maximum:** 20 mg/day. **ADULTS, CHILDREN WEIGHING MORE THAN 30 KG:** Initially, 5 mg twice daily for at least 7 days, then increase to 10 mg twice daily for at least 7 days, then increase to 20 mg twice daily. **Maximum:** 40 mg/day. **ELDERLY, HEPATIC IMPAIRMENT, CYP2C19 POOR METABOLIZERS:** Initially, 5 mg once daily for at least 7 days, then increase to 5 mg twice daily for at least 7 days, then increase to 10 mg twice daily. After 1 wk, may increase to 20 mg twice daily.

Dosage in Renal Impairment

No dose adjustment.

SIDE EFFECTS

Frequent (26%–10%): Sleepiness, URI, lethargy. **Occasional (9%–5%):** Drooling, nausea, vomiting, constipation, irritability, ataxia, insomnia, cough, fatigue. **Rare (4%–2%):** Psychomotor hyperactivity, UTI, decreased/increased appetite, dysarthria, pyrexia, dysphagia, bronchitis.

ADVERSE EFFECTS/TOXIC REACTIONS

May increase risk of suicidal behavior/ideation (less than 1%). Physical dependence can increase with higher doses or concomitant alcohol/drug abuse. Abrupt benzodiazepine withdrawal may present as profuse sweating, cramping, nausea, vomiting, muscle pain, convulsions, psychosis, hallucinations, aggression, tremor, anxiety, insomnia. Overdose may result in confusion, lethargy, diminished reflexes, respiratory depression, coma. **Antidote:** Flumazenil (see Appendix J for dosage). Decreased mobility may potentiate higher risk of pneumonia.

NURSING CONSIDERATIONS

BASELINE ASSESSMENT

Offer emotional support. Review history of seizure disorder (frequency, duration, intensity, level of consciousness [LOC]). Question history of alcohol use. Obtain baseline vital signs. Assess history of depression/suicidal ideation.

INTERVENTION/EVALUATION

Monitor for excess sedation, respiratory depression, suicidal ideation. Implement seizure precautions, observe frequently for seizure activity. Assist with ambulation if drowsiness, dizziness occurs. Evaluate for therapeutic response. Encourage turning, coughing, deep breathing for pts with decreased mobility or who are bedridden.

PATIENT/FAMILY TEACHING

• Avoid tasks that require alertness, motor skills until response to drug is established. • Do not abruptly discontinue medication. • If tapering, monitor for drug withdrawal symptoms. • Avoid alcohol. • Report depression, aggression, thoughts of suicide/self-harm, excessive drowsiness.

C

clofarabine

kloe-**far**-a-bine
(Clolar)
Do not confuse clofarabine with cladribine or clevidipine.

◆CLASSIFICATION

PHARMACOTHERAPEUTIC: Antimetabolite (purine analog). **CLINICAL:** Antineoplastic.

USES

Treatment of pediatric pts (1–21 yrs) with relapsed or refractory acute lymphoblastic leukemia (ALL). **OFF-LABEL:** Acute myeloid leukemia (AML) in adults 60 yrs or older. Treatment of relapsed/refractory ALL.

PRECAUTIONS

Contraindications: Hypersensitivity to clofarabine. **Cautions:** Dehydration, hypotension, concomitant nephrotoxic or hepatotoxic medications, renal/hepatic impairment.

ACTION

Metabolized intracellularly to clofarabine triphosphate. Inhibits ribonucleoside reductase, which inhibits DNA synthesis. Competes with DNA polymers, decreasing cell replication. **Therapeutic Effect:** Decreases cell replication, inhibits cell repair. Produces cell death.

PHARMACOKINETICS

Protein binding: 47%. Metabolized intracellularly. Primarily excreted in urine (40%–60% unchanged). **Half-life:** 5.2 hrs.

LIFESPAN CONSIDERATIONS

Pregnancy/Lactation: May cause fetal harm. Breastfeeding not recommended. **Children:** Safety and efficacy not established in pts younger than 1 yr. **Elderly:** No age-related precautions noted.

INTERACTIONS

DRUG: May decrease therapeutic effect of **BCG (intravesical), vaccines (live).** May increase adverse effects of **vaccines (live). HERBAL: Echinacea** may decrease therapeutic effect. **Herbals with hypertensive properties (e.g., licorice, yohimbe)** or **hypotensive properties (e.g., garlic, ginger, ginkgo biloba)** may alter effects. **FOOD:** None known. **LAB VALUES:** May increase serum creatinine, uric acid, ALT, AST, bilirubin.

AVAILABILITY (Rx)

Injection Solution: 1 mg/mL (20-mL vial).

ADMINISTRATION/HANDLING

IV

Reconstitution • Filter clofarabine through sterile, 0.2-micrometer syringe filter prior to dilution with D_5W or 0.9% NaCl to final concentration of 0.15–0.4 mg/mL.

Rate of administration • Administer over 1–2 hrs. • Continuously infuse IV fluids to decrease risk of tumor lysis syndrome, other adverse events.

Storage • Store at room temperature. • Use diluted solution within 24 hrs.

IV INCOMPATIBILITIES

Do not administer any other medication through same IV line.

INDICATIONS/ROUTES/DOSAGE

Acute Lymphoblastic Leukemia (ALL)

IV: CHILDREN 1–21 YRS: 52 mg/m^2 over 2 hrs once daily for 5 consecutive days; repeat q2–6wks following recovery or return to baseline organ function. (Subsequent cycles should begin no sooner than 14 days from day 1 of previous cycle and when ANC is 750 cells/mm^3 or greater.)

Dosage in Renal Impairment

Dosage is modified based on creatinine clearance.

Creatinine Clearance	Dosage
30–60 mL/min	Decrease dose by 50%
Less than 30 mL/min	Use with caution

C

Dosage in Hepatic Impairment

Baseline impairment: No dose adjustment. **Hepatotoxicity during treatment; Grade 3 or higher increase in bilirubin:** Discontinue. May restart at 25% dose reduction following recovery to baseline.

SIDE EFFECTS

Frequent (83%–20%): Vomiting, nausea, diarrhea, pruritus, headache, fever, dermatitis, rigors, abdominal pain, fatigue, tachycardia, epistaxis, anorexia, petechiae, limb pain, hypotension, anxiety, constipation, edema. **Occasional (19%–11%):** Cough, mucosal inflammation, erythema, flushing, hematuria, dizziness, gingival bleeding, injection site pain, respiratory distress, pharyngitis, back pain, palmar-plantar erythrodysesthesia syndrome, myalgia, oral candidiasis, hypertension, depression, irritability, arthralgia, anorexia. **Rare (10%):** Tremor, weight gain, drowsiness.

ADVERSE EFFECTS/TOXIC REACTIONS

Neutropenia occurred in 57% of pts; pericardial effusion in 35%; left ventricular systolic dysfunction in 27%; hepatomegaly, jaundice in 15%; pleural effusion, pneumonia, bacteremia in 10%; capillary leak syndrome in less than 10%.

NURSING CONSIDERATIONS

BASELINE ASSESSMENT

Question possibility of pregnancy. Obtain CBC, BMP, LFT, CrCl prior to therapy.

INTERVENTION/EVALUATION

Monitor CBC, renal function test, LFT, serum uric acid. Monitor respiratory status, cardiac function. Monitor daily pattern of bowel activity, stool consistency. Assess for GI disturbances. Assess skin for pruritus, dermatitis, petechiae, erythema on palms of hands and soles of feet. Assess for fever, sore throat; obtain blood cultures to detect evidence of infection. Ensure adequate hydration.

PATIENT/FAMILY TEACHING

• Do not have immunizations without physician's approval (drug lowers resistance). • Avoid contact with anyone who recently received a live virus vaccine. • Avoid crowds, those with infection. • Avoid pregnancy; pts of childbearing potential should use effective contraception. • Maintain strict oral hygiene and frequent handwashing. • Report fever, respiratory distress, prolonged nausea, vomiting, diarrhea, easy bruising.

clonazePAM

kloe-**naz**-e-pam
(KlonoPIN, Rivotril ✱)

■ **BLACK BOX ALERT** ■ Concomitant use with opioids may result in profound sedation, respiratory depression, coma, and death.

Do not confuse clonazePAM or KlonoPIN with cloBAZam, cloNIDine, cloZAPine, or LORazepam.

◆CLASSIFICATION

PHARMACOTHERAPEUTIC: Benzodiazepine (Schedule IV). **CLINICAL:** Anticonvulsant, antianxiety.

USES

Adjunct in treatment of Lennox-Gastaut syndrome (petit mal variant epilepsy); akinetic, myoclonic seizures; absence seizures (petit mal) unresponsive to succinimides. Treatment of panic disorder. **OFF-LABEL:** Burning mouth syndrome, REM sleep behavior disorder, essential tremor.

PRECAUTIONS

Contraindications: Hypersensitivity to clonazePAM. Active narrow-angle glaucoma, severe hepatic disease. **Cautions:** Renal/hepatic impairment, impaired gag reflex, chronic respiratory disease, elderly, debilitated pts, depression, pts at risk of suicide or drug dependence, concomitant use of other CNS depressants.

C

ACTION

Enhances activity of GABA; depresses nerve impulse transmission in motor cortex. **Therapeutic Effect:** Produces anxiolytic, anticonvulsant effects.

PHARMACOKINETICS

Route	Onset	Peak	Duration
PO	20–60 min	—	12 hrs or less

Well absorbed from GI tract. Protein binding: 85%. Metabolized in liver. Excreted in urine. Not removed by hemodialysis. **Half-life:** 18–50 hrs.

LIFESPAN CONSIDERATIONS

Pregnancy/Lactation: Crosses placenta. May be distributed in breast milk. Chronic ingestion during pregnancy may produce withdrawal symptoms, CNS depression in neonates. **Children:** Long-term use may adversely affect physical/mental development. **Elderly:** Not recommended in elderly due to anticholinergic effects, potential for sedation, orthostatic hypotension.

INTERACTIONS

DRUG: **Alcohol, other CNS depressants (e.g., lorazepam, morphine, zolpidem)** may increase CNS depressant effect. **Strong CYP3A4 inhibitors (e.g., clarithromycin, ketoconazole, ritonavir)** may increase concentration/effect. **Strong CYP3A4 inducers (e.g., carBAMazepine, phenytoin, rifAMPin)** may decrease concentration/effect. **HERBAL:** **Herbs with sedative properties (e.g., chamomile, kava kava, valerian)** may increase CNS depression. **St. John's wort** may decrease concentration/effects. **FOOD:** None known. **LAB VALUES:** None significant.

AVAILABILITY (Rx)

Tablets: 0.5 mg, 1 mg, 2 mg. **Tablets (Orally Disintegrating):** 0.125 mg, 0.25 mg, 0.5 mg, 1 mg, 2 mg.

ADMINISTRATION/HANDLING

PO

• Give without regard to food. • Swallow whole with water.

Orally Disintegrating Tablet

• Open pouch, peel back foil; do not push tablet through foil. • Remove tablet with dry hands, place in mouth. • Swallow with or without water. • Use immediately after removing from package.

INDICATIONS/ROUTES/DOSAGE

Seizures

PO: ADULTS, ELDERLY: Initial dose not to exceed 1.5 mg/day in 3 divided doses; may be increased in 0.5- to 1-mg increments every 3 days until seizures are controlled or adverse effects occur. **Maintenance:** 2–8 mg/day in 1–2 divided doses. **Maximum:** 20 mg/day. **CHILDREN 10 YRS AND OLDER OR WEIGHING 30 KG OR MORE:** Initially, 0.01–0.05 mg/kg/day in 2 or 3 doses (maximum initial dose: 0.05 mg 3 times/day). May increase in increments of 0.5–1 mg q3–7 days. **Maintenance:** 0.05–0.2 mg/kg/day in 2–3 divided doses. **Maximum:** 20 mg/day. **INFANTS, CHILDREN YOUNGER THAN 10 YRS OR WEIGHING LESS THAN 30 KG:** 0.01–0.03 mg/kg/day (maximum initial dose: 0.05 mg/kg/day) in 2–3 divided doses; may be increased by no more than 0.25–0.5 mg every 3 days until seizures are controlled or adverse effects occur. **Maintenance:** 0.1–0.2 mg/kg/day in 3 divided doses. **Maximum:** 0.2 mg/kg/day.

Panic Disorder

PO: ADULTS, ELDERLY: Initially, 0.25 mg twice daily. Increase in increments of 0.125–0.25 mg twice daily every 3 days. **Target dose:** 1 mg/day. **Maximum:** 4 mg/day. **Note:** Discontinue gradually by 0.125 mg twice daily q3days until completely withdrawn.

Dosage in Renal Impairment

Use caution.

Dosage in Hepatic Impairment

Mild to moderate impairment: Use with caution. **Severe impairment:** Contraindicated.

C

SIDE EFFECTS

Frequent (37%–11%): Mild, transient drowsiness; ataxia, behavioral disturbances (aggression, irritability, agitation), esp. in children. **Occasional (10%–5%):** Dizziness, ataxia, URI, fatigue. **Rare (4% or less):** Impaired memory, dysarthria, nervousness, sinusitis, rhinitis, constipation, allergic reaction.

ADVERSE EFFECTS/TOXIC REACTIONS

Abrupt withdrawal may result in pronounced restlessness, irritability, insomnia, hand tremors, abdominal/muscle cramps, diaphoresis, vomiting, status epilepticus. Overdose results in drowsiness, confusion, diminished reflexes, coma. **Antidote:** Flumazenil (see Appendix J for dosage).

NURSING CONSIDERATIONS

BASELINE ASSESSMENT

Review history of seizure disorder (frequency, duration, intensity, level of consciousness [LOC]). For panic attack, assess motor responses (agitation, trembling, tension), autonomic responses (cold/clammy hands, diaphoresis).

INTERVENTION/EVALUATION

Observe for excess sedation, respiratory depression, suicidal ideation. Assess children, elderly for paradoxical reaction, particularly during early therapy. Initiate seizure precautions, observe frequently for recurrence of seizure activity. Assist with ambulation if drowsiness, ataxia occur. For pts on long-term therapy, CBC, BMP, LFT should be performed periodically. Evaluate for therapeutic response: decreased intensity and frequency of seizures or, if used in panic attack, calm facial expression, decreased restlessness.

PATIENT/FAMILY TEACHING

• Avoid tasks that require alertness, motor skills until response to drug is established. • Do not abruptly discontinue medication after long-term therapy. • Strict maintenance of drug therapy is essential for seizure control. • Avoid alcohol. • Report depression, thoughts of suicide/self-harm, excessive drowsiness, GI symptoms, worsening or loss of seizure control.

cloNIDine

klon-i-deen
(Catapres, Catapres-TTS, Duraclon, Kapvay)

■ BLACK BOX ALERT ■ **Epidural:** Not to be used for perioperative, obstetric, or postpartum pain. Must dilute concentrated epidural injectable (500 mcg/mL) prior to use.

Do not confuse Catapres with Cataflam, or cloNIDine with clomiPHENE, clonazepam, KlonoPIN, or quiNIDine.

◆CLASSIFICATION

PHARMACOTHERAPEUTIC: Alpha$_2$-adrenergic agonist. **CLINICAL:** Antihypertensive.

USES

Immediate-Release, Transdermal Patch: Treatment of hypertension alone or in combination with other antihypertensive agents. **Kapvay:** Treatment of attention-deficit hyperactivity disorder (ADHD). **Epidural: (Additional)** Combined with opiates for relief of severe cancer pain. **OFF-LABEL:** Opioid or nicotine withdrawal, prevention of migraine headaches, treatment of diarrhea in diabetes mellitus, treatment of dysmenorrhea, menopausal flushing, alcohol dependence, glaucoma, cloZAPine-induced sialorrhea, Tourette's syndrome, insomnia in children.

PRECAUTIONS

Contraindications: Hypersensitivity to cloNIDine. **Epidural:** Contraindicated in pts with bleeding diathesis or infection at the injection site; pts receiving anticoagulation therapy. **Cautions:** Depression, elderly. Severe coronary insufficiency, recent MI, cerebrovascular disease, chronic renal impairment, preexisting bradycardia, sinus node dysfunction, conduction disturbances; concurrent use with digoxin, diltiaZEM, metoprolol, verapamil.

ACTION

Stimulates $alpha_2$-adrenergic receptors in the brainstem, reducing sympathetic outflow from the CNS. **Epidural:** Prevents pain signal transmission to brain and produces analgesia at pre- and post-alpha-adrenergic receptors in spinal cord. **ADHD:** Mechanism of action unknown. **Therapeutic Effect:** Reduces peripheral resistance; decreases B/P, heart rate. Produces analgesia.

PHARMACOKINETICS

Route	Onset	Peak	Duration
PO	0.5–1 hr	2–4 hrs	6–10 hrs

Well absorbed from GI tract. Transdermal best absorbed from chest and upper arm; least absorbed from thigh. Protein binding: 20%–40%. Metabolized in liver. Primarily excreted in urine. Minimally removed by hemodialysis. **Half-life:** 6–20 hrs (increased in renal impairment).

LIFESPAN CONSIDERATIONS

Pregnancy/Lactation: Crosses placenta. Distributed in breast milk. **Children:** More sensitive to effects; use caution. **Elderly:** Not recommended in elderly due to high risk of CNS adverse effects, orthostatic hypotension. Avoid as first-line antihypertensive.

INTERACTIONS

DRUG: **CNS depressants (e.g., alcohol, morphine, oxyCODONE, zolpidem)** may increase CNS depression. May increase AV blocking effect of **beta blockers (e.g., atenolol, carvedilol, metoprolol). Tricyclic antidepressants (e.g., amitriptyline, doxepin, nortriptyline)** may decrease effect (may require increased dose of cloNIDine). **Digoxin, diltiaZEM, metoprolol, verapamil** may increase risk of serious bradycardia. **HERBAL:** **Herbs with sedative properties (e.g., chamomile, kava kava, valerian)** may increase CNS depression. **Herbals with hypertensive properties (e.g., licorice, yohimbe)** or **hypotensive properties (e.g., garlic, ginger, ginkgo biloba)** may alter effects. **FOOD:** None known. **LAB VALUES:** None significant.

C

AVAILABILITY (Rx)

Injection Solution: ***(Duraclon):*** 100 mcg/mL, 500 mcg/mL. **Tablets:** ***(Catapres):*** 0.1 mg, 0.2 mg, 0.3 mg. **Transdermal Patch:** ***(Catapres-TTS):*** 2.5 mg (release at 0.1 mg/24 hrs), 5 mg (release at 0.2 mg/24 hrs), 7.5 mg (release at 0.3 mg/24 hrs).

Extended-Release Tablets: ***(Kapvay):*** 0.1 mg.

ADMINISTRATION/HANDLING

PO

• Give without regard to food. • Tablets may be crushed. • Give last oral dose just before bedtime. • Swallow extended-release tablets whole; do not break, crush, dissolve, or divide.

Transdermal

• Apply transdermal system to dry, hairless area of intact skin on upper arm or chest. • Rotate sites (prevents skin irritation). • Do not trim patch to adjust dose.

Epidural

• Must be administered only by medical personnel trained in epidural management.

IV INCOMPATIBILITIES

None known.

IV COMPATIBILITIES

Bupivacaine (Marcaine, Sensorcaine), fentaNYL (Sublimaze), heparin, ketamine (Ketalar), lidocaine, LORazepam (Ativan).

INDICATIONS/ROUTES/DOSAGE

Hypertension

PO: ADULTS: ***(Immediate-Release):*** Initially, 0.1 mg twice a day. Increase by

0.1 mg/day at wkly intervals. **Dosage range:** 0.2–0.6 mg/day in 2 divided doses. **ELDERLY:** Initially, 0.1 mg at bedtime. May increase gradually. **CHILDREN 12 YRS AND OLDER:** Initially, 0.2 mg/day in 2 divided doses. May increase gradually at 7-day intervals in 0.1 mg/day increments. **Usual Dose:** 0.2–0.6 mg/day. **Maximum:** 2.4 mg/day.

Transdermal: ADULTS, ELDERLY: Initially, system delivering 0.1 mg/24 hrs applied once q7days. May increase by 0.1 mg at 1- to 2-wk intervals. **Usual dosage range:** 0.1–0.3 mg once wkly.

Attention-Deficit Hyperactivity Disorder (ADHD)

Note: When discontinuing, taper gradually over 1–2 wks. ***(Extended-Release Tablets):*** Taper by 0.1 mg or less q3–7 days.

PO: CHILDREN WEIGHING 45 KG OR LESS: ***(Immediate-Release):*** Initially 0.05 mg/day at bedtime. May increase in increments of 0.05 mg/day q3–7days up to a maximum of 0.2 mg/day (27–40.5 kg), 0.3 mg/day (40.5–45 kg). **MORE THAN 45 KG:** ***(Immediate-Release):*** 0.1 mg at bedtime. May increase 0.1 mg/day q3–7 days. **Maximum:** 0.4 mg/day. ***(Extended-Release Tablet [Kapvay]):*** **CHILDREN 6 YRS AND OLDER:** Initially, 0.1 mg daily at bedtime. May increase in increments of 0.1 mg/day at wkly intervals (**maximum:** 0.4 mg/day). Doses should be taken twice daily with higher split dose given at bedtime.

Severe Pain

Epidural: ADULTS, ELDERLY: 30–40 mcg/hr. **CHILDREN:** Range: 0.5–2 mcg/kg/hr, not to exceed adult dose.

Dosage in Renal/Hepatic Impairment

No dose adjustment.

SIDE EFFECTS

Frequent (40%–10%): Dry mouth, drowsiness, dizziness, sedation, constipation. **Occasional (5%–1%): Tablets, Injection:** Depression, pedal edema, loss of appetite, decreased sexual function, itching eyes, dizziness, nausea, vomiting, nervousness. **Transdermal:** Pruritus, redness, or darkening of skin. **Rare (less than 1%):** Nightmares, vivid dreams, feeling of coldness in distal extremities (esp. the digits).

ADVERSE EFFECTS/TOXIC REACTIONS

Overdose produces profound hypotension, irritability, bradycardia, respiratory depression, hypothermia, miosis (pupillary constriction), arrhythmias, apnea. Abrupt withdrawal may result in rebound hypertension associated with nervousness, agitation, anxiety, insomnia, paresthesia, tremor, flushing, diaphoresis. May produce sedation in pts with acute CVA.

NURSING CONSIDERATIONS

BASELINE ASSESSMENT

Obtain B/P immediately before each dose is administered, in addition to regular monitoring (be alert to B/P fluctuations).

INTERVENTION/EVALUATION

Monitor B/P, pulse, mental status. Monitor daily pattern of bowel activity, stool consistency. If cloNIDine is to be withdrawn, discontinue concurrent beta-blocker therapy several days before discontinuing cloNIDine (prevents cloNIDine withdrawal hypertensive crisis). Slowly reduce cloNIDine dosage over 2–4 days.

PATIENT/FAMILY TEACHING

• Avoid tasks that require alertness, motor skills until response to drug is established. • To reduce hypotensive effect, rise slowly from lying to standing. • Skipping doses or voluntarily discontinuing drug may produce severe rebound hypertension. • Avoid alcohol. • If patch loosens during 7-day application period, secure with adhesive cover.

C

clopidogrel

TOP 100 HIGH ALERT

kloe-**pid**-oh-grel
(Plavix)

■ BLACK BOX ALERT ■ Diminished effectiveness in CYP2C19 metabolizers increases risk for cardiovascular events. Pts with CYP2C19*2 and/or CYP2C19*3 alleles may have reduced platelet inhibition.

Do not confuse Plavix with Elavil or Paxil.

◆CLASSIFICATION

PHARMACOTHERAPEUTIC: Thienopyridine derivative. **CLINICAL:** Antiplatelet.

USES

To reduce rate of MI and stroke (with aspirin) in pts with non–ST-segment elevation acute coronary syndrome (ACS), acute ST-elevation MI (STEMI); pts with history of recent MI or stroke, or established peripheral arterial disease (PAD). **OFF-LABEL:** Graft patency (saphenous vein), stable coronary artery disease (in combination with aspirin). Initial treatment of ACS in pts allergic to aspirin.

PRECAUTIONS

Contraindications: Hypersensitivity to clopidogrel. Active bleeding (e.g., peptic ulcer, intracranial hemorrhage). **Cautions:** Severe hepatic/renal impairment, pts at risk of increased bleeding (e.g., trauma), concurrent use of anticoagulants. Avoid concurrent use of CYP2C19 inhibitors (e.g., omeprazole).

ACTION

Active metabolite irreversibly blocks $P2Y_{12}$ component of ADP receptors on platelet surface, preventing activation of GPIIb/IIIa receptor complex. **Therapeutic Effect:** Inhibits platelet aggregation.

PHARMACOKINETICS

Route	Onset	Peak	Duration
PO	2 hrs	5–7 days (with repeated doses of 75 mg/day)	5 days after last dose

Rapidly absorbed. Protein binding: 98%. Metabolized in liver. Eliminated equally in the urine and feces. **Half-life:** 8 hrs.

LIFESPAN CONSIDERATIONS

Pregnancy/Lactation: Unknown if drug crosses placenta or is distributed in breast milk. **Children:** Safety and efficacy not established. **Elderly:** No age-related precautions noted.

INTERACTIONS

DRUG: May increase adverse effects of **apixaban, dabigatran, edoxaban, warfarin. Strong CYP2C19 inhibitors (e.g., fluvoxaMINE, FLUoxetine)** may decrease concentration/effect. **Chronic use of NSAIDs (e.g., diclofenac, meloxicam, naproxen)** may increase risk of GI bleeding. **HERBAL: Herbals with anticoagulant/antiplatelet properties (e.g., garlic, ginger, ginkgo biloba), glucosamine** may increase risk of bleeding. **FOOD: Grapefruit products** may decrease therapeutic effect. **LAB VALUES:** May increase serum bilirubin, ALT, AST, cholesterol, uric acid. May decrease neutrophil count, platelet count.

AVAILABILITY (Rx)

Tablets: 75 mg, 300 mg.

ADMINISTRATION/HANDLING

PO

- Give without regard to food. • Avoid grapefruit products.

INDICATIONS/ROUTES/DOSAGE

Recent MI, Stroke, PAD

PO: ADULTS, ELDERLY: 75 mg once daily.

C

Acute Coronary Syndrome (ACS), Unstable Angina/NSTEMI
PO: ADULTS, ELDERLY: Initially, loading dose of 300–600 mg, then 75 mg once daily (in combination with aspirin for up to 12 months, then aspirin indefinitely).

ACS (STEMI)
Note: Continue for at least 14 days up to 12 mos in absence of bleeding.
PO: ADULTS, ELDERLY 75 YRS OR YOUNGER: Initially 300-mg loading dose, then 75 mg once daily. **ELDERLY OLDER THAN 75 YRS:** 75 mg once daily.

ACS (PCI)
PO: ADULTS, ELDERLY: Initially, 600 mg, then 75 mg once daily (in combination with aspirin) for at least 12 months.

Dosage in Renal Impairment
No dose adjustment.

Dosage in Hepatic Impairment
Use caution.

SIDE EFFECTS

Frequent (15%): Skin disorders. **Occasional (8%–6%):** Upper respiratory tract infection, chest pain, flu-like symptoms, headache, dizziness, arthralgia. **Rare (5%–3%):** Fatigue, edema, hypertension, abdominal pain, dyspepsia, diarrhea, nausea, epistaxis, dyspnea, rhinitis.

ADVERSE EFFECTS/TOXIC REACTIONS

Agranulocytosis, aplastic anemia/pancytopenia, thrombotic thrombocytopenic purpura (TTP) occur rarely. Hepatitis, hypersensitivity reaction, anaphylactoid reaction have been reported.

NURSING CONSIDERATIONS

BASELINE ASSESSMENT

Obtain baseline chemistries, platelet count, PFA. Perform platelet counts before drug therapy, q2days during first wk of treatment, and wkly thereafter until therapeutic maintenance dose is reached. Abrupt discontinuation of drug therapy produces elevated platelet count within 5 days.

INTERVENTION/EVALUATION

Monitor platelet count for evidence of thrombocytopenia. Assess Hgb, Hct, for evidence of bleeding; serum ALT, AST, bilirubin, BUN, creatinine; signs/symptoms of hepatic insufficiency during therapy.

PATIENT/FAMILY TEACHING

• It may take longer to stop bleeding during drug therapy. • Report any unusual bleeding. • Inform physicians, dentists if clopidogrel is being taken, esp. before surgery is scheduled or before taking any new drug.

cloZAPine

kloe-za-peen
(Clozaril, Versacloz)

■ **BLACK BOX ALERT** ■
Significant risk of life-threatening agranulocytosis, increased risk of potentially fatal cardiovascular events, particularly myocarditis, in elderly pts with dementia-related psychosis. May cause severe orthostatic hypotension, bradycardia, syncope, cardiac arrest, dose-dependent seizures.
Do not confuse cloZAPine with clonazePAM, cloNIDine, or KlonoPIN, or Clozaril with Clinoril or Colazal.

◆CLASSIFICATION

PHARMACOTHERAPEUTIC: Second-generation (atypical) antipsychotic. **CLINICAL:** Antipsychotic.

USES

Management of severely ill schizophrenic pts who have failed to respond to other antipsychotic therapy. Treatment of recurrent suicidal behavior in schizophrenia or schizoaffective disorder. **OFF-LABEL:** Schizoaffective disorder, bipolar disorder, childhood psychosis, obsessive-compulsive disorder, agitation related to Alzheimer's dementia.

PRECAUTIONS

Contraindications: Hypersensitivity to cloZAPine. History of cloZAPine-induced agranulocytosis or severe granulocytopenia. **Cautions:** History of seizures, cardiovascular disease, myocarditis, respiratory/hepatic/renal impairment, alcohol withdrawal, high risk of suicide, paralytic ileus, myasthenia gravis, pts at risk for aspiration pneumonia, urinary retention, narrow-angle glaucoma, prostatic hypertrophy, xerostomia, visual disturbances, constipation, history of bowel obstruction, diabetes mellitus. History of long QT prolongation/ventricular arrhythmias; concomitant use of medications that prolong QT interval; hypokalemia, hypomagnesemia.

ACTION

Interferes with binding of DOPamine and serotonin receptor sites. **Therapeutic Effect:** Diminishes schizophrenic behavior.

PHARMACOKINETICS

Readily absorbed from GI tract. Protein binding: 97%. Metabolized in liver. Excreted in urine. **Half-life:** 12 hrs.

LIFESPAN CONSIDERATIONS

Pregnancy/Lactation: Crosses placenta. Avoid use during pregnancy. Distributed in breast milk. Breastfeeding not recommended. **Children:** Not recommended for use. **Elderly:** Avoid use in pts with dementia.

INTERACTIONS

DRUG: CNS depressants (e.g., alcohol, morphine, oxyCODONE, zolpidem) may increase CNS depression. **Anticholinergics (e.g., aclidinium, ipratropium, umeclidinium)** may increase anticholinergic effect. **Strong CYP3A4 inhibitors (e.g., clarithromycin, ketoconazole, ritonavir)** may increase concentration/effect. **Strong CYP3A4 inducers (e.g., carBAMazepine, phenytoin, rifAMPin)** may decrease concentration/effect. **Metoclopramide** may increase adverse effects. **HERBAL: St. John's wort** may decrease concentration/effect. **Herbals with hypotensive properties (e.g., garlic, ginger, ginkgo biloba)** may alter effects. **Herbals with sedative properties (e.g., chamomile, kava kava, valerian)** may increase CNS depression. **FOOD:** None known. **LAB VALUES:** May increase serum glucose, cholesterol (rare), triglycerides (rare).

AVAILABILITY (Rx)

Oral Suspension: ***(Versacloz):*** 50 mg/mL (100 mL). **Tablets:** ***(Clozaril):*** 25 mg, 50 mg, 100 mg, 200 mg. **Tablets:** ***(Orally Disintegrating):*** 12.5 mg, 25 mg, 100 mg, 150 mg, 200 mg.

ADMINISTRATION/HANDLING

PO

• Give without regard to food. • **Suspension:** Use oral syringes (provided). Shake well, administer dose immediately after preparing. Suspension stable for 100 days after initial bottle opening.

Orally Disintegrating Tablets

• Remove from foil blister; do not push tablet through foil. • Remove tablet with dry hands, place in mouth. • Allow to dissolve in mouth; swallow with saliva. • If dose requires splitting tablet, discard unused portion.

INDICATIONS/ROUTES/DOSAGE

Schizophrenic Disorders

◄ALERT► For initiation of therapy, must have WBC equal to or greater than 3,500 cells/mm^3 and ANC equal to or greater than 1,500 cells/mm^3. 1,000 cells/mm^3 or greater in pts with documented benign ethnic neutropenia (BEN). **PO: ADULTS:** Initially, 12.5 mg once or twice daily. May increase by 25–50 mg/day over 2 wks until target dose of 300–450 mg/day is achieved. May further increase by 50–100 mg/day no more than once or twice wkly. Range:

200–600 mg/day. **Maximum:** 900 mg/day. **ELDERLY:** Initially, 12.5 mg/day for 3 days, then 25 mg/day for 3 days. May further increase in increments of 12.5–25 mg daily q3days. **Mean dose:** 300 mg/day. **Maximum:** 700 mg/day.

Suicidal Behavior in Schizophrenia or Schizoaffective Disorder

PO: ADULTS: Initially, 12.5 mg 1–2 times/day. May increase in increments of 25–50 mg/day to a target dose of 300–450 mg/day after 2 wks. **Mean dose:** 300 mg/day. **Maximum:** 900 mg/day.

Dose Modification

Leukopenia/granulocytopenia: Mild: (WBC 3,000–3,500 cells/mm^3 and/or ANC 1,500–2,000 cells/mm^3): Continue treatment, monitor WBC and ANC twice wkly until WBC greater than 3,500 cells/mm^3 and ANC greater than 2,000 cells/mm^3. **Moderate: (WBC 2,000–3,000 cells/mm^3 and/or ANC greater than 1,000 cells/mm^3–1,500 cells/mm^3):** Interrupt therapy, monitor WBC and ANC daily until WBC greater than 3,000 cells/mm^3 and ANC greater than 1,500 cells/mm^3, then twice wkly until WBC greater than 3,500 cells/mm^3 and ANC greater than 2,000 cells/mm^3. **Severe: (WBC less than 2,000 cells/mm^3 and/or ANC less than 1,500 cells/mm^3):** Discontinue treatment. **Discontinue:** QTC interval greater than 500 msec, cardiomyopathy/myocarditis, hepatotoxicity, or neuroleptic malignant syndrome.

Dosage in Renal/Hepatic Impairment

No dose adjustment.

SIDE EFFECTS

Frequent (39%–14%): Drowsiness, salivation, tachycardia, dizziness, constipation. **Occasional (9%–4%):** Hypotension, headache, tremor, syncope, diaphoresis, dry mouth, nausea, visual disturbances, nightmares, restlessness, akinesia, agitation, hypertension, abdominal discomfort, heartburn, weight gain. **Rare:** Rigidity, confusion, fatigue, insomnia, diarrhea, rash.

ADVERSE EFFECTS/TOXIC REACTIONS

Seizures occur occasionally (3% of pts). Overdose produces CNS depression (sedation, delirium, coma), respiratory depression, hypersalivation. Blood dyscrasias, particularly agranulocytosis, mild leukopenia, may occur.

NURSING CONSIDERATIONS

BASELINE ASSESSMENT

Obtain baseline weight, glucose, Hgb A1c, WBC, absolute neutrophil count (ANC) before initiating treatment. Assess behavior, appearance, emotional status, response to environment, speech pattern, thought content.

INTERVENTION/EVALUATION

Monitor B/P for hypertension/hypotension. Assess pulse for tachycardia (common side effect). Monitor CBC for blood dyscrasias. Monitor ANC, WBC count every wk for first 6 mos, then biweekly for 6 mos. If CBC and ANC are normal after 12 mos, then monthly monitoring of CBC and ANC is recommended. Supervise suicidal-risk pt closely during early therapy (as depression lessens, energy level improves, increasing suicide potential). Assess for therapeutic response (interest in surroundings, improvement in self-care, increased ability to concentrate, relaxed facial expression).

PATIENT/FAMILY TEACHING

• Do not abruptly discontinue long-term drug therapy. • Avoid tasks that require alertness, motor skills until response to drug is established. • Drowsiness generally subsides during continued therapy. • Avoid alcohol, caffeine. • Report fever, sore throat, flu-like symptoms.

cobimetinib

koe-bi-**me**-ti-nib
(Cotellic)
Do not confuse cobimetinib with cabozantinib, imatinib, or trametinib.

◆CLASSIFICATION

PHARMACOTHERAPEUTIC: MEK inhibitor. **CLINICAL:** Antineoplastic.

USES

Treatment of pts with unresectable or metastatic melanoma with a BRAF V600E or V600K mutation, in combination with vemurafenib.

PRECAUTIONS

Contraindications: Hypersensitivity to cobimetinib. **Cautions:** Baseline anemia, lymphopenia, thrombocytopenia; cardiomyopathy, hepatic/renal impairment, HF, hypertension, ocular disorders; pts at risk for bleeding (history of gastrointestinal, genitourinary, intracranial, reproductive system bleeding), electrolyte imbalance. Not recommended in pts taking moderate or strong CYP3A inhibitors.

ACTION

Potent and selective inhibitor of mitogen-activated extracellular kinase (MEK) pathway. Reversibly inhibits MEK1 and MEK2, which are upstream regulators of the ERK pathway. The ERK pathway promotes cellular proliferation. MEK1 and MEK2 are part of the BRAF pathway. **Therapeutic Effect:** Increases apoptosis and reduces tumor growth.

PHARMACOKINETICS

Widely distributed. Metabolized in liver. Protein binding: 95%. Peak plasma concentration: 2.4 hrs. Steady state reached in 9 days. Eliminated in feces (76%), urine (18%). **Half-life:** 44 hrs.

LIFESPAN CONSIDERATIONS

Pregnancy/Lactation: Avoid pregnancy; may cause fetal harm/malformations. Females of reproductive potential should use effective contraception during treatment and up to 2 wks after discontinuation. Unknown if distributed in breast milk. Breastfeeding not recommended. May reduce fertility in females and males. **Children/Elderly:** Safety and efficacy not established.

INTERACTIONS

DRUG: **Strong CYP3A inhibitors (e.g., clarithromycin, ketoconazole, ritonavir), moderate CYP3A inhibitors (e.g., atazanavir, ciprofloxacin)** may increase concentration/effect. **Strong CYP3A inducers (e.g., carBAMazepine, rifampicin), moderate CYP3A inducers (e.g., bosentan, nafcillin)** may decrease concentration/effect. **HERBAL:** **St. John's wort** may decrease concentration/effect. **FOOD:** None known. **LAB VALUES:** Many increase serum alkaline phosphatase, ALT, AST, creatine phosphokinase, creatinine, GGT. May decrease Hct, Hgb, lymphocytes, platelets, RBCs; serum albumin, calcium, sodium. May increase or decrease serum potassium.

AVAILABILITY (Rx)

Tablets: 20 mg.

ADMINISTRATION/HANDLING

PO

• Give without regard to food. • If dose is missed or vomiting occurs during administration, give next dose at regularly scheduled time.

INDICATIONS/ROUTES/DOSAGE

Metastatic Melanoma

PO: ADULTS, ELDERLY: 60 mg (three 20-mg tablets) once daily for first 21 days of 28-day cycle (in combination with vemurafenib). Continue until disease progression or unacceptable toxicity.

C

Concomitant Use of CYP3A Inhibitors
Reduce dose to 20 mg once daily if short-term (14 days or less) use of moderate CYP3A inhibitors is unavoidable. May resume 60-mg once-daily dose once the short-term CYP3A inhibitor is discontinued. Use an alternative strong or moderate CYP3A inhibitor in pts already taking reduced dose of 20 mg or 40 mg daily.

Dose Modification
Based on Common Terminology Criteria for Adverse Events (CTCAE) grading 1–4. See prescribing information for vemurafenib for recommended dose modification.

Dose Reduction Schedule
First dose reduction: 40 mg once daily. **Second dose reduction:** 20 mg once daily. Permanently discontinue if unable to tolerate 20 mg once daily.

Cardiomyopathy
Asymptomatic decrease in left ventricular ejection fraction (LVEF) greater than 10% from baseline and less than institutional lower limit of normal (LLN): Withhold treatment for 2 wks, then reassess LVEF. Resume at next lower dose level if LVEF is at or above LLN and the decrease from baseline is 10% or less. Permanently discontinue if LVEF is less than LLN or the decrease from baseline LVEF is more than 10%. **Symptomatic decrease of LVEF from baseline:** Withhold treatment for up to 4 wks, then reassess LVEF. Resume at next lower dose level if symptoms resolve, LVEF is at or above LLN, and the decrease from baseline LVEF is 10% or less. Permanently discontinue if symptoms persist, LVEF is less than LLN, or the decrease from baseline LVEF is more than 10%.

Dermatologic Reactions
Grade 2 (intolerable); Grade 3 or 4: Withhold or reduce dose.

Hepatotoxicity or Hepatic Laboratory Abnormalities
First occurrence, Grade 4: Withhold treatment for up to 4 wks. If improved to Grade 0 or 1, resume at next lower dose level. If not improved to Grade 0 or 1 within 4 wks, permanently discontinue. **Recurrent Grade 4:** Permanently discontinue.

Hemorrhage
Grade 3: Withhold treatment for up to 4 wks. If not improved to Grade 0 or 1, resume at next lower dose level. If not improved within 4 wks, permanently discontinue. **Grade 4:** Permanently discontinue.

New Primary Malignancies (Cutaneous or Noncutaneous)
No dose adjustment.

Nonspecific Adverse Effects
Any intolerable Grade 2; any Grade 3: Withhold for up to 4 wks. If improved to Grade 0 or 1, resume at next lower dose level. If not improved within 4 wks, permanently discontinue. **First occurrence of any Grade 4:** Permanently discontinue.

Ocular Toxicities
Serious retinopathy: Withhold treatment for up to 4 wks. If signs and symptoms improve, resume at next lower dose level. If not improved or symptoms recur at the lower dose within 4 wks, permanently discontinue. **Retinal vein occlusion:** Permanently discontinue.

Photosensitivity
Grade 2 (intolerable); Grade 3 or 4: Withhold treatment for up to 4 wks. If improved to Grade 0 or 1, resume at next lower dose level. If not improved within 4 wks, permanently discontinue.

Rhabdomyolysis, CPK Level Elevations
Grade 4 CPK elevation or any CPK elevation with myalgia: Withhold treatment for up to 4 wks. If improved to Grade 3 or lower, resume at next lower dose level. If not improved within 4 wks, permanently discontinue.

Severe Hypersensitivity Reaction
Permanently discontinue.

C

Dosage in Renal Impairment

Mild to moderate impairment: No dose adjustment. **Severe impairment:** Not specified; use caution.

Dosage in Hepatic Impairment

Mild impairment: No dose adjustment. **Moderate to severe impairment:** Not specified; use caution.

SIDE EFFECTS

Frequent (60%–24%): Diarrhea, photosensitivity, sunburn, solar dermatitis, nausea, pyrexia, vomiting. **Occasional (16%–10%):** Acneiform dermatitis, stomatitis, aphthous stomatitis, mouth ulceration, mucosal inflammation, alopecia, hypertension, vision impairment, blurred vision, reduced visual acuity, hyperkeratosis, erythema, chills.

ADVERSE EFFECTS/TOXIC REACTIONS

Anemia, lymphopenia, thrombocytopenia is an expected response to therapy. New primary malignancies, including squamous cell carcinoma, keratoacanthoma, secondary-primary melanomas, were reported. Serious, sometimes fatal hemorrhagic events, including GI bleeding (4% of pts), intracranial bleeding (1% of pts), hematuria (2% of pts), reproductive system hemorrhage (2% of pts), have occurred. Other hemorrhagic events may include cerebral/conjunctival/intracranial/gingival/hemorrhoidal/ovarian/pulmonary/rectal/uterine/vaginal bleeding; ecchymosis, epistaxis. Grade 3 or 4 cardiomyopathy reported in 26% of pts. Grade 3 or 4 skin reactions including severe rash occurred in 16% of pts. Ocular toxicities, including retinopathy, chorioretinopathy, retinal detachment, reported in 26% of pts. Grade 3 or 4 CPK level elevations occurred in 14% of pts and may lead to rhabdomyolysis. Hepatotoxicity reported in 7%–11% of pts. Severe photosensitivity reported in 47% of pts.

NURSING CONSIDERATIONS

BASELINE ASSESSMENT

Confirm presence of BRAF V600E or V600K mutation in tumor specimen prior to initiation. Obtain baseline CBC, BMP, LFT, CPK; serum albumin, magnesium, phosphate, ionized calcium; urine pregnancy; vital signs. Obtain ophthalmologic exam with visual acuity; ECG, echocardiogram for LVEF. Assess skin for moles, lesions, papillomas. Verify use of effective contraception in females of reproductive potential. Receive full medication history, including herbal products. Question history as listed in Precautions. Assess hydration status.

INTERVENTION/EVALUATION

Monitor CBC, BMP, LFT, CPK; serum albumin, magnesium, phosphate, ionized calcium; vital signs. Assess skin for new lesions, dermal toxicities at least q2mos during treatment and for least 6 mos after discontinuation. Assess LVEF by echocardiogram 1 mo after initiation, then q3mos thereafter until discontinuation. If treatment interrupted due to change in LVEF, monitor LVEF at 2 wks, 4 wks, 10 wks, and 16 wks, and then as indicated. Conduct ophthalmologic examinations regularly, esp. with any new or worsening visual disturbances. Assess for eye pain, visual changes. Immediately report GI bleeding, hematuria, unusual reproductive system hemorrhage; symptoms of intracranial bleeding (aphasia, blindness, confusion, facial droop, hemiplegia, seizures). Monitor for hepatotoxicity; monitor for signs of rhabdomyolysis, such as dark-colored urine, flank pain, decreased urine output, muscle aches. Due to high risk of diarrhea, strictly monitor I&O.

PATIENT/FAMILY TEACHING

• Blood levels monitoring, cardiac function tests, eye exams, skin exams will be conducted frequently. • Treatment may lead to severe anemia, HF, kidney failure, new cancers, severe light sensitivity, liver dysfunction, skin toxicities (such as severe rash, peeling), vision changes. • Report bloody stools, bloody urine, unusual reproductive system bleeding, nosebleeds, coughing up blood; abdominal or flank pain, dark-colored urine, decreased urinary output; stroke-like symptoms; new skin moles or lesions, rash; eye pain, vision changes; heart problems such as shortness of breath, dizziness, fainting, palpitations. • Report any newly prescribed medications. • Avoid sunlight, tanning beds. Wear protective clothing, high-SPF sunscreen, and lip balm when outdoors. • Use contraception to avoid pregnancy. Do not breastfeed. Treatment may reduce fertility.

colchicine

HIGH ALERT

kol-chi-seen
(Colcrys, Gloperba, Mitigare)
Do not confuse colchicine with Cortrosyn.

CLASSIFICATION

PHARMACOTHERAPEUTIC: Alkaloid.
CLINICAL: Antigout.

USES

Prevention, treatment of acute gouty arthritis. Used to reduce frequency of recurrence of familial Mediterranean fever (FMF) in adults and children 4 yrs and older. **OFF-LABEL:** Treatment of biliary cirrhosis, recurrent pericarditis.

PRECAUTIONS

Contraindications: Hypersensitivity to colchicine. Concomitant use of a P-glycoprotein (e.g., cycloSPORINE) or strong CYP3A4 inhibitor (e.g., clarithromycin) in presence of renal or hepatic impairment. **Mitigare:** Pts with both renal/hepatic impairment. **Cautions:** Hepatic impairment, elderly, debilitated pts, renal impairment. Concomitant use of cycloSPORINE, diltiaZEM, verapamil, fibrates, statins may increase risk of myopathy.

ACTION

Disrupts cytoskeletal functions by preventing activation, degranulation, and migration of neutrophils associated with gout symptoms. In FMF, may interfere with intracellular assembly of inflammasome complex present in neutrophils and monocytes. **Therapeutic Effect:** Reduces inflammatory process.

PHARMACOKINETICS

Rapidly absorbed from GI tract. Oral bioavailability: 45%. Highest concentration is in liver, spleen, kidney. Protein binding: 30%–50%. Re-enters intestinal tract by biliary secretion and is reabsorbed from intestines. Partially metabolized in liver via CYP3A4. Eliminated primarily in feces. **Half-life:** 27–31 hrs.

LIFESPAN CONSIDERATIONS

Pregnancy/Lactation: Drug crosses placenta and is distributed in breast milk. **Children:** Safety and efficacy not established. **Elderly:** May be more susceptible to cumulative toxicity. Age-related renal impairment may increase risk of myopathy.

INTERACTIONS

DRUG: **CYP3A4 inhibitors (e.g., clarithromycin, ketoconazole, ritonavir), P-glycoprotein/ABCB1 inhibitors (e.g., amiodarone)** may increase concentration/effect. May increase concentration/effect; risk of adverse effects (myopathy) of **HMG-CoA inhibitors (statins) (e.g., atorvastatin).** **HERBAL:** None significant. **FOOD:** **Grapefruit products** may increase concentration/toxicity. **LAB VALUES:** May increase serum alkaline phosphatase, AST. May decrease platelet count.

AVAILABILITY (Rx)

Tablets: ***(Colcrys):*** 0.6 mg. **Capsule:** ***(Mitigare):*** 0.6 mg. **Oral Solution:** ***(Gloperba):*** 0.6 mg/5 mL.

ADMINISTRATION/HANDLING

PO

• Give without regard to food. • For FMF, give in 1 or 2 divided doses. • Give with adequate water and maintain fluid intake.

INDICATIONS/ROUTES/DOSAGE

Acute Gouty Arthritis (Colcrys)

PO: ADULTS, ELDERLY: Initially, 1.2 mg at first sign of gout flare, then 0.6 mg 1 hr later. **Maximum:** 1.8 mg within 1 hr. **Coadministration with strong CYP3A4 inhibitors:** Initially, 0.6 mg, then 0.3 mg dose 1 hr later. Do not repeat for at least 3 days. **Coadministration with moderate CYP3A4 inhibitors:** 1.2 mg once. Do not repeat for at least 3 days. **Coadministration with P-glycoprotein inhibitors:** 0.6 mg once. Do not repeat for at least 3 days.

Gout Prophylaxis (Colcrys, Mitigare)

Note: Duration of prophylaxis is 6 mos or 3 mos (pts without tophi) to 6 mos (pts with 1 or more tophi)

PO: ADULTS, ELDERLY: 0.6 mg 1–2 times/day. **Maximum:** 1.2 mg/day. **Coadministration with strong CYP3A4 inhibitors:** If dose is 0.6 mg 2 times/day, adjust dose to 0.3 mg once daily; if dose is 0.6 mg once daily, adjust dose to 0.3 mg every other day. **Coadministration with moderate CYP3A4 inhibitors:** If dose is 0.6 mg 2 times/day, adjust dose to 0.3 mg twice daily or 0.6 mg once daily; if dose is 0.6 mg once daily, adjust dose to 0.3 mg once daily. **Coadministration with P-glycoprotein inhibitors:** If dose is 0.6 mg 2 times/day, adjust dose to 0.3 mg once daily; if dose is 0.6 mg once daily, adjust dose to 0.3 mg every other day.

FMF (Colcrys)

PO: ADULTS, ELDERLY, CHILDREN OLDER THAN 12 YRS: 1.2–1.8 mg/day in 1–2 divided doses. Titrate dose in 0.6-mg increments. **Coadministration with strong CYP3A4 inhibitors: Maximum:** 0.6 mg once daily (or 0.3 mg twice daily). **Coadministration with moderate CYP3A4 inhibitors:** 1.2 mg/day (0.6 mg twice daily). **Coadministration with P-glycoprotein inhibitors:** 0.6 mg once daily (or 0.3 mg twice daily). **CHILDREN 6–12 YRS:** 0.9–1.8 mg/day in 1–2 divided doses. **CHILDREN 4–5 YRS:** 0.3–1.8 mg/day in 1–2 divided doses. **Note:** Increase or decrease dose by 0.3 mg/day, not to exceed maximum dose.

Pericarditis

PO: ADULTS, ELDERLY: 0.6 mg 2 times/day.

Dosage in Renal Impairment

Creatinine Clearance	Dosage
Less than 30 mL/min	
FMF	0.3 mg initially
Gout prophylaxis	0.3 mg/day
Gout flare	No reduction
HD	
FMF	0.3 mg as single dose
Gout prophylaxis	0.3 mg 2–4 times/wk

Dosage in Hepatic Impairment

Use caution.

SIDE EFFECTS

Frequent: Nausea, vomiting, abdominal discomfort. **Occasional:** Anorexia. **Rare:** Hypersensitivity reaction, including angioedema.

ADVERSE EFFECTS/TOXIC REACTIONS

Bone marrow depression (aplastic anemia, agranulocytosis, thrombocytopenia) may occur with long-term therapy. Overdose initially causes burning feeling in skin/throat; severe diarrhea, abdominal pain. Second stage manifests as fever, seizures, delirium, renal impairment (hematuria, oliguria). Third stage causes hair loss, leukocytosis, stomatitis.

NURSING CONSIDERATIONS

BASELINE ASSESSMENT

Obtain baseline laboratory studies. **Gout:** Assess involved joints for pain, mobility, edema. **Mediterranean fever:** Assess abdominal pain, fever, chills, erythema, swollen skin lesions.

INTERVENTION/EVALUATION

Discontinue medication immediately if GI symptoms occur. Encourage high fluid intake (3,000 mL/day). Monitor I&O (output should be at least 2,000 mL/day), CBC, hepatic/renal function tests. Monitor serum uric acid. Assess for therapeutic response: relief of pain, stiffness, swelling; increased joint mobility; reduced joint tenderness; improved grip strength.

PATIENT/FAMILY TEACHING

• Drink 8–10 (8-oz) glasses of fluid daily while taking medication. • Report skin rash, sore throat, fever, unusual bruising/bleeding, weakness, fatigue, numbness. • Stop medication as soon as gout pain is relieved or at first sign of nausea, vomiting, diarrhea. • Avoid grapefruit products.

conjugated estrogens

kon-joo-gate-ed **ess**-troe-jenz
(Premarin)

■ **BLACK BOX ALERT** ■ Risk of dementia may be increased in postmenopausal women. Do not use to prevent cardiovascular disease. May increase risk of endometrial carcinoma or invasive breast cancer in postmenopausal women.

Do not confuse Premarin with Primaxin, Provera, or Remeron.

FIXED-COMBINATION(S)

Duavee: conjugated estrogen/bazedoxifene (estrogen agonist/antagonist): 0.45 mg/20 mg.

◆CLASSIFICATION

PHARMACOTHERAPEUTIC: Estrogen. **CLINICAL:** Hormone.

USES

Management of moderate to severe vasomotor symptoms associated with menopause. Treatment of hypoestrogenism due to hypogonadism, castration, or primary ovarian failure. Prevention of osteoporosis in postmenopausal women. Palliative treatment of inoperable, progressive cancer of the prostate and breast in men, and of the breast in postmenopausal women. Abnormal uterine bleeding (injection only). Treatment of moderate to severe vulvar and vaginal atrophy due to menopause. **OFF-LABEL:** Prevention of estrogen deficiency–induced premenopausal osteoporosis. **Cream:** Prevention of nosebleeds.

PRECAUTIONS

Contraindications: Hypersensitivity to estrogens. Breast cancer (except in pts being treated for metastatic disease), hepatic disease, history of or current thrombophlebitis, undiagnosed abnormal vaginal bleeding, pregnancy, DVT or PE (current or history of), angioedema or anaphylactic reaction to estrogens, estrogen-dependent tumors. Known protein C, protein S, antithrombin deficiency or other thrombophilic disorder. **Cautions:** Asthma, epilepsy, migraine headaches, diabetes, cardiac/renal dysfunction, history of severe hypocalcemia, lupus erythematosus, porphyria, endometriosis, gallbladder disease, familial defects of lipoprotein metabolism. Hypoparathyroidism, history of cholestatic jaundice.

ACTION

Responsible for development and maintenance of female reproductive system and secondary sexual characteristics; modulates release of gonadotropin-releasing hormone, reduces follicle-stimulating hormone (FSH), luteinizing hormone (LH). **Therapeutic Effect:** Reduces elevated levels of gonadotropins, LH, and FSH.

PHARMACOKINETICS

Well absorbed from GI tract. Widely distributed. Protein binding: 50%–80%. Metabolized in liver. Primarily excreted in urine. **Half-life (total estrone):** 27 hrs.

LIFESPAN CONSIDERATIONS

Pregnancy/Lactation: Distributed in breast milk. May cause fetal harm. Breastfeeding not recommended. **Children:** Safety and efficacy not established. **Elderly:** No age-related precautions noted.

INTERACTIONS

DRUG: May decrease therapeutic effect of **anticoagulants (e.g., warfarin), anastrozole, exemestane.** **HERBAL:** **Herbals with estrogenic properties (e.g., fennel, red clover, ginseng)** may increase adverse effects. **FOOD:** **Grapefruit products** may increase concentration/toxicity. **LAB VALUES:** May increase serum glucose, HDL, calcium, triglycerides. May decrease serum cholesterol, LDH. May affect serum metapyrone testing, thyroid function tests.

AVAILABILITY (Rx)

Vaginal Cream: ***(Premarin):*** 0.625 mg/g. **Injection Powder for Reconstitution:** 25 mg. **Tablets:** 0.3 mg, 0.45 mg, 0.625 mg, 0.9 mg, 1.25 mg.

ADMINISTRATION/HANDLING

IV

Reconstitution • Reconstitute with Sterile Water for Injection. • Slowly add diluent, shaking gently. • Avoid vigorous shaking.
Rate of administration • Give slowly to prevent flushing reaction.
Storage • Refrigerate vials for IV use. • Use immediately following reconstitution.

PO

• Administer at same time each day. • Give with milk, food if nausea occurs.

IV INCOMPATIBILITIES

No information available on Y-site administration.

INDICATIONS/ROUTES/DOSAGE

Note: Cyclic administration is either 3 wks on, 1 wk off or 25 days on, 5 days off.

Vasomotor Symptoms Associated With Menopause
PO: ADULTS, ELDERLY: 0.3 mg/day cyclically or daily.

Vulvar and Vaginal Atrophy
PO: ADULTS, ELDERLY: 0.3 mg/day cyclically or daily.
Intravaginal: ADULTS, ELDERLY: 0.5–2 g/day cyclically.

Hypoestrogenism due to Hypogonadism
PO: ADULTS: 0.3–0.625 mg/day given cyclically. Dose may be titrated in 6- to 12-mo intervals. Progestin treatment should be added to maintain bone mineral density once skeletal maturity is achieved.

Hypoestrogenism due to Castration, Primary Ovarian Failure
PO: ADULTS: Initially, 1.25 mg/day cyclically. Adjust dosage, upward or downward, according to severity of symptoms and pt response. For maintenance, adjust dosage to lowest level that will provide effective control.

Postmenopausal Osteoporosis Prevention
PO: ADULTS, ELDERLY: 0.3 daily or cyclically.

Breast Cancer (Metastatic)
PO: ADULTS, ELDERLY: 10 mg 3 times/day for at least 3 mos.

Prostate Cancer (Advanced)
PO: ADULTS, ELDERLY: 1.25–2.5 mg 3 times/day.

Abnormal Uterine Bleeding
IV, IM: ADULTS: 25 mg; may repeat once in 6–12 hrs.

Dyspareunia
Intravaginal: ADULTS, ELDERLY: 0.5 g cyclically (21 days on, 7 days off) or 0.5 g twice weekly.

Dosage in Renal Impairment
No dose adjustment.

Dosage in Hepatic Impairment
Contraindicated.

SIDE EFFECTS

Frequent: Vaginal bleeding (spotting, breakthrough bleeding), breast pain/tenderness, gynecomastia. **Occasional:** Headache, hypertension, intolerance to contact lenses. **High doses:** Anorexia, nausea. **Rare:** Loss of scalp hair, depression.

ADVERSE EFFECTS/TOXIC REACTIONS

Prolonged administration may increase risk of breast, cervical, endometrial, hepatic, vaginal carcinoma; cerebrovascular disease, coronary heart disease, gallbladder disease, hypercalcemia.

NURSING CONSIDERATIONS

BASELINE ASSESSMENT

Question for hypersensitivity to estrogen, hepatic impairment, thromboembolic disorders associated with pregnancy, estrogen therapy. Assess frequency/severity of vasomotor symptoms. Review results of baseline mammogram in pts with breast cancer.

INTERVENTION/EVALUATION

Assess B/P periodically. Assess for edema; weigh daily. Monitor for loss of vision, diplopia, migraine, thromboembolic disorder, sudden onset of proptosis.

PATIENT/FAMILY TEACHING

• Avoid smoking due to increased risk of heart attack, blood clots. • Avoid grapefruit products. • Diet, exercise important part of therapy when used to retard osteoporosis. • Promptly report signs/symptoms of thromboembolic, thrombotic disorders: sudden severe headache, shortness of breath, vision/speech disturbance, weakness/numbness of an extremity, loss of coordination; pain in chest, groin, leg; abnormal vaginal bleeding, depression. • Teach female pts to perform breast self-exam. • Report weight gain of more than 5 lbs a wk. • Stop taking medication, contact physician if pregnancy is suspected.

copanlisib

koe-pan-lis-ib
(Aliqopa)
Do not confuse copanlisib with cabozantinib, cobimetinib, duvelisib, or idelalisib.

◆CLASSIFICATION

PHARMACOTHERAPEUTIC: Phosphatidylinositol 3-kinase inhibitor. **CLINICAL:** Antineoplastic.

USES

Treatment of adults with relapsed follicular lymphoma who have received at least two prior systemic therapies.

PRECAUTIONS

Contraindications: Hypersensitivity to copanlisib. **Cautions:** Baseline anemia, leukopenia, lymphopenia, neutropenia, thrombocytopenia; active infection, conditions predisposing to infection (e.g., diabetes, renal failure, immunocompromised pts, open wounds); history of diabetes, hypertension, pulmonary disease. Concomitant use of moderate CYP3A inhibitors.

ACTION

Inhibits phosphatidylinositol-3-kinase (PI3K) expressed on malignant B-cells. Inhibits signaling pathway of B-cell receptors, lymphoma cells lines, and CXCR12-mediated chemotaxis of malignant B-cells. **Therapeutic Effect:** Inhibits tumor cell growth and metastasis. Induces cellular death by apoptosis.

PHARMACOKINETICS

Widely distributed. Metabolized in liver. Protein binding: 84%. Excreted in feces (64%), urine (22%). **Half-life:** 39 hrs.

⌛ LIFESPAN CONSIDERATIONS

Pregnancy/Lactation: Avoid pregnancy; may cause fetal harm. Females of reproductive potential must use reliable form of contraception (failure rate less than 1% per yr) during treatment and for at least 1 mo after discontinuation. Unknown if distributed in breast milk. Breastfeeding not recommended during treatment and for at least 1 mo after discontinuation. May impair fertility in females and males of reproductive potential. **Males:** Must use condoms during treatment and up to 1 mo after treatment, despite prior history of vasectomy. **Children:** Safety and efficacy not established. **Elderly:** No age-related precautions noted.

INTERACTIONS

DRUG: **Strong CYP3A4 inhibitors (e.g., clarithromycin, ketoconazole, ritonavir)** may increase concentration/effect. **Strong CYP3A4 inducers (e.g., rifAMPin, phenytoin, carBAMazepine)** may decrease concentration/effect. May decrease effect of **BCG (intravesical).** May enhance adverse/toxic effects of **natalizumab, pimecrolimus, tacrolimus, vaccines (live).** **HERBAL:** **Echinacea, St. John's wort** may decrease concentration/effect. **FOOD:** **Grapefruit products** may increase concentration/effect. **LAB VALUES:** May increase serum glucose, lipase, triglycerides, uric acid. May decrease Hgb, lymphocytes, neutrophils, platelets, WBC; serum phosphate.

AVAILABILITY (Rx)

Injection, Lyophilized Solid for Reconstitution: 60 mg.

ADMINISTRATION/HANDLING

IV

Reconstitution • Reconstitute lyophilized solid using 4.4 mL of 0.9% NaCl for a vial concentration of 15 mg/mL. • Gently shake vial for 30 sec. • Allow vial to settle for 1 min (allowing bubbles to rise to surface). • If any contents are not completely dissolved, repeat gentle shaking and settling process. • Visually inspect for particulate matter or discoloration. Solution should appear colorless to slightly yellow in color. Do not use if solution is cloudy, discolored, or visible particles are observed. • For 60 mg dose, withdraw 4 mL of solution from vial. For 45 mg dose, withdraw 3 mL of solution from vial. For 30 mg dose, withdraw 2 mL of solution from vial. • Dilute solution in 100 mL of 0.9% NaCl. • Mix by gentle inversion.

Rate of administration • Infuse over 60 min.

Storage • Refrigerate unused vials. • May refrigerate reconstituted vial or diluted solution for up to 24 hrs. • If refrigerated, allow diluted solution to warm to room temperature before infusion. • Avoid direct sunlight.

IV COMPATIBILITIES/ INCOMPATIBILITIES

Reconstitute and dilute using only 0.9% NaCl. Do not infuse with other medications.

INDICATIONS/ROUTES/DOSAGE

Follicular Lymphoma

IV: ADULTS, ELDERLY: 60 mg on days 1, 8, and 15 of a 28-day cycle on an intermittent schedule (3 wks on, 1 wk off). Continue until disease progression or unacceptable toxicity.

Dose Modification

Based on Common Terminology Criteria for Adverse Events (CTCAE).

Hyperglycemia

Fasting serum blood glucose level equal to 160 mg/mL or greater (pre-dose): Withhold treatment until fasting serum glucose is 160 mg/mL or less. **Random/nonfasting blood glucose level equal to 200 mg/mL or greater:** Withhold treatment until random/nonfasting glucose is 200 mg/mL or less. **Serum blood glucose level equal to 500 mg/mL or greater (pre-dose or post-dose):** **First occurrence:** Withhold treatment until fasting glucose is 160 mg/mL or less, or until random/nonfasting glucose is 200 mg/mL or less. Then, reduce dose to 45 mg dose. **Subsequent**

occurrences: Withhold treatment until fasting glucose is 160 mg/mL or less, or until random/nonfasting glucose is 200 mg/mL or less. Then, reduce dose to 30 mg dose. If hyperglycemia persists at 30 mg dose, permanently discontinue.

Hypertension

B/P 150/90 mmHg or greater (pre-dose): Withhold treatment until two consecutive B/P measurements (at least 15 min apart) are less than 150/90 mmHg. **Non–life-threatening B/P 150/90 mmHg or greater (post-dose):** Continue at same dose if antihypertensive therapy is not indicated. If antihypertensive therapy is indicated, consider dose reduction from 60 mg to 45 mg, or from 45 mg to 30 mg. If B/P remains 150/90 mmHg or higher at 30 mg dose despite antihypertensive therapy, permanently discontinue. **Life-threatening B/P 150/90 mmHg or greater (post-dose):** Permanently discontinue.

Infection

Grade 3 or higher infection: Withhold treatment until resolved. **Suspected *Pneumocystis jiroveci* pneumonia (PJP) infection of any grade:** Withhold treatment. If PJP infection is confirmed, treat infection until resolved. Then, resume treatment at same dose with concomitant PJP preventative therapy.

Neutropenia

Absolute neutrophil count (ANC) less than 500 cells/mm³: Withhold treatment until ANC is 500 cells/mm³ or greater, then resume at same dose. **Recurrence of ANC 500 cells/mm³ or less:** Reduce dose to 45 mg.

Noninfectious Pneumonitis

Grade 2 noninfectious pneumonitis (NIP): Withhold treatment and treat NIP. Once recovered to Grade 1 or 0, reduce dose at 45 mg dose. If Grade 2 NIP recurs, permanently discontinue. **Grade 3 or higher noninfectious pneumonitis (NIP):** Permanently discontinue.

Severe Cutaneous Reactions

Grade 3 severe cutaneous reactions: Withhold treatment until resolved, then reduce dose from 60 mg to 45 mg, or from 45 mg to 30 mg. **Life-threatening severe cutaneous reactions:** Permanently discontinue.

Thrombocytopenia

Platelet count less than 25,000 cells/mm³: Withhold treatment until platelet count is 75,000 cells/mm³ or greater. If recovery occurs within 21 days, reduce dose from 60 mg to 45 mg, or from 45 mg to 30 mg. If recovery does not occur within 21 days, permanently discontinue.

Other Toxicities

Any other Grade 3 toxicities: Withhold treatment until resolved, then reduce dose from 60 mg to 45 mg, or from 45 mg to 30 mg.

Concomitant Use of Strong CYP3A Inhibitors

If strong CYP3A inhibitor cannot be discontinued, reduce dose to 45 mg.

Dosage in Renal Impairment

Mild to moderate impairment: No dose adjustment. **Severe impairment:** Not specified; use caution.

Dosage in Hepatic Impairment

Mild impairment: No dose adjustment. **Moderate to severe impairment:** Not specified; use caution.

SIDE EFFECTS

Frequent (36%): Fatigue, asthenia, diarrhea. **Occasional (15%–7%):** Rash, stomatitis, oropharyngeal erosion, oral pain, vomiting, mucosal inflammation, paresthesia, dysesthesia.

ADVERSE EFFECTS/TOXIC REACTIONS

Anemia, leukopenia, lymphopenia, neutropenia, thrombocytopenia are expected responses to therapy. Serious infections including bacterial/fungal/pneumococcal/viral pneumonia, bronchopulmonary aspergillosis, lung infection reported in 21% of pts. *Pneumocystis jiroveci* pneumonia reported in less than 1% of pts. Hyperglycemia reported 54% of pts. Blood glucose levels usually peaked 5–8 hrs after infusion. CTCAE Grade 3 hypertension occurred in 26% of pts. Noninfectious pneumonitis occurred in 5% of pts. Severe cutaneous reactions reported in 3% of pts.

NURSING CONSIDERATIONS

BASELINE ASSESSMENT

Obtain ANC, CBC, vital signs. Screen for active infection. Obtain pregnancy test in females of reproductive potential. Question current breastfeeding status. Confirm compliance of effective contraception. Question history of diabetes, hypertension, pulmonary disease. Pts with history of diabetes, hypertension should have adequate control prior to initiation. Receive full medication history and screen for interactions. Offer emotional support.

INTERVENTION/EVALUATION

Monitor ANC, CBC, platelet count periodically. Monitor blood glucose level prior to each treatment; B/P before and after each treatment. Be alert for infections, esp. lower respiratory tract infection such as *pneumocystis jiroveci* pneumonia, bacterial/fungal/pneumococcal/viral pneumonia (cough, dyspnea, hypoxia, pleuritic chest pain). Consider ABG, radiologic test if lung infection or pneumonitis suspected. If treatment-related toxicities occur, consider referral to specialist. Assess skin for cutaneous reactions.

PATIENT/FAMILY TEACHING

• Treatment may depress your immune system and reduce your ability to fight infection. Report symptoms of infection such as body aches, chills, cough, fatigue, fever. Avoid those with active infection. • Report symptoms of high blood sugar levels (confusion, excessive thirst/hunger, headache, frequent urination); high blood pressure (dizziness, headache, fainting); inflammation of the lung (excessive cough, difficulty breathing); toxic skin reactions (itching, peeling, rash, redness, swelling). • Use contraception to avoid pregnancy. Do not breastfeed. • Treatment may impair fertility. • Do not take newly prescribed medications unless approved by the prescriber who originally started treatment. • Do not ingest grapefruit products.

crizotinib

kriz-**o**-ti-nib
(Xalkori)

◆CLASSIFICATION

PHARMACOTHERAPEUTIC: Tyrosine kinase inhibitor. Anaplastic lymphoma kinase inhibitor. **CLINICAL:** Antineoplastic.

USES

Treatment of locally advanced or metastatic non–small-cell lung cancer (NSCLC) that is anaplastic lymphoma kinase (ALK) positive. Metastatic NSCLC in pts whose tumors are ROS1 positive.

PRECAUTIONS

Contraindications: Hypersensitivity to crizotinib. **Cautions:** Baseline hepatic impairment, congenital long QT interval syndrome. Pregnancy (avoid use). Concomitant use of CYP3A4 inducers/inhibitors, medications known to cause bradycardia, renal impairment.

ACTION

Inhibits receptor tyrosine kinases, including anaplastic lymphoma kinase (ALK), hepatocyte growth factor receptors (HGFR, c-Met), recepteur d'origine nantais (RON). ALK gene abnormalities due to mutation may result in expression of oncogenic fusion proteins. **Therapeutic Effect:** Inhibits tumor cell proliferation of cells expressing genetic alteration.

PHARMACOKINETICS

Well absorbed after PO administration. Peak plasma concentration: 4–6 hrs. Protein binding: 91%. Metabolized in liver. Excreted in feces (63%) and urine (22%). **Half-life:** 42 hrs.

LIFESPAN CONSIDERATIONS

Pregnancy/Lactation: Avoid pregnancy. May cause fetal harm. Contraception should be considered during therapy and for at least 12 wks after discontinuation. Do not initiate therapy until pregnancy status confirmed. Unknown if crosses placenta or distributed in breast milk. Nursing mothers must discontinue either nursing or drug therapy. **Children:** Safety and efficacy not established. **Elderly:** No age-related precautions noted.

INTERACTIONS

DRUG: **Strong CYP3A4 inhibitors (e.g., clarithromycin, ketoconazole, ritonavir)** may increase concentration/effect. **Strong CYP3A4 inducers (e.g., carBAMazepine, phenytoin, rifAMPin)** may decrease concentration/effect. May increase concentration/effect of **aprepitant, bosutinib, budesonide, cobimetinib, cycloSPORINE, ivabradine, neratinib, sirolimus, tacrolimus.** HERBAL: **St. John's wort** may decrease concentration/effect. FOOD: **Grapefruit products** may increase concentration/toxicity (potential for torsades, myelotoxicity). LAB VALUES: May increase serum ALT, AST, alkaline phosphatase, bilirubin. May decrease neutrophils, platelets, lymphocytes.

AVAILABILITY (Rx)

Capsules: 200 mg, 250 mg.

ADMINISTRATION/HANDLING

• May give without regard to food. • Avoid grapefruit products. • Do not break, crush, dissolve, or divide capsules.

INDICATIONS/ROUTES/DOSAGE

Non–Small-Cell Lung Cancer (ALK Positive), Metastatic NSCLC, ROS-1 Positive

PO: ADULTS: 250 mg twice daily. Continue until disease progression or unacceptable toxicity.

Dosage Modification

Interrupt and/or reduce to 200 mg twice daily based on graded protocol, including hematologic toxicity (Grade 4), elevated LFT with bilirubin elevation (Grade 1), QT prolongation (Grade 3). May reduce to 250 mg once daily if indicated. Discontinue treatment for QT prolongation (Grade 4), elevated LFT with bilirubin elevation (Grades 2, 3, 4), pneumonitis of any grade.

Hematologic Toxicity

Grade 3 toxicity (WBC 1,000–2,000 cells/mm^3, ANC 500–1,000 cells/mm^3, platelets 25,000–50,000 cells/mm^3), Grade 3 anemia: Withhold treatment until recovery to Grade 2 or less, then resume at same dosage. **Grade 4 toxicity (WBC less than 1,000 cells/mm^3, ANC less than 500 cells/mm^3, platelets less than 25,000 cells/mm^3), Grade 4 anemia:** Withhold treatment until recovery to Grade 2 or less, then resume at 200 mg twice daily. **Grade 4 toxicity on 200 mg twice daily:** Withhold treatment until recovery to Grade 2 or less, then resume at 250 mg once daily. **Recurrent Grade 4 toxicity on 250 mg once daily:** Permanently discontinue.

Cardiotoxicity

Grade 3 QTc prolongation on at least 2 separate ECGs: Withhold treatment until recovery to baseline or Grade 1 or less. Resume at 200 mg twice daily. **Recurrent Grade 3 QTc prolonga-**

tion on 200 mg twice daily: Withhold treatment until recovery to baseline or Grade 1 or less. Resume at 250 mg once daily. **Recurrent Grade 3 QTc prolongation on 250 mg once daily:** Permanently discontinue.

Bradycardia

Grades 2 or 3: Withhold until recovery to asymptomatic bradycardia or heart rate 60 or more beats/min, evaluate concomitant medications, then resume at 200 mg twice daily. **Grade 4 due to crizotinib:** Permanently discontinue. **Grade 4 associated with concurrent medications known to cause bradycardia/hypotension:** Withhold until recovery to asymptomatic bradycardia or heart rate 60 or more beats/min, and if concurrent medications can be stopped, resume at 250 mg once daily.

Pulmonary Toxicity

Permanently discontinue.

Dosage in Renal Impairment

CrCl less than 30 mL/min: 250 mg once daily.

Dosage in Hepatic Impairment

No dose adjustment (see dose for hepatotoxicity during treatment).

SIDE EFFECTS

Frequent (62%–27%): Diplopia, photopsia, photophobia, blurry vision, visual field defect, vitreous floaters, reduced visual acuity, nausea, diarrhea, vomiting, peripheral/localized edema, constipation. **Occasional (20%–4%):** Fatigue, decreased appetite, dizziness, neuropathy, paresthesia, dysgeusia, dyspepsia, dysphagia, esophageal obstruction/pain/spasm/ulcer, odynophagia, reflux esophagitis, rash, abdominal pain/tenderness, stomatitis, glossodynia, glossitis, cheilitis, mucosal inflammation, oropharyngeal pain/discomfort, bradycardia, headache, cough. **Rare (3%–1%):** Musculoskeletal chest pain, insomnia, dyspnea, arthralgia, nasopharyngitis, rhinitis, pharyngitis, URI, back pain, complex renal cysts, chest pain/tightness.

ADVERSE EFFECTS/TOXIC REACTIONS

Severe, sometimes fatal treatment-related pneumonitis, pneumonia, dyspnea, pulmonary embolism in less than 2% of pts was noted. Grade 3–4 elevation of hepatic enzymes, increased QT prolongation may require discontinuation. May cause thrombocytopenia, neutropenia, lymphopenia. Severe/worsening vitreous floaters, photopsia may indicate retinal hole, retinal detachment.

NURSING CONSIDERATIONS

BASELINE ASSESSMENT

Assess vital signs, O_2 saturation. Obtain baseline CBC with differential, serum chemistries, LFT, PT/INR, ECG; pregnancy test in females of reproductive potential. Obtain full medication history including vitamins, herbal products. Detection of ALK-positive NSCLC test needed prior to treatment. Assess history of tuberculosis, HIV, HF, bradyarrhythmias, electrolyte imbalance, medications that prolong QT interval. Assess visual acuity, history of vitreous floaters. Offer emotional support.

INTERVENTION/EVALUATION

Assess vital signs, O_2 saturation routinely. Monitor CBC with differential monthly, LFT, monthly; increase testing for Grades 2, 3, 4 adverse effects. Obtain ECG for bradycardia, electrolyte imbalance, chest pain, difficulty breathing. Monitor for bruising, hematuria, jaundice, right upper abdominal pain, weight loss, or acute infection (fever, diaphoresis, lethargy, oral mucosal changes, productive cough). Worsening cough, fever, or shortness of breath may indicate pneumonitis. Consider ophthalmological evaluation for vision changes. Reinforce birth control compliance.

C

PATIENT/FAMILY TEACHING

• Report urine changes, bloody or clay-colored stools, upper abdominal pain, nausea, vomiting, bruising, fever, cough, difficulty breathing. • Report history of liver abnormalities or heart problems, including long QT syndrome, syncope, palpitations, extremity swelling. • Immediately report any newly prescribed medications, suspected pregnancy, or vision changes, including light flashes, blurred vision, photophobia, or new or increased floaters. • Use contraception to avoid pregnancy. Do not breastfeed. • Avoid alcohol, grapefruit products.

cyclobenzaprine

sye-kloe-**ben**-za-preen
(Amrix, Fexmid)
Do not confuse cyclobenzaprine with cycloSERINE or cyproheptadine, or Flexeril with Floxin.

◆CLASSIFICATION

PHARMACOTHERAPEUTIC: Centrally acting muscle relaxant. **CLINICAL:** Skeletal muscle relaxant.

USES

Treatment of muscle spasm associated with acute, painful musculoskeletal conditions. **OFF-LABEL:** Treatment of muscle spasms associated with temporomandibular joint pain (TMJ).

PRECAUTIONS

Contraindications: Hypersensitivity to cyclobenzaprine. Acute recovery phase of MI, arrhythmias, HF, heart block, conduction disturbances, hyperthyroidism, use within 14 days of MAOIs. **Cautions:** Hepatic impairment, history of urinary hesitancy or retention, angle-closure glaucoma, increased intraocular pressure (IOP), elderly.

ACTION

Centrally acting skeletal muscle relaxant that reduces tonic somatic muscle activity at level of brainstem. Influences both alpha and gamma motor neurons. **Therapeutic Effect:** Relieves local skeletal muscle spasm.

PHARMACOKINETICS

Route	Onset	Peak	Duration
PO	1 hr	3–4 hrs	12–24 hrs

Well but slowly absorbed from GI tract. Protein binding: 93%. Metabolized in GI tract and liver. Primarily excreted in urine. **Half-life:** 8–37 hrs.

⌛ LIFESPAN CONSIDERATIONS

Pregnancy/Lactation: Unknown if drug crosses placenta or is distributed in breast milk. **Children:** Safety and efficacy not established. **Elderly:** Increased sensitivity to anticholinergic effects (e.g., confusion, urinary retention). Increased risk of falls, fractures. Not recommended.

INTERACTIONS

DRUG: **Alcohol, other CNS depressant medications (e.g., lorazepam, morphine, zolpidem)** may increase CNS depression. **MAOIs (e.g., phenelzine, selegiline)** may increase risk of hypertensive crisis, seizures. **Anticholinergics (e.g., aclidinium, ipratropium, umeclidinium)** may increase anticholinergic effect. **HERBAL:** **Herbals with sedative properties (e.g., chamomile, kava kava, valerian)** may increase CNS depression. **FOOD:** None known. **LAB VALUES:** None significant.

AVAILABILITY (Rx)

Tablets: 5 mg, 7.5 mg, 10 mg.

Capsules: ***(Extended-Release [Amrix]):*** 15 mg, 30 mg.

ADMINISTRATION/HANDLING

PO

• Give without regard to food. • Do not break, crush, dissolve, or divide extended-release capsule. • Give extended-release capsule at same time each day.

INDICATIONS/ROUTES/DOSAGE

◀ALERT▶ Do not use longer than 2–3 wks.

Acute, Painful Musculoskeletal Conditions

PO: ADULTS, ELDERLY, CHILDREN 15 YRS AND OLDER: Initially, 5 mg 3 times/day. May increase to 7.5–10 mg 3 times/day.

PO: *(Extended-Release)*: ADULTS: 15–30 mg once daily. Not recommended in elderly.

Dosage in Renal Impairment

No dose adjustment.

Dosage in Hepatic Impairment

Note: Extended-release capsule not recommended in hepatic impairment. **Mild impairment:** 5 mg 3 times/day. **Moderate to severe impairment:** Not recommended.

SIDE EFFECTS

Frequent (39%–11%): Drowsiness, dry mouth, dizziness. **Rare (3%–1%):** Fatigue, asthenia, blurred vision, headache, anxiety, confusion, nausea, constipation, dyspepsia, unpleasant taste.

ADVERSE EFFECTS/TOXIC REACTIONS

Overdose may result in visual hallucinations, hyperactive reflexes, muscle rigidity, vomiting, hyperpyrexia.

NURSING CONSIDERATIONS

BASELINE ASSESSMENT

Record onset, type, location, duration of muscular spasm. Check for immobility, stiffness, swelling.

INTERVENTION/EVALUATION

Assist with ambulation. Assess for therapeutic response: relief of pain; decreased stiffness, swelling; increased joint mobility; reduced joint tenderness; improved grip strength.

PATIENT/FAMILY TEACHING

• Avoid tasks that require alertness, motor skills until response to drug is established. • Drowsiness usually diminishes with continued therapy. • Avoid alcohol, other depressants while taking medication. • Avoid sudden changes in posture. • Sugarless gum, sips of water may relieve dry mouth.

cyclophosphamide HIGH ALERT

sye-kloe-**foss**-fa-mide
(Procytox ✦)

Do not confuse cyclophosphamide with cycloSPORINE or ifosfamide.

◆CLASSIFICATION

PHARMACOTHERAPEUTIC: Alkylating agent. **CLINICAL:** Antineoplastic.

USES

Treatment of acute lymphocytic, acute nonlymphocytic, chronic myelocytic, chronic lymphocytic leukemias; ovarian, breast carcinomas; neuroblastoma; retinoblastoma; Hodgkin's, non-Hodgkin's lymphomas; multiple myeloma; mycosis fungoides; nephrotic syndrome in children. **OFF-LABEL:** Treatment of adrenocortical, bladder, cervical, endometrial, prostatic, testicular carcinomas; Ewing's sarcoma; multiple sclerosis; non–small-cell, small-cell lung cancer; organ transplant rejection; osteosarcoma; ovarian germ cell, primary brain, trophoblastic tumors; rheumatoid arthritis; soft-tissue sarcomas; systemic dermatomyositis; systemic lupus erythematosus; Wilms' tumor.

PRECAUTIONS

Contraindications: Hypersensitivity to cyclophosphamide. Urinary outflow ob-

C

struction. **Cautions:** Severe leukopenia, thrombocytopenia, tumor infiltration of bone marrow, previous therapy with other antineoplastic agents, radiation, renal/hepatic/cardiac impairment, active UTI.

ACTION

Inhibits DNA, RNA protein synthesis by cross-linking with DNA, RNA strands. Cell cycle–phase nonspecific. **Therapeutic Effect:** Prevents cell growth. Potent immunosuppressant.

PHARMACOKINETICS

Well absorbed from GI tract. Protein binding: 10%–60%. Crosses blood-brain barrier. Metabolized in liver. Primarily excreted in urine. Removed by hemodialysis. **Half-life:** 3–12 hrs.

LIFESPAN CONSIDERATIONS

Pregnancy/Lactation: If possible, avoid use during pregnancy. Use of effective contraception during therapy and up to 1 yr after completion of therapy is recommended. May cause fetal malformations (limb abnormalities, cardiac anomalies, hernias). Distributed in breast milk. Breastfeeding not recommended. **Children:** No age-related precautions noted. **Elderly:** Age-related renal impairment may require dosage adjustment.

INTERACTIONS

DRUG: **CYP2D6 inducers (e.g., carBAMazepine, PHENobarbital)** may decrease concentration/effect. **Anthracycline agents (e.g., DOXOrubicin, epiRUBicin)** may increase risk of cardiomyopathy. **Live virus vaccines** may potentiate virus replication, increase vaccine side effects, decrease pt's antibody response to vaccine. **HERBAL:** Pts with an estrogen-dependent tumor should avoid **black cohosh, dong quai.** **FOOD:** None known. **LAB VALUES:** May increase serum uric acid.

AVAILABILITY (Rx)

Capsules: 25 mg, 50 mg. **Injection, Powder for Reconstitution:** 500 mg, 1 g, 2 g.

ADMINISTRATION/HANDLING

◄ALERT► May be carcinogenic, mutagenic, teratogenic. Handle with extreme care during preparation/administration.

IV

Reconstitution • Reconstitute each 100 mg with 5 mL Sterile Water for Injection, 0.9% NaCl, or D_5W to provide concentration of 20 mg/mL. • Shake to dissolve. • Allow to stand until clear.

Rate of administration • Infusion rates vary based on protocol. May give by direct IV injection, IV piggyback, or continuous IV infusion.

Storage • Reconstituted solution in 0.9% NaCl is stable for 24 hrs at room temperature or up to 6 days if refrigerated.

PO

• Give on an empty stomach. If GI upset occurs, give with food. • Do not cut or crush. • To minimize risk of bladder irritation, do not give at bedtime.

IV INCOMPATIBILITIES

Amphotericin B complex (Abelcet, AmBisome, Amphotec).

IV COMPATIBILITIES

Granisetron (Kytril), heparin, HYDROmorphone (Dilaudid), LORazepam (Ativan), morphine, ondansetron (Zofran), propofol (Diprivan).

INDICATIONS/ROUTES/DOSAGE

Note: Hematologic toxicity may require dose reduction.

Usual Dosage (Refer to Individual Protocols)

IV: **ADULTS, ELDERLY, CHILDREN:** (Single agent): 40–50 mg/kg in divided doses over 2–5 days or 10–15 mg/kg q7–10 days or 3–5 mg/kg twice wkly.

PO: ADULTS, ELDERLY, CHILDREN: 1–5 mg/kg/day.

Nephrotic Syndrome
PO: ADULTS, CHILDREN: 2 mg/kg/day for 60–90 days. **Maximum cumulative dose:** 168 mg/kg.

Dosage in Renal/Hepatic Impairment
No dose adjustment. Use caution.

SIDE EFFECTS

Expected: Marked leukopenia 8–15 days after initiation. **Frequent:** Nausea, vomiting (beginning about 6 hrs after administration and lasting about 4 hrs); alopecia (33%). **Occasional:** Diarrhea, darkening of skin/fingernails, stomatitis, headache, diaphoresis. **Rare:** Pain/redness at injection site.

ADVERSE EFFECTS/TOXIC REACTIONS

Myelosuppression (leukopenia, anemia, thrombocytopenia, hypoprothrombinemia) is an expected response to therapy. Expect leukopenia to resolve in 17–28 days. Anemia generally occurs after large doses or prolonged therapy. Thrombocytopenia may occur 10–15 days after drug initiation. Hemorrhagic cystitis occurs commonly in long-term therapy (esp. in children). Pulmonary fibrosis, cardiotoxicity noted with high doses. Amenorrhea, azoospermia, hyperkalemia may occur.

NURSING CONSIDERATIONS

BASELINE ASSESSMENT

Obtain CBC wkly during therapy or until maintenance dose is established, then at 2- to 3-wk intervals. Question history of urinary outlet flow obstruction, hepatic/renal impairment, active infections. Obtain pregnancy test in females of reproductive potential.

INTERVENTION/EVALUATION

Monitor CBC, serum BUN, creatinine, electrolytes, urine output. Monitor WBC counts closely during initial therapy. Monitor for hematologic toxicity (fever, sore throat, signs of local infection, unusual bruising/bleeding from any site), symptoms of anemia (excessive fatigue, weakness). Recovery from marked leukopenia due to myelosuppression can be expected in 17–28 days.

PATIENT/FAMILY TEACHING

• Encourage copious fluid intake, frequent voiding (assists in preventing cystitis) at least 24 hrs before, during, after therapy. • Do not have immunizations without physician's approval (drug lowers resistance). • Avoid contact with those who have recently received live virus vaccine. • Promptly report fever, sore throat, signs of local infection, difficulty or pain with urination, unusual bruising/bleeding from any site. • Hair loss is reversible, but new hair growth may have different color, texture. • Avoid pregnancy for up to 1 yr after completion of treatment.

cycloSPORINE

sye-kloe-**spor**-in
(Gengraf, Neoral, Restasis, SandIMMUNE)

BLACK BOX ALERT Only physicians experienced in management of immunosuppressive therapy and organ transplant pts should prescribe. Renal impairment may occur with high dosage. Increased risk of neoplasia, susceptibility to infections. May cause hypertension, nephrotoxicity. Psoriasis pts: Increased risk of developing skin malignancies. The modified/nonmodified formulations are not bioequivalent and cannot be used interchangeably without close monitoring.

Do not confuse cycloSPORINE with cycloSERINE or cyclophosphamide, Gengraf with ProGraf, Neoral with Neurontin or Nizoral, or SandIMMUNE with SandoSTATIN.

C

CLASSIFICATION

PHARMACOTHERAPEUTIC: Calcineurin inhibitor. **CLINICAL:** Immunosuppressant.

USES

Modified, Nonmodified: Prevents organ rejection of kidney, liver, heart in combination with steroid therapy and an antiproliferative immunosuppressive agent. **Nonmodified:** Treatment of chronic allograft rejection in those previously treated with other immunosuppressives. **Modified:** Treatment of severe, active rheumatoid arthritis, severe recalcitrant plaque psoriasis in nonimmunocompromised adults. **Ophthalmic:** Chronic dry eyes. **OFF-LABEL:** Allogenic stem cell transplants for prevention/treatment of graft-vs-host disease; focal segmental glomerulosclerosis, lupus nephritis, severe ulcerative colitis.

PRECAUTIONS

Contraindications: History of hypersensitivity to cycloSPORINE, polyoxyethylated castor oil; rheumatoid arthritis, psoriasis, uncontrolled hypertension, renal impairment, or malignancies in treatment of psoriasis or rheumatoid arthritis. **Cautions:** Hepatic/renal impairment. History of seizures. Avoid live vaccines.

ACTION

Inhibits cellular, humoral immune responses by inhibiting interleukin-2, a proliferative factor needed for T-cell activity. **Therapeutic Effect:** Prevents organ rejection, relieves symptoms of psoriasis, arthritis.

PHARMACOKINETICS

Variably absorbed from GI tract. Protein binding: 90%. Metabolized in liver. Eliminated primarily by biliary or fecal excretion. Not removed by hemodialysis. **Half-life:** Adults, 10–27 hrs; children, 7–19 hrs.

LIFESPAN CONSIDERATIONS

Pregnancy/Lactation: Readily crosses placenta. Distributed in breast milk. Breastfeeding not recommended. **Children:** No age-related precautions noted in transplant pts. **Elderly:** Increased risk of hypertension, increased serum creatinine.

INTERACTIONS

DRUG: May increase concentration/effects of **aliskiren, atorvastatin, dronedarone, lovastatin, pazopanib, simvastatin. Strong CYP3A4 inhibitors (e.g., clarithromycin, ketoconazole, ritonavir)** may increase concentration/effect. **Strong CYP3A4 inducers (e.g., carBAMazepine, phenytoin, rifAMPin)** may decrease concentration/effect. **Live virus vaccines** may potentiate virus replication, increase vaccine side effects, decrease pt's response to vaccine. **HERBAL: Echinacea** may decrease therapeutic effect. **FOOD: Grapefruit products** may increase absorption/immunosuppression, risk of toxicity. **LAB VALUES:** May increase serum BUN, alkaline phosphatase, amylase, bilirubin, creatinine, potassium, uric acid, ALT, AST. May decrease serum magnesium. **Therapeutic peak serum level:** 50–400 ng/mL; **toxic serum level:** greater than 400 ng/mL.

AVAILABILITY (Rx)

Capsules: ***(Gengraf, Neoral [Modified], SandIMMUNE [Nonmodified]):*** 25 mg, 50 mg, 100 mg. **Injection, Solution:** ***(SandIMMUNE):*** 50 mg/mL. **Ophthalmic Emulsion:** ***(Restasis):*** 0.05%. **Oral Solution:** ***(Gengraf, Neoral [Modified], SandIMMUNE [Nonmodified]):*** 100 mg/mL.

ADMINISTRATION/HANDLING

◀ALERT▶ Oral solution available in bottle form with calibrated liquid measuring device. Oral form should replace IV administration as soon as possible.

IV

Reconstitution • Dilute each mL (50 mg) concentrate with 20–100 mL 0.9% NaCl or D_5W (**maximum concentration:** 2.5 mg/mL).

Rate of administration • Infuse over 2–6 hrs. • Monitor pt continuously for hypersensitivity reaction (facial flushing, dyspnea).

Storage • Store parenteral form at room temperature. • Protect IV solution from light. • After diluted, stable for 6 hrs in PVC; 24 hrs in non-PVC or glass.

PO

• Administer consistently with relation to time of day and meals. • Oral solution may be mixed in glass container with milk, chocolate milk, orange juice, or apple juice (preferably at room temperature). Stir well. • Drink immediately. • Add more diluent to glass container. Mix with remaining solution to ensure total amount is given. • Dry outside of calibrated liquid measuring device before replacing cover. • Do not rinse with water. • Avoid refrigeration of oral solution (solution may separate). • Discard oral solution after 2 mos once bottle is opened.

Ophthalmic

• Invert vial several times to obtain uniform suspension. • Instruct pt to remove contact lenses before administration (may reinsert 15 min after administration). • May use with artificial tears.

IV INCOMPATIBILITIES

Acyclovir (Zovirax), amphotericin B complex (Abelcet, AmBisome, Amphotec), magnesium.

IV COMPATIBILITIES

Propofol (Diprivan).

INDICATIONS/ROUTES/DOSAGE

Note: The modified/nonmodified formulations are not bioequivalent and cannot be used interchangeably without close monitoring. Refer to institutional protocols. Dosing in clinical practice may differ greatly compared to manufacturer's labeling.

Transplantation, Prevention of Organ Rejection

Note: Initial dose given 4–12 hrs prior to transplant or postoperatively.

PO: ADULTS, ELDERLY, CHILDREN: Not modified: Initially, 10–12 mg/kg daily for 1–2 wks, then taper by 5% each wk to maintenance dose of 5–10 mg/kg daily. **Modified:** (dose dependent upon type of transplant). **Renal:** 6–12 mg/kg/day in 2 divided doses. **Hepatic:** 4–12 mg/kg/day in 2 divided doses. **Heart:** 4–10 mg/kg/day in 2 divided doses.

IV: ADULTS, ELDERLY, CHILDREN: Not modified: Initially, 5–6 mg/kg/dose daily. Switch to oral as soon as possible.

Rheumatoid Arthritis

PO: ADULTS, ELDERLY: Modified: Initially, 2.5 mg/kg a day in 2 divided doses. May increase by 0.5–0.75 mg/kg/day after 8 wks with additional increases made at 12 wks. **Maximum:** 4 mg/kg/day.

Psoriasis

PO: ADULTS, ELDERLY: Modified: Initially, 2.5 mg/kg/day in 2 divided doses. May increase by 0.5 mg/kg/day after 4 wks; additional increases may be made q2wks. **Maximum:** 4 mg/kg/day.

Dry Eye

Ophthalmic: ADULTS, ELDERLY: Instill 1 drop in each affected eye q12h.

Dosage in Renal Impairment

Modify dose if serum creatinine levels 25% or above pretreatment levels.

Dosage in Hepatic Impairment

Mild to moderate impairment: No dose adjustment. **Severe impairment:** Use caution.

SIDE EFFECTS

Frequent (26%–12%): Mild to moderate hypertension, hirsutism, tremor. **Occasional (4%–2%):** Acne, leg cramps, gingival hyperplasia (red, bleeding, tender gums), paresthesia, diarrhea, nausea, vomiting, headache. **Rare (less than 1%):** Hypersensitivity reaction, abdominal discomfort, gynecomastia, sinusitis.

ADVERSE EFFECTS/TOXIC REACTIONS

Mild nephrotoxicity occurs in 25% of renal transplants, 38% of cardiac transplants, 37% of liver transplants, generally 2–3 mos after transplantation (more severe toxicity may occur soon after transplantation). Hepatotoxicity occurs in 4% of renal, 7% of cardiac, and 4% of liver transplants, generally within first mo after transplantation. Both toxicities usually respond to dosage reduction. Severe hyperkalemia, hyperuricemia occur occasionally.

NURSING CONSIDERATIONS

BASELINE ASSESSMENT

Obtain BMP, LFT. If nephrotoxicity occurs, mild toxicity is generally noted 2–3 mos after transplantation; more severe toxicity noted early after transplantation; hepatotoxicity may be noted during first mo after transplantation.

INTERVENTION/EVALUATION

Diligently monitor serum BUN, creatinine, bilirubin, ALT, AST, LDH levels for evidence of hepatotoxicity/nephrotoxicity (mild toxicity noted by slow rise in serum levels; more overt toxicity noted by rapid rise in levels; hematuria also noted in nephrotoxicity). Monitor serum potassium for hyperkalemia. Encourage diligent oral hygiene (gingival hyperplasia). Monitor B/P for evidence of hypertension. **Note:** Reference ranges dependent on organ transplanted, organ function, cycloSPORINE toxicity. Trough levels should be obtained immediately prior to next dose. **Therapeutic serum level:** 50–400 ng/mL; **toxic serum level:** greater than 400 ng/mL.

PATIENT/FAMILY TEACHING

• Report severe headache, persistent nausea/vomiting, unusual swelling of extremities, chest pain. • Avoid grapefruit products (increases concentration/effects), St. John's wort (decreases concentration). • Do not take any newly prescribed or OTC medications unless approved by the prescriber who originally started treatment.

cytarabine HIGH ALERT

sye-**tar**-a-bine
(Ara-C, Cytosar-U ✱, Depo-Cyt ✱)

■ BLACK BOX ALERT ■ Must be administered by personnel trained in administration/handling of chemotherapeutic agents. **Conventional:** Potent myelosuppressant. High risk of multiple toxicities (GI, CNS, pulmonary, cardiac). **Liposomal:** Chemical arachnoiditis, manifested by profound nausea, vomiting, fever, may be fatal if untreated.

Do not confuse cytarabine with Cytoxan or vidarabine, or Cytosar with Cytoxan or Neosar.

◆CLASSIFICATION

PHARMACOTHERAPEUTIC: Antimetabolite. **CLINICAL:** Antineoplastic.

USES

Conventional: Remission induction in acute myeloid leukemia (AML), treatment of acute lymphoblastic leukemia (ALL) and chronic myeloid leukemia (CML), prophylaxis and treatment of meningeal leukemia. **Liposomal:** Treatment of lymphomatous meningitis. **OFF-LABEL: Ara-C:** Carcinomatous meningitis, Hodgkin's and non-Hodgkin's lymphomas, myelodysplastic syndrome.

PRECAUTIONS

Contraindications: Hypersensitivity to cytarabine. **Liposomal:** Active meningeal infection. **Cautions:** Renal/hepatic impairment, prior drug-induced bone marrow suppression.

ACTION

Inhibits DNA polymerase. Cell cycle–specific for S phase of cell division. **Therapeutic Effect:** Inhibits DNA synthesis. Potent immunosuppressive activity.

PHARMACOKINETICS

Widely distributed; moderate amount crosses blood-brain barrier. Protein binding: 15%. Primarily excreted in urine. **Half-life:** 1–3 hrs.

LIFESPAN CONSIDERATIONS

Pregnancy/Lactation: If possible, avoid use during pregnancy. May cause fetal malformations. Unknown if distributed in breast milk. Breastfeeding not recommended. **Children:** No age-related precautions noted. **Elderly:** Age-related renal impairment may require dosage adjustment.

INTERACTIONS

DRUG: May decrease therapeutic effect of **BCG (intravesical), vaccines (live).** May increase adverse effects of **vaccines (live).** May increase adverse effects of **natalizumab. HERBAL: Echinacea** may decrease therapeutic effect. **FOOD:** None known. **LAB VALUES:** May increase serum alkaline phosphatase, bilirubin, uric acid, AST.

AVAILABILITY (Rx)

Injection, Solution (Conventional): 20 mg/mL, 100 mg/mL. **Injection, Suspension (Liposomal):** 10 mg/mL.

ADMINISTRATION/HANDLING

◀ALERT▶ May give by subcutaneous, IV push, IV infusion, intrathecal routes at concentration not to exceed 100 mg/mL. May be carcinogenic, mutagenic, teratogenic (embryonic deformity). Handle with extreme care during preparation/administration. Liposomal for intrathecal use only.

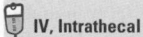

IV, Intrathecal

Reconstitution • Dilute with 250–1,000 mL D_5W or 0.9% NaCl for IV infusion. • **Intrathecal:** reconstitute vial with preservative-free 0.9% NaCl or pt's spinal fluid. Dose usually administered in 5–15 mL of solution, after equivalent volume of CSF removed. • **Liposomal:** No reconstitution required.

Rate of administration • Conventional: For IV infusion, give over 1–3 hrs or as continuous infusion.

Storage • Conventional: Store at room temperature. • Reconstituted solution is stable for 48 hrs at room temperature. • Use diluted solution within 24 hrs. • Discard if slight haze develops. • Liposomal: Refrigerate; use within 4 hrs following withdrawal from vial.

IV INCOMPATIBILITIES

Amphotericin B complex (Abelcet, AmBisome, Amphotec), ganciclovir (Cytovene), heparin, insulin (regular).

IV COMPATIBILITIES

Dexamethasone (Decadron), diphenhydrAMINE (Benadryl), filgrastim (Neupogen), granisetron (Kytril), HYDROmorphone (Dilaudid), LORazepam (Ativan), morphine, ondansetron (Zofran), potassium chloride, propofol (Diprivan).

INDICATIONS/ROUTES/DOSAGE

Usual Dosage for Induction (Conventional) (Refer to Individual Protocols)

IV: ADULTS, ELDERLY, CHILDREN: (Induction): 100 mg/m²/day continuous infusion for 7 days or 200 mg/m²/day continuous infusion (as 100 mg/m² over 12 hrs q12h) for 7 days.

Dosage in Renal/Hepatic Impairment

No dose adjustment.

SIDE EFFECTS

Frequent: IV (33%–16%): Asthenia, fever, pain, altered taste/smell, nausea, vomiting (risk greater with IV push than with continuous IV infusion). **Intrathecal (28%–11%):** Headache, asthenia, altered taste/smell, confusion, drowsiness, nausea, vomiting. **Occasional: IV (11%–7%):** Abnormal gait, drowsiness, constipation, back pain, urinary incontinence, peripheral edema, headache, confusion. **Intrathecal (7%–3%):** Peripheral edema, back pain, constipation, abnormal gait, urinary incontinence.

ADVERSE EFFECTS/TOXIC REACTIONS

Myelosuppression (leukopenia, anemia, thrombocytopenia, megaloblastosis, reticulocytopenia), occurring minimally after single IV dose. Leukopenia, anemia, thrombocytopenia should be expected with daily or continuous IV therapy. Cytarabine syndrome (fever, myalgia, rash, conjunctivitis, malaise, chest pain), hyperuricemia may occur. High-dose therapy may produce severe CNS, GI, pulmonary toxicity.

NURSING CONSIDERATIONS

BASELINE ASSESSMENT

Obtain baseline CBC, renal function, LFT. Leukocyte count decreases within 24 hrs after initial dose, continues to decrease for 7–9 days followed by brief rise at 12 days, decreases again at 15–24 days, then rises rapidly for next 10 days. Platelet count decreases 5 days after drug initiation to its lowest count at 12–15 days, then rises rapidly for next 10 days.

INTERVENTION/EVALUATION

Monitor BMP, LFT; serum uric acid. Monitor CBC for myelosuppression. Monitor for blood dyscrasias (fever, sore throat, signs of local infection, unusual bruising/bleeding from any site), symptoms of anemia (excessive fatigue, weakness). Monitor for signs of neuropathy (gait disturbances, handwriting difficulties, paresthesia).

PATIENT/FAMILY TEACHING

• Increase fluid intake (may protect against hyperuricemia). • Do not have immunizations without physician's approval (drug lowers resistance). • Avoid contact with those who have recently received live virus vaccine. • Promptly report fever, sore throat, signs of local infection, unusual bruising/bleeding from any site.

dabigatran

TOP 100

dab-i-**gah**-tran
(Pradaxa)

■ BLACK BOX ALERT ■ Risk of thrombotic events (e.g., stroke) is increased if discontinued for a reason other than pathological bleeding. Spinal or epidural hematoma may occur with neuraxial anesthesia.

◆CLASSIFICATION

PHARMACOTHERAPEUTIC: Direct thrombin inhibitor. **CLINICAL:** Anticoagulant.

USES

Indicated to reduce risk of stroke, systemic embolism in pts with nonvalvular atrial fibrillation. Treatment and reduction of risk of deep vein thrombosis (DVT) and pulmonary embolism (PE). Prophylaxis of DVT and PE in pts who have undergone hip replacement surgery.

PRECAUTIONS

Contraindications: Severe hypersensitivity to dabigatran. Active major bleeding, pts with mechanical prosthetic heart valves. **Cautions:** Renal impairment (CrCl 15–30 mL/min), moderate hepatic impairment, invasive procedures, spinal anesthesia, major surgery, pts with congenital or acquired bleeding disorders, elderly, concurrent use of medications that increase risk of bleeding, valvular heart disease.

ACTION

Reversible direct thrombin inhibitor that inhibits both free and fibrin-bound thrombin. **Therapeutic Effect:** Produces anticoagulation, preventing development of thrombus.

PHARMACOKINETICS

Metabolized in liver. Protein binding: 35%. Eliminated primarily in urine. **Half-life:** 12–17 hrs.

LIFESPAN CONSIDERATIONS

Pregnancy/Lactation: Unknown if distributed in breast milk. **Children:** Safety and efficacy not established in pts younger than 18 yrs. **Elderly:** Severe renal impairment may require dosage adjustment.

INTERACTIONS

DRUG: **Amiodarone, dronedarone, P-glycoprotein/ABCB1 inhibitors (e.g., amiodarone, colchicine, omeprazole)** may increase concentration/effect. **Antacids, P-glycoprotein (P-gp)/ABCB1 inducers (e.g., carBAMazepine, phenytoin)** may decrease concentration/effect. **Apixaban, edoxaban** may increase anticoagulant effect. **Aspirin, vorapaxar** may increase adverse effects. **HERBAL:** **Herbals with anticoagulant/antiplatelet properties (e.g., garlic, ginger, ginkgo biloba)** may increase effect. **St. John's wort** may decrease concentration/effect. **FOOD:** **High-fat meal** delays absorption approx. 2 hrs. **LAB VALUES:** May increase aPTT, PT, INR.

AVAILABILITY (Rx)

Capsules: 75 mg, 110 mg, 150 mg.

ADMINISTRATION/HANDLING

PO

- May be given without regard to food. Administer with water.
- Do not break, cut, open capsules.

INDICATIONS/ROUTES/DOSAGE

◀ALERT▶ Medication should be discontinued prior to invasive or surgical procedures.

Treatment/Prevention of DVT/PE

PO: ADULTS, ELDERLY: 150 mg twice daily (after at least 5–10 days of treatment with parenteral anticoagulants).

Nonvalvular Atrial Fibrillation

PO: ADULTS, ELDERLY: 150 mg twice daily (to reduce risk of stroke/systemic embolism).

Prophylaxis Following Hip Surgery
PO: ADULTS, ELDERLY: 110 mg on day one (1–4 hr postoperative and established hemostasis), then 220 mg daily for a minimum of 10–14 days up to 35 days.

Dosage in Renal Impairment
Nonvalvular atrial fibrillation: CrCl 15–30 mL/min: Reduce dose to 75 mg twice daily. **CrCl less than 15 mL/min, or HD:** Not recommended (HD removes ~60% over 2–3 hrs). **CrCl 30–50 mL/min with concomitant use of P-gp inhibitors:** Reduce dose to 75 mg twice daily if given with P-gp inhibitors dronedarone or ketoconazole (systemic). **CrCl less than 30 mL/min with concomitant use of P-gp inhibitors:** Avoid coadministration.
Treatment/Prevention of DVT/PE: CrCl less than or equal to 30 mL/min: Not specified. **CrCl less than 50 mL/min with concomitant use of P-gp inhibitors:** Avoid coadministration.
Prophylaxis following hip surgery: CrCl less than or equal to 30 mL/min: Not specified. **CrCl less than 50 mL/min with concomitant use of P-gp inhibitors:** Avoid coadministration.

Dosage in Hepatic Impairment
No dosage adjustment.

SIDE EFFECTS

Frequent (less than 16%): Dyspepsia (heartburn, nausea, indigestion), diarrhea, upper abdominal pain.

ADVERSE EFFECTS/TOXIC REACTIONS

Severe, sometimes fatal, hemorrhagic events, including intracranial hemorrhage, hemorrhagic stroke, GI bleeding, may occur. Hypersensitivity reactions, including anaphylaxis, reported in less than 1% of pts.

NURSING CONSIDERATIONS

BASELINE ASSESSMENT

Obtain CBC (esp. platelet count), BUN, serum creatinine; GFR, CrCl. Question history of mechanical heart valve, recent surgery; hepatic, renal impairment; recent spinal, epidural procedures; recent hemorrhagic events (intracranial hemorrhage, hemorrhagic stroke, GI/GU bleeding). Receive full medication history and screen for interactions. Screen for active bleeding.

INTERVENTION/EVALUATION

Obtain aPTT, platelet count if bleeding occurs. Assess for any signs of bleeding (hematuria, melena, bleeding from gums, petechiae, bruising), hematoma, hypotension, tachycardia, abdominal pain. Question for increase in discharge during menses. Use care when removing adhesives, tape. Monitor for symptoms of intracranial hemorrhage (altered mental status, aphasia, lethargy, hemiparesis, hemiplegia, seizures, vision changes).

PATIENT/FAMILY TEACHING

• Treatment may increase risk of bleeding. • Report dark or bloody urine, black or bloody stool, coffee-ground vomitus, bloody sputum, nosebleeds. • Stroke-like symptoms may indicate bleeding into the brain; report difficulty speaking, headache, numbness, paralysis, vision changes, seizures. • Do not chew, crush, open, or divide capsules. • Use electric razor, soft toothbrush to prevent bleeding. • Do not take newly prescribed medications, including OTC medications such as ibuprofen or naproxen, unless approved by physician who originally started treatment. • Stopping therapy may increase the risk of blood clots or stroke.

dabrafenib

da-**braf**-e-nib
(Tafinlar)
Do not confuse dabrafenib with dasatinib.

◆CLASSIFICATION

PHARMACOTHERAPEUTIC: BRAF kinase inhibitor. **CLINICAL:** Antineoplastic.

USES

Treatment of unresectable or metastatic melanoma with BRAF V600E mutation (single-agent therapy) or in pts with BRAF V600E or V600K mutations (in combination with trametinib). Adjuvant treatment of melanoma (in combination with trametinib) in pts with a BRAF V600E or BRAF V600K mutation, and lymph node involvement. Treatment of metastatic non–small-cell lung cancer (NSCLC) in combination with trametinib in pts with BRAF V600E mutation. Treatment of locally advanced or metastatic anaplastic thyroid cancer (in combination with trametinib) in pts with BRAF V600E mutation and with no satisfactory locoregional treatment options.

◀ALERT▶ Not indicated for treatment of wild-type BRAF melanomas, wild-type BRAF NSCLC, or wild-type BRAF anaplastic thyroid cancer.

PRECAUTIONS

Contraindications: Hypersensitivity to dabrafenib. **Cautions:** Diabetes, hepatic/renal impairment, dehydration, glucose-6-phosphate dehydrogenase (G6PD) deficiency, pts at increased risk for arrhythmias, HF.

ACTION

Selectively inhibits some mutant forms of protein kinase B-raf (BRAF). **Therapeutic Effect:** Inhibits tumor cell growth and survival.

PHARMACOKINETICS

Widely distributed. Metabolized in liver. Protein binding: 99.7%. Peak plasma concentration: 2 hrs. Excreted in feces (71%), urine (23%). **Half-life:** 8 hrs.

LIFESPAN CONSIDERATIONS

Pregnancy/Lactation: Avoid pregnancy; may cause fetal harm. Must use effective nonhormonal contraception during treatment and for at least 2 wks after discontinuation (intrauterine device, barrier methods). Unknown if distributed in breast milk. May impair fertility in females and males. **Children:** Safety and efficacy not established. **Elderly:** May have increased risk of adverse effects, skin lesions.

INTERACTIONS

DRUG: **Strong CYP2C8 inhibitors (e.g., gemfibrozil), strong CYP3A4 inhibitors (e.g., clarithromycin, ketoconazole, ritonavir)** may increase concentration/effect. **Strong CYP3A4 inducers (e.g., carBAMazepine, phenytoin, rifAMPin)** may decrease concentration/effect. May increase concentration/effects of **pazopanib, topotecan, voxilaprevir.** May decrease concentration/effect of **abemaciclib, axitinib, neratinib, olaparib, ranolazine.** May decrease effectiveness of **hormonal contraceptives.** **HERBAL:** **St. John's wort** may decrease concentration/effect. **FOOD:** **High-fat meals** may decrease absorption/effect. **LAB VALUES:** May increase serum glucose, alkaline phosphatase. May decrease serum phosphate, sodium.

AVAILABILITY (Rx)

Capsules: 50 mg, 75 mg.

ADMINISTRATION/HANDLING

PO

• Give at least 1 hr before or at least 2 hrs after meal. • Do not break, crush, open, or divide capsule. • Missed dose may be given up to 6 hrs before next dose.

INDICATIONS/ROUTES/DOSAGE

Melanoma, Metastatic/unresectable (With BRAF V600E mutation)

PO: **ADULTS, ELDERLY:** 150 mg twice daily (about 12 hrs apart). Continue until disease progression or unacceptable toxicity.

Melanoma (Metastatic/unresectable or adjuvant), NSCLC

PO: **ADULTS, ELDERLY:** 150 mg twice daily (in combination with trametinib). Continue until disease progression or unacceptable toxicity.

Dose Modification

Based on Common Terminology Criteria for Adverse Events (CTCAE).

Reduction Levels	Dose
1st dose reduction	100 mg twice daily
2nd dose reduction	75 mg twice daily
3rd dose reduction	50 mg twice daily

Cardiac

Symptomatic HF; absolute decrease in LVEF greater than 20% from baseline that is below the lower limit of normal: Withhold treatment until cardiac function improves, then resume at same dose.

D

Febrile Drug Reaction

Fever 101.3°F–104°F: Withhold treatment until resolved. Then resume at same dose (or at reduced dose level). **Fever greater than 104°F; fever associated with dehydration, hypotension, renal failure:** Withhold treatment until resolved, then resume at reduced dose level (or permanently discontinue).

Dermatologic Toxicity

Intolerable Grade 2 or any Grade 3 or 4 dermatologic toxicity: Withhold treatment for up to 3 wks. If improved, resume at reduced dose level. If not improved, permanently discontinue.

New Primary Malignancies

Noncutaneous RAS mutation-positive malignancies: Permanently discontinue.

Uveitis

Uveitis (including iritis and iridocyclitis): If mild to moderate uveitis does not improve with ocular therapy or if severe uveitis occurs, withhold treatment for up to 6 wks. If improved to Grade 1 or 0, resume at same dose (or at reduced dose level). If not improved, permanently discontinue.

Any Other Toxicity

Intolerable Grade 2 or any Grade 3 toxicity: Withhold treatment until improved to Grade 1 or 0, then resume at reduced dose level. If not improved, permanently discontinue. **First occurrence of any Grade 4 toxicity:** Withhold treatment until improved to Grade 1 or 0, then resume at reduced dose level (or permanently discontinue). **Recurrence of any Grade 4 toxicity:** Permanently discontinue.

Dosage in Renal Impairment

Mild to moderate impairment: No dosage adjustment. **Severe impairment:** Not specified; use caution.

Dosage in Hepatic Impairment

Mild impairment: No dosage adjustment. **Moderate to severe impairment:** Not specified; use caution.

SIDE EFFECTS

Frequent (37%–17%): Hyperkeratosis, headache, pyrexia, arthralgia, alopecia, rash. **Occasional (12%–10%):** Back pain, cough, myalgia, constipation, nasopharyngitis, fatigue.

ADVERSE EFFECTS/TOXIC REACTIONS

Cutaneous squamous cell carcinoma (cuSCC) and keratoacanthomas reported in 7% of pts (esp. elderly, prior skin cancer, chronic sun exposure). Skin reactions including palmar-plantar erythrodysesthesia syndrome (PPES), papilloma have occurred. May increase cell proliferation of wild-type BRAF melanoma or new malignant melanomas. Eye conditions including uveitis, iritis reported. Hyperglycemia reported in 6% of pts. Serious febrile drug reactions including hypotension, rigors, dehydration reported in 4% of pts. Pts with G6PD deficiency have increased risk of hemolytic anemia. Pancreatitis, interstitial nephritis, bullous rash reported in less than 10% of pts. Hemorrhagic events including GI bleeding, major organ bleeding may occur in pts receiving concomitant trametinib therapy. Cardiomyopathy with an absolute decrease in LVEF greater than 10% was reported.

NURSING CONSIDERATIONS

BASELINE ASSESSMENT

Obtain BMP, blood glucose level; pregnancy test in females of reproductive potential. Confirm BRAF V600 mutation status. Make note of current moles, lesions for future comparison. Conduct ophthalmologic exam, visual acuity.

Receive full medication history (including herbal products) and screen for interactions. Offer emotional support.

INTERVENTION/EVALUATION

Monitor serum electrolytes; serum blood glucose periodically (esp. in pts with diabetes). Obtain CBC if hemolytic anemia suspected in pts with G6PD deficiency. Monitor for signs of hyperglycemia. Assess skin for new moles, lesions q2 mos during treatment and at least 6 mos after discontinuation. Immediately report any vision changes, eye pain/swelling, febrile drug reactions, worsening renal function. Monitor I&Os. Consider echocardiogram in pts suspected of cardiomyopathy, decreased LVEF.

PATIENT/FAMILY TEACHING

• Treatment may increase risk of new cancers. • Do not breastfeed. • Avoid pregnancy; nonhormonal contraception should be used. • Report symptoms of high blood sugar levels (confusion, excessive thirst/hunger, headache, frequent urination); toxic skin reactions (itching, peeling, rash, redness, swelling); eye pain/swelling, vision changes; new moles or lesions of the skin. • Fevers may be complicated by low pressure, dehydration, or kidney failure. • Minimize exposure to sunlight. • Report bleeding of any kind. • Therapy may reduce your heart's ability to pump effectively; report difficulty breathing, chest pain, dizziness, palpitations, swelling of the legs or feet. • Do not take newly prescribed medications unless approved by the prescriber who originally started treatment.

dacomitinib

dak-oh-**mi**-ti-nib
(Vizimpro)
Do not confuse dacomitinib with afatinib, dabrafenib, dasatinib, erlotinib, gefitinib, or osimertinib.

◆CLASSIFICATION

PHARMACOTHERAPEUTIC: Tyrosine kinase inhibitor. Epidermal growth factor receptor (EGFR) inhibitor. **CLINICAL:** Antineoplastic.

USES

First-line treatment of metastatic non–small-cell lung cancer (NSCLC) with EGFR exon 19 deletion or exon 21 L858R substitution mutations.

PRECAUTIONS

Contraindications: Hypersensitivity to dacomitinib. **Cautions:** Baseline anemia, leukopenia; dehydration, diabetes, hepatic impairment; history of pulmonary disease.

ACTION

Irreversibly inhibits kinase activity of human EGFR family and certain EGFR mutations. **Therapeutic Effect:** Inhibits tumor cell growth and metastasis.

PHARMACOKINETICS

Widely distributed. Metabolized in liver. Protein binding: 98%. Peak plasma concentration: 6 hrs. Excreted in feces (79%), urine (3%). **Half-life:** 70 hrs.

LIFESPAN CONSIDERATIONS

Pregnancy/Lactation: Avoid pregnancy; may cause fetal harm. Females of reproductive potential should use effective contraception during treatment and for at least 17 days after discontinuation. Unknown if distributed in breast milk. Breastfeeding not recommended during treatment and for at least 17 days after discontinuation. **Children:** Safety and efficacy not established. **Elderly:** May have higher risk of Grade 3 and 4 toxic reactions; higher frequency of treatment interruptions or discontinuation.

INTERACTIONS

DRUG: **Histamine H_2 receptor antagonists (e.g., famotidine), proton pump inhibitors (e.g., omeprazole,**

pantoprazole) may decrease concentration/effect. May increase concentration/effects of **CYP2D6 substrates (e.g., amitriptyline, carvedilol, FLUoxetine, tamoxifen).** HERBAL: None significant. FOOD: None known. LAB VALUES: May increase **serum alkaline phosphatase, ALT, AST, bilirubin, creatinine, glucose.** May decrease **serum albumin, calcium, potassium, sodium, magnesium; Hgb, Hct, lymphocytes, RBC count.**

D

AVAILABILITY (Rx)

Tablets: 15 mg, 30 mg, 45 mg.

ADMINISTRATION/HANDLING

PO

• Give without regard to food. • If a dose is missed or vomiting occurs after administration, skip dose and give at next regularly scheduled time. • Give at least 6 hrs before or at least 10 hrs after H_2 receptor antagonists (e.g., famotidine).

INDICATIONS/ROUTES/DOSAGE

Non–Small-Cell Lung Cancer

PO: ADULTS, ELDERLY: 45 mg once daily. Continue until disease progression or unacceptable toxicity.

Reduction Schedule for Adverse Reactions

First dose reduction: 30 mg. **Second dose reduction:** 15 mg.

Dose Modification

Based on Common Terminology Criteria for Adverse Events (CTCAE).

Dermatologic Toxicity

Grade 2 skin reaction: Withhold treatment until improved to Grade 1 or 0, then resume at same dose level. **Recurrent or persistent Grade 2 skin reaction, Grade 3 or 4 skin reaction:** Withhold treatment until improved to Grade 1 or 0, then resume at reduced dose level.

GI Toxicity

Grade 2 diarrhea: Withhold treatment until improved to Grade 1 or 0, then resume at same dose level. **Recurrent Grade 2 diarrhea, Grade 3 or 4 diarrhea:** Withhold treatment until improved to Grade 1 or 0, then resume at reduced dose level.

Pulmonary Toxicity

Interstitial lung disease (ILD) of any grade: Permanently discontinue.

Other Toxicities

Any other Grade 3 or 4 toxic reactions: Withhold treatment until improved to Grade 2 or less, then resume at reduced dose level.

Dosage in Renal/Hepatic Impairment

Mild to moderate impairment: No dose adjustment. **Severe impairment:** Not specified; use caution.

SIDE EFFECTS

Frequent (87%–26%): Diarrhea, rash, paronychia, stomatitis, decreased appetite, dry skin, xerosis, decreased weight. **Occasional (23%–7%):** Alopecia, pruritus, cough, nasal disorder (inflammation, epistaxis, mucosal disorder, rhinitis), conjunctivitis, nausea, extremity pain, constipation, dyspnea, asthenia, musculoskeletal pain, mouth ulceration, insomnia, dermatitis, chest pain, fatigue, vomiting, dysgeusia. **Rare (2%–1%):** Keratitis, dehydration.

ADVERSE EFFECTS/TOXIC REACTIONS

Anemia, lymphopenia is an expected response to treatment. Nail reactions including nail infection, nail toxicity, onychoclasis, onycholysis, onychomadesis, paronychia reported in 64% of pts. CTCAE Grade 3 or 4 skin reactions occurred in 21% of pts. Upper respiratory tract infection reported in 12% of pts. Palmar-plantar erythrodysesthesia syndrome 15% of pts. Severe, sometimes fatal, ILD/pneumonitis reported in 1% of pts.

NURSING CONSIDERATIONS

BASELINE ASSESSMENT

Obtain ANC, CBC, LFTs; pregnancy test in females of reproductive potential. Question current breastfeeding status. Confirm compliance of effective contraception. Question history of hepatic impairment, pulmonary disease. Assess skin for open wounds, lesions. Assess hydration status. Receive full medication history and screen for interactions. Offer emotional support.

INTERVENTION/EVALUATION

Monitor CBC, LFTs as clinically indicated. Consider ABG, radiologic test if ILD/ pneumonitis (excessive cough, dyspnea, hypoxia) is suspected. Monitor daily pattern of bowel activity, stool consistency. Antidiarrheal medication may be needed to manage diarrhea. Assess skin for dermal toxicities, rash; nail toxicities. Monitor for symptoms of hyperglycemia (dehydration, confusion, excessive thirst, Kussmaul respirations, polyuria). Monitor I&Os, hydration status.

PATIENT/FAMILY TEACHING

• Treatment may cause severe diarrhea, which may require antidiarrheal medication. Report worsening of diarrhea or dehydration. • Drink plenty of fluids. • Use effective contraception to avoid pregnancy. Do not breastfeed. • Antacids may interfere with absorption. Take dacomitinib at least 6 hrs before or at least 10 hrs after antacid. • Avoid prolonged sun exposure/ tanning beds. Use high SPF sunscreen and lip balm to protect against sunburn. • Report symptoms of liver problems (abdominal pain, bruising, clay-colored stool, amber- or dark-colored urine, yellowing of the skin or eyes); inflammation of the lung (excessive cough, difficulty breathing, chest pain); toxic skin reactions (itching, peeling, rash, redness, swelling), high blood sugar levels (e.g., blurry vision, confusion, frequent urination, increased thirst, fruity breath).

dalfampridine

dal-**fam**-pri-deen
(Ampyra, Fampyra ✱)
Do not confuse Ampyra with anakinra, or dalfampridine with desipramine.

◆CLASSIFICATION

PHARMACOTHERAPEUTIC: Potassium channel blocker. **CLINICAL:** Multiple sclerosis agent.

USES

Indicated to improve ambulation in pts with MS.

PRECAUTIONS

Contraindications: Hypersensitivity to dalfampridine. History of seizures, moderate to severe renal impairment (CrCl equal to or less than 50 mL/min). **Cautions:** Mild renal impairment (CrCl equal to 51–80 mL/min).

ACTION

Improves conduction in demyelinated axons by delaying repolarization and prolonging duration of action potentials. **Therapeutic Effect:** Strengthens skeletal muscle fiber twitch activity; improves peripheral motor neurologic function.

PHARMACOKINETICS

Rapidly absorbed from GI tract. Minimally metabolized in liver. Primarily excreted in urine. **Half-life:** 5.2–6.5 hrs.

⧗ LIFESPAN CONSIDERATIONS

Pregnancy/Lactation: Unknown if drug crosses placenta or is distributed in breast milk. **Children:** Safety and efficacy not established. **Elderly:** Age-related renal impairment may require dosage adjustment.

INTERACTIONS

DRUG: None significant. **HERBAL:** None significant. **FOOD:** None known. **LAB VALUES:** May increase creatinine clearance.

AVAILABILITY (Rx)

Tablet, Film-Coated, Extended-Release: 10 mg.

ADMINISTRATION/HANDLING

PO

- May give without regard to food.
- Do not break, crush, dissolve, or divide tablets.

INDICATIONS/ROUTES/DOSAGE

Multiple Sclerosis

PO: ADULTS 18 YRS AND OLDER, ELDERLY: 10 mg twice daily. **Maximum:** 20 mg/day.

Dosage in Renal Impairment

CrCl 50 mL/min or less: Contraindicated.

Dosage in Hepatic Impairment

No dose adjustment.

SIDE EFFECTS

Frequent (9%–5%): Insomnia, dizziness, headache, nausea, asthenia, back pain. **Rare (4%–2%):** Paresthesia, nasopharyngitis, constipation, dyspepsia, pharyngolaryngeal pain.

ADVERSE EFFECTS/TOXIC REACTIONS

Urinary tract infection occurs in 12% of pts.

NURSING CONSIDERATIONS

BASELINE ASSESSMENT

Obtain CBC, BUN, creatinine clearance, serum chemistries prior to treatment and routinely thereafter. Conduct baseline neurologic exam. Assess motor function, gait, ability to ambulate.

INTERVENTION/EVALUATION

Monitor CBC, serum chemistries, renal function tests, particularly creatinine clearance. Monitor for urinary, respiratory infection. Assess for therapeutic response (improvement in walking as demonstrated by increase in walking speed).

PATIENT/FAMILY TEACHING

• Avoid tasks that require alertness, motor skills until response to drug is established. • Report difficulty in sleeping, dizziness, headache, nausea, back pain, loss of strength or energy. • Do not chew, crush, dissolve, or divide tablets. • Inform physician if ambulation does not improve or worsens.

dalteparin

HIGH ALERT

dal-te-par-in
(Fragmin)

■ BLACK BOX ALERT ■ Epidural or spinal anesthesia greatly increases potential for spinal or epidural hematoma, subsequent long-term or permanent paralysis.

Do not confuse dalteparin with heparin.

◆CLASSIFICATION

PHARMACOTHERAPEUTIC: Low molecular weight heparin. **CLINICAL:** Anticoagulant.

USES

Prevention of ischemic complications in pts with unstable angina or non–Q-wave MI. Prevention of deep vein thrombosis (DVT) in pts undergoing hip replacement surgery or in pts undergoing abdominal surgery who are at risk for thromboembolic complications (e.g., pts older than 40 yrs, obese, pts with malignancy, history of DVT or PE, surgery requiring general anesthesia and lasting more than 30 min). Extended treatment of symptomatic venous thromboembolism (VTE) to reduce recurrence of VTE in cancer pts. Prevention of DVT or pulmonary embolism in acutely ill pts with severely restricted mobility. Treatment of symptomatic venous thromboembolism (VTE) (e.g., DVT and/or PE) to reduce the recurrence of VTE in infants 1 mo or older, children, and adolescents.

PRECAUTIONS

Contraindications: Hypersensitivity to dalteparin, heparin, pork products; active major bleeding; concurrent heparin therapy; unstable angina; history of heparin-induced thrombocytopenia (HIT), or HIT with thrombosis; non–Q-wave MI; prolonged venous thromboembolism undergoing epidural/neuraxial anesthesia. **Cautions:** Conditions with increased risk for hemorrhage, bacterial endocarditis, renal/hepatic impairment, uncontrolled hypertension, history of recent GI ulceration/hemorrhage, peptic ulcer disease, pericarditis, preexisting thrombocytopenia, recent childbirth, concurrent use of aspirin.

ACTION

Antithrombin in presence of low molecular weight heparin inhibits factor Xa, thrombin. Only slightly influences platelet aggregation, PT, aPTT. **Therapeutic Effect:** Produces anticoagulation.

PHARMACOKINETICS

Route	Onset	Peak	Duration
SQ	N/A	4 hrs	N/A

Protein binding: less than 10%. **Half-life:** 3–5 hrs.

LIFESPAN CONSIDERATIONS

Pregnancy/Lactation: Use with caution, particularly during last trimester, immediate postpartum period (increased risk of maternal hemorrhage). Unknown if distributed in breast milk. **Children:** Safety and efficacy not established. **Elderly:** No age-related precautions noted.

INTERACTIONS

DRUG: NSAIDs (e.g., ibuprofen, ketorolac, naproxen) may increase risk of bleeding. May increase effect of **apixaban, dabigatran, edoxaban, rivaroxaban. HERBAL: Herbals with anticoagulant/antiplatelet properties (e.g., garlic, ginger, ginkgo biloba)** may increase risk of bleeding. **FOOD:** None known. **LAB VALUES:** May increase serum ALT, AST. May decrease serum triglycerides.

AVAILABILITY (Rx)

Injection, Solution: 2,500 units/0.2 mL, 5,000 units/0.2 mL, 7,500 units/0.3 mL, 10,000 units/mL, 12,500 units/0.5 mL, 15,000 units/0.6 mL, 18,000 units/0.72 mL.

ADMINISTRATION/HANDLING

SQ

• Visually inspect for particulate matter or discoloration. • Subcutaneously insert needle into abdomen, outer thigh, or upper arm region and inject solution. • Do not inject into areas of active skin disease or injury such as sunburns, rashes, inflammation, or infection. Rotate injection sites.

INDICATIONS/ROUTES/DOSAGE

Non-Orthopedic Surgery

SQ: ADULTS, ELDERLY: 5,000 units 12 hrs before surgery (or evening before), then 5,000 units once daily. Continue until fully ambulatory and VTE risk has diminished.

Total Hip Surgery

SQ: ADULTS, ELDERLY: 5,000 units once daily (initial dose 12 or more hrs pre-operative or 12 or more hrs post-operative once hemostasis achieved) for 10–14 days up to 35 days.

Unstable Angina, Non–Q-Wave MI

SQ: ADULTS, ELDERLY: 120 units/kg q12h for up to 5–8 days (**maximum:** 10,000 units/dose) given with aspirin. Discontinue dalteparin once clinically stable.

Venous Thromboembolism (Cancer pts)

SQ: ADULTS, ELDERLY: Initially (1 mo), 200 units/kg (**maximum:** 18,000 units) daily for 30 days. **Maintenance (2–6 mos):** 150 units/kg once daily (**maximum:** 18,000 units). If platelet count 50,000–100,000 cells/mm^3, reduce dose by 2,500 units until platelet count recovers to 100,000 cells/mm^3 or more. If platelet count less than 50,000 cells/mm^3, discontinue until platelet count recovers to more than 50,000 cells/mm^3.

Prevention of DVT, Acutely Ill Pt, Immobile Pt

SQ: ADULTS, ELDERLY: 5,000 units once daily. Continue for length of hospital stay or until pt is fully ambulatory and VTE risk has diminished.

Treatment, Symptomatic VTE (Children)

SQ: CHILDREN 8 YRS AND OLDER, ADOLESCENTS: 100 units/kg/dose q12h. **CHILDREN 2 YRS TO YOUNGER THAN 8 YRS:** 125 units/kg/dose q12h. **INFANTS TO CHILDREN YOUNGER THAN 2 YRS:** 150 units/kg/dose q12h.

Dosage in Renal Impairment

For CrCl less than 30 mL/min, monitor anti-Xa levels to determine appropriate dose.

Dosage in Hepatic Impairment

No dose adjustment.

SIDE EFFECTS

Occasional (7%–3%): Hematoma at injection site. **Rare (less than 1%):** Hypersensitivity reaction (chills, fever, pruritus, urticaria, asthma, rhinitis, lacrimation, headache); mild, local skin irritation.

ADVERSE EFFECTS/TOXIC REACTIONS

Overdose may lead to bleeding complications ranging from local ecchymoses to major hemorrhage. Thrombocytopenia occurs rarely.

NURSING CONSIDERATIONS

BASELINE ASSESSMENT

Obtain baseline coagulation studies, CBC, esp. platelet count. Determine baseline B/P. Screen for risk factors as listed in Precautions.

INTERVENTION/EVALUATION

Periodically monitor CBC, stool for occult blood (no need for daily monitoring in pts with normal presurgical coagulation parameters). Assess for any sign of bleeding (bleeding at surgical site, hematuria, blood in stool, bleeding from gums, petechiae, bruising/bleeding at injection sites). Monitor for DVT (extremity pain, swelling, redness), pulmonary embolism (chest pain, dyspnea, hypoxia, tachycardia).

PATIENT/FAMILY TEACHING

• Usual length of therapy is 5–10 days. • Do not take any OTC medication (esp. aspirin) without consulting physician. • Report bleeding, bruising, dizziness, light-headedness, rash, itching, fever, swelling, breathing difficulty. • Rotate injection sites daily. • Teach proper injection technique. • Monitor for symptoms of blood clots in the leg (extremity pain, swelling, redness) or blood clots in the lungs (chest pain, difficulty breathing, shortness of breath, fast heart rate).

dantrolene

dan-troe-leen
(Dantrium, Revonto, Ryanodex)

BLACK BOX ALERT Potential for hepatotoxicity.

Do not confuse Dantrium with danazol or Daraprim, or Revonto with Revatio.

◆CLASSIFICATION

PHARMACOTHERAPEUTIC: Calcium release blocker. **CLINICAL:** Skeletal muscle relaxant.

USES

PO: Treatment of spasticity associated with upper motor neuron disorder (e.g., spinal cord injuries, CVA, cerebral palsy, multiple sclerosis). Management of malignant hyperthermia (MH), prevention of MH in susceptible individuals.

Parenteral: Management of malignant hyperthermia. Prevention of malignant hyperthermia (preoperative/postoperative administration). OFF-LABEL: Neuroleptic malignant syndrome.

PRECAUTIONS

Contraindications: Hypersensitivity to dantrolene. **IV:** None. **PO:** When spasticity used to maintain posture/balance during locomotion or to obtain increased motor function. Active hepatic disease. **Cautions:** Cardiac/pulmonary impairment, history of previous hepatic disease.

ACTION

Interferes with release of calcium from sarcoplasmic reticulum of skeletal muscle. Prevents/reduces the increase in myoplasmic calcium ion concentration. **Therapeutic Effect:** Dissociates excitation-contraction coupling. Interferes with catabolic process associated with malignant hyperthermia.

PHARMACOKINETICS

Poorly absorbed from GI tract. Protein binding: High. Metabolized in liver. Primarily excreted in urine. **Half-life: IV:** 4–8 hrs; **PO:** 8.7 hrs.

LIFESPAN CONSIDERATIONS

Pregnancy/Lactation: Readily crosses placenta. Breastfeeding not recommended. **Children:** No age-related precautions noted in pts 5 yrs and older. **Elderly:** No precautions specified.

INTERACTIONS

DRUG: **CNS depressants (e.g., LORazepam, morphine, zolpidem)** may increase CNS depression with short-term use. **Strong CYP3A4 inducers (e.g., carBAMazepine, phenytoin, rifAMPin)** may decrease concentration/effect. HERBAL: **Herbals with sedative properties (e.g., chamomile, kava kava, valerian)** may increase CNS depression. **St. John's wort** may decrease concentration/effect. FOOD: None known. LAB VALUES: May alter serum ALT, AST.

AVAILABILITY (Rx)

Capsules: 25 mg, 50 mg, 100 mg. **Injection, Powder for Reconstitution:** 20-mg vial. **Injection Suspension:** 250 mg powder.

ADMINISTRATION/HANDLING

IV

Reconstitution • Reconstitute 20-mg vial with 60 mL Sterile Water for Injection (**not** Bacteriostatic Water for Injection). ***(Ryanodex):*** 250-mg vial with 5 mL Sterile Water for Injection.

Rate of administration • For therapeutic or emergency dose, give IV over 2–3 min. • For IV infusion, administer over 1 hr. • Diligently monitor for extravasation (high pH of IV preparation). May produce severe complications. ***(Ryanodex):*** Do not dilute; infuse into IV catheter or indwelling catheter. Infuse over 1 min.

Storage • Store at room temperature. • Use within 6 hrs after reconstitution. • Solution is clear, colorless. Discard if cloudy, precipitate forms.

PO

- Give without regard to food.

IV INCOMPATIBILITIES

D_5W, 0.9% NaCl.

INDICATIONS/ROUTES/DOSAGE

Spasticity

PO: ADULTS, ELDERLY: Initially, 25 mg once daily for 7 days; then 25 mg 3 times/day for 7 days; then 50 mg 3 times/day for 7 days; then 100 mg 3 times/day. **Maximum:** 400 mg/day. **CHILDREN:** Initially, 0.5 mg/kg/dose once daily for 7 days; then 0.5 mg/kg/dose 3 times/day for 7 days; then 1 mg/kg/dose 3 times/day for 7 days; then 2 mg/kg/dose 3 times/day. Some pts may require dosing 4 times/day. **Maximum:** 400 mg/day.

Perioperative Prophylaxis for Malignant Hyperthermic Crisis

PO: ADULTS, ELDERLY, CHILDREN: 4–8 mg/kg/day in 3–4 divided doses beginning

1–2 days before surgery; give last dose 3–4 hrs before surgery.
IV: ADULTS, ELDERLY, CHILDREN: 2.5 mg/kg about 1.25 hrs before surgery with additional doses as needed.

D

Management of Malignant Hyperthermic Crisis
IV: ADULTS, ELDERLY, CHILDREN: Initially, a minimum of 2.5 mg/kg rapid IV; may repeat up to total cumulative dose of 10 mg/kg. May follow with 1 mg/kg q4–6h (route not specified).

Dosage in Renal/Hepatic Impairment
No dose adjustment. Contraindicated with active hepatic disease.

SIDE EFFECTS

Frequent: Drowsiness, dizziness, weakness, general malaise, diarrhea (mild). **Occasional:** Confusion, diarrhea (severe), headache, insomnia, constipation, urinary frequency. **Rare:** Paradoxical CNS excitement or restlessness, paresthesia, tinnitus, slurred speech, tremor, blurred vision, dry mouth, nocturia, impotence, rash, pruritus.

ADVERSE EFFECTS/TOXIC REACTIONS

Risk of hepatotoxicity, most notably in females, pts 35 yrs and older, pts taking other hepatotoxic medications concurrently. Overt hepatitis noted most frequently between 3rd and 12th mo of therapy. Overdose results in vomiting, muscular hypotonia, muscle twitching, respiratory depression, seizures.

NURSING CONSIDERATIONS

BASELINE ASSESSMENT

Obtain baseline LFT. Record onset, type, location, duration of muscular spasm. Check for immobility, stiffness, swelling.

INTERVENTION/EVALUATION

Assist with ambulation. For pts on long-term therapy, hepatic/renal function tests, CBC should be performed periodically. Assess for therapeutic response: relief of pain, stiffness, spasm.

PATIENT/FAMILY TEACHING

• Drowsiness usually diminishes with continued therapy. • Avoid tasks that require alertness, motor skills until response to drug is established. • Avoid alcohol/other depressants. • Report continued weakness, fatigue, nausea, diarrhea, skin rash, itching, bloody/tarry stools.

dapagliflozin

dap-a-gli-**floe**-zin
(Farxiga)
Do not confuse dapagliflozin with canagliflozin, empagliflozin, or ertugliflozin. Farxiga with Fetzima.

FIXED-COMBINATIONS

Qtern: dapagliflozin/saxagliptin (an antidiabetic): 5 mg/5 mg, 10 mg/5 mg. **Qternmet XR:** dapagliflozin/saxagliptin/metformin (an antidiabetic): 2.5 mg/2.5 mg/1000 mg, 5 mg/2.5 mg/1000 mg, 5 mg/5 mg/1000 mg, 10 mg/5 mg/1000 mg. **Xigduo XR:** dapagliflozin/metformin (an antidiabetic): 2.5 mg/1000 mg, 5 mg/1000 mg, 10 mg/500 mg, 10 mg/1000 mg.

◆CLASSIFICATION

PHARMACOTHERAPEUTIC: Sodium-glucose cotransporter 2 (SGLT2) inhibitor. **CLINICAL:** Antidiabetic.

USES

Adjunctive treatment to diet and exercise to improve glycemic control in pts with type 2 diabetes mellitus. To reduce risk of hospitalization for HF in adults with type 2 diabetes mellitus and established cardiovascular disease or multiple cardiovascular risk factors. To reduce risk of cardiovascular death and hospitalization for HF in adults with HF with reduced ejection fraction (NYHA class II–IV).

PRECAUTIONS

Contraindications: Hypersensitivity to dapagliflozin; pts who are being treated for glycemic control without established cardiovascular disease or multiple cardiovascular risk factors with severe renal impairment (eGFR less than 30 mL/min); ESRD requiring dialysis. **Cautions:** Concomitant use of loop diuretics, other hypoglycemic agents (e.g., insulin, insulin secretagogues), baseline systolic hypotension, renal impairment, hypovolemia/dehydration, recent genital mycotic infection; pts at risk for diabetic ketoacidosis (insulin dose reduction, acute febrile illness, reduced calorie intake, surgery, alcohol abuse, history of pancreatitis). Not recommended in pts with active bladder cancer, diabetic ketoacidosis, type 1 diabetes mellitus.

ACTION

Inhibits SGLT2 in proximal renal tubule, reducing reabsorption of filtered glucose from tubular lumen and lowering renal threshold for glucose. Reduces reabsorption of sodium and increases delivery of sodium to the distal tubule. **Therapeutic Effect:** Increases urinary excretion of glucose; lowers serum glucose levels. Reduces cardiac preload and afterload; downregulates sympathetic activity.

PHARMACOKINETICS

Rapidly absorbed and widely distributed. Metabolized in liver. Protein binding: 91%. Peak plasma concentration: 2 hrs. Eliminated in urine (75%), feces (21%). Unknown if removed by hemodialysis. **Half-life:** 12.9 hrs.

LIFESPAN CONSIDERATIONS

Pregnancy/Lactation: Not recommended during second or third trimester. Unknown if distributed in breast milk. Breastfeeding not recommended. **Children:** Safety and efficacy not established in pts younger than 18 yrs. **Elderly:** May have increased risk for adverse reactions (dehydration, hypotension, syncope).

INTERACTIONS

DRUG: Insulin, insulin secretagogues (e.g., glyBURIDE) may increase risk of hypoglycemia. **HERBAL: Maitake** may increase hypoglycemic effect. **FOOD:** None known. **LAB VALUES:** May increase serum creatinine; low-density lipoprotein cholesterol (LDL-C); Hct. May decrease serum bicarbonate; eGFR. Expected to result in positive urine glucose test. May interfere with 1,5-anhydrogluitol (1,5-AG) assay.

AVAILABILITY (Rx)

Tablets: 5 mg, 10 mg.

ADMINISTRATION/HANDLING

PO

- Administer in the morning without regard to food.

INDICATIONS/ROUTES/DOSAGE

Type 2 Diabetes Mellitus (Glycemic control)

PO: ADULTS, ELDERLY: Initially, 5 mg once daily in AM. May increase to 10 mg once daily after 4–12 wks if needed for additional glycemic control.

Type 2 Diabetes Mellitus (Risk reduction for HF, cardiovascular disease)

PO: ADULTS, ELDERLY: 10 mg once daily.

Heart Failure (Risk reduction)

PO: ADULTS, ELDERLY: 10 mg once daily; 5 mg once daily may be needed in pts with acute renal dysfunction, volume depletion or hypotension.

Dose Modification

Concomitant use of insulin, insulin secretagogue: Consider lowering dose of insulin or insulin secretagogue to reduce hypoglycemic events.

D

Dosage in Renal Impairment
Type 2 Diabetes Mellitus (Glycemic control)
eGFR 45 mL/min or greater: No dose adjustment. **eGFR 30–44 mL/min:** Not recommended. **eGFR less than 30 mL/min, ESRD/dialysis:** Contraindicated.

Type 2 Diabetes Mellitus (Risk reduction for HF, cardiovascular disease)
eGFR 45 mL/min or greater: No dose adjustment. **eGFR 44 mL/min or less:** Insufficient data to recommend dose adjustment. **ESRD/dialysis:** Contraindicated.

HF (Risk reduction)
eGFR 30 mL/min or greater: No dose adjustment. **eGFR less than 30 mL/min:** Insufficient data to recommend dose adjustment. **ESRD/dialysis:** Contraindicated.

Dosage in Hepatic Impairment
Mild to moderate impairment: No dose adjustment. **Severe impairment:** No dose adjustment; use caution.

SIDE EFFECTS

Rare (3%–1%): Back pain, increased urination, nausea, constipation, extremity pain, discomfort with urination.

ADVERSE EFFECTS/TOXIC REACTIONS

Symptomatic hypotension (orthostatic hypotension, postural dizziness, syncope) may occur, esp. in pts who are elderly, use concomitant loop diuretics, or have baseline systolic hypotension. Intravascular volume depletion/contraction may cause acute kidney injury requiring dialysis. Fatal cases of ketoacidosis were reported. Hypoglycemic events were reported in pts using concomitant insulin, insulin secretagogues. Infections including influenza, nasopharyngitis, pyelonephritis, urosepsis, UTI, genital mycotic infections (male and female), upper respiratory tract infection may occur. Necrotizing fasciitis of the perineum (Fournier gangrene), a life-threatening necrotizing infection of the genital and perineum region that requires urgent surgical intervention, has been reported. Hypersensitivity reactions including anaphylaxis, angioedema, urticaria have occurred.

NURSING CONSIDERATIONS

BASELINE ASSESSMENT

Obtain BUN, serum creatinine, eGFR, CrCl, blood glucose level, Hgb A1c; B/P. Assess hydration status. Correct volume depletion prior to initiation. Assess pt's understanding of diabetes management, routine home glucose monitoring. Obtain dietary consult for nutritional education. Question history of renal impairment, type 1 diabetes, ketoacidosis. In pts with requiring surgery, consider suspending treatment at least 3 days prior to surgery.

INTERVENTION/EVALUATION

Monitor BUN, serum creatinine, eGFR, CrCl, blood glucose level, Hgb A1c; B/P periodically. Monitor for ketoacidosis (e.g., dehydration, confusion, extreme thirst, sweet-smelling breath, Kussmaul respirations, nausea), hypoglycemia (anxiety, confusion, diaphoresis, diplopia, dizziness, headache, hunger, perioral numbness, tachycardia, tremors), hyperglycemia (fatigue, Kussmaul respirations, polyphagia, polyuria, polydipsia, nausea, vomiting). Pts presenting with metabolic acidosis should be screened for ketoacidosis, regardless of serum glucose levels. Concomitant use of beta blockers (e.g., carvedilol, metoprolol) may mask symptoms of hypoglycemia. Monitor for acute kidney injury (dark-colored urine, flank pain, decreased urine output, muscle aches), infections (cough, fatigue, fever), urinary tract infections (dysuria, fever, flank pain, malaise), mycotic infections, Fournier gangrene (perineal necrosis). Screen for glucose-altering conditions (fever, increased activity or stress, surgical procedures). Monitor weight, I&Os. Monitor for hypersensitivity reactions (anaphylaxis, angioedema, urticaria).

PATIENT/FAMILY TEACHING

• Diabetes mellitus requires lifelong control. Diet and exercise are principal parts of treatment; do not skip or delay meals. Test blood sugar regularly. Monitor daily calorie intake. • When taking combination drug therapy or when glucose conditions are altered (excessive alcohol ingestion, insufficient carbohydrate intake, hormone deficiencies, critical illness), have a low blood sugar treatment available (e.g., glucagon, oral dextrose). • Genital itching or discharge may indicate yeast infection. • Report symptoms of perineal necrosis (e.g., discoloration, pain, swelling of the scrotum, penis, or perineum). • Therapy may increase risk for dehydration, low blood pressure, which may cause kidney failure. Report decreased urination, amber-colored urine, flank pain, fatigue, swelling of the hands or feet. Drink enough fluids to maintain adequate hydration. Pts with HF should be cautious of overhydration. • Report symptoms of UTI, kidney infection (back pain, pelvic pain, burning while urinating, cloudy or foul-smelling urine), allergic reactions (difficulty breathing, rash, wheezing; swelling of the face or tongue. • Go slowly from lying to standing. • Do not breastfeed.

DAPTOmycin

dap-toe-mye-sin
(Cubicin)
Do not confuse Cubicin with Cleocin, or DAPTOmycin with DACTINomycin.

◆CLASSIFICATION

PHARMACOTHERAPEUTIC: Cyclic lipopeptide antibacterial agent. **CLINICAL:** Antibiotic.

USES

Treatment of complicated skin/skin structure infections caused by susceptible strains of gram-positive pathogens, including *S. aureus* (methicillin susceptible and methicillin resistant [MRSA]), *S. pyogenes, S. agalactiae.* Treatment of *S. aureus* systemic infections caused by methicillin-susceptible and methicillin-resistant *S. aureus*. **OFF-LABEL:** Severe infections caused by MRSA or vancomycin-resistant *Enterococcus* (VRE); treatment of prosthetic joint infection caused by staphylococci or *Enterococcus*.

PRECAUTIONS

Contraindications: Hypersensitivity to daptomycin. **Cautions:** Severe renal impairment (CrCl less than 30 mL/min), concurrent use of other medications associated with myopathy (e.g., statins).

ACTION

Binds to bacterial membranes and causes rapid depolarization. Inhibits intracellular protein, DNA, RNA synthesis. **Therapeutic Effect:** Bactericidal.

PHARMACOKINETICS

Widely distributed. Protein binding: 90%. Primarily excreted unchanged in urine. Moderately removed by hemodialysis. **Half-life:** 7–8 hrs (increased in renal impairment).

⌛ LIFESPAN CONSIDERATIONS

Pregnancy/Lactation: Unknown if distributed in breast milk. **Children:** Pts younger than 12 mos of age may have increased risk of nervous/muscular system effects. **Elderly:** No age-related precautions noted.

INTERACTIONS

DRUG: **HMG-CoA reductase inhibitors (e.g., simvastatin)** may cause myopathy. **HERBAL:** None significant. **FOOD:** None known. **LAB VALUES:** May increase alkaline phosphatase, CPK, serum potassium. May alter LFT results.

AVAILABILITY (Rx)

Injection, Powder for Reconstitution: 500 mg/vial.

ADMINISTRATION/HANDLING

IV

Reconstitution • Reconstitute 500-mg vial with 10 mL 0.9% NaCl to provide a concentration of 50 mg/mL. May further dilute in 0.9% NaCl. • Do not shake or agitate vial.

Rate of administration • For IV injection, give over 2 min (concentration: 50 mg/mL). • For intermittent IV infusion (piggyback), infuse over 30 min.

Storage • Refrigerate intact vials. • Appears as pale yellow to light brown lyophilized cake. • Reconstituted solution is stable for 12 hrs at room temperature or up to 48 hrs if refrigerated. • Discard if particulate forms.

IV INCOMPATIBILITIES

Diluents containing dextrose. If same IV line is used to administer different drugs, flush line with 0.9% NaCl.

IV COMPATIBILITIES

0.9% NaCl, lactated Ringer's, aztreonam (Azactam), DOPamine, fluconazole (Diflucan), gentamicin, heparin, levoFLOXacin (Levaquin).

INDICATIONS/ROUTES/DOSAGE

Complicated Skin/Skin Structure Infections

IV: ADULTS, ELDERLY: 4–6 mg/kg every 24 hrs for 7–14 days.

Systemic Infections

IV: ADULTS, ELDERLY: 6–10 mg/kg once daily for 2–6 wks.

Dosage in Renal Impairment

CrCl less than 30 mL/min, hemodialysis (HD), peritoneal dialysis (PD): Dosage is 4 mg/kg q48h for skin and soft tissue infections; 6 mg/kg q48h for staphylococcal bacteremia. **HD:** Give dose after dialysis. **Continuous renal replacement therapy: Continuous venovenous hemodialysis (CVVHD):** 8 mg/kg q48h. **Continuous venovenous hemofiltration (CVVH) or continuous venovenous hemodiafiltration (CVVHDF):** 8 mg/kg q48h or 4–6 mg/kg q24h.

Dosage in Hepatic Impairment

No dose adjustment.

SIDE EFFECTS

Frequent (6%–5%): Constipation, nausea, peripheral injection site reactions, headache, diarrhea. **Occasional (4%–3%):** Insomnia, rash, vomiting. **Rare (less than 3%):** Pruritus, dizziness, hypotension.

ADVERSE EFFECTS/TOXIC REACTIONS

Myopathy (muscle pain/weakness, particularly in distal extremities) with CPK levels greater than 10 times ULN has occurred. Rhabdomyolysis may cause renal failure. Eosinophilic pneumonia, with symptoms including fever, hypoxia, respiratory insufficiency, pulmonary infiltrates was reported 2–4 wks after initiation. Antibiotic-associated colitis (abdominal cramps, fever, severe diarrhea), other superinfections may result from altered bacterial balance in GI tract. Persisting or relapsing *S. aureus* bacteremia/endocarditis, caused by reduced DAPTOmycin susceptibility, has occurred.

NURSING CONSIDERATIONS

BASELINE ASSESSMENT

Obtain CPK, blood cultures before first dose (therapy may begin before results are known). Question history of renal impairment. Screen for concomitant use of statins.

INTERVENTION/EVALUATION

Assess oral cavity for white patches on mucous membranes, tongue (thrush). Monitor for myopathy (muscle pain, weakness), CPK levels, renal function tests. Monitor daily pattern of bowel activity, stool consistency. Mild GI effects may be tolerable, but increasing severity may indicate onset of antibiotic-associated colitis. Be alert for superinfection: fever, vomiting, diarrhea, anal/

genital pruritus, oral mucosal changes (ulceration, pain, erythema). Monitor for dizziness; institute appropriate measures. Obtain repeat blood cultures in pts with persistent or relapsing *S. aureus* bacteremia/endocarditis or poor response to therapy.

PATIENT/FAMILY TEACHING

- Report rash, headache, nausea, dizziness, constipation, diarrhea, muscle pain, or any other new symptom.

daratumumab

dar-a-**toom**-ue-mab
(Darzalex)
Do not confuse daratumumab with adalimumab, ofatumumab, panitumumab, or necitumumab.

CLASSIFICATION

PHARMACOTHERAPEUTIC: Anti-CD38 monoclonal antibody. **CLINICAL:** Antineoplastic.

USES

Multiple myeloma (relapsed/refractory): Monotherapy for the treatment of pts with multiple myeloma who have received at least three prior lines of therapy including a proteasome inhibitor and an immunomodulatory agent or who are double-refractory to a proteasome inhibitor and an immunomodulatory agent. In combination with dexamethasone and either lenalidomide or bortezomib for treatment of multiple myeloma in pts who have received at least one prior therapy. In combination with pomalidomide and dexamethasone for treatment of multiple myeloma in pts who have received at least two prior therapies including lenalidomide and a proteasome inhibitor. **Multiple myeloma (newly diagnosed):** Treatment of newly diagnosed multiple myeloma in combination with bortezomib, melphalan, and predniSONE or in combination with lenalidomide and dexamethasone in pts ineligible for autologous stem cell transplant.

PRECAUTIONS

Contraindications: Hypersensitivity to daratumumab. **Cautions:** Obstructive pulmonary disorders (e.g., COPD, emphysema), baseline cytopenias, herpes zoster infection, elderly.

ACTION

Binds to cell surface glycoprotein CD38 on CD38-expressing tumor cells (highly expressed on myeloma cells). Inhibits tumor cell proliferation and induces apoptosis. **Therapeutic Effect:** Inhibits tumor cell growth and survival. Promotes tumor cell death.

PHARMACOKINETICS

Widely distributed. Metabolism not specified. Steady state reached approx. 5 mos into the q4wk dosing period (by 21st infusion). Elimination not specified. **Half-life:** 18 ± 9 days.

LIFESPAN CONSIDERATIONS

Pregnancy/Lactation: Avoid pregnancy; may cause fetal harm/malformations. Monoclonal antibodies are known to cross the placenta. Females of reproductive potential should use effective contraception during treatment and up to 3 mos after discontinuation. Unknown if distributed in breast milk. However, human immunoglobulin G is present in breast milk. **Children:** Safety and efficacy not established. **Elderly:** No age-related precautions noted.

INTERACTIONS

DRUG: May decrease therapeutic effect of **BCG intravesical.** **HERBAL:** None significant. **FOOD:** None known. **LAB VALUES:** Drug may be detected on both serum protein electrophoresis and immunofixation assays used to monitor multiple myeloma endogenous M protein. May affect the determination of complete response and disease progression of some pts with immunoglobulin G kappa myeloma protein. May cause positive Coombs' test. Expected to decrease Hgb, Hct, lymphocytes, neutrophils, platelets, RBCs.

AVAILABILITY (Rx)

Injection Solution: 100 mg/5 mL, 400 mg/20 mL.

ADMINISTRATION/HANDLING

IV

Preparation for administration • Calculate the dose required based on weight in kg. • Solution should appear colorless to pale yellow. Do not use if opaque particles, discoloration, or foreign particles are observed. • Remove a volume from the 0.9% NaCl infusion bag that is equal to the required volume of the dose solution. • Dilute in 1000 mL (first infusion) or 500 mL (subsequent infusions) 0.9% NaCl bag. • Mix by gentle inversion. Do not shake or agitate. • Infusion bags must be made of polyvinylchloride, polypropylene, polyethylene, or polyolefin blend. • Diluted solution may develop very small translucent to white proteinaceous particles; do not use if diluted solution is discolored or if visibly opaque or foreign particles are observed. • Discard used portions of vials.

Infusion guidelines • Prior to administration, premedicate with an IV corticosteroid, acetaminophen, and an IV or oral antihistamine approx. 60 min before each infusion (see manufacturer guidelines). • Infuse using an in-line, sterile, nonpyrogenic, low protein-binding polyethersulfone filter (0.22 or 0.2 μm). • Infuse via dedicated line using infusion pump. • Do not administer as IV push or bolus. • Infusion should be completed within 15 hrs. • If infusion cannot be completed for any reason, do not save unused portions for reuse. • Postinfusion, administer an oral corticosteroid on the first and second day after each infusion to reduce risk of delayed infusion reactions (see manufacturer guidelines). • In pts with a history of obstructive pulmonary disease, consider short-acting and long-acting bronchodilators and an inhaled corticosteroid postinfusion (may discontinue if no infusion reaction occurs after the first four infusions).

Rate of administration • **First infusion (1000 mL volume):** Infuse at 50 mL/hr for the first 60 min. Increase in increments of 50 mL/hr q1hr if no infusion reactions occur. **Maximum:** 200 mL/hr. • **Second infusion (500 mL volume):** Infuse at 50 mL/hr for the first 60 min. Increase in increments of 50 mL/hr q1hr if there were no Grade 1 or greater infusion reactions during the first 3 hrs of first infusion. **Maximum:** 200 mL/hr. • **Subsequent infusions (500 mL volume):** Infuse at 100 mL/hr if there were no Grade 1 or greater infusion reactions during a final infusion rate of greater than or equal to 100 mL/hr in the first two infusions. Increase in increments of 50 mL/hr q1hr if tolerated. **Maximum:** 200 mL/hr.

Storage • Refrigerate unused vials. • Do not shake. • May refrigerate diluted solution up to 24 hrs. • If diluted solution is refrigerated, allow solution to warm to room temperature before use. • Protect from light.

IV INCOMPATIBILITIES

Do not mix with other medications.

INDICATIONS/ROUTES/DOSAGE

Note: The initial dose (16 mg/kg on wk 1) may be divided over 2 consecutive days (8 mg/kg/day on days 1 and 2 of wk 1 of therapy) to facilitate administration.

Multiple Myeloma (Relapsed/refractory)

IV: ADULTS, ELDERLY: **(Monotherapy or combination with lenalidomide/dexamethasone or pomalidomide/dexamethasone): Wks 1–8:** 16 mg/kg once wkly. **Wks 9–24:** 16 mg/kg once q2wks. **Wk 25 and beyond:** 16 mg/kg once q4wks until disease progression. **(Combination with bortezomib/dexamethasone): Wks 1–9:** 16 mg/kg once wkly. **Wks 10–24:** 16 mg/

kg q3wks for 5 doses. **Wk 25 and beyond:** 16 mg/kg q4wks until disease progression.

Multiple Myeloma (Newly diagnosed)
IV: ADULTS, ELDERLY: **(In combination with bortezomib, melphalan and predniSONE): Wks 1–6:** 16 mg/kg once wkly. **Wks 7–54:** 16 mg/kg q3wks for 16 doses. **Wk 55 and beyond:** 16 mg/kg q4wks until disease progression. **(In combination with lenalidomide and low-dose dexamethasone): Wks 1–8:** 16 mg/kg once wkly for 8 doses. **Wks 9–24:** 16 mg/kg once q2wks for 8 doses. **Wks 25 and beyond:** 16 mg/kg once q4wks until disease progression.

Dose Modification
Infusion Reactions
Promptly interrupt infusion if any reaction occurs.
Grade 1 or 2 reaction: Once symptoms resolve, resume infusion at a decreased rate that is 50% (or less) of previous rate. If no further reactions are observed, may increase infusion rate as appropriate.
Grade 3 reaction: If symptoms resolve to Grade 2 or less, consider resuming infusion at a decreased rate that is 50% (or less) of previous rate. If no further reactions are observed, may increase rate as appropriate. If a Grade 3 reaction recurs, decrease rate as outlined earlier. If Grade 3 reaction occurs for a third time, permanently discontinue.
Grade 4 reaction: Permanently discontinue.

Dosage in Renal Impairment
No dose adjustment.

Dosage in Hepatic Impairment
Mild impairment: No dose adjustment.
Moderate to severe impairment: Not specified; use caution.

SIDE EFFECTS

Frequent (37%–14%): Fatigue, back pain, nausea, pyrexia, cough, nasal congestion, arthralgia, diarrhea, dyspnea, decreased appetite, extremity pain, constipation, vomiting. **Occasional (12%–10%):** Headache, musculoskeletal chest pain, chills, hypertension.

ADVERSE EFFECTS/TOXIC REACTIONS

Anemia, leukopenia, neutropenia, thrombocytopenia are expected responses to therapy. Infusion reactions occurred in approx. 50% of pts (mostly during first infusion). Infusion reactions can also occur with subsequent infusions (mainly during the infusion or within 4 hrs of completion). Severe infusion reactions may include cough, dyspnea, bronchospasm, hypertension, hypoxia, laryngeal edema, pulmonary edema, wheezing. Less common reactions may include chills, headache, hypotension, rash, nausea, pruritus, urticaria, vomiting. Infections including pneumonia, upper respiratory tract infection, nasopharyngitis reported in 20%–11% of pts. Herpes zoster reported in 3% of pts. Thrombocytopenia may increase risk of bleeding.

NURSING CONSIDERATIONS

BASELINE ASSESSMENT

Obtain CBC, blood type and screen; vital signs. Obtain pregnancy test in female pts of reproductive potential. Question history of COPD, emphysema, herpes infection; prior hypersensitivity reaction to any drug in treatment regimen; prior infusion reaction. Assess nutritional status. Screen for active infection. Offer emotional support.

INTERVENTION/EVALUATION

Monitor CBC, vital signs periodically. Administer in an environment equipped to monitor for and manage infusion reactions. If infusion reaction of any grade/severity occurs, immediately interrupt infusion and manage symptoms. Accurately record characteristics of infusion reactions (severity, type, time of onset). Reactions may affect future infusion rates. To prevent herpes zoster reactivation in pts with prior history, consider antiviral prophylaxis within 1 wk of starting treatment and continue for 3 mos following discontinuation. Monitor for

D

infection. Monitor daily pattern of bowel activity, stool consistency.

PATIENT/FAMILY TEACHING

• Treatment may depress your immune system and reduce your ability to fight infection. Report symptoms of infection such as body aches, chills, cough, fatigue, fever. Avoid those with active infection. • Use effective contraception to avoid pregnancy. Do not breastfeed. • Severe infusion reactions can occur at any time. Immediately report symptoms of infusion reactions such as chills, cough, difficulty breathing, headache, hives, itching, nausea, rash, stuffy or runny nose, throat tightness, vomiting, wheezing.

daratumumab/ hyaluronidase fihj

dar-a-**toom**-ue-mab **hye**-al-ure-**on**-i-dase
(Darzalex Faspro)
Do not confuse daratumumab with daclizumab, daratumumab, darolutamide, denosumab, dinutuximab, dupilumab, durvalumab, elotuzumab, rituximab/hyaluronidase, trastuzumab/hyaluronidase, or Darzalex Faspro with Darzalex.

◆CLASSIFICATION

PHARMACOTHERAPEUTIC: Anti-CD38 Monoclonal antibody. **CLINICAL:** Antineoplastic.

USES

Treatment of adults with multiple myeloma: in combination with bortezomib, melphalan, and prednisone in newly diagnosed pts who are ineligible for autologous stem cell transplant; in combination with lenalidomide and dexamethasone in newly diagnosed pts who are ineligible for autologous stem cell transplant and in pts with relapsed or refractory multiple myeloma who have received at least one prior therapy; in combination with bortezomib and dexamethasone in pts who have received at least one prior therapy; as monotherapy in pts who have received at least three prior lines of therapy including a proteasome inhibitor (PI) and an immunomodulatory agent or who are double refractory to a PI and an immunomodulatory agent.

PRECAUTIONS

Contraindications: Hypersensitivity to daratumumab, hyaluronidase. Combination treatment with lenalidomide in pregnant women. **Cautions:** Baseline cytopenias, active infection, obstructive pulmonary disorders (e.g., COPD, emphysema), herpes zoster infection, elderly; conditions predisposing to infection (e.g., diabetes, immunocompromised pts, renal failure, open wounds); history of hepatitis B infection.

ACTION

Daratumumab binds to cell surface glycoprotein CD38 on CD38-expressing tumor cells (highly expressed on myeloma cells). Inhibits tumor cell proliferation and induces apoptosis. Hyaluronidase increases permeability of subcutaneous tissue. **Therapeutic Effect:** Inhibits tumor cell growth and survival.

PHARMACOKINETICS

Widely distributed. Peak plasma concentration: 3 days. Eliminated by parallel and nonlinear saturable target mediated clearance. **Half-life:** 20 days.

⌛ LIFESPAN CONSIDERATIONS

Pregnancy/Lactation: Avoid pregnancy; may cause fetal harm. Females of reproductive potential must use effective contraception during treatment and for at least 3 mos after discontinuation. Unknown if distributed in breast milk; however, human immunoglobulin G (IgG) is present in breast milk.

Breastfeeding not recommend. **Children:** Safety and efficacy not established. **Elderly:** May have higher risk of infections, side effects.

INTERACTIONS

DRUG: May decrease effect of **BCG intravesical, vaccines (live).** May increase adverse/toxic effect of **natalizumab. Pimecrolimus, tacrolimus** may increase adverse/toxic effects. **HERBAL: Echinacea** may decrease therapeutic effect. **FOOD:** None known. **LAB VALUES:** May mask detection of antibodies to minor antigens. Drug may be detected on both serum protein electrophoresis and immunofixation assays used to monitor multiple myeloma endogenous M-protein. May affect the determination of complete response and disease progression of some pts with IgG kappa myeloma protein. May cause positive Coombs test. May increase serum glucose. May decrease serum calcium; Hgb, leukocytes, lymphocytes, neutrophils, platelets.

AVAILABILITY (Rx)

Injection Solution: Daratumumab 1,800 mg/hyaluronidase 30,000 units (120 mg/2,000 units/mL).

ADMINISTRATION/HANDLING

Subcutaneous

Premedication • Pretreat with acetaminophen 650–1000 mg PO, diphenhydramine 25–50 mg PO or IV, and a long- or intermediate-acting corticosteroid 1–3 hrs prior to each dose. • See manufacturer guidelines regarding premedication and postmedication corticosteroid therapy.

Preparation • Remove vial from refrigerator and allow solution to warm to room temperature. • Visually inspect for particulate matter or discoloration. Solution should appear colorless to yellow, clear to opalescent. Do not use if solution is cloudy, discolored, or visible particles are observed. • Withdraw 15 mL from vial into syringe. • To avoid clogging, immediately attach a new hypodermic needle or subcutaneous infusion set to syringe.

Administration • Insert needle subcutaneously into abdomen (only), approx. 3 inches (7.5 cm) to the right or left of navel and inject solution. • Do not inject into areas of active skin disease or injury such as sunburns, skin rashes, inflammation, skin infections, or active psoriasis. • Rotate injection sites. • Do not administer IV or intramuscularly. • If a dose is missed, administer as soon as possible and adjust dosing schedule to maintain dosing intervals.

Rate of administration • Inject over 3–5 minutes. • Decrease injection rate or interrupt administration if pain is experienced. If pain is not relieved by slowing or interrupting injection, may choose second injection site on opposite side of abdomen.

Storage • Refrigerate vials in original carton until time of use. • Protect from light. • Do not shake. • Do not freeze or expose to heating sources. • After vial is allowed to warm to room temperature, use within 24 hrs. • May store syringe containing solution at room temperature for up to 4 hrs.

INDICATIONS/ROUTES/DOSAGE

Multiple Myeloma

SQ: ADULTS: 1,800 mg/30,000 units/dose according to schedule. Continue until disease progression or unacceptable toxicity.

Dosing Schedule

Monotherapy or in combination with lenalidomide and dexamethasone: Give dose once weekly on wks 1–8, then once q2wks on wks 9–24, then once monthly on wk 25 and thereafter.

In combination with bortezomib, melphalan, prednisone: Give dose once weekly on wks 1–6, then once q3wks on wks 7–54, then once monthly on wk 55 and thereafter.

In combination with bortezomib and dexamethasone: Give dose once weekly on wks 1–9, then once q3wks on wks 10–24, then once monthly on wk 25 and thereafter.

D

Dose Modifications

Myelosuppression

Consider withholding treatment until neutropenia, thrombocytopenia improves.

Hypersensitivity Reactions

Permanently discontinue if anaphylaxis or Grade 4 administration-related reactions occur.

Dosage in Renal Impairment

Mild to severe impairment: No dose adjustment.

Dosage in Hepatic Impairment

Mild impairment: No dose adjustment. **Moderate to severe impairment:** Not specified; use caution.

SIDE EFFECTS

NOTE: Frequency and occurrence of side effects may vary based on treatment as monotherapy or in combination with other therapies. **Occasional (15%–6%):** Diarrhea, fatigue, pyrexia, back pain, injection site reaction, peripheral edema, arthralgia, musculoskeletal chest pain, constipation, vomiting, abdominal pain, decreased appetite, dehydration, insomnia, hypertension, hypotension, dizziness, neuropathy, paresthesia, pruritus, rash, cough, nausea, chills, dyspnea.

ADVERSE EFFECTS/TOXIC REACTIONS

NOTE: Frequency and occurrence of adverse reactions may vary based on treatment as monotherapy or in combination with other therapies. Myelosuppression (anemia, leukopenia, neutropenia, thrombocytopenia) has occurred. Grade 3 and 4 neutropenia was reported, esp. in pts with lower body weights. Severe systemic reactions including bronchospasm, dyspnea, hypertension, hypoxia, tachycardia wheezing reported in 10% of pts. Other systemic reactions including nasal congestion, cough, throat irritation, allergic rhinitis may occur. Anaphylactic reactions including chest pain, chills, hypotension, nausea, pruritus, pyrexia, vomiting were reported. Infections including upper respiratory tract infection (24% of pts), pneumonia (8% of pts); herpes zoster, UTI, influenza, sepsis (10% of pts) were reported. Atrial fibrillation reported in less than 10% of pts. May cause hepatitis B virus reactivation. Thrombocytopenia may increase risk of bleeding. Immunogenicity (auto-daratumumab antibodies) reported in 8% of pts.

NURSING CONSIDERATIONS

BASELINE ASSESSMENT

Obtain CBC, blood type and screen; pregnancy test in females of reproductive potential. Confirm compliance of effective contraception. Inform blood bank of treatment and possible treatment-related interference with serologic testing. In pts with COPD, inhaled corticosteroids and bronchodilators should be considered during the first 4 treatment doses. If pt does not experience a major systemic administration-related reaction after the first 4 doses, consider discontinuation of the additional inhaled corticosteroids and bronchodilators. To prevent herpes zoster reactivation in pts with a history of infection, initiate antiviral prophylaxis within 1 wk of initiation and continue for 3 mos after last dose. Question history of hepatitis B virus infection, COPD, emphysema, herpes zoster infection. Screen for active infection. Administer premedication and postmedication therapy per manufacturer guidelines. Offer emotional support.

INTERVENTION/EVALUATION

Monitor CBC periodically for myelosuppression. Diligently observe for hypersensitivity reactions throughout injection and treatment course; early detection is vital. If anaphylactic reaction occurs, initiate appropriate medical care (antipyretics, corticosteroids, oxygen therapy, IV hydration). Monitor for infections (cough, fever, fatigue), herpes zoster or hepatitis B virus reactivation; symptoms of hyperglycemia (blurred vision, confusion, excessive thirst, Kussmaul respirations, polyuria). If serious infection, sepsis occurs, initiate appropriate antimicrobial therapy. Monitor daily pattern of bowel activity, stool consistency. Encourage nutritional intake.

PATIENT/FAMILY TEACHING

• Treatment may depress your immune system and reduce your ability to fight infection. Report symptoms of infection such as body aches, burning with urination, chills, cough, fatigue, fever. Avoid those with active infection. Dormant chronic viral infections such as herpes zoster, hepatitis B infection can become reactivated. • Pretreatment and posttreatment with acetaminophen, antihistamines, or steroidal anti-inflammatories may help reduce allergic reactions. • Life-threatening anaphylaxis may occur. Immediately report serious allergic reactions of any kind, regardless of the time the dose was administered. • Report symptoms of bone marrow depression such as bruising, fatigue, fever, shortness of breath, weight loss; bleeding easily, bloody urine or stool. • Females of childbearing potential must use effective contraception during treatment and for at least 3 mos after last dose. Do not breastfeed. • Diarrhea is a common side effect. Drink plenty of fluids.

darbepoetin alfa

TOP 100

dar-be-poe-**e**-tin **al**-fa
(Aranesp)

BLACK BOX ALERT

Increased risk of serious cardiovascular events, thromboembolic events, mortality, time-to-tumor progression when administered to a target hemoglobin greater than 11 g/dL. Shortened overall survival and/or increased risk of tumor progression has been reported with breast, cervical, head/neck, NSCL cancers.

Do not confuse Aranesp with Aricept, or darbepoetin with dalteparin or epoetin.

◆CLASSIFICATION

PHARMACOTHERAPEUTIC: Erythropoiesis stimulating agent (ESA). **CLINICAL:** Hematopoietic agent.

USES

Treatment of anemia associated with chronic renal failure (including pts on dialysis and pts not on dialysis), treatment of anemia caused by concurrent myelosuppressive chemotherapy in pts planned to receive chemotherapy for minimum of 2 additional months. **OFF-LABEL:** Treatment of symptomatic anemia in myelodysplastic syndrome (MDS).

PRECAUTIONS

Contraindications: Hypersensitivity to darbepoetin. Pure red cell aplasia that begins after treatment with darbepoetin alfa or other erythropoietin protein medication. Uncontrolled hypertension. **Cautions:** History of seizures, hypertension. Not recommended in pts with mild to moderate anemia and HF or CAD.

ACTION

Stimulates division and differentiation of committed erythroid progenitor cells; induces release of reticulocytes from bone marrow into bloodstream. **Therapeutic Effect:** Induces erythropoiesis.

PHARMACOKINETICS

Well absorbed after SQ administration. **Half-life:** 48.5 hrs.

⌛ LIFESPAN CONSIDERATIONS

Pregnancy/Lactation: Unknown if drug crosses placenta or is distributed in breast milk. **Children:** Safety and efficacy not established. **Elderly:** Age-related renal impairment may require dosage adjustment.

D

INTERACTIONS

DRUG: **Contraceptives (e.g., estradiol, levonorgestrel), estrogens** may increase risk of thrombosis. **HERBAL:** None significant. **FOOD:** None known. **LAB VALUES:** May decrease serum ferritin, serum transferrin saturation.

AVAILABILITY (Rx)

Injection Solution: 25 mcg/mL, 40 mcg/mL, 60 mcg/mL, 100 mcg/mL, 200 mcg/mL, 300 mcg/mL. **Prefilled Syringe:** 10 mcg/0.4 mL, 25 mcg/0.42 mL, 40 mcg/0.4 mL, 60 mcg/0.3 mL, 100 mcg/0.5 mL, 150 mcg/0.3 mL, 200 mcg/0.4 mL, 300 mcg/0.6 mL, 500 mcg/mL.

ADMINISTRATION/HANDLING

IV

Preparation • Avoid excessive agitation of vial; do not shake (will cause foaming). Do not dilute.

Rate of administration • May be given as IV bolus.

Storage • Refrigerate. • Do not shake. Vigorous shaking may denature medication, rendering it inactive.

SQ

• Use 1 dose per vial; do not reenter vial. Discard unused portion.

IV INCOMPATIBILITIES

Do not mix with other medications.

INDICATIONS/ROUTES/DOSAGE

Anemia in Chronic Renal Failure

◀ALERT▶ Individualize dosing and use lowest dose to reduce need for RBC transfusions. **On Dialysis:** Initiate when Hgb less than 10 g/dL; reduce or stop dose when Hgb approaches or exceeds 11 g/dL. **Not on Dialysis:** Initiate when Hgb less than 10 g/dL and Hgb decline would likely result in RBC transfusion; reduce dose or stop if Hgb exceeds 10 g/dL.

IV, SQ: ADULTS, ELDERLY: On Dialysis: Initially, 0.45 mcg/kg once wkly or 0.75 mcg/kg once q2wks. **Not on Dialysis:** 0.45 mcg/kg q4wks.

Decrease dose by 25%: If Hgb approaches 12 g/dL or increases greater than 1 g/dL in any 2-wk period.

Increase dose by 25%: If Hgb does not increase by 1 g/dL after 4 wks of therapy and Hgb is below target range (with adequate iron stores). Do not increase dose more frequently than every 4 wks.

Note: If pt does not attain Hgb range of 10–12 g/dL after appropriate dosing over 12 wks, do not increase dose and use minimum effective dose to maintain Hgb level that will avoid red blood cell transfusions. Discontinue treatment if responsiveness does not improve.

Anemia Associated With Chemotherapy

◀ALERT▶ Initiate only if Hgb less than 10 g/dL and anticipated duration of myelosuppression is 2 months or longer. Titrate dose to maintain Hgb level and avoid RBC transfusions. Discontinue upon completion of chemotherapy.

SQ: ADULTS, ELDERLY: 2.25 mcg/kg once wkly or 500 mcg every 3 wks.

Increase dose: If Hgb does not increase by 1 g/dL after 6 wks and remains below 10 g/dL, increase dose to 4.5 mcg/kg once wkly. No dose adjustment if using q3wk dosing.

Decrease dose: Decrease dose by 40% if Hgb increases greater than 1 g/dL in any 2-wk period or Hgb reaches level that will avoid red blood cell transfusions.

Note: Withhold dose when Hgb exceeds a level needed to avoid RBC transfusions; resume at dose 40% lower when Hgb approaches a level where transfusions may be required.

Dosage in Renal/Hepatic Impairment

No dose adjustment.

SIDE EFFECTS

Frequent: Myalgia, hypertension/hypotension, headache, diarrhea. **Occasional:** Fatigue, edema, vomiting, reaction at injection site, asthenia, dizziness.

ADVERSE EFFECTS/TOXIC REACTIONS

Cardiovascular events, including CVA, MI, venous thromboembolism, vascular access device thrombosis, mortality, may occur when given to target hemoglobin greater than 11 g/dL or during rapid rise in hemoglobin. Hypersensitivity reactions, including anaphylaxis, may occur. Cases of anemia and pure red cell aplasia may occur in pts with chronic renal disease when given subcutaneously.

NURSING CONSIDERATIONS

BASELINE ASSESSMENT

Obtain CBC (esp. note Hgb, Hct). Assess B/P before drug administration. B/P often rises during early therapy in pts with history of hypertension. Assess serum iron (transferrin saturation should be greater than 20%), serum ferritin (greater than 100 ng/mL) before and during therapy. Consider supplemental iron therapy.

INTERVENTION/EVALUATION

Monitor CBC, reticulocyte count, serum BUN, creatinine, ferritin, potassium, phosphate. Monitor B/P aggressively for increase (25% of pts taking medication require antihypertension therapy, dietary restrictions).

PATIENT/FAMILY TEACHING

• Frequent blood tests needed to determine correct dose. • Report swollen extremities, breathing difficulty, extreme fatigue, or severe headache. • Avoid tasks requiring alertness, motor skills until response to drug is established.

darifenacin

dare-i-**fen**-a-sin
(Enablex)

◆CLASSIFICATION

PHARMACOTHERAPEUTIC: Muscarinic receptor antagonist. Anticholinergic agent. **CLINICAL:** Urinary antispasmodic.

USES

Management of symptoms of bladder overactivity (urge incontinence, urinary urgency/frequency).

PRECAUTIONS

Contraindications: Hypersensitivity to darifenacin. Pts with or at risk of uncontrolled narrow-angle glaucoma, gastric retention, urine retention. **Cautions:** Bladder outflow obstruction, hepatic impairment, nonobstructive prostatic hyperplasia, decreased GI motility (e.g., severe constipation, ulcerative colitis), GI obstructive disorders, controlled narrow-angle glaucoma, myasthenia gravis, concurrent use of strong CYP3A4 inhibitors. Hot weather and/or exercise.

ACTION

Acts as a direct antagonist at muscarinic receptor sites in cholinergically innervated organs; limits bladder contractions. **Therapeutic Effect:** Reduces symptoms of bladder irritability/overactivity (urge incontinence, urinary urgency/frequency), improves bladder capacity.

PHARMACOKINETICS

Well absorbed following PO administration. Protein binding: 98%. Metabolized in liver. Excreted in urine (60%), feces (40%). **Half-life:** 13–19 hrs.

⌛ LIFESPAN CONSIDERATIONS

Pregnancy/Lactation: Unknown if drug crosses placenta or is distributed in breast milk. **Children:** Safety and efficacy not established. **Elderly:** No age-related precautions noted.

INTERACTIONS

DRUG: **Strong CYP3A4 inhibitors (e.g., clarithromycin, ketoconazole, ritonavir)** may increase concentration/effect. **Strong CYP3A4 inducers (e.g., carBAMazepine, phenytoin, rifAMPin)** may decrease concentration/effect. **Anticholinergics (e.g., aclidinium, ipratropium, tiotropium, umeclidinium)** may increase anticholinergic effect. May increase concentration/effect of **thioridazine.** **HERBAL:** None significant. **FOOD:** None known. **LAB VALUES:** None known.

AVAILABILITY (Rx)

Tablets (Extended-Release): 7.5 mg, 15 mg.

ADMINISTRATION/HANDLING

PO

• Give without regard to food. • Administer extended-release tablets whole; do not break, crush, dissolve, or divide tablet.

INDICATIONS/ROUTES/DOSAGE

Overactive Bladder

PO: ADULTS, ELDERLY: Initially, 7.5 mg once daily. If response is not adequate after at least 2 wks, may increase to 15 mg once daily. Do not exceed 7.5 mg once daily in moderate hepatic impairment or concurrent use with strong or potent CYP3A4 inhibitors (e.g., clarithromycin, fluconazole, protease inhibitors).

Dosage in Renal Impairment

No dose adjustment.

Dosage Hepatic Impairment

Moderate impairment: Maximum: 7.5 mg. **Severe impairment:** Not recommended.

SIDE EFFECTS

Frequent (35%–21%): Dry mouth, constipation. **Occasional (8%–4%):** Dyspepsia, headache, nausea, abdominal pain. **Rare (3%–2%):** Asthenia, diarrhea, dizziness, ocular dryness.

ADVERSE EFFECTS/TOXIC REACTIONS

UTI occurs occasionally.

NURSING CONSIDERATIONS

BASELINE ASSESSMENT

Monitor voiding pattern, assess signs/symptoms of overactive bladder prior to therapy as baseline.

INTERVENTION/EVALUATION

Monitor I&O. Palpate bladder and use bladder scanner to assess for urine retention. Monitor daily pattern of bowel activity, stool consistency for evidence of constipation. Dry mouth may be relieved with sips of water. Assess for relief of symptoms of overactive bladder (urge incontinence, urinary frequency/urgency).

PATIENT/FAMILY TEACHING

• Swallow tablet whole; do not chew, crush, dissolve, or divide. • Increase fluid intake to reduce risk of constipation. • Avoid tasks that require alertness, motor skills until response to drug is established.

darolutamide

dar-oh-**loo**-ta-mide
(Nubeqa)
Do not confuse darolutamide with abiraterone, apalutamide, bicalutamide, dutasteride, enzalutamide, flutamide, or nilutamide.

CLASSIFICATION

PHARMACOTHERAPEUTIC: Androgen receptor inhibitor. **CLINICAL:** Antineoplastic.

USES

Treatment of nonmetastatic castration-resistant prostate cancer.

PRECAUTIONS

Contraindications: Hypersensitivity to darolutamide. **Cautions:** Hepatic/renal impairment, conditions predisposing to infection (e.g., diabetes, renal failure, immunocompromised pts, open wounds); history of cardiovascular disease (HF, ischemic heart disease). Avoid concomitant use of a combined G-gp and strong or moderate CYP3A4 inducer.

ACTION

Binds directly to ligands of androgen receptor, inhibiting androgen-receptor translocation and androgen receptor-mediated transcription. **Therapeutic Effect:** Decreases proliferation of prostate tumor cells, increases apoptosis (cellular death), resulting decreased tumor volume.

PHARMACOKINETICS

Widely distributed. Metabolized in liver to active metabolite. Protein binding: 92%. Peak plasma concentration: 4 hrs. Steady state reached in 2–5 days. Excreted in feces (32%), urine (63%). **Half-life:** 20 hrs.

LIFESPAN CONSIDERATIONS

Pregnancy/Lactation: Not indicated in female population. May cause fetal harm if administered in pregnant females. **Males:** Males with female partners of reproductive potential must use effective contraception during treatment and up to 1 wk after discontinuation. May impair fertility. **Children:** Safety and efficacy not established. **Elderly:** No age-related precautions noted.

INTERACTIONS

DRUG: May increase concentration of **alpelisib, cladribine, ozanimod, pazopanib, topotecan. Combined P-gp and strong or moderate CYP3A4 inducers (e.g., carBAMazepine, phenytoin, rifAMPin)** may decrease concentration/effect. **HERBAL:** None significant. **FOOD:** None known. **LAB VALUES:** May increase serum AST, bilirubin. May decrease neutrophils.

AVAILABILITY (Rx)

Tablets: 300 mg.

ADMINISTRATION/HANDLING

PO

• Give with food. • Swallow tablets whole; do not break, cut, crush, or divide.

INDICATIONS/ROUTES/DOSAGE

Note: Give concurrently with a gonadotropin-releasing hormone analog if pt had not received bilateral orchiectomy.

Nonmetastatic Castration-Resistant Prostate Cancer

PO: ADULTS, ELDERLY: 600 mg twice daily.

Dose Modification

Based on Common Terminology Criteria for Adverse Effects (CTCAE).

Any Grade 3 toxicity or intolerable side effect: Withhold treatment or reduce to 300 mg twice daily until symptoms improve. Doses less than 300 mg twice daily not recommended.

Dosage in Renal Impairment

Mild to moderate impairment: No dose adjustment. **Severe impairment (eGFR 15–29 mL/min) not undergoing HD:** 300 mg twice daily.

Dosage in Hepatic Impairment

Mild impairment: No dose adjustment. **Moderate impairment:** 300 mg twice daily. **Severe impairment:** Not specified; use caution.

SIDE EFFECTS

Occasional (16%–6%): Fatigue, asthenia, extremity pain. **Rare (3%–less than 1%):** Rash, hypertension, nausea, diarrhea.

ADVERSE EFFECTS/TOXIC REACTIONS

Cardiovascular events including ischemic heart disease (4% of pts), cardiac failure (2% of pts), cardiac arrest were reported. Other adverse effects may include hematuria, urinary retention, pneumonia.

NURSING CONSIDERATIONS

BASELINE ASSESSMENT

Pts should also receive a concomitant gonadotropin-releasing hormone analog or had a bilateral orchiectomy. Question history of hepatic/renal impairment, cardiac disease. Screen for active infection. Receive full medication history and screen for interactions. Offer emotional support.

D

INTERVENTION/EVALUATION

Monitor CBC periodically for neutropenia. Monitor for symptoms of HF (dyspnea, exercise intolerance, palpitations, peripheral edema), infection (cough, fever, fatigue).

PATIENT/FAMILY TEACHING

• Treatment may depress your immune system response and reduce your ability to fight infection. Report symptoms of infection such as body aches, chills, cough, fatigue, fever. Avoid those with active infection. • Report symptoms of liver problems (e.g., bruising, confusion; dark, amber-, orange-colored urine; right upper abdominal pain, yellowing of the skin or eyes); heart failure (e.g., chest pain, difficulty breathing, palpitations, swelling of extremities). • Males with female partners of childbearing potential must wear condoms during sexual activity. • There is a high risk of interactions with other medications. Do not take newly prescribed medications unless approved by prescriber who originally started therapy. • Avoid herbal supplements (esp. St. John's wort).

darunavir

TOP 100

dar-**ue**-na-veer
(Prezista)

FIXED-COMBINATION(S)

Prezcobix: Darunavir/cobicistat (antiretroviral booster): 800 mg/150 mg.

◆CLASSIFICATION

PHARMACOTHERAPEUTIC: Protease inhibitor (anti-HIV). **CLINICAL:** Antiretroviral.

USES

Treatment of HIV infection in combination with ritonavir and other antiretroviral agents in adults and children 3 yrs and older.

PRECAUTIONS

Contraindications: Hypersensitivity to darunavir. Concurrent therapy with alfuzosin, colchicine (in pts with renal and/or hepatic impairment), dihydroergotamine, dronedarone, elbasvir/grazoprevir, ergonovine, ergotamine, lovastatin, lurasidone, methylergonovine, oral midazolam, pimozide, ranolazine, rifAMPin, sildenafil (for treatment of PAH), simvastatin, St. John's wort, triazolam. **Cautions:** Diabetes, hemophilia, known sulfonamide allergy, hepatic impairment.

ACTION

Binds to site of HIV-I protease activity, inhibiting cleavage of viral precursors into functional proteins required for infectious HIV. **Therapeutic Effect:** Prevents formation of mature viral cells.

PHARMACOKINETICS

Readily absorbed following PO administration. Metabolized in liver. Protein binding: 95%. Excreted in feces (80%), urine (14%). Not significantly removed by hemodialysis. **Half-life:** 15 hrs.

⌛ LIFESPAN CONSIDERATIONS

Pregnancy/Lactation: Unknown if drug crosses placenta or is distributed in breast milk. Breastfeeding not recommended. **Children:** Safety and efficacy not established in pts younger than 3 yrs. **Elderly:** No age-related precautions noted.

INTERACTIONS

DRUG: May increase concentration/effects of **amiodarone, axitinib, bosutinib, budesonide, colchicine, dronedarone, eletriptan, ergot derivatives (e.g., ergotamine), fluticasone (nasal), lovastatin, midazolam, nimodipine, ranolazine, regorafenib, simvastatin, thioridazine. Strong CYP3A4 inducers (e.g., carBAMazepine, phenytoin, rifAMPin)** may decrease concentration/effect. **Strong CYP3A4 inhibitors (e.g.,**

carBAMazepine, ketoconazole, ritonavir) may increase concentration/effect. May decrease effects of **methadone, oral contraceptives.** HERBAL: **Garlic, St. John's wort** may lead to loss of virologic response, potential resistance to darunavir. FOOD: **Food** increases plasma concentration. LAB VALUES: May increase aPTT, PT, serum alkaline phosphatase, bilirubin, amylase, lipase, cholesterol, triglycerides, uric acid. May decrease lymphocytes/neutrophil count, platelets, WBC count; serum bicarbonate, albumin, calcium. May alter serum glucose, sodium.

AVAILABILITY (Rx)

Suspension, Oral: *(Prezista):* 100 mg/mL

Tablets: *(Prezista):* 75 mg, 150 mg, 600 mg, 800 mg.

ADMINISTRATION/HANDLING

PO

• Give with food (increases plasma concentration). • Coadministration with ritonavir required • Do not break, crush, dissolve, or divide film-coated tablets. • Shake suspension prior to each dose. Use provided oral dosing syringe.

INDICATIONS/ROUTES/DOSAGE

Note: Genotypic testing recommended in therapy-experienced pts.

HIV Infection, Treatment Experienced

PO: ADULTS, ELDERLY: **(With 1 or more darunavir resistance–associated substitution):** 600 mg administered twice daily with 100 mg ritonavir twice daily. **(With no darunavir resistance–associated substitutions):** 800 mg with 100 mg ritonavir or 150 mg cobicistat once daily.

HIV Infection, Treatment Naive

PO: ADULTS, ELDERLY: 800 mg administered with 100 mg ritonavir or 150 mg cobicistat once daily.

Usual Dosage During Pregnancy

PO: ADULTS: 600 mg administered twice daily with 100 mg ritonavir twice daily.

Usual Pediatric Dose

Treatment naive or treatment experienced with no darunavir resistance–associated substitutions: ***(Once-daily Dosing) (Suspension Only):*** WEIGHING 14 KG: 490 mg with 96 mg ritonavir. 13 KG: 455 mg with 80 mg ritonavir. 12 KG: 420 mg with 80 mg ritonavir. 11 KG: 385 mg with 64 mg ritonavir. 10 KG: 350 mg with 64 mg ritonavir. ***(Suspension or Tablets):*** WEIGHING 40 KG OR MORE: 800 mg with 100 mg ritonavir. 30–39 KG: 675 mg with 100 mg ritonavir. 15–29 KG: 600 mg with 100 mg ritonavir.

Treatment Experienced With 1 or More Darunavir Resistance–Associated Substitution

Use Tablet or Suspension

PO: CHILDREN WEIGHING 40 KG OR MORE: 600 mg twice daily with 100 mg ritonavir. WEIGHING 30–39 KG: 450 mg twice daily with 60 mg ritonavir. WEIGHING 15–29 KG: 375 mg twice daily with 48 mg ritonavir.

Use Oral Suspension Only

WEIGHING 14 KG TO LESS THAN 15 KG: 280 mg (48 mg ritonavir) twice daily. 13 KG TO LESS THAN 14 KG: 260 mg (40 mg ritonavir) twice daily. 12 KG TO LESS THAN 13 KG: 240 mg (40 mg ritonavir) twice daily. 11 KG TO LESS THAN 12 KG: 220 mg (32 mg ritonavir) twice daily. 10 KG TO LESS THAN 11 KG: 200 mg (32 mg ritonavir) twice daily.

Dosage in Renal Impairment

Mild to severe impairment: No dose adjustment.

Dosage in Hepatic Impairment

Mild to moderate impairment: No dose adjustment. **Severe impairment:** Not recommended.

SIDE EFFECTS

Frequent (19%–13%): Diarrhea, nausea, headache, nasopharyngitis. **Occasional** (3%–2%): Constipation, abdominal pain, vomiting. **Rare (less than 2%):** Allergic dermatitis, dyspepsia, flatulence, abdominal distention, anorexia, arthralgia, myalgia, paresthesia, memory impairment.

D

ADVERSE EFFECTS/TOXIC REACTIONS

Hyperglycemia, exacerbation of diabetes, diabetic ketoacidosis, new-onset diabetes have been reported in protease inhibitors. Drug-induced hepatotoxicity was reported, esp. in pts with advanced HIV disease, cirrhosis, hepatitis B or C virus infection, or pts taking multiple medications. May increase risk of bleeding in pts with history of hemophilia A or B. Immune reconstitution syndrome (inflammatory response to dormant opportunistic infections such as *Mycobacterium avium,* cytomegalovirus, PCP, tuberculosis, or acceleration of autoimmune disorders such as Graves' disease, polymyositis, Guillain-Barré) may occur. Skin reactions (including Stevens-Johnson syndrome, toxic epidermal necrolysis) occur rarely. Hypersensitivity reactions including anaphylaxis, angioedema, bronchospasm may occur.

NURSING CONSIDERATIONS

BASELINE ASSESSMENT

Obtain CD4+ count, viral load, HIV RNA level. Confirm HIV genotype. Question history of diabetes, hemophilia, hepatic impairment, prior hypersensitivity reactions. Receive full medication history (including herbal products); screen for contraindications/interactions. Offer emotional support.

INTERVENTION/EVALUATION

Monitor CD4+ count, viral load, HIV RNA level for treatment effectiveness. Monitor BMP, LFT, renal function, serum blood glucose periodically. An increase in serum creatinine greater than 0.4 mg/dL from baseline may indicate renal impairment. Closely monitor for GI discomfort. Monitor daily pattern of bowel activity, stool consistency. Monitor for hepatotoxicity (bruising, hematuria, jaundice, right upper abdominal pain, nausea, vomiting, weight loss), hypersensitivity reactions. Assess skin for rash, other skin reactions. Assess for immune reconstitution syndrome, opportunistic infections (onset of fever, oral mucosa changes, cough, other respiratory symptoms).

PATIENT/FAMILY TEACHING

• Treatment does not cure HIV infection, nor does it reduce risk of transmission. Practice safe sex with barrier methods or abstinence. • There is a high risk of drug interactions with other medications. Do not take newly prescribed medications unless approved by prescriber who originally started treatment. Do not take herbal products, esp. St. John's wort. • If amiodarone therapy cannot be withheld or stopped, immediately report symptoms of slow heart rate such as chest pain, confusion, dizziness, fainting, light-headedness, memory problems, palpitations, weakness. • Report any skin reactions. • Report any signs of decreased urine output, abdominal pain, yellowing of skin or eyes, darkened urine, clay-colored stools, weight loss. • As immune system strengthens, it may respond to dormant infections hidden within the body. Report any new fever, chills, body aches, cough, night sweats, shortness of breath. Antiretrovirals may cause excess body fat in the upper back, neck, breast, and trunk and may cause decreased body fat in legs, arms, and face. • Drug resistance can form if therapy is interrupted for even a short time; do not run out of supply. • Report symptoms of high blood sugar levels (confusion, excessive thirst/hunger, headache, frequent urination).

dasatinib

HIGH ALERT

da-**sa**-ti-nib
(Sprycel)
Do not confuse dasatinib with erlotinib, imatinib, or lapatinib.

◆CLASSIFICATION

PHARMACOTHERAPEUTIC: BCR-ABL tyrosine kinase inhibitor. **CLINICAL:** Antineoplastic.

USES

Chronic myeloid leukemia (CML): (Adults): Treatment of chronic, accelerated, myeloid or lymphoid blast phase of CML with resistance, intolerance to prior therapy, including imatinib. Treatment of Philadelphia chromosome–positive (Ph+) CML in chronic phase of newly diagnosed pt. **(Children):** Treatment of Ph+ CML in chronic phase. **Acute lymphoblastic leukemia:** Treatment of adults with Ph+ acute lymphoblastic leukemia (ALL) with resistance or intolerance to prior therapy, including imatinib. **(Children):** Treatment of newly diagnosed Ph+ ALL. **OFF-LABEL:** Post–stem cell transplant follow-up treatment of CML. Treatment of GI stromal tumor.

PRECAUTIONS

Contraindications: Hypersensitivity to dasatinib. **Cautions:** Hepatic impairment, myelosuppression (particularly thrombocytopenia), pts prone to fluid retention, pts at risk for QT interval prolongation or torsades de pointes (congenital long QT syndrome, medications that prolong QT interval, hypokalemia, hypomagnesemia); cardiovascular/pulmonary disease. Concomitant use of anticoagulants, CYP3A4 inducers/inhibitors may increase risk of pulmonary arterial hypertension.

ACTION

Reduces activity of proteins responsible for uncontrolled growth of leukemia cells by binding to most imatinib-resistant BCR-ABL mutations of pts with CML or ALL. **Therapeutic Effect:** Inhibits proliferation, tumor growth of CML and ALL cancer cell lines.

PHARMACOKINETICS

Extensively distributed in extravascular space. Protein binding: 96%. Metabolized in liver. Eliminated primarily in feces. **Half-life:** 3–5 hrs.

LIFESPAN CONSIDERATIONS

Pregnancy/Lactation: Has potential for severe teratogenic effects, fertility impairment. Breastfeeding not recommended. **Children:** Safety and efficacy not established in pts younger than 18 yrs. **Elderly:** No age-related precautions noted.

INTERACTIONS

DRUG: **CYP3A4 inhibitors (e.g., clarithromycin, ketoconazole, ritonavir)** may increase concentration/effect. **CYP3A4 inducers (e.g., carBAMazepine, phenytoin, rifAMPin)** may decrease concentration/effect. May decrease therapeutic effect of **BCG (intravesical), vaccines (live). H_2 antagonists (e.g., famotidine), proton pump inhibitors (e.g., omeprazole, pantoprazole)** may decrease concentration/effect. May increase adverse effects of **vaccines (live).** **HERBAL:** **Echinacea** may decrease therapeutic effect. **St. John's wort** may decrease concentration/effect. **FOOD:** **Grapefruit products** may increase concentration/toxicity (increased risk of torsades, myelotoxicity). **LAB VALUES:** May decrease WBC, platelets, Hgb, Hct, RBC; serum calcium, phosphates. May increase serum ALT, AST, bilirubin, creatinine.

AVAILABILITY (Rx)

Tablets (Film-Coated): 20 mg, 50 mg, 70 mg, 80 mg, 100 mg, 140 mg.

ADMINISTRATION/HANDLING

PO

• Give without regard to food. • Give with food or large glass of water if GI upset occurs. • Do not break, crush, dissolve, or divide film-coated tablets. • Do not give antacids either 2 hrs prior to or within 2 hrs after dasatinib administration.

INDICATIONS/ROUTES/DOSAGE

Note: CYP3A4 inhibitors: Consider decreasing dose from 100 mg to 20 mg or 140 mg to 40 mg. **CYP3A4 inducers:** Consider increasing dose with monitoring.

CML (Resistant or intolerant)

PO: ADULTS, ELDERLY: Chronic phase: 100 mg once daily. May increase to

140 mg once daily in pts not achieving cytogenetic response. **Accelerated or blast phase:** 140 mg once daily. May increase to 180 mg once daily in pts not achieving cytogenetic response.

Ph+ CML (Newly diagnosed in chronic phase)

PO: ADULTS, ELDERLY: 100 mg once daily. May increase to 140 mg/day in pts not achieving cytogenetic response. **CHILDREN (1 YR AND OLDER) WEIGHING 45 KG OR MORE:** 100 mg once daily. May increase to 120 mg once daily. **30–44 KG:** 70 mg once daily. May increase to 90 mg once daily. **20–29 KG:** 60 mg once daily. May increase to 70 mg once daily. **10–19 KG:** 40 mg once daily. May increase to 50 mg once daily.

Ph+ ALL

PO: ADULTS, ELDERLY: 140 mg once daily. May increase to 180 mg once daily in pts not achieving cytogenetic response. **CHILDREN WEIGHING 10 KG OR MORE, ADOLESCENTS WEIGHING 45 KG OR MORE:** 100 mg once daily. **30 TO LESS THAN 45 KG:** 70 mg once daily. **20 TO LESS THAN 30 KG:** 60 mg once daily. **10 TO LESS THAN 20 KG:** 40 mg once daily.

Dosage in Renal/Hepatic Impairment

No dose adjustment.

SIDE EFFECTS

Frequent (50%–32%): Fluid retention, diarrhea, headache, fatigue, musculoskeletal pain, fever, rash, nausea, dyspnea. **Occasional (28%–12%):** Cough, abdominal pain, vomiting, anorexia, asthenia, arthralgia, stomatitis, dizziness, constipation, peripheral neuropathy, myalgia. **Rare (less than 12%):** Abdominal distention, chills, weight increase, pruritus.

ADVERSE EFFECTS/TOXIC REACTIONS

Pleural effusion occurred in 8% of pts, febrile neutropenia in 7%, GI bleeding, pneumonia in 6%, thrombocytopenia in 5%, dyspnea in 4%; anemia, cardiac failure in 3%.

NURSING CONSIDERATIONS

BASELINE ASSESSMENT

Obtain CBC weekly for first mo, biweekly for second mo, and periodically thereafter. Monitor LFT before treatment begins and monthly thereafter. Obtain baseline weight. Offer emotional support.

INTERVENTION/EVALUATION

Monitor CBC weekly for first mo, biweekly for second mo, then periodically thereafter. Monitor LFT monthly. Weigh daily, monitor for unexpected rapid weight gain. Offer antiemetics to control nausea, vomiting. Monitor daily pattern of bowel activity, stool consistency. Assess oral mucous membranes for evidence of stomatitis. Monitor CBC for neutropenia, thrombocytopenia; monitor hepatic function tests for hepatotoxicity.

PATIENT/FAMILY TEACHING

• Avoid crowds, those with known infection. • Avoid contact with anyone who recently received live virus vaccine; do not receive vaccinations. • Antacids may be taken up to 2 hrs before or 2 hrs after taking dasatinib. • Avoid grapefruit products. • Do not chew, crush, dissolve, or divide tablets.

DAUNOrubicin

HIGH ALERT

daw-noe-**roo**-bi-sin
(Cerubidine, Vyxeos)

■ BLACK BOX ALERT ■ May cause cumulative, dose-related myocardial toxicity. Severe myelosuppression may lead to infection or hemorrhage. Must be administered by personnel trained in administration/handling of chemotherapeutic agents. Caution in pts with renal impairment or hepatic dysfunction. Extravasation may cause severe local tissue necrosis.

Do not confuse DAUNOrubicin with DACTINomycin, DOXOrubicin, epiRUBicin, IDArubicin, or valrubicin.

◆CLASSIFICATION

PHARMACOTHERAPEUTIC: Anthracycline topoisomerase II inhibitor. **CLINICAL:** Antineoplastic.

USES

Cerubidine: Treatment of leukemias (acute lymphocytic [ALL], acute myeloid [AML]) in combination with other agents. **Vyxeos:** Treatment of adults with newly diagnosed therapy-related AML or AML with myelodysplasia-related changes.

PRECAUTIONS

Contraindications: Hypersensitivity to DAUNOrubicin. **Cautions:** Preexisting heart disease or bone marrow suppression, hypertension, concurrent chemotherapeutic agents, elderly, infants, radiation therapy.

ACTION

Inhibits DNA and RNA synthesis by intercalation between DNA base pairs and by steric obstruction. Cell cycle–phase nonspecific. **Therapeutic Effect:** Inhibits tumor cell growth and survival.

PHARMACOKINETICS

Widely distributed. Protein binding: High. Does not cross blood-brain barrier. Metabolized in liver. Excreted in urine (40%); biliary excretion (40%). **Half-life:** 18.5 hrs; metabolite: 26.7 hrs.

LIFESPAN CONSIDERATIONS

Pregnancy/Lactation: Avoid pregnancy; may cause fetal harm. Breastfeeding not recommended. **Children:** Cardiotoxicity may be more frequent and occur at lower cumulative doses. **Elderly:** Cardiotoxicity may be more frequent; reduced bone marrow reserves require caution. Age-related renal impairment may require dosage adjustment.

INTERACTIONS

DRUG: **Bevacizumab, cyclophosphamide** may increase risk of cardiotoxicity. **Bone marrow depressants (e.g., cladribine)** may enhance myelosuppression. May decrease therapeutic effect of **BCG (intravesical). Live virus vaccines** may potentiate virus replication, increase vaccine side effects, decrease pt's antibody response to vaccine. **HERBAL:** **Echinacea** may decrease therapeutic effect. **FOOD:** None known. **LAB VALUES:** May increase serum alkaline phosphatase, bilirubin, uric acid, AST.

AVAILABILITY (Rx)

Injection Solution: *(Cerubidine):* 5 mg/mL. **Injection Suspension:** *(Vyxeos):* DAUNOrubicin 44 mg/cytarabine 100 mg

ADMINISTRATION/HANDLING

IV (Cerubidine)

Give by IV push or IV infusion.

Reconstitution • May further dilute with 100 mL D_5W or 0.9% NaCl.

Rate of administration • For IV push, withdraw desired dose into syringe containing 10–15 mL 0.9% NaCl. Inject over 1–5 min into tubing of rapidly infusing IV solution of D_5W or 0.9% NaCl. • For IV infusion, further dilute with 100 mL D_5W or 0.9% NaCl. Infuse over 15–30 min. • Extravasation produces immediate pain, severe local tissue damage. Aspirate as much infiltrated drug as possible, then infiltrate area with hydrocortisone sodium succinate injection (50–100 mg hydrocortisone) and/or isotonic sodium thiosulfate injection or ascorbic acid injection (1 mL of 5% injection). Apply cold compresses.

Storage • Refrigerate intact vials. • Protect from light. • Solutions prepared for infusion stable for 24 hrs at room temperature.

IV (Vyxeos)

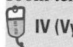

Reconstitution • Reconstitute each vial with 19 mL Sterile Water for Injection to a concentration of 2.2 mg/mL. • Swirl contents for 5 min while gently inverting vial q30sec. • Allow vial to rest for 15 min. • Dilute in 500 mL infusion bag containing NS or D_5W.

Rate of administration • Infuse

over 90 min. **Storage** • Refrigerate vials. • Protect from light. • Stable for up to 4 hrs when refrigerated.

IV INCOMPATIBILITIES

Allopurinol (Aloprim), aztreonam (Azactam), cefepime (Maxipime), dexamethasone (Decadron), heparin, piperacillin and tazobactam (Zosyn).

IV COMPATIBILITIES

Granisetron (Kytril), ondansetron (Zofran).

INDICATIONS/ROUTES/DOSAGE

◀ALERT▶ Refer to individual protocols. Cumulative dose should not exceed 550 mg/m^2 in adults (increased risk of cardiotoxicity) or 400 mg/m^2 in those receiving chest irradiation.

Acute Lymphocytic Leukemia

IV: ADULTS, ELDERLY: 45 mg/m^2 on days 1, 2, and 3 (in combination with vinCRIStine, predniSONE, asparaginase). **CHILDREN 2 YRS AND OLDER AND BODY SURFACE AREA 0.5 m^2 OR GREATER:** 25 mg/m^2 on day 1 of every wk for up to 4–6 cycles (in combination with vinCRIStine, predniSONE). **CHILDREN YOUNGER THAN 2 YRS, OR BODY SURFACE AREA LESS THAN 0.5 m^2:** 1 mg/kg/dose on day 1 of every wk for up to 4 to 6 cycles (in combination with vinCRIStine, predniSONE).

Acute Myeloid Leukemia

IV: ADULTS YOUNGER THAN 60 YRS: 45 mg/m^2 on days 1, 2, and 3 of induction course, then on days 1 and 2 of subsequent courses (in combination with cytarabine). **ADULTS 60 YRS AND OLDER:** 30 mg/m^2 on days 1, 2, and 3 of induction course, then on days 1 and 2 of subsequent courses (in combination with cytarabine).

AML (Vyxeos)

IV: ADULTS, ELDERLY: (Induction first cycle): DAUNOrubicin 44 mg/m^2 and cytarabine 100 mg/m^2 on days 1, 3, and 5. **(Induction second cycle):** Days 1 and 3 (may give 2–5 wks after 1st induction cycle). **(Consolidation):** DAUNOrubicin 29 mg/m^2 and cytarabine 65 mg/m^2 on days 1 and 3 (may give 1st consolidation cycle 5–8 wks after start of last induction and 2nd consolidation 5–8 wks after start of 1st consolidation cycle).

Dosage in Renal Impairment

Serum creatinine greater than 3 mg/dL: 50% of normal dose.

Dosage in Hepatic Impairment

Bilirubin 1.2–3 mg/dL: 75% of normal dose. **Bilirubin 3.1–5 mg/dL:** 50% of normal dose. **Bilirubin greater than 5 mg/dL:** DAUNOrubicin is not recommended for use in this pt population.

SIDE EFFECTS

Frequent: Complete alopecia (scalp, axillary, pubic), nausea, vomiting (beginning a few hrs after administration and lasting 24–48 hrs). **Occasional:** Diarrhea, abdominal pain, esophagitis, stomatitis, transverse pigmentation of fingernails, toenails. **Rare:** Transient fever, chills.

ADVERSE EFFECTS/TOXIC REACTIONS

Myelosuppression (severe leukopenia, anemia, thrombocytopenia) is expected. Decreases in platelet count, WBC count occur in 10–14 days, then return to normal level by third week. Cardiotoxicity including absolute decrease in LVEF, HF, death may occur, esp. in children and pts with preexisting cardiac disease. ECG findings and/or cardiomyopathy is manifested as HF (risk increases when cumulative dose exceeds 550 mg/m^2 in adults, 300 mg/m^2 in children 2 yrs and older, or total dosage greater than 10 mg/kg in children younger than 2 yrs). Pericarditis-myocarditis may occur. Secondary leukemias were reported in pts exposed to topoisomerase II inhibitors when used concomitantly with other antineoplastics or radiation therapy. Extravasation can cause severe local tissue necrosis.

NURSING CONSIDERATIONS

BASELINE ASSESSMENT

Obtain CBC, LFT; BUN, serum creatinine, CrCl, GFR in pts with renal impairment.

Obtain ECG before initiation, esp. in pts with cardiac disease. Antiemetics may be effective in preventing, treating nausea. Ensure patency of IV access. Obtain accurate height and weight for dose calculation. Offer emotional support.

INTERVENTION/EVALUATION

Obtain CBC frequently; BMP, LFT, serum uric acid periodically. Monitor daily pattern of bowel activity, stool consistency. Monitor for hematologic toxicity (fever, sore throat, signs of local infection, unusual bruising/bleeding from any site); symptoms of anemia (excessive fatigue, weakness). Diligently monitor for extravasation, tissue necrosis.

PATIENT/FAMILY TEACHING

• Urine may turn reddish color for 1–2 days after beginning therapy. • Hair loss is reversible, but new hair growth may have different color, texture. New hair growth resumes about 5 wks after last therapy dose • Maintain strict oral hygiene. • Do not have immunizations without physician's approval (drug lowers resistance). • Avoid contact with those who have recently received live virus vaccine. • Promptly report fever, sore throat, signs of local infection, unusual bruising/bleeding from any site, yellowing of whites of eyes/skin, difficulty breathing. • Report persistent nausea, vomiting. • Treatment may impair the heart's ability to pump blood effectively; report difficulty breathing, chest pain, palpitations, swelling of the legs or feet.

deferasirox

dee-**fur**-a-sir-ox
(Exjade, Jadenu)

BLACK BOX ALERT May cause renal/hepatic failure, hepatotoxicity, gastrointestinal hemorrhage.

Do not confuse deferasirox with deferoxamine.

◆CLASSIFICATION

PHARMACOTHERAPEUTIC: Iron-chelating agent. **CLINICAL:** Iron reduction agent.

USES

Treatment of chronic iron overload due to blood transfusions (transfusional hemosiderosis) in pts 2 yrs and older or due to non–transfusion-dependent thalassemia syndrome in pts 10 yrs and older.

PRECAUTIONS

Contraindications: Hypersensitivity to deferasirox. Platelet counts less than 50,000 cells/mm^3; poor performance status, high-risk myelodysplastic syndromes or advanced malignancies; CrCl less than 40 mL/min or serum creatinine greater than 2 times the upper limit of normal. **Cautions:** Renal/hepatic impairment, elderly, concurrent medications that may increase GI effects (e.g., NSAIDs).

ACTION

Selective for iron. Binds iron with high affinity in a 2:1 ratio. **Therapeutic Effect:** Induces iron excretion through the feces.

PHARMACOKINETICS

Well absorbed following PO administration. Protein binding: 99%. Metabolized in liver. Excreted in feces (84%), urine (8%). **Half-life:** 8–16 hrs.

⌛ LIFESPAN CONSIDERATIONS

Pregnancy/Lactation: Unknown if drug crosses placenta or is distributed in breast milk. **Children:** Not recommended for pts younger than 2 yrs. **Elderly:** No age-related precautions noted.

INTERACTIONS

DRUG: **Antacids containing aluminium** may decrease concentration/effects. May increase concentration/effect of **theophylline, tiZANidine.** **HERBAL:** None significant. **FOOD**: Bioavailability is variably increased when given with **food. LAB VALUES**: Decreases serum ferritin. May increase serum ALT, AST, creatinine; urine protein.

D

AVAILABILITY (Rx)

Packets, Sprinkle: ***(Jadenu):*** 90 mg, 180 mg, 360 mg. **Tablets:** ***(Jadenu):*** 90 mg, 180 mg, 360 mg. **Tablets, Soluble:** ***(Exjade):*** 125 mg, 250 mg, 500 mg.

ADMINISTRATION/HANDLING

PO

• Give on empty stomach 30 min before food. • Do not give simultaneously with aluminum-containing antacids, cholestyramine. • Tablets for suspension should not be chewed or swallowed whole. • Disperse tablet by stirring in water, apple juice, orange juice until fine suspension is achieved. • Dosage less than 1 g should be dispersed in 3.5 oz of liquid, dosage more than 1 g should be dispersed in 7 oz of liquid. If any residue remains in glass, resuspend with a small amount of liquid. • Give regular tablets whole with water.

INDICATIONS/ROUTES/DOSAGE

Iron Overload Due to Transfusions

PO: ADULTS, ELDERLY, CHILDREN 2 YRS AND OLDER: ***(Exjade):*** Initially, 20 mg/kg once daily. **Maintenance:** (Titrate to individual response and goals.) Adjust dosage by 5 or 10 mg/kg/day every 3–6 mos based on serum ferritin levels. Consider holding for serum ferritin less than 500 mcg/L. **Maximum:** 40 mg/kg once daily. ***(Jadenu):*** Initially, 14 mg/kg once daily. **Maintenance:** (Titrate to individual response and goals.) Adjust dosage by 3.5 or 7 mg/kg/day based on serum ferritin levels. Consider holding for serum ferritin less than 500 mcg/L. **Maximum:** 28 mcg/kg once daily.

Thalassemia Syndromes

PO: ADULTS, ELDERLY, CHILDREN 10 YRS AND OLDER: ***(Exjade):*** Initially, 10 mg/kg once daily. May increase to 20 mg/kg once daily after 4 wks if baseline iron is greater than 15 mg Fe/g dry wgt. ***(Jadenu):*** Initially, 7 mg/kg once daily. May increase to 14 mg/kg/day after 4 wks if baseline iron greater than 15 mg Fe/g dry wgt. **Maintenance:** ***(Exjade/Jadenu):*** Dose adjustments based on serum ferritin and hepatic iron concentrations.

Dosage in Renal Impairment

Note: See Contraindications.

ADULTS: For increase in serum creatinine greater than 33% on 2 consecutive measures, reduce daily dose by 10 mg/kg. **CHILDREN**: For increase in serum creatinine above age-appropriate upper limit of normal on 2 consecutive measures, reduce daily dose by 10 mg/kg. **CrCl 40–60 mL/min:** Reduce starting dose by 50%.

Dosage in Hepatic Impairment

For severe or persistent elevations in hepatic function tests, consider dose reduction or discontinuation. **Moderate impairment**: Reduce initial dose by 50%.

SIDE EFFECTS

Frequent (19%–10%): Fever, headache, abdominal pain, cough, nasopharyngitis, diarrhea, nausea, vomiting. **Occasional (9%–4%)**: Rash, arthralgia, fatigue, back pain, urticaria. **Rare (1%)**: Edema, sleep disorder, dizziness, anxiety.

ADVERSE EFFECTS/TOXIC REACTIONS

Bronchitis, pharyngitis, acute tonsillitis, ear infection occur occasionally. Hepatitis, auditory disturbances, ocular abnormalities occur rarely. Acute renal failure, cytopenias (e.g., agranulocytosis, neutropenia, thrombocytopenia) may occur.

NURSING CONSIDERATIONS

BASELINE ASSESSMENT

Obtain baseline serum CBC, ferritin, iron, creatinine, ALT, AST, urine protein, then monthly thereafter. Auditory, ophthalmic testing should be obtained before therapy and annually thereafter.

INTERVENTION/EVALUATION

Treatment should be interrupted if serum ferritin levels are consistently less than 500 mcg/L. Suspend treatment if severe rash occurs.

PATIENT/FAMILY TEACHING

• Take on empty stomach 30 min before food. • Do not chew or swallow soluble tablets; disperse tablet completely in water, apple juice, orange juice; drink resulting suspension immediately. • Do not take aluminum-containing antacids concurrently. • Report severe skin rash, changes in vision/hearing, or yellowing of skin/eyes.

denosumab

TOP 100

den-**oh**-sue-mab
(Prolia, Xgeva)
Do not confuse denosumab with daclizumab, or Prolia with Avandia or Zebeta.

CLASSIFICATION

PHARMACOTHERAPEUTIC: Monoclonal antibody (with affinity for RANKL). **CLINICAL:** Bone-modifying agent.

USES

Prolia: Treatment of osteoporosis in postmenopausal women at high risk for fracture. Treatment of glucocorticoid-induced osteoporosis in pts at high risk of fracture who are receiving an equivalent dose of 7.5 mg or more of predniSONE for duration of at least 6 mos. Treatment to increase bone mass in men at high risk for fractures; treatment of bone loss in men receiving androgen deprivation therapy for nonmetastatic prostate cancer and in women at high risk for fractures receiving adjuvant aromatase inhibitor therapy for breast cancer. **Xgeva:** Prevention of skeletal-related events (e.g., fracture, spinal cord compression) in pts with bone metastases from solid tumor or multiple myeloma. Treatment of giant cell tumor of bone in adults and skeletally mature adolescents. Treatment of hypercalcemia of malignancy refractory to bisphosphonate therapy. **OFF-LABEL:** Treatment of bone destruction caused by rheumatoid arthritis.

PRECAUTIONS

Contraindications: Hypersensitivity to denosumab. **Prolia:** Preexisting hypocalcemia, pregnancy. **Xgeva:** Preexisting hypocalcemia. **Cautions:** History of hypoparathyroidism, thyroid/parathyroid surgery, malabsorption syndromes, excision of small intestine, immunocompromised pts. Pts with severe renal impairment or receiving dialysis (greater risk for developing hypocalcemia). Pts with impaired immune system or immunosuppressive therapy.

ACTION

Binds to RANKL; blocks interaction between RANKL and RANK, preventing osteoclast formation. **Therapeutic Effect:** Decreases bone resorption; increases bone mass in osteoporosis; decreases skeletal-related events and tumor-induced bone destruction in solid tumors, multiple myeloma. Inhibits tumor growth.

PHARMACOKINETICS

Serum level detected 1 hr after administration. **Half-life:** 32 days.

LIFESPAN CONSIDERATIONS

Pregnancy/Lactation: Approved for use only in postmenopausal women.

Children: Approved for use only in postmenopausal women. **Elderly:** No age-related precautions noted.

INTERACTIONS

DRUG: May enhance adverse/toxic effect of **belimumab, immunosuppressants.** **HERBAL:** None significant. **FOOD:** None known. **LAB VALUES:** May decrease serum calcium. May increase serum cholesterol.

AVAILABILITY (Rx)

Injection, Solution: ***(Prolia):*** 60 mg/mL. ***(Xgeva):*** 120 mg/1.7 mL.

ADMINISTRATION/HANDLING

SQ

• Administer in upper arm, upper thigh, or abdomen.

Storage • Refrigerate. Use within 14 days once at room temperature. • Solution appears as clear, colorless to pale yellow.

INDICATIONS/ROUTES/DOSAGE

Note: Administer calcium and vitamin D to prevent/treat hypocalcemia.

Prolia

Androgen Deprivation, Bone Loss, Osteoporosis

SQ: ADULTS, ELDERLY: 60 mg every 6 mos.

Xgeva

Prevention of Skeletal-Related Events From Solid Tumors, Multiple Myeloma

SQ: ADULTS, ELDERLY: 120 mg q4wks.

Giant Cell Tumor of Bone, Hypercalcemia of Malignancy

SQ: ADULTS, ELDERLY, MATURE ADOLESCENTS: 120 mg q4wks with additional doses on days 8 and 15 of first mo of therapy.

Dosage in Renal/Hepatic Impairment

No dose adjustment.

SIDE EFFECTS

Frequent (35%–12%): Back pain, extremity pain. **Occasional (8%–5%):** Musculoskeletal pain, vertigo, peripheral edema, sciatica. **Rare (4%–2%):** Bone pain, upper abdominal pain, rash, insomnia, flatulence, pruritus, myalgia, asthenia, GI reflux.

ADVERSE EFFECTS/TOXIC REACTIONS

Increases risk of infection, specifically cystitis, upper respiratory tract infection, pneumonia, pharyngitis, herpes zoster (shingles) occur in 2%–6% of pts. Osteonecrosis of the jaw (OJN) was reported. Suppression of bone turnover, pancreatitis have been reported.

NURSING CONSIDERATIONS

BASELINE ASSESSMENT

Hypocalcemia must be corrected prior to treatment. Calcium 1,000 mg/day and vitamin D at least 400 international units/day should be given. Dental exam should be provided prior to treatment. Recommend baseline bone density scan.

INTERVENTION/EVALUATION

Monitor serum magnesium, calcium, ionized calcium, phosphate. In pts predisposed with hypocalcemia and disturbances of mineral metabolism, clinical monitoring of calcium, mineral levels is highly recommended. Adequately supplement all pts with calcium and vitamin D. Monitor for delayed fracture healing.

PATIENT/FAMILY TEACHING

• Report rash, new-onset eczema. • Seek prompt medical attention if signs, symptoms of severe infection (rash, itching, reddened skin, cellulitis) occur. • Report muscle stiffness, numbness, cramps, spasms (signs of hypocalcemia); swelling or drainage from jaw, mouth, or teeth.

desmopressin

des-moe-**press**-in
(DDAVP, DDAVP Rhinal Tube, Noctiva, Stimate)

◆CLASSIFICATION

PHARMACOTHERAPEUTIC: Synthetic vasopressin analog (hormone, posterior pituitary). **CLINICAL:** Antihemophilic. Hemostatic.

USES

Nasal, Parenteral: Antidiuretic replacement therapy in managing central cranial diabetes insipidus. Manage polyuria and polydipsia following head trauma or surgery in pituitary region. Maintain hemostasis and control bleeding in hemophilia A, von Willebrand's disease (type I). **PO:** Antidiuretic replacement therapy in managing central cranial diabetes insipidus, primary management of nocturnal enuresis, management of temporary polyuria, polydipsia following pituitary surgery or head trauma. **Intranasal:** Treatment of nocturia due to nocturnal polyuria in adults who awaken at least 2 times/night to void. **OFF-LABEL:** Uremic bleeding occurring with acute/chronic renal failure; prevent surgical bleeding in pts with uremia.

PRECAUTIONS

Contraindications: Hypersensitivity to desmopressin. Hyponatremia, history of hyponatremia, moderate to severe renal impairment. **Cautions:** Predisposition to thrombus formation; conditions with fluid, electrolyte imbalance; coronary artery disease; hypertensive cardiovascular disease, elderly pts, cystic fibrosis, HF, renal impairment, polydipsia. Avoid use in hemophilia A with factor VIII levels less than 5%; hemophilia B; severe type I, type IIB, platelet-type von Willebrand's disease.

ACTION

Increases cAMP in renal tubular cells, which increases water permeability, decreasing urine volume. Increases levels of von Willebrand factor, factor VIII, tissue plasminogen activator (tPA). **Therapeutic Effect:** Shortens activated partial thromboplastin time (aPTT), bleeding time. Decreases urinary output.

PHARMACOKINETICS

Route	Onset	Peak	Duration
PO	1 hr	2–7 hrs	8–12 hrs
IV	15–30 min	1.5–3 hrs	8–12 hrs
Intranasal	15 min–1 hr	1–5 hrs	8–12 hrs

Poorly absorbed after PO, nasal administration. Metabolism: Unknown. **Half-life: PO:** 1.5–2.5 hrs. **Intranasal:** 3.3–3.5 hrs. **IV:** 0.4–4 hrs.

⌛ LIFESPAN CONSIDERATIONS

Pregnancy/Lactation: Unknown if distributed in breast milk. **Children:** Caution in neonates, pts younger than 3 mos (increased risk of fluid balance problems). Careful fluid restrictions recommended in infants. **Elderly:** Increased risk of hyponatremia, water intoxication.

INTERACTIONS

DRUG: **CarBAMazepine, lamoTRIgine, NSAIDs (e.g., ibuprofen, ketorolac, naproxen), SSRIs (e.g., citalopram, sertraline), tricyclic antidepressants (e.g., amitriptyline, doxepin, nortriptyline)** may increase effect. **Demeclocycline, lithium** may decrease effect. **Corticosteroids (e.g., dexamethasone, predniSONE), loop diuretics (e.g., furosemide)** may increase hyponatremic effect. **HERBAL:** None significant. **FOOD:** None known. **LAB VALUES:** May decrease serum sodium.

AVAILABILITY (Rx)

Injection Solution: ***(DDAVP):*** 4 mcg/mL. **Nasal Solution:** ***(DDAVP Rhinal Tube 0.01%):*** 100 mcg/mL (10 mcg/spray). **Nasal Spray:** ***(Stimate):*** 1.5 mg/mL (150 mcg/spray). **Nasal Emulsion:** 1.66 mcg/0.1 mL. **Tablets:** ***(DDAVP):*** 0.1 mg, 0.2 mg.

ADMINISTRATION/HANDLING

IV

Reconstitution • For IV infusion, dilute in 10–50 mL 0.9% NaCl (10 mL for children 10 kg or less; 50 mL for adults, children greater than 10 kg).

Rate of administration • Infuse over 15–30 min.

Storage • Refrigerate.

SQ

• Withdraw dose from vial. Further dilution not required.

Intranasal

• Refrigerate DDAVP Rhinal Tube solution, Stimate nasal spray. • Rhinal Tube solution, Stimate nasal spray are stable for 3 wks at room temperature. • DDAVP nasal spray is stable at room temperature. • Calibrated catheter (rhinyle) is used to draw up measured quantity of desmopressin; with one end inserted in nose, pt blows on other end to deposit solution deep in nasal cavity. • For infants, young children, obtunded pts, air-filled syringe may be attached to catheter to deposit solution.

INDICATIONS/ROUTES/DOSAGE

Nocturia

Intranasal: ADULTS: 1.66 mcg in either nostril about 30 min before bedtime.

Primary Nocturnal Enuresis

PO: CHILDREN 6 YRS AND OLDER: 0.2–0.6 mg once before bedtime. Limit fluid intake 1 hr prior and at least 8 hrs after dose.

Central Cranial Diabetes Insipidus

◀ALERT▶ Fluid restriction should be observed.

PO: ADULTS, ELDERLY, CHILDREN 4 YRS AND OLDER: Initially, 0.05 mg twice daily. Titrate to desired response. Range: 0.1–1.2 mg/day in 2–3 divided doses.

IV, SQ: ADULTS, ELDERLY, CHILDREN 12 YRS AND OLDER: 2–4 mcg/day in 2 divided doses or one-tenth of maintenance intranasal dose.

Intranasal: ***(Use 100 mcg/mL concentration):*** **ADULTS, ELDERLY, CHILDREN OLDER THAN 12 YRS:** 10–40 mcg (0.1–0.4 mL) in 1–3 doses/day. Usual dose: 10 mcg 2 times/day. **CHILDREN 3 MOS–12 YRS:** Initially, 5 mcg (0.05 mL)/day. Range: 5–30 mcg (0.05–0.3 mL)/day as a single or 2 divided doses.

Hemophilia A, Von Willebrand's Disease (Type I)

IV infusion: ADULTS, ELDERLY, CHILDREN: 0.3 mcg/kg as slow infusion.

Intranasal: ***(Use 1.5 mg/mL concentration providing 150 mcg/spray):*** **ADULTS, ELDERLY, CHILDREN WEIGHING MORE THAN 50 KG:** 300 mcg; use 1 spray in each nostril. **ADULTS, ELDERLY, CHILDREN WEIGHING 50 KG OR LESS:** 150 mcg as a single spray. Repeat use based on clinical conditions/laboratory work.

Dosage in Renal Impairment

CrCl less than 50 mL/min: Not recommended.

Dosage in Hepatic Impairment

No dose adjustment.

SIDE EFFECTS

Occasional: IV: Pain, redness, swelling at injection site; headache, abdominal cramps, vulvular pain, flushed skin, mild B/P elevation, nausea with high dosages. **Nasal:** Rhinorrhea, nasal congestion, slight B/P elevation.

ADVERSE EFFECTS/TOXIC REACTIONS

Water intoxication, hyponatremia (headache, drowsiness, confusion, decreased urination, rapid weight gain, seizures, coma) may occur in overhydration. Children, elderly pts, infants are esp. at risk.

NURSING CONSIDERATIONS

BASELINE ASSESSMENT

Establish baselines for B/P, pulse, weight, serum electrolytes, urine specific gravity. Check lab values for factor VIII coagulant concentration for hemophilia A, von Willebrand's disease; bleeding times.

INTERVENTION/EVALUATION

Check B/P, pulse with IV infusion. Monitor pt weight, fluid intake; urine volume, urine specific gravity, osmolality, serum electrolytes for diabetes insipidus. Assess factor VIII antigen levels, aPTT, factor VIII activity level for hemophilia.

PATIENT/FAMILY TEACHING

• Avoid overhydration. • Follow guidelines for proper intranasal administration. • Report headache, shortness of breath, heartburn, nausea, abdominal cramps.

dexamethasone

dex-a-**meth**-a-sone
(Decadron, Dexamethasone Intensol, DexPak, Maxidex)
Do not confuse Decadron with Percodan, or dexamethasone with dextroamphetamine, or Maxidex with Maxzide.

FIXED-COMBINATION(S)

Ciprodex Otic: dexamethasone/ciprofloxacin (antibiotic): 0.1%/0.3%. **Dexacidin, Maxitrol:** dexamethasone/neomycin/polymyxin (anti-infectives): 0.1%/3.5 mg/10,000 units per g or mL.

◆CLASSIFICATION

PHARMACOTHERAPEUTIC: Glucocorticoid. **CLINICAL:** Anti-inflammatory. Antiemetic.

USES

Used primarily as an anti-inflammatory or immunosuppressant agent in a variety of diseases (e.g., allergic states, edematous states, neoplastic diseases, rheumatic disorders). **OFF-LABEL:** Antiemetic, treatment of croup, dexamethasone suppression test (indicator consistent with suicide and/or depression), accelerate fetal lung maturation. Treatment of acute mountain sickness, high-altitude cerebral edema.

PRECAUTIONS

Contraindications: Hypersensitivity to dexamethasone. Systemic fungal infections. **Cautions:** Thyroid disease, renal/hepatic impairment, cardiovascular disease, diabetes, glaucoma, cataracts, myasthenia gravis, pts at risk for seizures, osteoporosis, post-MI, elderly.

ACTION

Decreases inflammation by suppression of neutrophil migration, decreases production of inflammatory mediators. Reverses increased capillary permeability. Suppresses normal immune response. **Therapeutic Effect:** Decreases inflammation.

PHARMACOKINETICS

Rapidly absorbed from GI tract after PO administration. Widely distributed. Protein binding: High. Metabolized in liver. Primarily excreted in urine. Minimally removed by hemodialysis. **Half-life:** 3–4.5 hrs.

LIFESPAN CONSIDERATIONS

Pregnancy/Lactation: Crosses placenta. Distributed in breast milk. **Children:** Prolonged treatment with high-dose therapy may decrease short-term growth rate, cortisol secretion. **Elderly:** Higher risk for developing hypertension, osteoporosis.

INTERACTIONS

DRUG: **Amphotericin** may increase hypokalemia. **CYP3A4 inducers (e.g., carBAMazepine, phenytoin, rifAMPin)** may decrease concentration/effect. **CYP3A4 inhibitors (e.g., clarithromycin, ketoconazole, ritonavir), macrolide antibiotics** may increase concentration/effect. May decrease therapeutic effect of **aldesleukin**. May increase hyponatremic effect of **desmopressin**. **Live virus vaccines** may decrease pt's antibody response to vaccine, increase vaccine side effects, potentiate virus replication. **HERBAL:** **Echinacea** may increase immunosuppressant effect. **St. John's wort** may decrease concentration/effect. **FOOD:** Interferes with **calcium**

absorption. **LAB VALUES:** May increase serum glucose, lipids, sodium levels. May decrease serum calcium, potassium, thyroxine, WBC.

AVAILABILITY (Rx)

Elixir: 0.5 mg/5 mL. **Injection, Solution:** 4 mg/mL, 10 mg/mL. **Ophthalmic Solution:** 0.1%. **Ophthalmic Suspension:** 0.1%. **Solution, Oral:** 0.5 mg/5 mL. **Solution, Oral Concentrate:** ***(Dexamethasone Intensol):*** 1 mg/mL. **Tablets:** 0.5 mg, 0.75 mg, 1 mg, 1.5 mg, 2 mg, 4 mg, 6 mg.

ADMINISTRATION/HANDLING

IV

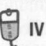

◄ALERT► Dexamethasone sodium phosphate may be given by IV push or IV infusion. Rapid injection may cause genital burning sensation in females.

• For IV push, give over 1–4 min if dose is less than 10 mg. • For IV infusion, mix with 50–100 mL 0.9% NaCl or D_5W and infuse over 15–30 min. • For neonates, solution must be preservative free. • IV solution must be used within 24 hrs.

IM

• Give deep IM, preferably in gluteus maximus.

PO

• Give with milk, food (to decrease GI effect).

Ophthalmic Solution, Suspension

• Place gloved finger on lower eyelid and pull out until a pocket is formed between eye and lower lid. • Place prescribed number of drops or 1/4 to 1/2 inch ointment into pocket. • Instruct pt to close eye gently for 1–2 min (so that medication will not be squeezed out of the sac). • Instruct pt to apply digital pressure to lacrimal sac at inner canthus for 1–2 min to minimize systemic absorption.

IV INCOMPATIBILITIES

Ciprofloxacin (Cipro), DAUNOrubicin (Cerubidine), IDArubicin (Idamycin), midazolam (Versed).

IV COMPATIBILITIES

Cimetidine (Tagamet), CISplatin (Platinol), cyclophosphamide (Cytoxan), cytarabine (Cytosar), DOCEtaxel (Taxotere), DOXOrubicin (Adriamycin), etoposide (VePesid), furosemide (Lasix), granisetron (Kytril), heparin, HYDROmorphone (Dilaudid), LORazepam (Ativan), morphine, ondansetron (Zofran), PACLitaxel (Taxol), palonosetron (Aloxi), potassium chloride, propofol (Diprivan).

INDICATIONS/ROUTES/DOSAGE

Usual Dosage Range

PO, IM, IV: ADULTS, ELDERLY: 4–20 mg/day as a single dose or in 2–4 divided doses. High dose: 0.4–0.8 mg/kg/day (usually not exceeding 40 mg/day).

Anti-Inflammatory

CHILDREN: 0.02–0.3 mg/kg/day in divided doses q6–12h.

Cerebral Edema

PO, IV, IM: CHILDREN: Loading dose of 1–2 mg/kg, then 1–1.5 mg/kg/day in divided doses q4–6h.

Nausea/Vomiting in Chemotherapy

Note: Refer to individual protocols and emetogenic potential.
CHILDREN: 2 mg q12h up to 6 mg/m^2/dose q6h.

Usual Ophthalmic Dosage, Ocular Inflammatory Conditions

ADULTS, ELDERLY, CHILDREN: ***(Solution):*** Initially, 2 drops q1h while awake and q2h at night for 1 day, then reduce to 3–4 times/day. ***(Suspension):*** 1–2 drops up to 4–6 times/day.

Dosage in Renal/Hepatic Impairment

No dose adjustment.

SIDE EFFECTS

Frequent: Inhalation: Cough, dry mouth, hoarseness, throat irritation. **Intranasal:** Burning, mucosal dryness. **Ophthalmic:** Blurred vision.

Systemic: Insomnia, facial edema (cushingoid appearance ["moon face"]), moderate abdominal distention, indigestion, increased appetite, nervousness, facial flushing, diaphoresis. **Occasional: Inhalation:** Localized fungal infection (thrush). **Intranasal:** Crusting inside nose, epistaxis, sore throat, ulceration of nasal mucosa. **Ophthalmic:** Decreased vision; lacrimation; eye pain; burning, stinging, redness of eyes; nausea; vomiting. **Systemic:** Dizziness, decreased/blurred vision. **Rare: Inhalation:** Increased bronchospasm, esophageal candidiasis. **Intranasal:** Nasal/pharyngeal candidiasis, eye pain. **Systemic:** Generalized allergic reaction (rash, urticaria); pain, redness, swelling at injection site; psychological changes; false sense of well-being; hallucinations; depression.

ADVERSE EFFECTS/TOXIC REACTIONS

Long-term therapy: Muscle wasting (esp. arms, legs), osteoporosis, spontaneous fractures, amenorrhea, cataracts, glaucoma, peptic ulcer disease, HF. **Ophthalmic:** Glaucoma, ocular hypertension, cataracts. **Abrupt withdrawal following long-term therapy:** Severe joint pain, severe headache, anorexia, nausea, fever, rebound inflammation, fatigue, weakness, lethargy, dizziness, orthostatic hypotension.

NURSING CONSIDERATIONS

BASELINE ASSESSMENT

Question for hypersensitivity to any corticosteroids. Obtain baselines for height, weight, B/P, serum glucose, electrolytes. Question medical history as listed in Precautions.

INTERVENTION/EVALUATION

Monitor I&O, daily weight, serum glucose. Assess for edema. Evaluate food tolerance. Report hyperacidity promptly. Check vital signs at least twice daily. Be alert to infection (sore throat, fever, vague symptoms). Monitor serum electrolytes, esp. for hypercalcemia, hypokalemia, paresthesia (esp. lower extremities, nausea/vomiting, irritability). Assess emotional status, ability to sleep. Abrupt withdrawal may cause adrenal insufficiency; taper dose gradually.

PATIENT/FAMILY TEACHING

• Do not change dose/schedule or stop taking drug. • **Must** taper off gradually under medical supervision. • Report fever, sore throat, muscle aches, sudden weight gain, edema, exposure to measles/chickenpox. • Severe stress (serious infection, surgery, trauma) may require increased dosage. • Avoid alcohol, limit caffeine.

dexmedetomidine

dex-med-e-**toe**-mye-deen
(Precedex)
Do not confuse Precedex with Percocet or Peridex.

◆CLASSIFICATION

PHARMACOTHERAPEUTIC: Alpha$_2$ agonist. **CLINICAL:** Sedative.

USES

Sedation of initially intubated, mechanically ventilated adults in intensive care setting. Use in nonintubated pts requiring sedation before and/or during surgical and other procedures. **OFF-LABEL:** Treatment of shivering, use in children. Awake craniotomy.

PRECAUTIONS

Contraindications: Hypersensitivity to dexmedetomidine. **Cautions:** Cardiac conduction delay disorders (e.g., AV block), bradycardia, hepatic impairment, hypovolemia, diabetes, hypotension, chronic hypertension, severe ventricular dysfunction, elderly, use of vasodilators or drugs decreasing heart rate.

ACTION

Selective alpha$_2$-adrenergic agonist. Inhibits norepinephrine release. **Therapeutic Effect:** Produces anesthetic, sedative effects.

PHARMACOKINETICS

Protein binding: 94%. Metabolized in liver. Excreted in urine (85%), feces (4%). **Half-life:** 2 hrs.

LIFESPAN CONSIDERATIONS

Pregnancy/Lactation: Unknown if distributed in breast milk. **Children:** Safety and efficacy not established. **Elderly:** May have increased risk of hypotension.

INTERACTIONS

DRUG: **Sedatives (e.g., midazolam, LORazepam), opioids (e.g., fentaNYL, morphine, HYDROmorphone), hypnotics (e.g., zolpidem, temazepam)** may increase CNS depression. **Antihypertensives (e.g., amLODIPine, cloNIDine, lisinopril, valsartan)** may increase risk of hypotension. **Beta blockers (e.g., carvedilol, metoprolol), calcium channel blockers (e.g., dilTIAZem, verapamil)** may increase risk of bradycardia, hypotension. **Tricyclic antidepressants (e.g., amitriptyline, doxepin)** may decrease antihypertensive effect. **HERBAL:** None significant. **FOOD:** None known. **LAB VALUES:** May increase serum alkaline phosphatase, ALT, AST, glucose, potassium. May decrease serum calcium, magnesium; Hgb, Hct, RBC.

AVAILABILITY (Rx)

Injection Solution: 80 mcg/20 mL, 200 mcg/2 mL vials, 4 mcg/mL solutions (50 mL, 100 mL).

ADMINISTRATION/HANDLING

IV

Reconstitution • Visually inspect for particulate matter or discoloration. Solution should appear clear, colorless. • Dilute 2 mL of dexmedetomidine with 48 mL 0.9% NaCl for a final concentration of 4 mcg/mL.

Rate of administration • Individualized, titrated to desired effect. Use controlled infusion pump.

Storage • Store at room temperature.

IV INCOMPATIBILITIES

Do not mix with any other medications.

IV COMPATIBILITIES

Amiodarone (Cordarone), bumetanide (Bumex), calcium gluconate, cisatracurium (Nimbex), dexamethasone, DOBUTamine, DOPamine, magnesium sulfate, norepinephrine (Levophed), propofol (Diprivan).

INDICATIONS/ROUTES/DOSAGE

ICU Sedation

IV: ADULTS: Loading dose of 1 mcg/kg over 10 min followed by maintenance infusion of 0.2–0.7 mcg/kg/hr. **ELDERLY:** May require decreased dosage.

Dosage in Renal Impairment

No dose adjustment.

Dosage in Hepatic Impairment

Use caution.

SIDE EFFECTS

Frequent (25%–12%): Hypotension, hypertension. **Occasional (9%–3%):** Nausea, constipation, bradycardia, pyrexia, dry mouth, vomiting, hypovolemia. **Rare (2%–less than 1%):** Agitation, hyperpyrexia, thirst, oliguria, wheezing.

ADVERSE EFFECTS/TOXIC REACTIONS

Significant bradycardia, sinus arrest, cardiac arrest, AV block, SVT, ventricular tachycardia may occur and may be fatal. Transient hypertension was reported during loading doses. Atrial fibrillation, hypoxia, pleural effusion may occur with too-rapid IV infusion. Bradycardia, hypotension may be more pronounced in pts with diabetes, hypovolemia, hypertension, or who are elderly. Acute respiratory distress syndrome (ARDS), respiratory failure, acidosis may occur with prolonged infusion time greater than 24 hrs.

NURSING CONSIDERATIONS

BASELINE ASSESSMENT

Obtain baseline B/P, heart rate. Recommend continuous cardiac monitoring during use. Assess mental status prior to initiation. Obtain full medication history; screen for medications known to cause hypotension, bradycardia, sedation. Question history of heart block, bradycardia, severe ventricular dysfunction; hepatic impairment.

INTERVENTION/EVALUATION

Assess cardiac monitor for arrhythmia, bradycardia, hypotension. Anticholinergic agents (e.g., glycopyrrolate, atropine) may be effective in treating drug-induced bradycardia. Monitor level of sedation; respiratory rate, rhythm. Monitor ventilator settings. Discontinue once pt is extubated.

PATIENT/FAMILY TEACHING

• B/P, heart will be continuously monitored during infusion. • If infusion is used for more than 6 hrs, agitation, nervousness, headaches may occur for up to 48 hrs. • Report other symptoms that may occur within 48 hrs (abdominal pain, confusion, constipation, dizziness, sweating, weakness, salt cravings, weight loss).

dextroamphetamine and amphetamine

TOP 100

dex-troe-am-**fet**-ah-meen/am-**fet**-ah-meen
(Adderall, Adderall-XR, Mydayis)

BLACK BOX ALERT High potential for abuse. Prolonged administration may lead to drug dependence. Severe cardiovascular events including CVA/MI reported.
Do not confuse Adderall with Inderal.

CLASSIFICATION

PHARMACOTHERAPEUTIC: Amphetamine (Schedule II). **CLINICAL:** CNS stimulant.

USES

Treatment of narcolepsy (immediate-release only); treatment of ADHD.

PRECAUTIONS

Contraindications: Hypersensitivity to dextroamphetamine, amphetamine, or sympathomimetics. Advanced arteriosclerosis, agitated mental states, glaucoma, history of alcohol or drug abuse, hypersensitivity to sympathomimetic amines, hyperthyroidism, moderate to severe hypertension, symptomatic cardiovascular disease, use of MAOIs within 14 days. **Cautions:** Elderly, debilitated pts, history of seizures, mild hypertension; history of drug abuse and misuse, drug-seeking behavior, dependency. Preexisting psychotic or bipolar disorder.

ACTION

Promotes release of primarily dopamine and norepinephrine from storage site in presynaptic nerve terminals. **Therapeutic Effect:** Increases motor activity, mental alertness; decreases drowsiness, fatigue; suppresses appetite.

PHARMACOKINETICS

Well absorbed following PO administration. Widely distributed including CNS. Metabolized in liver. Excreted in urine. Removed by hemodialysis. **Half-life:** 10–13 hrs.

LIFESPAN CONSIDERATIONS

Pregnancy/Lactation: Distributed in breast milk. **Children:** Safety and efficacy not established in pts younger than 3 yrs. **Elderly:** Age-related cardiovascular, cerebrovascular disease, hepatic/renal impairment may increase risk of side effects.

D

INTERACTIONS

DRUG: **MAOIs (e.g., phenelzine, selegiline)** may prolong, intensify effects. **HERBAL:** None significant. **FOOD:** None known. **LAB VALUES:** May increase plasma corticosteroid.

AVAILABILITY (Rx)

Tablets: ***(Adderall):*** 5 mg, 7.5 mg, 10 mg, 12.5 mg, 15 mg, 20 mg, 30 mg.

Capsules: ***(Extended-Release [Adderall-XR]):*** 5 mg, 10 mg, 15 mg, 20 mg, 25 mg, 30 mg. ***Mydayis:*** 12.5 mg, 25 mg, 37.5 mg, 50 mg.

ADMINISTRATION/HANDLING

PO

• Give immediate-release tablets at least 6 hrs before bedtime to prevent insomnia. • Extended-release capsules should be swallowed whole; do not break, crush, or cut. • Avoid afternoon doses to prevent insomnia. • May open capsules and sprinkle on applesauce. Instruct pt not to chew sprinkled beads; take immediately.

INDICATIONS/ROUTES/DOSAGE

Narcolepsy

PO: ADULTS, CHILDREN OLDER THAN 12 YRS: Initially, 10 mg/day. Increase by 10 mg/day at wkly intervals until therapeutic response is achieved. **Usual Range:** 20–60 mg/day given in 1–3 divided doses. **CHILDREN 6–12 YRS:** Initially, 5 mg/day. Increase by 5 mg/day at wkly intervals until therapeutic response is achieved. **Usual Range:** 5–60 mg/day given in 1–3 divided doses

ADHD

ADULTS, ELDERLY: ***(Adderall):*** Initially, 5 mg 1–2 times/day. May increase by 5-mg increments at wkly intervals. **Maximum:** 40 mg/day in 2–3 divided doses (usual intervals of 4–6 hrs). ***(Adderall-XR):*** Initially, 10–20 mg once daily in the morning. May increase in increments of 10–20 mg wkly. up to 60 mg/day. ***(Mydayis):*** Initially, 12.5 mg once daily in morning. May increase by 12.5 mg no sooner than once wkly. **Maximum:** 50 mg/day. **CHILDREN 13–17 YRS:** ***(Adderall):*** Initially, 5 mg 1–2 times/day. May increase by 5 mg at wkly intervals. **Maximum:** 40 mg/day in 1–3 divided doses (usual intervals of 4–6 hrs). ***(Adderall-XR):*** Initially, 10 mg once daily in the morning. May increase to 20 mg/day after 1 wk if symptoms are not controlled. May increase up to 60 mg/day. ***(Mydayis):*** Initially, 12.5 mg once daily in morning. May increase by 12.5 mg no sooner than once wkly. **Maximum:** 25 mg/day. **CHILDREN 6–12 YRS:** ***(Adderall):*** Initially, 5 mg 1–2 times/day. May increase in 5-mg increments at wkly intervals until optimal response is obtained. **Maximum:** 40 mg/day given in 1–3 divided doses (use intervals of 4–6 hrs between additional doses). ***(Adderall-XR):*** Initially, 5–10 mg once daily in the morning. May increase daily dose in 5- to 10-mg increments at wkly intervals. **Maximum:** 30 mg/day. **CHILDREN 3–5 YRS:** ***(Adderall):*** Initially, 2.5 mg/day given every morning. May increase daily dose in 2.5-mg increments at wkly intervals until optimal response is obtained. **Maximum:** 40 mg/day given in 1–3 divided doses (use intervals of 4–6 hrs between additional doses). Not recommended in children younger than 3 yrs.

Dosage in Renal/Hepatic Impairment

No dose adjustment.

SIDE EFFECTS

Frequent: Increased motor activity, talkativeness, nervousness, mild euphoria, insomnia. **Occasional:** Headache, chills, dry mouth, GI distress, worsening depression in pts who are clinically depressed, tachycardia, palpitations, chest pain, dizziness, decreased appetite.

ADVERSE EFFECTS/TOXIC REACTIONS

Overdose may produce skin pallor/flushing, arrhythmias, psychosis. Abrupt withdrawal after prolonged use of high doses may produce lethargy (may last for wks). Prolonged administration to children with ADHD may temporarily suppress normal weight/height pattern.

NURSING CONSIDERATIONS

BASELINE ASSESSMENT

Assess attention span, impulse control, interaction with others. Assess risk of drug abuse, misuse, drug-seeking behavior. Obtain baseline B/P. Assess sleep pattern.

INTERVENTION/EVALUATION

Monitor for CNS overstimulation, increase in B/P, growth rate, change in pulse rate, respirations, weight loss. Screen for misuse, abuse, drug-seeking behavior. **Narcolepsy:** Observe/document frequency of narcoleptic episodes. **ADHD:** Observe for improved attention span.

PATIENT/FAMILY TEACHING

• Normal dosage levels may produce tolerance to drug's anorexic mood-elevating effects within a few wks. • Dry mouth may be relieved with sugarless gum, sips of water. • Take early in day. • Do not break, chew, or crush extended-release capsules. • May mask extreme fatigue. • Report pronounced anxiety, dizziness, decreased appetite, dry mouth, new or worsening behavior, chest pain, palpitations. • Avoid alcohol, caffeine.

diazePAM

dye-**az**-e-pam
(Diastat, DiazePAM Intensol, Valium, Valtoco)

■ **BLACK BOX ALERT** ■ Concomitant use of benzodiazepines and opioids may result in profound sedation, respiratory depression, and death. Reserve for pts for whom alternative treatment options are inadequate.

Do not confuse diazePAM with diazoxide, dilTIAZem, Ditropan, or LORazepam, or Valium with Valcyte.

◆CLASSIFICATION

PHARMACOTHERAPEUTIC: Benzodiazepine (Schedule IV). **CLINICAL:** Antianxiety, skeletal muscle relaxant, anticonvulsant.

USES

Short-term relief of anxiety symptoms, relief of acute alcohol withdrawal. Adjunct for relief of acute musculoskeletal conditions, treatment of seizures (IV route used for termination of status epilepticus). **Gel:** Control of increased seizure activity in refractory epilepsy in pts on stable regimens. **OFF-LABEL:** Treatment of panic disorder. Short-term treatment of spasticity in children with cerebral palsy. Sedation for mechanically vented pts in ICU.

PRECAUTIONS

Contraindications: Hypersensitivity to diazepam. Acute narrow-angle glaucoma, untreated open-angle glaucoma, severe respiratory depression, severe hepatic insufficiency, sleep apnea syndrome, myasthenia gravis. Children younger than 6 mos (oral). **Cautions:** Pts receiving other CNS depressants or psychoactive agents, depression, history of drug and alcohol abuse, renal/hepatic impairment, respiratory disease, impaired gag reflex, concurrent use of strong CYP3A4 inhibitors or inducers.

ACTION

Depresses all levels of CNS by enhancing action of gamma-aminobutyric acid (GABA), a major inhibitory neurotransmitter in the brain. **Therapeutic Effect:** Produces anxiolytic effect, elevates seizure threshold, produces skeletal muscle relaxation.

PHARMACOKINETICS

Well absorbed from GI tract. Widely distributed. Protein binding: 98%. Excreted in urine. Minimally removed by hemodialysis. **Half-life:** 20–70 hrs (increased in hepatic dysfunction, elderly).

D

LIFESPAN CONSIDERATIONS

Pregnancy/Lactation: Crosses placenta. Distributed in breast milk. May increase risk of fetal abnormalities if administered during first trimester of pregnancy. Chronic ingestion during pregnancy may produce withdrawal symptoms, CNS depression in neonates. **Children/Elderly:** Use small initial doses with gradual increases to avoid ataxia, excessive sedation. Elderly at increased risk of impaired cognition, delirium, falls, fractures.

INTERACTIONS

DRUG: **Alcohol, CNS depressants (e.g., gabapentin, morphine, zolpidem)** may increase CNS depression. **CYP3A4 inducers (e.g., carBAMazepine, rifAMPin)** may decrease concentration. **CYP3A4 inhibitors (e.g., itraconazole, ketoconazole)** may increase concentration/effect. **OLANZapine** may increase adverse effects. HERBAL: **Herbals with sedative properties (e.g., chamomile, kava kava, valerian)** may increase CNS depression. **St. John's wort** may decrease concentration/effects. FOOD: **Grapefruit products** may increase concentration/effects. LAB VALUES: None significant. **Therapeutic serum level:** 0.5–2 mcg/mL; **toxic serum level:** greater than 3 mcg/mL.

AVAILABILITY (Rx)

Injection, Solution: 5 mg/mL. **Nasal:** 5 mg/0.1 mL, 7.5 mg/0.1 mL, 10 mg/0.1 mL. **Oral Concentrate:** ***(DiazePAM Intensol):*** 5 mg/mL. **Oral Solution:** 5 mg/5 mL. **Rectal Gel:** ***(Diastat):*** 2.5 mg, 10 mg, 20 mg. **Tablet:** ***(Valium):*** 2 mg, 5 mg, 10 mg.

ADMINISTRATION/HANDLING

IV

Rate of administration • Give by IV push into tubing of flowing IV solution as close as possible to vein insertion point. • Administer directly into large vein (reduces risk of thrombosis/phlebitis). Do not use small veins (e.g., wrist/dorsum of hand). • Administer IV at rate not exceeding 5 mg/min for adults. For children, give 1–2 mg/min (too-rapid IV may result in hypotension, respiratory depression). • Monitor respirations q5–15 min for 2 hrs.

Storage • Store at room temperature.

Intranasal

• Do not test or prime before use. • Administer one spray into one nostril.

IM

• Injection may be painful. Inject deeply into large muscle mass.

PO

• Give without regard to food. • Dilute oral concentrate with water, juice, carbonated beverages; may be mixed in semisolid food (applesauce, pudding). • Tablets may be crushed.

GEL

• Insert rectal tip and gently push plunger over 3 sec. Remove tip after 3 additional sec. • Buttocks should be held together for 3 sec after removal.

IV INCOMPATIBILITIES

Amphotericin B complex (Abelcet, AmBisome, Amphotec), cefepime (Maxipime), dilTIAZem (Cardizem), fluconazole (Diflucan), foscarnet (Foscavir), furosemide (Lasix), heparin, hydrocortisone (SOLU-Cortef), HYDROmorphone (Dilaudid), meropenem (Merrem IV), potassium chloride, propofol (Diprivan), vitamins.

IV COMPATIBILITIES

DOBUTamine (Dobutrex), fentaNYL, morphine.

INDICATIONS/ROUTES/DOSAGE

Anxiety (Acute/severe)

IM, IV, PO: ADULTS: 2–10 mg q3–6hrs PRN up to 40 mg/day based on response and tolerability.

Anxiety Disorders

PO: Initially, 2–5 mg once or twice daily. May gradually increase based on response and tolerability up to 40 mg/day in 2–4 divided doses.

D

Muscle Spasm, Spasticity/Rigidity

PO: ADULTS: Initially, 2 mg twice daily or 5 mg at bedtime. May gradually increase up to 40–60 mg/day in 3–4 divided doses based on response and tolerability. **ADOLESCENTS, CHILDREN, INFANTS 6 MOS AND OLDER:** Initially, 1–2.5 mg 3–4 times daily. May gradually increase as needed and tolerated.

Alcohol Withdraw

IV, PO: ADULTS: 5–20 mg PRN until appropriate sedation achieved. Dose and frequency determined by severity of withdrawal symptoms.

Status Epilepticus

IV: ADULTS: 5–10 mg as a single dose given at a maximum infusion rate of 5 mg/min. May repeat in 3–5 min if seizures do not subside. **INFANTS, CHILDREN:** 0.15–0.2 mg/kg over 2 min; may repeat after 5–10 min. **Maximum:** 10 mg/dose.

Acute Active Seizures

IV: ADULTS: 5–10 mg as a single dose. May repeat at 3- to 5-min intervals up to a total dose of 30 mg. **Intranasal:** 0.2 mg/kg as a single dose. May repeat once based on response and tolerability after 4 or more hrs. **Maximum dose:** 2 doses/episode. Do not use for more than 1 episode q5days or more than 5 episodes/mo.

Control of Increased Seizure Activity (Breakthrough seizures) in Pts With Refractory Epilepsy Who Are on Stable Regimens of Anticonvulsants

Note: Do not use gel for more than 5 episodes/mo or more than 1 episode q5days.

PO: ADULTS, ELDERLY: 2–10 mg 2–4 times/day.

Rectal gel: ADULTS, CHILDREN 12 YRS AND OLDER: 0.2 mg/kg; may be repeated in 4–12 hrs. **CHILDREN 6–11 YRS:** 0.3 mg/kg; may be repeated in 4–12 hrs. **Maximum:** 20 mg. **CHILDREN 2–5 YRS:** 0.5 mg/kg; may be repeated in 4–12 hrs. **Maximum:** 20 mg.

Dosage in Renal Impairment

Use caution.

Dosage in Hepatic Impairment

Use caution. Oral tablets contraindicated in severe hepatic impairment.

SIDE EFFECTS

Frequent: Pain with IM injection, drowsiness, fatigue, ataxia. **Occasional:** Slurred speech, orthostatic hypotension, headache, hypoactivity, constipation, nausea, blurred vision. **Rare:** Paradoxical CNS reactions (hyperactivity/nervousness in children, excitement/restlessness in elderly/debilitated pts) generally noted during first 2 wks of therapy, particularly in presence of uncontrolled pain.

ADVERSE EFFECTS/TOXIC REACTIONS

IV route may produce pain, swelling, thrombophlebitis, carpal tunnel syndrome. Abrupt or too-rapid withdrawal may result in pronounced restlessness, irritability, insomnia, hand tremor, abdominal/muscle cramps, diaphoresis, vomiting, seizures. Abrupt withdrawal in pts with epilepsy may produce increase in frequency/severity of seizures. Overdose results in drowsiness, confusion, diminished reflexes, CNS depression, coma. **Antidote:** Flumazenil (see Appendix J for dosage).

NURSING CONSIDERATIONS

BASELINE ASSESSMENT

Assess B/P, pulse, respirations immediately before administration. Assess risk of drug abuse, misuse, drug-seeking behavior. **Anxiety:** Assess autonomic response (cold, clammy hands; diaphoresis), motor response (agitation, trembling, tension). **Musculoskeletal spasm:** Record onset, type, location, duration of pain. Check for immobility, stiffness, swelling. **Seizures:** Review history of seizure disorder (length, intensity, frequency, duration, LOC). Observe frequently for recurrence of seizure activity.

INTERVENTION/EVALUATION

Monitor heart rate, respiratory rate, B/P, mental status. Assess children, elderly for paradoxical reaction, particularly during early therapy. Evaluate for therapeutic response (decrease in intensity/frequency of seizures; calm facial expression, decreased restlessness; decreased intensity of skeletal muscle pain). Screen for misuse, abuse, drug-seeking behavior. **Therapeutic serum level:** 0.5–2 mcg/mL; **toxic serum level:** greater than 3 mcg/mL.

PATIENT/FAMILY TEACHING

• Avoid alcohol. • Limit caffeine. • May cause drowsiness; avoid tasks that require alertness, motor skills until response to drug is established. • May be habit forming. • Avoid abrupt discontinuation after prolonged use.

diclofenac

dye-**kloe**-fen-ak
(Cambia, Flector, Voltaren Gel, Zipsor, Zorvolex)

■ BLACK BOX ALERT ■ Increased risk of serious cardiovascular thrombotic events, including myocardial infarction, CVA. Increased risk of severe GI reactions, including ulceration, bleeding, perforation of stomach, intestines. Contraindicated for treatment of perioperative pain in setting of CABG surgery.

Do not confuse Cataflam with Catapres, diclofenac with Diflucan or Duphalac, or Voltaren with traMADol, Ultram, or Verelan.

FIXED-COMBINATION(S)

Arthrotec: diclofenac/miSOPROStol (an antisecretory gastric protectant): 50 mg/200 mcg, 75 mg/200 mcg.

◆CLASSIFICATION

PHARMACOTHERAPEUTIC: NSAID (nonselective). **CLINICAL:** Analgesic, anti-inflammatory.

USES

PO: (Immediate-Release): Treatment of rheumatoid arthritis, osteoarthritis, mild to moderate acute pain, primary dysmenorrhea. **(Zipsor):** Mild to moderate pain. **(Zorvolex):** Mild to moderate pain, osteoarthritic pain. **(Delayed-Release):** Treatment of rheumatoid arthritis, osteoarthritis, ankylosing spondylitis. **(Extended-Release):** Treatment of rheumatoid arthritis, osteoarthritis. **Oral Solution (Cambia):** Treatment of migraine. **Powder for Oral Solution:** Acute treatment of migraine attacks with or without aura. **Topical Patch:** Treatment of acute pain due to minor strains, sprains, contusions. **OFF-LABEL:** Treatment of juvenile idiopathic arthritis.

PRECAUTIONS

Contraindications: Hypersensitivity to diclofenac. Pts experiencing asthma, urticaria after taking aspirin, other NSAIDs. Pts with moderate to severe renal impairment in perioperative period who are at risk for volume depletion (injection only); perioperative pain in setting of CABG surgery. **Cautions:** HF, hypertension, renal/hepatic impairment, hepatic porphyria, history of GI disease (e.g., bleeding, ulcers), concomitant use of aspirin or anticoagulants, elderly, debilitated pts.

ACTION

Reversibly inhibits cyclo-oxygenase-1 and -2 (COX-1 and COX-2) enzymes, resulting in decreased formation of prostaglandin precursors. **Therapeutic Effect:** Produces analgesic, antipyretic, anti-inflammatory effects.

PHARMACOKINETICS

Route	Onset	Peak	Duration
PO	30 min	2–3 hrs	Up to 8 hrs

Completely absorbed from GI tract. Protein binding: greater than 99%. Widely distributed. Metabolized in liver. Primarily excreted in urine. Minimally removed by hemodialysis. **Half-life:** 1.2–2 hrs.

⌛ LIFESPAN CONSIDERATIONS

Pregnancy/Lactation: Crosses placenta. Unknown if distributed in breast milk. Avoid use during third trimester (may adversely affect fetal cardiovascular system: premature closure of ductus arteriosus). **Children:** Safety and efficacy not established. **Elderly:** GI bleeding, ulceration more likely to cause serious adverse effects. Age-related renal impairment may increase risk of hepatic/renal toxicity; reduced dosage recommended.

INTERACTIONS

DRUG: **Aspirin, NSAIDs (e.g., ibuprofen, naproxen)** may increase risk of GI side effects/bleeding. May increase **cycloSPORINE** concentration/toxicity. **HERBAL:** **Herbals with anticoagulant/antiplatelet activity (e.g., garlic, ginger, ginkgo biloba)** may increase adverse effects. **FOOD:** None known. **LAB VALUES:** May increase urine protein, serum BUN, alkaline phosphatase, creatinine, LDH, potassium, ALT, AST. May decrease serum uric acid.

AVAILABILITY (Rx)

Transdermal Patch: ***(Flector):*** 1.3%. **Transdermal Gel:** ***(Voltaren):*** 1%. **Capsules:** ***(Zipsor):*** 25 mg. ***(Zorvolex):*** 18 mg, 35 mg. **Oral Solution:** ***(Cambia):*** 50-mg packets. **Tablets:** 50 mg.

Tablets: ***(Delayed-Release):*** 25 mg, 50 mg, 75 mg. **Tablets:** ***(Extended-Release):*** 100 mg.

ADMINISTRATION/HANDLING

PO

• Do not break, crush, dissolve, or divide enteric-coated tablets. • May give with food, milk, antacids if GI distress occurs. • ***(Cambia):*** Mix one packet in 1–2 oz water, stir well, and instruct pt to drink immediately.

Transdermal Patch

• Apply to intact skin; avoid contact with eyes. • Do not wear when bathing/showering. • Wash hands after handling.

INDICATIONS/ROUTES/DOSAGE

Osteoarthritis

PO: ***(Immediate-Release):*** **ADULTS, ELDERLY:** 50 mg 2–3 times/day.

PO: ***(Extended-Release):*** **ADULTS, ELDERLY:** 100 mg/day as a single dose. ***(Zorvolex):*** 35 mg 3 times/day.

PO: ***(Delayed-Release):*** **ADULTS, ELDERLY:** 50 mg 2–3 times/day or 75 mg twice daily.

Topical gel: **ADULTS, ELDERLY:** Apply 4 times/day.

Rheumatoid Arthritis (RA)

PO: ***(Immediate-Release):*** **ADULTS, ELDERLY:** 50 mg 3–4 times/day.

PO: ***(Extended-Release):*** **ADULTS, ELDERLY:** 100 mg once daily. May increase to 200 mg/day in 2 divided doses.

PO: ***(Delayed-Release):*** **ADULTS, ELDERLY:** 50 mg 3–4 times/day or 75 mg twice daily.

Ankylosing Spondylitis

PO: ***(Delayed-Release):*** **ADULTS, ELDERLY:** 25 mg 4 times/day and 25 mg at bedtime PRN.

Primary Dysmenorrhea

PO: ***(Immediate-Release):*** **ADULTS, ELDERLY:** 50 mg 3 times/day. May give 100 mg initially, then 50 mg 3 times/day.

Pain

PO: **ADULTS, ELDERLY:** ***(Immediate-Release):*** 100 mg once, then 50 mg 3 times/day. ***(Zipsor):*** 25 mg 4 times/day. ***(Zorvolex):*** 18–35 mg 3 times/day.

IV: 37.5 mg q6h prn. **Maximum:** 150 mg/day.

Topical Patch: ***(Flector):*** Apply 2 times/day.

Migraine (Oral solution)

PO: **ADULTS, ELDERLY:** 50 mg (one packet) once.

Dosage in Renal Impairment

Not recommended in severe impairment.

Dosage in Hepatic Impairment

May require dose adjustment. Use caution.

SIDE EFFECTS

Frequent (9%–4%): **PO:** Headache, abdominal cramps, constipation, diarrhea, nausea, dyspepsia. **Ophthalmic:** Burning, stinging on instillation, ocular

D

discomfort. **Occasional (3%–1%): PO:** Flatulence, dizziness, epigastric pain. **Ophthalmic:** Ocular itching, tearing. **Rare (less than 1%): PO:** Rash, peripheral edema, fluid retention, visual disturbances, vomiting, drowsiness.

ADVERSE EFFECTS/TOXIC REACTIONS

Overdose may result in acute renal failure. In pts treated chronically, peptic ulcer, GI bleeding, gastritis, severe hepatic reaction (jaundice), nephrotoxicity (hematuria, dysuria, proteinuria), severe hypersensitivity reaction (bronchospasm, angioedema) occur rarely.

NURSING CONSIDERATIONS

BASELINE ASSESSMENT

Obtain baseline B/P. **Anti-inflammatory:** Assess onset, type, location, duration of pain, inflammation. Inspect appearance of affected joints for immobility, deformities, skin condition.

INTERVENTION/EVALUATION

Monitor CBC, renal function, LFT, urine output, occult blood test, B/P. Monitor for headache, dyspepsia. Monitor daily pattern of bowel activity, stool consistency. Assess for therapeutic response: relief of pain, stiffness, swelling; increased joint mobility; reduced joint tenderness; improved grip strength.

PATIENT/FAMILY TEACHING

• Swallow tablets whole; do not chew, crush, dissolve, or divide. • Avoid aspirin, alcohol during therapy (increases risk of GI bleeding). • If GI upset occurs, take with food, milk. • Report skin rash, itching, weight gain, changes in vision, black stools, bleeding, jaundice, upper quadrant pain, persistent headache. • **Ophthalmic:** Do not use hydrogel soft contact lenses. • **Topical:** Avoid exposure to sunlight, sunlamps. • Report rash.

digoxin

HIGH ALERT

di-**jox**-in
(Digitek, Digox, Lanoxin)
Do not confuse digoxin with Desoxyn or doxepin, or Lanoxin with Lasix, Levoxyl, Levsinex, Lonox, or Mefoxin.

CLASSIFICATION

PHARMACOTHERAPEUTIC: Cardiac glycoside. **CLINICAL:** Antiarrhythmic.

USES

Treatment of mild to moderate HF. Control ventricular response rate in pts with chronic atrial fibrillation. **OFF-LABEL:** Fetal tachycardia with or without hydrops; decrease ventricular rate in supraventricular tachyarrhythmias.

PRECAUTIONS

Contraindications: Hypersensitivity to digoxin. Ventricular fibrillation. **Cautions:** Renal impairment, sinus nodal disease, acute MI (within 6 mos), second- or third-degree heart block (unless functioning pacemaker), concurrent use of strong inducers or inhibitors of P-glycoprotein (e.g., cyclosporine), hyperthyroidism, hypothyroidism, hypokalemia, hypocalcemia.

ACTION

HF: Inhibits sodium/potassium ATPase pump in myocardial cells. Promotes calcium influx. **Supraventricular arrhythmias:** Suppresses AV node conduction. **Therapeutic Effect: HF:** Increases contractility. **Supraventricular arrhythmias:** Increases effective refractory period/decreases conduction velocity, decreases ventricular heart rate of fast atrial arrhythmias.

PHARMACOKINETICS

Route	Onset	Peak	Duration
PO	0.5–2 hrs	2–8 hrs	3–4 days
IV	5–30 min	1–4 hrs	3–4 days

Readily absorbed from GI tract. Widely distributed. Protein binding: 30%. Partially metabolized in liver. Primarily excreted in urine. Minimally removed by hemodialysis. **Half-life:** 36–48 hrs (increased in renal impairment, elderly).

LIFESPAN CONSIDERATIONS

Pregnancy/Lactation: Crosses placenta. Distributed in breast milk. **Children:** Premature infants more susceptible to toxicity. **Elderly:** Age-related hepatic/renal impairment may require dosage adjustment. Increased risk of loss of appetite. Avoid use as first-line therapy for atrial fibrillation or HF.

INTERACTIONS

DRUG: Amiodarone may increase concentration/toxicity. **Beta blockers (e.g., metoprolol), calcium channel blockers (e.g., dilTIAZem)** may have additive effect on slowing AV nodal conduction. **Potassium-depleting diuretics (e.g., furosemide)** may increase toxicity due to hypokalemia. **Ketoconazole, vemurafenib** may increase concentration/effect. **Sucralfate** may decrease absorption/concentration. **HERBAL: Licorice** may increase adverse effects. **FOOD: Meals with increased fiber (bran) or high in pectin** may decrease absorption. **LAB VALUES:** None known.

AVAILABILITY (Rx)

Oral Solution: ***(Lanoxin):*** 50 mcg/mL. **Injection Solution:** ***(Lanoxin):*** 100 mcg/mL, 250 mcg/mL. **Tablets:** ***(Lanoxin):*** 62.5 mcg, 125 mcg, 187.5 mcg, 250 mcg.

ADMINISTRATION/HANDLING

◄ALERT► IM rarely used (produces severe local irritation, erratic absorption). If no other route possible, give deep into muscle followed by massage. Give no more than 2 mL at any one site.

IV

• May give undiluted or dilute with at least a 4-fold volume of Sterile Water for Injection or D_5W (less may cause precipitate). • Use immediately. • Give IV slowly over at least 5 min.

PO

• May give without regard to food. • Tablets may be crushed.

IV INCOMPATIBILITIES

Amphotericin B complex (Abelcet, AmBisome, Amphotec), fluconazole (Diflucan), foscarnet (Foscavir), propofol (Diprivan).

IV COMPATIBILITIES

DilTIAZem (Cardizem), furosemide (Lasix), heparin, insulin regular, lidocaine, midazolam (Versed), milrinone (Primacor), morphine, potassium chloride.

INDICATIONS/ROUTES/DOSAGE

Note: Loading dose not recommended in HF.

HF

PO: ADULTS, ELDERLY: 0.125–0.25 mg once daily.

Maintenance Dosage

	PO	IV/IM
Preterm infant	5–7.5 mcg/kg	4–6 mcg/kg
Full-term infant	8–10 mcg/kg	5–8 mcg/kg
1 mo–2 yrs	10–15 mcg/kg	9–15 mcg/kg
2–5 yrs	8–10 mcg/kg	6–9 mcg/kg
5–10 yrs	5–10 mcg/kg	4–8 mcg/kg
>10 yrs	2.5–5 mcg/kg	2–3 mcg/kg

Note: If age 11 yrs or older, give once daily. If 10 yrs or younger, give in equally divided doses twice daily.

Atrial Fibrillation

ADULTS, ELDERLY: Digitalizing dose (IV): Initially, 0.25–0.5 mg over several minutes. May repeat doses of 0.25 mg q6hrs up to a maximum of 1.5 mg over 24 hrs. **Maintenance dose (PO):** 0.125–0.25 mg once daily.

Dosage in Renal Impairment

Dosage adjustment is based on creatinine clearance. **Loading dose:** Decrease by 50% in end-stage renal disease.

D

Maintenance Dose

eGFR	Dosage
10–50 mL/min	25%–75% of usual dose or q36h (0.0625 mg q24–36hrs)
Less than 10 mL/min (HD, PD, CRRT)	10%–25% of usual dose or q48h (0.0625 mg q48h)

Dosage in Hepatic Impairment
No dose adjustment.

SIDE EFFECTS

Dizziness, headache, diarrhea, rash, visual disturbances.

ADVERSE EFFECTS/TOXIC REACTIONS

The most common early manifestations of digoxin toxicity are GI disturbances (anorexia, nausea, vomiting), neurologic abnormalities (fatigue, headache, depression, weakness, drowsiness, confusion, nightmares). Facial pain, personality change, ocular disturbances (photophobia, light flashes, halos around bright objects, yellow or green color perception) may occur. Sinus bradycardia, AV block, ventricular arrhythmias noted. **Antidote:** Digoxin immune FAB (see Appendix J for dosage).

NURSING CONSIDERATIONS

BASELINE ASSESSMENT

Assess apical pulse. If pulse is 60 or less/min (70 or less/min for children), withhold drug, contact physician. Blood samples are best taken 6–8 hrs after dose or just before next dose.

INTERVENTION/EVALUATION

Monitor pulse for bradycardia, ECG for arrhythmias for 1–2 hrs after administration (excessive slowing of pulse may be first clinical sign of toxicity). Assess for GI disturbances, neurologic abnormalities (signs of toxicity) q2–4h during loading dose (daily during maintenance). Monitor serum potassium, magnesium, calcium, renal function. **Therapeutic serum level:** 0.8–2 ng/mL; **toxic serum level:** greater than 2 ng/mL.

PATIENT/FAMILY TEACHING

• Follow-up visits, blood tests are an important part of therapy. • Follow guidelines to take apical pulse and report pulse of 60 or less/min (or as indicated by physician). • Wear/carry identification of digoxin therapy and inform dentist, other physician of taking digoxin. • Do not increase or skip doses. • Do not take OTC medications without consulting physician. • Report decreased appetite, nausea/vomiting, diarrhea, visual changes.

dilTIAZem

TOP 100

dil-**tye**-a-zem
(Apo-Diltiaz ✦, Cardizem, Cardizem CD, Cardizem LA, Cartia XT, Dilt-XR, Matzim LA, Taztia XT, Tiadylt ER, Tiazac)
Do not confuse Cardizem with Cardene or Cardene SR, Cartia XT with Procardia XL, dilTIAZem with Calan, diazePAM, or Dilantin, or Tiazac with Ziac.

FIXED-COMBINATION(S)

Teczem: dilTIAZem/enalapril (ACE inhibitor): 180 mg/5 mg.

◆CLASSIFICATION

PHARMACOTHERAPEUTIC: Calcium channel blocker. Non-dihydropyridine. **CLINICAL:** Antianginal, antihypertensive, class IV antiarrhythmic.

USES

PO: Treatment of angina due to coronary artery spasm (Prinzmetal's variant angina), chronic stable angina (effort-associated angina). Treatment of hypertension. **Parenteral:** Temporary control of rapid ventricular rate in atrial fibrillation/flutter. Rapid conversion of paroxysmal supraventricular tachycardia (PSVT) to normal sinus rhythm.

PRECAUTIONS

Contraindications: PO: Hypersensitivity to dilTIAZem, acute MI, pulmonary congestion, second- or third-degree AV block (except in presence of pacemaker), severe hypotension (less than 90 mm Hg, systolic), sick sinus syndrome (except in presence of pacemaker). **IV:** Hypersensitivity to dilTIAZem. Sick sinus syndrome or second- or third-degree block (except with functioning pacemaker), cardiogenic shock, administration of IV beta blocker within several hours, atrial fibrillation/flutter associated with accessory bypass tract, severe hypotension, ventricular tachycardia. **Cautions:** Renal/hepatic impairment, HF, concurrent use with beta blocker, hypertrophic obstructive cardiomyopathy.

ACTION

Inhibits calcium movement across cardiac, vascular smooth-muscle cell membranes (causes dilation of coronary arteries, peripheral arteries, arterioles) during depolarization. **Therapeutic Effect:** Relaxes coronary vascular smooth muscle, and coronary vasodilation increases myocardial oxygen delivery in pts with vasospastic angina.

PHARMACOKINETICS

Route	Onset	Peak	Duration
PO	0.5–1 hr	N/A	N/A
PO (extended-release)	2–3 hrs	N/A	N/A
IV	3 min	N/A	N/A

Well absorbed from GI tract. Protein binding: 70%–80%. Primarily excreted in urine. Not removed by hemodialysis. **Half-life:** 3–8 hrs.

LIFESPAN CONSIDERATIONS

Pregnancy/Lactation: Distributed in breast milk. **Children:** No age-related precautions noted. **Elderly:** Age-related renal impairment may require dosage adjustment.

INTERACTIONS

DRUG: Beta blockers (e.g., atenolol, carvedilol, metoprolol) may increase effects; risk of bradycardia. **Statins (e.g., atorvastatin, simvastatin), strong CYP3A4 inhibitors (e.g., clarithromycin, ketoconazole, ritonavir)** may increase concentration/effect. **Strong CYP3A4 inducers (e.g., carBAMazepine, phenytoin, rifAMPin)** may decrease concentration/effect. May increase concentration/effects of **bosutinib, budesonide. HERBAL: Ephedra, St. John's wort, yohimbe** may decrease concentration/effect. **Herbals with hypotensive properties (e.g., garlic, ginger, gingko biloba)** may increase effect. **St. John's wort** may decrease concentration. **FOOD: Grapefruit products** may increase concentration/effect. **LAB VALUES:** ECG: May increase PR interval.

AVAILABILITY (Rx)

Injection, Solution: 25 mg/5 mL, 50 mg/10 mL, 125 mg/25 mL. **Tablets, Immediate-Release:** 30 mg, 60 mg, 90 mg, 120 mg.

(Non-Crushable) **Capsules, Extended-Release, 24 Hour:** 120 mg, 180 mg, 240 mg, 300 mg, 360 mg, 420 mg. (Non-Crushable) **Capsules, Extended-Release, 12 Hour:** 60 mg, 90 mg, 120 mg. (Non-Crushable) **Tablets, Extended-Release, 24 Hour:** 120 mg, 180 mg, 240 mg, 300 mg, 360 mg, 420 mg.

ADMINISTRATION/HANDLING

IV

Reconstitution • Add 125 mg to 100 mL D_5W, 0.9% NaCl to provide concentration of 1 mg/mL.

Rate of administration • Infuse per dilution/rate chart provided by manufacturer.

Storage • Refrigerate vials. • After dilution, stable for 24 hrs.

PO

• Give immediate-release tablets before meals and at bedtime. • Tablets may be crushed. • Do not break, crush, dissolve, or divide sustained-release capsules or extended-release capsules or tablets. • Taztia XT capsules may be opened and mixed with applesauce; follow with glass of water. • Cardizem CD, Cardizem LA, Cartia XT, Matzim LA may be given without regard to food. • Dilacor XR, Dilt-XR to be given on empty stomach.

IV INCOMPATIBILITIES

AcetaZOLAMIDE (Diamox), acyclovir (Zovirax), ampicillin, ampicillin/sulbactam (Unasyn), diazePAM (Valium), furosemide (Lasix), heparin, insulin, nafcillin, phenytoin (Dilantin), rifAMPin (Rifadin), sodium bicarbonate.

IV COMPATIBILITIES

Albumin, aztreonam (Azactam), bumetanide (Bumex), ceFAZolin (Ancef), cefotaxime (Claforan), cefTAZidime (Fortaz), cefTRIAXone (Rocephin), cefuroxime (Zinacef), ciprofloxacin (Cipro), clindamycin (Cleocin), dexmedetomidine (Precedex), digoxin (Lanoxin), DOBUTamine (Dobutrex), DOPamine (Intropin), gentamicin, HYDROmorphone (Dilaudid), lidocaine, LORazepam (Ativan), metoclopramide (Reglan), metroNIDAZOLE (Flagyl), midazolam (Versed), morphine, multivitamins, nitroglycerin, norepinephrine (Levophed), potassium chloride, potassium phosphate, tobramycin (Nebcin), vancomycin (Vancocin).

INDICATIONS/ROUTES/DOSAGE

Angina

PO: ***(Immediate-Release):*** **ADULTS, ELDERLY:** Initially, 30 mg 4 times/day. Range: 240–360 mg/day.

PO: ***(24h Once Daily):*** **ADULTS, ELDERLY:** Initially, 120–180 mg once daily. May increase at 7- to 14-day intervals. Range: 240–360 mg.

Hypertension

PO: ***(Extended-Release Capsule [once-daily dosing]):*** Initially, 120–240 mg/day. May increase at 7- to 14-day intervals. Usual dose: 120–240 mg/day.

PO: ***(Extended-Release Capsule [twice-daily dosing]):*** **ADULTS, ELDERLY:** Initially, 60–120 mg twice daily. May increase at 7- to 14-day intervals. **Maintenance:** 120–180 mg twice daily.

Temporary Control of Rapid Ventricular Rate in Atrial Fibrillation/Flutter; Rapid Conversion of Paroxysmal Supraventricular Tachycardia to Normal Sinus Rhythm

IV bolus: ADULTS, ELDERLY: Initially, 0.25 mg/kg (average dose: 20 mg) actual body weight over 2 min. May repeat in 15 min at dose of 0.35 mg/kg (average dose: 25 mg) actual body weight. Subsequent doses individualized.

IV infusion: ADULTS, ELDERLY: After initial bolus injection, may begin infusion at 5–10 mg/hr; may increase by 5 mg/hr up to a maximum of 15 mg/hr. Continuous infusion longer than 24 hrs or infusion rate greater than 15 mg/hr are not recommended. Attempt conversion to PO therapy as soon as possible.

Dosage in Renal/Hepatic Impairment

Use with caution.

SIDE EFFECTS

Frequent (10%–5%): Peripheral edema, dizziness, light-headedness, headache, bradycardia, asthenia. **Occasional (5%–2%):** Nausea, constipation, flushing, ECG changes. **Rare (less than 2%):** Rash, micturition disorder (polyuria, nocturia, dysuria, frequency of urination), abdominal discomfort, drowsiness.

ADVERSE EFFECTS/TOXIC REACTIONS

Abrupt withdrawal may increase frequency, duration of angina, HF; second- or third-degree AV block occurs rarely. Overdose produces nausea, drowsiness, confusion, slurred speech, profound bradycardia. **Antidote:** Glucagon, insulin drip with continuous calcium infusion (see Appendix J for dosage).

NURSING CONSIDERATIONS

BASELINE ASSESSMENT

Record onset, type (sharp, dull, squeezing), radiation, location, intensity, duration of anginal pain, precipitating factors (exertion, emotional stress). Assess baseline renal/hepatic function tests. Assess B/P, apical pulse immediately before drug is administered. Obtain baseline ECG in pts with history of arrhythmia.

INTERVENTION/EVALUATION

Assist with ambulation if dizziness occurs. Assess for peripheral edema. Monitor pulse rate for bradycardia. Assess B/P, renal function, LFT, ECG with IV therapy. Question for asthenia, headache.

PATIENT/FAMILY TEACHING

• Do not abruptly discontinue medication. • Compliance with therapy regimen is essential to control anginal pain. • To avoid postural dizziness, go from lying to standing slowly. • Avoid tasks that require alertness, motor skills until response to drug is established. • Report palpitations, shortness of breath, pronounced dizziness, nausea, constipation. • Avoid alcohol (may increase risk of hypotension or vasodilation).

dimethyl fumarate TOP 100

dye-**meth**-il-**fue**-ma-rate
(Tecfidera)

Do not confuse dimethyl fumarate with dimethyl sulfoxide or monomethyl fumarate.

◆CLASSIFICATION

PHARMACOTHERAPEUTIC: Fumaric acid agent. **CLINICAL:** Multiple sclerosis agent. Immunomodulator.

USES

Treatment of relapsing-remitting multiple sclerosis.

PRECAUTIONS

Contraindications: Hypersensitivity to dimethyl fumarate. **Cautions:** Hepatic impairment (may increase hepatic transaminases, lymphopenia (may decrease lymphocyte count).

ACTION

Exact mechanism of action unknown. May include anti-inflammatory action and cytoprotective properties. **Therapeutic Effect:** Modifies disease progression.

PHARMACOKINETICS

Undergoes rapid hydrolysis into active metabolite, monomethyl fumarate. Peak concentration: 2–212 hrs. Protein binding: 27%–45%. Extensively metabolized by esterases. Primarily eliminated as exhaled carbon dioxide (60%). **Half-life:** 1 hr.

⌛ LIFESPAN CONSIDERATIONS

Pregnancy/Lactation: Unknown if distributed in breast milk. **Children:** Safety and efficacy not established. **Elderly:** No age-related precautions noted.

INTERACTIONS

DRUG: May decrease therapeutic effects; increase adverse effects of **vaccines (live).** **HERBAL:** None known. **FOOD:** None significant. **LAB VALUES:** May decrease lymphocytes. May increase serum ALT, AST; eosinophils; urine albumin.

AVAILABILITY (Rx)

Capsules, Delayed-Release: 120 mg, 240 mg.

ADMINISTRATION/HANDLING

PO

• Give capsule whole; do not break, crush, dissolve, or divide. • May give without regard to food. May give with food to decrease flushing reaction and GI effects. • Protect from light.

INDICATIONS/ROUTES/DOSAGE

Relapsing-Remitting Multiple Sclerosis

PO: ADULTS/ELDERLY: Initially, 120 mg twice daily for 7 days. Then, increase to 240 mg twice daily.

Dosage in Renal/Hepatic Impairment
No dose adjustment.

SIDE EFFECTS

Frequent (40%): Flushing. **Occasional (18%–5%):** Abdominal pain, diarrhea, nausea, vomiting, dyspepsia, pruritus, rash, erythema.

ADVERSE EFFECTS/TOXIC REACTIONS

Lymphopenia may increase risk for infection. Severe flushing may lead to noncompliance of therapy.

NURSING CONSIDERATIONS

BASELINE ASSESSMENT

Obtain baseline CBC, CMP, urine pregnancy if applicable. Question any plans of breastfeeding. Assess hydration status (urine output, skin turgor). Question history of hepatic impairment, lymphopenia. Assess baseline symptoms of MS (e.g., bladder/bowel dysfunction, cognitive impairment, depression, dysphagia, fatigue, gait disorder, numbness/tingling, pain, seizures, spasticity, tremors, weakness). Screen for active infection.

INTERVENTION/EVALUATION

Monitor CBC, LFT. Encourage PO intake. Offer antiemetics for nausea, vomiting. Question any episodes of noncompliance due to flushing, GI symptoms. Monitor for infectious process (fever, malaise, chills, body aches, cough). Conduct neurologic assessment. Assess for symptomatic improvement of MS.

PATIENT/FAMILY TEACHING

• Pts will most likely experience abdominal pain, diarrhea, nausea, and flushing. Side effects may decrease over time. • Take with meals to decrease flushing reaction. • Swallow capsule whole; do not chew, crush, dissolve, or divide. • Two dosage strengths will be provided for starting dose and maintenance dose. • Report any yellowing of skin or eyes, upper abdominal pain, bruising, dark-colored urine, fever, body aches, cough, dehydration.

dinutuximab

din-ue-**tux**-i-mab
(Unituxin)

■ BLACK BOX ALERT ■ Life-threatening infusion-related reactions have occurred. Administer required prehydration and premedication, including antihistamines, prior to each infusion. Treatment causes severe neuropathic pain. Administer IV opioids prior to each infusion and for 2 hrs following completion of infusion. Severe peripheral sensory neuropathy occurred in pts with neuroblastoma. Severe motor neuropathy was observed. Discontinue therapy if severe unresponsive pain, severe sensory neuropathy, or moderate to severe peripheral motor neuropathy occurs. **Do not confuse dinutuximab with brentuximab, cetuximab, riTUXimab, or siltuximab.**

◆CLASSIFICATION

PHARMACOTHERAPEUTIC: GD2-binding monoclonal antibody. **CLINICAL:** Antineoplastic.

USES

Used in combination with granulocyte-macrophage colony-stimulating factor (GM-CSF), interleukin-2 (IL-2), and 13-cis-retinoic acid for the treatment of pediatric pts with high-risk neuroblastoma who achieve at least a partial response to prior fine-line multiagent, multimodality therapy.

PRECAUTIONS

Contraindications: History of anaphylaxis to dinutuximab. **Cautions:** Active infection; baseline cytopenias; diabetes, dehydration, electrolyte imbalance, hepatic/renal impairment, peripheral or generalized edema; intolerance of opioids, antipyretics, antihistamines; history of arrhythmias, hypotension, neuropathy, optic disorders.

ACTION

Binds to glycolipid GD2 expressed on neuroblastoma cells and on normal cells of neuroectodermal origin, including CNS and peripheral nerves. Induces cell lysis of GD2-expressing cells through antibody-dependent cell-mediated cytotoxicity and complement-dependent cytotoxicity. **Therapeutic Effect:** Inhibits tumor cell growth and survival.

PHARMACOKINETICS

Widely distributed. Metabolism not specified. Protein binding: not specified. Elimination not specified. **Half-life:** 10 days.

LIFESPAN CONSIDERATIONS

Pregnancy/Lactation: Avoid pregnancy; may cause fetal harm, esp. in third trimester. Unknown if distributed in breast milk. However, human immunoglobulin G is present in human breast milk. Females of reproductive potential must use effective contraception during treatment and for at least 2 mos following discontinuation. **Children:** No age-related precautions noted. **Elderly:** Safety and efficacy not established.

INTERACTIONS

DRUG: May decrease therapeutic effect of **BCG (intravesical), vaccines (live).** May increase adverse effects of **belimumab, natalizumab, vaccines (live).** **HERBAL:** **Echinacea** may decrease therapeutic effect. **FOOD:** None known. **LAB VALUES:** May decrease Hgb, Hct, lymphocytes, neutrophils, platelets, RBCs; serum albumin, calcium, magnesium, phosphate, potassium, sodium. May increase serum ALT, AST, bilirubin, creatinine, glucose; urine protein.

AVAILABILITY (Rx)

Injection Solution: 17.5 mg/5 mL (3.5 mg/mL).

ADMINISTRATION/HANDLING

IV

Pretreatment Guidelines

Hydration • Administer bolus of 0.9% NaCl 10 mL/kg IV over 1 hr prior to initiation.

Analgesics • Administer morphine sulfate 50 mcg/kg IV immediately prior to initiation and then continue as morphine sulfate drip at rate of 20–50 mcg/kg/hr during and for 2 hrs following completion of infusion. • Administer additional doses of morphine sulfate 25–50 mcg/kg IV once every 2 hrs as needed for pain, followed by an increase in morphine infusion rate, if clinically stable. • Consider use of fentaNYL or HYDROmorphone if morphine sulfate not tolerated. • If pain is inadequately controlled with opioids, consider use of gabapentin or lidocaine in addition to IV morphine.

Antihistamines and antipyretics • Administer an antihistamine such as diphenhydrAMINE 0.5–1 mg/kg (maximum dose 50 mg) IV over 10–15 min, starting 20 min prior to initiation and as tolerated every 4–6 hrs during infusion. • Administer acetaminophen 10–15 mg/kg (maximum dose 650 mg) 20 minutes prior to each infusion and every 4–6 hrs as needed for fever/pain. • May administer ibuprofen 5–10 mg/kg every 6 hrs as needed for persistent fever/pain.

Preparation • Visually inspect for particulate matter or discoloration. Do not use if solution is cloudy or contains particulate matter. • Withdraw required volume from vial and inject into 100 mL 0.9% NaCl. • Mix by gentle inversion. Do not shake or agitate. • Discard unused portions of vial.

Rate of administration • Initiate infusion rate at 0.875 mg/m²/hr for 30 min via dedicated IV line. May gradually increase rate to maximum rate of 1.75/m²/hr as tolerated. • Do not infuse as IV push or bolus.

Storage • Refrigerate vials. • Protect from light by storing in outer carton. • May refrigerate diluted solution up to 4 hrs. • Discard diluted solution 24 hrs after preparation.

IV INCOMPATIBILITIES

Do not mix with other medications.

INDICATIONS/ROUTES/DOSAGE

Neuroblastoma

IV: PEDIATRIC: 17.5 mg/m²/day over 10–20 hrs for 4 consecutive days for maximum of 5 cycles (Tables 1 and 2).

D

TABLE 1 SCHEDULE OF DINUTUXIMAB ADMINISTRATION FOR CYCLES 1, 3, AND 5

Cycle Day	1 through 3	4	5	6	7	8 through 24*
dinutuximab		X	X	X	X	

*Cycles 2 and 4 are 32 days in duration.

TABLE 2 SCHEDULE OF DINUTUXIMAB ADMINISTRATION FOR CYCLES 2 AND 4

Cycle Day	1 through 7	8	9	10	11	12 through 32*
dinutuximab		X	X	X	X	

*Cycles 2 and 4 are 32 days in duration.

Dose Modification

Infusion-Related Reactions

Mild to moderate adverse reactions (transient rash, fever, rigors, or localized urticaria that respond promptly to symptomatic treatment): Decrease infusion rate to 50% of the previous rate. Once resolved, gradually increase infusion rate up to a maximum rate of 1.75 mg/m²/hr. **Prolonged or severe adverse reactions (mild bronchospasm without other symptoms, angioedema that does not affect the airway):** Immediately interrupt infusion. If symptoms resolve rapidly, restart infusion at 50% of the previous rate. **First recurrence of severe reaction:** Discontinue treatment until the following day. If symptoms resolve and continued treatment is still warranted, premedicate with hydrocortisone (per guidelines) and administer dinutuximab infusion at a rate of 0.875 mg/m²/hr in an intensive care unit. **Second recurrence of severe reaction:** Permanently discontinue.

Capillary Leak Syndrome

Moderate to severe, non–life-threatening capillary leak syndrome: Interrupt infusion. Once resolved, resume infusion rate at 50% of previous rate. **Life-threatening capillary leak syndrome:** Discontinue treatment for the current cycle. Once resolved, administer at 50% of the previous rate for subsequent cycles. **First recurrence:** Permanently discontinue.

Hypotension

Hypotension requiring medical intervention: Interrupt infusion. Once resolved, resume infusion rate at 50% of previous rate. If blood pressure remains stable for at least 2 hrs, increase infusion rate as tolerated up to maximum rate of 1.75 mg/m²/hr.

Infection

Severe systemic infection or sepsis: Discontinue treatment until infection resolves, then continue with subsequent cycles of treatment.

Neurologic Disorders of the Eye

Dilated pupil with sluggish reflex; other visual disturbances: Interrupt infusion. Once resolved, resume infusion rate at 50% of previous rate. **First recurrence or if accompanied by visual impairment:** Permanently discontinue.

Adverse Reactions Requiring Permanent Discontinuation (based on Common Terminology for Adverse Events [CTCAE])

Grade 3 or 4 anaphylaxis, serum sickness; Grade 3 pain unresponsive to maximum supportive measures; Grade 4 sensory neuropathy or Grade 3 sensory neuropathy that interferes with daily activities for more than 2 wks; Grade 2 peripheral motor neuropathy, subtotal or total vision loss; Grade 4 hyponatremia despite appropriate fluid management.

Dosage in Renal/Hepatic Impairment

Not specified; use caution.

SIDE EFFECTS

Frequent (85%–24%): Pain (abdominal, back, bladder, bone, chest, neck, facial, gingival, musculoskeletal, oropharyngeal, extremity), arthralgia, myalgia, neuralgia, proctalgia, pyrexia, hypotension, vomiting, diarrhea, urticaria, hypoxia. **Occasional (19%–10%):** Tachycardia, edema, hypertension, peripheral neuropathy, weight gain, nausea.

ADVERSE EFFECTS/TOXIC REACTIONS

Anemia, neutropenia, lymphopenia, thrombocytopenia are expected results of therapy. Severe bone marrow suppression occurred in up to 39% of pts. Serious infusion-related reactions, such as bronchospasm, dyspnea, facial and upper airway edema, hypotension, or stridor, may require urgent interventions, including bronchodilator therapy, blood pressure support, corticosteroids, infusion interruption, infusion rate reduction, or permanent treatment discontinuation. Severe infusion-related reactions were reported in 26% of pts. Infusion-related reactions usually occurred during or within 24 hrs of infusion completion. Other serious adverse effects may include: severe urticaria (13% of pts); anaphylaxis, cardiac arrest (1% or less of pts); pain despite pretreatment with analgesics including morphine sulfate infusion (85% of pts); Grade 3 pain (51% of pts); Grade 3 peripheral sensory/motor neuropathy (1% of pts); Grade 3–5 capillary leak syndrome (23% of pts); Grade 3 hypotension (16% of pts); Grade 3 or 4 bacteremia requiring IV antibiotics or other urgent interventions (13% of pts); sepsis (18% of pts); neurologic disorders of the eye, including blurred vision, photophobia, mydriasis, fixed or unequal pupils, optic nerve disorder, eyelid ptosis, papilledema (2%–13% of pts); Grade 3 or 4 electrolyte abnormalities, including hyponatremia, hypokalemia, hypocalcemia (37%–23% of pts); atypical hemolytic uremic syndrome resulting in anemia, electrolyte imbalance, hypertension, renal insufficiency. Bleeding events, including GI/rectal/renal/respiratory/urinary tract/catheter site hemorrhage, disseminated intravascular coagulation, epistaxis, hematemesis, hematochezia, hematuria, were reported. Immunogenicity (anti-dinutuximab antibodies) reported in 18% of pts.

NURSING CONSIDERATIONS

BASELINE ASSESSMENT

Obtain baseline CBC, BMP, LFT; serum magnesium, ionized calcium, prealbumin, phosphate triglyceride level; capillary blood glucose, urinalysis, urine protein, urine pregnancy test, vital signs. Verify that pts have adequate hematologic/hepatic/ophthalmic/respiratory/renal function and proper hydration status prior to start of each infusion. Ensure proper resuscitative equipment/medications are readily available. Obtain baseline visual acuity, pupillary response, neurologic status. Question history of anaphylaxis; intolerance of opioids, antipyretics, antihistamines. Screen for active infection. Offer emotional support.

INTERVENTION/EVALUATION

Frequently monitor CBC, BMP, LFT, other serum electrolytes, vital signs. Monitor I&O. Administer required prehydration and premedication with antihistamine, antipyretics, opioids prior to each infusion and during infusion as indicated. Diligently monitor for infusion-related reactions as listed in Adverse Effects/Toxic Reactions and institute medical support as needed. Monitor for bleeding events of any kind. Consider administration of naloxone if narcotic overdose is suspected. Routinely assess visual acuity, hydration status. Offer emotional support. Initiate fall precautions.

PATIENT/FAMILY TEACHING

• Serious infusion reactions, including anaphylaxis, difficulty breathing, facial swelling, itching, rash, and wheezing, may occur during or within 24 hrs of each infusion. • Immediately report any allergic reactions; bleeding of any kind; decreased urine output or dark urine; disorders of the eye including blurry vision, double vision, unequal pupil size, sensitivity to light, eyelid drooping; fever; palpitations; seizures (related to electrolyte imbalance); severe nerve pain or loss of motor function; signs of low blood pressure such as confusion, fainting, pallor; swelling of face, arms, or legs. • Moderate to severe generalized pain is an expected side effect. Medications for pain, fever, and mild allergic reactions will need to be provided before or during each infusion; report any intolerance to such medications. • Therapy is expected to lower blood counts/immune system and may increase risk of bleeding or infection. • Drink plenty of fluids. • Use effective contraception to avoid pregnancy. Do not breastfeed.

diphenhydrAMINE

dye-fen-**hye**-dra-meen
(Banophen, Benadryl, Benadryl Children's Allergy, Diphen, Diphenhist, Genahist, Nytol)
Do not confuse Benadryl with benazepril, Bentyl, or Benylin, or diphenhydrAMINE with desipramine, dicyclomine, or dimenhyDRINATE.

FIXED-COMBINATION(S)

Advil PM: diphenhydramine/ibuprofen (NSAID): 38 mg/200 mg. With calamine, an astringent, and camphor, a counterirritant **(Caladryl).**

◆CLASSIFICATION

PHARMACOTHERAPEUTIC: Histamine-1 antagonist, first generation. **CLINICAL:** Antihistamine, anticholinergic, antipruritic, antitussive, antiemetic, antidyskinetic.

USES

Treatment of allergic reactions, including nasal allergies and allergic dermatoses; parkinsonism, including drug-induced extrapyramidal symptoms; prevention/treatment of nausea, vomiting, or vertigo due to motion sickness; antitussive; short-term management of insomnia; adjunct to EPINEPHrine in treatment of anaphylaxis. Topical form used for relief of pruritus from insect bites, skin irritations.

PRECAUTIONS

Contraindications: Hypersensitivity to diphenhydrAMINE. Neonates or premature infants, breastfeeding. **Cautions:** Narrow-angle glaucoma, stenotic peptic ulcer, prostatic hypertrophy, pyloroduodenal/bladder neck obstruction, asthma, COPD, increased IOP, cardiovascular disease, hyperthyroidism, elderly.

ACTION

Competes with histamine for H-1 receptor site on effector cells in GI tract, blood vessels, respiratory tract. **Therapeutic Effect:** Produces anticholinergic, antipruritic, antitussive, antiemetic, antidyskinetic, sedative effects.

PHARMACOKINETICS

Route	Onset	Peak	Duration
PO	15–30 min	1–4 hrs	4–6 hrs
IV, IM	Less than 15 min	1–4 hrs	4–6 hrs

Well absorbed after PO, parenteral administration. Protein binding: 98%–99%. Widely distributed. Metabolized in liver. Primarily excreted in urine. **Half-life:** 1–4 hrs. Adults: 7–12 hrs, elderly: 9–18 hrs, children: 4–7 hrs.

⌛ LIFESPAN CONSIDERATIONS

Pregnancy/Lactation: Crosses placenta. Detected in breast milk (may produce irritability in breastfed infants). Increased risk of seizures in neonates, premature infants if used during third trimester of pregnancy. May prohibit lactation. **Children:** Not recommended in newborns, premature infants (increased risk of paradoxical reaction, seizures). **Elderly:** Potentially inappropriate due to potent anticholinergic effects. Increased risk for dizziness, sedation, confusion, hypotension, hyperexcitability.

INTERACTIONS

DRUG: **Alcohol, CNS depressants (e.g., LORazepam, morphine, zolpidem)** may increase CNS depressant effects. **Anticholinergics (e.g., aclidinium, ipratropium, tiotropium,**

umeclidinium) may increase anticholinergic effects. **HERBAL:** **Gotu kola, kava kava, valerian** may increase CNS depression. **FOOD:** None known. **LAB VALUES:** May suppress wheal/flare reactions to antigen skin testing unless drug is discontinued 4 days before testing.

AVAILABILITY (OTC)

Capsules: 25 mg, 50 mg. **Cream:** 1%, 2%. **Elixir:** 12.5 mg/5 mL. **Injection Solution:** 50 mg/mL. **Liquid:** 12.5 mg/5 mL. **Syrup:** 12.5 mg/5 mL. **Tablets:** 25 mg, 50 mg. **Tablets, Chewable:** 12.5 mg.

ADMINISTRATION/HANDLING

IV

• May be given undiluted. • Give IV injection over at least 1 min. **Maximum rate:** 25 mg/min.

IM

• Give deep IM into large muscle mass.

PO

• Give with food to decrease GI distress. • Scored tablets may be crushed.

IV INCOMPATIBILITIES

Allopurinol (Aloprim), cefepime (Maxipime), dexamethasone (Decadron), foscarnet (Foscavir).

IV COMPATIBILITIES

Atropine, cisplatin (Platinol), cyclophosphamide (Cytoxan), cytarabine (Ara-C), fentaNYL, glycopyrrolate (Robinul), heparin, hydrocortisone (SOLU-Cortef), HYDROmorphone (Dilaudid), hydrOXYzine (Vistaril), lidocaine, metoclopramide (Reglan), ondansetron (Zofran), potassium chloride, promethazine (Phenergan), propofol (Diprivan).

INDICATIONS/ROUTES/DOSAGE

Allergic Reaction

PO: **ADULTS, ELDERLY:** 25 mg q4–6h PRN or 50 mg q6h PRN. **IM, IV:** 10–50 mg/dose q6hrs PRN. **PO, IV, IM:** **CHILDREN:** 5 mg/kg/day in divided doses q6–8h. **Maximum:** 300 mg/day.

Motion Sickness

Note: When used for prophylaxis, give 30 min before motion.

PO: ***(Prophylaxis/Treatment):*** **ADULTS, ELDERLY:** 25 mg q4–6h PRN or 50 mg q6h PRN. **CHILDREN:** 5 mg/kg/day in 3–4 divided doses. **Maximum:** 300 mg/day. **IV/IM:** ***(Treatment):*** **ADULTS, ELDERLY:** 10–50 mg/dose. **CHILDREN:** 5 mg/kg/day in 4 divided doses. **Maximum:** 300 mg/day.

Nighttime Sleep Aid

PO: **ADULTS, ELDERLY, CHILDREN 12 YRS AND OLDER:** 25–50 mg at bedtime. **CHILDREN 2–11 YRS:** 1 mg/kg/dose. **Maximum Single Dose:** 50 mg.

Pruritus

Topical: **ADULTS, ELDERLY, CHILDREN 12 YRS AND OLDER:** Apply 1% or 2% cream or spray 3–4 times/day. **CHILDREN 2–11 YRS:** Apply 1% cream or spray 3–4 times/day.

Parkinsonism, Dystonic Reaction

PO: **ADULTS, ELDERLY:** 25 mg q4–6h PRN or 50 mg q6h PRN. **IM/IV:** 25–50 mg/dose.

Dosage in Renal/Hepatic Impairment

No dose adjustment.

SIDE EFFECTS

Frequent: Drowsiness, dizziness, muscle weakness, hypotension, urinary retention, thickening of bronchial secretions, dry mouth, nose, throat, lips; in elderly: sedation, dizziness, hypotension. **Occasional:** Epigastric distress, flushing, visual/hearing disturbances, paresthesia, diaphoresis, chills.

ADVERSE EFFECTS/TOXIC REACTIONS

Hypersensitivity reactions (eczema, pruritus, rash, cardiac disturbances, photosensitivity) may occur. Overdose symptoms may vary from CNS depression (sedation, apnea, hypotension, cardiovascular collapse, death) to severe paradoxical reactions (hallucinations, tremors, seizures). Children, infants, neonates may experience paradoxical reactions (restlessness, insomnia, euphoria, nervousness, tremors). Overdosage in children may result in hallucinations, seizures, death.

D

NURSING CONSIDERATIONS

BASELINE ASSESSMENT

If pt is having acute allergic reaction, obtain history of recently ingested foods, drugs, environmental exposure, emotional stress. Monitor B/P rate; depth, rhythm, type of respiration; quality, rate of pulse. Assess lung sounds for rhonchi, wheezing, rales.

INTERVENTION/EVALUATION

Monitor B/P, esp. in elderly (increased risk of hypotension). Monitor children closely for paradoxical reaction. Monitor for sedation.

PATIENT/FAMILY TEACHING

• Tolerance to antihistaminic effect generally does not occur; tolerance to sedative effect may occur. • Avoid tasks that require alertness, motor skills until response to drug is established. • Dry mouth, drowsiness, dizziness may be an expected response to drug. • Avoid alcohol.

diphenoxylate with atropine

dye-fen-**ox**-i-late **at**-roe-peen
(Lomotil)
Do not confuse Lomotil with LaMICtal, LamISIL, Lamotrigine, Lanoxin, or Lasix

FIXED-COMBINATION(S)

Lomotil: diphenoxylate/atropine (anticholinergic, antispasmodic): 2.5 mg/0.025 mg.

◆CLASSIFICATION

PHARMACOTHERAPEUTIC: Opioid/anticholinergic **(Schedule V). CLINICAL:** Antidiarrheal.

USES

Adjunctive treatment of acute, chronic diarrhea.

PRECAUTIONS

Contraindications: Hypersensitivity to diphenoxylate, atropine. Obstructive jaundice, diarrhea associated with pseudomembranous colitis or enterotoxin-producing bacteria. **Cautions:** Children (not recommended in children younger than 2 yrs): acute ulcerative colitis, renal/hepatic impairment.

ACTION

Acts locally and centrally on gastric mucosa. **Therapeutic Effect:** Reduces excessive GI motility and GI propulsion.

PHARMACOKINETICS

	Onset	Peak	Duration
Antidiarrheal	45–60 min	—	3–4 hrs

Well absorbed from GI tract. Metabolized in liver. Primarily eliminated in feces. **Half-life:** 2.5 hrs; metabolite: 12–24 hrs.

LIFESPAN CONSIDERATIONS

Pregnancy/Lactation: Unknown if drug crosses placenta or is distributed in breast milk. **Children:** Not recommended (increased susceptibility to toxicity, including respiratory depression). **Elderly:** More susceptible to anticholinergic effects, confusion, respiratory depression.

INTERACTIONS

DRUG: **Alcohol, CNS depressants (e.g., LORazepam, morphine, zolpidem)** may increase CNS depressant effects. **Anticholinergics (e.g., aclidinium, ipratropium, tiotropium, umeclidinium)** may increase effects of atropine. **MAOIs (e.g., phenelzine,**

selegiline) may precipitate hypertensive crisis. HERBAL: **Herbals with sedative properties (e.g., chamomile, kava kava, valerian)** may increase CNS depression. FOOD: None known. LAB VALUES: May increase serum amylase.

AVAILABILITY (Rx)

Liquid: *(Lomotil):* 2.5 mg diphenoxylate/0.025 mg atropine/5 mL. **Tablets:** *(Lomotil):* 2.5 mg diphenoxylate/0.025 mg atropine.

ADMINISTRATION/HANDLING

PO

• Give without regard to food. If GI irritation occurs, give with food. • Use liquid for children 2–12 yrs (use graduated dropper for administration of liquid medication).

INDICATIONS/ROUTES/DOSAGE

Diarrhea

PO: ADULTS, ELDERLY: Initially, 5 mg (2 tabs or 10 mL) 3–4 times/day. **Maximum:** 20 mg/day. Then reduce dose as needed.

Dosage in Renal/Hepatic Impairment

No dose adjustment. Use caution with severe renal/hepatic disease.

SIDE EFFECTS

Frequent: Drowsiness, light-headedness, dizziness, nausea. **Occasional:** Headache, dry mouth. **Rare:** Flushing, tachycardia, urinary retention, constipation, paradoxical reaction (marked by restlessness, agitation), blurred vision.

ADVERSE EFFECTS/TOXIC REACTIONS

Dehydration may predispose pt to diphenoxylate toxicity. Paralytic ileus, toxic megacolon (constipation, decreased appetite, abdominal pain with nausea/vomiting) occur rarely. Severe anticholinergic reaction (severe lethargy, hypotonic reflexes, hyperthermia) may result in severe respiratory depression, coma.

NURSING CONSIDERATIONS

BASELINE ASSESSMENT

Check baseline hydration status: skin turgor, mucous membranes for dryness, urinary status. Assess usual stool frequency, consistency.

INTERVENTION/EVALUATION

Encourage adequate fluid intake. Assess bowel sounds for peristalsis. Monitor daily pattern of bowel activity, stool consistency. Record time of evacuation. Assess for abdominal disturbances. Discontinue medication if abdominal distention occurs.

PATIENT/FAMILY TEACHING

• Avoid tasks that require alertness, motor skills until response to drug is established. • Avoid alcohol. • Report persistent fever, palpitations, diarrhea. • Report abdominal distention.

diroximel fumarate

dye-**rox**-i-mel **fyoo**-ma-rate
(Vumerity)
Do not confuse diroximel fumarate with dimethyl fumarate or monomethyl fumarate.

◆CLASSIFICATION

PHARMACOTHERAPEUTIC: Fumaric acid derivative. **CLINICAL:** Multiple sclerosis agent.

USES

Treatment of relapsing forms of multiple sclerosis (MS) in adults, to include clinically isolated syndrome, relapsing-remitting disease, and active secondary progressive disease.

PRECAUTIONS

Contraindications: Hypersensitivity reactions to diroximel fumarate or dimethyl fumarate. Concomitant use with dimethyl fumarate. **Cautions:** Baseline lymphopenia, hepatic/renal impairment; conditions

D

predisposing to infection (e.g., diabetes, renal failure, immunocompromised pts, open wounds); history of chronic opportunistic infections (esp. fungal/viral infections, tuberculosis).

D

ACTION

Exact mechanism of action unknown. May include anti-inflammatory action and cytoprotective properties via activation of the nuclear factor (erythroid-derived 2)–like-2 pathway. **Therapeutic Effect:** Modifies disease progression of MS.

PHARMACOKINETICS

Undergoes rapid hydrolysis by esterases into active metabolite, monomethyl fumarate. Protein binding: 27%–45%. Peak plasma concentration: 2.5–3 hrs. Primarily eliminated as exhaled carbon dioxide. **Half-life:** 1 hr.

⌛ LIFESPAN CONSIDERATIONS

Pregnancy/Lactation: Generally not initiated in pts considering a planned pregnancy or during pregnancy. Unknown if distributed in breast milk. **Children:** Safety and efficacy not established. **Elderly:** Not specified.

INTERACTIONS

DRUG: **Alcohol** may decrease concentration/effect. **Dimethyl or monomethyl fumarate** may increase adverse effects. HERBAL: None significant. FOOD: **High-fat, high-calorie meals** may reduce absorption/concentration. LAB VALUES: May increase serum ALT, AST, bilirubin; urine albumin. May decrease lymphocytes, eosinophils.

AVAILABILITY (Rx)

Capsules, Delayed-Release: 231 mg.

ADMINISTRATION/HANDLING

PO

• May take with or without food. Avoid high-fat, high-calorie meals. Meals should not be more than 700 calories and contain no more than 30 g of fat. • Administer capsule whole; do not crush, open, or sprinkle on food. • Avoid alcohol at same time of administration.

INDICATIONS/ROUTES/DOSAGE

Multiple Sclerosis (Relapsing)

PO: ADULTS: 231 mg twice daily for 7 days, then increase to a maintenance dose of 462 mg twice daily.

Dose Modifications

Unable to tolerate maintenance dose (GI effects, flushing): May reduce dose to 231 mg twice daily for up to 4 wks, then re-escalate dose to 462 mg twice daily. Consider permanent discontinuation if unable to tolerate return to maintenance dose.

Hepatotoxicity

Acute hepatic injury: Permanently discontinue if significant hepatic injury occurs.

Infections

Bacterial/fungal/viral infections: Consider withholding treatment until infection is resolved.

Lymphopenia

Lymphocyte count less than 500 cells/mm³ for greater than 6 mos: Consider withholding treatment until improved.

Dosage in Renal Impairment

Mild impairment: No dose adjustment. **Moderate to severe impairment:** Not recommended.

Dosage in Hepatic Impairment

Mild to severe impairment: Not specified; use caution.

SIDE EFFECTS

Frequent (40%): Flushing. **Occasional (18%–5%):** Abdominal pain, diarrhea, nausea, vomiting, pruritus, rash, erythema, dyspepsia.

ADVERSE EFFECTS/TOXIC REACTIONS

Hypersensitivity reactions including anaphylaxis, angioedema, dyspnea, urticaria were reported. Progressive multifocal leukoencephalopathy (PML), an opportunistic viral infection of the brain caused by the JC virus, may result in progressive permanent disability and death. Serious herpes zoster infections including disseminated herpes zoster, herpes zoster ophthalmicus, herpes zoster meningoencephalitis, herpes zoster meningomyelitis was reported. Other serious bacterial, fungal, viral infections may occur. Acute hepatic injury with serum aminotransferase greater than 5 times ULN and total bilirubin greater than 2 times ULN was reported. Severe flushing may lead to noncompliance of therapy.

NURSING CONSIDERATIONS

BASELINE ASSESSMENT

Obtain CBC (including lymphocyte count), LFT. Assess baseline symptoms of MS (e.g., bladder/bowel dysfunction, cognitive impairment, depression, dysphagia, fatigue, gait disorder, numbness/tingling, pain, seizures, spasticity, tremors, weakness). Screen for active infection.
Question history of hypersensitivity reactions, hepatic/renal impairment, herpes zoster infection, chronic infection.

INTERVENTION/EVALUATION

Obtain CBC (including lymphocyte count) 6 mos after initiation, then q6–12mos thereafter. Monitor LFT as clinically indicated. Pts with altered mental status, seizures, visual disturbances, generalized or unilateral weakness should be evaluated for herpes zoster meningoencephalitis, herpes zoster meningomyelitis, PML. If herpes zoster infection or other serious infection occurs, initiate treatment as appropriate. To reduce occurrence/severity of flushing, may administer non–enteric-coated aspirin (up to 325 mg) PO 30 min prior to dose. Question for noncompliance due to flushing, GI symptoms. Conduct neurologic assessment. Assess for symptomatic improvement of MS.

PATIENT/FAMILY TEACHING

• Treatment may depress your immune system and reduce your ability to fight infection. Report symptoms of infection such as body aches, burning with urination, chills, cough, fatigue, fever. Avoid those with active infection. Report travel plans to possible endemic areas. • PML, an opportunistic viral infection of the brain, may cause progressive, permanent disabilities or death. Report symptoms of PML or herpes zoster infection of the brain such as confusion, memory loss, paralysis, trouble speaking, vision loss, seizures, weakness. • GI symptoms (e.g., abdominal pain, diarrhea, nausea, vomiting, upset stomach), flushing are common side effects. • Take with meals to decrease flushing reaction. If taken with food, avoid high-fat, high-calorie meal or snack. Do not ingest alcohol with dose. • Report liver problems (abdominal pain, bruising, clay-colored stool, amber- or dark-colored urine, yellowing of the skin or eyes). • Allergic reactions such as difficulty breathing, hives, rash, swelling of the face or tongue, wheezing can happen at any time. If allergic reaction occurs, seek immediate medical attention.

DOBUTamine

HIGH ALERT

doe-**bue**-ta-meen

Do not confuse DOBUTamine with DOPamine.

◆CLASSIFICATION

PHARMACOTHERAPEUTIC: Adrenergic agonist. **CLINICAL:** Cardiac stimulant.

USES

Short-term management of cardiac decompensation.

PRECAUTIONS

Contraindications: Hypersensitivity to dobutamine. Hypertrophic cardiomyopathy with outflow obstruction. **Cautions:** Atrial fibrillation, hypovolemia, post-MI, concurrent use of MAOIs, elderly.

ACTION

Direct-action inotropic agent acting primarily on myocardial $beta_1$-adrenergic receptors. **Therapeutic Effect:** Enhances myocardial contractility, increases heart rate.

PHARMACOKINETICS

Route	Onset	Peak	Duration
IV	1–2 min	10 min	Length of infusion

Metabolized in liver. Primarily excreted in urine. Not removed by hemodialysis. **Half-life:** 2 min.

LIFESPAN CONSIDERATIONS

Pregnancy/Lactation: Unknown if drug crosses placenta or is distributed in breast milk. **Children/Elderly:** No age-related precautions noted.

INTERACTIONS

DRUG: **Sympathomimetics (e.g., norepinephrine, phenylephrine)** may increase effects. **HERBAL:** None significant. **FOOD:** None known. **LAB VALUES:** May decrease serum potassium.

AVAILABILITY (Rx)

Infusion (Ready-to-Use): 1 mg/mL (250 mL), 2 mg/mL (250 mL), 4 mg/mL (250 mL). **Injection Solution:** 12.5-mg/mL vial.

ADMINISTRATION/HANDLING

◀ALERT▶ Correct hypovolemia with volume expanders before DOBUTamine infusion. Pts with atrial fibrillation should be digitalized before infusion. Administer by IV infusion only.

IV

Reconstitution • Dilute vial in 0.9% NaCl or D_5W to maximum concentration of 5,000 mcg/mL (5 mg/mL).

Rate of administration • Use infusion pump to control flow rate. • Titrate dosage to individual response. • Infiltration causes local inflammatory changes. • Extravasation may cause dermal necrosis.

Storage • Store at room temperature. • Pink discoloration of solution (due to oxidation) does not indicate significant loss of potency if used within recommended time period. • Further diluted solution for infusion is stable for 48 hrs at room temperature, 7 days if refrigerated.

IV INCOMPATIBILITIES

Acyclovir (Zovirax), alteplase (Activase), amphotericin B complex (Abelcet, AmBisome, Amphotec), bumetanide (Bumex), cefepime (Maxipime), foscarnet (Foscavir), furosemide (Lasix), heparin, piperacillin/tazobactam (Zosyn), sodium bicarbonate.

IV COMPATIBILITIES

Amiodarone (Cordarone), calcium chloride, calcium gluconate, dilTIAZem (Cardizem), DOPamine (Intropin), enalapril (Vasotec), EPINEPHrine, famotidine (Pepcid), HYDROmorphone (Dilaudid), insulin (regular), lidocaine, LORazepam (Ativan), magnesium sulfate, midazolam (Versed), milrinone (Primacor), morphine, nitroglycerin, nitroprusside (Nipride), norepinephrine (Levophed), potassium chloride, propofol (Diprivan).

INDICATIONS/ROUTES/DOSAGE

◀ALERT▶ Dosage determined by severity of decompensation.

Cardiac Decompensation (Hemodynamic support)

IV infusion: ADULTS, ELDERLY: Initially, 0.5–2.5 mcg/kg/min. **Maintenance:** 2–20 mcg/kg/min titrated to desired response. May be infused at a rate of up to 40 mcg/kg/min to increase cardiac output. **NEONATES, INFANTS, CHILDREN, ADOLESCENTS:** Initially, 0.5–1 mcg/kg/min. Titrate gradually every few minutes until desired response. **Usual Range:** 2–20 mcg/kg/minute.

Dosage in Renal/Hepatic Impairment

No dose adjustment.

SIDE EFFECTS

Frequent (greater than 5%): Increased heart rate, B/P. **Occasional (5%–3%):** Pain at injection site. **Rare (3%–1%):** Nausea, headache, anginal pain, shortness of breath, fever.

ADVERSE EFFECTS/TOXIC REACTIONS

Overdose may produce severe tachycardia, severe hypertension.

NURSING CONSIDERATIONS

BASELINE ASSESSMENT

Pt must be on continuous cardiac monitoring. Determine weight (for dosage calculation). Obtain initial B/P, heart rate, respirations. Correct hypovolemia before drug therapy.

INTERVENTION/EVALUATION

Continuously monitor for cardiac rate, arrhythmias. Maintain accurate I&O; measure urinary output frequently. Assess serum potassium, plasma DOBUTamine (therapeutic range: 40–190 ng/mL). Monitor B/P continuously (hypertension risk greater in pts with preexisting hypertension). Check cardiac output, pulmonary wedge pressure/central venous pressure (CVP) frequently. Immediately notify physician of decreased urinary output, cardiac arrhythmias, significant increase in B/P, heart rate, or less commonly, hypotension.

DOCEtaxel

HIGH ALERT

doe-se-**tax**-el
(Taxotere)

■ BLACK BOX ALERT ■ Avoid use with serum bilirubin more than upper limit of normal (ULN) or serum ALT, AST more than 1.5 times ULN in conjunction with serum alkaline phosphatase more than 2.5 times ULN. Severe hypersensitivity reaction (rash, hypotension, bronchospasm, anaphylaxis) may occur. Fluid retention syndrome (pleural effusions, ascites, edema, dyspnea at rest) has been reported. Pts with abnormal hepatic function, receiving higher doses, and pts with non–small-cell lung carcinoma (NSCLC) and history of prior platinum treatment receiving DOCEtaxel dose of 100 mg/m^2 at higher risk for mortality. Avoid use with ANC less than 1,500 cells/mm^3.

Do not confuse DOCEtaxel with PACLitaxel or Taxotere with Taxol.

◆CLASSIFICATION

PHARMACOTHERAPEUTIC: Antimicrotubular, taxoid. **CLINICAL:** Antineoplastic.

USES

Treatment of locally advanced or metastatic breast carcinoma after failure of prior chemotherapy. Treatment of metastatic non–small-cell lung cancer (NSCLC). Treatment of metastatic prostate cancer, head and neck cancer (with predniSONE). Treatment of advanced gastric adenocarcinoma. **OFF-LABEL:** Bladder, esophageal, ovarian, small-cell lung carcinoma; soft tissue carcinoma, cervical cancer, Ewing's sarcoma, osteosarcoma.

PRECAUTIONS

Contraindications: Hypersensitivity to DOCEtaxel. History of severe hypersensitivity to drugs formulated with polysorbate 80, neutrophil count less than 1,500 cells/mm^3. **Cautions:** Hepatic impairment, myelosuppression, concomitant CYP3A4 inhibitors/inducers, fluid retention, pulmonary disease, HF, active infection.

ACTION

Promotes assembly of microtubules and inhibits depolymerization of tubulin, which stabilizes microtubules. **Therapeutic Effect:** Inhibits DNA, RNA, protein synthesis. Inhibits tumor cell growth and survival.

PHARMACOKINETICS

Widely distributed. Protein binding: 94%. Extensively metabolized in liver. Excreted in feces (75%), urine (6%). **Half-life:** 11.1 hrs.

⌛ LIFESPAN CONSIDERATIONS

Pregnancy/Lactation: May cause fetal harm. Unknown if distributed in breast milk.

D

Breastfeeding not recommended. **Children:** Safety and efficacy not established in pts younger than 16 yrs. **Elderly:** No age-related precautions noted.

INTERACTIONS

DRUG: **Strong CYP3A4 inhibitors (e.g., clarithromycin, ketoconazole, ritonavir)** may increase concentration/effect. **Strong CYP3A4 inducers (e.g., carBAMazepine, phenytoin, rifAMPin)** may decrease concentration/effect. **Live virus vaccines** may potentiate replication, increase vaccine side effects, decrease pt's antibody response to vaccine. HERBAL: **Echinacea** may decrease therapeutic effect. **St. John's wort** may decrease concentration/effect. FOOD: None known. LAB VALUES: May increase serum alkaline phosphatase, bilirubin, ALT, AST. Reduces neutrophil, platelet count, Hgb, Hct.

AVAILABILITY (Rx)

Injection Solution: 10 mg/mL, 20 mg/mL.

ADMINISTRATION/HANDLING

IV

Reconstitution (solution) • Withdraw dose and add to 250–500 mL 0.9% NaCl or D_5W in glass or polyolefin container to provide a final concentration of 0.3–0.74 mg/mL.

Rate of administration • Administer as a 1-hr infusion. • Monitor closely for hypersensitivity reaction (flushing, localized skin reaction, bronchospasm [may occur within a few min after beginning infusion]).

Storage • Store vials between 36°F–77°F. • Protect from bright light. • If refrigerated, stand vial at room temperature for 5 min before administering (do not store in PVC bags). • Diluted solution should be used within 4 hrs (including infusion time).

IV INCOMPATIBILITIES

Amphotericin B (Fungizone), methylPREDNISolone (SOLU), nalbuphine (Nubain).

IV COMPATIBILITIES

Bumetanide (Bumex), calcium gluconate, dexamethasone (Decadron), diphenhydrAMINE (Benadryl), DOBUTamine (Dobutrex), DOPamine (Intropin), furosemide (Lasix), granisetron (Kytril), heparin, HYDROmorphone (Dilaudid), LORazepam (Ativan), magnesium sulfate, mannitol, morphine, ondansetron (Zofran), palonosetron (Aloxi), potassium chloride.

INDICATIONS/ROUTES/DOSAGE

◀ALERT▶ Premedicate with oral corticosteroids (e.g., dexamethasone 16 mg/day for 5 days beginning day 1 before DOCEtaxel therapy); reduces severity of fluid retention, hypersensitivity reaction.

Breast Carcinoma

IV: ADULTS: Locally advanced or metastatic: 60–100 mg/m² given over 1 hr q3wks as a single agent. Operable, node positive: 75 mg/m² q3wks for 6 courses (in combination with DOXOrubicin and cyclophosphamide).

Non–Small-Cell Lung Carcinoma

IV: ADULTS: 75 mg/m² q3wks (as monotherapy or in combination with CISplatin).

Prostate Cancer

IV: ADULTS, ELDERLY: 75 mg/m² q3wks with concurrent administration of predniSONE.

Head/Neck Cancer

IV: ADULTS, ELDERLY: 75 mg/m² q3wks (in combination with CISplatin and fluorouracil) for 3–4 cycles, followed by radiation therapy.

Gastric Adenocarcinoma
IV: ADULTS, ELDERLY: 75 mg/m² q3wks (in combination with CISplatin and fluorouracil).

Dose Modification for Gastric or Head/ Neck Cancer

ALT, AST 2.5 to 5 times ULN and alkaline phosphatase less than or equal to 2.5 times ULN	80% of dose
ALT, AST 1.5 to 5 times ULN and alkaline phosphatase 2.5 to 5 times ULN	80% of dose
ALT, AST greater than 5 times ULN and/or alkaline phosphatase greater than 5 times ULN	Discontinue DOCEtaxel

Note: Toxicity includes febrile neutropenia, neutrophils less than 500 cells/mm³ for longer than 1 wk, severe cutaneous reactions. Also, for NSCLC, platelet nadir less than 25,000 cells/mm³, any CTCAE Grade 3 or 4 nonhematologic toxicity.

Breast Cancer
Reduce dose to 75 mg/m²; if toxicity persists, reduce to 55 mg/m².

Breast Cancer Adjuvant
Administer when neutrophils are less than 1,500 cells/mm³. If toxicity persists, or Grade 3 or 4 stomatitis, reduce dose to 60 mg/m².

Non–Small-Cell Lung Cancer
Monotherapy
Hold dose until toxicity resolves, then reduce dose to 55 mg/m². Discontinue if Grade 3 or 4 neuropathy occurs.
Combination Therapy
Reduce dose to 65 mg/m²; may further reduce to 50 mg/m² if needed.

Prostate Cancer
Reduce dose to 60 mg/m²; discontinue if toxicity persists.

Gastric or Head and Neck Cancer
Reduce dose to 60 mg/m²; if neutropenic toxicity persists, further reduce to 45 mg/m². For Grade 3 or 4 thrombocytopenia, reduce dose from 75 mg/m² to 60 mg/m²; discontinue if toxicity persists.

Dosage in Renal Impairment
No dose adjustment.

Dosage in Hepatic Impairment
Total bilirubin more than ULN, or ALT, AST more than 1.5 times ULN with alkaline phosphatase more than 2.5 times ULN: Use not recommended.

SIDE EFFECTS

Frequent (80%–19%): Alopecia, asthenia, hypersensitivity reaction (e.g., dermatitis), which is decreased in pts pretreated with oral corticosteroids; fluid retention, stomatitis, nausea, diarrhea, fever, nail changes, vomiting, myalgia. **Occasional:** Hypotension, edema, anorexia, headache, weight gain, infection (urinary tract, injection site, indwelling catheter tip), dizziness. **Rare:** Dry skin, sensory disorders (vision, speech, taste), arthralgia, weight loss, conjunctivitis, hematuria, proteinuria.

ADVERSE EFFECTS/TOXIC REACTIONS

In pts with normal hepatic function, neutropenia (ANC count less than 1,500 cells/mm³), leukopenia (WBC count less than 4,000 cells/mm³) occur in 96% of pts; anemia (hemoglobin level less than 11 g/dL) occurs in 90% of pts; thrombocytopenia (platelet count less than 100,000 cells/mm³) occurs in 8% of pts; infection occurs in 28% of pts. Neurosensory, neuromotor disturbances (distal paresthesia, weakness) occur in 54% and 13% of pts, respectively.

NURSING CONSIDERATIONS

BASELINE ASSESSMENT

Obtain baseline ANC, CBC, serum chemistries. Offer emotional support to pt, family. Antiemetics may be effective in preventing, treating nausea/vomiting.

Pt should be pretreated with corticosteroids to reduce fluid retention, hypersensitivity reaction. Offer emotional support.

INTERVENTION/EVALUATION

Frequently monitor blood counts, particularly ANC count (less than 1,500 cells/mm^3 requires discontinuation of therapy). Monitor LFT, serum uric acid levels. Observe for cutaneous reactions (rash with eruptions, mainly on hands, feet). Assess for extravascular fluid accumulation: rales in lungs, dependent edema, dyspnea at rest, pronounced abdominal distention (due to ascites).

PATIENT/FAMILY TEACHING

• Hair loss is reversible, but new hair growth may have different color or texture. • New hair growth resumes 2–3 mos after last therapy dose. • Maintain strict oral hygiene. • Do not have immunizations without physician's approval (drug lowers resistance). • Avoid those who have recently taken any live virus vaccine. • Report persistent nausea, diarrhea, respiratory difficulty, chest pain, fever, chills, unusual bleeding, bruising.

dofetilide

doe-**fet**-i-lide
(Tikosyn)

BLACK BOX ALERT Pt must be placed in a setting with continuous cardiac monitoring for minimum of 3 days and monitored by staff familiar with treatment of life-threatening arrhythmias.

◆CLASSIFICATION

PHARMACOTHERAPEUTIC: Potassium channel blocker. **CLINICAL:** Antiarrhythmic: Class III.

USES

Maintenance of normal sinus rhythm (NSR) in pts with chronic atrial fibrillation/atrial flutter of longer than 1-wk duration who have been converted to NSR. Conversion of atrial fibrillation/flutter to NSR.

PRECAUTIONS

Contraindications: Hypersensitivity to dofetilide. Congenital or acquired prolonged QT syndrome (do not use if baseline QT interval or QTc is greater than 440 msec), severe renal impairment, concurrent use of drugs that may prolong QT interval, hypokalemia, hypomagnesemia, concurrent use with verapamil, dolutegravir, itraconazole, ketoconazole, prochlorperazine, megestrol, cimetidine, hydroCHLOROthiazide, trimethoprim. Severe renal impairment (CrCl less than 20 mL/min). **Cautions:** Severe hepatic impairment, renal impairment, pts previously taking amiodarone, elderly. Concurrent use of other agents that prolong QT interval. Pts with sick sinus syndrome or second- or third-degree heart block unless functional pacemaker in place.

ACTION

Prolongs repolarization without affecting conduction velocity by blocking one or more time-dependent potassium currents. No effect on sodium channels, alpha-adrenergic, beta-adrenergic receptors. **Therapeutic Effect:** Terminates reentrant tachyarrhythmias, preventing reinduction.

PHARMACOKINETICS

Well absorbed following PO administration. 80% eliminated in urine as unchanged drug, 20% excreted as minimally active metabolites. Protein binding: 60%–70%. **Half-life:** 2–3 hrs.

⌛ LIFESPAN CONSIDERATIONS

Pregnancy/Lactation: Unknown if drug is distributed in breast milk. **Children:** No age-related precautions noted. **Elderly:** Age-related renal impairment may require dosage adjustment.

INTERACTIONS

DRUG: **Cimetidine, lamotrigine, ketoconazole, trimethoprim, verapamil**

may increase concentration/effect. **QT interval–prolonging medications (e.g., azithromycin, ceritinib, fingolimod, haloperidol, moxifloxacin)** may increase risk of QT interval prolongation. **HERBAL: Ephedra** may worsen arrhythmias. **FOOD:** None known. **LAB VALUES:** None significant.

AVAILABILITY (Rx)

Capsules: 125 mcg, 250 mcg, 500 mcg.

ADMINISTRATION/HANDLING

PO

• Give without regard to food. • Do not break, crush, or open capsules.

INDICATIONS/ROUTES/DOSAGE

◀ALERT▶ ECG interval measurements (esp. Qtc intervals), creatinine clearance, must be determined prior to first dose. Correct hypokalemia, hypomagnesemia prior to starting.

Antiarrhythmias

PO: ADULTS, ELDERLY: Initially, 500 mcg twice daily. Modify dose in response to QTc interval.

Dosage in Renal Impairment

Creatinine Clearance	Dosage
Greater than 60 mL/min	500 mcg twice daily
40–60 mL/min	250 mcg twice daily
20–39 mL/min	125 mcg twice daily
Less than 20 mL/min	Contraindicated

Dosage in Hepatic Impairment

No dose adjustment.

SIDE EFFECTS

Rare (less than 2%): Headache, chest pain, dizziness, dyspnea, nausea, insomnia, back/abdominal pain, diarrhea, rash.

ADVERSE EFFECTS/TOXIC REACTIONS

Angioedema, bradycardia, cerebral ischemia, facial paralysis, serious arrhythmias (ventricular, various forms of block) have been noted.

NURSING CONSIDERATIONS

BASELINE ASSESSMENT

Assess baseline serum electrolytes (esp. potassium, magnesium). Prior to initiating treatment, QTc intervals must be determined. Do not use if heart rate less than 50 beats/min. Provide continuous ECG monitoring, calculation of creatinine clearance, equipment for resuscitation available for minimum of 3 days. Anticipate proarrhythmic events.

INTERVENTION/EVALUATION

Assess for conversion of cardiac arrhythmias and absence of new arrhythmias. Constantly monitor ECG. Provide emotional support. Monitor renal function for electrolyte imbalance (prolonged or excessive diarrhea, sweating, vomiting, thirst).

PATIENT/FAMILY TEACHING

• Instruct pt on need for compliance and requirement for periodic monitoring of ECG and renal function. • Do not break, crush, or open capsule.

donepezil

doe-**nep**-e-zil
(Aricept RDT ♣, Aricept)
Do not confuse Aricept with Aciphex, Ascriptin, or Azilect.

FIXED-COMBINATION(S)

Namzaric: donepezil/memantine (NMDA receptor antagonist): 10 mg/14 mg, 10 mg/28 mg.

◆CLASSIFICATION

PHARMACOTHERAPEUTIC: Central acetylcholinesterase inhibitor. **CLINICAL:** Cholinergic.

USES

Treatment of mild, moderate, or severe dementia of Alzheimer's disease. **OFF-LABEL:** Treatment of behavioral syndromes in dementia, dementia associated with Parkinson's disease, Lewy body dementia.

PRECAUTIONS

Contraindications: History of hypersensitivity to donepezil, other piperidine derivatives. **Cautions:** Asthma, COPD, bradycardia, bladder outflow obstruction, history of ulcer disease, those taking concurrent NSAIDs, supraventricular cardiac conduction disturbances (e.g., sick sinus syndrome, Wolff-Parkinson-White syndrome), seizure disorder.

ACTION

Reversibly inhibits enzyme acetylcholinesterase, increasing concentration of acetylcholine at cholinergic synapses, enhancing cholinergic function in CNS. **Therapeutic Effect:** Slows progression of Alzheimer's disease.

PHARMACOKINETICS

Well absorbed after PO administration. Protein binding: 96%. Extensively metabolized. Eliminated in urine, feces. **Half-life:** 70 hrs.

LIFESPAN CONSIDERATIONS

Pregnancy/Lactation: Unknown if drug is distributed in breast milk. **Children:** Safety and efficacy not established. **Elderly:** No age-related precautions noted.

INTERACTIONS

DRUG: **Anticholinergic agents (e.g., glycopyrrolate, scopolamine)** may decrease therapeutic effect. May increase concentration/effects of **antipsychotic agents, beta blockers (e.g., atenolol, carvedilol, metoprolol), succinylcholine.** **HERBAL:** None significant. **FOOD:** None known. **LAB VALUES:** None significant.

AVAILABILITY (Rx)

Tablets: 5 mg, 10 mg, 23 mg. **Tablets (Orally Disintegrating):** 5 mg, 10 mg.

ADMINISTRATION/HANDLING

PO

• May be given at bedtime without regard to food. • Swallow tablets whole; do not break, crush, dissolve, or divide. • Follow dose with water.

INDICATIONS/ROUTES/DOSAGE

Alzheimer's Disease

PO: ADULTS, ELDERLY: For mild to moderate, initially 5 mg/day at bedtime. May increase at 4- to 6-wk intervals to 10 mg/day at bedtime. Range: 5–10 mg/day. For moderate to severe Alzheimer's, a dose of 23 mg once daily can be administered once pt has been taking 10 mg once daily for at least 3 mos. Range: 10–23 mg/day.

Dosage in Renal/Hepatic Impairment

No dose adjustment.

SIDE EFFECTS

Frequent (11%–8%): Nausea, diarrhea, headache, insomnia, nonspecific pain, dizziness. **Occasional (6%–3%):** Mild muscle cramps, fatigue, vomiting, anorexia, ecchymosis. **Rare (3%–2%):** Depression, abnormal dreams, weight loss, arthritis, drowsiness, syncope, frequent urination.

ADVERSE EFFECTS/TOXIC REACTIONS

Overdose may result in cholinergic crisis (severe nausea, increased salivation, diaphoresis, bradycardia, hypotension, flushed skin, abdominal pain, respiratory depression, seizures, cardiorespiratory collapse). Increasing muscle weakness may occur, resulting in death if muscles of respiration become involved. **Antidote:** Atropine sulfate 1–2 mg IV with subsequent doses based on therapeutic response.

NURSING CONSIDERATIONS

BASELINE ASSESSMENT

Assess cognitive function (e.g., memory, attention, reasoning). Obtain baseline vital signs. Assess history for peptic ulcer, urinary obstruction, asthma, COPD, seizure disorder, cardiac conduction disturbances.

INTERVENTION/EVALUATION

Monitor behavior, mood/cognitive function, activities of daily living. Monitor for cholinergic reaction (GI discomfort/cramping, feeling of facial warmth, excessive salivation/diaphoresis), lacrimation, pallor, urinary urgency, dizziness. Monitor for nausea, diarrhea, headache, insomnia.

PATIENT/FAMILY TEACHING

• Report nausea, vomiting, diarrhea, diaphoresis, increased salivary secretions, severe abdominal pain, dizziness. • May take without regard to food (best taken at bedtime). • Not a cure for Alzheimer's disease but may slow progression of symptoms.

DOPamine

HIGH ALERT

dope-a-meen

■ BLACK BOX ALERT ■ If extravasation occurs, infiltrate area with phentolamine (5–10 mL 0.9% NaCl) as soon as possible, no later than 12 hrs after extravasation.

Do not confuse DOPamine with DOBUTamine or Dopram.

◆CLASSIFICATION

PHARMACOTHERAPEUTIC: Sympathomimetic (adrenergic agonist). **CLINICAL:** Cardiac stimulant, vasopressor.

USES

Adjunct in treatment of shock (e.g., MI, trauma, renal failure, cardiac decompensation, open heart surgery), persisting after adequate fluid volume replacement. **OFF-LABEL:** Symptomatic bradycardia or heart block unresponsive to atropine or cardiac pacing.

PRECAUTIONS

Contraindications: Hypersensitivity to dopamine, sulfites. Pheochromocytoma, ventricular fibrillation. Uncorrected tachyarrhythmias. **Cautions:** Ischemic heart disease, occlusive vascular disease, hypovolemia, recent use of MAOIs (within 2–3 wks), ventricular arrhythmias, post-MI.

ACTION

Stimulates adrenergic and dopaminergic receptors. Effects are dose dependent. Lower dosage stimulates dopaminergic receptors, causing renal vasodilation. Higher doses stimulate both dopaminergic and $beta_1$-adrenergic receptors, causing cardiac stimulation and renal vasodilation. Higher doses stimulate alpha-adrenergic receptors, causing vasoconstriction, increased B/P. **Therapeutic Effect: Low dosage (1–5 mcg/kg/min):** Increases renal blood flow, urinary flow, sodium excretion. **Low to moderate dosage (5–10 mcg/kg/min):** Increases myocardial contractility, stroke volume, cardiac output. **High dosage (greater than 10 mcg/kg/min):** Increases peripheral resistance, vasoconstriction, B/P.

PHARMACOKINETICS

Route	Onset	Peak	Duration
IV	1–2 min	N/A	Less than 10 min

Widely distributed. Does not cross blood-brain barrier. Metabolized in liver, kidneys, plasma. Primarily excreted in urine. Not removed by hemodialysis. **Half-life:** 2 min.

⌛ LIFESPAN CONSIDERATIONS

Pregnancy/Lactation: Unknown if drug crosses placenta or is distributed in breast milk. **Children:** Recommended close hemodynamic monitoring (gangrene due to extravasation reported). **Elderly:** No age-related precautions noted.

D

INTERACTIONS

DRUG: **Ergot derivatives (e.g., ergotamine), MAOIs (e.g., phenelzine, selegiline), tricyclic antidepressants (e.g., amitriptyline)** may increase hypertensive effects. May increase hypotensive effect of **lurasidone.** **HERBAL:** None significant. **FOOD:** None known. **LAB VALUES:** None significant.

AVAILABILITY (Rx)

Injection Solution: 40 mg/mL. **Injection (Premix With Dextrose):** 0.8 mg/mL (250 mL, 500 mL), 1.6 mg/mL (250 mL, 500 mL), 3.2 mg/mL (250 mL).

ADMINISTRATION/HANDLING

◄ALERT► Fluid volume depletion must be corrected before administering DOPamine (may be used concurrently with fluid replacement).

IV

Reconstitution • Available prediluted in 250 or 500 mL D_5W or dilute in 250–500 mL 0.9% NaCl or D_5W, to maximum concentration of 3,200 mcg/mL (3.2 mg/mL).

Rate of administration • Administer into large vein (antecubital fossa, central line preferred) to prevent extravasation. • Use infusion pump to control flow rate. • Titrate drug to desired hemodynamic, renal response (optimum urinary flow determines dosage).

Storage • Do not use solutions darker than slightly yellow or discolored to yellow, brown, pink to purple (indicates decomposition of drug). • Stable for 24 hrs after dilution.

IV INCOMPATIBILITIES

Acyclovir (Zovirax), amphotericin B complex (Abelcet, AmBisome, Amphotec), cefepime (Maxipime), furosemide (Lasix), insulin, sodium bicarbonate.

IV COMPATIBILITIES

Amiodarone (Cordarone), calcium chloride, dexmedetomidine (Precedex), dilTIAZem (Cardizem), DOBUTamine (Dobutrex), enalapril (Vasotec), EPINEPHrine, heparin, HYDROmorphone (Dilaudid), labetalol (Trandate), levoFLOXacin (Levaquin), lidocaine, LORazepam (Ativan), methylPREDNISolone (Solu-Medrol), midazolam (Versed), milrinone (Primacor), morphine, niCARdipine (Cardene), nitroglycerin, norepinephrine (Levophed), piperacillin/tazobactam (Zosyn), potassium chloride, propofol (Diprivan).

INDICATIONS/ROUTES/DOSAGE

◄ALERT► Effects of DOPamine are dose dependent. Titrate to desired response. Doses greater than 20 mcg/kg/min may not have beneficial effect on BP and may increase risk of tachyarrhythmias.

Hemodynamic Support

IV infusion: ADULTS, ELDERLY, CHILDREN: Range: 2–20 mcg/kg/min. Titrate to desired response. May gradually increase by 5–10 mcg/kg/min increments. **Maximum:** 50 mcg/kg/min. **NEONATES:** 2–20 mcg/kg/min. Titrate gradually by 5–10 mcg/kg/min to desired response.

SIDE EFFECTS

Frequent: Headache, arrhythmias, tachycardia, anginal pain, palpitations, vasoconstriction, hypotension, nausea, vomiting, dyspnea. **Occasional:** Piloerection (goose bumps), bradycardia, widening of QRS complex.

ADVERSE EFFECTS/TOXIC REACTIONS

High doses may produce ventricular arrhythmias, tachycardia. Pts with occlusive vascular disease are at high risk for further compromise of circulation to extremities, which may result in gangrene. Tissue necrosis with sloughing may occur with extravasation of IV solution.

NURSING CONSIDERATIONS

BASELINE ASSESSMENT

Pt must be on continuous cardiac monitoring. Determine weight (for dosage calculation). Obtain initial B/P, heart rate, respirations. Assess patency of IV access.

INTERVENTION/EVALUATION

Continuously monitor for cardiac arrhythmias. Measure urinary output frequently. If extravasation occurs, immediately infiltrate affected tissue with 10–15 mL 0.9% NaCl solution containing 5–10 mg phentolamine mesylate. Monitor B/P, heart rate, respirations q15min during administration (more often if indicated). Assess cardiac output, pulmonary wedge pressure, or central venous pressure (CVP) frequently. Assess peripheral circulation (palpate pulses, note color/temperature of extremities). Immediately notify physician of decreased urinary output, cardiac arrhythmias, significant changes in B/P, heart rate, or failure to respond to increase or decrease in infusion rate, decreased peripheral circulation (cold, pale, mottled extremities). Taper dosage before discontinuing (abrupt cessation of therapy may result in marked hypotension). Be alert to excessive vasoconstriction (decreased urine output, increased heart rate, arrhythmias, disproportionate increase in diastolic B/P, decrease in pulse pressure); slow or temporarily stop infusion, notify physician.

doravirine/ lamivudine/ tenofovir

dor-a-**vir**-een/la-**miv**-ue-deen/ten-**oh**-foe-veer
(Delstrigo)

■ BLACK BOX ALERT ■ Severe exacerbations of hepatitis B virus (HBV) reported in pts coinfected with HIV-1 and HBV following discontinuation. If discontinuation occurs, monitor hepatic function for at least several mos. Initiate anti-HBV therapy if warranted.

Do not confuse doravirine/lamivudine/tenofovir (Delstrigo) with efavirenz/lamivudine/tenofovir (Symfi Lo), abacavir/dolutegravir/lamivudine (Triumeq), abacavir/lamivudine/zidovudine (Trizivir), bictegravir/emtricitabine/tenofovir (Biktarvy), efavirenz/emtricitabine/tenofovir (Atripla), or emtricitabine/lopinavir/ritonavir/tenofovir (Kaletra).

◆CLASSIFICATION

PHARMACOTHERAPEUTIC: Nonnucleoside reverse transcriptase inhibitor, nucleoside reverse transcriptase inhibitor, nucleotide reverse transcriptase inhibitor. **CLINICAL:** Antiretroviral agent (anti-HIV).

USES

Treatment of HIV-1 infection in adult pts with no antiretroviral treatment history.

PRECAUTIONS

Contraindications: Hypersensitivity to doravirine, lamivudine, or tenofovir. Concomitant use of strong CYP3A inducers (e.g., carBAMazepine, phenytoin, mitotane, rifAMPin, St. John's wort), enzalutamide. **Cautions:** Hyperlipidemia, psychiatric illness (e.g., depression, psychosis, suicidal ideation), renal/hepatic impairment; history of pathologic fracture, osteoporosis, osteopenia. Concomitant use of moderate CYP3A inducers. Not recommended in pts with CrCl less than 50 mL/min, end-stage renal disease requiring dialysis.

ACTION

Doravirine blocks noncompetitive HIV-1 reverse transcriptase (does not inhibit DNA polymerases or mitochondrial DNA polymerase). Lamivudine inhibits HIV reverse transcription via viral DNA chain termination. Tenofovir interferes with the HIV RNA-dependent DNA polymerase. **Therapeutic Effect:** Interferes with HIV-1 replication.

D

PHARMACOKINETICS

Widely distributed. Doravirine metabolized in liver. Tenofovir metabolized by enzymatic hydrolysis, mediated by macrophages and hepatocytes. Protein binding: (doravirine): 76%; (lamivudine): less than 36%, (tenofovir): less than 1%. Peak plasma concentration: (doravirine): 2 hrs; (tenofovir): 1 hr. Doravirine excreted primarily in urine (6%). Lamivudine excreted primarily in urine (71%). Tenofovir excreted primarily in urine (70%–80%). **Half-life:** (doravirine): 15 hrs; (lamivudine): 5–7 hrs; (tenofovir): 17 hrs.

LIFESPAN CONSIDERATIONS

Pregnancy/Lactation: Breastfeeding not recommended due to risk of postnatal HIV transmission. Unknown if doravirine is secreted in breast milk. Lamivudine, tenofovir is secreted in breast milk. **Children:** Safety and efficacy not established. **Elderly:** Not specified; use caution.

INTERACTIONS

DRUG: NSAIDS (e.g., ibuprofen, naproxen) may increase nephrotoxic effect of tenofovir. **Strong CYP3A inducers (e.g., carBAMazepine, phenytoin, rifAMPin), enzalutamide, mitotane** may decrease concentration/effect; use contraindicated. **Efavirenz, etravirine, nevirapine** may decrease concentration/effect of doravirine. **Hepatitis C antivirals (e.g., ledipasvir, sofosbuvir)** may increase concentration/effect of tenofovir. **Sorbitol** may decrease concentration/effect of lamivudine. Doravirine may decrease concentration of **ergonovine**. **HERBAL: St. John's wort** may decrease concentration/effect; use contraindicated. **FOOD:** None known. **LAB VALUES:** May increase serum alkaline phosphatase, amylase, ALT, AST, bilirubin, LDL cholesterol, GGT, creatine kinase, creatinine, lipase, triglycerides. May decrease serum potassium, phosphate; Hgb, Hct, RBCs.

AVAILABILITY (Rx)

Fixed-Dose Combination Tablets: (*doravirine/lamivudine/tenofovir [TDF]*): 100 mg/300 mg/300 mg.

ADMINISTRATION/HANDLING

PO

- Give without regard to food.

INDICATIONS/ROUTES/DOSAGE

HIV Infection

PO: ADULTS: 1 tablet once daily.

Dose Modification

Concomitant use of rifabutin: Give additional dose of doravirine 100 mg approx. 12 hrs after fixed-dose combination tablet.

Dosage in Renal Impairment

CrCl greater than 50 mL/min: No dose adjustment. CrCl less than 50 mL/min, ESRD requiring HD: Not recommended.

Dosage in Hepatic Impairment

Mild to moderate impairment: No dose adjustment. **Severe impairment:** Not specified; use caution.

SIDE EFFECTS

Occasional (7%–4%): Dizziness, nausea, abnormal dreams, insomnia. **Rare (3%–2%):** Diarrhea, somnolence, rash.

ADVERSE EFFECTS/TOXIC REACTIONS

May cause new or worsening renal failure including Fanconi syndrome (renal tubular injury, nonabsorption of essential electrolytes, acids, buffers in renal tubules). Renal tubular injury may lead to rhabdomyolysis, osteomalacia, muscle weakness, myopathy. May decrease bone mineral density, leading to pathologic fractures. Fatal lactic acidosis, severe hepatomegaly with steatosis (fatty liver) was reported. Fatal cases of hepatitis, fulminant hepatitis, hepatic injury requiring liver transplantation were reported. If therapy is discontinued, pts coinfected with hepatitis B or C virus have an increased risk for viral replication, worsening of hepatic function, and may experience hepatic decompensation and/or failure. Suicidal ideation, depression, suicide attempt were reported (primarily occurred in pts with prior psychiatric illness). May induce immune recovery syndrome (inflammatory response to dormant opportunistic infections such as *Mycobacterium avium*, cytomegalovirus, PCP, tuberculosis or acceleration of autoimmune disorders including Graves' disease, polymyositis, Guillain-Barre).

NURSING CONSIDERATIONS

BASELINE ASSESSMENT

Obtain LFT, BUN, serum creatinine, CrCl, eGFR, CD4+ count, viral load, HIV-1 RNA level; urine glucose, urine protein; pregnancy test in female pts of reproductive potential. Obtain serum phosphate level in pts with renal impairment. Test all pts for HBV infection. Receive full medication history (including herbal products) and screen for contraindications/interactions. Question history of hepatic/renal impairment, hyperlipidemia, hypersensitivity reactions, decreased mineral bone density, osteopenia, psychiatric illness. Offer emotional support.

INTERVENTION/EVALUATION

Monitor CD4+ count, viral load, HIV-1 RNA level for treatment effectiveness. Monitor LFT; assess for hepatic injury (bruising, hematuria, jaundice, right upper abdominal pain, nausea, vomiting, weight loss). If discontinuation of drug regimen occurs, monitor hepatic function for at least several mos. Initiate anti-HBV therapy if warranted. Obtain serum lactate level if lactic acidosis suspected (confusion, dyspnea, muscle cramps, tachypnea). Monitor renal function as clinically indicated. An increase of serum creatinine greater than 0.4 mg/dL from baseline may indicate renal impairment. Cough, dyspnea, fever, excess band cells on CBC may indicate acute infection (WBC count may be unreliable in pts with uncontrolled HIV infection). Assess skin for toxic skin reactions, rash. Screen for psychiatric symptoms (agitation, delusions, depression, paranoia, psychosis, suicidal ideation).

PATIENT/FAMILY TEACHING

• Treatment does not cure HIV infection nor reduce risk of transmission. Practice safe sex with barrier methods or abstinence. • Drug resistance can form if treatment is interrupted; do not run out of supply. • As immune system strengthens, it may respond to dormant infections hidden within the body. Report any new fever, chills, body aches, cough, night sweats, shortness of breath. • Fatal cases of liver inflammation or failure have occurred; report abdominal pain, clay-colored stools, yellowing of skin or eyes, weight loss. • Report symptoms of kidney inflammation or disease (decreased urine output, flank pain, darkened urine); toxic skin reactions (rash, pustules, skin eruptions). • Report any psychiatric symptoms (agitation, delusions, depression, mood alteration, paranoia, suicidal ideation). • Breastfeeding not recommended. • Decreased bone density may lead to pathologic fractures; report bone/extremity pain, suspected fractures. • Antiretrovirals may cause excess body fat in upper back, neck, breast, trunk, while also causing decreased body fat in legs, arms, face. • Do not take newly prescribed medications unless approved by prescriber who originally started treatment. • Do not take herbal products, esp. St. John's wort.

doxazosin

dox-a-**zoe**-sin
(Apo-Doxazosin ♣, Cardura, Cardura XL)

Do not confuse Cardura with Cardene, Cordarone, Coumadin, K-Dur, or Ridaura, or doxazosin with doxapram, doxepin, or DOXOrubicin.

◆CLASSIFICATION

PHARMACOTHERAPEUTIC: Alpha-adrenergic blocker. **CLINICAL:** Antihypertensive.

USES

Cardura: Treatment of mild to moderate hypertension. Used alone or in combination with other antihypertensives. Treatment of urinary outflow obstruction and/or obstruction and irritation associated with benign prostatic hyperplasia **(BPH)**. **Cardura XL:** Treatment of urinary outflow obstruction and/or obstruction and irritation associated with benign prostatic hyperplasia. **OFF-LABEL:** Pediatric hypertension. Facilitate distal ureteral stone expulsion. Erectile dysfunction in pts with BPH.

PRECAUTIONS

Contraindications: Hypersensitivity to doxazosin or other quinazolines (prazosin, terazosin). **Cautions:** Constipation, ileus, GI obstruction, hepatic impairment.

ACTION

Hypertension: Selectively blocks alpha$_1$-adrenergic receptors, decreasing peripheral vascular resistance. **BPH:** Inhibits postsynaptic alpha-adrenergic receptors in prostatic stromal and bladder neck tissues. **Therapeutic Effect: Hypertension:** Causes peripheral vasodilation, lowering B/P. **BPH:** Relaxes smooth muscle of bladder, prostate, reducing BPH symptoms.

PHARMACOKINETICS

Route	Onset	Peak	Duration
PO (antihypertensive)	1–2 hrs	2–6 hrs	24 hrs

Well absorbed from GI tract. Protein binding: 98%–99%. Metabolized in liver. Primarily eliminated in feces. Not removed by hemodialysis. **Half-life:** 19–22 hrs.

LIFESPAN CONSIDERATIONS

Pregnancy/Lactation: Unknown if drug crosses placenta or is distributed in breast milk. **Children:** Safety and efficacy not established. **Elderly:** May be more sensitive to hypotensive effects.

INTERACTIONS

DRUG: Strong CYP3A4 inducers (e.g., carBAMazepine, phenytoin, rifAMPin) may decrease concentration/effect. **Strong CYP3A4 inhibitors (e.g., clarithromycin, ketoconazole, ritonavir)** may increase concentration/effect. **HERBAL: St. John's wort** may decrease concentration/effect. **Yohimbe** may decrease antihypertensive effect. **FOOD:** None known. **LAB VALUES:** None significant.

AVAILABILITY (Rx)

Tablets: 1 mg, 2 mg, 4 mg, 8 mg.

Tablets, Extended-Release: 4 mg, 8 mg.

ADMINISTRATION/HANDLING

PO

• Give without regard to food. • Do not break, crush, dissolve, or divide extended-release tablet. • Immediate-release tablets given morning or evening; extended-release tablets given with morning meal.

INDICATIONS/ROUTES/DOSAGE

Hypertension

PO: ***(Immediate-Release):*** **ADULTS, ELDERLY:** Initially, 1 mg once daily. May increase to 2 mg once daily. Thereafter, may increase upward over several wks to a maximum of 16 mg/day.

Benign Prostatic Hyperplasia

PO: ***(Immediate-Release):*** **ADULTS, ELDERLY:** Initially, 1 mg/day. May titrate at intervals of 1–2 wks by doubling daily dose to 2 mg, 4 mg, and 8 mg. **Maximum:** 8 mg/day. ***(Extended-Release):*** Initially, 4 mg/day. May increase to 8 mg in 3–4 wks. **Note:** When switching to extended-release, omit evening dose prior to starting morning dose.

Dosage in Renal Impairment
No dose adjustment.

Dosage in Hepatic Impairment
Mild to moderate impairment: Use caution. **Severe Impairment:** Avoid use.

SIDE EFFECTS

Frequent (20%–10%): Dizziness, asthenia, headache, edema. **Occasional (9%–3%):** Nausea, pharyngitis, rhinitis, pain in extremities, drowsiness. **Rare (2%–1%):** Palpitations, diarrhea, constipation, dyspnea, myalgia, altered vision, anxiety.

ADVERSE EFFECTS/TOXIC REACTIONS

First-dose syncope (hypotension with sudden loss of consciousness) may occur 30–90 min after initial dose of 2 mg or greater, too-rapid increase in dosage, addition of another antihypertensive agent to therapy. First-dose syncope may be preceded by tachycardia (pulse rate 120–160 beats/min).

NURSING CONSIDERATIONS

BASELINE ASSESSMENT

Give first dose at bedtime. If initial dose is given during daytime, pt must remain recumbent for 3–4 hrs. Assess B/P, pulse immediately before each dose and q15–30min until B/P is stabilized (be alert to fluctuations).

INTERVENTION/EVALUATION

Monitor B/P, I&O. Monitor pulse diligently (first-dose syncope may be preceded by tachycardia). Assess for edema, headache. Assist with ambulation if dizziness, light-headedness occurs.

PATIENT/FAMILY TEACHING

• Full therapeutic effect may not occur for 3–4 wks. • May cause syncope (fainting); go from lying to standing slowly. • Avoid tasks that require alertness, motor skills until response to drug is established.

doxepin

dox-e-pin
(Prudoxin, Silenor, Sinequan ✱, Zonalon)

■ BLACK BOX ALERT ■ Increased risk of suicidal ideation and behavior in children, adolescents, young adults 18–24 yrs with major depressive disorder, other psychiatric disorders.

Do not confuse doxepin with digoxin, doxapram, doxazosin, Doxidan, or doxycycline, or SINEquan with SEROquel, or Singulair.

◆CLASSIFICATION

PHARMACOTHERAPEUTIC: Tricyclic. **CLINICAL:** Antidepressant, antianxiety, antineuralgic, antipruritic.

USES

Treatment of depression and/or anxiety. **Silenor (only):** Treatment of insomnia in pts with difficulty staying asleep. **Topical:** Treatment of pruritus associated with atopic dermatitis. **OFF-LABEL:** Treatment of neurogenic pain, treatment of anxiety.

PRECAUTIONS

Contraindications: Hypersensitivity to doxepin. Glaucoma, hypersensitivity to other tricyclic antidepressants, urinary retention, use of MAOIs within 14 days. **Cautions:** Cardiac/hepatic/renal disease, pts at risk for suicidal ideation, respiratory compromise, sleep apnea, history of bowel obstruction, increased IOP, glaucoma, history of seizures, history of urinary retention/obstruction, hyperthyroidism, prostatic hypertrophy, hiatal hernia, elderly.

ACTION

Increases synaptic concentrations of norepinephrine, serotonin by inhibiting reuptake. **Therapeutic Effect:** Produces antidepressant, anxiolytic effects.

D

PHARMACOKINETICS

PO: Rapidly absorbed from GI tract. Protein binding: 80%–85%. Metabolized in liver. Primarily excreted in urine. Not removed by hemodialysis. **Half-life:** 6–8 hrs. **Topical:** Absorbed through skin. Distributed to body tissues. Metabolized to active metabolite. Excreted in urine.

LIFESPAN CONSIDERATIONS

Pregnancy/Lactation: Crosses placenta. Distributed in breast milk. **Children:** Safety and efficacy not established in pts younger than 12 yrs. **Elderly:** Increased risk of toxicity (lower dosages recommended). Avoid doses greater than 6 mg/day due to anticholinergic effects, sedation, and orthostatic hypotension.

INTERACTIONS

DRUG: Alcohol, CNS depressants (e.g., LORazepam, morphine, zolpidem) may increase CNS, respiratory depression. **MAOIs (e.g., phenelzine, selegiline)** may increase risk of seizures, hyperpyrexia, hypertensive crisis (discontinue at least 2 wks prior to starting doxepin). **Anticholinergic agents (e.g., aclidinium, ipratropium, umeclidinium)** may increase anticholinergic effect. May increase QT interval-prolonging effect of **dronedarone. Strong CYP2D6 inhibitors (e.g., buPROPion, PARoxetine)** may increase concentration/effect. **HERBAL: Herbals with sedative properties (e.g., chamomile, kava kava, valerian)** may increase CNS depression. **St. John's wort** may decrease concentration/effect. **FOOD:** None known. **LAB VALUES:** May alter serum glucose, ECG readings. **Therapeutic serum level:** 110–250 ng/mL; **toxic serum level:** greater than 300 ng/mL.

AVAILABILITY (Rx)

Capsules: 10 mg, 25 mg, 50 mg, 75 mg, 100 mg, 150 mg. **Cream:** ***(Prudoxin, Zonalon):*** 5%. **Oral Concentrate:** 10 mg/mL. **Tablets:** ***(Silenor):*** 3 mg, 6 mg.

ADMINISTRATION/HANDLING

PO

• Give with food, milk if GI distress occurs. • Dilute concentrate in 4-oz glass of water, milk, or orange, tomato, prune, pineapple juice. Incompatible with carbonated drinks. • Give larger portion of daily dose at bedtime.

Topical

• Apply thin film of cream on affected areas of skin. • Do not use for more than 8 days. • Do not use occlusive dressing.

INDICATIONS/ROUTES/DOSAGE

Depression, Anxiety

Note: Gradually taper dose upon discontinuation of antidepressant therapy. **PO: ADULTS:** Initially, 25–50 mg/day at bedtime or in 2–3 divided doses. May increase gradually to usual dose of 100 mg–300 mg/day (single dose should not exceed 150 mg). **ELDERLY:** Initially, 10–25 mg at bedtime. May increase by 10–25 mg/day every 3–7 days.

Insomnia (Silenor only)

PO: ADULTS: 3–6 mg (give within 30 min of bedtime). **ELDERLY:** 3 mg (give within 30 min of bedtime). May increase to 6 mg once daily.

Pruritus Associated With Atopic Dermatitis

Topical: ADULTS, ELDERLY: Apply thin film 4 times/day at 3- to 4-hr intervals. Not recommended for more than 8 days.

Dosage in Renal Impairment

No dose adjustment.

Dosage in Hepatic Impairment

Use lower initial dose; adjust gradually. **Silenor:** Initially, 3 mg once daily.

SIDE EFFECTS

Frequent: PO: Orthostatic hypotension, drowsiness, dry mouth, headache, increased appetite, weight gain, nausea, unusual fatigue, unpleasant taste. **Topical:** Edema, increased pruritus, eczema, burning, tingling, stinging at application site, altered taste, dizziness, drowsiness, dry skin, dry mouth, fatigue, headache, thirst. **Occasional: PO:** Blurred vision, confusion, constipation, hallucinations, difficult urination, eye pain, irregular heartbeat, fine muscle tremors, nervousness, impaired sexual function, diarrhea, diaphoresis, heartburn, insomnia. **Silenor:** Nausea, upper respiratory infection. **Topical:** Anxiety, skin irritation/cracking, nausea. **Rare: PO:** Allergic reaction, alopecia, tinnitus, breast enlargement. **Topical:** Fever, photosensitivity.

ADVERSE EFFECTS/TOXIC REACTIONS

Abrupt or too-rapid withdrawal may result in headache, malaise, nausea, vomiting, vivid dreams. Overdose may produce confusion, severe drowsiness, agitation, tachycardia, arrhythmias, shortness of breath, vomiting.

NURSING CONSIDERATIONS

BASELINE ASSESSMENT

Assess B/P, pulse, ECG (those with history of cardiovascular disease). Obtain CBC, serum electrolyte tests before long-term therapy. Assess pt's appearance, behavior, level of interest, mood, suicidal ideation, sleep pattern.

INTERVENTION/EVALUATION

Monitor B/P, pulse, weight. Perform CBC, serum electrolyte tests periodically to assess renal/hepatic function. Monitor mental status, suicidal ideation. Supervise suicidal-risk pt closely during early therapy (as depression lessens, energy level improves, increasing suicide potential). Assess appearance, behavior, speech pattern, level of interest, mood. **Therapeutic serum level:** 110–250 ng/mL; **toxic serum level:** greater than 300 ng/mL.

PATIENT/FAMILY TEACHING

• Do not discontinue abruptly. • Change positions slowly to avoid dizziness. • Avoid tasks that require alertness, motor skills until response to drug is established. • Do not cover affected area with occlusive dressing after applying cream. • Avoid alcohol, limit caffeine. • May increase appetite. • Avoid exposure to sunlight/artificial light source. • Therapeutic effect may be noted within 2–5 days, maximum effect within 2–3 wks. • Report worsening depression, suicidal ideation, unusual changes in behavior (esp. at initiation of therapy or with changes in dosage).

D

DOXOrubicin HIGH ALERT

dox-o-**rue**-bi-sin
(Adriamycin, Caelyx ✱, Doxil, Lipodox-50)

■ **BLACK BOX ALERT** ■ May cause concurrent or cumulative myocardial toxicity. Acute allergic or anaphylaxis-like infusion reaction may be life-threatening. Severe myelosuppression may occur. Must be administered by personnel trained in administration/handling of chemotherapeutic agents. Secondary acute myelogenous leukemia and myelodysplastic syndrome have been reported. Potent vesicant.

Do not confuse DOXOrubicin with dactinomycin, DAUNOrubicin, doxazosin, epiRUBicin, IDArubicin, or valrubicin, or Adriamycin with Aredia or Idamycin.

◆CLASSIFICATION

PHARMACOTHERAPEUTIC: Anthracycline, topoisomerase II inhibitor. **CLINICAL:** Antineoplastic.

USES

Adriamycin: Treatment of acute lymphocytic leukemia (ALL), acute myeloid leukemia (AML), Hodgkin's lymphoma, malignant lymphoma; breast, gastric, small-cell lung, ovarian, epithelial, thyroid, bladder carcinomas; neuroblastoma, Wilms tumor, osteosarcoma, soft tissue sarcoma. **Doxil, Lipodox:** Treatment of AIDS-related Kaposi's sarcoma, advanced ovarian cancer. Used with bortezomib to treat multiple myeloma in pts who have not previously received bortezomib and have received at least one previous treatment. **OFF-LABEL: Adriamycin:** Multiple myeloma, endometrial carcinoma, uterine sarcoma; head and neck cancer, liver, kidney cancer. **Doxil:** Metastatic breast cancer, Hodgkin's lymphoma, cutaneous T-cell lymphomas, advanced soft tissue sarcomas, recurrent or metastatic cervical cancer, advanced or metastatic uterine sarcoma.

PRECAUTIONS

Contraindications: Hypersensitivity to DOXOrubicin. **Adriamycin:** Severe hepatic impairment, severe myocardial insufficiency, recent MI (within 4–6 wks), severe arrhythmias. Previous or concomitant treatment with high accumulative doses of DOXOrubicin, DAUNOrubicin, IDArubicin, or other anthracyclines or anthracenediones; severe, persistent drug-induced myelosuppression or baseline ANC count less than 1,500 cells/mm^3. **Doxil:** Breastfeeding (Canada). **Cautions:** Hepatic impairment. Cardiomyopathy, preexisting myelosuppression, severe HF. Pts who received radiation therapy.

ACTION

Inhibits DNA, RNA synthesis by binding with DNA strands. Liposomal encapsulation increases uptake by tumors, prolongs drug action, may decrease toxicity. **Therapeutic Effect:** Prevents cell division.

PHARMACOKINETICS

Widely distributed. Metabolized in liver. Protein binding: 74%–76%. Excreted in feces (40%), urine (5%–12%). **Half-life:** 20–48 hrs.

LIFESPAN CONSIDERATIONS

Pregnancy/Lactation: If possible, avoid use during pregnancy, esp. first trimester. Breastfeeding not recommended. **Children/Elderly:** Cardiotoxicity may be more frequent in pts younger than 2 yrs or older than 70 yrs.

INTERACTIONS

DRUG: CycloSPORINE may increase concentration/effect; risk of hematologic toxicity. **Bevacizumab, DAUNOrubicin** may increase risk of cardiotoxicity. **Bone marrow depressants (e.g., cladribine)** may increase myelosuppression. **Strong CYP3A4 inducers (e.g., carBAMazepine, phenytoin, rifAMPin)** may decrease concentration/effect. **Strong CYP3A4 inhibitors (e.g., clarithromycin, ketoconazole, ritonavir)** may increase concentration/effect. **Live virus vaccines** may potentiate virus replication, increase vaccine side effects, decrease pt's antibody response to vaccine. **HERBAL: St. John's wort** may decrease concentration/effect. **Echinacea** may decrease therapeutic effect. **FOOD:** None known. **LAB VALUES:** May cause ECG changes, increase serum uric acid. May decrease neutrophils, RBCs.

AVAILABILITY (Rx)

Injection, Powder for Reconstitution: 10 mg, 20 mg, 50 mg. **Injection Solution:** *(Adriamycin):* 2 mg/mL (5-mL, 10-mL, 25-mL, 100-mL vial). **Lipid Complex:** *(Doxil, Lipodox-50):* 2 mg/mL (10 mL, 25 mL).

ADMINISTRATION/HANDLING

◀ALERT▶ Wear gloves. If powder or solution comes into contact with skin, wash thoroughly. Avoid small veins; swollen/edematous extremities; areas overlying joints, tendons. • *(Doxil):* Do not use with in-line filter or mix with any diluent except D_5W. May be carcinogenic, mutagenic, teratogenic. Handle with extreme care during preparation/administration.

IV

Reconstitution • Dilute with 50–1,000 mL D_5W or 0.9% NaCl and give as continuous infusion. • *(Doxil):* Dilute each dose in 250 mL D_5W (doses greater than 90 mg in 500 mL D_5W).

Rate of administration • *(Adriamycin):* For IV push, administer into tubing of freely running IV infusion of D_5W or 0.9%

NaCl, preferably via butterfly needle over 3–5 min (avoids local erythematous streaking along vein and facial flushing). • Must test for flashback q30sec to be certain needle remains in vein during injection. IV piggyback over 15–60 min or continuous infusion. • Extravasation produces immediate pain, severe local tissue damage. Terminate administration immediately; withdraw as much medication as possible, obtain extravasation kit, follow protocol. • *(Doxil)*: Give as infusion over 60 min. Do not use in-line filter.

Storage • *(Adriamycin solution)*: Refrigerate vials. Solutions diluted in D_5W or 0.9% NaCl stable for 48 hrs at room temperature. • *(Doxil)*: Refrigerate unopened vials. After solution is diluted, use within 24 hrs.

IV INCOMPATIBILITIES

DOXOrubicin: Allopurinol (Aloprim), amphotericin B complex (Abelcet, AmBisome, Amphotec), cefepime (Maxipime), furosemide (Lasix), ganciclovir (Cytovene), heparin, piperacillin/tazobactam (Zosyn), propofol (Diprivan). **Doxil:** Do not mix with any other medications.

IV COMPATIBILITIES

Dexamethasone (Decadron), diphenhydrAMINE (Benadryl), granisetron (Kytril), HYDROmorphone (Dilaudid), LORazepam (Ativan), morphine, ondansetron (Zofran).

INDICATIONS/ROUTES/DOSAGE

◀ALERT▶ Refer to individual protocols.

Usual Dosage

IV: *(Adriamycin):* **ADULTS:** **(Single-agent therapy):** 60–75 mg/m² as a single dose every 21 days, 20 mg/m² once wkly. **(Combination therapy):** 40–75 mg/m² q21–28 days. Because of risk of cardiotoxicity, do not exceed cumulative dose of 550 mg/m² (400–450 mg/m² for those previously treated with related compounds or irradiation of cardiac region). **CHILDREN:** **(Single-agent therapy):** 60–75 mg/m² q3wks. **(Combination therapy):** 40–75 mg/m² q21–28 days.

Kaposi's Sarcoma

IV: *(Doxil, Lipodox):* **ADULTS:** 20 mg/m² q3wks infused over 30 min. Continue until disease progression or unacceptable toxicity.

Ovarian Cancer

IV: *(Doxil, Lipodox):* **ADULTS:** 50 mg/m² q4wks. Continue until disease progression or unacceptable toxicity.

Multiple Myeloma

IV: *(Doxil, Lipodox):* **ADULTS:** 30 mg/m²/dose on day 4 q3wks (in combination with bortezomib) for 8 cycles. Continue until disease progression or unacceptable toxicity.

Dosage in Renal Impairment

No dose adjustment.

Dose Modifications

Adriamycin

Neutropenic fever/Infection: Reduce dose to 75%. **ANC less than 1,000 cells/mm³:** Delay treatment until ANC 1,000 cells/mm³ or more. **Platelets less than 100,000/mm³:** Delay treatment until platelets 100,000 cells/mm³ or more.

Doxil

Adjustments for hand-foot syndrome, stomatitis, hematologic toxicities: Refer to manufacturer's guidelines.

Dosage in Hepatic Impairment

ADRIAMYCIN

Hepatic Function	Dosage
ALT, AST 2–3 times ULN	75% of normal dose
ALT, AST greater than 3 times ULN or bilirubin 1.2–3 mg/dL	50% of normal dose
Bilirubin 3.1–5 mg/dL	25% of normal dose
Bilirubin greater than 5 mg/dL	Not recommended

ULN = upper limit of normal.

DOXIL

Hepatic Function	Dosage
Bilirubin 1.2–3 mg/dL	50% of normal dose
Bilirubin greater than 3 mg/dL	25% of normal dose

SIDE EFFECTS

Frequent: Alopecia, nausea, vomiting, stomatitis, esophagitis (esp. if drug is given on several successive days), reddish urine. **Doxil:** Nausea. **Occasional:** Anorexia, diarrhea; hyperpigmentation of nailbeds, phalangeal, dermal creases. **Rare:** Fever, chills, conjunctivitis, lacrimation.

ADVERSE EFFECTS/TOXIC REACTIONS

Myelosuppression (anemia, leukopenia, thrombocytopenia) generally occurs within 10–15 days, returns to normal levels by third wk. Cardiotoxicity (either acute, manifested as transient ECG abnormalities, or chronic, manifested as HF) may occur.

NURSING CONSIDERATIONS

BASELINE ASSESSMENT

Obtain ANC, CBC before and at frequent intervals during therapy. Obtain ECG before therapy, LFT before each dose. Antiemetics may be effective in preventing, treating nausea. Offer emotional support.

INTERVENTION/EVALUATION

Monitor for stomatitis (burning or erythema of oral mucosa at inner margin of lips, difficulty swallowing). Observe IV injection site for infiltration, vein irritation. May lead to ulceration of mucous membranes within 2–3 days. Monitor hematologic status, renal/hepatic function studies, serum uric acid levels. Monitor daily pattern of bowel activity, stool consistency. Monitor for hematologic toxicity (fever, sore throat, signs of local infection, unusual bruising/bleeding from any site), symptoms of anemia (excessive fatigue, weakness).

PATIENT/FAMILY TEACHING

• Treatment may depress your immune system and reduce your ability to fight infection. Report symptoms of infection such as body aches, burning with urination, chills, cough, fatigue, fever. Avoid those with active infection. • Report symptoms of bone marrow depression (e.g., bruising, fatigue, fever, shortness of breath, weight loss; bleeding easily, bloody urine or stool). • Maintain strict oral hygiene. • Do not have immunizations without physician's approval (drug lowers resistance). • Avoid contact with those who have recently received live virus vaccine. • Report persistent nausea/vomiting. • Avoid alcohol (may cause GI irritation, a common side effect with liposomal DOXOrubicin).

doxycycline

TOP 100

dox-i-**sye**-kleen
(Acticlate, Adoxa, Apo-Doxy ✱, Avidoxy, Doryx, Doxy-100, Oracea, Vibramycin)
Do not confuse doxycycline with dicyclomine, doxepin, omadacycline, minocycline, tetracycline, or Monodox with Maalox, or Oracea with Orencia, or Vibramycin with Vancomycin or Vibativ, or Vibra-Tabs with Vibativ.

◆CLASSIFICATION

PHARMACOTHERAPEUTIC: Tetracycline. **CLINICAL:** Antibiotic.

USES

Treatment of susceptible infections due to *H. ducreyi, Pasteurella pestis, P. tularensis, Bacteroides* spp., *V. cholerae, Brucella* spp., *Rickettsiae, Y. pestis, Francisella tularensis, M. pneumoniae,* including brucellosis, chlamydia, cholera, granuloma inguinale, lymphogranuloma venereum, malaria prophylaxis, nongonococcal urethritis, pelvic inflammatory disease (PID), plague, psittacosis, relapsing fever, rickettsia infections, primary and secondary syphilis, tularemia. **(Oracea):** Treatment of inflammatory lesions in adults with rosacea. **OFF-LABEL:** Sclerosing agent for pleural effusion; vancomycin-resistant enterococci (VRE); alternative for MRSA, treatment of refractory periodontitis, juvenile periodontitis.

PRECAUTIONS

Contraindications: Hypersensitivity to doxycycline, other tetracyclines. **Cautions:** History or predisposition to oral candidiasis (Oracea); recent *Clostridium difficile* infection or antibiotic-associated colitis; history of pancreatitis. Avoid use during pregnancy, during tooth development in children. Avoid prolonged exposure to sunlight.

ACTION

Inhibits bacterial protein synthesis by binding to ribosomes. May cause alterations in the cytoplasmic membrane. **Therapeutic Effect:** Bacteriostatic.

PHARMACOKINETICS

Widely distributed. Partially inactivated in GI tract by chelate formation. Protein binding: greater than 90%. Peak plasma concentration: 1.5–4 hrs (immediate-release); 2.8–3 hrs (delayed-release). Excreted in feces (30%), urine (23%–40%). **Half-life:** 15–24 hrs.

LIFESPAN CONSIDERATIONS

Pregnancy/Lactation: Crosses placenta; distributed in breast milk. **Children:** May cause permanent discoloration of teeth, enamel hypoplasia. **Elderly:** No age-related precautions noted.

INTERACTIONS

DRUG: **Antacids containing aluminum, calcium, magnesium; laxatives containing magnesium, oral iron preparations** decrease absorption. **Barbiturates, carBAMazepine** may decrease concentration/effect. **Cholestyramine** may decrease absorption. **HERBAL:** None significant. **FOOD:** None known. **LAB VALUES:** May increase serum alkaline phosphatase, amylase, bilirubin, ALT, AST. May alter CBC.

AVAILABILITY (Rx)

Capsules: 40 mg, 50 mg, 75 mg, 100 mg, 150 mg. **Injection, Powder for Reconstitution:** 100 mg. **Oral Suspension:** 25 mg/5 mL. **Syrup:** 50 mg/5 mL. **Tablets:** 20 mg, 50 mg, 75 mg, 100 mg, 150 mg.

Tablets, Delayed-Release: 50 mg, 75 mg, 100 mg, 150 mg, 200 mg.

ADMINISTRATION/HANDLING

◄ALERT► Do not administer IM or SQ. Space doses evenly around clock.

IV

Reconstitution • Reconstitute each 100-mg vial with 10 mL Sterile Water for Injection for concentration of 10 mg/mL. • Further dilute each 100 mg with at least 100 mL D_5W, 0.9% NaCl, lactated Ringer's.

Rate of administration • Infuse over 1–4 hrs.

Storage • After reconstitution, IV infusion is stable for 12 hrs at room temperature or 72 hrs if refrigerated. • Protect from direct sunlight. Discard if precipitate forms.

PO

• Oral suspension is stable for 2 wks at room temperature. • Give with full glass of fluid. • Instruct pt to sit up for 30 min after taking to reduce risk of esophageal irritation and ulceration. • Give without regard to food. Oracea should be given 1 hr before or 2 hrs after meals. • Avoid concurrent use of antacids, milk; separate by 2 hrs.

IV INCOMPATIBILITIES

Allopurinol (Aloprim), heparin, piperacillin/tazobactam (Zosyn).

IV COMPATIBILITIES

Acyclovir (Zovirax), amiodarone (Cordarone), dexmedetomidine (Precedex), dilTIAZem (Cardizem), granisetron (Kytril), HYDROmorphone (Dilaudid), magnesium sulfate, meperidine

(Demerol), morphine, ondansetron (Zofran), propofol (Diprivan).

INDICATIONS/ROUTES/DOSAGE

Usual Dosage

PO: ADULTS, ELDERLY: 100–200 mg/day in 1–2 divided doses. **IV:** 100 mg q12h. **IV/PO: CHILDREN OLDER THAN 8 YRS:** 2.2 mg/kg/dose. (**Maximum:** 200 mg/day) in 1–2 divided doses.

Dosage in Renal/Hepatic Impairment

No dose adjustment.

SIDE EFFECTS

Frequent: Anorexia, nausea, vomiting, diarrhea, dysphagia, photosensitivity (may be severe). **Occasional:** Rash, urticaria.

ADVERSE EFFECTS/TOXIC REACTIONS

Superinfection (esp. fungal), benign intracranial hypertension (headache, visual changes) may occur. Hepatotoxicity, fatty degeneration of liver, pancreatitis occur rarely.

NURSING CONSIDERATIONS

BASELINE ASSESSMENT

Question for history of allergies, esp. to tetracyclines, sulfites.

INTERVENTION/EVALUATION

Monitor daily pattern of bowel activity, stool consistency. Assess skin for rash. Be alert for superinfection: fever, vomiting, diarrhea, anal/genital pruritus, oral mucosal changes (ulceration, pain, erythema).

PATIENT/FAMILY TEACHING

• Avoid unnecessary exposure to sunlight. • Do not take with antacids, iron products. • Complete full course of therapy. • After application of dental gel, avoid brushing teeth, flossing the treated areas for 7 days. • Report severe diarrhea. • May cause nausea, vomiting. If GI upset occurs, may take with small amount food; however, Oracea should be taken on an empty stomach.

dulaglutide

doo-la-**gloo**-tide
(Trulicity)

■ BLACK BOX ALERT ■ Contraindicated in pts with a personal/family history of medullary thyroid carcinoma (MTC) or in pts with multiple endocrine neoplasia syndrome type 2 (MEN2). Unknown if dulaglutide causes thyroid cell tumors in humans.

Do not confuse dulaglutide with albiglutide or liraglutide.

◆CLASSIFICATION

PHARMACOTHERAPEUTIC: GLP-1 receptor agonist. **CLINICAL:** Antidiabetic.

USES

Adjunct to diet and exercise to improve glycemic control in pts with type 2 diabetes mellitus.

PRECAUTIONS

Contraindications: Hypersensitivity to dulaglutide, other GLP-1 receptor agonists. Personal/family history of medullary thyroid carcinoma or multiple endocrine neoplasia syndrome type 2. **Cautions:** Pts with increased serum calcitonin, thyroid nodules, hx pancreatitis, renal/hepatic impairment. Not recommended in pts with severe GI disease, diabetic ketoacidosis, or type 1 diabetes.

ACTION

Activates GLP-1 receptors in pancreatic beta cells. **Therapeutic Effect:** Augments glucose-dependent insulin release, slows gastric emptying. Improves glycemic control.

PHARMACOKINETICS

Readily absorbed following SQ administration. Degraded into amino acids by general protein catabolism. Peak plasma concentration: 24–72 hrs. Steady state reached in 2–4 wks. Elimination not specified. **Half-life:** 5 days.

LIFESPAN CONSIDERATIONS

Pregnancy/Lactation: Unknown if distributed in breast milk. Must either discontinue drug or discontinue breastfeeding. **Children:** Safety and efficacy not established. **Elderly:** No age-related precautions noted.

INTERACTIONS

DRUG: Insulin, insulin secretagogues (e.g., glyBURIDE) may increase risk of hypoglycemia. **HERBAL:** None significant. **FOOD:** None known. **LAB VALUES:** Expected to decrease serum glucose, Hgb A1c. May increase amylase, lipase.

AVAILABILITY (Rx)

Prefilled Injector Pen or Syringe: 0.75 mg/0.5 mL, 1.5 mg/0.5 mL.

ADMINISTRATION/HANDLING

SQ

• Administer any time of day, without regard to food, on same day each week. • May change administration day if last dose was given more than 3 days prior. If dose missed, administer within 3 days of missed dose. If more than 3 days have passed after missed dose, wait until next regularly scheduled dose to administer.

Administration • Subcutaneously insert needle into abdomen, thigh, or upper arm region and inject solution. • Do not reuse needle. • Rotate injection sites each week.

Storage • Refrigerate unused pens/syringes; do not freeze. • May store at room temperature for up to 14 days. • Protect from light.

INDICATIONS/ROUTES/DOSAGE

Type 2 Diabetes Mellitus

SQ: ADULTS/ELDERLY: Initially, 0.75 mg once wkly. May increase to 1.5 mg once wkly after 4-8 wks. May further increase to 3 mg once wkly after at least 4 wks on 1.5 mg wkly dose. **Maximum:** 4.5 mg once wkly after at least 4 wks on 3 mg once wkly.

Dose Modification

Concomitant use with insulin secretagogue (e.g., sulfonylurea) or insulin: Consider reduced dose of insulin secretagogue or insulin based on glycemic goal.

Dosage in Renal Impairment

No dose adjustment.

Dosage in Hepatic Impairment

Use caution.

SIDE EFFECTS

Occasional (12%–6%): Nausea, diarrhea, vomiting, abdominal pain. **Rare (4% or less):** Decreased appetite, dyspepsia, fatigue, asthenia.

ADVERSE EFFECTS/TOXIC REACTIONS

May increase risk of acute renal failure or worsening of chronic renal impairment (esp. with dehydration), severe gastroparesis, pancreatitis, thyroid C-cell tumors. May increase risk of hypoglycemia when used with other hypoglycemic agents or insulin. Dyspnea, pruritus, rash may indicate hypersensitivity reaction. May prolong PR interval by 2–3 msec or may rarely cause first-degree AV block, tachycardia. Immunogenicity (antidulaglutide antibody formation) reported. Some pts with antibody formation also tested positive for antibodies to GLP-1 and human albumin.

NURSING CONSIDERATIONS

BASELINE ASSESSMENT

Obtain baseline fasting glucose level, Hgb A1c, BMP. Question history of medullary thyroid carcinoma, multiple endocrine neoplasia syndrome type 2, pancreatitis, renal impairment; first-degree AV block, PR interval prolongation. Receive full medication history and screen for use of other hypoglycemic agents or insulin. Assess pt's understanding of diabetes management, routine home glucose monitoring, medication self-administration. Assess hydration status.

INTERVENTION/EVALUATION

Monitor capillary blood glucose levels, Hgb A1c; renal function test in pts with renal impairment reporting severe GI reactions, including diarrhea, gastroparesis, vomiting. Screen for thyroid tumors (dysphagia, dyspnea, persistent hoarseness, neck mass). If tumor suspected, consider endocrinologist consultation. Clinical significance of serum calcitonin level or thyroid ultrasound with GLP-1–associated thyroid tumors is debated/unknown. Assess for hypoglycemia, hyperglycemia, hypersensitivity/allergic reaction. Screen for glucose-altering conditions: fever, stress, surgical procedures, trauma. Obtain dietary consult for nutritional education. Encourage PO intake.

PATIENT/FAMILY TEACHING

• Diabetes requires lifelong control. Diet and exercise are principal parts of treatment; do not skip or delay meals. Test blood sugar regularly. Monitor daily calorie intake. • When taking additional medications to lower blood sugar or when glucose demands are altered (fever, infection, stress, trauma), have low blood sugar treatment available (glucagon, oral dextrose). • Report suspected pregnancy or plans for breastfeeding. • Therapy may increase risk of thyroid cancer; report lumps or swelling of the neck; hoarseness, shortness of breath, trouble swallowing. • Persistent, severe abdominal pain that radiates to the back (with or without vomiting) may indicate acute pancreatitis. • Rash, itching, hives may indicate allergic reaction.

DULoxetine

TOP 100

du-**lox**-e-teen
(Cymbalta, Drizalma Sprinkle)

■ **BLACK BOX ALERT** ■ Increased risk of suicidal thinking and behavior in children, adolescents, young adults 18–24 yrs with major depressive disorder, other psychiatric disorders.

Do not confuse DULoxetine with FLUoxetine or PARoxetine.

◆CLASSIFICATION

PHARMACOTHERAPEUTIC: Serotonin norepinephrine reuptake inhibitor (SNRI). **CLINICAL:** Antidepressant.

USES

Treatment of major depression. Management of pain associated with diabetic neuropathy or chronic musculoskeletal pain. Treatment of generalized anxiety disorder. Treatment of fibromyalgia. **OFF-LABEL:** Treatment of stress urinary incontinence in women.

PRECAUTIONS

Contraindications: Hypersensitivity to DULoxetine. Uncontrolled narrow-angle glaucoma. Use of MAOI intended to treat psychiatric disorder (concurrent or within 14 days of discontinuing MAOI). Initiation of MAOI intended to treat psychiatric disorder within 5 days of discontinuing DULoxetine. Initiation of DULoxetine in pt receiving linezolid or IV methylene blue. **Cautions:** Renal impairment, history of alcoholism, chronic hepatic disease, history of mania, pts with suicidal ideation or behavior. Concurrent use with inhibitors of CYP1A2 or thioridazine, CNS depressants. Hypertension, controlled narrow-angle glaucoma, impaired GI motility. Concomitant use of NSAIDs (may increase risk of bleeding), history of seizures. Use of medications that lower seizure threshold; elderly; pts at high risk for suicide.

ACTION

Appears to inhibit serotonin and norepinephrine reuptake at CNS neuronal presynaptic membranes; is a less potent inhibitor of DOPamine reuptake. **Therapeutic Effect:** Produces antidepressant effect.

PHARMACOKINETICS

Well absorbed from GI tract. Protein binding: greater than 90%. Metabolized in liver. Excreted in urine (70%), feces (20%). **Half-life:** 8–17 hrs.

LIFESPAN CONSIDERATIONS

Pregnancy/Lactation: May produce neonatal adverse reactions (constant crying, feeding difficulty, hyperreflexia, irritability). Unknown if distributed in breast milk. Breastfeeding not recommended. **Children:** Safety and efficacy not established. **Elderly:** Caution required when increasing dosage.

INTERACTIONS

DRUG: Alcohol increases risk of hepatic injury. **CYP1A2** and **CYP2D6 inhibitors (e.g., FLUoxetine, fluvoxaMINE, PARoxetine)** may increase plasma concentration. **MAOIs** may cause serotonin syndrome (autonomic hyperactivity, coma, diaphoresis, excitement, hyperthermia, rigidity). **Aspirin, NSAIDs (e.g., ibuprofen, ketorolac, naproxen)** may increase risk of bleeding. May increase concentration, potential toxicity of **tricyclic antidepressants. HERBAL: Glucosamine, herbs with anticoagulant/antiplatelet properties (e.g., garlic, ginger, ginkgo biloba)** may increase effect. **FOOD:** None known. **LAB VALUES:** May increase serum bilirubin, ALT, AST, alkaline phosphatase.

AVAILABILITY (Rx)

Capsules (Delayed-Release, Enteric-Coated Pellets): 20 mg, 30 mg, 40 mg, 60 mg. **(Drizalma Sprinkle):** 20 mg, 30 mg, 40 mg, 60 mg delayed-release capsules.

ADMINISTRATION/HANDLING

ALERT Allow at least 14 days to elapse between use of MAOIs and DULoxetine.

PO

- Give without regard to food. Give with food, milk if GI distress occurs. • Do not break, crush, cut delayed-release capsules. • Contents of capsule may be sprinkled on applesauce or mixed in apple juice and swallowed (without chewing) immediately.

INDICATIONS/ROUTES/DOSAGE

Fibromyalgia

PO: ADULTS, ELDERLY: Initially, 30 mg/day for 1 wk. Increase to 60 mg/day.

Major Depressive Disorder

PO: ADULTS, ELDERLY: Initially, 40–60 mg/day in 1 or 2 divided doses. For doses greater than 60 mg/day, titrate in increments of 30 mg/day over 1 wk. **Maximum:** 120 mg/day.

Diabetic Neuropathy Pain

PO: ADULTS, ELDERLY: 60 mg once daily. **Maximum:** 60 mg/day. Consider lower dose with renal impairment or if tolerability is a concern.

Generalized Anxiety Disorder

PO: ADULTS, ELDERLY: Initially, 30–60 mg once daily. May increase up to 120 mg/day in 30-mg increments wkly. **CHILDREN 7–17 YRS:** Initially, 30 mg once daily. After 2 wks, may increase to 60 mg once daily. May further increase in increments of 30 mg/day at wkly intervals. **Maximum:** 120 mg/day.

Chronic Musculoskeletal Pain

PO: ADULTS, ELDERLY: 30 mg once daily for 1 wk, then increase to 60 mg once daily. **Maximum:** 60 mg/day.

Dosage in Renal Impairment

Mild to moderate impairment: No dose adjustment. **Severe impairment (GFR less than 30 mL/min):** Not recommended.

Dosage in Hepatic Impairment

Avoid use in pts with chronic hepatic disease or cirrhosis.

SIDE EFFECTS

Frequent (20%–11%): Nausea, dry mouth, constipation, insomnia. **Occasional (9%–5%):** Dizziness, fatigue, diarrhea, drowsiness, anorexia, diaphoresis, vomiting. **Rare (4%–2%):** Blurred vision, erectile dysfunction, delayed or failed ejaculation, anorgasmia, anxiety, decreased libido, hot flashes.

ADVERSE EFFECTS/TOXIC REACTIONS

May slightly increase heart rate. Colitis, dysphagia, gastritis, irritable bowel syndrome occur rarely.

NURSING CONSIDERATIONS

BASELINE ASSESSMENT

Assess appearance, behavior, speech pattern, level of interest, mood, sleep pattern, suicidal tendencies. Question pain level, intensity, location of pain.

INTERVENTION/EVALUATION

For pts on long-term therapy, serum chemistry profile to assess hepatic/renal function should be performed periodically. Supervise suicidal-risk pt closely during early therapy (as depression lessens, energy level improves, increasing suicide potential). Monitor B/P, mental status, anxiety, social functioning, serum glucose levels.

PATIENT/FAMILY TEACHING

• Therapeutic effect may be noted within 1–4 wks. • Do not abruptly discontinue medication. • Avoid tasks that require alertness, motor skills until response to drug is established. • Inform physician of intention of pregnancy or if pregnancy occurs. • Report anxiety, agitation, panic attacks, worsening of depression. • Avoid heavy alcohol intake (associated with severe hepatic injury).

dupilumab

doo-**pil**-ue-mab
(Dupixent)
Do not confuse dupilumab with belimumab, daclizumab, denosumab or durvalumab.

◆CLASSIFICATION

PHARMACOTHERAPEUTIC: Interleukin-4 alpha antagonist. Monoclonal antibody. **CLINICAL:** Antiasthmatic.

USES

Treatment of moderate to severe atopic dermatitis in adults and pediatric pts 6 yrs and older whose disease is not adequately controlled with topical prescription therapies or when those therapies are not advisable. May be used with or without corticosteroids. Add-on maintenance treatment of asthma in adults and pts 12 yrs and older with an eosinophilic phenotype or corticosteroid-dependent asthma. Add-on maintenance treatment in adults with inadequately controlled chronic rhinosinusitis with nasal polyposis.

PRECAUTIONS

Contraindications: Hypersensitivity to dupilumab. **Cautions:** History of herpes simplex infection, parasitic (helminth) infection. Avoid use of live vaccines.

ACTION

Binds to the IL-4Ra subunit inhibiting interleukin-4 (IL-4) and interleukin-13 (IL-13), signaling cytokine-induced responses, including release of proinflammatory cytokines. Mechanism of action in asthma not established. **Therapeutic Effect:** Reduces skin inflammation.

PHARMACOKINETICS

Widely distributed. Degraded into small peptides and amino acids via catabolic pathway. Peak plasma concentration: 7 days. Steady state reached by wk 16. Excretion/clearance: time to nondetectable concentration: 10 wks. **Half-life:** Not specified.

⌛ LIFESPAN CONSIDERATIONS

Pregnancy/Lactation: Unknown if distributed in breast milk. However, human immunoglobulin G (IgG) is present in breast milk and is known to cross the placenta. **Children:** Safety and efficacy not established. **Elderly:** No age-related precautions noted.

INTERACTIONS

DRUG: May enhance the adverse/toxic effects of **live virus vaccines, belimumab.** **HERBAL**: None significant. **FOOD**: None known. **LAB VALUES**: May increase eosinophils.

AVAILABILITY (Rx)

Injection, Solution: 200 mg/1.14 mL, 300 mg/2 mL in prefilled syringe. **Solution, Pen Injector**: 300 mg/2 mL (2 mL).

ADMINISTRATION/HANDLING

SQ

Preparation • Remove prefilled syringe from refrigerator and allow to warm to room temperature (approx. 45 min) with needle cap intact. • Visually inspect for particulate matter or discoloration. Solution should appear clear to slightly opalescent, colorless to pale yellow in color. Do not use if solution is cloudy, discolored, or if visible particles are observed.

Administration • Insert needle subcutaneously into upper arms, outer thigh, or abdomen, and inject solution. • Do not inject into areas of active skin disease or injury such as sunburns, skin rashes, inflammation, skin infections, or active psoriasis. • Rotate injection sites.

Storage • Refrigerate in original carton until time of use. • May be stored at room temperature for up to 14 days. • Protect from light. • Do not freeze or expose to external heat sources. • Do not shake.

INDICATIONS/ROUTES/DOSAGE

Atopic Dermatitis

SQ: ADULTS, ELDERLY: Initially, 600 mg (two 300-mg injections at different sites), then 300 mg every other week. If a dose is missed, administer within 7 days of missed dose, then resume normal schedule. If missed dose is not within 7 days, wait until next scheduled dose. **CHILDREN 6 YRS AND OLDER, ADOLESCENTS 17 YRS OR YOUNGER, WEIGHING 60 KG OR MORE**: Initially, 600 mg once (administered as two 300-mg injections), followed by a maintenance dose of 300 mg q2wks. **WEIGHING 30–59 KG**: Initially, 400 mg once (administered as two 200-mg injections), followed by a maintenance dose of 200 mg q2wks. **WEIGHING 15–29 KG**: Initially, 600 mg once (given as two 300-mg injections). **Maintenance**: 300 mg q4wks.

Asthma (Moderate to severe)

SQ: ADULTS, ELDERLY, CHILDREN 12 YRS AND OLDER: Initially, 400 mg (give as two 200-mg injections) or 600 mg (give as two 300-mg injections). **Maintenance:** 200 mg (following initial 400-mg dose) or 300 mg (following initial 600-mg dose) every other wk.

Asthma (Steroid-dependent or with atopic dermatitis)

SQ: ADULTS, ELDERLY, CHILDREN 12 YRS AND OLDER: Initially, 600 mg, then 300 mg every other wk.

Rhinosinusitis (Chronic) With Nasal Polyposis

SQ: ADULTS, ELDERLY: 300 mg every other wk. If a dose is missed, administer within 7 days of missed dose, then resume usual schedule. If a dose is missed by more than 7 days, skip dose and give at next regularly scheduled time.

Dosage in Renal/Hepatic Impairment

No dose adjustment (not studied).

SIDE EFFECTS

Occasional (10%): Injection site reactions, eye inflammation/irritation. **Rare (1%)**: Eye pruritus, dry eye.

ADVERSE EFFECTS/TOXIC REACTIONS

Hypersensitivity reactions including serum sickness (arthralgia, itching, glomerulonephritis, hypotension, lymphadenopathy, malaise, proteinuria, pyrexia, rash, shock, splenomegaly), urticaria reported in less than 1% of pts, which correlated with high antibody titers. Blepharitis, conjunctivitis (allergic, bacterial, giant papillary, viral), keratitis (ulcerative, allergic, atopic keratoconjunctivitis), herpes simplex infection (genital, otitis externa, herpes virus infection) may occur. Unknown if treatment will influence the immunologic response to helminth (parasite) infection. Immunogenicity (auto-dupilumab antibodies) reported in 7% of pts.

NURSING CONSIDERATIONS

BASELINE ASSESSMENT

Question history of herpes zoster infection, parasitic infection, hypersensitivity reaction. Question recent administration of live virus vaccine. Pts with preexisting helminth (parasite) infection should be treated prior to first dose. Inhaled or systemic corticosteroids should not be suddenly discontinued upon initiation. Conduct dermatologic exam; record characteristics of psoriatic lesions. Consider administration of age-appropriate immunizations (if applicable) before initiation. Assess pt's willingness to self-inject medication.

INTERVENTION/EVALUATION

Interrupt or discontinue treatment if hypersensitivity reaction, opportunistic infection (esp. parasite infection, herpes zoster infection), worsening of asthma-related symptoms (esp. in pts tapering off corticosteroids) occurs. Concomitant use of topical calcineurin inhibitors is allowed, but only for areas that remain problematic (face, neck, genitals, skin folds). Assess for improvement of skin lesions.

PATIENT/FAMILY TEACHING

• A healthcare provider will show you how to properly prepare and inject your medication. You must demonstrate correct preparation and injection techniques before using medication at home. • Inject medication into your outer thigh or abdomen; caregivers may also inject medication in the outer arm. • Immediately report allergic reactions such as difficulty breathing, itching, hives, rash, swelling of the face or tongue. • Report infections of any kind. • Do not stop corticosteroid therapy unless directed by prescriber. • Do not receive live vaccines. • Do not interrupt or stop asthma medications or treatments.

durvalumab

dur-**val**-ue-mab
(Imfinzi)
Do not confuse durvalumab with daclizumab, dupilumab, or nivolumab.

◆CLASSIFICATION

PHARMACOTHERAPEUTIC: Anti-programmed death ligand-1 (PD-L1). Monoclonal antibody. **CLINICAL:** Antineoplastic.

USES

Treatment of pts with locally advanced or metastatic urothelial carcinoma who have disease progression during or following platinum-containing chemotherapy or have disease progression within 12 mos of neoadjuvant or adjuvant treatment with platinum-containing chemotherapy. Treatment of unresectable stage III non–small-cell lung cancer (NSCLC) that has not progressed following concurrent platinum-based chemotherapy and radiation therapy. First-line treatment of adults with extensive stage small-cell lung cancer (ES-SCLC) in combination with etoposide and either CARBOplatin or CISplatin.

PRECAUTIONS

Contraindications: Hypersensitivity to durvalumab. **Cautions:** Active infection, conditions predisposing to infection (e.g., diabetes, immunocompromised pts, renal failure, open wounds); corticosteroid intolerance, baseline hematologic cytopenias, elderly pts, hepatic impairment, interstitial lung disease, renal insufficiency; history of autoimmune disorders (Crohn's disease, demyelinating polyneuropathy, Guillain-Barré syndrome, Hashimoto's thyroiditis, hyperthyroidism, myasthenia gravis, rheumatoid arthritis, Type 1 diabetes, vasculitis); diabetes, pancreatitis.

ACTION

Blocks programmed cell death ligand 1 (PD-L1) binding to PD-1 and CD80 (B7.1).

PD-L1 blockade increases T-cell activation allowing T-cells to kill tumor cells. Restores antitumor T-cell function. **Therapeutic Effect:** Inhibits tumor cell growth and metastasis.

PHARMACOKINETICS

Widely distributed. Metabolism not specified. Steady state reached in 16 wks. Excretion not specified. **Half-life:** 17 days.

LIFESPAN CONSIDERATIONS

Pregnancy/Lactation: Avoid pregnancy; may cause fetal harm. Females of reproductive potential should use effective contraception during treatment and for at least 3 mos after discontinuation. Unknown if distributed in breast milk; however, human immunoglobulin G (IgG) is present in breast milk and is known to cross the placenta. Breastfeeding not recommended during treatment and for at least 3 mos after discontinuation. **Children:** Safety and efficacy not established. **Elderly:** May have increased risk of toxic reactions; use caution.

INTERACTIONS

DRUG: May enhance adverse effects/toxicity of **belimumab**. **HERBAL:** None significant. **FOOD:** None known. **LAB VALUES:** May increase serum albumin, alkaline phosphatase, ALT, AST, bilirubin, calcium, creatinine, glucose, magnesium. May decrease serum sodium; Hgb, Hct, lymphocytes, neutrophils, RBCs. May increase or decrease serum potassium.

AVAILABILITY (Rx)

Injection: 120 mg/2.4 mL (50 mg/mL), 500 mg/10 mL (50 mg/mL).

ADMINISTRATION/HANDLING

IV

Preparation • Visually inspect vial for particulate matter or discoloration. Solution should appear clear to opalescent, colorless to slightly yellow in color. • Do not use if solution is cloudy, discolored, or if visible particles are observed. • Do not shake. • Withdraw proper volume from vial and dilute in 0.9% NaCl or D_5W to a final concentration of 1–15 mg/mL. • Gently invert to mix; do not shake. • Diluted solution should appear clear, colorless, and free of particles.

Rate of administration • Infuse over 60 min via dedicated IV line using a sterile, low protein-binding 0.2- or 0.22-micron in-line filter.

Storage • Refrigerate unused vials in original carton. • Protect from light. May refrigerate diluted solution for no more than 24 hrs or store at room temperature for no more than 4 hrs. If refrigerated, allow diluted solution to warm to room temperature before use. • Do not freeze or shake.

IV INCOMPATIBILITIES

Do not infuse with other medications.

INDICATIONS/ROUTES/DOSAGE

Urothelial Carcinoma

IV: ADULTS, ELDERLY: 10 mg/kg q2wks. Continue until disease progression or unacceptable toxicity.

NSCLC

IV: ADULTS, ELDERLY: 10 mg/kg q2wks. Continue until disease progression or unacceptable toxicity or maximum of 12 mos.

ES-SCLC

IV: ADULTS, ELDERLY: 1,500 mg q3wks prior to chemotherapy for 4 cycles, then q4wks as single therapy.

Dose Modification

Note: Withhold and/or discontinue durvalumab to manage adverse reactions. Based on severity of adverse reactions, withhold durvalumab and administer systemic corticosteroids. Initiate corticosteroid taper when adverse reactions improve to below Grade 1, and continue taper over at least 1 mo. If treatment is not permanently discontinued due to adverse reactions, resume therapy when adverse reactions return to Grade 1 or lower and the corticosteroid dose has been reduced to less than 10 mg predniSONE (or equivalent) per day. No dose reductions of durvalumab are recommended.

D

Colitis (GI toxicity)

Grade 2 diarrhea or colitis: Withhold dose. Start predniSONE 1–2 mg/kg/day (or equivalent) followed by taper. **Grade 3 or 4 diarrhea or colitis:** Permanently discontinue. Start predniSONE 1–2 mg/kg/day (or equivalent), followed by taper.

Dermatitis

Grade 2 rash or dermatitis (for greater than 1 wk); Grade 3 rash or dermatitis: Withhold dose. Consider starting predniSONE 1–2 mg/kg/day (or equivalent), followed by taper. **Grade 4 rash or dermatitis:** Permanently discontinue. Consider starting predniSONE 1–2 mg/kg/day (or equivalent), followed by taper.

Endocrinopathies

Grade 2–4 adrenal insufficiency (hypophysitis, hypopituitarism): Withhold dose until clinically stable. Start predniSONE 1–2 mg/kg/day (or equivalent), followed by taper. Consider hormone replacement therapy as clinically indicated. **Grade 2–4 hyperthyroidism:** Withhold dose until clinically stable and manage symptoms. **Grade 2–4 hypothyroidism:** Consider hormone replacement therapy. **Grade 2–4 type 1 diabetes:** Withhold dose until clinically stable. Start insulin therapy as clinically indicated.

Hepatotoxicity

Grade 2 hepatitis (serum ALT or AST greater than 3 and up to 5 times upper limit of normal [ULN] or serum bilirubin greater than 1.5 and up to 3 times ULN); Grade 3 hepatitis (serum ALT or AST less than or equal to 8 times ULN or serum bilirubin less than or equal to 5 times ULN): Withhold dose. Start predniSONE 1–2 mg/kg/day (or equivalent), followed by taper. **Grade 3 hepatitis (serum ALT or AST greater than 8 times ULN or serum bilirubin greater than 5 times ULN; transaminase elevation (concurrent serum ALT or AST greater than 3 times ULN and serum bilirubin greater than 2 times ULN) with no known cause:** Permanently discontinue. Start predniSONE 1–2 mg/kg/day (or equivalent), followed by taper.

Infection

Grade 3 or 4 infection: Withhold dose and manage symptoms. Start anti-infectives for suspected or confirmed infections.

Infusion-Related Reactions

Grade 1 or 2 infusion reactions: Interrupt or decrease rate of infusion. Consider premedication for subsequent infusions. **Grade 3 or 4 infusion reactions:** Permanently discontinue.

Nephritis (Renal toxicity during treatment)

Grade 2 nephritis (serum creatinine greater than 1.5 and up to 3 times ULN): Withhold dose. Start predniSONE 1–2 mg/kg/day (or equivalent), followed by taper. **Grade 3 nephritis (serum creatinine greater than 3 and up to 6 times ULN); Grade 4 nephritis (serum creatinine greater than 6 times ULN):** Permanently discontinue. Start predniSONE 1–2 mg/kg/day (or equivalent), followed by taper.

Other Toxic Reactions

Any other Grade 3 reactions: Withhold dose and manage symptoms. **Any other Grade 4 reactions:** Permanently discontinue. Start predniSONE 1–4 mg/kg/day (or equivalent), followed by taper.

Pneumonitis

Grade 2 pneumonitis: Withhold dose. Start predniSONE 1–2 mg/kg/day (or equivalent), followed by taper. **Grade 3 or Grade 4 pneumonitis:** Permanently discontinue. Start predniSONE 1–4 mg/kg/day (or equivalent) followed by taper.

Dosage in Renal/Hepatic Impairment (Prior to treatment initiation)

Not specified; use caution.

SIDE EFFECTS

Frequent (39%–19%): Fatigue, asthenia, malaise, back/musculoskeletal/neck pain, myalgia, constipation, decreased appetite. **Occasional (16%–11%):** Nausea, peripheral edema, scrotal edema, lymphedema, abdominal/flank pain, diarrhea, pyrexia, dyspnea, cough, dermatitis, dermatitis acneiform, dermatitis psoriasiform, psoriasis, maculopapular rash, pustular rash, eczema, erythema, erythema multiforme, erythematous rash, acne, lichen planus.

ADVERSE EFFECTS/TOXIC REACTIONS

Anemia, neutropenia, lymphopenia are expected responses to therapy. May cause severe, sometimes fatal immune-mediated reactions such as adrenal insufficiency (1% of pts), colitis (2% of pts), hepatitis (1% of pts), hypothyroidism (9% of pts), hyperthyroidism (6% of pts), hypophysitis, nephritis (less than 1% of pts), pneumonitis (2% of pts), type 1 diabetes (less than 1% of pts), rash (15% of pts); aseptic meningitis, hemolytic anemia, keratitis, myocarditis, myositis, thrombocytopenic purpura, uveitis. Urinary tract infections including candiduria, cystitis, urosepsis occurred in 15% of pts. Immunogenicity (auto-durvalumab antibodies) reported in 3% of pts.

NURSING CONSIDERATIONS

BASELINE ASSESSMENT

Obtain CBC, BMP, LFT, serum ionized calcium, magnesium; thyroid function test; pregnancy test in females of reproductive potential; vital signs. Question medical history as listed in Precautions; prior infusion reactions. Question intolerance to corticosteroids. Screen for active infection. Assess nutritional/hydration status. Conduct neurologic/dermatologic exam. Offer emotional support.

INTERVENTION/EVALUATION

Monitor CBC, BMP, LFT, serum ionized calcium, magnesium; thyroid function test periodically. Monitor for infusion reactions including angioedema, back or neck pain, dyspnea, flushing, pruritus, pyrexia, rash, syncope. Consider increasing corticosteroid dose if toxic effects worsen or do not improve. Assess skin for rash, lesions. Diligently monitor for immune-mediated adverse effects as listed in Adverse Effects/Toxic Reactions. If immune-mediated reactions occur, consider referral to specialist. Obtain CXR if interstitial lung disease, pneumonitis suspected. Interrupt or discontinue treatment if serious infection, opportunistic infection, sepsis occurs, and initiate appropriate antimicrobial therapy. If corticosteroid therapy is started, monitor capillary blood glucose and screen for corticosteroid side effects or intolerance. Report neurologic changes including nuchal rigidity with fever, positive Kernig's sign, positive Brudzinski's sign, altered mental status, seizures (related to aseptic meningitis). Strictly monitor I&O. Encourage fluid intake.

PATIENT/FAMILY TEACHING

• Treatment may depress your immune system and reduce your ability to fight infection. Report symptoms of infection such as body aches, chills, cough, fatigue, fever. Avoid those with active infection. • Use effective contraception to avoid pregnancy. Do not breastfeed. • Treatment may cause serious or life-threatening inflammatory reactions. Report symptoms of treatment-related inflammatory events in the following body systems: brain (confusion, headache, fever, rigid neck, seizures), colon (severe abdominal pain or diarrhea), eye (blurry vision, double vision, unequal pupil size, sensitivity to light, drooping eyelid), lung (chest pain, cough, shortness of breath), liver (bruising easily, amber-colored urine, clay-colored/tarry stools, yellowing of skin or eyes), nerves (severe nerve pain or loss of motor function), pituitary (persistent or unusual headache, dizziness, extreme weakness, fainting, vision changes), thyroid (trouble sleeping, high blood pressure, fast heart rate [overactive thyroid] or fatigue, goiter, weight gain [underactive thyroid]). Immediately report infusion reactions such as neck or back pain, dizziness, fever, flushing, itching, shortness of breath, swelling of the face. • Treatment may cause severe diarrhea. Drink plenty of fluids.

D

duvelisib

doo-ve-**lis**-ib
(Copiktra)

■ BLACK BOX ALERT ■ Fatal and/or serious infections, diarrhea, colitis, pneumonitis, cutaneous reactions have occurred. Monitor for infections, GI symptoms, pulmonary symptoms, infiltrates, cutaneous toxicities.

Do not confuse Copiktra with Cometriq; duvelisib with copanlisib, dabrafenib, dasatinib, durvalumab, or idelalisib.

◆CLASSIFICATION

PHARMACOTHERAPEUTIC: Phosphatidylinositol-3-kinase inhibitor. **CLINICAL:** Antineoplastic.

USES

Treatment of relapsed or refractory chronic lymphocytic leukemia (CLL) or small lymphocytic lymphoma (SLL) after at least two prior therapies. Treatment of relapsed or refractory follicular lymphoma after at least two prior systemic therapies.

PRECAUTIONS

Contraindications: Hypersensitivity to duvelisib. **Cautions:** Baseline anemia, leukopenia, lymphopenia, neutropenia, thrombocytopenia; active infection, conditions predisposing to infection (e.g., diabetes, renal failure, immunocompromised pts, open wounds), dehydration, hepatic impairment, history of pulmonary disease. Concomitant use of strong CYP3A inducers or CYP3A inhibitors.

ACTION

Inhibits phosphatidylinositol-3-kinase (PI3K) expressed on malignant B-cells. Inhibits signaling pathway of B-cell receptors, lymphoma cells lines, and CXCR12-mediated chemotaxis of malignant B cells. **Therapeutic Effect:** Inhibits tumor cell growth and metastasis.

PHARMACOKINETICS

Widely distributed. Metabolized in liver. Protein binding: 98%. Peak plasma concentration: 1–2 hrs. Excreted in feces (79%), urine (14%). **Half-life:** 4.7 hrs.

LIFESPAN CONSIDERATIONS

Pregnancy/Lactation: Avoid pregnancy; may cause fetal harm. Females of reproductive potential must use effective contraception during treatment and for at least 1 mo after discontinuation. Unknown if distributed in breast milk. Breastfeeding not recommended during treatment and for at least 1 mo after discontinuation. **Males:** Males with female partners of reproductive potential must use effective contraception during treatment and for at least 1 mo after discontinuation. May impair fertility. **Children:** Safety and efficacy not established. **Elderly:** No age-related precautions noted.

INTERACTIONS

DRUG: **Strong CYP3A4 inhibitors (e.g., clarithromycin, ketoconazole, ritonavir)** may increase concentration/effect. **Strong CYP3A4 inducers (e.g., carbamazepine, phenytoin, rifAMPin)** may decrease concentration/effect. May decrease efficacy of **BCG (intravesical), vaccines (live)**. May increase adverse effects of **vaccines (live)**. **HERBAL:** **St. John's wort** may decrease concentration/effect. **Echinacea** may decrease therapeutic effect. FOOD: **Grapefruit products** may increase concentration/effect. LAB VALUES: May increase serum alkaline phosphatase, amylase, ALT, AST, creatinine, lipase, potassium. May decrease serum albumin, calcium, sodium, phosphate; absolute neutrophil count (ANC), Hct, Hgb, leukocytes, lymphocytes, neutrophils, platelets, RBC count.

AVAILABILITY (Rx)

Capsules: 15 mg, 25 mg.

ADMINISTRATION/HANDLING

PO

• Give without regard to food. • Administer whole; do not break, cut, or open capsule. Capsule cannot be chewed. • If a dose is missed by no more than 6 hrs, administer as soon as possible. If a dose is missed by more than 6 hrs, skip dose and administer at next regularly scheduled time.

INDICATIONS/ROUTES/DOSAGE

Note: Recommend prophylactic therapy for *Pneumocystis jirovecii* pneumonia (PJP) during treatment and until absolute CD4+ T-cell count is greater than 200 cells/mm^3. To prevent cytomegalovirus (CMV) infection, recommend prophylactic antiviral therapy during treatment.

CLL, SLL, Follicular Lymphoma

PO: ADULTS, ELDERLY: 25 mg twice daily of 28-day cycle.

Reduction Schedule for Adverse Effects

First dose reduction: 15 mg. Unable to tolerate 15 mg dose: Permanently discontinue.

Dose Modification

Based on Common Terminology Criteria for Adverse Events (CTCAE).

Cutaneous Reactions

Grade 1 or 2 cutaneous reactions: Maintain dose and treat with supportive therapy. **Grade 3 cutaneous reactions:** Withhold treatment until resolved with supportive therapy, then resume at reduced dose. **Life-threatening or recurrent cutaneous reactions, Stevens-Johnson syndrome, toxic epidermal necrolysis, drug reaction with eosinophilia and systemic reaction:** Permanently discontinue.

Diarrhea or Colitis (noninfectious)

Grade 1 or 2 diarrhea that is responsive to antidiarrheal medication; asymptomatic Grade 1 colitis: Maintain dose and treat with antidiarrheal medication. **Grade 1 or 2 diarrhea that is not responsive to antidiarrheal medication:** Withhold treatment until resolved with supportive therapy. Once resolved, resume at reduced dose. **Grade 3 diarrhea, abdominal pain, hematochezia, stool with mucus, change in bowel habits, peritoneal signs:** Withhold treatment until resolved with supportive therapy, then resume at reduced dose. **Recurrent Grade 3 diarrhea; recurrent colitis (any grade):** Permanently discontinue.

Hepatotoxicity

Serum ALT/AST elevation 3–5 times upper limit of normal (ULN): Maintain dose. **Serum ALT/AST elevation greater than 5–20 times ULN:** Withhold treatment until serum ALT/AST less than 3 times ULN, then resume at same dose for first occurrence or at reduced dose for subsequent occurrence. **Serum ALT/AST elevation greater than 20 times ULN:** Permanently discontinue.

Infection

Grade 3 or higher infection: Withhold treatment until resolved, then resume at same or reduced dose. **PJP infection of any grade:** Withhold treatment and evaluate for confirmation. If PJP infection is confirmed, permanently discontinue. **Clinical CMV infection or viremia (confirmed with positive PCR test or antigen test):** Withhold treatment until resolved, then resume at same or reduced dose.

Neutropenia

ANC 500–1000 cells/mm³: Maintain dose. **ANC less than 500 cells/mm³:** Withhold treatment until ANC is greater than 500 cells/mm³, then resume at same dose for first occurrence or at reduced dose for subsequent occurrence.

Thrombocytopenia

Platelet count 25,000 to less than 50,000 cells/mm³ with Grade 1 bleeding: Maintain dose. **Platelet count 25,000 to less than 50,000 cells/mm³ with Grade 2 bleeding; platelet count less than 25,000 cells/mm³:** Withhold treatment until platelet count is greater than or equal to 25,000 cells/mm³ and bleeding has resolved (if applicable). Resume at same dose for first occurrence or at reduced dose for subsequent occurrence.

Pneumonitis (Noninfectious)

Grade 2 symptomatic pneumonitis: Withhold treatment and treat pneumonitis as appropriate. Once improved to Grade 1 or 0, resume at reduced dose. **Grade 3 pneumonitis; life-threatening or recurrent pneumonitis despite steroid therapy:** Permanently discontinue.

Concomitant Use With Strong CYP3A Inhibitors

If CYP3A inhibitor cannot be discontinued, reduce dose to 15 mg twice daily.

Dosage in Renal/Hepatic Impairment

Mild to severe impairment: Not specified; use caution.

SIDE EFFECTS

Frequent (50%–13%): Diarrhea, rash, fatigue, pyrexia, cough, nausea, musculoskeletal pain, abdominal pain, vomiting, mucositis, edema, decreased appetite, constipation. **Occasional (12%–10%):** Headache, dyspnea, arthralgia.

ADVERSE EFFECTS/TOXIC REACTIONS

Anemia, leukopenia, lymphopenia, lymphocytosis, neutropenia, thrombocytopenia are expected responses to therapy. Serious infections including pneumonia, bronchopulmonary aspergillosis, sepsis, lung infection reported in 31% of pts. *Pneumocystis jirovecii* pneumonia reported in less than 1% of pts. CMV infection/reactivation or viremia reported in 1% of pts. Fatal and/or severe diarrhea or colitis reported in 18% of pts. Serious cutaneous reactions including erythema, pruritus, rash, toxic skin eruption, skin peeling, exfoliation, keratinocyte necrosis occurred in 5% of pts. Fatal cases of toxic epidermal necrolysis, drug reaction with eosinophilia and systemic reaction have occurred. Noninfectious pneumonitis occurred in 5% of pts. Grade 3 or 4 hepatotoxicity reported in 2%–8% of pts. Grade 3 or 4 neutropenia reported in 42% of pts, which may greatly increase risk of infection.

NURSING CONSIDERATIONS

BASELINE ASSESSMENT

Obtain ANC, CBC, LFTs; pregnancy test in female pts of reproductive potential. Question current breastfeeding status. Confirm compliance of effective contraception. Screen for active infection. Recommend prophylaxis therapy for *Pneumocystis jirovecii* pneumonia during treatment and until absolute CD4+ T cell count is greater than 200 cells/mm³. To prevent CMV infection, recommend prophylactic antiviral therapy during treatment. Assess skin for open wounds, lesions. Assess hydration status. Question history of hepatic impairment, pulmonary disease. Receive full medication history and screen for interactions. Offer emotional support.

INTERVENTION/EVALUATION

Monitor ANC, CBC, LFT periodically. If blood dyscrasias occurs, monitor ANC, CBC wkly until improved. If hepatotoxicity occurs, monitor LFTs wkly until improved. Be alert for infections, esp. respiratory tract infection such as *Pneumocystis jirovecii* pneumonia, bacterial/fungal/pneumococcal/viral pneumonia (cough, dyspnea, hypoxia, pleuritic chest pain). If infection occurs, provide anti-infective therapy as appropriate. Consider ABG, radiologic test if ILD/pneumonitis (excessive cough, dyspnea, hypoxia) is suspected. If treatment-related toxicities occur, consider referral to specialist. Assess skin for cutaneous reactions, skin toxicities. Monitor for CMV reactivation (by PCR test or antigen test) at least monthly in pts who test positive for CMV. In pts who develop diarrhea, colitis, abdominal pain, or change in bowel habits, monitor daily pattern of bowel activity and stool consistency at least wkly until resolved with supportive therapies. In pts who develop cutaneous reactions, monitor at least wkly until resolved with supportive therapies. Monitor I&Os, hydration status.

PATIENT/FAMILY TEACHING

• Treatment may depress your immune system and reduce your ability to fight infection. Report symptoms of infection such as body aches, chills, cough, fatigue, fever. Avoid those with active infection. • Report symptoms of bone marrow depression such as bruising, fatigue, fever, shortness of breath, weight loss; bleeding easily, bloody urine or stool. • Report symptoms of liver problems (abdominal pain, bruising, clay-colored stool, amber- or dark-colored urine, yellowing of the skin or eyes); inflammation of the lung (excessive cough, difficulty breathing, chest pain); toxic skin reactions (itching, peeling, rash, redness, swelling). • Use effective contraception to avoid pregnancy. Do not breastfeed. • Treatment may cause severe diarrhea, which may require antidiarrheal medication. Report worsening of diarrhea or dehydration. Drink plenty of fluids. • Do not take newly prescribed medications unless approved by the prescriber who originally started treatment. • Do not ingest grapefruit products.

D

edoxaban

e-**dox**-a-ban
(Savaysa, Lixiana ✦)

■ BLACK BOX ALERT ■ Avoid use in nonvalvular atrial fibrillation pts with creatinine clearance (CrCl) greater than 95 mL/min (increased risk of ischemic stroke). Premature discontinuation of oral anticoagulant in the absence of alternative anticoagulation may increase risk of ischemic events. If treatment is discontinued for any reason other than pathologic bleeding or completion of course of therapy, consider coverage with another anticoagulant as described in transition guideline. Epidural or spinal hematomas may occur in pts who are receiving neuraxial anesthesia or undergoing spinal puncture, which may result in long-term or permanent paralysis. **Do not confuse edoxaban with apixaban or rivaroxaban.**

◆CLASSIFICATION

PHARMACOTHERAPEUTIC: Factor Xa inhibitor. **CLINICAL:** Anticoagulant.

USES

To reduce risk of stroke and systemic embolism (SE) in pts with nonvalvular atrial fibrillation (NVAF). Treatment of deep vein thrombosis (DVT) and pulmonary embolism (PE) following 5–10 days of initial therapy with a parenteral anticoagulant.

PRECAUTIONS

Contraindications: Hypersensitivity to edoxaban. Major active bleeding. **Cautions:** Elderly, pts at increased risk of bleeding (e.g., prior trauma, thrombocytopenia, severe uncontrolled hypertension; history of bleeding ulcers, upper or lower GI bleeding), recent surgery, renal/hepatic impairment. Avoid concomitant use with aspirin, heparin, low molecular weight heparin (LMWH), NSAIDs, P-gp inducers (e.g., rifAMPin). Not recommended in pts with CrCl greater than 95 mL/min (increased risk of ischemic stroke); mechanical heart valves; moderate to severe mitral stenosis.

ACTION

Selectively blocks active site of factor Xa, a key factor in the intrinsic and extrinsic pathway of blood coagulation cascade. Inhibits platelet activation and fibrin clot formation. **Therapeutic Effect:** Inhibits blood coagulation.

PHARMACOKINETICS

Readily absorbed and widely distributed. Peak plasma concentration: 1–2 hrs. Steady state reached within 3 days. Protein binding: 55%. Primarily excreted in urine (50%), biliary/intestinal excretion (remaining %). Not removed by hemodialysis. **Half-life:** 10–14 hrs.

⌛ LIFESPAN CONSIDERATIONS

Pregnancy/Lactation: Unknown if excreted in breast milk. **Children:** Safety and efficacy not established. **Elderly:** May have increased risk of bleeding due to age-related renal impairment.

INTERACTIONS

DRUG: **NSAIDs (e.g., ibuprofen, ketorolac, naproxen), fibrinolytic therapy (e.g., alteplase), aspirin** may increase concentration/effect; may increase risk of bleeding. **Strong CYP3A4 inducers (e.g., carBAMazepine, phenytoin, rifAMPin)** may decrease concentration/effect. **Apixaban, dabigatran, rivaroxaban** may increase anticoagulant effect. **HERBAL:** **Herbals with anticoagulant/antiplatelet properties (e.g., garlic, ginger, ginkgo biloba)** may increase risk of bleeding. **FOOD:** None known. **LAB VALUES:** May increase serum AST, ALT. May prolong aPTT, PT/INR.

AVAILABILITY (Rx)

Tablets: 15 mg, 30 mg, 60 mg.

ADMINISTRATION/HANDLING

PO

• Give without regard to food. • Do not administer within 2 hrs of removal of epidural or intrathecal catheters.

INDICATIONS/ROUTES/DOSAGE

Nonvalvular Atrial Fibrillation
PO: ADULTS, ELDERLY: 60 mg once daily.

DVT/PE
PO: ADULTS, ELDERLY WEIGHING MORE THAN 60 KG: 60 mg once daily following 5–10 days of initial therapy with a parenteral anticoagulant. **60 KG OR LESS:** 30 mg once daily.

Dose Modification
Body weight less than or equal to 60 kg or concomitant use of certain P-gp inhibitors: 30 mg once daily.

Dosage in Renal Impairment
(DVT/PE): CrCl 15–50 mL/min: 30 mg once daily. **CrCl less than 15 mL/min:** Not recommended. **(Nonvalvular atrial fibrillation): CrCl greater than 95 mL/min:** Not recommended. **CrCl 51–95 mL/min:** No dose adjustment. **CrCl 15–50 mL/min:** 30 mg once daily. **CrCl less than 15 mL/min:** Not recommended.

Dosage in Hepatic Impairment
Mild impairment: No dose adjustment. **Moderate to severe impairment:** Not recommended.

Discontinuation for Surgery or Other Interventions
Discontinue at least 24 hrs before invasive surgical procedures. May restart as soon as adequate hemostasis is achieved, noting that the time of onset of pharmacodynamic effect is 1–2 hrs.

Transition Guideline to Edoxaban
From warfarin or other vitamin K antagonists: Discontinue warfarin and start edoxaban when INR is less than or equal to 2.5. **From oral anticoagulants other than warfarin or other vitamin K antagonists:** Discontinue current oral anticoagulant and start edoxaban at the time of the next scheduled dose of the other oral anticoagulant. **From LMWH:** Discontinue LMWH and start edoxaban at the time of the next scheduled dose of LMWH. **From low unfractionated heparin:** Discontinue infusion and start edoxaban 4 hrs later.

Transition Guideline From Edoxaban to Other Anticoagulant
To Warfarin: Oral option: For pts taking edoxaban 60 mg, reduce to 30 mg and begin warfarin concomitantly. For pts taking edoxaban 30 mg, reduce dose to 15 mg and begin warfarin concomitantly. Once stable INR greater than or equal to 2, discontinue edoxaban and continue warfarin. **Parenteral option:** Discontinue edoxaban and administer parenteral anticoagulant and warfarin at the time of next scheduled edoxaban dose. Once stable INR greater than or equal to 2, discontinue parenteral anticoagulant and continue warfarin. **To non–vitamin K–dependent oral anticoagulant or parenteral anticoagulant:** Discontinue edoxaban and start other oral anticoagulant at the time of the next scheduled dose.

SIDE EFFECTS

Rare (4%): Rash.

ADVERSE EFFECTS/TOXIC REACTIONS

Hemorrhagic events including intracranial hemorrhage, hemorrhagic stroke, cutaneous/GI/GU/oral/pharyngeal/urethral/vaginal bleeding, epistaxis, epidural/spinal hematoma (esp. with epidural catheters, spinal trauma) were reported. Discontinuation in the absence of other adequate anticoagulants may increase the risk of ischemic events, stroke. May increase risk of epidural or spinal hematomas, which can lead to long-term or permanent paralysis. Protamine sulfate, vitamin K, tranexamic acid are not expected to reverse anticoagulant effect. Interstitial lung disease was reported in less than 1% of pts.

NURSING CONSIDERATIONS

BASELINE ASSESSMENT
Obtain baseline renal function test, esp. creatinine clearance; PT/INR in

pts transitioning on or off warfarin therapy. Do not initiate if CrCl greater than 95 mL/min. Question history of bleeding disorders, recent surgery, spinal procedures, intracranial hemorrhage, bleeding ulcers, open wounds, anemia, renal/hepatic impairment, trauma. Receive full medication history including herbal products.

E

INTERVENTION/EVALUATION

Monitor renal function test; occult urine/stool, urine output. Monitor for symptoms of hemorrhage: abdominal/back pain, headache, altered mental status, weakness, paresthesia, aphasia, vision changes, GI bleeding. Question for increase in menstrual bleeding/discharge. Assess peripheral pulses; skin for ecchymosis, petechiae. Assess urine output for hematuria.

PATIENT/FAMILY TEACHING

• Do not discontinue current blood thinning regimen or take any newly prescribed medication unless approved by prescriber who started anticoagulant therapy. • Suddenly stopping therapy may increase risk of stroke or blood clots. Refill prescriptions so that next scheduled dose is not missed. • Immediately report bleeding of any kind. • Avoid alcohol, aspirin, NSAIDs. • Consult physician before surgery/dental work. • Use electric razor, soft toothbrush to prevent bleeding. • Report any numbness, muscular weakness, signs of stroke (confusion, headache, one-sided weakness, trouble speaking), bloody stool or urine, nosebleeds. • Monitor changes in urine output.

elbasvir/grazoprevir

el-bas-vir/graz-**oh**-pre-vir
(Zepatier)

■ BLACK BOX ALERT ■ Hepatitis B virus reactivation may cause fulminant hepatitis, hepatic failure, and death.

Do not confuse elbasvir with daclatasvir, ombitasvir or grazoprevir with boceprevir or simeprevir.

◆CLASSIFICATION

PHARMACOTHERAPEUTIC: NS5A inhibitor/NS3/4A protease inhibitor.
CLINICAL: Antihepaciviral.

USES

Treatment of chronic hepatitis C virus genotypes 1 or 4 infection in adults, with or without ribavirin.

PRECAUTIONS

Contraindications: Hypersensitivity to elbasvir or grazoprevir, decompensated hepatic cirrhosis, moderate or severe hepatic impairment; concomitant use of organic anion transporting polypeptides 1B1/3 (OATP1B1/3) inhibitors, strong CYP3A inducers. Concomitant use of atazanavir, carBAMazepine, cycloSPORINE, darunavir, efavirenz, lopinavir, phenytoin, rifAMPin, saquinavir, St. John's wort, tipranavir. Any contraindications or hypersensitivity to ribavirin (if used with treatment regimen). **Cautions:** HIV infection, mild hepatic impairment. Safety and efficacy not established in pts with hepatitis B virus coinfection, liver transplant recipients.

ACTION

Elbasvir inhibits hepatitis C virus (HCV) NS5A protein, which is essential for viral RNA replication and virion assembly. Grazoprevir inhibits HCV NS3/4A protease needed for processing HCV-encoded polyproteins, which is essential for viral replication. **Therapeutic Effect:** Inhibits viral replication of hepatitis C virus.

PHARMACOKINETICS

Widely distributed. Metabolized in liver. Protein binding: elbasvir (99.9%), grazoprevir (98.8%). Peak plasma concentration: 3 hrs. Steady state reached in approx. 6 days. Excreted in feces (greater than 90%), urine (less than 1%). **Half-life:** elbasvir: 24 hrs; grazoprevir: 31 hrs.

LIFESPAN CONSIDERATIONS

Pregnancy/Lactation: Use caution in pregnancy. Unknown if distributed in breast milk. When used with ribavirin, breastfeeding and pregnancy are contraindicated during treatment and up to 6 mos after discontinuation. **Children:** Safety and efficacy not established. **Elderly:** May have increased risk of hepatotoxicity.

INTERACTIONS

DRUG: **Anticonvulsants (e.g., carBAMazepine, phenytoin), antimycobacterials (e.g., rifabutin, rifAMPin), efavirenz** may significantly decrease concentration/effect; use contraindicated. **Atazanavir, darunavir, cycloSPORINE** may significantly increase risk of hepatotoxicity; use contraindicated. **Moderate CYP3A inducers (e.g., amiodarone, dilTIAZem, fluconazole)** may decrease concentration/effect. **Elvitegravir/cobicistat/emtricitabine/tenofovir (disoproxil or alafenamide), ketoconazole** may increase concentration/effect. May increase concentration/effect of **atorvastatin, fluvastatin, HYDROcodone, lovastatin, niMODipine, rosuvastatin, simvastatin, tacrolimus.** HERBAL: **St. John's wort** may decrease concentration/effect; use contraindicated. FOOD: None known. LAB VALUES: May decrease Hgb. May increase serum ALT, bilirubin.

AVAILABILITY (Rx)

Fixed-Dose Combination Tablets: elbasvir 50 mg/grazoprevir 100 mg.

ADMINISTRATION/HANDLING

PO

- Give without regard to food.

INDICATIONS/ROUTES/DOSAGE

Note: NS5A resistance testing recommended in HCV genotype 1a infected pts prior to initiating treatment with Zepatier.

Chronic Hepatitis C Virus Infection

PO: ADULTS, ELDERLY: 1 tablet once daily (with or without ribavirin).

Treatment Regimen and Duration

PO: ADULTS, ELDERLY: **Genotype 1a: Treatment-naïve or peginterferon alfa (PegIFN)/ribavirin (RBV)–experienced without baseline NS5A polymorphisms:** 1 tablet once daily for 12 wks. **Genotype 1a: Treatment-naïve or PegIFN/RBV–experienced with baseline NS5A polymorphisms:** 1 tablet once daily with ribavirin for 16 wks. **Genotype 1b: Treatment-naïve or PegIFV/RBV–experienced:** 1 tablet once daily for 12 wks. **Genotype 1a or 1b: PegIFV/RBV/protease inhibitor–experienced:** 1 tablet once daily with ribavirin for 12 wks. **Genotype 4: Treatment-naïve:** 1 tablet once daily for 12 wks. **Genotype 4: PegIFN/RBV–experienced:** 1 tablet once daily with ribavirin for 16 wks.

Treatment-Induced Hepatotoxicity

Consider discontinuation in pts with persistent serum ALT elevation greater than 10 times upper limit of normal (ULN). Permanently discontinue if serum ALT elevation is accompanied with elevated alkaline phosphatase, conjugated bilirubin, prolonged INR, or signs of acute hepatic inflammation.

Dosage in Renal Impairment

No dose adjustment.

Dosage in Hepatic Impairment

Mild impairment: No dose adjustment. **Moderate to severe impairment:** Contraindicated.

SIDE EFFECTS

Occasional (11%–3%): Fatigue, headache, diarrhea, nausea, insomnia, dyspnea, rash, pruritus, irritability. **Rare (2%):** Abdominal pain, arthralgia.

ADVERSE EFFECTS/TOXIC REACTIONS

Serum ALT elevation up to 5 times ULN reported in 1% of pts. Serum bilirubin elevation greater than 2.5 times ULN occurred in 6% of pts. Serum ALT elevation occurred more frequently in the elderly, female pts, and pts of Asian ancestry.

NURSING CONSIDERATIONS

BASELINE ASSESSMENT

Obtain CBC, LFT, HCV-RNA level; pregnancy test in female pts of reproductive potential. Confirm hepatitis C genotype. In pts with HCV genotype 1a, recommend testing for the presence of NS5A resistance-associated polymorphisms prior to initiation. Receive full medication history including herbal products; screen for contraindications. Question history of chronic anemia, hepatitis B virus infection, HIV infection, liver transplantation.

INTERVENTION/EVALUATION

Obtain LFT at wk 8, then as clinically indicated. For pts receiving 16 wks of therapy, obtain additional LFT at wk 12. Monitor CBC periodically; HCV-RNA levels at wks 4, 8, 12, 16 and as clinically indicated. Monitor for hepatotoxicity. Assess for anemia-related dizziness, exertional dyspnea, fatigue, weakness, syncope. Encourage nutritional intake. Assess for decreased appetite, weight loss. Obtain monthly pregnancy tests in females of reproductive potential if treated with ribavirin.

PATIENT/FAMILY TEACHING

• Treatment may be used in combination with ribavirin (inform pt of side effects/toxic reactions). If therapy includes ribavirin, female pts of reproductive potential should avoid pregnancy during treatment and up to 6 mos after last dose. • Do not take newly prescribed medication unless approved by the doctor who originally started treatment. • Do not take herbal products, esp. St. John's wort. • Avoid alcohol, grapefruit products. • Report signs of treatment-induced liver injury such as abdominal pain, clay-colored stool, dark amber urine, decreased appetite, fatigue, weakness, yellowing of the skin or eyes. • Maintain proper nutritional intake.

eletriptan

el-e-**trip**-tan
(Relpax)

◆CLASSIFICATION

PHARMACOTHERAPEUTIC: Serotonin receptor agonist. **CLINICAL:** Antimigraine.

USES

Treatment of acute migraine headache with or without aura.

PRECAUTIONS

Contraindications: Hypersensitivity to eletriptan. Arrhythmias associated with conduction disorders, cerebrovascular syndrome including strokes and transient ischemic attacks (TIAs), coronary artery disease, hemiplegic or basilar migraine, ischemic heart disease, peripheral vascular disease including ischemic bowel disease, severe hepatic impairment, uncontrolled hypertension; use within 24 hrs of treatment with another 5-HT_1 agonist, an ergotamine-containing or ergot-type medication such as dihydroergotamine (DHE) or methysergide. Recent use (within 72 hrs) of strong CYP3A4 inhibitors (e.g., clarithromycin, ketoconazole, itraconazole, ritonavir). **Cautions:** Mild to moderate renal/hepatic impairment, controlled hypertension, history of CVA.

ACTION

Selective agonist for serotonin in cranial arteries; causes vasoconstriction and reduces inflammation. **Therapeutic Effect:** Relieves migraine headache.

PHARMACOKINETICS

Readily absorbed. Metabolized by liver. Excreted in urine. **Half-life:** 4.4 hrs (increased in hepatic impairment, elderly [older than 65 yrs]).

LIFESPAN CONSIDERATIONS

Pregnancy/Lactation: May decrease possibility of ovulation. Distributed in breast milk. **Children:** Safety and efficacy not established. **Elderly:** Increased risk of hypertension in those older than 65 yrs.

INTERACTIONS

DRUG: **Ergot derivatives (e.g., ergotamine)** may increase vasoconstrictive effect. **Strong CYP3A4 inhibitors (e.g., clarithromycin, ketoconazole, ritonavir)** may increase concentration/effect. **MAOIs (e.g., phenelzine, selegiline)** may cause serotonin syndrome. **HERBAL:** None significant. **FOOD:** None known. **LAB VALUES:** None significant.

AVAILABILITY (Rx)

Tablets: 20 mg, 40 mg.

ADMINISTRATION/HANDLING

PO

• Give without regard to food. • Do not break, crush, dissolve, or divide film-coated tablets.

INDICATIONS/ROUTES/DOSAGE

Acute Migraine Headache

PO: ADULTS, ELDERLY: Initially, 20–40 mg as a single dose. **Maximum:** 40 mg/dose. If headache improves but then returns, dose may be repeated after 2 hrs. **Maximum:** 80 mg/day.

Dosage in Renal/Hepatic Impairment

No dose adjustment. Not recommended in severe hepatic impairment.

SIDE EFFECTS

Occasional (6%–5%): Dizziness, drowsiness, asthenia, nausea. **Rare (3%–2%):** Paresthesia, headache, dry mouth, warm or hot sensation, dyspepsia, dysphagia.

ADVERSE EFFECTS/TOXIC REACTIONS

Cardiac reactions (ischemia, coronary artery vasospasm, MI), noncardiac vasospasm-related reactions (hemorrhage, CVA) occur rarely, particularly in pts with hypertension, obesity, diabetes, strong family history of coronary artery disease; smokers; males older than 40 yrs; postmenopausal women. May cause GI ischemia, bowel infarction, non–cardiac-related vasospasms including peripheral vascular ischemia, Raynaud's syndrome. Overuse may increase frequency, occurrence of headaches.

NURSING CONSIDERATIONS

BASELINE ASSESSMENT

Question characteristics of migraine headaches (onset, location, duration, possible precipitating symptoms). Obtain baseline B/P for evidence of uncontrolled hypertension (contraindication).

INTERVENTION/EVALUATION

Evaluate for relief of migraine headaches (photophobia, phonophobia, nausea, vomiting, pain, dizziness, fogginess). Monitor for cardiac arrhythmia, coronary events, hypertension, hypersensitivity reaction.

PATIENT/FAMILY TEACHING

• Take a single dose as soon as symptoms of an actual migraine attack appear. • Medication is intended to relieve migraine headaches, not to prevent or reduce number of attacks. • Avoid tasks that require alertness, motor skills until response to drug is established. • Immediately report palpitations, pain/tightness in chest/throat, sudden or severe abdominal pain, pain/weakness of extremities.

elexacaftor/tezacaftor/ivacaftor

e-lex-a-**kaf**-tor/tez-a-**kaf**-tor/eye-va-**kaf**-tor
(Trikafta)
Do not confuse elexacaftor/tezacaftor/ivacaftor (Trikafta)

with lumacaftor/ivacaftor (Orkambi).

◆CLASSIFICATION

PHARMACOTHERAPEUTIC: Cystic fibrosis transmembrane conductance regulator (CFTR) modulator. **CLINICAL:** Cystic fibrosis agent.

E

USES

Treatment of cystic fibrosis (CF) in pts aged 12 yrs and older who have at least one F508del mutation in the CFTR gene.

PRECAUTIONS

Contraindications: Hypersensitivity to elexacaftor, tezacaftor, ivacaftor. **Cautions:** Moderate hepatic impairment, concomitant use of CYP3A inhibitors. Avoid use of concomitant strong CYP3A inducers. Not recommended in severe hepatic impairment.

ACTION

Mutations in the CFTR gene (encodes the CFTR protein) are the cause of cystic fibrosis. The Phe508del mutation (most common CFTR mutation) causes abnormal CFTR trafficking, reducing the quantity of CFTR protein at the cell surface and disrupting channel gating. Elexacaftor and tezacaftor improve cellular processing/trafficking of Phe508del-CFTR, increasing CFTR at the cell surface. Ivacaftor increases chloride channel transport by augmenting channel gating. **Therapeutic Effect:** Improves lung/organ function, decreases respiratory exacerbations.

PHARMACOKINETICS

Widely distributed. Metabolized in liver. Protein binding: elexacaftor: greater than 99%, tezacaftor: 99%, ivacaftor: 99%. Peak plasma concentration: elexacaftor: 4–12 hrs, tezacaftor: 2–4 hrs, ivacaftor: 3–6 hrs. Steady state reached within 14 days (elexacaftor), 8 days (tezacaftor), 3–5 days (ivacaftor). Excretion: elexacaftor: feces (87%), urine (less than 1%); tezacaftor: feces (72%), urine (14%); ivacaftor: feces (89%), urine (7%). **Half-life:** elexacaftor: 29.8 ± 10.6 hrs, tezacaftor: 17.4 ± 3.66 hrs, ivacaftor: 15 ± 3.92 hrs.

⌛ LIFESPAN CONSIDERATIONS

Pregnancy/Lactation: Unknown if distributed in breast milk. Hormonal contraceptives may increase incidence of rash events. **Children:** Safety and efficacy not established in pts younger than 12 yrs. **Elderly:** Safety and efficacy not established.

INTERACTIONS

DRUG: Strong CYP3A4 inhibitors (e.g., clarithromycin, ketoconazole, ritonavir), moderate CYP3A inhibitors (e.g., erythromycin, fluconazole) may increase concentration/effect. **Strong CYP3A4 inducers (e.g., carBAMazepine, phenytoin, rifAMPin)** may decrease concentration/effect. May increase concentration of **afatinib, colchicine, conivaptan, idelalisib, pazopanib, rimegepant, topotecan. HERBAL: St. John's wort** may decrease concentration/effect. **FOOD: Grapefruit products** may increase concentration/effect. **LAB VALUES:** May increase serum ALT, AST, bilirubin, CPK. May decrease serum glucose.

AVAILABILITY (Rx)

Fixed-Dose Combination Tablets (copackaged with ivacaftor tablets): elexacaftor 100 mg/tezacaftor 50 mg/ivacaftor 75 mg per tablet; ivacaftor 150 mg.

ADMINISTRATION/HANDLING

PO

• Give with fat-containing food (e.g., eggs, butter, peanut butter, whole-milk dairy products [e.g., whole milk, cheese, yogurt]). • Administer tablets whole; do not break, crush, or divide. • If a morning dose is missed by more than 6 hrs, give as soon as possible, but do not give evening dose. If an evening dose is missed by more than 6 hrs, skip the evening dose and administer the morning dose at usual scheduled time. Do not give morning and evening doses at same time.

INDICATIONS/ROUTES/DOSAGE

Cystic Fibrosis

PO: ADULTS, CHILDREN 12 YRS AND OLDER: 2 fixed-dose combination tablets (elexacaftor 100 mg, tezacaftor 50 mg, ivacaftor 75 mg per tablet) in the morning and 1 tablet of ivacaftor (150 mg) in the evening (approx. 12 hrs apart).

Dose Modification

Concomitant Use of Moderate CYP3A Inhibitors

Note: Do not give evening dose of ivacaftor.

Dosing schedule for day 1: 2 fixed-dose combination tablets (elexacaftor 100 mg, tezacaftor 50 mg, ivacaftor 75 mg per tablet) in the morning. **Day 2:** 1 tablet of ivacaftor (150 mg) in the morning. **Day 3:** 2 fixed-dose combination tablets (elexacaftor 100 mg, tezacaftor 50 mg, ivacaftor 75 mg per tablet) in the morning. **Day 4:** 1 tablet of ivacaftor (150 mg) in the morning. Repeat the 4-day cycle thereafter.

Concomitant Use of Strong CYP3A Inhibitors

Note: Do not give evening dose of ivacaftor.

Dosing schedule for day 1: 2 fixed-dose combination tablets (elexacaftor 100 mg, tezacaftor 50 mg, ivacaftor 75 mg per tablet) in the morning. **Day 2 and 3:** No dose. **Day 4:** 2 fixed-dose combination tablets (elexacaftor 100 mg, tezacaftor 50 mg, ivacaftor 75 mg per tablet) in the morning. Repeat the 4-day cycle thereafter.

Hepatotoxicity

Serum ALT/AST greater than 5 times ULN, serum ALT/AST greater than 3 times ULN with bilirubin greater than 2 times ULN: Withhold treatment until resolved. Consider the risk versus benefit of resuming treatment.

Rash Events

Rash in females taking hormonal contraception: Consider withholding treatment and hormonal contraceptive until rash is resolved, then consider resuming treatment without hormonal contraceptive. If rash does not recur, may consider resuming hormonal contraceptive.

Dosage in Renal Impairment

Mild to moderate impairment: No dose adjustment. **Severe impairment, ESRD:** Not specified; use caution.

Dosage in Hepatic Impairment

Mild impairment: No dose adjustment. **Moderate impairment:** 2 fixed-dose combination tablets (elexacaftor 100 mg, tezacaftor 50 mg, ivacaftor 75 mg per tablet) in the morning only (do not give evening ivacaftor dose). **Severe impairment:** Not recommended.

SIDE EFFECTS

Occasional (17%–7%): Headache, abdominal pain, diarrhea, rash, nasal congestion, rhinorrhea, rhinitis. **Rare (5%–2%):** Flatulence, abdominal distention, dizziness, dysmenorrhea, acne, eczema, pruritus.

ADVERSE EFFECTS/TOXIC REACTIONS

Elevated transaminases may occur. Worsening of hepatic function was reported in pts with baseline hepatic impairment. Cataracts were reported in pediatric pts taking ivacaftor. Infections including upper respiratory tract infection (16% of pts), influenza (7% of pts), sinusitis (5% of pts), conjunctivitis, pharyngitis, tonsillitis, UTI were reported. Rash events were reported more frequently in females, which may be related to concomitant use of hormonal contraceptives.

NURSING CONSIDERATIONS

BASELINE ASSESSMENT

Obtain LFT. If pt's genotype is unknown, a CF mutation test should be obtained to confirm presence of at least one F508del mutation. Assess baseline symptoms of cystic fibrosis (abdominal discomfort/gas, persistent cough, inability to mobilize secretions, poor weight gain, lung infections, dyspnea). Question history of hepatic impairment. Receive full medication history and screen for drug interactions.

E

INTERVENTION/EVALUATION

Monitor LFT q3mos for 12 mos, then annually thereafter (or more frequently in pts with baseline hepatic impairment). Assess respiratory function, organ function for treatment effectiveness. Assess sputum production; ability to mobilize secretions. If concomitant use of strong or moderate CYP3A inhibitors is unavoidable, monitor for toxicities. Monitor for rash in females taking hormonal contraception.

PATIENT/FAMILY TEACHING

• Always take medication with fatty foods. • There is a high risk of interactions with other medications. Do not take newly prescribed medications unless approved by prescriber who originally started therapy. • Avoid vitamins, grapefruit products, herbal supplements (esp. St. John's wort). • Report symptoms of liver problems (e.g., bruising, confusion; dark, amber, orange-colored urine; right upper abdominal pain, yellowing of the skin or eyes). • Report vision changes, cataracts; signs of respiratory infection (e.g., cough, fever, shortness of breath). • Rashes are more common in female pts taking hormonal contraception.

elotuzumab

el-oh-**tooz**-ue-mab
(Empliciti)
Do not confuse elotuzumab with alemtuzumab, eculizumab, evolocumab, pertuzumab, gemtuzumab, trastuzumab.

◆CLASSIFICATION

PHARMACOTHERAPEUTIC: Anti-SLAMF7. Monoclonal antibody. **CLINICAL:** Antineoplastic.

USES

Treatment of multiple myeloma (in combination with lenalidomide and dexamethasone) in pts who have received one to three prior therapies or (in combination with pomalidomide and dexamethasone) in pts who have received at least two prior therapies including lenalidomide and a proteasome inhibitor.

PRECAUTIONS

Contraindications: Hypersensitivity to elotuzumab. **Cautions:** Diabetes, baseline cytopenias, hypertension; history of chronic opportunistic infections (esp. viral infections, fungal infections), conditions predisposing to infection (e.g., diabetes, kidney failure, open wounds). Concomitant use of medications known to cause bradycardia (e.g., antiarrhythmics, beta blockers, calcium channel blockers). Concomitant use of live vaccines not recommended during treatment and up to 3 mos after discontinuation. Avoid use during severe active infection.

ACTION

Binds to and specifically targets signaling lymphocytic activation molecule family member 7 (SLAMF7), a protein that is expressed on most myeloma and natural killer cells. Directly activates natural killer cells and facilitates cellular death. **Therapeutic Effect:** Inhibits tumor cell growth and metastasis.

PHARMACOKINETICS

Widely distributed. Metabolism not specified. Elimination not specified. **Half-life:** Not specified; 97% of steady-state concentration is expected to be eliminated within 82 days.

LIFESPAN CONSIDERATIONS

Pregnancy/Lactation: Avoid pregnancy; may cause fetal harm/malformations/fetal demise when used with lenalidomide. Unknown if distributed in breast milk. However, immunoglobulin G (IgG) is present in breast milk. Breastfeeding contraindicated when used with concomitant lenalidomide treatment. **Men:** Lenalidomide is present in semen. Recommend use of barrier methods during sexual activity. **Children:** Safety and efficacy not established. **Elderly:** No age-related precautions noted.

INTERACTIONS

DRUG: May increase immunosuppressant/toxic effects of **immunosuppressants (e.g., fingolimod, leflunomide, nivolumab). Roflumilast** may increase immunosuppressant effect. May enhance adverse/toxic effect of **live vaccines;** may decrease therapeutic effect of **vaccines. HERBAL:** Echinacea may decrease effect. **FOOD:** None known. **LAB VALUES:** May be detected on both serum protein electrophoresis and immunofixation assays used to monitor multiple myeloma endogenous M-protein. May affect the determination of complete response and disease progression of some pts with IgG kappa myeloma protein. Expected to decrease lymphocytes, leukocytes, platelets. May decrease serum albumin, bicarbonate, calcium. May increase serum alkaline phosphatase, ALT, AST, glucose, potassium.

AVAILABILITY (Rx)

Injection, Powder for Reconstitution: 300 mg, 400 mg.

ADMINISTRATION/HANDLING

IV

Reconstitution • Calculate the dose and number of vials required based on weight in kg. • Reconstitute the 300-mg vial with 13 mL of Sterile Water for Injection or the 400-mg vial with 17 mL of Sterile Water for Injection using an 18-g or lower (e.g., 17, 16, or 15) needle. • Gently roll vial upright to mix. To dissolve any powder left on top of vial or stopper, gently invert vial several times. • Do not shake or agitate. • The powder should dissolve in less than 10 min. • After dissolution, allow vials to stand for 5–10 min. • Visually inspect solution for particulate matter of discoloration. Solution should appear clear, colorless to slightly yellow. Discard if solution is cloudy or discolored or if foreign particles are observed. Each vial contains an overfill volume to allow for a specific withdrawal of 12 mL (300-mg vial) or 16 mL (400-mg vial). • Final concentration of withdrawn volume (without overfill) will equal 25 mg/mL. • Dilute in 230 mL of 0.9% NaCl or 5% Dextrose injection in polyvinyl chloride or polyolefin infusion bag. • Mix by gentle inversion; do not shake or agitate. • The volume may be adjusted in order to not exceed 5 mL/kg of pt weight at any given dose.

Infusion guidelines • Prior to administration, premedicate with dexamethasone, acetaminophen, antihistamine (H_1 antagonist, plus H_2 antagonist) approx. 45–90 min before each infusion (see manufacturer guidelines). • Use an in-line, sterile, nonpyrogenic, low protein-binding filter (0.2–1.2 mm). • Infuse via dedicated line using an infusion pump.

Rate of administration • **First infusion (cycle 1, dose 1):** Infuse at 0.5 mL/min for the first 30 min. If no infusion reactions occur, may increase to 1 mL/min for next 30 min. If tolerated, may increase to 2 mL/min. **Maximum rate:** 2 mL/min. • **Second infusion (cycle 1, dose 2):** Initiate at 1 mL/min for first 30 min if no infusion reactions occurred during first infusion. If tolerated, may increase to 2 mL/min until infusion completed. **Maximum rate:** 2 mL/min. • **Subsequent infusions (cycle 1, doses 3 and 4, all subsequent infusions):** Initiate at 2 mL/min until completion if no infusion reactions occurred during prior infusion. **Maximum rate:** 2 mL/min. In pts who have received four cycles of treatment, infusion rate may be increased to maximum rate of 5 mL/min.

Storage • Refrigerate intact vials until time of use. • Do not freeze or shake. • Refrigerate diluted solution up to 24 hrs. • May store at room temperature up to 8 hrs (of the total 24 hrs). • Diluted solution must be administered within 24 hrs of reconstitution. • Protect from light.

E

IV INCOMPATIBILITIES

Do not mix with other medications.

INDICATIONS/ROUTES/DOSAGE

Multiple Myeloma

Note: Premedicate with dexamethasone, H_1 or H_2 blocker, and acetaminophen 45–90 mins before infusion.

IV: ADULTS, ELDERLY: ***(In combination with lenalidomide and dexamethasone):*** **Cycles 1 and 2:** 10 mg/kg once wkly on days 1, 8, 15, 22 of 28-day cycle. **Cycles 3 and beyond:** 10 mg/kg once q2wks on days 1 and 15 of 28-day cycle. Continue until disease progression or unacceptable toxicity. ***(In combination with pomalidomide and dexamethasone):*** **Cycles 1 and 2:** 10 mg/kg once wkly on days 1, 8, 15, 22 of 28-day cycle. **Cycles 3 and beyond:** 20 mg/kg once q4wks on day 1 of 28-day cycle. Continue until disease progression or unacceptable toxicity.

Dose Modification

Infusion Reactions

Grade 2 or higher reaction: Interrupt infusion until symptoms improve. Once resolved to Grade 1 or 0, resume infusion at 0.5 mL/min. If tolerated, increase in increments of 0.5 mL/min q30mins back to previous rate. May further increase rate as indicated if no reaction recurs. If infusion reaction recurs, stop infusion and do not restart for that day.

Dosage in Renal/Hepatic Impairment

Not specified; use caution.

SIDE EFFECTS

Frequent (61%–20%): Fatigue, diarrhea, pyrexia, constipation, cough, peripheral neuropathy, decreased appetite. **Occasional (16%–10%):** Extremity pain, headache, vomiting, decreased weight, oropharyngeal pain, hypoesthesia, mood change, night sweats.

ADVERSE EFFECTS/TOXIC REACTIONS

All cases were reported in combination with lenalidomide and dexamethasone. Infusion reactions reported in 10% of pts. Most infusion reactions were Grade 3 and lower. Lymphopenia, leukopenia, thrombocytopenia are expected responses to therapy. Infections were reported in 81% of pts. Grade 3 or 4 infections occurred in 28% of pts. Nasopharyngitis (25% of pts), upper respiratory tract infection (23% of pts), opportunistic infection (22% of pts), herpes zoster (14% of pts), fungal infection (10% of pts), influenza; second primary malignancies, skin malignancies, solid tumors, malignant neoplasms; tachycardia, bradycardia, systolic or diastolic hypertension, hypotension; pulmonary embolism may occur. Hepatotoxicity with elevation of serum alkaline phosphatase greater than 2 times upper limit of normal (ULN), serum ALT/AST greater than 3 times ULN, total bilirubin greater than 2 times ULN reported in 3% of pts. Other adverse effects may include cataracts (12% of pts), hyperglycemia (89% of pts), hypersensitivity reaction (greater than 5% of pts). Immunogenicity (auto-elotuzumab antibodies) occurred in 19% of pts. Thrombocytopenia may increase risk of bleeding.

NURSING CONSIDERATIONS

BASELINE ASSESSMENT

Obtain CBC, BMP, LFT; serum ionized calcium; capillary blood glucose, vital signs; pregnancy test in female pts of reproductive potential. Obtain baseline ECG in pts concurrently using medications known to cause bradycardia. Question history of chronic opportunistic infections, diabetes, hepatic impairment, pulmonary embolism; prior infusion or hypersensitivity reactions. Screen for medications known to cause bradycardia, hyperglycemia. Screen for active infection. Offer emotional support.

INTERVENTION/EVALUATION

Obtain CBC, BMP, LFT, ionized calcium periodically. Administer in an environment equipped to monitor for and manage infusion reactions. If infusion reaction of any grade/severity occurs, immediately interrupt infusion and manage symptoms. Accurately record characteristics of infusion reactions (severity, type, time of onset). Infusion reactions may affect future infusion rates. Monitor HR, BP q30mins during infusion and for at least 2 hrs after completion in pts with prior hemodynamic reactions. Cough, dyspnea, hypoxia, tachycardia may indicate pulmonary embolism. Monitor for bradycardia, cataracts, hyperglycemia, hyperkalemia, hypersensitivity reaction, hepatotoxicity, neuropathy, tachycardia. Assess for new primary malignancies (solid tumors, skin cancers); skin for new lesions, moles. Monitor daily pattern bowel activity, stool consistency.

PATIENT/FAMILY TEACHING

• Treatment may depress your immune system and reduce your ability to fight infection. Report symptoms of infection such as body aches, chills, cough, fatigue, fever. Avoid those with active infection. • Therapy may decrease your heart rate, esp. in those taking medications that lower heart rate; report dizziness, chest pain, palpitations, or fainting. • Avoid pregnancy. Do not breastfeed. • Male pts should use condoms during sexual activity. • Treatment includes a steroid that may raise blood sugar levels; report dehydration, blurry vision, confusion, frequent urination, increased thirst, fruity breath. • Report allergic reactions of any kind. • Abdominal pain, easy bruising, clay-colored stools, dark-amber urine, fatigue, loss of appetite, yellowing of skin or eyes may indicate liver problem.

eluxadoline

el-ux-**ad**-oh-leen
(Viberzi)

◆CLASSIFICATION

PHARMACOTHERAPEUTIC: Mu-opioid receptor agonist. Schedule IV.
CLINICAL: GI agent.

USES

Treatment of irritable bowel syndrome with diarrhea (IBS-D) in adults.

PRECAUTIONS

Contraindications: Hypersensitivity to eluxadoline. Known or suspected biliary duct obstruction, sphincter of Oddi disease or dysfunction; pts without a gallbladder; severe hepatic impairment; severe constipation or sequelae from constipation, or known or suspected mechanical GI obstruction. History of alcoholism, alcohol abuse, alcohol addiction, or consumption of more than 3 alcoholic beverages/day. History of pancreatitis; structural disease of the pancreas, including known or suspected pancreatic duct obstruction. **Cautions:** Mild to moderate hepatic impairment, respiratory disease.

ACTION

Acts locally on mu opioid, delta opioid, and kappa opioid receptors involved with gut motility, pain sensations, and secretion of liquids within the digestive tract. **Therapeutic Effect:** Reduces abdominal pain and diarrhea (without causing constipation).

PHARMACOKINETICS

Metabolism not specified. Protein binding: 81%. Peak plasma concentration: 1.5 hrs. Primarily excreted in feces (82%), urine (less than 1%). **Half-life:** 3.7–6 hrs.

⌛ LIFESPAN CONSIDERATIONS

Pregnancy/Lactation: Unknown if distributed in breast milk. **Children:** Safety

and efficacy not established. **Elderly:** No age-related precautions noted.

INTERACTIONS

DRUG: OATP1B1 inhibitors (e.g., cycloSPORINE, ritonavir, rifAMPin), gemfibrozil may increase concentration/effect. **Drugs that cause constipation (e.g., alosetron, anticholinergics [e.g., diphenhydrAMINE], loperamide, opioids [e.g., morphine])** may increase risk of serious constipation-associated adverse effects. May increase concentration of **rosuvastatin**, increasing risk of myopathy/rhabdomyolysis. **HERBAL:** None significant. **FOOD: High-fat meals** may decrease absorption. **LAB VALUES:** May increase serum ALT, AST, lipase.

AVAILABILITY (Rx)

Tablets: 75 mg, 100 mg.

ADMINISTRATION/HANDLING

PO

• Administer with food. • If scheduled dose is missed, give next dose at the regular time; do not give 2 doses at once.

INDICATIONS/ROUTES/DOSAGE

Irritable Bowel Syndrome–Associated Diarrhea

PO: ADULTS, ELDERLY: 100 mg twice daily. May decrease to 75 mg twice daily if unable to tolerate 100-mg dose.

Dose Modification

Pts who are unable to tolerate 100-mg dose, or are receiving concomitant OATP1B1 inhibitors: 75 mg twice daily. **Pts who develop severe constipation for more than 4 days:** Permanently discontinue.

Dosage in Renal Impairment

Not specified; use caution.

Dosage in Hepatic Impairment

Mild to moderate impairment: 75 mg twice daily. **Severe impairment:** Contraindicated.

SIDE EFFECTS

Occasional (8%–4%): Constipation, nausea, abdominal pain (upper or lower), upper respiratory tract infection, vomiting. **Rare (3%–1%):** Abdominal distention, dizziness, flatulence, rash, urticaria, fatigue, sedation, somnolence, euphoric mood.

ADVERSE EFFECTS/TOXIC REACTIONS

May increase risk of sphincter of Oddi spasm (esp. in pts without a gallbladder), resulting in pancreatitis or hepatic enzyme elevation that may be associated with or without acute abdominal pain, or nausea/vomiting; 80% of pts reported sphincter of Oddi spasm within the first week of treatment. May also increase risk of pancreatitis that is not associated with sphincter of Oddi spasm. Infections including upper respiratory tract infection, bronchitis, nasopharyngitis, viral gastroenteritis were reported. May cause hypersensitivity reaction including asthma, bronchospasm, respiratory failure, wheezing. Recreational abuse may produce feelings of euphoria, which may lead to physical dependence.

NURSING CONSIDERATIONS

BASELINE ASSESSMENT

Obtain LFT in pts with baseline hepatic impairment. Receive full medication history and screen for interactions. Question pt's usual stool characteristics (color, frequency, consistency). Question history of alcoholism, biliary duct obstruction, cholecystectomy, mechanical GI obstruction, hepatic impairment, hypersensitivity reaction, pancreatic disease, respiratory disease, sphincter of Oddi disease or spasm. Assess hydration status.

INTERVENTION/EVALUATION

Monitor for abdominal pain that radiates to the back or shoulder, with or without nausea or vomiting (esp. during first few weeks of treatment). Obtain LFT, serum lipase level if acute pancreatitis, sphincter of Oddi spasm, biliary tract obstruction suspected. Monitor for hypersensitivity reaction including dyspnea, rash, wheezing. Observe and record daily pattern of bowel activity, stool consistency. Encourage PO intake. If an acute overdose occurs, a narcotic mu-opioid antagonist such as naloxone may be considered if reversal of overdose-related adverse effects is needed.

PATIENT/FAMILY TEACHING

• Therapy may cause inflammation of the pancreas (pancreatitis) or elevated liver-associated abdominal pain, esp. during the first few weeks of treatment. Report any new or worsening abdominal pain that radiates to the back or shoulder, with or without nausea/vomiting. • Avoid chronic or acute excessive use of alcohol; may increase risk of liver or pancreas injury. • If a dose is missed, take the next dose at the regular time; do not take 2 doses at once. • Report constipation lasting longer than 4 days. • Avoid medications that cause constipation (e.g., antidiarrheals, narcotics). • Report signs of allergic reaction; respiratory problems such as worsening of asthma, bronchitis, wheezing. • Drink plenty of fluids.

elvitegravir/cobicistat/emtricitabine/tenofovir

el-vye-**teg**-ra-veer/koe-**bik**-i-stat/em-trye-**sye**-ta-been/ten-**oh**-foe-veer (Stribild, Genvoya)

■ **BLACK BOX ALERT** ■
Serious, sometimes fatal, lactic acidosis and severe hepatomegaly with steatosis (fatty liver) have been reported. Severe exacerbations of hepatitis B virus (HBV) infection reported in pts coinfected with HIV-1 and HBV following discontinuation. If discontinuation of therapy occurs, monitor hepatic function for at least several mos. Initiate anti-HBV therapy if warranted.

Do not confuse elvitegravir/cobicistat/emtricitabine/tenofovir DF (Stribild) with elvitegravir/cobicistat/emtricitabine/tenofovir TAF (Genvoya), emtricitabine/rilpivirine/tenofovir (Complera), efavirenz/emtricitabine/tenofovir (Atripla), or emtricitabine/tenofovir (Truvada).

FIXED-COMBINATION(S)

Stribild: elvitegravir (an integrase inhibitor)/cobicistat (an antiretroviral booster, CYP3A inhibitor)/emtricitabine/tenofovir fumarate (DF) (an antiretroviral): 150 mg/150 mg/200 mg/300 mg. **Genvoya:** elvitegravir (an integrase inhibitor)/cobicistat (an antiretroviral booster, CYP3A inhibitor)/emtricitabine/tenofovir (TAF) (nucleoside analog reverse transcriptase inhibitors): 150 mg/150 mg/200 mg/10 mg.

◆CLASSIFICATION

PHARMACOTHERAPEUTIC: Integrase strand transfer inhibitor, antiretroviral booster, nucleoside reverse transcriptase inhibitor, nucleotide reverse transcriptase inhibitor. **CLINICAL:** Antiretroviral agent (anti-HIV).

USES

Stribild: Complete regimen for treatment of HIV-1 infection in adults and pediatric pts 12 yrs and older weighing at least 35 kg who have no antiretroviral treatment history or to replace the current antiretroviral regimen in those who are virologically suppressed (HIV-1 RNA less than 50 copies/mL) on a stable antiretroviral regimen for at least 6 mos with no history of treatment failure and no known substitutions associated with resistance to the individual drug components. **Genvoya:** Complete regimen for treatment of HIV-1 infection in adults and pediatric pts weighing at least 25 kg who have had no antiretroviral treatment history or to replace the current antiretroviral regimen in those who are virologically suppressed (HIV-1 RNA less than 50 copies/mL) on a stable antiretroviral regimen for at least 6 mos with no history of treatment failure and no known substitutions associated with resistance to the individual drug components.

PRECAUTIONS

Contraindications: Hypersensitivity to elvitegravir, cobicistat, emtricitabine, tenofovir. Concomitant use of alfuzosin, cisapride, ergot derivatives (e.g., ergotamine), lovastatin, nephrotoxic agents, other antiretrovirals, pimozide, rifampin, salmeterol, sildenafil (when used for pulmonary hypertension), simvastatin, St. John's wort; sedative/hypnotics (e.g., alprazolam, midazolam, triazolam, zolpidem) (may produce extreme sedation and/or respiratory depression). **Cautions:** Renal/hepatic impairment, history of pathological fracture, osteoporosis, osteopenia. Not recommended in pts with CrCl less than 70 mL/min (Stribild), severe hepatic impairment, suspected lactic acidosis; pts with CrCl less than 30 mL/min (Genvoya).

ACTION

Elvitegravir inhibits catalytic activity of HIV-1 integrase (prevents integration of pro-viral gene into human DNA). Cobicistat inhibits enzymes of CYP3A, boosting exposure of elvitegravir. Emtricitabine and tenofovir interfere with HIV viral RNA-dependent DNA polymerase activities. **Therapeutic Effect:** Interferes with HIV replication.

PHARMACOKINETICS

Widely distributed. Elvitegravir, cobicistat metabolized in liver. Emtricitabine phosphorylated by cellular enzymes. Tenofovir metabolized by enzymatic hydrolysis, mediated by macrophages and hepatocytes. Protein binding: (elvitegravir): greater than 99%; (cobicistat): 98%; (emtricitabine): less than 4%; (tenofovir): less than 1%. Elvitegravir excreted in feces (95%), urine (7%). Cobicistat excreted in feces (86%), urine (8%). Emtricitabine excreted in urine (70%), feces (14%). Tenofovir excreted primarily in urine (70–80%). **Half-life:** (emtricitabine): 13 hrs; (cobicistat): 4 hrs; (emtricitabine): 10 hrs; (tenofovir): 12–18 hrs.

⌛ LIFESPAN CONSIDERATIONS

Pregnancy/Lactation: Breastfeeding not recommended due to risk of postnatal HIV transmission. Emtricitabine, tenofovir are secreted in breast milk. Unknown if elvitegravir, cobicistat are secreted in breast milk. **Children:** Safety and efficacy not established in children younger than 12 yrs or weighing less than 35 kg (Stribild), children weighing less than 25 kg (Genvoya). **Elderly:** May have increased risk of adverse reactions/toxic reactions, osteopenia.

INTERACTIONS

DRUG: May increase concentration/effect of **axitinib, bortezomib, bosutinib, budesonide, cobimetinib, dabrafenib, eletriptan, everolimus, ibrutinib, irinotecan, lovastatin, lurasidone, neratinib, palbociclib, pazopanib, ranolazine, regorafenib, rivaroxaban, simvastatin, topotecan, vemurafenib, vorapaxar. CarBAMazepine, OXcarbazepine** may decrease concentration/effect of elvitegravir. **HERBAL: St. John's wort** may decrease concentration/effect of elvitegravir. **Red yeast** may increase risk of myopathy, rhabdomyolysis. **FOOD:** None known. **LAB VALUES:** May increase serum ALT, AST, amylase, bilirubin, BUN, cholesterol, creatine kinase (CK), creatinine, glucose, phosphorus, triglycerides; urine protein. May decrease CrCl, neutrophils.

AVAILABILITY (Rx)

Fixed-Dose Combination Tablets: ***(Stribild):*** elvitegravir/cobicistat/emtricitabine/tenofovir (DF): 150 mg/150 mg/200 mg/300 mg. ***(Genvoya):*** elvitegravir/cobicistat/emtricitabine/tenofovir (TAF): 150 mg/150 mg/200 mg/10 mg.

ADMINISTRATION/HANDLING

PO

• Give with food. • Administer at least 2 hrs before medications containing aluminum, magnesium (supplements, antacids, laxatives).

INDICATIONS/ROUTES/DOSAGE

HIV Infection

PO: ADULTS: ***(Stribild):*** 1 tablet once daily. **CHILDREN 12 YRS OR OLDER WEIGHING AT LEAST 35 KG:** 1 tablet once daily. ***(Genvoya):*** **PO: ADULTS:** 1 tablet once daily. **CHILDREN 12 YRS OR OLDER WEIGHING AT LEAST 25 KG:** 1 tablet once daily.

Dosage in Renal Impairment

(Stribild): **CrCl less than 70 mL/min before initiation:** Not recommended. **CrCl less than 50 mL/min during treatment:** Recommend discontinuation. ***(Genvoya):*** Not recommended in pts with CrCl less than 30 mL/min.

Dosage in Hepatic Impairment

Mild to moderate impairment: No dose adjustment. **Severe impairment:** Not recommended.

SIDE EFFECTS

Frequent (16%–12%): Nausea, asthenia, cough, diarrhea. **Occasional (10%–4%):** Headache, vomiting, abnormal dreams, abdominal pain, depression, paresthesia, fatigue, dyspepsia, arthralgia, neuropathy, hyperpigmentation. **Rare (3%–1%):** Dizziness, eczema, insomnia, flatulence, somnolence, pruritus, urticaria.

ADVERSE EFFECTS/TOXIC REACTIONS

May cause new or worsening renal failure including Fanconi syndrome (renal tubular injury, nonabsorption of essential electrolytes, acids, buffers in renal tubules). Renal tubular injury may lead to rhabdomyolysis, osteomalacia, muscle weakness, myopathy. May decrease bone mineral density, leading to pathological fractures. May cause redistribution/accumulation of body fat (lipodystrophy). Fatal lactic acidosis, severe hepatomegaly with steatosis (fatty liver) were reported. If therapy is discontinued, pts co-infected with hepatitis B or C virus have an increased risk for viral replication, worsening of hepatic function, and may experience hepatic decompensation and/or failure. May induce immune recovery syndrome (inflammatory response to dormant opportunistic infections, such as *Mycobacterium avium,* cytomegalovirus, PCP, tuberculosis, or acceleration of autoimmune disorders, including Graves' disease, polymyositis, Guillain-Barré). Allergic reactions including angioedema were reported.

NURSING CONSIDERATIONS

BASELINE ASSESSMENT

Obtain BUN, serum creatinine, CrCl, eGFR, CD4+ count, viral load, HIV-1 RNA level; urine glucose, urine protein. Obtain serum phosphate level in pts with renal impairment. Test all pts for HBV infection. Receive full medication history (including herbal products) and screen for contraindications/interactions. Concomitant use of other medications may need to be adjusted. Question history of diabetes, hyperlipidemia, decreased mineral bone density. Offer emotional support.

INTERVENTION/EVALUATION

Monitor CD4+ count, viral load, HIV-1 RNA level for treatment effectiveness. Monitor renal function as clinically indicated. An increase in serum creatinine greater than 0.4 mg/dL from baseline may indicate renal impairment. Obtain serum lactate level if lactic acidosis suspected. If other concomitant medications were not discontinued or adjusted, closely monitor for adverse effects/toxic reactions. Assess for hepatic injury (bruising, hematuria, jaundice, right upper abdominal pain, nausea, vomiting, weight loss). If discontinuation of drug regimen occurs, monitor hepatic function for at least several months. Initiate anti-HBV therapy if warranted. Monitor for immune recovery syndrome, esp. after initiating treatment. Cough, dyspnea, fever, excess band cells on CBC may indicate acute infection (WBC may be unreliable in pts with uncontrolled HIV infection). Monitor daily pattern of bowel activity, stool consistency; I&Os.

E

PATIENT/FAMILY TEACHING

• Treatment does not cure HIV infection nor reduce risk of transmission. Practice safe sex with barrier methods or abstinence. • Take with food (optimizes absorption). • Drug resistance can form if treatment is interrupted; do not run out of supply. • As immune system strengthens, it may respond to dormant infections hidden within the body. Report any new fever, chills, body aches, cough, night sweats, shortness of breath. • Report any signs of decreased urine output, abdominal pain, yellowing of skin or eyes, darkened urine, clay-colored stools, weight loss. • Lactating females should not breastfeed. • Decreased bone density may lead to pathological fractures; report bone/extremity pain, suspected fractures. • Antiretrovirals may cause excess body fat in upper back, neck, breast, trunk, while also causing decreased body fat in legs, arms, face. • Take dose at least 2 hrs before or at least 6 hrs after other medications containing aluminum, magnesium (supplements, antacids, laxatives). • Do not take newly prescribed medications, including OTC drugs, unless approved by doctor who originally started treatment.

empagliflozin

em-pa-gli-**floe**-zin
(Jardiance)
Do not confuse empagliflozin with canagliflozin, dapagliflozin, or ertugliflozin.

FIXED-COMBINATION(S)

Glyxambi: empagliflozin/linagliptin (an antidiabetic): 10 mg/5 mg, 25 mg/5 mg. **Synjardy:** Empagliflozin/metFORMIN (an antidiabetic): 5 mg/500 mg, 5 mg/1000 mg, 12.5 mg/500 mg, 12.5 mg/1000 mg. **Trijardy XR:** empagliflozin/linagliptin (an antidiabetic)/metformin (an antidiabetic): 10 mg/5 mg/1,000 mg; 25 mg/5 mg/1,000 mg; 5mg/ 2.5 mg/1,000 mg; 12.5 mg/2.5 mg/1,000 mg.

◆CLASSIFICATION

PHARMACOTHERAPEUTIC: Sodium-glucose co-transporter 2 (SGLT2) inhibitor. **CLINICAL:** Antidiabetic.

USES

Adjunctive treatment to diet and exercise to improve glycemic controls in pts with type 2 diabetes mellitus. Reduce risk of cardiovascular death in pts with type 2 diabetes and cardiovascular disease.

PRECAUTIONS

Contraindications: History of hypersensitivity to empagliflozin, other SGLT2 inhibitors, severe renal impairment (eGFR less than 30 mL/min), end-stage renal disease, dialysis. **Cautions:** Concomitant use of loop diuretics, other hypoglycemic agents (e.g., insulin, insulin secretagogues), baseline systolic hypotension, renal impairment, hypovolemia/dehydration, recent genital mycotic infection; pts at risk for diabetic ketoacidosis (insulin dose reduction, acute febrile illness, reduced calorie intake, surgery, alcohol abuse, history of pancreatitis). Not recommended in pts with active bladder cancer, diabetic ketoacidosis, type 1 diabetes mellitus.

ACTION

Inhibits SGLT2 in proximal renal tubule, reducing reabsorption of filtered glucose from tubular lumen and lowering renal threshold for glucose. Reduces reabsorption of sodium and increases delivery of sodium to the distal tubule. **Therapeutic Effect:** Increases urinary excretion of glucose; lowers serum glucose levels. Reduces cardiac preload and afterload; downregulates sympathetic activity.

PHARMACOKINETICS

Rapidly absorbed and widely distributed. Metabolized in liver. Peak plasma concentration: 1.5 hrs. Protein binding: 86%. Excreted in urine (54%) and feces (41%). **Half-life:** 12.4 hrs.

LIFESPAN CONSIDERATIONS

Pregnancy/Lactation: Avoid use during second or third trimester. Unknown if distributed in breast milk. Breastfeeding not recommended during treatment. **Children:** Safety and efficacy not established. **Elderly:** May have increased risk for adverse reactions (e.g., hypotension, syncope, dehydration).

INTERACTIONS

DRUG: **Insulin, insulin secretagogues (e.g., glyBURIDE)** may increase risk of hypoglycemia. **Loop diuretics (e.g., furosemide)** may increase risk of symptomatic hypotension. **HERBAL:** **Fenugreek, garlic, ginkgo, ginger, ginseng** may increase hypoglycemic effect. **FOOD:** None known. **LAB VALUES:** May increase serum creatinine; low-density lipoprotein cholesterol (LDL-C); Hct. May decrease serum bicarbonate; eGFR. Expected to result in positive urine glucose test. May interfere with 1,5-anhydrogluitol (1,5-AG) assay.

AVAILABILITY (Rx)

Tablets: 10 mg, 25 mg.

ADMINISTRATION/HANDLING

PO

- Give without regard to food in the morning.

INDICATIONS/ROUTES/DOSAGE

Type 2 Diabetes Mellitus, Reduce Risk of Cardiovascular Death

PO: ADULTS, ELDERLY: Initially, 10 mg once daily in the morning. May increase to 25 mg once daily.

Dosage in Renal Impairment

GFR 45 mL/min or greater: No dose adjustment. **GFR less than 45 mL/min:** Discontinue. Do not initiate.

Dosage in Hepatic Impairment

Mild to severe impairment: No dose adjustment.

SIDE EFFECTS

Rare (4%–1.1%): Increased urination, dyslipidemia, arthralgia, nausea.

ADVERSE EFFECTS/TOXIC REACTIONS

Symptomatic hypotension (orthostatic hypotension, postural dizziness, syncope) may occur, esp. in pts who are elderly, use concomitant loop diuretics, or have baseline systolic hypotension. Intravascular volume depletion/contraction may cause acute kidney injury requiring dialysis. Fatal cases of ketoacidosis were reported. Hypoglycemic events were reported in pts using concomitant insulin, insulin secretagogues. Infections including influenza, nasopharyngitis, pyelonephritis, urosepsis, UTI, genital mycotic infections (male and female), upper respiratory tract infection may occur. Necrotizing fasciitis of the perineum (Fournier gangrene), a life-threatening necrotizing infection of the genital and perineum region that requires urgent surgical intervention, has been reported. Hypersensitivity reactions including anaphylaxis, angioedema, urticaria have occurred.

NURSING CONSIDERATIONS

BASELINE ASSESSMENT

Obtain BUN, serum creatinine, eGFR, CrCl, blood glucose level, Hgb A1c; B/P. Assess hydration status. Correct volume depletion prior to initiation. Assess pt's understanding of diabetes management, routine home glucose monitoring. Obtain dietary consult for nutritional education. Question history of renal impairment, type 1 diabetes, ketoacidosis. In pts with requiring surgery, consider suspending treatment at least 3 days before surgery. Receive full medication history and screen for interactions.

E

INTERVENTION/EVALUATION

Monitor BUN, serum creatinine, eGFR, CrCl, blood glucose level, Hgb A1c; B/P periodically. Monitor for ketoacidosis (e.g., dehydration, confusion, extreme thirst, sweet-smelling breath, Kussmaul respirations, nausea), hypoglycemia (anxiety, confusion, diaphoresis, diplopia, dizziness, headache, hunger, perioral numbness, tachycardia, tremors), hyperglycemia (fatigue, Kussmaul respirations, polyphagia, polyuria, polydipsia, nausea, vomiting). Pts presenting with metabolic acidosis should be screened for ketoacidosis, regardless of serum glucose levels. Concomitant use of beta blockers (e.g., carvedilol, metoprolol) may mask symptoms of hypoglycemia. Monitor for acute kidney injury (dark-colored urine, flank pain, decreased urine output, muscle aches), infections (cough, fatigue, fever), urinary tract infections (dysuria, fever, flank pain, malaise), mycotic infections, Fournier gangrene (perineal necrosis). Screen for glucose-altering conditions (fever, increased activity or stress, surgical procedures). Monitor weight, I&Os. Monitor for hypersensitivity reactions (anaphylaxis, angioedema, urticaria).

PATIENT/FAMILY TEACHING

• Diabetes mellitus requires lifelong control. Diet and exercise are principal parts of treatment; do not skip or delay meals. Test blood sugar regularly. Monitor daily calorie intake. • When taking combination drug therapy or when glucose conditions are altered (excessive alcohol ingestion, insufficient carbohydrate intake, hormone deficiencies, critical illness), have a low blood sugar treatment available (e.g., glucagon, oral dextrose). • Genital itching or discharge may indicate yeast infection. • Report symptoms of perineal necrosis (e.g., discoloration, pain, swelling of the scrotum, penis, or perineum). • Therapy may increase risk for dehydration, low blood pressure, which may cause kidney failure. Report decreased urination, amber-colored urine, flank pain, fatigue, swelling of the hands or feet. Drink enough fluids to maintain adequate hydration. Pts with HF should be cautious of overhydration. • Report symptoms of UTI, kidney infection (back pain, pelvic pain, burning while urinating, cloudy or foul-smelling urine), allergic reactions (difficulty breathing, rash, wheezing; swelling of the face or tongue. • Go slowly from lying to standing. • Do not breastfeed.

emtricitabine/ tenofovir

em-trye-**sye**-ta-been/ten-**oh**-foe-veer (Truvada)

■ **BLACK BOX ALERT** ■ Serious, sometimes fatal, lactic acidosis and severe hepatomegaly with steatosis (fatty liver) have been reported. Severe exacerbations of hepatitis B virus (HBV) infection reported in pts co-infected with HIV-1 and HBV following discontinuation. If discontinuation of therapy occurs, monitor hepatic function for at least several mos. Initiate anti-HBV therapy if warranted. HIV-1 PrEP must only be prescribed to pts who are confirmed HIV-1 negative prior to initiation and who are screened periodically during use. Drug-resistant HIV-1 variants have occurred in pts with undetected acute HIV-1 infection. Do not initi-

ate HIV PrEP if symptoms of acute HIV-1 infection are present unless negative status is confirmed.
Do not confuse emtricitabine/tenofovir DF (Truvada) with bictegravir/emtricitabine/tenofovir (Biktarvy), elvitegravir/cobicistat/emtricitabine/tenofovir (Genvoya, Stribild), emtricitabine/rilpivirine/tenofovir (Complera), efavirenz/emtricitabine/tenofovir (Atripla) or emtricitabine/lopinavir/ritonavir/tenofovir (Kaletra).

FIXED-COMBINATION(S)

Truvada: emtricitabine/tenofovir (antiretrovirals).

◆CLASSIFICATION

PHARMACOTHERAPEUTIC: Nucleoside reverse transcriptase inhibitor, nucleoside reverse transcriptase inhibitor. **CLINICAL:** Antiretroviral agent (anti-HIV).

USES

Treatment of HIV-1 infection in adults and pediatric pts weighing at least 17 kg, in combination with other antiretrovirals. To reduce risk of sexually acquired HIV-1 in at-risk adults and adolescents weighing at least 35 kg, in combination with safer sex practices for pre-exposure prophylaxis (PrEP).

PRECAUTIONS

Contraindications: Hypersensitivity to emtricitabine, tenofovir. Use of HIV-1 PrEP in pts who are HIV-1 positive or unknown infection status. **Cautions:** Renal/hepatic impairment, history of pathological fracture, osteoporosis, osteopenia; depression, diabetes. Not recommended in pts with CrCl less than 30 mL/min, ESRD requiring dialysis (HIV-1 infection); pts with CrCl less than 60 mL/min (HIV-1 PrEP); suspected lactic acidosis.

ACTION

Emtricitabine and tenofovir interfere with HIV viral RNA-dependent DNA polymerase. **Therapeutic Effect:** Interferes with HIV replication.

PHARMACOKINETICS

Widely distributed. Emtricitabine phosphorylated by cellular enzymes. Tenofovir metabolized by enzymatic hydrolysis, mediated by macrophages and hepatocytes. Protein binding: (emtricitabine): less than 4%; (tenofovir): less than 1%. Peak plasma concentration: (emtricitabine): 1–2 hrs; (tenofovir): 1 hr. Emtricitabine excreted in urine (86%), feces (13%). Tenofovir excreted primarily in urine (70–80%). **Half-life:** (emtricitabine): 10 hrs; (tenofovir): 17 hrs.

⌛ LIFESPAN CONSIDERATIONS

Pregnancy/Lactation: Breastfeeding not recommended due to risk of postnatal HIV transmission. Emtricitabine, tenofovir are secreted in breast milk. **Children:** (HIV-1 infection): Safety and efficacy not established in pts weighing less than 17 kg. (HIV-1 PrEP): Adolescents may exhibit poor compliance with treatment; may benefit with more frequent visits/counseling. **Elderly:** Not specified; use caution.

INTERACTIONS

DRUG: **NSAIDs (e.g., ibuprofen, ketorolac, naproxen)** may enhance nephrotoxic effects of tenofovir. **Strong CYP3A4 inducers (e.g., carBAMazepine, phenytoin, rifAMPin)** may decrease concentration/effect. **HERBAL:** **St. John's wort** may decrease concentration/effect. **FOOD:** None known. **LAB VALUES:** May increase serum alkaline phosphatase, ALT/AST, amylase, cholesterol, creatine kinase (CK), creatinine, glucose, phosphorus, triglycerides; urine glucose. May decrease Hgb, neutrophils; CrCl.

AVAILABILITY (Rx)

Fixed-Dose Combination Tablets: ***(emtricitabine/tenofovir):*** 100 mg/150 mg,

133 mg/200 mg, 167 mg/250 mg, 200 mg/300 mg.

ADMINISTRATION/HANDLING

PO

- Give without regard to food.

INDICATIONS/ROUTES/DOSAGE

HIV-1 Prophylaxis (PrEP)

PO: ADULTS, ADOLESCENTS WEIGHING AT LEAST 35 KG: 1 tablet (200 mg/300 mg) once daily.

HIV-1 Infection (established)

PO: ADULTS, CHILDREN WEIGHING AT LEAST 35 KG: 1 tablet (200 mg/300 mg) once daily. **WEIGHING 28–34 KG:** 1 tablet (167 mg/250 mg) once daily. **WEIGHING 22–27 KG:** 1 tablet (133 mg/200 mg) once daily. **WEIGHING 17–21 KG:** 1 tablet (100 mg/150 mg) once daily.

Dosage in Renal Impairment

Mild impairment: CrCl 50–80 mL/min: No dose adjustment. **Moderate impairment: CrCl 30–49 mL/min:** Decrease frequency to q48h. **Severe impairment: CrCl less than 30 mL/min:** Not recommended.

Dosage in Hepatic Impairment

Mild to severe impairment: Not specified; use caution.

SIDE EFFECTS

Occasional (9%–5%): Fatigue, nausea, diarrhea, dizziness, rash (exfoliative, generalized, macular, maculo-papular, vesicular), pruritus, headache, insomnia. **Rare (2%):** Vomiting.

ADVERSE EFFECTS/TOXIC REACTIONS

If therapy is discontinued, pts co-infected with hepatitis B or C virus have an increased risk for viral replication, worsening of hepatic function, and may experience hepatic decompensation and/or failure. May cause new or worsening renal failure including Fanconi syndrome (renal tubular injury, nonabsorption of essential electrolytes, acids, buffers in renal tubules). Renal tubular injury may lead to rhabdomyolysis, osteomalacia, muscle weakness, myopathy. May decrease bone mineral density, leading to pathological fractures. May cause redistribution/accumulation of body fat (lipodystrophy). Fatal lactic acidosis, severe hepatomegaly with steatosis (fatty liver) were reported. May induce immune recovery syndrome (inflammatory response to dormant opportunistic infections, such as *Mycobacterium avium*, cytomegalovirus, PCP, tuberculosis, or acceleration of autoimmune disorders, including Graves' disease, polymyositis, Guillain-Barré). Use of HIV-1 PrEP in pts who are HIV-1 positive may develop HIV-1 resistance substitutions because prophylactic therapy is not a complete treatment regimen. Depression occurred in 9% of pts. Upper respiratory tract infection, sinusitis were reported in 8% of pts.

NURSING CONSIDERATIONS

BASELINE ASSESSMENT

Obtain BUN, serum creatinine, CrCl, eGFR; urine glucose, urine protein. Obtain CD4+ count, viral load, HIV-1 RNA level (if therapy used to treat known HIV-1 infection). Obtain serum phosphate level in pts with renal impairment. Test all pts for HBV infection. For HIV-1 PrEP, a negative HIV-1 test must be confirmed before initiation. If recent exposure is suspected (less than 1 mo) or if symptoms of acute HIV-1 infection are present (e.g., fatigue, fever, lymphadenopathy, myalgia, rash), delay initiation for at least 1 mo until HIV-1 status is confirmed. When considering HIV-1 PrEP, screen for high-risk factors including HIV-1 infected partners, sexual activity with high-prevalence area or social network and additional risk factors (e.g., drug or alcohol dependence, incarceration, noncompliant condom use, previous STD infections; sexual exchanges for food, money, shelter, drugs; sexual partners with unknown HIV-1 status who are at risk of infection). Question potential exposures (unprotected sexual activity, sexual activity with HIV-1 infected partner, breakage of condom). Question possibility of pregnancy. Question history of diabetes, depression, hyperlipidemia, decreased mineral bone density. Offer emotional support.

INTERVENTION/EVALUATION

Monitor CD4+ count, viral load, HIV-1 RNA level for treatment effectiveness (if therapy used to treat known HIV-1 infection). Monitor renal function as clinically indicated. An increase in serum creatinine greater than 0.4 mg/dL from baseline may indicate renal impairment. Obtain serum lactate level if lactic acidosis suspected. Assess for hepatic injury (bruising, hematuria, jaundice, right upper abdominal pain, nausea, vomiting, weight loss). If discontinuation of drug regimen occurs, monitor hepatic function for at least several months. Initiate anti-HBV therapy if warranted. Monitor for immune recovery syndrome, esp. after initiating treatment. Cough, dyspnea, fever, excess band cells on CBC may indicate acute infection (WBC may be unreliable in pts with uncontrolled HIV infection). Monitor daily pattern of bowel activity, stool consistency; I&Os. Monitor for symptoms of depression (fatigue, flat affect, irritability, feelings of sadness, hopelessness, suicidal ideation). For HIV-1 PrEP, test for HIV-1 infection at least q3mos. If symptoms of acute HIV-1 infection are present or screening indicates possible infection, consider conversion to full treatment regimen until an approved test has confirmed negative status.

PATIENT/FAMILY TEACHING

• Treatment does not cure HIV infection or reduce risk of transmission. Practice safe sex with barrier methods or abstinence. • Drug resistance can form if treatment is interrupted; do not run out of supply. • Report any signs of decreased urine output, abdominal pain, yellowing of skin or eyes, darkened urine, clay-colored stools, weight loss. • Lactating females should not breastfeed. • Decreased bone density may lead to pathological fractures; report bone/extremity pain, suspected fractures. • Antiretrovirals may cause excess body fat in upper back, neck, breast, trunk, while also causing decreased body fat in legs, arms, face. • Do not take newly prescribed medications, including OTC drugs, unless approved by doctor who originally started treatment.

• **HIV-1 Prep:** Despite preventative treatment, safer sex practices with condoms and risk reduction must be used. • A negative HIV test result must be obtained before initiation. • HIV status tests will be performed q3mos (or more frequently) after starting treatment. • If possible transmission or symptoms of HIV infection occur, therapy must be interrupted, and a complete HIV treatment regimen may be started until a negative HIV status test is confirmed. • Report symptoms of HIV infection such as diarrhea, fatigue, fever, myalgia, night sweats, rash, swelling of lymph nodes. • Immediately report breakage of condom, sexual activity with partner suspected of HIV infection, diagnosis of STD, sexual practices that increase risk for infection (inconsistent condom usage, multiple partners, alcohol/drug dependence; sex in exchange for money, shelter, food, drugs). • Stay compliant with preventative treatment regimen. Missing doses may increase risk of HIV transmission/infection.

enalapril

en-**al**-a-pril
(Epaned, Vasotec)

BLACK BOX ALERT May cause fetal injury. Discontinue as soon as possible once pregnancy is detected.

Do not confuse enalapril with Anafranil, Elavil, Eldepryl, lisinopril, or ramipril.

FIXED-COMBINATION(S)

Lexxel: enalapril/felodipine (calcium channel blocker): 5 mg/2.5 mg, 5 mg/5 mg. **Teczem:** enalapril/dilTIAZem (calcium channel blocker): 5 mg/180 mg. **Vaseretic:** enalapril/hydroCHLOROthiazide (diuretic): 5 mg/12.5 mg, 10 mg/25 mg.

◆CLASSIFICATION

PHARMACOTHERAPEUTIC: Angiotensin-converting enzyme (ACE) inhibitor. **CLINICAL:** Antihypertensive.

E

USES

Treatment of hypertension alone or in combination with other antihypertensives. Adjunctive therapy for symptomatic HF. **Epaned:** Treatment of hypertension in adults and children older than 1 mo. **OFF-LABEL:** Proteinuria in steroid-resistant nephrotic syndrome.

PRECAUTIONS

Contraindications: Hypersensitivity to enalapril. History of angioedema from previous treatment with ACE inhibitors. Idiopathic/hereditary angioedema. Concomitant use of aliskiren in pts with diabetes. Coadministration with or within 36 hrs of switching to or from a neprilysin inhibitor (e.g., sacubitril). **Cautions:** Renal impairment, hypertrophic cardiomyopathy with outflow tract obstruction; severe aortic stenosis; before, during, or immediately after major surgery. Concomitant use of potassium supplement; unstented unilateral or bilateral renal artery stenosis.

ACTION

Suppresses renin-angiotensin-aldosterone system (prevents conversion of angiotensin I to angiotensin II, a potent vasoconstrictor; may inhibit angiotensin II at local vascular, renal sites). Decreases plasma angiotensin II, increases plasma renin activity, decreases aldosterone secretion. **Therapeutic Effect:** In hypertension, reduces peripheral arterial resistance. In HF, increases cardiac output; decreases peripheral vascular resistance, B/P, pulmonary capillary wedge pressure, heart size.

PHARMACOKINETICS

Route	Onset	Peak	Duration
PO	1 hr	4–6 hrs	24 hrs
IV	15 min	1–4 hrs	6 hrs

Readily absorbed from GI tract. Prodrug undergoes hepatic biotransformation to enalaprilat. Protein binding: 50%–60%. Primarily excreted in urine. Removed by hemodialysis. **Half-life:** 11 hrs (increased in renal impairment).

⌛ LIFESPAN CONSIDERATIONS

Pregnancy/Lactation: Crosses placenta. Distributed in breast milk. May cause fetal/neonatal mortality, morbidity. **Children:** Safety and efficacy not established. **Elderly:** May be more susceptible to hypotensive effects.

INTERACTIONS

DRUG: **Aliskiren** may increase hyperkalemic effect. May increase potential for hypersensitivity reactions to **allopurinol. Angiotensin receptor blockers (e.g., losartan, valsartan)** may increase adverse effects. May increase adverse effects of **lithium, sacubitril.** **HERBAL:** **Herbals with hypertensive properties (e.g., licorice, yohimbe) or hypotensive properties (e.g., garlic, ginger, ginkgo biloba)** may alter effects. **FOOD:** None known. **LAB VALUES:** May increase serum BUN, alkaline phosphatase, bilirubin, creatinine, potassium, ALT, AST. May decrease serum sodium. May cause positive ANA titer.

AVAILABILITY (Rx)

Injection Solution: 1.25 mg/mL. **Oral Solution:** ***(Epaned):*** 1 mg/mL. **Tablets:** 2.5 mg, 5 mg, 10 mg, 20 mg.

ADMINISTRATION/HANDLING

IV

Reconstitution • May give undiluted or dilute with D_5W or 0.9% NaCl.

Rate of administration • For IV push, give undiluted over 5 min. • For IV piggyback, infuse over 10–15 min.

Storage • Store parenteral form at room temperature. • Use only clear, colorless solution. • Diluted IV solution is stable for 24 hrs at room temperature.

PO

• Give without regard to food. • Tablets may be crushed.

IV INCOMPATIBILITIES

Amphotericin B (Fungizone), amphotericin B complex (Abelcet, AmBisome, Amphotec), cefepime (Maxipime), phenytoin (Dilantin).

IV COMPATIBILITIES

Calcium gluconate, dexmedetomidine (Precedex), DOBUTamine (Dobutrex), DOPamine (Intropin), fentaNYL (Sublimaze), heparin, lidocaine, magnesium sulfate, morphine, nitroglycerin, potassium chloride, potassium phosphate, propofol (Diprivan).

INDICATIONS/ROUTES/DOSAGE

Hypertension

PO: ADULTS, ELDERLY: Initially, 2.5–5 mg/day (2.5 mg if pt taking a diuretic). May increase at 1–2 wk intervals. Range: 10–40 mg/day in 1–2 divided doses. **CHILDREN 1 MO–16 YRS:** Initially, 0.08 mg/kg once daily. Adjust dose based on pt response. **Maximum:** 5 mg/day. **NEONATES:** 0.04–0.1 mg/kg/day given q24h.

IV: ADULTS, ELDERLY: 0.625–1.25 mg q6h up to 5 mg q6h.

Adjunctive Therapy for HF

PO: ADULTS, ELDERLY: Initially, 2.5 mg twice daily. Titrate slowly at 1–2 wk intervals. Range: 5–40 mg/day in 2 divided doses. Target: 10–20 mg twice daily.

Dosage in Renal Impairment

CrCl greater than 30 mL/min: No dosage adjustment. **CrCl 30 mL/min or less: (HTN):** Initially, 2.5 mg/day. Titrate until B/P controlled. **(HF):** Initially, 2.5 mg twice daily. May increase by 2.5 mg/dose at greater than 4-day intervals. **Maximum:** 40 mg/day. **Hemodialysis:** Initially, 2.5 mg on dialysis days; adjust dose on non-dialysis days depending on B/P.

Dosage in Hepatic Impairment

No dose adjustment.

SIDE EFFECTS

Frequent (7%–5%): Headache, dizziness. **Occasional (3%–2%):** Orthostatic hypotension, fatigue, diarrhea, cough, syncope. **Rare (less than 2%):** Angina, abdominal pain, vomiting, nausea, rash, asthenia.

ADVERSE EFFECTS/TOXIC REACTIONS

Excessive hypotension ("first-dose syncope") may occur in pts with HF, severe salt or volume depletion. Angioedema (facial, lip swelling), hyperkalemia occur rarely. Agranulocytosis, neutropenia may be noted in pts with renal impairment, collagen vascular diseases (scleroderma, systemic lupus erythematosus). Nephrotic syndrome may be noted in those with history of renal disease.

NURSING CONSIDERATIONS

BASELINE ASSESSMENT

Obtain BUN, serum creatinine, CrCL. Receive full medication history, esp. potassium-sparing diuretics. Obtain B/P immediately before each dose (be alert to fluctuations). In pts with renal impairment, autoimmune disease, or taking drugs that affect leukocytes/immune response, CBC should be performed before beginning therapy, q2wks for 3 mos, then periodically thereafter.

INTERVENTION/EVALUATION

Assist with ambulation if dizziness occurs. Monitor B/P. Monitor daily pattern of bowel activity, stool consistency.

PATIENT/FAMILY TEACHING

• To reduce hypotensive effect, go from lying to standing slowly. • Several wks may be needed for full therapeutic effect of B/P reduction. • Skipping doses or voluntarily discontinuing drug may produce severe rebound hypertension. • Limit alcohol intake. • Report vomiting, diarrhea, diaphoresis, persistent cough, difficulty in breathing; swelling of face, lips, tongue.

enasidenib

en-a-**sid**-a-nib
(Idhifa)

■ BLACK BOX ALERT ■ May cause differentiation syndrome (a condition of life-threatening complications caused by chemotherapy), which can be fatal if not treated. If differentiation syndrome is suspected, consider treatment with a corticosteroid and hemodynamic monitoring.

Do not confuse enasidenib with cobimetinib, dabrafenib, encorafenib, ivosidenib, regorafenib, or trametinib.

◆CLASSIFICATION

PHARMACOTHERAPEUTIC: Isocitrate dehydrogenase-2 (IDH2) inhibitor. **CLINICAL:** Antineoplastic.

USES

Treatment of adults with relapsed or refractory acute myeloid leukemia (AML) with an isocitrate dehydrogenase-2 (IDH2) mutation.

PRECAUTIONS

Contraindications: Hypersensitivity to enasidenib. **Cautions:** Hepatic/renal impairment, dehydration; pts at high risk for tumor lysis syndrome (high tumor burden), conditions predisposing to infection (e.g., diabetes, renal failure, immunocompromised pts, open wounds).

ACTION

Inhibits isocitrate dehydrogenase-2 (IDH2) enzymes on mutant IDH2 variants, decreasing 2-hydroxyglutarate (2-HG) levels and restoring myeloid differentiation. **Therapeutic Effect:** Reduces blast counts; increases percentage of myeloid cells. Inhibits tumor growth and proliferation.

PHARMACOKINETICS

Widely distributed. Metabolized in liver. Protein binding: 99%. Peak plasma concentration: 4 hrs. Steady state reached in 29 days. Excreted in feces (89%), urine (11%). **Half-life:** 137 hrs.

⌛ LIFESPAN CONSIDERATIONS

Pregnancy/Lactation: Avoid pregnancy; may cause fetal harm. Females of reproductive potential and males with female partners of reproductive potential should use effective contraception during treatment and for at least 1 mo after discontinuation. Unknown if distributed in breast milk. Breastfeeding not recommended during treatment and for at least 1 mo after discontinuation. May impair fertility in both females and males of reproductive potential. **Children:** Safety and efficacy not established. **Elderly:** No age-related precautions noted.

INTERACTIONS

DRUG: None significant. **HERBAL:** None significant. **FOOD:** None known. **LAB VALUES:** May increase serum bilirubin; WBC. May decrease serum calcium, potassium, phosphorus.

AVAILABILITY (Rx)

Tablets: 50 mg, 100 mg.

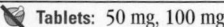

ADMINISTRATION/HANDLING

PO

• Give without regard to food. • Administer whole; do not cut, crush, or divide tablets.

INDICATIONS/ROUTES/DOSAGE

Acute Myeloid Leukemia

PO: ADULTS, ELDERLY: 100 mg once daily. Continue until disease progression or unacceptable toxicity. For pts without disease progression or unacceptable toxicity, treat for a minimum of 6 mos (allows time for clinical response).

Dose Modification

Based on Common Terminology Criteria for Adverse Events (CTCAE).

Differentiation Syndrome

If differentiation syndrome is suspected, treat with a systemic corticosteroid and hemodynamic monitoring. **Pulmonary failure requiring intubation or ventilation, renal dysfunction persisting greater than 48 hrs (despite treatment with a corticosteroid):** Withhold treatment until improved to Grade 2 or less, then resume at 100 mg once daily.

Hepatotoxicity

Serum bilirubin elevation greater than 3 times ULN for more than 2 wks (in the absence of transaminase elevation or other hepatic injury): Reduce dose to 50 mg once daily. If serum bilirubin improves to less than 2 times ULN, increase dose to 100 mg once daily.

Noninfectious Leukocytosis

WBC greater than 30,000 cells/mm^3: Consider therapy with hydroxyurea. If leukocytosis does not improve with hydroxyurea therapy, withhold enasidenib until WBC improves to less than 30,000/mm^3, then resume enasidenib at 100 mg once daily.

Any Other Toxicity

Any Grade 3 or 4 toxicity related to treatment (tumor lysis syndrome): Withhold treatment until resolved to Grade 2 or less, then resume at 50 mg once daily. If toxicities resolve to Grade 1 or 0, increase dose to 100 mg once daily.

Dosage in Renal Impairment

CrCl greater than 30 mL/min: No dose adjustment. **CrCl less than 30 mL/min:** Not specified; use caution.

Dosage in Hepatic Impairment

Mild impairment: No dose adjustment. **Moderate to severe impairment:** Not specified; use caution.

SIDE EFFECTS

Frequent (50%–25%): Nausea, diarrhea, vomiting, decreased appetite, dysgeusia.

ADVERSE EFFECTS/TOXIC REACTIONS

Life-threatening differentiation syndrome (bone pain, dyspnea, fever, lymphadenopathy, peripheral edema, plural/pericardial effusion, pulmonary infiltrates, rapid weight gain, respiratory distress; hepatic/renal/multi-organ dysfunction) reported in 14% of pts; may occur 10 days to 5 mos after initiation. Noninfectious leukocytosis reported in 12% of pts. Tumor lysis syndrome may present as acute renal failure, hypocalcemia, hyperuricemia, hyperphosphatemia. Acute respiratory distress syndrome, pulmonary edema occurred in less than 10% of pts.

NURSING CONSIDERATIONS

BASELINE ASSESSMENT

Obtain WBC; pregnancy test in females of reproductive potential. Verify presence of IDH2 mutations in the blood or bone marrow. Screen for active infection. Confirm compliance of effective contraception. Due to increased risk of tumor lysis syndrome, diarrhea, vomiting, assess adequate hydration before initiation. Offer emotional support.

INTERVENTION/EVALUATION

Monitor WBC for leukocytosis; BMP, serum calcium, phosphate, uric acid for tumor lysis syndrome (acute renal failure, electrolyte imbalance, cardiac arrhythmias, seizures) q2wks for the first 3 mos. Monitor LFT for transaminitis, hepatotoxicity periodically. If differentiation syndrome is suspected, consider treatment with a corticosteroid and hemodynamic monitoring. Once symptoms have resolved, taper corticosteroid therapy. Offer antiemetic if nausea occurs; antidiarrheal if diarrhea occurs. Monitor daily pattern of bowel activity, stool consistency. Ensure adequate hydration, nutrition. Monitor weight, I&Os.

PATIENT/FAMILY TEACHING

• Therapy may cause tumor lysis syndrome (a condition caused by the rapid breakdown of cancer cells), which can cause kidney failure and can be fatal. Report decreased urination, amber-colored urine, confusion, difficulty breathing, fatigue, fever, muscle or joint pain, palpitations, seizures, vomiting. • Treatment may cause differentiation syndrome (a condition of life-threatening complications caused by induction chemotherapy), which can be fatal. Report bone pain, difficulty breathing, fever, swelling of the lymph nodes or extremities, lung congestion or infection, organ dysfunction, rapid weight gain. • Use effective contraception to avoid pregnancy. Do not breastfeed. • Report treatment-induced liver toxicity such as bruising, confusion; amber, dark, orange-colored urine; right upper abdominal pain, yellowing of the skin or eyes. • Nausea, vomiting, diarrhea are common side effects. Drink plenty of fluids.

encorafenib

en-koe-**raf**-e-nib
(Braftovi)
Do not confuse encorafenib with binimetinib, cobimetinib, dabrafenib, dasatinib, erlotinib, trametinib, or vemurafenib, or Braftovi with Mektovi.

◆CLASSIFICATION

PHARMACOTHERAPEUTIC: BRAF kinase inhibitor. **CLINICAL:** Antineoplastic.

USES

Treatment of pts with unresectable or metastatic melanoma with a BRAF V600E or V600K mutation (in combination with binimetinib). Treatment of metastatic colorectal cancer (CRC) in adults with a BRAF V600E mutation (in combination with cetuximab) after prior therapy. **OFF-LABEL:** Treatment of colorectal cancer, metastatic, refractory (RAS wild-type, BRAF V600E-mutant).

PRECAUTIONS

Contraindications: Hypersensitivity to encorafenib. **Cautions:** Baseline anemia, leukopenia, lymphopenia, neutropenia; active infection; conditions predisposing to infection (e.g., diabetes, renal failure, immunocompromised pts, open wounds), diabetes, hepatic/renal impairment; pts at risk for QTc interval prolongation (congenital long QT syndrome, HF, mediations that prolong QTc interval, hypokalemia, hypomagnesemia): concomitant use of strong or moderate CYP3A inhibitors or strong or moderate CYP3A inducers.

ACTION

An ATP-competitive inhibitor of protein kinase BRAF, which suppresses the MAPK pathway. **Therapeutic Effect:** Inhibits tumor cell growth.

PHARMACOKINETICS

Widely distributed. Metabolized in liver. Protein binding: 86%. Peak plasma concentration: 2 hrs. Steady state reached in 15 days. Excreted in urine (47%), feces (47%). **Half-life:** 3.5 hrs.

⌛ LIFESPAN CONSIDERATIONS

Pregnancy/Lactation: Avoid pregnancy; may cause fetal harm. Female pts of reproductive potential must use effective nonhormonal contraception (e.g., barrier methods) during treatment and for at least 2 wks after discontinuation. Unknown if distributed in breast milk. Breastfeeding not recommended during treatment and for at least 2 wks after discontinuation. **Males:** May impair fertility. **Children:** Safety and efficacy not established. **Elderly:** No age-related precautions noted.

INTERACTIONS

DRUG: Strong CYP3A4 inhibitors (e.g., clarithromycin, ketoconazole), moderate CYP3A4 inhibitors (e.g., ciprofloxacin, dilTIAZem, fluconazole, verapamil) may increase concentration/effect. **Strong CYP3A4 inducers (e.g., carBAMazepine, phenytoin, rifAMPin)** may decrease concentration/effect. May decrease concentration/effect of **oral contraceptives. QT interval–prolonging medications (e.g., amiodarone, azithromycin, haloperidol, sotalol)** may increase risk of QTc interval prolongation. **HERBAL:** None significant. **FOOD: Grapefruit products** may increase concentration/effect; avoid use. **LAB VALUES:** May increase serum alkaline phosphatase, ALT, AST, creatinine, GGT, glucose, magnesium. May decrease serum sodium; Hct, Hgb, leukocytes, lymphocytes, neutrophils, RBCs.

AVAILABILITY (Rx)

Capsules: 75 mg.

ADMINISTRATION/HANDLING

PO

• Give without regard to food. • If a dose is missed or vomiting occurs after administration, give next dose at regularly scheduled time • Do not give a missed dose within 12 hrs of next dose. • Administer whole; do not break, cut, or open capsule. Capsule cannot be chewed.

INDICATIONS/ROUTES/DOSAGE

Metastatic Melanoma

PO: ADULTS, ELDERLY: 450 mg once daily (in combination with binimetinib). Continue until disease progression or unacceptable toxicity. If binimetinib withheld, reduce encorafenib dose to 300 mg until binimetinib is restarted.

Dose Reduction for Adverse Reactions (metastatic)

First dose reduction: 300 mg once daily. **Second dose reduction:** 225 mg once daily. **Unable to tolerate 225-mg dose:** Permanently discontinue.

Colorectal Cancer, Metastatic (with BRAF V600E mutation)

PO: ADULTS, ELDERLY: 300 mg once daily (in combination with cetuximab). Continue until disease progression or unacceptable toxicity.

Dose Reduction for Adverse Reactions (CRC)

First dose reduction: 225 mg once daily. **Second dose reduction:** 150 mg once daily. **Unable to tolerate 150-mg dose:** Permanently discontinue.

Dose Modification

Based on Common Terminology Criteria for Adverse Events (CTCAE). See prescribing information for binimetinib for recommended dose modification.

Dermatologic Reactions

Grade 2 skin reaction: If not improved within 2 wks, withhold treatment until improved to Grade 1 or 0, then resume at same dose. **Grade 3 skin reaction:** Withhold treatment until improved to Grade 1 or 0, then resume at same dose for first occurrence or at reduced dose for subsequent occurrence. **Grade 4 skin reaction:** Permanently discontinue.

Hepatotoxicity

Grade 2 serum ALT, AST elevation: Maintain dose. If not improved within 4 wks, withhold treatment until improved to Grade 1 or 0 (or to pretreatment baseline), then resume at same dose. **Grade 3 or 4 serum ALT, AST elevation:** See Other Adverse Reactions.

New Primary Malignancies

Noncutaneous RAS mutation–positive malignancies: Permanently discontinue.

QTc Interval Prolongation

QTcF interval greater than 500 msec and less than or equal to 60 msec from baseline: Withhold treatment until QTcF is less than or equal to 500 msec, then resume at reduced dose. **QTcF interval greater than 500 msec and greater than 60 msec from baseline:** Permanently discontinue.

Uveitis

Grade 1 or 2 uveitis that does not respond to ocular therapy; Grade 3 uveitis: Withhold treatment for up to 6 wks. If symptoms improve, resume at same or reduced dose. If not improved, permanently discontinue.

Other Adverse Reactions (Including hemorrhage)

Any recurrent Grade 2 reaction; first occurrence of any Grade 3 reaction: Withhold treatment for up to 4 wks. If improved to Grade 1 or 0 (or to pretreatment baseline), resume at reduced dose. If not improved, permanently discontinue. **First occurrence of any Grade 4 reaction:** Permanently discontinue or withhold treatment for up to 4 wks. If improved to Grade 1 or 0 (or to pretreatment baseline), resume at reduced dose. If not improved, permanently discontinue. **Recurrent Grade 3 reaction:** Consider permanent discontinuation. **Recurrent Grade 4 reaction:** Permanently discontinue.

Concomitant Use With CYP3A Inhibitors

If strong CYP3A inhibitor cannot be discontinued, reduce dose to one-third of the dose prior to use of strong CYP3A inhibitor. If moderate CYP3A inhibitor cannot be discontinued, reduce dose to one-half of the dose prior to use of moderate CYP3A inhibitor. If CYP3A inhibitor is discontinued for 3–5 half-lives, may resume dose prior to starting CYP3A inhibitor.

Dosage in Renal Impairment

Mild impairment: No dose adjustment. **Moderate to severe impairment:** Not specified; use caution.

Dosage in Hepatic Impairment

Mild to moderate impairment: No dose adjustment. **Severe impairment:** Not specified; use caution.

SIDE EFFECTS

Frequent (43%-14%): Fatigue, nausea, vomiting, abdominal pain, arthralgia, hyperkeratosis, myopathy, rash, headache, constipation, pyrexia, dry skin, dizziness, alopecia. **Occasional (13%–3%):** Pruritus, peripheral neuropathy, extremity pain, dysgeusia, acneiform dermatitis.

ADVERSE EFFECTS/TOXIC REACTIONS

Anemia, leukopenia, lymphopenia, neutropenia is an expected response to therapy. In pts receiving combination therapy, new primary cutaneous malignancies including cutaneous squamous cell carcinoma (including keratoacanthoma) (3% of pts), basal cell carcinoma (2% of pts) have occurred. In pts receiving single-agent therapy, new primary cutaneous malignancies including cutaneous squamous cell carcinoma (including keratoacanthoma) (8% of pts), basal cell carcinoma (1% of pts), new primary melanoma (5% of pts) have occurred. May increase potential for new primary noncutaneous malignancies associated with activation of RAS through mutation. May increase cellular proliferation of BRAF wild-type cells and activate MAP-kinase signaling. Serious hemorrhagic events including GI bleeding, rectal bleeding (4% of pts), hematochezia (3% of pts), hemorrhoidal hemorrhage (1% of pts) were reported. Fatal intracranial hemorrhage reported in 2% of pts in the setting of new or progressive brain metastasis. Uveitis, including iritis and iridocyclitis, occurred in 4% of pts. QTc interval prolongation reported in 1% of pts. Grade 3 or 4 dermatologic toxicities reported in 21% of pts when used as a single agent. Other reactions occurring in less than 10% of pts include facial paresis, pancreatitis, panniculitis, drug hypersensitivity.

NURSING CONSIDERATIONS

BASELINE ASSESSMENT

Obtain CBC, BMP, LFT; pregnancy test in female pts of reproductive potential. Confirm compliance of effective nonhormonal contraception. Correct hypokalemia, hypomagnesemia prior to and during treatment. Confirm presence of BRAF V600E or V600K mutation in tumor specimen. Perform full dermatologic exam; assess skin for moles, lesions, papillomas. Consider baseline ECG in pts at risk for QTc interval prolongation. Receive full medication history and screen for interactions (esp. QTc interval–prolonging medications). Question history of diabetes, hepatic/renal impairment, HF. Screen for active infection. Offer emotional support.

INTERVENTION/EVALUATION

Monitor CBC for anemia, leukopenia, lymphopenia, neutropenia; LFT for hepatotoxicity (bruising, hematuria, jaundice, right upper abdominal pain, nausea, vomiting, weight loss); serum potassium, magnesium in pts with QTc interval prolongation. Assess skin for new lesions, toxicities q2mos during treatment and up to 6 mos after discontinuation. Assess for eye pain/redness, visual changes at each office visit and at regular intervals. Monitor for toxicities if discontinuation of CYP3A inhibitor or CYP3A inducer is unavoidable. Monitor for signs of hyperglycemia (thirst, polyuria, confusion, dehydration). If QT interval–prolonging medications cannot be withheld, diligently monitor ECG for QT interval prolongation, cardiac arrhythmias. Monitor for GI bleeding, bloody stool; symptoms of intracranial bleeding (aphasia, blindness, confusion, facial droop, hemiplegia, seizures). Diligently screen for infections.

PATIENT/FAMILY TEACHING

• Treatment may depress your immune system and reduce your ability to fight infection. Report symptoms of infection such as body aches, chills, cough, fatigue, fever. Avoid those with active infection. • Expect frequent eye exams, skin exams. • Report any vision changes, eye redness. • Treatment may cause new skin cancers. Report new warts, moles. • Report symptoms of liver problems (bruising, confusion; dark, amber- or orange-colored urine; right upper abdominal pain, yellowing of the skin or eyes); hemorrhagic stroke (confusion, difficulty speaking, one-sided weakness or paralysis, loss of vision), GI bleeding such (bloody stools, rectal bleeding). • Use effective contraception to avoid pregnancy. Do not breastfeed. • Avoid grapefruit products, herbal supplements (esp. St. John's wort). • Report palpitations, chest pain, shortness of breath, dizziness, fainting; may indicate arrhythmia. •

enfortumab vedotin-ejfv

en-**fort**-ue-mab ve-**doe**-tin
(Padcev)
Do not confuse enfortumab with brentuximab vedotin, or elotuzumab.

◆CLASSIFICATION

PHARMACOTHERAPEUTIC: Anti-Nectin-4, antibody-drug conjugate (ADC), monoclonal antibody. **CLINICAL:** Antineoplastic.

USES

Treatment of adults with locally advanced or metastatic urothelial carcinoma who have previously received a programmed death receptor-1 (PD-1) or programmed death-ligand 1 (PD-L1) inhibitor and a platinum-containing chemotherapy in the neoadjuvant/adjuvant, locally advanced, or metastatic setting.

PRECAUTIONS

Contraindications: Hypersensitivity to enfortumab vedotin-ejfv. **Cautions:** Baseline cytopenias, diabetes, pts at risk for hyperglycemia (e.g., diabetes, chronic use of corticosteroids); conditions predisposing to infection (e.g., diabetes, renal failure, immunocompromised pts, open wounds); dermatologic disease; history of herpes zoster infection; concomitant use of CYP3A4 inhibitors. Not recommended in pts with moderate to severe hepatic impairment.

ACTION

Binds to and internalizes Nectin-4 antibody conjugated to a microtubule-disrupting agent, monomethyl auristatin E (MMAE). MMAE binds to and disrupts cellular microtubule network, causing cell cycle arrest and apoptosis (cellular death). **Therapeutic Effect:** Inhibits tumor cell growth.

PHARMACOKINETICS

Widely distributed. Metabolized via catabolism to small peptides, amino acids, unconjugated MMAE, unconjugated MMAE-related catabolites. Protein binding: 68%–82%. Peak plasma concentration: ADC: at end of infusion; MMAE: 2 days. Excreted in feces (17%), urine (6%). **Half-life:** ADC: 3.4 days; MMAE: 2.4 days.

LIFESPAN CONSIDERATIONS

Pregnancy/Lactation: Avoid pregnancy; may cause fetal harm. Females of reproductive potential must use effective contraception during treatment and for at least 2 mos after discontinuation. Unknown if distributed in breast milk. Breastfeeding not recommended during treatment and for at least 3 wks after discontinuation. May impair fertility. **Males:** Males with females of reproductive potential must use effective contraception during treatment and for at least 4 mos after discontinuation. **Children:** Safety and efficacy not established. **Elderly:** No age-related precautions noted.

INTERACTIONS

DRUG: **Strong CYP3A4 inhibitors (e.g., clarithromycin, ketoconazole, ritonavir)** may increase concentration/effect. **Strong CYP3A4 inducers (e.g., carBAMazepine, phenytoin, rifAMPin)** may decrease concentration/effect. **HERBAL:** None significant. **FOOD:** None known. **LAB VALUES:** May increase serum creatinine, glucose, lipase, uric acid. May decrease serum phosphate, potassium, sodium; Hgb, leukocytes, lymphocytes, neutrophils, platelets.

AVAILABILITY (Rx)

Injection, Powder for Reconstitution: 20 mg, 30 mg.

ADMINISTRATION/HANDLING

IV

Reconstitution • Must be prepared by personnel trained in aseptic manipulations and admixing of cytotoxic drugs. • Calculate the number of vials needed for reconstitution based on weight in kg. • Directing stream toward glass wall of vial, reconstitute 20-mg vial with 2.3 mL or 30-mg vial with 3.3 mL of Sterile Water for Injection to a final concentration of 10 mg/mL. • To prevent foaming, swirl vial gently until powder is completely dissolved. • Allow contents to settle until all bubbles are gone (at least 1 min). Do not shake or agitate. • Visually inspect for particulate matter or discoloration. Solution should appear clear to slightly opalescent, colorless to slightly yellow in color. Do not use if solution is cloudy or discolored or if visible particles are observed. • Dilute in infusion bag of 5% Dextrose, 0.9% NaCl, or lactated Ringer's to a final concentration of 0.3–4 mg/mL. • Do

not shake or agitate diluted solution. • Discard unused portions of vial.
Rate of administration • Give over 30 min via dedicated IV line. • Do not infuse as IV push or bolus.
Storage • Refrigerate unused vials in original carton. • May refrigerate reconstituted vials for up to 4 hrs. • May refrigerate diluted solution for up to 8 hrs. • Protect from light. • Do not shake, agitate, or freeze.

IV INCOMPATABILITIES

Do not mix with other medications or other infusion solutions that contain medications.

INDICATIONS/ROUTES/DOSAGE

Urothelial Carcinoma

IV: ADULTS, ELDERLY: 1.25 mg/kg (up to a maximum of 125 mg for pts weighing greater than or equal to 100 kg) on days 1, 8, and 15 of a 28-day cycle. Continue until disease progression or unacceptable toxicity.

Dose Reduction Schedule for Adverse Events

First dose reduction: 1 mg/kg up to 100 mg.
Second dose reduction: 0.75 mg/kg up to 75 mg.
Third dose reduction: 0.5 mg/kg up to 50 mg.

Dose Modification

Based on Common Terminology Criteria for Adverse Events (CTCAE).

Hyperglycemia

Serum blood glucose greater than 250 mg/dL: Withhold treatment until serum blood glucose level is less than or equal to 250 mg/dL, then resume at same dose.

Peripheral Neuropathy

Grade 2 peripheral neuropathy: Withhold treatment until improved to Grade 1 or 0, then resume at same dose. If neuropathy recurs, withhold treatment until improved to Grade 1 or 0, then resume at reduced dose level. **Grade 3 or 4 peripheral neuropathy:** Permanently discontinue.

Thrombocytopenia

Grade 2 or 3 thrombocytopenia: Withhold treatment until improved to Grade 1 or 0, then resume at same dose or reduced dose level. **Grade 4 thrombocytopenia:** Permanently discontinue.

Skin Toxicity

Grade 3 rash, pruritus, cutaneous reactions: Withhold treatment until improved to Grade 1 or 0, then resume at same dose or reduced dose level. **Grade 4 or recurrent Grade 3 rash, pruritus, cutaneous reactions:** Permanently discontinue.

Other Nonhematologic Toxicity

Grade 3 nonhematologic toxicity: Withhold treatment until improved to Grade 1 or 0, then resume at same dose or reduced dose level. **Grade 4 nonhematologic toxicity:** Permanently discontinue.

Dosage in Renal Impairment

Mild to severe impairment: No dose adjustment.

Dosage in Hepatic Impairment

Mild impairment: No dose adjustment. **Moderate to severe impairment:** Not recommended.

SIDE EFFECTS

Frequent (56%–26%): Fatigue, asthenia, decreased appetite, nausea, dysgeusia, diarrhea, dry eye, eye irritation, increased lacrimation, ocular discomfort, rash, erythema, skin exfoliation, urticaria, alopecia, dry skin, pruritus. **Occasional (18%):** Vomiting.

ADVERSE EFFECTS/TOXIC REACTIONS

Myelosuppression (anemia, leukopenia, lymphopenia, neutropenia) is an expected response to therapy. Fatal cases of hyperglycemia, diabetic ketoacidosis (DKA) were reported in pts regardless of history of diabetes. Grade 3 or 4 hyperglycemia was reported in 8% of pts, and more prevalent in pts with higher body mass index and in pts with elevated hemoglobin A1c. Peripheral neuropathy including hypoesthesia, gait disturbance, muscular weakness, paresthesia, peripheral motor/sensorimotor neuropathy reported in 49% of pts. Ocular disorders including keratitis, blurred vision, limbal stem cell deficiency, and other events associated with dry eyes have occurred. Grade 3 or 4 skin reactions including symmetrical drug-related intertriginous and flexural exanthema, bullous dermatitis, exfoliative dermatitis, palmar-plantar erythrodysesthesia (redness, swelling, numbness, skin sloughing of the hands and feet) reported in 10% of pts. Skin and soft tissue infusion site extravasation with secondary cellulitis, bullae, exfoliation reported in 1% of pts. Other serious reactions including UTI (6% of pts), cellulitis (5% of pts), febrile neutropenia (4% of pts), sepsis (3% of pts), acute kidney injury (3% of pts); acute respiratory failure, aspiration pneumonia, cardiac disorder (less than 1% of pts) may occur. GI events including colitis, enterocolitis were reported. Herpes zoster infection reported in 3% of pts. Immunogenicity (anti–enfortumab vedotin antibodies) reported in 1% of pts.

NURSING CONSIDERATIONS

BASELINE ASSESSMENT

Obtain weight in kilograms. Obtain CBC, LFT, blood glucose level, pregnancy test in females of reproductive potential. Verify compliance of effective contraception in females and males with female partners of reproductive potential. Obtain visual acuity. Screen for active infection. Question history of dermatological disease, hepatic impairment, optic disorders. Receive full medication history and screen for interactions. Offer emotional support.

INTERVENTION/EVALUATION

Monitor CBC, LFT, blood glucose levels periodically. Monitor for hyperglycemia (blurred vision, confusion, excessive thirst, Kussmaul respirations, polyuria); new onset or worsening peripheral neuropathy. Assess skin for dermatologic toxicities, palmar-plantar erythrodysesthesia. Consider topical corticosteroid if dermatologic effects occur. Consider artificial tears for dry eye prophylaxis. If symptoms do not resolve, consider treatment with topical steroids and referral to ophthalmologist. Monitor for drug toxicities if discontinuation or dose reduction of concomitant CYP3A inhibitor is unavoidable. If extravasation occurs, stop infusion and monitor for adverse reactions. Monitor daily pattern of bowel activity, stool consistency. Monitor for infections (cough, fatigue, fever). If serious infection, sepsis occurs, initiate appropriate antimicrobial therapy.

PATIENT/FAMILY TEACHING

• Treatment may depress your immune system and reduce your ability to fight infection. Report symptoms of infection such as body aches, burning with urination, chills, cough, fatigue, fever. Avoid those with active infection. • Report symptoms of bone marrow depression (e.g., bruising, fatigue, fever, shortness of breath, weight loss; bleeding easily, bloody urine or stool). • Report change of vision, blurry vision, dry eye symptoms not relieved by artificial tears. • Report symptoms of toxic skin reactions (e.g., itching, peeling, rash, redness, swelling); high blood sugar levels (e.g., blurred vision, excessive thirst/hunger, headache, frequent urination); or nervous system changes (e.g., altered memory, confusion, delirium, difficulty speaking, gait disturbance, numbness, tremors). • Females of childbearing potential must use effective contraception during treatment and for at least 2 mos after last dose. Do not breastfeed. Males with female partners of childbearing potential must use effective contraception during treatment and for at least 4 mos after last dose. • There is a high risk of interactions with other medications. Do not take any newly prescribed medications unless approved by prescriber who originally started treatment. Avoid grapefruit products, herbal supplements (esp. St. John's wort). • Diarrhea is a common side effect. Drink plenty of fluids.

enoxaparin

TOP 100 HIGH ALERT

en-**ox**-a-par-in
(Lovenox)

■ **BLACK BOX ALERT** ■ Epidural or spinal anesthesia greatly increases potential for spinal or epidural hematoma, subsequent long-term or permanent paralysis. **Do not confuse Lovenox with Lasix, Levaquin, Lotronex, or Protonix, or enoxaparin with dalteparin or heparin.**

◆CLASSIFICATION

PHARMACOTHERAPEUTIC: Low molecular weight heparin. **CLINICAL:** Anticoagulant.

USES

DVT prophylaxis following hip or knee replacement surgery, abdominal surgery, or pts with severely restricted mobility during acute illness. Treatment of acute coronary syndrome (ACS): unstable angina, non–Q-wave MI, acute ST-segment elevation MI (STEMI). Treatment of DVT with or without pulmonary embolism (PE) (inpatient); without PE (outpatient). **OFF-LABEL:** DVT prophylaxis following moderate-risk general surgery, gynecologic surgery; management of venous thromboembolism (VTE) during pregnancy. Bariatric surgery, mechanical heart valve to bridge anticoagulation, percutaneous coronary intervention (PCI) adjunctive therapy.

PRECAUTIONS

Contraindications: Hypersensitivity to enoxaparin. Active major bleeding, concurrent heparin therapy, hypersensitivity to heparin, pork products. History of heparin-induced thrombocytopenia (HIT) in past 100 days or in the presence of circulating antibodies. **Cautions:** Conditions with increased risk of hemorrhage, platelet defects, renal impairment (renal failure), elderly, uncontrolled arterial hypertension, history of recent GI ulceration or hemorrhage. When neuraxial anesthesia (epidural or spinal anesthesia) or spinal puncture is used, pts anticoagulated or scheduled to be anticoagulated with enoxaparin for prevention of thromboembolic complications are at risk for developing an epidural or spinal hematoma that can result in long-term or permanent paralysis. Bacterial endocarditis, hemorrhagic stroke, history of heparin-induced thrombocytopenia (HIT), severe hepatic disease.

ACTION

Enhances the inhibition rate of clotting proteases by antithrombin III. Impairs normal hemostasis and inhibition of factor Xa. **Therapeutic Effect:** Produces anticoagulation. Does not significantly influence PT, aPTT.

PHARMACOKINETICS

Route	Onset	Peak	Duration
SQ	N/A	3–5 hrs	12 hrs

Well absorbed after SQ administration. Excreted primarily in urine. Not removed by hemodialysis. **Half-life:** 4.5–7 hrs.

LIFESPAN CONSIDERATIONS

Pregnancy/Lactation: Use with caution, particularly during third trimester, immediate postpartum period (increased risk of maternal hemorrhage). Unknown if distributed in breast milk. Pregnant women with mechanical heart valves (and their fetuses) may have increased risk of bleeding. **Children:** Safety and efficacy not established in pts younger than 1 mo. **Elderly:** May be more susceptible to bleeding.

E

INTERACTIONS

DRUG: **Anticoagulants (e.g., apixaban, dabigatran, edoxaban, rivaroxaban), antiplatelets (e.g., aspirin, clopidogrel, ticagrelor), NSAIDs (ibuprofen, ketorolac, naproxen), thrombolytics (e.g., alteplase), warfarin** may increase anticoagulant effect; risk of bleeding. **HERBAL:** **Herbals with anticoagulant/antiplatelet activity (e.g., garlic, ginger, ginkgo biloba)** may increase adverse effects. **FOOD:** None known. **LAB VALUES:** Increases serum alkaline phosphatase, ALT, AST. May decrease Hgb, Hct, platelets, RBCs.

AVAILABILITY (Rx)

Injection Solution: 30 mg/0.3 mL, 40 mg/0.4 mL, 60 mg/0.6 mL, 80 mg/0.8 mL, 100 mg/mL, 120 mg/0.8 mL, 150 mg/mL in prefilled syringes.

ADMINISTRATION/HANDLING

◀ALERT▶ Do not mix with other injections, infusions. Do not give IM.

SQ

Preparation • Visually inspect for particulate matter or discoloration. Solution should appear clear, colorless to pale yellow in color. Do not use if solution is cloudy, discolored, or if visible particles are observed.
Administration • Flick syringe so that the air bubble rises toward the plunger. • Insert needle subcutaneously into abdomen or outer thigh and inject solution (including air bubble). • Do not inject into areas of active skin disease or injury such as sunburns, skin rashes, inflammation, skin infections, or active psoriasis. • Rotate injection sites.
Storage • Store at room temperature.

INDICATIONS/ROUTES/DOSAGE

Prevention of Deep Vein Thrombosis (DVT) After Hip and Knee Surgery

SQ: ADULTS, ELDERLY: **Knee surgery:** 30 mg twice daily, generally for 10 days or up to 35 days, with initial dose given 12 hrs or more pre-operatively or 12 hrs or more post-operatively once hemostasis achieved. **Hip surgery: (Once daily):** An initial dose of 40 mg, given 12 hrs or more pre-operatively or 12 hrs or more post-operatively once hemostasis achieved. Following hip surgery, recommend continuing 40 mg once daily for at least 10 days or up to 35 days post-op. **(Twice daily):** 30 mg q12h with initial dose, 12 hrs or more pre-operatively or 12 hrs or more post-operatively once hemostasis achieved and q12h for at least 10 days or up to 35 days.

Prevention of DVT After Non-Orthopedic Surgery

SQ: ADULTS, ELDERLY: 40 mg/day for 7–10 days, with initial dose given 2 hrs before abdominal surgery or approximately 12 hrs before other surgeries.

Prevention of DVT After Bariatric Surgery

BMI 50 kg/m^2 or less: 40 mg q12h. **BMI greater than 50 kg/m^2:** 60 mg q12h.

Prevention of Long-Term DVT in Nonsurgical Acute Illness

SQ: ADULTS, ELDERLY: 40 mg once daily; continue until risk of DVT has diminished (usually 6–11 days).

Prevention of Ischemic Complications of Unstable Angina, Non–Q-Wave MI (With oral aspirin therapy)

SQ: ADULTS, ELDERLY: 1 mg/kg q12h (with oral aspirin).

STEMI

SQ: ADULTS YOUNGER THAN 75 YRS: 30 mg IV once plus 1 mg/kg q12h (**maximum:** 100 mg first 2 doses only). **ADULTS 75 YRS OR OLDER:** 0.75 mg/kg (**maximum:** 75 mg first 2 doses only) q12h.

Acute DVT

SQ: ADULTS, ELDERLY: (inpatient): 1 mg/kg q12h or 1.5 mg/kg once daily. **(outpatient):** 1 mg/kg q12h.

Usual Pediatric Dosage

SQ: CHILDREN 2 MOS AND OLDER: 0.5 mg/kg q12h (prophylaxis); 1 mg/kg q12h (treatment). **NEONATES, INFANTS YOUNGER THAN 2 MOS:** 0.75/mg/kg/dose q12h (prophylaxis); 1.5 mg/kg/dose q12h (treatment).

Dosage in Renal Impairment

Elimination is decreased when CrCl is less than 30 mL/min. Monitor and adjust dosage as necessary.

Use	Dosage
Abdominal surgery, pts with acute illness	30 mg once/day
Hip, knee surgery	30 mg once/day
DVT, angina, MI	1 mg/kg once/day
STEMI: (younger than 75 yrs)	30 mg IV once plus 1 mg/kg q24h
STEMI (75 yrs or older)	1 mg/kg q24h
NSTEMI	1 mg/kg q24h

Dosage in Hepatic Impairment

Use caution.

SIDE EFFECTS

Occasional (4%–1%): Injection site hematoma, nausea, peripheral edema.

ADVERSE EFFECTS/TOXIC REACTIONS

May lead to bleeding complications ranging from local ecchymoses to major hemorrhage. May cause heparin-induced thrombocytopenia (HIT). **Antidote:** IV injection of protamine sulfate (1% solution) equal to dose of enoxaparin injected. 1 mg protamine sulfate neutralizes 1 mg enoxaparin. One additional dose of 0.5 mg protamine sulfate per 1 mg enoxaparin may be given if aPTT tested 2–4 hrs after first injection remains prolonged.

NURSING CONSIDERATIONS

BASELINE ASSESSMENT

Obtain baseline CBC. Note platelet count. Question medical history as listed in Precautions. Ensure that pt has not received spinal anesthesia, spinal procedures. Assess for active bleeding. Assess pt's willingness to self-inject medication. Assess potential risk of bleeding.

INTERVENTION/EVALUATION

Periodically monitor CBC, platelet count, stool for occult blood (no need for daily monitoring in pts with normal presurgical coagulation parameters). A decrease in the platelet count of more than 50% from baseline may indicate heparin-induced thrombocytopenia. Ensure active hemostasis of puncture site following PCI. Assess for any sign of bleeding (bleeding at surgical site, hematuria, blood in stool, bleeding from gums, petechiae, bruising, bleeding from injection sites).

PATIENT/FAMILY TEACHING

• Usual length of therapy is 7–10 days. • A healthcare provider will show you how to properly prepare and inject your medication. You must demonstrate correct preparation and injection techniques before using medication at home. • Do not discontinue current blood thinning regimen or take any newly prescribed medications unless approved by the prescriber who originally started treatment. • Suddenly stopping therapy may increase the risk of blood clots or stroke. • Report bleeding of any kind (bloody urine, stool; nosebleeds; increased menstrual bleeding). If bleeding occurs, it may take longer to stop bleeding. • Immediately report signs of stroke (confusion, headache, numbness, one-sided weakness, trouble speaking, loss of vision). • Minor blunt force trauma to the head, chest, or abdomen can be life-threatening. • Do not take aspirin, herbal supplements, OTC nonsteroidal anti-inflammatories (may increase risk of bleeding). • Consult physician before any surgery/dental work. • Use electric razor, soft toothbrush to prevent bleeding.

entecavir

en-**tek**-a-veer
(Baraclude, Apo-Entecavir ✱)

■ BLACK BOX ALERT ■ Serious, sometimes fatal hypersensitivity reaction, lactic acidosis, severe hepatomegaly with steatosis (fatty liver) have occurred. May cause HIV resistance in chronic hepatitis B pts. Severe acute exacerbations of hepatitis B virus infection may occur upon discontinuation of entecavir.

◆ CLASSIFICATION

PHARMACOTHERAPEUTIC: Reverse transcriptase inhibitor, nucleoside. **CLINICAL:** Antihepadnaviral agent.

USES

Treatment of chronic hepatitis B virus (HBV) infection in adults and children 2 yrs and older with evidence of active viral replication and evidence of either persistent transaminase elevations or histologically active disease or evidence of decompensated hepatic disease. **OFF-LABEL:** HBV reinfection prophylaxis, post–liver transplant, HIV/HBV coinfection.

PRECAUTIONS

Contraindications: Hypersensitivity to entecavir. **Cautions:** Renal impairment, pts receiving concurrent therapy that may reduce renal function. Pts at risk for hepatic disease. Cross resistance may develop with lamivudine.

ACTION

Inhibits hepatitis B viral polymerase, an enzyme blocking reverse transcriptase activity. **Therapeutic Effect:** Interferes with viral DNA synthesis.

PHARMACOKINETICS

Poorly absorbed from GI tract. Protein binding: 13%. Extensively distributed into tissues. Partially metabolized in liver. Excreted primarily in urine. **Half-life:** 5–6 days (increased in renal impairment).

⌛ LIFESPAN CONSIDERATIONS

Pregnancy/Lactation: Unknown if drug crosses placenta or is distributed in breast milk. **Children:** Safety and efficacy not established in pts younger than 16 yrs. **Elderly:** Age-related renal impairment may require dosage adjustment.

INTERACTIONS

DRUG: **Cladribine** may decrease therapeutic effect. **HERBAL:** None significant. **FOOD:** **Food** delays absorption, decreases concentration. **LAB VALUES:** May increase serum amylase, lipase, bilirubin, ALT, AST, creatinine, glucose. May decrease serum albumin; platelets.

AVAILABILITY (Rx)

Oral Solution: 0.05 mg/mL. **Tablets:** 0.5 mg, 1 mg.

ADMINISTRATION/HANDLING

PO

• Administer tablets on an empty stomach (at least 2 hrs after a meal and 2 hrs before the next meal). • Do not dilute, mix oral solution with water or any other liquid. • Each bottle of oral solution is accompanied by a dosing spoon. Before administering, hold spoon in vertical position, fill it gradually to mark corresponding to prescribed dose.

Storage • Store tablets, oral solution at room temperature.

INDICATIONS/ROUTES/DOSAGE

Chronic Hepatitis B Virus Infection (No previous nucleoside treatment)

PO: ADULTS, ELDERLY, CHILDREN 16 YRS AND OLDER: 0.5 mg once daily. **CHILDREN 2 YRS AND OLDER, WEIGHING MORE THAN 30 KG:** 0.5 mg once daily (tablet or solution). **27–30 KG:** 0.45 mg once daily (solution). **24–26 KG:** 0.4 mg once daily (solution). **21–23 KG:** 0.35 mg once daily (solution). **18–20 KG:** 0.3 mg once daily (solution). **15–17 KG:** 0.25 mg once daily (solution). **12–14 KG:** 0.2 mg once daily (solution). **10–11 KG:** 0.15 mg once daily (solution).

Chronic Hepatitis B Virus Infection (Receiving lamiVUDine, known lamiVUDine resistance, decompensated liver disease)

PO: ADULTS, ELDERLY, CHILDREN 16 YRS AND OLDER: 1 mg once daily. **CHILDREN 2 YRS AND OLDER, WEIGHING MORE THAN 30 KG:** 1 mg once daily (tablet or solution). **27–30 KG:** 0.9 mg once daily (solution). **24–26 KG:** 0.8 mg once daily (solution). **21–23 KG:** 0.7 mg once daily (solution). **18–20 KG:** 0.6 mg once daily (solution). **15–17 KG:** 0.5 mg once daily (solution). **12–14 KG:** 0.4 mg once daily (solution). **10–11 KG:** 0.3 mg once daily (solution).

Dosage in Renal Impairment

Creatinine Clearance	Dosage
50 mL/min and greater	0.5 mg once daily
30–49 mL/min	0.25 mg once daily
10–29 mL/min	0.15 mg once daily
9 mL/min and less	0.05 mg once daily

Dosage in Hepatic Impairment

No dose adjustment.

SIDE EFFECTS

Occasional (4%–3%): Headache, fatigue. **Rare (less than 1%):** Diarrhea, dyspepsia, nausea, vomiting, dizziness, insomnia.

ADVERSE EFFECTS/TOXIC REACTIONS

Lactic acidosis, severe hepatomegaly with steatosis have been reported. Severe, acute exacerbations of hepatitis B virus infection have been reported in pts who have discontinued therapy; reinitiation of antihepatitis B therapy may be required. Hematuria occurs occasionally. May cause development of HIV resistance if HIV untreated.

NURSING CONSIDERATIONS

BASELINE ASSESSMENT

Obtain HIV status. Obtain LFT before beginning therapy and at periodic intervals during therapy. Offer emotional support. Obtain full medication history.

INTERVENTION/EVALUATION

Hepatic function should be monitored closely with both clinical and laboratory follow-up for at least several mos in pts who discontinue antihepatitis B therapy. For pts on therapy, closely monitor serum amylase, lipase, bilirubin, ALT, AST, creatinine, glucose, albumin; platelet count. Assess for evidence of GI discomfort.

PATIENT/FAMILY TEACHING

• Take medication at least 2 hrs after a meal and 2 hrs before the next meal. • Avoid transmission of hepatitis B infection to others through sexual contact, blood contamination. • Immediately report unusual muscle pain, abdominal pain with nausea/vomiting, cold feeling in extremities, dizziness (signs and symptoms signaling onset of lactic acidosis).

entrectinib

en-**trek**-ti-nib
(Rozlytrek)

Do not confuse entrectinib with alectinib, enasidenib, encorafenib, erdafitinib, erlotinib, fedratinib, or larotrectinib.

◆Classification

PHARMACOTHERAPEUTIC: Tropomyosin receptor kinase (TRK) inhibitor. **CLINICAL:** Antineoplastic.

USES

Treatment of adults with metastatic non–small-cell lung cancer (NSCLC) whose tumors are ROS1 positive. Treatment of adult and pediatric pts (12 yrs and older) with solid tumors that have a neurotrophic receptor tyrosine kinase (NTRK) gene fusion without a known acquired resistance mutation; are metastatic or where surgical resection is likely to result in severe morbidity; and have no satisfactory alternative treatment or that have progressed following treatment.

PRECAUTIONS

Contraindications: Hypersensitivity to entrectinib. **Cautions:** Baseline cytopenias, hepatic impairment, cardiac disease (cardiomyopathy, HF), conditions predisposing to infection (e.g., diabetes, immunocompromised pts, renal failure, open wounds), pts at risk for bone fractures (e.g., fall risk, osteoporosis, chronic use of corticosteroids), pts at risk for QTc interval prolongation, cardiac arrhythmias (congenital long QT syndrome, HF, concomitant use of QT interval–prolonging medications, hypokalemia, hypomagnesemia); pts at high risk for suicide ideation and behavior (e.g., history of depression, mood disorder, psychiatric disorder). History of hyperuricemia, gout. Avoid concomitant use of moderate or strong CYP3A inhibitors/inducers.

ACTION

Inhibits activation of tropomyosin receptor kinase (TRK) proteins encoded by NTRK gene fusions. Inhibits proto-oncogenic tyrosine-protein kinase ROS1 and anaplastic lymphoma kinase (ALK). **Therapeutic Effect:** Inhibits tumor cell proliferation.

PHARMACOKINETICS

Widely distributed. Metabolized in liver. Protein binding: 99%. Peak plasma concentration: 4–6 hrs. Excreted in feces (83%), urine (3%). **Half-life:** 20–40 hrs.

LIFESPAN CONSIDERATIONS

Pregnancy/Lactation: Avoid pregnancy; may cause fetal harm. Females of reproductive potential should use effective contraception during treatment and for at least 5 wks after discontinuation. Unknown if distributed in breast milk. Breastfeeding not recommended during treatment and up to 7 days after discontinuation. **Males:** Males with female partners of reproductive potential should use effective contraception during treatment and for at least 3 mos after discontinuation. **Children:** Safety and efficacy not established in pts younger than 12 yrs. **Elderly:** Safety and efficacy not established.

INTERACTIONS

DRUG: **Strong CYP3A4 inhibitors (e.g., clarithromycin, ketoconazole, ritonavir), moderate CYP3A4 inhibitors (e.g., fluconazole, verapamil)** may increase concentration/effect. **Strong CYP3A4 inducers (e.g., carBAMazepine, phenytoin, rifAMPin), moderate CYP3A inducers (e.g., bosentan, nafcillin)** may decrease concentration/effect. May increase QT interval–prolonging effect of **amiodarone, azithromycin, ciprofloxacin, haloperidol, methadone, sotalol.** **HERBAL:** None significant. **FOOD:** **Grapefruit products** may increase concentration/effect. **LAB VALUES:** May increase serum alkaline phosphatase, ALT, AST, amylase, creatinine, lipase, potassium, sodium, uric acid. May decrease serum albumin, calcium, phosphate; Hgb, RBC, lymphocytes, neutrophils.

AVAILABILITY (Rx)

Capsules: 100 mg, 200 mg.

ADMINISTRATION/HANDLING

PO

• Give without regard to food. Administer capsules whole; do not break, cut, or open. • Capsules cannot be chewed. • If a dose is missed, give as soon as possible unless next dose is due within 12 hrs. • If vomiting occurs immediately after administration, repeat the dose.

INDICATIONS/ROUTES/DOSAGE

NSCLC (ROS1-Positive)

PO: ADULTS: 600 mg once daily. Continue until disease progression or unacceptable toxicity.

Solid Tumors (NTRK gene fusion positive)
PO: ADULTS: 600 mg once daily. Continue until disease progression or unacceptable toxicity. **CHILDREN WITH BODY SURFACE AREA (BSA) GREATER THAN 1.5 m²:** 600 mg once daily. Continue until disease progression or unacceptable toxicity. **BSA 1.11–1.5 m²:** 500 mg once daily. **BSA 0.91–1.1 m²:** 400 mg once daily.

Dose Reduction Schedule

Dose Reduction for Adverse Reactions	Adults/ Children 12 yrs and Older With BSA Greater Than 1.5 m²	Children 12 yrs and Older With BSA 1.11–1.5 m²	Children 12 yrs and Older With BSA 0.91–1.1 m²:
First reduction	400 mg once daily	400 mg once daily	300 mg once daily
Second reduction	200 mg once daily	200 mg onoc daily	200 mg once daily

Permanently discontinue if unable to tolerate two dose reductions.

Dose Modification
Based on Common Terminology Criteria for Adverse Events (CTCAE).
Cardiotoxicity
Grade 2 or 3 HF: Withhold treatment until improved to Grade 1 or 0, then resume at reduced dose level. **Grade 4 HF:** Permanently discontinue. **QTc interval greater than 500 msec:** Withhold treatment until QTc interval recovers to baseline. Resume at the same dose if risk factors for QT interval prolongation are identified and corrected. Resume at a reduced dose if risk factors for QT interval prolongation risk factors are not identified. **Torsades de pointes, polymorphic ventricular tachycardia, symptoms of serious arrhythmia:** Permanently discontinue.

Central Nervous System (CNS) Toxicity
Intolerable Grade 2 CNS effects: Withhold treatment until improved to Grade 1 or baseline, then resume at same dose or reduced dose level. **Grade 3 CNS effects:** Withhold treatment until improved to Grade 1 or baseline, then resume at reduced dose level. **Grade 4 CNS effects:** Permanently discontinue.

Hematologic Toxicity
Grade 3 or 4 anemia or neutropenia: Withhold treatment until improves to Grade 2 or less, then resume at the same or reduced dose.

Hepatotoxicity
Grade 3 hepatotoxicity: Withhold treatment until improved to Grade 1 or baseline. Resume at same dose if resolved within 4 wks. Permanently discontinue if not resolved within 4 wks. **Recurrence of Grade 3 hepatotoxicity:** Resume at reduced dose if resolved within 4 wks. **Grade 4 hepatotoxicity:** Withhold treatment until improved to Grade 1 or baseline. Resume at reduced dose if resolved within 4 wks. Permanently discontinue if not resolved within 4 wks or if Grade 4 hepatotoxicity recurs. **Serum ALT/AST greater than 3 times ULN with bilirubin greater than 1.5 times ULN (without cholestasis or hemolysis):** Permanently discontinue.

Hyperuricemia
Grade 4 or symptomatic hyperuricemia: Start urate-lowering medication. Withhold treatment until improved, then resume or same or reduced dose.

Ocular Toxicity
Grade 2 (or greater) vision disorders: Withhold treatment until improved or stabilized, then resume at the same or reduced dose.

Other Toxicities
Any other Grade 3 or 4 toxicity: Withhold treatment until toxicity improves to Grade 1 or baseline, then resume at the same or reduced dose if resolved within 4 wks. Permanently discontinue if not resolved within 4 wks or if Grade 4 toxicity recurs.

E

Concomitant Use of CYP3A Inhibitor
If strong CYP3A inhibitor cannot be avoided, reduce entrectinib dose to 100 mg. If moderate CYP3A inhibitor cannot be avoided, reduce entrectinib dose to 200 mg. If strong or moderate CYP3A inhibitor is discontinued for 3–5 half-lives, resume entrectinib dose prior to use of CYP3A inhibitor.

E

Dosage in Renal Impairment
Mild to moderate impairment: No dose adjustment. **Severe impairment:** Not specified; use caution.

Dosage in Hepatic Impairment
Mild impairment: No dose adjustment. **Moderate to severe impairment:** Not specified; use caution.

SIDE EFFECTS

Frequent (48%–21%): Fatigue, asthenia, constipation, dysgeusia, edema (facial, generalized, localized, peripheral), dizziness, vertigo, postural dizziness, diarrhea, nausea, dysesthesia, paresthesia, hyperesthesia, hypoesthesia, dysesthesia, oral hypoesthesia, dyspnea, myalgia, musculoskeletal pain, increased weight, cough, vomiting, pyrexia, arthralgia. **Occasional (18%–10%):** Headache, hypotension, abdominal pain, sleep disorder, hypersomnia, insomnia, somnolence, decreased appetite, muscular weakness, back pain, rash, extremity pain, dysphagia, dehydration. **Rare (4%):** Hypoxia, syncope.

ADVERSE EFFECTS/TOXIC REACTIONS

Myelosuppression (anemia, lymphopenia, neutropenia) is an expected response to therapy. HF reported in 3% of pts. Median onset of HF was approx. 2 mos. Myocarditis in the absence of HF reported in less than 1% of pts. CNS effects including altered mental status, aphasia, amnesia, ataxia, balance disorder, cognitive impairment, confusion, delirium, disturbance in attention, hallucinations, memory impairment, peripheral neuropathy reported in 27% of pts. Mood disorders including affect lability, affective disorder, agitation, anxiety, depression, euphoria, irritability, mood swings, psychomotor dysfunction, suicide reported in 10% of pts. Bone fractures (hip, femoral, bilateral femoral neck, tibial shaft) reported in 5% of adults and 23% of pediatric pts. Hepatotoxicity (serum ALT/AST elevation) reported in 36%–42% of pts; Grade 3 or 4 transaminase elevation reported in 3% of pts. Hyperuricemia reported in 9% of pts. QTc interval prolongation of greater than 60 msec (3% of pts) and greater than 500 msec (less than 1% of pts) has occurred. Ocular toxicities including adhesions, blindness, blurry vision, cataract, corneal erosion, diplopia, visual impairment, photophobia, photopsia, retinal hemorrhage, vitreous detachment, vitreous floaters may occur. Infections including respiratory tract infection, lung infection, pneumonia (10% of pts), UTI (13% of pts), sepsis were reported. Other reactions may include pulmonary embolism, falls, GI perforation.

NURSING CONSIDERATIONS

BASELINE ASSESSMENT

Obtain CBC, LFT, serum magnesium, uric acid level; pregnancy test in females of reproductive potential. Verify use of effective contraception in females of reproductive potential. Confirm presence of NTRK gene fusion or ROS1 rearrangements in tumor specimen. Assess risk of QT interval prolongation, fractures, falls. Question history of cardiac disease, HF, gout, hyperuricemia; depression, mood disorder, suicidal ideation and behavior. Obtain ECG; echocardiogram for baseline LVEF. Screen for active infection. Receive full medication history and screen for interactions. Offer emotional support.

INTERVENTION/EVALUATION

Monitor CBC, uric acid level periodically. Monitor LFT for hepatotoxicity (bruising, hematuria, jaundice, right upper abdominal pain, nausea, vomiting, weight loss) q2wks for 1 mo, then monthly thereafter.

Monitor for symptoms of HF (dyspnea, edema, fatigue, palpitations). Assess LVEF by echocardiogram if cardiotoxicity, HF is suspected. Monitor ECG periodically. Diligently assess for suicidal ideation and behavior; new-onset or worsening of anxiety, depression, mood disorder. Consult mental health professional if mood disorder is suspected. Monitor for symptoms of tumor lysis syndrome (acute renal failure, electrolyte imbalance, hyperuricemia, cardiac arrhythmias, seizures); bone fractures (pain, deformity, changes in mobility), hyperuricemia (joint pain/inflammation/redness), PE (chest pain, dyspnea, tachycardia); infections (cough, fatigue, fever). If serious infection or sepsis occurs, initiate appropriate antimicrobial therapy. Assess for visual changes at each office visit. If change of vision occurs, consider referral to ophthalmologist. Assess for CNS effects. Monitor for toxicities if discontinuation of CYP3A inhibitor is unavoidable. If QT interval–prolonging medications cannot be withheld, diligently monitor ECG for QT interval prolongation, cardiac arrhythmias. Monitor daily pattern of bowel activity, stool consistency, I&Os.

PATIENT/FAMILY TEACHING.

• Treatment may depress your immune system and reduce your ability to fight infection. Report symptoms of infection such as body aches, burning with urination, chills, cough, fatigue, fever. Avoid those with active infection. • Report symptoms of bone marrow depression such as bruising, fatigue, fever, shortness of breath, weight loss; bleeding easily, bloody urine or stool. • Therapy may cause vision changes or decrease the heart's ability to pump blood effectively. • Report symptoms of liver problems (bruising, confusion; dark, amber-, orange-colored urine; right upper abdominal pain, yellowing of the skin or eyes); HF (shortness of breath, palpitations; swelling of legs, ankle, feet); bone fractures (e.g., pain, deformity, changes in mobility), gout (joint pain/swelling/redness/warmth), nervous system changes (altered memory, confusion, delirium, difficulty speaking, gait disturbance, numbness, tremors), lung embolism (difficulty breathing, chest pain, rapid heart rate). • Seek immediate medical attention if thoughts of suicide, new onset or worsening of anxiety, depression, or changes in mood occurs. • Avoid tasks that require alertness, motor skills until response to drug is established. • Use effective contraception. Do not breastfeed. • There is a high risk of interactions with other medications. Do not take any newly prescribed medications unless approved by prescriber who originally started treatment. Avoid grapefruit products, herbal supplements. • Diarrhea is a common side effect. Drink plenty of fluids.

enzalutamide

en-za-**loo**-ta-mide
(Xtandi)
Do not confuse enzalutamide with bicalutamide, flutamide, or nilutamide.

CLASSIFICATION

PHARMACOTHERAPEUTIC: Antiandrogen renal inhibitor. **CLINICAL:** Antineoplastic.

USES

Treatment of metastatic castration-resistant prostate cancer. Treatment of castration-sensitive prostate cancer.

PRECAUTIONS

Contraindications: Hypersensitivity to enzalutamide. Women who are pregnant or may become pregnant (not indicated in female population). **Cautions:** History of seizure disorder, underlying brain injury with loss of consciousness, tran-

E

sient ischemic attack within past 12 mos, CVA, brain metastases, brain arteriovenous abnormality, ischemic heart disease; pts at risk for fractures (e.g., osteoporosis, osteopenia), falls; conditions predisposing to infection (e.g., diabetes, renal failure, immunocompromised pts, open wounds), use of concurrent medications that may lower seizure threshold.

E

ACTION

Inhibits androgen binding to androgen receptors in target tissue, and inhibits interaction with DNA. **Therapeutic Effect:** Decreases proliferation, induces cell death of prostate cancer cells.

PHARMACOKINETICS

Readily absorbed in GI tract. Maximum plasma concentration achieved in 0.5–3 hrs. Metabolized in liver. Protein binding: (97%–98%). Primarily excreted in urine. **Half-life:** 5.8 days (Range: 2.8–10.2 days).

LIFESPAN CONSIDERATIONS

Pregnancy/Lactation: Not used in female population. **Children:** Safety and efficacy not established. **Elderly:** No age-related precautions noted.

INTERACTIONS

DRUG: Strong CYP2C8, CYP3A4 inhibitors (e.g., gemfibrozil, itraconazole) may increase concentration/effect. **CYP3A4 inducers (e.g., carBAMazepine, phenytoin, rifAMPin)** may decrease concentration/effect. **Drugs that lower seizure threshold (e.g., buPROPion, cloZAPine, haloperidol, traMADol)** may increase risk of seizures. May decrease concentration/effect of **cycloSPORINE, ergot derivatives (e.g., ergotamine), fosphenytoin, phenytoin, sirolimus, tacrolimus. HERBAL: St. John's wort** may decrease concentration/effect. **FOOD:** None known. **LAB VALUES:** May increase serum ALT, AST, bilirubin. May decrease Hgb, Hct, platelets, WBC count.

AVAILABILITY (Rx)

Capsules: 40 mg.

ADMINISTRATION/HANDLING

PO

- May give with or without food. Take at same time each day. Swallow whole.
- Do not break, crush, dissolve, or open capsules.

INDICATIONS/ROUTES/DOSAGE

Metastatic Castration-Resistant or Castration-Sensitive Prostate Cancer

PO: ADULTS, ELDERLY: 160 mg (4 × 40 mg capsules) given once daily.

Dose Modification

If CTCAE Grade 3 or greater toxicity or an intolerable side effect occurs, withhold treatment for 1 week or until symptoms improve to Grade 2 or less, then resume at same dose or a reduced dose (120 mg or 80 mg). **Concurrent use of strong CYP2C8 inhibitors:** Avoid use (if possible). If concurrent use is necessary, reduce the enzalutamide dose to 80 mg once daily. **Concurrent use of strong CYP3A4 inducers:** Increase dose to 240 mg once daily.

Dosage in Renal/Hepatic Impairment

No dose adjustment.

SIDE EFFECTS

Common (51%): Asthenia. **Frequent (26%–15%):** Back pain, diarrhea, arthralgia, hot flashes, peripheral edema, musculoskeletal pain. **Occasional (12%–6%):** Headache, dizziness, insomnia, hematuria, paresthesia, anxiety, hypertension. **Rare (4%–2%):** Mental impairment disorders (includes amnesia, memory impairment, cognitive disorder, attention deficit), hematuria (includes pollakiuria, pruritus, dry skin).

ADVERSE EFFECTS/TOXIC REACTIONS

Upper respiratory tract infection occurs in 11% of pts; lower respiratory tract and lung infection (includes pneumonia, bronchitis) occur in slightly less (9% of pts). Spinal cord compression and cauda equina syndrome occur in 7% of pts. Life-threatening ischemic heart disease reported in 3% of pts. May increase risk of cardiovascular disease. Fall and fractures were reported. Reversible posterior leukoencephalopathy syndrome (RPLS) may present as aphasia, altered mental status, paralysis, vision loss, weakness. Hypersensitivity reactions including angioedema, anaphylaxis may occur. May increase risk of seizures.

NURSING CONSIDERATIONS

BASELINE ASSESSMENT

Obtain LFT. Assess risk for falls/fractures. Screen for active infection. Question history of seizures, ischemic heart disease, cerebrovascular disease. Optimize cardiovascular risk factors (diabetes, hypertension, dyslipidemia) to reduce risk of treatment-induced ischemic heart disease. Obtain full medication history and screen for interactions. Offer emotional support.

INTERVENTION/EVALUATION

Monitor LFT periodically. Monitor B/P for hypertension. Obtain echocardiogram if ischemic heart disease (dyspnea, edema, exercise intolerance, palpitations) is suspected. Monitor for hypersensitivity reactions, seizure activity. Monitor for infections (cough, fatigue, fever). RPLS should be considered in pts with altered mental status, confusion, headache, seizures, visual disturbances. Altered gait, paralysis, numbness/weakness/pain of extremities may indicate spinal cord compression or cauda equina syndrome. Question incidence of falls.

PATIENT/FAMILY TEACHING

• Treatment may depress your immune system and reduce your ability to fight infection. Report symptoms of infection such as body aches, burning with urination, chills, cough, fatigue, fever. Avoid those with active infection. • There is a high risk of interactions with other medications. Do not take any newly prescribed medications unless approved by prescriber who originally started treatment. Avoid herbal supplements (esp. St. John's wort). • Treatment may increase risk of falls/fractures, seizures. • Life-threatening heart disease may occur. Report difficulty breathing, palpitations, swelling of ankles or feet. • Nervous system changes including confusion, seizures, headache, blurry vision, trouble speaking may indicate life-threatening brain dysfunction/swelling. • Sexually active men must wear condom during treatment and for 1 wk after treatment due to potential risks to fetus. • Women who are pregnant or are planning pregnancy may not touch medication without gloves.

EPINEPHrine

HIGH ALERT

ep-i-**nef**-rin
(Adrenalin, EpiPen, EpiPen Jr., Twinject ✱)
Do not confuse EPINEPHrine with ePHEDrine.

FIXED-COMBINATION(S)

LidoSite: EPINEPHrine/lidocaine (anesthetic): 0.1%/10%.

◆CLASSIFICATION

PHARMACOTHERAPEUTIC: Sympathomimetic (alpha-, beta-adrenergic agonist). **CLINICAL:** Antiglaucoma, bronchodilator, cardiac stimulant, antiallergic, antihemorrhagic, priapism reversal agent.

USES

Treatment of allergic reactions (including anaphylactic reactions). Treatment of hypotension associated with septic shock. Added to local anesthetics to decrease systemic absorption and increase duration of activity of local anesthetic. Decreases superficial hemorrhage. **OFF-LABEL:** Ventricular fibrillation or pulseless ventricular tachycardia unresponsive to initial defibrillatory shocks; pulseless electrical activity, asystole, hypotension unresponsive to volume resuscitation; bradycardia/hypotension unresponsive to atropine or pacing; inotropic support.

PRECAUTIONS

Contraindications: Hypersensitivity to EPINEPHrine. **Note:** There are no absolute contraindications with injectable EPINEPHrine in a life-threatening situation. **IV:** Narrow-angle glaucoma, thyrotoxicosis, diabetes, hypertension, other cardiovascular disorders. **Inhalation:** Concurrent use or within 2 wks of MAOIs. **Cautions:** Elderly, diabetes mellitus, hypertension, Parkinson's disease, thyroid disease, cerebrovascular or cardiovascular disease, concurrent use of tricyclic antidepressants. History of prostate enlargement, urinary retention.

ACTION

Stimulates alpha-adrenergic receptors (vasoconstriction, pressor effects), $beta_1$-adrenergic receptors (cardiac stimulation), $beta_2$-adrenergic receptors (bronchial dilation, vasodilation). **Therapeutic Effect:** Relaxes smooth muscle of bronchial tree, produces cardiac stimulation, dilates skeletal muscle vasculature.

PHARMACOKINETICS

Route	Onset	Peak	Duration
IM	5–10 min	20 min	1–4 hrs
SQ	5–10 min	20 min	1–4 hrs
Inhalation	3–5 min	20 min	1–3 hrs

Well absorbed after parenteral administration; minimally absorbed after inhalation. Metabolized in liver, other tissues, sympathetic nerve endings. Excreted in urine. Ophthalmic form may be systemically absorbed as a result of drainage into nasal pharyngeal passages. Mydriasis occurs within several min and persists several hrs; vasoconstriction occurs within 5 min and lasts less than 1 hr.

LIFESPAN CONSIDERATIONS

Pregnancy/Lactation: Crosses placenta. Distributed in breast milk. **Children/Elderly:** No age-related precautions noted.

INTERACTIONS

DRUG: May decrease effects of **beta blockers (e.g., carvedilol, metoprolol). Digoxin, sympathomimetics (e.g., dopamine, norepinephrine)** may increase risk of cardiac arrhythmias. **Ergonovine, methergine, oxytocin** may increase vasoconstriction. **MAOIs (e.g., phenelzine, selegiline), tricyclic antidepressants (e.g., amitriptyline, doxepin, nortriptyline)** may increase cardiovascular effects. **HERBAL: Ephedra, yohimbe** may increase CNS stimulation. **FOOD:** None known. **LAB VALUES:** May decrease serum potassium.

AVAILABILITY (Rx)

Injection, Solution (Prefilled Syringes): *(EpiPen):* 0.3 mg/0.3 mL. *(EpiPen Jr.):* 0.15 mg/0.3 mL. *(Twinject):* 0.15 mg/0.15 mL. **Injection, Solution:** 0.1 mg/mL (1:10,000), 1 mg/mL (1:1,000).

Solution for Oral Inhalation: *(Adrenalin):* 2.25% (0.5 mL).

ADMINISTRATION/HANDLING

IV

Reconstitution • For injection, dilute each 1 mg of 1:1,000 solution with 10 mL 0.9% NaCl to provide 1:10,000 solution and inject each 1 mg or fraction thereof over 1 min or more (except in cardiac arrest). • For infusion, further dilute

with 250–500 mL D_5W. Maximum concentration 64 mcg/mL.
Rate of administration • For IV infusion, give at 1–10 mcg/min (titrate to desired response).
Storage • Store parenteral forms at room temperature. • Do not use if solution appears discolored or contains a precipitate.

SQ
• Shake ampule thoroughly. • Use tuberculin syringe for injection into lateral deltoid region. • Massage injection site (minimizes vasoconstriction effect). Use only 1:1,000 solution.

Nebulizer
• No more than 10 drops Adrenalin Chloride solution 1:100 should be placed in reservoir of nebulizer. • Place nozzle just inside pt's partially opened mouth. • As bulb is squeezed once or twice, instruct pt to inhale deeply, drawing vaporized solution into lungs. • Rinse mouth with water immediately after inhalation (prevents mouth/throat dryness). • When nebulizer is not in use, replace stopper, keep in upright position.

IV INCOMPATIBILITIES
Ampicillin, pantoprazole (Protonix), sodium bicarbonate.

IV COMPATIBILITIES
Calcium chloride, calcium gluconate, dexmedetomidine (Precedex), dilTIAZem (Cardizem), DOBUTamine (Dobutrex), DOPamine (Intropin), fentaNYL (Sublimaze), heparin, HYDROmorphone (Dilaudid), LORazepam (Ativan), midazolam (Versed), milrinone (Primacor), morphine, nitroglycerin, norepinephrine (Levophed), potassium chloride, propofol (Diprivan).

INDICATIONS/ROUTES/DOSAGE
Hypersensitivity Reactions (including anaphylaxis)
IM, SQ: ADULTS, ELDERLY: 0.2–0.5 mg (0.2–0.5 mL of 1 mg/mL solution). May repeat q5–15 min if anaphylaxis persists. CHILDREN: 0.01 mg/kg (0.01 mL/kg of a 1 mg/mL solution) q5–15 min. **Maximum:** 0.3–0.5 mg q5–15 min.

Hypotension (Shock)
IV infusion: ADULTS, ELDERLY: Initially, 0.1-0.5 mcg/kg/min. Titrate to desired response. ADOLESCENTS, CHILDREN, INFANTS: Initially, 0.1–1 mcg/kg/min. Titrate to desired response.

Cardiac Arrest
IV: ADULTS, ELDERLY: Initially, 1 mg. May repeat q3–5min as needed. CHILDREN: Initially, 0.01 mg/kg (0.1 mL/kg of a 0.1 mg/mL solution). May repeat q3–5min as needed.
Endotracheal: ADULTS, ELDERLY: 2–2.5 mg q3–5min as needed. CHILDREN: 0.1 mg/kg (0.1 mL/kg of a 1 mg/mL solution). May repeat q3–5min as needed. **Maximum single dose:** 2.5 mg.

Dosage in Renal/Hepatic Impairment
No dose adjustment.

SIDE EFFECTS
Frequent: **Systemic:** Tachycardia, palpitations, anxiety. **Ophthalmic:** Headache, eye irritation, watering of eyes. **Occasional:** **Systemic:** Dizziness, light-headedness, facial flushing, headache, diaphoresis, increased B/P, nausea, trembling, insomnia, vomiting, fatigue. **Ophthalmic:** Blurred/decreased vision, eye pain. **Rare:** **Systemic:** Chest discomfort/pain, arrhythmias, bronchospasm, dry mouth/throat.

ADVERSE EFFECTS/TOXIC REACTIONS
Excessive doses may cause acute hypertension, arrhythmias. Prolonged/excessive use may result in metabolic acidosis due to increased serum lactic acid. Metabolic acidosis may cause disorientation, fatigue, hyperventilation, headache, nausea, vomiting, diarrhea.

NURSING CONSIDERATIONS

INTERVENTION/EVALUATION

Monitor changes of B/P, HR. Assess lung sounds for rhonchi, wheezing, rales. Monitor ABGs. In cardiac arrest, adhere to ACLS protocols.

PATIENT/FAMILY TEACHING

• Avoid excessive use of caffeine. • Report any new symptoms (tachycardia, shortness of breath, dizziness) immediately: may be systemic effects.

eplerenone

ep-**ler**-e-none
(Inspra)
Do not confuse Inspra with Spiriva.

◆CLASSIFICATION

PHARMACOTHERAPEUTIC: Aldosterone receptor antagonist. **CLINICAL:** Antihypertensive.

USES

Treatment of hypertension alone or in combination with other antihypertensive agents. Treatment of HF following acute myocardial infarction (AMI).

PRECAUTIONS

Contraindications: Hypersensitivity to eplerenone. Concurrent use with strong CYP3A4 inhibitors (e.g., ketoconazole, itraconazole), CrCl less than 30 mL/min, serum potassium level greater than 5.5 mEq/L at initiation. Use in pts with Addison's disease. **Hypertension (Additional):** Type 2 diabetes with microalbuminuria; CrCl less than 50 mL/min; serum creatinine greater than 2 mg/dL in men, greater than 1.8 mg/dL in women; concomitant use of potassium supplements or potassium-sparing diuretics. **Cautions:** Hyperkalemia, HF, post-MI, diabetes, mild renal impairment.

ACTION

Binds to mineralocorticoid receptors in kidney, heart, blood vessels, brain, blocking binding of aldosterone. **Therapeutic Effect:** Reduces B/P. Prevents myocardial and vascular fibrosis.

PHARMACOKINETICS

Absorption unaffected by food. Protein binding: 50%. Metabolized in liver. Excreted in urine (67%), feces (32%). Not removed by hemodialysis. **Half-life:** 4–6 hrs.

LIFESPAN CONSIDERATIONS

Pregnancy/Lactation: Unknown if drug crosses placenta or is distributed in breast milk. **Children:** Safety and efficacy not established. **Elderly:** No age-related precautions noted.

INTERACTIONS

DRUG: **ACE inhibitors (e.g., enalapril, lisinopril), angiotensin II antagonists (e.g., losartan, valsartan), potassium-sparing diuretics (e.g., spironolactone), potassium supplements** increase risk of hyperkalemia. May increase the hyperkalemic effect of **cycloSPORINE, tacrolimus. Strong CYP3A4 inhibitors (e.g., clarithromycin, ketoconazole, ritonavir)** may increase concentration/effect. **Strong CYP3A4 inducers (e.g., carBAMazepine, phenytoin, rifAMPin)** may decrease concentration/effect. **NSAIDs (e.g., diclofenac, meloxicam, naproxen)** may decrease antihypertensive effect. **HERBAL:** None significant. **FOOD:** **Grapefruit products** may increase potential for hyperkalemia, arrhythmias. **LAB VALUES:** May increase serum potassium, ALT, AST, cholesterol, triglycerides, serum creatinine, uric acid. May decrease serum sodium.

AVAILABILITY (Rx)

Tablets: 25 mg, 50 mg.

ADMINISTRATION/HANDLING

• Do not break, crush, dissolve, or divide film-coated tablets. • May give without regard to food.

INDICATIONS/ROUTES/DOSAGE

Hypertension

PO: ADULTS, ELDERLY: Initially, 50 mg once daily. If 50 mg once daily produces an inadequate B/P response, may increase dosage to 50 mg twice daily. If pt is concurrently receiving CYP3A4 inhibitors (e.g., erythromycin, verapamil, or fluconazole), reduce initial dose to 25 mg once daily. **Maximum:** 50 mg/day.

HF Following MI

PO: ADULTS, ELDERLY: Initially, 25 mg once daily. If tolerated, titrate up to 50 mg once daily within 4 wks.

Dosage Adjustment for Serum Potassium Concentrations in HF

Less than 5 mEq/L: Increase dose from 25 mg daily to 50 mg daily or increase dose from 25 mg every other day to 25 mg daily. **5–5.4 mEq/L:** No adjustment needed. **5.5–5.9 mEq/L:** Decrease dose from 50 mg daily to 25 mg daily or from 25 mg daily to 25 mg every other day. Decrease dose from 25 mg every other day to withhold medication. **6 mEq/L or greater:** Withhold medication until potassium is less than 5.5 mEq/L, then restart at 25 mg every other day.

Dosage in Renal Impairment

Contraindicated in pts with hypertension with CrCl less than 50 mL/min or serum creatinine greater than 2 mg/dL in males or greater than 1.8 mg/dL in females. All other indications, CrCl less than 30 mL/min, use is contraindicated.

Dosage in Hepatic Impairment

No dose adjustment.

SIDE EFFECTS

Rare (3%–1%): Dizziness, diarrhea, cough, fatigue, flu-like symptoms, abdominal pain.

ADVERSE EFFECTS/TOXIC REACTIONS

Hyperkalemia may occur, particularly in pts with type 2 diabetes mellitus and microalbuminuria.

NURSING CONSIDERATIONS

BASELINE ASSESSMENT

Obtain serum potassium level. Obtain B/P, apical pulse immediately before each dose, in addition to regular monitoring (be alert to fluctuations). If excessive reduction in B/P occurs, place pt in supine position, feet slightly elevated.

INTERVENTION/EVALUATION

Monitor serum potassium. Assist with ambulation if dizziness occurs. Assess B/P for hypertension/hypotension. Assess for evidence of flu-like symptoms.

PATIENT/FAMILY TEACHING

• Avoid tasks that require alertness, motor skills until response to drug is established (possible dizziness effect). • Hypertension requires lifelong control. • Avoid exercising during hot weather (risk of dehydration, hypotension). • Do not use salt substitutes containing potassium.

epoetin alfa

TOP 100

e-**poe**-e-tin **al**-fa
(Epogen, Eprex ✱, Procrit, Retacrit)

■ BLACK BOX ALERT ■ Increased risk of serious cardiovascular events, thromboembolic events, mortality, time-to-tumor progression in pts with head and neck cancer, metastatic breast cancer, non–small-cell lung cancer when administered to a target hemoglobin of more than 11 g/dL. Increases rate of deep vein thrombosis in perioperative pts not receiving anticoagulant therapy.

Do not confuse epoetin with darbepoetin, or Epogen with Neupogen.

◆CLASSIFICATION

PHARMACOTHERAPEUTIC: Erythropoiesis-stimulating agent (ESA). **CLINICAL:** Erythropoietin.

E

USES

Treatment of anemia in pts receiving or who have received myelosuppressive chemotherapy for a planned minimum of 2 mos of chemotherapy; pts with chronic renal failure to decrease need for RBC transfusion; HIV-infected pts on zidovudine (AZT) therapy when endogenous erythropoietin levels are 500 Units/mL or less; pts scheduled for elective noncardiac, nonvascular surgery, reducing need for allogenic blood transfusions when perioperative Hgb is greater than 10 or less than or equal to 13 g/dL and high risk for blood loss. **OFF-LABEL:** Anemia in myelodysplastic syndromes.

PRECAUTIONS

Contraindications: Hypersensitivity to epoetin. Pure red cell aplasia that begins after treatment, uncontrolled hypertension. **Cautions:** History of seizures or controlled hypertension. **Cancer pts:** Tumor growth, shortened survival may occur when Hgb levels of 11 g/dL or greater are achieved with epoetin alfa. **Chronic renal failure pts:** Increased risk for serious cardiovascular reactions (e.g., stroke, MI) when Hgb levels greater than 11 g/dL are achieved with epoetin alfa.

ACTION

Stimulates division, differentiation of erythroid progenitor cells in bone marrow. **Therapeutic Effect:** Induces erythropoiesis, releases reticulocytes from bone marrow into blood, where they mature into erythrocytes.

PHARMACOKINETICS

Well absorbed after SQ administration. Following administration, an increase in reticulocyte count occurs within 10 days, and increases in Hgb, Hct, and RBC count are seen within 2–6 wks. **Half-life:** 4–13 hrs.

LIFESPAN CONSIDERATIONS

Pregnancy/Lactation: Unknown if drug crosses placenta or is distributed in breast milk. **Children:** Safety and efficacy not established in pts 12 yrs and younger. **Elderly:** No age-related precautions noted.

INTERACTIONS

DRUG: None significant. **HERBAL:** None significant. **FOOD:** None known. **LAB VALUES:** May increase serum BUN, phosphorus, potassium, creatinine, uric acid, sodium. May decrease bleeding time, iron concentration, serum ferritin.

AVAILABILITY (Rx)

Injection Solution: ***(Epogen, Procrit):*** 2,000 units/mL, 3,000 units/mL, 4,000 units/mL, 10,000 units/mL, 20,000 units/mL, 40,000 units/mL.

ADMINISTRATION/HANDLING

◀ALERT▶ Avoid excessive agitation of vial; do not shake (foaming).

IV

Reconstitution • No reconstitution necessary.

Rate of administration • May be given as an IV bolus.

Storage • Refrigerate. • Vigorous shaking may denature medication, rendering it inactive.

SQ

• Mix in syringe with bacteriostatic 0.9% NaCl with benzyl alcohol 0.9% (bacteriostatic saline) at a 1:1 ratio (benzyl alcohol acts as local anesthetic; may reduce injection site discomfort). • Use 1 dose per vial; do not reenter vial. Discard unused portion.

IV INCOMPATIBILITIES

Do not mix injection form with other medications.

INDICATIONS/ROUTES/DOSAGE

Anemia Associated With Chemotherapy

◀ALERT▶ Begin therapy only if Hgb less than 10 g/dL and anticipated duration of myelosuppressive chemotherapy is greater than 2 mos. Use minimum effective dose to maintain Hgb level that will avoid

red blood cell transfusions. Discontinue upon completion of chemotherapy.
SQ: ADULTS, ELDERLY: Initially, 150 units/kg 3 times/wk (commonly used dose of 10,000 units 3 times/wk) or 40,000 units once wkly. **IV: CHILDREN 5 YRS AND OLDER:** 600 units/kg once wkly. **Maximum:** 40,000 units.
Increase dose: ADULTS, ELDERLY: If Hgb does not increase by greater than 1 g/dL and remains below 10 g/dL after initial 4 wks, may increase to 300 units/kg 3 times/wk or 60,000 units once wkly. **CHILDREN:** If Hgb does not increase by greater than 1 g/dL and remains less than 10 g/dL after initial 4 wks of once-wkly dosing, may increase dose to 900 units/kg/wk. **Maximum:** 60,000 units once wkly.
Decrease dose: Decrease dose by 25% if Hgb increases greater than 1 g/dL in any 2-wk period or Hgb level reaches level that will avoid red blood cell transfusions.

Reduction of Allogenic Blood Transfusions in Elective Surgery
SQ: ADULTS, ELDERLY: 300 units/kg/day for 10 days before and 4 days after surgery or 600 units/kg once weekly for 4 doses given 21, 14, 7 days before surgery and on the day of surgery.

Anemia in Chronic Renal Failure
◀ALERT▶ Individualize dose, using lowest dose to reduce need for RBC transfusions. **ON DIALYSIS:** Initiate when Hgb less than 10 g/dL; reduce dose or discontinue if Hgb approaches or exceeds 11 g/dL. **NOT ON DIALYSIS:** Initiate when Hgb less than 10 g/dL; reduce dose or stop if Hgb exceeds 10 g/dL.
IV, SQ: ADULTS, ELDERLY: 50–100 units/kg 3 times/wk. **CHILDREN:** 50 units/kg 3 times/wk. **Maintenance: Decrease dose by 25%:** If Hgb increases greater than 1 g/dL in any 2-wk period. **Increase dose by 25%:** If Hgb does not increase by greater than 1 g/dL after 4 wks of therapy. Do not increase dose more frequently than every 4 wks. **Note:** If pt does not attain adequate response after appropriate dosing over 12 wks, do not continue to increase dose, and use minimum effective dose to maintain Hgb level that will avoid red blood cell transfusions.

HIV Infection in Pts Treated with Zidovudine (AZT)
IV, SQ: ADULTS: Initially, 100 units/kg 3 times/wk for 8 wks; may increase by 50–100 units/kg 3 times/wk. Evaluate response q4–8wks thereafter. Adjust dosage by 50–100 units/kg 3 times/wk. If dosages larger than 300 units/kg 3 times/wk are not eliciting response, it is unlikely pt will respond. **Maintenance:** Titrate to maintain desired Hgb level. Hgb levels should not exceed 12 g/dL. If Hgb greater than 12 g/dL, resume treatment with 25% dose reduction when Hgb drops below 11 g/dL. Discontinue if Hgb increase not attained with 300 units/kg for 8 wks.

Dosage in Renal/Hepatic Impairment
No dose adjustment.

SIDE EFFECTS

Pts Receiving Chemotherapy
Frequent (20%–17%): Fever, diarrhea, nausea, vomiting, edema. **Occasional (13%–11%):** Asthenia, shortness of breath, paresthesia. **Rare (5%–3%):** Dizziness, trunk pain.

Pts With Chronic Renal Failure
Frequent (24%–11%): Hypertension, headache, nausea, arthralgia. **Occasional (9%–7%):** Fatigue, edema, diarrhea, vomiting, chest pain, skin reactions at administration site, asthenia, dizziness.

Pts With HIV Infection Treated With AZT
Frequent (38%–15%): Fever, fatigue, headache, cough, diarrhea, rash, nausea. **Occasional (14%–9%):** Shortness of breath, asthenia, skin reaction at injection site, dizziness.

ADVERSE EFFECTS/TOXIC REACTIONS

Hypertensive encephalopathy, thrombosis, cerebrovascular accident, MI, seizures occur rarely. Hyperkalemia occurs occasionally in pts with chronic renal failure, usually in those who do not comply with medication regimen, dietary guidelines, frequency of dialysis regimen.

NURSING CONSIDERATIONS

BASELINE ASSESSMENT

Assess B/P before initiation (80% of pts with chronic renal failure have history of hypertension). B/P often rises during early therapy in pts with history of hypertension. Consider that all pts eventually need supplemental iron therapy. Assess serum iron (should be greater than 20%), serum ferritin (should be greater than 100 ng/mL) before and during therapy. Establish baseline CBC (esp. note Hct).

INTERVENTION/EVALUATION

Assess CBC routinely (esp. Hgb, Hct). Monitor aggressively for increased B/P (25% of pts require antihypertensive therapy, dietary restrictions). Monitor temperature, esp. in cancer pts on chemotherapy and zidovudine-treated HIV pts. Monitor serum BUN, uric acid, creatinine, phosphorus, potassium, esp. in chronic renal failure pts.

PATIENT/FAMILY TEACHING

• Frequent laboratory assessments needed to determine correct dosage. • Immediately report any severe headache. • Avoid potentially hazardous activity during first 90 days of therapy (increased risk of seizures in pts with chronic renal failure during first 90 days). • Specific dietary regimen must be maintained.

eprosartan

ep-roe-**sar**-tan
(Teveten ✦)

■ **BLACK BOX ALERT** ■ May cause fetal injury, mortality. Discontinue as soon as possible once pregnancy is detected.

FIXED-COMBINATION(S)

Teveten HCT: eprosartan/hydroCHLOROthiazide (a diuretic): 400 mg/12.5 mg.

◆CLASSIFICATION

PHARMACOTHERAPEUTIC: Angiotensin II receptor antagonist. **CLINICAL:** Antihypertensive.

USES

Treatment of hypertension (alone or in combination with other medications).

PRECAUTIONS

Contraindications: Hypersensitivity to eprosartan. Concomitant use with aliskiren in pts with diabetes. **Cautions:** Unstented unilateral/bilateral renal artery stenosis, preexisting renal insufficiency. Concomitant use of potassium-sparing medications (e.g., spironolactone), potassium supplements, pts who are volume depleted.

ACTION

Potent vasodilator. Blocks vasoconstrictor, aldosterone-secreting effects of angiotensin II, inhibiting binding of angiotensin II to AT_1 receptors. **Therapeutic Effect:** Causes vasodilation, decreases peripheral resistance, decreases B/P.

PHARMACOKINETICS

Rapidly absorbed after PO administration. Protein binding: 98%. Minimally metabolized in liver. Primarily excreted via urine, biliary system. Minimally removed by hemodialysis. **Half-life:** 5–9 hrs.

⌛ LIFESPAN CONSIDERATIONS

Pregnancy/Lactation: Has caused fetal and neonatal morbidity and mortality. Potential for adverse effects on breastfeeding infant. Breastfeeding not recommended. **Children:** Safety and efficacy not established. **Elderly:** No age-related precautions noted.

INTERACTIONS

DRUG: **Aliskiren** may increase hyperkalemic effect. May increase adverse/toxicity of **ACE inhibitors (e.g., benazepril, lisinopril).** **HERBAL:** **Herbals with**

hypertensive properties (e.g., licorice, yohimbe) or hypotensive properties (e.g., garlic, ginger, ginkgo biloba) may alter effects. **FOOD:** None known. **LAB VALUES:** May increase serum BUN, alkaline phosphatase, bilirubin, creatinine, ALT, AST. May decrease Hgb, Hct.

AVAILABILITY (Rx)

Tablets: 400 mg, 600 mg.

ADMINISTRATION/HANDLING

PO

• Give without regard to food. • Do not break, crush, dissolve, or divide tablets.

INDICATIONS/ROUTES/DOSAGE

Hypertension

PO: ADULTS, ELDERLY: Initially, 600 mg once daily. Titrate up to 800 mg/day in 1-2 divided doses.

Dosage in Renal Impairment

Mild impairment: No dose adjustment. **Moderate to severe impairment: Maximum:** 600 mg/day.

Dosage in Hepatic Impairment

No dose adjustment. **Severe impairment: Maximum:** 600 mg/day.

SIDE EFFECTS

Occasional (5%–2%): Headache, cough, dizziness. **Rare (less than 2%):** Muscle pain, fatigue, diarrhea, upper respiratory tract infection, dyspepsia.

ADVERSE EFFECTS/TOXIC REACTIONS

Overdosage may manifest as hypotension, tachycardia. Bradycardia occurs less often.

NURSING CONSIDERATIONS

BASELINE ASSESSMENT

Obtain B/P, apical pulse immediately before each dose, in addition to regular monitoring (be alert to fluctuations). Question for history of hepatic/renal impairment, renal artery stenosis. Obtain urine pregnancy test. Assess medication history (esp. diuretics).

INTERVENTION/EVALUATION

Monitor B/P, pulse, serum BUN, creatinine, electrolytes, urinalysis.

PATIENT/FAMILY TEACHING

• Avoid pregnancy. • Avoid tasks that require alertness, motor skills until response to drug is established. • Restrict sodium, alcohol intake. • Follow diet, control weight. • Do not stop taking medication; hypertension requires lifelong control. • Check B/P regularly. • Do not chew, crush, dissolve, or divide tablets; take whole.

eptinezumab-jjmr

ep-ti-**nez**-ue-mab
(Vyepti)

Do not confuse eptinezumab with eptifibatide, galcanezumab, fremanezumab, obinutuzumab, or trastuzumab, or Vyepti with Vyleesi or Vyzulta.

◆CLASSIFICATION

PHARMACOTHERAPEUTIC: Calcitonin gene–related peptide (CGRP) ligand, humanized immunoglobulin G1 (IgG1) monoclonal antibody. **CLINICAL:** Migraine prophylaxis agent.

USES

Preventative treatment of migraines in adults.

PRECAUTIONS

Contraindications: Hypersensitivity to eptinezumab-jjmr. **Cautions:** None known.

ACTION

Binds to and inhibits calcitonin gene–related peptide (CGRP) receptor. **Therapeutic Effect:** Reduces occurrence of acute or chronic migraine headaches.

E

PHARMACOKINETICS

Widely distributed. Metabolized and eliminated via proteolytic degradation into small peptides, amino acids. Steady state reached after first dose. **Half-life:** 27 days.

LIFESPAN CONSIDERATIONS

Pregnancy/Lactation: Unknown if distributed in breast milk. However, human immunoglobulin G (IgG) is present in breast milk. **Children:** Safety and efficacy not established. **Elderly:** Safety and efficacy not established.

INTERACTIONS

DRUG: None known. **HERBAL:** None significant. **FOOD:** None known. **LAB VALUES:** None known.

AVAILABILITY (RX)

Injection Solution: 100 mg.

ADMINISTRATION/HANDLING

IV.

Preparation • Visually inspect for particulate matter or discoloration. Solution should appear clear to slightly opalescent, colorless to brownish-yellow in color. Do not use if solution is cloudy or discolored or if visible particles are observed. • Withdraw 1 mL from vial (or 1 mL from each 3 single-dose vials for 300-mg dose) into syringe and dilute into 100-mL bag containing 0.9% NaCl. Infusion bag must be made of polyvinyl chloride (PVC), polyethylene, or polyolefin. • Mix by gentle inversion. • Do not shake or agitate.

Rate of administration • Infuse over 30 min using 0.2–0.22 micron filter via dedicated IV line. • Do not administer as IV push or bolus.

Postinfusion Guidelines • After infusion is complete, flush IV line with 20 mL 0.9% NaCl.

Storage • Refrigerate vials in original carton until time of use. • Protect from light. • Do not shake. • Do not freeze or expose to heating sources. • Store diluted solution at room temperature for up to 8 hrs.

IV INCOMPATABILITIES

Do not infuse or mix with other medications.

INDICATIONS/ROUTES/DOSAGE

Migraine Headaches

IV: ADULTS: 100 mg once q3mos. **Maximum:** 300 mg once q3mos.

Dosage in Renal Impairment

Mild to severe impairment: No dose adjustment.

Dosage in Hepatic Impairment

Mild to severe impairment: No dose adjustment.

SIDE EFFECTS

Occasional (8%–6%): Nasopharyngitis.

ADVERSE EFFECTS/TOXIC REACTIONS

Hypersensitivity reactions including angioedema, facial flushing, urticaria, rash may occur. Immunogenicity (auto-eptinezumab antibodies) reported in 18%–20% of pts.

NURSING CONSIDERATIONS

BASELINE ASSESSMENT

Question characteristics of migraine headaches (onset, location, duration, possible precipitating symptoms). Question for hypersensitivity reactions.

INTERVENTION/EVALUATION

Evaluate for relief of migraine headaches (photophobia, phonophobia, nausea, vomiting, pain, dizziness, fogginess). Monitor for hypersensitivity reactions.

PATIENT/FAMILY TEACHING

• Allergic reactions such as itching, rash, swelling of the face or tongue can happen at any time. If allergic reaction occurs, seek immediate medical attention. • Consult healthcare provider if pregnancy occurs or for any plans to breastfeed.

erdafitinib

er-da-fi-ti-nib
(Balversa)
Do not confuse erdafitinib with enasidenib, encorafenib, erlotinib or gefitinib, or Balversa with Balziva.

◆CLASSIFICATION

PHARMACOTHERAPEUTIC: Fibroblast growth factor receptor (FGFR) inhibitor. Tyrosine kinase inhibitor. **CLINICAL:** Antineoplastic.

USES

Treatment of adult pts with locally advanced or metastatic urothelial carcinoma that has susceptible FGFR3 or FGFR2 genetic mutation alterations and progressed during or following at least one line of prior platinum-containing chemotherapy including within 12 mos of neoadjuvant or adjuvant platinum-containing chemotherapy.

PRECAUTIONS

Contraindications: Hypersensitivity to erdafitinib. **Cautions:** Baseline hemoglobinemia, neutropenia, leukopenia, thrombocytopenia; conditions predisposing to infection (e.g., diabetes, renal failure, immunocompromised pts, open wounds), hepatic/renal impairment, optic disorders, pts at risk for hyperphosphatemia (hypoparathyroidism, concomitant use of phosphorus-containing medications, chronic kidney disease), CYP2C9 poor metabolizers (pts with CYP2C9*3/*3 genotype); concomitant use of CYP3A inhibitors or inducers, CYP2C9 inducers or inhibitors, CYP34A substrates, OAT2 substrates, or P-gp substrates.

ACTION

Binds to and inhibits fibroblast growth factor receptor (FGFR) enzyme activity. Decreases FGFR-related signaling and cell viability. **Therapeutic Effect:** Inhibits tumor cell growth and metastasis. Induces cellular death of tumor cells.

PHARMACOKINETICS

Widely distributed. Metabolized in liver. Protein binding: 99.8%. Peak plasma concentration: 2.5 hrs. Steady state reached in 2 wks. Excreted in feces (69%), urine (19%). **Half-life:** 59 hrs.

LIFESPAN CONSIDERATIONS

Pregnancy/Lactation: Avoid pregnancy; may cause fetal harm. Females and males with female partners of reproductive potential should use effective contraception during treatment and up to 1 mo after discontinuation. Unknown if distributed in breast milk. Breastfeeding not recommended during treatment and for at least 1 mo after discontinuation. May impair fertility in female pts. **Children:** Safety and efficacy not established. **Elderly:** No age-related precautions noted.

INTERACTIONS

DRUG: **Strong CYP3A4 inhibitors (e.g., clarithromycin, ketoconazole), moderate CYP3A inhibitors (e.g., ciprofloxacin, dilTIAZem, fluconazole, verapamil)** may increase concentration/effect. **Strong CYP3A4 inducers (e.g., carBAMazepine, phenytoin, rifAMPin)** may decrease concentration/effect. **Phosphate-altering drugs (e.g., ergocalciferol, K-phos, PhosLo, Renagel)** may alter phosphate level; may affect dose modifications. **HERBAL:** **St. John's wort** may decrease concentration/effect. **FOOD:** **Phosphorus-containing foods (e.g., dairy products, deli meats, nuts, peanut butter)** may increase serum phosphate; may affect dose modifications. Restrict phosphate intake to 600–800 mg daily. **LAB VALUES:** May increase serum alkaline phosphatase, ALT, AST, calcium, creatinine, glucose, potassium. May decrease serum albumin, sodium; Hgb, leukocytes, neutrophils, platelets. May increase or decrease serum phosphate.

AVAILABILITY (Rx)

Tablets: 3 mg, 4 mg, 5 mg.

ADMINISTRATION/HANDLING

E

PO

• Give without regard to food. Administer tablets whole; do not break, cut, crush, or divide. Tablets should not be chewed. • If a dose is missed, give as soon as possible. If vomiting occurs after administration, give next dose at regularly scheduled time.

INDICATIONS/ROUTES/DOSAGE

Note: Assess serum phosphate levels 14–21 days after therapy initiation. Restrict phosphate intake to 600–800 mg daily

Urothelial Carcinoma

PO: ADULTS, ELDERLY: Initially, 8 mg once daily. After 14–21 days, increase dose to 9 mg once daily if serum phosphate is less than 5.5 mg/dL and there are no ocular toxicities or Grade 2 (or higher) adverse reactions. Continue until disease progression or unacceptable toxicity.

Dose Reduction Schedule for Adverse Reactions

Dose	First Dose Reduction	Second Dose Reduction	Third Dose Reduction	Fourth Dose Reduction	Fifth Dose Reduction
9 mg	8 mg	6 mg	5 mg	4 mg	Discontinue
8 mg	6 mg	5 mg	4 mg	Discontinue	N/A

Dose Modification

Based on Common Terminology Criteria for Adverse Events (CTCAE).

Hyperphosphatemia

Serum phosphate 5.6–6.9 mg/dL (1.8–2.3 mmol/L): Maintain dose. **7–9 mg/dL (2.3–2.9 mmol/L):** Withhold treatment until serum phosphate is less than 5.5 mg/dL (or baseline), then resume at same dose. May reduce dose if hyperphosphatemia lasts greater than 1 wk. **Greater than 9 mg/dL and less than 10 mg/dL (greater than 2.9 mmol/L):** Withhold treatment until serum phosphate is less than 5.5 mg/dL (or baseline), then resume at next lower dose level. **Greater than 10 mg/dL (greater than 3.2 mmol/L); significant change of baseline renal function; Grade 3 hypercalcemia:** Withhold treatment until serum phosphate is less than 5.5 mg/dL (or baseline), then resume at 2 lower dose levels.

Serious Retinopathy/Retinal Pigment Epithelial Detachment

Asymptomatic; clinical of diagnostic observation: Withhold treatment until resolved. Resume at next lower dose level if resolved within 4 wks. Consider re-escalation of dose if symptoms do not recur for 1 mo. If stable but not resolved for 2 consecutive eye exams, resume at next lower dose level. **Visual acuity 20/40 (or better) or greater than or equal to 3 lines of decreased vision from baseline:** Withhold treatment until resolved. Resume at next lower dose level if resolved within 4 wks. **Visual acuity worse than 20/40 or greater than 3 lines of decreased vision from baseline:** Withhold treatment until resolved. Resume at 2 lower dose levels if resolved within 4 wks. Consider permanent discontinuation if recurrent. **Visual acuity 20/200 or worse in affected eye:** Permanently discontinue.

Other Adverse Reactions

Any Grade 3 reaction: Withhold treatment until improved to Grade 1 or 0, then resume at next lower dose level. **Any Grade 4 reaction:** Permanently discontinue.

Dosage in Renal Impairment

Mild to moderate impairment: No dose adjustment. **Severe impairment:** Not specified; use caution.

Dosage in Hepatic Impairment

Mild impairment: No dose adjustment. **Moderate to severe impairment:** Not specified; use caution.

SIDE EFFECTS

Frequent (56%–20%): Stomatitis, fatigue, asthenia, lethargy, malaise, diarrhea, dry mouth, onycholysis, onychoclasis, nail disorder, nail dystrophy, nail ridging, decreased appetite, dysgeusia, constipation, dry eye, alopecia, abdominal pain, nausea, musculoskeletal pain, back/chest/neck pain. **Occasional (17%–10%):** Blurry vision, decreased weight, cachexia, pyrexia, vomiting, nail discoloration, oropharyngeal pain, arthralgia, increased lacrimation, dyspnea.

ADVERSE EFFECTS/TOXIC REACTIONS

Hemoglobinemia, leukopenia, neutropenia, thrombocytopenia are expected responses to therapy. Ocular toxicities including serious retinopathy/retinal pigment epithelial detachment reported in 25% of pts. Ocular disorders including keratitis, foreign body sensation, corneal erosion reported in 28% of pts. Grade 3 serious retinopathy/retinal pigment epithelial detachment reported in 3% of pts. Hyperphosphatemia reported in 76% of pts with 32% of pts requiring oral phosphate binders. Palmar-plantar erythrodysesthesia syndrome reported in 26% of pts. Hematuria reported in 11% of pts. Infections including paronychia (17% of pts), urinary tract infection (17% of pts), conjunctivitis (11% of pts) may occur.

NURSING CONSIDERATIONS

BASELINE ASSESSMENT

Obtain CBC, BMP, LFTs, serum phosphate level; pregnancy test in female pts of reproductive potential. Confirm presence of susceptible FGFR genetic alterations in tumor specimens. Verify compliance of effective contraception in female pts and male pts with female partners of reproductive potential. Obtain visual acuity. Screen for active infection. Question history of hepatic/renal impairment, optic disorders. Receive full medication history and screen for interactions. Offer emotional support.

INTERVENTION/EVALUATION

Monitor CBC, BMP, LFTs, serum ionized calcium periodically. Obtain serum phosphate level 14–21 days after initiation. Restrict phosphorus intake to 600–800 mg daily. If serum phosphate is greater than 7 mg/dL, consider administration of an oral phosphate binder until serum phosphate is less than 5.5 mg/dL. Obtain weekly serum phosphate levels in pts who develop hyperphosphatemia. Monitor for symptoms of hyperphosphatemia, which may mimic symptoms of hypocalcemia (facial twitching, muscle cramps, numbness of hand, feet, lips; seizures). Assess skin for dermal toxicities. Monthly ophthalmologic exams (including visual acuity, slit lamp examination, fundoscopy, optical coherence tomography) should be performed by a specialist for the first 4 mos, then q3mos thereafter, or emergently if new symptoms occur. Obtain urinalysis if UTI is suspected (dysuria, fever, foul-smelling or cloudy urine, urinary frequency). Diligently monitor for infections.

PATIENT/FAMILY TEACHING

• Treatment may depress your immune system and reduce your ability to fight infection. Report symptoms of infection such as body aches, burning with urination, chills, cough, fatigue, fever. Avoid those with active infection. • Report symptoms of bone marrow depression such as bruising, fatigue, fever, shortness of breath, weight loss; bleeding easily, bloody urine or stool. • Expect frequent eye exams, skin exams. Immediately report vision changes of any kind. • Use effective contraception to avoid pregnancy. Do not breastfeed. • Limit intake of phosphorus-containing food unless blood tests verify acceptable phosphate levels. • Report liver problems such as bruising, confusion, dark or amber-colored urine, right upper abdominal pain, or yellowing of the skin or eyes; symptoms of UTI (burning with urination, fever, urinary frequency, foul-smelling or cloudy urine). • There is a high risk of interactions with other medications. Do not take any newly prescribed medications unless approved by prescriber who originally started treatment. • Avoid grapefruit products, herbal supplements (esp. St. John's wort).

erenumab-aooe

e-**ren**-ue-mab-aooe
(Aimovig)
Do not confuse erenumab with aducanumab or secukinumab.

CLASSIFICATION

PHARMACOTHERAPEUTIC: Calcitonin gene-related peptide (CGRP) receptor antagonist. Monoclonal antibody. **CLINICAL:** Migraine prophylaxis agent.

USES

Preventative treatment of migraines in adults.

PRECAUTIONS

Contraindications: Hypersensitivity to erenumab-aooe. **Cautions:** Latex allergy (when handling needle cap).

ACTION

Binds to and inhibits calcitonin gene-related peptide (CGRP) receptor. **Therapeutic Effect:** Reduces occurrence of acute or chronic migraine headaches.

PHARMACOKINETICS

Widely distributed. Peak plasma concentration: 6 days. Steady state reached by 3 mos of dosing. Eliminated mainly via proteolytic degradation. **Half-life:** 28 days.

LIFESPAN CONSIDERATIONS

Pregnancy/Lactation: Unknown if distributed in breast milk. **Children:** Safety and efficacy not established. **Elderly:** Not specified.

INTERACTIONS

DRUG: May enhance the adverse/toxic effect of **belimumab. HERBAL:** None significant. **FOOD:** None known. **LAB VALUES:** None known.

AVAILABILITY (Rx)

Injection Solution: 70 mg/1 mL, 140 mg/mL in prefilled syringe or autoinjector.

ADMINISTRATION/HANDLING

SQ

Preparation • Remove prefilled syringe or autoinjector from refrigerator and allow solution to warm to room temperature (approx. 30 min) with needle cap intact. • Visually inspect for particulate matter or discoloration. Solution should appear clear, colorless to slightly yellow in color. Do not use if solution is cloudy, discolored, or visible particles are observed.
Administration • Insert needle subcutaneously into upper arm, outer thigh, or abdomen and inject solution. • Do not inject into areas of active skin disease or injury such as sunburns, skin rashes, inflammation, skin infections, or active psoriasis. • Do not administer IV or intramuscularly. • Rotate injection sites.
Storage • Refrigerate prefilled syringes in original carton until time of use. • May store at room temperature for up to 7 days. Once warmed to

room temperature, do not place back into refrigerator. • Do not freeze or expose to heating sources. • Do not shake. • Protect from light.

INDICATIONS/ROUTES/DOSAGE

Acute or Chronic Migraine Headaches

SQ: ADULTS: 70 mg once monthly. May increase to 140 mg once monthly if 70 mg dose is ineffective.

Dosage in Renal Impairment

Mild to moderate impairment: No dose adjustment. **Severe impairment:** Not specified; use caution.

Dosage in Hepatic Impairment

Not specified; use caution.

SIDE EFFECTS

Occasional (6%–1%): Injection site pain/erythema, constipation, cramps, muscle spasm.

ADVERSE EFFECTS/TOXIC REACTIONS

Immunogenicity (auto-erenumab antibodies) occurred in 6.2% of pts.

NURSING CONSIDERATIONS

BASELINE ASSESSMENT

Question characteristics of migraine headaches (onset, location, duration, possible precipitating symptoms). Question history of latex allergy. Assess pt's willingness to self-inject medication.

INTERVENTION/EVALUATION

Evaluate for relief of migraine headaches (photophobia, phonophobia, nausea, vomiting, pain, dizziness, fogginess).

PATIENT/FAMILY TEACHING

• Latex needle cap may cause a skin reaction in pts with a latex allergy if direct skin contact is made. • A healthcare provider will show you how to properly prepare and inject medication. You must demonstrate correct preparation and injection techniques before using medication at home.

eriBULin

er-i-bue-lin
(Halaven)
Do not confuse eriBULin with epiRUBicin or erlotinib.

◆CLASSIFICATION

PHARMACOTHERAPEUTIC: Microtubule inhibitor. **CLINICAL:** Antineoplastic.

USES

Treatment of metastatic breast cancer in pts who previously received at least 2 chemotherapeutic regimens for treatment. Treatment of metastatic or unresectable liposarcoma in pts who received a prior anthracycline-containing regimen.

PRECAUTIONS

Contraindications: Hypersensitivity to eriBULin. **Cautions:** Pts at risk for QT interval prolongation (e.g., congenital long QT syndrome, QT interval–prolonging medications, hypokalemia, hypomagnesemia); hepatic/renal impairment, moderate to severe neuropathy, HF; conditions predisposing to infection (e.g., diabetes, renal failure, immunocompromised pts, open wounds).

ACTION

Inhibits growth phase of microtubule by inhibiting formation of mitotic spindles. Causes mitotic blockage and arrests the cell cycle. **Therapeutic Effect:** Blocks cells in mitotic phase of cell division, leading to tumor cell death.

PHARMACOKINETICS

Widely distributed. Metabolism is negligible. Protein binding: 49%–65%. Excreted in feces (82%), urine (9%). **Half-life:** 40 hrs.

⌛ LIFESPAN CONSIDERATIONS

Pregnancy/Lactation: Avoid pregnancy; may cause fetal harm. Females of reproductive potential must use effective contraception during treatment and for at least 2 wks after discontinuation. Unknown if distributed in breast milk. **Males:** Males with female partners of reproductive potential must use effective contraception during treatment and for at least 3.5 mos after discontinuation. May impair fertility. **Children:** Safety and efficacy not established in pts younger than 18 yrs. **Elderly:** No age-related precautions noted.

INTERACTIONS

DRUG: May decrease levels/effects of **BCG (intravesical). May increase QT interval–prolonging effect of amiodarone, azithromycin, ciprofloxacin, haloperidol. HERBAL:** None significant. **FOOD:** None known. **LAB VALUES:** May decrease WBC, Hgb, Hct, platelet count, potassium. May increase ALT.

AVAILABILITY (Rx)

Injection, Solution: 1 mg/2 mL (0.5 mg/mL).

ADMINISTRATION/HANDLING

IV

Reconstitution • May administer undiluted or dilute in 100 mL 0.9% NaCl.

Rate of administration • Administer over 2–5 min.

Storage • Store at room temperature. • Once diluted, syringe or diluted solution may be stored for up to 4 hrs at room temperature or up to 24 hrs if refrigerated.

IV INCOMPATIBILITIES

Do not dilute with D_5W or administer through IV line containing solutions with dextrose or in same IV line with other medications.

INDICATIONS/ROUTES/DOSAGE

Metastatic Breast Cancer, Liposarcoma

IV: ADULTS, ELDERLY: 1.4 mg/m² over 2–5 min on days 1 and 8 of 21-day cycle.

Dosage in Renal Impairment

Mild impairment: No dose adjustment.

Moderate to severe impairment: CrCl 15–49 mL/min: 1.1 mg/m²/dose.

Dosage in Hepatic Impairment

Mild impairment: 1.1 mg/m²/dose. **Moderate impairment:** 0.7 mg/m²/dose. **Severe impairment:** Use not recommended.

Recommended Dose Delays

Do not administer day 1 or day 8 of treatment for any of the following: ANC less than 1,000 cells/mm³, platelets less than 75,000 cells/mm³, Grade 3 or 4 nonhematologic toxicities. Day 8 dose may be delayed for maximum of 1 wk. If toxicities do not resolve or improve to Grade 2 severity by day 15, omit dose. If toxicities resolve or improve to Grade 2 severity by day 15, continue treatment at reduced dose and initiate next cycle no sooner than 2 wks later. Do not re-escalate dose after it has been reduced.

SIDE EFFECTS

Common (54%–35%): Fatigue, asthenia, alopecia, peripheral sensory neuropathy, nausea. **Frequent (25%–18%):** Constipation, arthralgia/myalgia, decreased weight, anorexia, pyrexia, headache, diarrhea, vomiting. **Occasional (16%–9%):** Back pain, dyspnea, cough, bone pain, extremity pain, urinary tract infection, oral mucosal inflammation.

ADVERSE EFFECTS/TOXIC REACTIONS

Neutropenia occurs in 82% of pts, with 57% developing Grade 3 neutropenia. Severe neutropenia (ANC less than 500 cells/mm³) lasting more than 1 wk occurred in 12%. Anemia occurs in 58% of pts. Peripheral neuropathy occurs in 8% of pts. Prolonged QTc interval may be noted on or after day 8 of treatment.

NURSING CONSIDERATIONS

BASELINE ASSESSMENT

Obtain CBC (prior to each dose); pregnancy test in females of reproductive potential. Screen for active infection, QT interval–prolonging medications. Offer emotional support.

INTERVENTION/EVALUATION

Monitor for infections (cough, fatigue, fever). Monitor for symptoms of neuropathy (burning sensation, hyperesthesia, hypoesthesia, paresthesia, discomfort, neuropathic pain). Assess hands, feet for erythema. Monitor CBC for evidence of neutropenia, thrombocytopenia. Assess mouth for stomatitis (erythema, ulceration, mucosal burning).

PATIENT/FAMILY TEACHING

• Treatment may depress your immune system response and reduce your ability to fight infection. Report symptoms of infection such as body aches, chills, cough, fatigue, fever. Avoid those with active infection. • Report symptoms of bone marrow depression such as bruising, fatigue, fever, shortness of breath, weight loss; bleeding easily, bloody urine or stool. • Report liver problems (abdominal pain, bruising, clay-colored stool, amber- or dark-colored urine, yellowing of the skin or eyes), kidney problems (decreased urine output, flank pain, darkened urine). • Use effective contraception to avoid pregnancy. Do not breastfeed.

erlotinib

HIGH ALERT

er-**loe**-ti-nib
(Tarceva)

Do not confuse erlotinib with dasatinib, eriBULin, gefitinib, imatinib, or lapatinib.

◆CLASSIFICATION

PHARMACOTHERAPEUTIC: Epidermal growth factor receptor (EGFR) inhibitor; tyrosine kinase inhibitor. **CLINICAL:** Antineoplastic.

USES

Treatment of locally advanced or metastatic non–small-cell lung cancer (NSCLC) after failure of at least one prior chemotherapy regimen (as monotherapy). First-line treatment of locally advanced, unresectable, or metastatic pancreatic cancer (in combination with gemcitabine).

PRECAUTIONS

Contraindications: Hypersensitivity to erlotinib. **Cautions:** Severe hepatic/renal impairment, cardiovascular disease. Concurrent use of strong CYP3A4 inhibitors and inducers or CYP1A2 inhibitors, pts at risk for GI perforation (e.g., peptic ulcer disease, diverticular disease), conditions predisposing to infection (e.g., diabetes, renal failure, immunocompromised pts, open wounds).

ACTION

Reversibly inhibits overall epidermal growth factor receptor (EGFR)–tyrosine kinase activity. Inhibits intracellular phosphorylation. **Therapeutic Effect:** Produces tumor cell death.

PHARMACOKINETICS

Widely distributed. Metabolized in liver. Protein binding: 93%. Excreted in feces (83%), urine (8%). **Half-life:** 24–36 hrs.

LIFESPAN CONSIDERATIONS

Pregnancy/Lactation: Unknown if drug crosses placenta or is distributed in breast milk. **Children:** Safety and efficacy not established. **Elderly:** No age-related precautions noted.

INTERACTIONS

DRUG: Strong CYP3A4 inhibitors (e.g., clarithromycin, ketoconazole, ritonavir) may increase concentration/effects. **Strong CYP3A4 inducers (e.g., carBAMazepine, phenytoin, rifAMPin)** may decrease concentration/effect. **Antacids, proton pump inhibitors (e.g., omeprazole, pan-**

toprazole), H_2 antagonists (e.g., raNITIdine) may decrease absorption/effect. **Warfarin** may increase risk of bleeding. **Statins (e.g., atorvastatin, simvastatin)** may increase risk of myopathy, rhabdomyolysis. **HERBAL: St. John's wort** may decrease concentration/effect. **FOOD: Grapefruit products** may increase potential for myelotoxicity. **LAB VALUES:** May increase serum bilirubin, ALT, AST.

AVAILABILITY (Rx)

Tablets: 25 mg, 100 mg, 150 mg.

ADMINISTRATION/HANDLING

PO

• Give at least 1 hr before or 2 hrs after ingestion of food. • Avoid grapefruit products. • May dissolve in 3–4 oz water and give orally or via feeding tube. • Give 10 hrs after or 2 hrs before H_2 antagonists (e.g., famotidine), proton pump inhibitors (e.g., omeprazole, pantoprazole).

INDICATIONS/ROUTES/DOSAGE

NSCLC

PO: ADULTS, ELDERLY: 150 mg/day until disease progression or unacceptable toxicity occurs.

Pancreatic Cancer

PO: ADULTS, ELDERLY: 100 mg/day, in combination with gemcitabine, until disease progression or unacceptable toxicity occurs.

Dose Modification

Permanently discontinue treatment in pts with interstitial lung disease (ILD); severe hepatotoxicity that does not significantly improve or resolve within 3 wks; GI perforation; severe bullous, blistering, or exfoliative skin conditions; corneal perforation or severe ulceration. Withhold treatment and consider discontinuation in pts with preexisting hepatic impairment or biliary obstruction for doubling or tripling of transaminase values over baseline; severe renal toxicity, acute or worsening ocular disorders. Withhold treatment in pts with severe rash or persistent diarrhea not responsive to medical management; Grade 3 or 4 keratitis or Grade 2 keratitis lasting longer than 2 wks; or pt being investigated for ILD. Once improved to Grade 1 or 0, then resume at reduced 50-mg dose increments.

Dosage in Renal Impairment

Interrupt dosing for Grade 3 or 4 renal toxicity during treatment.

Dosage in Hepatic Impairment

Use extreme caution. Reduce starting dose to 75 mg and individualize dose escalation if tolerated.

SIDE EFFECTS

Frequent (85%–21%): Rash, diarrhea, decreased appetite, fatigue, cough, dyspnea, pyrexia, nausea, dry skin. **Occasional (19%–11%):** Back pain, chest pain, mucosal inflammation, stomatitis, pruritus, cough, headache, paronychia, arthralgia, musculoskeletal pain.

ADVERSE EFFECTS/TOXIC REACTIONS

Severe, life-threatening pneumonitis, ILD, respiratory failure reported in 9% of pts. Life-threatening hepatorenal syndrome reported in less 1% of pts. Fatal cases of GI perforation; blistering, and exfoliative skin reactions, including Stevens-Johnson syndrome/toxic epidermal necrolysis; ocular disorders including dry eye, keratoconjunctivitis, keratitis, leading to corneal perforation or ulceration, were reported. CVA reported in 3% of pts. Microangiopathic hemolytic anemia with thrombocytopenia was reported. Fatal hemorrhagic events were reported in pts taking concomitant warfarin. Myopathy, rhabdomyolysis was reported in pts taking concomitant statin therapy. Depression reported in 19% of pts.

NURSING CONSIDERATIONS

BASELINE ASSESSMENT

Obtain CBC, BMP, LFT; pregnancy test in females of reproductive potential. Confirm compliance of effective contraception. Question history of CVA, optic disorders, pulmonary disease, hepatic/renal impairment, GI perforation. Screen for active infection. Receive full medication history and screen for interactions. Offer emotional support.

INTERVENTION/EVALUATION

Monitor CBC, LFT, renal function periodically. An increase of serum creatinine greater than 0.4 mg/dL from baseline may indicate renal impairment. Consider ABG, radiologic test if ILD/pneumonitis (excessive cough, dyspnea, fever, hypoxia) is suspected. Consider treatment with corticosteroids if ILD/pneumonitis is confirmed. Monitor for infections (cough, fatigue, fever). If serious infection occurs, initiate appropriate antimicrobial therapy. Monitor daily pattern of bowel activity, stool consistency. Abdominal pain, fever, melena may indicate GI perforation. Monitor for toxic skin reactions, rash. Assess for symptoms of CVA (aphasia, blindness, confusion, facial droop, hemiplegia, seizures). Monitor for ocular toxicities. Monitor for depression.

PATIENT/FAMILY TEACHING

• Treatment may depress your immune system response and reduce your ability to fight infection. Report symptoms of infection such as body aches, chills, cough, fatigue, fever. Avoid those with active infection. • Report symptoms of lung inflammation (excessive coughing, difficulty breathing, chest pain); liver problems (abdominal pain, bruising, clay-colored stool, amber or dark colored urine, yellowing of the skin or eyes), eye problems (dry eye, eye pain/swelling/redness), kidney problems (decreased urine output, flank pain, darkened urine); toxic skin reactions (rash, skin eruptions), stroke (confusion, difficulty speaking, one-sided weakness or paralysis, loss of vision), intestinal tear (abdominal pain, bloody stool, fever). • Use effective contraception to avoid pregnancy. Do not breastfeed. • There is a high risk of interactions with other medications. Do not take newly prescribed medications unless approved by prescriber who originally started treatment. • Report changes in mood, depression.

ertapenem

er-ta-**pen**-em
(INVanz)
Do not confuse ertapenem with doripenem, imipenem, or meropenem, or INVanz with AVINza.

◆CLASSIFICATION

PHARMACOTHERAPEUTIC: Carbapenem. **CLINICAL:** Antibiotic.

USES

Treatment of susceptible infections due to *S. aureus* (methicillin-susceptible only), *S. agalactiae, S. pneumoniae* (penicillin-susceptible only), *S. pyogenes, E. coli, H. influenzae* (beta-lactamase negative strains only), *K. pneumoniae, M. catarrhalis, Bacteroides* spp., *C. clostridioforme, Peptostreptococcus* spp., including moderate to severe intra-abdominal, skin/skin structure infections; community-acquired pneumonia; complicated UTI; acute pelvic infection; adult diabetic foot infections without osteomyelitis. Prevention of surgical site infection. **OFF-LABEL:** Treatment of IV catheter–related bloodstream infection; prosthetic joint infection.

PRECAUTIONS

Contraindications: Hypersensitivity to ertapenem. History of anaphylactic hypersensitivity to beta-lactams (e.g., imipenem, meropenem), hypersensitivity to amide-type local anesthetics (e.g., lidocaine) (IM use only). **Cautions:** Hypersensitivity to penicillins, cephalosporins, renal impairment, CNS disorders (brain lesions or history of seizure disorder), elderly.

E

ACTION

Penetrates bacterial cell wall of microorganisms, binds to penicillin-binding proteins, inhibiting cell wall synthesis. **Therapeutic Effect:** Produces bacterial cell death.

PHARMACOKINETICS

Almost completely absorbed after IM administration. Protein binding: 85%–95%. Widely distributed. Primarily excreted in urine (80%), feces (10%). Removed by hemodialysis. **Half-life:** 4 hrs.

LIFESPAN CONSIDERATIONS

Pregnancy/Lactation: Distributed in breast milk. **Children:** Safety and efficacy not established in pts younger than 18 yrs. **Elderly:** Advanced or end-stage renal insufficiency may require dosage adjustment.

INTERACTIONS

DRUG: **Probenecid** may increase concentration/effect. May decrease concentration/effect of **valproic acid, BCG (intravesical).** **HERBAL:** None significant. **FOOD:** None known. **LAB VALUES:** May increase serum alkaline phosphatase, ALT, AST, bilirubin, BUN, creatinine, glucose, PT, aPTT, sodium. May decrease platelet count, Hgb, Hct, WBC.

AVAILABILITY (Rx)

Injection, Powder for Reconstitution: 1 g.

ADMINISTRATION/HANDLING

IV

Reconstitution • Dilute 1-g vial with 10 mL 0.9% NaCl or Bacteriostatic Water for Injection. • Shake well to dissolve. • Further dilute with 50 mL 0.9% NaCl (**maximum concentration:** 20 mg/mL).

Rate of administration • Give by intermittent IV infusion (piggyback). Do not give IV push. • Infuse over 30 min.

Storage • Solution appears colorless to yellow (variation in color does not affect potency). • Discard if solution contains precipitate. • Reconstituted solution is stable for 6 hrs at room temperature or 24 hrs if refrigerated.

IM

• Reconstitute with 3.2 mL 1% lidocaine HCl injection (without EPINEPHrine). • Shake vial thoroughly. • Inject deep in large muscle mass (gluteal or lateral part of thigh). • Administer suspension within 1 hr after preparation.

IV INCOMPATIBILITIES

Do not mix or infuse with any other medications. Do not use diluents or IV solutions containing dextrose.

IV COMPATIBILITIES

Heparin, potassium chloride, tigecycline (Tygacil), Sterile Water for Injection, 0.9% NaCl.

INDICATIONS/ROUTES/DOSAGE

Usual Dosage Range

IM, IV: ADULTS, ELDERLY, CHILDREN 13 YRS AND OLDER: 1 g/day. **CHILDREN 3 MOS–12 YRS:** 15 mg/kg 2 times/day. **Maximum:** 500 mg/dose.

Dosage in Renal Impairment

CrCl 30 mL/min or less	500 mg once daily
Hemodialysis	If daily dose given within 6h prior to HD, give 150 mg dose after HD.
Peritoneal dialysis	500 mg once daily

Dosage in Hepatic Impairment

No dose adjustment.

SIDE EFFECTS

Frequent (10%–6%): Diarrhea, nausea, headache. **Occasional (5%–2%):** Altered mental status, insomnia, rash, abdominal pain, constipation, chest pain, vomiting, edema, fever. **Rare (less than 2%):** Dizziness, cough, oral candidiasis, anxiety, tachycardia, phlebitis at IV site.

ADVERSE EFFECTS/TOXIC REACTIONS

Antibiotic-associated colitis, other superinfections (abdominal cramps, severe watery diarrhea, fever) may result from altered bacterial balance in GI tract. Anaphylactic reactions have been reported. Seizures may occur in pts with CNS disorders (brain lesions, history of seizures), bacterial meningitis, severe renal impairment.

NURSING CONSIDERATIONS

BASELINE ASSESSMENT

Question for history of allergies, particularly to beta-lactams, penicillins, cephalosporins. Inquire about history of seizures.

INTERVENTION/EVALUATION

Monitor WBC count. Monitor renal/hepatic function. Monitor daily pattern of bowel activity, stool consistency. Monitor for nausea, vomiting. Evaluate hydration status. Evaluate for inflammation at IV injection site. Assess skin for rash. Observe mental status; be alert to tremors, possible seizures. Assess sleep pattern for evidence of insomnia.

PATIENT/FAMILY TEACHING

- Report tremors, seizures, rash, prolonged diarrhea, chest pain, other new symptoms.

ertugliflozin

er-too-gli-**floe**-zin
(Steglatro)

Do not confuse ertugliflozin with canagliflozin, dapagliflozin, or empagliflozin.

FIXED-COMBINATIONS

Segluromet: ertugliflozin/metformin (an antidiabetic): 2.5 mg/500 mg. **Steglujan:** ertugliflozin/sitagliptin (an antidiabetic): 5 mg/100 mg.

◆CLASSIFICATION

PHARMACOTHERAPEUTIC: Sodium-glucose cotransporter 2 (SGLT2) inhibitor. **CLINICAL:** Antidiabetic.

USES

Adjunctive treatment to diet and exercise to improve glycemic control in pts with type 2 diabetes mellitus.

PRECAUTIONS

Contraindications: Hypersensitivity to ertugliflozin, other SGLT2 inhibitors; severe renal impairment (eGFR less than 30 mL/min), ESRD, dialysis. **Cautions:** Concurrent use of diuretics, other hypoglycemic medications; mild to moderate renal impairment (CrCl less than 30 mL/min), hypovolemia (anemia, dehydration), elderly; pts with low systolic B/P, hyperlipidemia. Pts at risk for lower leg amputation (diabetic foot ulcers, peripheral vascular disease, neuropathy). History of genital mycotic infection. Not recommended in pts with diabetic ketoacidosis, type 1 diabetes mellitus.

ACTION

Inhibits SGLT2 in proximal renal tubule, reducing reabsorption of filtered glucose from tubular lumen and lowering renal threshold for glucose. **Therapeutic Effect:** Increases urinary excretion of glucose, lowers serum glucose levels.

PHARMACOKINETICS

Readily absorbed. Metabolized in liver by glucuronidation. Protein binding: 94%. Peak plasma concentration: 1 hr. Excreted in urine (50%), feces (41%). **Half-life:** 17 hrs.

⌛ LIFESPAN CONSIDERATIONS

Pregnancy/Lactation: Not recommended in second or third trimester. Unknown if distributed in breast milk. Breastfeeding not recommended. **Children:** Safety and efficacy not established.

Elderly: May have increased risk for adverse reactions (dehydration, hypotension, syncope).

INTERACTIONS

DRUG: **Insulin, insulin secretagogues (e.g., glyBURIDE)** may increase risk of hypoglycemia. **Loop diuretics (e.g., furosemide)** may increase risk of symptomatic hypotension. **HERBAL:** **Fenugreek, garlic, ginkgo, ginger, ginseng** may increase hypoglycemic effect. None significant. **FOOD:** None known. **LAB VALUES:** May increase low-density lipoprotein cholesterol (LDL-C), serum creatinine phosphate; Hgb. May decrease eGFR.

AVAILABILITY (Rx)

Tablets: 5 mg, 15 mg.

ADMINISTRATION/HANDLING

PO

- Give without regard to food in the morning.

INDICATIONS/ROUTES/DOSAGE

Type 2 Diabetes Mellitus

PO: ADULTS, ELDERLY: Initially, 5 mg once daily in the morning. May increase dose based on tolerability. **Maximum:** 15 mg/day.

Dosage in Renal Impairment

eGFR greater than 60 mL/min: No dose adjustment. **eGFR 30–59 mL/min:** Not recommended. **eGFR less than 30 mL/min:** Contraindicated.

Dosage in Hepatic Impairment

Mild to moderate impairment: No dose adjustment. **Severe impairment:** Not specified; use caution.

SIDE EFFECTS

Rare (2%–less than 1%): Headache, increased urination, nasopharyngitis, back pain, decreased weight, thirst, dry mouth, polydipsia, dry throat.

ADVERSE EFFECTS/TOXIC REACTIONS

Symptomatic hypotension (orthostatic hypotension, postural dizziness, syncope) may occur, esp. in pts who are elderly, use diuretics, or have low systolic B/P. Fatal cases of ketoacidosis have occurred. Intravascular volume depletion/contraction may cause acute kidney injury requiring dialysis. Hypoglycemic events were reported, esp. in pts using concomitant hypoglycemic medications that cause hypoglycemia. Infections including urosepsis, pyelonephritis, UTI, genital mycotic infections (male and female), upper respiratory tract infection may occur. May increase risk of lower limb amputations. Necrotizing fasciitis of the perineum (Fournier gangrene), a life-threatening necrotizing infection of the genital and perineum region that requires urgent surgical intervention, has been reported.

NURSING CONSIDERATIONS

BASELINE ASSESSMENT

Obtain BUN, serum creatinine, eGFR, CrCl; capillary blood glucose, Hgb A1c; B/P. Correct volume-depletion before initiation. Assess pt's understanding of diabetes management, routine home glucose monitoring. Receive full medication history and screen for interactions. Question history of renal impairment. Screen for risks of lower limb amputation (e.g., peripheral vascular disease, diabetic foot ulcers, neuropathy).

INTERVENTION/EVALUATION

Obtain BUN, serum creatinine, eGFR, CrCl; capillary blood glucose, Hgb A1c periodically. Monitor for symptoms of ketoacidosis (e.g., dehydration, confusion, extreme thirst, fruity breath, Kussmaul respirations, nausea). Pts presenting with metabolic acidosis should be screened for ketoacidosis, regardless of serum glucose levels. Assess for hypoglycemia (anxiety, confusion, diaphoresis, diplopia, dizziness, headache, hunger, perioral numbness, tachycardia, tremors); hyperglycemia (fatigue, Kussmaul respirations, polyphagia, polyuria, polydipsia, nausea, vomiting). Concomitant use of beta blockers (e.g., carvedilol, metoprolol) may mask symptoms of hypoglycemia. Monitor for acute kidney injury (dark-colored urine, flank pain, decreased urine output, muscle aches), UTI (dysuria, fever, flank pain, malaise), mycotic infections, Fournier gangrene (perineal necrosis). Screen for glucose-altering conditions: fever, increased activity or stress, surgical procedures. Obtain dietary consult for nutritional education. Encourage fluid intake. Monitor weight, I&Os.

PATIENT/FAMILY TEACHING

• Diabetes mellitus requires lifelong control. Diet and exercise are principal parts of treatment; do not skip or delay meals. • Test blood sugar regularly. • Monitor daily calorie intake. • When taking combination drug therapy or when glucose demands are altered (fever, infection, trauma, stress), have low blood sugar treatment readily available (glucagon, oral dextrose). • Go slowly from lying to standing to prevent dizziness. • Genital itching may indicate yeast infection. • Therapy may increase risk for dehydration/low blood pressure, which may cause kidney failure. Immediately report decreased urination, amber-colored urine, flank pain, fatigue, swelling of the hands or feet. • Report symptoms of UTI, kidney infection (e.g., burning while urinating, cloudy or foul-smelling urine, pelvic pain, back pain), perineal necrosis (e.g., discoloration, pain, swelling of the scrotum, penis, or perineum). • Do not breastfeed.

erythromycin

er-**ith**-roe-**mye**-sin
(Akne-Mycin, EES, Erybid ✱, Eryc, EryDerm, EryPed, Ery-Tab, Erythrocin)

Do not confuse Eryc with Emcyt, or erythromycin with azithromycin or clarithromycin.

FIXED-COMBINATION(S)

Eryzole, Pediazole: erythromycin/sulfiSOXAZOLE (sulfonamide): 200 mg/600 mg per 5 mL.

◆CLASSIFICATION

PHARMACOTHERAPEUTIC: Macrolide. **CLINICAL:** Antibiotic, anti-acne.

USES

Treatment of susceptible infections due to *S. pyogenes, S. pneumoniae, S. aureus, M. pneumoniae, Legionella, Chlamydia, N. gonorrhoeae, E. histolytica,* including syphilis, nongonococcal urethritis, diphtheria, pertussis, chancroid, *Campylobacter* gastroenteritis. **Topical:** Treatment of acne vulgaris. **Ophthalmic:** Prevention of gonococcal ophthalmia neonatorum, superficial ocular infections. **OFF-LABEL: Systemic:** Treatment of acne vulgaris, chancroid, *Campylobacter* enteritis, gastroparesis, Lyme disease, preoperative gut sterilization. **Topical:** Treatment of minor bacterial skin infections. **Ophthalmic:** Treatment of blepharitis, conjunctivitis, keratitis, chlamydial trachoma.

PRECAUTIONS

Contraindications: Hypersensitivity to erythromycin. Concomitant administration with ergot derivatives, lovastatin, pimozide, simvastatin. **Cautions:** Elderly, myasthenia gravis, strong CYP3A4 inhibitor, hepatic impairment, pts with prolonged QT intervals, uncorrected hypokalemia or hypomagnesemia, concurrent use of class IA or III antiarrhythmics.

ACTION

Penetrates bacterial cell membranes, reversibly binds to bacterial ribosomes, inhibiting RNA-dependent protein synthesis. **Therapeutic Effect:** Bacteriostatic.

PHARMACOKINETICS

Variably absorbed from GI tract (depending on dosage form used). Protein binding: 70%–90%. Widely distributed. Metabolized in liver. Primarily eliminated in feces by bile. Not removed by hemodialysis. **Half-life:** 1.4–2 hrs (increased in renal impairment).

LIFESPAN CONSIDERATIONS

Pregnancy/Lactation: Crosses placenta. Distributed in breast milk. Erythromycin estolate may increase hepatic enzymes in pregnant women. **Children/Elderly:** No age-related precautions noted. High dosage in pts with decreased hepatic/renal function increases risk of hearing loss.

INTERACTIONS

DRUG: May increase concentration/effect of **bosutinib, budesonide, busPIRone, cycloSPORINE, calcium channel blockers (e.g., dilTIAZem, verapamil), statins (e.g., atorvastatin, simvastatin). Amiodarone, dronedarone, fluconazole** may increase QT interval–prolonging effect. **Strong CYP3A4 inducers (e.g., carBAMazepine, phenytoin, rifAMPin)** may decrease concentration/effect. **HERBAL: St. John's wort** may decrease concentration. **FOOD:** None known. **LAB VALUES:** May increase serum alkaline phosphatase, bilirubin, ALT, AST.

AVAILABILITY (Rx)

Gel, Topical: 2%. **Injection, Powder for Reconstitution:** 500 mg. **Ointment, Ophthalmic:** 0.5%. **Ointment, Topical:** ***(Akne-Mycin):*** 2%. **Oral Suspension:** ***(EES, EryPed):*** 200 mg/5 mL, 400 mg/5 mL. **Tablet as Base:** 250 mg, 500 mg. **Tablet as Ethylsuccinate:** ***(EES):*** 400 mg.

Capsules, Delayed-Release: 250 mg. **Tablets, Delayed-Release (Ery-Tab):** 250 mg, 333 mg, 500 mg.

ADMINISTRATION/HANDLING

IV

Reconstitution • Reconstitute each 500 mg with 10 mL Sterile Water for Injection without preservative to provide a concentration of 50 mg/mL. • Further dilute with 100–250 mL D_5W or 0.9% NaCl to maximum concentration of 5 mg/mL.

Rate of administration • For intermittent IV infusion (piggyback), infuse over 20–60 min.

Storage • Store parenteral form at room temperature. • Initial reconstituted solution in vial is stable for 2 wks refrigerated or 24 hrs at room temperature. • Diluted IV solution stable for 8 hrs at room temperature or 24 hrs if refrigerated. • Discard if precipitate forms.

PO

• May give with food to decrease GI upset. Do not give with milk or acidic beverages. • Oral suspension is stable for 35 days at room temperature. • Do not crush delayed-release capsules, tablets.

Ophthalmic

• Place gloved finger on lower eyelid and pull out until a pocket is formed between eye and lower lid. • Place 1/4–1/2 inch of ointment into pocket. • Instruct pt to close eye gently for 1–2 min (so that medication will not be squeezed out of the sac) and to roll eyeball to increase contact area of drug to eye.

IV INCOMPATIBILITIES

Fluconazole (Diflucan), furosemide (Lasix), heparin, metoclopramide (Reglan).

IV COMPATIBILITIES

Amiodarone (Cordarone), dilTIAZem (Cardizem), HYDROmorphone (Dilaudid), lidocaine, LORazepam (Ativan), magnesium sulfate, midazolam (Versed), morphine, multivitamins, potassium chloride.

INDICATIONS/ROUTES/DOSAGE

Usual Dosage Range

PO: ADULTS, ELDERLY: ***(Base):*** 250–500 mg q6–12h. **Maximum:** 4 g/day. **CHILDREN:** 30–50 mg/kg/day in divided doses q6–8h. **Maximum:** 2 g/day. *(Ethylsuccinate):* ADULTS, ELDERLY: 400–800 mg q6–12h. **Maximum:** 4 g/day. CHILDREN: 30–50 mg/kg/day in divided doses q6–8h. **Maximum:** 2 g/day. NEONATES: 10 mg/kg/dose q8–12h.

IV: ADULTS, ELDERLY: 15–20 mg/kg/day divided q6h. **Maximum:** 4 g/day. CHILDREN, INFANTS: 15–20 mg/kg/day divided q6h. **Maximum:** 4 g/day. NEONATES: 10 mg/kg/dose q8–12h.

Dosage in Renal/Hepatic Impairment

No dose adjustment.

SIDE EFFECTS

Frequent: **IV:** Abdominal cramping/discomfort, phlebitis/thrombophlebitis. **Topical:** Dry skin (50%). Occasional: Nausea, vomiting, diarrhea, rash, urticaria. Rare: **Ophthalmic:** Sensitivity reaction with increased irritation, burning, itching, inflammation. **Topical:** Urticaria.

ADVERSE EFFECTS/TOXIC REACTIONS

Antibiotic-associated colitis, other superinfections (abdominal cramps, severe watery diarrhea, fever), reversible cholestatic hepatitis may occur. High dosage in pts with renal impairment may lead to reversible hearing loss. Anaphylaxis occurs rarely. Ventricular arrhythmias, prolonged QT interval occur rarely with IV form.

NURSING CONSIDERATIONS

BASELINE ASSESSMENT

Question for history of allergies (particularly erythromycins), hepatitis. Receive full medication history and screen for interactions.

INTERVENTION/EVALUATION

Monitor daily pattern of bowel activity, stool consistency. Assess skin for rash. Assess for hepatotoxicity (malaise, fever, abdominal pain, GI disturbances). Be alert for superinfection: fever, vomiting, diarrhea, anal/genital pruritus, oral mucosal changes (ulceration, pain, erythema). Check for phlebitis (heat, pain, red streaking over vein). Monitor for high-dose hearing loss.

PATIENT/FAMILY TEACHING

• Continue therapy for full length of treatment. • Doses should be evenly spaced. • Take medication with 8 oz water 1 hr before or 2 hrs following food or beverage. • **Ophthalmic:** Report burning, itching, inflammation. • **Topical:** Report excessive skin dryness, itching, burning. • Improvement of acne may not occur for 1–2 mos; maximum benefit may take 3 mos; therapy may last mos or yrs. • Use caution if using other topical acne preparations containing peeling or abrasive agents, medicated or abrasive soaps, cosmetics containing alcohol (e.g., astringents, aftershave lotion).

E

escitalopram

es-sye-**tal**-o-pram
(Cipralex ✱, Lexapro)

BLACK BOX ALERT Increased risk of suicidal ideation and behavior in children, adolescents, young adults 18–24 yrs with major depressive disorder, other psychiatric disorders.

◆CLASSIFICATION

PHARMACOTHERAPEUTIC: Selective serotonin reuptake inhibitor. CLINICAL: Antidepressant.

USES

Treatment of major depressive disorder. Treatment of generalized anxiety disorder (GAD). OFF-LABEL: Seasonal affective disorder (SAD) in children and adolescents, pervasive developmental disorders (e.g., autism), vasomotor symptoms associated with menopause.

PRECAUTIONS

Contraindications: Hypersensitivity to escitalopram. Use of MAOI intended to treat psychiatric disorders (concurrent or within 14 days of discontinuing either escitalopram or MAOI). Initiation in pts receiving linezolid or IV methylene blue. Concurrent use with pimozide.

Cautions: Hepatic/renal impairment, history of seizure disorder, concurrent use of CNS depressants, pts at high risk of suicide, concomitant aspirin, NSAIDs, warfarin (may potentiate bleeding risk), elderly, metabolic disease; recent history of MI, cardiovascular disease.

ACTION

Blocks uptake of neurotransmitter serotonin at neuronal presynaptic membranes, increasing its availability at postsynaptic receptor sites. **Therapeutic Effect:** Antidepressant effect.

PHARMACOKINETICS

Readily absorbed. Protein binding: 56%. Primarily metabolized in liver. Primarily excreted in feces, with a lesser amount eliminated in urine. **Half-life:** 35 hrs.

LIFESPAN CONSIDERATIONS

Pregnancy/Lactation: Distributed in breast milk. **Children:** May cause increased anticholinergic effects or hyperexcitability. **Elderly:** More sensitive to anticholinergic effects (e.g., dry mouth), more likely to experience dizziness, sedation, confusion, hypotension, hyperexcitability.

INTERACTIONS

DRUG: **Alcohol, CNS depressants (e.g., LORazepam, morphine, zolpidem)** may increase CNS depression. **Linezolid, aspirin, NSAIDs (e.g., ibuprofen, ketorolac, naproxen), warfarin** may increase risk of bleeding. **MAOIs (e.g., phenelzine, selegiline)** may cause serotonin syndrome (autonomic hyperactivity, diaphoresis, excitement, hyperthermia, rigidity, neuroleptic malignant syndrome, coma). **SUMAtriptan** may cause weakness, hyperreflexia, poor coordination. **Strong CYP3A4 inducers (e.g., carBAMazepine, phenytoin, rifAMPin)** may decrease concentration/effect. **HERBAL:** **St. John's wort** may decrease concentration/effect. **FOOD:** None known. **LAB VALUES:** May decrease serum sodium.

AVAILABILITY (Rx)

Oral Solution: 5 mg/5 mL.

Tablets: 5 mg, 10 mg, 20 mg.

ADMINISTRATION/HANDLING

PO

- Give without regard to food.
- Do not break, crush, dissolve, or divide tablets.

INDICATIONS/ROUTES/DOSAGE

Depression

PO: **ADULTS:** Initially, 10 mg once daily in the morning or evening. May increase to 20 mg after a minimum of 1 wk. **ELDERLY:** 10 mg/day. **ADOLESCENTS 12–17 YRS:** Initially, 10 mg once daily. May increase to 20 mg/day after at least 3 wks. **Maximum:** 20 mg once daily. Recommended: 10 mg once daily.

Generalized Anxiety Disorder

PO: **ADULTS:** Initially, 10 mg once daily in morning or evening. May increase to 20 mg after minimum of 1 wk. **ELDERLY:** 10 mg/day.

Dosage in Renal Impairment

Mild to moderate impairment: No dose adjustment. **Severe impairment:** Use caution in pts with CrCl less than 20 mL/min.

Dosage in Hepatic Impairment

10 mg/day.

SIDE EFFECTS

Frequent (21%–11%): Nausea, dry mouth, drowsiness, insomnia, diaphoresis. **Occasional (8%–4%):** Tremor, diarrhea, abnormal ejaculation, dyspepsia, fatigue, anxiety, vomiting, anorexia. **Rare (3%–2%):** Sinusitis, sexual dysfunction, menstrual disorder, abdominal pain, agitation, decreased libido.

ADVERSE EFFECTS/TOXIC REACTIONS

Overdose manifested as dizziness, drowsiness, tachycardia, confusion, seizures.

NURSING CONSIDERATIONS

BASELINE ASSESSMENT

For pts on long-term therapy, LFT, renal function tests, blood counts should be performed periodically. Observe, record behavior. Assess psychological status, thought content, sleep pattern, appearance, interest in environment.

INTERVENTION/EVALUATION

Supervise suicidal-risk pt closely during early therapy (as depression lessens, energy level improves, suicide potential increases). Assess appearance, behavior, speech pattern, level of interest, mood. Monitor for suicidal ideation (esp. at beginning of therapy or when doses are increased or decreased), social interaction, mania, panic attacks.

PATIENT/FAMILY TEACHING

• Do not stop taking medication or increase dosage. • Avoid alcohol. • Avoid tasks that require alertness, motor skills until response to drug is established. • Report worsening depression, suicidal ideation, unusual changes in behavior.

esketamine

es-ket-a-meen

(Spravato)

BLACK BOX ALERT May cause sedation, dissociative or perceptual changes after administration. Monitor for at least 2 hrs after each treatment session. Assess if pt is clinically stable before discharge from healthcare setting. Due to high risk of abuse, monitor for symptoms of drug abuse and misuse (drug-seeking behavior, dependency). May increase risk of suicidal thoughts and behavior.

Do not confuse esketamine with amphetamine, ketamine, or ergotamine, or Spravato with Steglatro.

Classification

PHARMACOTHERAPEUTIC: N-methyl-*D*-aspartate (NMDA) receptor antagonist (Schedule III). **CLINICAL:** Antidepressant.

USES

Treatment of adults with treatment-resistant depression (in combination with an oral antidepressant). Treatment of adults with depressive symptoms with major depressive disorder (MDD) with acute suicidal ideation and behavior (in combination with an oral antidepressant).

PRECAUTIONS

Contraindications: Hypersensitivity to esketamine, ketamine. Aneurysmal vascular disease, arteriovenous malformation. History of intracerebral hemorrhage. **Cautions:** Hypertension, hepatic impairment, pts at high risk for suicide and ideation; history of drug abuse and misuse, drug-seeking behavior, dependency. History of hypertensive encephalopathy. Not indicated as an anesthetic agent.

ACTION

Exact mechanism unknown. Antagonizes NMDA receptor, an ionotropic glutamine receptor. Noresketamine (major circulating metabolite) demonstrates activity at the same receptor with less affinity. **Therapeutic Effect:** Decreases effects of depression.

PHARMACOKINETICS

Metabolized in liver. Protein binding: 43%–45%. Peak plasma concentration: 20–40 min. Excreted in urine (less than 1%) as unchanged drug. **Half-life:** 7–12 hrs; (metabolite): 8 hrs.

LIFESPAN CONSIDERATIONS

Pregnancy/Lactation: Avoid pregnancy, may cause fetal harm. Distributed in breast milk. Breastfeeding not recommended. **Children:** Safety and efficacy not established. **Elderly:** No age-related precautions noted.

INTERACTIONS

DRUG: **Alcohol, CNS depressants (e.g., LORazepam, morphine, zolpidem)** may increase sedative effects. **Stimulants (e.g., amphetamines, methylphenidate,**

modafinil), MAOIs (e.g., phenelzine, selegiline) may increase hypertensive effects. **HERBAL: Herbals with sedative properties (e.g., chamomile, kava kava, valerian)** may increase CNS depression. **FOOD:** None known. **LAB VALUES:** None known.

AVAILABILITY (RX)

Nasal Spray: Two-spray device containing 28 mg/inhalation.

ADMINISTRATION/HANDLING

Intranasal

Guidelines • Must be administered in a healthcare setting under the direct supervision of a healthcare provider. Due to nausea/vomiting, pts should avoid eating food at least 2 hrs prior to dose and avoid drinking liquids at least 30 min prior to dose. • Do not prime device before use (will result in waste of dose). Use two devices for 56-mg dose or three devices for 84-mg dose with a 5-min rest between doses. • Place pt in supine position with head of bed at 45 degrees during administration.

Administration • Instruct pt to clear nasal passages as much as possible before use. • Insert tip into one nostril, pointing toward nasal turbines, away from nasal septum. Pump medication into one nostril while pt holds other nostril closed and gently sniffs dose. • Repeat steps with a 5-min rest period between next dose.

INDICATIONS/ROUTES/DOSAGE

Depression (Treatment-resistant)

Intranasal: ADULTS: Induction phase (wks 1–4): Give twice wkly on wks 1–4. **Starting dose on day 1:** 56 mg. **Subsequent doses:** 56 mg (or 84 mg based on efficacy and tolerability). **Maintenance:** 56 mg or 84 mg once wkly on wks 5–8, then 56 mg or 84 mg q2wks (or once wkly) on wk 9 and thereafter.

MDD With Acute Suicidal Ideation and Behavior

INTRANASAL: ADULTS: 84 mg twice wkly for 4 wks. May reduce to 56 mg twice wkly based on tolerability. After 4 wks, assess need for continued therapy.

Dosage in Renal Impairment

Mild to severe impairment: Not specified; use caution.

Dosage in Hepatic Impairment

Mild to moderate impairment: No dose adjustment. **Severe impairment:** Not recommended.

SIDE EFFECTS

Frequent (31%–18%): Anxiety, agitation, fear, irritability, nervousness, tension, dizziness, sedation, somnolence, hypersomnia, vertigo, nausea, headache, dysgeusia, hypoesthesia. **Occasional (11%–5%):** Lethargy, fatigue, increased blood pressure, vomiting, insomnia, nasal discomfort, throat irritation, diarrhea, dry mouth, feeling drunk. **Rare (3%–2%):** Constipation, abnormal feeling, hyperhidrosis, euphoria, dysarthria, tremor, mental impairment, pollakiuria, oropharyngeal pain, tachycardia, extrasystoles.

ADVERSE EFFECTS/TOXIC REACTIONS

Disassociation and perceptual changes including derealization, depersonalization, diplopia, hallucinations, photophobia, visual impairment; distortion of time, space, illusion reported in 61%–84% of pts. May increase risk of suicidal thoughts and behavior, esp. in pts with major depressive disorder. An increase of systolic B/P greater than or equal to 40 mm Hg and/or diastolic B/P greater than or equal to 25 mm Hg reported in 8%–19% of pts. A substantial increase in B/P can occur with any dose, regardless of prior tolerated doses. Ulcerative or interstitial cystitis, long-term cognitive impairment may occur with repeated misuse and abuse.

NURSING CONSIDERATIONS

BASELINE ASSESSMENT

Obtain pregnancy test in females of reproductive potential. Assess B/P prior to each dose. If systolic B/P is greater than 140 mm Hg or diastolic B/P is greater than 90 mm Hg, consider risk and benefit of treatment. Do not administer if an increase of B/P or intracranial pressure is a serious risk. Concomitant nasal corticosteroids or decongestants on dosing days should be administered at least 1 hr prior to dose. Question history of hypertension, vascular aneurysms, cerebrovascular conditions, hepatic impairment. Assess risk of drug abuse, misuse, drug-seeking behavior. If a treatment session is missed or symptoms of depression worsen, consider returning to prior dosing schedule (e.g., q2wks to once wkly or once wkly to twice wkly).

INTERVENTION/EVALUATION

Monitor for increased B/P, CNS effects after dose. May discharge pt from healthcare setting if clinically stable for at least 2 hrs and B/P has decreased to acceptable level. Pts with moderate hepatic impairment may need to be monitored for longer than 2 hrs after administration. Monitor for nausea, vomiting after administration. Diligently screen for suicidal ideation and behavior; new onset or worsening of anxiety, depression, mood disorder. Screen for misuse, abuse, drug-seeking behavior. Monitor for ulcerative or interstitial cystitis (bladder/pelvic pain or pressure, nocturia, urgency). Assess for improvement of depression (improved emotion, self-image, interest in activities; decreased agitation, loneliness, self-harm).

PATIENT/FAMILY TEACHING

• Seek immediate medical attention if thoughts of suicide, new-onset or worsening of anxiety, depression, or changes in mood occurs. • Nervous system changes including altered perception, euphoria, delirium, difficulty speaking, distortion of time may occur. Avoid tasks that require alertness, motor skills until next day after a restful sleep. • Treatment may increase blood pressure. Avoid stimulants. • Do not eat food for at least 2 hrs before dose. Avoid liquids at least 30 min before dose. • Avoid pregnancy; treatment may cause fetal harm. Do not breastfeed.

esmolol

HIGH ALERT

es-moe-lol
(Brevibloc)
Do not confuse Brevibloc with Bumex or Buprenex, or esmolol with Osmitrol.

◆CLASSIFICATION

PHARMACOTHERAPEUTIC: Beta$_1$-adrenergic blocker. **CLINICAL:** Antiarrhythmic, antihypertensive.

USES

Rapid, short-term control of ventricular rate in supraventricular tachycardia (SVT), atrial fibrillation or flutter; treatment of tachycardia and/or hypertension (esp. intraop or postop). Treatment of noncompensatory sinus tachycardia. **OFF-LABEL:** Postoperative hypertension or SVT in children. Arrhythmia and/or rate control in ACS, intubation, thyroid storm, pheochromocytoma, electroconvulsive therapy.

PRECAUTIONS

Contraindications: Hypersensitivity to esmolol. Cardiogenic shock, uncompensated cardiac failure, second- or third-degree heart block (except in pts with pacemaker), severe sinus bradycardia, sick sinus syndrome, IV administration of calcium blockers in close proximity to esmolol, pulmonary hypertension. **Cautions:** Compensated HF; concurrent use of digoxin, verapamil, dilTIAZem. Diabetes, myasthenia gravis, renal impairment, history of anaphylaxis to allergens. Hypovolemia, hypertension, bronchospastic disease, peripheral vascular disease, Raynaud's disease.

E

ACTION

Selectively blocks $beta_1$-adrenergic receptors. **Therapeutic Effect:** Slows sinus heart rate, decreases cardiac output, reducing B/P.

PHARMACOKINETICS

Rapidly metabolized primarily by esterase in cytosol of red blood cells. Protein binding: 55%. Less than 1%–2% excreted in urine. **Half-life:** 9 min.

LIFESPAN CONSIDERATIONS

Pregnancy/Lactation: Crosses placenta; distributed in breast milk. **Children:** Safety and efficacy not established. **Elderly:** No age-related precautions noted.

INTERACTIONS

DRUG: **Alpha-2 agonists (e.g., norepinephrine), calcium channel blockers (e.g., dilTIAZem, verapamil), dronedarone, rivastigmine** may increase the bradycardic effect. May increase bradycardic effect of **fingolimod.** May increase vasoconstricting effect of **ergot derivatives (e.g., ergotamine).** **HERBAL:** **Herbals with hypotensive properties (e.g., garlic, ginger, gingko biloba)** may increase effect. **Herbals with hypertensive properties (e.g., yohimbe)** may decrease effect. **FOOD:** None known. **LAB VALUES:** None significant.

AVAILABILITY (Rx)

Injection Solution: 10 mg/mL (10 mL, 250 mL), 20 mg/mL (100 mL).

ADMINISTRATION/HANDLING

◀ALERT▶ Give by IV infusion. Avoid butterfly needles, very small veins (can cause thrombophlebitis).

IV

Rate of administration • Administer by controlled infusion device; titrate to tolerance and response. • Infuse IV loading dose over 1–2 min. • Hypotension (systolic B/P less than 90 mm Hg) is greatest during first 30 min of IV infusion.

Storage • Use only clear and colorless to light yellow solution. • Discard solution if discolored or precipitate forms.

IV INCOMPATIBILITIES

Amphotericin B complex (Abelcet, AmBisome, Amphotec), furosemide (Lasix).

IV COMPATIBILITIES

Amiodarone (Cordarone), dexmedetomidine (Precedex), dilTIAZem (Cardizem), DOPamine (Intropin), heparin, magnesium, midazolam (Versed), potassium chloride, propofol (Diprivan).

INDICATIONS/ROUTES/DOSAGE

Rate Control in Supraventricular Arrhythmias

IV: ADULTS, ELDERLY: Initially, loading dose of 500 mcg/kg/min for 1 min, followed by 50 mcg/kg/min for 4 min. If optimum response is not attained in 5 min, give second loading dose of 500 mcg/kg/min for 1 min, followed by infusion of 100 mcg/kg/min for 4 min. A third (and final) loading dose can be given and infusion increased by 50 mcg/kg/min, up to 200 mcg/kg/min, for 4 min. Once desired response is attained, increase infusion by no more than 25 mcg/kg/min. Infusion usually administered over 24–48 hrs in most pts. Range: 50–200 mcg/kg/min (average dose 100 mcg/kg/min).

Intraop/Postop Tachycardia Hypertension (Immediate control)

IV: ADULTS, ELDERLY: Initially, 1,000 mcg/kg over 30 sec, then 150 mcg/kg/min infusion up to 300 mcg/kg/min.

Dosage in Renal/Hepatic Impairment

No dose adjustment.

SIDE EFFECTS

Generally well tolerated, with transient, mild side effects. **Frequent:** Hypotension (systolic B/P less than 90 mm Hg) manifested as dizziness, nausea, diaphoresis, headache, cold extremities, fatigue. **Occasional:** Anxiety, drowsiness, flushed skin, vomiting, confusion, inflammation at injection site, fever.

ADVERSE EFFECTS/TOXIC REACTIONS

Overdose may produce profound hypotension, bradycardia, dizziness, syncope, drowsiness, breathing difficulty, bluish fingernails or palms of hands, seizures. May potentiate insulin-induced hypoglycemia in diabetic pts.

NURSING CONSIDERATIONS

BASELINE ASSESSMENT

Assess B/P, apical pulse immediately before drug is administered (if pulse is 60 or less/min or systolic B/P is 90 mm Hg or less, withhold medication, contact physician).

INTERVENTION/EVALUATION

Monitor B/P for hypotension, ECG, heart rate, respiratory rate, development of diaphoresis, dizziness (usually first sign of impending hypotension). Assess pulse for quality, irregular rate, bradycardia, extremities for coldness. Assist with ambulation if dizziness occurs. Assess for nausea, diaphoresis, headache, fatigue.

esomeprazole

es-o-**mep**-ra-zole
(NexIUM, NexIUM 24 HR, Nexium IV)
Do not confuse esomeprazole with ARIPiprazole or omeprazole, or NexIUM with NexAVAR.

FIXED-COMBINATION(S)

Vimovo: esomeprazole/naproxen (NSAID): 20 mg/375 mg, 20 mg/500 mg.

◆CLASSIFICATION

PHARMACOTHERAPEUTIC: Proton pump inhibitor. **CLINICAL:** Gastric acid inhibitor.

USES

PO: Short-term treatment (4–8 wks) of erosive esophagitis; maintenance treatment of healing of erosive esophagitis; symptomatic gastroesophageal reflux disease (GERD). Treatment of pathologic hypersecretory conditions, including Zollinger-Ellison syndrome. Used in triple therapy with amoxicillin and clarithromycin for treatment of *H. pylori* infection in pts with duodenal ulcer. Reduces risk of NSAID-induced gastric ulcer. **OTC:** Treatment of frequent heartburn (2 or more days/wk). **IV:** Treatment of GERD with erosive esophagitis. Reduce risk of ulcer rebleeding postprocedures.

PRECAUTIONS

Contraindications: Hypersensitivity to esomeprazole, other proton pump inhibitors. **Cautions:** May increase risk of hip, wrist, spine fractures; hepatic impairment; elderly; Asian populations. Concurrent use of CYP3A4 inducers (e.g., rifAMPin).

ACTION

Inhibits H^+/K^+-ATPase on surface of gastric parietal cells. **Therapeutic Effect:** Reduces gastric acid secretion.

PHARMACOKINETICS

Well absorbed after PO administration. Protein binding: 97%. Extensively metabolized in liver. Primarily excreted in urine. **Half-life:** 1–1.5 hrs.

LIFESPAN CONSIDERATIONS

Pregnancy/Lactation: Unknown if drug crosses placenta or is distributed in breast milk. **Children:** Safety and efficacy not established. **Elderly:** No age-related precautions noted.

E

INTERACTIONS

DRUG: May decrease concentration/effect of **acalabrutinib, cefuroxime, erlotinib, neratinib, pazopanib. Strong CYP2C19 inducers (e.g., FLUoxetine)** may decrease concentration/effect. **CYP3A4 inducers (e.g., carBAMazepine, phenytoin, rifAMPin)** may decrease concentration/effect. **HERBAL: St. John's wort** may decrease concentration/effect. **FOOD:** None known. **LAB VALUES:** None significant.

AVAILABILITY (Rx)

Injection, Powder for Reconstitution: 20 mg, 40 mg. **Oral Suspension, Delayed-Release Packets:** 2.5 mg, 5 mg, 10 mg, 20 mg, 40 mg.

Capsules ***(Delayed-Release: [NexIUM]):*** 20 mg, 40 mg. ***[Nexium 24 HR]:*** 20 mg. **Tablets:** ***(Delayed-Release):*** 20 mg.

ADMINISTRATION/HANDLING

IV

Reconstitution • For IV push, add 5 mL of 0.9% NaCl to esomeprazole vial.

Infusion • For IV infusion, dissolve contents of one vial in 50 mL 0.9% NaCl, or D_5W.

Rate of administration • For IV push, administer over not less than 3 min. For intermittent infusion (piggyback) infuse over 10–30 min. • Flush line with 0.9% NaCl, or D_5W, both before and after administration.

Storage • Use only clear and colorless to very slightly yellow solution. • Discard solution if particulate forms. • IV infusion stable for 12 hrs in 0.9% NaCl or lactated Ringer's; 6 hrs in D_5W.

PO (Capsules)

• Give 1 hr or more before eating (best before breakfast). • Do not crush, cut capsule; administer whole. • For pts with difficulty swallowing capsules, open capsule and mix pellets with 1 tbsp applesauce. Swallow immediately without chewing.

PO (Oral Suspension)

• Empty contents into 5 mL water for 2.5 mg, 5 mg; 15 mL for 10 mg, 20 mg, 40 mg and stir. • Let stand 2–3 min to thicken. • Stir and drink within 30 min.

IV INCOMPATIBILITIES

Do not mix esomeprazole with any other medications through the same IV line or tubing.

IV COMPATIBILITIES

Ceftaroline (Teflaro), doripenem (Doribax).

INDICATIONS/ROUTES/DOSAGE

Erosive Esophagitis

PO: ADULTS, ELDERLY, CHILDREN 12 YRS AND OLDER: 20–40 mg once daily for 4–8 wks. May continue for additional 4–8 wks. **CHILDREN 1–11 YRS, WEIGHING 20 KG OR MORE:** 10–20 mg/day for up to 8 wks. **WEIGHING LESS THAN 20 KG:** 10 mg/day for up to 8 wks. **CHILDREN 1–11 MOS, WEIGHING MORE THAN 7.5 KG–12 KG:** 10 mg/day for up to 6 wks. **6–7.5 KG:** 5 mg/day for up to 6 wks. **3–5 KG:** 2.5 mg/day for up to 6 wks.

Maintenance Therapy for Erosive Esophagitis

PO: ADULTS, ELDERLY: 20 mg/day.

Treatment of NSAID-Induced Gastric Ulcers

PO: ADULTS, ELDERLY: 20 mg/day for 8 wks.

Prevention of NSAID-Induced Gastric Ulcer

PO: ADULTS, ELDERLY: 20–40 mg once daily for up to 6 mos.

Gastroesophageal Reflux Disease (GERD)
IV: ADULTS, ELDERLY: 20 or 40 mg once daily for up to 10 days. **CHILDREN 1–17 YRS, WEIGHING 55 KG OR MORE:** 20 mg once daily; **1–17 YRS, WEIGHING LESS THAN 55 KG:** 10 mg once daily; **1 MO TO LESS THAN 1 YR:** 0.5 mg/kg once daily.
PO: ADULTS, ELDERLY, CHILDREN, 12–17 YRS: 20 mg once daily for up to 8 wks. **CHILDREN 1–11 YRS:** 10 mg/day for up to 8 wks.

Zollinger-Ellison Syndrome
PO: ADULTS, ELDERLY: 40 mg 2 times/day. Doses up to 240 mg/day have been used.

Duodenal Ulcer Caused by *Helicobacter pylori*
PO: ADULTS, ELDERLY: 20-40 mg twice daily (as part of multidrug regimen).

Heartburn (OTC)
PO: ADULTS, ELDERLY: 20 mg/day for 14 days. May repeat after 4 mos if needed.

Dosage in Renal Impairment
No dose adjustment.

Dosage in Hepatic Impairment
Mild to moderate impairment: No dose adjustment. **Severe impairment:** Doses should not exceed 20 mg/day.

SIDE EFFECTS

Frequent (7%): Headache. **Occasional (3%–2%):** Diarrhea, abdominal pain, nausea. **Rare (less than 2%):** Dizziness, asthenia, vomiting, constipation, rash, cough.

ADVERSE EFFECTS/TOXIC REACTIONS

Pancreatitis, hepatotoxicity, interstitial nephritis occur rarely.

NURSING CONSIDERATIONS

BASELINE ASSESSMENT

Assess epigastric/abdominal pain. Question history of hepatic impairment, pathologic bone fractures.

INTERVENTION/EVALUATION

Evaluate for therapeutic response (relief of GI symptoms). Question if GI discomfort, nausea, diarrhea occur. Monitor for occult blood, observe for hemorrhage in pts with peptic ulcer.

PATIENT/FAMILY TEACHING

• Report headache. • Take at least 1 hr before eating. • If swallowing capsules is difficult, open capsule and mix pellets with 1 tbsp applesauce. Swallow immediately without chewing.

E

estradiol

es-tra-**dye**-ole
(Alora, Climara, Delestrogen, Depo-Estradiol, Divigel, Dotti, Elestrin, Estrogel, Evamist, Femring, Menostar, Minivelle, Vivelle-Dot)

BLACK BOX ALERT Increased risk of dementia when given to women 65 yrs and older. Use of estrogen without progestin increases risk of endometrial cancer in postmenopausal women with intact uterus. Increased risk of invasive breast cancer in postmenopausal women using conjugated estrogens with medroxyPROGESTERone. Do not use to prevent cardiovascular disease or dementia.

Do not confuse Alora with Aldara, or Estraderm with Testoderm.

FIXED-COMBINATION(S)

Activella: estradiol/norethindrone (hormone): 1 mg/0.5 mg. **Climara PRO:** estradiol/levonorgestrel (progestin): 0.045 mg/24 hr, 0.015 mg/24 hr. **Combi-patch:** estradiol/norethindrone (hormone): 0.05 mg/0.14 mg, 0.05 mg/0.25 mg. **Femhrt:** estradiol/norethindrone (hormone): 5 mcg/1 mg. **Lunelle:** estradiol/medroxyprogesterone (progestin): 5 mg/25 mg per 0.5 mL.

◆CLASSIFICATION

PHARMACOTHERAPEUTIC: Estrogen derivative. **CLINICAL:** Estrogen, antineoplastic.

USES

Treatment of moderate to severe vasomotor symptoms associated with menopause, vulvar and vaginal atrophy associated with menopause, hypoestrogenism (due to castration, hypogonadism, primary ovarian failure), metastatic breast cancer (palliation) in men and postmenopausal women, advanced prostate cancer (palliation), prevention of osteoporosis in postmenopausal women.

PRECAUTIONS

Contraindications: Hypersensitivity to estradiol, angioedema, hepatic dysfunction or disease, undiagnosed abnormal vaginal bleeding, active or history of arterial thrombosis, estrogen-dependent cancer (known, suspected, or history of), known or suspected breast cancer (except for pts being treated for metastatic disease), pregnancy, thrombophlebitis or thromboembolic disorders (current or history of), known protein C, protein S, antithrombin deficiency or other known thrombophilic disorder. **Cautions:** Renal insufficiency, diabetes mellitus, endometriosis, severe hypocalcemia, hyperlipidemias, asthma, epilepsy, migraines, SLE, hypertension, hypocalcemia, hypothyroidism, history of jaundice due to past estrogen use or pregnancy, cardiovascular disease, obesity, porphyria, severe hypocalcemia.

ACTION

Modulates pituitary secretion of gonadotropins; follicle-stimulating hormone (FSH), luteinizing hormone (LH). **Therapeutic Effect:** Promotes normal growth/development of female sex organs. Reduces elevated levels of FSH, LH.

PHARMACOKINETICS

Well absorbed from GI tract. Widely distributed. Protein binding: 50%–80%. Metabolized in liver. Primarily excreted in urine. **Half-life:** Unknown.

LIFESPAN CONSIDERATIONS

Pregnancy/Lactation: Contraindicated during pregnancy. Breastfeeding not recommended. **Children:** Caution in pts for whom bone growth is not complete (may accelerate epiphyseal closure). **Elderly:** May increase risk of new-onset dementia.

INTERACTIONS

DRUG: **CYP3A4 inducers (e.g., carBAMazepine, rifAMPin)** may decrease concentration/effects. **CYP3A4 inhibitors (e.g., clarithromycin, ketoconazole, ritonavir)** may increase concentration/effect. May decrease therapeutic effect of **anastrozole, exemestane.** **HERBAL:** **Herbals with estrogenic properties (e.g., dong quai, ginkgo biloba, ginseng, red clover)** may increase adverse effects. **St. John's wort** may decrease concentration/effects of estrogens. **FOOD:** None known. **LAB VALUES:** May increase serum glucose, calcium, HDL, triglycerides. May decrease serum cholesterol, LDL. May affect metapyrone testing, thyroid function tests.

AVAILABILITY (Rx)

Cream, Topical: 0.4%, 0.6%. **Emulsion, Topical:** ***(Estrasorb):*** 4.35 mg estradiol/1.74 g pouch (contents of 2 pouches deliver estradiol 0.05 mg/day). **Gel, Topical:** ***(Divigel):*** 0.1% (0.25-g packet delivers estradiol 0.25 mg, 0.5-g packet delivers estradiol 0.5 mg, 1-g packet delivers 1 mg). ***(Elestrin):*** 0.06% delivers 0.52 mg estradiol/actuation. ***(Estrogel):*** 0.06% delivers 0.75 mg/actuation. **Injection (Cypionate):** ***Depo-Estradiol:*** 5 mg/mL. **(Valerate):** ***Delestrogen:*** 10 mg/mL, 20 mg/mL, 40 mg/mL. **Tablets:** 0.5 mg, 1 mg, 2 mg. **Topical Spray:** ***(Evamist):*** 1.53 mg/spray. **Transdermal System:** ***(Alora):*** twice wkly: 0.025 mg/24 hrs, 0.05 mg/24 hrs, 0.075 mg/24 hrs, 0.1 mg/24 hrs. ***(Climara):*** once wkly: 0.025 mg/24 hrs, 0.0375 mg/24 hrs, 0.05 mg/24 hrs, 0.06 mg/24 hrs, 0.075 mg/24 hrs, 0.1 mg/24 hrs. ***(Menostar):*** once wkly: 0.014 mg/24 hrs. ***(Minivelle, Vivelle-Dot):*** twice wkly: 0.025 mg/24 hrs, 0.0375 mg/24 hrs, 0.05 mg/24 hrs, 0.075 mg/24 hrs, 0.1 mg/24 hrs. **Vaginal Cream:** ***(Estrace):*** 0.1 mg/g. **Vaginal Ring:** ***(Estring):*** 2 mg (releases 7.5 mcg/day over 90 days). ***(Femring):*** 0.05 mg/day (total estradiol 12.4 mg release 0.05 mg/day over 3 mos); 0.1 mg/day (total estradiol 24.8 mg-release 0.1 mg/day over 3 mos). **Vaginal Tablet:** ***(Vagifem):*** 10 mcg.

ADMINISTRATION/HANDLING

IM

• Rotate vial to disperse drug in solution. • Inject deep IM in large muscle mass.

PO

• Administer at same time each day.
• Administer with food.

Transdermal

• Remove old patch; select new site (buttocks are alternative application site). • Peel off protective strip to expose adhesive surface. • Apply to clean, dry, intact skin on trunk of body (area with as little hair as possible). • Press in place for at least 10 sec (do not apply to breasts or waistline).

Vaginal

• Apply at bedtime for best absorption. • Insert end of filled applicator into vagina, directed slightly toward sacrum; push plunger down completely. • Avoid skin contact with cream (prevents skin absorption).

INDICATIONS/ROUTES/DOSAGE

Prostate Cancer

IM: ***(Delestrogen):*** **ADULTS, ELDERLY:** 30 mg or more q1–2wks.
PO: ADULTS, ELDERLY: 1–2 mg tid for at least 3 mos.

Breast Cancer (Metastatic)

PO: ADULTS, ELDERLY: 10 mg 3 times/day for at least 3 mos.

Osteoporosis Prophylaxis in Postmenopausal Females

PO: ADULTS, ELDERLY: 0.5 mg/day cyclically (3 wks on, 1 wk off).
Transdermal: ***(Climara):*** **ADULTS, ELDERLY:** Initially, 0.025 mg/24 hrs wkly; adjust dose as needed.
Transdermal: ***(Alora, Minivelle, Vivelle-Dot):*** **ADULTS, ELDERLY:** Initially, 0.025 mg/24 hrs patch twice wkly; adjust dose as needed.
Transdermal: ***(Menostar):*** **ADULTS, ELDERLY:** 0.014 mg/24 hrs patch wkly.

Female Hypoestrogenism

PO: ADULTS, ELDERLY: 1–2 mg/day; adjust dose as needed.
IM: ***(Depo-Estradiol):*** **ADULTS, ELDERLY:** 1.5–2 mg monthly.
IM: ***(Delestrogen):*** **ADULTS, ELDERLY:** 10–20 mg q4wks.
Transdermal: ***(Alora):*** Initially, 0.05 mg/day twice wkly. ***(Climara):*** 0.025 mg/day once wkly. ***(Vivelle-Dot):*** 0.025 mg/day twice wkly.

Vasomotor Symptoms Associated With Menopause

PO: ADULTS, ELDERLY: 0.5–2 mg/day cyclically (3 wks on, 1 wk off); adjust dose as needed.
IM: ***(Depo-Estradiol):*** **ADULTS, ELDERLY:** 1–5 mg q3–4wks.
IM: ***(Delestrogen):*** **ADULTS, ELDERLY:** 10–20 mg q4wks.
Topical emulsion: ***(Estrasorb):*** **ADULTS, ELDERLY:** 3.48 g (contents of 2 pouches) once daily in the morning.
Topical gel: ***(Estrogel):*** **ADULTS, ELDERLY:** 1.25 g/day.
Transdermal spray: ***(Evamist):*** Initially, 1 spray daily. May increase to 2–3 sprays daily.
Transdermal: ***(Climara):*** **ADULTS, ELDERLY:** 0.025 mg/24 hrs wkly. Adjust dose as needed.
Transdermal: ADULTS, ELDERLY: ***(Alora):*** 0.05 mg/24 hrs twice wkly. ***(Vivelle-Dot):*** 0.0375 mg/24 hrs twice wkly.

Vaginal ring: ***(Femring):*** **ADULTS, ELDERLY:** 0.05 mg. May increase to 0.1 mg if needed.

Vulvar and Vaginal Atrophy Associated With Menopause

IM: ***(Delestrogen):*** **ADULTS, ELDERLY:** 10–20 mg q4wks.
Vaginal ring: ***(Femring):*** Initially 0.05 mg. Usual dose: 0.05–0.1 mg q3mos.
PO: ***(Estrace):*** 0.5–1 mg/day 3 wks on and 1 wk off.
Topical gel: ***(Estrogel):*** 1.25 g/day at same time each day.
Transdermal: ***(Alora, Climara, Vivelle-Dot):*** See dose in availability section).
Vaginal ring: ***(Estring):*** **ADULTS, ELDERLY:** 2 mg. Ring to remain in place for 90 days.
Vaginal cream: ***(Estrace):*** Insert 2–4 g/day intravaginally for 2 wks, then reduce dose to half of initial dose for 2 wks, then maintenance dose of 1 g 1–3 times/wk.
Vaginal tablet: ***(Vagifem):*** **ADULTS, ELDERLY:** Initially, 1 tablet/day for 2 wks. **Maintenance:** 1 tablet twice wkly.

Dosage in Renal Impairment
No dose adjustment.

Dosage in Hepatic Impairment
Contraindicated.

SIDE EFFECTS

Frequent: Anorexia, nausea, swelling of breasts, peripheral edema marked by swollen ankles and feet. **Transdermal:** Skin irritation, redness. **Occasional:** Vomiting (esp. with high doses), headache (may be severe), intolerance to contact lenses, hypertension, glucose intolerance, brown spots on exposed skin. **Vaginal:** Local irritation, vaginal discharge, changes in vaginal bleeding (spotting, breakthrough, prolonged bleeding). **Rare:** Chorea (involuntary movements), hirsutism (abnormal hairiness), loss of scalp hair, depression.

ADVERSE EFFECTS/TOXIC REACTIONS

Prolonged administration increases risk of gallbladder disease, thromboembolic disease, breast/cervical/vaginal/endometrial/hepatic carcinoma. Cholestatic jaundice occurs rarely.

NURSING CONSIDERATIONS

BASELINE ASSESSMENT

Assess frequency/severity of vasomotor symptoms. Question medical history as listed in Precautions. Question for possibility of pregnancy (contraindicated).

INTERVENTION/EVALUATION

Monitor B/P, weight, serum calcium, glucose, LFT. Monitor for loss of vision, sudden onset of proptosis, diplopia, migraine, thromboembolic disorders.

PATIENT/FAMILY TEACHING

• Limit alcohol, caffeine. • Avoid grapefruit products. • Immediately report sudden headache, vomiting, disturbance of vision/speech, numbness/weakness of extremities, chest pain, calf pain, shortness of breath, severe abdominal pain, mental depression, unusual bleeding. • Avoid smoking. • Report abnormal vaginal bleeding. • Never place patch on breast or waistline.

eszopiclone

TOP 100

e-**zop**-i-klone
(Lunesta)
Do not confuse Lunesta with Neulasta.

◆CLASSIFICATION

PHARMACOTHERAPEUTIC: Nonbenzodiazepine (Schedule IV). **CLINICAL:** Hypnotic.

USES

Treatment of insomnia.

PRECAUTIONS

Contraindications: Hypersensitivity to eszopiclone. **Cautions:** Hepatic impairment, compromised respiratory function, COPD, sleep apnea, clinical depression, suicidal ideation, history of drug dependence; concomitant CNS depressants, strong CYP3A4 inhibitors (e.g., ketoconazole); elderly.

ACTION

May interact with GABA-receptor complexes at binding domains located close to or allosterically coupled to benzodiazepine receptors. **Therapeutic Effect:** Prevents insomnia, difficulty maintaining normal sleep.

PHARMACOKINETICS

Rapidly absorbed following PO administration. Protein binding: 52%–59%. Metabolized in liver. Excreted in urine. **Half-life:** 5–6 hrs.

LIFESPAN CONSIDERATIONS

Pregnancy/Lactation: Unknown if drug crosses placenta or is distributed in breast milk. **Children:** Safety and efficacy not established. **Elderly:** Pts with impaired motor or cognitive performance may require dosage adjustment.

INTERACTIONS

DRUG: **CYP3A4 inhibitors (e.g., clarithromycin, ketoconazole, ritonavir)** may increase concentration/toxicity. **Strong CYP3A4 inducers (e.g., carBAMazepine, phenytoin, rifAMPin)** may decrease concentration/effect. **CNS depressants (e.g., alcohol, morphine, oxyCODONE, zolpidem)** may increase CNS depression. **HERBAL:** **Herbals with sedative properties (e.g., chamomile, kava kava, valerian)** may increase CNS depression. **St. John's wort** may decrease concentration/effect. **FOOD:** Onset of action may be reduced if taken with or immediately after a **high-fat meal.** **LAB VALUES:** None known.

AVAILABILITY (Rx)

Tablets, Film-Coated: 1 mg, 2 mg, 3 mg.

ADMINISTRATION/HANDLING

PO

• Should be administered immediately before bedtime. • Do not give with or immediately following a high-fat or heavy meal. • Do not break, crush, dissolve, or divide tablet.

INDICATIONS/ROUTES/DOSAGE

Insomnia

PO: ADULTS: 1 mg before bedtime. **Maximum:** 3 mg. **Concurrent use with CYP3A4 inhibitors (e.g., clarithromycin, erythromycin, azole antifungals):** 1 mg before bedtime; if needed, dose may be increased to 2 mg. **ELDERLY, DEBILITATED PTS:** Initially, 1 mg before bedtime. **Maximum:** 2 mg.

Sleep Maintenance Difficulty

PO: ADULTS: 2 mg before bedtime.

Dosage in Renal Impairment

No dose adjustment.

Dosage in Hepatic Impairment

Use caution. Initially, 1 mg immediately before bedtime. **Maximum:** 2 mg.

SIDE EFFECTS

Frequent (34%–21%): Unpleasant taste, headache. **Occasional (10%–4%):** Drowsiness, dry mouth, dyspepsia, dizziness, nervousness, nausea, rash, pruritus, depression, diarrhea. **Rare (3%–2%):** Hallucinations, anxiety, confusion, abnormal dreams, decreased libido, neuralgia.

ADVERSE EFFECTS/TOXIC REACTIONS

Chest pain, peripheral edema occur occasionally.

NURSING CONSIDERATIONS

BASELINE ASSESSMENT

Assess B/P, pulse, respirations. Raise bed rails, provide call light. Provide environment conducive to sleep (quiet environment, low or no lighting). Question usual sleep patterns. Initiate fall precautions. Screen for other conditions affecting sleep (e.g., stress, depression, hyperactivity, drug abuse).

INTERVENTION/EVALUATION

Assess sleep pattern of pt. Evaluate for therapeutic response (decrease in number of nocturnal awakenings, increase in length of sleep).

PATIENT/FAMILY TEACHING

• Take only when experiencing insomnia. Do not take when insomnia is not present. • Do not break, chew, crush, dissolve, or divide tablet. Take whole. • Avoid alcohol. • At least 8 hrs must be devoted for sleep time before daily activity begins. • Take immediately before bedtime. • Report insomnia that worsens or persists longer than 7–10 days, abnormal thoughts or behavior, memory loss, anxiety.

etanercept

TOP 100

e-**tan**-er-sept
(Enbrel, Enbrel SureClick, Enbrel Mini)

BLACK BOX ALERT Serious, potentially fatal infections, including bacterial sepsis, tuberculosis, have occurred. Lymphomas, other malignancies may occur (reported in children/adolescents).

Do not confuse Enbrel with Levbid.

CLASSIFICATION

PHARMACOTHERAPEUTIC: Protein, TNF inhibitor. **CLINICAL:** Antiarthritic.

USES

Treatment of moderate to severely active rheumatoid arthritis (RA). Treatment of moderately to severely active polyarticular juvenile idiopathic arthritis (JIA), ankylosing spondylitis (AS), psoriatic arthritis. Treatment of chronic, moderate to severe plaque psoriasis. **OFF-LABEL:** Treatment of acute graft-versus-host disease.

PRECAUTIONS

Contraindications: Hypersensitivity to etanercept. Serious active infection or sepsis. **Cautions:** History of recurrent infections, conditions predisposing to infection (e.g., diabetes, renal failure, immunocompromised pts, open wounds). History of HF, decreased left ventricular function, significant hematologic abnormalities; moderate to severe alcoholic hepatitis, elderly, preexisting or recent-onset CNS demyelinating disorder.

ACTION

Binds to tumor necrosis factor (TNF), blocking its interaction with cell surface receptors. Elevated levels of TNF, involved in inflammatory processes and the resulting joint pathology of rheumatoid arthritis, JIA, AS, and plaque psoriasis. **Therapeutic Effect:** Relieves symptoms of arthritis, psoriasis, spondylitis.

PHARMACOKINETICS

Well absorbed after SQ administration. **Half-life:** 72–132 hrs.

LIFESPAN CONSIDERATIONS

Pregnancy/Lactation: Unknown if distributed in breast milk. **Children:** No age-related precautions noted in pts 4 yrs and older. **Elderly:** No age-related precautions noted.

INTERACTIONS

DRUG: Anakinra, anti-TNF agents, baricitinib, pimecrolimus, rituximab, tacrolimus (topical), tocilizumab may increase adverse/toxic effects. May increase concentration, adverse/toxic effects of **belimumab, natalizumab, tofacitinib.** Use of **live virus vaccines** may potentiate virus replication, increase vaccine side effect, decrease pt's antibody response to vaccine. **HERBAL:** **Echinacea** may decrease effects. **FOOD:** None known. **LAB VALUES:** May increase serum alkaline phosphatase, ALT, AST, bilirubin.

AVAILABILITY (Rx)

Injection Solution (Cartridge): 50 mg/mL. **Injection, Solution (Prefilled Syringe):** 25 mg/0.5 mL, 50 mg/mL. **Injection, Solution (Autoinjector):** 50 mg/mL. **Solution, Reconstituted:** 25 mg.

ADMINISTRATION/HANDLING

◀ALERT▶ Do not add other medications to solution. Do not use filter during reconstitution or administration.

SQ

• Refrigerate prefilled syringes. • Inject into thigh, abdomen, upper arm. Rotate injection sites. • Give new injection at least 1 inch from an old site and never into area where skin is tender, bruised, red, hard. • Once reconstituted, may be stored in vial for up to 14 days refrigerated.

INDICATIONS/ROUTES/DOSAGE

Rheumatoid Arthritis (RA), Psoriatic Arthritis, Ankylosing Spondylitis

SQ: ADULTS, ELDERLY: 25 mg twice wkly given 72–96 hrs apart or 50 mg once wkly. **Maximum:** 50 mg/wk.

Juvenile Rheumatoid Arthritis (JIA)

SQ: CHILDREN 2–17 YRS: (63 kg or greater): 50 mg once wkly. (Less than 63 kg): 0.8 mg/kg once wkly. **Maximum:** 50 mg/dose.

Plaque Psoriasis

SQ: ADULTS, ELDERLY: 50 mg twice wkly (give 3–4 days apart) for 3 mos. (25 mg or 50 mg once wkly have also been used.) **Maintenance:** 50 mg once wkly. **CHILDREN 4–17 YRS:** 0.8 mg/kg once wkly. **Maximum:** 50 mg/wk.

Dosage in Renal/Hepatic Impairment

No dose adjustment.

SIDE EFFECTS

Frequent (37%): Injection site erythema, pruritus, pain, swelling; abdominal pain, vomiting (more common in children than adults). **Occasional (16%–4%):** Headache, rhinitis, dizziness, pharyngitis, cough, asthenia, abdominal pain, dyspepsia. **Rare (less than 3%):** Sinusitis, allergic reaction.

ADVERSE EFFECTS/TOXIC REACTIONS

Infection (pyelonephritis, cellulitis, osteomyelitis, wound infection, leg ulcer, septic arthritis, diarrhea, bronchitis, pneumonia) occurs in 29%–38% of pts. Rare adverse effects include heart failure, hypertension, hypotension, pancreatitis, GI hemorrhage.

NURSING CONSIDERATIONS

BASELINE ASSESSMENT

Assess onset, type, location, duration of pain, inflammation. If significant exposure to varicella virus has occurred during treatment, therapy should be temporarily discontinued and treatment with varicella-zoster immune globulin should be considered. Screen for active infection. Question history as listed in Precautions. Question travel history. Screen for active infection.

INTERVENTION/EVALUATION

Assess for improvement of joint swelling, pain, tenderness. Monitor erythrocyte sedimentation rate (ESR), C-reactive protein level, CBC with differential, platelet count. Observe for signs of infection.

PATIENT/FAMILY TEACHING

• A healthcare provider will show you how to properly prepare and inject medication. You must demonstrate correct preparation and injection techniques before using medication at home. • Treatment may depress your immune system response and reduce your ability to fight infection. Report symptoms of infection such as body aches, chills, cough, fatigue, fever. Avoid those with active infection. • Report travel plans to endemic areas. • Injection site reaction generally occurs in first mo of treatment and decreases in frequency during continued therapy. • Do not receive live vaccines during treatment. • Report persistent fever, bruising, bleeding, pallor.

etoposide, VP-16 HIGH ALERT

e-**toe**-poe-side
(Etopophos, Toposar, VePesid 🍁)

BLACK BOX ALERT Severe myelosuppression with resulting infection, bleeding may occur. Must be administered by personnel trained in administration/handling of chemotherapeutic agents.

Do not confuse etoposide with etidronate, or VePesid with Pepcid or Versed.

◆CLASSIFICATION

PHARMACOTHERAPEUTIC: Topoisomerase II inhibitor. **CLINICAL:** Antineoplastic.

USES

Treatment of refractory testicular tumors, small-cell lung carcinoma. **OFF-LABEL:** Acute lymphocytic, acute nonlymphocytic leukemias; Ewing's and Kaposi's sarcoma; Hodgkin's and non-Hodgkin's lymphomas; endometrial, gastric, non–small-cell lung carcinomas; multiple myeloma; myelodysplastic syndromes; neuroblastoma; osteosarcoma; ovarian germ cell tumors; primary brain, gestational trophoblastic tumors; soft tissue sarcomas; Wilms tumor.

PRECAUTIONS

Contraindications: Hypersensitivity to etoposide. **Cautions:** Hepatic/renal impairment, myelosuppression, elderly, pts with low serum albumin.

ACTION

Induces single- and double-stranded breaks in DNA. Cell cycle–dependent and phase-specific; most effective in S and G_2 phases of cell division. **Therapeutic Effect:** Inhibits, alters DNA synthesis.

PHARMACOKINETICS

Variably absorbed from GI tract. Rapidly distributed, low concentrations in CSF. Protein binding: 97%. Metabolized in liver. Primarily excreted in urine. Not removed by hemodialysis. **Half-life:** 3–12 hrs.

⌛ LIFESPAN CONSIDERATIONS

Pregnancy/Lactation: If possible, avoid use during pregnancy, esp. first trimester. May cause fetal harm. Breastfeeding not recommended. **Children:** Safety and efficacy not established. **Elderly:** Age-related renal impairment may require dosage adjustment.

INTERACTIONS

DRUG: **Bone marrow depressants (e.g., cladribine)** may increase myelosuppression. **Live-virus vaccines** may potentiate virus replication, increase vaccine side effects, decrease pt's antibody response to vaccine. **Strong CYP3A4 inducers (e.g., carBAMazepine, phenytoin, rifAMPin)** may decrease concentration/effect. **HERBAL:** **St. John's wort** may decrease concentration. **FOOD:** None known. **LAB VALUES:** Expected decrease of leukocytes, platelets, RBC, Hgb, Hct.

AVAILABILITY (Rx)

Capsules: 50 mg. **Injection, Powder for Reconstitution:** ***(Etopophos):*** 100 mg. **Injection Solution:** ***(Toposar):*** 20 mg/mL (5 mL, 25 mL, 50 mL).

ADMINISTRATION/HANDLING

◀ALERT▶ Administer by slow IV infusion. Wear gloves when preparing solution. If powder or solution comes in contact with skin, wash immediately and thoroughly with soap, water. May be carcinogenic, mutagenic, teratogenic. Handle with extreme care during preparation, administration.

IV

Reconstitution • *(Toposar)* Dilute to a concentration of 0.2–0.4 mg/mL in D_5W or 0.9% NaCl. • *(Etopophos)* Reconstitute each 100 mg with 5–10 mL Sterile Water for Injection, D_5W, or 0.9% NaCl to provide concentration of 20 mg/mL or 10 mg/mL, respectively. • May give without further dilution or further dilute to concentration as low as 0.1 mg/mL with 0.9% NaCl or D_5W.

Rate of administration • *(Toposar)* Infuse slowly, at least 30–60 min (rapid IV may produce marked hypotension) at a rate not to exceed 100 mg/m²/hr. • Monitor for anaphylactic reaction during infusion (chills, fever, dyspnea, diaphoresis, lacrimation, sneezing, throat, back, chest pain). • *(Etopophos)* May give over as little as 5 min up to 210 min.

Storage • *(Toposar)* Store injection at room temperature before dilution. • Concentrate for injection is clear, yellow. • Diluted solution is stable at room temperature for 96 hrs at 0.2 mg/mL, 24 hrs at 0.4 mg/mL. • Discard if crystallization occurs. • *(Etopophos)* Refrigerate vials. • Stable at room temperature for 24 hrs or for 7 days if refrigerated after reconstitution.

PO

Storage • Refrigerate gelatin capsules.

IV INCOMPATIBILITIES

VePesid: Cefepime (Maxipime), filgrastim (Neupogen). **Etopophos:** Amphotericin B (Fungizone), cefepime (Maxipime), chlorproMAZINE (Thorazine), methylPREDNISolone (Solu-Medrol), prochlorperazine (Compazine).

IV COMPATIBILITIES

VePesid: CARBOplatin (Paraplatin), CISplatin (Platinol), cytarabine (Cytosar), DAUNOrubicin (Cerubidine), DOXOrubicin (Adriamycin), granisetron (Kytril), mitoXANTRONE (Novantrone), ondansetron (Zofran). **Etopophos:** CARBOplatin (Paraplatin), CISplatin (Platinol), cytarabine (Cytosar), dacarbazine (DTIC-Dome), DAUNOrubicin (Cerubidine), dexamethasone (Decadron), diphenhydrAMINE (Benadryl), DOXOrubicin (Adriamycin), granisetron (Kytril), magnesium sulfate, mannitol, mitoXANTRONE (Novantrone), ondansetron (Zofran), potassium chloride.

INDICATIONS/ROUTES/DOSAGE

◀ALERT▶ Dosage individualized based on clinical response, tolerance to adverse effects. Treatment repeated at 3- to 4-wk intervals. Refer to individual protocols.

Refractory Testicular Tumors

IV: ADULTS: 50–100 mg/m²/day on days 1–5, or 100 mg/m²/day on days 1, 3, 5 (as combination therapy). Give q3–4wks for 3–4 courses.

Small-Cell Lung Carcinoma

PO: ADULTS: Twice the IV dose rounded to nearest 50 mg. Give once daily for doses 200 mg or less, in divided doses for dosages greater than 200 mg.

IV: ADULTS: 35 mg/m²/day for 4 consecutive days up to 50 mg/m²/day for 5 consecutive days q3–4wks (as combination therapy).

Dosage in Renal Impairment

Creatinine Clearance	Dosage
15–50 mL/min	75% of normal dose
Less than 15 mL/min	Consider further dose reduction

E

E

Dosage in Hepatic Impairment
No dose adjustment.

SIDE EFFECTS

Frequent (66%–43%): Mild to moderate nausea/vomiting, alopecia. **Occasional (13%–6%):** Diarrhea, anorexia, stomatitis. **Rare (2% or less):** Hypotension, peripheral neuropathy.

ADVERSE EFFECTS/TOXIC REACTIONS

Myelosuppression manifested as hematologic toxicity, principally anemia, leukopenia (occurring 7–14 days after drug administration), thrombocytopenia (occurring 9–16 days after administration), and, to lesser extent, pancytopenia. Bone marrow recovery occurs by day 20. Hepatotoxicity occurs occasionally. Amenorrhea, angioedema, cortical blindness (transient), cyanosis, dysphagia, erythema, esophagitis, extravasation (induration/necrosis), hyperpigmentation, hypersensitivity reaction, pneumonitis, heart disease (ischemic), laryngospasm, maculopapular rash, malaise, metabolic acidosis, mucositis, MI, optic neuritis, ovarian failure, pruritic erythematous rash, pruritus, pulmonary fibrosis, radiation-recall phenomenon (dermatitis), reversible posterior leukoencephalopathy syndrome (RPLS), seizure, Stevens-Johnson syndrome, tongue edema, toxic epidermal necrolysis, toxic megacolon reported in less than 1 % of pts.

NURSING CONSIDERATIONS

BASELINE ASSESSMENT

Obtain CBC before and at frequent intervals during therapy. Antiemetics readily control nausea, vomiting. Screen for active infection. Offer emotional support.

INTERVENTION/EVALUATION

Monitor CBC, B/P, hepatic/renal function tests. Monitor daily pattern of bowel activity, stool consistency. Monitor for hematologic toxicity (fever, sore throat, signs of local infection, unusual bruising/bleeding from any site), symptoms of anemia (excessive fatigue, weakness). Assess for paresthesia (peripheral neuropathy). Monitor for infection (cough, fatigue, fever).

PATIENT/FAMILY TEACHING

• Treatment may depress your immune system response and reduce your ability to fight infection. Report symptoms of infection such as body aches, chills, cough, fatigue, fever. Avoid those with active infection. • Avoid pregnancy. • Promptly report fever, sore throat, signs of local infection, unusual bruising or bleeding from any site, burning or pain with urination, numbness in extremities, yellowing of skin or eyes.

everolimus

TOP 100

e-**veer**-oh-li-mus
(Afinitor, Afinitor Disperz, Zortress)

BLACK BOX ALERT Immunosuppressant (may result in infection, malignancy including lymphoma or skin cancer); increased risk of nephrotoxicity in renal transplants (avoid standard doses of cycloSPORINE); increased risk of renal arterial or venous thrombosis in renal transplants.

Do not confuse Afinitor with Lipitor, or everolimus with sirolimus, tacrolimus, or temsirolimus.

CLASSIFICATION

PHARMACOTHERAPEUTIC: mTOR kinase inhibitor. **CLINICAL:** Antineoplastic, immunosuppressant.

USES

Afinitor: Treatment of advanced renal cell carcinoma after failure of treatment with SUNItinib or SORAfenib. Treatment of subependymal giant cell astrocytoma (SEGA) associated with tuberous sclerosis. Treatment of progressive neuroendocrine tumors of pancreatic origin and progressive, well-differentiated, nonfunctional neuroendocrine tumors of GI or lung origin. Treatment of advanced hormone receptor–positive, HER2-negative breast cancer in postmenopausal women. Treatment of tuberous sclerosis complex (TSC) not requiring immediate surgery. **Afinitor Disperz:** Treatment of SEGA associated with TSC requiring intervention but that cannot be curatively resected. Treatment of TSC-associated partial-onset seizures. **Zortress:** Prophylaxis of organ rejection after kidney/liver transplant at low to moderate immunologic risk. **OFF-LABEL:** Relapsed or refractory Waldenström's macroglobulinemia. Treatment of progressive advanced carcinoid tumors.

PRECAUTIONS

Contraindications: Hypersensitivity to everolimus, sirolimus, other rapamycin derivatives. **Cautions:** Conditions predisposing to infection (e.g., diabetes, renal failure, immunocompromised pts, open wounds). Hereditary galactose intolerance; renal/hepatic impairment; hyperlipidemia; concurrent use of CYP3A4 inducers and inhibitors. Medications known to cause angioedema.

ACTION

Binds to the FK binding protein to form a complex that inhibits activation of mTOR. Inhibits vascular endothelial growth factor (VEGF). **Therapeutic Effect:** Reduces cell proliferation, produces cell death. Has antiproliferative and antiangiogenic properties.

PHARMACOKINETICS

Peak concentration occurs in 1–2 hrs following administration, with steady-state levels achieved in 2 wks. Undergoes extensive hepatic metabolism. Protein binding: 74%. Eliminated in feces (80%), urine (5%). **Half-life:** 30 hrs.

LIFESPAN CONSIDERATIONS

Pregnancy/Lactation: Avoid pregnancy during treatment and for up to 8 wks after discontinuation. Breastfeeding not recommended during treatment and for up to 2 wks after discontinuation. May cause fetal harm. Unknown if distributed in breast milk. **Children:** Safety and efficacy not established. **Elderly:** No age-related precautions noted.

INTERACTIONS

DRUG: **CYP3A4 inhibitors (e.g., clarithromycin, ketoconazole, ritonavir)**, **P-gp inhibitors (e.g., cycloSPORINE)** may increase concentration /effect. **CYP3A4 inducers (e.g., carBAMazepine, phenytoin, rifAMPin)** may decrease concentration/effect. **HERBAL:** **Echinacea** may decrease therapeutic effect. **St. John's wort** may decrease concentration/effect. **FOOD:** **High-fat meals** may reduce plasma concentration. **Grapefruit products** may increase concentration/effect (potential for myelotoxicity, nephrotoxicity). **LAB VALUES:** May increase serum BUN, creatinine, glucose, triglycerides, lipids. May decrease neutrophils, Hgb, platelets.

AVAILABILITY (Rx)

Tablets: ***(Zortress):*** 0.25 mg, 0.5 mg, 0.75 mg, 1 mg. **Tablets:** ***(Afinitor):*** 2.5 mg, 5 mg, 7.5 mg, 10 mg. **Tablets for Oral Suspension:** ***(Afinitor Disperz):*** 2 mg, 3 mg, 5 mg.

ADMINISTRATION/HANDLING

• Give without regard to food. • Swallow tablets whole; do not crush/cut Afinitor or Zortress. • If pt unable to swallow Afinitor tablets, may disperse in water with gentle stirring; give immediately. • Administer Afinitor Disperz as suspension only. Disperse in water until dissolved. • Avoid direct contact of dispersed tablet or oral solution with skin or mucous membranes.

INDICATIONS/ROUTES/DOSAGE

◀ALERT▶ If pt requires coadministration of a strong CYP3A4 inducer (e.g., carBAMazepine, dexamethasone, PHENobarbital, phenytoin, rifabutin, rifAMPin), consider doubling the dose. If strong inducer is discontinued, reduce everolimus to dose used prior to initiation. If moderate CYP3A4 inhibitors are required, reduce dose by 50%.

E

Renal Carcinoma, Neuroendocrine Tumors, Breast Cancer, TSC

PO: ADULTS, ELDERLY: *(Afinitor):* 10 mg once daily. **Coadministration with CYP3A4 inhibitors or P-gp inhibitors:** 2.5 mg once daily. May increase to 5 mg/day. **Coadministration with CYP3A4 inducers:** Increase by 5-mg increments up to 20 mg/day.

Renal Transplant Rejection Prophylaxis

PO: ADULTS, ELDERLY: *(Zortress):* Initially, 0.75 mg 2 times/day. Adjust dose at 4- to 5-day intervals based on serum concentration, tolerability, and response. Give in combination with basiliximab and concurrently with reduced doses of cycloSPORINE and corticosteroids.

Liver Transplant Rejection Prophylaxis (Begin at least 30 days post-transplant)

PO: ADULTS, ELDERLY: *(Zortress):* Initially, 1 mg 2 times/day. Adjust dose at 4- to 5-day intervals based on serum concentration, tolerability, and response.

SEGA

PO: ADULTS, ELDERLY: Initially, 4.5 mg/m^2 once daily, titrated to attain trough concentration of 5–15 ng/mL. **If trough greater than 15 ng/mL:** reduce dose by 2.5 mg/day (tablets) or 2 mg/day (tablets for oral suspension). **If trough less than 15 ng/mL:** increase dose by 2.5 mg/day (tablets) or 2 mg/day (tablets for oral suspension).

Tsc-Associated Partial-Onset Seizures

PO: ADULTS, ELDERLY, CHILDREN 2 YRS AND OLDER: Initially, 5 mg/m^2 once daily, titrated to attain trough concentration of 5–15 ng/mL. Maximum dose increment at any titration must not exceed 5 mg.

Dosage in Renal Impairment

No dose adjustment.

Dosage in Hepatic Impairment

	Mild	Moderate	Severe
Breast Cancer PNET, RCC, renal angiomyolipoma	7.5 mg/day or 5 mg/day	5 mg/day or 2.5 mg/day	2.5 mg/day
Liver/Renal transplant	Reduce dose by 33%	Reduce dose by 50%	Reduce dose by 50%
SEGA	No change	No change	Initial dose 2.5 mg/m^2/day

SIDE EFFECTS

Common (44%–26%): Stomatitis, asthenia. Diarrhea, cough, rash, nausea. **Frequent (25%–20%):** Peripheral edema, anorexia, dyspnea, vomiting, pyrexia. **Occasional (19%–10%):** Mucosal inflammation, headache, epistaxis, pruritus, dry skin, epigastric distress, extremity pain. **Rare (less than 10%):** Abdominal pain, insomnia, dry mouth, dizziness, paresthesia, eyelid edema, hypertension, nail disorder, chills.

ADVERSE EFFECTS/TOXIC REACTIONS

Noninfectious pneumonitis characterized as hypoxia, pleural effusion, cough, or dyspnea was reported in 14% of pts; Grade 3 noninfectious pneumonitis reported in 4%. Localized and systemic infections, including pneumonia, other bacterial infections, and invasive fungal infections, have occurred due to everolimus immunosuppressive properties. Renal failure occurs in 3% of pts.

NURSING CONSIDERATIONS

BASELINE ASSESSMENT

Assess medical history, esp. renal function, use of other immunosuppressants. Obtain

CBC, BMP, LFT before treatment begins and routinely thereafter. Screen for active infection. Offer emotional support.

INTERVENTION/EVALUATION

Offer antiemetics to control nausea, vomiting. Monitor daily pattern of bowel activity, stool consistency. Assess skin for evidence of rash, edema. Monitor CBC, particularly Hgb, platelet, neutrophil count; BUN, creatinine, LFT. Monitor for shortness of breath, fatigue, hypertension. Monitor for infection (cough, fatigue, fever).

PATIENT/FAMILY TEACHING

• Treatment may depress your immune system and reduce your ability to fight infection. Report symptoms of infection such as body aches, burning with urination, chills, cough, fatigue, fever. Avoid those with active infection. • Report symptoms of bone marrow depression (e.g., bruising, fatigue, fever, shortness of breath, weight loss; bleeding easily, bloody urine or stool). • Avoid direct contact of crushed tablets with skin or mucous membrane (wash thoroughly if contact occurs). • Avoid grapefruit products.

exemestane

HIGH ALERT

ex-e-**mes**-tane
(Aromasin)
Do not confuse Aromasin with Arimidex, or exemestane with estramustine.

◆CLASSIFICATION

PHARMACOTHERAPEUTIC: Aromatase inhibitor. **CLINICAL:** Antineoplastic.

USES

Treatment of advanced breast cancer in postmenopausal women whose disease has progressed following tamoxifen therapy. Adjuvant treatment of postmenopausal women with estrogen receptor–positive early breast cancer after 2–3 yrs of tamoxifen therapy for completion of 5 consecutive yrs of adjuvant hormonal therapy. **OFF-LABEL:** Reduces risk of invasive breast cancer in postmenopausal women; treatment of endometrial cancer, uterine sarcoma.

PRECAUTIONS

Contraindications: Hypersensitivity to exemestane. **Cautions:** Not indicated for use in premenopausal women. Concomitant use of estrogen-containing agents, strong CYP3A4 inducers.

ACTION

Inactivates aromatase, the principal enzyme that converts androgens to estrogens in both premenopausal and postmenopausal women, lowering circulating estrogen level. **Therapeutic Effect:** Inhibits growth of breast cancers stimulated by estrogens.

PHARMACOKINETICS

Rapidly absorbed after PO administration. Protein binding: 90%. Distributed extensively into tissues. Metabolized in liver. Excreted in urine and feces. **Half-life:** 24 hrs.

LIFESPAN CONSIDERATIONS

Pregnancy/Lactation: Indicated for postmenopausal women. **Children:** Not indicated for use in this pt population. **Elderly:** No age-related precautions noted.

INTERACTIONS

DRUG: **CYP3A4 inducers (e.g., PHENobarbital, rifAMPin)** may decrease concentration/effect. **Estrogen derivatives** may decrease therapeutic effect. **HERBAL:** **St. John's wort** may decrease concentration. **FOOD:** None known. **LAB VALUES:** May increase serum alkaline phosphatase, ALT, AST.

AVAILABILITY (Rx)

Tablets: 25 mg.

ADMINISTRATION/HANDLING

PO

• Give after meals.

INDICATIONS/ROUTES/DOSAGE

Breast Cancer (Early)

PO: POSTMENOPAUSAL WOMEN: 25 mg once daily after a meal (following 2–3 yrs tamoxifen therapy) for total duration of 5 yrs of endocrine therapy (in absence of recurrence or contralateral breast cancer).

E

Breast Cancer (Advanced)

PO: POSTMENOPAUSAL WOMEN: 25 mg once daily after a meal. 50 mg/day when used concurrently with potent CYP3A4 inducers (e.g., rifAMPin, phenytoin). Continue until tumor progression.

Dosage in Renal/Hepatic Impairment

No dose adjustment.

SIDE EFFECTS

Frequent (22%–10%): Fatigue, nausea, depression, hot flashes, pain, insomnia, anxiety, dyspnea. **Occasional (8%–5%):** Headache, dizziness, vomiting, peripheral edema, abdominal pain, anorexia, flu-like symptoms, diaphoresis, constipation, hypertension. **Rare (4%):** Diarrhea.

ADVERSE EFFECTS/TOXIC REACTIONS

MI has been reported.

NURSING CONSIDERATIONS

BASELINE ASSESSMENT

Question history of cardiac disease. Receive full medication history and screen for interactions. Offer emotional support.

INTERVENTION/EVALUATION

Monitor for onset of depression. Assess sleep pattern. Monitor for and assist with ambulation if dizziness occurs. Assess for headache. Offer antiemetic for nausea/vomiting.

PATIENT/FAMILY TEACHING

• Report if nausea, hot flashes become unmanageable. • Avoid tasks that require alertness, motor skills until response to drug is established. • Best taken after meals and at same time each day.

exenatide HIGH ALERT

ex-**en**-a-tide
(Bydureon, Bydureon BCise, Byetta, 5 mcg Pen, 10 mcg Pen)

BLACK BOX ALERT (Bydureon): Risk of thyroid C-cell tumors.

◆CLASSIFICATION

PHARMACOTHERAPEUTIC: Glucagon-like peptide-1 (GLP-1) receptor agonist. **CLINICAL:** Antidiabetic.

USES

Adjunct to diet, exercise to improve glycemic control in pts with type 2 diabetes mellitus.

PRECAUTIONS

Contraindications: Hypersensitivity to exenatide. Bydureon only: History of medullary thyroid carcinoma. Pts with multiple endocrine neoplasia syndrome type 2 (MEN2). **Cautions:** Diabetic ketoacidosis, type 1 diabetes mellitus. Pts with renal transplantation or moderate renal impairment. Not recommended in severe renal impairment, severe GI disease, pancreatitis.

ACTION

Stimulates release of insulin from beta cells of pancreas, mimics enhancement of glucose-dependent insulin secretion, suppresses elevated glucagon secretion, slows gastric emptying (central action increases satiety). **Therapeutic Effect:** Improves glycemic control by increasing postmeal insulin secretion, decreasing postmeal glucagon levels, delaying gastric emptying, and increasing satiety.

PHARMACOKINETICS

Minimal systemic metabolism. Eliminated by glomerular filtration with subsequent proteolytic degradation. **Half-life:** 2.4 hrs.

⌛ LIFESPAN CONSIDERATIONS

Pregnancy/Lactation: Unknown if distributed in breast milk. **Children:** Safety

and efficacy not established. **Elderly:** No age-related precautions noted.

INTERACTIONS

DRUG: May decrease concentration/effect of **oral contraceptives.** May increase hypoglycemic effect of **insulin, sulfonylureas (e.g., glyburide).** **HERBAL:** None significant. **FOOD:** None known. **LAB VALUES:** None known.

AVAILABILITY (Rx)

Injection, Solution (Prefilled Pen): *(Byetta):* 10 mcg/0.04 mL (2.4 mL); 5 mcg/0.02 mL (1.2 mL). **Pen Injector:** *(Bydureon):* 2 mg. **Injection Prefilled Single-Dose Auto-injector:** *(Bydureon BCise):* 2 mg in 0.85 ml vehicle.

ADMINISTRATION/HANDLING

SQ

• May be given in thigh, abdomen, upper arm. • Rotation of injection sites is essential; maintain careful injection site record. • Give within 60 min before morning and evening meals. Give suspension immediately after powder is suspended.

Storage • Refrigerate prefilled pens. • Discard if freezing occurs. • May be stored at room temperature after first use. • Discard pen 30 days after initial use. • *(Bydureon BCise):* Remove from refrigerator 15 min prior to mixing. To mix, shake vigorously for at least 15 sec.

INDICATIONS/ROUTE/DOSAGE

Diabetes Mellitus

SQ: ADULTS, ELDERLY: (Byetta) 5 mcg per dose given twice daily within the 60-min period before the morning and evening meals. Dose may be increased to 10 mcg twice daily after 1 mo of therapy. (Bydureon): 2 mg once q7days any time of day, with or without meals.

Dosage in Renal Impairment

Mild impairment: No dose adjustment. **Moderate impairment:** Use caution. **Severe impairment: CrCl less than 30 mL/min or ESRD:** Not recommended.

Dosage in Hepatic Impairment

No dose adjustment.

SIDE EFFECTS

(Byetta): **Frequent (44%):** Nausea. **Occasional (13%–6%):** Diarrhea, vomiting, dizziness, anxiety, dyspepsia. **Rare (less than 6%):** Weakness. *(Bydureon):* **5% or greater:** Nausea, diarrhea, headache, constipation, vomiting, dyspepsia, injection site pruritus or nodule.

ADVERSE EFFECTS/TOXIC REACTIONS

With concurrent sulfonylurea, hypoglycemia occurs in 36% when given a 10-mcg dose of exenatide, 16% when given a 5-mcg dose. May cause acute pancreatitis.

NURSING CONSIDERATIONS

BASELINE ASSESSMENT

Check serum glucose before administration. Discuss lifestyle to determine extent of learning, emotional needs. Ensure follow-up instruction if pt or family does not thoroughly understand diabetes management, glucose-testing technique. At least 1 mo should elapse to assess response to drug before new dose adjustment is made.

INTERVENTION/EVALUATION

Monitor serum glucose, food intake, renal function. Assess for hypoglycemia (cool wet skin, tremors, dizziness, anxiety, headache, tachycardia, numbness in mouth, hunger, diplopia), hyperglycemia (polyuria, polyphagia, polydipsia, nausea, vomiting, dim vision, fatigue, deep rapid breathing). Be alert to conditions that alter glucose requirements (fever, increased activity or stress, surgical procedure).

PATIENT/FAMILY TEACHING

• Diabetes mellitus requires lifelong control. • Prescribed diet and exercise are principal parts of treatment. Do not skip, delay meals. • Continue to adhere to dietary instructions, regular exercise program, regular testing of serum glucose. • When taking combination drug therapy or when glucose conditions are altered (excessive alcohol ingestion, insufficient carbohydrate intake, hormone deficiencies, critical illness), have a low blood sugar treatment available (e.g., glucagon, oral dextrose). • Report any unexplained severe abdominal pain with or without nausea or vomiting.

E

ezetimibe

TOP 100

e-**zet**-i-mib
(Ezetrol, Zetia)
Do not confuse Zetia with Zebeta or Zestril.

FIXED-COMBINATION(S)

Liptruzet: ezetimibe/atorvastatin (statin): 10 mg/10 mg, 10 mg/20 mg, 10 mg/40 mg, 10 mg/80 mg. **Vytorin:** ezetimibe/simvastatin (statin): 10 mg/10 mg, 10 mg/20 mg, 10 mg/40 mg, 10 mg/80 mg.

◆CLASSIFICATION

PHARMACOTHERAPEUTIC: Antihyperlipidemic. **CLINICAL:** Anticholesterol agent.

USES

Adjunct to diet for treatment of primary hypercholesterolemia (monotherapy or in combination with HMG-CoA reductase inhibitors [statins]), homozygous sitosterolemia, homozygous familial hypercholesterolemia (combined with atorvastatin or simvastatin). Mixed hyperlipidemia (in combination with fenofibrate).

PRECAUTIONS

Contraindications: Hypersensitivity to ezetimibe. Concurrent use of an HMG-CoA reductase inhibitor (atorvastatin, fluvastatin, lovastatin, pravastatin, simvastatin) in pts with active hepatic disease or unexplained persistent elevations in serum transaminase; pregnancy and breastfeeding (when used with a statin). **Cautions:** Severe renal or mild hepatic impairment. Not recommended in those with moderate or severe hepatic impairment.

ACTION

Inhibits cholesterol absorption in brush border of small intestine, leading to decrease in delivery of intestinal cholesterol to liver. Reduces hepatic cholesterol stores and increases clearance of cholesterol from the blood. **Therapeutic Effect:** Reduces total serum cholesterol, LDL, triglycerides; increases HDL.

PHARMACOKINETICS

Well absorbed following PO administration. Protein binding: greater than 90%. Metabolized in small intestine and liver. Excreted in feces (78%), urine (11%). **Half-life:** 22 hrs.

⌛ LIFESPAN CONSIDERATIONS

Pregnancy/Lactation: Unknown if drug crosses placenta or is distributed in breast milk. **Children:** Safety and efficacy not established in pts 10 yrs or younger. **Elderly:** Age-related mild hepatic impairment may require dosage adjustment.

INTERACTIONS

DRUG: Bile acid sequestrants (e.g., cholestyramine) may decrease absorption/effect. May increase concentration/effect of **cycloSPORINE. Fenofibrate and derivatives, gemfibrozil** may increase adverse effects. **HERBAL:** None significant. **FOOD:** None known. **LAB VALUES:** May increase serum alkaline phosphatase, bilirubin, ALT, AST.

AVAILABILITY (Rx)

Tablets: 10 mg.

ADMINISTRATION/HANDLING

• Give without regard to food. • May give at same time as statins. Give at least 2 hrs before or 4 hrs after bile acid sequestrants.

INDICATIONS/ROUTES/DOSAGE

Hypercholesterolemia

PO: ADULTS, ELDERLY, CHILDREN 10 YRS AND OLDER: Initially, 10 mg once daily, given with or without food. If pt is also receiving a bile acid sequestrant, give ezetimibe at least 2 hrs before or at least 4 hrs after bile acid sequestrant.

Dosage in Renal Impairment

No dose adjustment.

Dosage in Hepatic Impairment

Mild impairment: No dose adjustment. **Moderate to severe impairment:** Not recommended.

SIDE EFFECTS

Occasional (4%–3%): Back pain, diarrhea, arthralgia, sinusitis, abdominal pain. **Rare (2%):** Cough, pharyngitis, fatigue, depression.

ADVERSE EFFECTS/TOXIC REACTIONS

Hepatitis, hypersensitivity reaction, myopathy, rhabdomyolysis occur rarely.

NURSING CONSIDERATIONS

BASELINE ASSESSMENT

Obtain diet history, esp. fat consumption. Obtain serum cholesterol, triglycerides, hepatic function tests, blood counts during initial therapy and periodically during treatment. Treatment should be discontinued if hepatic enzyme levels persist more than 3 times normal limit. Receive full medication history and screen for interactions. Question history of hepatic/renal impairment.

INTERVENTION/EVALUATION

Monitor daily pattern of bowel activity, stool consistency. Question pt for signs/symptoms of back pain, abdominal disturbances. Monitor serum cholesterol, triglycerides for therapeutic response.

PATIENT/FAMILY TEACHING

• Periodic laboratory tests are essential part of therapy. • Do not stop medication without consulting physician. • Report muscular or bone pain. • May take at same time as statins. Take at least 2 hrs before or 4 hrs after cholestyramine, colestipol, colesevelam.

famciclovir

fam-**sye**-klo-veer
(Apo-Famciclovir ✱, Famvir ✱)
Do not confuse famciclovir with acyclovir, ganciclovir, or valGANciclovir; or Famvir with Femara.

◆CLASSIFICATION

PHARMACOTHERAPEUTIC: Synthetic nucleoside. **CLINICAL:** Antiviral.

USES

Treatment of acute herpes zoster (shingles) in immunocompetent pts, treatment and suppression of recurrent genital herpes in immunocompetent pts, treatment of recurrent mucocutaneous herpes simplex in HIV-infected pts. Treatment of recurrent herpes labialis (cold sores) in immunocompetent pts.

PRECAUTIONS

Contraindications: Hypersensitivity to famciclovir, penciclovir. **Cautions:** Renal impairment. Avoid use in galactose intolerance, severe lactose deficiency, or glucose-galactose malabsorption syndromes.

ACTION

Inhibits HSV-2 polymerase, inhibiting herpes viral DNA synthesis and replication. **Therapeutic Effect:** Suppresses replication of herpes simplex virus, varicella-zoster virus. Shortens healing time of herpes zoster lesions. Reduces symptom severity of genital herpes.

PHARMACOKINETICS

Rapidly absorbed. Protein binding: 20%–25%. Rapidly metabolized to penciclovir by enzymes in GI tract, liver, plasma. Excreted unchanged in urine. Removed by hemodialysis. **Half-life:** 2–3 hrs (increased in severe renal failure).

⌛ LIFESPAN CONSIDERATIONS

Pregnancy/Lactation: Unknown if excreted in breast milk. **Children:** Safety and efficacy not established. **Elderly:** Age-related renal impairment may require dosage adjustment.

INTERACTIONS

DRUG: None significant. **HERBAL:** None significant. **FOOD:** None known. **LAB VALUES:** May increase serum ALT, AST, amylase, bilirubin, lipase. May decrease neutrophils, platelets.

AVAILABILITY (Rx)

Tablets: 125 mg, 250 mg, 500 mg.

ADMINISTRATION/HANDLING

PO

• Give without regard to food. • Give with food to decrease GI distress.

INDICATIONS/ROUTES/DOSAGE

Herpes Zoster (Shingles)

PO: ADULTS: 500 mg q8h for 7 days. Begin as soon as possible after diagnosis and within 72 hrs of rash onset. **(HIV pts):** 500 mg 3 times/day for 7–10 days.

Genital Herpes Simplex (Initial)

PO: ADULTS: 250 mg 3 times/day for 7–10 days. **(HIV pts):** 500 mg twice daily for 5-10 days.

Genital Herpes Simplex (Recurrence)

PO: ADULTS: 125 mg 2 times/day for 5 days; or 500 mg once, then 250 mg 2 times/day for 2 days. **(HIV pts):** 500 mg twice daily for 5-10 days.

Genital Herpes Simplex (Suppression)

PO: ADULTS: 250 mg twice daily for up to 1 yr. **(HIV pts):** 500 mg twice daily continued indefinitely.

Herpes Labialis (Cold sores)
PO: ADULTS, ELDERLY: (Immunocompetent): 1,500 mg as a single dose. Initiate at first sign or symptoms. **(HIV pts):** 500 mg 2 times/day for 5–10 days.

Dosage in Renal Impairment
Dosage and frequency are modified based on creatinine clearance and disease process.

Creatinine Clearance	Herpes Zoster	Recurrent Genital Herpes (single-day regimen)	Recurrent Genital Herpes (suppression)	Recurrent Herpes Labialis Treatment (single-day regimen)	Recurrent Orolabial or Genital Herpes in HIV Pts
40–59 mL/min	500 mg q12h	500 mg q12h	—	750 mg	—
20–39 mL/min	500 mg q24h	500 mg	125 mg q12h	500 mg	500 mg q24h
Less than 20 mL/min	250 mg q24h	250 mg	125 mg q24h	250 mg	250 mg q24h
Hemodialysis	250 mg after each hemodialysis session	250 mg after each hemodialysis session	125 mg after each hemodialysis session	250 mg after each hemodialysis session	250 mg after each hemodialysis session

Dosage in Hemodialysis Pts
Herpes zoster: 250 mg after each dialysis treatment. **Genital herpes:** 125 mg after each dialysis treatment.

Dosage in Hepatic Impairment
No dose adjustment.

SIDE EFFECTS

Frequent (23%–12%): Headache, nausea. **Occasional (10%–2%):** Dizziness, drowsiness, paresthesia (esp. feet), diarrhea, vomiting, constipation, decreased appetite, fatigue, fever, pharyngitis, sinusitis, pruritus. **Rare (less than 2%):** Insomnia, abdominal pain, dyspepsia, flatulence, back pain, arthralgia.

ADVERSE EFFECTS/TOXIC REACTIONS

Urticaria, severe skin rash, hallucinations, confusion (delirium, disorientation occur predominantly in elderly) has been reported.

NURSING CONSIDERATIONS

BASELINE ASSESSMENT

Obtain baseline chemistry tests, esp. renal function. Question history of galactose intolerance, severe lactose deficiency, glucose-galactose malabsorption, renal impairment. Assess herpetic lesions.

INTERVENTION/EVALUATION

Evaluate cutaneous lesions. Be alert to neurologic effects: headache, dizziness. Provide analgesics, comfort measures. Monitor renal function, hepatic enzymes, CBC.

PATIENT/FAMILY TEACHING

• Do not touch lesions with fingers to avoid spreading infection to new site. • **Genital herpes:** Continue therapy for full length of treatment. • Avoid contact with lesions during duration of outbreak to prevent cross-contamination. • Use condoms during sexual activity. • Report if lesions recur or do not improve. • Avoid tasks that require alertness, motor skills until response to drug is established.

famotidine

fa-**moe**-ta-deen
(Acid Reducer Maximum Strength, Apo-Famotidine ✱, Pepcid)

Do not confuse famotidine with cimetidine, ranitidine, fluoxetine, or furosemide.

FIXED-COMBINATION(S)

Duexis: famotidine/ibuprofen (an NSAID): 26.6 mg/800 mg. **Pepcid Complete:** famotidine/calcium chloride/magnesium hydroxide (antacids): 10 mg/800 mg/165 mg.

F

◆CLASSIFICATION

PHARMACOTHERAPEUTIC: H_2 receptor antagonist. **CLINICAL:** Antiulcer, gastric acid secretion inhibitor.

USES

Treatment of active duodenal ulcer. Prevention, maintenance of duodenal ulcer recurrence. Treatment of active gastric ulcer. Treatment of gastroesophageal reflux disease (GERD) and esophagitis due to GERD. OTC formulation for relief of heartburn, acid indigestion, sour stomach. **OFF-LABEL:** *H. pylori* eradication, risk reduction of duodenal ulcer recurrence (part of multidrug regimen), stress ulcer prophylaxis in critically ill pts, relief of gastritis.

PRECAUTIONS

Contraindications: Hypersensitivity to famotidine, other H_2 antagonists. **OTC:** Avoid use in pts with dysphagia, odynophagia, hematemesis, melena, hematochezia, renal impairment. **Cautions:** Renal/hepatic impairment, elderly, thrombocytopenia.

ACTION

Inhibits histamine action of H_2 receptors of parietal cells. **Therapeutic Effect:** Inhibits gastric acid secretion (fasting, nocturnal, or stimulated by food, caffeine, insulin).

PHARMACOKINETICS

Route	Onset	Peak	Duration
PO	1 hr	1–4 hrs	10–12 hrs
IV	0.5 hr	0.5–3 hrs	10–12 hrs

Rapidly, incompletely absorbed from GI tract. Protein binding: 15%–20%. Partially metabolized in liver. Primarily excreted in urine. Not removed by hemodialysis. **Half-life:** 2.5–3.5 hrs (increased in renal impairment).

⌛ LIFESPAN CONSIDERATIONS

Pregnancy/Lactation: Unknown if drug crosses placenta or is distributed in breast milk. **Children:** No age-related precautions noted. **Elderly:** Confusion more likely to occur, esp. in pts with renal/hepatic impairment.

INTERACTIONS

DRUG: May decrease absorption of **atazanavir, cefuroxime, itraconazole, ketoconazole.** May decrease concentration/effect of **neratinib, pazopanib.** May increase concentration/effect of **risedronate.** **HERBAL:** None significant. **FOOD:** None known. **LAB VALUES:** Interferes with skin tests using allergen extracts. May increase serum alkaline phosphatase, ALT, AST. May decrease platelet count.

AVAILABILITY (Rx)

Infusion, Premix: 20 mg in 50 mL 0.9% NaCl. **Injection, Solution:** 10 mg/mL (2-mL vial). **Powder for Oral Suspension:** 40 mg/5 mL. **Tablets:** 10 mg, 20 mg, 40 mg.

ADMINISTRATION/HANDLING

IV

Reconstitution • For IV push, dilute 20 mg with 5–10 mL 0.9% NaCl. • For intermittent IV infusion (piggyback), dilute with 50–100 mL D_5W, or 0.9% NaCl.

Rate of administration • Give IV push over at least 2 min. • Infuse piggyback over 15–30 min.

Storage • Refrigerate unused vials. • IV solution appears clear, colorless. • After dilution, IV solution is stable for 48 hrs if refrigerated.

PO

• Store tablets, suspension at room temperature. • Following reconstitution, oral suspension is stable for 30 days at room temperature. • Give without regard to meals. • Shake suspension well before use.

IV INCOMPATIBILITIES

Amphotericin B complex (Abelcet, AmBisome, Amphotec), piperacillin/tazobactam (Zosyn).

IV COMPATIBILITIES

Calcium gluconate, dexamethasone (Decadron), dexmedetomidine (Precedex), DOBUTamine (Dobutrex), DOPamine (Intropin), DOXOrubicin (Adriamycin), furosemide (Lasix), heparin, HYDROmorphone (Dilaudid), insulin (regular), lidocaine, LORazepam (Ativan), magnesium sulfate, midazolam (Versed), morphine, nitroglycerin, norepinephrine (Levophed), ondansetron (Zofran), potassium chloride, potassium phosphate, propofol (Diprivan).

INDICATIONS/ROUTES/DOSAGE

Duodenal Ulcer

PO: ADULTS, ELDERLY: ADOLESCENTS, CHILDREN WEIGHING MORE THAN 40 KG (Tablets): 20 mg twice daily for 6 wks. **CHILDREN 1–16 YRS:** 1 mg/kg/day in 2 divided doses. **Maximum:** 40 mg 2 times/day. **CHILDREN 3 MOS–11 MOS:** 0.5 mg/kg/dose twice daily. **CHILDREN YOUNGER THAN 3 MOS, NEONATES:** 0.5 mg/kg/dose once daily.

Gastric Ulcer

PO: ADULTS, ELDERLY: ADOLESCENTS, CHILDREN WEIGHING MORE THAN 40 KG (Tablets, Acute therapy): 40 mg/day at bedtime for up to 8 wks. **CHILDREN (Suspension):** 0.5 mg/kg/day at bedtime or divided twice daily. **Maximum:** 40 mg/day.

Gastroesophageal Reflux Disease (GERD)

Note: A proton pump inhibitor is recommended for more severe or more frequent initial symptoms (with or without evidence of erosive esophagitis).

PO: ADULTS, ELDERLY (mild/intermittent symptoms without evidence of erosive esophagitis): Initially, 10 mg twice daily. May increase to 20 mg twice daily after 2–4 wks if symptoms persist. If symptoms still persist, may continue as needed.

Acid Indigestion, Heartburn (OTC Use)

PO: ADULTS, ELDERLY, CHILDREN 12 YRS AND OLDER: 10–20 mg q12h. May take 15–60 min before eating. **Maximum:** 40 mg/day.

Usual Parenteral Dosage

IV: ADULTS, ELDERLY, CHILDREN OLDER THAN 12 YRS: 20 mg q12h. **CHILDREN 1–12 YRS:** 0.25–0.5 mg/kg q12h. **Maximum:** 40 mg/day (20 mg/dose).

Dosage in Renal Impairment

Creatinine Clearance	Dosage
Less than 50 mL/min	50% normal dose or increase dosing interval to 48 hrs

Dosage in Hepatic Impairment

No dose adjustment.

SIDE EFFECTS

Occasional (5%): Headache. **Rare (2% or less):** Confusion, constipation, diarrhea, dizziness.

ADVERSE EFFECTS/TOXIC REACTIONS

Agranulocytosis, pancytopenia, thrombocytopenia occur rarely.

NURSING CONSIDERATIONS

BASELINE ASSESSMENT

Assess epigastric/abdominal pain. Verify platelet count in critically ill pts.

INTERVENTION/EVALUATION

Monitor daily pattern of bowel activity, stool consistency. Monitor for headache. Assess for confusion in elderly. Consider interrupting treatment in pts who develop thrombocytopenia.

PATIENT/FAMILY TEACHING

• Report headache. • Avoid excessive amounts of coffee, aspirin. • Report persistent symptoms of heartburn, acid indigestion, sour stomach.

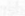

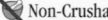

fam-trastuzumab deruxtecan-nxki

fam tras-**tu**-zoo-mab de-**rux**-the-can (Enhertu)

BLACK BOX ALERT Serious and fatal cases of interstitial lung disease (ILD), pneumonitis were reported. Monitor for symptoms of ILD, pneumonitis including cough, dyspnea, fever, worsening of respiratory symptoms. Permanently discontinue in pts with grade 2 (or higher) ILD, pneumonitis occurs. Treatment may cause fetal harm. Recommend effective contraception.

Do not confuse fam-trastuzumab deruxtecan-nxki with ado-trastuzumab emtansine, brentuximab vedotin, pertuzumab, trastuzumab (or biosimilars), or trastuzumab/hyaluronidase.

◆CLASSIFICATION

PHARMACOTHERAPEUTIC: Human epidermal growth factor receptor 2 (HER2)–directed; Antibody drug conjugate; topoisomerase inhibitor. Humanized IgG1 monoclonal antibody. **CLINICAL:** Antineoplastic.

USES

Treatment of adults with unresectable or metastatic HER2-positive breast cancer who have received two or more prior anti-HER2–based regimens in the metastatic setting.

PRECAUTIONS

Contraindications: Hypersensitivity to fam-trastuzumab deruxtecan-nxki, trastuzumab. **Cautions:** Baseline cytopenias, hepatic impairment, pulmonary disease, cardiovascular disease, HF; conditions predisposing to infection (e.g., diabetes, renal failure, immunocompromised pts, open wounds). Do not substitute with trastuzumab or ado-trastuzumab.

ACTION

Composed of a cleavable tetrapeptide-based linker (trastuzumab) and cytotoxic topoisomerase I inhibitor, DXd (an exatecan derivative). Binds to HER2 receptor and undergoes internalization and intracellular linker cleavage by lysosomal enzymes, resulting in DNA damage and apoptosis (cellular death). **Therapeutic Effect:** Inhibits tumor cell growth.

PHARMACOKINETICS

Widely distributed. Degrades into small peptides and amino acids via catabolic pathway. DXd is metabolized in liver. Protein binding: 97%. Excretion not specified. **Half-life:** 5.7 days, (DXd): 5.8 days.

⌛ LIFESPAN CONSIDERATIONS

Pregnancy/Lactation: Avoid pregnancy; may cause fetal harm. Females of reproductive potential should use effective contraception during treatment and for at least 7 mos after discontinuation. Unknown if distributed in breast milk. Breastfeeding not recommended during treatment and for at least 7 mos after discontinuation. **Males:** Males with female partners of reproductive potential should use effective contraception during treatment and for at least 4 mos after discontinuation. May impair fertility. **Children:** Safety and efficacy not established. **Elderly:** No age-related precautions noted.

INTERACTIONS

DRUG: May decrease effect of **BCG (intravesical).** May increase cardiotoxic effects of **anthracyclines (e.g., DOXOrubicin). Cladribine, dipyrone** may increase myelosuppressive effect. **HERBAL:** None significant. **FOOD:** None known. **LAB VALUES:** May increase serum ALT, AST. May decrease serum potassium; Hgb, Hct, leukocytes, lymphocytes, neutrophils, platelets, RBCs, WBCs.

AVAILABILITY (Rx)

Injection, Powder for Reconstitution: 100 mg.

ADMINISTRATION/HANDLING

IV

Reconstitution • Must be prepared by personal trained in aseptic manipulations and admixing of cytotoxic drugs. • Calculate the number of vials needed for reconstitution based on weight in kg. • Direct stream toward glass wall of vial. • Reconstitute 100 mg vial with 5 mL of Sterile Water for Injection to a final concentration of 20 mg/mL. • Swirl vial gently until powder is completely dissolved. Do not shake or agitate. • Visually inspect for particulate matter or discoloration. Solution should appear clear and colorless to light yellow in color. Do not use if solution is cloudy, discolored, or if visible particles are observed. • Dilute in 100 mL infusion bag of D_5W. Infusion bag must be made of polyvinyl chloride (PVC) or polyolefin. • Mix by gentle inversion. • Do not shake or agitate diluted solution.

Infusion guidelines • If diluted solution was refrigerated, allow solution to warm to room temperature before infusion. • Infuse via dedicated IV line using an infusion set made of polyolefin or polybutadiene, and a 0.2 or 0.22 micron in-line filter made of polyethersulfone or polysulfone. • Do not administer as IV push or bolus. • If a dose is missed, do not wait until next cycle; administer as soon as possible. Adjust schedule to maintain q3wk cycle.

Rate of administration • Give initial infusion over 90 min. Give subsequent infusions over 30 min if prior infusions were tolerated. May slow or interrupt infusion if infusion reactions occur.

Storage • Refrigerate unused vials in original carton. • May refrigerate reconstituted vials for up to 24 hrs. • May refrigerate diluted solution for up to 24 hrs or store at room temperature for up to 4 hrs. • Protect from light. • Do not shake, agitate, or freeze.

IV INCOMPATABILITIES

Do not mix with solutions containing NaCl or other medications.

INDICATIONS/ROUTES/DOSAGE

Breast Cancer (HER2-Positive)

IV: ADULTS: 5.4 mg/kg q3wks (21-day cycle) until disease progression or unacceptable toxicity.

Dose Reduction for Adverse Events

Note: Do not re-escalate if a dose reduction is made.
First dose reduction: 4.4 mg/kg.
Second dose reduction: 3.2 mg/kg.
Unable to tolerate 3.2 mg/kg: Permanently discontinue.

Dose Modification

Based on Common Terminology Criteria for Adverse Events (CTCAE).

Interstitial Lung Disease (ILD)

Grade 1 ILD/pneumonitis (asymptomatic): Withhold treatment until resolved. If resolved within 28 days, resume at same dose. If resolved in greater than 28 days, resume at reduced dose level.
Grade 2 ILD/pneumonitis (symptomatic): Permanently discontinue.

Neutropenia

Grade 3 neutropenia (500–999 cells/mm³): Withhold treatment until improved to grade 2 or less, then resume at same dose. **Grade 4 neutropenia (less than 500 cells/mm³):** Withhold treatment until improved to grade 2 or less, then resume at reduced dose level. **Febrile neutropenia (less than 1,000 cells/mm³ and temperature greater than 38.3°C or sustained temperature 38°C for more than 1 hr):** Withhold treatment until resolved, then resume at reduced dose level.

Left Ventricular Dysfunction

Left ventricular ejection fraction (LVEF) greater than 45% and an

absolute decrease from baseline of 10%–20%: Maintain the same dose. **LVEF 40%–45% and an absolute decrease from baseline of less than 10%:** Maintain same dose and assess LVEF within 3 wks. **LVEF 4%–45% and an absolute decrease from baseline of 10%–20%:** Withhold treatment and assess LVEF within 3 wks. If LVEF improves to within 10% from baseline, resume at same dose. If LVEF does not improve to within 10% from baseline, permanently discontinue. **LVEF less than 40% or an absolute decrease from baseline of greater than 20%:** Withhold treatment and assess LVEF within 3 wks. If LVEF of less than 40% or an absolute decrease from baseline of greater than 20% is confirmed, permanently discontinue. **Symptomatic HF:** Permanently discontinue.

Dosage in Renal Impairment

Mild to moderate impairment: No dose adjustment. **Severe impairment:** Not specified; use caution.

Dosage in Hepatic Impairment

Mild to moderate impairment: No dose adjustment. **Severe impairment:** Not specified; use caution.

SIDE EFFECTS

Frequent (79%–29%): Nausea, fatigue, asthenia, vomiting, alopecia, constipation, decreased appetite, diarrhea. **Occasional (20%–10%):** Cough, abdominal pain, headache, stomatitis, aphthous ulcer, mouth ulceration, oral mucosa erosion/blistering, dyspnea, dyspepsia, dry eye, rash, dizziness.

ADVERSE EFFECTS/TOXIC REACTIONS

Myelosuppression (anemia, leukopenia, lymphopenia, neutropenia, thrombocytopenia) is an expected response to therapy, but more severe reactions including severe neutropenia, febrile neutropenia may be life-threatening. Grade 3 or 4 neutropenia reported in 16% of pts. Severe, life-threatening pneumonitis, ILD, respiratory failure reported in 9% of pts. Epistaxis reported in 13% of pts. Upper respiratory tract infections reported in 15% of pts. Immunogenicity (auto–fam-trastuzumab deruxtecan-nxki antibodies) reported in less than 1 % of pts.

NURSING CONSIDERATIONS

BASELINE ASSESSMENT

Obtain CBC; pregnancy test in females of reproductive potential. Confirm compliance of effective contraception. Confirm HER2-positive status. Obtain weight in kilograms. Assess LVEF by echocardiogram. Question history of hepatic impairment, pulmonary disease, cardiovascular disease, HF. Screen for active infection. Assess hydration/nutritional status. Offer emotional support.

INTERVENTION/EVALUATION

Monitor CBC for myelosuppression prior to each dose. Consider ABG, radiologic test if ILD/pneumonitis (excessive cough, dyspnea, fever, hypoxia) is suspected. Consider treatment with corticosteroids if ILD/pneumonitis is confirmed. Assess LVEF by echocardiogram at regular intervals. If treatment is withheld due to change in LVEF, monitor LVEF within 3 wks. Monitor for infections (cough, fatigue, fever). If serious infection occurs, initiate appropriate antimicrobial therapy. Monitor daily pattern of bowel activity, stool consistency. Offer antiemetic if nausea/vomiting occurs.

PATIENT/FAMILY TEACHING

• Treatment may depress your immune system response and reduce your ability to fight infection. Report symptoms of infection such as body aches, chills, cough, fatigue, fever. Avoid those with active infection. • Report symptoms of bone marrow depression (e.g., bruising, fatigue, fever, shortness of breath, weight loss; bleeding easily, bloody urine or stool). • Report symptoms of lung inflammation (excessive coughing, difficulty breathing, chest pain); heart failure (e.g., chest pain, difficulty breathing, palpitations, swelling of extremities). • Treatment may reduce the heart's ability to pump effectively; expect routine echocardiograms. • Use effective contraception to avoid pregnancy. Do not breastfeed. • Nausea/vomiting is a common side effect. • Maintain proper hydration and nutrition.

febuxostat

fe-**bux**-oh-stat
(Uloric)
Do not confuse febuxostat with panobinostat or Femstat.

◆CLASSIFICATION

PHARMACOTHERAPEUTIC: Xanthine oxidase inhibitor. **CLINICAL:** Antigout agent.

USES

Chronic management of hyperuricemia in pts with gout. Not recommended for treatment of asymptomatic hyperuricemia.

PRECAUTIONS

Contraindications: Hypersensitivity to febuxostat. Concomitant use with azaTHIOprine, mercaptopurine. **Cautions:** Severe renal/hepatic impairment, history of heart disease or stroke. Hypersensitivity to allopurinol. Pts at risk for urate formation.

ACTION

Decreases uric acid production by selectively inhibiting the enzyme xanthine oxidase. **Therapeutic Effect:** Reduces uric acid concentrations in serum and urine.

PHARMACOKINETICS

Well absorbed from GI tract. Widely distributed. Protein binding: 99%. Metabolized in liver. Excreted in urine (49%), feces (45%). Removed by hemodialysis. **Half-life:** 5–8 hrs.

⌛ LIFESPAN CONSIDERATIONS

Pregnancy/Lactation: Unknown if drug crosses placenta or is distributed in breast milk. **Children:** Safety and efficacy not established. **Elderly:** No age-related precautions noted.

INTERACTIONS

DRUG: May increase concentration, toxicity of **azaTHIOprine, mercaptopurine, theophylline.** **HERBAL:** None significant. **FOOD:** None known. **LAB VALUES:** May increase serum alkaline phosphatase, ALT, AST, LDH, amylase, sodium, potassium, cholesterol, triglycerides, BUN, creatinine. May decrease platelets, Hgb, Hct, neutrophils. May prolong prothrombin time.

AVAILABILITY (Rx)

Tablets: 40 mg, 80 mg.

ADMINISTRATION/HANDLING

PO

• Give without regard to food or antacids.

INDICATIONS/ROUTES/DOSAGE

◀ALERT▶ Recommended concomitant NSAID or colchicine with initiation of therapy and continue for up to 6 mos to prevent exacerbations of gout.

Hyperuricemia

PO: ADULTS, ELDERLY: Initially, 40 mg once daily. If pt does not achieve serum uric acid level less than 6 mg/dL after 2 wks with 40 mg, may give 80 mg once daily. **Maximum:** 120 mg/day.

Dosage in Renal/Hepatic Impairment

Mild to moderate impairment: No dose adjustment. **Severe impairment:** Use caution.

SIDE EFFECTS

Rare (1%): Nausea, arthralgia, rash, dizziness.

ADVERSE EFFECTS/TOXIC REACTIONS

Hepatic function abnormalities occur in 6% of pts. May increase risk of thromboembolic events including CVA, MI.

NURSING CONSIDERATIONS

BASELINE ASSESSMENT

Assess renal function, LFT; concomitant use with azaTHIOprine, mercaptopurine, theophylline (contraindicated).

INTERVENTION/EVALUATION

Discontinue medication immediately if rash appears. Encourage high fluid intake (3,000 mL/day). Monitor I&O (output should be at least 2,000 mL/day). Monitor CBC, serum uric acid, renal function, LFT. Assess urine for cloudiness, unusual color, odor. Assess for therapeutic response (reduced joint tenderness, swelling, redness, limitation of motion). Monitor for symptoms of CVA, MI.

PATIENT/FAMILY TEACHING

• Encourage drinking 8–10 (8-oz) glasses of fluid daily while taking medication. • Report rash, chest pain, shortness of breath, symptoms suggestive of stroke. • Gout attacks may occur for several months after starting treatment (medication is not a pain reliever). • Continue taking even if gout attack occurs.

fenofibrate

TOP 100

fen-o-**fye**-brate
(Antara, Fenoglide, Fibricor, Lipofen, Lipidil EZ ✦, Tricor, Triglide, Trilipix)
Do not confuse Tricor with Fibricor or Tracleer.

◆CLASSIFICATION

PHARMACOTHERAPEUTIC: Fibric acid derivative. **CLINICAL:** Antihyperlipidemic.

USES

Adjunct to diet for reduction of low-density lipoprotein cholesterol (LDL-C), total cholesterol, triglycerides (types IV and V hyperlipidemia), apo-lipoprotein B, and to increase high-density lipoprotein cholesterol (HDL-C) in pts with primary hypercholesterolemia, mixed dyslipidemia. Adjunctive therapy to diet for treatment of severe hypertriglyceridemia (Fredrickson types IV and V).

PRECAUTIONS

Contraindications: Hypersensitivity to fenofibrate. Active hepatic disease, preexisting gallbladder disease, severe renal/hepatic dysfunction (including primary biliary cirrhosis, unexplained persistent hepatic function abnormality), breastfeeding. End-stage renal disease (ESRD). **Cautions:** Anticoagulant therapy (e.g., warfarin), history of hepatic disease, venous thromboembolism, mild to moderate renal impairment, substantial alcohol consumption, statin or colchicine therapy (increased risk of myopathy, rhabdomyolysis), elderly.

ACTION

Downregulates apoprotein C-III and upregulates synthesis of apoprotein A-I, fatty acid transport protein, and lipoprotein lipase, increasing VLDL catabolism. **Therapeutic Effect:** Decreases triglycerides, VLDL levels, modestly increases HDL.

PHARMACOKINETICS

Well absorbed from GI tract. Absorption increased when given with food. Protein binding: 99%. Metabolized in liver. Excreted in urine (60%), feces (25%). Not removed by hemodialysis. **Half-life:** 10–35 hrs.

⌛ LIFESPAN CONSIDERATIONS

Pregnancy/Lactation: Safety in pregnancy not established. Breastfeeding not recommended. **Children:** Safety and efficacy not established. **Elderly:** No age-related precautions noted.

INTERACTIONS

DRUG: Potentiates effects of **anticoagulants (e.g., warfarin). Bile acid sequestrants** may impede absorption. **CycloSPORINE** may increase concentration, risk of nephrotoxicity. **Colchicine, HMG-CoA reductase inhibitors (statins)** may increase risk of severe myopathy, rhabdomyolysis, acute renal failure. **HERBAL:** None significant. **FOOD: All foods** increase absorption. **LAB VALUES:** May increase serum creatine kinase (CK), ALT, AST. May decrease Hgb, Hct, WBC; serum uric acid.

AVAILABILITY (Rx)

Capsules: 30 mg, 43 mg, 50 mg, 67 mg, 90 mg, 130 mg, 134 mg, 150 mg, 200 mg. **Capsules, Delayed-Release:** 45 mg, 135 mg. **Tablets:** 35 mg, 40 mg, 48 mg, 54 mg, 105 mg, 120 mg,145 mg, 160 mg.

ADMINISTRATION/HANDLING

PO

• Give Fenoglide, Lipofen, Lofibra with meals. • Antara, Fibricor, Tricor, Triglide, and Trilipix may be given without regard to food. Antara, Fenoglide, Lipofen: Swallow whole; do not open (capsules), crush, dissolve, or cut.

INDICATIONS/ROUTES/DOSAGE

Hypertriglyceridemia

PO: ***(Antara):*** **ADULTS, ELDERLY:** 30–90 mg/day. ***(Fenofibrate):*** **ADULTS, ELDERLY:** 43–130 mg/day. ***(Fenoglide):*** **ADULTS, ELDERLY:** 40–120 mg/day with meals. ***(Fibricor):*** **ADULTS, ELDERLY:** 35–105 mg/day. ***(Lipofen):*** **ADULTS, ELDERLY:** 50–150 mg/day with meals. ***(Lofibra):*** **ADULTS, ELDERLY:** (micronized) 67–200 mg/day with meals; (tablets): 54-160 mg/day. ***(Tricor):*** **ADULTS, ELDERLY:** 48–145 mg/day. ***(Triglide):*** **ADULTS, ELDERLY:** 160 mg/day. ***(Trilipix):*** **ADULTS, ELDERLY:** 45–135 mg/day.

Hypercholesterolemia, Mixed Hyperlipidemia

PO: ***(Antara):*** **ADULTS, ELDERLY:** 90 mg/day. ***(Fenofibrate):*** **ADULTS, ELDERLY:** 130 mg/day. ***(Fenoglide):*** **ADULTS, ELDERLY:** 120 mg/day with meals. ***(Fibricor):*** **ADULTS, ELDERLY:** 105 mg/day. ***(Lipofen):*** **ADULTS, ELDERLY:** 150 mg/day with meals. ***(Lofibra):*** **ADULTS, ELDERLY:** (micronized) 200 mg/day with meals; (tablets): 160 mg/day. ***(Tricor):*** **ADULTS, ELDERLY:** 145 mg/day. ***(Triglide):*** **ADULTS, ELDERLY:** 160 mg/day. ***(Trilipix):*** **ADULTS, ELDERLY:** 135 mg/day.

Dosage in Renal Impairment

Monitor renal function before adjusting dose. Decrease dose or increase dosing interval for pts with renal failure.

Initial doses:	Antara: 30 mg/day	Lofibra: 67 mg/day
	Fenoglide: 40 mg/day	Tricor: 48 mg/day
	Lipofen: 50 mg/day	Triglide: 50 mg/day

Dosage in Hepatic Impairment

Contraindicated.

SIDE EFFECTS

Frequent (8%–4%): Pain, rash, headache, asthenia, fatigue, flu-like symptoms, dyspepsia, nausea/vomiting, rhinitis. **Occasional (3%–2%):** Diarrhea, abdominal pain, constipation, flatulence, arthralgia, decreased libido, dizziness, pruritus. **Rare (less than 2%):** Increased appetite, insomnia, polyuria, cough, blurred vision, eye floaters, earache.

ADVERSE EFFECTS/TOXIC REACTIONS

May increase cholesterol excrtion into bile, leading to cholelithiasis. Pancreatitis, hepatitis, thrombocytopenia, agranulocytosis occur rarely.

NURSING CONSIDERATIONS

BASELINE ASSESSMENT

Obtain diet history, esp. fat consumption. Obtain serum cholesterol, triglycerides, LFT, CBC during initial therapy and periodically during treatment. Treatment should be discontinued if hepatic enzyme levels persist greater than 3 times normal limit. Question medical history as listed in Precautions.

INTERVENTION/EVALUATION

For pts on concurrent therapy with HMG-CoA reductase inhibitors, monitor for complaints of myopathy (muscle pain, weakness). Monitor serum creatine kinase (CK). Monitor serum cholesterol, triglyceride for therapeutic response.

PATIENT/FAMILY TEACHING

• Report severe diarrhea, constipation, nausea. • Report skin rash/irritation, insomnia, muscle pain, tremors, dizziness.

fentaNYL

TOP 100 HIGH ALERT

fen-ta-nil
(Abstral, Actiq, Duragesic, Fentora, Ionsys, Lazanda, Sublimaze, Subsys)

BLACK BOX ALERT Physical and psychological dependence may occur with prolonged use. Must be alert to abuse, misuse, or diversion. May cause life-threatening hypoventilation, respiratory depression, or death. Use with strong or moderate CYP3A4 inhibitors may result in potentially fatal respiratory depression. **Buccal:** Tablet and lozenge contain enough medication to potentially be fatal to children. **Transdermal patch:** Serious or life-threatening hypoventilation has occurred. Limit use to children 2 yrs of age and older. Exposure to direct heat source increases drug release, resulting in overdose/death.

Do not confuse fentaNYL with alfentanil or SUFentanil.

CLASSIFICATION

PHARMACOTHERAPEUTIC: Opioid, narcotic agonist (Schedule II). **CLINICAL:** Analgesic.

USES

Injection: (FentaNYL): Pain relief, preop medication; adjunct to general or regional anesthesia. **Abstral:** Treatment of breakthrough pain in cancer pts 18 yrs of age and older. **Actiq:** Treatment of breakthrough pain in chronic cancer or AIDS-related pain. **Duragesic:** Management of chronic pain *(transdermal)*. **Fentora:** Breakthrough pain in pts on chronic opioids. **Ionsys:** Short-term management of acute postoperative pain in adults. **Lazanda:** Management of breakthrough pain in cancer. **Onsolis:** Breakthrough pain in pts with cancer currently receiving opioids and tolerant to opioid therapy. **Subsys:** Treatment of breakthrough cancer pain.

PRECAUTIONS

Contraindications: Hypersensitivity to fentaNYL. **Transdermal device (additional):** Significant respiratory depression, acute/severe bronchial asthma, paralytic ileus, GI obstruction. **Transdermal patch (additional):** Significant respiratory depression, acute/severe bronchial asthma, paralytic ileus, short-term therapy for acute or postoperative pain, pts who are not opioid tolerant. **Transmucosal buccal, buccal films, lozenges, sublingual tablets/spray, nasal spray (additional):** Management of acute or postoperative pain, pts who are not opioid tolerant. GI obstruction, significant respiratory depression (Actiq, Fentora only), acute or severe bronchial asthma. **Cautions:** Bradycardia; renal, hepatic, respiratory disease; head injuries; altered LOC; biliary tract disease; acute pancreatitis; cor pulmonale; significant COPD; increased ICP; use of MAOIs within 14 days; elderly; morbid obesity; history of drug abuse and misuse, drug-seeking behavior, dependency.

ACTION

Binds to opioid receptors in CNS, reducing stimuli from sensory nerve endings; inhibits ascending pain pathways. **Therapeutic Effect:** Alters pain reception, increases pain threshold.

PHARMACOKINETICS

Route	Onset	Peak	Duration
IV	1–2 min	3–5 min	0.5–1 hr
IM	7–15 min	20–30 min	1–2 hrs
Transdermal	6–8 hrs	24 hrs	72 hrs
Transmucosal	5–15 min	20–30 min	1–2 hrs

Well absorbed after IM or topical administration. Transmucosal form absorbed through buccal mucosa and GI tract. Protein binding: 80%–85%. Metabolized in liver. Primarily excreted by biliary system.

Half-life: 2–4 hrs IV; 17 hrs transdermal; 6.6 hrs transmucosal.

LIFESPAN CONSIDERATIONS

Pregnancy/Lactation: Readily crosses placenta. Unknown if distributed in breast milk. May prolong labor if administered in latent phase of first stage of labor or before cervical dilation of 4–5 cm has occurred. Respiratory depression may occur in neonate if mother received opiates during labor. **Children:** Neonates more susceptible to respiratory depressant effects. Patch: Safety and efficacy not established in pts younger than 12 yrs. **Elderly:** May be more susceptible to respiratory depressant effects. Age-related renal impairment may require dosage adjustment.

INTERACTIONS

DRUG: **Strong CYP3A4 inhibitors (e.g., clarithromycin, ketoconazole, ritonavir), cimetidine** may increase concentration/effect; risk for respiratory depression. **Strong CYP3A4 inducers (e.g., carBAMazepine, phenytoin, rifAMPin)** may decrease concentration/effect. **Alcohol, CNS depressants (e.g., LORazepam, haloperidol, zolpidem)** may increase CNS depression. May increase serotonergic effect of **MAOIs (e.g., phenelzine, selegiline).** HERBAL: **Herbals with sedative properties (e.g., chamomile, kava kava, valerian)** may increase CNS depression. **St. John's wort** may decrease concentration/effect. FOOD: None known. LAB VALUES: May increase serum amylase, lipase.

AVAILABILITY (Rx)

Buccal Tablet: ***(Fentora):*** 100 mcg, 200 mcg, 400 mcg, 600 mcg, 800 mcg. **Buccal Soluble Film:** ***(Onsolis):*** 200 mcg, 400 mcg, 600 mcg, 800 mcg, 1,200 mcg. **Injection Solution:** 50 mcg/mL. **Nasal Spray:** ***(Lazanda):*** 100 mcg/spray, 300 mcg/spray, 400 mcg/spray. **Sublingual Tablets:** ***(Abstral):*** 100 mcg, 200 mcg, 300 mcg, 400 mcg, 600 mcg, 800 mcg. **Sublingual Spray:** ***(Subsys):*** 100 mcg, 200 mcg, 400 mcg, 600 mcg, 800 mcg. **Transdermal Patch:** ***(Duragesic):*** 12 mcg/hr, 25 mcg/hr, 50 mcg/hr, 75 mcg/hr, 100 mcg/hr. **Transmucosal Lozenges:** ***(Actiq):*** 200 mcg, 400 mcg, 600 mcg, 800 mcg, 1,200 mcg, 1,600 mcg.

ADMINISTRATION/HANDLING

IV

Rate of administration • Give by slow IV injection (over 1–2 min). • Too-rapid injection increases risk of severe adverse reactions (skeletal/thoracic muscle rigidity resulting in apnea, laryngospasm, bronchospasm, peripheral circulatory collapse, anaphylactoid effects, cardiac arrest).

Storage • Store parenteral form at room temperature. • Opiate antagonist (naloxone) should be readily available.

Transdermal

• Apply to hairless area of intact skin of upper torso. • Use flat, nonirritated site. • Firmly press evenly and hold for 30 sec, ensuring that adhesion is in full contact with skin and that edges are completely sealed. • Use only water to cleanse site before application (soaps, oils may irritate skin). • Rotate sites of application. • Carefully fold used patches so that system adheres to itself; discard in toilet. • If patch becomes loose, cover with a transparent adhesive dressing; if patch comes off, apply new patch, rotating sites (this starts a new dosing interval). Normal exposure to water may loosen the adhesive.

Buccal Film

• Wet inside of cheek. • Place film inside mouth with pink side of unit against cheek. • Press film against cheek and hold for 5 sec. • Leave in place until dissolved (15–30 min). • Do not chew, swallow, cut film. • Liquids may be given after 5 min of application; food after film dissolves.

Buccal Tablets

• Place tablet above a rear molar between upper cheek and gum. • Dissolve over 30 min. • Swallow remaining pieces with water. • Do not split tablet.

Sublingual Spray

• Open blister pack with scissors immediately prior to use. • Spray contents underneath tongue.

Sublingual Tablets

• Place under tongue. • Dissolves rapidly. • Do not suck, chew, or swallow tablet.

Nasal

• Prime device before use by spraying into pouch. • Insert nozzle about 12 inch into nose, pointing toward bridge of nose, tilting bottle slightly. • Press down firmly until hearing a "click" and number on counting window advances by one. Do not blow nose for at least 30 min following administration.

Transmucosal

• Suck lozenge vigorously. • Allow to dissolve over 15 min. • Do not chew.

IV INCOMPATIBILITIES

Azithromycin (Zithromax), pantoprazole (Protonix), phenytoin (Dilantin).

IV COMPATIBILITIES

Atropine, bupivacaine (Marcaine, Sensorcaine), cloNIDine (Duraclon), dexmedetomidine (Precedex), dilTIAZem (Cardizem), diphenhydrAMINE (Benadryl), DOBUTamine (Dobutrex), DOPamine (Intropin), droperidol (Inapsine), heparin, HYDROmorphone (Dilaudid), ketorolac (Toradol), LORazepam (Ativan), metoclopramide (Reglan), midazolam (Versed), milrinone (Primacor), morphine, nitroglycerin, norepinephrine (Levophed), ondansetron (Zofran), potassium chloride, propofol (Diprivan).

INDICATIONS/ROUTES/DOSAGE

Note: Doses titrated to desired effect dependent upon degree of analgesia, pt status.

Acute Pain Management (FentaNYL)

IM/IV: ADULTS, ELDERLY: 25–50 mcg or 0.35–0.5 mcg/kg q30–60 min as needed.

Continuous IV Infusion (FentaNYL)

ADULTS, ELDERLY: After initial loading dose (25–100 mcg), begin infusion at 25–50 mcg/hr. Titrate q30–60 min to clinical effect. Usual dose range: 50–200 mcg/hour. Weight-based dosing range: 0.7–10 mcg/kg/hr.

Usual Buccal Dose (Fentora)

ADULTS, ELDERLY: Initially, 100 mcg. Titrate dose up to 800 mcg single dose, providing adequate analgesia with tolerable side effects.

Usual Buccal Soluble Film Dose (Onsolis)

Note: All pts must initiate with 200 mcg. **ADULTS, ELDERLY:** Initially, 200 mcg up to 1,200 mcg. **Maximum:** No more than 4 doses/day; separate by at least 2 hrs.

Usual Nasal Dose (Lazanda)

Nasal: ADULTS, ELDERLY: Initially, 100 mcg. Titrate from 100 mcg to 200 mcg to 300 mcg to 400 mcg to 600 mcg to 800 mcg **(maximum).** Wait at least 2 hrs between doses; no more than 4 doses in 24 hrs.

Usual Sublingual Tablet Dose (Abstral)

ADULTS, ELDERLY: Initially, 100 mcg, then titrate to 400 mcg in 100 mcg increments, then in 200 mcg increments to 600 mcg up to 800 mcg. Wait at least 2 hrs between doses; no more than 4 doses in 24 hrs.

Usual Sublingual Spray Dose (Subsys)

ADULTS, ELDERLY: Initially, 100 mcg. May repeat with same dose in 30 min if pain not relieved. Must wait at least 4 hours before treating another episode of pain. May titrate to 200 mcg to 400 mcg to 600 mcg to 800 mcg to 1200 mcg to 1600 mcg.

Usual Transdermal Dose (Duragesic)

ADULTS, ELDERLY, CHILDREN 12 YRS AND OLDER: Initially, 12–25 mcg/hr. May increase after 3 days. Do not titrate more frequently than q3days following initial application or q6days thereafter.

Usual Transmucosal Dose (Actiq)

ADULTS, CHILDREN: 200–1200 mcg for breakthrough pain. Limit to 4 applications/day. Titrate to provide adequate analgesia while minimizing adverse effects.

Dosage in Renal/Hepatic Impairment
Injection: No dose adjustment.
Transdermal patch: **Mild to moderate impairment:** Reduce dose by 50%. **Severe impairment:** Not recommended.

SIDE EFFECTS

Frequent: **IV:** Postop drowsiness, nausea, vomiting. **Transdermal (10%–3%):** Headache, pruritus, nausea, vomiting, diaphoresis, dyspnea, confusion, dizziness, drowsiness, diarrhea, constipation, decreased appetite. **Occasional:** **IV:** Postop confusion, blurred vision, chills, orthostatic hypotension, constipation, difficulty urinating. **Transdermal (3%–1%):** Chest pain, arrhythmias, erythema, pruritus, syncope, agitation, skin irritations.

ADVERSE EFFECTS/TOXIC REACTIONS

Overdose or too-rapid IV administration may produce severe respiratory depression, skeletal/thoracic muscle rigidity (may lead to apnea, laryngospasm, bronchospasm, cold/clammy skin, cyanosis, coma). Tolerance to analgesic effect may occur with repeated use. **Antidote:** Naloxone (see Appendix J for dosage). Abrupt stoppage of prolonged high-dose, continuous infusions may induce opiate withdrawal. Concomitant use with benzodiazepines may result in profound sedation, respiratory depression, coma, and death.

NURSING CONSIDERATIONS

BASELINE ASSESSMENT

Resuscitative equipment, opiate antagonist (naloxone 0.5 mcg/kg) should be available for initial use. Establish baseline B/P, respirations. Assess type, location, intensity, duration of pain. Determine daily morphine equivalency in cancer pts who are being transitioned to chronic therapy. Assess risk of drug abuse, misuse, drug-seeking behavior.

INTERVENTION/EVALUATION

Assist with ambulation. Encourage postop pt to turn, cough, deep breathe q2h. Monitor respiratory rate, B/P, heart rate, oxygen saturation. Assess for relief of pain. In pts with prolonged high-dose, continuous infusions (critical care, ventilated pts), consider weaning drip gradually or transition to a fentanyl patch to decrease symptoms of opiate withdrawal. Screen for misuse, abuse, drug-seeking behavior.

PATIENT/FAMILY TEACHING

• Avoid alcohol; do not take other medications without consulting physician. • Avoid tasks that require alertness, motor skills until response to drug is established. • Teach pt proper transdermal, buccal, lozenge administration. • **Transdermal:** Avoid saunas (increases drug release time). • Use as directed to avoid overdosage; potential for physical dependence with prolonged use. • Report constipation, absence of pain relief. • Taper slowly after long-term use.

F

ferric carboxymaltose

fer-ik kar-box-ee-**mawl**-tose
(Injectafer)

ferric gluconate

fer-ick **gloo**-koe-nate
(Ferrlecit)

ferrous fumarate

fer-us **fue**-ma-rate
(Ferrocite, Palafer ✱)

ferrous gluconate

fer-us **gloo**-koe-nate
(Apo-Ferrous Gluconate ✱, Ferate)

ferrous sulfate

fer-us **sul**-fate
(Fer-In-Sol, Fer-Iron, Slow-Fe)

ferumoxytol

fer-ue **mox**-i-tol
(Feraheme)

◆CLASSIFICATION

PHARMACOTHERAPEUTIC: Enzymatic mineral. **CLINICAL:** Iron preparation.

USES

Ferric carboxymaltose, ferumoxytol: Treatment of iron deficiency in adults. **Ferrous fumarate, gluconate, sulfate:** Prevention, treatment of iron-deficiency anemia. **Ferric gluconate:** Treatment of iron-deficiency anemia in combination with erythropoietin in HD pts.

PRECAUTIONS

Contraindications: Hypersensitivity to iron salts. Hemochromatosis, hemolytic anemias. **Cautions:** Peptic ulcer, regional enteritis, ulcerative colitis, pts receiving frequent blood transfusions.

ACTION

Essential component in formation of Hgb, myoglobin, enzymes. Promotes effective erythropoiesis and transport, utilization of oxygen. **Therapeutic Effect:** Prevents iron deficiency.

PHARMACOKINETICS

Absorbed in duodenum and upper jejunum. Ten percent absorbed in pts with normal iron stores; increased to 20%–30% in pts with inadequate iron stores. Primarily bound to serum transferrin. Excreted in urine, sweat, sloughing of intestinal mucosa, menses. **Half-life:** 6 hrs.

LIFESPAN CONSIDERATIONS

Pregnancy/Lactation: Crosses placenta; distributed in breast milk. **Children/Elderly:** No age-related precautions noted.

INTERACTIONS

DRUG: Antacids may decrease absorption of ferrous compounds. May decrease absorption of **bisphosphonates (e.g., risedronate), cefdinir, quinolones, tetracyclines. HERBAL:** None significant. **FOOD: Cereal, coffee, dietary fiber, eggs, milk, tea** decrease absorption. **LAB VALUES:** May increase serum bilirubin, iron. May decrease serum calcium.

AVAILABILITY (OTC)

Ferric Carboxymaltose
Injection, Solution: 750 mg/15 mL.

Ferric Gluconate
Injection, Solution: 12.5 mg/mL.

Ferrous Fumarate
Tablets: 90 mg (29.5 mg elemental iron), 324 mg (106 mg elemental iron).

Ferrous Gluconate
Tablets: 240 mg (27 mg elemental iron) (Fergon), 325 mg (36 mg elemental iron).

Ferrous Sulfate
Oral Solution: 75 mg/mL (15 mg/mL elemental iron). **Tablets:** 325 mg (65 mg elemental iron). **Syrup:** 300 mg/5 mL (60 mg elemental iron per 5 mL).

Tablets (Timed-Release): 160 mg (50 mg elemental iron). **Ferumoxytol:** 510 mg/17 mL.

ADMINISTRATION/HANDLING

PO

• Store all forms (tablets, capsules, suspension, drops) at room temperature. • Ideally, give between meals with water or juice but may give with meals if GI discomfort occurs. • Transient staining of mucous membranes, teeth occurs with liquid iron preparation. To avoid staining, place liquid on back of tongue with dropper or straw. • Do not give with milk or milk products. • Do not break, crush, dissolve, or divide timed-release tablets.

INDICATIONS/ROUTES/DOSAGE

Iron-Deficiency Anemia

Dosage is expressed in terms of milligrams of elemental iron. Assess degree of anemia, pt weight, presence of any bleeding. Expect to use periodic hematologic determinations as guide to therapy. **IV:** ***(Ferric Carboxymaltose):*** **ADULTS, ELDERLY: (50 KG OR GREATER):** 750 mg on day 1; repeat dose after at least 7 days. **(LESS THAN 50 KG):** 15 mg/kg on day 1; repeat dose after at least 7 days. ***(Ferric Gluconate):*** **ADULTS, ELDERLY:** 125 mg/dose. Usual dose: 1,000 mg given over 8 sessions. ***(Ferumoxytol):*** **ADULTS, ELDERLY:** 510 mg (as IV infusion). May repeat dose 3–8 days after initial dose.

PO: ***(Ferrous Fumarate):*** **ADULTS, ELDERLY:** 65–200 mg/day in 2–3 divided doses. **CHILDREN:** 3–6 mg/kg/day in 2–3 divided doses. ***(Ferrous Gluconate):*** **ADULTS, ELDERLY:** 65–200 mg/day in 2–3 divided doses. **CHILDREN:** 3–6 mg/kg/day in 2–3 divided doses. ***(Ferrous Sulfate):*** **ADULTS, ELDERLY:** 65–200 mg/day in 2–3 divided doses. **CHILDREN:** 3–6 mg/kg/day in 2–3 divided doses.

IV: ***(Iron Dextran):*** **ADULTS, ELDERLY, CHILDREN WEIGHING MORE THAN 15 KG:** Dose in mL (50 mg elemental iron/mL) = 0.0442 (desired Hgb less observed Hgb) × lean body weight (in kg) + (0.26 × lean body weight). Give 2 mL or less once daily until total dose reached. **IV: ADULTS, ELDERLY, CHILDREN WEIGHING MORE THAN 15 KG:** Dose in mL (50 mg elemental iron/mL) = 0.0442 (desired Hgb less observed Hgb) × lean body weight (in kg) + (0.26 × lean body weight). Give 2 mL or less once daily until total dose reached. **CHILDREN WEIGHING 5–15 KG:** Dose in mL (50 mg elemental iron/mL) = 0.0442 (desired Hgb less observed Hgb) × body weight (in kg) + (0.26 × body weight). Give 2 mL or less once daily until total dose reached.

IV: ADULTS, ELDERLY (HEMODIALYSIS-DEPENDENT PTS): 5 mL iron sucrose (100 mg elemental iron) delivered during dialysis; administer 1–3 times/wk to total dose of 1,000 mg in 10 doses. Give no more than 3 times/wk. **CHILDREN 2 YRS AND OLDER:** 0.5 mg/kg/dose (**maximum:** 100 mg) q2wks for 6 doses. **(PERITONEAL DIALYSIS–DEPENDENT PTS):** Two infusions of 300 mg over 90 min 14 days apart, followed by a single 400-mg dose over 2.5 hrs 14 days later. **CHILDREN 2 YRS AND OLDER:** 0.5 mg/kg/dose (**maximum:** 100 mg) q4wks for 3 doses. **(NON–DIALYSIS-DEPENDENT PTS):** 200 mg over 2–5 min on 5 different occasions within 14 days. **CHILDREN 2 YRS AND OLDER:** 0.5 mg/kg/dose (**maximum:** 100 mg) q4wks for 3 doses.

Prevention of Iron Deficiency

PO: ***(Ferrous Fumarate):*** **ADULTS, ELDERLY:** 30–60 mg/day. **CHILDREN: (5–12 yrs):** 30–60 mg/day. **(2–4 yrs):** 30 mg/day. **(6 mos–1 yr):** 10–12.5 mg/day. ***(Ferrous Gluconate):*** **ADULTS, ELDERLY:** 30–60 mg/day. **CHILDREN: (5–12 yrs):** 30–60 mg/day. **(2–4 yrs):** 30 mg/day. **(6 mos–1 yr):** 10–12.5 mg/day. ***(Ferrous Sulfate):*** **ADULTS, ELDERLY:** 30–60 mg/day. **CHILDREN: (5–12 yrs):** 30–60 mg/day. **(2–4 yrs):** 30 mg/day. **(6 mos–1 yr):** 10–12.5 mg/day.

SIDE EFFECTS

Occasional: Mild, transient nausea. **Rare:** Heartburn, anorexia, constipation, diarrhea.

ADVERSE EFFECTS/TOXIC REACTIONS

Large doses may aggravate existing GI tract disease (peptic ulcer, regional enteritis, ulcerative colitis). Severe iron poisoning occurs most often in children, manifested as vomiting, severe abdominal pain, diarrhea, dehydration, followed by hyperventilation, pallor, cyanosis, cardiovascular collapse.

NURSING CONSIDERATIONS

BASELINE ASSESSMENT

Assess nutritional status, dietary history. Question history of hemochromatosis, hemolytic anemia, ulcerative colitis. Question use of antacids, calcium supplements.

INTERVENTION/EVALUATION

Monitor serum iron, total iron-binding capacity, reticulocyte count, Hgb, ferritin. Monitor daily pattern of bowel activity, stool consistency. Assess for clinical improvement, record relief of iron-deficiency symptoms (fatigue, irritability, pallor, paresthesia of extremities, headache).

PATIENT/FAMILY TEACHING

• Expect stool color to darken. • Oral liquid may stain teeth. • To prevent mucous membrane and teeth staining with liquid preparation, use dropper or straw and allow solution to drop on back of tongue. • If GI discomfort occurs, take after meals or with food. • Do not take within 2 hrs of other medication or eggs, milk, tea, coffee, cereal. • Do not take antacids or OTC calcium supplements.

fesoterodine

fes-oh-**ter**-oh-deen
(Toviaz)
Do not confuse fesoterodine with fexofenadine or tolterodine.

◆CLASSIFICATION

PHARMACOTHERAPEUTIC: Muscarinic receptor antagonist. **CLINICAL:** Anticholingergic.

USES

Treatment of overactive bladder with symptoms including urinary incontinence, urgency, frequency.

PRECAUTIONS

Contraindications: Hypersensitivity to fesoterodine. Gastric retention, uncontrolled narrow-angle glaucoma, urinary retention. **Cautions:** Severe renal impairment, severe hepatic impairment, clinically significant bladder outflow obstruction (risk of urinary retention), GI obstructive disorders (e.g., pyloric stenosis [risk of gastric retention], treated narrow-angle glaucoma, myasthenia gravis, concurrent therapy with strong CYP3A4 inhibitors, elderly, use in hot weather.

ACTION

Exhibits antimuscarinic activity by interceding via cholinergic muscarinic receptors, thereby mediating urinary bladder contraction. **Therapeutic Effect:** Decreases urinary frequency, urgency.

PHARMACOKINETICS

Well absorbed following PO administration. Protein binding: 50%. Rapidly and extensively hydrolyzed to its active metabolite. Primarily excreted in urine. **Half-life:** 7 hours.

LIFESPAN CONSIDERATIONS

Pregnancy/Lactation: Unknown if distributed in breast milk. **Children:** Safety and efficacy not established. **Elderly:** Increased incidence of antimuscarinic adverse events, including dry mouth, constipation, dyspepsia; increase in residual urine, dizziness, urinary tract infections higher in pts 75 yrs of age and older.

INTERACTIONS

DRUG: **CYP3A4 inhibitors (e.g., clarithromycin, ketoconazole, ritonavir)** may increase concentration/effect. **Aclidinium, ipratropium, tiotropium, umeclidinium** may increase anticholinergic effect. **Strong CYP3A4 inducers (e.g., carBAMazepine, phenytoin, rifAMPin)** may decrease concentration/effect. **HERBAL:** **St. John's wort** may decrease concentration/effect. **FOOD:** None known. **LAB VALUES:** May increase serum ALT, GGT.

AVAILABILITY (Rx)

Tablets, Extended-Release: 4 mg, 8 mg.

ADMINISTRATION/HANDLING

PO

• May be administered with or without food. • Swallow whole; do not break, crush, dissolve, or divide tablet.

INDICATIONS/ROUTES/DOSAGE

Overactive Bladder

PO: **ADULTS, ELDERLY:** Initially, 4 mg once daily. May increase to 8 mg once daily.

Maximum dose for pts with concurrent use of strong CYP3A4 inhibitors (e.g., erythromycin, ketoconazole) is 4 mg once daily.

Dosage in Renal Impairment

PO: ADULTS, ELDERLY: Maximum: 4 mg with CrCl less than 30 mL/min.

Dosage in Hepatic Impairment

Mild to moderate impairment: No dose adjustment. **Severe impairment:** Not recommended.

SIDE EFFECTS

Frequent (34%–18%): Dry mouth. **Occasional (6%–3%):** Constipation, urinary tract infection, dry eyes. **Rare (2% or less):** Nausea, dysuria, back pain, rash, insomnia, peripheral edema.

ADVERSE EFFECTS/TOXIC REACTIONS

Severe anticholinergic effects including abdominal cramps, facial warmth, excessive salivation/lacrimation, diaphoresis, pallor, urinary urgency, blurred vision.

NURSING CONSIDERATIONS

BASELINE ASSESSMENT

Assess urinary pattern (e.g., urinary frequency, urgency). Question history as listed in Precautions. Receive full medication history.

INTERVENTION/EVALUATION

Assist with ambulation if dizziness occurs. Question for visual changes. Monitor incontinence, postvoid residuals. Monitor daily pattern of bowel activity, stool consistency.

PATIENT/FAMILY TEACHING

• May produce constipation and urinary retention. • Blurred vision may occur; use caution until drug effects have been determined. • Heat prostration (due to decreased sweating) can occur if used in a hot environment. • Do not ingest grapefruit products.

fexofenadine

fex-oh-**fen**-a-deen
(Allegra Allergy, Allegra Allergy Children's)
Do not confuse Allegra with Viagra, or fexofenadine with fesoterodine.

FIXED-COMBINATION(S)

Allegra-D 12 Hour: fexofenadine/pseudoephedrine (sympathomimetic): 60 mg/120 mg. **Allegra-D 24 Hour:** fexofenadine/pseudoephedrine (sympathomimetic): 180 mg/240 mg.

◆CLASSIFICATION

PHARMACOTHERAPEUTIC: Histamine H_1 antagonist (second generation). **CLINICAL:** CLINICAL: Antihistamine.

USES

Relief of symptoms associated with hayfever or other upper respiratory allergies (e.g., runny nose, sneezing, itching of nose/throat).

PRECAUTIONS

Contraindications: Hypersensitivity to fexofenadine. **Cautions:** Renal impairment, hypertension (if drug combined with pseudoephedrine). Orally disintegrating tablet not recommended in children younger than 6 yrs.

ACTION

Competes with histamine-1 receptor site on effector cells in GI tract, blood vessels, and respiratory tract. **Therapeutic Effect:** Relieves hayfever/upper respiratory symptoms.

PHARMACOKINETICS

	Onset	Peak	Duration
PO	60 min	—	12 hrs or greater

Rapidly absorbed after PO administration. Protein binding: 60%–70%. Does not cross blood-brain barrier. Minimally metabolized. Excreted in feces (80%), urine (11%). Not removed by hemodialysis. **Half-life:** 14.4 hrs (increased in renal impairment).

LIFESPAN CONSIDERATIONS

Pregnancy/Lactation: Unknown if drug crosses placenta or is distributed in breast milk. **Children:** Safety and efficacy not established in pts younger than 12 yrs. **Elderly:** No age-related precautions noted.

INTERACTIONS

DRUG: **Aluminum- and magnesium-containing antacids** may decrease absorption. **Aclidinium, ipratropium, tiotropium, umeclidinium** may increase anticholinergic effect. **CNS depressants (e.g., alcohol, morphine, oxyCODONE, zolpidem)** may increase CNS depression. May increase concentrations of **erythromycin, ketoconazole.** **HERBAL:** **Herbals with sedative properties (e.g., chamomile, kava kava, valerian)** may increase CNS depression. **FOOD:** **Grapefruit products** may decrease concentration/effect. **LAB VALUES:** May suppress wheal, flare reactions to antigen skin testing unless drug is discontinued at least 4 days before testing.

AVAILABILITY (Rx)

Oral Suspension: 30 mg/5 mL. **Tablets:** 60 mg, 180 mg. **Tablets (Orally Disintegrating):** 30 mg.

ADMINISTRATION/HANDLING

PO

• Give without regard to food. • Avoid giving with fruit juices (apple, grapefruit, orange). Administer with water only. • Shake suspension well before use.

PO (Orally Disintegrating Tablet)

• Take on empty stomach. • Remove from blister pack; immediately place on tongue. • May take with or without liquid. • Do not split or cut.

INDICATIONS/ROUTES/DOSAGE

Hayfever, Upper Respiratory Symptoms

PO: ADULTS, ELDERLY, CHILDREN 12 YRS AND OLDER: 60 mg twice daily or 180 mg once daily. **CHILDREN 2–11 YRS:** 30 mg twice daily.

Dosage in Renal Impairment

PO: ADULTS, ELDERLY, CHILDREN 12 YRS AND OLDER: 60 mg once daily. **CHILDREN 2–11 YRS:** 30 mg once daily. **CHILDREN 6 MOS–LESS THAN 2 YRS:** 15 mg once daily.

CrCl	Adults	Children
>50 mL/min	No adjustment	No adjustment
10–50 mL/min	60 mg q12–24h	60 mg q24h
<10 mL/min	30 mg q24h	30 mg q24h

Dosage in Hepatic Impairment

No dose adjustment.

SIDE EFFECTS

Rare (less than 2%): Drowsiness, headache, fatigue, nausea, vomiting, abdominal distress, dysmenorrhea.

ADVERSE EFFECTS/TOXIC REACTIONS

Hypersensitivity reaction occurs rarely.

NURSING CONSIDERATIONS

BASELINE ASSESSMENT

Assess severity of congestion, rhinitis, urticaria, watery eyes. Monitor rate, depth, rhythm, type of respiration; quality, rate of pulse. Assess lung sounds for rhonchi, wheezing, rales.

INTERVENTION/EVALUATION

Assess for therapeutic response; relief from allergy: itching, red, watery eyes, rhinorrhea, sneezing.

PATIENT/FAMILY TEACHING

• Avoid tasks that require alertness, motor skills until response to drug is established. • Avoid alcohol during antihistamine therapy. • Coffee, tea may help reduce drowsiness. • Do not take with any fruit juices.

fidaxomicin

fye-**dax**-oh-**mye**-sin
(Dificid)
Do not confuse fidaxomicin with azithromycin, clindamycin, erythromycin, gentamicin, plazomicin, or tobramycin.

◆CLASSIFICATION

PHARMACOTHERAPEUTIC: Macrolide. **CLINICAL:** Antibiotic.

USES

Treatment of *Clostridioides difficile*–associated diarrhea in adults and children 6 mos and older.

PRECAUTIONS

Contraindications: Hypersensitivity to fidaxomicin. **Cautions:** History of anemia, neutropenia, macrolide allergy.

ACTION

Binds to ribosomal sites of susceptible organisms, inhibiting RNA-dependent protein synthesis by RNA polymerase. **Therapeutic Effect:** Bactericidal against *C. difficile.*

PHARMACOKINETICS

Minimal systemic absorption following PO administration. Mainly confined to GI tract. Excreted primarily in feces (92%). **Half-life:** 9 hrs.

⌛ LIFESPAN CONSIDERATIONS

Pregnancy/Lactation: Unknown if distributed in breast milk. **Children:** Safety and efficacy not established in pts younger than 6 mos. **Elderly:** No age-related precautions noted.

INTERACTIONS

DRUG: None significant. **HERBAL:** None known. **FOOD:** None significant. **LAB VALUES:** May increase serum alkaline phosphatase, ALT, AST, bilirubin. May decrease serum bicarbonate; platelets.

AVAILABILITY (Rx)

Tablets: 200 mg.

ADMINISTRATION/HANDLING

- Give without regard to food.

INDICATIONS/ROUTES/DOSAGE

***Clostridioides Difficile*–Associated Diarrhea**
PO: ADULTS: 200 mg twice daily for 10 days. **ADOLESCENTS, CHILDREN, INFANTS 6 MOS AND OLDER: (WEIGHING 12.5 KG OR MORE):** 200 mg twice daily for 10 days. **(9 KG TO LESS THAN 12.5 KG):** ***Oral suspension:*** 160 mg twice daily for 10 days. **(7 KG TO LESS THAN 9 KG):** 120 mg twice daily for 10 days. **(4 KG TO LESS THAN 7 KG):** 80 mg twice daily for 10 days.

Dosage in Renal/Hepatic Impairment
No dose adjustment.

SIDE EFFECTS

Occasional (13%–6%): Pyrexia, nausea, vomiting, abdominal pain. **Rare (less than 2%):** Abdominal distension, abdominal tenderness, dyspepsia, dysphagia, flatulence, hyperglycemia.

ADVERSE EFFECTS/TOXIC REACTIONS

Hypersensitivity reactions including angioedema, dyspnea, pruritus, rash were reported. May increase risk of development of drug-resistant bacteria or superinfection when used in the absence of proven or strongly suspected *C. difficile* infection. GI hemorrhage reported in 4% of pts. Other reactions include drug eruption, metabolic acidosis.

NURSING CONSIDERATIONS

BASELINE ASSESSMENT

Verify positive *C. difficile* toxin test before initiating treatment. Initiate contact precautions. Obtain baseline CBC, electrolytes, renal function, fecal occult blood test. Assess bowel sounds, stool characteristics (color, frequency, consistency). Assess hydration status.

INTERVENTION/EVALUATION

Monitor for volume loss, dehydration, hypotension, abdominal pain, pyrexia. Encourage nutrition/fluid intake. Monitor daily pattern of bowel activity, stool consistency. Routinely assess bowel sounds. Screen for intestinal obstruction (increased nausea, abdominal pain, hyperactive bowel sounds) and consider radiologic test if suspected. Monitor for hypersensitivity reactions, GI bleeding (melena, rectal bleeding).

PATIENT/FAMILY TEACHING

• It is essential to complete drug therapy despite improvement of symptoms. Early discontinuation may result in antibacterial resistance and increased risk of recurrent infection. • Report GI bleeding; symptoms of bowel obstruction (e.g., abdominal pain, fever, nausea, vomiting). Report allergic reactions such as itching, rash; swelling of the face or tongue. • *C. difficile* infection is extremely contagious to others. Wash hands frequently with soap and water, esp. after bowel movements. *C. difficile* spores can live on objects for months. Use bleach products to cleanse bathroom, doorknobs, other high-touch surfaces. If possible, use a separate bathroom away from others. • Drink plenty of fluids.

filgrastim

TOP 100

fil-**gras**-tim

(Granix, Neupogen, Nivestym, Zarxio)

Do not confuse Neupogen with Epogen, Neulasta, Neumega, or Nutramigen.

◆CLASSIFICATION

PHARMACOTHERAPEUTIC: Hematopoietic agent. **CLINICAL:** Granulocyte colony-stimulating factor (G-CSF).

USES

Granix: Decreases duration of severe neutropenia in adults and children 1 mo and older with nonmyeloid malignancies receiving chemotherapy associated with severe neutropenia, fever. **Neupogen, Zarxio:** Reduces neutropenia duration, sequelae in pts with nonmyeloid malignancies having myeloablative therapy followed by bone marrow transplant (BMT). Mobilization of hematopoietic progenitor cells into peripheral blood for collection by apheresis. Treatment of chronic, severe neutropenia. Decreases incidence of infection in pts with malignancies receiving chemotherapy associated with increased incidence of severe neutropenia with fever. Reduces time to neutrophil recovery/duration of fever after induction/consolidation chemotherapy in AML pts. **Neupogen:** Increases survival in pts acutely exposed to myelosuppressive doses of radiation. **OFF-LABEL:** Treatment of AIDS-related neutropenia in pts receiving zidovudine; drug-induced neutropenia; anemia in myelodysplastic syndrome; hepatitis C virus infection treatment-associated neutropenia.

PRECAUTIONS

Contraindications: Hypersensitivity to filgrastim. **Neupogen, Zarxio (additional):** History of serious allergic reaction to human granulocyte colony-stimulating factors. **Cautions:** Malignancy with myeloid characteristics (due to G-CSF's potential to act as growth factor), gout, psoriasis, neutrophil count greater than 50,000 cells/mm^3, sickle cell disease, concomitant use of other drugs that may result in thrombocytopenia. Do not use 24 hrs before or after cytotoxic chemotherapy.

ACTION

Stimulates production, maturation, activation of neutrophils. **Therapeutic Effect:** Increases migration and cytotoxicity of neutrophils.

PHARMACOKINETICS

Readily absorbed. Onset of action: 24 hrs (plateaus in 3–5 days). WBC return to normal in 4–7 days. Not removed by hemodialysis. **Half-life:** 3.5 hrs.

LIFESPAN CONSIDERATIONS

Pregnancy/Lactation: Unknown if drug crosses placenta or is distributed in breast milk. **Children/Elderly:** No age-related precautions noted.

INTERACTIONS

DRUG: May increase concentration/effects of **bleomycin, cyclophosphamide, topotecan.** **HERBAL:** None significant. **FOOD:** None known. **LAB VALUES:** May increase LDH, leukocyte alkaline phosphatase (LAP) scores, serum alkaline phosphatase, uric acid.

AVAILABILITY (Rx)

Injection Solution: ***(Neupogen):*** 300 mcg/mL, 480 mcg/1.6 mL **Injection, Prefilled Syringe:** ***(Granix, Neupogen, Zarxio):*** 300 mcg/0.5 mL, 480 mcg/0.8 mL.

ADMINISTRATION/HANDLING

◀ALERT▶ May be given by SQ injection, short IV infusion (15–30 min), or continuous IV infusion. Do not dilute with normal saline.

IV

Reconstitution • Allow vial to warm to room temperature (approx. 30 min). • Visually inspect for particulate matter or discoloration. • Dilute in D_5W from concentration of 300 mcg/mL to 5 mcg/mL (do not dilute to a final concentration less than 5 mcg/mL). Diluted solutions of 5–15 mcg/mL should have addition of albumin to a final concentration of 2 mg/mL. • Do not dilute with saline.

Rate of administration • For intermittent infusion (piggyback), infuse over 15–30 min. • For continuous infusion, give single dose over 4–24 hrs. • In all situations, flush IV line with D_5W before and after administration.

Storage • Refrigerate vials and syringes. • Stable for up to 24 hrs at room temperature (provided vial contents are clear and contain no particulate matter).

SQ

• Aspirate syringe before injection (avoid intra-arterial administration).

Storage • Store in refrigerator, but remove before use and allow to warm to room temperature.

IV INCOMPATIBILITIES

Amphotericin (Fungizone), cefepime (Maxipime), cefotaxime (Claforan), cefOXitin (Mefoxin), ceftizoxime (Cefizox), cefTRIAXone (Rocephin), clindamycin (Cleocin), DACTINomycin (Cosmegen), etoposide (VePesid), fluorouracil, furosemide (Lasix), heparin, mannitol, methylPREDNISolone (Solu-Medrol), mitoMYcin (Mutamycin), prochlorperazine (Compazine).

IV COMPATIBILITIES

Bumetanide (Bumex), calcium gluconate, HYDROmorphone (Dilaudid), LORazepam (Ativan), morphine, potassium chloride.

INDICATIONS/ROUTES/DOSAGE

◀ALERT▶ Begin therapy at least 24 hrs after last dose of chemotherapy and at least 24 hrs after bone marrow infusion. Dosing based on actual body weight.

Chemotherapy-Induced Neutropenia

IV or SQ infusion, SQ injection: ***(Neupogen and biosimilars):*** **ADULTS, ELDERLY, CHILDREN:** Initially, 5 mcg/kg/day. May increase by 5 mcg/kg for each chemotherapy cycle based on duration/severity of neutropenia; continue for up to 14 days or until absolute neutrophil count (ANC) reaches 10,000 cells/mm^3.

Granix

SQ: ADULTS, ELDERLY: 5 mcg/kg/day. Continue until nadir has passed and neutrophil count recovered to normal range.

Bone Marrow Transplant

IV or SQ infusion: ***(Neupogen and biosimilars):*** **ADULTS, ELDERLY, CHILDREN:** 10 mcg/kg/day. Administer >24 hrs after chemotherapy or bone marrow transfusion. Adjust dosage daily during period of neutrophil recovery based on neutrophil response.

Mobilization of Progenitor Cells

IV or SQ infusion: ***(Neupogen and biosimilars):*** **ADULTS:** 10 mcg/kg/day in donors beginning at least 4 days before first leukapheresis and continuing until last leukapheresis (usually for 6–7 days). Discontinue for WBC greater than 100,000 cells/mm^3.

Chronic Neutropenia, Congenital Neutropenia

SQ: ***(Neupogen and biosimilars):*** **ADULTS, CHILDREN:** Initially, 6 mcg/kg/dose twice daily. Adjust dose based on ANC/clinical response.

Idiopathic or Cyclic Chronic Neutropenia

SQ: ***(Neupogen and biosimilars):*** **ADULTS, CHILDREN:** Initially, 5 mcg/kg/dose once daily. Adjust dose based on ANC/clinical response.

Radiation Injury Syndrome

SQ: ***(Neupogen only):*** **ADULTS, ELDERLY:** 10 mcg/kg once daily. Continue until ANC remains greater than 1,000 cells/mm^3 for 3 consecutive CBCs or ANC exceeds 10,000 cells/mm^3 after radiation-induced nadir.

Dosage in Renal/Hepatic Impairment

No dose adjustment.

SIDE EFFECTS

Frequent (57%–11%): Nausea/vomiting, mild to severe bone pain (more frequent with high-dose IV form, less frequent with low-dose SQ form), alopecia, diarrhea, fever, fatigue. **Occasional (9%–5%):** Anorexia, dyspnea, headache, cough, rash. **Rare (less than 5%):** Psoriasis, hematuria, proteinuria, osteoporosis.

ADVERSE EFFECTS/TOXIC REACTIONS

Long-term administration occasionally produces chronic neutropenia, splenomegaly. Acute respiratory distress syndrome, alveolar hemorrhage and hemoptysis (pts undergoing peripheral blood progenitor cell collection mobilization), capillary leak syndrome, cutaneous vasculitis, glomerulonephritis, leukocytosis, MI, thrombocytopenia, sickle cell crisis, splenic rupture may occur.

NURSING CONSIDERATIONS

BASELINE ASSESSMENT

Obtain CBC prior to initiation and twice wkly thereafter.

INTERVENTION/EVALUATION

In septic pts, be alert for adult respiratory distress syndrome. Closely monitor those with preexisting cardiac conditions. Monitor B/P (transient decrease in B/P may occur), temperature, CBC with differential, platelet count, serum uric acid, hepatic function tests.

PATIENT/FAMILY TEACHING

- Report fever, chills, severe bone pain, chest pain, palpitations, difficulty breathing; left upper abdominal pain/tightness; flank pain.

finasteride

fin-**as**-ter-ide

(Propecia, Proscar)

Do not confuse finasteride with furosemide, or Proscar with ProSom, Provera, or PROzac.

◆CLASSIFICATION

PHARMACOTHERAPEUTIC: 5-alpha-reductase inhibitor. **CLINICAL:** Benign prostatic hyperplasia agent.

USES

Proscar: Treatment (monotherapy) of symptomatic benign prostatic hyperplasia (BPH) to improve symptoms, reduce risk of acute urinary retention, or reduce the need for surgery, including transurethral resection of the prostate (TURP) and prostatectomy. Used in combination with an alpha-blocker (e.g., doxazosin) to reduce risk of symptomatic progression. **Propecia:** Treatment of male pattern hair loss. **OFF-LABEL:** Treatment of female hirsutism.

PRECAUTIONS

Contraindications: Hypersensitivity to finasteride, pregnancy or women of childbearing potential. **Cautions:** Hepatic impairment, urinary outflow obstruction, urinary retention. Women who are attempting to conceive should avoid exposure to crushed or broken tablets.

ACTION

Inhibits 5-alpha reductase, an intracellular enzyme that converts testosterone into dihydrotestosterone (DHT) in prostate gland, resulting in decreased serum DHT. **Therapeutic Effect:** Reduces size of prostate gland.

PHARMACOKINETICS

Route	Onset	Peak	Duration
PO (reduction of DHT)	8 hrs	—	24 hrs

Rapidly absorbed from GI tract. Protein binding: 90%. Widely distributed. Metabolized in liver. **Half-life:** 6–8 hrs. Onset of clinical effect: 3–6 mos of continued therapy.

LIFESPAN CONSIDERATIONS

Pregnancy/Lactation: Physical handling of tablet by those who are or may become pregnant may produce abnormalities of external genitalia of male fetus. **Children:** Not indicated for use in children. **Elderly:** No age-related precautions noted.

INTERACTIONS

DRUG: None significant. **HERBAL: St. John's wort** may decrease concentration. Avoid concurrent use with **saw palmetto** (not adequately studied). **FOOD:** None known. **LAB VALUES:** Decreases serum prostate-specific antigen (PSA) level, even in presence of prostate cancer. Decreases dihydrotestosterone (DHT). Increases follicle-stimulating hormone (FSH), luteinizing hormone (LH), testosterone.

AVAILABILITY (Rx)

Tablets: 1 mg (Propecia), 5 mg (Proscar).

ADMINISTRATION/HANDLING

PO

• Do not break, crush, dissolve, or divide film-coated tablets. • Give without regard to food.

INDICATIONS/ROUTES/DOSAGE

Benign Prostatic Hyperplasia (BPH)

PO: ADULTS, ELDERLY: ***(Proscar):*** 5 mg once daily. Use as single agent or in combination with doxazosin (6–12 mos of treatment usually needed to assess benefit).

Hair Loss

PO: ADULTS: ***(Propecia):*** 1 mg/day (Continue for at least 12 mos to assess full benefit).

Dosage in Renal Impairment

No dose adjustment.

Dosage in Hepatic Impairment

Use caution.

SIDE EFFECTS

Rare (4%–2%): Gynecomastia, sexual dysfunction (impotence, decreased libido, decreased volume of ejaculate).

ADVERSE EFFECTS/TOXIC REACTIONS

Hypersensitivity reaction, circumoral swelling, testicular pain occur rarely.

NURSING CONSIDERATIONS

BASELINE ASSESSMENT

Digital rectal exam, serum prostate-specific antigen (PSA) determination should be performed in pts with benign prostatic hyperplasia (BPH) before initiating therapy and periodically thereafter. Assess usual urinary characteristics (frequency, ability to empty bladder, urinary flow). Assess degree of urinary retention with bladder scan.

INTERVENTION/EVALUATION

Diligently monitor I&O, esp. in pts with large residual urinary volume, severely diminished urinary flow, or obstructive uropathy. Obtain periodic bladder scan to assess treatment effectiveness (or to assess for acute urinary retention).

PATIENT/FAMILY TEACHING

• Treatment may cause impotence, decreased volume of ejaculate. • May not notice improved urinary flow even if prostate gland shrinks. • Must take medication longer than 6 mos, and it is unknown if medication decreases need for surgery. • Because of potential risk to male fetus, women who are or may become pregnant should not handle tablets or be exposed to pt's semen. • Immediately report inability to urinate or severe bladder pain.

fingolimod

TOP 100

fin-**goe**-li-mod
(Gilenya)

◆CLASSIFICATION

PHARMACOTHERAPEUTIC: Sphingosine 1-phosphate (S1P) receptor modulator. **CLINICAL:** Multiple sclerosis agent.

USES

Treatment of pts 10 yrs and older with relapsing forms of multiple sclerosis (MS) to reduce frequency of clinical exacerbations, delay accumulation of physical disability.

PRECAUTIONS

Contraindications: Hypersensitivity to fingolimod. Sick sinus syndrome, second-degree or higher conduction block (unless pt has functioning pacemaker). Baseline QT interval 500 msec or greater. Concurrent use of class Ia or III antiarrhythmic. Recent (within 6 mos) MI, unstable angina, stroke, TIA, decompensated requiring hospitalization or NYHA class III/IV HF. **Cautions:** Concomitant use of antiarrhythmics, beta blockers, calcium channel blockers, immunosuppressants, immune modulators, antineoplastics, QT interval–prolonging medications (e.g., amiodarone, ciprofloxacin); bradycardia, severe hepatic impairment, ischemic heart disease, diabetes, hypokalemia, hypomagnesemia; history of syncope, uveitis; pts at risk for developing bradycardia or heart block.

ACTION

Blocks capacity of lymphocytes to move out from lymph nodes, reducing number of lymphocytes available to the CNS. **Therapeutic Effect:** May involve reduction of lymphocyte migration into central nervous system, which reduces central inflammation.

PHARMACOKINETICS

Metabolized by the enzyme sphingosine kinase to active metabolite. Highly distributed in red blood cells (85%). Minimally metabolized in liver. Protein binding: 99.7%. Primarily excreted in urine. **Half-life:** 6–9 days.

⧗ LIFESPAN CONSIDERATIONS

Pregnancy/Lactation: May cause fetal harm. Unknown if distributed in breast milk. **Children:** Safety and efficacy not established in pts younger than 18 yrs. **Elderly:** Age-related severe hepatic impairment may increase risk of adverse reactions.

INTERACTIONS

DRUG: **Beta blockers (e.g., carvedilol, metoprolol), calcium channel blockers (e.g., dilTIAZem, verapamil), ceritinib, esmolol** may increase risk of bradycardia. May increase effects of **QT interval–prolonging medications (e.g., amiodarone, azithromycin, ciprofloxacin, haloperidol).** May increase toxic effects of **leflunomide, natalizumab.** May decrease effect of **nivolumab, sipuleucel-T.** May increase immunosuppressive effect of **tofacitinib, other immunosuppressants.** May decrease therapeutic effect of **vaccines,** increase toxic effects of **live vaccines.** **HERBAL:** **Echinacea** may decrease therapeutic effect. **FOOD:** None known. **LAB VALUES:** Expect decrease in neutrophil count. May increase serum alkaline phosphatase, ALT, AST, bilirubin, triglycerides. May reduce diagnostic effect of *Coccidioides immitis* skin test.

AVAILABILITY (Rx)

Capsules: 0.25 mg, 0.5 mg.

ADMINISTRATION/HANDLING

PO

- May give without regard to food.

INDICATIONS/ROUTES/DOSAGE

Multiple Sclerosis

PO: ADULTS 18 YRS AND OLDER, ELDERLY: 0.5 mg once daily. **CHILDREN 10 YRS AND OLDER, ADOLESCENTS WEIGHING MORE THAN 40 KG:** 0.5 mg once daily. **WEIGHING 40 KG OR LESS:** 0.25 mg once daily.

Dosage in Renal/Hepatic Impairment

Mild to moderate impairment: No dose adjustment. **Severe impairment:** Use caution.

SIDE EFFECTS

Frequent (25%–10%): Headache, diarrhea, back pain, cough. **Occasional (8%–5%):** Dyspnea, clinical depression, dizziness, hypertension, migraine, paresthesia, decreased weight. **Rare (4%–2%):** Blurred vision, alopecia, eye pain, asthenia, eczema, pruritus.

ADVERSE EFFECTS/TOXIC REACTIONS

May increase risk of infections (influenza, herpes viral infection, bronchitis, sinusitis, gastroenteritis, ear infection) in 13%–4% of pts. Pts with diabetes or history of uveitis are at increased risk for developing macular edema. Cases of skin cancer, lymphoma, basal cell carcinoma have been reported. Progressive multifocal leukoencephalopathy (PML) (weakness, paralysis, vision loss, aphasia, cognition impairment) may occur. Neurotoxicity, posterior reversible encephalopathy may evolve into cerebral hemorrhage, CVA. May increase risk of hypertension.

NURSING CONSIDERATIONS

BASELINE ASSESSMENT

Obtain baseline CBC, serum chemistries prior to initial treatment. At initial treatment (within first 4–6 hrs after dose), medication reduces heart rate, AV conduction, followed by progressive increase after first day of treatment. Obtain baseline vitals, with particular attention to pulse rate. Perform ophthalmologic evaluation prior to treatment and 3–4 mos after initiation of treatment. Question medical history as listed in Precautions. Obtain full medication history and screen for interactions.

INTERVENTION/EVALUATION

Monitor for bradycardia for 6 hrs after first dose, then as appropriate. Periodically monitor CBC, serum chemistries, particularly lymphocyte count (expected to decrease approximately 80% from baseline with continued treatment). Monitor for signs of systemic or local infection. Diligently monitor for hypersensitivity reaction, neurological changes, symptoms of posterior reversible encephalopathy (altered mental status, seizures, visual disturbances), PML, QT interval prolongation. Assess for new skin lesions, malignancies. Conduct ophthalmologic exams q3–4 mos after initiation, during treatment, and with any changes in vision.

PATIENT/FAMILY TEACHING

• Obtain regular eye examinations during and for 2 mos following treatment. • Use effective methods of contraception during and for 3 mos following treatment. • Im-

F

mediately report neurological changes such as confusion, severe headache, seizure activity, vision changes, trouble speaking, one-sided weakness, paralysis. • Treatment may increase risk of certain cancers; report new skin lesions, fever, chills, night sweats, generalized weakness, weight loss, or pain or swelling of the lymph nodes. • Report allergic reactions such as itching, rash, swelling of the face or tongue. • Report symptoms of infection, visual changes, yellowing of skin, eyes, dark urine. • Due to high risk for drug interactions, do not take newly prescribed medication unless approved by prescriber who originally started treatment.

F

fluconazole

flu-**kon**-a-zole
(Diflucan)
Do not confuse Diflucan with diclofenac, Diprivan, or disulfiram, or fluconazole with itraconazole, ketoconazole, omeprazole, or pantoprazole.

◆CLASSIFICATION

PHARMACOTHERAPEUTIC: Synthetic azole. **CLINICAL:** Antifungal agent.

USES

Antifungal prophylaxis in pts undergoing bone marrow transplant; candidiasis (esophageal, oropharyngeal, urinary tract, vaginal); systemic *Candida* infections (e.g., candidemia); treatment of cryptococcal meningitis. **OFF-LABEL:** Cryptococcal pneumonia, candidal intertrigo.

PRECAUTIONS

Contraindications: Hypersensitivity to fluconazole. Concomitant administration of QT-prolonging medications (e.g., erythromycin, pimozide). **Cautions:** Hepatic/renal impairment, hypokalemia, hypersensitivity to other triazoles (e.g., itraconazole, terconazole), imidazoles (e.g., butoconazole, ketoconazole). Medications or conditions known to cause arrhythmias.

ACTION

Interferes with fungal cytochrome P-450 activity, an enzyme necessary for ergosterol formation (principal sterol in fungal cell membrane). **Therapeutic Effect:** Directly damages fungal membrane, altering its function. Fungistatic.

PHARMACOKINETICS

Well absorbed from GI tract. Widely distributed, including to CSF. Protein binding: 11%. Partially metabolized in liver. Excreted unchanged primarily in urine. Partially removed by hemodialysis. **Half-life:** 20–30 hrs (increased in renal impairment).

⌛ LIFESPAN CONSIDERATIONS

Pregnancy/Lactation: Secreted in human breast milk. Use caution in breastfeeding females. **Children:** No age-related precautions noted. **Elderly:** Age-related renal impairment may require dosage adjustment.

INTERACTIONS

DRUG: May increase concentration/effect of **budesonide, calcium channel blockers (e.g., amlodipine, nifedipine, verapamil), cyclosporine, ivabradine, methadone, rifabutin, sirolimus, tacrolimus, tofacitinib.** May decrease effect of ***Saccharomyces boulardii.*** May increase concentration/effect, risk of myopathy of **HMG-CoA reductase inhibitors (e.g., atorvastatin, simvastatin).** **HERBAL:** None significant. **FOOD:** None known. **LAB VALUES:** May increase serum alkaline phosphatase, bilirubin, ALT, AST.

AVAILABILITY (Rx)

Injection, Solution, Pre-Mix: 200 mg (100 mL), 400 mg (200 mL). **Powder**

for Oral Suspension: 10 mg/mL, 40 mg/mL. **Tablets:** 50 mg, 100 mg, 150 mg, 200 mg.

ADMINISTRATION/HANDLING

IV

Rate of administration • Do not exceed maximum flow rate of 200 mg/hr.
Storage • Store at room temperature. • Do not remove from outer wrap until ready to use. • Squeeze inner bag to check for leaks. • Do not use parenteral form if solution is cloudy, precipitate forms, seal is not intact, or it is discolored. • Do not add supplementary medication.

PO

• Give without regard to food.

IV INCOMPATIBILITIES

Amphotericin B (Fungizone), amphotericin B complex (Abelcet, AmBisome, Amphotec), ampicillin (Polycillin), calcium gluconate, cefotaxime (Claforan), cefTRIAXone (Rocephin), cefuroxime (Zinacef), chloramphenicol (Chloromycetin), clindamycin (Cleocin), co-trimoxazole (Bactrim), diazePAM (Valium), digoxin (Lanoxin), erythromycin (Erythrocin), furosemide (Lasix), haloperidol (Haldol), hydrOXYzine (Vistaril), imipenem and cilastatin (Primaxin).

IV COMPATIBILITIES

Dexmedetomidine (Precedex), dilTIAZem (Cardizem), DOBUTamine (Dobutrex), DOPamine (Intropin), heparin, lipids, LORazepam (Ativan), midazolam (Versed), propofol (Diprivan).

INDICATIONS/ROUTES/DOSAGE

ALERT PO and IV therapy equally effective; IV therapy recommended for pts intolerant of drug or unable to take orally. Oral suspension stable for 14 days at room temperature or refrigerated.

Usual Dosage

Note: Duration and dose dependent on location/severity of infection.
PO/IV: ADULTS, ELDERLY: 150 mg once or **loading dose:** 200–800 mg. **Maintenance dose:** 200–800 mg once daily. **ADOLESCENTS, CHILDREN, INFANTS: Loading dose:** 6–12 mg/kg. **Maintenance dose:** 3–12 mg/kg once daily. **Maximum:** 600 mg/day. **NEONATES:** Initially, 25 mg/kg on day 1, then 12 mg/kg once daily.

Dosage in Renal Impairment

After a loading dose of 400 mg, daily dosage is based on creatinine clearance.

Creatinine Clearance	Dosage
Greater than 50 mL/min	100%
50 mL/min or less	50%
Dialysis	50%
CCRT	400–800 mg as loading dose
CVVH	then 200–800 mg/day
CVVHDF	400–800 mg as loading dose, then 400–800 mg/day

Dosage in Hepatic Impairment

Use caution.

SIDE EFFECTS

Occasional (4%–1%): Hypersensitivity reaction (chills, fever, pruritus, rash), dizziness, drowsiness, headache, constipation, diarrhea, nausea, vomiting, abdominal pain.

ADVERSE EFFECTS/TOXIC REACTIONS

Exfoliative skin disorders, serious hepatic injury, blood dyscrasias (eosinophilia, thrombocytopenia, anemia, leukopenia) have been reported rarely. May increase risk of QT prolongation, torsades de pointes. Skin disorders including Stevens-Johnson syndrome, toxic epidermal necrolysis may occur.

NURSING CONSIDERATIONS

BASELINE ASSESSMENT

Obtain CBC, LFT; serum potassium in critically ill pts. Receive full medication history and screen for interactions. Assess areas of infection. Assess infected area.

INTERVENTION/EVALUATION

Monitor hepatic function in critically ill pts. Assess for hypersensitivity reaction (chills, fever). Report rash, itching promptly. Monitor daily pattern of bowel activity, stool consistency. Assess for dizziness; provide assistance as needed.

PATIENT/FAMILY TEACHING

• Report dark urine, pale stool, jaundiced skin or sclera of eyes, rash, pruritus. • Pts with oropharyngeal infections should maintain fastidious oral hygiene. • Consult physician before taking any other medication.

fluorouracil, 5-FU HIGH ALERT

flure-oh-**ue**-ra-sil
(Adrucil, Carac, Efudex, Fluoroplex, Tolak)

BLACK BOX ALERT Must be administered by personnel trained in administration/handling of chemotherapeutic agents.

Do not confuse Efudex with Efidac.

◆CLASSIFICATION

PHARMACOTHERAPEUTIC: Antimetabolite. **CLINICAL:** Antineoplastic.

USES

Parenteral: Treatment of carcinoma of colon, rectum, breast, stomach (gastric), pancreas. **Topical:** Treatment of multiple actinic or solar keratoses, superficial basal cell carcinomas. **OFF-LABEL: Parenteral:** Treatment of carcinoma of bladder, cervical, endometrial, head/neck, anal, esophageal, renal cell, unknown primary cancer.

PRECAUTIONS

Contraindications: Hypersensitivity to fluorouracil. Myelosuppression, poor nutritional status, potentially serious infections. **Cautions:** History of high-dose pelvic irradiation, hepatic/renal impairment, palmar-plantar erythrodysesthesia syndrome (hand and foot syndrome), previous use of alkylating agents. Pts with widespread metastatic marrow involvement.

ACTION

Blocks formation of thymidylic acid. Cell cycle–specific for S phase of cell division. **Therapeutic Effect:** Inhibits DNA, RNA synthesis. **Topical:** Destroys rapidly proliferating cells.

PHARMACOKINETICS

Widely distributed. Crosses blood-brain barrier. Metabolized in liver. Primarily excreted by lungs as carbon dioxide. Removed by hemodialysis. **Half-life:** 16 min.

LIFESPAN CONSIDERATIONS

Pregnancy/Lactation: If possible, avoid use during pregnancy, esp. first trimester. May cause fetal harm. Unknown if distributed in breast milk. Breastfeeding not recommended. **Children:** No age-related precautions noted. **Elderly:** Age-related renal impairment may require dosage adjustment.

INTERACTIONS

DRUG: Bone marrow depressants (e.g., cladribine) may increase risk of myelosuppression. **Live virus vaccines** may potentiate virus replication, increase vaccine side effects, decrease pt's antibody response to vaccine. **HERBAL: Echinacea** may decrease effects. **FOOD:** None known. **LAB VALUES:** May decrease serum albumin. **Topical:** May cause eosinophilia, leukocytosis, thrombocytopenia, toxic granulation.

AVAILABILITY (Rx)

Cream, Topical: ***(Carac):*** 0.5%. ***(Tolak):*** 4%, ***(Efudex):*** 5%. ***(Fluoroplex):*** 1%. **Injection**

Solution: *(Adrucil):* 50 mg/mL. **Solution, Topical:** *(Efudex):* 2%, 5%.

ADMINISTRATION/HANDLING

◄ALERT► Give by IV injection or IV infusion. Do not add to other IV infusions. Avoid small veins, swollen/edematous extremities, areas overlying joints, tendons. May be carcinogenic, mutagenic, teratogenic. Handle with extreme care during preparation/administration.

IV

Reconstitution • IV push does not need to be diluted or reconstituted. • Inject through Y-tube or 3-way stopcock of free-flowing solution. • For IV infusion, further dilute with 50–1,000 mL D_5W or 0.9% NaCl.

Rate of administration • Give IV push slowly over 1–2 min. • IV infusion is administered over 30 min–24 hrs (refer to individual protocols). • Extravasation produces immediate pain, severe local tissue damage.

Storage • Store at room temperature. • Solution appears colorless to faint yellow. Slight discoloration does not adversely affect potency or safety. • If precipitate forms, redissolve by heating, shaking vigorously; allow to cool to body temperature. • Diluted solutions stable for 72 hrs at room temperature.

IV INCOMPATIBILITIES

Amphotericin B complex (Abelcet, AmBisome, Amphotec), filgrastim (Neupogen), ondansetron (Zofran), vinorelbine (Navelbine).

IV COMPATIBILITIES

Granisetron (Kytril), heparin, HYDROmorphone (Dilaudid), leucovorin, morphine, potassium chloride, propofol (Diprivan).

INDICATIONS/ROUTES/DOSAGE

Note: Refer to individual protocols.

Usual Range

IV bolus: ADULTS, ELDERLY: 200–1000 mg/m²/day for 1–21 days or 500–600 mg/m²/dose q3–4wks.

IV infusion: ADULTS, ELDERLY: 15 mg/kg/day or 500 mg/m²/day over 4 hrs for 5 days or 800–1200 mg/m² over 24–120 hrs.

Multiple Actinic or Solar Keratoses

Topical: ***(Carac 0.5%):*** **ADULTS, ELDERLY:** Apply once daily for up to 4 wks. ***(Efudex 5%):*** **ADULTS, ELDERLY:** Apply twice daily for 2–4 wks. ***(Fluoroplex 1%):*** Apply twice daily for 2–6 wks. ***(Tolak 4%):*** Apply once daily for 4 wks.

Basal Cell Carcinoma

Topical: *(Efudex 5%):* **ADULTS, ELDERLY:** Apply twice daily for 3–6 wks up to 10–12 wks.

Dosage in Renal Impairment

No dose adjustment.

Dosage in Hepatic Impairment

Use extreme caution.

SIDE EFFECTS

Parenteral: Frequent (greater than 10%): Alopecia, dermatitis, anorexia, diarrhea, esophagitis, dyspepsia, stomatitis. **Occasional (10%–1%):** Cardiotoxicity (angina, ECG changes), skin dryness, epithelial fissuring, nausea, vomiting, excessive lacrimation, blurred vision. **Rare (less than 1%):** Headache, photosensitivity, somnolence, allergic reaction, dyspnea, hypotension, MI, pulmonary edema. **Topical: Occasional:** Erythema, skin ulceration, pruritus, hyperpigmentation, dermatitis, insomnia, stomatitis, irritability, photosensitivity, excessive lacrimation, blurred vision.

ADVERSE EFFECTS/TOXIC REACTIONS

Earliest sign of toxicity (4–8 days after beginning therapy) is stomatitis (dry mouth, burning sensation, mucosal erythema, ulceration at inner margin of lips). Most common dermatologic toxicity is pruritic rash (generally on extremities, less frequently on trunk). Leukopenia (WBC less than 3500 cells/mm³) generally occurs within 9–14 days after drug administration but may occur as late as 25th day. Thrombocytopenia (platelets less than 100,000 cells/mm^3) occasionally occurs within 7–17 days after administration. Pancytopenia, agranulocytosis occur rarely.

NURSING CONSIDERATIONS

BASELINE ASSESSMENT

Obtain CBC with differential, renal function, LFT and monitor during therapy. Question history of hypersensitivity reaction, hepatic/renal impairment.

INTERVENTION/EVALUATION

Monitor for rapidly falling WBC, platelet count; intractable diarrhea, GI bleeding (bright red or tarry stool). Assess oral mucosa for stomatitis. Drug should be discontinued if intractable diarrhea, stomatitis, GI bleeding occurs. Assess skin for rash.

PATIENT/FAMILY TEACHING

• Maintain strict oral hygiene. • Report signs/symptoms of infection (cough, fatigue, fever), unusual bruising/bleeding, visual changes, nausea, vomiting, diarrhea, chest pain, palpitations. • Avoid sunlight, artificial light sources; wear protective clothing, sunglasses, sunscreen. • **Topical:** Apply only to affected area. • Do not use occlusive coverings. • Be careful near eyes, nose, mouth. • Wash hands thoroughly after application. • Treated areas may be unsightly for several weeks after therapy.

FLUoxetine

floo-**ox**-e-teen
(PROzac, Sarafem)

BLACK BOX ALERT Increased risk of suicidal thinking and behavior in children, adolescents, young adults 18–24 yrs of age with major depressive disorder, other psychiatric disorders.

Do not confuse FLUoxetine with DULoxetine, famotidine, fluvastatin, fluvoxaMINE, furosemide, or PARoxetine, or PROzac with Paxil, PriLOSEC, Prograf, Proscar, or ProSom, or Sarafem with Serophene.

FIXED-COMBINATION(S)

Symbyax: FLUoxetine/OLANZapine (an antipsychotic): 25 mg/6 mg, 25 mg/12 mg, 50 mg/6 mg, 50 mg/12 mg.

◆CLASSIFICATION

PHARMACOTHERAPEUTIC: Selective serotonin reuptake inhibitor (SSRI). **CLINICAL:** Antidepressant.

USES

Treatment of major depressive disorder (MDD), obsessive-compulsive disorder (OCD), binge-eating and vomiting in moderate to severe bulimia nervosa, premenstrual dysphoric disorder (PMDD), panic disorder with or without agoraphobia. Treatment of resistant or bipolar 1 depression (with OLANZapine). **OFF-LABEL:** Treatment of fibromyalgia, posttraumatic stress disorder (PTSD), Raynaud's phenomena, social anxiety disorder, selective mutism.

PRECAUTIONS

Contraindications: Hypersensitivity to FLUoxetine. Use of MAOIs within 5 wks of discontinuing FLUoxetine or within 14 days of discontinuing MAOIs. Initiation in pts receiving linezolid or methylene blue. Use with pimozide or thioridazine. **Note:** Do not initiate thioridazine until 5 wks after discontinuing fluoxetine. **Cautions:** Seizure disorder, cardiac dysfunction (e.g., history of MI), diabetes, pts at risk for QT interval prolongation, cardiac arrhythmias (congenital long QT syndrome, HF, QT interval–prolonging medications, hypokalemia, hypomagnesemia), renal/hepatic impairment, pts at high risk for suicide, in pts where weight loss is undesirable, elderly. Pts at risk of acute narrow-angle glaucoma or with increased intraocular pressure.

ACTION

Selectively inhibits serotonin uptake in CNS, enhancing serotonergic function. **Therapeutic Effect:** Relieves depression; reduces obsessive-compulsive, bulimic behavior.

PHARMACOKINETICS

Well absorbed from GI tract. Crosses blood-brain barrier. Protein binding: 94%. Metabolized in liver. Primarily excreted in urine. Not removed by hemodialysis. **Half-life:** 2–3 days; metabolite, 7–9 days.

LIFESPAN CONSIDERATIONS

Pregnancy/Lactation: Unknown whether drug crosses placenta or is distributed in breast milk. **Children:** May be more sensitive to behavioral side effects (e.g., insomnia, restlessness). **Elderly:** No age-related precautions noted.

INTERACTIONS

DRUG: **NSAIDs (e.g., ibuprofen, ketorolac, naproxen), antiplatelets (e.g., clopidogrel), anticoagulants (e.g., warfarin)** may increase risk of bleeding. **Alcohol, other CNS depressants (e.g., LORazepam, morphine, zolpidem)** may increase CNS depression. **MAOIs (e.g., phenelzine, selegiline)** may produce serotonin syndrome and neuroleptic malignant syndrome. **Strong CYP2D6 inhibitors (e.g., bupropion)** may increase concentration/effect. May decrease concentration/effect of **tamoxifen. QT interval–prolonging medications (e.g., amiodarone, azithromycin, ciprofloxacin, haloperidol, methadone, sotalol)** may increase risk of QT interval prolongation. May increase adverse effects of **tricyclic antidepressants (e.g., amitriptyline).** HERBAL: **Herbals with sedative properties (e.g., chamomile, kava kava, valerian)** may increase CNS depression. **St. John's wort** may decrease concentration/effect. FOOD: None known. LAB VALUES: May decrease serum sodium. May increase serum ALT, AST.

AVAILABILITY (Rx)

Capsules: 10 mg, 20 mg, 40 mg. **Oral Solution:** 20 mg/5 mL. **Tablets:** 10 mg, 20 mg, 60 mg.

Capsules (Delayed-Release): 90 mg.

ADMINISTRATION/HANDLING

PO

• Give without regard to food, but give with food, milk if GI distress occurs. • **Bipolar disorder:** Give once daily in evening. • **Depression, OCD:** Give once daily in morning or twice daily (morning and noon). • **Bulimia:** Give once daily in morning.

F

INDICATIONS/ROUTES/DOSAGE

ALERT Use lower or less frequent doses in pts with renal/hepatic impairment, pts with concurrent disease or multiple medications, the elderly. Decrease gradually to minimize withdrawal symptoms and to allow for detection of re-emerging symptoms.

Depression

PO: ADULTS, ELDERLY: Initially, 20 mg each morning. May increase after several wks by 20 mg/day. **Maximum:** 80 mg/day as single or 2 divided doses. *(Weekly):* 90 mg/wk, begin 7 days after last dose of 20 mg in pts maintained on 20 mg/day. **CHILDREN 8–18 YRS:** Initially, 10–20 mg/day. Lower-weight children may be started at 10 mg/day and increased to 20 mg/day after several wks if needed.

Panic Disorder

PO: ADULTS, ELDERLY: Initially, 5–10 mg/day. After 3–7 days, may increase dose in 5–10 mg increments at intervals of at least 1 wk to usual dose of 20–40 mg/day. **Maximum:** 60 mg/day.

Bulimia Nervosa

PO: ADULTS: Initially, 20 mg/day. May increase by 20 mg increments at intervals of at least 1 wk. **Maximum:** 60 mg/day.

Obsessive-Compulsive Disorder (OCD)

PO: ADULTS, ELDERLY: Initially, 10–20 mg once daily. May increase by 20 mg increments at intervals of at least 1 wk. Range: 40–80 mg/day. **Maximum:** 120 mg/day. **CHILDREN 7–18 YRS:** Initially, 10 mg/day. May increase to 20 mg/day after 2 wks. Range: 20–60 mg/day.

Depression Associated With Bipolar Disorder

PO: ADULTS, ELDERLY, CHILDREN 10–17 YRS: ***(With Olanzapine):*** Initially, 20 mg/day in evening. May increase gradually in 10–20 mg increments. Range: 20–50 mg/day.

Premenstrual Dysphoric Disorder (PMDD) (Sarafem)

PO: ADULTS: (Continuous daily dosing): Initially, 10 mg once daily. Increase to 20 mg/day over first month. In a subsequent menstrual cycle, a further increase to 30 mg/day may be necessary. **(Intermittent dosing):** Initially, 10 mg once daily during luteal phase of menstrual cycle only. Over first month, may increase to 20 mg once daily during luteal phase. In a subsequent menstrual cycle, a further increase to 30 mg/day during luteal phase may be necessary.

Dosage in Renal/Hepatic Impairment

Use caution.

SIDE EFFECTS

Frequent (greater than 10%): Headache, asthenia, insomnia, anxiety, drowsiness, nausea, diarrhea, decreased appetite. **Occasional (9%–2%):** Dizziness, tremor, fatigue, vomiting, constipation, dry mouth, abdominal pain, nasal congestion, diaphoresis, rash. **Rare (less than 2%):** Flushed skin, light-headedness, impaired concentration.

ADVERSE EFFECTS/TOXIC REACTIONS

May increase risk of suicide. Agitation, coma, diarrhea, delirium, hallucinations, hyperreflexia, hyperthermia, tachycardia, seizures may indicate life-threatening serotonin syndrome.

NURSING CONSIDERATIONS

BASELINE ASSESSMENT

Assess appearance, behavior, mood, suicidal tendencies. For pts on long-term therapy, baseline renal function, LFT, blood counts should be performed at baseline and periodically thereafter.

INTERVENTION/EVALUATION

Supervise suicidal-risk pt closely during early therapy (as depression lessens, energy level improves, increasing suicide potential). Monitor mental status, anxiety, social functioning, appetite, nutritional intake. Monitor daily pattern of bowel activity, stool consistency. Assess skin for rash. Monitor serum LFT, glucose, sodium; weight.

PATIENT/FAMILY TEACHING

• Maximum therapeutic response may require 4 or more wks of therapy. • Do not abruptly discontinue medication. • Avoid tasks that require alertness, motor skills until response to drug is established. • Avoid alcohol. • To avoid insomnia, take last dose of drug before 4 PM. • Seek immediate medical attention if thoughts of suicide, new-onset or worsening of anxiety, depression, or changes in mood occur.

fluticasone

TOP 100

floo-**tik**-a-sone

(Arnuity Ellipta, Cutivate, Flonase, 🍁 Flonase Allergy Relief, Flovent Diskus, Xhance, Flonase Sensimist)

Do not confuse Cutivate with Ultravate, or Flonase with Flovent, Beconase.

FIXED-COMBINATION(S)

Advair, Advair Diskus, Advair HFA: fluticasone/salmeterol (bronchodilator): 100 mcg/50 mcg, 250 mcg/50 mcg, 500 mcg/50 mcg. **Breo Ellipta:** fluticasone/vilanterol (bronchodilator): 100 mcg/25 mcg. **Dymista:** fluticasone/azelastine (an antihistamine): 50 mcg/137 mcg per spray. **Trelegy Ellipta:** fluticasone/umeclidinium (anticholinergic)/vilanterol (bronchodilator): 100 mcg/62.5 mcg/25 mcg.

◆CLASSIFICATION

PHARMACOTHERAPEUTIC: Corticosteroid. **CLINICAL:** Anti-inflammatory, antipruritic.

USES

Nasal: Management of nasal symptoms of perennial nonallergic rhinitis in adults and children 4 yrs and older. Management of seasonal and perennial allergic rhinitis in adults, children 2 yrs and older. **(Xhance):** Treatment of nasal polyps in pts 18 yrs and older. **(OTC):** Relief of hayfever/other upper respiratory allergies. **Topical:** Relief of inflammation/pruritus associated with steroid-responsive disorders (e.g., contact dermatitis, eczema), atopic dermatitis. **Inhalation:** Maintenance treatment of bronchial asthma as prophylactic therapy.

PRECAUTIONS

Contraindications: Hypersensitivity to fluticasone. (Arnuity Ellipta, Flovent Diskus): Severe hypersensitivity to milk proteins or lactose. **Inhalation:** Primary treatment of status asthmaticus, acute exacerbation of asthma, other acute asthmatic conditions. **Cautions:** Untreated systemic ocular herpes simplex; untreated fungal, bacterial infection; active or quiescent tuberculosis. Thyroid disease, cardiovascular disease, diabetes, glaucoma, hepatic/renal impairment, cataracts, myasthenia gravis, seizures, GI disease, risk for osteoporosis, untreated localized infection of nasal mucosa. Following acute MI; concurrent use with strong CYP3A4 inhibitors.

ACTION

Direct local effect as potent vasoconstrictor, anti-inflammatory. **Therapeutic Effect:** Prevents, controls inflammation.

PHARMACOKINETICS

Inhalation/intranasal: Protein binding: 91%. Metabolized in liver. Excreted in urine. **Half-life:** 3–7.8 hrs. **Topical:** Amount absorbed depends on affected area and skin condition (absorption increased with fever, hydration, inflamed or denuded skin).

⌛ LIFESPAN CONSIDERATIONS

Pregnancy/Lactation: Unknown if drug crosses placenta or is distributed in breast milk. **Children:** Safety and efficacy not established in pts younger than 4 yrs. Children 4 yrs and older may experience growth suppression with prolonged or high doses. **Elderly:** No age-related precautions noted.

INTERACTIONS

DRUG: **Strong CYP3A4 inhibitors (e.g., clarithromycin, ketoconazole, ritonavir)** may increase concentration/effect. **HERBAL:** **Echinacea** may decrease concentration/effects. **FOOD:** None known. **LAB VALUES:** None significant.

AVAILABILITY (Rx)

Aerosol for Oral Inhalation: ***(Flovent HFA):*** 44 mcg/inhalation, 110 mcg/inhalation, 220 mcg/inhalation. **Cream:** ***(Cutivate):*** 0.05%. **Ointment:** ***(Cutivate):*** 0.005%. **Powder for Oral Inhalation:** ***(Flovent Diskus):*** 50 mcg/blister, 100 mcg/blister, 250 mcg/blister. ***(Arnuity Ellipta):*** 50 mcg/actuation, 100 mcg/actuation, 200 mcg/actuation. **Suspension Intranasal Spray:** ***(Flonase Allergy Relief):*** 50 mcg/inhalation. ***(Flonase Sensimist):*** 27.5 mcg/spray. ***(Xhance):*** 93 mcg/actuation.

ADMINISTRATION/HANDLING

Inhalation

Flovent HFA

• Shake container well. Prime before first use. Instruct pt to exhale completely. Place mouthpiece fully into mouth, inhale, and hold breath as long as possible before exhaling. • Allow 30–60 seconds between inhalations. • Rinsing mouth after each use decreases dry mouth, hoarseness.

Flovent Diskus

• Do not shake or prime before use. Place mouthpiece fully into mouth, inhale quickly and deeply, remove device, and hold breath up to 10 seconds.

Arnuity Ellipta

• Do not shake or prime before use; put mouthpiece between lips, breathe deeply and slowly through the mouth, remove inhaler, and hold breath for 3–4 seconds.

Intranasal

• Instruct pt to clear nasal passages as much as possible before use (topical nasal decongestants may be needed 5–15 min before use). • Tilt head slightly forward. • Insert spray tip into 1 nostril, pointing toward inflamed nasal turbinates, away from nasal septum. • Pump medication into 1 nostril while pt holds other nostril closed, concurrently inspires through nose.

INDICATIONS/ROUTES/DOSAGE

Nonallergic Rhinitis

Intranasal: *(Flonase):* **ADULTS, ELDERLY:** Initially, 200 mcg (2 sprays in each nostril once daily or 1 spray in each nostril q12h). **Maintenance:** 1 spray in each nostril once daily. May increase to 100 mcg (2 sprays) in each nostril. **Maximum:** 200 mcg/day. **CHILDREN 4 YRS AND OLDER:** Initially, 100 mcg (1 spray in each nostril once daily). **Maximum:** 200 mcg/day (2 sprays each nostril). *(Flonase Sensimist):* **ADULTS, ELDERLY, CHILDREN 12 YRS AND OLDER:** 110 mcg (2 sprays in each nostril) once daily. **Maintenance:** 55 mcg (1 spray in each nostril) once daily. **CHILDREN 2–11 YRS:** 55 mcg (1 spray in each nostril) once daily.

Allergic Rhinitis

(Flonase Sensimist): **ADULTS, ELDERLY, CHILDREN 12 YRS AND OLDER:** 110 mcg (2 sprays in each nostril) once daily. **Maintenance:** 55 mcg (1 spray in each nostril) once daily. **CHILDREN 2–11 YRS:** 55 mcg (1 spray in each nostril) once daily.

Usual Topical Dosage

Note: Ointment for adults only.

Topical: ADULTS, ELDERLY, CHILDREN 3 MOS AND OLDER: Apply sparingly to affected area once or twice daily.

Nasal Polyps

(Xhance): **ADULTS, ELDERLY:** 93 mcg (1 spray) per nostril twice daily. May increase to 2 sprays twice daily.

Maintenance Treatment of Asthma

Inhalation powder: *(Arnuity Ellipta):* **ADULTS, ELDERLY, CHILDREN 12 YRS AND OLDER:** 100–200 mcg once daily. **Maximum:** 200 mcg/day. **CHILDREN 5–11 YRS:** 50 mcg once daily. *(Flovent Diskus):* **ADULTS, ELDERLY, CHILDREN 12 YRS AND OLDER:** Initially, 100 mcg twice daily. **Maximum:** 500 mcg twice daily. *(Flovent HFA):* **ADULTS, ELDERLY, CHILDREN 12 YRS AND OLDER:** 88 mcg twice daily. **Maximum:** 440 mcg twice daily. **USUAL PEDIATRIC DOSE (4–11 YRS):** *(Flovent Diskus):* Initially, 50 mcg twice daily. May increase to 100 mcg twice daily. *(Flovent HFA):* 88 mcg twice daily.

Dosage in Renal/Hepatic Impairment

No dose adjustment. *(Arnuity Ellipta):* Use caution in hepatic impairment.

SIDE EFFECTS

Frequent: Inhalation: Throat irritation, hoarseness, dry mouth, cough, temporary wheezing, oropharyngeal candidiasis (particularly if mouth is not rinsed with water after each administration). **Intranasal:** Mild nasopharyngeal irritation, nasal burning, stinging, dryness, rebound congestion, rhinorrhea, altered sense of taste. **Occasional: Inhalation:** Oral candidiasis. **Intranasal:** Nasal/pharyngeal candidiasis, headache. **Topical:** Stinging, burning of skin.

ADVERSE EFFECTS/TOXIC REACTIONS

None known.

NURSING CONSIDERATIONS

BASELINE ASSESSMENT

Establish baseline history of skin disorder, asthma, rhinitis. Question hypersensitivity, esp. milk products or lactose. Question medical history as listed in Precautions.

INTERVENTION/EVALUATION

Monitor rate, depth, rhythm, type of respiration; quality/rate of pulse. Assess lung sounds for rhonchi, wheezing, rales. Assess oral mucous membranes for evidence of candidiasis. Monitor growth in pediatric pts. **Topical:** Assess involved area for therapeutic response to irritation.

PATIENT/FAMILY TEACHING

• Pts receiving bronchodilators by inhalation concomitantly with steroid inhalation therapy should use bronchodilator several min before corticosteroid aerosol (enhances penetration of steroid into bronchial tree). • Do not change dose/schedule or stop taking drug; must taper off gradually under medical supervision. • Maintain strict oral hygiene. • Rinse mouth with water immediately after inhalation (prevents mouth/throat dryness, oral fungal infection). • Increase fluid intake (decreases lung secretion viscosity). • **Intranasal:** Clear nasal passages before use. • Report if no improvement in symptoms or if sneezing/nasal irritation occurs. • Improvement noted in several days. • **Topical:** Rub thin film gently into affected area. • Use only for prescribed area and no longer than ordered. • Avoid contact with eyes.

fluvoxaMINE

floo-**vox**-a-meen
(Luvox ✤)

■ BLACK BOX ALERT ■ Increased risk of suicidal ideation and behavior in children, adolescents, young adults 18–24 yrs with major depressive disorder, other psychiatric disorders.
Do not confuse fluvoxaMINE with flavoxATE or FLUoxetine, or Luvox with Lasix, Levoxyl, or Lovenox.

◆CLASSIFICATION

PHARMACOTHERAPEUTIC: Selective serotonin reuptake inhibitor. **CLINICAL:** Antidepressant.

USES

Immediate-Release: Treatment of obsessive-compulsive disorder (OCD) in adults and children 8–17 yrs of age. **Extended-Release:** Treatment of OCD in adults. **OFF-LABEL:** Treatment of social anxiety disorder (SAD), posttraumatic stress disorder (PTSD).

PRECAUTIONS

Contraindications: Hypersensitivity to fluvoxaMINE. Use of MAOIs concurrently or within 14 days of discontinuing MAOIs or fluvoxaMINE. Concomitant use with alosetron, pimozide, ramelteon, thioridazine, or tiZANidine. Initiation of fluvoxaMINE in pts receiving linezolid or methylene blue. **Cautions:** Renal/hepatic impairment, elderly, impaired platelet aggregation; concurrent use of NSAIDs, aspirin; seizure disorder; pts that are volume depleted; third trimester of pregnancy; pts with high suicide risk; risk of bleeding or receiving concurrent anticoagulant therapy. May precipitate a shift to mania or hypomania in pts with bipolar disorder.

ACTION

Selectively inhibits neuronal reuptake of serotonin. **Therapeutic Effect:** Relieves depression, symptoms of obsessive-compulsive disorder (OCD).

PHARMACOKINETICS

Well absorbed following PO administration. Protein binding: 77%. Metabolized in liver. Excreted in urine. **Half-life:** 15–20 hrs.

⌛ LIFESPAN CONSIDERATIONS

Pregnancy/Lactation: Unknown if drug crosses the placenta; distributed in breast milk. **Children:** Safety and efficacy not established in pts younger than 8 yrs. **Elderly:** Potential for reduced serum clearance; maintain caution.

INTERACTIONS

DRUG: MAOIs (e.g., phenelzine, selegiline) may increase risk of serotonin syndrome (hyperthermia, rigidity, myoclonus). **Tricyclic antidepressants (e.g., amitriptyline)** may increase concentration/effect. **Alcohol** may increase adverse effects. May increase concentration/effects of **ramelteon, thioridazine, tiZANidine.** HERBAL: **Herbals with anticoagulant/antiplatelet properties (e.g., garlic, ginger, ginkgo biloba), glucosamine** may increase effect. FOOD: **Grapefruit products** may increase concentration/effect. LAB VALUES: May decrease serum sodium.

AVAILABILITY (Rx)

Tablets: 25 mg, 50 mg, 100 mg.

Capsules (Extended-Release): 100 mg, 150 mg.

ADMINISTRATION/HANDLING

• Do not break, crush, dissolve, or divide extended-release capsules. • May give with or without food.

INDICATIONS/ROUTES/DOSAGE

Obsessive-Compulsive Disorder (OCD)

PO: ***(Immediate-Release):*** **ADULTS:** Initially, 50 mg at bedtime; may increase by 50 mg every 4–7 days. Dosages greater than 100 mg/day should be given in 2 divided doses with larger dose given at bedtime. Usual dose: 100–300 mg/day. **Maximum:** 300 mg/day. ***(Extended-Release):*** Initially, 100 mg once daily at bedtime. May increase by 50 mg at no less than 1-wk intervals. Range: 100–300 mg/day. **Maximum:** 300 mg/day. **CHILDREN 8–17 YRS:** ***(Immediate-Release):*** Initially, 25 mg at bedtime; may increase by 25 mg every 4–7 days. Dosages greater than 50 mg/day should be given in 2 divided doses with larger dose given at bedtime. **Maximum:** **(CHILDREN 8–11 YRS):** 200 mg/day. **(CHILDREN 12–17 YRS):** 300 mg/day.

Dosage in Renal/Hepatic Impairment

No dose adjustment.

SIDE EFFECTS

Frequent (40%–21%): Nausea, headache, drowsiness, insomnia. **Occasional (14%–8%):** Dizziness, diarrhea, dry mouth, asthenia, dyspepsia, constipation, abnormal ejaculation. **Rare (6%–3%):** Anorexia, anxiety, tremor, vomiting, flatulence, urinary frequency, sexual dysfunction, altered taste.

ADVERSE EFFECTS/TOXIC REACTIONS

Agitation, coma, diarrhea, delirium, hallucinations, hyperreflexia, hyperthermia, tachycardia, seizures may indicate life-threatening serotonin syndrome.

NURSING CONSIDERATIONS

BASELINE ASSESSMENT

Obtain LFT. Receive full medication history in screen for interactions, esp. contraindicated use of concomitant medications. Question history of seizure disorder. Assess hydration status.

INTERVENTION/EVALUATION

Supervise suicidal-risk pt closely during early therapy (as depression lessens, energy level improves, increasing suicide potential). Assess appearance, behavior, speech pattern, level of interest, mood. Assist with ambulation if dizziness, drowsiness occurs. Monitor daily pattern of bowel activity, stool consistency.

PATIENT/FAMILY TEACHING

• Maximum therapeutic response may require 4 wks or more of therapy. • Dry mouth may be relieved by sugarless gum, sips of water. • Do not abruptly discontinue medication. • Avoid tasks that require alertness, motor skills until response to drug is established. • Seek immediate medical attention if thoughts of suicide, new-onset or worsening of anxiety, depression, or changes in mood occur.

folic acid

foe-lik **as**-id

Do not confuse folic acid with folinic acid.

CLASSIFICATION

PHARMACOTHERAPEUTIC: Vitamin, water soluble. **CLINICAL:** Nutritional supplement.

USES

Treatment of megaloblastic and macrocytic anemias due to folate deficiency. Treatment of anemias due to folate deficiency in pregnant women. Folate supplementation during periconceptual period decreases risk of neural tube defects.

PRECAUTIONS

Contraindications: Hypersensitivity to folic acid. **Cautions:** Anemias (aplastic, normocytic, pernicious, refractory) when anemia present with vitamin B_{12} deficiency.

ACTION

Stimulates production of platelets, WBCs in folate-deficiency anemia. Necessary for formation of coenzymes in many metabolic pathways. Necessary for erythropoiesis. **Therapeutic Effect:** Essential for nucleoprotein synthesis, maintenance of normal erythropoiesis.

PHARMACOKINETICS

PO form almost completely absorbed from GI tract (upper duodenum). Protein binding: High. Metabolized in liver. Excreted in urine. Removed by hemodialysis.

LIFESPAN CONSIDERATIONS

Pregnancy/Lactation: Distributed in breast milk. **Children/Elderly:** No age-related precautions noted.

INTERACTIONS

DRUG: None significant. **HERBAL: Green tea** may increase concentration. **FOOD:** None known. **LAB VALUES:** May decrease vitamin B_{12} concentration.

AVAILABILITY (Rx)

Capsules: 0.8 mg, 5 mg, 20 mg. **Injection Solution:** 5 mg/mL. **Tablets:** 0.4 mg (OTC), 0.8 mg (OTC), 1 mg.

ADMINISTRATION/HANDLING

PO

- May give without regard to food.

IV

May give 5 mg or less undiluted over at least 1 min, or dilute with 50 mL 0.9% NaCl or D_5W and infuse over 30 min.

INDICATIONS/ROUTES/DOSAGE

Anemia

IM/IV/SQ/PO: ADULTS, ELDERLY, CHILDREN 4 YRS AND OLDER: 1–5 mg/day. **CHILDREN YOUNGER THAN 4 YRS:** Up to 0.3 mg/day. **INFANTS:** 0.1 mg/day. **PREGNANT/LACTATING FEMALES:** 0.8 mg/day.

Prevention of Neural Tube Defects

PO: FEMALES OF CHILDBEARING AGE: 400–800 mcg/day. **FEMALES AT HIGH RISK OR FAMILY HISTORY OF NEURAL TUBE DEFECTS:** 4 mg/day.

SIDE EFFECTS

None known.

ADVERSE EFFECTS/TOXIC REACTIONS

Allergic hypersensitivity occurs rarely with parenteral form. Oral folic acid is nontoxic.

NURSING CONSIDERATIONS

BASELINE ASSESSMENT

Pernicious anemia should be ruled out with Schilling test and vitamin B_{12} blood level before initiating therapy (may produce irreversible neurologic damage). Resistance to treatment may occur if decreased hematopoiesis, alcoholism, antimetabolic drugs, deficiency of vitamin B_6, B_{12}, C, E is evident.

INTERVENTION/EVALUATION

Assess for therapeutic improvement: improved sense of well-being, relief from iron deficiency symptoms (fatigue, shortness of breath, sore tongue, headache, pallor).

PATIENT/FAMILY TEACHING

- Eat foods rich in folic acid, including fruits, vegetables, organ meats.

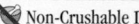

F

fondaparinux

HIGH ALERT

fon-**dap**-a-rin-ux
(Arixtra)

BLACK BOX ALERT Epidural or spinal anesthesia greatly increases potential for spinal or epidural hematoma, subsequent long-term or permanent paralysis.

F

CLASSIFICATION

PHARMACOTHERAPEUTIC: Factor Xa inhibitor. **CLINICAL:** Antithrombotic.

USES

Prevention of venous thromboembolism in pts undergoing total hip replacement, hip fracture surgery, knee replacement surgery, abdominal surgery. Treatment of acute deep vein thrombosis (DVT), acute pulmonary embolism in conjunction with warfarin. **OFF-LABEL:** Prophylaxis of DVT in pts with history of heparin-induced thrombocytopenia (HIT), acute symptomatic superficial vein thrombosis of the legs.

PRECAUTIONS

Contraindications: Hypersensitivity to fondaparinux, active major bleeding, bacterial endocarditis, prophylaxis treatment in pts with body weight less than 50 kg, severe renal impairment (CrCl less than 30 mL/min), thrombocytopenia associated with antiplatelet antibody formation in presence of fondaparinux. **Cautions:** Conditions with increased risk of bleeding, bacterial endocarditis, active ulcerative GI disease, hemorrhagic stroke; shortly after brain, spinal, or ophthalmologic surgery; concurrent platelet inhibitors, severe uncontrolled hypertension, history of CVA, history of heparin-induced thrombocytopenia, renal/hepatic impairment, elderly, indwelling epidural catheter use.

ACTION

Factor Xa inhibitor that selectively binds to antithrombin and increases its affinity for factor Xa, inhibiting factor Xa, stopping blood coagulation cascade. **Therapeutic Effect:** Indirectly prevents formation of thrombin and subsequently fibrin clot.

PHARMACOKINETICS

Well absorbed after SQ administration. Undergoes minimal, if any, metabolism. Highly bound to antithrombin III. Distributed mainly in blood and to a minor extent in extravascular fluid. Excreted unchanged in urine. Removed by hemodialysis. **Half-life:** 17–21 hrs (increased in renal impairment).

LIFESPAN CONSIDERATIONS

Pregnancy/Lactation: Use with caution, particularly during third trimester, immediate postpartum period (increased risk of maternal hemorrhage). Unknown if excreted in breast milk. **Children:** Safety and efficacy not established. **Elderly:** Age-related renal impairment may increase risk of bleeding.

INTERACTIONS

DRUG: **Anticoagulants (e.g., heparin, warfarin), aspirin, NSAIDs (e.g., ibuprofen, ketorolac, naproxen)** may increase risk of bleeding. May increase effect of **apixaban, dabigatran, edoxaban, rivaroxaban.** **HERBAL:** **Herbals with anticoagulant/antiplatelet properties (e.g., garlic, ginger, ginkgo biloba)** may increase effect. **FOOD:** None known. **LAB VALUES:** May cause reversible increases in serum creatinine, ALT, AST. May decrease Hgb, Hct, platelet count.

AVAILABILITY (Rx)

Injection, Solution: 2.5 mg/0.5 mL, 5 mg/0.4 mL, 7.5 mg/0.6 mL, 10 mg/0.8 mL.

ADMINISTRATION/HANDLING

SQ

• Parenteral form appears clear, colorless. Discard if discoloration or particulate matter is noted. • Store at room temperature. • Do not expel air bubble from prefilled syringe before injection. • Insert needle subcutaneously into upper arm, outer thigh, or abdomen and inject solution. • Do not inject into areas of active skin disease or injury such as sunburns, rashes, inflammation, skin infections, or active psoriasis. • Rotate injection sites.

INDICATIONS/ROUTES/DOSAGE

◄ALERT► For SQ administration only.

Prevention of Venous Thromboembolism

SQ: ADULTS WEIGHING 50 KG OR MORE: 2.5 mg once daily for 5–9 days after surgery (up to 10 days following abdominal surgery; optimal duration in orthopedic surgery is unknown, but usually given for a minimum of 10-14 days and extended for up to 35 days. Initial dose should be given no earlier than 6–8 hrs after surgery. Initiate dose once hemostasis established. **WEIGHING LESS THAN 50 KG:** Contraindicated.

Treatment of Venous Thromboembolism, Pulmonary Embolism

Note: Start warfarin on first treatment day and continue fondaparinux until INR reaches 2 to 3 for at least 24 hr. Usual duration of fondaparinux: 5–9 days.

SQ: ADULTS, ELDERLY WEIGHING MORE THAN 100 KG: 10 mg once daily. **ADULTS, ELDERLY WEIGHING 50–100 KG:** 7.5 mg once daily. **ADULTS, ELDERLY WEIGHING LESS THAN 50 KG:** 5 mg once daily.

Dosage in Renal Impairment

CrCl greater than 50 mL/min: No dose adjustment. **CrCl 30–50 mL/min:** Use caution (50% dose reduction or use of low-dose heparin). **CrCl less than 30 mL/min:** Contraindicated.

Dosage in Hepatic Impairment

Mild to moderate impairment: No dose adjustment. **Severe impairment:** Use caution.

SIDE EFFECTS

Frequent (19%–11%): Anemia, fever, nausea. **Occasional (10%–4%):** Edema, constipation, rash, vomiting, insomnia, increased wound drainage, hypokalemia. **Rare (less than 4%):** Dizziness, hypotension, confusion, urinary retention, injection site hematoma, diarrhea, dyspepsia, headache.

ADVERSE EFFECTS/TOXIC REACTIONS

Accidental overdose may lead to bleeding complications ranging from local ecchymoses to major hemorrhage. Thrombocytopenia occurs rarely.

NURSING CONSIDERATIONS

BASELINE ASSESSMENT

Assess CBC, renal function test. Evaluate potential risk for bleeding. Question history of recent surgery, trauma, intracranial hemorrhage, GI bleeding. Question medical history as listed in Precautions. Ensure that pt has not received spinal anesthesia, spinal procedures.

INTERVENTION/EVALUATION

Periodically monitor CBC, esp. platelet count, stool for occult blood (no need for daily monitoring in pts with normal presurgical coagulation parameters). Assess for any signs of bleeding: bleeding at surgical site, hematuria, blood in stool, bleeding from gums, petechiae, ecchymosis, bleeding from injection sites. Monitor B/P, pulse; hypotension, tachycardia may indicate bleeding, hypovolemia.

PATIENT/FAMILY TEACHING

• Usual length of therapy is 5–9 days. • Do not take any OTC medication (esp. aspirin, NSAIDs). • Report swelling of hands/feet, unusual back pain, unusual bleeding/bruising, weakness. Treatment may increase risk of bleeding into the brain; report confusion, one-sided weakness, trouble speaking, seizures. Treatment may increase risk of GI bleeding; report bloody stool, vomiting up blood; dark, tarry stools.

F

fosinopril

foe-**sin**-oh-pril

■ BLACK BOX ALERT ■ May cause fetal injury, mortality. Discontinue as soon as possible once pregnancy is detected.

Do not confuse fosinopril with Fosamax or lisinopril, or Monopril with Accupril, minoxidil, moexipril, or ramipril.

◆CLASSIFICATION

PHARMACOTHERAPEUTIC: ACE inhibitor. **CLINICAL:** Antihypertensive.

F

USES

Treatment of hypertension. Adjunctive treatment of HF.

PRECAUTIONS

Contraindications: Hypersensitivity to fosinopril. History of angioedema from previous treatment with ACE inhibitors. Concomitant use with aliskiren in pts with diabetes. **Cautions:** Renal/hepatic impairment, pts with sodium depletion or on diuretic therapy, dialysis, hypovolemia, hypertrophic cardiomyopathy with outflow tract obstruction, hyperkalemia, concomitant use of potassium supplements, unstented unilateral/bilateral renal stenosis, diabetes, severe aortic stenosis. Before, during, or immediately after major surgery.

ACTION

Suppresses renin-angiotensin-aldosterone system (prevents conversion of angiotensin I to angiotensin II, a potent vasoconstrictor; may inhibit angiotensin II at local vascular, renal sites). Decreases plasma angiotensin II, increases plasma renin activity, decreases aldosterone secretion. **Therapeutic Effect:** Reduces B/P.

PHARMACOKINETICS

Route	Onset	Peak	Duration
PO	1 hr	2–6 hrs	24 hrs

Slowly absorbed from GI tract. Protein binding: 97%–98%. Metabolized in liver and GI mucosa. Primarily excreted in urine. Minimal removal by hemodialysis. **Half-life:** 11.5 hrs.

⌛ LIFESPAN CONSIDERATIONS

Pregnancy/Lactation: Crosses placenta. Distributed in breast milk. May cause fetal or neonatal mortality or morbidity. **Children:** Safety and efficacy not established. Neonates, infants may be at increased risk for oliguria, neurologic abnormalities. **Elderly:** May be more sensitive to hypotensive effects.

INTERACTIONS

DRUG: **Potassium-sparing diuretics (e.g., spironolactone), potassium supplements** may cause hyperkalemia. May increase **lithium** concentration/toxicity. **Antacids** may decrease absorption. **Aliskiren** may increase hyperkalemic effect. May increase potential for allergic reactions to **allopurinol. Angiotensin receptor blockers (ARBs)(e.g., losartan, valsartan)** may increase adverse effects. May increase adverse effects of **lithium, sacubitril.** **HERBAL:** **Herbals with hypertensive properties (e.g., licorice, yohimbe) or hypotensive properties (e.g., garlic, ginger, ginkgo biloba)** may alter effects. **FOOD:** None known. **LAB VALUES:** May increase serum BUN, alkaline phosphatase, bilirubin, creatinine, potassium, ALT, AST. May decrease serum sodium. May cause positive antinuclear antibody titer (ANA).

AVAILABILITY (Rx)

Tablets: 10 mg, 20 mg, 40 mg.

ADMINISTRATION/HANDLING

PO

• Give without regard to food. • Tablets may be crushed.

INDICATIONS/ROUTES/DOSAGE

Hypertension

PO: ADULTS, ELDERLY: Initially, 10 mg once daily. **Maintenance:** 10–40 mg once daily. **Maximum:** 80 mg once daily. CHILDREN 6–16 YRS WEIGHING MORE THAN 50 KG: Initially, 5 mg once daily. **Maximum:** 40 mg once daily. WEIGHING 50 KG OR LESS: Initially, 0.1 mg/kg once daily. May increase up to a maximum of 0.6 mg/kg not to exceed 40 mg/day.

HF

PO: ADULTS, ELDERLY: Initially, 10 mg once daily. May increase dose over several wks. **Maintenance:** 20–40 mg once daily. **Maximum:** 40 mg once daily.

Dosage in Renal Impairment

Reduce initial dose to 5 mg in pts with HF.

Dosage in Hepatic Impairment

No dose adjustment.

SIDE EFFECTS

Frequent (12%–9%): Dizziness, cough. **Occasional (4%–2%):** Hypotension, nausea, vomiting, upper respiratory tract infection.

ADVERSE EFFECTS/TOXIC REACTIONS

Excessive hypotension ("first-dose syncope") may occur in pts with HF, severely salt/volume depleted. Angioedema (swelling of face/lips), hyperkalemia occur rarely. Agranulocytosis, neutropenia may be noted in pts with renal impairment, collagen vascular disease (scleroderma, systemic lupus erythematosus). Nephrotic syndrome may be noted in those with history of renal disease.

NURSING CONSIDERATIONS

BASELINE ASSESSMENT

Obtain B/P immediately before each dose. Renal function tests should be performed before beginning therapy. In pts with renal impairment, autoimmune disease, or taking drugs that affect leukocytes or immune response, CBC, differential count should be performed before therapy begins and q2wks for 3 mos, then periodically thereafter. Question medical history as listed in Precautions. Question history of hypersensitivity reaction, angioedema.

INTERVENTION/EVALUATION

Monitor B/P. Assess for urinary frequency. Auscultate lung sounds for rales, wheezing in pts with HF. Monitor renal function tests, CBC, urinalysis for proteinuria. Observe for angioedema (swelling of face, lips, tongue). Monitor serum potassium in those on concurrent diuretic therapy.

PATIENT/FAMILY TEACHING

• Report any sign of infection (sore throat, fever). • Several wks may be needed for full therapeutic effect of B/P reduction. • Skipping doses or voluntarily discontinuing drug may produce severe rebound hypertension. • To reduce hypotensive effect, go from lying to standing slowly. • Immediately report swelling of face, lips, tongue, difficulty breathing, vomiting, excessive perspiration, persistent cough. • Avoid potassium salt substitutes.

fosphenytoin

fos-**fen**-i-toyn
(Cerebyx)
Do not confuse Cerebyx with CeleBREX or CeleXA, or fosphenytoin with fospropofol.

◆CLASSIFICATION

PHARMACOTHERAPEUTIC: Hydantoin. CLINICAL: Anticonvulsant.

USES

Control of generalized tonic-clonic status epilepticus convulsive status epilepticus. Prevention, treatment of seizures occurring during neurosurgery. Short-term substitution for oral phenytoin.

PRECAUTIONS

Contraindications: Hypersensitivity to fosphenytoin, phenytoin, other hydantoins. Adams-Stokes syndrome; second- or third-degree AV block; sinus bradycardia;

SA block; concurrent use of delavirdine. History of hepatotoxicity attributed to fosphenytoin or phenytoin. **Cautions:** Porphyria, diabetes, hypothyroidism, hypotension, severe myocardial insufficiency, renal/hepatic disease, hypoalbuminemia.

ACTION

Stabilizes neuronal membranes, limits spread of seizure activity by increasing efflux or decreasing influx of sodium ions across cell membranes in the motor cortex during nerve impulse generation. **Therapeutic Effect:** Decreases seizure activity.

PHARMACOKINETICS

Completely absorbed after IM administration. Protein binding: 95%–99%. Rapidly and completely hydrolyzed to phenytoin after IM or IV administration. Time of complete conversion to phenytoin: 4 hrs after IM injection; 2 hrs after IV infusion. **Half-life:** 8–15 min (for conversion to phenytoin). (Phenytoin: 12–29 hrs.)

LIFESPAN CONSIDERATIONS

Pregnancy/Lactation: May increase frequency of seizures during pregnancy. Increased risk of congenital malformations. Unknown if excreted in breast milk. **Children:** Safety and efficacy not established. **Elderly:** Lower dosage recommended.

INTERACTIONS

DRUG: **Alcohol, other CNS depressants (e.g., LORazepam, morphine, zolpidem)** may increase CNS depression. May decrease concentration/effect of **apixaban, axitinib, dabigatran, dronedarone, itraconazole, ivabradine, nimodipine, rivaroxaban.** **HERBAL:** **Herbals with sedative properties (e.g., chamomile, kava kava, valerian)** may increase CNS depression. **FOOD:** None known. **LAB VALUES:** May increase serum glucose, GGT, alkaline phosphatase.

AVAILABILITY (Rx)

Injection Solution: 100 mg PE/2 mL, 500 mg PE/10 mL.

ADMINISTRATION/HANDLING

IV

Reconstitution • Dilute in D_5W or 0.9% NaCl to a concentration ranging from 1.5–25 mg PE/mL.

Rate of administration • Administer at rate less than 150 mg PE/min (decreases risk of hypotension, arrhythmias). Children: 2 mg PE/kg/min. **Maximum:** 150 mg PE/min.

Storage • Refrigerate. • Do not store at room temperature for longer than 48 hrs. • After dilution, solution is stable for 8 hrs at room temperature or 24 hrs if refrigerated.

IV INCOMPATIBILITIES

Midazolam (Versed).

IV COMPATIBILITIES

LORazepam (Ativan), PHENobarbital, potassium chloride.

INDICATIONS/ROUTES/DOSAGE

◄ALERT► 150 mg fosphenytoin yields 100 mg phenytoin. Dosage, concentration solution, infusion rate of fosphenytoin are expressed in terms of phenytoin equivalents (PE).

Status Epilepticus

IV: **ADULTS:** **Loading dose:** 20 mg PE/kg infused at rate of 100–150 mg PE/min. May give an additional 5–10 mg PE/kg 10 min after loading dose. **Maximum total loading dose:** 30 mg PE/kg. **Maintenance dose:** Initially, 4–7 mg PE/kg/day (usual daily dose: 300–400 mg PE) given in 2–4 divided doses. **ADOLESCENTS, CHILDREN:** **Loading dose:** 10–15 mg PE/kg at a rate of 1–2 mg PE/kg/min (or 150 mg PE/min, whichever rate is slower). **Maintenance dose:** 2–4 mg PE/kg given 12 hrs after loading dose, then q12h (4–8 mg PE/kg/day in divided doses) at a rate of 1–2 mg PE/kg/min (or 100 mg PE/min, whichever rate is slower).

Short-Term Substitution for Oral Phenytoin

IV, IM: **ADULTS:** May substitute for oral phenytoin at same total daily dose.

Dosage in Renal/Hepatic Impairment
No dose adjustment.

SIDE EFFECTS

Frequent: Dizziness, paresthesia, tinnitus, pruritus, headache, drowsiness. **Occasional:** Morbilliform rash.

ADVERSE EFFECTS/TOXIC REACTIONS

Toxic fosphenytoin serum concentration may produce ataxia (muscular incoordination), nystagmus (rhythmic oscillation of eyes), diplopia, lethargy, slurred speech, nausea, vomiting, hypotension. As drug level increases, extreme lethargy may progress to coma.

NURSING CONSIDERATIONS

BASELINE ASSESSMENT

Review history of seizure disorder (intensity, frequency, duration, LOC). Initiate seizure precautions. Obtain vital signs, medication history (esp. use of phenytoin, other anticonvulsants). Observe clinically.

INTERVENTION/EVALUATION

Monitor ECG, cardiac function, respiratory function, B/P during and immediately following infusion (10–20 min). Discontinue if skin rash appears. Interrupt or decrease rate if hypotension, arrhythmias occur. Monitor free and total Dilantin levels (2 hrs after IV infusion or 4 hrs after IM injection).

PATIENT/FAMILY TEACHING

• If noncompliance is cause of acute seizures, discuss and address reasons for noncompliance. • Avoid tasks that require alertness, motor skills until response to drug is established.

frovatriptan

froe-va-**trip**-tan
(Frova)

◆CLASSIFICATION

PHARMACOTHERAPEUTIC: Serotonin 5-HT_1 receptor agonist. **CLINICAL:** Antimigraine.

USES

Acute treatment of migraine headache with or without aura in adults.

PRECAUTIONS

Contraindications: Hypersensitivity to frovatriptan. Management of basilar or hemiplegic migraine, cerebrovascular or peripheral vascular disease, coronary artery disease, ischemic heart disease (angina pectoris, history of MI, silent ischemia, Prinzmetal's angina), severe hepatic impairment (Child-Pugh Grade C), uncontrolled hypertension, use within 24 hrs of ergotamine-containing preparations or another serotonin receptor agonist. **Cautions:** Mild to moderate hepatic impairment, history of seizures or structural brain lesions.

ACTION

Selective agonist for serotonin in cranial arteries causing vasoconstriction and reduction of inflammation. **Therapeutic Effect:** Relieves migraine headache.

PHARMACOKINETICS

Well absorbed after PO administration. Protein binding: 15%. Metabolized in liver. Eliminated in feces (62%), urine (32%). **Half-life:** 26 hrs (increased in hepatic impairment).

LIFESPAN CONSIDERATIONS

Pregnancy/Lactation: Unknown if excreted in breast milk. **Children:** Safety and efficacy not established. **Elderly:** Not recommended in this population.

INTERACTIONS

DRUG: **Ergotamine-containing medications** may produce vasospastic reaction. May increase adverse effect of **SUMAtriptan.** **Antiemetics** ($\textbf{5-HT}_3$ **antagonists**), **antiparkinson agents (MAOIs)**, **linezolid**, **metOLazone**, **opioid agonists** may increase serotonergic effect. **HERBAL:** None significant. **FOOD:** None known. **LAB VALUES:** None significant.

AVAILABILITY (Rx)

Tablets: 2.5 mg.

ADMINISTRATION/HANDLING

PO

• Give with fluids as soon as symptoms appear. • Do not break, crush, dissolve, or divide film-coated tablets.

INDICATIONS/ROUTES/DOSAGE

Acute Migraine Headache

PO: ADULTS, ELDERLY: Initially, 2.5 mg. If headache improves but then returns, dose may be repeated after at least 2 hrs. **Maximum:** 7.5 mg/day.

Dosage in Renal Impairment

No dose adjustment.

Dosage in Hepatic Impairment

Mild to moderate impairment: No dose adjustment. **Severe impairment:** Use caution.

SIDE EFFECTS

Occasional (8%–4%): Dizziness, paresthesia, fatigue, flushing. **Rare (3%–2%):** Hot/cold sensation, dry mouth, dyspepsia.

ADVERSE EFFECTS/TOXIC REACTIONS

Cardiac reactions (ischemia, coronary artery vasospasm, MI), noncardiac vasospasm-related reactions (cerebral hemorrhage, CVA) occur rarely, particularly in pts with hypertension, obesity, smokers, diabetes, strong family history of coronary artery disease; males older than 40 yrs; postmenopausal women.

NURSING CONSIDERATIONS

BASELINE ASSESSMENT

Question history of peripheral vascular disease, renal/hepatic impairment, possibility of pregnancy, cardiac disease. Question regarding onset, location, duration of migraine, possible precipitating factors.

INTERVENTION/EVALUATION

Assess for relief of migraine headache, potential for photophobia, phonophobia (sound sensitivity), nausea, vomiting.

PATIENT/FAMILY TEACHING

• Take a single dose as soon as symptoms of an actual migraine attack appear. • Medication is intended to relieve migraine headaches, not to prevent or reduce number of attacks. • Avoid tasks that require alertness, motor skills until response to drug is established. • Immediately report palpitations, pain, tightness in chest or throat, sudden or severe abdominal pain, pain or weakness of extremities.

furosemide

HIGH ALERT

fur-**oh**-se-myde
(Apo-Furosemide, Lasix)

■ BLACK BOX ALERT ■ Large doses can lead to profound diuresis with water and electrolyte depletion.

Do not confuse furosemide with famotidine, finasteride, fluconazole, FLUoxetine, loperamide, or torsemide, or Lasix with Lidex, Lovenox, Luvox, or Luxiq.

CLASSIFICATION

PHARMACOTHERAPEUTIC: Loop diuretic. **CLINICAL:** Diuretic. Antihypertensive.

USES

Treatment of edema associated with HF and renal/hepatic disease; acute pulmonary edema.

PRECAUTIONS

Contraindications: Hypersensitivity to furosemide. Anuria. **Cautions:** Hepatic cirrhosis, hepatic coma, severe electrolyte depletion, systemic lupus erythematosus. Pts with prostatic hyperplasia/urinary stricture.

ACTION

Inhibits reabsorption of sodium, chloride in ascending loop of Henle and proximal/distal renal tubules. **Therapeutic Effect:** Increases excretion of water, sodium, chloride, magnesium, calcium.

PHARMACOKINETICS

Route	Onset	Peak	Duration
PO	30–60 min	1–2 hrs	6–8 hrs
IV	5 min	20–60 min	2 hrs
IM	30 min	N/A	N/A

Moderately absorbed from GI tract. Protein binding: greater than 98%. Partially metabolized in liver. Primarily excreted in urine (nonrenal clearance increases in severe renal impairment). Not removed by hemodialysis. **Half-life:** 30–90 min (increased in renal/hepatic impairment, neonates).

LIFESPAN CONSIDERATIONS

Pregnancy/Lactation: Crosses placenta. Distributed in breast milk. **Children:** Half-life increased in neonates; may require increased dosage interval. **Elderly:** May be more sensitive to hypotensive, electrolyte effects, developing circulatory collapse, thromboembolic effect. Age-related renal impairment may require dosage adjustment.

INTERACTIONS

DRUG: **Bile acid sequestrants (e.g., cholestyramine), sucralfate** may decrease absorption/effect. May increase hyponatremic effect of **desmopressin.** May increase QT interval–prolonging effect of **dofetilide. Amphotericin B, nephrotoxic ototoxic medications (e.g., lisinopril, IV contrast dye, vancomycin)** may increase risk of nephrotoxicity, ototoxicity. May increase risk of **lithium** toxicity. **Other medications causing hypokalemia (e.g., HCTZ, laxatives)** may increase risk of hypokalemia. **HERBAL:** **Herbals with hypertensive properties (e.g., licorice, yohimbe) or hypotensive properties (e.g., garlic, ginger, ginkgo biloba)** may alter effects. **FOOD:** None known. **LAB VALUES:** May increase serum glucose, BUN, uric acid. May decrease serum calcium, chloride, magnesium, potassium, sodium.

AVAILABILITY (Rx)

Injection Solution: 10 mg/mL (2 mL, 4 mL, 10 mL). **Oral Solution:** 10 mg/mL, 40 mg/5 mL. **Tablets:** 20 mg, 40 mg, 80 mg.

F

ADMINISTRATION/HANDLING

IV

Rate of administration • May give undiluted but is compatible with D_5W or 0.9% NaCl. • May be diluted for infusion to 1–2 mg/mL (**Maximum:** 10 mg/mL). • Administer each 40 mg or fraction by IV push over 1–2 min. Do not exceed administration rate of 4 mg/min for short-term intermittent infusion.

Storage • Solution appears clear, colorless. • Discard yellow solutions. • Stable for 24 hrs at room temperature when mixed with 0.9% NaCl or D_5W.

IM

• Temporary pain at injection site may be noted.

PO

• Administer on empty stomach. • Give with food to avoid GI upset, preferably with breakfast (may prevent nocturia). • Food may decrease diuretic effect.

IV INCOMPATIBILITIES

Ciprofloxacin (Cipro), dilTIAZem (Cardizem), DOBUTamine (Dobutrex), DOPamine (Intropin), DOXOrubicin (Adriamycin), droperidol (Inapsine), esmolol (Brevibloc), famotidine (Pepcid), filgrastim (Neupogen), fluconazole (Diflucan), gemcitabine (Gemzar), gentamicin (Garamycin), IDArubicin (Idamycin), labetalol (Trandate), metoclopramide (Reglan), midazolam (Versed), milrinone (Primacor), niCARdipine (Cardene), ondansetron (Zofran), quiNIDine, thiopental (Pentothal), vinBLAStine (Velban), vinCRIStine (Oncovin), vinorelbine (Navelbine).

IV COMPATIBILITIES

Amiodarone (Cordarone), bumetanide (Bumex), calcium gluconate, cimetidine (Tagamet), dexmedetomidine (Precedex), heparin, HYDROmorphone (Dilaudid), lidocaine, lipids, morphine, nitroglycerin, norepinephrine (Levophed), potassium chloride, propofol (Diprivan).

F

INDICATIONS/ROUTES/DOSAGE

Edema, HF

PO: ADULTS, ELDERLY: Initially, 20–40 mg once, then titrate as needed. May titrate up to 600 mg/day in severe edematous states. **CHILDREN:** Initially, 0.5–2 mg/kg/dose. May increase by 1–2 mg/kg/dose at 6–8 hr intervals. **Maximum:** 6 mg/kg/day (not to exceed maximum adult dose of 600 mg/day). **NEONATES:** 1 mg/kg/dose 1–2 times/day.

IV: ADULTS, ELDERLY: 20–40 mg once, then titrate as needed. **Maximum single dose:** 200 mg. **CHILDREN:** Initially, 0.5–2 mg/kg/dose. May increase by 1 mg/kg/dose no sooner than 2 hrs after previous dose. **Maximum:** 6 mg/kg/dose. (Not to exceed maximum adult dose of 200 mg/dose.) **NEONATES:** 1–2 mg/kg/dose q12–24h.

IV infusion: ADULTS, ELDERLY: Bolus loading dose of 40–100 mg over 1–2 min, followed by initial infusion rate of 5 mg/hr; repeat loading dose before increasing infusion rate. **Maximum:** 40 mg/hr. **CHILDREN:** Bolus loading dose of 0.1 mg/kg, then initial infusion rate of 0.05–0.4 mg/kg/hr; titrate to desired effect. **NEONATES:** Initially, 0.1–0.2 mg/kg/hr. May increase by 0.1 mg/kg/hr q12–24h. **Maximum:** 0.4 mg/kg/hr.

Dosage in Renal Impairment

Avoid use in oliguric states.

Dosage in Hepatic Impairment

No dose adjustment. Decreased effect, increased sensitivity to hypokalemia/volume depletion in cirrhosis.

SIDE EFFECTS

Expected: Increased urinary frequency/volume. **Frequent:** Nausea, dyspepsia, abdominal cramps, diarrhea or constipation, electrolyte disturbances. **Occasional:** Dizziness, light-headedness, headache, blurred vision, paresthesia, photosensitivity, rash, fatigue, bladder spasm, restlessness, diaphoresis. **Rare:** Flank pain.

ADVERSE EFFECTS/TOXIC REACTIONS

Vigorous diuresis may lead to profound water loss/electrolyte depletion, resulting in hypokalemia, hyponatremia, dehydration. Sudden volume depletion may result in increased risk of thrombosis, circulatory collapse, sudden death. Acute hypotensive episodes may occur, sometimes several days after beginning therapy. Ototoxicity (deafness, vertigo, tinnitus) may occur, esp. in pts with severe renal impairment. Can exacerbate diabetes mellitus, systemic lupus erythematosus, gout, pancreatitis. Blood dyscrasias have been reported.

NURSING CONSIDERATIONS

BASELINE ASSESSMENT

Check vital signs, esp. B/P, pulse, for hypotension before administration. Assess baseline renal function, serum electrolytes, esp. serum sodium, potassium. Assess skin turgor, mucous membranes for hydration status; observe for edema. Obtain baseline weight. Initiate I&O monitoring. Auscultate lung sounds. In pts with hepatic cirrhosis and ascites, consider giving initial doses in a hospital setting.

INTERVENTION/EVALUATION

Monitor B/P, vital signs, serum electrolytes, I&O, weight. Note extent of diuresis. Watch for symptoms of electrolyte imbalance: Hypokalemia may result in changes in muscle strength, tremor, muscle cramps, altered mental status, cardiac arrhythmias; hyponatremia may result in confusion, thirst, cold/clammy skin. Consider potassium supplementation if hypokalemia occurs.

PATIENT/FAMILY TEACHING

• Expect increased frequency, volume of urination. • Report palpitations, signs of electrolyte imbalances (noted previously), hearing abnormalities (sense of fullness in ears, tinnitus). • Eat foods high in potassium such as whole grains (cereals), legumes, meat, bananas, apricots, orange juice, potatoes (white, sweet), raisins. • Avoid sunlight, sunlamps.

F

gabapentin

ga-ba-**pen**-tin
(Gralise, Horizant, Neurontin)
Do not confuse Neurontin with Motrin, Neoral, nitrofurantoin, Noroxin, or Zarontin.

◆CLASSIFICATION

PHARMACOTHERAPEUTIC: Gamma-aminobutyric acid analogue. **CLINICAL:** Anticonvulsant, antineuralgic.

G

USES

Neurontin: Adjunct in treatment of partial seizures (with or without secondary generalized seizures) in children 3 yrs and older and adults. Management of postherpetic neuralgia (PHN). **Horizant:** Treatment of moderate to severe primary restless legs syndrome (RLS), PHN. **Gralise:** Management of PHN. **OFF-LABEL:** Treatment of neuropathic pain, diabetic peripheral neuropathy, vasomotor symptoms, fibromyalgia, postoperative pain adjunct.

PRECAUTIONS

Contraindications: Hypersensitivity to gabapentin. **Cautions:** Severe renal impairment, elderly, history of suicidal behavior; substance abuse.

ACTION

Binds to gabapentin binding sites in brain and may modulate release of excitatory neurotransmitters, which participates in epileptogenesis and nociception. **Therapeutic Effect:** Reduces seizure activity, neuropathic pain.

PHARMACOKINETICS

Well absorbed from GI tract (not affected by food). Protein binding: less than 5%. Widely distributed. Crosses blood-brain barrier. Primarily excreted unchanged in urine. Removed by hemodialysis. **Half-life:** 5–7 hrs (increased in renal impairment, elderly).

⌛ LIFESPAN CONSIDERATIONS

Pregnancy/Lactation: Crosses placenta, excreted in breast milk. **Children:** Safety and efficacy not established in pts 3 yrs and younger. **Elderly:** Age-related renal impairment may require dosage adjustment.

INTERACTIONS

DRUG: **CNS depressants (e.g., alcohol, morphine, tapentadol, zolpidem)** may increase CNS depression. **HERBAL:** **Herbals with sedative properties (e.g., chamomile, kava kava, valerian)** may increase CNS depression. **FOOD:** None known. **LAB VALUES:** May alter serum glucose; WBC count. May increase serum alkaline phosphatase, ALT, AST, bilirubin.

AVAILABILITY (Rx)

Capsules: 100 mg, 300 mg, 400 mg. **Oral Solution:** 250 mg/5 mL. **Tablets:** 600 mg, 800 mg. **Tablets:** ***(Gralise):*** 300 mg, 600 mg.

Tablets: ***(Extended-Release [Horizant]):*** 300 mg, 600 mg.

ADMINISTRATION/HANDLING

PO

Immediate-release/solution • Give without regard to meals; may give with food to avoid, reduce GI upset. • Swallow extended-release tablets whole; do not break, crush, dissolve, or divide. Take with evening meal.

INDICATIONS/ROUTES/DOSAGE

Note: When given 3 times/day, maximum time between doses should not exceed 12 hrs. If treatment is discontinued or anticonvulsant therapy is added, do so gradually over at least 1 wk (reduces risk of loss of seizure control).

Adjunctive Therapy for Seizure Control

PO: ADULTS, ELDERLY, CHILDREN 13 YRS AND OLDER: Initially, 300 mg 3 times/day. May titrate dosage. Range: 900–1,800 mg/day in 3 divided doses. **Maximum:** 3,600 mg/day. **CHILDREN 3–12 YRS:** Initially, 10–15 mg/kg/day in 3 divided doses. May titrate up to 25–35 mg/kg/day (for children

5–12 yrs) and 40 mg/kg/day (for children 3–4 yrs). **Maximum:** 50 mg/kg/day.

Adjunctive Therapy for Neuropathic Pain
PO: ADULTS, ELDERLY: ***(Immediate-Release):*** Initially, 100–300 mg 1–3 times/day. May increase up to 1,200 mg 3 times/day. ***(Extended-Release):*** Initially, 300 mg at bedtime. May increase up to target dose of 900–3,600 mg once daily.

Postherpetic Neuralgia
PO: ADULTS, ELDERLY: ***(Neurontin):*** 300 mg once on day 1, 300 mg twice daily on day 2, and 300 mg 3 times/day on day 3 as needed. Range: 1,800–3,600 mg/day. ***(Gralise):*** 300 mg once on day 1; 600 mg once on day 2; 900 mg once daily on days 3–6; 1,200 mg once daily on days 7–10; 1,500 mg once daily on days 11–14; then 1,800 mg once daily. ***(Horizant):*** 600 mg once daily in AM for 3 days, then increase to 600 mg twice daily.

RLS
PO: ADULTS, ELDERLY: ***(Horizant):*** 600 mg once daily at about 5 PM.

Dosage in Renal Impairment
Dosage and frequency are modified based on creatinine clearance.

Dosage in Hepatic Impairment
No dose adjustment.

SIDE EFFECTS

Frequent (19%–10%): Fatigue, drowsiness, dizziness, ataxia. **Occasional (8%–3%):** Nystagmus, tremor, diplopia, rhinitis, weight gain, peripheral edema. **Rare (less than 2%):** Anxiety, dysarthria, memory loss, dyspepsia, pharyngitis, myalgia.

ADVERSE EFFECTS/TOXIC REACTIONS

Abrupt withdrawal may increase seizure frequency, increase risk of suicidal behavior/thoughts. Overdosage may result in slurred speech, drowsiness, lethargy, diarrhea. Drug reaction with eosinophilia and systemic symptoms (multiorgan hypersensitivity) was reported. Hypersensitivity reaction, including anaphylaxis and angioedema, can occur at any time.

NURSING CONSIDERATIONS

BASELINE ASSESSMENT

Review history of seizure disorder (type, onset, intensity, frequency, duration, LOC). Assess location, intensity of neuralgia/neuropathic pain. Question history of renal impairment.

INTERVENTION/EVALUATION

Provide safety measures as needed. Monitor seizure frequency/duration, renal function, weight, behavior in children. Monitor for signs/symptoms of depression, suicidal tendencies, other unusual behavior; hypersensitivity reaction.

PATIENT/FAMILY TEACHING

• Use only as prescribed; do not abruptly stop taking drug (may increase seizure frequency). • Avoid tasks that require alertness, motor skills until response to drug is established. • Avoid alcohol. • Report suicidal ideation, depression, unusual behavioral changes (esp. with

Creatinine Clearance	Neurontin Dosage (Immediate-Release)	Gralise Dosage (Extended-Release)	Horizant Dosage	
			RLS	PHN
30–59 mL/min	200–700 mg q12h	600–1,800 mg once/day	300–600 mg/day	Same
16–29 mL/min	200–700 mg once daily	Not recommended	300 mg/day	Same
Less than 16 mL/min	100–300 mg once daily	Not recommended	300 mg q48h	Same
Hemodialysis	125–350 mg following HD	Not recommended	Not recommended	300–600 mg following HD

changes in dosage), worsening of seizure activity or loss of seizure control. • Seek medical attention for allergic reactions including difficulty breathing, coughing, wheezing, throat tightness, swelling of face or tongue.

galantamine

gal-**an**-ta-meen
(Razadyne, Razadyne ER)
Do not confuse Razadyne with Rozerem.

G

CLASSIFICATION

PHARMACOTHERAPEUTIC: Acetylcholinesterase inhibitor (central). **CLINICAL:** Antidementia.

USES

Treatment of mild to moderate dementia of Alzheimer's type. **OFF-LABEL:** Diabetic neuropathy, neuropathic pain, postoperative pain (adjunct), hot flashes.

PRECAUTIONS

Contraindications: Hypersensitivity to galantamine. **Cautions:** Moderate renal/hepatic impairment (not recommended in severe impairment), history of ulcer disease, asthma, COPD, bladder outflow obstruction, supraventricular cardiac conduction conditions (except with pacemaker), seizure disorder, concurrent medications that slow cardiac conduction through SA or AV node. Elderly with low body weight and/or serious co-morbidities.

ACTION

Elevates acetylcholine concentrations in cerebral cortex by slowing degeneration of acetylcholine released by still intact cholinergic neurons. May increase serotonin/glutamate levels. **Therapeutic Effect:** Slows progression of Alzheimer's disease.

PHARMACOKINETICS

Rapidly, completely absorbed from GI tract. Protein binding: 18%. Distributed to blood cells; binds to plasma proteins, mainly albumin. Metabolized in liver. Excreted in urine. **Half-life:** 7 hrs.

LIFESPAN CONSIDERATIONS

Pregnancy/Lactation: Unknown if crosses placenta or is distributed in breast milk. **Children:** Not prescribed for this pt population. **Elderly:** No age-related precautions noted, but use is not recommended in pts with severe hepatic/renal impairment (CrCl less than 9 mL/min).

INTERACTIONS

DRUG: Anticholinergic agents (e.g., hyoscyamine, glycopyrrolate) may decrease levels/effects. **Strong CYP3A4 inhibitors (e.g., clarithromycin, ketoconazole, ritonavir)** may increase concentration/effect. May increase bradycardiac effect of **beta blockers (e.g., carvedilol, metoprolol).**
HERBAL: None significant. **FOOD:** None known. **LAB VALUES:** None significant.

AVAILABILITY (Rx)

Oral Solution: 4 mg/mL. **Tablets:** ***(Razadyne):*** 4 mg, 8 mg, 12 mg.
Capsules: ***(Extended-Release [Razadyne ER]):*** 8 mg, 16 mg, 24 mg.

ADMINISTRATION/HANDLING

PO

• Give tablet or solution with morning and evening meals. • Mix oral solution with nonalcoholic beverage, take immediately. • Extended-release capsule should be given with breakfast. Swallow whole. Do not break, crush, cut, or divide.

INDICATIONS/ROUTES/DOSAGE

Note: If therapy interrupted for 3 or more days, restart at lowest dose; then increase gradually.

Alzheimer's Disease

PO: ***(Immediate-Release Tablets, Oral Solution):*** **ADULTS, ELDERLY:** Initially, 4 mg twice daily (8 mg/day). After a minimum of 4 wks (if well tolerated), may increase to 8 mg twice daily (16 mg/day). After another 4 wks, may increase to 12 mg twice daily (24 mg/day). Range: 16–24 mg/day in 2 divided doses.

PO: ***(Extended-Release):*** **ADULTS, ELDERLY:** Initially, 8 mg once daily for 4 wks; then increase to 16 mg once daily for 4 wks or longer. If tolerated, may increase to 24 mg once daily. Range: 16–24 mg once daily.

Dosage in Renal/Hepatic Impairment

Moderate impairment: Maximum dosage is 16 mg/day. **Severe impairment:** Not recommended.

SIDE EFFECTS

Frequent (17%–7%): Nausea, vomiting, diarrhea, anorexia, weight loss. **Occasional (5%–4%):** Abdominal pain, insomnia, depression, headache, dizziness, fatigue, rhinitis. **Rare (less than 3%):** Tremors, constipation, confusion, cough, anxiety, urinary incontinence.

ADVERSE EFFECTS/TOXIC REACTIONS

Overdose may cause cholinergic crisis (increased salivation, lacrimation, urination, defecation, bradycardia, hypotension, muscle weakness). Treatment aimed at generally supportive measures, use of anticholinergics (e.g., atropine). Toxic skin reactions including Stevens-Johnson syndrome, acute generalized exanthematous pustulosis, erythema multiforme were reported. Vagotonic effects may cause bradycardia, heart block.

NURSING CONSIDERATIONS

BASELINE ASSESSMENT

Assess cognitive, behavioral, functional deficits of pt. Obtain baseline serum renal function, LFT. Question history as listed in Precautions, esp. cardiac conduction disorders.

INTERVENTION/EVALUATION

Monitor cognitive, behavioral, functional status of pt. Evaluate ECG, periodic rhythm strips in pts with underlying arrhythmias. Assess for evidence of GI disturbances (nausea, vomiting, diarrhea, anorexia, weight loss). Monitor for toxic skin reactions; cardiac effects (bradycardia).

PATIENT/FAMILY TEACHING

• Take with meals (reduces risk of nausea). • Avoid tasks that require alertness, motor skills until response to drug is established. • Report persistent GI disturbances, excessive salivation, diaphoresis, excessive tearing, excessive fatigue, insomnia, depression, dizziness, increased muscle weakness, palpitations.

ganciclovir

gan-**sye**-kloe-veer
(Cytovene)

■ **BLACK BOX ALERT** ■ Toxicity presents as neutropenia, thrombocytopenia, anemia. Studies suggest carcinogenic and teratogenic effects, inhibition of spermatogenesis. May cause birth defects.

Do not confuse Cytovene with Cytosar, or ganciclovir with famciclovir or acyclovir.

◆CLASSIFICATION

PHARMACOTHERAPEUTIC: Synthetic nucleoside. **CLINICAL:** Antiviral.

USES

Treatment of cytomegalovirus (CMV) retinitis in immunocompromised pts (e.g., HIV), prophylaxis of CMV infection in transplant pts. **OFF-LABEL:** CMV retinitis.

PRECAUTIONS

Contraindications: Hypersensitivity to acyclovir, ganciclovir, valganciclovir. **Cautions:** Neutropenia, thrombocytopenia, renal impairment, children (long-term safety not determined due to potential for long-term carcinogenic, adverse reproductive effects), pregnancy. Absolute neutrophil count less than 500 cells/mm^3, platelet count less than 25,000 cells/mm^3.

ACTION

Competes with viral DNA polymerase and incorporation into growing viral DNA chains. **Therapeutic Effect:** Interferes with DNA synthesis, viral replication.

PHARMACOKINETICS

Widely distributed (including CSF and ocular tissue). Protein binding: 1%–2%. Excreted primarily in urine. Removed by hemodialysis. **Half-life:** 1.7–5.8 hrs (increased in renal impairment).

LIFESPAN CONSIDERATIONS

Pregnancy/Lactation: Avoid pregnancy. Females of reproductive potential should use effective contraception during treatment and for 30 days after discontinuation; male pts should use a barrier contraceptive during and for at least 90 days after discontinuation. Do not breastfeed. May resume breastfeeding no sooner than 72 hrs after the last dose. **Children:** Safety and efficacy not established in pts younger than 12 yrs. **Elderly:** Age-related renal impairment may require dosage adjustment.

INTERACTIONS

DRUG: **Bone marrow depressants** may increase myelosuppression. **Imipenem** may increase risk for seizures. **HERBAL:** None significant. **FOOD:** None known. **LAB VALUES:** May increase serum alkaline phosphatase, ALT, AST, bilirubin, BUN, creatinine.

AVAILABILITY (Rx)

Injection, Powder for Reconstitution: ***(Cytovene):*** 500 mg. **Solution, Intravenous:** 500 mg/250 mL, 50 mg/mL (10 mL).

ADMINISTRATION/HANDLING

IV

Reconstitution • Reconstitute 500-mg vial with 10 mL Sterile Water for Injection to provide concentration of 50 mg/mL; do **not** use Bacteriostatic Water (contains parabens, which are incompatible with ganciclovir). • Further dilute with 100 mL D_5W, 0.9% NaCl to provide a concentration of 10 mg/mL or less for infusion.

Rate of administration • Administer only by IV infusion over at least 1 hr. • Do not give by IV push or rapid IV infusion (increases risk of toxicity). Flush line with 0.9% NaCl before and after administration.

Storage • Store vials at room temperature. Do not refrigerate. • Reconstituted solution in vial is stable for 12 hrs at room temperature. • After dilution, use within 24 hrs. • Discard if precipitate forms, discoloration occurs. • Avoid exposure to skin, eyes, mucous membranes. • Use latex gloves, safety glasses during preparation/handling of solution. • Avoid inhalation. • If solution contacts skin or mucous membranes, wash thoroughly with soap and water; rinse eyes thoroughly with plain water.

IV INCOMPATIBILITIES

Aldesleukin (Proleukin), amifostine (Ethyol), aztreonam (Azactam), cefepime (Maxipime), cytarabine (ARA-C), DOXOrubicin (Adriamycin), fludarabine (Fludara), foscarnet (Foscavir), gemcitabine (Gemzar), ondansetron (Zofran), piperacillin and tazobactam (Zosyn), sargramostim (Leukine), vinorelbine (Navelbine).

IV COMPATIBILITIES

Amphotericin B, enalapril (Vasotec), filgrastim (Neupogen), fluconazole (Diflucan), granisetron (Kytril), propofol (Diprivan).

INDICATIONS/ROUTES/DOSAGE

Cytomegalovirus (CMV) Retinitis

IV: ADULTS, CHILDREN 3 MOS AND OLDER: 5 mg/kg/dose q12h for 14–21 days, then 5 mg/kg/day as a single daily dose or 6 mg/kg 5 days/wk as maintenance therapy.

Prevention of CMV in Transplant Pts

IV: ADULTS, CHILDREN: 5 mg/kg/dose q12h for 7–14 days, then 5 mg/kg/day as a single daily dose or 6 mg/kg 5 days/wk. Duration dependent on clinical condition and degree of immunosuppression.

Congenital CMV

IV: NEONATES: 6 mg/kg/dose q12h for 6 wks (if HIV positive, longer duration may be considered).

Dosage in Renal Impairment

Dosage and frequency are modified based on creatinine clearance (see table).

Creatinine Clearance	Dosage	
	IV Induction	IV Maintenance
50–69 mL/min	2.5 mg/kg q12h	2.5 mg/kg q24h
25–49 mL/min	2.5 mg/kg q24h	1.25 mg/kg q24h
10–24 mL/min	1.25 mg/kg q24h	0.625 mg/kg q24h
Less than 10 mL/min	1.25 mg/kg 3 times/wk	0.625 mg/kg 3 times/wk
Hemodialysis (give after HD on HD days)	1.25 mg/kg q48–72h	0.625 mg/kg q48–72h
Peritoneal dialysis	1.25 mg/kg 3 times/wk	0.625 mg/kg 3 times/wk
Continuous renal replacement therapy		
Continuous venovenous hemofiltration	2.5 mg/kg q24h	1.25 mg/kg q24h
Continuous venovenous hemodialysis/continuous venovenous hemodiafiltration	2.5 mg/kg q12h	2.5 mg/kg q24h

Dosage in Hepatic Impairment
No dose adjustment.

SIDE EFFECTS

Frequent (41%–13%): Diarrhea, fever, nausea, abdominal pain, vomiting. **Occasional (11%–6%):** Diaphoresis, infection, paresthesia, flatulence, pruritus. **Rare (4%–2%):** Headache, stomatitis, dyspepsia, phlebitis.

ADVERSE EFFECTS/TOXIC REACTIONS

Hematologic toxicity occurs commonly: leukopenia (41%–29% of pts), anemia (25%–19% of pts). Intraocular implant occasionally results in visual acuity loss, vitreous hemorrhage, retinal detachment. GI hemorrhage occurs rarely.

NURSING CONSIDERATIONS

BASELINE ASSESSMENT

Obtain CBC, BMP, LFT in critically ill pts. Perform baseline ophthalmic exam. Obtain specimens for support of differential diagnosis (urine, feces, blood, throat) since retinal infection is usually due to hematogenous dissemination.

INTERVENTION/EVALUATION

Monitor I&O, ensure adequate hydration (minimum 1,500 mL/24 hrs). Diligently evaluate hematology reports for neutropenia, thrombocytopenia, leukopenia. Obtain periodic ophthalmic examinations. Question pt regarding visual acuity, therapeutic improvement, complications. Assess for rash, pruritus.

PATIENT/FAMILY TEACHING

• Ganciclovir provides suppression, not cure, of cytomegalovirus (CMV) retinitis. • Frequent blood tests, eye exams are necessary during therapy due to toxic nature of drug. • May temporarily or permanently inhibit sperm production in men, suppress fertility in women. • Barrier contraception should be used during and for 90 days after therapy due to mutagenic potential.

gefitinib

ge-fi-ti-nib
(Iressa)
Do not confuse gefitinib with erlotinib, dasatinib, imatinib, or lapatinib.

◆CLASSIFICATION

PHARMACOTHERAPEUTIC: Epidermal growth factor receptor (EGFR) inhibitor. Tyrosine kinase inhibitor. **CLINICAL:** Antineoplastic.

USES

First-line treatment of metastatic non–small-cell lung cancer (NSCLC) whose tumors have epidermal growth factor receptor (EGFR) exon 19 deletions or exon 21 substitution mutations.

PRECAUTIONS

Contraindications: Hypersensitivity to gefitinib. **Cautions:** Hepatic impairment, lung disease, ocular disease, concurrent administration of CYP3A4 inducers and inhibitors.

G

ACTION

Reversibly inhibits epidermal growth factor receptor–tyrosine kinase (EGFR-TK), a key driver in tumor cell growth. EGFR is expressed on cell surfaces of cancer cells. **Therapeutic Effect:** Inhibits tumor cell proliferation and survival.

PHARMACOKINETICS

Slowly absorbed following PO administration. Peak plasma levels in 3–7 hrs. Protein binding: 90%. Metabolized in liver. Excreted primarily in feces (86%). **Half-life:** 48 hrs.

LIFESPAN CONSIDERATIONS

Pregnancy/Lactation: Avoid pregnancy. Use effective contraception during treatment and for at least 2 wks after discontinuation. Unknown if crosses placenta or distributed in breast milk. Must either discontinue breastfeeding or discontinue therapy. **Children:** Safety and efficacy not established. **Elderly:** No age-related precautions noted.

INTERACTIONS

DRUG: **CYP3A4 inhibitors (e.g., clarithromycin, ketoconazole, ritonavir)** may increase concentration. **CYP3A4 inducers (e.g., carBAMazepine, phenytoin, rifAMPin)** may decrease concentration. **H_2 antagonists (e.g., famotidine), proton pump inhibitors (e.g., pantoprazole)** may decrease concentration. May increase bleeding risk with **warfarin. Antacids** may decrease concentration/effect. **HERBAL:** **St. John's wort** may decrease concentration/effect. **FOOD:** Avoid grapefruit products. **LAB VALUES:** May increase serum AST, ALT, bilirubin, urine protein.

AVAILABILITY (Rx)

Tablets: 250 mg.

ADMINISTRATION/HANDLING

• May give without regard to food. • Avoid grapefruit products. • Do not crush or cut. Swallow whole or administer as dispersion in water. Gently swirl glass for up to 20 min and immediately ingest once dispersed.

INDICATIONS/ROUTES/DOSAGE

NSCLC

PO: ADULTS, ELDERLY: 250 mg once daily, with or without food. Continue until disease progression or unacceptable toxicity.

Concomitant Use of CYP3A4 Inducers

Consider increasing dose to 500 mg once daily if use of CYP3A4 is unavoidable. If CYP3A4 inducer is discontinued, reduce dose to 250 mg 7 days after discontinuation.

Dosage in Renal Impairment

No dose adjustment.

Dosage in Hepatic Impairment

Mild impairment: No dose adjustment. **Moderate to severe impairment:** Use with caution.

SIDE EFFECTS

Frequent (47%–15%): Skin reactions (e.g., acne, pruritus, rash, xeroderma), diarrhea, decreased appetite, vomiting. **Occasional (7%–5%):** Stomatitis, conjunctivitis, blepharitis, dry eye, nail disorders (e.g., infection).

ADVERSE EFFECTS/TOXIC REACTIONS

Hepatotoxicity, interstitial lung disease, gastrointestinal perforation, severe or persistent diarrhea, ocular disorders including keratitis, bullous and exfoliative skin disorders.

NURSING CONSIDERATIONS

BASELINE ASSESSMENT

Obtain CBC with differential, serum chemistries, LFT, thyroid function test, PT/INT (if taking warfarin), EGFR mutation serostatus. Question possibility of pregnancy or plans of breastfeeding. Receive full medication history including vitamins, minerals, herbal products. Assess visual acuity.

INTERVENTION/EVALUATION

Assess vital signs, oxygen saturation routinely. Routinely monitor CBC with differential, LFT. Worsening cough, fever, or shortness of breath may indicate interstitial lung disease. Consider ophthalmologic evaluation for vision changes. Monitor for bruising, hematuria, jaundice, right upper abdominal pain, weight loss, or acute infection (fever, diaphoresis, lethargy, productive cough). Monitor for skin lesions.

PATIENT/FAMILY TEACHING

• Report urine changes, bloody or clay-colored stools, upper abdominal pain, nausea, vomiting, bruising, fever, cough, difficulty breathing. • Immediately report any newly prescribed medications, suspected pregnancy, vision changes (eye pain, bleeding, sensitivity to light), or persistent diarrhea, dehydration. • Avoid alcohol. • Avoid grapefruit products.

gemcitabine HIGH ALERT

jem-**sye**-ta-been

Do not confuse gemcitabine with gemtuzumab.

◆CLASSIFICATION

PHARMACOTHERAPEUTIC: Antimetabolite. **CLINICAL:** Antineoplastic.

USES

Metastatic breast cancer in combination with PACLitaxel. Treatment of locally advanced (stage II, III) or metastatic (stage IV) adenocarcinoma of pancreas. In combination with CISplatin for treatment of locally advanced or metastatic non–small-cell lung cancer (NSCLC). Treatment of advanced ovarian cancer (in combination with CARBOplatin) that has relapsed. **OFF-LABEL:** Treatment of biliary tract carcinoma, bladder carcinoma, germ cell tumors (e.g., testicular), Hodgkin's lymphoma, non-Hodgkin's lymphoma, cervical cancer.

PRECAUTIONS

Contraindications: Hypersensitivity to gemcitabine. **Cautions:** Renal/hepatic impairment, baseline cytopenias, elderly, concurrent radiation therapy, impaired pulmonary function.

ACTION

Inhibits ribonucleotide reductase, the enzyme necessary for catalyzing DNA synthesis. Cell-cycle specific for the S-phase. **Therapeutic Effect:** Produces death of cells undergoing DNA synthesis.

PHARMACOKINETICS

Not extensively distributed after IV infusion (increased with length of infusion). Protein binding: less than 10%. Metabolized intracellularly by nucleoside kinases. Excreted primarily in urine. **Half-life:** Influenced by duration of infusion. Infusion 1 hr or less: 42–94 min; infusion 3–4 hrs: 4–10.5 hrs.

⧖ LIFESPAN CONSIDERATIONS

Pregnancy/Lactation: Avoid pregnancy; may cause fetal harm. Females of reproductive potential must use effective contraception during treatment and for at least 6 mos after discontinuation. Breastfeeding not recommended during treatment and for at least 1 wk after discontinuation. **Males:** Males with female partners of reproductive potential must use effective contraception during treatment and for at least 3 mos after last dose. May impair fertility. **Children:** Safety and efficacy not established. **Elderly:** Increased risk of hematologic toxicity.

INTERACTIONS

DRUG: Bone marrow depressants (e.g., cladribine) may increase risk of myelosuppression. **Live virus vaccines** may potentiate virus replication, increase vaccine side effects, decrease pt's antibody response to vaccine. **HERBAL: Echinacea** may decrease therapeutic effect. **FOOD:** None known. **LAB VALUES:** May increase serum BUN, alkaline phosphatase, bilirubin, creatinine, ALT, AST. May decrease Hgb, Hct, leukocyte count, platelet count.

AVAILABILITY (Rx)

Injection, Powder for Reconstitution: 200-mg, 1-g, 2-g vials. **Injection, Solution:** 38 mg/mL, 100 mg/mL.

ADMINISTRATION/HANDLING

IV

Reconstitution • Use gloves when handling/preparing. • Reconstitute with 0.9% NaCl injection without preservative to provide concentration of 38 mg/mL. • Shake to dissolve. Further diluted with 50–500 mL 0.9% NaCl to a concentration as low as 0.1 mg/mL.

Rate of administration • Infuse over 30 min. • Infusion time greater than 60 min increases toxicity.

Storage • Store at room temperature (refrigeration may cause crystallization). • Reconstituted vials or diluted solutions are stable for 24 hrs at room temperature. Do not refrigerate.

IV INCOMPATIBILITIES

Acyclovir (Zovirax), amphotericin B (Fungizone), cefotaxime (Claforan), furosemide (Lasix), ganciclovir (Cytovene), imipenem/cilastatin (Primaxin), irinotecan (Camptosar), methotrexate, methylPREDNISolone (SOLU-Medrol), mitoMYcin (Mutamycin), piperacillin/tazobactam (Zosyn), prochlorperazine (Compazine).

IV COMPATIBILITIES

Bumetanide (Bumex), calcium gluconate, dexamethasone (Decadron), diphenhydrAMINE (Benadryl), DOBUTamine (Dobutrex), DOPamine (Intropin), granisetron (Kytril), heparin, hydrocortisone (Solu-CORTEF), LORazepam (Ativan), ondansetron (Zofran), potassium chloride.

INDICATIONS/ROUTES/DOSAGE

◄ALERT► Dosage is individualized based on clinical response, tolerance to adverse effects. When used in combination therapy, consult specific protocols for optimum dosage, sequence of drug administration. See manufacturer guidelines regarding dose modifications.

Breast Cancer (Metastatic)

IV: ADULTS, ELDERLY: (in combination with PACLitaxel): 1,250 mg/m^2 over 30 min on days 1 and 8 of each 21-day cycle.

Non–Small-Cell Lung Cancer (NSCLC) (Inoperable, locally advanced, or metastatic)

IV: ADULTS, ELDERLY, CHILDREN: (in combination with CISplatin): 1,000 mg/m^2 on days 1, 8, and 15, repeated every 28 days; or 1,250 mg/m^2 on days 1 and 8. Repeat every 21 days.

Ovarian Cancer (Advanced)

IV: ADULTS, ELDERLY: (in combination with CARBOplatin): 1,000 mg/m^2 on days 1 and 8 of each 21-day cycle.

Pancreatic Cancer (Locally advanced or metastatic)

IV: ADULTS: 1,000 mg/m^2 once wkly for up to 7 wks (or until toxicity necessitates decreasing dosage or withholding the dose), followed by 1 wk of rest. Subsequent cycles should consist of once-wkly dose for 3 consecutive wks out of every 4 wks (days 1, 8,15 q28days).

Dosage in Renal/Hepatic Impairment

No dose adjustment.

Dosage Reduction

Pancreatic Cancer, Non–Small-Cell Lung Cancer

Dosage adjustments should be based on granulocyte count and platelet count, as follows:

Absolute Granulocyte Counts (cells/mm^3)	Platelet Count (cells/mm^3)	% of Full Dose
1,000	100,000	100
500–999	50,000–99,000	75
Less than 500 or	Less than 50,000	Hold

Breast Cancer Absolute Granulocyte Counts (cells/mm³)	Platelet Count (cells/mm³)	% of Full Dose
Equal to or greater than 1,200 and	Greater than 75,000	100
1,000–1,199 or	50,000–75,000	75
700–999 and	Equal to or greater than 50,000	50
Less than 700 or	Less than 50,000	Hold

Ovarian Cancer Absolute Granulocyte Counts (cells/mm³)	Platelet Count (cells/mm³)	% of Full Dose
1,500 or greater and	100,000 or greater	100
1,000–1,499 and/or	75,000–99,999	50
Less than 1,000 and/or	Less than 75,000	Hold

SIDE EFFECTS

Frequent (69%–20%): Nausea, vomiting, generalized pain, fever, mild to moderate pruritic rash, mild to moderate dyspnea, constipation, peripheral edema. **Occasional (19%–10%):** Diarrhea, petechiae, alopecia, stomatitis, infection, drowsiness, paresthesia. **Rare:** Diaphoresis, rhinitis, insomnia, malaise.

ADVERSE EFFECTS/TOXIC REACTIONS

Myelosuppression (anemia, neutropenia, thrombocytopenia) is an expected response to therapy. Severe, life-threatening toxicity may occur when given during or within 7 days of radiation therapy. Prolongation of infusion time beyond 60 min or doses given more frequently than every wk may increase risk of asthenia, hypotension, severe flu-like symptoms. Pulmonary toxicity including pneumonitis, pulmonary fibrosis, pulmonary edema, acute respiratory distress syndrome (ARDS) was reported. Life-threatening hemolytic uremic syndrome may lead to renal failure, dialysis, and death. Drug-induced hepatic injury, including hepatic failure and death, has occurred. Posterior reversible encephalopathy syndrome, a dysfunction of the brain caused by swelling, may evolve into an ischemic CVA or cerebral hemorrhage. May cause capillary leak syndrome.

NURSING CONSIDERATIONS

BASELINE ASSESSMENT

Obtain CBC, BMP, LFT; pregnancy test in females of reproductive potential. Confirm compliance of effective contraception. Screen for active infection. Drug should be suspended or dosage modified if myelosuppression is detected. Question history of pulmonary disease, hepatic/renal impairment. Offer emotional support.

INTERVENTION/EVALUATION

Monitor CBC with differential prior to each dose; LFT, renal function periodically. An increase of serum creatinine greater than 0.4 mg/dL from baseline may indicate renal impairment. Monitor pulmonary status, pulse oximeter readings. Consider ABG, radiologic test if ILD/pneumonitis (excessive cough, dyspnea, fever, hypoxia) is suspected. Consider treatment with corticosteroids if ILD/pneumonitis is confirmed. Monitor for infections (cough, fatigue, fever). If serious infection occurs, initiate appropriate antimicrobial therapy. Monitor daily pattern of bowel activity, stool consistency. Assess skin for rash. RPLS should be considered in pts with altered mental status, confusion, headache, seizures, visual disturbances.

PATIENT/FAMILY TEACHING

• Treatment may depress your immune system response and reduce your ability to fight infection. Report symptoms of infection such as body aches, chills, cough, fatigue, fever. Avoid those with active infection. • Report symptoms of lung inflammation (excessive coughing, difficulty breathing, chest pain); liver problems (abdominal pain, bruising, clay-colored stool, amber- or dark-colored urine, yellowing of the skin or eyes), kidney problems (decreased urine output, flank pain, darkened urine). • Therapy may cause kidney failure, requiring treatment with dialysis. • Nervous system changes including confusion, headache, seizures may indicate life-threatening brain dysfunction/swelling. • Use effective contraception to avoid pregnancy. Do not breastfeed.

gemfibrozil

jem-**fye**-broe-zil
(Lopid)
Do not confuse Lopid with Levbid, Lipitor, Lodine, or Slo-Bid.

◆CLASSIFICATION

PHARMACOTHERAPEUTIC: Fibric acid derivative. **CLINICAL:** Antihyperlipidemic.

USES

Treatment of hypertriglyceridemia in Fredrickson types IV and V hyperlipidemia in pts who are at greater risk for pancreatitis and those who have not responded to dietary intervention. Reduce risk of coronary heart disease (CHD) development in Fredrickson type IIb pts without symptoms who have decreased HDL, increased LDL, increased triglycerides.

PRECAUTIONS

Contraindications: Hypersensitivity to gemfibrozil. Hepatic impairment (including primary biliary cirrhosis), preexisting gallbladder disease, severe renal impairment, concurrent use with dasabuvir, repaglinide or simvastatin. **Cautions:** Concurrent use with statins, mild to moderate renal impairment. anticoagulant therapy (e.g., warfarin).

ACTION

Exact mechanism of action unknown. Can inhibit lipolysis of fat in adipose tissue, decrease hepatic uptake of free fatty acids (reduces hepatic triglyceride production), or inhibit hepatic secretion of very low-density lipoprotein (VLDL). **Therapeutic Effect:** Lowers serum cholesterol, triglycerides (decreases VLDL, LDL; increases HDL).

PHARMACOKINETICS

Well absorbed from GI tract. Protein binding: 99%. Metabolized in liver. Primarily excreted in urine. Not removed by hemodialysis. **Half-life:** 1.5 hrs.

⌛ LIFESPAN CONSIDERATIONS

Pregnancy/Lactation: Unknown if drug crosses placenta or is distributed in breast milk. Decision to discontinue breastfeeding or drug should be based on potential for serious adverse effects. **Children:** Not recommended in pts younger than 2 yrs (cholesterol necessary for normal development). **Elderly:** Age-related renal impairment may require dosage adjustment.

INTERACTIONS

DRUG: **Statins (e.g., atorvastatin, simvastatin)** may increase risk for myopathy/rhabdomyolysis. May increase effects of **repaglinide, warfarin. Bile acid–binding resins (e.g., colestipol)** may decrease concentration. May increase adverse effects of **ezetimibe.** **HERBAL:** None significant. **FOOD:** None known. **LAB VALUES:** May increase serum alkaline phosphatase, bilirubin, creatine kinase, LDH, ALT, AST. May decrease Hgb, Hct, leukocyte counts, serum potassium.

AVAILABILITY (Rx)

Tablets: 600 mg.

ADMINISTRATION/HANDLING

PO

• Give 30 min before morning and evening meals.

INDICATIONS/ROUTES/DOSAGE

Hyperlipidemia/Hypertriglyceridemia

PO: ADULTS, ELDERLY: 600 mg twice daily 30 min before breakfast and dinner.

Dosage in Renal Impairment

Use caution. Contraindicated in severe impairment.

Dosage in Hepatic Impairment
Contraindicated.

SIDE EFFECTS

Frequent (20%): Dyspepsia. **Occasional (10%–2%):** Abdominal pain, diarrhea, nausea, vomiting, fatigue. **Rare (less than 2%):** Constipation, acute appendicitis, vertigo, headache, rash, pruritus, altered taste.

ADVERSE EFFECTS/TOXIC REACTIONS

Cholelithiasis, cholecystitis, acute appendicitis, pancreatitis, malignancy occur rarely.

NURSING CONSIDERATIONS

BASELINE ASSESSMENT

Obtain diet history, esp. fat/alcohol consumption. Obtain serum triglyceride, cholesterol, LFT. Question history of hepatic/renal impairment, cholecystectomy. Receive full medication history and screen for contraindications.

INTERVENTION/EVALUATION

Monitor LDL, VLDL, serum triglycerides, cholesterol for therapeutic response. Monitor daily pattern of bowel activity, stool consistency. Assess for rash, pruritus. Assess for abdominal pain, esp. right upper quadrant or epigastric pain suggestive of adverse gallbladder effects. Monitor serum glucose in pts receiving insulin, oral antihyperglycemics.

PATIENT/FAMILY TEACHING

• Follow special diet (important part of treatment). • Take before meals. • Periodic lab tests are essential part of therapy. • Report pronounced dizziness, blurred vision, abdominal pain, diarrhea, nausea, vomiting.

gentamicin

jen-ta-**mye**-sin

BLACK BOX ALERT Aminoglycoside antibiotics may cause neurotoxicity, nephrotoxicity. Risk of ototoxicity directly proportional to dosage, duration of treatment; ototoxicity usually is irreversible, precipitated by tinnitus, vertigo. May cause fetal harm if given during pregnancy.

Do not confuse gentamicin with azithromycin, clindamycin, fidaxomicin, plazomicin, tobramycin, or vancomycin.

CLASSIFICATION

PHARMACOTHERAPEUTIC: Aminoglycoside. **CLINICAL:** Antibiotic.

G

USES

Parenteral: Treatment of infections susceptible to *Pseudomonas, Proteus, Serratia,* and other gram-negative organisms and gram-positive *Staphylococcus* including skin/skin structure, bone, joint, respiratory tract, intra-abdominal, complicated urinary tract, acute pelvic infections; burns; septicemia; meningitis. **Ophthalmic:** Ophthalmic infections caused by susceptible bacteria. **OFF-LABEL:** Surgical (preoperative) prophylaxis.

PRECAUTIONS

Contraindications: Hypersensitivity to gentamicin, other aminoglycosides (cross-sensitivity) or their components. **Cautions:** Elderly, neonates due to renal insufficiency or immaturity, neuromuscular disorders (potential for respiratory depression), vestibular or cochlear impairment, renal impairment, hypocalcemia, myasthenia gravis. Pediatric pts on extracorporeal membrane oxygenation.

ACTION

Interferes with bacterial protein synthesis. Binds to 30S ribosomal subunit, causing a defective cell membrane. **Therapeutic Effect:** Bactericidal.

PHARMACOKINETICS

Rapid, complete absorption after IM administration. Protein binding: less than 30%. Widely distributed (does not cross blood-brain barrier, low concentrations in CSF). Excreted unchanged in urine. Removed by hemodialysis. **Half-life:** 2–4 hrs (increased in renal impairment, neonates; decreased in cystic fibrosis, burn, or febrile pts).

LIFESPAN CONSIDERATIONS

Pregnancy/Lactation: Readily crosses placenta; unknown if distributed in breast milk. **Children:** Caution in neonates: Immature renal function increases half-life and toxicity. **Elderly:** Age-related renal impairment may require dosage adjustment.

G

INTERACTIONS

DRUG: **Nephrotoxic (e.g., furosemide, IV contrast dye), ototoxic medications (e.g., CISplatin, cycloSPORINE, foscarnet, furosemide, mannitol)** may increase risk of nephrotoxicity, ototoxicity. **HERBAL:** None significant. **FOOD:** None known. **LAB VALUES:** May increase serum BUN, creatinine, bilirubin, LDH, ALT, AST. May decrease serum calcium, magnesium, potassium, sodium. **Therapeutic serum level:** peak: 4–10 mcg/mL; trough: 0.5–2 mcg/mL. **Toxic serum level:** peak: greater than 10 mcg/mL; trough: greater than 2 mcg/mL.

AVAILABILITY (Rx)

Injection, Infusion: 60 mg/50 mL, 80 mg/50 mL, 80 mg/100 mL, 100 mg/50 mL, 100 mg/100 mL, 120 mg/100 mL. **Injection, Solution:** 40 mg/mL. **Ointment, Ophthalmic:** 0.3%. **Solution, Ophthalmic:** ***(Gentak):*** 0.3%.

ADMINISTRATION/HANDLING

IV

Reconstitution • Dilute with 50–100 mL D_5W or 0.9% NaCl. Amount of diluent for infants, children depends on individual needs.

Rate of administration • Infuse over 30–60 min for adults, older children; over 60–120 min for infants, young children.

Storage • Store vials at room temperature. • Solution appears clear or slightly yellow. • Intermittent IV infusion (piggyback) is stable for 48 hrs at room temperature or refrigerated. • Discard if precipitate forms.

IM

• To minimize discomfort, give deep IM slowly. • Less painful if injected into gluteus maximus than lateral aspect of thigh.

Ophthalmic

• Place gloved finger on lower eyelid and pull out until a pocket is formed between eye and lower lid. • Place prescribed number of drops or ointment into pocket. Instruct pt to close eye gently for 1–2 min (so that medication will not be squeezed out of the sac). • **Solution:** Instruct pt to apply digital pressure to lacrimal sac at inner canthus for 1 min to minimize systemic absorption. • **Ointment:** Instruct pt to roll eyeball to increase contact area of drug to eye. • Remove excess solution or ointment around eye with tissue.

IV INCOMPATIBILITIES

Allopurinol (Aloprim), amphotericin B complex (Abelcet, AmBisome, Amphotec), furosemide (Lasix), heparin, hetastarch (Hespan), IDArubicin (Idamycin), indomethacin (Indocin), propofol (Diprivan).

IV COMPATIBILITIES

Amiodarone (Cordarone), dexmedetomidine (Precedex), dilTIAZem (Cardizem), enalapril (Vasotec), filgrastim (Neupogen), HYDROmorphone (Dilaudid), insulin, LORazepam (Ativan), magnesium sulfate, midazolam (Versed), morphine, multivitamins.

INDICATIONS/ROUTES/DOSAGE

◀ALERT▶ Space parenteral doses evenly around the clock. Peak, trough levels are determined periodically to maintain desired serum concentrations and minimize risk of toxicity. Target peak concentrations based on indication and site of infection (e.g., 4–6 mcg/mL for UTI; 7–10 mcg/mL for serious infection). Trough concentrations should be less than 2 mcg/mL.

Usual Parenteral Dosage

IM, IV: ADULTS, ELDERLY: (Conventional): 3–5 mg/kg/day in divided doses q8h. **(Once Daily):** 5–7 mg/kg/dose q24h. **ADOLESCENTS, CHILDREN, INFANTS:** 2–2.5 mg/kg/dose q8h.

NEONATES (WEIGHING MORE THAN 2 KG): PNA 8–28 days: 4–5 mg/kg/dose q24h; **PNA 7 days or less:** 4 mg/kg/dose q24h. **(1–2 KG): PNA 8–28 days:** 5 mg/kg/dose q36h; **PNA 7 days or less:** 5 mg/kg/dose q48h. **(WEIGHING LESS THAN 1 KG): PNA 15–28 days:** 5 mg/kg/dose q36h; **PNA 14 days or less:** 5 mg/kg/dose q48h.

Hemodialysis (HD)

Note: Administer after HD on dialysis days.

Loading dose: 2–3 mg/kg, then 1 mg/kg q48–72h for mild UTI or synergy (consider redose for pre- or post-HD concentrations less than 1 mg/L); 1–1.5 mg/kg q48–72h for moderate to severe UTI (consider redose for pre-HD concentration less than 1.5–2 mg/L or post-HD concentrations less than 1 mg/L); 1.5–2 mg/kg q48–72h for systemic gram-negative rod infection (consider redose for pre-HD concentration less than 3–5 mg/L or post-HD concentrations less than 2 mg/L).

Continuous Renal Replacement Therapy (CRRT)

Loading dose: 2–3 mg/kg, then 1 mg/kg q24–36h for mild UTI or synergy (redose when concentration less than 1 mg/L); 1–1.5 mg/kg q24–36h for moderate to severe UTI (redose when concentration less than 1.5–2 mg/L); 1.5–2.5 mg/kg q24–48h for systemic gram-negative infection (redose when concentration less than 3–5 mg/L).

Usual Ophthalmic Dosage

Ophthalmic ointment: ADULTS, ELDERLY: Apply 12-inch strip to conjunctival sac 2–3 times/day.

Ophthalmic solution: ADULTS, ELDERLY, CHILDREN: 1–2 drops q2–4h up to 2 drops/hr.

Dosage in Renal Impairment

Adults

Creatinine Clearance	Conventional Dosage	Once-Daily Dosage
Greater than 60 mL/mil	q8h	q24h
41–60 mL/min	q12h	q36h
20–40 mL/min	q24h	q48h
Less than 20 mL/min	Loading dose, then monitor levels to determine dosage interval	Monitor levels

Children

Creatinine Clearance	Conventional Dosage
Greater than 50 mL/min	q8h
30–50 mL/min	q12–18h
10–29 mL/min	q18–24h
Less than 10 mL/min	q48–72h

Dosage in Hepatic Impairment

Monitor plasma concentrations.

SIDE EFFECTS

Occasional: IM: Pain, induration at injection site. **IV:** Phlebitis, thrombophlebitis, hypersensitivity reactions (fever, pruritus, rash, urticaria). **Ophthalmic:** Burning, tearing, itching, blurred vision. **Rare:** Alopecia, hypertension, fatigue.

ADVERSE EFFECTS/TOXIC REACTIONS

Nephrotoxicity may be reversible if drug is stopped at first sign of symptoms. Irreversible ototoxicity (tinnitus, dizziness, diminished hearing), neurotoxicity (headache, dizziness, lethargy, tremor, visual disturbances) occur occasionally. Risk increases with higher dosages, prolonged therapy, or if solution is applied directly to mucosa. Superinfections, particularly with fungi, may result from bacterial imbalance via any route of administration. Ophthalmic application may cause paresthesia of conjunctiva, mydriasis.

NURSING CONSIDERATIONS

BASELINE ASSESSMENT

Dehydration must be treated before beginning parenteral therapy. Establish baseline hearing acuity. Question for history of allergies, esp. aminoglycosides, sulfites (parabens for topical/ophthalmic routes). Screen for risk of acute kidney injury, esp. pts at risk for renal failure (baseline renal insufficiency, elderly, HF, hypertension, septic shock).

G

INTERVENTION/EVALUATION

Monitor I&O (maintain hydration), urinalysis, BUN, creatinine. Be alert to ototoxic, neurotoxic symptoms (see Adverse Effects/Toxic Reactions). Check IM injection site for induration. Evaluate IV site for phlebitis (heat, pain, red streaking over vein). Assess for rash (**Ophthalmic:** redness, burning, itching, tearing). Be alert for superinfection (genital/anal pruritus, changes in oral mucosa, diarrhea). When treating pts with neuromuscular disorders, assess respiratory response carefully. **Therapeutic serum level:** peak: 4–10 mcg/mL; peak levels are 2–3 times greater with once-daily dosing; trough: 0.5–2 mcg/mL. **Toxic serum level:** peak: greater than 10 mcg/mL; trough: greater than 2 mcg/mL.

PATIENT/FAMILY TEACHING

• Discomfort may occur with IM injection. • Blurred vision, tearing may occur briefly after each ophthalmic dose. • Report any hearing, visual, balance, urinary problems, even after therapy is completed. • **Ophthalmic:** Report if tearing, redness, irritation continues.

gilteritinib

gil-te-**ri**-ti-nib
(Xospata)

■ BLACK BOX ALERT ■ Life-threatening and/or fatal differentiation syndrome with symptoms including fever, dyspnea, hypoxia, pulmonary infiltrates, pleural or pericardial effusion, rapid weight gain or peripheral edema, hypotension, renal dysfunction may occur. Initiate corticosteroid therapy and hemodynamic monitoring in pts suspected of differentiation syndrome until symptoms resolve.

Do not confuse gilteritinib with gefitinib, Gilotrif, or glasdegib.

◆CLASSIFICATION

PHARMACOTHERAPEUTIC: FMS-like tyrosine kinase 3 (FLT3) inhibitor. Tyrosine kinase inhibitor. **CLINICAL:** Antineoplastic.

USES

Treatment of adults who have relapsed or refractory acute myeloid leukemia (AML) with an FMS-like tyrosine kinase 3 (FLT3) mutation.

PRECAUTIONS

Contraindications: Hypersensitivity to gilteritinib. **Cautions:** Baseline neutropenia, hypotension; active infection, cardiac disease, hepatic/renal impairment, electrolyte imbalance, conditions predisposing to infection (e.g., diabetes, renal failure, immunocompromised pts, open wounds); pts at risk for QTc interval prolongation (congenital long QT syndrome, HF, QT interval–prolonging medications, hypokalemia, hypomagnesemia); concomitant use of P-gp inhibitors, strong CYP3A inhibitors, strong CYP3A inducers; history of GI perforation, pancreatitis.

ACTION

Inhibits multiple tyrosine kinases including FLT3 receptor signaling and proliferation in cells expressing FLT3 mutation. **Therapeutic Effect:** Induces apoptosis in mutant-expressing leukemic cells.

PHARMACOKINETICS

Widely distributed. Metabolized in liver. Protein binding: 94%. Peak plasma concentration: 4–6 hrs. Steady state reached in 15 days. Excreted in feces (65%), urine (16%). **Half-life:** 113 hrs.

LIFESPAN CONSIDERATIONS

Pregnancy/Lactation: Avoid pregnancy; may cause fetal harm. Females of reproductive potential must use effective contraception during treatment and for at least 6 mos after discontinuation. Unknown if distributed in breast milk. Breastfeeding not recommended during treatment and for at least 2 mos after discontinuation. **Males:** Males with female partners of reproductive potential must use effective contraception during treatment and for at least 4 mos after discontinuation. **Children:** Safety and efficacy not established. **Elderly:** No age-related precautions noted.

INTERACTIONS

DRUG: Strong CYP3A4 inhibitors (e.g., clarithromycin, ketoconazole) may increase concentration/effect. **CYP3A4 inducers** used concomitantly with **P-gp inducers, strong CYP3A4 inducers (e.g., carBAMazepine, phenytoin, rifAMPin)** may decrease concentration/effect. **QT interval–prolonging medications (e.g., amiodarone, azithromycin, citalopram, escitalopram, haloperidol, sotalol)** may increase risk of QTc interval prolongation. May decrease therapeutic effect of **selective serotonin receptor inhibitors (SSRIs) (e.g., escitalopram, FLUoxetine, sertraline). HERBAL: St. John's wort** may decrease concentration/effect. **FOOD: High-fat meals** may delay absorption. **LAB VALUES:** May increase serum alkaline phosphatase, ALT, AST, creatine kinase, triglycerides. May decrease serum calcium, phosphate, sodium; neutrophils.

AVAILABILITY (Rx)

Tablets: 40 mg.

ADMINISTRATION/HANDLING

PO

• Give without regard to meals. • Administer whole; do not break, cut, crush, or divide tablets. • Tablets cannot be chewed. • If vomiting occurs after administration, give next dose at regularly scheduled time. • If a dose is missed, administer as soon as possible. • Do not give a missed dose within 12 hrs of next dose.

INDICATIONS/ROUTES/DOSAGE

Acute Myeloid Leukemia

PO: ADULTS: 120 mg once daily for at least 6 mos. Continue until disease progression or unacceptable toxicity.

Dose Modification

Based on Common Terminology Criteria for Adverse Events (CTCAE).

Differentiation Syndrome

Withhold treatment if symptoms are severe and persist for more than 48 hrs after initiation of corticosteroids. Resume treatment when symptoms improve to Grade 2 or less.

QT Interval Prolongation

QTc interval greater than 500 msec: Withhold treatment until QTc interval returns to within 30 msec of baseline or 480 msec or less, then resume at reduced dose of 80 mg.
QTc interval increased by greater than 30 msec on ECG on day 8 of cycle 1: Confirm with ECG on day 9. If confirmed, consider reducing dose to 80 mg.

Other Adverse Reactions

Any Grade 3 or higher toxicity: Withhold treatment until improved to Grade 1, then resume at reduced dose of 80 mg.

Pancreatitis

Withhold treatment until pancreatitis is resolved, then resume at reduced dose of 80 mg.

Reversible Posterior Leukoencephalopathy Syndrome

Permanently discontinue.

Dosage in Renal Impairment

Mild to moderate impairment: No dose adjustment. **Severe impairment:** Not specified; use caution.

Dosage in Hepatic Impairment

Mild to moderate impairment: No dose adjustment. **Severe impairment:** Not specified; use caution.

SIDE EFFECTS

Frequent (50%–21%): Myalgia, arthralgia, pain (back, bone, chest, extremity, musculoskeletal, neck), asthenia, fatigue, malaise, fever, mucositis, edema (face, generalized, localized, peripheral), rash, diarrhea, dyspnea, nausea, cough, constipation, eye disorder, headache, dizziness, hypotension, vomiting. **Occasional (18%–11%):** Abdominal pain, neuropathy, insomnia, dysgeusia.

ADVERSE EFFECTS/TOXIC REACTIONS

Life-threatening and/or fatal differentiation syndrome, a condition with rapid proliferation and differentiation of myeloid cells, reported in 3% of pts. Reversible posterior leukoencephalopathy syndrome reported in 1% of pts. QT interval prolongation with QTc interval greater than 500 msec (1% of pts) and QTc interval greater than 60 msec from baseline (7% of pts) have occurred. Pancreatitis reported in 4% of pts. Other significant adverse effects may include renal impairment (21% of pts), cardiac failure (4% of pts), pericardial effusion (4% of pts), pericarditis (2% of pts), large intestine perforation (1% of pts).

NURSING CONSIDERATIONS

BASELINE ASSESSMENT

Obtain CBC, BMP, LFT, CPK; ECG; pregnancy test in female pts of reproductive potential. Replete electrolytes if applicable. Confirm presence of FLT3-positive mutation. Screen for active infection. Confirm compliance of effective contraception. Question history of cardiac/hepatic/renal disease, GI perforation, pancreatitis. Assess risk for QT interval prolongation. Receive full medication history and screen for interactions. Offer emotional support.

INTERVENTION/EVALUATION

Monitor CBC, BMP, LFT, CPK at least wkly for 4 wks, then every other week for 4 wks, then monthly until discontinuation. If QT interval–prolonging medications cannot be withheld, diligently monitor ECG; serum potassium, magnesium for QT interval prolongation, cardiac arrhythmias. An increase of serum creatinine greater than 0.4 mg/dL from baseline may indicate renal impairment. Obtain ECG on days 8 and 15 of cycle 1 and prior to the start of next two subsequent cycles. Monitor B/P for hypotension, esp. in pts taking antihypertensives. Monitor for symptoms of differentiation syndrome (dyspnea, fever hypotension, hypoxia, pulmonary infiltrates, pleural or pericardial effusion, rapid weight gain or peripheral edema, renal dysfunction, or concomitant febrile neutropenic dermatosis). If differentiation syndrome is suspected, initiate corticosteroids and hemodynamic monitoring until symptoms resolve for at least 3 days. Reversible posterior leukoencephalopathy syndrome should be considered in pts with altered mental status, headache, seizures, visual disturbances. Report abdominal pain, fever, melena (may indicate GI perforation). Monitor daily pattern of bowel activity, stool consistency. Assess skin for toxic skin reactions, rash. Monitor for pancreatitis (severe, steady abdominal pain often radiating to the back [with or without vomiting]). Ensure adequate hydration, nutrition.

PATIENT/FAMILY TEACHING

• Treatment may depress your immune system response and reduce your ability to fight infection. Report symptoms of infection such as body aches, chills, cough, fatigue, fever. Avoid those with active infection. • Report symptoms of bone marrow depression such as bruising, fatigue, fever, shortness of breath, weight loss; bleeding easily, bloody urine or stool. • Treatment may cause life-threatening differentiation syndrome as early as 2 days after starting therapy. Report difficulty breathing, fever, low blood pressure, rapid weight gain, swelling of the hands or feet, decreased urine output. • Nervous system changes including confusion, headache, seizures may indicate life-threatening brain dysfunction/swelling. • Use effective contraception to avoid pregnancy. Do not breastfeed. • Report liver problems (abdominal pain, bruising, clay-colored stool, amber- or dark-colored urine, yellowing of the skin or eyes); heart problems (chest tightness, dizziness, fainting, palpitations, shortness of breath skin), kidney problems (decreased urine output, flank pain, darkened urine); toxic skin reactions (rash, skin eruptions). • Persistent, severe abdominal pain that radiates to the back (with or without vomiting) may indicate acute inflammation of the pancreas. • There is a high risk of interactions with other medications. Do not take newly prescribed medications unless approved by prescriber who originally started treatment. • Do not take herbal products or ingest grapefruit products. • Report dizziness, chest pain, fainting, palpitations, shortness of breath); may indicate heart arrhythmia.

glasdegib

glas-**deg**-ib
(Daurismo)

BLACK BOX ALERT May cause severe birth defects, embryo-fetal death in pregnant females. Obtain pregnancy test in females of reproductive potential prior to initiation. Females of reproductive potential must use effective contraception during treatment and for at least 30 days after discontinuation. Due to potential exposure through semen, males with female partners of reproductive potential or a pregnant partner must use effective contraception (e.g., condoms) during treatment and for at least 30 days after discontinuation despite prior vasectomy.

Do not confuse glasdegib with gefitinib, gilteritinib, sonidegib, or vismodegib.

CLASSIFICATION

PHARMACOTHERAPEUTIC: Hedgehog pathway inhibitor. **CLINICAL:** Antineoplastic.

USES

Treatment of newly diagnosed acute myeloid leukemia in adults who are 75 yrs or older or who have comorbidities that preclude use of intensive induction chemotherapy (in combination with low-dose cytarabine).

PRECAUTIONS

ALERT Do not donate blood products or sperm during treatment and for at least 30 days after discontinuation. **Contraindications:** Hypersensitivity to glasdegib. **Cautions:** Baseline neutropenia, thrombocytopenia; active infection, cardiac disease, hepatic/renal impairment, electrolyte imbalance; conditions predisposing to infection (e.g., diabetes, renal failure, immunocompromised pts, open wounds); pts at risk for QTc interval prolongation, cardiac arrhythmias (congenital long QT syndrome, HF, QT interval–prolonging medications, hypokalemia, hypomagnesemia); concomitant use of anticoagulants, strong CYP3A inhibitors, strong CYP3A inducers.

ACTION

Blocks translocation of Smoothened (SMO) into cilia, preventing SMO-mediated activation of downstream Hedgehog targets. **Therapeutic Effect:** Inhibits tumor cell growth and reduces the number of blast cells in marrow.

PHARMACOKINETICS

Widely distributed. Metabolized in liver. Protein binding: 91%. Peak plasma concentration: 1.3–1.8 hrs. Steady state reached in 8 days. Excreted in urine (49%), feces (42%). **Half-life:** 17.4 hrs.

LIFESPAN CONSIDERATIONS

Pregnancy/Lactation: Avoid pregnancy; may cause fetal harm. Females of reproductive potential must use effective contraception during treatment and for at least 30 days after discontinuation. Unknown if distributed in breast milk. Breastfeeding not recommended during treatment and for at least 30 days after discontinuation. **Males:** May impair fertility. Males with female partners of reproductive potential or a pregnant partner must use effective contraception during treatment and for at least 30 days after discontinuation despite prior vasectomy. **Children:** Safety and efficacy not established. **Elderly:** No age-related precautions noted.

INTERACTIONS

DRUG: Strong CYP3A4 inhibitors (e.g., clarithromycin, ketoconazole) may increase concentration/effect. **Strong CYP3A4 inducers (e.g., carBAMazepine, phenytoin, rifAMPin)** may decrease concentration/effect. **QT interval–prolonging medications (e.g., amiodarone, azithromycin, haloperidol, sotalol)** may increase risk of QT interval prolongation. **HERBAL: St. John's wort** may decrease concentration/effect. **FOOD:** None known. **LAB VALUES:** May increase serum alkaline phosphatase, ALT, AST, bilirubin, CPK, creatinine, potassium. May decrease Hgb, neutrophils, platelets; serum calcium, magnesium, phosphate.

AVAILABILITY (Rx)

Tablets: 25 mg, 100 mg.

ADMINISTRATION/HANDLING

PO

• Give without regard to meals. • Administer whole; do not break, cut, crush, or divide tablets. • Tablets cannot be chewed. • If vomiting occurs after administration, give next dose at regularly scheduled time. • If a dose is missed, administer as soon as possible. • Do not give a missed dose within 12 hrs of next dose.

INDICATIONS/ROUTES/DOSAGE

Acute Myeloid Leukemia

PO: ADULTS, ELDERLY: 100 mg once daily on days 1–28 (in combination with cytarabine 20 mg SQ twice daily on days 1–10 of each 28-day cycle) for a minimum of 6 cycles. Continue until disease progression or unacceptable toxicity.

Dose Modification

Based on Common Terminology Criteria for Adverse Events (CTCAE).

Neutropenia

Neutrophils less than 500 cells/mm³ for more than 42 days in absence of disease: Permanently discontinue glasdegib and cytarabine.

Nonhematologic Toxicity

Any Grade 3 nonhematologic toxicity: Withhold treatment (including cytarabine) until improved to Grade 1 or 0, then resume at same dose or reduce to 50 mg (resume cytarabine at same dose or reduce to 15 mg or 10 mg). If toxicity recurs, permanently discontinue glasdegib and cytarabine. If recurrent toxicity is only related to glasdegib, then cytarabine may be continued. **Any Grade 4 nonhematologic toxicity:** Permanently discontinue glasdegib and cytarabine.

QT Interval Prolongation (On at least two separate ECGs)

QTc interval 481–500 msec: Assess and replete electrolyte levels. Assess and adjust concomitant use of medications known to cause QTc interval prolongation. When QTc interval prolongation improves to 480 msec or less, monitor ECG at least wkly for 2 wks. **QTc interval greater 500 msec:** Withhold treatment. Assess and replete electrolyte levels. Assess and adjust concomitant use of medications known to cause QTc interval prolongation. When QTc interval returns to within 30 msec of baseline or 480 msec or less, resume at reduced dose of 50 mg. **QTc interval prolongation with life-threatening arrhythmia:** Permanently discontinue.

Thrombocytopenia

Platelets less than 10,000 cells/mm³ for more than 42 days in absence of disease: Permanently discontinue glasdegib and cytarabine.

Dosage in Renal Impairment

Mild to moderate impairment: No dose adjustment. **Severe impairment:** Not specified; use caution.

Dosage in Hepatic Impairment

Mild impairment: No dose adjustment. **Moderate to severe impairment:** Not specified; use caution.

SIDE EFFECTS

Frequent (36%–18%): Fatigue, asthenia, edema, pain (back, bone, chest, musculoskeletal, neck), myalgia, arthralgia, nausea, dyspnea, mucositis, decreased appetite, dysgeusia, rash, constipation, pyrexia, diarrhea, cough, vomiting, dizziness. **Occasional (15%–12%):** Muscle spasm, headache, toothache, alopecia.

ADVERSE EFFECTS/TOXIC REACTIONS

Anemia, neutropenia, thrombocytopenia is an expected response to therapy. Cardiac arrhythmias including atrial fibrillation, ventricular fibrillation, ventricular tachycardia may occur. QT interval prolongation with QTc interval greater than 500 msec (5% of pts) and QTc interval greater than 60 msec from baseline (4% of pts) have occurred. Bleeding events including disseminated intravascular coagulation, epistaxis, hemoptysis, hemorrhage (cerebral, eye, conjunctival, GI, retinal, tracheal), thrombotic thrombocytopenic purpura, subdural hematoma reported in 30% of pts. Febrile neutropenia reported in 31% of pts. Renal insufficiency including acute kidney injury, oliguria, renal failure reported in 19% of pts. Infections including pneumonia (19% of pts), sepsis (7% of pts) may occurred.

NURSING CONSIDERATIONS

BASELINE ASSESSMENT

Obtain CBC, BMP, LFT, CK, ECG; pregnancy test in female pts of reproductive potential. Replete electrolytes if applicable. Screen for active infection. Confirm compliance of effective contraception. Receive full medication history and screen for interactions. Assess risk for QT interval prolongation. Question history of cardiac/pulmonary/renal disease, cardiac arrhythmias. Offer emotional support.

INTERVENTION/EVALUATION

Monitor CBC, BMP, LFT at least wkly for 1 mo, then monitor electrolytes, BUN, serum creatinine, GFR, CrCl monthly thereafter. An increase of serum creatinine greater than 0.4 mg/dL from baseline may indicate renal impairment. Obtain ECG approx. 1 wk after initiation, then monthly for 2 mos (or more frequently if indicated). If QT interval–prolonging medications cannot be withheld, diligently monitor ECG; serum potassium, magnesium for QT interval prolongation, cardiac arrhythmias. Obtain CK level if muscle aches or spasms occur. Serum CK level elevations usually occur before muscle symptoms are reported. Diligently monitor for infections, febrile neutropenia. Monitor for bleeding events of any kind; symptoms of intracranial bleeding (aphasia, blindness, confusion, facial droop, hemiplegia, seizures). Assess skin for toxic skin reactions, rash.

PATIENT/FAMILY TEACHING

• Treatment may depress your immune system response and reduce your ability to fight infection. Report symptoms of infection such as body aches, chills, cough, fatigue, fever. Avoid those with active infection. • Report symptoms of bone marrow depression such as bruising, fatigue, fever, shortness of breath, weight loss; bleeding easily, bloody urine or stool. • Do not donate blood or blood products during treatment and for at least 30 days after last dose. • Treatment may cause muscle damage, which may lead to kidney failure. Report musculoskeletal symptoms such as muscle pain/spasms/tenderness/weakness. • Report liver problems (abdominal pain, bruising, clay-colored stool, amber- or dark-colored urine, yellowing of the skin or eyes), hemorrhagic stroke (confusion, difficulty speaking, one-sided weakness or paralysis, loss of vision), kidney problems (decreased urine output, flank pain, darkened urine), skin reactions (rash, skin eruptions), bleeding of any kind. • Report dizziness, chest pain, fainting, palpitations, shortness of breath); may indicate heart arrhythmia. • Use effective contraception to avoid pregnancy. Do not breastfeed. • There is a high risk of interactions with other medications. Do not take

G

newly prescribed medications unless approved by prescriber who originally started treatment. • Avoid grapefruit products, herbal supplements (esp. St. John's wort).

glatiramer

TOP 100

gla-**tir**-a-mer
(Copaxone, Glatopa, Glatect ✱)
Do not confuse Copaxone with Compazine.

◆CLASSIFICATION

PHARMACOTHERAPEUTIC: Immunosuppressive. **CLINICAL:** Neurologic agent for multiple sclerosis.

USES

Treatment of relapsing, remitting multiple sclerosis.

PRECAUTIONS

Contraindications: Hypersensitivity to glatiramer, mannitol. **Cautions:** Pts exhibiting immediate postinjection reaction (flushing, chest pain, palpitations, anxiety, dyspnea, urticaria); conditions predisposing to infection (e.g., diabetes, renal failure, immunocompromised pts, open wounds); history of chronic opportunistic infections (esp. fungal/viral infections, tuberculosis).

ACTION

Induces/activates T-lymphocyte suppressor cells specific to myelin antigens. May also interfere with the antigen-presenting function of immune cells. **Therapeutic Effect:** Slows progression of multiple sclerosis.

PHARMACOKINETICS

Substantial fraction of glatiramer is hydrolyzed locally. Some fraction of injected material enters lymphatic circulation, reaching regional lymph nodes; some may enter systemic circulation intact.

⌛ LIFESPAN CONSIDERATIONS

Pregnancy/Lactation: Unknown if distributed in breast milk. **Children/Elderly:** Safety and efficacy not established.

INTERACTIONS

DRUG: May decrease therapeutic effect of **BCG (intravesical), vaccines (live).** May increase toxic/adverse effects of **live vaccines**. **HERBAL:** **Echinacea** may decrease effects. **FOOD:** None known. **LAB VALUES:** None significant.

AVAILABILITY (Rx)

Injection Solution: ***(Copaxone, Glatopa):*** 20 mg/mL in prefilled syringes, 40 mg/mL in prefilled syringes.

ADMINISTRATION/HANDLING

SQ

Preparation • If refrigerated, allow solution to warm to room temperature (approx. 20 min) with needle cap intact. • Visually inspect for particulate matter or discoloration. Solution should appear clear, colorless to slightly yellow in color. Do not use if solution is cloudy, discolored, or visible particles are observed.

Administration • Insert needle subcutaneously into upper arm, outer thigh, hip, or abdomen and inject solution. • Do not inject into areas of active skin disease or injury such as sunburns, skin rashes, inflammation, skin infections, or active psoriasis. • Rotate injection sites. • Do not administer IV or intramuscularly.

Storage • Refrigerate prefilled syringes in original carton until time of use. • Protect from intense light. • Do not freeze or expose to heating sources. • May store at room temperature for 30 days.

INDICATIONS/ROUTES/DOSAGE

Multiple Sclerosis

Note: Dose forms 20 mg/mL and 40 mg/mL are not interchangeable.

SQ: ADULTS, ELDERLY: 20 mg once daily or 40 mg 3 times/wk at least 48 hrs apart.

Dosage in Renal/Hepatic Impairment
No dose adjustment.

SIDE EFFECTS

Expected (73%–40%): Pain, erythema, inflammation, pruritus at injection site, asthenia. **Frequent (27%–18%):** Arthralgia, vasodilation, anxiety, hypertonia, nausea, transient chest pain, dyspnea, flu-like symptoms, rash, pruritus. **Occasional (17%–10%):** Palpitations, back pain, diaphoresis, rhinitis, diarrhea, urinary urgency. **Rare (less than 9%):** Anorexia, fever, neck pain, peripheral edema, ear pain, facial edema, vertigo, vomiting.

ADVERSE EFFECTS/TOXIC REACTIONS

Immediate postinjection reactions including anxiety, chest pain, dyspnea, flushing, palpitations, tachycardia, throat constriction may occur. Transient chest pain (not associated with immediate postinjection reactions) have occurred. Localized lipoatrophy, skin necrosis reported in 2% of pts. Severe hepatic injury, hepatic failure may occur.

NURSING CONSIDERATIONS

BASELINE ASSESSMENT

Assess baseline symptoms of MS (e.g., bladder/bowel dysfunction, cognitive impairment, depression, dysphagia, fatigue, gait disorder, numbness/tingling, pain, seizures, spasticity, tremors, weakness). Screen for active infection.

INTERVENTION/EVALUATION

Monitor LFT as clinically indicated. Monitor for immediate postreaction symptoms; injection site reactions, necrosis. Conduct neurologic assessment. Assess for symptomatic improvement of MS.

PATIENT/FAMILY TEACHING

• A healthcare provider will show you how to properly prepare and inject your medication. You must demonstrate correct preparation and injection techniques before using medication at home. • Treatment may depress your immune system and reduce your ability to fight infection. Report symptoms of infection such as body aches, burning with urination, chills, cough, fatigue, fever. Avoid those with active infection. • Report travel plans to possible endemic areas. • Report liver problems (abdominal pain, bruising, clay-colored stool, amber- or dark-colored urine, yellowing of the skin or eyes). • Immediate injections reactions such as anxiety, chest pain, difficulty breathing, fast heart rate, flushing, palpitations, throat constriction may occur.

glecaprevir/ pibrentasvir

glec-**a**-pre-vir/pi-**brent**-as-vir
(Mavyret)

BLACK BOX ALERT Test all pts for hepatitis B virus (HBV) infection before initiation. HBV reactivation was reported in HCV/HBV co-infected pts who were undergoing or had completed treatment with HCV direct-acting antivirals and were not receiving HBV antiviral therapy. HBV reactivation may cause fulminant hepatitis, hepatic failure, and death.

Do not confuse glecaprevir with boceprevir, grazoprevir, fosamprenavir, paritaprevir, simeprevir, telaprevir, or voxilaprevir, or pibrentasvir with daclatasvir, ledipasvir, ombitasvir, or velpatasvir.

FIXED-COMBINATION(S)

Mavyret: glecaprevir/pibrentasvir: 100 mg/40 mg.

◆CLASSIFICATION

PHARMACOTHERAPEUTIC: NS3/4A protease inhibitor, NS5A protein inhibitor. **CLINICAL:** Antihepaciviral.

USES

Treatment of adults and pediatric pts 12 yrs and older or weighing 45 kg or more with chronic hepatitis C virus (HCV) infection without cirrhosis or with compensated cirrhosis who have genotype 1, 2, 3, 4, 5, or 6 infection. Treatment of adults and pediatric pts 12 yrs and older or weighing 45 kg or more with HCV genotype 1 infection who have previously been treated with an HCV regimen containing an NS5A inhibitor or an NS5A protease inhibitor, but not both.

PRECAUTIONS

Contraindications: Hypersensitivity to glecaprevir, pibrentasvir. Concomitant use with atazanavir, rifampin. Severe hepatic impairment. **Cautions:** HIV infection, hepatic disease unrelated to HCV infection, HBV infection. Concomitant use of P-gp substrates or inhibitors, BCRP substrates, CYP3A4 inducers. Not recommended in pts with moderate hepatic impairment.

ACTION

Glecaprevir inhibits NS3/4A protease, necessary for proteolytic cleavage of HCV-encoded polyprotein. Pibrentasvir inhibits the HCV NS5A protein, essential for viral replication. **Therapeutic Effect:** Inhibits viral replication of HCV.

PHARMACOKINETICS

Widely distributed. Glecaprevir metabolized in liver. Pibrentasvir metabolism not specified. Protein binding: (glecaprevir): 98%; (pibrentasvir): greater than 99%. Peak plasma concentration: 5 hrs. Glecaprevir excreted in feces (92%), urine (1%). Pibrentasvir primarily excreted in feces (97%). **Half-life:** (glecaprevir): 6 hrs; (pibrentasvir): 13 hrs.

LIFESPAN CONSIDERATIONS

Pregnancy/Lactation: Unknown if distributed in breast milk. **Children:** Safety and efficacy not established. **Elderly:** No age-related precautions noted.

INTERACTIONS

DRUG: **Atazanavir, cycloSPORINE, darunavir, efavirenz, irinotecan** may increase concentration of glecaprevir/pibrentasvir. Glecaprevir/pibrentasvir may increase concentration of **afatinib, atorvastatin, digoxin, lovastatin, simvastatin, topotecan, venetoclax, voxilaprevir. CYP3A4 inducers (e.g., carBAMazepine, phenytoin, rifAMPin)** may decrease concentration/effect. **Ethinyl estradiol–containing hormonal contraceptives** may increase risk of hepatotoxicity. **HERBAL: St. John's wort** may decrease concentration/effect. **FOOD:** None known. **LAB VALUES:** May increase serum bilirubin.

AVAILABILITY (Rx)

Fixed-Dose Combination Tablets: glecaprevir/pibrentasvir: 100 mg/40 mg.

ADMINISTRATION/HANDLING

PO

• Give with food. • If dose is missed, administer as soon as possible if no more than 18 hrs have passed since the last dose. If more than 18 hrs have passed, skip the missed dose and administer the next dose at regularly scheduled time.

INDICATIONS/ROUTES/DOSAGE

Hepatitis C Virus Infection

PO: ADULTS, ELDERLY: 3 tablets once daily (total dose: glecaprevir 300 mg and pibrentasvir 120 mg).

Treatment Regimen and Duration

Treatment-Naïve HCV Genotype 1, 2, 3, 4, 5, or 6

Without cirrhosis: glecaprevir/pibrentasvir for 8 wks. **With compensated cirrhosis:** glecaprevir/pibrentasvir for 8 wks.

Treatment-Experienced Genotype 1

Prior treatment with NS5A inhibitor (without NS3/4A protease inhibitor) without cirrhosis or with compensated cirrhosis: glecaprevir/pibrentasvir for 16 wks. **Prior treatment with NS3/4A protease inhibitor (without NS5A inhibitor) without cirrhosis or with compensated cirrhosis:** glecaprevir/pibrentasvir for 12 wks. **Prior treatment with peginterferon, ribavirin,**

sofosbuvir without cirrhosis: glecaprevir/pibrentasvir for 8 wks. **Prior treatment with peginterferon, ribavirin, sofosbuvir with compensated cirrhosis:** glecaprevir/pibrentasvir for 12 wks.

Treatment-Experienced Genotype 2, 4, 5, or 6
Prior treatment with peginterferon, ribavirin, sofosbuvir without cirrhosis: glecaprevir/pibrentasvir for 8 wks. **Prior treatment with peginterferon, ribavirin, sofosbuvir with compensated cirrhosis:** glecaprevir/pibrentasvir for 12 wks.

Treatment-Experienced Genotype 3
Prior treatment with peginterferon, ribavirin, sofosbuvir without cirrhosis or with compensated cirrhosis: glecaprevir/pibrentasvir for 16 wks.

Liver/Kidney Transplant Recipients
Recommend glecaprevir/pibrentasvir for 12 wks. A treatment duration of 16 wks is recommended in pts with HCV genotype 1 who are treatment-experienced (prior treatment with NS5A inhibitor [without NS3/4A protease inhibitor]) or in pts with HCV genotype 3 who are treatment-experienced (prior treatment with peginterferon, ribavirin, sofosbuvir).

Dosage in Renal Impairment
Mild to severe impairment: No dose adjustment.

Dosage in Hepatic Impairment
Mild impairment: No dose adjustment. **Moderate impairment:** Not recommended. **Severe impairment:** Contraindicated.

SIDE EFFECTS

Frequent (16%–11%): Headache, fatigue. **Occasional (9%–7%):** Nausea, diarrhea, pruritus.

ADVERSE EFFECTS/TOXIC REACTIONS

HBV reactivation was reported in pts co-infected with HBV/HVC. HBV reactivation may result in fulminant hepatitis, hepatic failure, death.

NURSING CONSIDERATIONS

BASELINE ASSESSMENT

Obtain LFT, HCV-RNA level. Confirm hepatitis C virus genotype. Test all pts for hepatitis B virus infection. Initiate anti-HBV therapy if warranted. Question history of hepatic disease unrelated to HCV infection, HIV infection; liver/kidney transplantation; concomitant use of other antiretroviral therapy. Receive full medication history and screen for interactions (esp. atazanavir, rifampin).

INTERVENTION/EVALUATION

Periodically monitor HCV-RNA level for treatment effectiveness (or upon completion of treatment). Closely monitor for exacerbation of hepatitis or HBV reactivation. Monitor for rhabdomyolysis (muscle weakness, myalgia, myopathy, decreased urinary output) in pts taking HMG-CoA reductase inhibitors.

PATIENT/FAMILY TEACHING

• Take with food. • There is a high risk of drug interactions with other medications. Do not take newly prescribed medications unless approved by prescriber who originally started treatment. Do not take herbal products. • Pts taking statins (lipid medication) may have an increased risk of rhabdomyolysis, a breakdown of muscle tissue that can cause kidney failure. Report flank pain, muscle pain, darkened urine, decreased urinary output. • Ethinyl estradiol–containing hormonal contraceptives may increase risk of liver injury and are not recommended.

glimepiride

HIGH ALERT

glye-**mep**-ir-ide
(Amaryl)
Do not confuse Amaryl with Altace, Amerge, or Reminyl, or Avandaryl with Benadryl, or glimepiride with glipiZIDE or glyBURIDE.

G

FIXED-COMBINATION(S)

Avandaryl: glimepiride/rosiglitazone (an antidiabetic): 1 mg/4 mg, 2 mg/4 mg, 4 mg/4 mg.
Duetact: glimepiride/pioglitazone (an antidiabetic): 2 mg/30 mg, 4 mg/30 mg.

◆CLASSIFICATION

PHARMACOTHERAPEUTIC: Sulfonylurea. **CLINICAL:** Antidiabetic agent.

G

USES

Adjunct to diet, exercise in the management of type 2 diabetes mellitus.

PRECAUTIONS

Contraindications: Hypersensitivity to glimepiride, sulfonamides. Diabetic ketoacidosis (with or without coma). **Cautions:** Renal/hepatic impairment, glucose-altering conditions (fever, trauma, infection), G6PD deficiency, elderly, malnourished. Allergy to sulfa.

ACTION

Stimulates release of insulin from beta cells of pancreas, decreases glucose output from liver, increases insulin sensitivity at peripheral sites. **Therapeutic Effect:** Lowers serum glucose.

PHARMACOKINETICS

Route	Onset	Peak	Duration
PO	N/A	2–3 hrs	24 hrs

Completely absorbed from GI tract. Protein binding: greater than 99%. Metabolized in liver. Excreted in urine (60%), feces (40%). **Half-life:** 5–9.2 hrs.

⌛ LIFESPAN CONSIDERATIONS

Pregnancy/Lactation: Avoid pregnancy. Unknown if distributed in breast milk. **Children:** Safety and efficacy not established. **Elderly:** Hypoglycemia may be difficult to recognize. Age-related renal impairment may increase sensitivity to glucose-lowering effect.

INTERACTIONS

DRUG: **Beta blockers (e.g., carvedilol, metoprolol)** may increase hypoglycemic effect, mask signs of hypoglycemia. **Cimetidine, ciprofloxacin, fluconazole, raNITIdine, large doses of salicylates** may increase effect. **RifAMPin** may decrease concentration/effect. **Thiazolidinediones (e.g., pioglitazone)** may increase hypoglycemic effect. **HERBAL:** **Herbals with hypoglycemic properties (e.g., fenugreek)** may increase risk of hypoglycemia. **FOOD:** **Alcohol** may cause rare disulfiram reaction. **LAB VALUES:** May increase LDH concentrations, serum alkaline phosphatase, ALT, AST, bilirubin, C-peptide.

AVAILABILITY (Rx)

Tablets: 1 mg, 2 mg, 4 mg.

ADMINISTRATION/HANDLING

PO

- Give with breakfast or first main meal.

INDICATIONS/ROUTES/DOSAGE

Diabetes Mellitus

PO: ADULTS: Initially, 1–2 mg once daily with breakfast or first main meal. May increase by 1–2 mg q1–2wks, based on serum glucose response. **Maximum:** 8 mg/day. **ELDERLY:** Avoid use.

Dosage in Renal Impairment

Initially, 1 mg/day, then titrate dose based on fasting serum glucose levels.

Dosage in Hepatic Impairment

No dose adjustment (not studied).

SIDE EFFECTS

Rare (less than 3%): Altered taste, dizziness, drowsiness, weight gain, constipation, diarrhea, heartburn, nausea, vomiting, stomach fullness, headache, photosensitivity, peeling of skin, pruritus, rash.

ADVERSE EFFECTS/TOXIC REACTIONS

Overdose or insufficient food intake may produce hypoglycemia (esp. with increased glucose demands). GI hemorrhage, cholestatic hepatic jaundice, leukopenia, thrombocytopenia, pancytopenia, agranulocytosis, aplastic or hemolytic anemia occur rarely.

NURSING CONSIDERATIONS

BASELINE ASSESSMENT

Check serum glucose level. Discuss lifestyle to determine extent of learning, emotional needs. Ensure follow-up instruction if pt or family does not thoroughly understand diabetes management or serum glucose testing technique.

INTERVENTION/EVALUATION

Monitor serum glucose level, food intake. Assess for hypoglycemia (cool/wet skin, tremors, dizziness, anxiety, headache, tachycardia, perioral numbness, hunger, diplopia), hyperglycemia (polyuria, polyphagia, polydipsia, nausea, vomiting, dim vision, fatigue, deep or rapid breathing). Be alert to conditions that alter glucose requirements (fever, increased activity or stress, trauma, surgical procedure).

PATIENT/ FAMILY TEACHING

• Diabetes mellitus requires lifelong control. Diet and exercise are principal parts of treatment; do not skip or delay meals. Test blood sugar regularly. Monitor daily calorie intake. • When taking combination drug therapy or when glucose conditions are altered (excessive alcohol ingestion, insufficient carbohydrate intake, hormone deficiencies, critical illness), have a low blood sugar treatment available (e.g., glucagon, oral dextrose).

glipiZIDE

HIGH ALERT

glip-i-zide
(Glucotrol, Glucotrol XL)
Do not confuse glipiZIDE with glimepiride or glyBURIDE, or Glucotrol with Glucophage or Glucotrol XL.

FIXED-COMBINATION(S)

GlipiZIDE/metFORMIN (an antidiabetic): 2.5 mg/250 mg, 2.5 mg/500 mg, 5 mg/500 mg.

◆CLASSIFICATION

PHARMACOTHERAPEUTIC: Sulfonylurea. **CLINICAL:** Antidiabetic agent.

USES

Adjunct to diet, exercise in management of type 2 diabetes mellitus.

PRECAUTIONS

Contraindications: Hypersensitivity to glipiZIDE, sulfonamides. Diabetic ketoacidosis with or without coma, type 1 diabetes mellitus. **Cautions:** Elderly, malnourished, concomitant use of beta blockers, pts with G6PD deficiency, hepatic/renal impairment. Avoid use of extended-release tablets in pts with stricture/narrowing of GI tract.

ACTION

Stimulates release of insulin from beta cells of pancreas, decreases glucose output from liver, increases insulin sensitivity at peripheral sites. **Therapeutic Effect:** Lowers serum glucose.

PHARMACOKINETICS

Route	Onset	Peak	Duration
PO	15–30 min	2–3 hrs	12–24 hrs
Extended-release	2–3 hrs	6–12 hrs	24 hrs

Well absorbed from GI tract. Protein binding: 92%–99%. Metabolized in liver. Excreted in urine. **Half-life:** 2–4 hrs.

⌛ LIFESPAN CONSIDERATIONS

Pregnancy/Lactation: Agents other than glipizide are recommended to treat diabetes in pregnant women. GlipiZIDE given within 1 mo of delivery may produce neonatal hypoglycemia. Drug crosses placenta. Distributed in breast milk. **Children:** Safety and efficacy not established. **Elderly:** Hypoglycemia may be difficult to recognize. Age-related renal impairment may increase sensitivity to glucose-lowering effect.

INTERACTIONS

DRUG: **Betablockers (e.g., carvedilol, metoprolol)** may increase hypoglycemic effect, mask signs of hypoglycemia. **RifAMPin** may decrease concentration/effect. **Thiazolidinediones (e.g., pioglitazone)** may increase hypoglycemic effect. HERBAL: **Herbals with hypoglycemic properties (e.g., fenugreek)** may increase risk of hypoglycemia. FOOD: None known. LAB VALUES: May increase serum alkaline phosphatase, LDH, ALT, AST, bilirubin, C-peptide.

AVAILABILITY (Rx)

Tablets: 5 mg, 10 mg. Tablets: *(Extended-Release):* 2.5 mg, 5 mg, 10 mg.

ADMINISTRATION/HANDLING

PO

• Give immediate-release tablets 30 min before meals. Give extended-release tablets with breakfast. • Do not crush, cut, dissolve, or divide extended-release tablets.

INDICATIONS/ROUTES/DOSAGE

Diabetes Mellitus

PO: ADULTS: *(Immediate-Release):* Initially, 2.5 mg/day. Adjust dosage in 2.5- to 5-mg increments at intervals of 1–2 wks. **Maximum effective dose:** 20 mg/day. *(Extended-Release):* Initially, 2.5–5 mg/day. May increase dose no more frequently than q7days. **Maximum dose:** 20 mg/day. ELDERLY: *(Immediate-Release):* Initially, 2.5 mg/day. May increase by 2.5–5 mg/day q1–2wks. Maintenance dose should be conservative to avoid hypoglycemia. *(Extended-Release):* Initially, 2.5 mg/day. Maintenance dose should be conservative to avoid hypoglycemia.

Dosage in Renal Impairment

For creatinine clearance of 50 mL/min or less, reduce dose by 50%.

Dosage in Hepatic Impairment

(Immediate-Release): Initial dose: 2.5 mg/day.

SIDE EFFECTS

Rare (less than 3%): Altered taste, dizziness, drowsiness, weight gain, constipation, diarrhea, heartburn, nausea, vomiting, headache, photosensitivity, peeling of skin, pruritus, rash.

ADVERSE EFFECTS/TOXIC REACTIONS

Overdose or insufficient food intake may produce hypoglycemia (esp. with increased glucose demands). GI hemorrhage, cholestatic hepatic jaundice, leukopenia, thrombocytopenia, pancytopenia, agranulocytosis, aplastic or hemolytic anemia occur rarely.

NURSING CONSIDERATIONS

BASELINE ASSESSMENT

Check serum glucose level. Discuss lifestyle to determine extent of learning, emotional needs. Ensure follow-up instruction if pt or family does not thoroughly understand diabetes management or serum glucose testing technique.

INTERVENTION/EVALUATION

Monitor serum glucose level, food intake. Assess for hypoglycemia (cool/wet skin, tremors, dizziness, anxiety, headache, tachycardia, perioral numbness, hunger, diplopia), hyperglycemia (polyuria, polyphagia, polydipsia, nausea, vomiting, dim vision, fatigue, deep or rapid breathing). Be alert to conditions that alter glucose requirements (fever, increased activity or stress, trauma, surgical procedure).

PATIENT/ FAMILY TEACHING

• Diabetes mellitus requires lifelong control. Diet and exercise are principal parts of treatment; do not skip or delay meals. Test blood sugar regularly. Monitor daily calorie intake. • When taking combination drug therapy or when glucose conditions are altered (excessive alcohol ingestion, insufficient carbohydrate intake, hormone deficiencies, critical illness), have a low blood sugar treatment available (e.g., glucagon, oral dextrose)

glyBURIDE

TOP 100 HIGH ALERT

glye-bue-ride
(DiaBeta ✱, Euglucon ✱, Glynase)
Do not confuse DiaBeta with Zebeta, glyBURIDE with glimepiride, glipiZIDE, or Glucotrol.

FIXED-COMBINATION(S)

Glucovance: glyBURIDE/metFORMIN (an antidiabetic): 1.25 mg/250 mg, 2.5 mg/500 mg, 5 mg/500 mg.

◆CLASSIFICATION

PHARMACOTHERAPEUTIC: Sulfonylurea. **CLINICAL:** Antidiabetic agent.

USES

Adjunct to diet, exercise in management of stable, mild to moderately severe type 2 diabetes mellitus.

PRECAUTIONS

Contraindications: Hypersensitivity to glyBURIDE. Diabetic ketoacidosis with or without coma, type 1 diabetes mellitus, concurrent use with bosentan. **Cautions:** Stress, elderly, debilitated pts, malnourished, severe hepatic/renal impairment, G6PD deficiency, adrenal and/or pituitary insufficiency.

ACTION

Stimulates release of insulin from beta cells of pancreas, decreases glucose output from liver, increases insulin sensitivity at peripheral sites. **Therapeutic Effect:** Lowers serum glucose level.

PHARMACOKINETICS

Route	Onset	Peak	Duration
PO	0.25–1 hr	1–2 hrs	12–24 hrs

Well absorbed from GI tract. Protein binding: 99%. Metabolized in liver. Primarily excreted in urine. Not removed by hemodialysis. **Half-life:** 5–16 hrs.

LIFESPAN CONSIDERATIONS

Pregnancy/Lactation: Crosses placenta. Distributed in breast milk. May produce neonatal hypoglycemia if given within 2 wks of delivery. **Children:** Safety and efficacy not established. **Elderly:** Hypoglycemia may be difficult to recognize. Age-related renal impairment may increase sensitivity to glucose-lowering effect.

INTERACTIONS

DRUG: **Beta blockers (e.g., carvedilol, metoprolol)** may increase hypoglycemic effect, mask signs of hypoglycemia. **RifAMPin** may decrease concentration/effect. **Thiazolidinediones (e.g., pioglitazone)** may increase hypoglycemic effect. **HERBAL:** **Herbals with hypoglycemic properties (e.g., fenugreek)** may increase risk of hypoglycemia. **FOOD:** None known. **LAB VALUES:** May increase serum alkaline phosphatase, LDH, ALT, AST, bilirubin, C-peptide.

AVAILABILITY (Rx)

Tablets: 1.25 mg, 2.5 mg, 5 mg. **Tablets, Micronized:** 1.5 mg, 3 mg, 6 mg.

ADMINISTRATION/HANDLING

PO

- May give with food at same time each day.

INDICATIONS/ROUTES/DOSAGE

Diabetes Mellitus

PO: *(Tablets):* **ADULTS:** Initially, 1.25–5 mg. May increase by 2.5 mg/day at wkly intervals. **Maintenance:** 1.25–20 mg/day as single or divided doses. **Maximum:** 20 mg/day. **ELDERLY:** Avoid use.

PO: *(Tablets, Micronized):* **ADULTS:** Initially 0.75–3 mg/day. May increase by 1.5 mg/day at wkly intervals. **Maintenance:** 0.75–12 mg/day as a single dose or in divided doses. **Maximum:** 12 mg/day. **ELDERLY:** Avoid use.

Dosage in Renal Impairment

Not recommended for pts with creatinine clearance less than 60 mL/min.

Dosage in Hepatic Impairment

No dose adjustment.

SIDE EFFECTS

Rare (less than 3%): Altered taste, dizziness, drowsiness, weight gain, constipation, diarrhea, heartburn, nausea, vomiting, headache, photosensitivity, peeling of skin, pruritus, rash.

ADVERSE EFFECTS/TOXIC REACTIONS

Overdose or insufficient food intake may produce hypoglycemia (esp. in pts with increased glucose demands). Cholestatic jaundice, leukopenia, thrombocytopenia, pancytopenia, agranulocytosis, aplastic or hemolytic anemia occur rarely.

NURSING CONSIDERATIONS

BASELINE ASSESSMENT

Check serum glucose level. Discuss lifestyle to determine extent of learning, emotional needs. Ensure follow-up instruction if pt or family does not thoroughly understand diabetes management or glucose testing technique.

INTERVENTION/EVALUATION

Monitor serum glucose level, food intake. Assess for hypoglycemia (cool/wet skin, tremors, dizziness, anxiety, headache, tachycardia, perioral numbness, hunger, diplopia); hyperglycemia (polyuria, polyphagia, polydipsia, nausea, vomiting, dim vision, fatigue, deep or rapid breathing). Be alert to conditions that alter glucose requirements (fever, increased activity or stress, trauma, surgical procedure).

PATIENT/ FAMILY TEACHING

• Diabetes mellitus requires lifelong control. Diet and exercise are principal parts of treatment; do not skip or delay meals. Test blood sugar regularly. Monitor daily calorie intake. • When taking combination drug therapy or when glucose conditions are altered (excessive alcohol ingestion, insufficient carbohydrate intake, hormone deficiencies, critical illness), have a low blood sugar treatment available (e.g., glucagon, oral dextrose).

golimumab

goe-**lim**-ue-mab
(Simponi, Simponi Aria)

■ BLACK BOX ALERT ■ Tuberculosis (TB), invasive fungal infections, other opportunistic infections reported. Discontinue treatment if active infection or sepsis occurs. Test for TB prior to and during treatment, regardless of initial result; if positive, start treatment for TB prior to initiating therapy. Lymphoma, other malignancies reported in pts treated with tumor necrosis factor blockers.

Do not confuse Simponi (SQ) with Simponi Aria (IV)

◆CLASSIFICATION

PHARMACOTHERAPEUTIC: Monoclonal antibody. Tumor necrosis factor (TNF) blocking agent. **CLINICAL:** Antipsoriatic agent, antirheumatic, disease-modifying agent.

USES

Simponi, Simponi Aria: Used alone or in combination with methotrexate for the treatment of adults and children 2 yrs of age and older with active psoriatic arthritis. Used in combination with methotrexate for the treatment of adult pts with moderately to severely active rheumatoid arthritis. Used alone or in combination with methotrexate for the treatment of adult pts with active ankylosing spondylitis. Treatment of active polyarticular juvenile idiopathic arthritis in children 2 yrs of age and older. **Simponi: (Additional)** Treatment of moderate to severe active ulcerative colitis in pts with corticosteroid dependence or who are refractory/intolerant to aminosalicylates, oral steroids, azathioprine, or 6-mercaptopurine.

PRECAUTIONS

Contraindications: Hypersensitivity to golimumab. **Cautions:** Elderly, concomitant immunosuppressants, comorbid conditions predisposing to infections (e.g., diabetes). Residence or travel from areas of endemic mycosis; tuberculosis, underlying hematologic disorders, preexisting or recent-onset demyelinating disorders (e.g., multiple sclerosis, polyneuropathy), pts with HF or decreased left ventricular function. Avoid concomitant use with live vaccines, abatacept, or anakinra (increased incidence of serious infections). Do not start during an active infection.

ACTION

Binds specifically to tumor necrosis factor (TNF) alpha, blocking its interaction with cell surface TNF receptors. **Therapeutic Effect:** Alters biologic activity of TNF alpha, reduces inflammation, may alter pathophysiology of rheumatoid arthritis.

PHARMACOKINETICS

Serum concentration reaches steady state by wk 12. Elimination pathway not specified. **Half-life:** 12–14 days.

LIFESPAN CONSIDERATIONS

Pregnancy/Lactation: Unknown if distributed in breast milk. Must either discontinue drug or discontinue breastfeeding. **Children:** Safety and efficacy not established. **Elderly:** May have increased risk of serious infections, malignancy.

INTERACTIONS

DRUG: **Anakinra, anti-TNF agents, baricitinib, pimecrolimus, riTUXimab, tacrolimus (topical), tocilizumab** may increase adverse effects. May decrease therapeutic effect of **BCG (intravesical), vaccines (live).** May increase levels, adverse effects of **belimumab, natalizumab, tofacitinib, vaccines (live).** **HERBAL:** **Echinacea** may decrease effects. **FOOD:** None known. **LAB VALUES:** May increase ALT, AST. May decrease Hgb, leukocytes, neutrophils, platelets.

AVAILABILITY (Rx)

Injection Solution: ***(Simponi):*** 50 mg/0.5 mL, 100 mg/mL in single-dose prefilled autoinjector or prefilled syringe. **Injection Solution:** ***(Simponi Aria):*** 50 mg/4 mL per single-use vial (12.5 mg/mL).

ADMINISTRATION/HANDLING

Simponi SQ

• Remove prefilled syringe or autoinjector from refrigerator. Allow to sit at room temperature for 30 min; do not warm in any other way. • Avoid areas where skin is scarred, tender, bruised, red, scaly, hard. Recommended injection site is front of middle thighs, although lower abdomen 2 inches below navel or outer, upper arms are acceptable. • Inject within 5 min after cap has been removed.

Autoinjector

• Push open end of autoinjector firmly against skin at 90-degree angle. • Do not pull autoinjector away from skin until a first "click" sound is heard and then a second "click" sound (injection is finished and needle is pulled back). This usually takes 3 to 6 sec but may take up to 15 sec for the second "click" to be heard. If autoinjector is pulled away from skin before injection is completed, full dose may not be administered.

Prefilled Syringe

• Gently pinch skin and hold firmly. Use a quick, dart-like motion to insert needle into pinched skin at a 45-degree angle.

Storage • Refrigerate; do not freeze. Do not shake. • Solution appears slightly opalescent, colorless to light yellow. Discard if cloudy or contains particulate.

Simponi Aria

◀ALERT▶ Use in-line 0.22-micron filter.

IV

Reconstitution • Calculate dosage and number of vials needed based on pt weight. • Visually inspect for particulate matter. • Dilute in 100 mL 0.9% NaCl. • Prior to mixing, withdraw and discard volume of 0.9% NaCl equal to the volume of patient-dosed solution. • Slowly inject solution into bag and gently mix. • Do not shake.

Rate of administration • Infuse over 30 min using an in-line low protein-binding 0.22-micron filter.

Storage • Refrigerate vials, prefilled syringes • Vial solution should be colorless to light yellow and opalescent. • It is normal for solution to develop fine translucent particles since drug is a protein. • Do not use if opaque particles, discoloration, or other foreign particles are present. • May store diluted solution at room temperature up to 4 hrs.

IV INCOMPATIBILITIES

Do not infuse concomitantly with other drugs.

INDICATIONS/ROUTES/DOSAGE

Active Psoriatic Arthritis

Note: Use alone or in combination with methotrexate or other nonbiologic DMARD.

SQ: *(Simponi):* **ADULTS, ELDERLY:** 50 mg once monthly.

IV infusion: *(Simponi Aria):* **ADULTS, ELDERLY:** 2 mg/kg at wk 0, 4 then q8wks thereafter. **CHILDREN, ADOLESCENTS:** 80 mg/m^2/dose at wks 0, 4, then q8wks thereafter.

Moderate to Severe Active Rheumatoid Arthritis (With methotrexate)

SQ: *(Simponi):* **ADULTS, ELDERLY:** 50 mg once monthly.

IV infusion: *(Simponi Aria):* **ADULTS, ELDERLY:** 2 mg/kg at wk 0 and wk 4. Then, decrease frequency to q8wks.

Active Ankylosing Spondylitis

Note: Use alone or in combination with methotrexate or other nonbiologic DMARD.

SQ: *(Simponi):* **ADULTS, ELDERLY:** 50 mg once monthly.

IV infusion: *(Simponi Aria):* **ADULTS, ELDERLY:** 2 mg/kg at wk 0, 4 then q8wks thereafter.

Ulcerative Colitis

SQ: *(Simponi):* **ADULTS, ELDERLY:** Initially, 200 mg, then 100 mg 2 wks later, and then 100 mg q4wks thereafter.

Polyarticular Juvenile Idiopathic Arthritis

IV: *(Simponi Aria):* **CHILDREN, ADOLESCENTS:** 80 mg/m^2/dose at wks 0, 4, then q8wks thereafter.

Dosage in Renal/Hepatic Impairment

No dose adjustment.

SIDE EFFECTS

Frequent (13%): Laryngitis, nasopharyngitis, pharyngitis, rhinitis, upper respiratory tract infection. **Occasional (3%–2%):** Bronchitis, hypertension, rash, pyrexia. **Rare (less than 1%):** Dizziness, paresthesia, constipation.

ADVERSE EFFECTS/TOXIC REACTIONS

Neutropenia, lymphopenia may increase risk of infection. New-onset psoriasis, exacerbation of preexisting psoriasis have been reported. Serious infections including sepsis, pneumonia, cellulitis, TB, invasive fungal infections reported. May increase risk of lymphoma, melanoma, new malignancies. New onset or exacerbation of CNS demyelinating disorders, including multiple sclerosis, or worsening of HF have occurred. Viral reactivation of herpes zoster, HIV, hepatitis B virus infection may occur. Pts who receive TNF blockers have risk of autoantibody formation (immunogenicity). Hypersensitivity reactions including anaphylaxis reported. May induce lupus-like symptoms (butterfly rash, new joint pain, peripheral edema, UV sensitivity).

NURSING CONSIDERATIONS

BASELINE ASSESSMENT

Obtain CBC, LFT; pregnancy test in females of reproductive potential. Do not initiate therapy if active infection suspected. Evaluate for active TB and test for latent infection prior to and during treatment. Induration of 5 mm or greater with tuberculin skin test should be considered a positive result when assessing for latent TB. Antifungal therapy should be considered for those who reside or travel to regions where mycoses are endemic. Question history of anemia, HF, CNS disorders, hepatic impairment, HIV, malignancies. Assess skin for moles, lesions. Receive full medication history including herbal products.

INTERVENTION/EVALUATION

Monitor CBC, LFT every 4–8 wks, then periodically. Screen pts for TB (night sweats, hemoptysis, weight loss, fever) regardless of baseline tuberculin skin test result. Monitor hepatitis B virus carriers during treatment and several mos after treatment. If any viral reactivation occurs, interrupt treatment and consider antiviral therapy. Discontinue treatment if acute infection, opportunistic infection, or sepsis occurs, and initiate appropriate antimicrobial therapy. Routinely assess skin for new lesions. Peripheral edema, difficulty breathing, coarse crackles on lung auscultation, elevated BNP may indicate worsening HF. Monitor for hypersensitivity reactions.

PATIENT/FAMILY TEACHING

• Treatment may depress your immune system and reduce your ability to fight infection. Report symptoms of infection such as body aches, chills, cough, fatigue, fever. Avoid those with active infection. • Do not receive live vaccines. • Report history of HIV, fungal infections, HF, hepatitis B, multiple sclerosis, TB, or close relatives who have active TB. Report travel plans to possible endemic areas. Blood levels, TB screening will be routinely monitored. • Hives, swelling of face, difficulty breathing may indicate allergic reaction. • Do not breastfeed. • Abdominal pain, yellowing of skin or eyes, dark-amber urine, clay-colored stools, fatigue, loss of appetite may indicate liver problems. • Decreased platelet count may increase risk of bleeding. • Swelling of hands or feet, difficulty breathing may indicate HF.

goserelin

HIGH ALERT

goe-se-**rel**-in
(Zoladex, Zoladex LA ✱)

◆CLASSIFICATION

PHARMACOTHERAPEUTIC: Gonadotropin-releasing hormone analogue. **CLINICAL:** Antineoplastic.

USES

Treatment of locally confined prostate cancer. Palliative treatment of advanced carcinoma of prostate as alternative when orchiectomy, estrogen therapy is either not indicated or unacceptable. In combination with an antiestrogen before and during radiation therapy for early stages of prostate cancer. Management of endometriosis. Treatment of advanced breast cancer in premenopausal and perimenopausal women. Endometrial thinning before ablation for dysfunctional uterine bleeding.

PRECAUTIONS

Contraindications: Hypersensitivity to goserelin, GnRH, GnRH agonist analogues. Pregnancy (except when used for palliative treatment of advanced breast cancer). **Cautions:** Women of childbearing potential until pregnancy has been excluded. Pts at risk for decreased bone density; diabetes.

ACTION

Initially, stimulates release of luteinizing hormone (LH) and follicle-stimulating hormone (FSH) from anterior pituitary. Chronic administration causes a sustained suppression of pituitary gonadotropins. **Therapeutic Effect:** In females, reduces ovarian, uterine, mammary gland size; regresses hormone-responsive tumors. In males, decreases testosterone level, reduces growth of abnormal prostate tissue.

PHARMACOKINETICS

Protein binding: 27%. Metabolized in liver. Excreted in urine. **Half-life:** 4.2 hrs (male); 2.3 hrs (female).

⌛ LIFESPAN CONSIDERATIONS

Pregnancy/Lactation: Crosses placenta; unknown if distributed in breast milk. **Children:** Safety and efficacy not established. **Elderly:** No age-related precautions noted.

INTERACTIONS

DRUG: **Medications prolonging the QT interval (e.g., amiodarone, azithromycin, ceritinib, haloperidol,**

moxifloxacin) may increase risk of QT interval prolongation, cardiac arrhythmias. **HERBAL:** None significant. **FOOD:** None known. **LAB VALUES:** May increase serum prostatic acid phosphatase, testosterone, calcium; Hgb A1c.

AVAILABILITY (Rx)

Injection, Implant: ***(Zoladex):*** 3.6 mg, 10.8 mg.

G

ADMINISTRATION/HANDLING

SQ Implant

• Administer implant by inserting needle at 30- to 45-degree angle into anterior abdominal wall below the navel line. Do not attempt to eliminate air bubbles or aspirate prior to injection. Do not penetrate into muscle or peritoneum.

INDICATIONS/ROUTES/DOSAGE

Prostatic Carcinoma, Advanced

SQ: ADULTS OLDER THAN 18 YRS, ELDERLY: 3.6 mg every 28 days or 10.8 mg q12wks subcutaneously into upper abdominal wall.

Prostate Carcinoma, Locally Confined

SQ: ADULTS, ELDERLY: (in combination with an antiestrogen and radiotherapy, begin 8 wks prior to radiotherapy): 3.6 mg once. 28 days after initial dose, give 3.6 mg q28days for 4 doses or 10.8 mg one time.

Breast Carcinoma, Endometriosis

SQ: ADULTS: 3.6 mg every 28 days (6 mos for endometriosis). Subcutaneously into upper abdominal wall.

Endometrial Thinning

SQ: ADULTS: 3.6 mg subcutaneously into upper abdominal wall as a single dose or in 2 doses 4 wks apart.

Endometriosis

SQ: ADULTS: 3.6 mg every 28 days for 6 mos.

Dosage in Renal/Hepatic Impairment

No dose adjustment.

SIDE EFFECTS

Frequent (60%–13%): Headache, hot flashes, depression, diaphoresis, sexual dysfunction, impotence, lower urinary tract symptoms. **Occasional (10%–5%):** Pain, lethargy, dizziness, insomnia, anorexia, nausea, rash, upper respiratory tract infection, hirsutism, abdominal pain. **Rare:** Pruritus.

ADVERSE EFFECTS/TOXIC REACTIONS

Arrhythmias, HF, hypertension occur rarely. Ureteral obstruction, spinal cord compression have been observed (immediate orchiectomy may be necessary). Hypersensitivity reactions, including anaphylaxis, may occur. Hyperglycemia, new-onset diabetes occurred in men taking GnRH antagonists. Increased risk of MI, sudden cardiac death was reported. Injection site injuries including hematoma, hemorrhage, hemorrhagic shock may require blood transfusion or surgical intervention.

NURSING CONSIDERATIONS

BASELINE ASSESSMENT

Question history of diabetes, cardiovascular disease, recent MI, prior hypersensitivity reaction. Receive full medication history; screen for QT interval–prolonging medications, anticoagulant medications. Screen for conditions predisposing to QT interval prolongation. In males, question history of urethral obstruction, urinary retention, spinal cord compression, spinal stenosis. Obtain urine pregnancy. If applicable, obtain bone density test.

INTERVENTION/EVALUATION

Monitor pt closely for worsening signs/symptoms of prostatic cancer, esp. during first mo of therapy.

PATIENT/FAMILY TEACHING

• Use nonhormonal methods of contraception during therapy. • Report suspected pregnancy or if regular menstruation does not cease. • Breakthrough menstrual bleeding may occur if dose is missed. • Immediately report sudden weakness, paralysis, numbness, tingling; difficulty urinating, bladder distention. • Do not take newly prescribed medications unless approved by prescriber who originally started treatment. • Severe bleeding may occur at the injection site, esp. in pts who take blood-thinning medication. • Pts with heart disease are at an increased risk of heart attack or sudden death.

granisetron

gra-**nis**-e-tron
(Sancuso, Sustol)

Do not confuse granisetron with alosetron, cilansetron, dolasetron, ondansetron, or palonosetron.

♦CLASSIFICATION

PHARMACOTHERAPEUTIC: Selective serotonin receptor antagonist ($5\text{-}HT_3$). **CLINICAL:** Antiemetic.

USES

Prevention of nausea/vomiting associated with emetogenic cancer therapy and cancer radiation therapy. **OFF-LABEL:** Prevention, treatment of postop nausea, vomiting. Breakthrough treatment of chemotherapy-associated nausea/vomiting.

PRECAUTIONS

Contraindications: Hypersensitivity to granisetron. Hypersensitivity to other $5\text{-}HT_3$ receptor antagonists. **Cautions:** Congenital QT prolongation, concomitant administration of medications that prolong QT interval, electrolyte abnormalities, cumulative high-dose anthracycline therapy. Following abdominal surgery or in chemotherapy-induced nausea, vomiting (may mask progressive ileus or gastric distention), hepatic disease.

ACTION

Selectively blocks serotonin stimulation at receptor sites centrally in chemoreceptor trigger zone, peripherally on vagal nerve terminals. **Therapeutic Effect:** Prevents nausea/vomiting.

PHARMACOKINETICS

Route	Onset	Peak	Duration
IV	1–3 min	N/A	24 hrs

Rapidly, widely distributed to tissues. Protein binding: 65%. Metabolized in liver. Excreted in urine (48%), feces (38%). **Half-life:** 10–12 hrs (increased in elderly).

LIFESPAN CONSIDERATIONS

Pregnancy/Lactation: Unknown if distributed in breast milk. **Children:** Safety and efficacy not established in pts younger than 2 yrs. **Elderly:** No age-related precautions noted.

INTERACTIONS

DRUG: **QT interval–prolonging medications (e.g., amiodarone, azithromycin, ceritinib, haloperidol, moxifloxacin)** may increase risk of QT interval prolongation, cardiac arrhythmias. **SSRIs (e.g., escitalopram, PARoxetine, sertraline), SNRIs (e.g., DULoxetine, venlafaxine)** may increase risk of serotonin syndrome. **HERBAL:** None significant. **FOOD:** None known. **LAB VALUES:** May increase serum ALT, AST.

AVAILABILITY (Rx)

Injection: ***(Extended-Release [Sustol]):*** 10 mg/0.4 mL single-dose syringe. **Injection Solution:** 1 mg/mL. **Tablets:** 1 mg. **Transdermal Patch:** ***(Sancuso):*** 52-cm^2 patch containing 34.3 mg granisetron delivering 3.1 mg/24 hrs.

ADMINISTRATION/HANDLING

IV

Reconstitution • May be given undiluted or dilute with 20–50 mL 0.9% NaCl or D_5W. Do not mix with other medications.

Rate of administration • May give undiluted as IV push over 30 sec. • For IV piggyback, infuse over 5–10 min depending on volume of diluent used.

Storage • Appears as a clear, colorless solution. • Store at room temperature. • After dilution, stable for 3 days at room temperature or 7 days if refrigerated. • Inspect for particulates, discoloration.

PO

• Give 30 min to 1 hr prior to initiating chemotherapy.

SQ

Administer in skin of back of upper arm, abdomen (at least 1 inch away from umbilicus). Avoid areas of compromised skin. Administer over 20–30 sec.

Transdermal

• Apply to clean, dry intact skin on upper outer arm. • Remove immediately from pouch before application. • Do not cut patch.

IV INCOMPATIBILITIES

Amphotericin B (Fungizone).

IV COMPATIBILITIES

Allopurinol (Aloprim), bumetanide (Bumex), calcium gluconate, CARBOplatin (Paraplatin), CISplatin (Platinol), cyclophosphamide (Cytoxan), cytarabine (Ara-C), dacarbazine (DTIC-Dome), dexamethasone (Decadron), dexmedetomidine (Precedex), diphenhydrAMINE (Benadryl), DOCEtaxel (Taxotere), DOXOrubicin (Adriamycin), etoposide (VePesid), gemcitabine (Gemzar), magnesium, mitoXANTRONE (Novantrone), PACLitaxel (Taxol), potassium.

INDICATIONS/ROUTES/DOSAGE

Prevention of Chemotherapy-Induced Nausea/Vomiting

PO: ADULTS, ELDERLY: 2 mg up to 1 hr before chemotherapy or 1 mg up to 1 hr before chemotherapy, with a second dose 12 hrs later.

IV: ADULTS, ELDERLY, CHILDREN 2 YRS AND OLDER: 10 mcg/kg/dose (**Maximum:** 1 mg/dose) within 30 min of chemotherapy. **Maximum:** 1 mg.

SQ: ADULTS, ELDERLY: In combination with dexamethasone: 10 mg at least 30 min before chemotherapy. Do not repeat more frequently than 7 days.

Transdermal: ADULTS, ELDERLY: Apply 24–48 hrs prior to chemotherapy. Remove minimum 24 hrs after completion of chemotherapy. May be worn up to 7 days, depending on chemotherapy duration.

Prevention of Radiation-Induced Nausea/Vomiting

PO: ADULTS, ELDERLY: 2 mg once daily, given 1 hr before radiation therapy.

Postop Nausea/Vomiting

IV: ADULTS, ELDERLY: 0.35–3 mg (5–20 mcg/kg) given at end of surgery.

Dosage in Renal/Hepatic Impairment

No dose adjustment. ***(Sustol):*** **Moderate impairment:** No more frequently than 14 days. **Severe impairment:** Not recommended.

SIDE EFFECTS

Frequent (21%–14%): Headache, constipation, asthenia. **Occasional** (8%–6%): Diarrhea, abdominal pain. **Rare** (less than 2%): Altered taste, fever.

ADVERSE EFFECTS/TOXIC REACTIONS

Hypersensitivity reaction, hypertension, hypotension, arrhythmias (sinus bradycardia, atrial fibrillation, AV block, ventricular ectopy), ECG abnormalities occur rarely. Increased risk of serotonin syndrome reported in pts taking concomitant serotonergic drugs (e.g., SSRIs, SNRIs). May prolong QTc interval.

NURSING CONSIDERATIONS

BASELINE ASSESSMENT

Assess hydration status. Ensure that granisetron is given within 30 min of starting chemotherapy. Receive full medication history and screen for interactions. Screen for QT interval–prolonging conditions.

INTERVENTION/EVALUATION

Monitor for therapeutic effect. Assess for headache. Monitor for dehydration due to recurrent vomiting. Monitor daily pattern of bowel activity, stool consistency.

PATIENT/FAMILY TEACHING

• Granisetron is effective shortly following administration; prevents nausea/vomiting. • Transitory taste disorder may occur.

guselkumab

gue-sel-**koo**-mab
(Tremfya)
Do not confuse guselkumab with golimumab, infliximab, secukinumab.

CLASSIFICATION

PHARMACOTHERAPEUTIC: Interleukin-23 inhibitor. Monoclonal antibody. **CLINICAL:** Antipsoriasis agent.

USES

Treatment of moderate to severe plaque psoriasis in adult pts who are candidates for systemic therapy or phototherapy. Treatment of active psoriatic arthritis in adults.

PRECAUTIONS

Contraindications: Hypersensitivity to guselkumab. **Cautions:** Hepatic impairment, active infection until resolved, history of chronic or recurrent infections, conditions predisposing to infection (e.g., diabetes, immunocompromised pts, open wounds), prior tuberculosis exposure (do not give to pts with active TB infection). Concomitant use of live vaccines not recommended.

ACTION

Selectively binds to interleukin-23 receptor reducing levels of IL-17A, IL-17F, IL-22. IL-23 is a cytokine that is involved in inflammatory and immune responses. **Therapeutic Effect:** Inhibits release of proinflammatory cytokines and chemokines.

PHARMACOKINETICS

Widely distributed. Degraded into small peptides and amino acids via catabolic pathways. Peak plasma concentration: 5.5 days. Elimination not specified. **Half-life:** 15–18 days.

LIFESPAN CONSIDERATIONS

Pregnancy/Lactation: Unknown if distributed in breast milk; however, human immunoglobulin G (IgG) is present in breast milk and is known to cross placenta. **Children:** Safety and efficacy not established. **Elderly:** No age-related precautions noted.

INTERACTIONS

DRUG: May enhance adverse/toxic effects, diminish therapeutic effects of **natalizumab, vaccines (live)**. May decrease therapeutic effect of **BCG (intravesical)**. **HERBAL:** **Echinacea** may decrease effect. **FOOD:** None known. **LAB VALUES:** May increase serum ALT, AST.

AVAILABILITY (Rx)

Injection, Solution: 100 mg/mL in pen-injector, prefilled syringe.

ADMINISTRATION/HANDLING

SQ

Preparation • Remove prefilled syringe from refrigerator and allow to warm to room temperature (approx. 30 min) with needle cap intact. • Visually inspect for particulate matter or discoloration. Solution should appear clear, colorless to slightly yellow in color; may contain small translucent particles. Do not use if solution is cloudy, discolored, or if large particles are observed. • Discard unused portions.

Administration • Insert needle subcutaneously into back of upper arms, front of thighs, or into lower abdomen (except for 2 inches around navel), and inject solution. • Do not inject into areas of the skin where it is tender, bruised, red, hard, thick, scaly, or affected by psoriasis. • Rotate injection sites.

G

Storage • Refrigerate prefilled syringes in original carton until time of use. • Do not freeze. • Do not shake. • Protect from light.

INDICATIONS/ROUTES/DOSAGE

Plaque Psoriasis

SQ: ADULTS, ELDERLY: 100 mg at wk 0, wk 4, and then q8wks thereafter.

Psoriatic Arthritis

SQ: ADULTS, ELDERLY: 100 mg at wks 0 and 4, then q8wks thereafter. May administer alone or in combination with conventional disease-modifying antirheumatic drugs (e.g., methotrexate).

Dosage in Renal/Hepatic Impairment

Not specified; use caution.

SIDE EFFECTS

Occasional (5%–2%): Headache, tension headache, arthralgia, diarrhea.

ADVERSE EFFECTS/TOXIC REACTIONS

May increase risk of tuberculosis infection. Other infections including upper respiratory tract infection, nasopharyngitis, pharyngitis, viral upper respiratory tract infection (14% of pts), gastroenteritis, viral gastroenteritis (1% of pts), tinea infections (1% of pts), herpes simplex virus (1% of pts) may occur. Mild to moderate elevated serum ALT, AST reported in 3% of pts. Immunogenicity (auto-guselkumab antibodies) occurred in 6% of pts.

NURSING CONSIDERATIONS

BASELINE ASSESSMENT

Obtain LFT in pts with hepatic impairment. Question history of hepatic impairment, herpes zoster infection, parasitic infection. Screen for active infection. Pts should be evaluated for active tuberculosis and tested for latent infection prior to initiating treatment and periodically during therapy. Induration of 5 mm or greater with tuberculin skin testing should be considered a positive test result when assessing if treatment for latent tuberculosis is necessary. Conduct dermatologic exam; record characteristics of psoriatic lesions. Assess pt's willingness to self-inject medication.

INTERVENTION/EVALUATION

Monitor LFT periodically. Monitor for symptoms of tuberculosis, including those who tested negative for latent tuberculosis infection prior to initiating therapy. Interrupt or discontinue treatment if serious infection, opportunistic infection, or sepsis occurs, and initiate appropriate antimicrobial therapy. Assess skin for improvement of lesions.

PATIENT/FAMILY TEACHING

• A health care provider will show you how to properly prepare and inject your medication. You must demonstrate correct preparation and injection techniques before using medication at home. • Treatment may depress your immune system response and reduce your ability to fight infection. Report symptoms of infection such as body aches, chills, cough, fatigue, fever. Avoid those with active infection. • Do not receive live vaccines. • Expect frequent tuberculosis screening. Report travel plans to possible endemic areas. • Report liver problems such as abdominal pain, bruising, clay-colored stool, yellowing of the skin or eyes.

haloperidol

hal-o-**per**-i-dol
(Haldol, Haldol Decanoate, Novo-Peridol ✱)

■ **BLACK BOX ALERT** ■ Increased risk of mortality in elderly pts with dementia-related psychosis with use of injections.

Do not confuse Haldol with Halcion or Stadol.

◆CLASSIFICATION

PHARMACOTHERAPEUTIC: First-generation (typical) antipsychotic. **CLINICAL:** Antipsychotic, antiemetic, antidyskinetic.

USES

Treatment of schizophrenia, Tourette's disorder (controls tics and vocal utterances), severe behavioral problems in children with combative explosive hyperexcitability without immediate provocation. Management of psychotic disorder, short-term treatment of hyperactive children. **OFF-LABEL:** Treatment of nonschizophrenic psychosis, alcohol dependence, psychosis/agitation related to Alzheimer's dementia, emergency sedation of severely agitated/psychotic pts.

PRECAUTIONS

Contraindications: Hypersensitivity to haloperidol, CNS depression, coma, Parkinson's disease. **Cautions:** Renal/hepatic impairment, cardiovascular disease, history of seizures, prolonged QT syndrome, medications that prolong QT interval, hypothyroidism, thyrotoxicosis, electrolyte imbalance (e.g., hypokalemia, hypomagnesemia), EEG abnormalities, narrow–angle glaucoma, elderly, pts at risk for pneumonia, decreased GI motility, urinary retention, BPH, visual disturbances, myelosuppression. Pts at risk for orthostatic hypotension (e.g., cerebrovascular disease).

ACTION

Nonselectively blocks postsynaptic DOPamine receptors in brain. **Therapeutic Effect:** Produces tranquilizing effect. Strong extrapyramidal, antiemetic effects; weak anticholinergic, sedative effects.

PHARMACOKINETICS

Readily absorbed from GI tract. Protein binding: 92%. Metabolized in liver. Excreted in urine. Not removed by hemodialysis. **Half-life:** 20 hrs.

⌛ LIFESPAN CONSIDERATIONS

Pregnancy/Lactation: Crosses placenta. Distributed in breast milk. **Children:** More susceptible to dystonias; not recommended in pts younger than 3 yrs. **Elderly:** More susceptible to orthostatic hypotension, anticholinergic effects, sedation; increased risk for extrapyramidal effects. Decreased dosage recommended.

INTERACTIONS

DRUG: **Alcohol, other CNS depressants (e.g., diphenhydrAMINE, gabapentin, LORazepam, morphine)** may increase CNS depression. **CYP3A4 inducers (e.g., carBAMazepine, phenytoin, rifAMPin)** may decrease concentration. **Medications prolonging QT interval (e.g., amiodarone, ciprofloxacin, ondansetron)** may increase risk of QT prolongation. **Aclidinium, ipratropium, tiotropium, umeclidinium** may increase anticholinergic effect. **Metoclopramide may increase adverse effects.** **HERBAL:** **Herbals with sedative properties (e.g., chamomile, kava, kava, valerian)** may increase CNS depression. **St. John's wort** may decrease concentration/effect. **FOOD:** None known. **LAB VALUES:** None significant. **Therapeutic serum level:** 0.2–1 mcg/mL; **toxic serum level:** Greater than 1 mcg/mL.

AVAILABILITY (Rx)

Injection, Oil: ***(Decanoate):*** 50 mg/mL, 100 mg/mL. **Injection, Solution:** ***(Lactate):*** 5 mg/mL. **Oral Concentrate:** 2 mg/mL. **Tablets:** 0.5 mg, 1 mg, 2 mg, 5 mg, 10 mg, 20 mg.

ADMINISTRATION/HANDLING

IV

◀ALERT▶ Only haloperidol lactate is given IV.

Note: For IV administration, ECG monitoring for QT prolongation/arrhythmias is recommended.

Reconstitution • May give undiluted. • May add to 50–100 mL of D_5W.

Rate of administration • Give IV push at rate of 5 mg/min. • Infuse IV piggyback over 30 min. • For IV infusion, up to 25 mg/hr has been used (titrated to pt response).

Storage • Discard if precipitate forms, discoloration occurs. • Store at room temperature; do not freeze. • Protect from light.

IM

Parenteral administration • Pt should remain recumbent for 30–60 min to minimize hypotensive effect. • Prepare Decanoate IM injection using 21-gauge needle. • Do not exceed maximum volume of 3 mL per IM injection site. • Inject slow, deep IM into upper outer quadrant of gluteus maximus.

PO

• Give without regard to food. • Scored tablets may be crushed. • Dilute oral concentrate with water or juice. • Avoid skin contact with oral concentrate; may cause contact dermatitis.

IV INCOMPATIBILITIES

Allopurinol (Aloprim), amphotericin B complex (Abelcet, AmBisome, Amphotec), cefepime (Maxipime), fluconazole (Diflucan), foscarnet (Foscavir), heparin, nitroprusside (Nipride), piperacillin/tazobactam (Zosyn).

IV COMPATIBILITIES

DOBUTamine (Dobutrex), DOPamine (Intropin), fentaNYL (Sublimaze), HYDROmorphone (Dilaudid), lidocaine, LORazepam (Ativan), midazolam (Versed), morphine, nitroglycerin, norepinephrine (Levophed), propofol (Diprivan).

INDICATIONS/ROUTES/DOSAGE

Usual Dosage

IV: ***(Lactate):*** **ADULTS, ELDERLY:** Initially, 2–10 mg/day in 1–3 divided doses. Adjust dose based on response and tolerability. **Maximum:** 30 mg/day. **ADOLESCENTS, CHILDREN, INFANTS:** 0.05–0.15 mg/kg. May repeat. **Maximum Dose:** 5 mg. ***(Decanoate):*** **ADULTS, ELDERLY:** Initially, 10–20 times stabilized oral dose. **Maximum Initial Dose:** 100 mg (doses greater the 100 mg should be given as 2 separate injections 3–7 days apart). **Maintenance:** 10–15 times daily oral dose. **Maximum:** 450 mg q4wks.

PO: ADULTS, ELDERLY: Initially, 2–10 mg/day in 1–3 divided doses. Adjust dose based on response and tolerability. **Maximum:** 30 mg/day. **CHILDREN WEIGHING MORE THAN 40 KG, ADOLESCENTS:** 0.5–15 mg/day in 2–3 divided doses. May increase at no less than 5–7 days. **Maximum:** 15 mg/day. **CHILDREN 3–12 YRS, WEIGHING 15–40 KG:** Initially, 0.5 mg/day in 2–3 divided doses. May increase by 0.5 mg q5–7days. Range: 0.05–0.15 mg/kg/day in 2–3 divided doses. **Maximum:** 15 mg/day.

Tourette's Disorder

PO: CHILDREN 3–12 YRS, WEIGHING 15–40 KG: Initially, 0.5 mg/day in 2–3 divided doses. May increase by 0.25–0.5 mg/day every 5–7 days to usual dose of 0.75–3 mg/day in divided doses. **CHILDREN WEIGHING MORE THAN 40 KG, ADOLESCENTS:** Initially, 0.25–0.5 mg/day in 2–3 divided doses. May increase as needed every 5–7 days to usual dose of 1–4 mg/day.

Dosage in Renal/Hepatic Impairment

No dose adjustment.

SIDE EFFECTS

Frequent: Blurred vision, constipation, orthostatic hypotension, dry mouth, swelling or soreness of female breasts, peripheral edema. **Occasional:** Allergic reaction, difficulty urinating, decreased thirst, dizziness, diminished sexual function, drowsiness, nausea, vomiting, photosensitivity, lethargy.

ADVERSE EFFECTS/TOXIC REACTIONS

Extrapyramidal symptoms (EPS) appear to be dose related and typically occur in first few days of therapy. Marked drowsiness/lethargy, excessive salivation, fixed stare may be mild to severe in intensity. Less frequently noted are severe akathisia (motor restlessness), acute dystonias: torticollis (neck muscle spasm), opisthotonos (rigidity of back muscles), oculogyric crisis (rolling back of eyes). Tardive dyskinesia (tongue protrusion, puffing of cheeks, chewing/puckering of the mouth) may occur during long-term therapy or after drug discontinuance and may be irreversible. Elderly female pts have greater risk of developing this reaction. May increase risk of QT interval prolongation, cardiac arrhythmias.

NURSING CONSIDERATIONS

BASELINE ASSESSMENT

Assess behavior, appearance, emotional status, response to environment, speech pattern, thought content. Assess mental status. Screen for comorbidities as listed in Precautions (esp. seizure disorder, long QT syndrome).

INTERVENTION/EVALUATION

Monitor B/P, heart rate/rhythm. Monitor ECG, QT interval. Supervise suicidal-risk pts closely during early therapy (as depression lessens, energy level improves, increasing suicide potential). Monitor for rigidity, tremor, mask-like facial expression, fine tongue movement. Assess for therapeutic response (interest in surroundings, improvement in self-care, increased ability to concentrate, relaxed facial expression). **Therapeutic serum level:** 0.2–1 mcg/mL; **toxic serum level:** greater than 1 mcg/mL.

PATIENT/FAMILY TEACHING

• Full therapeutic effect may take up to 6 wks. • Do not abruptly withdraw from long-term drug therapy. • Sugarless gum, sips of water may relieve dry mouth. • Drowsiness generally subsides during continued therapy. • Avoid tasks that require alertness, motor skills until response to drug is established. • Avoid alcohol. • Report muscle stiffness, lip puckering, tongue protrusion, restlessness. • Avoid overheating, dehydration, exposure to sunlight (increased risk of heatstroke).

heparin

HIGH ALERT

hep-a-rin
(Hepalean Leo ✦)
Do not confuse heparin with Hespan.

◆CLASSIFICATION

PHARMACOTHERAPEUTIC: Blood modifier. **CLINICAL:** Anticoagulant.

USES

Prophylaxis and treatment of thromboembolic disorders and thromboembolic complications associated with atrial fibrillation; anticoagulant for extracorporeal and dialysis procedures; maintain patency of IV devices. Prevents clotting in arterial and cardiac surgery. **OFF-LABEL:** STEMI, non-STEMI, unstable angina, anticoagulant used during percutaneous coronary intervention.

PRECAUTIONS

Contraindications: Hypersensitivity to heparin. Severe thrombocytopenia, uncontrolled active bleeding (unless secondary to disseminated intravascular coagulation [DIC]), history of heparin-induced thrombocytopenia (HIT), heparin-induced thrombocytopenia with thrombosis (HITT), or pts who test positive for HIT antibody. **Cautions:** Allergy to pork. Pts at risk for bleeding (e.g., congenital/acquired bleeding disorders, active GI ulcerative disease, hemophilia, concomitant platelet inhibitors, severe hypertension, menses, recent lumbar puncture or spinal anesthesia; recent major surgery, trauma). Use of preservative-free heparin recommended in neonates, infants, pregnant or nursing mothers.

ACTION

Potentiates action of antithrombin III. Interferes with blood coagulation by blocking conversion of prothrombin to thrombin and fibrinogen to fibrin. **Therapeutic Effect:** Prevents further extension of existing thrombi or new clot formation. No effect on existing clots.

PHARMACOKINETICS

Well absorbed following SQ administration. Protein binding: Very high. Metabolized in liver. Removed from circulation via uptake by reticuloendothelial system. Primarily excreted in urine. Not removed by hemodialysis. **Half-life:** 1–6 hrs.

H

LIFESPAN CONSIDERATIONS

Pregnancy/Lactation: Use with caution, particularly during last trimester, immediate postpartum period (increased risk of maternal hemorrhage). Does not cross placenta. Not distributed in breast milk. **Children:** No age-related precautions noted. Benzyl alcohol preservative may cause gasping syndrome in infants. **Elderly:** More susceptible to hemorrhage. Age-related renal impairment may increase risk of bleeding.

INTERACTIONS

DRUG: **Anticoagulants (e.g., apixaban, dabigatran, rivaroxaban, warfarin)** may increase anticoagulant effect; risk of bleeding. **platelet aggregation inhibitors (e.g., aspirin), thrombolytics (e.g., tissue plasminogen activator [TPA])** may increase risk of bleeding. **HERBAL:** **Herbals with anticoagulant/antiplatelet properties (e.g., garlic, ginger, ginkgo biloba)** may increase risk of bleeding. **FOOD:** None known. **LAB VALUES:** May increase free fatty acids, serum ALT, AST; aPTT. May decrease serum cholesterol.

AVAILABILITY (Rx)

Injection Solution: 10 units/mL, 100 units/mL, 1,000 units/mL, 5,000 units/mL, 5,000 units/0.5 mL. **Premix Solution for Infusion:** 25,000 units/250 mL infusion, 25,000 units/500 mL infusion.

ADMINISTRATION/HANDLING

◀ALERT▶ Do not give by IM injection (pain, hematoma, ulceration, erythema).

IV

◀ALERT▶ Used in full-dose therapy. Intermittent IV dosage produces higher incidence of bleeding abnormalities. Continuous IV route preferred.

Reconstitution • Premix solution requires no reconstitution.

Rate of administration • Infuse and titrate per protocol using infusion pump.

Storage • Store at room temperature.

SQ

◀ALERT▶ Used in low-dose therapy. • After withdrawal of heparin from vial, change needle before injection (prevents leakage along needle track). • Inject above iliac crest or in abdominal fat layer. Do not inject within 2 inches of umbilicus or any scar tissue. • Withdraw needle rapidly, apply prolonged pressure at injection site. Do not massage or apply heat/cold to injection site. • Rotate injection sites.

IV INCOMPATIBILITIES

Amiodarone (Cordarone), amphotericin B complex (Abelcet, AmBisome, Amphotec), ciprofloxacin (Cipro), dacarbazine (DTIC), diazePAM (Valium), DOBUTamine (Dobutrex), DOXOrubicin (Adriamycin), filgrastim (Neupogen), gentamicin (Garamycin), haloperidol (Haldol), IDArubicin (Idamycin), labetalol (Trandate), niCARdipine (Cardene), phenytoin (Dilantin), quiNIDine, tobramycin (Nebcin), vancomycin (Vancocin).

IV COMPATIBILITIES

Ampicillin/sulbactam (Unasyn), aztreonam (Azactam), calcium gluconate, ceFAZolin (Ancef), cefTAZidime (Fortaz), cefTRIAXone (Rocephin), dexmedetomidine (Precedex), digoxin (Lanoxin), dilTIAZem (Cardizem), DOPamine (Intropin), enalapril (Vasotec), famotidine (Pepcid), fentaNYL (Sublimaze), furosemide (Lasix), HYDROmorphone (Dilaudid), insulin, lidocaine, LORazepam (Ativan), magnesium sulfate, methylPREDNISolone (Solu-Medrol), midazolam (Versed), milrinone (Primacor), morphine, nitroglycerin, norepinephrine (Levophed), oxytocin (Pitocin), piperacillin/tazobactam (Zosyn), procainamide (Pronestyl), propofol (Diprivan).

INDICATIONS/ROUTES/DOSAGE

Line Flushing

IV: ADULTS, ELDERLY, CHILDREN: 100 units as needed. **INFANTS WEIGHING LESS THAN 10 KG:** 10 units as needed.

Atrial Fibrillation

IV infusion: ADULTS, ELDERLY: 60–80 units/kg bolus **Maximum:** 5,000 units), then 12–18 units/kg/hr **Maximum:** 1,000 units/hr). Adjust infusion rate to maintain anticoagulation target based on institutional protocol.

Acute Coronary Syndrome

IV infusion: ADULTS, ELDERLY: 60 units/kg bolus (**Maximum:** 4,000 units), then 12 units/kg/hr (**Maximum:** 1,000 units/hr as continuous infusion). Adjust infusion rate to maintain anticoagulation target based on institutional protocol.

Treatment of DVT/PE

IV Infusion: ADULTS, ELDERLY: 80 units/kg bolus (**Maximum:** 5,000 units), then 18 units/kg/hr. Adjust infusion rate to maintain anticoagulation target based on institutional protocol.

Usual Infant/Neonatal Dose

IV infusion: 75units/kgbolusover10min, then initial maintenance dose of 28 units/kg/hr. Adjust dose according to aPTT per protocol.

Usual Adolescent/Children Dose

IV infusion: 75 units/kg bolus over 10 min, then initial maintenance dose of 20 units/kg/hr. Adjust infusion rate to maintain anticoagulation target based on institutional protocol.

Thromboembolic Prophylaxis

SQ: ADULTS, ELDERLY: 5,000 units q8–12h.

Dosage in Renal/Hepatic Impairment

No dose adjustment.

SIDE EFFECTS

Occasional: Pruritus, burning (particularly on soles of feet) caused by vasospastic reaction. **Rare:** Pain, cyanosis of extremity 6–10 days after initial therapy lasting 4–6 hrs, hypersensitivity reaction (chills, fever, pruritus, urticaria, asthma, rhinitis, lacrimation, headache).

ADVERSE EFFECTS/TOXIC REACTIONS

Bleeding complications ranging from local ecchymoses to major hemorrhage (cutaneous/GI/genitourinary/intracranial/nasal/oral/pharyngeal/urethral/vaginal bleeding) occur more frequently in high-dose therapy, intermittent IV infusion, women 60 yrs and older. HIT can cause life-threatening thromboembolism such as CVA, MI, DVT, pulmonary embolism, renal artery thrombosis, mesenteric thrombosis. **Antidote:** Protamine sulfate 1–1.5 mg IV for every 100 units heparin SQ within 30 min of overdose, 0.5–0.75 mg for every 100 units heparin SQ if within 30–60 min of overdose, 0.25–0.375 mg for every 100 units heparin SQ if 2 hrs have elapsed since overdose, 25–50 mg if heparin was given by IV infusion.

NURSING CONSIDERATIONS

BASELINE ASSESSMENT

Obtain CBC, PT/INR, aPTT. Cross-check dose with coworker. Assess for bleeding risk. Question history of recent trauma, head injuries, GI/GU bleeding. Ensure that pt has not received spinal anesthesia, spinal procedures.

INTERVENTION/EVALUATION

Monitor CBC, PT/INR daily. Obtain aPTT 6 hrs after initiation or any change in dosage (or per clinical standards) until maintenance dose is established, then check aPTT q24hrs (or per clinical standards). In long-term therapy, monitor 1–2 times/mo. Diligently assess for bleeding. If platelet count decreases more than 50% from baseline, obtain stat HIT antibody test. If HIT antibody positive, discontinue heparin and consider treatment with direct thrombin inhibitor (e.g., argatroban); avoid all heparin products and place heparin allergy on chart. Monitor urine and stool for occult blood. Assess for decrease in B/P, increase in pulse rate, complaint of abdominal/back pain, severe headache (may be evidence of hemorrhage). Question for increase in amount of discharge during menses. Assess peripheral pulses; skin for ecchymosis, petechiae. Check for excessive bleeding from minor cuts, scratches. Assess gums for erythema, gingival bleeding. Assess urine output for hematuria. Avoid IM injections due to potential for hematomas. When converting to warfarin (Coumadin) therapy, monitor PT/INR results (will be 10%–20% higher while heparin is given concurrently).

PATIENT/FAMILY TEACHING

• Use electric razor, soft toothbrush to prevent bleeding. • Report red or dark urine, black or red stool, coffee-ground vomitus, blood-tinged mucus from cough, signs of stroke, nosebleeds, or increase in menstruation. • Do not use any OTC medication without physician approval (may interfere with platelet aggregation). • Wear or carry identification that notes anticoagulant therapy. • Inform dentist, other physicians of heparin therapy. • Limit alcohol.

hydrALAZINE

hye-**dral**-a-zeen
(Apresoline ✤)
Do not confuse hydrALAZINE with hydrOXYzine.

FIXED-COMBINATION(S)

Apresazide: hydrALAZINE/hydroCHLOROthiazide (a diuretic): 25 mg/25 mg, 50 mg/50 mg, 100 mg/50 mg. **BiDil:** hydrALAZINE/isosorbide (a nitrate): 37.5 mg/20 mg.

◆CLASSIFICATION

PHARMACOTHERAPEUTIC: Vasodilator. **CLINICAL:** Antihypertensive.

USES

Management of moderate to severe hypertension. **OFF-LABEL:** Hypertension secondary to eclampsia, preeclampsia. Treatment of HF with reduced ejection fraction, postoperative hypertension.

PRECAUTIONS

Contraindications: Hypersensitivity to hydrALAZINE. Coronary artery disease, mitral valvular rheumatic heart disease. **Cautions:** Advanced renal impairment, cerebrovascular accident, suspected coronary artery disease. Pts with mitral valvular disease, positive ANA titer, pulmonary hypertension.

ACTION

Direct vasodilating effects on arterioles. **Therapeutic Effect:** Decreases B/P, systemic vascular resistance.

PHARMACOKINETICS

Route	Onset	Peak	Duration
PO	20–30 min	N/A	Up to 8 hrs
IV	5–20 min	N/A	1–4 hrs

Well absorbed from GI tract. Widely distributed. Protein binding: 85%–90%. Metabolized in liver. Primarily excreted in urine. Not removed by hemodialysis. **Half-life:** 3–7 hrs (increased in renal impairment).

⌛ LIFESPAN CONSIDERATIONS

Pregnancy/Lactation: Drug crosses placenta. Unknown if distributed in breast milk. Thrombocytopenia, leukopenia, petechial bleeding, hematomas have occurred in newborns (resolved within 1–3 wks). **Children:** No age-related precautions noted. **Elderly:** More sensitive to hypotensive effects. Age-related renal impairment may require dosage adjustment.

INTERACTIONS

DRUG: Diuretics (e.g., furosemide, HCTZ), other antihypertensives (e.g., amLODIPine, cloNIDine, lisinopril, valsartan) may increase hypotensive effect. **HERBAL: Herbals with hypertensive properties (e.g., licorice,**

yohimbe) or hypotensive properties (e.g., garlic, ginger, ginkgo biloba) may alter effects. FOOD: Any **foods** may increase absorption. LAB VALUES: May produce positive direct Coombs' test.

AVAILABILITY (Rx)

Injection Solution: 20 mg/mL. **Tablets:** 10 mg, 25 mg, 50 mg, 100 mg.

ADMINISTRATION/HANDLING

IV

Rate of administration • May give undiluted. • Administer slowly: maximum rate 5 mg/min (0.2 mg/kg/min for children).

Storage • Store at room temperature.

PO

• Best given with food at regularly spaced meals. • Tablets may be crushed.

IV INCOMPATIBILITIES

Ampicillin (Polycillin), furosemide (Lasix).

IV COMPATIBILITIES

DOBUTamine (Dobutrex), heparin, hydrocortisone (Solu-Cortef), nitroglycerin, potassium chloride.

INDICATIONS/ROUTES/DOSAGE

Hypertension

PO: ADULTS, ELDERLY: Initially, 10 mg 4 times/day for first 2–4 days. May increase to 25 mg 4 times/day balance of first wk. May increase by 10–25 mg/dose gradually q2–5 days to 50 mg 4 times/day. Usual range: 100–200 mg/day in 2–3 divided doses. **CHILDREN:** Initially, 0.75 mg/kg/day in 2–4 divided doses. May increase over 3–4 wks. **Maximum:** 7.5 mg/kg/day in 2–4 divided doses. **Maximum daily dose:** 200 mg/day in divided doses.

IV, IM: ADULTS, ELDERLY: Initially, 10–20 mg/dose q4–6h. May increase to 40 mg/dose. **CHILDREN:** Initially, 0.1–0.2 mg/kg/dose q4–6h. Usual range: 0.2–0.6 mg/kg/dose q4–6h. as needed. **Maximum dose:** 20 mg.

Dosage in Renal Impairment

Dosage interval is based on creatinine clearance.

Creatinine Clearance	Dosage
10–50 mL/min	q8h
Less than 10 mL/min	q12–24h

Dosage in Hepatic Impairment

No dose adjustment.

SIDE EFFECTS

Occasional: Headache, anorexia, nausea, vomiting, diarrhea, palpitations, tachycardia, angina pectoris. **Rare:** Constipation, ileus, edema, peripheral neuritis (paresthesia), dizziness, muscle cramps, anxiety, hypersensitivity reactions (rash, urticaria, pruritus, fever, chills, arthralgia), nasal congestion, flushing, conjunctivitis.

ADVERSE EFFECTS/TOXIC REACTIONS

High dosage may produce lupus erythematosus–like reaction (fever, facial rash, muscle/joint aches, glomerulonephritis, splenomegaly). Severe orthostatic hypotension, skin flushing, severe headache, myocardial ischemia, cardiac arrhythmias may develop. Profound shock may occur with severe overdosage.

NURSING CONSIDERATIONS

BASELINE ASSESSMENT

Obtain B/P, pulse immediately before each dose, in addition to regular monitoring (be alert to fluctuations).

INTERVENTION/EVALUATION

Monitor B/P, pulse. Monitor for headache, palpitations, tachycardia. Assess for peripheral edema of hands, feet.

PATIENT/FAMILY TEACHING

• To reduce hypotensive effect, go from lying to standing slowly. • Report muscle/joint aches, fever (lupus-like reaction), flu-like symptoms. • Limit alcohol use.

hydroCHLOROthiazide

hye-dro-**klor**-oh-**thy**-ah-zide
(Urozide 🍁)
Do not confuse Microzide with Maxzide.

FIXED-COMBINATION(S)

Accuretic: hydroCHLOROthiazide/quinapril (an angiotensin-converting enzyme [ACE] inhibitor): 12.5 mg/10 mg, 12.5 mg/20 mg, 25 mg/20 mg. **Aldactazide:** hydroCHLOROthiazide/spironolactone (a potassium-sparing diuretic): 25 mg/25 mg, 50 mg/50 mg. **Aldoril:** hydroCHLOROthiazide/methyldopa (an antihypertensive): 15 mg/250 mg, 25 mg/250 mg, 30 mg/500 mg, 50 mg/500 mg. **Amturnide:** hydroCHLOROthiazide/aliskiren (renin inhibitor)/amLODIPine (calcium channel blocker): 12.5 mg/150 mg/5 mg, 12.5 mg/300 mg/5 mg, 25 mg/300 mg/5 mg, 12.5 mg/300 mg/10 mg, 25 mg/300 mg/10 mg. **Apresazide:** hydroCHLOROthiazide/hydrALAZINE (a vasodilator): 25 mg/25 mg, 50 mg/50 mg, 50 mg/100 mg. **Atacand HCT:** hydroCHLOROthiazide/candesartan (an angiotensin II receptor antagonist): 12.5 mg/16 mg, 12.5 mg/32 mg. **Avalide:** hydroCHLOROthiazide/irbesartan (an angiotensin II receptor antagonist): 12.5 mg/150 mg, 12.5 mg/300 mg, 25 mg/300 mg. **Benicar HCT:** hydroCHLOROthiazide/olmesartan (an angiotensin II receptor antagonist): 12.5 mg/20 mg, 12.5 mg/40 mg, 25 mg/40 mg. **Capozide:** hydroCHLOROthiazide/captopril (an ACE inhibitor): 15 mg/25 mg, 15 mg/50 mg, 25 mg/25 mg, 25 mg/50 mg. **Diovan HCT:** hydroCHLOROthiazide/valsartan (an angiotensin II receptor antagonist): 12.5 mg/80 mg, 12.5 mg/160 mg. **Dutoprol:** hydroCHLOROthiazide/metoprolol (a beta blocker): 12.5 mg/25 mg, 12.5 mg/50 mg, 12.5 mg/100 mg. **Dyazide/Maxide:** hydroCHLOROthiazide/triamterene (a potassium-sparing diuretic): 25 mg/37.5 mg, 25 mg/50 mg, 50 mg/75 mg. **Exforge HCT:** hydroCHLOROthiazide/amLODIPine (a calcium channel blocker)/valsartan (an angiotensin II receptor blocker): 12.5 mg/5 mg/160 mg, 25 mg/5 mg/160 mg, 12.5 mg/10 mg/160 mg, 25 mg/10 mg/160 mg, 25 mg/10 mg/320 mg. **Hyzaar:** hydroCHLOROthiazide/losartan (an angiotensin II receptor antagonist): 12.5 mg/50 mg, 12.5 mg/100 mg, 25 mg/100 mg. **Inderide:** hydroCHLOROthiazide/propranolol (a beta blocker): 25 mg/40 mg, 25 mg/80 mg, 50 mg/80 mg, 50 mg/120 mg, 50 mg/160 mg. **Lopressor HCT:** hydroCHLOROthiazide/metoprolol (a beta blocker): 25 mg/50 mg, 25 mg/100 mg, 50 mg/100 mg. **Lotensin HCT:** hydroCHLOROthiazide/benazepril (an ACE inhibitor): 6.25 mg/5 mg, 12.5 mg/10 mg, 12.5 mg/20 mg, 25 mg/20 mg. **Micardis HCT:** hydroCHLOROthiazide/telmisartan (an angiotensin II receptor antagonist): 12.5 mg/40 mg, 12.5 mg/80 mg. **Moduretic:** hydroCHLOROthiazide/aMILoride (a potassium-sparing diuretic): 50 mg/5 mg. **Normozide:** hydroCHLOROthiazide/labetalol (a beta blocker): 25 mg/100 mg, 25 mg/300 mg. **Prinzide/Zestoretic:** hydroCHLOROthiazide/lisinopril (an ACE inhibitor): 12.5 mg/10 mg, 12.5 mg/20 mg, 25 mg/20 mg. **Tekturna HCT:** hydroCHLOROthiazide/aliskiren (a renin inhibitor): 12.5 mg/150 mg, 25 mg/300 mg. **Teveten HCT:** hydroCHLOROthiazide/eprosartan (an angiotensin II receptor antagonist): 12.5 mg/600 mg, 25 mg/600 mg. **Timolide:** hydroCHLOROthiazide/timolol (a beta blocker): 25 mg/10 mg. **Tribenzor:** hydroCHLOROthiazide/olmesartan/amLODIPine: 12.5 mg/20 mg/5 mg, 12.5 mg/40 mg/5 mg, 25 mg/40 mg/5 mg, 12.5 mg/40 mg/10 mg, 25 mg/40 mg/10 mg. **Uniretic:** hydroCHLOROthiazide/moexipril (an ACE inhibitor): 12.5 mg/7.5

mg, 25 mg/15 mg. **Vaseretic:** hydroCHLOROthiazide/enalapril (an ACE inhibitor): 12.5 mg/5 mg, 25 mg/10 mg. **Ziac:** hydroCHLOROthiazide/bisoprolol (a beta blocker): 6.25 mg/5 mg, 6.25 mg/10 mg.

◆CLASSIFICATION

PHARMACOTHERAPEUTIC: Sulfonamide derivative. Thiazide diuretic. **CLINICAL:** Antihypertensive.

USES

Treatment of mild to moderate hypertension, edema in HF, hepatic cirrhosis, renal dysfunction (e.g., nephrotic syndrome). **OFF-LABEL:** Treatment of calcium nephrolithiasis.

PRECAUTIONS

Contraindications: Hypersensitivity to hydroCHLOROthiazide. Anuria, history of hypersensitivity to sulfonamides or thiazide diuretics. **Cautions:** Severe renal/hepatic impairment, prediabetes or diabetes, elderly or debilitated, history of gout, moderate to high serum cholesterol, hypercalcemia, hypokalemia.

ACTION

Inhibits sodium reabsorption in distal renal tubules, causing excretion of sodium, potassium, hydrogen ions, water. **Therapeutic Effect:** Promotes diuresis; reduces B/P.

PHARMACOKINETICS

Route	Onset	Peak	Duration
PO (diuretic)	2 hrs	4–6 hrs	6–12 hrs

Variably absorbed from GI tract. Primarily excreted unchanged in urine. Not removed by hemodialysis. **Half-life:** 5.6–14.8 hrs.

⌛ LIFESPAN CONSIDERATIONS

Pregnancy/Lactation: Crosses placenta. Small amount distributed in breast milk. Breastfeeding not recommended. **Children:** No age-related precautions noted, except jaundiced infants may be at risk for hyperbilirubinemia. **Elderly:** May be more sensitive to hypotensive, electrolyte effects. Age-related renal impairment may require dosage adjustment.

INTERACTIONS

DRUG: **Bile acid sequestrants (e.g., cholestyramine, colestipol), antihypertensives (e.g., amLODIPine, cloNIDine, lisinopril, valsartan)** may increase hypotensive effect. May increase risk of **digoxin** toxicity. May increase risk of **lithium** toxicity. **HERBAL:** **Herbals with hypertensive properties (e.g., licorice, yohimbe) or hypotensive properties (e.g., garlic, ginger, ginkgo biloba)** may alter effects. **Licorice** may increase hypokalemic effect. **FOOD:** None known. **LAB VALUES:** May increase serum glucose, cholesterol, LDL, bilirubin, calcium, creatinine, uric acid, triglycerides. May decrease urinary calcium, serum magnesium, potassium, sodium.

AVAILABILITY (Rx)

Capsules: 12.5 mg. **Tablets:** 12.5 mg, 25 mg, 50 mg.

ADMINISTRATION/HANDLING

PO

• May take with or without food. If GI upset occurs, give with food or milk, preferably with breakfast (may prevent nocturia). • Give last dose no later than 6 PM unless instructed otherwise.

INDICATIONS/ROUTES/DOSAGE

Edema

PO: ADULTS: Initially, 25–100 mg/day in 1–2 divided doses. Adjust dose based on response and tolerability. **Maximum:** 200 mg/day in 1–2 divided doses.

Hypertension

PO: ADULTS: Initially, 12.5–25 mg once daily. May increase up to 50 mg once daily.

Usual Elderly Dose

PO: ADULTS: Initially, 12.5 mg once daily. Titrate in increments of 12.5 mg as necessary. **Maximum:** 50 mg/day in 1–2 divided doses.

Usual Pediatric Dosage (Edema/HTN)

PO: CHILDREN 2–12 YRS: 1–2 mg/kg/day. **Maximum:** 100 mg/day. **CHILDREN 6 MOS–2 YRS:** 1–2 mg/kg/day in 1–2 divided doses. **Maximum:** 37.5 mg/day. **CHILDREN YOUNGER THAN 6 MOS:** 1–2 mg/kg/day in 1–2 divided doses. **Maximum:** 37.5 mg/day.

Dosage in Renal Impairment

Creatinine clearance less than 30 mL/min: Generally not effective. Avoid use with creatinine clearance less than 10 mL/min.

Dosage in Hepatic Impairment

Use caution.

SIDE EFFECTS

Expected: Increased urinary frequency (diminishes with continued use), urine volume. **Frequent:** Potassium depletion. **Occasional:** Orthostatic hypotension, headache, GI disturbances, photosensitivity.

ADVERSE EFFECTS/TOXIC REACTIONS

Vigorous diuresis may lead to profound water loss/electrolyte depletion, resulting in hypokalemia, hyponatremia, dehydration. Acute hypotensive episodes may occur. Hyperglycemia may occur during prolonged therapy. Pancreatitis, blood dyscrasias, pulmonary edema, allergic pneumonitis, dermatologic reactions occur rarely. Overdose can lead to lethargy, coma without changes in electrolytes or hydration.

NURSING CONSIDERATIONS

BASELINE ASSESSMENT

Check vital signs, esp. B/P for hypotension, before administration. Assess baseline electrolytes, esp. for hypokalemia. Evaluate skin turgor, mucous membranes for hydration status. Evaluate for peripheral edema. Assess muscle strength, mental status. Note skin temperature, moisture. Obtain baseline weight. Monitor I&O.

INTERVENTION/EVALUATION

Continue to monitor B/P, vital signs, electrolytes, I&O, daily weight. Note extent of diuresis. Watch for changes from initial assessment (hypokalemia may result in weakness, tremor, muscle cramps, nausea, vomiting, altered mental status, tachycardia; hyponatremia may result in confusion, thirst, cold/clammy skin). Be esp. alert for potassium depletion in pts taking digoxin (cardiac arrhythmias). Potassium supplements are frequently ordered. Check for constipation (may occur with exercise diuresis).

PATIENT/FAMILY TEACHING

• Expect increased frequency (diminishes with continued use), volume of urination. • To reduce hypotensive effect, go from lying to standing slowly. • Eat foods high in potassium, such as whole grains (cereals), legumes, meat, bananas, apricots, orange juice, potatoes (white, sweet), raisins. • Protect skin from sun, ultraviolet light (photosensitivity may occur).

HYDROcodone TOP 100 HIGH ALERT

hye-droe-**koe**-done
(Hycodan ✱, Hysingla ER, Robidone ✱, Zohydro ER)

■ **BLACK BOX ALERT** ■ Risk of opioid addiction, abuse, and misuse. Serious, life-threatening, or fatal respiratory depression may occur. Accidental ingestion by children can result in fatal overdose. Prolonged use during pregnancy may result in opioid withdrawal syndrome. Concomitant use of CYP3A4 inhibitors may increase concentration/effect. Discontinuation of CYP3A4 inducers may increase concentration/effect. Concomitant use of CNS depressants (e.g., benzodiazepines) may result in profound sedation, respiratory depression, coma, or death.

Do not confuse Hycodan with Vicodin.

FIXED-COMBINATION(S)

Hycet: HYDROcodone/acetaminophen: 7.5 mg/325 mg per 15 mL. **Hycodan:** HYDROcodone/homatropine (an anticholinergic): 5 mg/1.5 mg. **Hycotuss, Vitussin:** HYDROcodone/guaiFENesin (an expectorant): 5 mg/100 mg. **Norco:** HYDROcodone/acetaminophen: 5 mg/325 mg, 7.5 mg/325 mg, 10 mg/325 mg. **Reprexain CIII:** HYDROcodone/ibuprofen (an NSAID): 5 mg/200 mg. **Rezira:** HYDROcodone/pseudoephedrine (a nasal decongestant): 5 mg/60 mg per 5 mL. **Tussend:** HYDROcodone/pseudoephedrine (a sympathomimetic)/guaiFENesin (an expectorant): 2.5 mg/30 mg/100 mg per 5 mL. **Vicodin:** HYDROcodone/acetaminophen: 5 mg/300 mg. **Vicodin ES:** HYDROcodone/acetaminophen: 7.5 mg/300 mg. **Vicodin HP:** HYDROcodone/acetaminophen: 10 mg/300 mg. **Vicoprofen:** HYDROcodone/ibuprofen (an NSAID): 7.5 mg/200 mg. **Xodol:** HYDROcodone/acetaminophen: 5 mg/300 mg, 7.5 mg/300 mg, 10 mg/300 mg. **Zutripro:** HYDROcodone/chlorpheniramine (an antihistamine)/pseudoephedrine (a nasal decongestant): 5 mg/4 mg/60 mg.

◆ CLASSIFICATION

PHARMACOTHERAPEUTIC: Opioid agonist (Schedule III). **CLINICAL:** Narcotic analgesic.

USES

Relief of moderate to moderately severe pain. **Hysingla ER, Zohydro ER:** Around-the-clock management of moderate to severe chronic pain.

PRECAUTIONS

Contraindications: Hypersensitivity to HYDROcodone. Significant respiratory depression, acute or severe bronchial asthma or hypercarbia, GI obstruction including paralytic ileus (known or suspected). **Cautions:** Adrenal insufficiency, biliary tract disease, pancreatitis, CNS depression/coma, acute alcoholism, hypothyroidism; severe renal, hepatic, or pulmonary impairment; urinary stricture, prostatic hypertrophy, seizures, elderly, debilitated, other CNS depressants, history of drug abuse and misuse, drug-seeking behavior, dependency.

ACTION

Binds with opioid receptors in CNS. **Therapeutic Effect:** Reduces intensity of incoming pain stimuli from sensory nerve endings, altering pain perception, emotional response to pain; suppresses cough reflex.

PHARMACOKINETICS

Route	Onset	Peak	Duration
PO (analgesic)	10–20 min	30–60 min	4–6 hrs
PO (antitussive)	N/A	N/A	4–6 hrs

Well absorbed from GI tract. Metabolized in liver. Primarily excreted in urine. **Half-life:** 3.8 hrs (increased in elderly).

LIFESPAN CONSIDERATIONS

Pregnancy/Lactation: Readily crosses placenta. Distributed in breast milk. May prolong labor if administered in latent phase of first stage of labor or before cervical dilation of 4–5 cm has occurred. Respiratory depression may occur in neonate if mother received opiates during labor. Regular use of opiates during pregnancy may produce withdrawal symptoms (irritability, excessive crying, tremors, hyperactive reflexes, fever, vomiting, diarrhea, yawning, sneezing, seizures) in the neonate. **Children:** Pts younger than 2 yrs may be more susceptible to respiratory depression. **Elderly:** May be more susceptible to respiratory depression, may cause paradoxical excitement. Age-related renal impairment, prostatic hypertrophy or obstruction may increase risk of urinary retention; dosage adjustment recommended.

INTERACTIONS

DRUG: **CNS depressants (e.g., alcohol, morphine, oxyCODONE, zolpidem)** may increase CNS depression. **MAOIs (e.g., phenelzine, selegiline)** may increase adverse effects. **CYP3A4 inhibitors (e.g., clarithromycin, ketoconazole, ritonavir)** may increase or prolong opioid effects. HERBAL: **Herbals with sedative properties (e.g., chamomile, kava, kava, valerian)** may increase CNS depression. **St. John's wort** may decrease concentration/effect. FOOD: None known. LAB VALUES: May increase serum amylase, lipase.

AVAILABILITY (Rx)

Capsules: *(Extended-Release [Zohydro ER]):* 10 mg, 15 mg, 20 mg, 30 mg, 40 mg, 50 mg. *Tablets: (Extended-Release [Hysingla ER]):* 20 mg, 30 mg, 40 mg, 60 mg, 80 mg, 100 mg, 120 mg.

ADMINISTRATION/HANDLING

PO

• Give without regard to food. • Extended-release capsules/tablets must be swallowed whole. Do not cut, crush, or dissolve.

INDICATIONS/ROUTES/DOSAGE

Analgesia (Combination products)

PO: ADULTS, CHILDREN WEIGHING 50 KG OR MORE: Initially, 2.5–10 mg q3–4h as needed. ADULTS, CHILDREN WEIGHING LESS THAN 50 KG: Initially, 0.1–0.2 mg/kg q4–6h as needed. ELDERLY: 2.5–5 mg q4–6h.

Analgesia (Extended-release)

PO: ADULTS, ELDERLY: *(Zohydro ER):* Initially, 10 mg q12h. May increase by 10 mg q12h q3–7 days to achieve adequate analgesia. *(Hysingla ER):* Initially, 20 mg q24h. May titrate in increments of 10–20 mg q3–5 days to achieve adequate analgesia.

Dosage in Renal Impairment

No dose adjustment.

Dosage in Hepatic Impairment

Use caution.

SIDE EFFECTS

Frequent: Lethargy, hypotension, diaphoresis, facial flushing, dizziness, drowsiness. Occasional: Urine retention, blurred vision, constipation, dry mouth, headache, nausea, vomiting, difficult/painful urination, euphoria, dysphoria.

ADVERSE EFFECTS/TOXIC REACTIONS

Overdose results in respiratory depression, skeletal muscle flaccidity, cold/clammy skin, cyanosis, extreme drowsiness progressing to seizures, stupor, coma. Tolerance to analgesic effect, physical dependence may occur with repeated use. Prolonged duration of action, cumulative effect may occur in those with hepatic/renal impairment. Concomitant use with benzodiazepines may result in profound sedation, respiratory depression, coma, and death. **Antidote:** Naloxone (see Appendix J).

NURSING CONSIDERATIONS

BASELINE ASSESSMENT

Obtain vital signs. If respirations are 12/min or less (20/min or less in children), withhold medication, contact physician. Assess risk of drug abuse, misuse, drug-seeking behavior. **Analgesic:** Assess onset, type, location, duration of pain. Effect of medication is reduced if full pain recurs before next dose. **Antitussive:** Assess type, severity, frequency of cough.

INTERVENTION/EVALUATION

Palpate bladder for urinary retention. Monitor daily pattern of bowel activity, stool consistency. Initiate deep breathing and coughing exercises, particularly in pts with pulmonary impairment. Assess for clinical improvement; record onset of relief of pain, cough. Screen for misuse, abuse, drug-seeking behavior.

PATIENT/FAMILY TEACHING

• Go from lying to standing slowly to avoid orthostatic hypotension. • Avoid tasks that require alertness, motor skills until response to drug is established. • Avoid alcohol. • Tolerance or dependence may occur with prolonged use at high dosages. • Report nausea, vomiting, constipation, shortness of breath, difficulty breathing. • Taper slowly after long-term use.

hydrocortisone

hye-droe-**kor**-ti-sone
(Anusol HC, Colocort, Cortaid, SOLU-Cortef, Cortenema, Preparation H, Proctocort, Cortef)
Do not confuse hydrocortisone with hydroCHLOROthiazide, HYDROcodone, or hydroxychloroquine, Cortef with Coreg, or SOLU-Cortef with SOLU-medrol.

FIXED-COMBINATION(S)

Cortisporin: hydrocortisone/neomycin/polymyxin (an anti-infective): 5 mg/10,000 units/5 mg, 10 mg/10,000 units/5 mg. **Lipsovir:** hydrocortisone/acyclovir (an antiviral): 1%/5%.

CLASSIFICATION

PHARMACOTHERAPEUTIC: Corticosteroid. **CLINICAL:** Glucocorticoid.

USES

Systemic: Management of adrenocortical insufficiency, anti-inflammatory, immunosuppressive. **Topical:** Inflammatory dermatoses, adjunctive treatment of ulcerative colitis, atopic dermatitis, inflamed hemorrhoids. **OFF-LABEL:** Management of septic shock. Treatment of thyroid storm.

PRECAUTIONS

Contraindications: Hypersensitivity to hydrocortisone. Systemic fungal infections. Use in premature infants. Administration of live or attenuated virus vaccines. IM administration in idiopathic thrombocytopenia purpura. **Cautions:** Thyroid dysfunction, cirrhosis, hypertension, osteoporosis, thromboembolic tendencies or thrombophlebitis, HF, seizure disorders, diabetes, respiratory tuberculosis, untreated systemic infections, renal/hepatic impairment, acute MI, myasthenia gravis, glaucoma, cataracts, increased intraocular pressure, elderly, immunocompromised pts (e.g., diabetes, renal failure, open wounds).

ACTION

Inhibits accumulation of inflammatory cells at inflammation sites, phagocytosis, lysosomal enzyme release, synthesis and/or release of mediators of inflammation. Reverses increased capillary permeability. **Therapeutic Effect:** Prevents/suppresses cell-mediated immune reactions. Decreases/prevents tissue response to inflammatory process.

PHARMACOKINETICS

Route	Onset	Peak	Duration
IV	N/A	4–6 hrs	8–12 hrs

Well absorbed after IM administration. Widely distributed. Metabolized in liver. **Half-life:** Plasma, 1.5–2 hrs; biologic, 8–12 hrs.

LIFESPAN CONSIDERATIONS

Pregnancy/Lactation: Crosses placenta; distributed in breast milk. May produce cleft palate if used chronically during first trimester. Breastfeeding not recommended. **Children:** Prolonged treatment or high dosages may decrease short-term growth rate, cortisol secretion. **Elderly:** May be more susceptible to developing hypertension or osteoporosis.

INTERACTIONS

DRUG: May increase hypokalemic effects of **diuretics (e.g., furosemide). CYP3A4 inducers (e.g., carBAMazepine, phenytoin, rifAMPin)** may decrease effects. **Live virus vaccines** may decrease pt's antibody response to vaccine, increase vaccine side effects, potentiate virus replication. May decrease therapeutic effect of **aldesleukin, BCG (intravesical).** May increase hyponatremic effect of **desmopressin.** HERBAL: **St. John's wort** may decrease concentration/effect. **Echinacea** may decrease therapeutic effect. FOOD: None known. LAB VALUES: May increase serum glucose, lipids, sodium. May decrease serum calcium, potassium, thyroxine; WBC count.

AVAILABILITY (Rx)

Cream, Rectal: ***(Anusol HC, Preparation H Hydrocortisone):*** 1%, 2.5%. **Cream, Topical:** 0.5%, 1%, 2.5%. **Injection, Powder for Reconstitution:** ***(Solu-Cortef):*** 100 mg, 250 mg, 500 mg, 1 g. **Ointment, Topical:** 0.5%, 1%, 2.5%. **Suppository** ***(Anusol HC):*** 25 mg. **Suspension, Rectal:** ***(Colocort, Cortenema):*** 100 mg/60 mL. **Tablets:** ***(Cortef):*** 5 mg, 10 mg, 20 mg.

ADMINISTRATION/HANDLING

IV

Hydrocortisone Sodium Succinate

Reconstitution • Initially, reconstitute vial per manufacturer's instructions. • May further dilute with D_5W or 0.9% NaCl. For IV push, dilute to 50 mg/mL; for intermittent infusion, dilute to 1 mg/mL. **Note:** 100–3,000 mg may be added to 50 mL D_5W or 0.9% NaCl.

Rate of administration • Administer IV push over 3–5 min (over 10 min for doses 500 mg or greater). Give intermittent infusion over 20–30 min.

Storage • Store at room temperature. • Once reconstituted, stable for 3 days at room temperature. Once further diluted with 0.9% NaCl or D_5W, stability is concentration dependent: 1 mg/mL (24 hrs), 2–60 mg/mL (4 hrs).

PO

• Give with food or milk if GI distress occurs.

Rectal

• Shake homogeneous suspension well. • Instruct pt to lie on left side with left leg extended, right leg flexed. • Gently insert applicator tip into rectum, pointed slightly toward navel (umbilicus). Slowly instill medication.

Topical

• Gently cleanse area before application. • Use occlusive dressings only as ordered. • Apply sparingly; rub into area thoroughly.

IV INCOMPATIBILITIES

Ciprofloxacin (Cipro), diazePAM (Valium), midazolam (Versed), phenytoin (Dilantin).

IV COMPATIBILITIES

Amphotericin, calcium gluconate, cefepime (Maxipime), digoxin (Lanoxin), dilTIAZem (Cardizem), diphenhydrAMINE (Benadryl), DOPamine (Intropin), insulin, lidocaine, LORazepam (Ativan), magnesium sulfate, morphine, norepinephrine (Levophed), procainamide (Pronestyl), potassium chloride, propofol (Diprivan).

INDICATIONS/ROUTES/DOSAGE

Acute Adrenal Insufficiency

IV: ADULTS, ELDERLY: 100 mg IV bolus, then 25–75 mg q6h for 24 hrs (or 200 mg/24h as continuous infusion), then taper slowly. INFANTS, CHILDREN, ADOLESCENTS: 50–100 mg/m^2 once, then 50–100 mg/m^2/day in 4 divided doses.

Anti-inflammation, Immunosuppression

IV, IM: ADULTS, ELDERLY: 100–500 mg/dose at intervals of 2 hrs, 4 hrs, or 6 hrs. CHILDREN: 1–5 mg/kg/day in divided doses q12h.

PO: ADULTS, ELDERLY: 20–240 mg/day in divided doses. CHILDREN: 2.5–10 mg/kg/day in divided doses q6–8h.

Adjunctive Treatment of Ulcerative Colitis

Rectal: ***(Enema):*** ADULTS, ELDERLY: 100 mg 1 or 2 times/day. Continue for 3–4 wks. Once improved, may taper gradually to a nightly regimen.

(Rectal Foam): **ADULTS, ELDERLY:** 1 applicator 1–2 times/day. Continue for 3–4 wks. Once improved, may taper gradually to a nightly regimen.

Usual Topical Dose
ADULTS, ELDERLY: Apply sparingly 2–4 times/day.

Dosage in Renal/Hepatic Impairment
No dose adjustment.

SIDE EFFECTS

Frequent: Insomnia, heartburn, anxiety, abdominal distention, diaphoresis, acne, mood swings, increased appetite, facial flushing, delayed wound healing, increased susceptibility to infection, diarrhea or constipation. **Occasional:** Headache, edema, change in skin color, frequent urination. **Topical:** Pruritus, redness, irritation. **Rare:** Tachycardia, allergic reaction (rash, hives), psychological changes, hallucinations, depression. **Topical:** Allergic contact dermatitis, purpura. **Systemic:** Absorption more likely with use of occlusive dressings or extensive application in young children.

ADVERSE EFFECTS/TOXIC REACTIONS

Long-term therapy: Hypocalcemia, hypokalemia, muscle wasting (esp. arms, legs), osteoporosis, spontaneous fractures, amenorrhea, cataracts, glaucoma, peptic ulcer, HF. **Abrupt withdrawal after long-term therapy:** Nausea, fever, headache, sudden severe joint pain, rebound inflammation, fatigue, weakness, lethargy, dizziness, orthostatic hypotension.

NURSING CONSIDERATIONS

BASELINE ASSESSMENT

Obtain baseline weight, B/P, serum glucose, cholesterol, electrolytes. Screen for infections including fungal infections, TB, viral skin lesions. Question medical history as listed in Precautions.

INTERVENTION/EVALUATION

Assess for edema. Be alert to infection (reduced immune response): sore throat, fever, vague symptoms. Monitor daily pattern of bowel activity, stool consistency. Monitor electrolytes, B/P, weight, serum glucose. Monitor for hypocalcemia (muscle twitching, cramps), hypokalemia (weakness, paresthesia [esp. lower extremities], nausea/vomiting, irritability, ECG changes). Assess emotional status, ability to sleep.

PATIENT/FAMILY TEACHING

- Report fever, sore throat, muscle aches, sudden weight gain, swelling, visual disturbances, behavioral changes.
- Do not take aspirin or any other medication without consulting physician.
- Limit caffeine; avoid alcohol.
- Inform dentist, other physicians of cortisone therapy now or within past 12 mos.
- **Topical:** Apply after shower or bath for best absorption.
- Do not cover or use occlusive dressings unless ordered by physician; do not use tight diapers, plastic pants, coverings.
- Avoid contact with eyes.

HYDROmorphone HIGH ALERT

hye-droe-**mor**-fone
(Dilaudid, Hydromorph Contin ✦)

BLACK BOX ALERT High abuse potential, life-threatening respiratory depression risk. Other opioids, alcohol, CNS depressants increase risk of potentially fatal respiratory depression. Highly concentrated form (Dilaudid HP, 10 mg/mL) not to be interchanged with less concentrated form (Dilaudid); overdose, death may result. Exalgo: For use in opioid-tolerant pts. Do not crush, break, chew, or dissolve. Swallow whole.

Do not confuse Dilaudid with Demerol or Dilantin, or HYDROmorphone with HYDROcodone or morphine.

◆CLASSIFICATION

PHARMACOTHERAPEUTIC: Opioid agonist (Schedule II). **CLINICAL:** Narcotic analgesic.

USES

Relief of moderate to severe pain. Extended-release tablet (Exalgo): Around the clock, continuous analgesia for extended period.

PRECAUTIONS

Contraindications: Hypersensitivity to HYDROmorphone. Acute or severe bronchial asthma, severe respiratory depression. GI obstruction including paralytic ileus (known or suspected). **Additional Product-Specific Contraindications:** **Dilaudid HP injection:** Opioid-intolerant pts. **Extended-Release Tablets:** Opioid-intolerant pts, preexisting GI surgery/diseases causing GI narrowing. **Cautions:** Severe hepatic, renal, respiratory disease; hypothyroidism, adrenal cortical insufficiency, seizures, acute alcoholism, head injury, intracranial lesions, increased intracranial pressure, prostatic hypertrophy, Addison's disease, urethral stricture, pancreatitis, biliary tract disease, cardiovascular disease, morbid obesity, delirium tremens, toxic psychosis, pts with CNS depression or coma, pts with depleted blood volume, obstructive bowel disorder; history of drug abuse and misuse, drug-seeking behavior, dependency.

ACTION

Binds to opioid receptors in CNS, reducing intensity of pain stimuli from sensory nerve endings. **Therapeutic Effect:** Alters perception, emotional response to pain; suppresses cough reflex.

PHARMACOKINETICS

Route	Onset	Peak	Duration
PO	30 min	90–120 min	4 hrs
IV	10–15 min	15–30 min	2–3 hrs
IM	15 min	30–60 min	4–5 hrs
SQ	15 min	30–90 min	4 hrs
Rectal	15–30 min	N/A	N/A

Well absorbed from GI tract after IM administration. Widely distributed. Metabolized in liver. Excreted in urine. **Half-life:** 2.6–4 hrs.

LIFESPAN CONSIDERATIONS

Pregnancy/Lactation: Readily crosses placenta. Unknown if distributed in breast milk. May prolong labor if administered in latent phase of first stage of labor or before cervical dilation of 4–5 cm has occurred. Respiratory depression may occur in neonate if mother receives opiates during labor. Regular use of opiates during pregnancy may produce withdrawal symptoms in the neonate (irritability, excessive crying, tremors, hyperactive reflexes, fever, vomiting, diarrhea, yawning, sneezing, seizures). **Children:** Pts younger than 2 yrs may be more susceptible to respiratory depression. **Elderly:** May be more susceptible to respiratory depression, may cause paradoxical excitement. Age-related renal impairment, prostatic hypertrophy or obstruction may increase risk of urinary retention; dosage adjustment recommended.

INTERACTIONS

DRUG: **CNS depressants (e.g., alcohol, morphine, LORazepam, zolpidem)** may increase CNS depression. **MAOIs (e.g., phenelzine, selegiline)** may increase adverse effects. **HERBAL:** **Herbals with sedative properties (e.g., chamomile, kava, kava, valerian)** may increase CNS depression. **FOOD:** None known. **LAB VALUES:** May increase serum amylase, lipase.

AVAILABILITY (Rx)

Injection, Solution: 1 mg/mL, 2 mg/mL, 4 mg/mL, 10 mg/mL. **Liquid, Oral:** 1 mg/mL. **Suppository:** 3 mg. **Tablets:** 2 mg, 4 mg, 8 mg.

Tablets: ***(Extended-Release):*** 8 mg, 12 mg, 16 mg, 32 mg.

ADMINISTRATION/HANDLING

IV

◀ALERT▶ High-concentration injection (10 mg/mL) should be used only in pts tolerant to opiate agonists, currently receiving high doses of another opiate agonist for severe, chronic pain due to cancer. **Reconstitution** • May give undiluted. • May further dilute with 5 mL Sterile Water for Injection or 0.9% NaCl.

Rate of administration • Administer IV push very slowly (over 2–3 min). • Rapid IV increases risk of severe adverse reactions (chest wall rigidity, apnea, peripheral circulatory collapse, anaphylactoid effects, cardiac arrest).
Storage • Store at room temperature; protect from light. • Slight yellow discoloration of parenteral form does not indicate loss of potency.

IM, SQ
• Subcutaneously or intramuscularly insert needle and inject solution. Pulling back the plunger before IM injection may ensure that drug is not delivered directly into bloodstream (however, this topic is currently debated). • Administer slowly; rotate injection sites. • Pts with circulatory impairment experience higher risk of overdosage due to delayed absorption of repeated administration.

PO
• Give without regard to food. • Tablets may be crushed. • Extended-release tablets must be swallowed whole; do not break, crush, dissolve, or divide.

Rectal
• Refrigerate suppositories. • Moisten suppository with cold water before inserting well up into rectum.

IV INCOMPATIBILITIES

Amphotericin B complex (Abelcet, AmBisome, Amphotec), ceFAZolin (Ancef, Kefzol), diazePAM (Valium), PHENobarbital, phenytoin (Dilantin).

IV COMPATIBILITIES

Dexmedetomidine (Precedex), dilTIAZem (Cardizem), diphenhydrAMINE (Benadryl), DOBUTamine (Dobutrex), DOPamine (Intropin), fentaNYL (Sublimaze), furosemide (Lasix), heparin, LORazepam (Ativan), magnesium sulfate, metoclopramide (Reglan), midazolam (Versed), milrinone (Primacor), morphine, propofol (Diprivan).

INDICATIONS/ROUTES/DOSAGE

Analgesia (Acute, moderate to severe)
PO: ADULTS: ***(Immediate-Release):*** Initially 2–4 mg q4–6h as needed (tablets) or 2.5–10 mg q3–6h as needed (liquid). **ELDERLY:** Use with caution; initiating at the low end of the dosage range is recommended. **CHILDREN, ADOLESCENTS WEIGHING MORE THAN 50 KG:** 1–2 mg q3–4h as needed. **CHILDREN OLDER THAN 6 MOS WEIGHING LESS THAN 50 KG:** 0.03–0.08 mg/kg/dose q3–4h as needed.
IV (For use in opiate-naive pts): ADULTS: 0.2–1 mg q2–3h (pts with prior opioid exposure may require higher doses). **ELDERLY:** 0.2 mg q2–3h PRN or 0.25–0.5 mg q3–4 PRN. **CHILDREN, ADOLESCENTS WEIGHING MORE THAN 50 KG:** 0.2–0.6 mg/dose q2–4h as needed. **CHILDREN WEIGHING 50 KG OR LESS:** 0.015 mg/kg/dose q3–6h as needed.
Rectal: ADULTS, ELDERLY: 3 mg q6–8h.

Patient-Controlled Analgesia (PCA)
IV: ADULTS, ELDERLY: Loading dose: 0.4 mg. Demand dose: 0.1–0.4. Lockout interval: 10 min.
Epidural: ADULTS, ELDERLY: Bolus dose of 0.4–1 mg; infusion rate: 0.03–0.3 mg/hr; demand dose: 0.02–0.05 mg. Lockout interval: 10–15 min.

Continuous Infusion
IV infusion: ADULTS, ELDERLY: 0.5–3 mg/hr.

Dosage in Renal/Hepatic Impairment
Decrease initial dose; use with caution.

SIDE EFFECTS

Frequent: Drowsiness, dizziness, hypotension (including orthostatic hypotension), decreased appetite. **Occasional:** Confusion, diaphoresis, facial flushing, urinary retention, constipation, dry mouth, nausea, vomiting, headache, pain at injection site. **Rare:** Allergic reaction, depression.

ADVERSE EFFECTS/TOXIC REACTIONS

Overdose results in respiratory depression, skeletal muscle flaccidity, cold/

clammy skin, cyanosis, extreme drowsiness progressing to seizures, stupor, coma. Tolerance to analgesic effect, physical dependence may occur with repeated use. Prolonged duration of action, cumulative effect may occur in those with hepatic/renal impairment. Concomitant use with benzodiazepines may result in profound sedation, respiratory depression, coma, and death. **Antidote:** Naloxone (see Appendix J).

NURSING CONSIDERATIONS

BASELINE ASSESSMENT

Obtain vital signs. If respirations are 12/min or less (20/min or less in children), withhold medication, contact physician. Assess risk of drug abuse, misuse, drug-seeking behavior. **Analgesic:** Assess onset, type, location, duration of pain. Effect of medication is reduced if full pain recurs before next dose. **Antitussive:** Assess type, severity, frequency of cough. Screen for misuse, abuse, drug-seeking behavior.

INTERVENTION/EVALUATION

Monitor vital signs; assess for pain relief, cough. To prevent pain cycles, instruct pt to request pain medication as soon as discomfort begins. Monitor daily pattern of bowel activity, stool consistency (esp. in long-term use). Initiate deep breathing and coughing exercises, particularly in pts with pulmonary impairment. Assess for clinical improvement; record onset of relief of pain, cough. Screen for misuse, abuse, drug-seeking behavior.

PATIENT/FAMILY TEACHING

• Avoid alcohol. • Avoid tasks that require alertness/motor skills until response to drug is established. • Tolerance or dependence may occur with prolonged use at high dosages. • Change positions slowly to avoid orthostatic hypotension. • Do not chew, crush, dissolve, or divide extended-release tablets.

hydrOXYzine

hye-**drox**-ee-zeen

(Atarax ✱, Novo-Hydroxyzin ✱, Vistaril)

Do not confuse hydrOXYzine with hydrALAZINE or hydroxyurea, or Vistaril with Restoril, Versed, or Zestril.

◆CLASSIFICATION

PHARMACOTHERAPEUTIC: Histamine H_1 antagonist (first generation). **CLINICAL:** Antihistamine, antianxiety, antispasmodic, antiemetic, antipruritic.

USES

Antiemetic, treatment of anxiety/agitation, antipruritic.

PRECAUTIONS

Contraindications: Hypersensitivity to hydrOXYzine. Early pregnancy; SQ, IV administration; pts with prolonged QT interval. **Cautions:** Narrow-angle glaucoma, prostatic hypertrophy, bladder neck obstruction, asthma, COPD, elderly.

ACTION

Competes with histamine for receptor sites in GI tract, blood vessels, respiratory tract. **Therapeutic Effect:** Produces anxiolytic, anticholinergic, antihistaminic, analgesic effects; relaxes skeletal muscle; controls nausea, vomiting.

PHARMACOKINETICS

Route	Onset	Peak	Duration
PO	15–30 min	N/A	4–6 hrs

Well absorbed from GI tract and after parenteral administration. Metabolized in liver. Primarily excreted in urine. Not removed by hemodialysis. **Half-life:** 3–7 hrs (increased in elderly, hepatic impairment).

⌛ LIFESPAN CONSIDERATIONS

Pregnancy/Lactation: Unknown if drug crosses placenta or is distributed in breast milk. **Children:** Not recommended in newborns or premature infants (increased risk of anticholinergic effects). Paradoxical excitement may occur. **Elderly:** Increased risk of dizziness, sedation, confusion. Hypotension, hyperexcitability may occur.

INTERACTIONS

DRUG: **QT interval–prolonging medications (e.g., amiodarone, azithromycin, ceritinib, haloperidol, moxifloxacin)** may increase risk of QT interval prolongation, torsades de pointes. **CNS depressants (e.g., alcohol, morphine, oxyCODONE, zolpidem)** may increase CNS depression. **Aclidinium, ipratropium, tiotropium, umeclidinium** may increase anticholinergic effect. **HERBAL:** **Herbals with sedative properties (e.g., chamomile, kava, kava, valerian)** may increase CNS depression. **FOOD:** None known. **LAB VALUES:** May cause false-positive urine 17-hydroxycorticosteroid determinations.

AVAILABILITY (Rx)

Oral Solution: 10 mg/5 mL. **Syrup:** 10 mg/5 mL. **Tablets:** 10 mg, 25 mg, 50 mg.

Capsules: 25 mg, 50 mg, 100 mg.

ADMINISTRATION/HANDLING

PO

• May give without regard to food. • Shake oral suspension well. • Scored tablets may be crushed; do not break, crush, or open capsule.

INDICATIONS/ROUTES/DOSAGE

Anxiety

Note: Initiate elderly dose at the lower end of recommended dosage.

PO: **ADULTS, ELDERLY:** 50–100 mg 4 times/day or 37.5–75 mg/day in divided doses. **CHILDREN 6 YRS AND OLDER:** 12.5–25 mg 3–4 times/day. **CHILDREN YOUNGER THAN 6 YRS:** 12.5 mg 3–4 times/day.

Pruritus

PO: **ADULTS, ELDERLY:** 25 mg 3–4 times/day. **CHILDREN 6 YRS AND OLDER:** 12.5–25 mg 3–4 times/day. **CHILDREN YOUNGER THAN 6 YRS:** 12.5 mg 3–4 times/day.

Dosage in Renal/Hepatic Impairment

No dose adjustment. Change dosing interval to q24h in pts with primary biliary cirrhosis.

SIDE EFFECTS

Side effects are generally mild, transient. **Frequent:** Drowsiness, dry mouth, marked discomfort with IM injection. **Occasional:** Dizziness, ataxia, asthenia, slurred speech, headache, agitation, increased anxiety. **Rare:** Paradoxical reactions (hyperactivity, anxiety in children; excitement, restlessness in elderly or debilitated pts) generally noted during first 2 wks of therapy, particularly in presence of uncontrolled pain.

ADVERSE EFFECTS/TOXIC REACTIONS

Hypersensitivity reaction (wheezing, dyspnea, chest tightness) may occur. QT interval prolongation, torsades de pointes have been reported. Acute generalized exanthematous pustulosis (AGEP) may occur.

NURSING CONSIDERATIONS

BASELINE ASSESSMENT

Anxiety: Offer emotional support. Assess motor responses (agitation, trembling, tension), autonomic responses (cold/clammy hands, diaphoresis). **Antiemetic:** Assess for dehydration (poor skin turgor, dry mucous membranes, longitudinal furrows in tongue).

INTERVENTION/EVALUATION

For pts on long-term therapy, CBC, BMP, LFT should be performed periodically. Monitor lung sounds for signs of hypersensitivity reaction. Monitor serum electrolytes in pts with severe vomiting. Assess for paradoxical reaction, particularly during early therapy. Assist with ambulation if drowsiness, light-headedness occur. Obtain ECG if palpitations occur or cardiac arrhythmia is suspected. Assess skin for rash, pustules.

PATIENT/FAMILY TEACHING

• Marked discomfort may occur with IM injection. • Sugarless gum, sips of water may relieve dry mouth. • Drowsiness usually diminishes with continued therapy. • Avoid tasks that require alertness, motor skills until response to drug is established. • Treatment may cause life-threatening heart arrhythmias; report chest pain, difficulty breathing, palpitations, passing out. Do not take newly prescribed medications unless approved by prescriber who originally started treatment.

H

ibandronate

eye-**ban**-droe-nate
(Boniva)

◆CLASSIFICATION

PHARMACOTHERAPEUTIC: Bisphosphonate. **CLINICAL:** Calcium regulator.

USES

Treatment/prevention of osteoporosis in postmenopausal women. **OFF-LABEL:** Hypercalcemia of malignancy; reduces bone pain and skeletal complications from metastatic bone disease due to breast cancer.

PRECAUTIONS

Contraindications: Hypersensitivity to ibandronate, other bisphosphonates; oral tablets in pts unable to stand or sit upright for at least 60 min; pts with abnormalities of the esophagus that would delay emptying (e.g., stricture, achalasia), hypocalcemia. **Cautions:** GI diseases (duodenitis, dysphagia, esophagitis, gastritis, ulcers [drug may exacerbate these conditions]), renal impairment with CrCl less than 30 mL/min.

ACTION

Inhibits bone resorption via activity on osteoclasts or osteoclast precursors. **Therapeutic Effect:** Reduces rate of bone resorption, resulting in indirect increased bone mineral density.

PHARMACOKINETICS

Absorbed in upper GI tract. Extent of absorption impaired by food, beverages (other than plain water). Protein binding: 85%–99%. Rapidly binds to bone. Unabsorbed portion excreted in urine. **Half-life: PO:** 37–157 hrs; **IV:** 5–25 hrs.

LIFESPAN CONSIDERATIONS

Pregnancy/Lactation: May cause fetal harm/malformations. Unknown if distributed in breast milk. Breastfeeding not recommended. **Children:** Safety and efficacy not established. **Elderly:** No age-related precautions noted.

INTERACTIONS

DRUG: Antacids, calcium, magnesium may decrease concentration/effect. **Aspirin, NSAIDs (e.g., ibuprofen, ketorolac, naproxen)** may increase adverse effects. **HERBAL:** None significant. **FOOD: Beverages (other than plain water), dietary supplements, dairy products, food** interfere with absorption. **LAB VALUES:** May decrease serum alkaline phosphatase. May increase serum cholesterol.

AVAILABILITY (Rx)

Injection Solution: 3 mg/3 mL syringe.
Tablets: 150 mg.

ADMINISTRATION/HANDLING

PO

• Give 60 min before first food or beverage of the day, on an empty stomach with 6–8 oz plain water (not mineral water) while pt is standing or sitting in upright position. • Pt cannot lie down for 60 min following administration. • Instruct pt to swallow whole; do not break, crush, dissolve, or divide tablet (potential for oropharyngeal ulceration).

IV

• Give over 15–30 sec. • Give over 1 hr for metastatic bone disease; over 1–2 hrs for hypercalcemia of malignancy.

INDICATIONS/ROUTES/DOSAGE

Note: May consider discontinuing after 3–5 yrs in pts at low risk for fracture. Consider supplemental calcium and vitamin D if dietary intake is inadequate.

Osteoporosis

PO (Prevention/Treatment): ADULTS, ELDERLY: 150 mg once monthly.
IV (Treatment): ADULTS, ELDERLY: 3 mg q3mos.

Dosage in Renal Impairment

Not recommended for pts with CrCl less than 30 mL/min.

Dosage in Hepatic Impairment
No dose adjustment.

SIDE EFFECTS

Frequent (13%–6%): Back pain, dyspepsia, peripheral discomfort, diarrhea, headache, myalgia. **IV:** Abdominal pain, dyspepsia, constipation, nausea, diarrhea. **Occasional (4%–3%):** Dizziness, arthralgia, asthenia. **Rare (2% or less):** Vomiting, hypersensitivity reaction.

ADVERSE EFFECTS/TOXIC REACTIONS

Upper respiratory infection occurs occasionally. Overdose results in hypocalcemia, hypophosphatemia, significant GI disturbances.

NURSING CONSIDERATIONS

BASELINE ASSESSMENT

Obtain serum calcium, vitamin D level. Hypocalcemia, vitamin D deficiency must be corrected before beginning therapy. Obtain results of bone density study.

INTERVENTION/EVALUATION

Monitor serum calcium, phosphate. Monitor renal function tests.

PATIENT/FAMILY TEACHING

• Expected benefits occur only when medication is taken with full glass (6–8 oz) of plain water, first thing in the morning and at least 60 min before first food, beverage, medication of the day. Any other beverage (mineral water, orange juice, coffee) significantly reduces absorption of medication. • Do not chew, crush, dissolve, or divide tablets; swallow whole. • Do not lie down for at least 60 min after taking medication (potentiates delivery to stomach, reduces risk of esophageal irritation). • Report swallowing difficulties, pain when swallowing, chest pain, new/worsening heartburn. • Consider weight-bearing exercises; modify behavioral factors (e.g., cigarette smoking, alcohol consumption). • Calcium and vitamin D supplements should be taken if dietary intake inadequate.

ibrutinib

eye-**broo**-ti-nib
(Imbruvica)
Do not confuse ibrutinib with axitinib, dasatinib, erlotinib, gefitinib, imatinib, nilotinib, PONATinib, SORAfenib, SUNItinib, or vandetanib.

◆CLASSIFICATION

PHARMACOTHERAPEUTIC: Bruton tyrosine kinase inhibitor. **CLINICAL:** Antineoplastic.

USES

Treatment of pts with mantle cell lymphoma (MCL) who have received at least one prior therapy, chronic lymphocytic leukemia and small lymphocytic lymphoma (CLL/SLL) (as monotherapy or in combination with bendamustine and riTUXimab or with obinutuzumab), CLL/SLL with 17p deletion, treatment of Waldenstrom's macroglobulinemia (WM) (as monotherapy or in combination with rituximab). Marginal zone lymphoma (MZL) requiring systemic therapy and having received at least one prior anti-CD-20–based therapy. Treatment of chronic graft-versus-host disease (CGVHD) after failure of at least one line of systemic therapy.

PRECAUTIONS

Contraindications: Hypersensitivity to ibrutinib. **Cautions:** Hepatic/renal impairment, elderly, pregnancy, history of GI disease (e.g., bleeding, ulcers); pts at high risk for tumor lysis syndrome (high tumor burden).

ACTION

Inhibits enzymatic activity of Bruton's tyrosine kinase (BTK), a signaling molecule that promotes malignant B-cell proliferation and survival. **Therapeutic Effect:** Decreases malignant B-cell proliferation and survival.

PHARMACOKINETICS

Readily absorbed following PO. Metabolized in liver. Peak plasma concentration: 1–2 hrs. Protein binding: 97%. Excreted in feces (80%), urine (10%). **Half-life:** 4–6 hrs.

LIFESPAN CONSIDERATIONS

Pregnancy/Lactation: May cause fetal harm. Avoid pregnancy. Unknown if distributed in breast milk. Must either discontinue drug or discontinue breastfeeding. **Children:** Safety and efficacy not established. **Elderly:** Increased risk of cardiac events (atrial fibrillation, hypertension), infections (pneumonia, cellulitis), GI events (diarrhea, dehydration, bleeding).

INTERACTIONS

DRUG: **Strong CYP3A4 inhibitors (e.g., ketoconazole, clarithromycin)** may increase plasma concentration/effect; avoid use. **Strong CYP3A4 inducers (e.g., carBAMazepine, rifAMPin, phenytoin)** may decrease plasma concentration/effect; avoid use. **Anticoagulants (e.g., warfarin), antiplatelets (e.g., aspirin, clopidogrel), NSAIDs** may increase risk of bleeding. May decrease the therapeutic effect of **BCG (intravesical), vaccines (live).** May increase adverse/toxic effects of **natalizumab, vaccines (live).** HERBAL: **St. John's wort** may decrease concentration/effect. FOOD: **Grapefruit products, Seville oranges** may increase concentration/effect. **Bitter orange** may increase concentration/effect. LAB VALUES: May decrease Hgb, Hct, neutrophils, platelets.

AVAILABILITY (Rx)

Capsules: 70 mg, 140 mg. **Tablets:** 140 mg, 280 mg, 420 mg, 560 mg.

ADMINISTRATION/HANDLING

PO

• Give with water. • Swallow capsules/tablets whole. Do not break, cut, or open capsules. Do not break, cut, crush, or divide tablets. Capsules/tablets cannot be chewed.

INDICATIONS/ROUTES/DOSAGE

MCL, MZL

PO: ADULTS, ELDERLY: 560 mg once daily. Continue until disease progression or unacceptable toxicity.

WM, CGVHD

PO: ADULTS, ELDERLY: 420 mg once daily. Continue until disease progression or unacceptable toxicity.

CLL/SLL

PO: ADULTS, ELDERLY: 420 mg once daily (as monotherapy, or in combination with rituximab or obinutuzumab, or in combination with bendamustine and rituximab). Continue until disease progression or unacceptable toxicity.

Dose Modification

Based on Common Terminology Criteria for Adverse Events (CTCAE).

Any Grade 3 or Greater Nonhematologic Event, Grade 3 or Greater Neutropenia with Infection or Fever, or Any Grade 4 Hematologic Toxicities

Interrupt treatment until resolution to Grade 1 or baseline, then restart at initial dose. If toxicity recurs, interrupt treatment until resolution to Grade 1 or baseline, then reduce dose to 420 mg daily (one capsule less). If toxicity recurs, interrupt treatment until resolution to Grade 1 or baseline, then reduce dose to 280 mg once daily (one capsule less). If toxicity still occurs at 280 mg dose, discontinue treatment.

Concomitant Use of Moderate CYP3A4 Inhibitors (e.g., fluconazole, dilTIAZem, verapamil)

Start at reduced dose of 140 mg daily. If toxicity occurs, either discontinue treatment or find alternate agent with less CYP3A inhibition.

Concomitant Short-Term Use of Strong CYP3A4 Inhibitors (7 days or less) (e.g., antifungals, antibiotics)

Interrupt treatment until strong CYP3A medications no longer needed.

I

Concomitant Chronic Use of Strong CYP3A4 Inhibitors or Inducers

Treatment not recommended.

Dosage in Renal Impairment

No dose adjustment.

Dosage in Hepatic Impairment

Mild impairment: Decrease dose to 140 mg. **Moderate to severe impairment:** Avoid use.

SIDE EFFECTS

Frequent (51%–23%): Diarrhea, fatigue, musculoskeletal pain, peripheral edema, nausea, bruising, dyspnea, constipation, rash, abdominal pain, vomiting. **Occasional (21%–11%):** Decreased appetite, cough, pyrexia, stomatitis, asthenia, dizziness, muscle spasms, dehydration, headache, dyspepsia, petechiae, arthralgia.

ADVERSE EFFECTS/TOXIC REACTIONS

Anemia, lymphopenia, neutropenia, thrombocytopenia are expected responses to therapy. Severe myelosuppression (Grade 3–4 CTCAE) reported in 41% of pts: neutropenia (29%), thrombocytopenia (17%), anemia (9%). Infections including upper respiratory tract infection, UTI, pneumonia, skin infection, sinusitis were reported. Hemorrhagic events including epistaxis, GI bleeding, hematuria, intracranial hemorrhage, subdural hematoma reported in 5% of pts. Serious and fatal cases of renal toxicity reported: increased serum creatinine 1.5 times upper limit of normal (ULN) (67% of pts), increased serum creatinine 1.53 times ULN (9% of pts). Second primary malignancies including skin cancer (4%), other carcinomas (1%) occurred. Fatal cardiac arrhythmias (ventricular tachycardia, atrial fibrillation, atrial flutter) may occur. Tumor lysis syndrome may present as acute renal failure, hypocalcemia, hyperuricemia, hyperphosphatemia.

NURSING CONSIDERATIONS

BASELINE ASSESSMENT

Obtain baseline vital signs, CBC, serum chemistries, LFT, PT/INR if on anticoagulants. Question history of arrhythmias, HF, GI bleed, hepatic/renal impairment, peripheral edema, pulmonary disease. Obtain negative pregnancy test before initiating treatment. Assess hydration status. Receive full medication history including herbal products. Assess skin for open/unhealed wounds, lesions, moles. Assess risk of tumor lysis syndrome. Conduct baseline neurologic exam. Offer emotional support.

INTERVENTION/EVALUATION

Monitor CBC monthly; LFT, serum chemistries, renal function routinely. Monitor stool frequency, consistency, characteristics. Immediately report hemorrhagic events: epistaxis, hematuria, hemoptysis, melena. Monitor serum uric acid level if tumor lysis syndrome (acute renal failure, electrolyte imbalance, cardiac arrhythmias, seizures) is suspected. Obtain ECG for arrhythmias, dyspnea, palpitations. Screen for possible intracranial hemorrhage: altered mental status, aphasia, hemiparesis, unequal pupils, homonymous hemianopsia (blindness of one half of vision on same side of both eyes). Monitor for renal toxicity (anuria, hypertension, generalized edema, flank pain). Assess skin for new lesions.

PATIENT/FAMILY TEACHING

• Treatment may depress your immune system response and reduce your ability to fight infection. Report symptoms of infection such as body aches, chills, cough, fatigue, fever. Avoid those with active infection. • Report symptoms of bone marrow depression such as bruising, fatigue, fever, shortness of breath, weight loss; bleeding easily, bloody urine or stool. • Report palpitations, chest pain, shortness of breath, dizziness, fainting; may indicate arrhythmia. • Therapy may cause life-threatening tumor lysis syndrome (a condition caused by the rapid breakdown of cancer cells), which can cause kidney failure. Report decreased urination, amber-colored urine; confusion, difficulty breathing, fatigue, fever, muscle or joint pain, palpitations, seizures, vomiting. • Report any black/tarry stools, bruising, nausea, RUQ abdominal pain, yellowing of skin or eyes, palpitations, nose bleeds, blood in urine or stool, decreased urine output. • Avoid alcohol. • Do not take herbal products. • Do not ingest grapefruit products. • Severe diarrhea may lead to dehydration. • Contact physician before any planned surgical/dental procedures. • Immediately report neurological changes: confusion, one-sided paralysis, difficulty speaking, partial blindness. • Do not receive live vaccines. • Do not break, crush, or open capsule.

ibuprofen

eye-bue-**pro**-fen
(Advil, Caldolor, Motrin, NeoProfen)

BLACK BOX ALERT Increased risk of serious cardiovascular thrombotic events, including myocardial infarction, CVA. Contraindicated in setting of CABG surgery. Increased risk of severe GI reactions, including ulceration, bleeding, perforation.

Do not confuse Motrin with Neurontin or Advil with Aleve.

FIXED-COMBINATION(S)

Children's Advil Cold: ibuprofen/pseudoephedrine (a nasal decongestant): 100 mg/15 mg per 5 mL. **Combunox:** ibuprofen/oxyCODONE (a narcotic analgesic): 400 mg/5 mg. **Duexis:** ibuprofen/famotidine (an H_2 antagonist): 800 mg/26.6 mg. **Reprexain CIII:** ibuprofen/HYDROcodone (a narcotic analgesic): 200 mg/5 mg. **Vicoprofen:** ibuprofen/HYDROcodone (a narcotic analgesic): 200 mg/7.5 mg.

CLASSIFICATION

PHARMACOTHERAPEUTIC: NSAID. **CLINICAL:** Antirheumatic, analgesic, antipyretic, antidysmenorrheal, vascular headache suppressant.

USES

Oral: Treatment of fever, inflammatory disease, and rheumatoid disorders, osteoarthritis, mild to moderate pain, primary dysmenorrhea. **Caldolor:** Mild to moderate pain; severe pain in combination with an opioid analgesic; fever. **NeoProfen:** To close a clinically significant patent ductus arteriosus (PDA) in premature infants weighing between 500 and 1,500 g who are no more than 32 wks gestational age when usual medical management is ineffective. **OFF-LABEL:** Treatment of cystic fibrosis, pericarditis. Juvenile idiopathic arthritis.

PRECAUTIONS

Contraindications: History of hypersensitivity to ibuprofen, aspirin, other NSAIDs. Treatment of perioperative pain in coronary artery bypass graft (CABG) surgery. Aspirin triad (bronchial asthma, aspirin intolerance, rhinitis). **NeoProfen:** Preterm neonates with proven or suspected untreated infection, elevated total bilirubin, congenital heart disease in whom patency of the patent ductus arteriosus is necessary for satisfactory pulmonary or systemic blood flow (e.g., pulmonary atresia), bleeding, thrombocytopenia, coagulation defects, proven or suspected necrotizing enterocolitis, significant renal impairment. **Cautions:** Pts with fluid retention, HF, dehydration, coagulation disorders, concurrent use with aspirin, anticoagulants, steroids; history of GI disease (e.g., bleeding, ulcers), smoking, use of alcohol, elderly, debilitated pts, hepatic/renal impairment, asthma.

ACTION

Reversibly inhibits COX-1 and COX-2 enzymes, resulting in decreased formation

I

of prostaglandin precursors. **Therapeutic Effect:** Produces analgesic, anti-inflammatory effects; decreases fever.

PHARMACOKINETICS

Route	Onset	Peak	Duration
PO (analgesic)	0.5 hr	N/A	4–6 hrs
PO (antirheumatic)	2 days	1–2 wks	N/A

Rapidly absorbed from GI tract. Protein binding: 90%–99%. Metabolized in liver. Primarily excreted in urine. Not removed by hemodialysis. **Half-life:** 2–4 hrs.

LIFESPAN CONSIDERATIONS

Pregnancy/Lactation: Unknown if drug crosses placenta or is distributed in breast milk. Avoid use during third trimester (may adversely affect fetal cardiovascular system: premature closure of ductus arteriosus). **Children:** Safety and efficacy not established in pts younger than 6 mos. **Elderly:** GI bleeding, ulceration more likely to cause serious adverse effects. Age-related renal impairment may increase risk of hepatic/renal toxicity; reduced dosage recommended.

INTERACTIONS

DRUG: May decrease effects of **antihypertensives (e.g., amLODIPine, lisinopril, valsartan), diuretics (e.g., furosemide). Aspirin, other salicylates** may increase risk of GI side effects, bleeding. May increase effect of **apixaban, dabigatran, edoxaban, rivaroxaban, warfarin. Bile acid sequestrants (e.g., cholestyramine)** may decrease absorption/effect. May increase nephrotoxic effect of **cycloSPORINE.** May increase concentration, risk of toxicity of **lithium, methotrexate.** **HERBAL:** **Glucosamine, herbs with anticoagulant/antiplatelet properties (e.g., garlic, ginger, ginseng, ginkgo biloba)** may increase concentration/effect. **FOOD:** None known. **LAB VALUES:** May prolong bleeding time. May alter serum glucose level. May increase serum BUN, creatinine, potassium, ALT, AST. May decrease serum calcium, glucose; Hgb, Hct, platelets.

AVAILABILITY (Rx)

Capsules: 200 mg. **Injection, Solution:** ***(NeoProfen):*** 10 mg/mL. ***(Caldolor):*** 100 mg/mL. **Suspension, Oral:** 100 mg/5 mL. **Suspension, Oral Drops:** 40 mg/mL. **Tablets:** 200 mg, 400 mg, 600 mg, 800 mg. **Tablets, Chewable:** 100 mg.

ADMINISTRATION/HANDLING

IV (Caldolor)

Reconstitution • Dilute with D_5W or 0.9% NaCl to final concentration of 4 mg/mL or less.

Rate of administration • Infuse over at least 30 min.

Storage • Store at room temperature. • Stable for 24 hrs after dilution.

IV (NeoProfen)

Reconstitution • Dilute to appropriate volume with D_5W or 0.9% NaCl. • Discard any remaining medication after first withdrawal from vial.

Rate of administration • Administer via IV port nearest the insertion site. • Infuse continuously over 15 min.

Storage • Store at room temperature. • Stable for 30 min after dilution.

PO

• Give with food, milk, antacids if GI distress occurs.

INDICATIONS/ROUTES/DOSAGE

Fever

PO: ADULTS, ELDERLY: 200–400 mg q4–6h prn. **CHILDREN 12 YRS AND OLDER, ADOLESCENTS:** 200–400 mg q4-6h prn. **Maximum daily dose:** 1,200 mg/day. **CHILDREN 6 MOS AND OLDER:**

Weight		Dosage	
kg	lbs	Age	(mg)
5.4–8.1	12–17	6–11 mos	50
8.2–10.8	18–23	12–23 mos	75
10.9–16.3	24–35	2–3 yrs	100
16.4–21.7	36–47	4–5 yrs	150

Weight		Dosage	
kg	lbs	Age	(mg)
21.8–27.2	48–59	6–8 yrs	200
27.3–32.6	60–71	9–10 yrs	250
32.7–43.2	72–95	11 yrs	300

IV: ADULTS, ELDERLY: 400 mg q4–6h or 100–200 mg q4h prn. **Maximum:** 3.2 g/day. **CHILDREN 12–17 YRS:** 400 mg q4–6h prn. **Maximum:** 2,400 mg/day. **CHILDREN 6 MOS–11 YRS:** 10 mg/kg q4–6h prn. **Maximum dose:** 400 mg. **Maximum:** 40 mg/kg up to 2,400 mg/day.

Osteoarthritis, Rheumatoid Disorders
PO: ADULTS, ELDERLY: 400–800 mg 3–4 times/day. **Maximum:** 3.2 g/day.

Pain
PO: ADULTS, ELDERLY: 200–400 mg q4–6h prn. **Maximum:** 3,200 mg/day. **CHILDREN 12 YRS AND OLDER, ADOLESCENTS:** 200-400 mg q4-6h prn. **Maximum daily dose:** 1,200 mg/day. **CHILDREN 6 MOS–11 YRS:** See chart under Fever dosing.
IV: ADULTS, ELDERLY: 400–800 mg q6h prn. **Maximum:** 3.2 g/day. **CHILDREN, ADOLESCENTS: (12–17 yrs):** 400 mg q4–6h prn. **Maximum:** 2,400 mg/day. **(6 MOS–12 YRS):** 10 mg/kg (**maximum dose:** 400 mg) q4–6h prn. **Maximum:** 40 mg/kg/day or 2,400 mg, whichever is less.

Primary Dysmenorrhea
PO: ADULTS: 200–800 mg q4–6h prn. **Maximum:** 2,400 mg/day.

Patent Ductus Arteriosus (PDA)
IV: INFANTS: Initially, 10 mg/kg followed by 2 doses of 5 mg/kg at 24 hrs and 48 hrs. All doses based on birth weight.

Dosage in Renal Impairment
Hold if anuria or oliguria evident. Avoid use in severe impairment.

Dosage in Hepatic Impairment
Avoid use in severe impairment.

SIDE EFFECTS

Occasional (9%–3%): Nausea, vomiting, dyspepsia, dizziness, rash. **Rare (less than 3%):** Diarrhea or constipation, flatulence, abdominal cramps or pain, pruritus, increased B/P.

ADVERSE EFFECTS/TOXIC REACTIONS

Overdose may result in metabolic acidosis. Rare reactions with long-term use include peptic ulcer, GI bleeding, gastritis, severe hepatic reaction (cholestasis, jaundice), nephrotoxicity (dysuria, hematuria, proteinuria, nephrotic syndrome), severe hypersensitivity reaction (particularly in pts with systemic lupus erythematosus or other collagen diseases). **NeoProfen:** Hypoglycemia, hypocalcemia, respiratory failure, UTI, edema, atelectasis may occur. **Caldolor:** Abdominal pain, anemia, cough, dizziness, dyspnea, edema, hypertension, nausea, vomiting have been reported.

NURSING CONSIDERATIONS

BASELINE ASSESSMENT

Assess onset, type, location, duration of pain, inflammation. Inspect appearance of affected joints for immobility, deformities, skin condition. Assess temperature. Question medical history as listed in Precautions.

INTERVENTION/EVALUATION

Monitor for evidence of nausea, dyspepsia. Assess skin for rash. Observe for bleeding, bruising, occult blood loss. Evaluate for therapeutic response: relief of pain, stiffness, swelling; increased joint mobility; reduced joint tenderness; improved grip strength. Monitor for fever.

PATIENT/FAMILY TEACHING

• Avoid aspirin, alcohol during therapy (increases risk of GI bleeding). • If GI upset occurs, take with food, milk, antacids. • May cause dizziness. • Report ringing in ears, persistent stomach pain, respiratory difficulty, unusual bruising/bleeding, swelling of extremities, chest pain/palpitations.

I

idelalisib

eye-**del**-a-**lis**-ib
(Zydelig)

■ **BLACK BOX ALERT** ■ Fatal and/or serious hepatotoxicity may occur. Monitor LFT prior to and during treatment. Fatal and/or serious and severe diarrhea or colitis may occur. Monitor for GI symptoms. Fatal and serious pneumonitis may occur. Monitor for pulmonary symptoms and bilateral interstitial infiltrates. Interrupt, then reduce or discontinue treatment if hepatotoxicity, severe diarrhea, or pneumonitis occurs. Fatal and serious intestinal perforation may occur. Discontinue if perforation suspected.

I

◆CLASSIFICATION

PHARMACOTHERAPEUTIC: Phosphatidylinositol 3-kinase inhibitor. **CLINICAL:** Antineoplastic.

USES

Treatment of relapsed chronic lymphocytic leukemia (CLL), in combination with riTUXimab, in pts for whom riTUXimab alone would not be considered appropriate therapy due to other comorbidities. Treatment of relapsed follicular B-cell non-Hodgkin's lymphoma (FL) or relapsed small lymphocytic lymphoma (SLL) in pts who have received at least two prior systemic therapies.

PRECAUTIONS

Contraindications: History of serious allergic reactions to idelalisib (e.g., anaphylaxis, toxic epidermal necrolysis). **Cautions:** Baseline anemia, leukopenia, neutropenia, thrombocytopenia; GI bleeding, hepatic impairment. Pts with active infection, high tumor burden. Avoid concomitant use of hepatotoxic or promotility medications.

ACTION

Inhibits phosphatidylinositol 3-kinase, which is highly expressed in malignant lymphoid B cells. Inhibits several cell-signaling pathways, including B-cell receptor signaling and CXCR4 and CXCR5 signaling, which are involved in trafficking B cells to lymph nodes and bone marrow. **Therapeutic Effect:** Inhibits tumor cell growth and metastasis.

PHARMACOKINETICS

Readily absorbed. Metabolized in liver. Protein binding: 84%. Peak plasma concentration: 1.5 hrs. Excreted in feces (78%), urine (14%). **Half-life:** 8.3 hrs.

⌛ LIFESPAN CONSIDERATIONS

Pregnancy/Lactation: May cause fetal harm; avoid pregnancy. Use effective contraception during treatment and for at least 1 mo after discontinuation. Unknown if distributed in breast milk. Must either discontinue drug or discontinue breastfeeding. **Children:** Safety and efficacy not established. **Elderly:** May have increased risk of side effects/adverse reactions.

INTERACTIONS

DRUG: **Strong CYP3A4 inducers (e.g., carBAMazepine, rifAMPin, phenytoin)** may decrease concentration/effect. **Strong CYP3A4 inhibitors (clarithromycin, ketoconazole, ritonavir)** may increase concentration/effect. May increase adverse effects of **natalizumab, vaccines (live).** May decrease therapeutic effect of **BCG (intravesical), vaccines (live).** **HERBAL:** **St. John's wort** may decrease concentration/effect. **Echinacea** may decrease therapeutic effect. **FOOD:** None known. **LAB VALUES:** May increase serum ALT, AST, bilirubin, GGT; triglycerides. May decrease Hgb, neutrophils, platelets, serum sodium. May increase or decrease lymphocytes, serum glucose.

AVAILABILITY (Rx)

Tablets: 100 mg, 150 mg.

ADMINISTRATION/HANDLING

PO

• Give without regard to food. • Swallow tablets whole.

INDICATIONS/ROUTES/DOSAGE

Chronic Lymphocytic Leukemia (in combination with riTUXimab), Follicular B-cell Non-Hodgkin's Lymphoma, Small Lymphocytic Lymphoma

PO: ADULTS/ELDERLY: 150 mg twice daily. Continue until disease progression or unacceptable toxicity.

Dose Modification

Hepatotoxicity

Elevated serum ALT, AST 3–5 times upper limit of normal (ULN): Maintain dose. **5–20 times ULN:** Monitor serum ALT, AST wkly. Withhold until ALT, AST less than 1 time ULN, then resume at 100 mg twice daily. **Greater than 20 times ULN:** Permanently discontinue.

Elevated Serum Bilirubin

1.5–3 times ULN: Monitor serum bilirubin wkly. Maintain dose. **3–10 times ULN:** Monitor serum bilirubin wkly. Withhold until bilirubin less than 1 time ULN, then resume at 100-mg dose. **Greater than 10 times ULN:** Permanently discontinue.

Diarrhea

Moderate diarrhea: Maintain dose. **Severe diarrhea or hospitalization:** Withhold until resolved, then resume at 100-mg dose. **Life-threatening diarrhea:** Permanently discontinue.

Neutropenia

ANC 1,000–1,500 cells/mm^3: Maintain dose. **ANC 500–1,000 cells/mm^3:** Monitor ANC wkly and maintain dose. **ANC less than 500 cells/mm^3:** Permanently discontinue.

Thrombocytopenia

Platelets 50,000–75,000 cells/mm^3: Maintain dose. **Platelets 25,000–50,000 cells/mm^3:** Monitor platelet count wkly and maintain dose. **Platelets less than 25,000 cells/mm^3:** Monitor platelet count wkly. Withhold until platelets greater than 25,000 cells/mm^3, then resume at 100-mg dose.

Pneumonitis

Any symptoms: Permanently discontinue.

Dosage in Renal Impairment

No dose adjustment.

Dosage in Hepatic Impairment

Use caution. See dose modification.

SIDE EFFECTS

CLL

Frequent (35%–21%): Pyrexia, nausea, diarrhea, chills. **Occasional (10%–5%):** Headache, vomiting, generalized pain, arthralgia, stomatitis, gastric reflux, nasal congestion.

Non-Hodgkin's Lymphoma

Frequent (47%–21%): Diarrhea, fatigue, nausea, cough, pyrexia, abdominal pain, rash. **Occasional (17%–10%):** Dyspnea, decreased appetite, vomiting, asthenia, night sweats, insomnia, headache, peripheral edema.

ADVERSE EFFECTS/TOXIC REACTIONS

Thrombocytopenia, neutropenia, leukopenia, lymphopenia are expected responses to therapy, but more severe reactions, including bone marrow failure, febrile neutropenia, may occur. Fatal and/or serious events including hepatotoxicity (14% of pts), severe diarrhea or colitis (14% of pts), hypersensitivity reactions (including anaphylaxis), pneumonitis, intestinal perforation were reported. Neutropenia occurred in 31% of pts, which may greatly increase risk of infection. Severe skin reactions including toxic epidermal necrolysis, generalized rash, exfoliative rash were reported. Other infections may include bronchitis, *C. difficile* colitis, pneumonia, sepsis, UTI. Fatal and/or serious intestinal perforation may occur.

NURSING CONSIDERATIONS

BASELINE ASSESSMENT

Obtain ANC, CBC, BMP, pregnancy test in females of reproductive potential. Receive full medication history including herbal products. Question history of hypersensitivity reaction or acute skin reactions to drug class. Perform full dermatologic exam with routine assessment. Offer emotional support.

INTERVENTION/EVALUATION

Monitor CBC frequently. Any interruption of therapy or dosage change may require wkly lab monitoring until symptoms resolve. Obtain *C. difficile* toxin PCR if severe diarrhea occurs. Screen for acute cutaneous reactions, allergic reactions, other acute infections (sepsis, UTI), hepatic impairment, pulmonary events (dyspnea, pneumonitis, pneumonia), or tumor lysis syndrome (electrolyte imbalance, uric acid nephropathy, acute renal failure). Monitor strict I&O, hydration status, stool frequency and consistency.

PATIENT/FAMILY TEACHING

• Treatment may depress your immune system response and reduce your ability to fight infection. Report symptoms of infection such as body aches, chills, cough, fatigue, fever. Avoid those with active infection. • Report symptoms of bone marrow depression such as bruising, fatigue, fever, shortness of breath, weight loss; bleeding easily, bloody urine or stool. • Avoid pregnancy; do not breastfeed. • Report abdominal pain, amber or bloody urine, bruising, black/tarry stools, persistent diarrhea, yellowing of skin or eyes. • Avoid alcohol. • Immediately report difficult breathing, severe coughing, chest tightness. • Therapy may cause severe allergic reactions, intestinal tearing, or skin rashes or severe diarrhea related to an infected colon. • Do not take any over-the-counter medications including herbal products unless approved by your doctor.

ifosfamide HIGH ALERT

eye-**fos**-fa-mide
(Ifex)

■ BLACK BOX ALERT ■ Hemorrhagic cystitis may occur. Severe myelosuppressant. May cause CNS toxicity, including confusion, coma. Must be administered by personnel trained in administration/handling of chemotherapeutic agents. May cause severe nephrotoxicity, resulting in renal failure.

Do not confuse ifosfamide with cyclophosphamide.

◆CLASSIFICATION

PHARMACOTHERAPEUTIC: Alkylating agent. **CLINICAL:** Antineoplastic.

USES

Treatment of germ cell testicular carcinoma (used in combination with other chemotherapy agents and with concurrent mesna for prophylaxis of hemorrhagic cystitis). **OFF-LABEL:** Small-cell lung, non–small-cell lung, ovarian, cervical, bladder cancer; soft tissue sarcomas, Hodgkin's, non-Hodgkin's lymphomas; osteosarcoma; head and neck, Ewing's sarcoma.

PRECAUTIONS

Contraindications: Hypersensitivity to ifosfamide. Urinary outflow obstruction. **Cautions:** Renal/hepatic impairment, compromised bone marrow reserve, active urinary tract infection, preexisting cardiac disease, prior radiation therapy, conditions predisposing to infection (e.g., diabetes, renal failure, immunocompromised pts, open wounds). Avoid use in pts with WBCs less than 2,000 cells/mm^3 and platelets less than 50,000 cells/mm^3.

ACTION

Inhibits DNA, protein synthesis by cross-linking with DNA strands, preventing cell growth. **Therapeutic Effect:** Produces cellular death (apoptosis).

PHARMACOKINETICS

Metabolized in liver. Protein binding: negligible. Crosses blood-brain barrier (to a limited extent). Primarily excreted in urine. Removed by hemodialysis. **Half-life:** 11–15 hrs (high dose); 4–7 hrs (low dose).

LIFESPAN CONSIDERATIONS

Pregnancy/Lactation: If possible, avoid use during pregnancy, esp. first trimester. Males must use effective contraception and not conceive a child during treatment and for at least 6 months after discontinuation. May cause fetal harm. Distributed in breast milk. Breastfeeding not recommended. **Children:** Not intended for this pt population. **Elderly:** Age-related renal impairment may require dosage adjustment.

INTERACTIONS

DRUG: **Bone marrow depressants (e.g., cladribine)** may increase myelosuppression. **Live virus vaccines** may potentiate virus replication, increase vaccine side effects, decrease pt's antibody response to vaccine. **HERBAL:** **Echinacea** may decrease therapeutic effect. **FOOD:** None known. **LAB VALUES:** May increase serum BUN, bilirubin, creatinine, uric acid, ALT, AST.

AVAILABILITY (Rx)

Injection, Powder for Reconstitution: *(Ifex)*: 1 g, 3 g. **Injection, Solution:** 50 mg/mL.

ADMINISTRATION/HANDLING

◀ALERT▶ Hemorrhagic cystitis occurs if mesna is not given concurrently. Mesna should always be given with ifosfamide.

IV

Reconstitution • Reconstitute vial with Sterile Water for Injection or Bacteriostatic Water for Injection to provide concentration of 50 mg/mL. Shake to dissolve. • Further dilute with 50–1,000 mL D_5W or 0.9% NaCl to provide concentration of 0.6–20 mg/mL.

Rate of administration • Infuse over minimum of 30 min. • Give with at least 2,000 mL PO or IV fluid (prevents bladder toxicity). • Give with protectant against hemorrhagic cystitis (i.e., mesna).

Storage • Store vials of powder at room temperature. • Refrigerate vials of solution. • After reconstitution with Bacteriostatic Water for Injection, vials and diluted solutions stable for 24 hrs if refrigerated.

IV INCOMPATIBILITIES

Cefepime (Maxipime), methotrexate.

IV COMPATIBILITIES

Granisetron (Kytril), ondansetron (Zofran).

INDICATIONS/ROUTES/DOSAGE

◀ALERT▶ Dosage individualized based on clinical response, tolerance to adverse effects. When used in combination therapy, consult specific protocols for optimum dosage, sequence of drug administration.

Germ Cell Testicular Carcinoma

IV: ADULTS: 1,200 mg/m²/day for 5 consecutive days. Repeat q3wks or after recovery from hematologic toxicity. Administer with mesna and hydration (to prevent bladder toxicity).

Dosage in Renal/Hepatic Impairment

Use caution.

SIDE EFFECTS

Frequent (83%–58%): Alopecia, nausea, vomiting. **Occasional (15%–5%):** Confusion, drowsiness, hallucinations, infection. **Rare (less than 5%):** Dizziness, seizures, disorientation, fever, malaise, stomatitis (mucosal irritation, glossitis, gingivitis).

ADVERSE EFFECTS/TOXIC REACTIONS

Hemorrhagic cystitis with hematuria, dysuria occurs frequently if protective agent (mesna) is not used. Myelosuppression (leukopenia, thrombocytopenia) occurs frequently. Pulmonary toxicity, hepatotoxicity, nephrotoxicity, cardiotoxicity, CNS toxicity (confusion, hallucinations, drowsiness, coma) may require discontinuation of therapy. Secondary malignancies including lymphoma, thyroid cancer, sarcoma were reported. Veno-occlusive hepatic disease may occur. May impair healing of wounds.

NURSING CONSIDERATIONS

BASELINE ASSESSMENT

Obtain urinalysis before each dose. If hematuria occurs (greater than 10 RBCs per field), therapy should be withheld until resolution occurs. Obtain WBC, platelet count, Hgb before each dose. Offer emotional support.

INTERVENTION/EVALUATION

Monitor hematologic studies, urinalysis, renal function, LFT. Assess for fever, sore throat, signs of local infection, unusual bruising/bleeding from any site, symptoms of anemia (excessive fatigue, weakness). Monitor for toxicities.

PATIENT/FAMILY TEACHING

• Treatment may depress your immune system response and reduce your ability to fight infection. Report symptoms of infection such as body aches, chills, cough, fatigue, fever. Avoid those with active infection. • Drink plenty of fluids (protects against cystitis). • Do not have immunizations without physician's approval (drug lowers resistance). • Avoid contact with those who have recently received live virus vaccine. • Avoid crowds, those with infections. • Report unusual bleeding/bruising, fever, chills, sore throat, joint pain, sores in mouth or on lips, yellowing skin or eyes.

iloperidone

eye-loe-**per**-i-doan
(Fanapt, Fanapt Titration Pack)

BLACK BOX ALERT Elderly pts with dementia-related psychosis are at increased risk for mortality due to cerebrovascular events.

Do not confuse iloperidone with amiodarone or dronedarone.

◆CLASSIFICATION

PHARMACOTHERAPEUTIC: Second-generation (atypical) antipsychotic. **CLINICAL:** Antipsychotic.

USES

Acute treatment of schizophrenia in adults.

PRECAUTIONS

Contraindications: Hypersensitivity to iloperidone. **Cautions:** Cardiovascular disease (HF, history of MI, ischemia, cardiac conduction abnormalities), cerebrovascular disease (increases risk of CVA in pts with dementia, seizure disorders). Pts at risk for orthostatic hypotension. Pts with bradycardia, hypokalemia, hypomagnesemia may be at greater risk for torsades de pointes. History of seizures, conditions lowering seizure threshold, high risk of suicide, risk of aspiration pneumonia, congenital QT syndrome, concurrent use of medications that prolong QT interval, decreased GI motility, urinary retention, BPH, xerostomia, visual problems, hepatic impairment, narrow-angle glaucoma, diabetes, elderly.

ACTION

Mixed combination of DOPamine type 2 (D_2) and serotonin type 2 ($5\text{-}HT_2$) antagonisms (thought to improve negative symptoms of psychosis). **Therapeutic Effect:** Diminishes symptoms of schizophrenia and reduces incidence of extrapyramidal side effects.

PHARMACOKINETICS

Steady-state concentration occurs in 3–4 days. Well absorbed from GI tract (unaffected by food). Protein binding: 95%. Metabolized in liver. Primarily excreted in urine, with a lesser amount excreted in feces. **Half-life:** 18–33 hrs.

⌛ LIFESPAN CONSIDERATIONS

Pregnancy/Lactation: Unknown if drug crosses placenta or is excreted in breast milk. Breastfeeding not recommended. **Children:** Safety and efficacy not established. **Elderly:** More susceptible to postural hypotension. Increased risk of cerebrovascular events, mortality, including stroke in elderly pts with psychosis.

INTERACTIONS

DRUG: **Alcohol, CNS depressants (e.g., diphenhydrAMINE, LORazepam, morphine)** may increase CNS depression. **Strong CYP3A4 inhibitors (e.g., clarithromycin, ketoconazole, ritonavir), strong CYP2D6 inhibitors (e.g., FLUoxetine, PARoxetine)** may increase concentration/ effect. **Medications causing prolongation of QT interval (e.g., amiodarone, dofetilide, sotalol)** may increase effects on cardiac conduction, leading to malignant arrhythmias (torsades de pointes). HERBAL: **Herbals with sedative properties (e.g., chamomile, kava kava, valerian)** may increase CNS depression. FOOD: None known. LAB VALUES: May increase serum prolactin levels.

AVAILABILITY (Rx)

Tablets: 1 mg, 2 mg, 4 mg, 6 mg, 8 mg, 10 mg, 12 mg.

ADMINISTRATION/HANDLING

PO

• Give without regard to food. • Tablets may be crushed.

INDICATIONS/ROUTES/DOSAGE

Note: Titrate to the proper dose range with dosage adjustments not to exceed 2 mg twice daily (4 mg/day).

Schizophrenia

PO: ADULTS: To avoid orthostatic hypotension, begin with 1 mg twice daily, then adjust dosage to 2 mg twice daily, 4 mg twice daily, 6 mg twice daily, 8 mg twice daily, 10 mg twice daily, and 12 mg twice daily on days 2, 3, 4, 5, 6, and 7, respectively, to reach target daily dose of 12–24 mg/day in 2 divided doses. **Note:** Reduce dose by 50% when receiving strong CYP2D6 or CYP3A4 inhibitors or poor metabolizers of CYP2D6 (see Interactions).

Dosage in Renal Impairment

No dose adjustment.

Dosage in Hepatic Impairment

Mild impairment: No adjustment. **Moderate impairment:** Use caution. **Severe impairment:** Not recommended.

SIDE EFFECTS

Frequent (20%–12%): Dizziness, drowsiness, tachycardia. **Occasional** (10%–4%): Nausea, dry mouth, nasal congestion, weight increase, diarrhea, fatigue, orthostatic hypotension. **Rare** (3%–1%): Arthralgia, musculoskeletal stiffness, abdominal discomfort, nasopharyngitis, tremor, hypotension, rash, ejaculatory failure, dyspnea, blurred vision, lethargy.

ADVERSE EFFECTS/TOXIC REACTIONS

Extrapyramidal disorders, including tardive dyskinesia (protrusion of tongue, puffing of cheeks, chewing/puckering of the mouth), occur in 4% of pts. Upper respiratory infection occurs in 3% of pts. QT interval prolongation may produce torsades de pointes, a form of ventricular tachycardia. Neuroleptic malignant syndrome (e.g., hyperpyrexia, muscle rigidity, altered mental status, irregular pulse or B/P) has been noted.

NURSING CONSIDERATIONS

BASELINE ASSESSMENT

Assess pt's behavior, appearance, emotional status, response to environment, speech pattern, thought content. ECG should be obtained to assess for QT prolongation before instituting medication. Question medical history as listed in Precautions.

INTERVENTION/EVALUATION

Monitor for orthostatic hypotension; assist with ambulation. Monitor for fine tongue movement (may be first sign of tardive dyskinesia, possibly irreversible). Monitor serum potassium, magnesium in pts at risk for electrolyte disturbances. Assess for therapeutic response (greater interest in surroundings, improved self-care, increased ability to concentrate, relaxed facial expression).

PATIENT/FAMILY TEACHING

• Avoid tasks that require alertness, motor skills until response to drug is established. • Be alert to symptoms of orthostatic hypotension; slowly go from lying to standing. • Report if feeling faint, if experiencing heart palpitations, or if fever or muscle rigidity occurs. • Report extrapyramidal symptoms (e.g., involuntary muscle movements, tics) immediately.

imatinib

TOP 100 HIGH ALERT

im-**at**-in-ib
(Gleevec)

Do not confuse imatinib with dasatinib, erlotinib, lapatinib, nilotinib, SORAfenib, or SUNItinib.

◆CLASSIFICATION

PHARMACOTHERAPEUTIC: BCR-ABL tyrosine kinase inhibitor. **CLINICAL:** Antineoplastic.

USES

Newly diagnosed chronic-phase Philadelphia chromosome positive chronic myeloid leukemia (Ph+ CML) in children and adults. Pts in blast crisis, accelerated phase, or chronic phase Ph+ CML who have already failed interferon therapy. Adults with relapsed or refractory Ph+ acute lymphoblastic leukemia (ALL). Treatment in children with Ph+ ALL. Adults with myelodysplastic/myeloproliferative disease (MDS/MPD) associated with platelet-derived growth factor receptor (PDGFR) gene rearrangements. Adults with aggressive systemic mastocytosis (ASM) without mutation of the D816V c-Kit or unknown mutation status of the c-Kit. Adults with hypereosinophilic syndrome (HES) and/or chronic eosinophilic leukemia (CEL) with positive, negative, or unknown FIP1L1-PDGFR fusion kinase. Adults with dermatofibrosarcoma protuberans (DFSP) that is unresectable, recurrent, and/or metastatic. Pts with malignant gastrointestinal stromal tumors (GIST) that are unresectable and/or metastatic. Prevention of cancer recurrence in pts following surgical removal of GIST. **OFF-LABEL:** Treatment of desmoid tumors (soft tissue sarcoma). Post–stem cell transplant (allogeneic), follow-up treatment in recurrent CML. Treatment of advanced or metastatic melanoma.

PRECAUTIONS

Contraindications: Hypersensitivity to imatinib. **Cautions:** Hepatic/renal impairment, thyroidectomy pts, hypothyroidism, gastric surgery pts. Pts in whom fluid accumulation is poorly tolerated (e.g., HF, hypertension, pulmonary disease).

ACTION

Inhibits Bcr-Abl tyrosine kinase, an enzyme created by Philadelphia chromosome abnormality found in pts with chronic myeloid leukemia. **Therapeutic Effect:** Blocks tumor cell proliferation and induces cellular death (apoptosis).

PHARMACOKINETICS

Well absorbed after PO administration. Protein binding: 95%. Metabolized in liver. Eliminated in feces (68%), urine (13%). **Half-life:** 18 hrs; metabolite, 40 hrs.

⌛ LIFESPAN CONSIDERATIONS

Pregnancy/Lactation: May cause fetal harm. Breastfeeding not recommended. **Children:** Safety and efficacy not established. **Elderly:** Increased frequency of fluid retention.

INTERACTIONS

DRUG: **CYP3A4 inducers (e.g., carBAMazepine, phenytoin, rifAMPin)** may decrease concentration/effect. **CYP3A4 inhibitors (e.g., clarithromycin, ketoconazole, ritonavir)** may increase concentration/effect. **Bone marrow depressants (e.g., cladribine)** may increase myelosuppression. **Live virus vaccines** may potentiate virus replication, increase vaccine side effects, decrease pt's antibody response to vaccine. May decrease effect of **warfarin.** HERBAL: **Echinacea** may decrease therapeutic effect. **St. John's wort** decreases concentration. FOOD: **Grapefruit products** may increase concentration. LAB VALUES: May increase serum bilirubin, ALT, AST, creatinine. May decrease platelet count, RBC, WBC count; serum potassium, albumin, calcium.

AVAILABILITY (Rx)

Tablets: 100 mg, 400 mg.

ADMINISTRATION/HANDLING

PO

• Give with a meal and large glass of water. • Tablets may be dispersed in water or apple juice (stir until dissolved; give immediately). Do not crush or chew tablets.

INDICATIONS/ROUTES/DOSAGE

Ph+ Chronic Myeloid Leukemia (CML) (Chronic phase)

PO: ADULTS, ELDERLY: 400 mg once daily; may increase to 600 mg/day. **Maximum:** 800 mg. **CHILDREN:** 340 mg/m^2/day. **Maximum:** 600 mg.

Ph+ CML (Accelerated phase)

PO: ADULTS, ELDERLY: 600 mg once daily. May increase to 800 mg/day in 2 divided doses (400 mg twice daily). **CHILDREN:** 340 mg/m^2/day. **Maximum:** 600 mg.

Ph+ Acute Lymphoblastic Leukemia (ALL)

PO: ADULTS, ELDERLY: 600 mg once daily.

Gastrointestinal Stromal Tumors (GIST) (Following complete resection)

PO: ADULTS, ELDERLY: 400 mg once daily for 3 yrs.

GIST (Unresectable)

PO: ADULTS, ELDERLY: 400 mg once daily. May increase up to 400 mg twice daily.

Aggressive Systemic Mastocytosis (ASM) With Eosinophilia

PO: ADULTS, ELDERLY: Initially, 100 mg/day. May increase up to 400 mg/day.

ASM Without Mutation of the D816V C-Kit or Unknown Mutation Status of C-Kit

PO: ADULTS, ELDERLY: 400 mg once daily.

Dermatofibrosarcoma Protuberans (DFSP)

PO: ADULTS, ELDERLY: 400 mg twice daily.

Hypereosinophilic Syndrome (HES)/ Chronic Eosinophilic Leukemia (CEL)

PO: ADULTS, ELDERLY: 400 mg once daily.

HES/CEL With Positive or Unknown FIP1L1-PDGFR Fusion Kinase

PO: ADULTS, ELDERLY: Initially, 100 mg/day. May increase up to 400 mg/day.

Myelodysplastic/Myeloproliferative Disease (MDS/MPD)

PO: ADULTS, ELDERLY: 400 mg once daily.

Usual Dosage for Children (2 yrs and older)

Ph+ CML (Chronic Phase, Recurrent, or Resistant)

PO: 340 mg/m^2/day. **Maximum:** 600 mg/day.

Ph+ CML (Chronic Phase, Newly Diagnosed, Ph+ ALL)

PO: 340 mg/m^2/day. **Maximum:** 600 mg/day.

I

Dosage With Strong CYP3A4 Inducers
Increase dose by 50% with careful monitoring.

Dosage in Renal Impairment

Creatinine Clearance	Maximum Dose
40–59 mL/min	600 mg
20–39 mL/min	400 mg
Less than 20 mL/min	100 mg

Dosage in Hepatic Impairment
Mild to moderate impairment: No adjustment. **Severe impairment:** Reduce dosage by 25%.

SIDE EFFECTS

Frequent (68%–24%): Nausea, diarrhea, vomiting, headache, fluid retention, rash, musculoskeletal pain, muscle cramps, arthralgia. **Occasional (23%–10%):** Abdominal pain, cough, myalgia, fatigue, fever, anorexia, dyspepsia, constipation, night sweats, pruritus, dizziness, blurred vision, somnolence. **Rare (less than 10%):** Nasopharyngitis, petechiae, asthenia, epistaxis.

ADVERSE EFFECTS/TOXIC REACTIONS

Severe fluid retention (pleural effusion, pericardial effusion, pulmonary edema, ascites), hepatotoxicity occur rarely. Neutropenia, thrombocytopenia are expected responses to the therapy. Respiratory toxicity is manifested as dyspnea, pneumonia. Heart damage (left ventricular dysfunction, HF) may occur.

NURSING CONSIDERATIONS

BASELINE ASSESSMENT

Obtain CBC, BMP, LFT; pregnancy test in females of reproductive potential. Screen for active infection. Offer emotional support.

INTERVENTION/EVALUATION

Monitor for unexpected, rapid weight gain. Offer antiemetics to control nausea, vomiting. Monitor daily pattern of bowel activity, stool consistency. Monitor CBC wkly for first mo, biweekly for second mo, periodically thereafter for evidence of neutropenia, thrombocytopenia; assess hepatic function tests for hepatotoxicity. Monitor renal function, serum electrolytes. Duration of neutropenia or thrombocytopenia ranges from 2–4 wks.

PATIENT/FAMILY TEACHING

• Treatment may depress your immune system response and reduce your ability to fight infection. Report symptoms of infection such as body aches, chills, cough, fatigue, fever. Avoid those with active infection. • Take with food and a full glass of water. • Avoid grapefruit products. • Report chest pain, swelling of extremities, weight gain greater than 5 lb, easy bruising/bleeding. • Avoid tasks that require alertness, motor skills until response to drug is established.

immune globulin IV (IGIV)

im-**mune** **glob**-u-lin
(Asceniv, Bivigam, Carimune NF, Flebogamma DIF, Gammagard Liquid, Gammagard S/D, Gammaplex, Gamunex-C, Hizentra, Octagam 5%, Privigen)

BLACK BOX ALERT Acute renal impairment characterized by increased serum creatinine, oliguria, acute renal failure, osmotic nephrosis, particularly pts with any degree of renal insufficiency, diabetes mellitus, volume depletion, sepsis, and those older than age 65 yrs. Thrombosis may occur (administer at the minimum dose and minimum infusion rate; ensure adequate hydration).

◆CLASSIFICATION

PHARMACOTHERAPEUTIC: Immune globulin, blood product. **CLINICAL:** Immunizing agent.

USES

Treatment of pts with primary humoral immunodeficiency syndromes, acute/chronic immune idiopathic thrombocytopenic purpura (ITP), prevention of coronary artery aneurysms associated with Kawasaki disease, prevention of recurrent bacterial infections in pts with hypogammaglobulinemia associated with B-cell chronic lymphocytic leukemia (CLL). Treatment of chronic inflammatory demyelinating polyneuropathies. Provide passive immunity in pts with hepatitis A, measles, rubella, varicella. **OFF-LABEL:** Guillain-Barré syndrome; myasthenia gravis; prevention of acute infections in immunosuppressed pts; prevention, treatment of infection in high-risk, preterm, low-birth-weight neonates; treatment of multiple sclerosis, HIV-associated thrombocytopenia.

PRECAUTIONS

Contraindications: Hypersensitivity to immune globulin. Selective IgA deficiency, hyperprolinemia (Hizentra, Privigen), severe thrombocytopenia, coagulation disorders where IM injections contraindicated. Hypersensitivity to corn (Octagam); infants/neonates for whom sucrose or fructose tolerance has not been established (Gammaplex). **Cautions:** Cardiovascular disease, history of thrombosis, renal impairment.

ACTION

Replacement therapy for primary/secondary immunodeficiencies and lgG antibodies against bacteria, viral antigens; interferes with receptors on cells of reticuloendothelial system for autoimmune cytopenias/idiopathic thrombocytopenia purpura (ITP); increases antibody titer and antigen-antibody reaction potential. **Therapeutic Effect:** Provides passive immunity replacement for immunodeficiencies, increases antibody titer.

PHARMACOKINETICS

Evenly distributed between intravascular and extravascular space. **Half-life:** 21–23 days.

LIFESPAN CONSIDERATIONS

Pregnancy/Lactation: Unknown if drug crosses placenta or is distributed in breast milk. **Children/Elderly:** No age-related precautions noted.

INTERACTIONS

DRUG: **Live virus vaccines** may increase vaccine side effects, potentiate virus replication, decrease pt's antibody response to vaccine. **HERBAL:** None significant. **FOOD:** None known. **LAB VALUES:** None significant.

AVAILABILITY (Rx)

Injection, Powder for Reconstitution: ***(Carimune NF):*** 3 g, 6 g, 12 g. ***(Gammagard S/D):*** 5 g, 10 g. **Injection, Solution:** ***(Asceniv, Bivigam 10%, Flebogamma DIF 5%, 10%, Gammagard Liquid 10%, Gammaplex 5%, Gamunex-C 10%, Octagam 5%, Privigen 10%).***

ADMINISTRATION/HANDLING

IV

◀ALERT▶ Monitor vital signs, B/P diligently during and immediately after IV administration (precipitous fall in B/P may indicate anaphylactic reaction). Stop infusion immediately. EPINEPHrine should be readily available.

Reconstitution • Reconstitute only with diluent provided by manufacturer. • Discard partially used or turbid preparations.

Rate of administration • Give by infusion only. • After reconstitution, administer via separate tubing. • Rate of infusion varies with product used.

Storage • Refer to individual IV preparations for storage requirements, stability after reconstitution.

IV INCOMPATIBILITIES

Do not mix with any other medications.

INDICATIONS/ROUTES/DOSAGE

Primary Immunodeficiency Syndrome

IV: ADULTS, ELDERLY, CHILDREN: ***(Privigen):*** 200–800 mg/kg q3–4wks. ***(Carimune NF):*** 400–800 mg/kg q3–4 wks. ***(Flebogamma DIF, Gammagard, Gamunex-C, Octagam):*** 300–600 mg/kg/q3–4wks. ***(Asceniv, Bivigam, Gammaplex):*** 300–800 mg/kg q3–4wks.

Idiopathic Thrombocytopenic Purpura (ITP)

IV: ADULTS, ELDERLY, CHILDREN: ***(Carimune NF):*** 400 mg/kg/day for 2–5 days. **Maintenance:** 400–1,000 mg/kg/dose to maintain platelet count or control bleeding. ***(Gammagard):*** 1,000 mg/kg: up to 3 total doses may be given on alternate days based on pt response and/or platelet count. ***(Gammaplex, Octagam, Flebogamma DIF):*** 1,000 mg/kg once daily for 2 consecutive days.

Kawasaki Disease

Note: Must be used with aspirin.

IV: CHILDREN: ***(Gammagard):*** 1,000 mg/kg as single dose or 400 mg/kg/day for 4 consecutive days. Begin within 7 days of onset of fever. **American Heart Association guidelines:** 2,000 mg/kg as a single dose given over 10–12 hrs within 10 days of disease onset.

Chronic Lymphocytic Leukemia (CLL)

IV: ADULTS, ELDERLY, CHILDREN: ***(Gammagard):*** 400 mg/kg/dose q3–4wks.

Chronic Inflammatory Demyelinating Polyneuropathy

IV: ADULTS, ELDERLY, CHILDREN: ***(Gamunex-C):*** **Loading Dose:** 2 g/kg divided over 2–4 days (consecutive). **Maintenance:** 1 g/kg/day q3wks or 500 mg/kg for 2 consecutive days q3wks. ***(Privigen):*** **Loading Dose:** 2 g/kg in divided doses over 2–5 consecutive days. **Maintenance:** 1 g/kg q3wks or 500 mg/kg for 2 consecutive days q3wks.

Dosage in Renal Impairment

Caution when giving IV.

Dosage in Hepatic Impairment

No dose adjustment.

SIDE EFFECTS

Frequent: Tachycardia, backache, headache, arthralgia, myalgia. **Occasional:** Fatigue, wheezing, injection site rash/pain, leg cramps, urticaria, bluish color of lips/nailbeds, light-headedness.

ADVERSE EFFECTS/TOXIC REACTIONS

Anaphylactic reactions occur rarely, but incidence increases with repeated injections. EPINEPHrine should be readily available. Overdose may produce chest tightness, chills, diaphoresis, dizziness, facial flushing, nausea, vomiting, fever, hypotension. Hypersensitivity reaction (anxiety, arthralgia, dizziness, flushing, myalgia, palpitations, pruritus) occurs rarely.

NURSING CONSIDERATIONS

BASELINE ASSESSMENT

Question history of cardiac disease, thrombosis. Have EPINEPHrine readily available. Pt should be well hydrated prior to administration.

INTERVENTION/EVALUATION

Control rate of IV infusion carefully; too-rapid infusion increases risk of precipitous fall in B/P, signs of anaphylaxis (facial flushing, chest tightness, chills, fever, nausea, vomiting, diaphoresis). Assess pt closely during infusion, esp. first hr; monitor vital signs continuously. Stop infusion if aforementioned signs noted. For treatment of idiopathic thrombocytopenic purpura (ITP), monitor platelet count.

PATIENT/FAMILY TEACHING

• Explain rationale for therapy. • Report sudden weight gain, fluid retention, edema, decreased urine output, shortness of breath.

indomethacin

in-doe-**meth**-a-sin
(Indocin, Tivorbex)

BLACK BOX ALERT Increased risk of serious cardiovascular thrombotic events, including myocardial infarction, CVA. Increased risk of severe GI reactions, including ulceration, bleeding, perforation.

Do not confuse Indocin with Imodium, Minocin, or Vicodin.

CLASSIFICATION

PHARMACOTHERAPEUTIC: NSAID. **CLINICAL:** Anti-inflammatory, analgesic.

USES

Indocin: Treatment of active stages of rheumatoid arthritis, osteoarthritis, ankylosing spondylitis, acute gouty arthritis. Relieves acute bursitis, tendinitis. **Tivorbex:** Treatment of mild to moderate acute pain in adults. **IV:** For closure of hemodynamically significant patent ductus arteriosus of premature infants weighing between 500 and 1,750 g when 48-hr usual medical management is ineffective. **OFF-LABEL:** Management of preterm labor.

PRECAUTIONS

Contraindications: Hypersensitivity to aspirin, indomethacin, other NSAIDs. Perioperative pain in setting of CABG surgery. History of asthma, urticaria, allergic reactions after taking aspirin, other NSAIDs. **Suppositories:** History of proctitis, recent rectal bleeding. **Injection:** In preterm infants with untreated/systemic infection or congenital heart disease where patency of PDA necessary for pulmonary or systemic blood flow; bleeding, thrombocytopenia, coagulation defects, necrotizing enterocolitis, significant renal dysfunction. **Cautions:** Cardiac dysfunction, fluid retention, HF, hypertension, renal/hepatic impairment, epilepsy; concurrent aspirin, steroids, anticoagulant therapy. Treatment of juvenile rheumatoid arthritis in children. History of GI disease (bleeding or ulcers), elderly, debilitated, asthma, depression, Parkinson's disease.

ACTION

Reversibly inhibits COX-1 and COX-2 enzymes. Produces antipyretic, analgesic, anti-inflammatory effects by inhibiting prostaglandin synthesis. **Therapeutic Effect:** Reduces inflammatory response, fever, intensity of pain. Closure of patent ductus arteriosus.

PHARMACOKINETICS

Route	Onset	Peak	Duration
PO	30 min	—	4–6 hrs

Well absorbed from GI tract. Protein binding: 99%. Metabolized in liver. Excreted in urine. **Half-life:** 4.5 hrs.

LIFESPAN CONSIDERATIONS

Pregnancy/Lactation: Crosses placenta; distributed in breast milk. Avoid use during third trimester. **Children:** Safety and efficacy not established in those younger than 14 yrs. **Elderly:** Increased risk of serious adverse effects; GI bleeding, ulceration.

INTERACTIONS

DRUG: May increase risk of bleeding; adverse effects of **apixaban, dabigatran, edoxaban, rivaroxaban. Bile acid sequestrants (e.g., cholestyramine)** may decrease absorption/effect. May increase nephrotoxic effect of **cycloSPORINE.** May increase concentration/effect of **lithium.** May decrease effect of **loop diuretics (e.g., bumetanide, furosemide). HERBAL: Glucosamine, herbals with anticoagulant/antiplatelet properties (e.g., garlic, ginger, ginseng, ginkgo biloba)** may increase concentration/effect. **FOOD:** None known. **LAB VALUES:** May prolong bleeding time. May alter serum glucose. May increase serum BUN, creatinine, potassium, ALT, AST. May decrease serum sodium, platelet count, leukocytes.

AVAILABILITY (Rx)

Capsules: 25 mg, 50 mg. ***(Tivorbex):*** 20 mg. **Injection, Powder for Reconstitution:** ***(Indocin IV):*** 1 mg. **Oral Suspension:** ***(Indocin):*** 25 mg/5 mL. **Suppository:** 50 mg.

Capsules, Extended-Release: 75 mg.

ADMINISTRATION/HANDLING

IV

Reconstitution • To 1-mg vial, add 1–2 mL preservative-free Sterile Water for Injection or 0.9% NaCl to provide concentration of 1 mg/mL or 0.5 mg/mL, respectively. • Do not further dilute.

Rate of administration • Administer over 20–30 min.

Storage • Use IV solution immediately following reconstitution. • IV solution appears clear; discard if cloudy or precipitate forms. • Discard unused portion.

PO

• Give after meals or with food, antacids. • Do not break, crush, or open extended-release capsule. Swallow whole.

IV INCOMPATIBILITIES

Amino acid injection, calcium gluconate, DOBUTamine (Dobutrex), DOPamine (Intropin), gentamicin (Garamycin), tobramycin (Nebcin).

IV COMPATIBILITIES

Insulin, potassium.

INDICATIONS/ROUTES/DOSAGE

Moderate to Severe Rheumatoid Arthritis (RA), Osteoarthritis, Ankylosing Spondylitis

PO: ADULTS, ELDERLY, CHILDREN OLDER THAN 14 YRS: ***(Immediate-Release):*** Initially, 25 mg 2–3 times/day; increased by 25–50 mg/wk up to 150–200 mg/day. ***(Extended-Release):*** Initially, 75 mg once daily. May increase to 75 mg twice daily. **Maximum:** 150 mg/day. **CHILDREN 2 YRS AND OLDER:** ***(Immediate-Release):*** 1–2 mg/kg/day in 2–4 divided doses. **Maximum:** 4 mg/kg/day not to exceed 150–200 mg/day.

Acute Gouty Arthritis

PO, rectal: ADULTS, ELDERLY: ***(Immediate-Release):*** 50 mg 3 times/day for 5–7 days until pain is tolerable, then rapidly reduce dose to complete cessation of medication.

Acute Bursitis, Tendonitis

PO: ADULTS, ELDERLY: ***(Immediate-Release):*** 75–150 mg/day in 3–4 divided doses for 7–14 days. ***(Extended-Release):*** 75–150 mg/day in 1–2 doses/day for 7–14 days.

Acute Pain

PO: ADULTS, ELDERLY: ***(Tivorbex):*** 20 mg 3 times/day or 40 mg 2–3 times/day.

Patent Ductus Arteriosus

IV: NEONATES: Initially, 0.2 mg/kg. Subsequent doses are based on age, as follows: **NEONATES OLDER THAN 7 DAYS:** 0.25 mg/kg for 2nd and 3rd doses. **NEONATES 2–7 DAYS:** 0.2 mg/kg for 2nd and 3rd doses. **NEONATES YOUNGER THAN 48 HRS:** 0.1 mg/kg for 2nd and 3rd doses. In general, dosing interval is 12 hrs if urine output is greater than 1 mL/kg/hr after prior dose, 24 hrs if urine output is less than 1 mL/kg/hr but greater than 0.6 mL/kg/hr. Dose is held if urine output is less than 0.6 mL/kg/hr or if neonate is anuric.

Dosage in Renal Impairment

Mild to moderate impairment: No dose adjustment. **Severe impairment:** Not recommended.

Dosage in Hepatic Impairment

Use caution.

SIDE EFFECTS

Frequent (11%–3%): Headache, nausea, vomiting, dyspepsia, dizziness. **Occasional (less than 3%):** Depression, tinnitus, diaphoresis, drowsiness, constipation, diarrhea. **Patent ductus arteriosus:** Bleeding abnormalities. **Rare:** Hypertension, confusion, urticaria, pruritus, rash, blurred vision.

ADVERSE EFFECTS/TOXIC REACTIONS

Paralytic ileus, ulceration of esophagus, stomach, duodenum, small intestine may occur. Pts with renal impairment may develop hyperkalemia with worsening of renal impairment. May aggravate depression or other psychiatric disturbances, epilepsy, parkinsonism. Nephrotoxicity (dysuria, hematuria, proteinuria, nephrotic syndrome) occurs rarely. Metabolic acidosis/alkalosis, bradycardia occur rarely in neonates with patent ductus arteriosus.

NURSING CONSIDERATIONS

BASELINE ASSESSMENT

Assess onset, type, location, duration of pain, fever, inflammation. Inspect appearance of affected joints for immobility, deformities, skin condition. Question medical history as listed in Precautions.

INTERVENTION/EVALUATION

Monitor serum BUN, creatinine, potassium, LFT. Monitor for evidence of nausea, dyspepsia. Assist with ambulation if dizziness occurs. Evaluate for therapeutic response: relief of pain, stiffness, swelling; increased joint mobility; reduced joint tenderness; improved grip strength. Observe for weight gain, edema, bleeding, bruising. In neonates, also monitor heart rate, heart sounds for murmur, B/P, urine output, ECG, serum sodium, glucose, platelets.

PATIENT/FAMILY TEACHING

• Avoid aspirin, alcohol during therapy (increases risk of GI bleeding). • If GI upset occurs, take with food, milk. • Avoid tasks that require alertness, motor skills until response to drug is established. • Report ringing in ears, persistent stomach pain, unusual bruising/bleeding.

inFLIXimab

TOP 100

in-**flix**-i-mab
(Remicade, Inflectra, Renflexis)

BLACK BOX ALERT Risk of severe/fatal opportunistic infections (tuberculosis, sepsis, fungal), reactivation of latent infections. Rare cases of very aggressive, usually fatal hepatosplenic T-cell lymphoma reported in adolescents, young adults with Crohn's disease. **Do not confuse inFLIXimab with riTUXimab, or Remicade with Reminyl.**

CLASSIFICATION

PHARMACOTHERAPEUTIC: Tumor necrosis factor (TNF) blocking agent. Monoclonal antibody. **CLINICAL:** Antirheumatic, disease-modifying, GI, immunosuppressant agent.

USES

In combination with methotrexate, reduces signs/symptoms, inhibits progression of structural damage, improves physical function in moderate to severe active rheumatoid arthritis (RA). Treatment of psoriatic arthritis. Reduces signs/symptoms, induces and maintains remission in moderate to severe active Crohn's disease. Reduces number of draining enterocutaneous/rectovaginal fistulas, maintains fistula closure in fistulizing Crohn's disease. Reduces sign/symptoms of active ankylosing spondylitis. Treatment of chronic severe plaque psoriasis in pts who are candidates for systemic therapy. Reduces sign/symptoms, induces and maintains clinical remission and mucosal healing, eliminates corticosteroid use in moderate to severe active ulcerative colitis.

PRECAUTIONS

Contraindications: Hypersensitivity to inFLIXimab. Moderate to severe HF (doses greater than 5 mg/kg should be avoided). Sensitivity to murine proteins, sepsis, serious active infection. **Cautions:** Hematologic abnormalities, history of COPD, preexisting or recent-onset CNS demyelinating disorders, seizures, mild HF, history of recurrent infections, conditions predisposing pt to infections (e.g., diabetes), pts exposed to tuberculosis, elderly pts, chronic hepatitis B virus infection.

ACTION

Binds to tumor necrosis factor (TNF), inhibiting functional activity of TNF (induction of proinflammatory cytokines, enhanced leukocytic migration, activation of neutrophils/eosinophils). **Therapeutic Effect:** Prevents disease and allows diseased joints to heal.

PHARMACOKINETICS

Absorbed into GI tissue; primarily distributed in vascular compartment. **Half-life:** 8–9.5 days.

LIFESPAN CONSIDERATIONS

Pregnancy/Lactation: Unknown if distributed in breast milk. **Children:** Safety and efficacy not established. **Elderly:** Use cautiously due to higher rate of infection.

INTERACTIONS

DRUG: **Anakinra, anti-TNF agents, baricitinib, pimecrolimus, riTUXimab, tacrolimus (topical), tocilizumab** may increase adverse effects. May decrease therapeutic effect of **BCG (intravesical), vaccines (live).** May increase levels, adverse effects of **belimumab, natalizumab, tofacitinib, vaccines (live).** **HERBAL:** **Echinacea** may decrease effects. **FOOD:** None known. **LAB VALUES:** May increase serum alkaline phosphatase, ALT, AST, bilirubin.

AVAILABILITY (Rx)

Injection, Powder for Reconstitution: 100 mg.

ADMINISTRATION/HANDLING

IV

Reconstitution • Reconstitute each vial with 10 mL Sterile Water for Injection, using 21-gauge or smaller needle. Direct stream of Sterile Water for Injection to glass wall of vial. • Swirl vial gently to dissolve contents (do not shake). • Allow solution to stand for 5 min and inject into 250-mL bag 0.9% NaCl; gently mix. Concentration should range between 0.4 and 4 mg/mL. • Begin infusion within 3 hrs after reconstitution.

Rate of administration • Administer IV infusion over at least 2 hrs using a low protein-binding filter.

Storage • Refrigerate vials. • Solution should appear colorless to light yellow and opalescent; do not use if discolored or if particulate forms.

IV INCOMPATIBILITIES

Do not infuse in same IV line with other agents.

INDICATIONS/ROUTES/DOSAGE

◀ALERT▶ Premedicate with antihistamines, acetaminophen, steroids to prevent/manage infusion reactions.

Rheumatoid Arthritis (RA)

IV infusion: **ADULTS, ELDERLY:** **In combination with methotrexate:** 3 mg/kg followed by additional doses at 2 and 6 wks after first infusion, then q8wks thereafter. Range: 3–10 mg/kg repeated at 4- to 8-wk intervals.

Crohn's Disease

IV infusion: **ADULTS, ELDERLY, CHILDREN 6 YRS AND OLDER:** 5 mg/kg followed by additional doses at 2 and 6 wks after first infusion, then q8wks thereafter. For adults who respond then lose response, consideration may be given to treatment with 10 mg/kg.

Ankylosing Spondylitis
IV infusion: ADULTS, ELDERLY: 5 mg/kg followed by additional doses at 2 and 6 wks after first infusion, then q6wks thereafter.

Psoriatic Arthritis
IV infusion: ADULTS, ELDERLY: 5 mg/kg followed by additional doses at 2 and 6 wks after first infusion, then q8wks thereafter. May be used with or without methotrexate.

Plaque Psoriasis
IV infusion: ADULTS, ELDERLY: 5 mg/kg followed by additional doses at 2 and 6 wks after first infusion, then q8wks thereafter.

Ulcerative Colitis
IV infusion: ADULTS, ELDERLY, CHILDREN 6 YRS AND OLDER: 5 mg/kg followed by additional doses at 2 and 6 wks after first infusion, then q8wks thereafter.

Dosage in Renal/Hepatic Impairment
No dose adjustment.

SIDE EFFECTS

Frequent (22%–10%): Headache, nausea, fatigue, fever. **Occasional (9%–5%):** Fever/chills during infusion, pharyngitis, vomiting, pain, dizziness, bronchitis, rash, rhinitis, cough, pruritus, sinusitis, myalgia, back pain. **Rare (4%–1%):** Hypotension or hypertension, paresthesia, anxiety, depression, insomnia, diarrhea, UTI.

ADVERSE EFFECTS/TOXIC REACTIONS

Serious infections, including sepsis, occur rarely. Potential for hypersensitivity reaction, lupus-like syndrome, severe hepatic reaction, HF.

NURSING CONSIDERATIONS

BASELINE ASSESSMENT

Evaluate baseline hydration status (skin turgor urinary status). Question history of CNS disorders, COPD, HF. Screen for active infection. Pts should be evaluated for active tuberculosis and tested for latent infection prior to initiating treatment and periodically during therapy. Induration of 5 mm or greater with tuberculin skin test should be considered a positive test result when assessing if treatment for latent tuberculosis is necessary. Verify that pt has not received live vaccines prior to initiation.

INTERVENTION/EVALUATION

Monitor urinalysis, erythrocyte sedimentation rate (ESR), B/P. Monitor for signs of infection. Monitor daily pattern of bowel activity, stool consistency. **Crohn's disease:** Monitor C-reactive protein, frequency of stools. Assess for abdominal pain. **Rheumatoid arthritis (RA):** Monitor C-reactive protein. Assess for decreased pain, swollen joints, stiffness.

PATIENT/FAMILY TEACHING

• Report persistent fever, cough, abdominal pain, swelling of ankles/feet. • Treatment may depress your immune system and reduce your ability to fight infection. • Report symptoms of infection such as body aches, chills, cough, fatigue, fever. Avoid those with active infection. • Do not receive live vaccines. • Expect frequent tuberculosis screening. • Report travel plans to possible endemic areas.

inotuzumab ozogamicin

in-oh-**tooz**-ue-mab **oh**-zoe-ga-**mye**-sin
(Besponsa)

■ **BLACK BOX ALERT** ■ Hepatotoxicity, including fatal hepatic veno-occlusive disease may occur, esp. in pts who underwent hematopoietic stem cell transplant (HSCT) or underwent HSCT conditioning

I

regimens containing two alkylating agents and had a total bilirubin level greater than ULN. Other risk factors for hepatic veno-occlusive disease may include advanced age, prior hepatic disease, later salvage lines, greater number of treatment cycles. Permanently discontinue in pts who develop hepatic veno-occlusive disease. LFT elevations may require treatment interruption, dose reduction, or permanent discontinuation. Increased occurrence of post-HSCT nonrelapse mortality was reported.

Do not confuse inotuzumab with ado-trastuzumab, alemtuzumab, atezolizumab, benralizumab, dinutuximab, elotuzumab, gemtuzumab, ipilimumab, obinutuzumab, pertuzumab, trastuzumab.

◆CLASSIFICATION

PHARMACOTHERAPEUTIC: Anti-CD22. Antibody drug conjugate (ADC). Monoclonal antibody. **CLINICAL:** Antineoplastic.

USES

Treatment of adults with relapsed or refractory B-cell precursor acute lymphoblastic leukemia (ALL).

PRECAUTIONS

Contraindications: Hypersensitivity to inotuzumab. Administration of live vaccines. **Cautions:** Conditions predisposing to infection (e.g., diabetes, immunocompromised pts, renal failure, open wounds), elderly. Pts at risk for hepatic veno-occlusive disease (e.g., advanced age, prior HSCT, prior hepatic disease (e.g., cirrhosis, hepatitis), later salvage lines, greater number of treatment cycles). Pts at risk for QT interval prolongation or torsades de pointes (congenital long QT syndrome, medications that prolong QT interval, hypokalemia, hypomagnesemia). Pts at risk for hemorrhage (e.g., history of intracranial/GI bleeding, coagulation disorders, recent trauma; concomitant use of anticoagulants, antiplatelets, NSAIDS). Pts at risk for tumor lysis syndrome (high tumor burden).

ACTION

Binds to and internalizes ADC-CD22 complex in CD22-expressing tumor cells, promoting cellular release of N-acetyl-gamma-calicheamicin dimethyl hydrazide (a cytotoxic agent). Activation of N-acetyl-gamma-calicheamicin dimethyl hydrazide induces breakage of double-strand DNA, resulting in cell cycle arrest and apoptosis. **Therapeutic Effect:** Inhibits tumor cell growth and metastasis in ALL.

PHARMACOKINETICS

Widely distributed. N-acetyl-gamma-calicheamicin dimethyl hydrazide metabolized by nonenzymatic reduction. Protein binding: 97%. Steady state reached by treatment cycle 4. Excretion not specified. **Half-life:** 12.3 days.

⌛ LIFESPAN CONSIDERATIONS

Pregnancy/Lactation: Avoid pregnancy; may cause fetal harm. Unknown if distributed in breast milk. Females of reproductive potential must use effective contraception during treatment and for at least 8 mos after discontinuation. Males with female partners of reproductive potential must use effective contraception during treatment and for at least 5 mos after discontinuation. Breastfeeding not recommended during treatment and for at least 2 mos after discontinuation. May impair fertility in females. **Children:** Safety and efficacy not established. **Elderly:** No age-related precautions noted.

INTERACTIONS

DRUG: **QT interval–prolonging medications (e.g., amiodarone, azithromycin, ciprofloxacin, haloperidol, sotalol)** may increase risk of QT interval prolongation, torsades de pointes. May diminish therapeutic effect of **nivolumab.** May increase adverse effects of **natalizumab, vaccines (live).** May decrease therapeutic effect of **BCG (intravesical),**

vaccines (live). HERBAL: Echinacea may decrease concentration/effect. **FOOD:** None known. **LAB VALUES:** May decrease Hgb, leukocytes, lymphocytes, neutrophils, platelets. May increase serum alkaline phosphatase, ALT, amylase AST, bilirubin, GGT, lipase, uric acid. May decrease diagnostic effect of *Coccidioides immitis* skin test.

AVAILABILITY (Rx)

Injection, Powder for Reconstitution: 0.9 mg.

ADMINISTRATION/HANDLING

IV

Premedication • Premedicate with a corticosteroid, antipyretic, and antihistamine before each dose.

Reconstitution • Must be prepared by personnel trained in aseptic manipulations and admixing of cytotoxic drugs. • Calculate the number of vials required for dose. • Reconstitute each vial with 4 mL Sterile Water for Injection for a final concentration of 0.25 mg/mL that delivers 3.6 mL (0.9 mg). • Gently swirl vial until completely dissolved. • Do not shake or agitate. • Visually inspect for particulate matter or discoloration. Solution should appear clear to opalescent, colorless to slightly yellow in color. Do not use if solution is cloudy or discolored, or if visible particles are observed. • Calculate required volume of reconstituted solution according to body surface area. • Dilute in 50 mL 0.9% NaCl polyvinyl chloride (PVC) infusion bag made of (DEHP or non-DEHP), polyolefin, or ethylene vinyl acetate. • Mix by gently inversion. Do not shake or agitate. • Discard unused portions.

Rate of administration • Infuse over 60 min via dedicated IV line. • In-line filters are not required. However, if an in-line filter is used, filters made of polyethersulfone (PES), polyvinylidene fluoride (PVDF), or hydrophilic polysulfone (HPS) are recommended. Do not use filters made of nylon or mixed cellulose ester (MCE). • Do not administer as IV push or bolus.

Storage • Refrigerate unused vials in original carton. • Protect vial, reconstituted solution, diluted solution from light. • Do not freeze. • Reconstitution solution must be diluted within 4 hrs. • Diluted solution may be stored at room temperature for up to 4 hrs or refrigerated for up to 3 hrs. • If refrigerated, allow diluted solution to warm to room temperature (approx. 1 hr). • Infusion must be completed within 8 hrs of reconstitution.

INDICATIONS/ROUTES/DOSAGE

ALL (Relapsed or refractory)

IV: ADULTS, ELDERLY: Induction cycle 1: 0.8 mg/m^2 on day 1, then 0.5 mg/m^2 on day 8 and day 15 of 21-day cycle (total cycle dose: 1.8 mg/m^2 per cycle, given in 3 divided doses). May extend duration of induction cycle to 28 days if pt achieves complete remission (CR), complete remission with incomplete hematologic recovery (CRi), or to allow time for recovery of toxicity. **Subsequent cycles in pts with CR or CRi:** 0.5 mg/m^2 on days 1, 8, and 15 of 28-day cycle (total cycle dose: 1.5 mg/m^2 per cycle, given in 3 divided doses). **Subsequent cycles in pts who have not achieved CR or CRi:** 0.8 mg/m^2 on day 1, then 0.5 mg/m^2 on day 8 and day 15 of 28-day cycle (total cycle dose: 1.8 mg/m^2 per cycle, given in 3 divided doses). Recommend discontinuation in pts who do not achieve CR or CRi within 3 cycles. **Proceeding to HCST:** Treatment duration of 2 cycles. May consider a third cycle in pts who do not achieve CR or Cri and minimal residual disease after 2 cycles. **Not proceeding to HCST:** May consider up to a maximum of 6 cycles.

Dose Modification

Note: Doses within a treatment cycle (e.g., day 8, day 15) do not require interruption if related to neutropenia or thrombocytopenia. Treatment interruptions within a cycle are recommended for nonhematological toxicities. Do not re-escalate reduced doses that are related to toxicity.

Duration of Dose Interruption (Nonhematological toxicities)
Less than 7 days within a cycle: Interrupt the next dose (ensure a minimum of 6 days between doses). **7 days or more:** Skip the next dose within the cycle. **14 days or more:** Once toxicity is adequately resolved, decrease total dose of subsequent cycle by 25%. May further reduce to 2 doses per cycle for subsequent cycles if further dose modification is required. If unable to tolerate a total dose reduction of 25%, followed by a reduction to 2 doses per cycle, permanently discontinue. **More than 28 days:** Consider permanent discontinuation.

Hematologic Toxicities
ANC greater than or equal to 1,000 cells/mm^3 (prior to treatment): If ANC decreases, interrupt next cycle until ANC is greater than or equal to 1,000 cells/mm^3. Discontinue treatment if ANC is less than 1,000 cells/mm^3 for more than 28 days (and related to treatment). **Platelet count greater than or equal to 50,000 cells/mm^3 (prior to treatment):** If platelet count decreases, interrupt next cycle until platelet count is greater than or equal to 50,000 cells/mm^3. Discontinue treatment if platelet count is less than 50,000 cells/mm^3 for more than 28 days (and related to treatment). **ANC less than 1,000 cells/mm^3 and/or platelet count less than 50,000 cells/mm^3 (prior to treatment):** If ANC or platelet count decreases, interrupt next cycle until one of following occurs: ANC and platelet count recover to at least baseline of the prior cycle; ANC is greater than or equal to 1,000 cells/mm^3 and platelet count is greater than or equal to 50,000 cells/mm^3; disease is improved or stable, and the decrease of ANC and platelet count is not related to treatment.

Hepatotoxicity
Serum ALT/AST greater than 2.5 times ULN and serum bilirubin greater than 1.5 times ULN: Interrupt treatment until serum ALT/AST is less than or equal to 2.5 times ULN and serum bilirubin is less than 1.5 times ULN prior to each dose (unless related to Gilbert's syndrome or hemodialysis). Permanently discontinue if serum ALT/AST does not recover to less than or equal to 2.5 times ULN or serum bilirubin does not recover to less than 1.5 times ULN. **Hepatic veno-occlusive disease, severe liver injury:** Permanently discontinue.

Other Nonhematologic Toxicities
Any CTCAE Grade 2 nonhematologic toxicities: Withhold treatment until recovery to Grade 1 or pretreatment grade levels before each dose.

Dosage in Renal Impairment
Mild impairment: No dose adjustment to initial dose. **Severe to moderate impairment:** Not specified; use caution.

Dosage in Hepatic Impairment
Mild to moderate impairment: No dose adjustment to initial dose. **Severe impairment, ESRD, HD:** Use caution.

SIDE EFFECTS

Frequent (35%–17%): Fatigue, asthenia, headache, migraine, sinus headache, pyrexia, nausea, abdominal pain, esophageal pain, abdominal tenderness, hepatic pain. **Occasional (16%–11%):** Constipation, vomiting, stomatitis, aphthous ulcer, mucosal inflammation, mouth ulceration, oral pain, oropharyngeal pain, chills.

ADVERSE EFFECTS/TOXIC REACTIONS

Anemia, leukopenia, lymphopenia, neutropenia, thrombocytopenia are expected responses to therapy, but more severe reactions, including bone marrow failure, febrile neutropenia, may be life-threatening. Hemorrhagic events including contusion, ecchymosis, epistaxis, gingival bleeding, hematemesis, hematochezia, hematotympanum, hematuria, metrorrhagia, subdural hematoma, postprocedural hematoma, hemorrhagic shock, hemorrhage (conjunctival, gastric, GI, hemorrhoidal, intra-abdominal, intracranial, lip, mesenteric, mouth, muscle, rectal, SQ, vaginal) have occurred. Hepatotoxicity, including fatal hepatic veno-occlusive disease, may occur, esp. in pts who underwent HSCT or underwent HSCT conditioning regimens containing two alkylating agents and had a total bilirubin level greater than ULN. An increased occurrence of post-HSCT nonrelapse mortality was reported. Serious, sometimes fatal, infections including neutropenic sepsis, pneumonia, sepsis, pseudomonal sepsis occurred in 5% of pts. Tumor lysis syndrome may present as acute renal failure, hypocalcemia, hyperuricemia, hyperphosphatemia. May cause QT interval prolongation, esp. in pts with history of long QTc prolongation or in pts taking medications known to prolong QT interval. Immunogenicity (anti-inotuzumab antibodies) occurred in 3% of pts.

NURSING CONSIDERATIONS

BASELINE ASSESSMENT

Obtain ANC, CBC, LFT; ECG before each dose. Calculate body surface area. Obtain pregnancy test in females of reproductive potential. Screen for active infection. Assess risk for bleeding, hemorrhage, hepatic veno-occlusive disease, infection, QT prolongation. Due to risk of tumor lysis syndrome, assess adequate hydration before initiation. Receive full medication history and screen for interactions. Offer emotional support.

INTERVENTION/EVALUATION

Monitor ANC, CBC for myelosuppression. Monitor ECG for QT interval prolongation. LFTs should be obtained before each dose and correlated with symptoms of hepatic veno-occlusive disease (ascites, serum bilirubin elevation, hepatomegaly, rapid weight gain). Diligently monitor pts who underwent HSCT or are planning HSCT. Monitor for infusion-related reactions (e.g., chills, dyspnea, fever, rash) during infusion and for at least 1 hr after infusion is completed. If infusion-related reaction occurs during administration, interrupt infusion and provide medical support. Severe reactions may require administration of antihistamines, corticosteroids. Permanently discontinue treatment if severe or life-threatening reactions occur. Be alert for serious infection, opportunistic infection, sepsis (fever, decreased urinary output, hypotension, tachycardia, tachypnea). If infection occurs, provide anti-infective therapy as appropriate. Monitor for hemorrhagic events including intracranial hemorrhage (altered mental status, aphasia, blindness, hemiparesis, unequal pupils, seizures), GI bleeding (hematemesis, melena, rectal bleeding), epistaxis. Tumor lysis syndrome may present as acute renal failure, hypocalcemia, hyperuricemia, hyperphosphatemia. Monitor daily pattern of bowel activity, stool consistency.

PATIENT/FAMILY TEACHING

• Treatment may depress your immune system response and reduce your ability to fight infection. Report symptoms of infection such as body aches, chills, cough, fatigue, fever. Avoid those with active infection. • Report symptoms of bone marrow depression such as bruising, fatigue, fever, shortness of breath, weight loss; bleeding easily, bloody urine or stool. • Therapy may cause life-threatening tumor lysis syndrome (a condition caused by the rapid breakdown of cancer cells), which can cause kidney failure. Report decreased urination, amber-colored urine; confusion, difficulty breathing, fatigue, fever, muscle or joint pain, palpitations, seizures, vomiting. • Avoid pregnancy using effective contraception. Treatment may cause fetal harm. Do not breastfeed during treatment and for at least 2 mos after last dose. • Life-threatening bleeding may occur; report bloody stool, bloody urine; rectal bleeding, nosebleeds, vomiting up blood; symptoms of hemorrhagic stroke (confusion, blindness, difficulty speaking, paralysis, seizures). • Do not take any newly prescribed medications unless approved by doctor who originally started treatment. • Report symptoms of long QT syndrome such as chest pain, dizziness, fainting, palpitations, shortness of breath. • Report liver problems such as abdominal pain, bruising, clay-colored stool, amber or dark-colored urine, yellowing of the skin or eyes. • Pts who have had HSCT or are planning HSCT have an increased risk of mortality.

I

insulin

TOP 100 HIGH ALERT

in-su-lin

Do not confuse NovoLOG with HumaLOG or NovoLIN.

■ BLACK BOX ALERT ■ (Afrezza): Acute bronchospasms reported in pts with asthma and COPD.

FIXED-COMBINATION(S)

HumaLOG Mix 75/25: lispro suspension 75% and lispro solution 25%. **HumuLIN Mix 50/50:** NPH 50% and regular 50%. **HumuLIN 70/30, NovoLIN 70/30:** NPH 70% and rapid-acting regular 30%. **NovoLOG Mix 70/30:** aspart suspension 70% and aspart solution 30%. **Ryzodeg 70/30:** degludec suspension 70% and aspart solution 30%. **Soliqua 100/33:** glargine 100 units/mL and lixisenatide (a glucagon-like peptide 1 [GLP-1] receptor agonist) 33 mcg/mL. **Xultophy 100/3.6:** degludec 100 units/mL and liraglutide (a GLP-1 receptor agonist) 3.6 mg/mL.

◆CLASSIFICATION

PHARMACOTHERAPEUTIC: Exogenous insulin. **CLINICAL:** Antidiabetic.

USES

Treatment of type 1 diabetes (insulin-dependent) and type 2 diabetes (non–insulin-dependent) to improve glycemic control. **OFF-LABEL: Insulin aspart, insulin lispro, insulin regular:** Gestational diabetes, mild to moderate diabetic ketoacidosis, mild to moderate hyperosmolar hyperglycemic state. **Insulin NPH:** Gestational diabetes.

PRECAUTIONS

Contraindications: Hypersensitivity to insulin, use during episodes of hypoglycemia. **Afrezza only:** Chronic lung disease. **Cautions:** Pts at risk for hypokalemia; renal/hepatic impairment, elderly. **Afrezza only:** Must be used with a long-acting insulin in type 1 diabetes. Not recommended for use in diabetic ketoacidosis or in smokers. Pts with active lung cancer, history of lung cancer, or at risk for lung cancer.

ACTION

Acts via specific receptor to regulate metabolism of carbohydrates, protein, and fats. Acts on liver, skeletal muscle, and adipose tissue. **Liver:** Stimulates hepatic glycogen synthesis, synthesis of fatty acids. **Muscle:** Increases protein, glycogen synthesis. **Adipose tissue:** Stimulates lipoproteins to provide free fatty acids, triglyceride synthesis. **Therapeutic Effect:** Controls serum glucose levels.

PHARMACOKINETICS

Rapid-Acting

	Onset (min)	Peak (hrs)	Duration (hrs)
Fiasp	12–18	1.5–2.2	5–7
Aspart (NovoLOG)	10–20	1–3	3–5
Glulisine (Apidra)	5–15	0.75–1.25	2–4
Insulin Human (Afrezza)	15–30	1	2
Lispro (HumaLOG)	15–30	0.5–2.5	3–6.5

Short-Acting

	Onset (min)	Peak (hrs)	Duration (hrs)
Regular (HumuLIN R)	30–60	1–5	6–10
Regular (NovoLIN R)	30–60	1–5	6–10

Intermediate-Acting

	Onset (hrs)	Peak (hrs)	Duration (hrs)
NPH (HumuLIN N)	1–2	6–14	16–24+
NPH (NovoLIN N)	1–2	6–14	16–24+

Long-Acting

	Onset (hrs)	Peak (hrs)	Duration (hrs)
Degludec (Tresiba)	0.5–1.5	12	42
Detemir (Levemir)	3–4	3–9	6–23
Glargine (Lantus)	3–4	No peak	24
Glargine (Toujeo)	Over 6	No peak	Over 24

LIFESPAN CONSIDERATIONS

Pregnancy/Lactation: Insulin is the drug of choice for diabetes in pregnancy; close medical supervision is needed. Following delivery, insulin needs may drop for 24–72 hrs, then rise to prepregnancy levels. Not distributed in breast milk; lactation may decrease insulin requirements. **Children:** No age-related precautions noted. **Elderly:** Decreased vision, fine motor tremors may lead to inaccurate self-dosing.

INTERACTIONS

DRUG: **Alcohol** may increase risk of hypoglycemia. **Beta blockers (e.g., carvedilol, metoprolol)** may alter effects; may mask signs, prolong periods of hypoglycemia. **glucagon-like peptide 1 (GLP-1) agents (e.g., liraglutide), dipeptidyl peptidase (DPP)-4 agents (e.g., linagliptin), thiazolidinediones (e.g., pioglitazone), pramlintide** may increase hypoglycemic effect. **HERBAL:** **Herbals with hypoglycemic properties (e.g., fenugreek)** may increase hypoglycemic effect. **FOOD:** None known. **LAB VALUES:** May decrease serum magnesium, phosphate, potassium.

AVAILABILITY (Rx)

Rapid-Acting

Inhalation Powder: ***(Afrezza):*** 4 units, 8 units, 12 units as single-use inhalation cartridges. ***Aspart (NovoLOG):*** 100 units/mL *vial, 3-mL cartridge, 3-mL Flex-Pen.* ***Glulisine (Apidra):*** 100 units/mL vial, 3-mL cartridge. ***Lispro (HumaLOG):*** 100 units/mL vial, 3-mL cartridge, 3-mL pen.

Short-Acting

Regular: ***(HumuLIN R):*** 100 units/mL vial, U-500 Kwik Pen. **Regular:** ***(NovoLIN R):*** 100 units/mL vial, 3-mL cartridge, 3-mL Innolet prefilled syringe.

Intermediate-Acting

NPH: ***(HumuLIN N):*** 100 units/mL vial, 3-mL pen. **NPH:** ***(NovoLIN N):*** 100 units/mL vial, 3-mL cartridge, 3-mL Innolet prefilled syringe.

Long-Acting

Detemir: ***(Levemir):*** 100 units/mL vial, 3-mL Flex-Pen. **Glargine:** ***(Lantus):*** 100 units/mL vial, 3-mL cartridge. **Glargine:** ***(Toujeo SoloStar):*** 300 units/mL. ***(Basaglar KwikPen):*** 100 units/mL.

Intermediate- and Short-Acting Mixtures: HumuLIN 50/50, HumuLIN 70/30, HumaLOG Mix 75/25, HumaLOG Mix 50/50, NovoLIN 70/30, NovoLOG Mix 70/30. **Solution, IV** ***(Myxredlin):*** 100 units/100 mL in NaCl 0.9% (100 mL).

ADMINISTRATION/HANDLING

IV

Regular and Insulin Glulisine

- *(Apidra):* Use only if solution is clear.
- May give undiluted.

Rapid-Acting

• ***(Afrezza):*** Administer using a single inhalation/cartridge. Give at beginning of a meal. • ***(Aspart [NovoLOG]):*** May give SQ, IV infusion. • Can mix with NPH (draw aspart into syringe first; inject immediately after mixing). • After first use, stable at room temperature for 28 days. • Administer 5–10 min before meals. • ***Glulisine (Apidra):*** May mix with NPH (draw glulisine into syringe first; inject immediately after mixing). • After first use, stable at room temperature for 28 days. • Administer 15 min before or within 20 min after starting a meal. • ***(Lispro [HumaLOG]):*** For SQ use only. • May mix with NPH. Stable for 28 days at room temperature; syringe is stable for 14 days if refrigerated. • After first use, stable at room temperature for 28 days. • Administer 15 min before or immediately after meals.

Short-Acting

Regular • ***(HumuLIN R, NovoLIN R):*** May give SQ, IM, IV. • May mix with NPH for immediate use or for storage for future use. Stable for 1 mo at room temperature, 3 mos if refrigerated. • Can mix with Sterile Water for Injection or 0.9% NaCl. • After first use, stable at room temperature for 28 days. • Administer 30 min before meals.

Intermediate-Acting

NPH • ***(HumuLIN N, NovoLIN N):*** For SQ use only. • May mix with aspart (NovoLOG) or lispro (HumaLOG). Draw aspart or lispro first and use immediately. • May mix with regular (HumuLIN R, NovoLIN R) insulin. Draw regular insulin first, use immediately or may store for future use (up to 28 days). • After first use, stable at room temperature for 28 days. • Administer 15 min before meals when mixed with aspart or lispro; 30 min before meals when mixed with regular insulin.

Long-Acting

• ***(Degludec [Tresiba]):*** For SQ use only. • Do not mix with other insulins. • After first use, stable at room temperature for 56 days. • May take once daily any time of day. • ***(Detemir [Levemir]):*** For SQ use only. • Do not mix with other insulins. • After first use, stable at room temperature for 42 days. • Evening dose given at dinner or at bedtime. Twice-daily regimens can be given 12 hrs after morning dose. • ***(Glargine [Lantus, Toujeo]):*** For SQ use only. • Do not mix with other insulins. • After first use, stable at room temperature for 28 days. • Administer once daily at same time. Meal timing is not applicable.

SQ

• Check serum glucose concentration before administration; dosage highly individualized. • SQ injections may be given in thigh, abdomen, upper arm, buttocks, upper back if there is adequate adipose tissue. • Rotation of injection sites is essential; maintain careful record. • Prefilled syringes should be stored in vertical or oblique position to avoid plugging; plunger should be pulled back slightly and syringe rocked to remix solution before injection.

IV INCOMPATIBILITIES

DilTIAZem (Cardizem), DOPamine (Intropin), nafcillin (Nafcil).

IV COMPATIBILITIES

Amiodarone (Cordarone), ampicillin/sulbactam (Unasyn), ceFAZolin (Ancef), digoxin (Lanoxin), DOBUTamine (Dobutrex), famotidine (Pepcid), gentamicin, heparin, magnesium sulfate, metoclopramide (Reglan), midazolam (Versed), milrinone (Primacor), morphine, nitroglycerin, potassium chloride, propofol (Diprivan), vancomycin (Vancocin).

INDICATIONS/ROUTES/DOSAGE

Note: Insulin requirements vary dramatically among pts, requiring dosage adjustment.

Type 1 Diabetes

Multiple daily injections, guided by glucose monitoring or continuous SQ insulin infusions, is standard of care. **Usual initial dose:** 0.4–0.5 unit/kg/day in divided doses. **Usual maintenance:** 0.4–1 units/kg/day in divided doses.

Type 2 Diabetes

Initially, 4–6 units or 0.1 units/kg given before largest meal of day. Adjust dose by 2 units q3days to reach fasting glucose target (while avoiding hypoglycemia). General goal is to achieve Hgb A1c less than 7% using safe medication titration. Dual therapy (metformin and a second antihyperglycemic agent) is recommended in pts who fail to achieve glycemic goals after 3 mos with lifestyle interventions and metformin monotherapy. ***(Afrezza):*** Dosage based on metabolic needs, blood glucose results, glycemic goal control.

Dosage in Renal Impairment

Creatinine Clearance	Dose
10–50 mL/min	75% normal dose
Less than 10 mL/min	25%–50% normal dose

Dosage in Hepatic Impairment

Insulin requirement may be reduced.

SIDE EFFECTS

Occasional: Localized redness, swelling, itching (due to improper insulin injection technique), allergy to insulin cleansing solution. **Infrequent:** Somogyi effect (rebound hyperglycemia) with chronically excessive insulin dosages. Systemic allergic reaction (rash, angioedema, anaphylaxis), lipodystrophy (depression at injection site due to breakdown of adipose tissue), lipohypertrophy (accumulation of SQ tissue at injection site due to inadequate site rotation). **Rare:** Insulin resistance.

ADVERSE EFFECTS/TOXIC REACTIONS

Severe hypoglycemia (due to hyperinsulinism) may occur with insulin overdose, decrease/delay of food intake, excessive exercise, pts with brittle diabetes. Diabetic ketoacidosis may result from stress, illness, omission of insulin dose, long-term poor insulin control.

NURSING CONSIDERATIONS

BASELINE ASSESSMENT

Obtain serum glucose level, Hgb A1c. Discuss lifestyle to determine extent of learning, emotional needs. If given IV, obtain serum chemistries (esp. serum potassium).

INTERVENTION/EVALUATION

Assess for hypoglycemia (refer to pharmacokinetics table for peak times and duration): cool, wet skin, tremors, dizziness, headache, anxiety, tachycardia, numbness in mouth, hunger, diplopia. Assess sleeping pt for restlessness, diaphoresis. Check for hyperglycemia: polyuria (excessive urine output), polyphagia (excessive food intake), polydipsia (excessive thirst), nausea/vomiting, dim vision, fatigue, deep and rapid breathing (Kussmaul respirations). Be alert to conditions altering glucose requirements: fever, trauma, increased activity/stress, surgical procedure.

PATIENT/FAMILY TEACHING

• Instruct on proper technique for drug administration, testing of glucose, signs/symptoms of hypoglycemia and hyperglycemia. • Diet and exercise are essential parts of treatment; do not skip/delay meals. • Carry candy, sugar packets, other sugar supplements for immediate response to hypoglycemia. • Wear or carry medical alert identification. • Check with physician when insulin demands are altered (e.g., fever, infection, trauma, stress, heavy physical activity). • Do not take other medication without consulting physician. • Weight control, exercise, hygiene (including foot care), not smoking are integral parts of therapy. • Protect skin, limit sun exposure. • Inform dentist, physician, surgeon of medication before any treatment is given.

I

interferon alfa-2b HIGH ALERT

in-ter-**feer**-on
(Intron-A)

■ BLACK BOX ALERT ■ May cause or aggravate fatal or life-threatening autoimmune disorders, ischemia, neuropsychiatric symptoms (profound depression, suicidal thoughts/behaviors), infectious disorders.

Do not confuse interferon alfa-2b with interferon alfa-2a, interferon alfa-n3, or peginterferon alfa-2b, or Intron with Peg-Intron.

FIXED-COMBINATION(S)

Rebetron: interferon alfa-2b/ribavirin (an antiviral): 3 million units/200 mg.

◆CLASSIFICATION

PHARMACOTHERAPEUTIC: Biologic response modifier, immunomodulator. **CLINICAL:** Antineoplastic.

USES

Treatment of hairy cell leukemia, condylomata acuminata (genital, venereal warts), malignant melanoma, AIDS-related Kaposi's sarcoma, chronic hepatitis C virus infection (including children 3 yrs of age and older), chronic hepatitis B virus infection (including children 1 yr and older), follicular non-Hodgkin's lymphoma. **OFF-LABEL:** Treatment of bladder, cervical, renal carcinoma; chronic myelocytic leukemia; laryngeal papillomatosis; multiple myeloma; cutaneous T-cell lymphoma; mycosis fungoides; West Nile virus.

PRECAUTIONS

Contraindications: Hypersensitivity to interferon alfa-2b. Decompensated hepatic disease, autoimmune hepatitis. **In combination with ribavirin:** Women who are pregnant, men with pregnant partners, pts with hemoglobinemias (e.g., sickle cell anemia), CrCl less than 50 mL/min). **Cautions:** Renal/hepatic impairment, seizure disorder, compromised CNS function, cardiac diseases, myelosuppression, concurrent use of medications causing myelosuppression, pulmonary impairment, multiple sclerosis, diabetes, thyroid disease, coagulopathy, hypertension, preexisting eye disorders, history of psychiatric disorders. History of autoimmune disorders, MI, arrhythmias, cardiac abnormalities.

ACTION

Binds to a specific receptor on cell membrane to initiate intracellular activity, including suppression of cell proliferation, augmenting specific cytotoxicity of lymphocytes and increasing phagocyte activity. **Therapeutic Effect:** Prevents rapid growth of malignant cells; inhibits hepatitis virus.

PHARMACOKINETICS

Well absorbed after IM, SQ administration. Undergoes proteolytic degradation during reabsorption in kidneys. **Half-life:** 2–3 hrs.

⌛ LIFESPAN CONSIDERATIONS

Pregnancy/Lactation: If possible, avoid use during pregnancy. Breastfeeding not recommended. **Children:** Safety and efficacy not established. **Elderly:** Neurotoxicity, cardiotoxicity may occur more frequently. Age-related renal impairment may require dosage adjustment.

INTERACTIONS

DRUG: **Bone marrow depressants (e.g., cladribine)** may increase myelosuppression. May increase concentration/effect of **tiZANidine.** **HERBAL:** None significant. **FOOD:** None known. **LAB VALUES:** May increase PT, aPTT, LDH, serum alkaline phosphatase, ALT, AST. May decrease Hgb, Hct, leukocyte, platelet counts.

AVAILABILITY (Rx)

Injection, Powder for Reconstitution: 10 million units, 18 million units, 50 million units.

Injection, Solution: 6 million units/mL, 10 million units/mL.

ADMINISTRATION/HANDLING

IV

Reconstitution • Prepare immediately before use. • Reconstitute with diluent provided by manufacturer. • Withdraw desired dose and further dilute with 100 mL 0.9% NaCl to provide final concentration of at least 10 million international units/100 mL.

Rate of administration • Administer over 20 min.

Storage • Refrigerate unopened vials. • Following reconstitution, stable for 24 hrs if refrigerated.

IM, SQ

IM • Rotate sites. Preferred sites are anterior thigh, deltoid, and superolateral buttock. Administer in evening (if possible).

SQ • Reconstitute with recommended amount of Sterile Water for Injection. Agitate gently; do not shake. Rotate sites. Preferred sites are anterior thigh, abdomen (except around navel), outer upper arm.

IV INCOMPATIBILITIES

D_5W. Do not mix with other medications via Y-site administration.

IV COMPATIBILITIES

0.9% NaCl, lactated Ringer's.

INDICATIONS/ROUTES/DOSAGE

Hairy Cell Leukemia

IM, SQ: ADULTS: 2 million units/m^2 3 times/wk on alternating days for up to 6 mos. May continue treatment for sustained response. If severe adverse reactions occur, modify dose or temporarily discontinue drug. Discontinue for disease progression or failure to respond after 6 months.

Condylomata Acuminata

Intralesional: ADULTS: 1 million units/lesion 3 times/wk on alternating days for 3 wks. May administer a second course at 12–16 wks. Use only 10 million–unit vial, and reconstitute with no more than 1 mL diluent. **Maximum:** 5 lesions per treatment.

AIDS-Related Kaposi's Sarcoma

IM, SQ: ADULTS: 30 million units/m^2 3 times/wk on alternating days. Use only 50 million–unit vials. Continue until disease progression or maximal response achieved after 16 wks. If severe adverse reactions occur, modify dose or temporarily discontinue drug.

Chronic Hepatitis B Virus Infection

IM, SQ: ADULTS: 30–35 million units wkly, either as 5 million units/day or 10 million units 3 times/wk for 16 wks.

SQ: CHILDREN 1–17 YRS: 3 million units/m^2 3 times/wk for 1 wk, then 6 million units/m^2 3 times/wk for 16–24 wks. **Maximum:** 10 million units 3 times/wk.

Malignant Melanoma

IV: ADULTS: **Induction:** Initially, 20 million units/m^2 5 times/wk for 4 wks. **Maintenance:** 10 million units subcutaneously 3 times/wk for 48 wks.

Follicular Non-Hodgkin's Lymphoma

SQ: ADULTS: 5 million units 3 times/wk for up to 18 mos.

Dosage in Renal Impairment

Do not use when combined with ribavirin.

Dosage in Hepatic Impairment
No dose adjustment (see Contraindications).

SIDE EFFECTS

Frequent: Flu-like symptoms (fever, fatigue, headache, myalgia, anorexia, chills), rash (hairy cell leukemia, Kaposi's sarcoma only). **Pts with Kaposi's sarcoma:** All previously mentioned side effects plus depression, dyspepsia, dry mouth or thirst, alopecia, rigors. **Occasional:** Dizziness, pruritus, dry skin, dermatitis, altered taste. **Rare:** Confusion, leg cramps, back pain, gingivitis, flushing, tremor, anxiety, eye pain.

ADVERSE EFFECTS/TOXIC REACTIONS

Hypersensitivity reactions occur rarely. Severe flu-like symptoms appear dose-related.

NURSING CONSIDERATIONS

BASELINE ASSESSMENT

CBC, blood chemistries, urinalysis, renal function, LFT should be performed before initial therapy and routinely thereafter.

INTERVENTION/EVALUATION

Offer emotional support. Monitor all levels of clinical function (numerous side effects). Encourage PO intake, particularly during early therapy. Monitor for worsening depression, suicidal ideation, associated behaviors.

PATIENT/FAMILY TEACHING

• Clinical response occurs in 1–3 mos. • Flu-like symptoms tend to diminish with continued therapy. • Some symptoms may be alleviated or minimized by bedtime doses. • Do not have immunizations without physician's approval (drug lowers resistance). • Avoid contact with those who have recently received live virus vaccine. • Avoid tasks that require alertness, motor skills until response to drug is established. • Sips of tepid water may relieve dry mouth. • Report depression, thoughts of suicide, unusual behavior.

TOP 100

interferon beta-1a

in-ter-**feer**-on
(Avonex, Rebif)
Do not confuse Avonex with Avelox, or interferon beta-1a with interferon beta-1b.

◆CLASSIFICATION

PHARMACOTHERAPEUTIC: Biologic response modifier. **CLINICAL:** Multiple sclerosis agent.

USES

Treatment of relapsing multiple sclerosis to slow progression of physical disability, decrease frequency of clinical exacerbations.

PRECAUTIONS

Contraindications: Hypersensitivity to natural or recombinant interferon, human albumin (only for albumin-containing products). **Cautions:** Depression, severe psychiatric disorders, hepatic impairment, increased serum ALT at baseline, alcohol abuse, cardiovascular disease, seizure disorders, myelosuppression.

ACTION

Exact mechanism unknown. Alters expression and response to surface antigens and may enhance immune cell activity. **Therapeutic Effect:** Slows progression of multiple sclerosis.

PHARMACOKINETICS

Peak serum levels attained 3–15 hrs after IM administration. Biologic markers increase within 12 hrs and remain elevated for 4 days. **Half-life:** 10 hrs (Avonex); 69 hrs (Rebif).

⌛ LIFESPAN CONSIDERATIONS

Pregnancy/Lactation: Has abortifacient potential. Unknown if distributed in breast milk. **Children:** Safety and efficacy not established. **Elderly:** No information available.

INTERACTIONS

DRUG: None significant. **HERBAL:** None significant. **FOOD:** None known. **LAB VALUES:** May increase serum glucose, BUN, alkaline phosphatase, bilirubin, calcium, ALT, AST. May decrease Hgb, neutrophil, platelet, WBC.

AVAILABILITY (Rx)

Injection, Powder for Reconstitution: ***(Avonex):*** 30 mcg. **Injection Solution, Prefilled Syringe:** ***(Rebif):*** 22 mcg/0.5 mL, 44 mcg/0.5 mL. ***(Avonex):*** 30 mcg/0.5 mL. **Titration Pack, Prefilled Syringe:** ***(Rebif):*** 8.8 mcg/0.2 mL, 22 mcg/0.5 mL.

ADMINISTRATION/HANDLING

IM (Avonex) Syringe

• Refrigerate syringe. • Allow to warm to room temperature before use. • May store up to 7 days at room temperature.

IM (Avonex) Vial

• Refrigerate vials (may store at room temperature up to 30 days). • Following reconstitution, may refrigerate again but use within 6 hrs if refrigerated. • Reconstitute 30-mcg MicroPin (6.6 million international units) vial with 1.1 mL diluent (supplied by manufacturer). • Gently swirl to dissolve medication; do not shake. • Discard if discolored or particulate forms. • Discard unused portion (contains no preservative).

SQ (Rebif)

• Refrigerate. May store at room temperature up to 30 days. Avoid heat, light. • Administer at same time of day 3 days each wk. Separate doses by at least 48 hrs.

INDICATIONS/ROUTES/DOSAGE

Relapsing Multiple Sclerosis

IM: ***(Avonex):*** **ADULTS:** 30 mcg once wkly.

SQ: ***(Rebif):*** **ADULTS: Target dose 44 mcg 3 times/wk:** Initially, 8.8 mcg 3 times/wk for 2 wks, then 22 mcg 3 times/wk for 2 wks, then 44 mcg 3 times/wk thereafter. **Target dose 22 mcg 3 times/wk:** Initially, 4.4 mcg 3 times/wk for 2 wks, then 11 mcg 3 times/wk for 2 wks, then 22 mcg 3 times/wk thereafter.

Dosage in Renal Impairment

No dose adjustment.

Dosage in Hepatic Impairment (Rebif)

Use with caution in pts with history of active hepatic disease or ALT more than 2.5 times upper limit of normal (ULN).

SIDE EFFECTS

Frequent (67%–11%): Headache, flu-like symptoms, myalgia, upper respiratory tract infection, depression with suicidal ideation, generalized pain, asthenia, chills, sinusitis, infection. **Occasional (9%–4%):** Abdominal pain, arthralgia, chest pain, dyspnea, malaise, syncope. **Rare (3%):** Injection site reaction, hypersensitivity reaction.

ADVERSE EFFECTS/TOXIC REACTIONS

Anemia occurs in 8% of pts. Hepatic failure has been reported.

NURSING CONSIDERATIONS

BASELINE ASSESSMENT

Obtain CBC, BMP, LFT. Assess home situation for support of therapy.

INTERVENTION/EVALUATION

Assess for headache, flu-like symptoms, myalgia. Periodically monitor lab results, re-evaluate injection technique. Assess for depression, suicidal ideation.

PATIENT/FAMILY TEACHING

• Do not change schedule, dosage without consulting physician. • Follow guidelines for reconstitution of product and administration, including aseptic technique. • Use puncture-resistant container for used needles, syringes; dispose of used needles, syringes properly. • Injection site reactions may occur. These do not require discontinuation of therapy, but type and extent should be carefully noted. Report flu-like symptoms (fever, chills, fatigue, muscle aches).

interferon beta-1b TOP 100

in-ter-**feer**-on
(Betaseron, Extavia)
Do not confuse interferon beta-1b with interferon beta-1a.

◆CLASSIFICATION

PHARMACOTHERAPEUTIC: Biologic response modifier. **CLINICAL:** Multiple sclerosis agent.

USES

Reduces frequency of clinical exacerbations in pts with relapsing-remitting multiple sclerosis (recurrent attacks of neurologic dysfunction).

PRECAUTIONS

Contraindications: Hypersensitivity to albumin, interferon. **Cautions:** Depression, severe psychiatric disorders, hepatic/renal impairment, alcohol abuse, cardiovascular disease, seizure disorders, myelosuppression, pulmonary disease.

ACTION

Exact mechanism unknown. Immunomodulator effects include enhanced suppression of T-cell activity, reduced pro-inflammatory cytokines, reduced movement of lymphocytes into CNS. **Therapeutic Effect:** Improves MRI lesions, decreases relapse rate and disease severity in multiple sclerosis.

PHARMACOKINETICS

Slowly absorbed following SQ administration. **Half-life:** 8 min–4.3 hrs.

⌛ LIFESPAN CONSIDERATIONS

Pregnancy/Lactation: Spontaneous abortions reported. Discontinuation of the drug before conception is recommended. Unknown if distributed in breast milk. **Children:** Safety and efficacy not established. **Elderly:** No information available.

INTERACTIONS

DRUG: None significant. **HERBAL:** None significant. **FOOD:** None known. **LAB VALUES:** May increase bilirubin, ALT, AST. May decrease neutrophil, lymphocyte, WBC.

AVAILABILITY (Rx)

Injection, Powder for Reconstitution: 0.3 mg.

ADMINISTRATION/HANDLING

SQ

• Store vials at room temperature. • After reconstitution, stable for 3 hrs if refrigerated. • Use within 3 hrs of reconstitution. • Discard if discolored or precipitate forms. • Reconstitute 0.3-mg (9.6 million international units) vial with 1.2 mL diluent (supplied by manufacturer) to provide concentration of 0.25 mg/mL (8 million units/mL). • Gently swirl to dissolve medication; do not shake. • Withdraw 1 mL solution and inject subcutaneously into arms, abdomen, hips, thighs using 27-gauge needle. • Discard unused portion (contains no preservative).

INDICATIONS/ROUTES/DOSAGE

Relapsing-Remitting Multiple Sclerosis
SQ: ADULTS: Initially, 0.0625 mg (0.25 mL) every other day; gradually increase by 0.0625 mg every 2 wks. Target dose: 0.25 mg every other day.

Dosage in Renal/Hepatic Impairment
No dose adjustment.

SIDE EFFECTS

Frequent (85%–21%): Injection site reaction, headache, flu-like symptoms, fever, asthenia, myalgia, sinusitis, diarrhea, dizziness, altered mental status, constipation, diaphoresis, vomiting. **Occasional (15%–4%):** Malaise, drowsiness, alopecia.

ADVERSE EFFECTS/TOXIC REACTIONS

Seizures occur rarely.

NURSING CONSIDERATIONS

BASELINE ASSESSMENT

Obtain CBC, BMP, LFT. Assess home situation for support of therapy.

INTERVENTION/EVALUATION

Periodically monitor lab results, re-evaluate injection technique. Assess for nausea (high incidence). Monitor sleep pattern. Monitor daily pattern of bowel activity, stool consistency. Assist with ambulation if dizziness occurs. Monitor food intake.

PATIENT/FAMILY TEACHING

• Report flu-like symptoms (fever, chills, fatigue, muscle aches); occur commonly but decrease over time. • Wear sunscreen, protective clothing if exposed to sunlight, ultraviolet light until tolerance known.

ipilimumab

ip-i-**lim**-ue-mab
(Yervoy)

■ **BLACK BOX ALERT** ■ Severe and fatal immune-mediated adverse reactions due to T-cell activation and proliferation are capable of involving any organ system. Specific reactions include enterocolitis, hepatitis, dermatitis, neuropathy, endocrinopathy. Majority of immune-mediated reactions may initially manifest during treatment or weeks to months after treatment. Permanently discontinue treatment and initiate high-dose corticosteroid therapy for severe immune-mediated adverse reactions. Assess all pts for signs/symptoms of enterocolitis, hepatitis, dermatitis (including toxic epidermal necrolysis), neuropathy, endocrinopathy, and evaluate clinical chemistries, including hepatic function tests and thyroid tests at baseline and before each treatment.

◆CLASSIFICATION

PHARMACOTHERAPEUTIC: Human cytotoxic T-lymphocyte antigen 4 (CTLA-4)–blocking antibody. Monoclonal antibody. **CLINICAL:** Antineoplastic.

USES

Treatment of unresectable or metastatic melanoma in adults and children 12 yrs of age and older. Adjuvant treatment of pts with cutaneous melanoma with pathologic involvement of regional lymph nodes and who have undergone complete resection, including total lymphadenectomy. Treatment of metastatic colorectal cancer (in combination with nivolumab). Treatment of advanced renal cell carcinoma (in combination with nivolumab).

PRECAUTIONS

Contraindications: Hypersensitivity to ipilimumab. **Cautions:** Hepatic impairment, chronic peripheral neuropathy, thyroid/adrenal/pituitary dysfunction, autoimmune disorders (ulcerative colitis, Crohn's disease, lupus, sarcoidosis).

ACTION

Augments T-cell activation and proliferation. Binds to cytotoxic T-lymphocyte–associated antigen 4 (CTLA-4) and blocks interaction of CTLA-4 with its ligands, allowing for enhanced T-cell activation and proliferation. **Therapeutic Effect:** May indirectly mediate T-cell immune responses against tumors.

PHARMACOKINETICS

Metabolized in liver. Steady state reached by third dose. **Half-life:** 14.7 days.

LIFESPAN CONSIDERATIONS

Pregnancy/Lactation: May cause fetal harm. Use effective contraception during treatment and for at least 3 mos after discontinuation. Unknown if distributed in breast milk. Discontinue drug or discontinue breastfeeding. **Children:** Safety and efficacy not established. **Elderly:** No age-related precautions noted.

INTERACTIONS

DRUG: May increase hepatotoxic effect of **vemurafenib.** **HERBAL:** None significant. **FOOD:** None known. **LAB VALUES:** May increase serum ALT, AST, bilirubin; eosinophils.

AVAILABILITY (Rx)

Injection, Solution: 5 mg/mL (10 mL, 40 mL vials).

ADMINISTRATION/HANDLING

IV

◄ALERT► Use sterile, nonpyrogenic, low protein-binding in-line filter. Use dedicated line only.

Reconstitution • Calculate number of vials needed for injection. • Inspect for particulate matter or discoloration. • Allow vials to stand at room temperature for approximately 5 min. • Withdraw proper volume and transfer to infusion bag. Dilute in NaCl or D_5W with final concentration ranging from 1–2 mg/mL. • Mix diluted solution by gentle inversion. Do not shake or agitate.

Rate of administration • Infuse over 90 min. Flush with 0.9% NaCl or D_5W at end of infusion.

Storage • Solution should be translucent to white or pale yellow with amorphous particles. • Discard vial if cloudy or discolored. • Refrigerate vials until time of use. • May store diluted solution either under refrigeration or at room temperature for no more than 24 hrs.

INDICATIONS/ROUTES/DOSAGE

Metastatic Melanoma

IV: ADULTS, CHILDREN 12 YRS AND OLDER: 3 mg/kg q3wks for maximum of 4 doses. Doses may be delayed due to toxicity, but all doses must be given within 16 wks of initial dose.

◄ALERT► Pts presenting with severe immune-mediated adverse reactions must immediately discontinue drug therapy and start predniSONE 1 mg/kg/day.

Cutaneous Melanoma

IV: ADULTS: 10 mg/kg q3wks for 4 doses, then 10 mg/kg q12wks for up to 3 yrs. If toxicity occurs, doses are omitted (not delayed).

Colorectal Cancer

IV: ADULTS, CHILDREN 12 YRS AND OLDER: 1 mg/kg q3wks for up to 4 combination doses, followed by nivolumab monotherapy. Continue until disease progression or unacceptable toxicity.

Renal Cell Cancer

IV: ADULTS: 1 mg/kg q3wks for up to 4 combination doses, followed by nivolumab monotherapy. Continue until disease progression or unacceptable toxicity.

Dosage Modification

Hold scheduled dose for moderate immune-mediated adverse reactions. Pts with complete or partial resolution of adverse reactions and who are receiving less than 7.5 mg/day of predniSONE may resume scheduled doses. Permanently discontinue for persistent moderate adverse reactions or inability to reduce corticosteroid dose to 7.5 mg/day, failure to complete full treatment course in 16 wks, any severe or life-threatening adverse reactions.

Hepatotoxicity

ALT/AST greater than 2.5 times upper limit of normal (ULN) or bilirubin greater than 1.5–3 times ULN: Withhold treatment. **ALT/AST greater than 5 times ULN or bilirubin greater than 3 times ULN:** Permanently discontinue.

Dosage in Renal/Hepatic Impairment

No dose adjustment.

SIDE EFFECTS

Frequent (42%): Fatigue. **Occasional** (32%–29%): Diarrhea, pruritus, rash, colitis.

ADVERSE EFFECTS/TOXIC REACTIONS

Severe and fatal immune-mediated adverse reactions have occurred. Enterocolitis (7% of pts) may present with fever, ileus, abdominal pain, GI bleeding, intestinal perforation, severe dehydrating diarrhea. Endocrinopathies (4% of pts), including hypopituitarism, adrenal insufficiency, hypogonadism, hypothyroidism, may present with fatigue, headache, mental status change, unusual bowel habits, hypotension and may require emergent hormone replacement therapy. Dermatitis including toxic epidermal necrolysis (2% of pts) may present with full-thickness ulceration or necrotic, bullous, hemorrhagic manifestations. Hepatotoxicity (1% of pts), defined as LFT greater than 2.5–5 times ULN, may present with right upper abdominal pain, jaundice, black/tarry stools, bruising, dark-colored urine, nausea, vomiting. Neuropathy (1% of pts), including Guillain-Barré syndrome or myasthenia gravis, may present with weakness, sensory alterations, paresthesia, paralysis. Other serious adverse reactions such as pneumonitis, meningitis, nephritis, eosinophilia, pericarditis, myocarditis, angiopathy, temporal arteritis, vasculitis, polymyalgia rheumatica, conjunctivitis, blepharitis, episcleritis, scleritis, leukocytoclastic vasculitis, erythema multiforme, psoriasis, pancreatitis, arthritis, autoimmune thyroiditis reported. Anti-ipilimumab antibodies reported in 1.1% of pts. All severe immune-mediated adverse reactions require immediate high-dose corticosteroid therapy.

NURSING CONSIDERATIONS

BASELINE ASSESSMENT

Obtain CBC, BMP, LFT; pregnancy test in females of reproductive potential. Screen for history of hepatic impairment, chronic neuropathy, thyroid/adrenal/pituitary dysfunction, autoimmune disorders. Screen for active infection. Receive full medication history including herbal products.

INTERVENTION/EVALUATION

Monitor vital signs, LFT, thyroid panel before each dose. Continue focused assessment and screen for life-threatening immune-mediated adverse reactions. If adverse reactions occur, immediately notify physician and initiate proper treatment. Report suspected pregnancy. Obtain CBC, blood cultures for fever, suspected infection. ECG for palpitations, chest pain, difficulty breathing, dizziness. If predniSONE therapy initiated, monitor capillary blood glucose and screen for side effects.

PATIENT/FAMILY TEACHING

• Serious and fatal adverse reactions indicate inflammation to certain systems: intestines (diarrhea, dark/tarry stools, abdominal pain), liver (yellowing of the skin, dark-colored urine, right upper quadrant pain, bruising), skin (rash, mouth sores, blisters, ulcers), nerves (weakness, numbness, tingling, difficulty breathing, paralysis), hormonal glands (headaches, weight gain, palpitations, changes in mood or behavior, dizziness), eyes (blurry vision, double vision, eye pain/redness). • PredniSONE therapy may be started if adverse reactions occur. • May cause fetal harm, stillbirth, premature delivery. • Report any chest pain, palpitations, fever, swollen glands, stomach pain, vomiting, or any sign of adverse reactions.

ipratropium TOP 100

ip-ra-**troe**-pee-um
(Atrovent HFA, Apo-Ipravent ✱)
Do not confuse Atrovent with Alupent or Serevent, or ipratropium with tiotropium.

FIXED-COMBINATION(S)

Combivent, DuoNeb: ipratropium/albuterol (a bronchodilator): *Aerosol:* 18 mcg/90 mcg per actuation. *Solution:* 0.5 mg/2.5 mg per 3 mL.

◆CLASSIFICATION

PHARMACOTHERAPEUTIC: Anticholinergic. **CLINICAL:** Bronchodilator.

USES

Inhalation, Nebulization: Maintenance treatment of bronchospasm due to COPD, including bronchitis, emphysema. Not indicated for immediate bronchospasm relief. **Nasal Spray:** Symptomatic relief of rhinorrhea associated with the common cold and allergic/nonallergic rhinitis.
OFF-LABEL: Acute asthma (exacerbation).

PRECAUTIONS

Contraindications: History of hypersensitivity to ipratropium, atropine. **Cautions:** Narrow-angle glaucoma, prostatic hypertrophy, bladder neck obstruction, myasthenia gravis.

ACTION

Blocks action of acetylcholine at parasympathetic sites in bronchial smooth muscle. Application to nasal mucosa inhibits serous/seromucous gland secretions. **Therapeutic Effect:** Causes bronchodilation, inhibits nasal secretions.

PHARMACOKINETICS

Route	Onset	Peak	Duration
Inhalation	1–3 min	1.5–2 hrs	Up to 4 hrs
Nasal	5 min	1–4 hrs	4–8 hrs

Minimal systemic absorption after inhalation. Metabolized in liver (systemic absorption). Primarily excreted in feces. **Half-life:** 1.5–4 hrs (nasal).

LIFESPAN CONSIDERATIONS

Pregnancy/Lactation: Unknown if distributed in breast milk. **Children/Elderly:** No age-related precautions noted.

INTERACTIONS

DRUG: **Anticholinergics (e.g., aclidinium, ipratropium, tiotropium, umeclidinium), medications with anticholinergic properties** may increase toxicity. **HERBAL:** None significant. **FOOD:** None known. **LAB VALUES:** None significant.

AVAILABILITY (Rx)

Aerosol for Oral Inhalation: ***(Atrovent HFA):*** 17 mcg/actuation. **Solution, Intranasal Spray:** 0.03%; 0.06%. **Solution for Nebulization:** 0.02% (500 mcg).

ADMINISTRATION/HANDLING

Inhalation

• Do not shake. Prime before first use or if not used for more than 3 days. • Instruct pt to exhale completely, place mouthpiece between lips, inhale deeply through mouth while fully depressing top of canister. Hold breath as long as possible before exhaling slowly. • Allow at least 1 minute between inhalations. • Rinse mouth with water immediately after inhalation (prevents mouth/throat dryness).

Nebulization

• May be administered with or without dilution in 0.9% NaCl. • Stable for 1 hr when mixed with albuterol. • Give over 5–15 min.

Nasal

• Store at room temperature. • Initial pump priming requires 7 actuations of pump. • If used regularly as recommended, no further priming is required. If not used for more than 4 hrs, pump will require 2 actuations, or if not used for more than 7 days, the pump will require 7 actuations to reprime.

INDICATIONS/ROUTES/DOSAGE

Bronchodilator for COPD

Inhalation: **ADULTS, ELDERLY, CHILDREN OLDER THAN 12 YRS:** 2 inhalations 4 times/day. **Maximum:** 12 inhalations per 24 hrs.
Nebulization: **ADULTS, ELDERLY, CHILDREN OLDER THAN 12 YRS:** 500 mcg (1 unit dose vial) 3–4 times/day (doses 6–8 hrs apart).

Asthma Exacerbation

Note: Should be given in combination with a short-acting beta-adrenergic agonist.
Inhalation: **ADULTS, ELDERLY, CHILDREN OLDER THAN 12 YRS:** 8 inhalations q20min as needed for up to 3 hrs. **CHILDREN 6–12 YRS:** 4–8 inhalations q20min as needed for up to 3 hrs. **CHILDREN 5 YRS OR YOUNGER:** 2 inhalations q20 min for 1 hr.
Nebulization: **ADULTS, ELDERLY, CHILDREN OLDER THAN 12 YRS:** 500 mcg q20min for 3 doses, then as needed. **CHILDREN 6–12 YRS:** 250–500 mcg q20min for 3 doses, then as needed. **CHILDREN 5 YRS OR YOUNGER:** 250 mcg q20 min for 1 hr.

Rhinorrhea (Perennial allergic/nonallergic rhinitis)

Intranasal: ***(0.03%):*** **ADULTS, ELDERLY, CHILDREN 6 YRS AND OLDER:** 2 sprays (21 mcg/spray) per nostril 2–3 times/day. Total dose: 168–252 mcg/day.

Rhinorrhea (Common cold)

Intranasal: ***(0.06%):*** **ADULTS, ELDERLY, CHILDREN 12 YRS AND OLDER:** 2 sprays (42 mcg/spray) per nostril 3–4 times/day for up to 4 days. Total dose: 504–672 mcg/day. **CHILDREN 5–11 YRS:** 2 sprays per nostril 3 times/day for up to 4 days. Total dose: 504 mcg/day.

Rhinorrhea (Seasonal allergy)
Intranasal: *(0.06%):* **ADULTS, ELDERLY, CHILDREN 5 YRS AND OLDER:** 2 sprays (42 mcg/spray) per nostril 4 times/day for up to 3 wks. Total dose: 672 mcg/day.

Dosage in Renal/Hepatic Impairment
No dose adjustment.

SIDE EFFECTS

Frequent: Inhalation (6%–3%): Cough, dry mouth, headache, nausea. **Nasal:** Dry nose/mouth, headache, nasal irritation. **Occasional: Inhalation (2%):** Dizziness, transient increased bronchospasm. **Rare (less than 1%): Inhalation:** Hypotension, insomnia, metallic/unpleasant taste, palpitations, urinary retention. **Nasal:** Diarrhea, constipation, dry throat, abdominal pain, nasal congestion.

ADVERSE EFFECTS/TOXIC REACTIONS

Worsening of angle-closure glaucoma, acute eye pain, hypotension occur rarely.

NURSING CONSIDERATIONS

BASELINE ASSESSMENT

Auscultate lung sounds. Question history of glaucoma, urinary retention, myasthenia gravis.

INTERVENTION/EVALUATION

Monitor rate, depth, rhythm, type of respiration; quality, rate of pulse. Assess lung sounds for rhonchi, wheezing, rales. Monitor ABGs. Observe for retractions (clavicular, sternal, intercostal), hand tremor. Evaluate for clinical improvement (quieter, slower respirations, relaxed facial expression, cessation of retractions). Monitor for improvement of rhinorrhea.

PATIENT/ FAMILY TEACHING

• Increase fluid intake (decreases lung secretion viscosity). • Do not take more than 2 inhalations at any one time (excessive use may produce paradoxical bronchoconstriction, decreased bronchodilating effect). • Rinsing mouth with water immediately after inhalation may prevent mouth and throat dryness. • Avoid excessive use of caffeine derivatives (chocolate, coffee, tea, cola, cocoa).

irbesartan

ir-be-**sar**-tan
(Avapro)

BLACK BOX ALERT May cause fetal injury, mortality if used during second or third trimester of pregnancy. Discontinue as soon as possible once pregnancy is detected.
Do not confuse Avapro with Anaprox.

FIXED-COMBINATION(S)

Avalide: irbesartan/hydroCHLOROthiazide (a diuretic): 150 mg/12.5 mg, 300 mg/12.5 mg, 300 mg/25 mg.

◆CLASSIFICATION

PHARMACOTHERAPEUTIC: Angiotensin II receptor antagonist. **CLINICAL:** Antihypertensive.

USES

Treatment of hypertension alone or in combination with other antihypertensives. Treatment of diabetic nephropathy in pts with type 2 diabetes. **OFF-LABEL:** Reduce proteinuria in children with chronic kidney disease.

PRECAUTIONS

Contraindications: Hypersensitivity to irbesartan. Concomitant use with aliskiren in pts with diabetes. **Cautions:** Renal impairment, unstented unilateral or bilateral renal artery stenosis, dehydration, HF, idiopathic or hereditary angioedema or angioedema associated with ACE inhibitor therapy.

ACTION

Blocks vasoconstriction, aldosterone-secreting effects of angiotensin II, inhibiting binding of angiotensin II to AT_1 receptors. **Therapeutic Effect:** Produces vasodilation, decreases peripheral resistance, decreases B/P.

PHARMACOKINETICS

Route	Onset	Peak	Duration
PO	—	1–2 hrs	Greater than 24 hrs

Rapidly, completely absorbed after PO administration. Protein binding: 90%. Metabolized in liver. Excreted in feces (80%), urine (20%). Not removed by hemodialysis. **Half-life:** 11–15 hrs.

LIFESPAN CONSIDERATIONS

Pregnancy/Lactation: Unknown if distributed in breast milk. May cause fetal or neonatal morbidity or mortality. **Children:** Safety and efficacy not established. **Elderly:** No age-related precautions noted.

INTERACTIONS

DRUG: **Aliskiren** may increase hyperkalemic effect. May increase adverse of **ACE inhibitors (e.g., benazepril, lisinopril). NSAIDs (e.g., ibuprofen, ketorolac, naproxen)** may decrease antihypertensive effect. **HERBAL:** **Herbals with hypertensive properties (e.g., licorice, yohimbe) or hypotensive properties (e.g., garlic, ginger, ginkgo biloba)** may alter effects. **FOOD:** None known. **LAB VALUES:** May slightly increase serum BUN, creatinine. May decrease Hgb.

AVAILABILITY (Rx)

Tablets: 75 mg, 150 mg, 300 mg.

ADMINISTRATION/HANDLING

PO

- Give without regard to food.

INDICATIONS/ROUTES/DOSAGE

Hypertension

PO: ADULTS, ELDERLY, CHILDREN 13 YRS AND OLDER: Initially, 75–150 mg/day. May increase to 300 mg/day. **CHILDREN 6–12 YRS:** Initially, 75 mg/day. May increase to 150 mg/day.

Diabetic Nephropathy

PO: ADULTS, ELDERLY: 300 mg once daily.

Dosage in Renal/Hepatic Impairment

No dose adjustment.

SIDE EFFECTS

Occasional (9%–3%): Upper respiratory tract infection, fatigue, diarrhea, cough. **Rare (2%–1%):** Heartburn, dizziness, headache, nausea, rash.

ADVERSE EFFECTS/TOXIC REACTIONS

Overdose may manifest as hypotension, syncope, tachycardia. Bradycardia occurs less often.

NURSING CONSIDERATIONS

BASELINE ASSESSMENT

Obtain B/P, pulse immediately before each dose in addition to regular monitoring (be alert to fluctuations). Question possibility of pregnancy. Assess medication history (esp. diuretic therapy).

INTERVENTION/EVALUATION

Maintain hydration (offer fluids frequently). Assess for evidence of upper respiratory infection. Assist with ambulation if dizziness occurs. Monitor B/P, pulse. Assess for hypotension.

PATIENT/ FAMILY TEACHING

• May cause fetal or neonatal morbidity or mortality. • Report any sign of infection (sore throat, fever). • Avoid exercising during hot weather (risk of dehydration, hypotension).

irinotecan

eye-ri-noe-**tee**-kan
(Camptosar, Onivyde)

■ BLACK BOX ALERT ■ **(Camptosar, Onivyde):** Can induce both early and late forms of severe diarrhea. Early diarrhea (during or shortly after administration) accompanied by salivation, rhinitis, lacrimation, diaphoresis, flushing. Late diarrhea (occurring more than 24 hrs after administration) can be prolonged and life-threatening. **(Camptosar):**

May produce severe, profound myelosuppression. Administer under supervision of experienced cancer chemotherapy physician. **(Onivyde):** Severe, life-threatening, or fatal neutropenic fever/sepsis occurred. Withhold for ANC below 1,500 cells/mm^3 or neutropenic fever. Monitor blood cell counts.

◆CLASSIFICATION

PHARMACOTHERAPEUTIC: Topoisomerase-I inhibitor. **CLINICAL:** Antineoplastic.

USES

Camptosar: Treatment of metastatic carcinoma of colon or rectum. **Onivyde:** Treatment of metastatic adenocarcinoma of the pancreas (in combination with 5-fluorouracil and leucovorin) after disease progression following gemcitabine-based therapy. **OFF-LABEL:** Non–small-cell lung cancer; small-cell lung cancer; CNS tumor; cervical, gastric, pancreatic, ovarian, esophageal cancer; Ewing's sarcoma; brain tumor.

PRECAUTIONS

Contraindications: Hypersensitivity to irinotecan. **Cautions:** Pt previously receiving pelvic, abdominal irradiation (increased risk of myelosuppression), pts older than 65 yrs, hepatic dysfunction, hyperbilirubinemia, renal impairment, preexisting pulmonary disease, conditions predisposing to infection (e.g., diabetes, renal failure, immunocompromised pts, open wounds).

ACTION

Binds reversibly with topoisomerase I, an enzyme that relieves torsional strain in DNA by inducing reversible single-strand breaks. Prevents religation of these single-stranded breaks, resulting in damage to double-strand DNA, cell death. **Therapeutic Effect:** Produces cytotoxic effect on cancer cells.

PHARMACOKINETICS

Metabolized in liver. Protein binding: 95% (metabolite). Excreted in urine and eliminated by biliary route. **Half-life:** 6–12 hrs; metabolite, 10–20 hrs.

LIFESPAN CONSIDERATIONS

Pregnancy/Lactation: Avoid pregnancy; may cause fetal harm. Females of reproductive potential must use effective contraception during treatment and for at least 6 mos after discontinuation. Breastfeeding not recommended during treatment and for at least 7 days after discontinuation. May impair fertility. **Males:** Males with female partners of reproductive potential must use effective contraception during treatment and for at least 3 mos after discontinuation. May impair fertility. **Children:** Safety and efficacy not established. **Elderly:** Risk of diarrhea significantly increased.

INTERACTIONS

DRUG: **Strong CYP3A4 inducers (e.g., carBAMazepine, phenytoin, rifAMPin)** may decrease concentration/effect. **Strong CYP3A4 inhibitors (e.g., clarithromycin, ketoconazole, ritonavir)** may increase concentration/effect. May decrease the therapeutic effect of **BCG (intravesical), vaccines (live).** May increase adverse effects of **vaccines (live). UGT1A1 inhibitors (e.g., erlotinib, nilotinib)** may increase concentration/effect. **HERBAL:** **St. John's wort** may decrease concentration/effect. **FOOD:** None known. **LAB VALUES:** May increase serum alkaline phosphatase, AST. May decrease Hgb, leukocytes, platelets.

AVAILABILITY (Rx)

Injection Solution: ***(Conventional):*** 20 mg/mL (2 mL, 5 mL, 15 mL, 25 mL). ***(Liposomal):*** 43 mg/10 mL.

ADMINISTRATION/HANDLING

IV

Camptosar

Reconstitution • Dilute in D_5W (preferred) or 0.9% NaCl to concentration of 0.12–2.8 mg/mL.

Rate of administration • Administer all doses as IV infusion over 30–90 min. • Assess for extravasation (flush

site with Sterile Water for Injection, apply ice if extravasation occurs).
Storage • Store vials at room temperature, protect from light. • Solution diluted with D_5W is stable for 24 hrs at room temperature or 48 hrs if refrigerated. • Solution diluted with 0.9% NaCl is stable for 24 hrs at room temperature. • Do not refrigerate solution if diluted with 0.9% NaCl.

Onivyde
Reconstitution • Withdraw dose from vial and dilute with 500 mL D_5W or 0.9% NaCl. Mix gently.
Rate of administration • Infuse over 90 min.
Storage • Refrigerate vials; do not freeze. • Protect from light. • Stable for 4 hrs at room temperature or 24 hrs refrigerated.

IV INCOMPATIBILITIES

Gemcitabine (Gemzar).

INDICATIONS/ROUTES/DOSAGE

Carcinoma of the Colon, Rectum (Camptosar)
IV: ***(Single-Agent Therapy):*** **ADULTS, ELDERLY: (WEEKLY REGIMEN):** Initially, 125 mg/m^2 once wkly for 4 wks, followed by a rest period of 2 wks. Additional courses may be repeated q6wks. Dosage may be adjusted in 25–50 mg/m^2 increments/decrements to as high as 150 mg/m^2 or as low as 50 mg/m^2. **(3-WEEK REGIMEN):** 350 mg/m^2 q3wks. Dosage may be adjusted to as low as 200 mg/m^2 in decrements of 25–50 mg/m^2.
(In Combination With Leucovorin and 5-Fluorouracil):(Leucovorin given immediately following irinotecan, then 5-fluorouracil immediately following leucovorin.) **REGIMEN 1:** 125 mg/m^2 on days 1, 8, 15, 22. Dose may be adjusted to 100 mg/m^2, then 75 mg/m^2, then decrements of approximately 20%. **REGIMEN 2:** 180 mg/m^2 on days 1, 15, 29. Dose may be adjusted to 150 mg/m^2, then 120 mg/m^2, then decrements of approximately 20%.

Pancreatic Cancer (Onivyde)
IV Infusion: ADULTS, ELDERLY: 70 mg/m^2 once q2wks (in combination with leucovorin and 5-fluorouracil). Reduce initial starting dose to 50 mg/m^2 in pts homozygous for the UGT1A1*28 allele. May increase dose to 70 mg/m^2 as tolerated.

Dosage in Renal Impairment
No dose adjustment.

Dosage in Hepatic Impairment

Serum Bilirubin	Dose
Greater than ULN to 2 mg/dL:	Reduce dose one level
Greater than 2 mg/dL:	Not recommended

SIDE EFFECTS

Expected (64%–32%): Nausea, alopecia, vomiting, diarrhea. **Frequent (29%–22%):** Constipation, fatigue, fever, asthenia, skeletal pain, abdominal pain, dyspnea. **Occasional (19%–16%):** Anorexia, headache, stomatitis, rash.

ADVERSE EFFECTS/TOXIC REACTIONS

Myelosuppression is an expected response to therapy, but more severe reactions including febrile neutropenia may be life threatening. Pts who are homozygous for the UGT1A1*28 allele are at increased risk for neutropenia. Hypersensitivity reactions including anaphylaxis may occur. Fatal pulmonary toxicities, interstitial pulmonary disease were reported. Diarrhea may cause severe dehydration, renal failure, which can be fatal. Cholinergic reactions including rhinitis, increased salivation, miosis, lacrimation, diaphoresis, flushing, and intestinal hyperperistalsis may occur.

NURSING CONSIDERATIONS

BASELINE ASSESSMENT

Obtain CBC (prior to each dose), LFT; pregnancy test in females of reproductive potential. Due to risk of severe dehydration related to diarrhea, ensure adequate hydration prior to each dose. Question history pulmonary disease, hepatic/renal impairment. Screen for active infection. Receive full medication history and screen for interactions. Premedicate with antiemetics on day of treatment, starting at least 30 min before administration. Offer emotional support.

INTERVENTION/EVALUATION

Monitor CBC as indicated. Monitor pulmonary status, pulse oximeter readings. Consider ABG, radiologic test if ILD/pneumonitis (excessive cough, dyspnea, fever, hypoxia) is suspected. Consider treatment with corticosteroids if ILD/pneumonitis is confirmed. Monitor for infections (cough, fatigue, fever). If serious infection occurs, initiate appropriate antimicrobial therapy. Monitor daily pattern of bowel activity, stool consistency. Severe diarrhea may be life-threatening. Monitor for hypersensitivity reactions, anaphylaxis. Assess skin for rash.

PATIENT/ FAMILY TEACHING

• Treatment may depress your immune system response and reduce your ability to fight infection. Report symptoms of infection such as body aches, chills, cough, fatigue, fever. Avoid those with active infection. • Report symptoms of lung inflammation (excessive coughing, difficulty breathing, chest pain); liver problems (abdominal pain, bruising, clay-colored stool, amber- or dark-colored urine, yellowing of the skin or eyes). • Diarrhea may cause severe dehydration, which can be life-threatening. Report diarrhea of any severity. • Allergic reactions, including anaphylaxis, can occur. • Use effective contraception to avoid pregnancy. Do not breastfeed. • There is a high risk of interactions with other medications. Do not take newly prescribed medications unless approved by prescriber who originally started treatment. • Report diarrhea, vomiting, fever, light-headedness, dizziness. • Do not have immunizations without physician's approval (drug lowers resistance). • Avoid contact with those who have recently received live virus vaccine. • Avoid crowds, those with infections.

isatuximab-irfc

eye-sa-**tux**-i-mab
(Sarclisa)

Do not confuse isatuximab with daratumumab, dinutuximab, elotuzumab, ipilimumab, ixabepilone, ixazomib or rituximab.

◆CLASSIFICATION

PHARMACOTHERAPEUTIC: Anti-CD38 immunoglobulin G1–derived monoclonal antibody. **CLINICAL:** Antineoplastic.

USES

Treatment of multiple myeloma (in combination with pomalidomide and dexamethasone) in adults who have received at least two prior therapies including lenalidomide and a proteasome inhibitor.

PRECAUTIONS

Contraindications: Hypersensitivity to isatuximab. **Cautions:** Baseline cytopenias, conditions predisposing to infection (e.g., diabetes, renal failure, immunocompromised pts, open wounds).

ACTION

Binds to and inhibits cell surface glycoprotein CD38 on CD38-expressing tumor cells (highly expressed on myeloma cells). Promotes antibody-dependent cellular phagocytosis and cell-mediated cytotoxicity. Suppresses CD38-positive T-regulatory cells and activates natural killer cells in the absence of CD38-positive target tumor cells. **Therapeutic Effect:** Inhibits tumor cell growth.

PHARMACOKINETICS

Widely distributed. Metabolized into small peptides via catabolic pathway. Steady state reached in 8 wks. **Half-life:** Not specified.

I

LIFESPAN CONSIDERATIONS

Pregnancy/Lactation: Avoid pregnancy; may cause fetal harm. Females of reproductive potential must use effective contraception during treatment and for at least 5 mos after discontinuation. Unknown if distributed in breast milk. However, human immunoglobulin G (IgG) is present in breast milk and is known to cross the placenta. Breastfeeding not recommended. **Children:** Safety and efficacy not established. **Elderly:** No age-related precautions noted.

INTERACTIONS

DRUG: May decrease effect of **BCG intravesical, vaccines (live).** May increase adverse/toxic effect of **leflunomide, natalizumab. Cladribine, upadacitinib** may enhance the immunosuppressive effect. **Pimecrolimus, tacrolimus (topical)** may increase adverse/toxic effects **HERBAL:** **Echinacea** may decrease therapeutic effect. **FOOD:** None known. **LAB VALUES:** May mask detection of antibodies to minor antigens. Drug may be detected on both serum protein electrophoresis and immunofixation assays used to monitor multiple myeloma endogenous M-protein. May affect the determination of complete response and disease progression of some pts with IgG kappa myeloma protein. May cause positive Coombs test. May decrease Hgb, Hct, lymphocytes, neutrophils, platelets, RBCs.

AVAILABILITY (Rx)

Injection Solution: 100 mg/5 mL (20 mg/mL), 500 mg/25 mg/mL (20 mg/mL).

ADMINISTRATION/HANDLING

IV

Premedication • Give dexamethasone 40 mg PO or IV (20 mg PO or IV in pts 75 yrs or older), acetaminophen 650–1000 mg PO (or equivalent), an H_2 antagonist, and diphenhydramine 25–50 mg PO or IV (or equivalent) approx. 15–60 min prior to infusion. Diphenhydramine IV is preferred for the first 4 treatments.

Infusion guidelines • Infusion bag must be made of polyolefins, polyethylene, polypropylene, polyvinyl chloride (PVC) with di-(2-ethylhexyl) phthalate (DEHP), or ethyl vinyl acetate (EVA). • Infuse via dedicated IV line with a 0.22 micron in-line filter. • Do not administer as IV push or bolus. • Do not administer with other infusions. • If a dose is missed, give as soon as possible and adjust schedule to maintain treatment interval.

Preparation • Must be prepared by personnel trained in aseptic manipulations and admixing of cytotoxic drugs. • Calculate the number of vials needed for dose based on weight in kg. • Visually inspect for particulate matter or discoloration. Solution should appear clear to slightly opalescent, colorless to slightly yellow in color. Do not use if solution is cloudy, discolored, or if visible particles are observed. • Remove a volume from a 250 mL NaCl or D_5W infusion bag that is equal to the required volume of vial for dose. • Dilute in 250 mL NaCl or D_5W infusion bag. • Gently invert to mix. Do not shake or agitate.

Rate of administration • **First infusion:** Infuse at 25 mL/hr for 60 min. May increase rate in increments of 25 mL/hr q30min up to a maximum rate of 150 mL/hr if no infusion reactions occur. • **Second infusion:** Infuse at 50 mL/hr for the first 30 min. May increase rate in increments of 100 mL/hr q30min up to a maximum rate of 200 mL/hr if no infusion reactions occur. • **Subsequent infusions:** Infuse at 200 mL/hr if previous infusion rates were tolerated. **Maximum rate:** 200 mL/hr.

Infusion reactions • If Grade 1 or 2 infusion-related reactions occur, interrupt infusion and treat symptoms. If symptoms improve, resume infusion at half of the initial infusion rate. If symptoms do not recur after 30 min, may increase to initial rate, and then follow usual titration protocol. • Permanently discontinue in pts with a Grade 3 or 4 infusion-related reaction or if symptoms do not improve or recur after interrupting infusion.

Storage • Refrigerate unused vials in original carton. • Protect from light. • May refrigerate diluted solution for up to 48 hrs or store at room temperature for up to 8 hrs. • Do not shake, agitate, or freeze.

IV INCOMPATABILITIES

Do not mix with solutions containing other medications.

INDICATIONS/ROUTES/DOSAGE

Multiple Myeloma

IV: ADULTS: Cycle 1: 10 mg/kg on days 1, 8, 15, and 22 of a 28-day cycle (in combination with pomalidomide and dexamethasone). **Cycle 2 and thereafter:** 10 mg/kg on days 1 and 15 of 28-day cycle (in combination with pomalidomide and dexamethasone). Continue until disease progression or unacceptable toxicity. If hematological toxicity occurs, may consider withholding treatment until blood counts improve.

Dose Modification

Neutropenia

Grade 4 neutropenia: Withhold treatment until neutrophil count improves to 1000 cells/mm^3, then resume at same dose.

Dosage in Renal Impairment

Mild to severe impairment: No dose adjustment.

Dosage in Hepatic Impairment

Mild impairment: No dose adjustment. **Moderate to severe impairment:** Not specified; use caution.

SIDE EFFECTS

Frequent (26%): Diarrhea. **Occasional (17%–12%):** Dyspnea, nausea, vomiting.

ADVERSE EFFECTS/TOXIC REACTIONS

Myelosuppression (anemia, lymphopenia, neutropenia, thrombocytopenia) is an expected response to therapy, but more severe reactions including severe neutropenia, febrile neutropenia may be life threatening. Grade 3 or 4 neutropenia reported in 85% of pts. Infusion-related reactions including chills, cough, dyspnea, nausea reported in 39% of pts. Grade 3 or 4 infusion reactions including dyspnea, hypertension, bronchospasm reported in 1% of pts. Infections including pneumonia (bronchopulmonary aspergillosis, *Haemophilus* pneumonia, influenza, *Pneumocystis jiroveci* pneumonia; bacterial/candidal/streptococcal/viral pneumonia), respiratory tract infections (bronchiolitis, bronchitis, viral bronchitis, nasopharyngitis, laryngitis, pharyngitis, parainfluenza virus infection, rhinitis, tracheitis, bacterial infection), UTI were reported. Secondary malignancies including skin squamous cell carcinoma, breast angiosarcoma, myelodysplastic syndrome were reported.

NURSING CONSIDERATIONS

BASELINE ASSESSMENT

Obtain CBC, blood type and screen; pregnancy test in females of reproductive potential. Confirm compliance of effective contraception. Inform blood bank of treatment and possible treatment-related interference with serologic testing. Administer in an environment equipped to monitor for and manage infusion-related reactions. Obtain weight in kilograms. Screen for active infection. Question for prior infusion-related reactions before each infusion. Offer emotional support.

INTERVENTION/EVALUATION

Monitor CBC periodically for myelosuppression. Monitor vital sign during infusion. If infusion-related reaction occurs, interrupt infusion and manage symptoms. Infusion reactions were usually reported during the first infusion. Most infusion reactions resolve on the same day of administration. Monitor for infections (cough, fatigue, fever), new malignancies. If serious infection occurs, initiate appropriate antimicrobial therapy. Monitor daily pattern of bowel activity, stool consistency. Offer antiemetic if nausea/vomiting occurs.

PATIENT/FAMILY TEACHING

• Treatment may depress your immune system and reduce your ability to fight infection. Report symptoms of infection such as body aches, burning with urination, chills, cough, fatigue, fever. Avoid those with active infection. • Report symptoms of bone marrow depression (e.g., bruising, fatigue, fever, shortness of breath, weight loss; bleeding easily, bloody urine or stool). • Immediately report symptoms of infusion-related reactions such as chills, cough, difficulty breathing, nausea, throat tightness. • Pretreatment with acetaminophen, antihistamines, steroidal anti-inflammatories may help reduce infusion reactions. • Due to pretreatment with a corticosteroid, pts with diabetes may experience a transient rise in blood sugar levels. • Use effective contraception to avoid pregnancy. Do not breastfeed. • Treatment may cause new cancers.

isavuconazonium

eye-sa-vue-**kon**-a-**zoe**-nee-um
(Cresemba)

◆CLASSIFICATION

PHARMACOTHERAPEUTIC: Azole antifungal derivative. **CLINICAL:** Antifungal.

USES

Treatment of invasive aspergillosis and invasive mucormycosis in pts 18 yrs and older.

PRECAUTIONS

Contraindications: Hypersensitivity to isavuconazonium or isavuconazole, concomitant use of strong CYP3A inhibitors (e.g., ketoconazole, high-dose ritonavir), strong CYP3A inducers (e.g., carBAMazepine, rifAMPin, St. John's wort), history of short QT syndrome. **Cautions:** Renal/hepatic impairment, hypersensitivity to other azoles. Pts at risk for acute pancreatitis; concomitant use of nephrotoxic medications; pts at risk for hypokalemia, hypomagnesemia. Concomitant use of medications that prolong QT interval.

ACTION

Isavuconazonium is the prodrug of isavuconazole. Interferes with fungal cytochrome activity, decreasing ergosterol synthesis, inhibiting fungal cell membrane formation. **Therapeutic Effect:** Damages fungal cell wall membrane.

PHARMACOKINETICS

Widely distributed. Metabolized in liver. Protein binding: greater than 99%. Peak plasma concentration: 2–3 hrs. Excreted in feces (46%), urine (46%). **Half-life:** 130 hrs.

⌛ LIFESPAN CONSIDERATIONS

Pregnancy/Lactation: May cause fetal harm. Avoid pregnancy. Breastfeeding not recommended. **Children:** Safety and efficacy not established. **Elderly:** No age-related precautions noted.

INTERACTIONS

DRUG: **Strong CYP3A4 inhibitors (e.g., clarithromycin, ketoconazole, ritonavir)** may increase concentration/effect. **Strong CYP3A4 inducers (e.g., carBAMazepine, rifAMPin)** may decrease concentration/effect. May increase concentration/effects of **cycloSPORINE, digoxin, eplerenone, estrogen, everolimus, midazolam, mycophenolate sirolimus, tacrolimus.** May decrease therapeutic effect of ***Saccharomyces boulardii.*** **HERBAL:** **St. John's wort** may decrease concentration/effect. **FOOD:** None known. **LAB VALUES:** May increase serum alkaline phosphatase, ALT, AST, bilirubin. May decrease serum potassium, magnesium.

AVAILABILITY (Rx)

Injection Powder: 372 mg/vial (equivalent to 200 mg isavuconazole). **Capsules:** 186 mg (equivalent to 100 mg isavuconazole).

ADMINISTRATION/HANDLING

IV

Reconstitution • Reconstitute vial with 5 mL Sterile Water for Injection. • Gently shake until completely dissolved. • Visually inspect for particulate matter or discoloration. Solution may contain visible translucent to white particles. • Inject reconstituted solution into 250 mL 0.9% NaCl or 5% Dextrose injection. • Gently invert bag to mix. Do not shake or agitate. Do not use pneumatic transport system. • Diluted solution may also contain visible translucent to white particles (which will be removed by in-line filter).

Administration • Do not give as IV push or bolus. Flush IV line with 0.9% NaCl or 5% Dextrose injection prior to and after infusion.

Rate of administration • Infuse over 60 min (minimum) using 0.2- to 1.2-micron in-line filter.

Storage • Diluted solution may be stored at room temperature up to 6 hrs or refrigerated up to 24 hrs. • Do not freeze.

PO

• Give without regard to food. • Do not cut, crush, divide, or open capsules.

INDICATIONS/ROUTES/DOSAGE

Note: 372 mg is equivalent to 200 mg isavuconazole. Duration of therapy: minimum of 6–12 wks.

Invasive Aspergillosis, Invasive Mucormycosis

IV: ADULTS, ELDERLY: Loading dose: 372 mg q8h for 6 doses (48 hrs). **Maintenance:** 372 mg once daily. Start maintenance dose 12–24 hrs after last loading dose. **PO: ADULTS, ELDERLY: Loading dose:** 372 mg (2 capsules) q8h for 6 doses (48 hrs). **Maintenance:** 372 mg (2 capsules) once daily. Start maintenance dose 12–24 hrs after last loading dose.

Dosage in Renal Impairment

No dose adjustment.

Dosage in Hepatic Impairment

Mild to moderate impairment: No dose adjustment. **Severe impairment:** Not specified; use caution.

SIDE EFFECTS

Frequent (28%–17%): Nausea, vomiting, diarrhea, abdominal pain, headache, dyspnea. **Occasional (15%–6%):** Peripheral edema, constipation, fatigue, insomnia, back pain, delirium, agitation, confusion, disorientation, chest pain, rash, pruritus, hypotension, anxiety, dyspepsia, injection site reaction, decreased appetite.

ADVERSE EFFECTS/TOXIC REACTIONS

Severe hepatic injury including cholestasis, hepatitis, hepatic failure reported in pts with underlying medical conditions (e.g., hematologic malignancies). Infusion-related reactions including chills, dizziness, dyspnea, hypoesthesia, hypotension, paresthesia may occur. Acute respiratory failure, renal failure, Stevens-Johnson syndrome, serious hypersensitivity reaction (including anaphylaxis) were reported.

NURSING CONSIDERATIONS

BASELINE ASSESSMENT

Obtain LFT. Confirm negative pregnancy test before initiating treatment. Specimens for fungal culture, histopathology should be obtained prior to initiating therapy. Receive full medication history and screen for interactions/contraindications. Question history of hypersensitivity reaction, hepatic impairment.

INTERVENTION/EVALUATION

Monitor LFT periodically. Monitor for infusion-related reactions, hypersensitivity reactions, anaphylaxis. Monitor I&O. Report worsening of hepatic/renal function.

PATIENT/FAMILY TEACHING

• Swallow capsule whole; do not chew, crush, cut, or open capsules. • Use effective contraception to avoid pregnancy. • Do not take herbal products such as St. John's wort. • Report liver problems such as upper abdominal pain, bleeding, dark or amber-colored urine, nausea, vomiting, or yellowing of the skin or eyes. • Report decreased urinary output, extremity swelling, dark-colored urine; skin changes such as rash, skin bubbling, or sloughing.

I

isoniazid

eye-soe-**nye**-a-zid
(Isotamine 🍁)

■ BLACK BOX ALERT ■ Severe, potentially fatal hepatitis may occur.

FIXED-COMBINATION(S)

Rifamate: isoniazid/rifAMPin (antitubercular): 150 mg/300 mg.
Rifater: isoniazid/pyrazinamide/rifAMPin (antitubercular): 50 mg/300 mg/120 mg.

◆CLASSIFICATION

PHARMACOTHERAPEUTIC: Isonicotinic acid derivative. **CLINICAL:** Antitubercular.

USES

Treatment of susceptible active tuberculosis due to *Mycobacterium tuberculosis*. Treatment of latent tuberculosis caused by *Mycobacterium tuberculosis*.

PRECAUTIONS

Contraindications: Hypersensitivity to isoniazid (including drug-induced hepatitis), acute hepatic disease, hepatic injury or severe adverse reactions with previous isoniazid therapy. **Cautions:** Chronic hepatic disease, alcoholism, severe renal impairment. Pregnancy, pts at risk for peripheral neuropathy, HIV infection, history of hypersensitivity reactions to latent TB infection medications.

ACTION

Inhibits mycolic acid synthesis. Causes disruption of bacterial cell wall, loss of acid-fast properties in susceptible mycobacteria. **Therapeutic Effect:** Bactericidal against actively growing intracellular, extracellular susceptible mycobacteria.

PHARMACOKINETICS

Note: Isoniazid is metabolized by acetylation. The rate of acetylation is genetically determined (e.g., 50% of black and Caucasian pts are slow inactivators; Eskimo and Asian pts are rapid inactivators. Slower inactivation may lead to higher blood levels and increased adverse effects.
Readily absorbed from GI tract. Protein binding: 10%–15%. Widely distributed (including to CSF). Metabolized in liver. Primarily excreted in urine. Removed by hemodialysis. **Half-life:** (Fast acetylators): 30–100 min; (slow acetylators): 2–5 hrs.

⌛ LIFESPAN CONSIDERATIONS

Pregnancy/Lactation: Prophylaxis usually postponed until after delivery. Crosses placenta. Distributed in breast milk. **Children:** No age-related precautions noted. **Elderly:** More susceptible to developing hepatitis.

INTERACTIONS

DRUG: May increase concentration/effect of **carBAMazepine, fosphenytoin, lomitapide, phenytoin. Hepatotoxic medications (e.g., acetaminophen, rifAMPin)** may increase risk of hepatotoxicity. May decrease **ketoconazole** concentration. **HERBAL:** None significant. FOOD: **Foods containing tyramine** may cause hypertensive crisis. LAB VALUES: May increase serum bilirubin, ALT, AST.

AVAILABILITY (Rx)

Solution, Injection: 100 mg/mL. **Syrup, Oral:** 50 mg/5 mL. **Tablets:** 100 mg, 300 mg.

ADMINISTRATION/HANDLING

PO

• Give 1 hr before or 2 hrs following meals (may give with food to decrease GI upset, but will delay absorption). • Administer at least 1 hr before antacids, esp. those containing aluminum.

INDICATIONS/ROUTES/DOSAGE

Active Tuberculosis (in combination with one or more antituberculars)

IM/PO: ADULTS, ELDERLY, CHILDREN WEIGHING 40 KG OR MORE: 5 mg/kg once daily. **Usual dose:** 300 mg. **CHILDREN WEIGHING LESS THAN 40 KG:** 10–15 mg/kg once daily. **Maximum:** 300 mg.
Note: Give isoniazid with rifAMPin, pyrazinamide, and with or without ethambutol for 8 wks, then give with rifAMPin for 18 wks.

Latent Tuberculosis

Note: Give for 9 mos.
IM/PO: ADULTS, ELDERLY, CHILDREN 12 YRS AND OLDER: 5 mg/kg once daily (**Maximum:** 300 mg) or 15 mg/kg twice wkly (**Maximum:** 900 mg). **CHILDREN YOUNGER THAN 12 YRS:** 10–20 mg/kg/day as a single daily dose. **Maximum:** 300 mg/day or 20–40 mg/kg 2 times/wk. **Maximum:** 900 mg/dose.

Dosage in Renal Impairment

No dose adjustment.

Dosage in Hepatic Impairment

Use caution. Contraindicated with acute hepatic disease.

SIDE EFFECTS

Frequent: Nausea, vomiting, diarrhea, abdominal pain. **Rare:** Pain at injection site, hypersensitivity reaction.

ADVERSE EFFECTS/TOXIC REACTIONS

Neurotoxicity (ataxia, paresthesia), optic neuritis, hepatotoxicity occur rarely.

NURSING CONSIDERATIONS

BASELINE ASSESSMENT

Question for history of hypersensitivity reactions, hepatic injury or disease, sensitivity to nicotinic acid or chemically related medications. Ensure collection of specimens for culture, sensitivity. Evaluate initial LFT.

INTERVENTION/EVALUATION

Monitor LFT, assess for hepatitis: anorexia, nausea, vomiting, weakness, fatigue, dark urine, jaundice (withhold concurrent INH therapy and inform physician promptly). Assess for paresthesia of extremities (pts esp. at risk for neuropathy may be given pyridoxine prophylactically: malnourished, elderly, diabetics, pts with chronic hepatic disease [including alcoholics]). Be alert for fever, skin eruptions (hypersensitivity reaction).

PATIENT/FAMILY TEACHING

• Do not skip doses; continue to take isoniazid for full length of therapy (6–24 mos). • Take preferably 1 hr before or 2 hrs following meals (with food if GI upset). • Avoid alcohol during treatment. • Do not take any other medications, including antacids, without consulting physician. • Must take isoniazid at least 1 hr before antacid. • Avoid tuna, sauerkraut, aged cheeses, smoked fish (consult list of tyramine-containing foods), which may cause hypertensive reaction (red/itching skin, palpitations, light-headedness, hot or clammy feeling, headache). • Report any new symptom, immediately for vision difficulties, nausea/vomiting, dark urine, yellowing of skin/eyes (jaundice), fatigue, paresthesia of extremities.

isosorbide dinitrate

eye-soe-**sor**-bide
(ISDN ✱, Dilatrate-SR, Isordil)

isosorbide mononitrate

(Apo-ISMN ✱, Imdur ✱)
Do not confuse Imdur with Imuran, Inderal, or K-Dur, Isordil with Inderal, Isuprel, or Plendil.

FIXED-COMBINATION(S)

BiDil: isosorbide dinitrate/hydrALAZINE (a vasodilator): 20 mg/37.5 mg.

◆CLASSIFICATION

PHARMACOTHERAPEUTIC: Nitrate. **CLINICAL:** Antianginal.

USES

Dinitrate: Prevention of angina pectoris due to coronary artery disease. **Mononitrate:** Treatment (immediate-release only) and prevention of angina pectoris due to coronary artery disease.

PRECAUTIONS

Contraindications: Hypersensitivity to nitrates, concurrent use of sildenafil, tadalafil, vardenafil, or riociguat. **Cautions:** Inferior wall MI, head trauma, increased intracranial pressure (ICP), orthostatic hypotension, blood volume depletion from diuretic therapy, systolic B/P less than 90 mm Hg, hypertrophic cardiomyopathy, alcohol consumption.

ACTION

Forms free radical nitric oxide which activates intracellular cyclic guanosine monophosphate, leading to smooth muscle relaxation. **Therapeutic Effect:** Relaxes vascular smooth muscle of arterial, venous vasculature. Decreases preload, afterload, cardiac oxygen demand.

PHARMACOKINETICS

Route	Onset	Peak	Duration
Dinitrate			
Sublingual	3 min	N/A	1–2 hrs
PO	45–60 min	N/A	up to 8 hrs
Mononitrate			
PO (extended-release)	30–60 min	N/A	12–24 hrs

Dinitrate poorly absorbed and metabolized in liver to its active metabolite isosorbide mononitrate. Mononitrate well absorbed after PO administration. Primarily excreted in urine. **Half-life:** Dinitrate, 1–4 hrs; mononitrate, 4 hrs.

⌛ LIFESPAN CONSIDERATIONS

Pregnancy/Lactation: Unknown if drug crosses placenta or is distributed in breast milk. **Children:** Safety and efficacy not established. **Elderly:** May be more sensitive to hypotensive effects. Age-related renal impairment may require dosage adjustment.

INTERACTIONS

DRUG: **Alcohol, riociguat, sildenafil, tadalafil, vardenafil** may potentiate hypotensive effects (concurrent use of these agents is contraindicated). **Strong CYP3A4 inhibitors (e.g., clarithromycin, ketoconazole, ritonavir)** may increase concentration/effect. **HERBAL:** **St. John's wort** may decrease concentration/effect. **FOOD:** None known. **LAB VALUES:** May increase urine catecholamine, urine vanillylmandelic acid levels.

AVAILABILITY (Rx)

Dinitrate
Tablets: 5 mg, 10 mg, 20 mg, 30 mg, 40 mg.

Capsules, Extended-Release: 40 mg.

Mononitrate
Tablets: 10 mg, 20 mg.

Tablets, Extended-Release: 30 mg, 60 mg, 120 mg.

ADMINISTRATION/HANDLING

PO
- Best if taken on an empty stomach.
- Do not administer around the clock.

• Oral tablets may be crushed. • Do not crush/break sustained-, extended-release form.

INDICATIONS/ROUTES/DOSAGE

Angina

Note: Dinitrate used only for prevention. **PO:** ***(Isosorbide Dinitrate) (Immediate-Release):*** **ADULTS, ELDERLY:** Initially, 5–20 mg 2–3 times/day. **Maintenance:** 10–40 mg (or between 5–80 mg) 2–3 times/day. ***(Sustained-Release):*** **ADULTS, ELDERLY:** 40 mg 1–2 times/day. A nitrate-free interval of greater than 18 hrs is recommended. **Maximum:** 160 mg/day. **PO:** ***(Isosorbide Mononitrate) (Immediate-Release):*** **ADULTS, ELDERLY:** 20 mg twice daily given 7 hrs apart to decrease tolerance development. In pts with small stature, may start at 5 mg twice daily and titrate to at least 10 mg twice daily in first 2–3 days of therapy. ***(Sustained-Release):*** Initially, 30–60 mg/day in morning as a single dose. May increase dose at 3-day intervals to 120 mg once daily. **Maximum daily single dose:** 240 mg.

Dosage in Renal/Hepatic Impairment

No dose adjustment.

SIDE EFFECTS

Frequent: Headache (may be severe) occurs mostly in early therapy, diminishes rapidly in intensity, usually disappears during continued treatment. **Sublingual:** Burning, tingling at oral point of dissolution. **Occasional:** Transient flushing of face/neck, dizziness, weakness, orthostatic hypotension, nausea, vomiting, restlessness. GI upset, blurred vision, dry mouth.

ADVERSE EFFECTS/TOXIC REACTIONS

Discontinue if blurred vision occurs. Severe orthostatic hypotension manifested by syncope, pulselessness, cold/clammy skin, diaphoresis has been reported. Tolerance may occur with repeated, prolonged therapy, but may not occur with extended-release form. Minor tolerance with intermittent use of sublingual tablets. High dosage tends to produce severe headache.

NURSING CONSIDERATIONS

BASELINE ASSESSMENT

Record onset, type (sharp, dull, squeezing), radiation, location, intensity, duration of anginal pain; precipitating factors (exertion, emotional stress). If headache occurs during management therapy, administer medication with meals.

INTERVENTION/EVALUATION

Assist with ambulation if light-headedness, dizziness occurs. Assess for facial/neck flushing. Monitor number of anginal episodes, orthostatic B/P.

PATIENT/FAMILY TEACHING

• Do not chew, crush, dissolve, or divide sublingual, extended-release, sustained-release forms. • Take sublingual tablets while sitting down. • Go from lying to standing slowly (prevents dizziness effect). • Take oral form on empty stomach (however, if headache occurs during management therapy, take medication with meals). • Dissolve sublingual tablet under tongue; do not swallow. • Avoid alcohol (intensifies hypotensive effect). • If alcohol is ingested soon after taking nitrates, possible acute hypotensive episode (marked drop in B/P, vertigo, pallor) may occur. • Report signs/symptoms of hypotension, angina.

itraconazole

it-ra-**kon**-a-zole
(Sporanox, Tolsura)

BLACK BOX ALERT Serious cardiovascular events, including HF, ventricular tachycardia, torsades de pointes, death, have occurred due to concurrent use with colchicine (pts with renal/hepatic impairment), dofetilide, dronedarone, eplerenone, ergot alkaloids, felodipine, fesoterodine, irinotecan, ivabradine, levomethadyl, lovastatin, lurasidone, methadone, midazolam (oral), pimozide, quiNIDine, ranolazine, simvastatin, solifenacin, ticagrelor, or triazolam.

Negative inotropic effects observed following IV administration. Contraindicated for treatment of onychomycosis in pts with HF, ventricular dysfunction.

Do not confuse itraconazole with fluconazole, ketoconazole, miconazole, posaconazole, voriconazole, or Sporanox with Suprax or Topamax.

CLASSIFICATION

PHARMACOTHERAPEUTIC: Azole-derivative antifungal. **CLINICAL:** Antifungal.

I

USES

Oral capsules: Treatment of aspergillosis, blastomycosis, esophageal and oropharyngeal candidiasis, empiric treatment in febrile neutropenia, histoplasmosis, onychomycosis. **Oral solution:** Treatment of oral and esophageal candidiasis. **Oral tablet:** Treatment of onychomycosis of toenail.

PRECAUTIONS

Contraindications: Hypersensitivity to itraconazole, other azoles. Treatment of onychomycosis in pts with evidence of ventricular dysfunction (e.g., HF or history of HF); concurrent use of dofetilide, dronedarone, eplerenone, ergot derivatives, felodipine, irinotecan, lovastatin, lurasidone, methadone, midazolam (oral), pimozide, ranolazine, simvastatin, ticagrelor, triazolam, quiNIDine; concurrent use with colchicine, fesoterodine, solifenacin in pts with renal/hepatic impairment; treatment of onychomycosis in women who are pregnant or are intending to become pregnant. **Cautions:** Preexisting hepatic impairment (not recommended in pts with active hepatic disease, elevated LFTs), renal impairment, pts with risk factors for HF (e.g., COPD, myocardial ischemia).

ACTION

Inhibits synthesis of ergosterol (vital component of fungal cell formation). **Therapeutic Effect:** Damages fungal cell membrane, altering its function. Fungistatic.

PHARMACOKINETICS

Moderately absorbed from GI tract. Absorption is increased when taken with food. Protein binding: 99%. Widely distributed, primarily in fatty tissue, liver, kidneys. Metabolized in liver. Primarily excreted in urine. Not removed by hemodialysis. **Half-life:** 16–26 hrs.

LIFESPAN CONSIDERATIONS

Pregnancy/Lactation: Distributed in breast milk. **Children:** Safety and efficacy not established. **Elderly:** Age-related renal impairment may require dosage adjustment.

INTERACTIONS

DRUG: May increase concentration/toxicity of **aliskiren, calcium channel–blocking agents (e.g., felodipine, NIFEdipine), cycloSPORINE, digoxin, dofetilide, eplerenone, ergot alkaloids, HMG-CoA reductase inhibitors (e.g., lovastatin, simvastatin), midazolam, sirolimus, tacrolimus, warfarin. Strong CYP3A4 inhibitors (e.g., clarithromycin, ketoconazole, ritonavir)** may increase concentration/effect. **Strong CYP3A4 inducers (e.g., carbamazepine, phenytoin, rifampin)** may decrease concentration/effect. May inhibit metabolism of **DOCEtaxel, vinca alkaloids. Antacids, H2 antagonists, proton pump inhibitors** may decrease absorption. **HERBAL: St. John's wort** may decrease concentration/effect. **FOOD: Grapefruit products** may alter absorption. **LAB VALUES:** May increase serum alkaline phosphatase, bilirubin, ALT, AST, LDH. May decrease serum potassium.

AVAILABILITY (Rx)

Capsules: ***(Sporanox)***: 100 mg. ***(Tolsura)***: 65 mg. **Oral Solution:** ***(Sporanox)***: 10 mg/mL.

ADMINISTRATION/HANDLING

PO

• Give capsules with food (increases absorption). • Give solution on empty stomach. Swish vigorously in mouth, then swallow.

INDICATIONS/ROUTES/DOSAGE

Note: Capsules/tablets are not bioequivalent with oral solution.

Blastomycosis, Histoplasmosis

PO: ADULTS, ELDERLY: ***(Sporanox [Oral Solution or Capsule]):*** 200 mg 3 times/day for 3 days, then 200 mg twice daily. ***(Tolsura):*** 130 mg once daily; if no improvement or evidence of progressive fungal infection, increase dose in 65 mg increments to a maximum of 260 mg/day given in 2 divided doses. For life-threatening infections, give a loading dose of 130 mg 3 times/day for the first 3 days of treatment. Treatment should be continued for 3 mos or greater.

Aspergillosis

PO: ADULTS, ELDERLY: ***(Sporanox [Oral Solution]):*** 200 mg 2 times/day for minimum of 6–12 wks. ***(Tolsura):*** 130 mg 1–2 times/day. For life-threatening infections, give a loading dose of 130 mg 3 times/day for the first 3 days of treatment. Treatment should be continued for at least 3 mos.

Esophageal Candidiasis

PO: ADULTS, ELDERLY: ***(Oral Solution):*** Swish 100–200 mg (10–20 mL) in mouth for several seconds, then swallow once daily for a minimum of 3 wks. Continue for 2 wks after resolution of symptoms. **Maximum:** 200 mg/day.

Oropharyngeal Candidiasis

PO: ADULTS, ELDERLY: 200 mg (10 mL) oral solution, swish and swallow once daily for up to 28 days.

Onychomycosis (Fingernail)

PO: ADULTS, ELDERLY: ***(Capsule):*** 200 mg twice daily for 7 days, off for 21 days, repeat 200 mg twice daily for 7 days.

Onychomycosis (Toenail)

PO: ADULTS, ELDERLY: ***(Tablet):*** 200 mg once daily for 12 wks.

Dosage in Renal/Hepatic Impairment

Use caution.

SIDE EFFECTS

Frequent (11%–9%): Nausea, rash. **Occasional (5%–3%):** Vomiting, headache, diarrhea, hypertension, peripheral edema, fatigue, fever. **Rare (2% or less):** Abdominal pain, dizziness, anorexia, pruritus.

ADVERSE EFFECTS/TOXIC REACTIONS

Hepatitis (anorexia, abdominal pain, unusual fatigue/weakness, jaundiced skin/sclera, dark urine) occurs rarely.

NURSING CONSIDERATIONS

BASELINE ASSESSMENT

Obtain LFT. Assess allergies. Receive full medication history (numerous contraindications/cautions).

INTERVENTION/EVALUATION

Monitor for hepatotoxicity (abdominal pain, jaundice, nausea, vomiting). Monitor LFT in pts with preexisting hepatic impairment.

PATIENT/ FAMILY TEACHING

• Take capsules with food, liquids if GI distress occurs. • Therapy will continue for at least 3 mos, until lab tests, clinical presentation indicate infection is controlled. • Report liver problems (abdominal pain, bruising, clay-colored stool, amber- or dark-colored urine, yellowing of the skin or eyes). • Avoid grapefruit products.

ivabradine

eye-**vab**-ra-deen
(Corlanor)

◆CLASSIFICATION

PHARMACOTHERAPEUTIC: Hyperpolarization-activated cyclic nucleotide-gated (HCN) channel blocker.

CLINICAL: Reduces risk of worsening HF.

USES

To reduce the risk of hospitalization for worsening HF in pts with stable, symptomatic chronic HF with left ventricular ejection fraction less than or equal to 35%, who are in sinus rhythm with a resting heart rate greater than or equal to 70 bpm, and either are on maximally tolerated dose of beta blockers or have a contraindication to beta blocker use.

PRECAUTIONS

Contraindications: Hypersensitivity to ivabradine. Acute decompensated HF, B/P less than 90/50 mm Hg, sick sinus syndrome; sinoatrial block or third-degree AV block (unless a functional pacemaker is present), resting heart rate less than 60 bpm prior to initiation, severe hepatic impairment, pacemaker dependence (heart rate maintained exclusively by a pacemaker), concomitant use of strong CYP3A4 inhibitors. **Cautions:** History of atrial fibrillation, hypertension. Avoid concomitant use of dilTIAZem or verapamil. Avoid use in pts with second-degree heart block (unless a functioning pacemaker is present). Pts at risk for bradycardia. Not recommended with pacemakers set to rate of 60 bpm or greater.

ACTION

Reduces spontaneous pacemaker activity of the cardiac sinus node by blocking HCN channels that are responsible for cardiac current, which regulates heart rate. Does not affect ventricular repolarization or myocardial contractility. Also inhibits retinal current involved in reducing bright light in retina. **Therapeutic Effect:** Reduces heart rate.

PHARMACOKINETICS

Widely distributed. Metabolized in liver and intestines. Protein binding: 70%. Peak plasma concentration: 1 hr. Eliminated in feces, urine (% not specified). **Half-life:** 6 hrs.

⌛ LIFESPAN CONSIDERATIONS

Pregnancy/Lactation: May cause fetal harm. Females of reproductive potential should use effective contraception. Unknown if distributed in breast milk. If treatment is decided to be absolutely necessary, pregnant pts should be closely monitored for destabilizing HF, esp. during the first trimester. Pregnant women with chronic HF in the third trimester should be closely monitored for preterm birth. **Children:** Safety and efficacy not established. **Elderly:** No age-related precautions noted.

INTERACTIONS

DRUG: **DilTIAZem, verapamil** may increase concentration/effect; may further increase risk of bradycardia. **Strong CYP3A4 inhibitors (e.g., clarithromycin, ketoconazole, ritonavir)** may increase concentration/effect. **Strong CYP3A4 inducers (e.g., carBAMazepine, phenytoin, rifAMPin)** may decrease concentration/effect. **HERBAL:** **St. John's wort** may decrease concentration/effect. **FOOD:** **Grapefruit products** may increase concentration/effect. **LAB VALUES:** None significant.

AVAILABILITY (Rx)

Tablets: 5 mg, 7.5 mg.

ADMINISTRATION/HANDLING

PO

- Give with meals. May divide 5-mg tablet, providing 2.5-mg dose.

INDICATIONS/ROUTES/DOSAGE

HF

PO: ADULTS, ELDERLY: Initially, 5 mg twice daily for 14 days, then adjust dose to resting heart rate of 50–60 bpm. Further adjustments based on resting heart rate and tolerability. **Maximum:** 7.5 mg twice daily. (See Dose Modification). **Pts with history of conduction defects, pts in whom bradycardia could lead to**

hemodynamic compromise: Initiate therapy at 2.5 mg twice daily.

Dose Modification

Adjust dose to maintain a resting heart between 50–60 bpm as follows:

Heart Rate	Dose Adjustment
Greater than 60 bpm	Increase by 2.5 mg (given twice daily) up to maximum dose of 7.5 mg daily.
50–60 bpm	Maintain dose.
Less than 50 bpm or symptomatic bradycardia	Decrease by 2.5 mg (given twice daily); if current dose is 2.5 mg twice daily, permanently discontinue.

Dosage in Renal Impairment

Mild to moderate impairment: CrCl 15 mL/min or greater: No dose adjustment. **Severe impairment: CrCl less than 15 mL/min:** Use caution.

Dosage in Hepatic Impairment

Mild to moderate impairment: No dose adjustment. **Severe impairment:** Contraindicated.

SIDE EFFECTS

Occasional (10%–3%): Bradycardia, hypertension, phosphenes (visual disturbances, luminous phenomena), visual brightness.

ADVERSE EFFECTS/TOXIC REACTIONS

May increase risk of atrial fibrillation (8.3% of pts). Bradycardia, sinus arrest, or heart block may occur. Bradycardia occurred in 10% of pts. Risk factors for bradycardia may include sinus node dysfunction, conduction defects (e.g., first- or second-degree AV block, bundle branch block), ventricular dyssynchrony, or use of negative chronotropic drugs. Phosphenes, a transient enhanced brightness in the visual field (which may include halos, stroboscopic or kaleidoscopic effect, colored bright lights, or multiple images) may occur. Phosphenes are usually triggered by sudden variations in light intensity and generally occur within the first 2 mos of treatment. Other adverse reactions such as angioedema, diplopia, erythema, hypotension, pruritus, rash, syncope, urticaria, vertigo, visual impairment occur rarely. Overdose may lead to severe and prolonged bradycardia requiring temporary cardiac pacing or infusion of IV beta-stimulating agents.

NURSING CONSIDERATIONS

BASELINE ASSESSMENT

Obtain heart rate, B/P. Confirm negative pregnancy test before initiating therapy. Receive full medication history and screen for interactions. Screen for contraindications as listed in Precautions. Question history of atrial fibrillation, bradycardia, hypertension.

INTERVENTION/EVALUATION

Monitor heart rate, B/P. Diligently monitor for atrial fibrillation, bradycardia, syncope. If symptomatic bradycardia occurs, temporary cardiac pacing or infusion of beta-stimulating agents may be warranted. Monitor for hypersensitivity reaction. Monitor for visual changes. Initiate fall precautions.

PATIENT/FAMILY TEACHING

• Take medication with meals. • Avoid grapefruit products, herbal supplements such as St. John's wort. • Use effective contraception to avoid pregnancy. • Report symptoms of low heart rate such as confusion, dizziness, fatigue, fainting, low blood pressure, pallor. • Report symptoms of atrial fibrillation such as chest pressure, palpitations, shortness of breath. • Treatment may cause luminous phenomena (phosphenes), a transient visual brightness that may include halos, light sensitivity, or colored bright lights. • Avoid tasks that require alertness, motor skills until response to drug is established. • Report allergic reactions such as hives, itching, rash, tongue swelling.

I

ivosidenib

eye-voe-**sid**-e-nib
(Tibsovo)

■ BLACK BOX ALERT ■ Life-threatening and/or fatal differentiation syndrome with symptoms including fever, dyspnea, hypoxia, pulmonary infiltrates, pleural or pericardial effusion, rapid weight gain or peripheral edema, hypotension, renal dysfunction may occur. Initiate corticosteroid therapy and hemodynamic monitoring in pts suspected of differentiation syndrome until symptoms resolve.

Do not confuse ivosidenib with enasidenib, ibrutinib, idelalisib, imatinib, or ixazomib.

CLASSIFICATION

PHARMACOTHERAPEUTIC: Isocitrate dehydrogenase-1 (IDH1) inhibitor. **CLINICAL:** Antineoplastic.

I

USES

Treatment of acute myeloid leukemia (AML) with a susceptible IDH1 mutation in adults with newly diagnosed AML who are 75 yrs or older or who have comorbidities that preclude use of intensive induction chemotherapy. Treatment of AML with a susceptible IDH1 mutation in adults with relapsed or refractory AML.

PRECAUTIONS

Contraindications: Hypersensitivity to ivosidenib. **Cautions:** Baseline leukopenia, hypotension; active infection, cardiac disease, hepatic/renal impairment, electrolyte imbalance; conditions predisposing to infection (e.g., diabetes, renal failure, immunocompromised pts, open wounds); pts at risk for QTc interval prolongation, cardiac arrhythmias (congenital long QT syndrome, HF, QT interval–prolonging medications, hypokalemia, hypomagnesemia); concomitant use strong or moderate CYP3A inhibitors, strong CYP3A inducers; dehydration; pts at high risk for tumor lysis syndrome (high tumor burden).

ACTION

Inhibits IDH1 enzymes on mutant IDH1 variants, decreasing 2-hydroxyglutarate (2-HG) levels and restoring myeloid differentiation. **Therapeutic Effect:** Reduces blast counts; increases percentage of myeloid cells. Inhibits tumor growth and proliferation.

PHARMACOKINETICS

Widely distributed. Metabolized in liver. Protein binding: 92%–96%. Peak plasma concentration: 3 hrs. Steady state reached in 14 days. Excreted in feces (77%), urine (17%). **Half-life:** 93 hrs.

LIFESPAN CONSIDERATIONS

Pregnancy/Lactation: Avoid pregnancy; may cause fetal harm. Unknown if distributed in breast milk. Breastfeeding not recommended during treatment and for at least 30 days after discontinuation. **Children:** Safety and efficacy not established. **Elderly:** No age-related precautions noted.

INTERACTIONS

DRUG: **Strong CYP3A4 inhibitors (e.g., clarithromycin, ketoconazole), moderate CYP3A4 inhibitors (e.g., erythromycin, dilTIAZem, fluconazole)** may increase concentration/effect. **Strong CYP3A4 inducers (e.g., carBAMazepine, phenytoin, rifAMPin)** may decrease concentration/effect. **QT interval–prolonging medications (e.g., amiodarone, azithromycin, citalopram, clarithromycin, escitalopram, haloperidol)** may increase risk of QTc interval prolongation. May increase QT prolongation effect of **dronedarone. May decrease effect of oral contraceptives.** **HERBAL:** **St. John's wort** may decrease concentration/effect. **FOOD:** **High-fat meals** may increase concentration/effect. **LAB VALUES:** May increase serum alkaline phosphatase, ALT, AST, bilirubin, creatinine, uric acid. May decrease Hgb, WBCs; serum magnesium, phosphate, potassium, sodium.

AVAILABILITY (Rx)

Tablets: 250 mg.

ADMINISTRATION/HANDLING

PO

• Give without regard to low-fat food. • Do not give with a high-fat meal. • Administer whole; do not break, cut, crush, or divide tablets. • Tablets cannot be chewed. • If vomiting occurs after administration, give next dose at regularly scheduled time. • If a dose is missed, administer as soon as possible • Do not give a missed dose within 12 hrs of next dose.

INDICATIONS/ROUTES/DOSAGE

Acute Myeloid Leukemia

PO: ADULTS, ELDERLY: 500 mg once daily for at least 6 mos. Continue until disease progression or unacceptable toxicity.

Dose Modification

Based on Common Terminology Criteria for Adverse Events (CTCAE).

Differentiation Syndrome

Withhold treatment if symptoms are severe and persist for more than 48 hrs after initiation of corticosteroids. Resume treatment when symptoms improve to Grade 2 or less.

Guillain-Barré Syndrome

Permanently discontinue.

Noninfectious Leukocytosis

WBC count greater than 25,000 cells/mm³ or absolute increase in total WBC count greater than 15,000 cells/mm³ from baseline: If indicated, treat with hydroxyurea and leukapheresis. Taper hydroxyurea after leukocytosis improves or resolves. If leukocytosis does not improve with hydroxyurea, withhold treatment until resolved, then resume at same dose.

QT Interval Prolongation

QTc interval 481–500 msec: Withhold treatment. Assess and replete electrolyte levels. Assess and adjust concomitant use of medications known to cause QTc interval prolongation. When QTc interval prolongation improves to 480 msec or less, resume at same dose and monitor ECG at least wkly for 2 wks. **QTc interval greater than 500 msec:** Withhold treatment. Assess and replete electrolyte levels. Assess and adjust concomitant use of medications known to cause QTc interval prolongation. When QTc interval returns to within 30 msec of baseline or 480 msec or less, resume at reduced dose of 250 mg. **QTc interval prolongation with life-threatening arrhythmia:** Permanently discontinue.

Other Adverse Reactions

Any Grade 3 or higher toxicity: Withhold treatment until improved to Grade 2, then resume at reduced dose of 250 mg. May increase to 500 mg if toxicities further improve to Grade 1 or 0. **Recurrent Grade 3 or higher toxicity:** Permanently discontinue.

Concomitant Use of CYP3A4 Inhibitor

If concomitant CYP3A4 inhibitor cannot be discontinued, reduce ivosidenib dose to 250 mg. If CYP3A inhibitor is discontinued for 3–5 half-lives, increase ivosidenib dose to 500 mg.

Dosage in Renal Impairment

Mild to moderate impairment: No dose adjustment. **Severe impairment:** Not specified; use caution.

Dosage in Hepatic Impairment

Mild to moderate impairment: No dose adjustment. **Severe impairment:** Not specified; use caution.

SIDE EFFECTS

Frequent (39%–18%): Fatigue, asthenia, arthralgia, diarrhea, dyspnea, edema, nausea, abdominal pain, mucositis, rash, pyrexia, cough, constipation, vomiting, decreased appetite, myalgia. **Occasional (16%–12%):** Chest pain, headache, neuropathy, hypotension.

ADVERSE EFFECTS/TOXIC REACTIONS

Anemia, leukopenia is an expected response to therapy. Life-threatening and/or fatal differentiation syndrome, a condition with rapid proliferation and differentiation of myeloid cells, reported in 19%–25% of pts. QT interval prolongation with QTc interval greater than 500 msec (9% of pts) and QTc interval greater than 60 msec from baseline (14% of pts) have occurred. Guillain-Barré syndrome occurred in less than 1% of pts. Noninfectious leukocytosis reported in 12% of pts. Tumor lysis syndrome may present as acute renal failure, hypocalcemia, hyperuricemia, hyperphosphatemia.

NURSING CONSIDERATIONS

BASELINE ASSESSMENT

Obtain CBC, BMP, LFT; ECG; pregnancy test in female pts of reproductive potential. Replete electrolytes if applicable. Confirm presence of IDH1 mutations in the blood or bone marrow. Assess adequate hydration prior to initiation due to increased risk of tumor lysis syndrome, diarrhea, vomiting. Screen for active infection. Receive full medication history and screen for interactions. Concomitant use of other medications may need to be adjusted. Assess risk for QT interval prolongation, tumor lysis syndrome. Question history of cardiac/hepatic/renal disease, cardiac arrhythmias. Offer emotional support.

INTERVENTION/EVALUATION

Monitor CBC, BMP, LFT at least wkly for 4 wks, then every other wk for 4 wks, then monthly until discontinuation. Monitor CK levels wkly for at least 4 wks. An increase of serum creatinine greater than 0.4 mg/dL from baseline may indicate renal impairment. Monitor serum uric acid level if tumor lysis syndrome (acute renal failure, electrolyte imbalance, cardiac arrhythmias, seizures) is suspected. Monitor ECG at least wkly for 3 wks, then monthly until discontinuation. If QT interval–prolonging medications cannot be withheld, diligently monitor ECG; serum potassium, magnesium for QT interval prolongation, cardiac arrhythmias. Monitor B/P for hypotension, esp. in pts taking antihypertensives. Monitor for symptoms of differentiation syndrome (dyspnea, fever hypotension, hypoxia, pulmonary infiltrates, pleural or pericardial effusion, rapid weight gain or peripheral edema, renal dysfunction, or concomitant febrile neutropenic dermatosis). If differentiation syndrome is suspected, initiate corticosteroids and hemodynamic monitoring until symptoms resolve for at least 3 days. Monitor for symptoms of Guillain-Barré syndrome (dysphagia, dysarthria, dyspnea, motor weakness, paresthesia, sensory alterations). Diligently monitor for infection. Assess skin for skin reactions, rash. Monitor daily pattern of bowel activity, stool consistency. Ensure adequate hydration, nutrition.

PATIENT/FAMILY TEACHING

• Treatment may depress your immune system response and reduce your ability to fight infection. Report symptoms of infection such as body aches, chills, cough, fatigue, fever. Avoid those with active infection. • Report symptoms of bone marrow depression such as bruising, fatigue, fever, shortness of breath, weight loss; bleeding easily, bloody urine or stool. • Report palpitations, chest pain, shortness of breath, dizziness, fainting; may indicate arrhythmia. • Therapy may cause life-threatening tumor lysis syndrome (a condition caused by the rapid breakdown of cancer cells), which can cause kidney failure. Report decreased urination, amber-colored urine; confusion, difficulty breathing, fatigue, fever, muscle or joint pain, palpitations, seizures, vomiting. • Treatment may cause life-threatening differentiation syndrome as early as 2 days after starting therapy. Report difficulty breathing, fever, low blood pressure, rapid weight gain, swelling of the hands or feet, decreased urine output. • Report liver problems (abdominal pain, bruising, clay-colored stool, amber- or dark-colored urine, yellowing of the skin or eyes), kidney problems (decreased urine output, flank pain, darkened urine), skin reactions (rash, skin eruptions). • There is a high risk of interactions with other medications. Do not take newly prescribed medications unless approved by prescriber who originally started treatment. • Avoid grapefruit products, herbal supplements (esp. St. John's wort). • Report suspected pregnancy. Do not breastfeed. • Drink plenty of fluids. • Avoid high-fat meals during administration.

ixabepilone

ix-ab-**ep**-i-lone
(Ixempra)

BLACK BOX ALERT Combination therapy with capecitabine is contraindicated in pts with serum ALT or AST greater than 2.5 times upper limit of normal (ULN) or bilirubin greater than 1 times ULN due to increased risk of toxicity, neutropenia-related mortality.

◆ CLASSIFICATION

PHARMACOTHERAPEUTIC: Epothilone microtubule inhibitor, antimitotic agent. **CLINICAL:** Antineoplastic.

USES

Combination therapy with capecitabine for treatment of metastatic or locally advanced breast cancer in pts after failure of anthracycline, taxane therapy. As monotherapy, treatment of metastatic or locally advanced breast cancer in pts after failure of anthracycline, taxane, and capecitabine therapy. **OFF-LABEL:** Treatment of endometrial cancer.

PRECAUTIONS

Contraindications: Hypersensitivity to ixabepilone. Severe hypersensitivity reaction (Grade 3 or 4) to Cremophor, baseline neutrophil count less than 1,500 cells/mm^3 or platelet count less than 100,000 cells/mm^3. **Combination Capecitabine Therapy:** Serum ALT or AST greater than 2.5 times the upper limit of normal, bilirubin greater than 1 times the upper limit of normal. **Cautions:** Diabetes, existing moderate to severe neuropathy, history of cardiovascular disease. **Monotherapy:** Serum ALT or AST greater than 5 times upper limit of normal bilirubin greater than 3 times upper limit of normal.

I

ACTION

Binds directly on microtubules during active stage of G2 and M phases of cell cycle, preventing formation of microtubules, an essential part of the process of separation of chromosomes. **Therapeutic Effect:** Blocks cells in mitotic phase of cell division, leading to cell death.

PHARMACOKINETICS

Metabolized in liver. Protein binding: 77%. Excreted in feces (65%), urine (21%). **Half-life:** 52 hrs.

⌛ LIFESPAN CONSIDERATIONS

Pregnancy/Lactation: May cause fetal harm. Unknown if distributed in breast milk. **Children:** Safety and efficacy not established. **Elderly:** Higher incidence of severe adverse reactions in those older than 65 yrs.

INTERACTIONS

DRUG: **Strong CYP3A4 Inhibitors (e.g., clarithromycin, ketoconazole, ritonavir)** may increase concentration/effect. **Strong CYP3A4 inducers (e.g., carBAMazepine, phenytoin, rifAMPin)** may decrease concentration/effect. **HERBAL:** **St. John's wort**

may decrease concentration/effect. **FOOD:** **Grapefruit products** may increase concentration/effect. **LAB VALUES:** May increase serum ALT, AST, bilirubin. May decrease WBCs, Hgb, platelets.

AVAILABILITY (Rx)

Injection, Solution: Kit: 15-mg kit supplied with diluent for Ixempra, 8 mL; 45 mg supplied with diluent for Ixempra, 23.5 mL.

ADMINISTRATION/HANDLING

IV

Reconstitution • Withdraw diluent and slowly inject into vial. • Gently swirl and invert until powder is completely dissolved. • Further dilute with 250 mL lactated Ringer's. • Solution may be stored in vial for a maximum of 1 hr at room temperature. • Final concentration for infusion must be between 0.2 mg/mL and 0.6 mg/mL. • Mix infusion bag by manual rotation.

Rate of administration • Administer through an in-line filter of 0.2 to 1.2 microns. • Infuse over 3 hrs. Administration must be completed within 6 hrs of reconstitution.

Storage • Refrigerate kit. • Prior to reconstitution, kit should be removed from refrigerator and allowed to stand at room temperature for approximately 30 min. • When vials are initially removed from refrigerator, a white precipitate may be observed in the diluent vial. • This precipitate will dissolve to form a clear solution once diluent warms to room temperature. • Once diluted with lactated Ringer's, solution is stable at room temperature and room light for a maximum of 6 hrs.

INDICATIONS/ROUTES/DOSAGE

◄ALERT► An H_1 antagonist (diphenhydrAMINE 50 mg PO or equivalent) and an H_2 antagonist (famotidine 20–40 mg PO or equivalent) must be given prior to beginning treatment with ixabepilone. Pts who experienced a previous hypersensitivity reaction to ixabepilone require pretreatment with corticosteroids (e.g., dexamethasone 20 mg IV 30 min before infusion, or PO 1 hr before infusion) in addition to pretreatment with H_1 and H_2 antagonists.

Breast Cancer (Monotherapy or in combination with capecitabine)

IV: ADULTS, ELDERLY: 40 mg/m^2 infused over 3 hrs q3 wks. **Maximum:** 88 mg. Continue until disease progression or unacceptable toxicity.

Monotherapy Dosage Adjustments for Hepatic Impairment

Mild Hepatic Impairment (ALT and AST less than 2.5 times upper limit of normal [ULN] and bilirubin less than 1 Time ULN)

IV: ADULTS, ELDERLY: 40 mg/m^2 infused over 3 hrs q3 wks.

Mild Hepatic Impairment (ALT and AST greater than 2.5 times ULN and less than 10 times ULN and bilirubin greater than 1 time ULN and less than 1.5 times ULN)

IV: ADULTS, ELDERLY: 32 mg/m^2 infused over 3 hrs q3 wks.

Moderate Hepatic Impairment (ALT and AST less than 10 times ULN and bilirubin greater than 1.5 times ULN and less than 3 times ULN)

IV infusion: ADULTS, ELDERLY: 20–30 mg/m^2 infused over 3 hrs q3 wks (initiate at 20 mg/m^2; may increase up to a maximum of 30 mg/m^2 in subsequent cycles if tolerated).

Dosage With Strong CYP3A4 Inhibitors/Inducers

Inhibitors: Consider dose reduction to 20 mg/m^2. **Inducers:** Consider dose increase to 60 mg/m^2.

Dosage in Renal Impairment

No dose adjustment.

Dose Modification

Dosage adjustment based on grade of neuropathy, hematologic conditions.

Hematologic

Neutrophils less than 500 cells/mm^3 for 7 days or longer: Reduce dose by 20%. **Neutropenic fever:** Reduce dose by 20%. **Platelets less than 25,000 cells/mm^3 (less than 50,000 cells/mm^3 with bleeding):** Reduce dose by 20%.

Neuropathy

Grade 2 for 7 days or longer or Grade 3 for less than 7 days: Reduce dose by 20%. **Grade 3 for 7 days or longer:** Discontinue treatment. **Grade 3 (other than neuropathy):** Reduce dose by 20%. **Grade 4:** Discontinue treatment.

SIDE EFFECTS

Common (62%): Peripheral sensory neuropathy. **Frequent (56%–46%):** Fatigue, asthenia, myalgia, arthralgia, alopecia, nausea. **Occasional (29%–11%):** Vomiting, stomatitis, mucositis, diarrhea, musculoskeletal pain, anorexia, constipation, abdominal pain, headache. **Rare (9%–5%):** Skin rash, nail disorder, edema, hand-foot syndrome (blistering/rash/peeling of skin on palms of hands, soles of feet), pyrexia, dizziness, pruritus, gastroesophageal reflux disease (GERD), hot flashes, taste disorder, insomnia.

ADVERSE EFFECTS/TOXIC REACTIONS

Neuropathy occurs early during treatment; 75% of new onset or worsening neuropathy occurred during first 3 cycles. Diabetics may be at increased risk for severe neuropathy manifested as Grade 4 neutropenia. Neutropenia, leukopenia occur commonly; anemia, thrombocytopenia occur rarely. Hypersensitivity reactions including bronchospasm, flushing, rash, dyspnea may occur. Severe hypersensitivity reactions may require emergent intervention (e.g., epinephrine, corticosteroids).

NURSING CONSIDERATIONS

BASELINE ASSESSMENT

Obtain CBC, BMP, LFT; pregnancy in females of reproductive potential. Offer emotional support.

INTERVENTION/EVALUATION

Monitor for symptoms of neuropathy (burning sensation, hyperesthesia, hypoesthesia, paresthesia, discomfort, neuropathic pain). Assess skin for erythema. Monitor CBC for evidence of neutropenia, thrombocytopenia; LFT for hepatotoxicity. Assess mouth for stomatitis, mucositis. If hypersensitivity reactions occur, provide immediate supportive measures.

PATIENT/FAMILY TEACHING

• Treatment may depress your immune system response and reduce your ability to fight infection. Report symptoms of infection such as body aches, chills, cough, fatigue, fever. Avoid those with active infection. • Report allergic reactions such as bronchospasm, difficulty breathing, flushing.

ixazomib

ix-**az**-oh-mib
(Ninlaro)
Do not confuse ixazomib with bortezomib, carfilzomib, idelalisib, or ixekizumab.

◆CLASSIFICATION

PHARMACOTHERAPEUTIC: Proteasome inhibitor. **CLINICAL:** Antineoplastic.

USES

Treatment of multiple myeloma (in combination with lenalidomide and dexamethasone) in pts who have received at least 1 prior therapy.

PRECAUTIONS

Contraindications: Severe hypersensitivity to ixazomib. **Cautions:** Baseline neutropenia, thrombocytopenia; hepatic/renal impairment, chronic peripheral edema, predisposing factors to infection (e.g., diabetes, renal failure, open wounds). Concomitant use of strong CYP3A inducers not recommended.

ACTION

Reversibly inhibits activity of beta 5 subunit of the 20S proteasome, leading to cell cycle arrest and tumor cell death (apoptosis). **Therapeutic Effect:** Inhibits tumor cells growth and metastasis.

PHARMACOKINETICS

Well absorbed following oral administration. Widely distributed. Metabolized in liver. Protein binding: 99%. Peak plasma concentration: 1 hr. Excreted in urine (62%), feces (22%). Not removed by hemodialysis. **Half-life:** 9.5 days.

LIFESPAN CONSIDERATIONS

Pregnancy/Lactation: Avoid pregnancy; may cause fetal harm/malformations. Female and male pts of reproductive potential should use effective contraception during treatment and up to 3 mos after discontinuation. Unknown if distributed in breast milk. Breastfeeding not recommended. **Children:** Safety and efficacy not established. **Elderly:** No age-related precautions noted.

INTERACTIONS

DRUG: **Strong CYP3A inducers (e.g., carBAMazepine, phenytoin, rifAMPin)** may decrease concentration/effect; avoid use. May decrease effect of **oral contraceptives.** **HERBAL:** **St. John's wort** may decrease concentration/effect. **FOOD:** **High-fat meals** may decrease absorption/concentration. **LAB VALUES:** Expected to decrease neutrophils, platelets.

AVAILABILITY (Rx)

Capsules: 2.3 mg, 3 mg, 4 mg.

ADMINISTRATION/HANDLING

PO

• Capsule contents are hazardous; use cytotoxic precautions during handling and disposal. • Administer capsule whole; do not break, cut, crush, or open. • Give at least 1 hr before or 2 hrs after food. • Give on the same day each wk and at the same time that day. If a dose is missed, do not administer within 72 hrs of next scheduled dose. • If vomiting occurs after dosing, do not readminister; give dose at next scheduled time.

INDICATIONS/ROUTES/DOSAGE

Multiple Myeloma

Note: ANC should be 1,000 cells/mm^3 or greater, platelets 75,000 cells/mm^3 or greater, nonhematologic toxicities at baseline or Grade 1 or less prior to initiating a new cycle of therapy.

PO: ADULTS, ELDERLY: 4 mg once wkly on days 1, 8, and 15 of 28-day cycle, in combination with lenalidomide 25 mg daily (on days 1–21 of 28-day cycle) and dexamethasone 40 mg (on days 1, 8, 15, and 22 of 28-day cycle). Continue until disease progression or unacceptable toxicity.

Dose Reduction Schedule

Initial dose: 4 mg. **First dose reduction:** 3 mg. **Second dose reduction:** 2.3 mg. **Unable to tolerate 2.3-mg dose:** Permanently discontinue.

Dose Modification

Based on Common Terminology Criteria for Adverse Events (CTCAE).

Thrombocytopenia

Platelet count less than 30,000 cells/mm^3: Withhold ixazomib and lenalidomide until platelet count is 30,000 cells/mm^3 or greater, then resume ixazomib at the same dose and resume lenalidomide at reduced dose level (see manufacturer guidelines). **Recurrence of platelet count less than 30,000 cells/mm^3:** Withhold ixazomib and lenalidomide until platelet count is 30,000 cells/mm^3 or greater, then resume ixazomib at reduced dose level and resume lenalidomide at the same dose. **Additional occurrences:** Alternate dose modification of ixazomib and lenalidomide.

Neutropenia

Absolute neutrophil count (ANC) less than 500 cells/mm^3: Withhold ixazomib and lenalidomide until ANC is 500 cells/mm^3 or greater, then resume ixazomib at the same dose and resume lenalidomide at reduced dose level (see manufacturer guidelines). **Recurrence of ANC less than 500 cells/mm^3:** Withhold ixazomib and lenalidomide until ANC is 500 cells/mm^3 or greater, then resume ixazomib at reduced dose level and resume lenalidomide at the same dose. **Additional occurrences:** Alternate dose modification of ixazomib and lenalidomide.

Rash

Grade 2 or 3 rash: Withhold lenalidomide until resolved to Grade 1 or 0, then resume lenalidomide at next lower dose level (see manufacturer guidelines) and resume ixazomib at the same dose. **Recurrence of Grade 2 or 3 rash:** Withhold ixazomib and lenalidomide until recovery to Grade 1 or 0, then resume ixazomib at reduced dose level and resume lenalidomide at the same dose. **Grade 4 rash:** Permanently discontinue. **Additional occurrences:** Alternate dose modification of ixazomib and lenalidomide.

Peripheral Neuropathy

Grade 1 (with pain) or Grade 2: Withhold ixazomib until resolved to baseline or improved to Grade 1 or 0 without pain (at prescriber's discretion), then resume ixazomib at the same dose. **Grade 2 (with pain) or Grade 3:** Withhold ixazomib until resolved to baseline or improved to Grade 1 or 0 without pain (at prescriber's discretion), then resume ixazomib at reduced dose level. **Grade 4:** Permanently discontinue.

Any Other Nonhematologic Toxicity

Grade 3 or 4: Withhold ixazomib until resolved to baseline or improved to Grade 1 or 0 (at physician's discretion), then resume ixazomib at reduced dose level.

Dosage in Renal Impairment

Mild to moderate impairment: Not specified; use caution. **Severe impairment (CrCl less than 30 mL/min), end-stage renal disease:** Reduce starting dose to 3 mg.

Dosage in Hepatic Impairment

Mild impairment: No dose adjustment. **Moderate to severe impairment:** Reduce starting dose to 3 mg.

SIDE EFFECTS

Frequent (42%–26%): Diarrhea, constipation, nausea. **Occasional (22%–5%):** Vomiting, back pain, blurry vision, dry eye.

ADVERSE EFFECTS/TOXIC REACTIONS

Neutropenia, thrombocytopenia are expected responses to therapy. Thrombocytopenia reported in 78% of pts; neutropenia in 67% of pts. Severe diarrhea may lead to discontinuation of treatment. Peripheral neuropathy reported in 28% of pts (sensory neuropathies were the most common type). Peripheral edema occurred in 28% of pts. Dermatologic toxicities including maculopapular and macular rash may occur. Infectious processes including upper respiratory tract infection (19% of pts), conjunctivitis (6% of pts) may occur. Other toxic reactions including neutrophilic dermatosis, posterior reversible encephalopathy, Stevens-Johnson syndrome, thrombotic thrombocytopenic purpura, transverse myelitis, treatment-induced hepatotoxicity, tumor lysis syndrome, occur rarely.

NURSING CONSIDERATIONS

BASELINE ASSESSMENT

Obtain ANC, CBC (esp. platelet count), renal function test (in pts with renal impairment), LFT; pregnancy test in female pts of reproductive potential. Screen for active infection. Question history of peripheral neuropathy, peripheral edema, hepatic/renal impairment, current hemodialysis status. Receive full medication history and screen for interactions. Assess hydration status. Obtain baseline visual acuity. Obtain dietary consult for nutritional support. Offer emotional support.

INTERVENTION/EVALUATION

Monitor ANC, platelet count at least monthly, more frequently during first 3 cycles; LFT in pts with hepatic impairment. Consider concomitant granulocyte colony-stimulating factor (e.g., filgrastim, pegfilgrastim) in pts with neutropenia. Monitor for dehydration, electrolyte imbalance if diarrhea occurs. Offer antiemetics for nausea, antidiarrheals for diarrhea. Monitor for infection (esp. in pts with neutropenia); dermal toxicity, skin rashes, petechiae; peripheral neuropathy (with or without pain); peripheral edema. Monitor daily pattern bowel activity, stool consistency. Monitor for side effects of dexamethasone (e.g., hyperglycemia, weight loss, decreased appetite), lenalidomide (see prescribing information). Reversible posterior leukoencephalopathy syndrome should be considered in pts with altered mental status, confusion, headache, seizures, visual disturbances. Obtain visual acuity if vision becomes blurry.

PATIENT/FAMILY TEACHING

• Treatment may depress your immune system and reduce your ability to fight infection. Report symptoms of infection such as body aches, chills, cough, fatigue, fever. Avoid those with active infection. • Use effective contraception to avoid pregnancy. Do not breastfeed. • Do not take ixazomib and dexamethasone at the same time. Take dexamethasone with food to minimize GI upset. • Do not expose the capsule contents to the skin or eyes. If eyes are exposed to the capsule powder, thoroughly flush eyes with water. If skin is exposed to the capsule powder, thoroughly wash skin with soap and water. • Treatment may cause nerve pain; extreme sensitivity to touch; muscle weakness; or prickling, tingling, numbness in your hands and feet. • Report neurologic changes such as blurry vision, confusion, headache, seizures; may indicate life-threatening brain swelling. • Treatment may increase risk of bleeding. • Do not take herbal supplements, esp. St. John's wort.

ixekizumab

ix-ee-**kiz**-ue-mab
(Taltz)
Do not confuse ixekizumab with daclizumab, eculizumab, gevokizumab, secukinumab, or ustekinumab.

◆CLASSIFICATION

PHARMACOTHERAPEUTIC: Human interleukin-17A antagonist. Monoclonal antibody. **CLINICAL:** Antipsoriasis agent.

USES

Treatment of moderate to severe plaque psoriasis in adults and children 6 yrs and older who are candidates for systemic therapy or phototherapy. Treatment of active psoriatic arthritis in adults. Treatment of active ankylosing spondylitis. Treatment of active nonradiographic axial spondyloarthritis with objective signs of inflammation in adults.

PRECAUTIONS

Contraindications: Hypersensitivity to ixekizumab. **Cautions:** Baseline neutropenia, thrombocytopenia; inflammatory bowel disease (Crohn's disease, ulcerative colitis), HIV infection, concomitant immunosuppressant therapy, conditions predisposing to infection (e.g., diabetes, renal failure, open wounds), pts who have been exposed to tuberculosis. Concomitant use of live vaccines not recommended.

ACTION

Selectively binds to and inhibits interaction of interleukin-17A receptor, a naturally occurring cytokine that is involved in inflammatory and immune response. **Therapeutic Effect:** Alters biologic immune response; inhibits release of proinflammatory cytokines and chemokines.

PHARMACOKINETICS

Widely distributed. Degraded into small peptides and amino acids via catabolic pathway. Peak plasma concentration: 4 days. Steady state reached in 8–10 wks. Elimination not specified. **Half-life:** 13 days.

LIFESPAN CONSIDERATIONS

Pregnancy/Lactation: Unknown if distributed in breast milk. However, human immunoglobulin G is present in breast milk and is known to cross placenta. **Children:** Safety and efficacy not established in pts younger than 6 yrs. **Elderly:** No age-related precautions noted.

INTERACTIONS

DRUG: May decrease therapeutic response of **BCG (intravesical), live vaccines**. May enhance the adverse/toxic effects of **belimumab, natalizumab, live vaccines. HERBAL: Echinacea** may decrease effect. **FOOD:** None known. **LAB VALUES:** May decrease neutrophils, platelets. May decrease diagnostic effect of *Coccidioides immitis* skin test.

AVAILABILITY (Rx)

Auto-injector Pen: 80 mg/mL. **Prefilled Syringe:** 80 mg/mL.

ADMINISTRATION/HANDLING

SQ

• Follow instructions for preparation according to manufacturer guidelines. • Remove auto-injector or prefilled syringe from refrigerator and allow to warm to room temperature (approx. 30 min) with needle cap intact. • Visually inspect for particulate matter or discoloration. Solution should appear clear, colorless to slightly yellow in color. Do not use if solution is cloudy, discolored, or if visible particles are observed.

Administration • Insert needle subcutaneously into upper arms, outer thigh, or abdomen, and inject solution. • Do not inject into areas of active skin disease or injury such as sunburns, skin rashes, inflammation, skin infections, or active psoriasis. • Rotate injection sites.

Storage • Refrigerate until time of use. • Do not freeze. • Do not shake. • Protect from light.

INDICATIONS/ROUTES/DOSAGE

Ankylosing Spondylitis

SQ: ADULTS, ELDERLY: 160 mg (two 80-mg injections) once, then 80 mg q4wks. May give alone or in combination with conventional disease-modifying antirheumatic drugs, corticosteroids, NSAIDs, and/or analgesics.

Plaque Psoriasis

SQ: ADULTS, ELDERLY: Initially, 160 mg (two injections of 80 mg) once, then 80 mg at wks 2, 4, 6, 8, 10, 12, then 80 mg once q4wks. **ADOLESCENTS, CHILDREN 6 YRS AND OLDER: (WEIGHING 50 KG OR MORE):** 160 mg (two 80-mg injections) once, then 80 mg q4wks. **(25–50 KG):** 80 mg once, then 40 mg q4wks. **(LESS THAN 25 KG):** 40 mg once, then 20 mg q4wks.

Psoriatic Arthritis

Note: For pts with coexisting plaque psoriasis, use dosage for plaque psoriasis.

SQ: ADULTS, ELDERLY: 160 mg (two 80-mg injections) once, then 80 mg q4wks. May give alone or in combination with conventional disease-modifying antirheumatic drugs (e.g., methotrexate).

Nonradiographic Axial Spondyloarthritis

SQ: ADULTS, ELDERLY: 80 mg q4wks.

Dosage in Renal/Hepatic Impairment

Not specified; use caution.

SIDE EFFECTS

Occasional (17%): Injection site reactions (pain, erythema). **Rare (2%):** Nausea.

ADVERSE EFFECTS/TOXIC REACTIONS

May increase risk of infection including tuberculosis. Infections including upper respiratory tract infection (14% of pts), nasopharyngitis (14% of pts), tinea infections (2% of pts) have occurred. Cytopenias including neutropenia (11% of pts), thrombocytopenia (3% of pts) were reported. May cause exacerbation of Crohn's disease and ulcerative colitis. Hypersensitivity reactions, including angioedema, occur rarely. Immunogenicity (auto-ixekizumab antibodies) occurred in less than 9% of pts.

NURSING CONSIDERATIONS

BASELINE ASSESSMENT

Obtain CBC in pts with known history of neutropenia, thrombocytopenia. Screen for active infection. Pts should be evaluated for active tuberculosis and tested for latent infection prior to initiating treatment and periodically during therapy. Induration of 5 mm or greater with tuberculin skin testing should be considered a positive test result when assessing if treatment for latent tuberculosis is necessary. Consider administration of age-appropriate immunizations (if applicable) before initiation. Question history of Crohn's disease, ulcerative colitis, hypersensitivity reaction. Conduct dermatologic exam; record characteristics of psoriatic lesions.

INTERVENTION/EVALUATION

Monitor for symptoms of tuberculosis, including pts who tested negative for latent tuberculosis infection prior to initiating therapy. Interrupt or discontinue treatment if serious infection, opportunistic infection, or sepsis occurs, and initiate appropriate antimicrobial therapy. Assess skin for improvement of lesions. Monitor for hypersensitivity reaction, symptoms of inflammatory bowel disease.

PATIENT/FAMILY TEACHING

• A healthcare provider will show you how to properly prepare and inject your medication. You must demonstrate correct preparation and injection techniques before using medication at home. • Treatment may depress your immune system response and reduce your ability to fight infection. Report symptoms of infection such as body aches, chills, cough, fatigue, fever. Avoid people with active infection. • Do not receive live vaccines. • Expect frequent tuberculosis screening. • Report travel plans to possible endemic areas. • Immediately report difficulty breathing, itching, hives, rash, swelling of the face or tongue; may indicate allergic reaction. • Treatment may cause worsening of Crohn's disease or cause inflammatory bowel disease. Report abdominal pain, diarrhea, weight loss.

ketorolac

kee-**toe**-role-ak
(Acular, Acular LS, Acuvail, Apo-Ketorolac ✱, Sprix, Toradol ✱)

BLACK BOX ALERT Increased risk of serious cardiovascular thrombotic events, including myocardial infarction, CVA. Increased risk of severe GI reactions, including ulceration, bleeding, perforation.

Do not confuse Acular with Acthar or Ocular, ketorolac with Ketalar, or Toradol with Foradil, Inderal, TEGretol, or traMADol.

◆CLASSIFICATION

PHARMACOTHERAPEUTIC: NSAID. **CLINICAL:** Analgesic, intraocular anti-inflammatory.

USES

PO, Injection, Nasal: Short-term (5 days or less) relief of mild to moderate pain. **Ophthalmic:** Relief of ocular itching due to seasonal allergic conjunctivitis. Treatment postop for inflammation following cataract extraction, pain following incisional refractive surgery. **OFF-LABEL:** Prevention, treatment of ocular inflammation (ophthalmic form).

PRECAUTIONS

Contraindications: Hypersensitivity to ketorolac, aspirin, or other NSAIDs. Intracranial bleeding, hemorrhagic diathesis, incomplete hemostasis, high risk of bleeding; concomitant use of aspirin, NSAIDs, probenecid, or pentoxifylline; labor and delivery, advanced renal impairment or risk of renal failure, active or history of peptic ulcer disease, chronic inflammation of GI tract, recent or history of GI bleeding/ulceration. Perioperative pain in setting of CABG surgery. Prophylaxis before major surgery. **Cautions:** Hepatic impairment, history of GI tract disease, asthma, coagulation disorders, receiving anticoagulants, fluid retention, HF, renal impairment, inflammatory bowel disease, smoking, use of alcohol, elderly, debilitated.

ACTION

Inhibits COX-1 and COX-2 enzymes, resulting in decreased prostaglandin synthesis; reduces prostaglandin levels in aqueous humor. **Therapeutic Effect:** Produces analgesic, antipyretic, anti-inflammatory effect; reduces intraocular inflammation.

PHARMACOKINETICS

Well absorbed (100%) following oral administration. Protein binding: 99%. Metabolized in liver. Primarily excreted in urine. Not removed by hemodialysis. **Half-life:** 5–9 hrs (increased in renal impairment, in elderly).

⌛ LIFESPAN CONSIDERATIONS

Pregnancy/Lactation: Unknown if distributed in breast milk. Avoid use during third trimester (may adversely affect fetal cardiovascular system: premature closure of ductus arteriosus). **Children:** Safety and efficacy not established, but doses of 0.5 mg/kg have been used. **Elderly:** GI bleeding, ulceration more likely to cause serious adverse effects. Age-related renal impairment may increase risk of hepatic/renal toxicity; decreased dosage recommended.

INTERACTIONS

DRUG: May decrease effects of **antihypertensives (e.g., amLODIPine, lisinopril), diuretics (e.g., furosemide, HCTZ). Aspirin, NSAIDs, other salicylates** may increase risk of GI side effects, bleeding. May increase risk of bleeding with **heparin, oral anticoagulants (e.g., warfarin).** May increase concentration, risk of toxicity of **lithium.** May increase effect of **apixaban, dabigatran, edoxaban, rivaroxaban. Bile acid sequestrants (e.g., cholestyramine)** may decrease absorption/effect. May increase nephrotoxic effect of **cycloSPORINE.** **HERBAL: Glucosamine, herbs with anticoagulant/antiplatelet properties (e.g., garlic, ginger, ginseng, ginkgo**

biloba) may increase concentration/effect. **FOOD**: None known. **LAB VALUES**: May prolong bleeding time. May increase serum ALT, AST, BUN, potassium, creatinine.

AVAILABILITY (Rx)

Injection Solution: 15 mg/mL, 30 mg/mL. **Nasal Spray**: ***(Sprix)***: 1.7-g bottle provides 8 sprays (15.75 mg/spray). **Ophthalmic Solution**: ***(Acular LS)***: 0.4%, ***(Acuvail)***: 0.45%, ***(Acular)***: 0.5%. **Tablets**: 10 mg.

ADMINISTRATION/HANDLING

IV

• Give undiluted as IV push. • Give over at least 15 sec.

IM

• Give deep IM slowly into large muscle mass.

PO

• Give with food, milk, antacids if GI distress occurs.

Ophthalmic

• Place gloved finger on lower eyelid and pull out until pocket is formed between eye and lower lid. Place prescribed number of drops into pocket. • Instruct pt to close eye gently for 1–2 min (so that medication will not be squeezed out of the sac) and to apply digital pressure to lacrimal sac at inner canthus for 1 min to minimize system absorption.

IV INCOMPATIBILITIES

Promethazine (Phenergan).

IV COMPATIBILITIES

FentaNYL (Sublimaze), HYDROmorphone (Dilaudid), morphine, nalbuphine (Nubain).

INDICATIONS/ROUTES/DOSAGE

Note: Total duration is 5 days (parenteral and oral). Do not increase dose/frequency; supplement with low-dose opioids if needed.

Pain Management

Note: Avoid use in the elderly.

PO: **ADULTS**: Initially, 20 mg (10 mg for elderly), then 10 mg q4–6h. **Maximum:** 40 mg/24 hrs.

IM: **ADULTS**: 60 mg once or 30 mg q6h. **Maximum:** 120 mg/24 hrs. **PTS WITH RENAL IMPAIRMENT, PTS WEIGHING LESS THAN 50 KG**: 30 mg once or 15 mg q6h. **Maximum:** 60 mg/24 hrs.

IV: **ADULTS**: 30 mg once or 30 mg q6h. **Maximum:** 120 mg/24 hrs. **PTS WITH RENAL IMPAIRMENT, PTS WEIGHING LESS THAN 50 KG**: 15 mg once or 15 mg q6h. **Maximum:** 60 mg/24 hrs.

Nasal spray: ADULTS WEIGHING 50 KG OR MORE: One spray (15.75 mg) in each nostril (total dose: 31.5 mg) q6-8h. **Maximum dose:** Four sprays (126 mg/day). **ADULTS WEIGHING LESS THAN 50 KG**: One spray (15.75 mg) in each nostril (total dose: 15.75 mg) q6-8h. **Maximum dose:** Four sprays (63 mg/day).

Allergic Conjunctivitis

Ophthalmic: ADULTS, ELDERLY, CHILDREN 2 YRS AND OLDER: 1 drop (0.5%) 4 times/day.

Cataract Extraction

Ophthalmic: ADULTS, ELDERLY: 1 drop (0.5%) 4 times/day. Begin 24 hrs after surgery and continue for 2 wks.

Corneal Refractive Surgery

Ophthalmic: ADULTS, ELDERLY: 1 drop (0.4%) 4 times/day for up to 4 days after surgery.

Dosage in Renal Impairment

See dosage section.

Dosage in Hepatic Impairment

Use caution.

SIDE EFFECTS

Frequent (17%–12%): Headache, nausea, abdominal cramps/pain, dyspepsia. **Occasional (9%–3%)**: Diarrhea. **Nasal:** Nasal discomfort, rhinalgia, increased lacrimation, throat irritation, rhinitis. **Ophthalmic:** Transient stinging, burning. **Rare (3%–1%):** Constipation, vomiting, flatulence, stomatitis. **Ophthalmic:** Ocular irritation, allergic reactions (manifested by pruritus, stinging), superficial ocular infection, keratitis.

ADVERSE EFFECTS/TOXIC REACTIONS

Peptic ulcer, GI bleeding, gastritis, severe hepatic reaction (cholestasis, jaundice) occur rarely. Nephrotoxicity (glomerular nephritis, interstitial nephritis, nephrotic syndrome) may occur in pts with preexisting renal impairment. Acute hypersensitivity reaction (fever, chills, joint pain) occurs rarely.

NURSING CONSIDERATIONS

BASELINE ASSESSMENT

Assess onset, type, location, duration of pain. Obtain baseline renal/hepatic function tests.

INTERVENTION/EVALUATION

Monitor renal function, LFT, urinary output. Monitor daily pattern of bowel activity, stool consistency. Observe for occult blood loss. Assess for therapeutic response: relief of pain, stiffness, swelling; increased joint mobility; reduced joint tenderness; improved grip strength. Monitor for bleeding (may also occur with ophthalmic route due to systemic absorption).

PATIENT/FAMILY TEACHING

• Avoid aspirin, alcohol. • Report abdominal pain, bloody stools, or vomiting blood. • If GI upset occurs, take with food, milk. • **Ophthalmic:** Transient stinging, burning may occur upon instillation. • Do not administer while wearing soft contact lenses.

K

labetalol

la-**bayt**-a-lol
(Trandate 🍁)
Do not confuse labetalol with atenolol, betaxolol, metoprolol or propranolol, or Trandate with traMADol or TRENtal.

FIXED-COMBINATION(S)

Normozide: labetalol/hydroCHLOROthiazide (a diuretic): 100 mg/25 mg, 200 mg/25 mg, 300 mg/25 mg.

◆CLASSIFICATION

PHARMACOTHERAPEUTIC: Alpha-, beta-adrenergic blocker. **CLINICAL:** Antihypertensive.

L

USES

Management of hypertension. IV for severe hypertension. **OFF-LABEL:** Management of preeclampsia, severe hypertension in pregnancy, hypertension during acute ischemic stroke, pediatric hypertension.

PRECAUTIONS

Contraindications: Hypersensitivity to labetalol. Bronchial asthma, history of obstructive airway disease, cardiogenic shock, uncompensated HF, second- or third-degree heart block (except in pts with functioning pacemaker), severe bradycardia, conditions associated with severe, prolonged hypotension. **Cautions:** Compensated HF, severe anaphylaxis to allergens, myasthenia gravis, psychiatric disease, hepatic impairment, pheochromocytoma, diabetes; concurrent use with digoxin, verapamil, or dilTIAZem; arterial obstruction, elderly. Pts with peripheral vascular disease, Raynaud's disease.

ACTION

Blocks alpha-1, beta-1, beta-2 (large doses) adrenergic receptor sites. **Therapeutic Effect:** Decreases peripheral vascular resistance, B/P.

PHARMACOKINETICS

Route	Onset	Peak	Duration
PO	0.5–2 hrs	2–4 hrs	8–12 hrs
IV	2–5 min	5–15 min	2–4 hrs

Incompletely absorbed from GI tract. Bioavailability: 25%. Protein binding: 50%. Metabolized in liver. Primarily excreted in urine. Not removed by hemodialysis. **Half-life:** 6–8 hrs.

⌛ LIFESPAN CONSIDERATIONS

Pregnancy/Lactation: Drug crosses placenta. Small amount distributed in breast milk. **Children:** Safety and efficacy not established. **Elderly:** Age-related peripheral vascular disease may increase susceptibility to decreased peripheral circulation. May have increased risk of orthostatic hypotension.

INTERACTIONS

DRUG: May decrease effects of **beta$_2$-adrenergic agonists (e.g., arformoterol, salmeterol), theophylline. Dronedarone, rivastigmine** may increase bradycardic effect. May increase bradycardic effect of **fingolimod. HERBAL: Herbals with hypertensive properties (e.g., licorice, yohimbe) or hypotensive properties (e.g., garlic, ginger, ginkgo biloba)** may alter effects. **FOOD:** None known. **LAB VALUES:** May increase serum antinuclear antibody titer (ANA), BUN, LDH, alkaline phosphatase, bilirubin, creatinine, potassium, triglycerides, lipoprotein, uric acid, ALT, AST.

AVAILABILITY (Rx)

Injection Solution: 5 mg/mL. **Tablets:** 100 mg, 200 mg, 300 mg.

ADMINISTRATION/HANDLING

IV

◀ALERT▶ Prolonged duration of action: Monitor several hrs after administration. Excessive administration may result in prolonged hypotension and/or bradycardia.

Reconstitution • For IV infusion, dilute in D_5W to provide concentration of 1–2 mg/mL.
Rate of administration • For IV push, administer at a rate of 10 mg/min. • For IV infusion, administer at rate of 2 mg/min initially. Rate is adjusted according to B/P. • Monitor B/P immediately before and q5–10min during IV administration (maximum effect occurs within 5 min).
Storage • Store at room temperature. • After dilution, IV solution is stable for 72 hrs. • Solution appears clear, colorless to light yellow. • Discard if discolored or precipitate forms.

PO
• Give without regard to food. • Tablets may be crushed.

IV INCOMPATIBILITIES

Amphotericin B complex (Abelcet, AmBisome, Amphotec), ceftaroline (Teflaro), cefTRIAXone (Rocephin), furosemide (Lasix), heparin, nafcillin (Nafcil).

IV COMPATIBILITIES

Amiodarone (Cordarone), calcium gluconate, dexmedetomidine (Precedex), dilTIAZem (Cardizem), DOBUTamine (Dobutrex), DOPamine (Intropin), enalapril (Vasotec), fentaNYL (Sublimaze), HYDROmorphone (Dilaudid), lidocaine, LORazepam (Ativan), magnesium sulfate, midazolam (Versed), milrinone (Primacor), morphine, nitroglycerin, norepinephrine (Levophed), potassium chloride, potassium phosphate, propofol (Diprivan).

INDICATIONS/ROUTES/DOSAGE

Hypertension
PO: ADULTS, ELDERLY: Initially, 100 mg twice daily. Adjust in increments of 100 mg twice daily q2–3days. Usual dose: 200–800 mg/day in 2 divided doses. May require up to 2,400 mg/day. **CHILDREN:** 1–3 mg/kg/day in 2 divided doses. **Maximum:** 10–12 mg/kg/day up to 1,200 mg/day.

Severe Hypertension, Hypertensive Crisis
IV: ADULTS: Initially, 10–20 mg (bolus over 1–2 min). Additional doses of 20–80 mg may be given at 10-min intervals until target BP reached. **CHILDREN:** 0.2–1 mg/kg/dose. **Maximum:** 40 mg/dose.
IV infusion: ADULTS: Initially, 0.5–2 mg/min up to 10 mg/min. **CHILDREN:** 0.25–3 mg/kg/hr. **Maximum:** 3 mg/kg/hr.

Dosage in Renal Impairment
No dose adjustment.

Dosage in Hepatic Impairment
Use caution.

SIDE EFFECTS

Frequent (20%–11%): Drowsiness, dizziness, excessive fatigue. **Occasional (10% or less):** Dyspnea, peripheral edema, depression, anxiety, constipation, diarrhea, nasal congestion, weakness, diminished sexual function, transient scalp tingling, insomnia, nausea, vomiting, abdominal discomfort. **Rare:** Altered taste, dry eyes, increased urination, paresthesia.

ADVERSE EFFECTS/TOXIC REACTIONS

May precipitate, aggravate HF due to decreased myocardial stimulation. Abrupt withdrawal may precipitate myocardial ischemia, producing chest pain, diaphoresis, palpitations, headache, tremor. May mask signs, symptoms of acute hypoglycemia (tachycardia, B/P changes) in diabetic pts. Rapid reduction of blood pressure may cause CVA, optic nerve infarction, ischemic changes on ECG. May cause severe orthostatic hypotension.

NURSING CONSIDERATIONS

BASELINE ASSESSMENT
Assess renal function, LFT. Assess B/P, heart rate immediately before drug administration (if pulse is 60/min or less or systolic B/P is lower than 90 mm Hg, withhold medication, contact physician). Question history of bradycardia, HF, second- or third-degree heart block, myasthenia gravis.

INTERVENTION/EVALUATION
Monitor B/P for hypotension; heart rate. Monitor ECG for cardiac arrhythmias.

L

Assist with ambulation if dizziness occurs. Assess for evidence of HF: dyspnea (particularly on exertion or lying down), night cough, peripheral edema, distended neck veins. Monitor I&O (increase in weight, decrease in urine output may indicate HF).

PATIENT/FAMILY TEACHING

• Do not discontinue drug except upon advice of physician (abrupt discontinuation may precipitate HF). • Slowly go from lying to standing. • Compliance with therapy regimen is essential to control hypertension, arrhythmias. • Avoid tasks that require alertness, motor skills until response to drug is established. • Report shortness of breath, excessive fatigue, weight gain, prolonged dizziness, headache. • Do not use nasal decongestants, OTC cold preparations (stimulants) without physician approval. • Limit alcohol.

L

lacosamide

la-**koe**-sa-myde
(Vimpat)
Do not confuse lacosamide with zonisamide, or Vimpat with Venofer, Vfend, or Vimovo.

◆CLASSIFICATION

PHARMACOTHERAPEUTIC: Succinimide **(Schedule V). CLINICAL:** Anticonvulsant.

USES

Monotherapy or adjunctive therapy for treatment of partial-onset seizures in pts 4 yrs and older.

PRECAUTIONS

Contraindications: Hypersensitivity to lacosamide. **Cautions:** Renal/hepatic impairment, cardiac conduction problems (e.g., marked first-degree AV block, second-degree or higher AV block, sick sinus syndrome without pacemaker), myocardial ischemia, HF, pts at risk of suicide.

ACTION

Selectively enhances slow inactivation of sodium channels, stabilizing hyperexcitable neuronal membranes and inhibits neuronal firing. **Therapeutic Effect:** Reduces seizure frequency.

PHARMACOKINETICS

Readily absorbed. Protein binding: 15%. Peak plasma concentration: 1–4 hrs after oral dosing and is reached at the end of IV infusion. Primarily excreted in urine. Steady-state reached in 3 days. Removed by hemodialysis. **Half-life:** 13 hrs.

LIFESPAN CONSIDERATIONS

Pregnancy/Lactation: Use in pregnancy if benefits outweigh risk. Unknown if distributed in breast milk. **Children:** Safety and efficacy not established in pts younger than 17 yrs. **Elderly:** No age-related precautions noted.

INTERACTIONS

DRUG: None significant. **HERBAL:** None significant. **FOOD:** None known. **LAB VALUES:** May increase serum ALT; proteinuria.

AVAILABILITY (Rx)

Injection Solution: 10 mg/mL (20 mL). **Oral Solution:** 10 mg/mL.

Tablets: 50 mg, 100 mg, 150 mg, 200 mg.

ADMINISTRATION/HANDLING

PO

• Give without regard to food. • Do not break, crush, dissolve, or divide film-coated tablets. • Oral solution should be administered with a calibrated measuring device. • Discard any unused portion after 7 wks.

IV

• Appears as a clear, colorless solution. • Discard unused portion or if precipitate or discoloration is present. May give without further dilution. • If mixing with diluent, may be stored for 24 hrs at room temperature. Infuse over 30–60 min.

IV COMPATIBILITIES

0.9% NaCl, D_5W, lactated Ringer's.

INDICATIONS/ROUTES/DOSAGE

Note: IV dose is same as oral dose. May give undiluted or mixed in compatible diluent and infused over 30–60 min.

Partial-Onset Seizures

Monotherapy

PO/IV: ADULTS, ELDERLY: Initially, 100 mg twice daily. May increase by 50 mg twice daily at wkly intervals. **Maintenance:** 150–200 mg twice daily. CHILDREN 4–17 YRS, WEIGHING 50 KG OR MORE: Initially, 50 mg twice daily. May increase by 50 mg twice daily at wkly intervals. **Maintenance:** 150–200 mg twice daily. WEIGHING 30–49 KG: Initially, 1 mg/kg/dose twice daily. May increase by 1 mg/kg/dose twice daily at wkly intervals. **Maintenance:** 2–4 mg/kg/dose twice daily. WEIGHING 11–29 KG: Initially, 1 mg/kg/dose twice daily. May increase by 1 mg/kg/dose twice daily at wkly intervals. **Maintenance:** 3–6 mg/kg/dose twice daily.

Adjunctive Therapy

PO/IV: ADULTS, ELDERLY: Initially, 50 mg twice daily. May increase by 50 mg twice daily at wkly intervals. **Maintenance:** 100–200 mg twice daily. **Maximum:** 400 mg/day. CHILDREN 4–17 YRS, WEIGHING 50 KG OR MORE: Initially, 50 mg twice daily. **Maintenance:** 100–200 mg twice daily. WEIGHING 30–49 KG: Initially, 1 mg/kg/dose twice daily. **Maintenance:** 2–4 mg/kg/dose twice daily. WEIGHING 11–29 KG: Initially, 1 mg/kg/dose twice daily. **Maintenance:** 3–6 mg/kg/dose twice daily.

Switch From IV to PO

When switching from IV to PO form, use same equivalent daily dosage and frequency as IV administration.

Switch From PO to IV

When switching from PO to IV form, initial total daily IV dosage should be equivalent to total daily dosage and frequency of PO form and should be infused IV over 30–60 min.

Dosage in Renal Impairment

Use caution when titrating. **Mild to moderate impairment:** No dose adjustment. **Severe impairment, end-stage renal disease: Maximum:** 300 mg/day.

Dosage in Hepatic Impairment

Use caution when titrating. **Mild to moderate impairment: Maximum:** 300 mg/day. **Severe impairment:** Not recommended.

SIDE EFFECTS

Frequent (31%–13%): Dizziness, headache. **Occasional** (11%–5%): Nausea, double vision, vomiting, fatigue, blurred vision, ataxia, tremor, nystagmus. **Rare** (4%–2%): Vertigo, diarrhea, gait disturbances, memory impairment, depression, pruritus, injection site discomfort.

ADVERSE EFFECTS/TOXIC REACTIONS

Increased risk of suicidal ideation, behavior. PR interval prolongation, AV block, ventricular tachyarrhythmias may occur. Sudden discontinuation may increase risk of seizures. Drug reaction with eosinophilia and systemic symptoms (DRESS), also known as multiorgan hypersensitivity, has been reported. DRESS may present with facial swelling, eosinophilia, fever, lymphadenopathy, rash, which may be associated with other organ systems, such as hepatitis, hematologic abnormalities, myocarditis, nephritis. Psychiatric conditions (aggression, agitation, hallucinations, psychotic disorder) may occur. Leukopenia, anemia, thrombocytopenia occur rarely.

NURSING CONSIDERATIONS

BASELINE ASSESSMENT

Review history of seizure disorder (intensity, frequency, duration, level of consciousness). Initiate seizure precautions. Renal function, LFT, CBC should be performed before therapy begins and periodically during therapy. Question history of cardiac conduction disorders, depression, suicidal ideation and behavior.

L

INTERVENTION/EVALUATION

Observe for recurrence of seizure activity. Assess for clinical improvement (decrease in intensity/frequency of seizures). Assist with ambulation if dizziness occurs. Assess for suicidal ideation, depression, behavioral changes. Drug should be withdrawn gradually (over a minimum of 1 wk) to minimize potential for increased seizure frequency. Monitor ECG for QT prolongation. Monitor for symptoms of DRESS; cardiac effects.

PATIENT/FAMILY TEACHING

• Strict maintenance of drug therapy is essential for seizure control. • Avoid tasks that require alertness, motor skills until response to drug is established. • Do not abruptly discontinue medication (may cause seizures; symptoms of withdrawal syndrome). • Treatment may affect the electrical properties of the heart; report palpitations, loss of consciousness. • Seek immediate medical attention if thoughts of suicide, new-onset or worsening of anxiety, depression, or changes in mood occurs. • Avoid alcohol, nervous system depressants. • Report symptoms of drug-induced hypersensitivity syndrome (e.g., fever, swollen face/lymph nodes; skin rash/peeling/inflammation).

lactulose

lak-tyoo-lose
(Constulose, Enulose, Generlac, Kristalose)
Do not confuse lactulose with lactose.

◆CLASSIFICATION

PHARMACOTHERAPEUTIC: Lactose derivative. **CLINICAL:** Hyperosmotic laxative, ammonia detoxicant.

USES

Prevention, treatment of portal-systemic encephalopathy (including hepatic precoma, coma); treatment of constipation.

PRECAUTIONS

Contraindications: Hypersensitivity to lactulose. Pts requiring a low-galactose diet. **Cautions:** Diabetes, hepatic impairment, dehydration.

ACTION

Inhibits diffusion of NH_3 into blood by converting NH_3 to NH_4^+; enhances diffusion of NH_3 from blood to gut, where it is converted to NH_4^+; produces osmotic effect in colon, resulting in colon distention, promoting peristalsis. **Therapeutic Effect:** Promotes increased peristalsis, bowel evacuation; decreases serum ammonia concentration.

PHARMACOKINETICS

Poorly absorbed from GI tract. Extensively metabolized in colon. Primarily excreted in feces.

⧗ LIFESPAN CONSIDERATIONS

Pregnancy/Lactation: Unknown if drug crosses placenta or is distributed in breast milk. **Children:** Avoid use in pts younger than 6 yrs (usually unable to describe symptoms). **Elderly:** No age-related precautions noted.

INTERACTIONS

DRUG: None significant. **HERBAL:** None significant. **FOOD:** None known. **LAB VALUES:** May decrease serum potassium (GI loss).

AVAILABILITY (Rx)

Packets: ***(Kristalose):*** 10 g, 20 g. **Solution, Oral:** 10 g/15 mL.

ADMINISTRATION/HANDLING

PO

• Store solution at room temperature. • Solution appears pale yellow to yellow, viscous liquid. Cloudiness, darkened solution does not indicate potency loss. • Drink water, juice, milk with each dose (aids stool softening, increases palatability). • Mix packets with 4 oz water.

Rectal

• Lubricate anus with petroleum jelly before enema insertion. • Insert carefully (prevents damage to rectal wall) with nozzle toward navel. • Squeeze container until entire dose expelled. • Instruct pt to retain 30–60 min in divided doses. • **Maximum:** 60 mL/day (40 g/day).

INDICATIONS/ROUTES/DOSAGE

Constipation

PO: ADULTS, ELDERLY: 15–30 mL or 1–2 packets (10–20 g)/day, up to 60 mL or 4 packets (40 g)/day. **CHILDREN:** 1.5–3 mL/kg/day (1–2 g/kg/day) in 1–2 divided doses. **Maximum:** 60 mL/day.

Prevention of Portal-Systemic Encephalopathy

ADULTS, ELDERLY: 30–45 mL (20–30 g) 3–4 times/day. Adjust dose q1–2 days to produce 2–3 soft stools/day. **CHILDREN:** 40–90 mL/day (26.7–60 g/day) in divided doses 3–4 times/day. **INFANTS:** 2.5–10 mL/day (1.7–6.7 g/day) in 3–4 divided doses. Adjust dose q1–2 days to produce 2–3 soft stools/day.

Treatment of Portal-Systemic Encephalopathy

PO: ADULTS, ELDERLY: Initially, 30–45 mL (20–30 g) every hr to induce rapid laxation. Then, 30–45 mL 3–4 times/day. Adjust dose q1–2days to produce 2–3 soft stools/day.

Rectal Administration (As retention enema)

200 g (300 mL) diluted with 700 mL water or NaCl via rectal balloon catheter. Retain 30–60 min q4–6h. (Transition to oral prior to stopping rectal administration.)

Dosage in Renal/Hepatic Impairment

No dose adjustment.

SIDE EFFECTS

Occasional: Abdominal cramping, flatulence, increased thirst, abdominal discomfort. **Rare:** Nausea, vomiting.

ADVERSE EFFECTS/TOXIC REACTIONS

Severe diarrhea may cause dehydration, electrolyte imbalance. Long-term use may result in laxative dependence, chronic constipation, loss of normal bowel function.

NURSING CONSIDERATIONS

BASELINE ASSESSMENT

Obtain serum ammonia level in pts being treated for hyperammonemia. Question usual stool pattern, frequency, characteristics. Conduct neurological exam in pts with elevated serum ammonia levels, symptoms of encephalopathy. Assess hydration status.

INTERVENTION/EVALUATION

Monitor serum ammonia level in pts being treated for hyperammonemia. Encourage adequate fluid intake. Assess bowel sounds for peristalsis. Monitor daily pattern of bowel activity, stool consistency; record time of evacuation. Monitor serum electrolytes in pts with prolonged, frequent, excessive use of medication. Monitor encephalopathic pts for symptom improvement (alertness, orientation, ability to follow commands).

PATIENT/FAMILY TEACHING

• Evacuation occurs in 24–48 hrs of initial dose. • Institute measures to promote defecation: increase fluid intake, exercise, high-fiber diet. • Drink plenty of fluids. • If therapy was started to treat high ammonia levels, notify physician if worsening of confusion, lethargy, weakness occurs.

lamoTRIgine

la-**moe**-tri-jeen
(LaMICtal, LaMICtal ODT, LaMICtal XR, Subvenite)

BLACK BOX ALERT Severe, potentially life-threatening skin rashes have been reported, including Stevens-Johnson syndrome. Risk increased with coadministration with valproic acid and rapid-dose titration.

Do not confuse LaMICtal with labetalol, LamISIL, or Lomotil, or lamoTRIgine with labetalol, levETIRAcetam, lamiVUDine, or levothyroxine.

◆CLASSIFICATION

PHARMACOTHERAPEUTIC: Phenyltriazine. **CLINICAL:** Anticonvulsant.

USES

Immediate-Release: Adjunctive therapy in adults and children 2 yrs of age and older with generalized tonic-clonic seizures, partial seizures, and generalized seizures of Lennox-Gastaut syndrome. Conversion to monotherapy in adults treated with another enzyme-inducing antiepileptic drug (EIAED) (e.g., valproic acid, carBAMazepine, phenytoin, PHENobarbital, or primidone as the single antiepileptic drug). Long-term maintenance treatment of bipolar disorder. Treatment of pts 2 yrs and older with primary generalized tonic-clonic seizures. **Extended-Release:** Adjunctive therapy for primary generalized tonic-clonic and partial-onset seizures in pts 13 yrs and older. Conversion to monotherapy in pts 13 yrs and older with partial seizures receiving treatment with a single antiepileptic drug (AED).

L

PRECAUTIONS

Contraindications: Hypersensitivity to lamoTRIgine. **Cautions:** Renal/hepatic impairment, pts at high risk of suicide, pts taking estrogen-containing oral contraceptives, history of adverse hematologic reaction.

ACTION

Inhibits voltage-sensitive sodium channels, stabilizing neuronal membranes. Inhibits release of glutamide (an excitatory amino acid). **Therapeutic Effect:** Reduces frequency of seizure activity. Delays time to occurrence of acute mood episodes (mania, depression, hypomania).

⌛ LIFESPAN CONSIDERATIONS

Pregnancy/Lactation: Distributed in breast milk. Breastfeeding not recommended. Increased fetal risk of oral cleft formation has been noted with use during pregnancy. **Children:** Safety and efficacy not established in pts younger than 18 yrs with bipolar disorder or in pts younger than 13 yrs with epilepsy. **Elderly:** Age-related renal impairment may require dosage adjustment.

INTERACTIONS

DRUG: CarBAMazepine, PHENobarbital, primidone, phenytoin, rifAMPin may decrease concentration/effect. **Valproic acid** may increase concentration/effects. May increase adverse effects of **carBAMazepine, dofetilide. Estrogen (contraceptive)** may decrease concentration/effect. **CNS depressants (e.g., alcohol, morphine, zolpidem)** may increase CNS depression. **HERBAL: Herbals with sedative properties (e.g., chamomile, kava kava, valerian)** may increase CNS depression. **FOOD:** None known. **LAB VALUES:** None significant.

AVAILABILITY (Rx)

Tablets: 25 mg, 100 mg, 150 mg, 200 mg. **Tablets, Chewable:** 5 mg, 25 mg. **Tablets, Orally Disintegrating:** 25 mg, 50 mg, 100 mg, 200 mg.

Tablets, Extended-Release: 25 mg, 50 mg, 100 mg, 200 mg, 250 mg, 300 mg.

ADMINISTRATION/HANDLING

PO

• Give without regard to food. • Chewable tablets may be dispensed in water or diluted fruit juice, or swallowed whole. • Extended-release tablets must be swallowed whole; do not break, crush, dissolve, or divide. • Place orally disintegrating tablet on tongue, allow to dissolve. Pt must not break, cut, or chew. Can be swallowed without regard to food or water.

INDICATIONS/ROUTES/DOSAGE

Lennox-Gastaut, Primary Generalized Tonic-Clonic Seizures, Partial Seizures

PO: ADULTS, ELDERLY, CHILDREN OLDER THAN 12 YRS: Initially, 25 mg/day for 2 wks, then increase to 50 mg/day for 2 wks. After 4 wks, may increase by 50 mg/day at 1- to 2-wk intervals. **Maintenance:** 225–375 mg/day in 2 divided doses. **CHILDREN**

2–12 YRS: **Note:** Only whole tablets should be used for dosing. Round dose down to nearest whole tablet. Initially, 0.3 mg/kg/day in 1–2 divided doses for 2 wks, then increase to 0.6 mg/kg/day in 1–2 divided doses for 2 wks. After 4 wks, may increase by 0.6 mg/kg/day at 1- to 2-wk intervals. **Maintenance:** 4.5–7.5 mg/kg/day in 2 divided doses. **Maximum:** 300 mg/day in 2 divided doses.

Adjusted Dosage With Antiepileptic Drugs Containing Valproic Acid

PO: ADULTS, ELDERLY, CHILDREN OLDER THAN 12 YRS: Initially, 12.5–25 mg every other day for 2 wks, then increase to 25 mg/day for 2 wks. After 4 wks, may increase by 25–50 mg/day at 1- to 2-wk intervals. **Maintenance:** 100–400 mg/day in 2 divided doses (100–200 mg/day when taking lamoTRIgine with valproic acid alone). **CHILDREN 2–12 YRS:** **Note:** Only whole tablets should be used for dosing. Round dose down to nearest whole tablet. Initially, 0.15 mg/kg/day in 1–2 divided doses for 2 wks, then increase to 0.3 mg/kg/day in 1–2 divided doses for 2 wks. After 4 wks, may increase by 0.3 mg/kg/day at 1- to 2-wk intervals. **Maintenance:** 1–5 mg/kg/day in 2 divided doses. **Maximum:** 200 mg/day in 2 divided doses.

Adjusted Dosage With EIAED Without Valproic Acid

PO: ADULTS, ELDERLY, CHILDREN OLDER THAN 12 YRS: Initially, 50 mg/day for 2 wks, then increase to 100 mg/day in 2 divided doses for 2 wks. After 4 wks, may increase by 100 mg/day at 1- to 2-wk intervals. **Maintenance:** 300–500 mg/day in 2 divided doses. **CHILDREN 2–12 YRS:** **Note:** Only whole tablets should be used for dosing. Round dose down to nearest whole tablet. Initially, 0.6 mg/kg/day in 1–2 divided doses for 2 wks, then increase to 1.2 mg/kg/day in 1–2 divided doses for 2 wks. After 4 wks, may increase by 1.2 mg/kg/day at 1- to 2-wk intervals. **Maintenance:** 5–15 mg/kg/day in 2 divided doses. **Maximum:** 400 mg/day in 2 divided doses.

Usual Maintenance Range for Extended-Release Tablets

PTS TAKING VALPROIC ACID: 200–250 mg once daily. **PTS TAKING EIAED WITHOUT VALPROIC ACID:** 400–600 mg once daily. **PTS NOT TAKING EIAED:** 300–400 mg once daily.

Conversion to Monotherapy for Pts Receiving EIAEDs

PO: ADULTS, ELDERLY, CHILDREN 16 YRS AND OLDER: 500 mg/day in 2 divided doses. Titrate to desired dose while maintaining EIAED at fixed level, then withdraw EIAED by 20% each wk over a 4-wk period.

Conversion to Monotherapy for Pts Receiving Valproic Acid

PO: ADULTS, ELDERLY, CHILDREN 16 YRS AND OLDER: Titrate lamoTRIgine to 200 mg/day, maintaining valproic acid dose. Maintain lamoTRIgine dose and decrease valproic acid to 500 mg/day, no greater than 500 mg/day, then maintain 500 mg/day for 1 wk. Increase lamoTRIgine to 300 mg/day and decrease valproic acid to 250 mg/day. Maintain for 1 wk, then discontinue valproic acid and increase lamoTRIgine by 100 mg/day each wk until maintenance dose of 500 mg/day reached.

Bipolar Disorder

PO: ADULTS, ELDERLY: Initially, 25 mg/day for 2 wks, then 50 mg/day for 2 wks, then 100 mg/day for 1 wk, then 200 mg/day beginning with wk 6.

Bipolar Disorder in Pts Receiving EIAEDs

PO: ADULTS, ELDERLY: 50 mg/day for 2 wks, then 100 mg/day for 2 wks, then 200 mg/day for 1 wk, then 300 mg/day for 1 wk, then up to usual maintenance dose 400 mg/day in divided doses.

Bipolar Disorder in Pts Receiving Valproic Acid

PO: ADULTS, ELDERLY: 25 mg/day every other day for 2 wks, then 25 mg/day for 2 wks, then 50 mg/day for 1 wk, then 100 mg/day. **Usual maintenance dose with valproic acid:** 100 mg/day.

Usual Dosage for LaMICtal XR

Adjunct therapy: Range: 200–600 mg/day.

L

Conversion to monotherapy: Range: 250–500 mg/day.

Discontinuation Therapy

◀ALERT▶ A dosage reduction of approximately 50%/wk over at least 2 wks is recommended.

Dosage in Renal Impairment

◀ALERT▶ Decreased dosage may be effective in pts with significant renal impairment.

Dosage in Hepatic Impairment

Mild impairment: No dose adjustment. **Moderate to severe impairment without ascites:** Reduce dose by 25%. **Severe impairment with ascites:** Reduce dose by 50%.

L

SIDE EFFECTS

Frequent (38%–14%): Dizziness, headache, diplopia, ataxia, nausea, blurred vision, drowsiness, rhinitis. **Occasional (10%–5%):** Rash, pharyngitis, vomiting, cough, flu-like symptoms, diarrhea, dysmenorrhea, fever, insomnia, dyspepsia. **Rare:** Constipation, tremor, anxiety, pruritus, vaginitis, hypersensitivity reaction.

ADVERSE EFFECTS/TOXIC REACTIONS

Abrupt withdrawal may increase seizure frequency. Serious rashes, including Stevens-Johnson syndrome, have been reported. May increase risk of suicidal thoughts and behavior. Hemophagocytic lymphohistiocytosis, a life-threatening syndrome of extreme systemic inflammation characterized by hepatosplenomegaly, lymphadenopathy, fever, rash, organ dysfunction, has occurred. Life-threatening eosinophilia and systemic symptoms (DRESS) may occur. May increase risk of aseptic meningitis. Abrupt withdrawal may increase frequency of seizures.

NURSING CONSIDERATIONS

BASELINE ASSESSMENT

Review history of seizure disorder (type, onset, intensity, frequency, duration, LOC), medication history (esp. other anticonvulsants), other medical conditions (e.g., renal impairment). Initiate seizure precautions. Assess baseline mood, behavior. Question history of suicidal ideation and behavior.

INTERVENTION/EVALUATION

Report occurrence of rash (drug discontinuation may be necessary). Assist with ambulation if dizziness, ataxia occurs. Assess for clinical improvement (decreased intensity/frequency of seizures). Assess for visual abnormalities, headache. Monitor for suicidal ideation, depression, behavioral changes. Monitor for symptoms of DRESS.

PATIENT/ FAMILY TEACHING

• Take medication only as prescribed; do not abruptly discontinue medication after long-term therapy. • Avoid alcohol. • Avoid tasks that require alertness, motor skills until response to drug is established. • Carry identification card/bracelet to note anticonvulsant therapy. • Strict maintenance of drug therapy is essential for seizure control. • Report any rash, fever, swelling of glands, worsening depression, suicidal ideation, unusual changes in behavior, worsening of seizure control. • May cause photosensitivity reaction; avoid exposure to sunlight, ultraviolet light.

lansoprazole

lan-**soe**-pra-zole
(Prevacid, Prevacid Solu-Tab, Prevacid 24HR)

Do not confuse lansoprazole with ARIPiprazole or dexlansoprazole, or Prevacid with Pravachol, PriLOSEC, or Prinivil.

FIXED-COMBINATION(S)

Prevacid NapraPac: lansoprazole/naproxen (an NSAID): 15 mg/375 mg, 15 mg/500 mg. **Prevpac:** Combination card containing amoxicillin 500 mg (4 capsules), lansoprazole 30 mg (2 capsules), clarithromycin 500 mg (2 tablets).

◆CLASSIFICATION

PHARMACOTHERAPEUTIC: Proton pump inhibitor. **CLINICAL:** Antiulcer agent.

USES

Short-term treatment (4 wks and less) of healing, symptomatic relief of active duodenal ulcer; short-term treatment (8 wks and less) for healing, symptomatic relief of erosive esophagitis. Long-term treatment of pathologic hypersecretory conditions, including Zollinger-Ellison syndrome. Short-term treatment (8 wks and less) of active benign gastric ulcer, *H. pylori*–associated duodenal ulcer (part of multidrug regimen), maintenance treatment for healed duodenal ulcer. Treatment of gastroesophageal reflux disease (GERD), NSAID-associated gastric ulcer. Reduce risk of NSAID-associated gastric ulcer in pts with history of gastric ulcer requiring NSAIDs. **OTC:** Relief of frequent heartburn (2 or more days/wk). **IV:** Short-term treatment of erosive esophagitis. **OFF-LABEL:** Stress ulcer prophylaxis in critically ill.

PRECAUTIONS

Contraindications: Hypersensitivity to lansoprazole, other proton pump inhibitors. Concomitant use with rilpivirine. **Cautions:** Hepatic impairment. May increase risk of hip, wrist, spine fractures; GI infections.

ACTION

Inhibits the (H^+, K^+)–ATPase enzyme system, blocking the final step in gastric acid secretion. **Therapeutic Effect:** Suppresses gastric acid secretion.

PHARMACOKINETICS

Rapid, complete absorption (food may decrease absorption) once drug has left stomach. Protein binding: 97%. Distributed primarily to gastric parietal cells. Metabolized in liver. Excreted in bile and urine. Not removed by hemodialysis. **Half-life:** 1.5 hrs (increased in hepatic impairment, elderly).

⌛ LIFESPAN CONSIDERATIONS

Pregnancy/Lactation: Unknown if distributed in breast milk. **Children:** Safety and efficacy not established. **Elderly:** No age-related precautions noted but doses greater than 30 mg not recommended.

INTERACTIONS

DRUG: May decrease concentration/effect of **atazanavir.** May increase effect of **warfarin.** May decrease effect of **clopidogrel, risedronate.** May decrease concentration/effects of **acalabrutinib, cefuroxime, erlotinib, neratinib, pazopanib. Strong CYP2C19 inducers (e.g., fluoxetine), strong CYP3A4 inducers (e.g., carBAMazepine, phenytoin, rifAMPin)** may decrease concentration/effect. **HERBAL: St. John's wort** may decrease concentration/effect. **FOOD: Food** may decrease absorption. **LAB VALUES:** May increase serum LDH, alkaline phosphatase, bilirubin, cholesterol, creatinine, ALT, AST, triglycerides, uric acid; Hgb, Hct. May produce abnormal albumin/globulin ratio, electrolyte balance, platelet, RBC, WBC count.

AVAILABILITY (Rx)

Tablets, Orally Disintegrating: 15 mg, 30 mg.

Capsules, Delayed-Release: 15 mg, 30 mg.

ADMINISTRATION/HANDLING

PO

• Best if taken before breakfast • Do not cut/crush delayed-release capsules. • If pt has difficulty swallowing capsules, open capsules, sprinkle granules on 1 tbsp of applesauce, give immediately. Do not crush or allow pt to chew granules.

PO (Solu-Tab)

• Place tablet on tongue; allow to dissolve, then swallow. • May give via oral syringe or nasogastric tube. • May dissolve in 4 mL (15 mg) or 10 mL (30 mg) water.

INDICATIONS/ROUTES/DOSAGE

Duodenal Ulcer

PO: ADULTS, ELDERLY: 15 mg/day, for up to 4 wks. **Maintenance:** 15 mg/day.

Erosive Esophagitis

PO: ADULTS, ELDERLY: 30 mg/day, for up to 8 wks. If healing does not occur within 8 wks may give for additional 8 wks. **Maintenance:** 15 mg/day. **CHILDREN 1–11 YRS, WEIGHING MORE THAN 30 KG:** 30 mg/day for up to 12 wks; **WEIGHING 30 KG OR LESS:** 15 mg/day for up to 12 wks.

Gastric Ulcer

PO: ADULTS: 30 mg/day for up to 8 wks.

NSAID Gastric Ulcer

PO: ADULTS, ELDERLY: Healing: 30 mg/day for up to 8 wks. **Prevention:** 15 mg/day for up to 12 wks.

Gastroesophageal Reflux Disease (GERD)

PO: ADULTS: 15 mg/day for up to 8 wks. **CHILDREN 12–17 YRS:** 30 mg/day up to 8 wks. **CHILDREN 1–11 YRS, WEIGHING MORE THAN 30 KG:** 30 mg/day for up to 8 wks; **WEIGHING 30 KG OR LESS:** 15 mg/day for up to 8 wks.

***H. Pylori* Infection**

PO: ADULTS, ELDERLY: (triple drug therapy including amoxicillin, clarithromycin) 30 mg q12h for 10–14 days or (with amoxicillin) 30 mg 3 times/day for 14 days.

Pathologic Hypersecretory Conditions (Including Zollinger-Ellison syndrome)

PO: ADULTS, ELDERLY: Initially, 60 mg/day. Individualize dosage according to pt needs and for as long as clinically indicated. Administer doses greater than 120 mg/day in divided doses.

Heartburn (OTC)

PO: ADULTS, ELDERLY: 15 mg once daily for 14 days. May repeat q4mos.

Dosage in Renal Impairment

No dose adjustment.

Dosage in Hepatic Impairment

Consider dose reduction in severe impairment.

SIDE EFFECTS

Occasional (3%–2%): Diarrhea, abdominal pain, rash, pruritus, altered appetite. **Rare (1%):** Nausea, headache.

ADVERSE EFFECTS/TOXIC REACTIONS

Bilirubinemia, eosinophilia, hyperlipidemia occur rarely. May increase risk of *C. difficile* infection. Chronic use may increase risk of osteoporosis, fractures.

NURSING CONSIDERATIONS

BASELINE ASSESSMENT

Assess for epigastric/abdominal pain, evidence of GI bleeding.

INTERVENTION/EVALUATION

Assess for therapeutic response (relief of GI symptoms). Question if diarrhea, abdominal pain, nausea occurs. Obtain *C. difficile* PCR test in pts with persistent diarrhea, fever, abdominal pain.

PATIENT/ FAMILY TEACHING

• Do not chew, crush delayed-release capsules. • For pts who have difficulty swallowing capsules, open capsules, sprinkle granules on 1 tbsp of applesauce, swallow immediately.

lapatinib

la-**pa**-tin-ib
(Tykerb)

BLACK BOX ALERT Hepatotoxicity (serum ALT or AST more than 3 times upper limit of normal [ULN] and total bilirubin more than 2 times ULN), possibly severe, has occurred.

Do not confuse lapatinib with dasatinib, erlotinib, or imatinib.

◆CLASSIFICATION

PHARMACOTHERAPEUTIC: Epidermal growth factor receptor (EGFR) inhibitor. Tyrosine kinase inhibitor. **CLINICAL:** Antineoplastic.

USES

Combination treatment with capecitabine for the treatment of human epidermal growth receptor type 2 (HER2)–overexpressing advanced or metastatic breast cancer in pts who have received prior therapy including an anthracycline, a taxane, and trastuzumab. Combination treatment with letrozole for treatment of postmenopausal women with *HER2*-overexpressing hormone receptor–positive metastatic breast cancer for whom hormonal therapy is indicated. **OFF-LABEL:** Treatment (in combination with trastuzumab) of *HER2*-overexpressing metastatic breast cancer that progressed on prior trastuzumab-containing therapy. Treatment of *HER2*-overexpressing metastatic breast cancer with brain metastasis.

PRECAUTIONS

Contraindications: Hypersensitivity to lapatinib. **Cautions:** Baseline cytopenias, conditions predisposing to infection (e.g., diabetes, renal failure, immunocompromised pts, open wounds), hepatic impairment, cardiac disease, HF; pts at risk for QT interval prolongation (congenital long QT syndrome, HF, medications that prolong QT interval, hypokalemia, hypomagnesemia); History of treatment with anthracyclines, chest wall irradiation. Avoid concurrent use with strong CYP3A4 inhibitors or inducers.

ACTION

Inhibitory action against kinases targeting intracellular components of epidermal growth factor receptor ErbB1 and a second receptor, human epidermal receptor (HER2 [ErbB2]). **Therapeutic Effect:** Inhibits tumor cell growth and metastasis.

PHARMACOKINETICS

Route	Onset	Peak	Duration
PO	30 min	4 hrs	—

Steady-state level reached within 6–7 days. Incomplete and variable oral absorption. Undergoes extensive metabolism. Protein binding: 99%. Minimally excreted in feces and plasma. **Half-life:** 24 hrs.

LIFESPAN CONSIDERATIONS

Pregnancy/Lactation: Avoid pregnancy; may cause fetal harm. Females and males with female partners of reproductive potential must use effective contraception during treatment and for at least 1 wk after discontinuation. Breastfeeding not recommended during treatment and for at least 1 wk after discontinuation. **Children:** Safety and efficacy not established. **Elderly:** No age-related precautions noted.

INTERACTIONS

DRUG: **QT interval–prolonging medications (e.g., amiodarone, azithromycin, ceritinib, haloperidol, moxifloxacin)** may increase risk of QT interval prolongation, cardiac arrhythmias. **CYP3A4 inhibitors (e.g., clarithromycin, ketoconazole, ritonavir), dexamethasone** may increase concentration/effect. **CYP3A4 inducers (e.g., carBAMazepine, phenytoin, rifAMPin)** may decrease concentration/effect. **HERBAL:** **St. John's wort** decreases concentration/effect. **FOOD:** **Grapefruit products** may increase concentration/effect. (potential for torsades, myelotoxicity). **LAB VALUES:** May increase serum ALT, AST, bilirubin. May decrease neutrophils, Hgb, platelets.

AVAILABILITY (Rx)

Tablets: 250 mg.

ADMINISTRATION/HANDLING

PO

- Do not break, crush, dissolve, or divide film-coated tablets. • Give at least 1 hr before or 1 hr after food. Take full dose at same time each day.

INDICATIONS/ROUTES/DOSAGE

Breast Cancer

PO: ADULTS, ELDERLY: With capecitabine: 1,250 mg (5 tablets) once daily. **With letrozole:** 1,500 mg once daily continuously with letrozole. Continue until disease progresses or unacceptable toxicity.

Dose Modification

Cardiac Toxicity

Discontinue with decreased left ventricular ejection fraction Grade 2 or higher, or in pts with an ejection fraction that drops to lower limit of normal. May be started at a reduced dose (1,000 mg/day) at a minimum of 2 wks when ejection fraction returns to normal and pt is asymptomatic.

Pulmonary Toxicity

Discontinue with symptoms indicative of interstitial lung disease or pneumonitis Grade 3 or higher.

Severe Hepatic Impairment

With capecitabine: 750 mg/day. **With letrozole:** 1,000 mg/day.

CYP3A4 Inhibitors/Inducers

Concomitant use of CYP3A4 inhibitors may require dose reduction of lapatinib (e.g., decrease to 500 mg/day with careful monitoring); CYP3A4 inducers may require dose increase of lapatinib (e.g., increase to 4,500 mg with capecitabine or 5,500 mg with letrozole).

L

Dosage in Renal Impairment

No dose adjustment.

Dosage in Hepatic Impairment

Mild to moderate impairment: No dose adjustment. **Severe impairment:** See dose modification.

SIDE EFFECTS

Common (65%–44%): Diarrhea, hand-foot syndrome (blistering/rash/peeling of skin on palms of hands, soles of feet), nausea. **Frequent (28%–26%):** Rash, vomiting. **Occasional (15%–10%):** Mucosal inflammation, stomatitis, extremity pain, back pain, dry skin, insomnia.

ADVERSE EFFECTS/TOXIC REACTIONS

May cause cardiac toxicity, decreased LVEF, ILD/pneumonitis. Life-threatening hepatotoxicity may occur days to several mos after initiation. Grade 3 or 4 diarrhea reported in less than 10% and less than 15% of pts, respectively. Concentration-dependent QT interval prolongation may occur. Life-threatening cutaneous reactions including erythema multiforme, Stevens-Johnson syndrome, toxic epidermal necrolysis were reported.

NURSING CONSIDERATIONS

BASELINE ASSESSMENT

Obtain CBC, BMP, LFT, ECG; pregnancy test in females of reproductive potential. Confirm compliance of effective contraception. Assess LVEF by echocardiogram. Confirm HER2-positive status. Question history pulmonary disease, hepatic/renal impairment, cardiac disease, HF. Screen for active infection. Assess hydration status. Receive full medication history and screen for interactions. Offer emotional support.

INTERVENTION/EVALUATION

Monitor CBC for myelosuppression; LFT for hepatotoxicity (abdominal pain, nausea, jaundice, weight loss); ECG for QT interval prolongation. Monitor serum electrolytes if severe diarrhea occurs. Diarrhea must be treated promptly. Consider ABG, radiologic test if ILD/pneumonitis (excessive cough, dyspnea, fever, hypoxia) is suspected. Consider treatment with corticosteroids if ILD/pneumonitis is confirmed. Assess LVEF by echocardiogram as clinically indicated. Monitor for infections (cough, fatigue, fever). If serious infection occurs, initiate appropriate antimicrobial therapy. Monitor daily pattern of bowel activity, stool consistency. Monitor for toxicities if discontinuation or dose reduction of strong CYP3A4 inhibitor is avoidable. Assess skin for cutaneous toxicities.

PATIENT/FAMILY TEACHING

• Treatment may depress your immune system response and reduce your ability to fight infection. Report symptoms of infection such as body aches, chills, cough, fatigue, fever. Avoid those with active infection. • Report symptoms of bone marrow depression (e.g., bruising, fatigue, fever, shortness of breath, weight loss; bleeding easily, bloody urine or stool). • Report symptoms of lung inflammation (excessive coughing, difficulty breathing, chest pain);

heart failure (e.g., chest pain, difficulty breathing, palpitations, swelling of extremities); liver problems (abdominal pain, bruising, clay-colored stool, amber- or dark-colored urine, yellowing of the skin or eyes). • Treatment may reduce the heart's ability to pump effectively; expect routine echocardiograms. • Use effective contraception to avoid pregnancy. Do not breastfeed. • Diarrhea is a common side effect. • Maintain proper hydration and nutrition. • There is a high risk of interactions with other medications. Do not take newly prescribed medications unless approved by prescriber who originally started treatment.

larotrectinib

lar-oh-**trek**-ti-nib
(Vitrakvi)
Do not confuse larotrectinib with alectinib, lapatinib, lenvatinib, or lorlatinib.

◆CLASSIFICATION

PHARMACOTHERAPEUTIC: Tropomyosin receptor kinase (TRK) inhibitor. Tyrosine kinase inhibitor. **CLINICAL:** Antineoplastic.

USES

Treatment of adult and pediatric pts with solid tumors that have a neurotrophic receptor tyrosine kinase *(NTRK)* gene fusion without a known acquired resistance mutation; are metastatic or where surgical resection is likely to result in severe morbidity; and have no satisfactory alternative treatment or that have progressed following treatment.

PRECAUTIONS

Contraindications: Hypersensitivity to larotrectinib. **Cautions:** Baseline anemia, neutropenia; hepatic impairment, active infection, conditions predisposing to infection (e.g., diabetes, renal failure, immunocompromised pts, open wounds); concomitant use of strong CYP3A inhibitors, strong CYP3A inducers.

ACTION

Inhibits activation of tropomyosin receptor kinase (TRK) proteins resulting from *NTRK* gene fusions, deletion of protein regulatory domain, or in cells with overexpression of TRK proteins. **Therapeutic Effect:** Inhibits tumor cell proliferation.

PHARMACOKINETICS

Widely distributed. Metabolized in liver. Protein binding: 70%. Excreted in feces (58%), urine (39%). **Half-life:** 2.9 hrs.

⧖ LIFESPAN CONSIDERATIONS

Pregnancy/Lactation: Avoid pregnancy; may cause fetal harm. Females and males with female partners of reproductive potential must use effective contraception during treatment and for at least 1 wk after discontinuation. Unknown if distributed in breast milk. Breastfeeding not recommended during treatment and for at least 1 wk after discontinuation. May impair fertility. **Children:** May have increased risk of increased weight, neutropenia. **Elderly:** Not specified; use caution.

INTERACTIONS

DRUG: Strong CYP3A4 inhibitors (e.g., clarithromycin, ketoconazole) may increase concentration/effect. **Strong CYP3A4 inducers (e.g., carBAMazepine, phenytoin, rifAMPin)** may decrease concentration/effect. **HERBAL: St. John's wort** may decrease concentration/effect. **FOOD: Grapefruit products** may increase concentration/effect. **LAB VALUES:** May increase serum alkaline phosphatase, ALT, AST. May decrease serum albumin; Hgb, neutrophils, RBCs.

AVAILABILITY (Rx)

Capsules: 25 mg, 100 mg. **Solution, Oral:** 20 mg/mL.

ADMINISTRATION/HANDLING

PO

• Give without regard to food. • Capsules/oral solution may be used interchangeably. • If vomiting occurs after administration, give next dose at regularly scheduled time. • Do not give a missed dose within 6 hrs of next dose. **Capsules:** Administer capsules whole with water; do not break, cut, or open. • Capsules cannot be chewed. **Solution, Oral:** Refrigerate glass bottle. Do not freeze. • Discard unused contents after 90 days of first opening bottle. • See manufacturer guidelines regarding preparation and administration of oral solution.

INDICATIONS/ROUTES/DOSAGE

L

Solid Tumors

PO: ADULTS, CHILDREN WITH BODY SURFACE AREA OF AT LEAST 1 m²: 100 mg twice daily. Continue until disease progression or unacceptable toxicity. **CHILDREN WITH BODY SURFACE AREA LESS THAN 1 m²:** 100 mg/m² twice daily. Continue until disease progression or unacceptable toxicity.

Dose Reduction Schedule

Dose Reduction for Adverse Reactions	Adults/Children With Body Surface Area of at Least 1 m²	Children With Body Surface Area Less Than 1 m²
First	75 mg twice daily	75 mg/m² twice daily
Second	50 mg twice daily	50 mg/m² twice daily
Third	100 mg once daily	25 mg/m² twice daily

Dose Modification

Based on Common Terminology Criteria for Adverse Events (CTCAE).

Any Grade 3 or 4 Adverse Reaction

Note (includes hepatotoxicity and neurotoxicity): Withhold treatment until resolved or improved to Grade 1, then resume at reduced dose level. If not resolved within 4 wks, permanently discontinue.

Concomitant Use of Strong CYP3A4 Inhibitor

If strong CYP3A4 inhibitor cannot be discontinued, reduce larotrectinib dose by 50%. If strong CYP3A inhibitor is discontinued for 3–5 half-lives, resume larotrectinib dose prior to use of strong CYP3A4 inhibitor.

Concomitant Use of Strong CYP3A4 Inducer

If strong CYP3A4 inducer cannot be discontinued, double the larotrectinib dose. If strong CYP3A inducer is discontinued for 3–5 half-lives, resume larotrectinib dose prior to use of strong CYP3A4 inducer.

Dosage in Renal Impairment

Mild to severe impairment: No dose adjustment.

Dosage in Hepatic Impairment

Mild impairment: No dose adjustment. **Moderate to severe impairment:** Reduce starting dose by 50%.

SIDE EFFECTS

Frequent (37%–15%): Fatigue, nausea, dizziness, cough, vomiting, constipation, diarrhea, pyrexia, dyspnea, increased weight, peripheral edema. **Occasional (14%–11%):** Arthralgia, myalgia, muscular weakness, headache, abdominal pain, decreased appetite, back pain, extremity pain, nasal congestion, hypertension.

ADVERSE EFFECTS/TOXIC REACTIONS

Anemia, neutropenia is an expected response to therapy. Neurotoxic events including delirium, dysarthria, dizziness, gait disturbance, memory impairment, paresthesia, tremor occurred in 53% of pts. Grade 4 encephalopathy reported in less than 1% of pts. Hepatotoxicity with transaminase elevations of any grade reported in 45%. Grade 3 hepatotoxicity reported in 6% of pts. Falls reported in 10% of pts.

NURSING CONSIDERATIONS

BASELINE ASSESSMENT

Obtain CBC, LFT; pregnancy test in females of reproductive potential. Confirm presence of NTRK gene fusion in tumor specimen. Screen for active infection. Confirm compliance of effective contraception. Question history of hepatic impairment. Receive full medication history and screen for interactions. Initiate fall precautions. Offer emotional support.

INTERVENTION/EVALUATION

Monitor CBC for anemia, neutropenia periodically; LFT for hepatotoxicity (bruising, hematuria, jaundice, right upper abdominal pain, nausea, vomiting, weight loss) q2wks for 4 wks, then monthly thereafter (or as clinically indicated). Monitor for neurotoxicities. If concomitant use of strong CYP3A inhibitor or strong CYP3A inducer is unavoidable, monitor for drug toxicities. Diligently screen for infections.

PATIENT/FAMILY TEACHING

• Treatment may depress your immune system response and reduce your ability to fight infection. Report symptoms of infection such as body aches, chills, cough, fatigue, fever. Avoid those with active infection. • Nervous system changes including altered memory, confusion, delirium, difficulty speaking, gait disturbance, numbness, tremors may occur. Avoid tasks that require alertness, motor skills if neurologic effects are occurring. • Use effective contraception to avoid pregnancy. Do not breastfeed. • Report liver problems (abdominal pain, bruising, clay-colored stool, amber- or dark-colored urine, yellowing of the skin or eyes). • There is a high risk of interactions with other medications. Do not take newly prescribed medications unless approved by prescriber who originally started treatment. • Avoid grapefruit products, herbal supplements (esp. St. John's wort).

ledipasvir/sofosbuvir

le-**dip**-as-vir/soe-**fos**-bue-vir (Harvoni)

■ **BLACK BOX ALERT** ■ Test all pts for hepatitis B virus (HBV) infection prior to initiation. HBV reactivation was reported in HCV/HBV coinfected pts who were undergoing or had completed treatment with HCV direct-acting antivirals and were not receiving HBV antiviral therapy. HBV reactivation may cause fulminant hepatitis, hepatic failure, and death.

Do not confuse ledipasvir with daclatasvir, elbasvir, or ombitasvir, or sofosbuvir with dasabuvir.

◆ CLASSIFICATION

PHARMACOTHERAPEUTIC: Combination nucleotide analog NS5A inhibitor and nucleotide analog NS5B polymerase inhibitor. **CLINICAL:** Antihepaciviral.

USES

Treatment of chronic hepatitis C virus (HCV) in adults and children 12 yrs and older or weighing at least 35 kg with genotype 1, 4, 5, or 6 infection without cirrhosis or with compensated cirrhosis; genotype 1 infection in adults with decompensated cirrhosis, in combination with ribavirin; genotype 1 or 4 infection in adults who are liver transplant recipients without cirrhosis or with compensated cirrhosis, in combination with ribavirin.

PRECAUTIONS

Note: If used with ribavirin, the Contraindications and Cautions for the use of ribavirin also apply.
Contraindications: Hypersensitivity to ledipasvir, sofosbuvir. **Cautions:** Advanced hepatic disease, HIV infection, hepatitis B virus infection. Concomitant use of amiodarone (with or without beta blockers) in pts with underlying cardiac disease. Concomitant use of P-glycoprotein (P-gp) inducers not recommended.

L

ACTION

Ledipasvir inhibits HCV NS5A protein, essential for viral replication. Sofosbuvir is converted to its active form and inhibits NS5B RNA-dependent RNA polymerase, also essential for viral replication. **Therapeutic Effect:** Inhibits viral replication of HCV.

PHARMACOKINETICS

Widely absorbed. Ledipasvir is metabolized by oxidative processes. Sofosbuvir is metabolized in liver. Protein binding: 99.8% (ledipasvir), 61%–65% (sofosbuvir). Peak plasma concentration: 4–4.5 hrs (ledipasvir), 0.8–1 hr (sofosbuvir). Ledipasvir is excreted in feces (87%) and urine (1%). Sofosbuvir is excreted in urine (80%), feces (14%). **Half-life:** 47 hrs (ledipasvir), 0.4 hr (sofosbuvir).

L

⌛ LIFESPAN CONSIDERATIONS

Pregnancy/Lactation: Unknown if ledipasvir or sofosbuvir is distributed in breast milk. When administered with ribavirin, therapy is contraindicated in pregnant women and in men whose female partners are pregnant. **Children:** Safety and efficacy not established in pts younger than 12 yrs of age or weight less than 35 kg. **Elderly:** No age-related precautions noted.

INTERACTIONS

DRUG: May enhance bradycardic effect of **amiodarone**. May increase concentration of **rosuvastatin. Aluminum- or magnesium-containing antacids, H_2-receptor antagonists (e.g., famotidine), proton pump inhibitors (e.g., omeprazole), anticonvulsants (e.g., carBAMazepine), antimycobacterials (e.g., rifAMPin)** may decrease concentration/effects. **HERBAL:** None significant. **FOOD:** None known. **LAB VALUES:** May increase serum bilirubin.

AVAILABILITY (Rx)

Tablets, Fixed-Dose Combination: 90 mg (ledipasvir)/400 mg (sofosbuvir).

ADMINISTRATION/HANDLING

PO

• Give without regard to food.

INDICATIONS/ROUTES/DOSAGE

Hepatitis C Virus Infection

PO: ADULTS, ELDERLY, CHILDREN 12 YRS OF AGE AND OLDER, WEIGHING 35 KG OR MORE: 1 tablet (ledipasvir/sofosbuvir) once daily. See manufacturer guidelines for treatment with ribavirin.

Treatment Regimen and Duration for Adults

Genotype 1

Treatment-naïve without cirrhosis or with compensated cirrhosis (Child-Pugh A): Ledipasvir/sofosbuvir for 12 wks. Treatment for 8 wks may be considered in treatment-naïve genotype 1 pts without cirrhosis who have HCV-RNA level less than 6 million international units/mL prior to initiation. **Treatment-experienced without cirrhosis:** Ledipasvir/sofosbuvir for 12 wks. **Treatment-experienced with compensated cirrhosis (Child-Pugh A):** Ledipasvir/sofosbuvir for 24 wks. Ledipasvir/sofosbuvir plus ribavirin for 12 wks may be considered in treatment-experienced genotype 1 pts with cirrhosis who are eligible for ribavirin. **Treatment-naïve and treatment-experienced with decompensated cirrhosis (Child-Pugh B or C):** Ledipasvir/sofosbuvir plus ribavirin for 12 wks.

Genotype 1 or 4

Treatment-naïve and treatment-experienced liver transplant recipients without cirrhosis or with compensated cirrhosis (Child-Pugh A): Ledipasvir/sofosbuvir plus ribavirin for 12 wks.

Treatment Regimen and Duration for Children

Genotype 1

Treatment-naïve without cirrhosis or with compensated cirrhosis (Child-Pugh A): Ledipasvir/sofosbuvir for 12 wks. **Treatment-experienced without cirrhosis:** Ledipasvir/sofosbuvir for 12 wks. **Treatment-experienced with compensated cirrhosis (Child-Pugh A):** Ledipasvir/sofosbuvir for 24 wks.

Genotype 4, 5, or 6

Treatment-naïve and treatment-experienced without cirrhosis or with compensated cirrhosis (Child-Pugh A): Ledipasvir/sofosbuvir for 12 wks.

Dosage in Renal Impairment

Mild to moderate impairment: No dose adjustment. **Severe impairment:** Not specified; use caution.

Dosage in Hepatic Impairment

No dose adjustment.

SIDE EFFECTS

Occasional (16%–4%): Fatigue, headache, nausea, diarrhea. **Rare (3%):** Insomnia. **Ribavirin: Frequent (31%–29%):** Asthenia, headache. **Occasional (18%–5%):** Fatigue, myalgia, irritability, dizziness. **Rare (3%):** Dyspnea.

ADVERSE EFFECTS/TOXIC REACTIONS

HBV reactivation was reported in pts co-infected with HBV/HCV; may result in fulminant hepatitis, hepatic failure, death. Cardiac arrest, symptomatic bradycardia, pacemaker implantation was reported in pts taking concomitant amiodarone. Bradycardia usually occurred within hrs to days, but may occur up to 2 wks after initiation. Pts with underlying cardiac disease, advanced hepatic disease, or pts taking concomitant beta blockers are at an increased risk for bradycardia when used concomitantly with amiodarone. Psychiatric disorders including depression may occur.

NURSING CONSIDERATIONS

BASELINE ASSESSMENT

Obtain LFT, HCV-RNA level; pregnancy test in females of reproductive potential; CBC for pts treated with ribavirin. Confirm HCV genotype. Test all pts for HBV infection prior to initiation. Receive full medication history and screen for contraindications/interactions, esp. concomitant use of amiodarone. Question for history of chronic anemia, HBV infection, HIV infection, liver transplantation.

INTERVENTION/EVALUATION

Periodically monitor LFT, HCV-RNA level for treatment effectiveness. Closely monitor for exacerbation of hepatitis or HBV reactivation. If unable to discontinue amiodarone, consider inpatient cardiac monitoring for at least 48 hrs, followed by outpatient or self-monitoring of heart rate for at least 2 wks after initiation. Cardiac monitoring is also recommended in pts who discontinue amiodarone just prior to initiation. In females of reproductive potential who are taking concomitant ribavirin, reinforce birth control compliance and obtain monthly pregnancy tests. Monitor for new-onset or worsening of depression

PATIENT/FAMILY TEACHING

• Pts who take amiodarone (an antiarrhythmic) during therapy may require inpatient and outpatient cardiac monitoring (and in some cases pacemaker implantation) due to an increased risk of slow heart rate or cardiac arrest. If amiodarone therapy cannot be withheld or stopped, immediately report symptoms of slow heart rate such as chest pain, confusion, dizziness, fainting, light-headedness, memory problems, palpitations, weakness. • Treatment may be used in combination with ribavirin (inform pt of contraindications/adverse effects of ribavirin therapy). If therapy includes treatment with ribavirin, use effective contraception to avoid pregnancy. Do not breastfeed. • There is a high risk of interactions with other medications. Do not take newly prescribed medications unless approved by prescriber who originally started treatment. • Do not take herbal products. • Avoid alcohol. • Report signs of depression.

L

leflunomide

lee-**floo**-noe-myde
(Apo-Leflunomide ✦, Arava)

BLACK BOX ALERT Do not use during pregnancy. Women of childbearing potential must be counseled regarding fetal risk, use of reliable contraceptives confirmed, possibility of pregnancy excluded. Severe hepatic injury may occur.

◆CLASSIFICATION

PHARMACOTHERAPEUTIC: Disease-modifying agent. **CLINICAL:** Anti-rheumatic.

USES

Treatment of active rheumatoid arthritis (RA). Improve physical function in pts with rheumatoid arthritis. **OFF-LABEL:** Treatment of cytomegalovirus (CMV) disease. Prevention of acute/chronic rejection in recipients of solid organ transplants.

PRECAUTIONS

Contraindications: Hypersensitivity to leflunomide. Pregnancy or plans for pregnancy. Severe hepatic impairment. Concomitant use with teriflunomide. **Cautions:** Hepatic/renal impairment, hepatitis B or C virus infection, pts with immunodeficiency or bone marrow dysplasias, breast-feeding mothers, conditions predisposing to infection (e.g., diabetes, renal failure, immunocompromised pts, open wounds), latent TB, significant hematologic abnormalities, diabetes, concomitant use of neurotoxic medications, elderly pts.

ACTION

Inhibits pyrimidine synthesis, resulting in antiproliferative and anti-inflammatory effects. **Therapeutic Effect:** Reduces signs/symptoms of RA, retards structural damage.

PHARMACOKINETICS

Widely distributed. Metabolized in liver. Protein binding: greater than 99%. Excreted in feces (68%), urine (23%). Not removed by hemodialysis. **Half-life:** 16 days.

⌛ LIFESPAN CONSIDERATIONS

Pregnancy/Lactation: Can cause fetal harm. Contraindicated in pregnancy. Unknown if distributed in breast milk. Breastfeeding not recommended. **Children:** Safety and efficacy not established. **Elderly:** No age-related precautions noted.

INTERACTIONS

DRUG: **RifAMPin** may increase concentration/effect. **Hepatotoxic medications (e.g., acetaminophen, ketoconazole, simvastatin)** may increase risk of side effects, hepatotoxicity. May decrease the therapeutic effect of **BCG (intravesical), nivolumab, vaccines (live).** May increase adverse effects of **natalizumab, vaccines (live).** **HERBAL:** **Echinacea** may decrease effects. **FOOD:** None known. **LAB VALUES:** May increase serum ALT, AST, alkaline phosphatase, bilirubin.

AVAILABILITY (Rx)

Tablets: 10 mg, 20 mg.

ADMINISTRATION/HANDLING

PO

- Give without regard to food.

INDICATIONS/ROUTES/DOSAGE

Rheumatoid Arthritis (RA)

PO: ADULTS, ELDERLY: Initially, 100 mg/day for 3 days, then 10–20 mg/day. (Loading dose may be omitted in pts at increased risk of hepatic or hematologic toxicity.)

Dosage in Renal Impairment

No dose adjustment.

Dosage in Hepatic Impairment

ALT 2–3 times upper limit of normal (ULN): Not recommended. **Persistent ALT level greater than 3 times ULN:** Discontinue and initiate accelerated drug elimination. Cholestyramine 8 g 3 times/day for 11 days or activated charcoal 50 g q12h for 11 days.

SIDE EFFECTS

Frequent (20%–10%): Diarrhea, respiratory tract infection, alopecia, rash, nausea.

ADVERSE EFFECTS/TOXIC REACTIONS

Pancytopenia, agranulocytosis, leukopenia, neutropenia, thrombocytopenia may occur, esp. in pts taking concomitant methotrexate, other immunosuppresants. Severe hepatic injury, fatal hepatic failure, acute hepatic necrosis, colitis, pancreatitis may occur. Severe infections including aspergillosis, *Pneumocystis jiroveci* pneumonia, tuberculosis, sepsis were reported. Cutaneous skin reactions including Stevens-Johnson syndrome, toxic epidermal necrolysis, drug reaction with eosinophilia and systemic symptoms (DRESS), vasculitis, cutaneous lupus erythematosus, psoriasis were reported. May increase risk of malignancies, lymphoproliferative disorders, peripheral neuropathy. Other reactions may include interstitial lung disease (ILD), pneumonitis, thrombophlebitis.

NURSING CONSIDERATIONS

BASELINE ASSESSMENT

Obtain CBC, LFT; pregnancy test in females of reproductive potential. Confirm compliance of effective contraception. Assess onset, location, duration of pain and inflammation. Inspect appearance of affected joints for immobility, deformities. Evaluate for active TB and test for latent infection prior to and during treatment. Induration of 5 mm or greater with purified protein derivative (PPD) is considered a positive result when assessing for latent TB. Consider treatment with antimycobacterial therapy in pts with latent TB. Question history pulmonary disease, hepatic impairment, chronic infections (hepatitis B or C virus, HIV, latent TB. Screen for active infection. Receive full medication history and screen for interactions.

INTERVENTION/EVALUATION

Monitor CBC, LFT periodically. Monitor for TB regardless of baseline PPD. Monitor for hepatotoxicity (abdominal pain, jaundice, nausea, vomiting, weight loss). Consider ABG, radiologic test if ILD/pneumonitis (excessive cough, dyspnea, fever, hypoxia) is suspected. Consider treatment with corticosteroids if ILD/pneumonitis is confirmed. Monitor for infections (cough, fatigue, fever). Assess skin for cutaneous toxicities. Assess for therapeutic response: relief of pain, stiffness, swelling; increased joint mobility; reduced joint tenderness; improved grip strength.

PATIENT/FAMILY TEACHING

• Treatment may depress your immune system response and reduce your ability to fight infection. Report symptoms of infection such as body aches, chills, cough, fatigue, fever. Avoid those with active infection. • Expect routine tuberculosis screening. Report any travel plans to possible endemic areas. • Do not receive live vaccines. • Report liver problems (bruising, confusion, dark- or amber-colored urine, right upper abdominal pain, or yellowing of the skin or eyes), lung inflammation (excessive coughing, difficulty breathing, chest pain). • Treatment may cause reactivation of chronic viral infections, new cancers. • Use effective contraception to avoid pregnancy.

lenalidomide

len-a-**lid**-o-myde
(Revlimid)

BLACK BOX ALERT Analogue to thalidomide. High potential for significant birth defects. Hematologic toxicity (thrombocytopenia, neutropenia) occurs in 80% of pts. Greatly increases risk for DVT, pulmonary embolism in multiple myeloma pts.

Do not confuse lenalidomide with thalidomide.

◆CLASSIFICATION

PHARMACOTHERAPEUTIC: Angiogenesis inhibitor. **CLINICAL:** Antineoplastic.

USES

Treatment of low- to intermediate-risk myelodysplastic syndrome (MDS) in pts with deletion 5q cytogenetic abnormality with transfusion-dependent anemia. Treatment of multiple myeloma (in combination with dexamethasone). Treatment of pts with mantle cell lymphoma that has relapsed or progressed after 2 prior therapies (one of which included bortezomib). Maintenance treatment for multiple myeloma (following autologous stem cell transplant). Treatment of previously treated follicular lymphoma (in combination with rITUXimab). Treatment of previously treated marginal zone lymphoma (in combination with riTUXimab). **OFF-LABEL:** Systemic amyloidosis, lower-risk myelodysplastic syndrome, non-Hodgkin's lymphoma. Relapsed or refractory chronic lymphocytic leukemia (CLL).

PRECAUTIONS

Contraindications: Hypersensitivity to lenalidomide. Pregnancy, women capable of becoming pregnant. **Cautions:** Renal/hepatic impairment, conditions predisposing to infection (e.g., diabetes, renal failure, immunocompromised pts, open wounds). History of arterial thromboembolic events, hypertension, hyperlipidemia. Avoid use in pts with glucose intolerance, lactase deficiency.

ACTION

Inhibits secretion of pro-inflammatory cytokines, increases secretion of anti-inflammatory cytokines. Enhances cell-mediated immunity by stimulation of T cells. **Therapeutic Effect:** Inhibits myeloma cell growth; induces cell cycle arrest and cell death.

PHARMACOKINETICS

Well absorbed following PO administration. Protein binding: 30%. Excreted in urine. **Half-life:** 3 hrs (increased in renal impairment).

LIFESPAN CONSIDERATIONS

Pregnancy/Lactation: Contraindicated in women who are or may become pregnant, who are not using two reliable forms of contraception, or who are not abstinent. Can cause severe birth defects, fetal death. Unknown if distributed in breast milk; breastfeeding not recommended. **Children:** Safety and efficacy not established. **Elderly:** Age-related renal impairment may require caution in dosage selection. Risk of toxic reactions greater in those with renal insufficiency.

INTERACTIONS

DRUG: May increase toxic effects of **abatacept, anakinra, bisphosphonate derivatives, canakinumab, leflunomide, natalizumab, nivolumab, rilonacept, tofacitinib, vedolizumab**. May increase immunosuppressive effects of **certolizumab, fingolimod, ocrelizumab**. **Denosumab, dipyrone, pimecrolimus** may increase risk of toxicity. May decrease therapeutic effect of **nivolumab. Dexamethasone, erythropoiesis-stimulating agents, estrogens** may increase risk of thrombosis. **Ocrelizumab, roflumilast, tocilizumab** may increase immunosuppressive effects. May increase concentration effect of **digoxin**. May increase adverse effects/decrease therapeutic of **vaccines (live). HERBAL: Echinacea** may decrease therapeutic effect. **FOOD:** None known. **LAB VALUES:** May decrease WBC count, Hgb, Hct platelets, troponin I, serum creatinine, sodium, T_3, T_4. May decrease serum bilirubin, glucose, potassium, magnesium.

AVAILABILITY (Rx)

Capsules: 2.5 mg, 5 mg, 10 mg, 15 mg, 20 mg, 25 mg.

ADMINISTRATION/HANDLING

• Store at room temperature. • Do not break, crush, dissolve, or divide capsules. • Swallow whole with water.

INDICATIONS/ROUTES/DOSAGE

Myelodysplastic Syndrome

PO: ADULTS, ELDERLY: 10 mg once daily. Continue until disease progression or unacceptable toxicity.

Dosage Adjustments for Myelodysplastic Syndrome

Platelets

Thrombocytopenia within 4 wks with 10 mg/day: Baseline platelets 100,000 cells/mm^3 or greater: If platelets less than 50,000 cells/mm^3, hold treatment. Resume at 5 mg/day when platelets return to 50,000 cells/mm^3 or greater. **Baseline platelets less than 100,000 cells/mm^3:** If platelets fall to 50% of baseline, hold treatment. Resume at 5 mg/day if baseline is 60,000 cells/mm^3 or greater and platelets return to 50,000 cells/mm^3 or greater. Resume at 5 mg/day if baseline is less than 60,000 cells/mm^3 and platelets return to 30,000 cells/mm^3 or greater.

Thrombocytopenia after 4 wks with 10 mg/day: If platelets less than 30,000 cells/mm^3 OR less than 50,000 cells/mm^3 with platelet transfusion, hold treatment. Resume at 5 mg/day when platelets return to 30,000 cells/mm^3 or greater.

Thrombocytopenia developing with 5 mg/day: If platelets less than 30,000 cells/mm^3 OR less than 50,000 cells/mm^3 with platelet transfusion, hold treatment. Resume at 5 mg every other day when platelets return to 30,000 cells/mm^3 or greater.

Neutrophils

Neutropenia within 4 wks with 10 mg/day: Baseline absolute neutrophil count (ANC) 1,000/mcl or greater: If ANC less than 750 cells/mm^3, hold treatment. Resume at 5 mg/day when ANC 1,000 cells/mm^3 or greater. **Baseline ANC less than 1,000 cells/mm^3:** If ANC less than 500 cells/mm^3, hold treatment. Resume at 5 mg/day when ANC 500 cells/mm^3 or greater.

Neutropenia after 4 wks with 10 mg/day: If ANC less than 500 cells/mm^3 for 7 days or longer or associated with fever, hold treatment. Resume at 5 mg/day when ANC 500 cells/mm^3 or greater.

Neutropenia developing with 5 mg/day: If ANC less than 500 cells/mm^3 for 7 days or longer or associated with fever, hold treatment. Resume at 5 mg every other day when ANC 500 cells/mm^3 or greater.

Follicular Lymphoma, Marginal Zone Lymphoma

PO: ADULTS, ELDERLY: 20 mg once daily for 21 days of 28-day cycle (in combination with riTUXimab) for up to 12 cycles.

Mantle Cell Lymphoma

PO: ADULTS, ELDERLY: 25 mg once daily on days 1–21 of repeated 28-day cycle. Continue until disease progression or unacceptable toxicity.

Multiple Myeloma

PO: ADULTS, ELDERLY: 25 mg/day on days 1–21 of repeated 28-day cycle (in combination with dexamethasone). Continue until disease progression or unacceptable toxicity. If eligible for transplant, HSCT mobilization should occur within 4 cycles of lenalidomide-containing therapy.

Multiple Myeloma Following Auto-HSCT

PO: ADULTS, ELDERLY: 10 mg once daily continuously on days 1–28 of repeated 28-day cycle. If tolerated, may increase to 15 mg once daily after 3 cycles.

Dosage Adjustments for Multiple Myeloma

Thrombocytopenia: If platelets fall to less than 30,000 cells/mm^3, hold treatment, monitor CBC. Resume at 15 mg/day when platelets 30,000 cells/mm^3 or greater. For each subsequent fall to less than 30,000 cells/mm^3, hold treatment and resume at 5 mg/day less than previous dose when platelets return to 30,000 cells/mm^3 or greater. Do not dose to less than 5 mg/day.

Neutropenia: If neutrophils fall to less than 1,000 cells/mm^3, hold treatment, add G-CSF, follow CBC wkly. Resume at 25 mg/day when neutrophils return to 1,000 cells/mm^3 and neutropenia is the only toxicity. Resume at 15 mg/day if

L

other toxicity is present. For each subsequent fall to less than 1,000 cells/mm^3, hold treatment and resume at 5 mg/day less than previous dose when neutrophils return to 1,000 cells/mm^3 or greater. Do not dose to less than 5 mg/day.

Dosage in Renal Impairment	Creatinine Clearance 30–59 mL/min	Creatinine Clearance Less Than 30 mL/min (Non-dialysis dependent)	Creatinine Clearance Less Than 30 mL/min (Dialysis dependent)
Myelodysplastic syndrome	5 mg once daily	2.5 mg once daily	2.5 mg once daily (give after dialysis)
Multiple myeloma	10 mg once daily	15 mg q48h	5 mg once daily (give after dialysis)

Dosage in Hepatic Impairment
No dose adjustment.

SIDE EFFECTS

Frequent (49%–31%): Diarrhea, pruritus, rash, fatigue. **Occasional (24%–12%):** Constipation, nausea, arthralgia, fever, back pain, peripheral edema, cough, dizziness, headache, muscle cramps, epistaxis, asthenia, dry skin, abdominal pain. **Rare (10%–5%):** Extremity pain, vomiting, generalized edema, anorexia, insomnia, night sweats, myalgia, dry mouth, ecchymosis, rigors, depression, dysgeusia, palpitations.

ADVERSE EFFECTS/TOXIC REACTIONS

Significant increased risk of deep vein thrombosis (DVT), pulmonary embolism. Thrombocytopenia occurs in 62% of pts, neutropenia in 59% of pts, and anemia in 12% of pts. Upper respiratory infection (nasopharyngitis, pneumonia, sinusitis, bronchitis, rhinitis), UTI occur occasionally. Cellulitis, peripheral neuropathy, hypertension, hypothyroidism occur in approximately 6% of pts.

NURSING CONSIDERATIONS

BASELINE ASSESSMENT

Obtain CBC. Due to high potential for human birth defects/fetal death, female pts must avoid pregnancy 4 wks before therapy, during therapy, during dose interruptions, and 4 wks following therapy. Two reliable forms of contraception must be used even if pt has history of infertility unless it is due to hysterectomy or menopause that has occurred for at least 24 consecutive mos. Confirm two negative pregnancy tests before therapy initiation. Screen for risk of arterial, venous thrombosis. Offer emotional support.

INTERVENTION/EVALUATION

Monitor CBC, BMP, serum magnesium as appropriate. Perform pregnancy tests on women of childbearing potential: wkly during the first 4 wks, then at 4-wk intervals in pts with regular menstrual cycles or q2wks in pts with irregular menstrual cycles. Monitor for hematologic toxicity; obtain CBC wkly during first 8 wks of therapy and at least monthly thereafter. Observe for symptoms of thromboembolism (shortness of breath, chest pain, extremity pain, swelling, stroke-like symptoms).

PATIENT/FAMILY TEACHING

• Two reliable forms of birth control must be used at least 4 wks before, during, and for 4 wks following therapy. • A pregnancy test must be performed within 10–14 days and 24 hrs before therapy begins. • Males must always use a latex or synthetic condom during any sexual contact with females of childbearing potential even if they have undergone a successful vasectomy. • Avoid crowds; avoid those with active infection. • Treatment may cause blood clots in the arms, legs, or lungs; report arm or leg pain/swelling, difficulty breathing, chest pain.

lenvatinib

len-va-ti-nib
(Lenvima)
Do not confuse lenvatinib with dasatinib, ibrutinib, imatinib.

◆CLASSIFICATION

PHARMACOTHERAPEUTIC: Vascular endothelial growth factor (VEGF) inhibitor. Tyrosine kinase inhibitor. **CLINICAL:** Antineoplastic.

USES

Treatment of locally recurrent or metastatic, progressive, radioactive iodine–refractory differentiated thyroid cancer. Treatment of advanced renal cell carcinoma (RCC) in combination with everolimus after one course of another antineoplastic. First-line treatment of unresectable hepatocellular carcinoma (HCC). Treatment of advanced endometrial carcinoma (in combination with pembrolizumab).

PRECAUTIONS

Contraindications: Hypersensitivity to lenvatinib. **Cautions:** Electrolyte imbalance (hypokalemia, hypomagnesemia), hepatic/renal impairment, conditions predisposing to infection (e.g., diabetes, renal failure, immunocompromised pts, open wounds). History of cardiac dysfunction (HF, pulmonary edema, right or left ventricular dysfunction), GI perforation/hemorrhage, hypertension, long QT interval syndrome, medications that prolong QT interval, thromboembolic events (e.g., CVA, DVT), pituitary/thyroid disease.

ACTION

Inhibits tyrosine kinase receptor activity of vascular endothelial growth factor (VEGF) receptors. Inhibits tumor angiogenesis, growth, progression. **Therapeutic Effect:** Decreases tumor cell growth, slows cancer progression.

PHARMACOKINETICS

Readily absorbed. Metabolized in liver. Protein binding: 98%–99%. Peak plasma concentration: 1–4 hrs. Excreted in feces (64%), urine (25%). Not removed by dialysis. **Half-life:** 28 hrs.

⌛ LIFESPAN CONSIDERATIONS

Pregnancy/Lactation: Avoid pregnancy; may cause fetal harm. Females of reproductive potential must use effective contraception during treatment for at least 2 wks after discontinuation. Potentially distributed in breast milk. May reduce fertility in both female and male pts. **Children:** Safety and efficacy not established. **Elderly:** No age-related precautions noted.

INTERACTIONS

DRUG: **Strong CYP3A4 inhibitors (e.g., clarithromycin, ketoconazole, ritonavir)** may increase concentration/effect. May increase QT-prolonging effect of **amiodarone, citalopram, clarithromycin, moxifloxacin, nilotinib, quetiapine, ribociclib, thioridazine.** **HERBAL:** None significant. **FOOD:** None known. **LAB VALUES:** May increase serum alkaline phosphatase, ALT/AST, amylase, bilirubin, cholesterol, creatinine, lipase. May decrease serum albumin, glucose, magnesium; platelets. May increase or decrease serum calcium, potassium.

AVAILABILITY (Rx)

Capsules: 4 mg, 10 mg.

ADMINISTRATION/HANDLING

PO

• Give without regard to food. • Do not cut, crush, divide, or open capsules. • Should be swallowed whole. May be dissolved with 15 mL water or apple juice by first adding whole capsule to liquid; leave for 10 min, stir for 3 min, then administer. Then add 15 mL to glass, swirl, swallow additional liquid.

L

INDICATIONS/ROUTES/DOSAGE

Thyroid Cancer

PO: ADULTS, ELDERLY: 24 mg once daily. Continue until disease progression or unacceptable toxicity.

RCC

PO: ADULTS, ELDERLY: 18 mg once daily (in combination with everolimus). Continue until disease progression or unacceptable toxicity.

HCC

PO: ADULTS, ELDERLY: (60 KG OR GREATER): 12 mg once daily. **(LESS THAN 60 KG):** 8 mg once daily. Continue until disease progression or unacceptable toxicity.

Endometrial Carcinoma (Advanced)

PO: ADULTS, ELDERLY: 20 mg once daily (in combination with pembrolizumab). Continue until disease progression or unacceptable toxicity.

Dose Modification

Based on Common Terminology Criteria for Adverse Events (CTCAE).

Adverse Reaction	Modification	Adjusted Dose (Thyroid cancer)
First occurrence	Interrupt until resolved to Grade 0 or 1 or baseline	20 mg once daily
Second occurrence	Interrupt until resolved to Grade 0 or 1 or baseline	14 mg once daily
Third occurrence	Interrupt until resolved to Grade 0 or 1 or baseline	10 mg once daily

Adjusted dose for RCC is lower. 14 mg for first occurrence, 10 mg for second occurrence, 8 mg for third occurrence.

Arterial Thrombotic Event

Discontinue treatment.

Cardiac Dysfunction/Hemorrhagic Event

PO: ADULTS, ELDERLY: Interrupt treatment for Grade 3 event until improved to Grade 0 to 1 or baseline. Either resume at reduced dose or discontinue (depending on the severity and persistence). Discontinue for Grade 4 event.

GI Perforation/Fistula Formation

Discontinue treatment.

Hypertension

PO: ADULTS, ELDERLY: Interrupt treatment for Grade 3 hypertension that persists despite optimal antihypertensive therapy. Resume at reduced dose when hypertension is controlled at less than or equal to Grade 2. Discontinue for life-threatening hypertension.

Proteinuria

PO: ADULTS, ELDERLY: Interrupt treatment for greater than or equal to 2 g proteinuria/24 hrs. Resume at reduced dose when proteinuria less than 2 g/24 hrs. Discontinue if nephrotic syndrome occurs.

QT Prolongation

PO: ADULTS, ELDERLY: Interrupt treatment for Grade 3 or greater. Resume at reduced dose when QT prolongation resolved to Grade 0 or 1 or baseline.

Renal Failure/Impairment or Hepatotoxicity

PO: ADULTS, ELDERLY: Interrupt treatment for Grade 3 or 4 renal failure/impairment or hepatotoxicity until resolved to Grade 0 or 1 or baseline. Either resume at reduced dose or discontinue (depending on the severity and persistence). Discontinue if hepatic failure occurs.

Reversible Posterior Leukoencephalopathy Syndrome (RPLS)

PO: ADULTS, ELDERLY: Interrupt treatment until fully resolved. Resume at reduced dose or discontinue (depending on the severity and persistence of neurologic symptoms).

Other Adverse Reactions

PO: ADULTS, ELDERLY: Reduce dose according to dose modification table. Due to limited data, there are no recommendations on resuming treatment in pts with Grade 4 adverse events that resolve.

Dosage in Renal/Hepatic Impairment

Mild to moderate impairment: No dose adjustment. **Severe impairment:** 14 mg once daily.

SIDE EFFECTS

Frequent (73%–29%): Hypertension, diarrhea, fatigue, asthenia, malaise, arthralgia, myalgia, decreased appetite, weight decreased, nausea, stomatitis, glossitis, mouth ulceration, mucosal inflammation, headache, vomiting, dysphonia, abdominal pain, constipation. **Occasional (25%–7%):** Oral pain, glossodynia, cough, peripheral edema, rash, dysgeusia, dry mouth, dizziness, dyspepsia, insomnia, alopecia, hypotension, dehydration, hyperkeratosis.

ADVERSE EFFECTS/TOXIC REACTIONS

Serious adverse effects may include arterial thromboembolic events (5% of pts); cardiac dysfunction (7% of pts); dental and oral infections including gingivitis, parotitis, pericoronitis, periodontitis, sialoadenitis, tooth abscess, tooth infection (10% of pts); GI perforation/fistula formation (2% of pts); hemorrhagic events (35% of pts); hepatotoxicity (4% of pts); hypertension (73% of pts); Grade 3 or greater hypocalcemia (9% of pts); impairment of thyroid-stimulating hormone (57% of pts); palmar-plantar erythrodysesthesia (32% of pts); proteinuria (34% of pts); QT interval prolongation (9% of pts); renal failure (14% of pts); urinary tract infection (11% of pts). Reverse posterior leukoencephalopathy occurs rarely. The median onset of hypertension was 16 days. The most frequently reported hemorrhagic event was epistaxis. The primary risk factor for renal failure was dehydration and hypovolemia related to diarrhea and vomiting.

NURSING CONSIDERATIONS

BASELINE ASSESSMENT

Obtain CBC, BMP, LFT; urinalysis for proteinuria. Confirm negative pregnancy status before initiating treatment. Receive full medication history and screen for interactions. Question history of cardiac/pituitary/thyroid disease, CVA/DVT, hypertension, hepatic/renal impairment, long QT interval syndrome. Assess oral cavity for lesions, poor dentation. Ensure that B/P is controlled prior to initiation. Assess hydration status. Offer emotional support.

INTERVENTION/EVALUATION

Monitor B/P after 1 wk, then q2wks for the first 2 mos, then at least monthly thereafter. Monitor LFT every 2 wks for the first 2 mos, then at least monthly thereafter. Monitor for proteinuria periodically. If urine dipstick proteinuria is greater than or equal to 2+, obtain a 24 hr urine protein test. Monitor blood calcium levels at least monthly and replace as needed depending on severity, presence of ECG changes, persistence of hypocalcemia. Monitor and correct other electrolyte abnormalities as needed. Initiate medical management for nausea, vomiting, diarrhea prior to any interruption or dose reduction. Reversible posterior leukoencephalopathy syndrome should be considered in pts with altered mental status, confusion, headache, seizures, visual disturbances. Immediately report abdominal pain, GI bleeding, hemoptysis (may indicate GI perforation/fistula formation). Obtain cardiac echocardiogram, ECG if cardiac decompensation is suspected.

PATIENT/FAMILY TEACHING

- Report liver problems such as upper abdominal pain, bruising, dark or amber-colored urine, nausea, vomiting, or

L

yellowing of the skin or eyes; heart problems such as chest tightness, dizziness, fainting, palpitations, shortness of breath; kidney problems such as dark-colored urine, decreased urine output, extremity swelling, flank pain; skin changes such as rash, skin bubbling, sloughing. • Neurologic changes including blurry vision, confusion, headache, one-sided weakness, seizures, trouble speaking may indicate high blood pressure crisis, stroke, or life-threatening brain swelling. • Report mouth ulceration, jaw pain. • Swallow capsules whole; do not chew, crush, cut, or open capsules. • Treatment may increase risk of GI bleeding, nosebleeds. • Drink plenty of fluids. • Use effective contraception to avoid pregnancy. Do not breastfeed.

L

letrozole

let-roe-zole

(Femara)

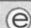

Do not confuse Femara with Famvir, Femhrt, or Provera, or letrozole with anastrozole.

CLASSIFICATION

PHARMACOTHERAPEUTIC: Aromatase inhibitor, hormone. **CLINICAL:** Antineoplastic.

USES

First-line treatment of hormone receptor–positive or hormone receptor unknown locally advanced or metastatic breast cancer. Treatment of advanced breast cancer in postmenopausal women with disease progression following antiestrogen therapy. Postsurgical treatment for postmenopausal women with hormone receptor–positive early breast cancer. Extended treatment of early breast cancer after 5 yrs of tamoxifen. **OFF-LABEL:** Treatment of ovarian (epithelial), endometrial cancer.

PRECAUTIONS

Contraindications: Hypersensitivity to letrozole, other aromatase inhibitors. Use in women who are or may become pregnant. **Cautions:** Hepatic impairment, hyperlipidemia.

ACTION

Decreases circulating estrogen by inhibiting aromatase, an enzyme that catalyzes the final step in estrogen production (inhibits conversion of androgens to estrogens). **Therapeutic Effect:** Inhibits growth of breast cancers stimulated by estrogens.

PHARMACOKINETICS

Rapidly, completely absorbed. Metabolized in liver. Primarily excreted in urine. Unknown if removed by hemodialysis. **Half-life:** Approximately 2 days.

LIFESPAN CONSIDERATIONS

Pregnancy/Lactation: Unknown if distributed in breast milk. May cause fetal harm. **Children:** Safety and efficacy not established. **Elderly:** No age-related precautions noted.

INTERACTIONS

DRUG: **Tamoxifen** may reduce concentration. **HERBAL:** None significant. **FOOD:** None known. **LAB VALUES:** May increase serum calcium, cholesterol, GGT, ALT, AST, bilirubin.

AVAILABILITY (Rx)

Tablets: 2.5 mg.

ADMINISTRATION/HANDLING

PO

- Give without regard to food.

INDICATIONS/ROUTES/DOSAGE

Breast Cancer (Advanced)

PO: ADULTS, ELDERLY: 2.5 mg/day. Continue until tumor progression is evident.

Breast Cancer (Early–adjuvant treatment)

PO: ADULTS, ELDERLY: (Postmenopausal): 2.5 mg/day for planned duration of 5 yrs. Discontinue at relapse.

Breast Cancer (Early–extended adjuvant treatment)

PO: ADULTS, ELDERLY: (Postmenopausal): 2.5 mg/day for planned duration of 5 yrs (after 5 yrs of tamoxifen). Discontinue at relapse.

Dosage in Renal Impairment

No dose adjustment.

Dosage in Severe Hepatic Impairment

PO: ADULTS, ELDERLY: 2.5 mg every other day.

SIDE EFFECTS

Frequent (21%–9%): Musculoskeletal pain (back, arm, leg), nausea, headache. **Occasional (8%–5%):** Constipation, arthralgia, fatigue, vomiting, hot flashes, diarrhea, abdominal pain, cough, rash, anorexia, hypertension, peripheral edema. **Rare (4%–1%):** Asthenia, drowsiness, dyspepsia, weight gain, pruritus.

ADVERSE EFFECTS/TOXIC REACTIONS

Pleural effusion, pulmonary embolism, bone fracture, thromboembolic disorder, MI occur rarely.

NURSING CONSIDERATIONS

BASELINE ASSESSMENT

Obtain baseline CBC, chemistries, renal function, LFT. Obtain pregnancy test prior to beginning therapy. Offer emotional support.

INTERVENTION/EVALUATION

Assist with ambulation if asthenia, dizziness occurs. Assess for headache. Offer antiemetic for nausea, vomiting. Monitor CBC, thyroid function, electrolytes, renal function, LFT. Monitor for evidence of musculoskeletal pain; offer analgesics for pain relief.

PATIENT/FAMILY TEACHING

• Report if nausea, asthenia, hot flashes become unmanageable. • Discuss importance of negative pregnancy test prior to beginning therapy; discuss nonhormonal methods of birth control. • Explain possible risk to fetus if pt is or becomes pregnant before or during therapy.

leucovorin

loo-**koe**-vor-in

Do not confuse leucovorin with Leukeran.

◆CLASSIFICATION

PHARMACOTHERAPEUTIC: Rescue agent (chemotherapy). **CLINICAL:** Antidote.

USES

Treatment of megaloblastic anemias when folate deficient. Palliative treatment of advanced colon cancer (with fluorouracil). IV rescue therapy after high-dose methotrexate for osteosarcoma or orally to diminish toxicity and impaired methotrexate elimination. **OFF-LABEL:** Adjunctive cofactor therapy in methanol toxicity. Prevents pyrimethamine hematologic toxicity in HIV-positive pts.

PRECAUTIONS

Contraindications: Hypersensitivity to leucovorin. Pernicious anemia, other megaloblastic anemias secondary to vitamin B_{12} deficiency. **Cautions:** Renal impairment.

ACTION

Actively competes with methotrexate for same transport processes into cells, displaces methotrexate from intracellular binding sites, and restores active folate stores necessary for DNA/RNA synthesis. **Therapeutic Effect:** Reverses toxic effects of folic acid antagonists. Reverses folic acid deficiency.

PHARMACOKINETICS

Readily absorbed from GI tract. Widely distributed. Metabolized in liver, intestinal mucosa. Primarily excreted in urine. **Half-life:** 15 min; metabolite, 30–35 min.

LIFESPAN CONSIDERATIONS

Pregnancy/Lactation: Unknown if drug crosses placenta or is distributed in breast milk. **Children:** May increase risk of seizures by counteracting anticonvulsant effects of **barbiturates, hydantoins. Elderly:** Age-related renal impairment may require dosage adjustment when used for rescue from effects of high-dose methotrexate therapy.

INTERACTIONS

DRUG: May decrease effects of **trimethoprim, anticonvulsants (e.g., phenytoin).** May increase **5-fluorouracil** toxicity/effects when taken in combination. **HERBAL:** None significant. **FOOD:** None known. **LAB VALUES:** May decrease platelets, WBCs (when used in combination with 5-fluorouracil).

AVAILABILITY (Rx)

Injection, Powder for Reconstitution: 50 mg, 100 mg, 200 mg, 350 mg, 500 mg. **Injection, Solution:** 10 mg/mL. **Tablets:** 5 mg, 10 mg, 15 mg, 25 mg.

ADMINISTRATION/HANDLING

IV

ALERT Strict adherence to timing of 5-fluorouracil following leucovorin therapy must be maintained.

Reconstitution • Reconstitute each 50-mg vial with 5 mL Sterile Water for Injection or Bacteriostatic Water for Injection containing benzyl alcohol to provide concentration of 10 mg/mL. • Due to benzyl alcohol in 1-mg ampule and in Bacteriostatic Water for Injection, reconstitute doses greater than 10 mg/m^2 with Sterile Water for Injection. • Further dilute with 100–1,000 mL D_5W or 0.9% NaCl.

Rate of administration • Do not exceed 160 mg/min if given by IV infusion (due to calcium content).

Storage • Store powdered vials for parenteral use at room temperature. • Refrigerate solution for injection vials. • Injection appears as clear, yellowish solution. • Use immediately if reconstituted with Sterile Water for Injection; stable for 7 days if reconstituted with Bacteriostatic Water for Injection. Diluted solutions stable for 24 hrs at room temperature or 4 days refrigerated.

PO

- Scored tablets may be crushed.

IV INCOMPATIBILITIES

Amphotericin B complex (Abelcet, AmBisome, Amphotec), droperidol (Inapsine), foscarnet (Foscavir).

IV COMPATIBILITIES

CISplatin (Platinol AQ), cyclophosphamide (Cytoxan), DOXOrubicin (Adriamycin), etoposide (VePesid), filgrastim (Neupogen), 5-fluorouracil, gemcitabine (Gemzar), granisetron (Kytril), heparin, methotrexate, metoclopramide (Reglan), mitoMYcin (Mutamycin), piperacillin and tazobactam (Zosyn), vinBLAStine (Velban), vinCRIStine (Oncovin).

INDICATIONS/ROUTES/DOSAGE

Rescue in High-Dose Methotrexate Therapy

PO, IV, IM: ADULTS, ELDERLY, CHILDREN: 15 mg (approximately 10 mg/m^2) started 24 hrs after starting methotrexate infusion; continue q6h for 10 doses, until methotrexate level is less than 0.05 micromole/L. Additional dose adjusted based on methotrexate levels.

Folic Acid Antagonist Overdose

PO: ADULTS, ELDERLY, CHILDREN: 5–15 mg/day.

Megaloblastic Anemia Secondary to Folate Deficiency

IM/IV: ADULTS, ELDERLY, CHILDREN: 1 mg or less per day.

Colon Cancer

ALERT For rescue therapy in cancer chemotherapy, refer to specific protocols used for optimal dosage and sequence of leucovorin administration.

IV: ADULTS, ELDERLY: ***(In Combination With 5-Fluorouracil):*** 200 mg/m² daily for 5 days. Repeat course at 4-wk intervals for 2 courses, then 4- to 5-wk intervals or 20 mg/m² daily for 5 days. Repeat course at 4-wk intervals for 2 courses, then 4- to 5-wk intervals.

Dosage in Renal/Hepatic Impairment
No dose adjustment.

SIDE EFFECTS

Frequent: When combined with chemotherapeutic agents: diarrhea, stomatitis, nausea, vomiting, lethargy, malaise, fatigue, alopecia, anorexia. **Occasional:** Urticaria, dermatitis.

ADVERSE EFFECTS/TOXIC REACTIONS

Excessive dosage may negate chemotherapeutic effects of folic acid antagonists. Anaphylaxis occurs rarely. Diarrhea may cause rapid clinical deterioration.

NURSING CONSIDERATIONS

BASELINE ASSESSMENT

Obtain baseline CBC, LFT, renal function. Give as soon as possible, preferably within 1 hr, for treatment of accidental overdosage of folic acid antagonists.

INTERVENTION/EVALUATION

Monitor for vomiting (may need to change from oral to parenteral therapy). Observe elderly, debilitated closely due to risk for severe toxicities. Assess CBC, BMP, LFT.

PATIENT/FAMILY TEACHING

• Explain purpose of medication in treatment of cancer. • Report allergic reaction, vomiting.

leuprolide ⓔ

loo-proe-lide
(Eligard, Lupron ✱, Lupron Depot, Lupron Depot-Ped)

◆CLASSIFICATION

PHARMACOTHERAPEUTIC: Gonadotropin-releasing hormone (GnRH) analogue. **CLINICAL:** Antineoplastic.

USES

Palliative treatment of advanced prostate carcinoma. Management of endometriosis. Treatment of anemia caused by uterine leiomyomata (fibroids). Treatment of central precocious puberty. **OFF-LABEL:** Treatment of breast cancer, infertility.

PRECAUTIONS

Contraindications: Hypersensitivity to leuprolide, GnRH, GnRH-agonist analogue. Pregnancy or women who may become pregnant, breastfeeding (Lupron Depot 3.75 mg and 11.25 mg), abnormal, undiagnosed vaginal bleeding (Lupron Depot 3.75 mg and 11.25 mg). 22.5 mg, 30 mg, 45 mg Lupron Depot and Eligard (all strengths) not indicated for use in women. **Cautions:** History of psychiatric illness, QTc prolongation or medications that prolong QTc interval, preexisting cardiac disease, chronic alcohol use, steroid therapy, seizures or medications that decrease seizures threshold.

ACTION

Inhibits gonadotropin secretion; produces an initial increase in LH and FSH, causing a transient increase in testosterone (males) and estrone/estradione in premenopausal women. Continuous administration results in decreased levels of testosterone (male) and estrogen (females). **Therapeutic Effect:** Produces pharmacologic castration, decreases growth of abnormal prostate tissue in males; causes endometrial tissue to become inactive, atrophic in females; decreases rate of pubertal development in children with central precocious puberty.

PHARMACOKINETICS

Rapidly, well absorbed after SQ administration. Absorbed slowly after IM administration. Protein binding: 43%–49%. **Half-life:** 3–4 hrs.

LIFESPAN CONSIDERATIONS

Pregnancy/Lactation: Depot: Contraindicated in pregnancy. May cause spontaneous abortion. **Children:** Long-term safety not established. **Elderly:** No age-related precautions noted.

INTERACTIONS

DRUG: QT interval–prolonging medications (e.g., amiodarone, azithromycin, ceritinib, haloperidol, moxifloxacin) may increase risk of QT interval prolongation, cardiac arrhythmias. **HERBAL:** None significant. **FOOD:** None known. **LAB VALUES:** May increase serum prostatic acid phosphatase (PAP). Initially increases, then decreases serum testosterone. May increase serum ALT, AST, alkaline phosphatase, glucose, LDH, LDL, cholesterol, triglycerides. May decrease platelets, WBC.

L

AVAILABILITY (Rx)

Injection Depot Formulation: ***(Eligard):*** 7.5 mg, 22.5 mg, 30 mg, 45 mg. ***(Lupron Depot-Ped):*** 7.5 mg, 11.25 mg (3-month), 11.25 (monthly), 15 mg, 30 mg. ***(Lupron Depot):*** 3.75 mg, 11.25 mg, 22.5 mg, 30 mg, 45 mg. **Injection Solution:** 5 mg/mL.

ADMINISTRATION/HANDLING

◀ALERT▶ May be carcinogenic, mutagenic, teratogenic. Handle with extreme care during preparation/administration.

IM

• ***(Lupron Depot):*** Store at room temperature. • Protect from light, heat. • Do not freeze vials. • Reconstitute only with diluent provided. Follow manufacturer's instructions for mixing. • Do not use needles less than 22 gauge; use syringes provided by the manufacturer (0.5-mL low-dose insulin syringes may be used as an alternative). • Administer immediately.

• ***(Eligard):*** Refrigerate. • Allow to warm to room temperature before reconstitution. • Follow manufacturer's instructions for mixing. • Following reconstitution, administer within 30 min.

SQ

• ***(Lupron):*** Refrigerate vials. • Injection appears clear, colorless. • Discard if discolored or precipitate forms. • Administer into deltoid muscle, anterior thigh, abdomen.

INDICATIONS/ROUTES/DOSAGE

Advanced Prostatic Carcinoma

IM: ***(Lupron Depot):*** **ADULTS, ELDERLY:** 7.5 mg q1mo, 22.5 mg q3mos, 30 mg q4mos, or 45 mg q6mos.

SQ: ***(Eligard):*** **ADULTS, ELDERLY:** 7.5 mg every mo, 22.5 mg q3mos, 30 mg q4mos, or 45 mg q6mos.

SQ: ***(Lupron):*** **ADULTS, ELDERLY:** 1 mg/day.

Endometriosis

IM: ***(Lupron Depot):*** **ADULTS, ELDERLY:** 3.75 mg/mo for up to 6 mos or 11.25 mg q3mos for up to 2 doses.

Uterine Leiomyomata

IM: ***(with iron [Lupron Depot]):*** **ADULTS, ELDERLY:** 3.75 mg/mo for up to 3 mos or 11.25 mg as a single injection.

Precocious Puberty

IM: ***(Lupron Depot-Ped):*** **CHILDREN WEIGHING MORE THAN 37.5 KG:** 15 mg q1mo. **WEIGHING 25 KG TO 37.5 KG:** 11.25 mg q1mo. **WEIGHING 25 KG OR LESS:** 7.5 mg q1mo. Titrate dose upward by 3.75 mg/mo if down regulation not achieved. **LUPRON DEPOT-PED (3 MOS):** 11.25 mg or 30 mg q12wks.

SQ: ***(Lupron):*** **CHILDREN:** Initially, 50 mcg/kg/day. Titrate upward by 10 mcg/kg/day if down regulation is not achieved.

Dosage in Renal/Hepatic Impairment

No dose adjustment.

SIDE EFFECTS

Frequent: Hot flashes (ranging from mild flushing to diaphoresis), migraines, hyperhidrosis. **Females:** Amenorrhea, spotting. **Occasional:** Arrhythmias, palpitations, blurred vision, dizziness, edema, headache, burning, pruritus, swelling at injection site, nausea, insomnia, weight gain. **Females:** Deepening voice, hirsutism, decreased libido, increased breast tenderness, vaginitis, altered mood. **Males:** Constipation, decreased testicle size, gynecomastia, impotence, decreased appetite, angina. **Rare: Males:** Thrombophlebitis.

ADVERSE EFFECTS/TOXIC REACTIONS

Occasionally, signs/symptoms of prostatic carcinoma worsen 1–2 wks after initial dosing (subsides during continued therapy). Increased bone pain and, less frequently, dysuria, hematuria, weakness, paresthesia of lower extremities may be noted. MI, pulmonary embolism occur rarely.

NURSING CONSIDERATIONS

BASELINE ASSESSMENT

Question for possibility of pregnancy before initiating therapy. Obtain serum testosterone, prostatic acid phosphates (PAP) periodically during therapy. Question medical history as listed in Precautions. Offer emotional support.

INTERVENTION/EVALUATION

Monitor for arrhythmias, palpitations. Assess for peripheral edema. Assess sleep pattern. Monitor for visual difficulties. Assist with ambulation if dizziness occurs. Offer antiemetics if nausea occurs. Serum testosterone, PAP should increase during first wk of therapy. Serum testosterone then should decrease to baseline level or less within 2 wks, PAP within 4 wks.

PATIENT/ FAMILY TEACHING

• Hot flashes tend to decrease during continued therapy. • Temporary exacerbation of signs/symptoms of disease may occur during first few wks of therapy. • Use contraceptive measures. • Report persistent, regular menstruation; pregnancy. • Avoid tasks that require alertness, motor skills until response to drug is established (potential for dizziness).

levalbuterol

lee-val-**bue**-ter-ole
(Xopenex, Xopenex HFA, Xopenex Concentrate)
Do not confuse Xopenex with Xanax.

◆CLASSIFICATION

PHARMACOTHERAPEUTIC: Beta$_2$ agonist. **CLINICAL:** Bronchodilator.

USES

Treatment, prevention of bronchospasm due to reversible obstructive airway disease.

PRECAUTIONS

Contraindications: History of hypersensitivity to albuterol or levalbuterol. **Cautions:** Cardiovascular disorders (cardiac arrhythmias, HF), seizures, hypertension, hyperthyroidism, diabetes, glaucoma, hypokalemia.

ACTION

Stimulates beta$_2$-adrenergic receptors in lungs, resulting in relaxation of bronchial smooth muscle. **Therapeutic Effect:** Relieves bronchospasm, reduces airway resistance.

PHARMACOKINETICS

Route	Onset	Peak	Duration
Inhalation	5–10 min	1.5 hrs	5–6 hrs
Nebulization	10–17 min	1.5 hrs	5–8 hrs

Half-life: 3.3–4 hrs.

⌛ LIFESPAN CONSIDERATIONS

Pregnancy/Lactation: Crosses placenta. Unknown if distributed in breast milk. **Pregnancy Category C. Children:** Safety and efficacy not established in pts younger than 12 yrs. **Elderly:** Lower initial dosages recommended.

INTERACTIONS

DRUG: **Beta blockers (e.g., carvedilol, metoprolol)** antagonize effects; may produce severe bronchospasm. **MAOIs (e.g., phenelzine, tranylcypromine), tricyclic antidepressants (e.g., amitriptyline, desipramine)** may potentiate cardiovascular effects. **Diuretics (e.g., furosemide, HCTZ)** may increase hypokalemia. **Linezolid** may enhance the hypertensive effect. May increase adverse effects of **loxapine.** **HERBAL:** None significant. **FOOD:** None known. **LAB VALUES:** May decrease serum potassium.

L

AVAILABILITY (Rx)

Inhalation Aerosol: 45 mcg/activation. **Solution for Nebulization:** 0.31 mg in 3-mL vials, 0.63 mg in 3-mL vials, 1.25 mg in 3-mL vials, 1.25 mg in 0.5-mL vials.

ADMINISTRATION/HANDLING

Nebulization

• No diluent necessary. • Protect from light, excessive heat. Store at room temperature. • Once foil is opened, use within 2 wks. • Use within 1 wk and protect from light after removal from pouch • Discard if solution is not colorless. • Do not mix with other medications. • Concentrated solution (1.25 mg in 0.5 mL) should be diluted with 2.5 mL 0.9% NaCl prior to use. • Give over 5–15 min.

Inhalation

• Shake well before inhalation. • Prime before initial use or if not used for more than 3 days. • Following first inhalation, wait 2 min before inhaling second dose (allows for deeper bronchial penetration). • Rinsing mouth with water immediately after inhalation prevents mouth/throat dryness.

INDICATIONS/ROUTES/DOSAGE

Treatment/Prevention of Bronchospasm

Nebulization: ADULTS, ELDERLY, CHILDREN 12 YRS AND OLDER: Initially, 0.63 mg 3 times/day 6–8 hrs apart. May increase to 1.25 mg 3 times/day with close monitoring. **CHILDREN 5–11 YRS:** Initially, 0.31 mg 3 times/day. **Maximum:** 0.63 mg 3 times/day. **CHILDREN 4 YRS OR YOUNGER:** 0.31–1.25 mg q4–6h as needed.

Inhalation: ADULTS, ELDERLY, CHILDREN 4 YRS AND OLDER: 1–2 inhalations q4–6h.

Acute Asthma Exacerbation

Nebulization: ADULTS, ELDERLY, CHILDREN 12 YRS AND OLDER: 1.25–2.5 mg q20min for 3 doses, then 1.25–5 mg q1–4h as needed. **CHILDREN YOUNGER THAN 12 YRS:** 0.075 mg/kg (minimum dose: 1.25 mg) q20min for 3 doses, then 0.075–0.15 mg/kg (Maximum: 5 mg dose) q1–4h as needed.

Inhalation: ADULTS, ELDERLY, CHILDREN 12 YRS AND OLDER: 4–8 puffs q20min for up to 4 hrs, then q1–4h. **CHILDREN YOUNGER THAN 12 YRS:** 4–8 puffs q20min for 3 doses, then q1–4h.

Dosage in Renal/Hepatic Impairment

No dose adjustment.

SIDE EFFECTS

Occasional (11%–4%): Nervousness, tremor, rhinitis, flu-like illness. **Rare (less than 3%):** Tachycardia, dizziness, anxiety, viral infection, dyspepsia, dry mouth, headache, chest pain.

ADVERSE EFFECTS/TOXIC REACTIONS

Excessive sympathomimetic stimulation may produce palpitations, premature heart contraction, tachycardia, chest pain, slight increase in B/P followed by substantial decrease, chills, diaphoresis, blanching of skin. Too-frequent or excessive use may decrease bronchodilating effectiveness, lead to severe, paradoxical bronchoconstriction.

NURSING CONSIDERATIONS

BASELINE ASSESSMENT

Assess lung sounds, pulse, B/P, oxygen saturation. Note color, amount of sputum.

INTERVENTION/EVALUATION

Monitor rate, depth, rhythm, type of respiration; quality/rate of pulse, ECG, serum potassium. Assess lung sounds for wheezing (bronchoconstriction). Observe for paradoxical bronchospasm.

PATIENT/ FAMILY TEACHING

• Increase fluid intake (decreases lung secretion viscosity). • Rinsing mouth with water immediately after inhalation may prevent mouth/throat dryness. • Avoid excessive use of caffeine derivatives (chocolate, coffee, tea, cola, cocoa). • Report if palpitations, tachycardia, chest pain, tremors, dizziness, headache occurs or shortness of breath is not relieved.

levETIRAcetam

lee-ve-tye-**ra**-se-tam
(Keppra, Keppra XR, Roweepra, Roweepra XR, Spritam)
Do not confuse Keppra with Kaletra, Keflex, or Keppra XR, or levETIRAcetam with levo-FLOXacin.

◆CLASSIFICATION

PHARMACOTHERAPEUTIC: Pyrrolidine derivative. **CLINICAL:** Anticonvulsant.

USES

Adjunctive therapy in treatment of partial-onset, myoclonic, and/or primary generalized tonic-clonic seizures.

PRECAUTIONS

Contraindications: Hypersensitivity to levETIRAcetam. **Cautions:** Renal impairment, pts with depression at high risk for suicide.

ACTION

Exact mechanism unknown. May inhibit voltage-dependent calcium channels, facilitate GABA inhibitory transmission, reduce potassium current, or bind to synaptic proteins that modulate neurotransmitter release. **Therapeutic Effect:** Prevents seizure activity.

PHARMACOKINETICS

Rapidly absorbed and widely distributed. Protein binding: less than 10%. Metabolized primarily by enzymatic hydrolysis. Primarily excreted in urine as unchanged drug. **Half-life:** 6–8 hrs.

LIFESPAN CONSIDERATIONS

Pregnancy/Lactation: Distributed in breast milk. Breastfeeding not recommended. **Children:** Safety and efficacy not established in children 4 yrs or younger. **Elderly:** Age-related renal impairment may require dosage adjustment.

INTERACTIONS

DRUG: CNS depressants (e.g., alcohol, morphine, zolpidem) may increase CNS depression. **HERBAL: Herbals with sedative properties (e.g., chamomile, kava kava, valerian)** may increase CNS depression. **FOOD:** None known. **LAB VALUES:** May decrease Hgb, Hct, RBC, WBC.

AVAILABILITY (Rx)

Injection, Solution: 100 mg/mL. **Oral Solution:** 100 mg/mL. **Tablets:** 250 mg, 500 mg, 750 mg, 1,000 mg.

Tablets, Extended-Release: 500 mg, 750 mg. **Tablets (ODT):** 250 mg, 500 mg, 750 mg, 1,000 mg.

ADMINISTRATION/HANDLING

IV

Rate of infusion • Infuse over 15 min.
Reconstitution • Dilute with 100 mL 0.9% NaCl or D_5W.
Storage • Store at room temperature. • Stable for 24 hrs following dilution.

PO

• Give without regard to food. • **Oral Solution:** Use a calibrated measuring device. • **Tablet (immediate-release,**

extended-release): Administer tablet whole; do not cut, break, or crush. • **Tablet (ODT):** Place whole tablet on tongue and follow with sip of liquid. Swallowing allowed only after tablet has disintegrated. • Use oral solution for pts weighing 20 kg or less. • Use tablets or oral solution for pts weighing more than 20 kg.

IV COMPATIBILITIES

DiazePAM (Valium), LORazepam (Ativan), valproate (Depacon).

INDICATIONS/ROUTES/DOSAGE

Partial-Onset Seizures

IV/PO: ADULTS, ELDERLY, CHILDREN 17 YRS AND OLDER: ***(Immediate-Release Tablets, Oral Solution, Tablets for Oral Suspension):*** Initially, 500 mg q12h. May increase by 1,000 mg/day q2wks. **Maximum:** 3,000 mg/day in 2 divided doses. ***(Extended-Release Tablets):*** 1,000 mg once daily. May increase in increments of 1,000 mg/day q2wks. **Maximum:** 3,000 mg once daily.

IV/PO: CHILDREN 4–16 YRS: ***(Oral Solution, Tablets):*** 20 mg/kg/day in 2 divided doses. May increase q2wks by 10 mg/kg/dose up to 60 mg/kg/day in 2 divided doses. **Maximum:** 3,000 mg/day. ***(Tablets):*** **WEIGHING MORE THAN 40 KG:** 500 mg twice daily. May increase q2wks by 500 mg/dose. **Maximum:** 1,500 mg twice daily. **20–40 KG:** 250 mg twice daily. May increase q2wks by 250 mg/dose. **Maximum:** 750 mg twice daily. **CHILDREN 6 MOS TO YOUNGER THAN 4 YRS:** ***(Oral Solution):*** 20 mg/kg/day in 2 divided doses. May increase q2wks by 10 mg/kg/dose. **Maximum:** 50 mg/kg/day in 2 divided doses. **CHILDREN 1 MO TO YOUNGER THAN 6 MOS:** ***(Oral Solution):*** 14 mg/kg/day in 2 divided doses. May increase q2wks by 7 mg/kg/dose. **Maximum:** 42 mg/kg/day in 2 divided doses.

Myoclonic Seizures

PO, IV: CHILDREN 16 YRS AND OLDER: ***(Immediate-Release Tablets, Oral Solution, Tablets for Oral Suspension):*** Initially, 500 mg q12h. May increase by 1,000 mg/day q2wks. **Maximum:** 3,000 mg/day in 2 divided doses. **CHILDREN 6–15 YRS:** Initially, 10 mg/kg twice daily. May increase by 10 mg/kg/dose q2wks up to recommended dose of 30 mg/kg twice daily.

Tonic-Clonic Seizures

PO, IV: ADULTS, ELDERLY, CHILDREN 16 YRS AND OLDER: ***(Immediate-Release Tablets, Oral Solution, Tablets for Oral Suspension):*** Initially, 500 mg twice daily. May increase by 1,000 mg/day q2wks up to recommended dose of 1,500 mg 2 times/day. **CHILDREN 6–15 YRS:** Initially, 10 mg/kg twice daily. May increase by 20 mg/kg/day q2wks up to recommended dose of 30 mg/kg 2 times/day.

Dosage in Renal Impairment

Dosage is modified based on creatinine clearance. **Note: CrCl less than 50 mL/min:** Not recommended with Keppra XR.

Creatinine Clearance	Dosage (Immediate-Release, IV)	Dosage (Extended-Release)
Greater than 80 mL/min:	500–1,500 mg q12h	1,000–3,000 mg q24h
50–80 mL/min:	500–1,000 mg q12h	1,000–2,000 mg q24h
30–49 mL/min:	250–750 mg q12h	500–1,500 mg q24h
Less than 30 mL/min:	250–500 mg q12h	500–1,000 mg q24h
End-stage renal disease using dialysis:	500–1,000 mg q24h; after dialysis, a 250- to 500–mg supplemental dose is recommended	NA
CRRT	250–750 mg q12h	

Dosage in Hepatic Impairment

No dose adjustment.

SIDE EFFECTS

Frequent (15%–10%): Drowsiness, asthenia, headache, infection. **Occasional (9%–3%):** Dizziness, pharyngitis, pain, depression, anxiety, vertigo, rhinitis, anorexia. **Rare (less than 3%):** Amnesia, emotional lability, cough, sinusitis, anorexia, diplopia.

ADVERSE EFFECTS/TOXIC REACTIONS

Acute psychosis, agitation, delirium, impulsivity have been reported. Sudden discontinuance increases risk of seizure activity. Serious dermatological reactions, including Stevens-Johnson syndrome and toxic epidermal necrolysis, have been reported.

NURSING CONSIDERATIONS

BASELINE ASSESSMENT

Review history of seizure disorder (intensity, frequency, duration, LOC). Initiate seizure precautions. Question prior hypersensitivity reaction. Obtain renal function test.

INTERVENTION/EVALUATION

Observe for recurrence of seizure activity. Assess for clinical improvement (decrease in intensity/frequency of seizures). Monitor renal function tests. Observe for suicidal ideation, depression, behavioral changes. Assist with ambulation if dizziness occurs.

PATIENT/ FAMILY TEACHING

• Drowsiness usually diminishes with continued therapy. • Avoid tasks that require alertness, motor skills until response to drug is established. • Avoid alcohol. • Do not abruptly discontinue medication (may precipitate seizures). • Strict maintenance of drug therapy is essential for seizure control. • Report mood swings, hostile behavior, suicidal ideation, unusual changes in behavior.

levoFLOXacin TOP 100

lee-voe-**flox**-a-sin
(Iquix, Levaquin, Quixin)

BLACK BOX ALERT May increase risk of tendonitis, tendon rupture. (Risk increased with concurrent corticosteroids, organ transplant, pts older than 60 yrs.) May exacerbate myasthenia gravis. **Do not confuse Levaquin with Levoxyl, Levsin/SL, or Lovenox, or levoFLOXacin with levETIRAcetam or levothyroxine.**

◆CLASSIFICATION

PHARMACOTHERAPEUTIC: Fluoroquinolone. **CLINICAL:** Antibiotic.

USES

Treatment of susceptible infections due to *S. pneumoniae, S. aureus, E. faecalis, H. influenzae, M. catarrhalis, Serratia marcescens, K. pneumoniae, E. coli, P. mirabilis, P. aeruginosa, C. pneumoniae, Legionella pneumophila, Mycoplasma pneumoniae,* including acute bacterial exacerbation of chronic bronchitis, acute bacterial sinusitis, community-acquired pneumonia, nosocomial pneumonia, complicated and uncomplicated UTI, acute pyelonephritis, complicated and uncomplicated mild to moderate skin/skin structure infections, prostatitis. Inhalation anthrax (postexposure); plague. **Ophthalmic:** Treatment of superficial infections to conjunctiva (0.5%), cornea (1.5%). **OFF-LABEL:** Urethritis, traveler's diarrhea, diverticulitis, enterocolitis, Legionnaire's disease, peritonitis. Treatment of prosthetic joint infection.

PRECAUTIONS

Contraindications: Hypersensitivity to levoFLOXacin, other fluoroquinolones. **Cautions:** Known or suspected CNS disorders, seizure disorder, renal impairment, bradycardia, rheumatoid arthritis, elderly, myasthenia gravis, severe cerebral arteriosclerosis, pts at risk for QT interval prolongation (congenital long QT syndrome, HF, medications that prolong QT interval, hypokalemia, hypomagnesemia), diabetes, pts at risk for tendon rupture, tendonitis (e.g., renal failure, concomitant use of corticosteroids, organ transplant recipient, rheumatoid arthritis, elderly, strenuous physical activity or exercise).

ACTION

Inhibits DNA enzyme gyrase in susceptible microorganisms, interfering with bacterial cell replication, repair. **Therapeutic Effect:** Bactericidal.

PHARMACOKINETICS

Well absorbed after PO, IV administration. Protein binding: 50%. Widely distributed. Excreted unchanged in urine. Partially removed by hemodialysis. **Half-life:** 6–8 hrs.

LIFESPAN CONSIDERATIONS

Pregnancy/Lactation: Distributed in breast milk. Avoid use in pregnancy. **Children:** Safety and efficacy not established. **Elderly:** Age-related renal impairment may require dosage adjustment.

L

INTERACTIONS

DRUG: May decrease therapeutic effect of **BCG (intravesical). Antacids; calcium, magnesium, iron preparations; sucralfate, zinc** decrease absorption. **NSAIDs (e.g., ibuprofen, ketorolac, naproxen)** may increase risk of CNS stimulation, seizures. **Medications that prolong QT interval (e.g., amiodarone, haloperidol, sotalol)** may increase risk of arrhythmias. May increase effects of **warfarin. HERBAL:** None significant. **FOOD:** None known. **LAB VALUES:** May alter serum glucose.

AVAILABILITY (Rx)

Infusion Premix: 250 mg/50 mL, 500 mg/100 mL, 750 mg/150 mL. **Injection, Solution:** 25 mg/mL. **Ophthalmic Solution:** 0.5%. **Oral Solution:** 25 mg/mL. **Tablets:** 250 mg, 500 mg, 750 mg.

ADMINISTRATION/HANDLING

IV

Reconstitution • For infusion using single-dose vial, withdraw desired amount (10 mL for 250 mg, 20 mL for 500 mg). Dilute each 10 mL (250 mg) with minimum 40 mL 0.9% NaCl, D_5W, providing a concentration of 5 mg/mL.

Rate of administration • Administer no less than 60 min for 250 mg or 500 mg; 90 min for 750 mg.

Storage • Available in single-dose 20-mL (500-mg) vials and premixed with D_5W, ready to infuse. • Diluted vials stable for 72 hrs at room temperature, 14 days if refrigerated.

PO

• Do not administer antacids (aluminum, magnesium), sucralfate, iron, or multivitamin preparations with zinc within 2 hrs of administration (significantly reduces absorption). • Give tablets without regard to food. • Give oral solution 1 hr before or 2 hrs after meals.

Ophthalmic

• Place a gloved finger on lower eyelid and pull out until a pocket is formed between eye and lower lid. • Place prescribed number of drops into pocket. • Instruct pt to close eye gently (so that medication will not be squeezed out of the sac) and to apply digital pressure to lacrimal sac for 1–2 min to minimize systemic absorption.

IV INCOMPATIBILITIES

Furosemide (Lasix), heparin, insulin, nitroglycerin, propofol (Diprivan).

IV COMPATIBILITIES

Dexmedetomidine (Precedex), DOBUTamine (Dobutrex), DOPamine (Intropin), fentaNYL (Sublimaze), lidocaine, lorazepam (Ativan), magnesium, morphine.

INDICATIONS/ROUTES/DOSAGE

Usual Dosage Range

PO, IV: **ADULTS, ELDERLY:** 250–500 mg q24h; 750 mg q24h for severe or complicated infections.

Bacterial Conjunctivitis

Ophthalmic: **ADULTS, ELDERLY, CHILDREN 1 YR AND OLDER:** 1–2 drops q2h for 2 days while awake (up to 8 times/day), then 1–2 drops q4h while awake up to 4 times/day.

Dosage in Renal Impairment

Normal renal function dosage of 250 mg/day:

Creatinine Clearance	Dosage
20–49 mL/min	No change
10–19 mL/min	250 mg initially, then 250 mg q48h

Normal renal function dosage of 500 mg/day:

Creatinine Clearance	Dosage
50–80 mL/min	No change
20–49 mL/min	500 mg initially, then 250 mg q24h
10–19 mL/min	500 mg initially, then 250 mg q48h

For pts undergoing dialysis, 500 mg initially, then 250 mg q48h.

Normal renal function dosage of 750 mg/day:

Creatinine Clearance	Dosage
50–80 mL/min	No change
20–49 mL/min	Initially, 750 mg, then 750 mg q48h
10–19 mL/min	Initially, 750 mg, then 500 mg q48h
Dialysis	500 mg q48h (administer after dialysis on dialysis days)
Continuous renal replacement therapy	
CVVH	500–750 mg once, then 250 mg q24h
CVVHD	500–750 mg once, then 250–500 mg q24h
CVVHDT	500–750 mg once, then 250–750 mg q24h

Dosage in Hepatic Impairment

No dose adjustment.

SIDE EFFECTS

Occasional (3%–1%): Diarrhea, nausea, abdominal pain, dizziness, drowsiness, headache. **Ophthalmic:** Local burning/discomfort, margin crusting, crystals/scales, foreign body sensation, ocular itching, altered taste. **Rare (less than 1%):** Flatulence; pain, inflammation, swelling in calves, hands, shoulder; chest pain, difficulty breathing, palpitations, edema, tendon pain. **Ophthalmic:** Corneal staining, keratitis, allergic reaction, eyelid swelling, tearing, reduced visual acuity.

ADVERSE EFFECTS/TOXIC REACTIONS

Antibiotic-associated colitis, other superinfections (abdominal cramps, severe watery diarrhea, fever) may occur. Superinfection (genital/anal pruritus, ulceration/changes in oral mucosa, moderate to severe diarrhea) may occur from altered bacterial balance in GI tract. Hypersensitivity reactions, including photosensitivity (rash, pruritus, blisters, edema, sensation of burning skin), have occurred in pts receiving fluoroquinolones. May increase risk of tendonitis, tendon rupture, peripheral neuropathy; CNS effects including agitation, anxiety, confusion, depression, dizziness, hallucinations, nightmares, paranoia, tremors, vertigo. May exacerbate muscle weakness in pts with myasthenia gravis.

NURSING CONSIDERATIONS

BASELINE ASSESSMENT

Question for hypersensitivity to levoFLOXacin, other fluoroquinolones. Question history as listed in Precautions. Receive full medication history, and screen for interactions, esp. medications that prolong QT interval. Obtain baseline ECG.

INTERVENTION/EVALUATION

Monitor serum glucose, renal function, LFT. Monitor daily pattern of bowel activity, stool consistency. Promptly report hypersensitivity reaction: skin rash, urticaria, pruritus, photosensitivity. Be alert for superinfection: fever, vomiting, diarrhea, anal/genital pruritus, oral mucosal changes (ulceration, pain, erythema). Monitor for muscle weakness, voice dystonia in pts with myasthenia gravis; pain, swelling, bruising, popping of tendons.

PATIENT/FAMILY TEACHING

• It is essential to complete drug therapy despite symptom improvement. Early discontinuation may result in antibacterial resistance or increase risk of recurrent infection. • Report any episodes of diarrhea, esp. the first few mos after final dose. Frequent diarrhea, fever, abdominal pain, blood-streaked stool may indicate infectious diarrhea, which may be contagious to others. • Severe allergic reactions, such as hives, palpitations, rash, shortness of breath, tongue swelling, may occur. • Tendon inflammation/swelling, tendon rupture may occur; report bruising, pain, swelling in tendon areas or snapping, popping of tendons. • Immediately report nervous system problems such as anxiety, confusion, dizziness, nervousness, nightmares, thoughts of suicide, seizures, tremors, trouble sleeping. • Treatment may cause heart problems such as low heart rate, palpitations; permanent nerve damage such as burning, numbness, tingling, weakness. • Do not take aluminum- or magnesium-containing antacids, multivitamins, zinc or iron products at least 2 hrs before or 6 hrs after dose. • Drink plenty of fluids.

L

levothyroxine

TOP 100

lee-voe-thy-**rox**-een
(Eltroxin ✱, Euthyrox, Levoxyl, Synthroid, Tirosint, Unithroid)

BLACK BOX ALERT Ineffective, potentially toxic for weight reduction. High doses increase risk of serious, life-threatening toxic effects, especially when used with some anorectic drugs.

Do not confuse levothyroxine with lamoTRIgine, Lanoxin, levoFLOXacin or liothyronine, or Levoxyl with Lanoxin, Levaquin, or Luvox, or Synthroid with Symmetrel.

FIXED-COMBINATION(S)

With liothyronine, T_3 **(Thyrolar).**

◆CLASSIFICATION

PHARMACOTHERAPEUTIC: Synthetic isomer of thyroxine. **CLINICAL:** Thyroid hormone (T_4).

USES

PO: Treatment of hypothyroidism, pituitary thyroid-stimulating hormone (TSH) suppression. **IV:** Myxedema coma. **OFF-LABEL:** Management of hemodynamically unstable potential organ donors.

PRECAUTIONS

Contraindications: Hypersensitivity to levothyroxine. Acute MI, untreated subclinical or overt thyrotoxicosis, uncorrected adrenal insufficiency. **Capsule:** Inability to swallow capsules. **Cautions:** Elderly pts, angina pectoris, hypertension, other cardiovascular disease, adrenal insufficiency, myxedema, diabetes mellitus and insipidus, swallowing disorders.

ACTION

Converts to T_3, then binds to thyroid receptor proteins exerting metabolic effects through control of DNA transcription and protein synthesis. **Therapeutic Effect:** Involved in normal metabolism, growth and development. Increases basal metabolic rate, enhances gluconeogenesis, stimulates protein synthesis.

PHARMACOKINETICS

Variable, incomplete absorption from GI tract. Protein binding: greater than 99%. Widely distributed. Deiodinated in peripheral tissues, minimal metabolism in liver. Eliminated by biliary excretion. **Half-life:** 6–7 days.

⌛ LIFESPAN CONSIDERATIONS

Pregnancy/Lactation: Does not cross placenta. Minimal distribution in breast milk. **Children:** No age-related precautions noted. Caution in neonates in interpreting thyroid function tests. **Elderly:** May be more sensitive to thyroid effects; individualized dosage recommended.

INTERACTIONS

DRUG: **Cholestyramine, colestipol, aluminum-** and **magnesium-containing antacids, calcium, iron** may decrease absorption (do not administer within 4 hrs). **Estrogens** may decrease therapeutic effect. May enhance effects of **oral anticoagulants (e.g., warfarin).** HERBAL: None significant. FOOD: None known. LAB VALUES: None known.

AVAILABILITY (Rx)

Capsules: ***(Tirosint):*** 13 mcg, 25 mcg, 50 mcg, 75 mcg, 88 mcg, 100 mcg, 112 mcg, 125 mcg, 137 mcg, 150 mcg. **Injection, Powder for Reconstitution:** 100 mcg, 200 mcg, 500 mcg. **Solution, Oral** ***(Tirosint):*** 13 mcg/mL, 25 mcg/mL, 50 mcg/mL, 75 mcg/mL, 88 mcg/mL 100 mcg/mL, 112 mcg/mL, 125 mcg/mL, 137 mcg/mL, 150 mcg/mL, 175 mcg/mL, 200 mcg/mL. **Tablets:** 25 mcg, 50 mcg, 75 mcg, 88 mcg, 100 mcg, 112 mcg, 125 mcg, 137 mcg, 150 mcg, 175 mcg, 200 mcg, 300 mcg.

ADMINISTRATION/HANDLING

◀ALERT▶ Do not interchange brands (known issues with bioequivalence between manufacturers).

IV

Reconstitution • Reconstitute 200-mcg or 500-mcg vial with 5 mL 0.9% NaCl to provide concentration of 40 or 100 mcg/mL, respectively; shake until clear.
Rate of administration • Use immediately; discard unused portions. • Give each 100 mcg or less over 1 min.
Storage • Store vials at room temperature.

PO

• Administer in the morning on an empty stomach, 30 min before food. • Administer before breakfast to prevent insomnia. • Tablets may be crushed. • Take 4 hrs apart from antacids, iron, calcium supplements.

IV INCOMPATIBILITIES

Do not use or mix with other IV solutions.

INDICATIONS/ROUTES/DOSAGE

Note: Doses based on clinical response and laboratory parameters. IV dose is 75–80% of oral dose once daily.

Hypothyroidism

Note: Adjust dose q3–6wks based on clinical response and serum TSH and/or free T4 concentrations.

PO: ADULTS 60 YRS OR YOUNGER WITHOUT EVIDENCE OF CORONARY HEART DISEASE: 1.6 mcg/kg/day as single daily dose. ADULTS OLDER THAN 60 YRS WITHOUT EVIDENCE OF CORONARY HEART DISEASE: Initially, 25–50 mcg once daily. ADULTS WITH CARDIAC DISEASE: Initially, 12.5–50 mcg/day. Adjust dose by 12.5–25 mcg/day at 6–8-wk intervals. CHILDREN OLDER THAN 12 YRS, GROWTH AND PUBERTY INCOMPLETE: 2–3 mcg/kg/day. CHILDREN 6–12 YRS: 4–5 mcg/kg/day. CHILDREN 1–5 YRS: 5–6 mcg/kg/day. CHILDREN 6–12 MOS: 6–8 mcg/kg/day. CHILDREN 3–5 MOS: 8–10 mcg/kg/day. CHILDREN YOUNGER THAN 3 MOS: 10–15 mcg/kg/day.

Myxedema Coma

IV: ADULTS, ELDERLY: Initially, 200–400 mcg, then 50–100 mcg once daily until able to tolerate PO administration.

Pituitary Thyroid-Stimulating Hormone (TSH) Suppression

PO: ADULTS, ELDERLY: Initially, 1.6–2 mcg/kg/day immediately after surgery. Adjust dose after 6 wks based on TSH suppression goals.

Dosage in Renal/Hepatic Impairment

No dose adjustment.

SIDE EFFECTS

Occasional: Reversible hair loss at start of therapy in children. **Rare:** Dry skin, GI intolerance, rash, urticaria, pseudotumor cerebri, severe headache in children.

ADVERSE EFFECTS/TOXIC REACTIONS

Excessive dosage produces signs/symptoms of hyperthyroidism (weight loss, palpitations, increased appetite, tremors, anxiety, tachycardia, hypertension, headache, insomnia, menstrual irregularities). Cardiac arrhythmias occur rarely. Long-term therapy may decrease bone mineral density.

NURSING CONSIDERATIONS

BASELINE ASSESSMENT

Obtain TSH, T_3, T_4, weight, vital signs. Signs/symptoms of diabetes, diabetes insipidus, adrenal insufficiency, hypopituitarism. Treat with adrenocortical steroids before thyroid therapy in coexisting hypothyroidism and hypoadrenalism.

INTERVENTION/EVALUATION

Monitor pulse for rate, rhythm (report pulse greater than 100 or marked increase). Observe for tremors, anxiety. Assess appetite, sleep pattern. **Children: (Undertreatment):** May decrease intellectual development, linear growth. **(Overtreatment):** Adversely affects brain maturation, accelerates bone age. Monitor thyroid function tests.

PATIENT/ FAMILY TEACHING

• Do not discontinue therapy; replacement for hypothyroidism is lifelong. • Follow-up office visits, thyroid function tests are essential. • Take medication at the same time each day, preferably in the morning. • Monitor pulse for rate, rhythm; report irregular rhythm or pulse rate over 100 beats/min. • Promptly report chest pain, weight loss, anxiety, tremors, insomnia. • Children may have reversible hair loss, increased aggressiveness during first few mos of therapy. • Full therapeutic effect may take 1–3 wks.

lidocaine TOP 100

lye-doe-kane
(Lidoderm, Xylocaine)

FIXED-COMBINATION(S)

EMLA: lidocaine/prilocaine (an anesthetic): 2.5%/2.5%. **LidoSite:** lidocaine/EPINEPHrine (a sympathomimetic): 10%/0.1%. **Lidocaine with EPINEPHrine:** lidocaine/EPINEPHrine (a sympathomimetic): 2%/1:50,000, 1%/1:100,000, 1%/1:200,000, 0.5%/1:200,000. **Synéra:** lidocaine/tetracaine (an anesthetic): 70 mg/70 mg.

◆CLASSIFICATION

PHARMACOTHERAPEUTIC: Amide anesthetic. **CLINICAL:** Class 1B antiarrhythmic, anesthetic.

USES

Antiarrhythmic: Rapid control of acute ventricular arrhythmias following MI, cardiac catheterization, cardiac surgery. **Local anesthetic:** Infiltration/nerve block for dental/surgical procedures, childbirth. **Topical anesthetic:** Local skin disorders (minor burns, insect bites, prickly heat, skin manifestations of chickenpox, abrasions). Mucous membranes (local anesthesia of oral, nasal, laryngeal mucous membranes; local anesthesia of respiratory, urinary tracts; relief of discomfort of pruritus ani, hemorrhoids, pruritus vulvae). **Dermal patch:** Relief of chronic pain in postherpetic neuralgia, allodynia (painful hypersensitivity).

PRECAUTIONS

Contraindications: Hypersensitivity to lidocaine. Adams-Stokes syndrome, hypersensitivity to amide-type local anesthetics, supraventricular arrhythmias, Wolff-Parkinson-White syndrome. Severe degree of SA, AV, or intraventricular heart block (except in pts with functioning pacemaker). **Cautions:** Hepatic disease, marked hypoxia, severe respiratory depression, hypovolemia, incomplete heart. History of malignant hyperthermia, shock, elderly pts, HF.

ACTION

Anesthetic: Inhibits conduction of nerve impulses. **Therapeutic Effect:** Causes temporary loss of feeling/sensation. **Antiarrhythmic:** Suppresses automaticity of conduction tissue; increases electrical stimulation threshold of ventricle, His-Purkinje system; and spontaneous depolarization of ventricle during diastole. Blocks initiation/conduction of nerve impulses by decreasing neuronal membrane's permeability to sodium ions. **Therapeutic Effect:** Inhibits ventricular arrhythmias.

PHARMACOKINETICS

Route	Onset	Peak	Duration
IV	30–90 sec	N/A	10–20 min
Local anesthetic	2.5 min	N/A	30–60 min

Completely absorbed after IV administration. Protein binding: 60%–80%. Widely distributed. Metabolized in liver. Primarily excreted in urine. Minimally removed by hemodialysis. **Half-life:** 1–2 hrs.

LIFESPAN CONSIDERATIONS

Pregnancy/Lactation: Crosses placenta. Distributed in breast milk. **Children:** No age-related precautions noted. **Elderly:** More sensitive to adverse effects. Dose, rate of infusion should be reduced. Age-related renal impairment may require dosage adjustment.

INTERACTIONS

DRUG: **Strong CYP3A4 inhibitors (e.g., clarithromycin, ketoconazole, ritonavir), CYP1A2 inhibitors (e.g., ciprofloxacin)** may increase concentration/effect. **Strong CYP3A4 inducers (e.g., carBAMazepine, phenytoin, rifAMPin)** may decrease concentration/effect. **HERBAL:** **St. John's wort** may decrease concentration/effect. **FOOD:** None known. **LAB VALUES:** IM lidocaine may increase creatine kinase (CK) level. **Therapeutic serum level:** 1.5–6 mcg/mL; **toxic serum level:** greater than 6 mcg/mL.

AVAILABILITY (Rx)

Cream, Topical: 4%. **Infusion Premix:** 0.4% (4 mg/mL in 250 mL, 500 mL); 0.8% (8 mg/mL in 250 mL, 500 mL). **Injection, Solution:** 0.5% (5 mg/mL), 1% (10 mg/mL), 2% (20 mg/mL). **Jelly, Topical:** 2%. **Solution, Topical:** 4%. **Solution, Viscous:** 2%. **Transdermal, Topical:** ***(Lidoderm):*** 4%, 5%.

ADMINISTRATION/HANDLING

◀ALERT▶ Resuscitative equipment, drugs (including O_2) must always be readily available when administering lidocaine by any route.

IV

◀ALERT▶ Use only lidocaine without preservative, clearly marked **for IV use.** **Reconstitution** • For IV infusion, prepare solution by adding 2 g to 250–500 mL D_5W or 0.9% NaCl to provide concentration of 8 mg/mL or 4 mg/mL, respectively. • Commercially available preparations of 0.4% and 0.8% may be used for IV infusion. **Maximum concentration:** 4 g/250 mL (16 mg/mL).
Rate of administration • For IV push, use 1% (10 mg/mL) or 2% (20 mg/mL). • Administer IV push at rate of 25–50 mg/min. • Administer for IV infusion at rate of 1–4 mg/min (1–4 mL); use volume control IV set.
Storage • Store premix solutions at room temperature.

Topical

• Not for ophthalmic use. • For skin disorders, apply directly to affected area or put on gauze or bandage, which is then applied to the skin. • For mucous membrane use, apply to desired area per manufacturer's insert. • Administer lowest dosage possible that still provides anesthesia.

Dermal Patch
Avoid exposing to external heat source. Patch should not get wet (do not wear while bathing/swimming). Patch may be cut to appropriate size.

IV INCOMPATIBILITIES

Amphotericin B complex (Abelcet, AmBisome, Amphotec).

IV COMPATIBILITIES

Amiodarone (Cordarone), calcium gluconate, dexmedetomidine (Precedex), digoxin (Lanoxin), dilTIAZem (Cardizem), DOBUTamine (Dobutrex), DOPamine (Intropin), enalapril (Vasotec), furosemide (Lasix), heparin, insulin, nitroglycerin, potassium chloride.

L

INDICATIONS/ROUTES/DOSAGE

Ventricular Arrhythmias
IV: ADULTS, ELDERLY: Initially, 1–1.5 mg/kg. Refractory ventricular tachycardia, fibrillation: Repeat dose at 0.5–0.75 mg/kg q10–15min after initial dose for a maximum of 3 doses. Total dose not to exceed 3 mg/kg. Follow with continuous infusion (1–4 mg/min) after return of circulation. Reappearance of arrhythmia during infusion: 0.5 mg/kg, reassess infusion. CHILDREN, INFANTS: Initially, 1 mg/kg (**Maximum:** 100 mg). May repeat second dose of 0.5–1 mg/kg if start of infusion longer than 15 min. **Maintenance:** 20–50 mcg/kg/min as IV infusion.

Local Anesthesia
Infiltration, nerve block: ADULTS: Local anesthetic dosage varies with procedure, degree of anesthesia, vascularity, duration. **Maximum:** 4.5 mg/kg or 300 mg. Do not repeat within 2 hrs.

Topical Local Anesthesia
Topical: ADULTS, ELDERLY: Apply to affected areas as needed.

Treatment of Localized Pain
◀ALERT▶ Transdermal patch may contain conducting metal (e.g., aluminum). Remove patch prior to MRI.

Topical: ***(Dermal Patch):*** ADULTS, ELDERLY: Apply to intact skin over most painful area. **Maximum:** Up to 3 patches at a time for up to 12 hrs in a 24-hr period.

Dosage in Renal Impairment
No dose adjustment.

Dosage in Hepatic Impairment
Use caution.

SIDE EFFECTS

CNS effects generally dose-related and of short duration. **Occasional:** **Infiltration/nerve block:** Pain at injection site. **Topical:** Burning, stinging, tenderness at application site. **Rare:** Generally associated with high dose: Drowsiness, dizziness, disorientation, light-headedness, tremors, apprehension, euphoria, sensation of heat, cold, numbness; blurred or double vision, tinnitus, nausea.

ADVERSE EFFECTS/TOXIC REACTIONS

Serious adverse reactions to lidocaine are uncommon, but high dosage by any route may produce cardiovascular depression, bradycardia, hypotension, arrhythmias, heart block, cardiovascular collapse, cardiac arrest. Potential for malignant hyperthermia, CNS toxicity may occur, esp. with regional anesthesia use, progressing rapidly from mild side effects to tremors, drowsiness, seizures, vomiting, respiratory depression. Methemoglobinemia (evidenced by cyanosis) has occurred following topical application of lidocaine for teething discomfort and laryngeal anesthetic spray.

NURSING CONSIDERATIONS

BASELINE ASSESSMENT

Question for hypersensitivity to lidocaine, amide anesthetics. Obtain baseline B/P, pulse, respiratory rate, ECG, serum electrolytes.

INTERVENTION/EVALUATION

Monitor ECG, vital signs during and following drug administration for cardiac performance. If ECG shows arrhythmias, prolongation of PR interval or QRS complex, inform physician immediately. Assess pulse for rhythm, rate, quality. Assess B/P for evidence of hypotension. Monitor for therapeutic serum level (1.5–6 mcg/mL). For lidocaine given by all routes, monitor vital signs, LOC. Drowsiness should be considered a warning sign of high serum levels of lidocaine. **Therapeutic serum level:** 1.5–6 mcg/mL; **toxic serum level:** greater than 6 mcg/mL.

PATIENT/ FAMILY TEACHING

• **Local anesthesia:** Due to loss of feeling/sensation, protective measures may be needed until anesthetic wears off (no ambulation, including special positions for some regional anesthesia). • **Oral mucous membrane anesthesia:** Do not eat, drink, chew gum for 1 hr after application (swallowing reflex may be impaired, increasing risk of aspiration; numbness of tongue, buccal mucosa may lead to bite trauma). • **IV infusions:** Report dizziness, numbness, double vision, nausea, pain/burning, respiratory difficulty. • **Topical:** Report irritation, pain, numbness, swelling, blurred vision, tinnitus, respiratory difficulty.

linaclotide

lin-a-**kloe**-tide
(Constella ✦, Linzess)

■ **BLACK BOX ALERT** ■ Contraindicated in pediatric pts 6 yrs of age and younger. Avoid use in pediatric patients 7 yrs through 17 yrs old.

◆CLASSIFICATION

PHARMACOTHERAPEUTIC: Guanylate cyclase-C (cGMP) agonist. **CLINICAL:** GI agent.

USES

Treatment of irritable bowel syndrome with constipation (IBS-C), chronic idiopathic constipation (CIC) in adults.

PRECAUTIONS

Contraindications: Hypersensitivity to linaclotide. Pediatric pts 6 yrs and younger, known or suspected mechanical GI obstruction. **Cautions:** Diarrhea.

ACTION

Binds on the luminal surface of GI epithelium. Increases cGMP, which stimulates chloride and bicarbonate into intestinal lumen. **Therapeutic Effect:** Increases intestinal fluid, accelerates transit.

PHARMACOKINETICS

Metabolized within GI tract. Minimal distribution beyond GI tissue. Minimal systemic absorption. **Half-life:** N/A.

LIFESPAN CONSIDERATIONS

Pregnancy/Lactation: Unknown if distributed in breast milk. **Children:** Avoid use in pediatric pts 7–17 yrs. Contraindicated in pediatric pts 6 yrs and younger. **Elderly:** No age-related precautions noted.

INTERACTIONS

DRUG: None significant. **HERBAL:** None significant. **FOOD:** None known. **LAB VALUES:** None significant.

AVAILABILITY (Rx)

Capsules: 72 mcg, 145 mcg, 290 mcg.

ADMINISTRATION/HANDLING

PO

• Give on empty stomach at least 30 min prior to first meal of day. • Do not break or crush. • For pts with swallowing difficulty, capsule may be opened and sprinkled on applesauce or into 30 mL bottled water.

INDICATIONS/ROUTES/DOSAGE

Irritable Bowel Syndrome With Constipation

PO: ADULTS 18 YRS AND OLDER, ELDERLY: 290 mcg once daily.

Chronic Idiopathic Constipation

PO: ADULTS 18 YRS AND OLDER, ELDERLY: 72–145 mcg once daily.

Dosage in Renal/Hepatic Impairment
No dose adjustment.

SIDE EFFECTS

Frequent (16%): Diarrhea (may begin within first 2 wks of initiation of treatment). **Occasional (7%–2%):** Abdominal pain, flatulence, headache, abdominal distention. **Rare (1% and Less):** Gastroesophageal reflux, vomiting.

ADVERSE EFFECTS/TOXIC REACTIONS

Severe diarrhea reported in 2% of pts. Viral gastroenteritis reported in 3% of pts. Fecal incontinence, dehydration reported in 1% of pts. Dose reduced or suspended secondary to diarrhea, other GI adverse reaction.

NURSING CONSIDERATIONS

BASELINE ASSESSMENT

Encourage adequate fluid intake. Assess bowel sounds for peristalsis. Assess for abdominal disturbances.

INTERVENTION/EVALUATION

For pts with irritable bowel syndrome, assess for improvement in symptoms (relief from bloating, cramping, urgency, abdominal discomfort). Monitor daily bowel activity, stool consistency. Monitor serum electrolytes in pts with prolonged, frequent, or excessive use of medication.

PATIENT/FAMILY TEACHING

• Institute measures to promote defecation: increase fluid intake, exercise, high-fiber diet. • Report new/worsening episodes of abdominal pain, severe diarrhea. • Do not break, crush, or open capsule. Take whole.

linagliptin

lin-a-**glip**-tin
(Tradjenta)
Do not confuse linagliptin with SAXagliptin or SITagliptin.

FIXED-COMBINATION(S)

Glyxambi: linagliptin/empagliflozin (an antidiabetic): 5 mg/10 mg, 5 mg/25 mg. **Jentadueto:** linagliptin/metFORMIN (an antidiabetic): 2.5 mg/500 mg; 2.5 mg/850 mg; 2.5 mg/1,000 mg. **Jentadueto XR:** linagliptin/metFORMIN (extended-release): 2.5 mg/1,000 mg; 5 mg/1,000 mg. **Trijardy XR:** empagliflozin (an antidiabetic)/linagliptin (an antidiabetic)/metformin (an antidiabetic): 10 mg/5 mg/1,000 mg; 25 mg/5 mg/1,000 mg; 5mg/2.5 mg/1,000 mg; 12.5 mg/2.5 mg/1,000 mg.

◆CLASSIFICATION

PHARMACOTHERAPEUTIC: Dipeptidyl peptidase-4 (DDP-4) inhibitor (gliptin). **CLINICAL:** Antidiabetic agent.

USES

Adjunctive treatment to diet and exercise to improve glycemic control in pts with type 2 diabetes alone or in combination with other antidiabetic agents.

PRECAUTIONS

Contraindications: Hypersensitivity to linagliptin, other DD4 inhibitors. **Cautions:** Concurrent use of other hypoglycemics. Not recommended for use in type 1 diabetes, diabetic ketoacidosis, history of pancreatitis, HF.

ACTION

Prolongs active incretin levels by inhibiting DDP-4 enzyme. **Therapeutic Effect:** Incretin hormones increase insulin synthesis/release from pancreatic beta cells and decrease glucagon secretion from pancreatic alpha cells. Lowers serum glucose levels.

PHARMACOKINETICS

Rapidly absorbed following PO administration. Peak plasma concentration: 1.5 hrs. Extensive tissue distribution. Protein binding: 70%–99%. Minimal metabolism (90% excreted as unchanged metabolite). Excreted primarily in enterohepatic system (80%), urine (5%). **Half-life:** 12 hrs.

LIFESPAN CONSIDERATIONS

Pregnancy/Lactation: Unknown if distributed in breast milk. **Children:** Safety and efficacy not established. **Elderly:** No age-related precautions noted.

INTERACTIONS

DRUG: **Strong CYP3A4 inducers (e.g., carBAMazepine, phenytoin, rifAMPin)** may decrease concentration/effect. **Antidiabetic agents (e.g., insulin, metFORMIN, SAXagliptin, SITagliptin, sulfonylureas)** may increase risk of hypoglycemia. HERBAL: **Ginseng, ginger, other herbs with hypoglycemic activity** may increase risk of hypoglycemia. **St. John's wort** may decrease concentration/effect. FOOD: None known. LAB VALUES: Decreases serum glucose. May increase serum uric acid.

AVAILABILITY (Rx)

Tablets: 5 mg.

ADMINISTRATION/HANDLING

PO

- May give without regard to food.

INDICATIONS/ROUTES/DOSAGE

Note: Dose reduction of insulin and/or insulin secretagogues may be needed.

Type 2 Diabetes Mellitus

PO: ADULTS, ELDERLY: 5 mg once daily.

Dosage in Renal/Hepatic Impairment

No dose adjustment.

SIDE EFFECTS

Occasional (5%): Nasopharyngitis. Rare (less than 2%): Cough, headache.

ADVERSE EFFECTS/TOXIC REACTIONS

Hypoglycemia reported in 7% of pts. Concomitant use of hypoglycemic medication may increase hypoglycemic risk. Pancreatitis, hypersensitivity reactions (angioedema, rash, urticaria, pruritus, bronchospasm) occur rarely.

NURSING CONSIDERATIONS

BASELINE ASSESSMENT

Check blood glucose, hemoglobin A1c level. Assess pt's understanding of diabetes management, routine glucose monitoring. Receive full medication history including herbal products.

INTERVENTION/EVALUATION

Monitor blood glucose, hemoglobin A1c level. Assess for hypoglycemia (diaphoresis, tremors, dizziness, anxiety, headache, tachycardia, perioral numbness, hunger, diplopia, difficulty concentrating), hyperglycemia (polyuria, polyphagia, polydipsia, nausea, vomiting, fatigue, Kussmaul breathing). Screen for glucose-altering conditions: fever, increased activity or stress, surgical procedures. Dietary consult for nutritional education.

PATIENT/FAMILY TEACHING

• Diabetes requires lifelong control. • Diet and exercise are principal parts of treatment; do not skip or delay meals. • Test blood glucose regularly. • When taking combination drug therapy or when glucose demands are altered (excessive alcohol ingestion, insufficient carbohydrate intake, hormone deficiencies, critical illness), have hypoglycemic treatment available (glucagon, oral dextrose). • Monitor daily calorie intake.

L

linezolid

lin-**ez**-oh-lid
(Apo-Linezolid ✦, Zyvox, Zyvoxam ✦)

Do not confuse Zyvox with Zosyn or Zovirax.

◆CLASSIFICATION

PHARMACOTHERAPEUTIC: Oxazolidinone. CLINICAL: Antibiotic.

USES

Treatment of susceptible infections due to aerobic and facultative, gram-positive microorganisms, including *E. faecium* (vancomycin-resistant strains only), *S. aureus* (including methicillin-resistant strains), *S. agalactiae, S. pneumoniae* (including multidrug-resistant strains), *S. pyogenes*. Treatment of pneumonia (community-acquired and hospital-acquired), skin, soft tissue infections (including diabetic foot infections), bacteremia caused by susceptible vancomycin-resistant (VRE) organisms. **OFF-LABEL:** Treatment of prosthetic joint infection. Septic arthritis.

PRECAUTIONS

Contraindications: Hypersensitivity to linezolid. Concurrent use or within 2 wks of MAOIs. **Cautions:** History of seizures, preexisting myelosuppression, medications that may cause bone marrow depression, uncontrolled hypertension, pheochromocytoma, carcinoid syndrome, untreated hyperthyroidism, diabetes, chronic infection; concurrent use of SSRIs, SNRIs, tricyclic antidepressants, triptans, buPROPion.

ACTION

Inhibits bacterial protein synthesis by binding to bacterial ribosomal RNA sites, preventing formation of a functional initiation complex that is essential for bacterial translation. **Therapeutic Effect:** Bacteriostatic against enterococci, staphylococci; bactericidal against streptococci.

PHARMACOKINETICS

Rapidly, extensively absorbed after PO administration. Protein binding: 31%. Metabolized in liver by oxidation. Excreted in urine. **Half-life:** 4–5.4 hrs.

LIFESPAN CONSIDERATIONS

Pregnancy/Lactation: Unknown if distributed in breast milk. **Children:** Safety and efficacy not established. **Elderly:** No age-related precautions noted.

INTERACTIONS

DRUG: **Adrenergic medications (sympathomimetics)** may increase effects. **SSRIs (e.g., escitalopram,** PARoxetine, **sertraline), SNRIs (e.g.,** DULoxetine, **venlafaxine)** may increase risk of serotonin syndrome. **Alcohol, carBAMazepine, maprotiline, tapentadol** may increase adverse effects. **HERBAL:** Supplements containing **caffeine, tyrosine,** or **tryptophan** may precipitate hypertensive crisis. **FOOD:** Excessive amounts of **tyramine-containing foods, beverages** may cause significant hypertension. **LAB VALUES:** May decrease Hgb, neutrophils, platelets, WBC. May increase serum ALT, AST, alkaline phosphatase, amylase, bilirubin, BUN, creatinine, LDH, lipase.

AVAILABILITY (Rx)

Injection Premix: 2 mg/mL in 100-mL, 300-mL bags. **Powder for Oral Suspension:** 100 mg/5 mL. **Tablets:** 600 mg.

ADMINISTRATION/HANDLING

IV

Rate of administration • Infuse over 30–120 min. • Should be administered without further dilution.

Storage • Store at room temperature. • Protect from light. • Yellow color does not affect potency.

PO

• Give without regard to food. • Use suspension within 21 days after reconstitution. Gently invert 3–5 times before administration. • Do not shake.

IV INCOMPATIBILITIES

Amphotericin B complex (Abelcet, AmBisome, Amphotec), co-trimoxazole (Bactrim), diazePAM (Valium), erythromycin (Erythrocin), pentamidine (Pentam IV), phenytoin (Dilantin).

IV COMPATIBILITIES

Calcium gluconate, dexmedetomidine (Precedex), heparin, magnesium, potassium chloride.

INDICATIONS/ROUTES/DOSAGE

Vancomycin-Resistant Infections (VRE)

PO, IV: ADULTS, ELDERLY, CHILDREN OLDER THAN 11 YRS: 600 mg q12h. **CHILDREN 11 YRS AND YOUNGER:** 10 mg/kg q8–12h. **Maximum:** 600 mg/dose.

Pneumonia, Complicated Skin/Skin Structure Infections

PO, IV: ADULTS, ELDERLY, CHILDREN OLDER THAN 11 YRS: 600 mg q12h. **CHILDREN 11 YRS AND YOUNGER:** 10 mg/kg q8h. **Maximum:** 600 mg/dose.

Uncomplicated Skin/Skin Structure Infections

PO: ADULTS, ELDERLY: 600 mg q12h. **CHILDREN OLDER THAN 11 YRS:** 600 mg q12h. **CHILDREN 5–11 YRS:** 10 mg/kg/dose q12h. **Maximum:** 600 mg/dose. **CHILDREN YOUNGER THAN 5 YRS:** 10 mg/kg q8h. **Maximum:** 600 mg/dose.

Usual Neonate Dosage

PO, IV: NEONATES: 10 mg/kg/dose q8–12h.

Dosage in Renal/Hepatic Impairment

No dose adjustment. Administer after HD on dialysis days.

SIDE EFFECTS

Occasional (9%–2%): Diarrhea, nausea, vomiting, insomnia, constipation, rash, dizziness, fever, headache. **Rare (less than 2%):** Altered taste, vaginal candidiasis, fungal infection, tongue discoloration.

ADVERSE EFFECTS/TOXIC REACTIONS

Thrombocytopenia, myelosuppression occur rarely. Antibiotic-associated colitis, other superinfections (abdominal cramps, severe watery diarrhea, fever) may result from altered bacterial balance in GI tract.

NURSING CONSIDERATIONS

BASELINE ASSESSMENT

Obtain appropriate culture specimens for sensitivity testing prior to therapy. Obtain baseline CBC, chemistries. Question medical history as listed in Precautions. Receive full medication history and screen for interactions.

INTERVENTION/EVALUATION

Monitor daily pattern of bowel activity, stool consistency. Mild GI effects may be tolerable, but increasing severity may indicate onset of antibiotic-associated colitis. Be alert for superinfection: fever, vomiting, diarrhea, anal/genital pruritus, oral mucosal changes (ulceration, pain, erythema). Monitor CBC, platelets, Hgb, chemistries.

PATIENT/ FAMILY TEACHING

• Continue therapy for full length of treatment. • Doses should be evenly spaced. • May cause GI upset (may take with food, milk). • Excessive amounts of tyramine-containing foods (red wine, aged cheese) may cause severe reaction (severe headache, neck stiffness, diaphoresis, palpitations). • Avoid alcohol. • Report persistent diarrhea, nausea, vomiting.

liraglutide

TOP 100

leer-a-**gloo**-tide
(Saxenda, Victoza)

BLACK BOX ALERT Causes dose-dependent and treatment duration–dependent thyroid C-cell tumors, including medullary thyroid cancer.

FIXED-COMBINATION(S)

Xultophy: liraglutide 3.6 mg/mL and insulin degludec 100 units/mL.

◆CLASSIFICATION

PHARMACOTHERAPEUTIC: Antihyperglycemic (glucagon-like peptide-1 [GLP-1]) receptor agonist. **CLINICAL:** Antidiabetic agent.

USES

Saxenda: Adjunct to diet and increased physical activity for chronic weight

L

management in adults with body mass index (BMI) of 30 kg/m^2 or greater, or 27 kg/m^2 or greater, with at least one co-morbid condition (e.g., hypertension, diabetes, dyslipidemia). **Victoza:** Adjunct to diet and exercise to improve glycemic control in adults and children 10 yrs of age and older with type 2 diabetes. Reduce risk of major cardiovascular events (e.g., MI, stroke) in adults with type 2 diabetes and established cardiovascular (CV) disease.

PRECAUTIONS

Contraindications: Hypersensitivity to liraglutide. Personal or family history of medullary thyroid carcinoma (MTC), pts with multiple endocrine neoplasia syndrome type 2 (MEN2). **Saxenda:** Pregnancy. **Cautions:** History of pancreatitis, cholelithiasis, alcohol abuse, renal/hepatic impairment. History of angioedema to other GLP-1 receptor agonists. Do not use in type 1 diabetes or diabetic ketoacidosis. Medications requiring a narrow therapeutic index or requiring rapid GI absorption.

ACTION

Stimulates release of insulin from pancreatic beta cells, mimics enhancement of glucose-dependent insulin secretion, decreases inappropriate glucagon secretion, slows gastric emptying, decreases food intake. **Therapeutic Effect:** Improves glycemic control by increasing postmeal insulin secretion, emptying, increasing satiety.

PHARMACOKINETICS

Maximum concentration achieved in 8–12 hrs. Protein binding: 98%. Metabolized to large proteins without a specific organ as major route of elimination. **Half-life:** 13 hrs.

LIFESPAN CONSIDERATIONS

Pregnancy/Lactation: Unknown if distributed in breast milk. **Children:** Safety and efficacy not established. **Elderly:** No age-related precautions noted.

INTERACTIONS

DRUG: May increase hypoglycemic effect of **insulin, sulfonylureas. HERBAL:** None significant. **FOOD:** None known. **LAB VALUES:** Decreases glucose serum levels (when used in combination with insulin secretagogues [e.g., sulfonylureas]).

AVAILABILITY (Rx)

SQ, Solution (Prefilled Pen): ***(Victoza):*** 18 mg/3 mL. ***(Saxenda):*** 18 mg/3 mL. Delivers doses of 0.6 mg, 1.2 mg, 1.8 mg, 2.4 mg, or 3 mg.

ADMINISTRATION/HANDLING

• Insert needle subcutaneously into upper arms, outer thigh, or abdomen, and inject solution. • Do not inject into areas of active skin disease or injury such as sunburns, skin rashes, inflammation, skin infections, or active psoriasis. • Rotate injection sites.

Storage • Refrigerate prefilled pens. • Discard if freezing occurs. • Discard pen 30 days after initial use.

INDICATIONS/ROUTES/DOSAGE

Diabetes (Victoza) With or Without CV Disease

SQ: ADULTS, ELDERLY, CHILDREN 10 YRS AND OLDER: Initial dose: 0.6 mg once daily for at least 1 wk. (**Note:** This dose is intended to reduce GI symptoms during initial titration; it is not effective for glycemic control.) After 1 wk, increase dose to 1.2 mg. If 1.2-mg dose does not result in acceptable glycemic control, dose can be increased to 1.8 mg.

Weight Management (Saxenda)

SQ: ADULTS, ELDERLY: Initially, 0.6 mg once daily for 1 week. Increase wkly by 0.6 mg/day to a target dose of 3 mg once daily. **Note:** Evaluate change in body weight after 12 wks at maximum tolerated dose or 16 wks after initiation. Discontinue if less than 4%–5% of baseline weight not achieved.

Dosage in Renal/Hepatic Impairment

Use caution.

SIDE EFFECTS

Frequent (greater than 13%): Headache, nausea, diarrhea, liraglutide antibody resistance. **Occasional (13%–6%):** Diarrhea, vomiting, dizziness, nervousness, dyspepsia. **Rare (less than 6%):** Weakness, decreased appetite.

ADVERSE EFFECTS/TOXIC REACTIONS

Serious hypoglycemia may occur when used concurrently with insulin analogue (e.g., sulfonylurea); consider lowering dose.

NURSING CONSIDERATIONS

BASELINE ASSESSMENT

Check blood glucose concentration before administration. Discuss pt's lifestyle to determine extent of learning, emotional needs. Ensure follow-up instruction if pt/family does not thoroughly understand diabetes management or glucose testing technique. Dose is gradually increased to improve GI tolerance.

INTERVENTION/EVALUATION

Monitor blood glucose level, food intake. Assess for hypoglycemia (cool wet skin, tremors, dizziness, anxiety, headache, tachycardia, numbness in mouth, hunger, diplopia) or hyperglycemia (polyuria, polyphagia, polydipsia, nausea, vomiting, dim vision, fatigue, deep rapid breathing). Be alert to conditions that alter glucose requirements (fever, increased activity/stress, surgical procedures). Consider lowering dose of insulin analogue to reduce risk of hypoglycemia.

PATIENT/FAMILY TEACHING

• A health care provider will show you how to properly prepare and inject your medication. You must demonstrate correct preparation and injection techniques before using medication at home. • Diabetes requires lifelong control. • Prescribed diet, exercise are principal parts of treatment; do not skip/delay meals. • Continue following dietary instructions, regular exercise program, regular testing of blood glucose level. • Serious hypoglycemia may occur when used concurrently with insulin analogue (e.g., sulfonylurea). • Have source of glucose available to treat symptoms of low blood sugar.

TOP 100

lisdexamfetamine

lis-dex-am-**fet**-a-meen
(Vyvanse)

BLACK BOX ALERT Potential for drug abuse dependency exists. Assess for abuse potential and monitor for abuse potential/dependence.

Do not confuse lisdexamfetamine with dextroamphetamine, or Vyvanse with Glucovance, Vivactil, or Vytorin.

◆CLASSIFICATION

PHARMACOTHERAPEUTIC: Amphetamine (Schedule II). **CLINICAL:** CNS stimulant.

USES

Treatment of attention-deficit/hyperactivity disorder (ADHD), moderate to severe binge eating disorder (BED).

PRECAUTIONS

Contraindications: Hypersensitivity to lisdexamfetamine, amphetamine products. Concurrent use or within 2 wks of use of MAOI. **Cautions:** Hyperthyroidism, glaucoma, agitated states, cardiovascular conditions (hypertension, recent MI, ventricular arrhythmias), elderly, psychiatric/seizures, preexisting psychosis or bipolar disorder, Tourette syndrome. Avoid use in pts with serious structural cardiac abnormalities, cardiomyopathy, arrhythmias, CAD; history of drug abuse and misuse, drug-seeking behavior, dependency.

ACTION

Exact mechanism unknown. Enhances action of DOPamine, norepinephrine by blocking reuptake from synapses, increasing levels in extraneuronal space. **Therapeutic Effect:** Improves attention span in ADHD. Reduces severity of BED.

PHARMACOKINETICS

Rapidly absorbed. Converted to dextroamphetamine. Excreted in urine. **Half-life:** Less than 1 hr.

LIFESPAN CONSIDERATIONS

Pregnancy/Lactation: Has potential for fetal harm. Distributed in breast milk. **Children:** Safety and efficacy not established in pts younger than 6 yrs. **Elderly:** No age-related precautions noted.

INTERACTIONS

DRUG: MAOIs (e.g., phenelzine, selegiline) may increase hypertensive effect. May decrease sedative effect of **antihistamines (e.g., diphenhydrAMINE).** May decrease hypotensive effects of **antihypertensives (e.g., amLODIPine, lisinopril, valsartan). Haloperidol, lithium, urinary acidifying agents (e.g., ammonium chloride, sodium acid phosphate)** may decrease therapeutic effect. May decrease concentration/effect of **PHENobarbital, phenytoin. Tricyclic antidepressants (e.g., amitriptyline, doxepin)** may increase stimulatory effects. **HERBAL:** None significant. **FOOD:** None known. **LAB VALUES:** May increase plasma corticosteroid.

AVAILABILITY (Rx)

Capsules: 10 mg, 20 mg, 30 mg, 40 mg, 50 mg, 60 mg, 70 mg. **Tablets, Chewable:** 10 mg, 20 mg, 30 mg, 40 mg, 50 mg, 60 mg.

ADMINISTRATION/HANDLING

PO

• May be given in the morning without regard to food. • Administer capsule whole; pt must not chew. • Capsules may be opened and dissolved in water and taken immediately. • **Chewable tablets**: Tablets must be chewed thoroughly before swallowing.

INDICATIONS/ROUTES/DOSAGE

ADHD

Note: Assess for cardiac disease and risk of abuse before initiating.

PO: ADULTS, CHILDREN 6 YRS AND OLDER: Initially, 30 mg once daily in the morning. May increase dosage in increments of 10 or 20 mg/day at 3- to 7-day intervals until optimal response obtained. **Maximum:** 70 mg/day.

BED

PO: ADULTS, ELDERLY: Initially, 30 mg once daily in morning. May increase by 20 mg/day at wkly intervals to a target dose of 50–70 mg once daily. **Maximum:** 70 mg/day.

Dosage in Renal Impairment

CrCl 30 mL/min or greater: Maximum: 70 mg/day. **CrCl 15–29 mL/min: Maximum:** 50 mg/day. **CrCl less than 15 mL/min or end-stage renal disease: Maximum:** 30 mg/day.

Dosage in Hepatic Impairment

No dose adjustment.

SIDE EFFECTS

Frequent (39%): Decreased appetite. **Occasional (19%–9%):** Insomnia, upper abdominal pain, headache, irritability, vomiting, weight decrease. **Rare (6%–2%):** Nausea, dry mouth, dizziness, rash, affect change, fatigue, tic.

ADVERSE EFFECTS/TOXIC REACTIONS

Abrupt withdrawal following prolonged administration of high dosage may produce extreme fatigue (may last for wks). Prolonged administration to children with ADHD may produce a suppression of weight and/or height patterns. May produce cardiac irregularities, psychotic syndrome.

NURSING CONSIDERATIONS

BASELINE ASSESSMENT

Assess attention span, impulse control, interaction with others. Question history of cardiomyopathy, glaucoma, hypertension, hyperthyroidism, psychiatric disorder, renal impairment. Receive full medication history and screen for interactions. Assess for drug-seeking behavior; risk of drug abuse and misuse.

INTERVENTION/EVALUATION

Monitor for CNS stimulation, increase in B/P, weight loss, pulse, sleep pattern, appetite; palpitations, cardiac arrhythmia. Observe for signs of hostility, aggression, depression. Screen for drug abuse and misuse, drug-seeking behavior.

PATIENT/FAMILY TEACHING

• Take early in day. • May mask extreme fatigue. • Report pronounced dizziness, decreased appetite, dry mouth, weight loss, new or worsened psychiatric problems, palpitations, dyspnea. • Suddenly stopping treatment may cause extreme fatigue that can last for wks. Discontinuance must be done under the close supervision of health care professional.

lisinopril

TOP 100

lye-**sin**-o-pril
(Prinivil, Qbrelis, Zestril)

BLACK BOX ALERT May cause fetal injury, mortality. Discontinue as soon as possible once pregnancy is detected.

Do not confuse lisinopril with fosinopril, Lipitor, or RisperDAL, or Prinivil with Plendil, Pravachol, Prevacid, PriLOSEC, Proventil, or Restoril, or Zestril with Desyrel, Restoril, Vistaril, Zetia, Zostrix, or Zyprexa.
Do not confuse lisinopril's combination form Zestoretic with PriLOSEC.

FIXED-COMBINATION(S)

Prinzide/Zestoretic: lisinopril/hydroCHLOROthiazide (a diuretic): 10 mg/12.5 mg, 20 mg/12.5 mg, 20 mg/25 mg.

◆CLASSIFICATION

PHARMACOTHERAPEUTIC: ACE inhibitor. **CLINICAL:** Antihypertensive.

USES

Treatment of hypertension in adults and children 6 yrs and older. Adjunctive therapy to reduce signs/symptoms of systolic HF. Treatment of acute MI within 24 hrs in hemodynamically stable pts to improve survival.

PRECAUTIONS

Contraindications: Hypersensitivity to lisinopril, other ACE inhibitors. History of angioedema from treatment with ACE inhibitors, idiopathic or hereditary angioedema. Concomitant use with aliskiren in pts with diabetes. Coadministration with or within 36 hrs of switching to or from a neprilysin inhibitor (e.g., sacubitril). **Cautions:** Renal impairment, unstented unilateral/bilateral renal artery stenosis, volume depletion, ischemic heart disease, cerebrovascular disease, severe aortic stenosis, hypertrophic cardiomyopathy, HF, systolic B/P less than 100, dialysis, hyponatremia; before, during, or immediately after major surgery. Concomitant use of potassium supplements.

ACTION

Competitive inhibitor of angiotensin-converting enzyme (ACE) (prevents conversion of angiotensin I to angiotensin II, a potent vasoconstrictor; may inhibit angiotensin II at local vascular, renal sites). Decreases plasma angiotensin II, increases plasma renin activity, decreases aldosterone secretion. **Therapeutic Effect:** Reduces blood pressure.

PHARMACOKINETICS

Route	Onset	Peak	Duration
PO	1 hr	6 hrs	24 hrs

Incompletely absorbed from GI tract. Protein binding: 25%. Primarily excreted unchanged in urine. Removed by hemodialysis. **Half-life:** 12 hrs (increased in renal impairment).

LIFESPAN CONSIDERATIONS

Pregnancy/Lactation: Crosses placenta. Unknown if distributed in breast milk. **Children:** Safety and efficacy not established. **Elderly:** May be more sensitive to hypotensive effects.

INTERACTIONS

DRUG: **Aliskiren** may increase hyperkalemic effect. May increase potential for allergic reactions to **allopurinol. Angiotensin receptor blockers (e.g., losartan, valsartan)** may increase adverse effects. May increase adverse effects of **lithium, sacubitril.** **HERBAL:** **Herbals with hypertensive properties (e.g., licorice, yohimbe) or hypotensive properties (e.g., garlic, ginger, ginkgo biloba)** may alter effects. **FOOD:** None known. **LAB VALUES:** May increase serum BUN, alkaline phosphatase, bilirubin, creatinine, potassium, ALT, AST. May decrease serum sodium. May cause positive ANA titer.

AVAILABILITY (Rx)

Solution, Oral: ***(Qbrelis):*** 1 mg/mL. **Tablets:** 2.5 mg, 5 mg, 10 mg, 20 mg, 30 mg, 40 mg.

ADMINISTRATION/HANDLING

PO

• Give without regard to food. • Tablets may be crushed.

INDICATIONS/ROUTES/DOSAGE

Hypertension

PO: ADULTS: Initially, 5–10 mg once daily. Evaluate response q4–6wks and titrate dose in 1-step increments prn (e.g., increase the daily dose by doubling), up to 40 mg once daily. **ELDERLY:** Initially, 2.5–5 mg once daily. Evaluate response q4–6wks and titrate dose in 1-step increments prn (e.g., increase the daily dose by doubling), up to 40 mg once daily. **CHILDREN 6 YRS OR OLDER:** Initially, 0.07 mg/kg once daily (up to 5 mg). Titrate at 1- to 2-wk intervals. **Maximum:** 0.6 mg/kg/day or 40 mg/day.

HF

PO: ADULTS, ELDERLY: Initially, 2.5–5 mg/day. May increase by no more than 10 mg/day at intervals of at least 2 wks to a target dose of 20–40 mg once daily.

Acute MI (to improve survival)

PO: ADULTS, ELDERLY: Initially, 2.5–5 mg, then titrate slowly to 10 mg/day or higher, if tolerated. **Maximum:** 40 mg/day.

Dosage in Renal Impairment

CrCl less than 30 mL/min: Not recommended in children. Titrate to pt's needs after giving the following initial dose:

Hypertension

Creatinine Clearance	Initial Dose
10–30 mL/min	5 mg
Less than 10 mL/min or Dialysis	2.5 mg

HF

CrCl less than 30 mL/min or serum creatinine greater than 3 mg/dL: Initial dose: 2.5 mg.

Acute MI

CrCl 30 mL/min or less: Initial dose: 2.5 mg.

Dosage in Hepatic Impairment

No dose adjustment.

SIDE EFFECTS

Frequent (12%–5%): Headache, dizziness, postural hypotension. **Occasional (4%–2%):** Chest discomfort, fatigue, rash, abdominal pain, nausea, diarrhea, upper respiratory infection. **Rare (1% or less):** Palpitations, tachycardia, peripheral edema, insomnia, paresthesia, confusion, constipation, dry mouth, muscle cramps.

ADVERSE EFFECTS/TOXIC REACTIONS

Excessive hypotension (first-dose syncope) may occur in pts with HF, severe salt/volume depletion. Angioedema (swelling of face and lips), hyperkalemia occur rarely. Agranulocytosis, neutropenia may be noted in pts with collagen vascular disease (scleroderma, systemic lupus erythematosus). Nephrotic syndrome may be noted in pts with history of renal disease.

NURSING CONSIDERATIONS

BASELINE ASSESSMENT

Obtain BMP (esp. serum BUN, creatinine, sodium, potassium; CrCl, GFR). Obtain B/P, apical pulse immediately before each dose in addition to regular monitoring (be alert to fluctuations). In pts with renal impairment, autoimmune disease, taking drugs that affect leukocytes or immune response, CBC and differential count should be performed before beginning therapy and q2wks for 3 mos, then periodically thereafter. Question history of aortic stenosis, cardiac disease, cardiomyopathy, renal impairment or stenosis.

INTERVENTION/EVALUATION

Monitor B/P, renal function tests, serum potassium. Assess for edema. Monitor I&O; weigh daily. Monitor daily pattern of bowel activity, stool consistency. Assist with ambulation if dizziness occurs.

PATIENT/ FAMILY TEACHING

• To reduce hypotensive effect, go from lying to standing slowly. • Limit alcohol intake. • Report vomiting, diarrhea, diaphoresis, swelling of face/lips/tongue, difficulty in breathing, persistent cough. • Limit salt intake. • Maintain adequate hydration. • Report decreased urinary output, dark-colored urine, swelling of the hands and feet. • Immediately report allergic reactions, esp. life-threatening swelling of the face or tongue.

lithium

lith-ee-um
(Carbolith ✱, Lithobid, Lithane ✱, Lithmax ✱)

■ **BLACK BOX ALERT** ■ Lithium toxicity is closely related to serum lithium levels and can occur at therapeutic doses. Routine determination of serum lithium levels is essential during therapy.

Do not confuse Lithobid with Levbid or Lithostat.

◆CLASSIFICATION

PHARMACOTHERAPEUTIC: Mood-stabilizing agent. **CLINICAL:** Antimanic.

USES

Management of bipolar disorder. Treatment of mania in pts with bipolar disorder. **OFF-LABEL:** Augmenting agent for depression.

PRECAUTIONS

Contraindications: Hypersensitivity to lithium. Severely debilitated pts, severe cardiovascular disease, concurrent use with diuretics, severe dehydration, severe renal disease, severe sodium depletion or dehydration. **Cautions:** Mild to moderate cardiovascular disease, thyroid disease, elderly, mild to moderate renal impairment, medications altering sodium excretion, pregnancy, pts at risk for suicide, hypovolemia, pts receiving neuromuscular blocking agents.

ACTION

Exact mechanism unknown. Alters cation transport across cell membrane in nerve/muscle cells; influences reuptake of serotonin/norepinephrine. **Therapeutic Effect:** Stabilizes mood, reducing episodes of mania.

PHARMACOKINETICS

Rapidly, completely absorbed from GI tract. Protein binding: None. Primarily excreted unchanged in urine. Removed by hemodialysis. **Half-life:** 18–24 hrs (increased in elderly).

LIFESPAN CONSIDERATIONS

Pregnancy/Lactation: Freely crosses placenta. Distributed in breast milk. **Children:** May increase bone formation or density (alter parathyroid hormone concentrations). **Elderly:** More susceptible to develop lithium-induced goiter or clinical hypothyroidism, CNS toxicity. Increased thirst, urination noted more frequently; lower dosage recommended.

INTERACTIONS

DRUG: **Diuretics (e.g., furosemide, hydroCHLOROthiazide), NSAIDs (e.g., ibuprofen, naproxen, ketorolac), metroNIDAZOLE, ACE inhibitors (e.g., enalapril, lisinopril), angiotensin II antagonists (e.g., losartan, valsartan), SSRIs (e.g., escitalopram, PARoxetine, sertraline), calcium channel blockers (e.g., amLODIPine, dilTIAZem, verapamil)** may increase lithium concentration, risk of toxicity. May increase neurotoxic effect of **tricyclic antidepressants (e.g., amitriptyline). MAOIs (e.g., phenelzine, selegiline)** may increase adverse effects. **HERBAL:** None significant. **FOOD:** None known. **LAB VALUES:** May increase serum glucose, immunoreactive parathyroid hormone, calcium. **Therapeutic serum level:** 0.6–1.2 mEq/L; **toxic serum level:** greater than 1.5 mEq/L.

AVAILABILITY (Rx)

Capsules: 150 mg, 300 mg, 600 mg. **Oral Solution:** 8 mEq/5 mL (equivalent to 300 mg lithium carbonate). **Tablets:** 300 mg.

Tablets (Extended-Release): 300 mg, 450 mg.

ADMINISTRATION/HANDLING

PO

• Administer with meals, milk to decrease GI upset. • Do not break, crush, dissolve, or divide extended-release tablets.

INDICATIONS/ROUTES/DOSAGE

◄ALERT► During acute phase, a therapeutic serum lithium concentration of 0.6–1.2 mEq/L is required. For long-term control, desired level is 0.8–1 mEq/L. Monitor serum drug concentration, clinical response to determine proper dosage.

Usual Dosage

PO: ADULTS, ELDERLY, CHILDREN OLDER THAN 12 YRS: Initially, 600–900 mg. May increase by 300–600 mg increments q1–5days based on response and tolerability. Usual dose: 900–1,800 mg /day in 1–3 divided doses.

Dosage in Renal Impairment

Creatinine Clearance	Dosage
10–50 mL/min	50%–75% normal dose
Less than 10 mL/min	25%–50% normal dose
End-stage renal disease with HD	Dose after HD

Dosage in Hepatic Impairment

No dose adjustment.

SIDE EFFECTS

◄ALERT► Side effects are dose related and seldom occur at lithium serum levels less than 1.5 mEq/L. **Occasional:** Fine hand tremor, polydipsia, polyuria, mild nausea. **Rare:** Weight gain, bradycardia, tachycardia, acne, rash, muscle twitching, peripheral cyanosis, pseudotumor cerebri (eye pain, headache, tinnitus, vision disturbances).

ADVERSE EFFECTS/TOXIC REACTIONS

Lithium serum concentration of 1.5–2.0 mEq/L may produce vomiting, diarrhea, drowsiness, confusion, incoordination, coarse hand tremor, muscle twitching, T-wave depression on ECG. Lithium serum concentration of 2.0–2.5 mEq/L may result in ataxia, giddiness, tinnitus, blurred vision, clonic movements, severe hypotension. Acute toxicity may be characterized by seizures, oliguria, circulatory failure, coma, death.

NURSING CONSIDERATIONS

BASELINE ASSESSMENT

Question history of cardiac/thyroid disease, renal impairment. Assess hydration status. Assess mental status (e.g., mood, behavior). Serum lithium levels should be tested q3–4days during initial phase of therapy, q1–2mos thereafter, and wkly if there is no improvement of disorder or adverse effects occur.

INTERVENTION/EVALUATION

Clinical assessment of therapeutic effect, tolerance to drug effect is necessary for correct dosing-level management. Assess behavior, appearance, emotional status, response to environment, speech pattern, thought content. Monitor serum lithium concentrations, CBC with differential, urinalysis, creatinine clearance. Monitor renal, hepatic, thyroid, cardiovascular function; serum electrolytes. Assess for increased urinary output, persistent thirst. Report polyuria, prolonged vomiting, diarrhea, fever to physician (may need to temporarily reduce or discontinue dosage). Monitor for signs of lithium toxicity. Assess for therapeutic response (interest in surroundings, improvement in self-care, increased ability to concentrate, relaxed facial expression). Monitor lithium levels q3–4days at initiation of therapy (then q1–2mos). Obtain lithium levels 8–12 hrs postdose. **Therapeutic serum level:** 0.6–1.2 mEq/L; **toxic serum level:** greater than 1.5 mEq/L.

PATIENT/ FAMILY TEACHING

• Limit alcohol, caffeine intake. • Avoid tasks requiring coordination until CNS effects of drug are known. • May cause dry mouth. • Maintain adequate salt, fluid intake (avoid dehydration). • Report vomiting, diarrhea, muscle weakness, tremors, drowsiness, ataxia. • Monitoring of serum level is necessary to determine proper dose.

lixisenatide

lix-i-sen-a-tide
(Adlyxin)
Do not confuse lixisenatide with exenatide, liraglutide.

FIXED-COMBINATION(S)

Soliqua: lixisenatide 33 mcg/mL and insulin glargine 100 units/mL.

◆CLASSIFICATION

PHARMACOTHERAPEUTIC: Antihyperglycemic (glucagon-like peptide-1 [GLP-1]) receptor agonist. **CLINICAL:** Antidiabetic agent.

USES

Adjunct to diet and exercise to improve glycemic controls in pts with type 2 diabetes mellitus.

PRECAUTIONS

Contraindications: Hypersensitivity to lixisenatide. **Cautions:** Renal impairment, severe gastroparesis, history of pancreatitis. Not recommended in pts with diabetic ketoacidosis, type 1 diabetes mellitus. Not a substitute for insulin. Medications with narrow therapeutic index or requiring rapid GI absorption.

ACTION

Increases glucose-dependent insulin secretion; decreases inappropriate glucagon secretion. Slows gastric emptying. **Therapeutic Effect:** Improves glycemic control by lowering fasting glucose and postprandial blood glucose.

PHARMACOKINETICS

Widely distributed. Protein binding: not specified. Peak plasma concentration: 1–3.5 hrs. Eliminated through glomerulus filtration and proteolytic degradation. **Half-life:** 3 hrs.

LIFESPAN CONSIDERATIONS

Pregnancy/Lactation: Unknown if distributed in breast milk. **Children:** Safety and efficacy not established. **Elderly:** No age-related precautions noted.

INTERACTIONS

DRUG: May increase hypoglycemic effect when added to **insulin, sulfonylureas (e.g., glipiZIDE, glyBURIDE).** May decrease concentration/effect of **oral contraceptives. Oral contraceptive** should be taken 1 hr before or 11 hrs after lixisenatide. **HERBAL:** None significant. **FOOD:** None known. **LAB VALUES:** Expected to decrease serum glucose, Hgb A1c.

AVAILABILITY (Rx)

Prefilled Injector Pens: 10 mcg/0.2 mL, 20 mcg/0.2 mL.

ADMINISTRATION/HANDLING

SQ

Preparation • Follow instructions for preparation according to manufacturer guidelines. • Visually inspect for particulate matter or discoloration. Solution should appear clear and colorless. • Do not use if solution is cloudy or discolored or if visible particles are observed.

Administration • Administer within 1 hr before the first meal of the day, preferably the same time each day. If a dose is missed, administer within 1 hr prior to next meal. • Insert needle subcutaneously into upper arms, outer thigh, or abdomen, and inject solution. • Do not inject into areas of active skin disease or injury such as sunburns, skin rashes, inflammation, skin infections, or active psoriasis. • Rotate injection sites.

Storage • Refrigerate unused injector pens. • Once injector pen is activated, store at room temperature for up to 14 days. • Do not freeze. • Protect from light.

INDICATIONS/ROUTES/DOSAGE

Type 2 Diabetes Mellitus

SQ: ADULTS, ELDERLY: 10 mcg once daily for 14 days. Increase to 20 mcg once daily on day 15. **Maintenance:** 20 mcg once daily.

Dosage in Renal Impairment

Use caution.

Dosage in Hepatic Impairment

No dose adjustment.

SIDE EFFECTS

Frequent (25%–10%): Nausea, vomiting. **Occasional (9%–1%):** Headache, diarrhea, dizziness, dyspepsia, constipation, abdominal distention, abdominal pain.

ADVERSE EFFECTS/TOXIC REACTIONS

May increase risk of acute renal failure or worsening of chronic renal impairment (esp. in pts with vomiting, dehydration). May increase risk of hypoglycemia when used with other hypoglycemic agents or insulin. Anaphylaxis reported in less than 1% of pts. Other hypersensitivity reactions including angioedema, bronchospasm, laryngeal edema occur rarely. Acute pancreatitis, hemorrhagic or necrotizing pancreatitis were reported. Immunogenicity (auto-lixisenatide antibodies) occurred in 70% of pts.

NURSING CONSIDERATIONS

BASELINE ASSESSMENT

Obtain baseline fasting glucose level, Hgb A1c; BMP. Question history of renal impairment, gastroparesis, hypersensitivity reaction. Screen for use of other hypoglycemic agents or insulin. Assess pt's understanding of diabetes management, routine home glucose monitoring, medication self-administration. Assess hydration status. Obtain dietary consult for nutritional education.

INTERVENTION/EVALUATION

Monitor capillary blood glucose levels, Hgb A1c; renal function test (esp. in pts with renal impairment who report diarrhea, gastroparesis, vomiting). Assess for hypoglycemia (anxiety, confusion, diaphoresis, diplopia, dizziness, headache, hunger, perioral numbness, tachycardia, tremors), hyperglycemia (confusion, fatigue, Kussmaul breathing, nausea, polyuria, vomiting). Screen for glucose-altering conditions (fever, stress, surgical procedures, trauma). Monitor for hypersensitivity reactions; abdominal pain that radiates to the back. Encourage fluid intake. Monitor I&O.

PATIENT/FAMILY TEACHING

- Diabetes requires lifelong control. Diet and exercise are principal parts of treatment; do not skip or delay meals. • Test blood sugar regularly. • Monitor daily calorie intake. • When taking additional medications to lower blood sugar or when glucose demands are altered (excessive alcohol ingestion, insufficient carbohydrate intake, hormone deficiencies, critical illness), have low blood sugar treatment available (glucagon, oral dextrose).
- Persistent, severe abdominal pain that radiates to the back (with or without vomiting) may indicate acute pancreatitis. • Report allergic reactions of any kind, esp. difficulty breathing, itching, rash, swelling of the face or throat. • Oral contraceptives should be taken at least 1 hr before or 11 hrs after dose. • Therapy may cause acute kidney injury or kidney failure; report decreased urine output, amber-colored urine, flank pain.

loperamide

loe-**per**-a-myde
(Imodium A-D)
Do not confuse Imodium with Indocin, or loperamide with furosemide.

FIXED-COMBINATION(S)

Imodium Advanced: loperamide/simethicone (an antiflatulent): 2 mg/125 mg.

◆CLASSIFICATION

PHARMACOTHERAPEUTIC: Antidiarrheal agent. **CLINICAL:** Antidiarrheal.

USES

Controls, provides symptomatic relief of acute nonspecific diarrhea in pts 2 yrs and older; chronic diarrhea associated with inflammatory bowel disease in adults; reduces volume of ileostomy discharge. **OTC:** Control symptoms of diarrhea, including traveler's diarrhea. **OFF-LABEL:** Chemotherapy-induced diarrhea, irinotecan-induced delayed diarrhea.

L

PRECAUTIONS

Contraindications: Hypersensitivity to loperamide. Abdominal pain without diarrhea; children younger than 2 yrs; acute dysentery, acute ulcerative colitis, bacterial enterocolitis caused by invasive organisms, including *Salmonella, Shigella, Campylobacter;* pseudomembranous colitis associated with broad-spectrum antibiotic use. **Cautions:** Hepatic impairment, use in young children. Avoid use when inhibition of peristalsis is undesirable (e.g., potential for ileus, megacolon). Avoid use in pts with risk factors for QT prolongation.

ACTION

Directly affects intestinal wall muscles through opioid receptor. **Therapeutic Effect:** Slows intestinal motility, prolongs transit time of intestinal contents by reducing fecal volume, diminishing loss of fluid, electrolytes, increasing viscosity, bulk of stool. Increases tone of anal sphincter.

PHARMACOKINETICS

Poorly absorbed from GI tract. Protein binding: 97%. Metabolized in liver. Excreted in feces (30%), urine (less than

2%). Not removed by hemodialysis. **Half-life:** 9–14 hrs.

LIFESPAN CONSIDERATIONS

Pregnancy/Lactation: Unknown if drug crosses placenta or is distributed in breast milk. **Children:** Not recommended for pts younger than 2 yrs (infants younger than 3 mos more susceptible to CNS effects). **Elderly:** May mask dehydration, electrolyte depletion.

INTERACTIONS

DRUG: May increase concentration/effects of **QT-prolonging agents (e.g., amiodarone, haloperidol, sotalol). Ranolazine** may increase levels/effects. **HERBAL:** None significant. **FOOD:** None known. **LAB VALUES:** None significant.

L

AVAILABILITY (Rx)

Capsules: 2 mg. **Liquid:** 1 mg/7.5 mL. **Suspension, Oral:** 1 mg/7.5 mL. **Tablet:** 2 mg.

ADMINISTRATION/HANDLING

Liquid

- When administering to children, use accompanying plastic dropper to measure the liquid.

INDICATIONS/ROUTES/DOSAGE

Acute Diarrhea

PO: ***(Capsules):*** **ADULTS, ELDERLY:** Initially, 4 mg, then 2 mg after each unformed stool. **Maximum:** 16 mg/day. **ADOLESCENTS, CHILDREN 12 YRS AND OLDER:** Initially, 4 mg, then 2 mg after each subsequent loose stool. **Maximum:** 8 mg/day. **9–11 YRS WEIGHING 27.1–43 KG:** Initially, 2 mg, then 1 mg after each subsequent loose stool. **Maximum:** 6 mg/day. **6–8 YRS WEIGHING 21–27 KG:** Initially 2 mg, then 1 mg after each subsequent loose stool. **Maximum:** 4 mg/day. **2–5 YRS WEIGHING 13–20 KG:** Initially, 1 mg, then 1 mg after each subsequent loose stool. **Maximum:** 3 mg/day.

Chronic Diarrhea

PO: ADULTS, ELDERLY: Initially, 4 mg, then 2 mg after each unformed stool until diarrhea is controlled. Average maintenance dose: 4–8 mg/day. **Maximum:** 16 mg/day.

Traveler's Diarrhea

PO: ADULTS, ELDERLY: Initially, 4 mg, then 2 mg after each loose bowel movement (LBM). **Maximum:** 16 mg/day (OTC: 8 mg/day).

Dosage in Renal/Hepatic Impairment

No dose adjustment.

SIDE EFFECTS

Rare: Dry mouth, drowsiness, abdominal discomfort, allergic reaction (rash, pruritus).

ADVERSE EFFECTS/TOXIC REACTIONS

Toxicity results in constipation, GI irritation (nausea, vomiting), CNS depression. Activated charcoal is used to treat loperamide toxicity.

NURSING CONSIDERATIONS

BASELINE ASSESSMENT

Do not administer if GI bleeding, mechanical obstruction is suspected. Investigate cause of diarrhea (infectious vs. noninfectious). The use of antidiarrheals in the presence of *C. difficile*–associated diarrhea or other diarrhea caused by bacteria is controversial (drug may inhibit expulsion of toxic bacteria while elderly and debilitated pts are at an increased risk of mortality due to dehydration).

INTERVENTION/EVALUATION

Encourage adequate fluid intake. Assess bowel sounds for peristalsis. Monitor daily pattern of bowel activity, stool consistency. Withhold drug, notify physician promptly in event of abdominal pain, distention, fever.

PATIENT/FAMILY TEACHING

- Do not exceed prescribed dose. • May cause dry mouth. • Avoid alcohol. • Avoid tasks that require alertness, motor skills until response to drug is established. • Report diarrhea lasting more than 3 days, abdominal pain with distention, new-onset fever.

loratadine

lor-**at**-a-deen
(Alavert, Claritin, Claritin Reditabs, Loradamed)
Do not confuse loratadine with clonidine, or Claritin with clarithromycin.

FIXED-COMBINATION(S)

Alavert Allergy and Sinus, Claritin-D: loratadine/pseudoephedrine (a sympathomimetic): 5 mg/120 mg, 10 mg/240 mg.

◆ CLASSIFICATION

PHARMACOTHERAPEUTIC: H_1 antagonist, second generation. **CLINICAL:** Antihistamine.

USES

Relief of nasal, non-nasal symptoms of seasonal allergic rhinitis (hay fever). Treatment of itching due to hives (urticaria).

PRECAUTIONS

Contraindications: Hypersensitivity to loratadine. **Cautions:** Renal/hepatic impairment.

ACTION

Competes with histamine for H_1 receptor sites on effector cells. **Therapeutic Effect:** Prevents allergic responses mediated by histamine (e.g., rhinitis, urticaria, pruritus).

PHARMACOKINETICS

Route	Onset	Peak	Duration
PO	1–3 hrs	8–12 hrs	Longer than 24 hrs

Rapidly, almost completely absorbed from GI tract. Protein binding: 97%; metabolite, 73%–77%. Distributed mainly to liver, lungs, GI tract, bile. Metabolized in liver. Excreted in urine (40%) and feces (40%). Not removed by hemodialysis. **Half-life:** 8.4 hrs; metabolite, 28 hrs (increased in elderly, hepatic impairment).

⌛ LIFESPAN CONSIDERATIONS

Pregnancy/Lactation: Distributed in breast milk. **Children:** Safety and efficacy not established in pts younger than 2 yrs. **Elderly:** More sensitive to anticholinergic effects (e.g., dry mouth, nose, throat).

INTERACTIONS

DRUG: **Aclidinium, ipratropium, tiotropium, umeclidinium** may increase anticholinergic effect. **HERBAL:** **Herbals with sedative properties (e.g., chamomile, kava kava, valerian)** may increase CNS depression. **FOOD:** **All foods** delay absorption. **LAB VALUES:** May suppress wheal, flare reactions to antigen skin testing unless drug is discontinued 4 days before testing.

AVAILABILITY (Rx)

Capsule: 10 mg. **Solution, Oral:** 5 mg/5 mL. **Syrup:** 5 mg/5 mL. **Tablets:** 10 mg. **Tablets, Chewable:** 5 mg. **Tablets, Orally Disintegrating:** 5 mg, 10 mg.

ADMINISTRATION/HANDLING

PO

- May take without regard for food.

Orally Disintegrating Tablets

• Place under tongue. • Disintegration occurs within seconds, after which tablet contents may be swallowed with or without water.

INDICATIONS/ROUTES/DOSAGE

Allergic Rhinitis

PO: **ADULTS, ELDERLY, CHILDREN 6 YRS AND OLDER:** 10 mg once daily or 5 mg twice daily. **CHILDREN 2–5 YRS:** 5 mg once daily.

Urticaria

PO: **ADULTS, ELDERLY, ADOLESCENTS:** Initially, 10 mg once daily. May increase to 10

L

mg twice daily. **CHILDREN 2–12 YRS:** 5 mg once daily.

Dosage in Renal Impairment (CrCl less than 30 mL/min)

PO: ADULTS, ELDERLY, CHILDREN 6 YRS AND OLDER: 10 mg every other day. **CHILDREN 2–5 YRS:** No dose adjustment.

Dosage in Hepatic Impairment

No dose adjustment.

SIDE EFFECTS

Frequent (12%–8%): Headache, fatigue, drowsiness. **Occasional (3%):** Dry mouth, nose, throat. **Rare:** Photosensitivity.

ADVERSE EFFECTS/TOXIC REACTIONS

None significant.

NURSING CONSIDERATIONS

BASELINE ASSESSMENT

Assess lung sounds for wheezing; skin for urticaria, other allergy symptoms.

INTERVENTION/EVALUATION

For upper respiratory allergies, increase fluids to decrease viscosity of secretions, offset thirst, replenish loss of fluids from increased diaphoresis. Monitor symptoms for therapeutic response.

PATIENT/FAMILY TEACHING

• Drink plenty of water (may cause dry mouth). • Avoid alcohol. • Avoid tasks that require alertness, motor skills until response to drug is established (may cause drowsiness). • May cause photosensitivity reactions (avoid direct exposure to sunlight).

LORazepam

lor-**az**-e-pam

(Ativan, LORazepam Intensol)

BLACK BOX ALERT Concomitant use of benzodiazepines and opioids may result in profound sedation, respiratory depression, coma, and death. Reserve concomitant prescribing of these drugs for use in pts for whom alternative treatment options are inadequate. Limit dosages and durations to the minimum required. Follow pts for signs and symptoms of respiratory depression and sedation.

Do not confuse Ativan with Ambien or Atarax, or LORazepam with ALPRAZolam, diazePAM, Lovaza, temazepam, or zolpidem.

CLASSIFICATION

PHARMACOTHERAPEUTIC: Benzodiazepine (Schedule IV). **CLINICAL:** Antianxiety, sedative-hypnotic, antiemetic, skeletal muscle relaxant, amnesiac, anticonvulsant, antitremor.

USES

PO: Management of anxiety disorders, short-term relief of symptoms of anxiety, anxiety associated with depressive symptoms. **IV:** Status epilepticus, preanesthesia for amnesia, sedation. **OFF-LABEL:** Treatment of alcohol withdrawal, psychogenic catatonia, partial complex seizures, agitation (IV administration only), antiemetic for chemotherapy; rapid tranquilization of agitated pt, status epilepticus in children.

PRECAUTIONS

Contraindications: Hypersensitivity to LORazepam, other benzodiazepines. Acute narrow-angle glaucoma, severe respiratory depression (except during mechanical ventilation). **Cautions:** Neonates, renal/hepatic impairment, compromised pulmonary function, depression, concomitant use of CNS depressants; pts at high risk for suicidal ideation and behavior; history of drug abuse and misuse, drug-seeking behavior, dependency.

ACTION

Enhances action of inhibitory neurotransmitter gamma-aminobutyric acid

(GABA) in CNS, affecting memory, motor, sensory, cognitive function. **Therapeutic Effect:** Produces anxiolytic, anticonvulsant, sedative, muscle relaxant, antiemetic effects.

PHARMACOKINETICS

Route	Onset	Peak	Duration
PO	30–60 min	N/A	6–8 hrs
IV	5–20 min	N/A	6–8 hrs
IM	20–30 min	N/A	6–8 hrs

Well absorbed after PO, IM administration. Protein binding: 85%. Widely distributed. Metabolized in liver. Primarily excreted in urine. Not removed by hemodialysis. **Half-life:** 10–20 hrs.

LIFESPAN CONSIDERATIONS

Pregnancy/Lactation: May cross placenta. May be distributed in breast milk. May increase risk of fetal abnormalities if administered during first trimester of pregnancy. Chronic ingestion during pregnancy may produce fetal toxicity, withdrawal symptoms, CNS depression in neonates. **Children:** Safety and efficacy not established in pts younger than 12 yrs. **Elderly:** Use small initial doses with gradual increases to avoid ataxia, excessive sedation, or paradoxical CNS restlessness, excitement. May be more susceptible to cognitive impairment, delirium, falls, fractures.

INTERACTIONS

DRUG: **Valproic acid** may increase concentration/effects. **Alcohol, other CNS depressants (e.g., morphine, PHENobarbital, zolpidem)** may increase CNS depression. **HERBAL:** **Herbals with sedative properties (e.g., chamomile, kava kava, valerian)** may increase CNS depression. **FOOD:** None known. **LAB VALUES:** None significant. **Therapeutic serum level:** 50–240 ng/mL; **toxic serum level:** unknown.

AVAILABILITY (Rx)

Injection Solution: 2 mg/mL, 4 mg/mL. **Oral Solution:** ***(Lorazepam Intensol):*** 2 mg/mL. **Tablets:** 0.5 mg, 1 mg, 2 mg.

ADMINISTRATION/HANDLING

IV

Reconstitution • Dilute with equal volume of Sterile Water for Injection, D_5W, or 0.9% NaCl.

Rate of administration • Give by IV push into tubing of free-flowing IV infusion (0.9% NaCl, D_5W) at a rate not to exceed 2 mg/min.

Storage • Refrigerate parenteral form. • Do not use if discolored or precipitate forms. • Avoid freezing.

IM

• Give deep IM into large muscle mass.

PO

• Give with food. • Tablets may be crushed. • Dilute oral solution in water, juice, soda, or semisolid food.

IV INCOMPATIBILITIES

Aztreonam (Azactam), ondansetron (Zofran).

IV COMPATIBILITIES

Bumetanide (Bumex), cefepime (Maxipime), dexmedetomidine (Precedex), dilTIAZem (Cardizem), DOBUTamine (Dobutrex), DOPamine (Intropin), heparin, labetalol (Normodyne, Trandate), milrinone (Primacor), norepinephrine (Levophed), piperacillin and tazobactam (Zosyn), potassium, propofol (Diprivan).

INDICATIONS/ROUTES/DOSAGE

Anxiety

PO: **ADULTS, ELDERLY:** Initially, 0.5–2 mg q4–6h as needed up to 10 mg/day. **ADOLESCENTS, CHILDREN 12 YRS AND OLDER:** 0.25–2 mg/dose 2–3 times/day. **Maximum dose:** 2 mg.

Status Epilepticus

IV: **ADULTS, ELDERLY:** 4 mg given at maximum rate of 2 mg/min. May repeat in 3–5 min. **ADOLESCENTS, CHILDREN, INFANTS:** 0.05–0.1mg/kg. **Maximum:** 4mg. May repeat in 3–5 min. A nonben-

L

zodiazepine, antiseizure agent should be given to prevent recurrence of seizures.

Dosage in Renal/Hepatic Impairment
PO: No dose adjustment.
IM, IV: Mild to moderate impairment: Use caution. Not recommended in severe impairment.

SIDE EFFECTS

Frequent (16%–7%): Drowsiness, dizziness. **Rare (less than 4%):** Weakness, ataxia, headache, hypotension, nausea, vomiting, confusion, injection site reaction.

ADVERSE EFFECTS/TOXIC REACTIONS

Abrupt or too-rapid withdrawal may result in pronounced restlessness, irritability, insomnia, hand tremor, abdominal cramping, muscle cramps, diaphoresis, vomiting, seizures. Overdose results in drowsiness, confusion, diminished reflexes, coma. **Antidote:** Flumazenil (see Appendix J for dosage).

NURSING CONSIDERATIONS

BASELINE ASSESSMENT

Offer emotional support to anxious pt. Pt must remain recumbent following parenteral administration to reduce hypotensive effect. Assess motor responses (agitation, trembling, tension), autonomic responses (cold or clammy hands, diaphoresis). Assess for drug-seeking behavior; risk of drug abuse and misuse.

INTERVENTION/EVALUATION

Monitor B/P, respiratory rate, heart rate. Diligently screen for suicidal ideation and behavior; new-onset or worsening of anxiety, depression, mood disorder. Screen for drug abuse and misuse, drug-seeking behavior. Assess for paradoxical reaction, particularly during early therapy. Evaluate for therapeutic response: calm facial expression, decreased restlessness, insomnia, decrease in seizure-related symptoms. **Therapeutic serum level:** 50–240 ng/mL; **toxic serum level:** N/A.

PATIENT/FAMILY TEACHING

• Drowsiness usually subsides during continued therapy. • Avoid tasks that require alertness, motor skills until response to drug is established. • Smoking reduces drug effectiveness. • Do not abruptly discontinue medication after long-term therapy. • Do not use alcohol, CNS depressants. • Contraception recommended for long-term therapy. • Seek immediate medical attention if thoughts of suicide, new-onset or worsening of anxiety, depression, or changes in mood occur.

lorlatinib

lor-**la**-ti-nib
(Lorbrena)
Do not confuse lorlatinib with alectinib, brigatinib, ceritinib, crizotinib, erlotinib, lapatinib, neratinib, lenvatinib, loratadine, or lorazepam.

◆CLASSIFICATION

PHARMACOTHERAPEUTIC: Anaplastic lymphoma kinase inhibitor. Tyrosine kinase inhibitor. **CLINICAL:** Antineoplastic.

USES

Treatment of pts with anaplastic lymphoma kinase (ALK)–positive metastatic non–small-cell lung cancer (NSCLC) whose disease has progressed on crizotinib and at least one other ALK inhibitor for metastatic disease; or progressed on alectinib as the first ALK inhibitor therapy for metastatic disease; or progressed on ceritinib as the first ALK inhibitor therapy for metastatic disease.

PRECAUTIONS

Contraindications: Hypersensitivity to lorlatinib. Concomitant use of strong CYP3 inducers. **Cautions:** Baseline cytopenias, hyperlipidemia, cardiac or pulmonary disease, hepatic impairment, concomitant use of strong or moderate CYP3A inhibitors, moderate CYP3A inducers; pt at risk for atrioventricular (AV) block (idiopathic cardiac conduction disorders, ischemic heart disease, increased vagal tone, concomitant use of antiarrhythmics, beta blockers, calcium channel blockers); history of anxiety, depression, suicidal ideation and behavior, mood disorder.

ACTION

Inhibits ALK phosphorylation, ALK downstream signaling proteins, multiple mutant forms of ALK (activity against ALK, ROS1, TYK1, FER, FPS, TRKA, TRKB, TRKC, FAK, FAK2, and ACK). Also has activity against cells expressing EML4-ALK. **Therapeutic Effect:** Expresses antitumor activity against ALK mutant forms in NSCLC in pts who have progressed with alectinib, ceritinib, or crizotinib.

PHARMACOKINETICS

Widely distributed. Metabolized in liver. Protein binding: 66%. Peak plasma concentration: 1.2–2 hrs. Excreted in urine (48%), feces (41%). **Half-life:** 24 hrs.

⌛ LIFESPAN CONSIDERATIONS

Pregnancy/Lactation: Avoid pregnancy; may cause fetal harm. Females of reproductive potential must use effective nonhormonal contraception during treatment and for at least 6 mos after discontinuation. Hormonal contraception may become ineffective with treatment. Unknown if distributed in breast milk. Breastfeeding not recommended during treatment and for at least 7 days after discontinuation. **Males:** Males with female partners of reproductive potential must use barrier methods during treatment and for at least 3 mos after discontinuation. May impair fertility. **Children:** Safety and efficacy not established. **Elderly:** No age-related precautions noted.

INTERACTIONS

DRUG: **Strong CYP3A4 inhibitors (e.g., clarithromycin, ketoconazole)** may increase concentration/effect. **Strong CYP3A4 inducers (e.g., carBAMazepine, phenytoin, rifAMPin)** may decrease concentration/effect; use contraindicated due to risk of severe hepatotoxicity. **Moderate CYP3A inducers (e.g., bosentan, nafcillin)** may decrease concentration/effect. **HERBAL:** **St. John's wort** may decrease concentration/effect; use contraindicated. **FOOD:** None known. **LAB VALUES:** May increase serum alkaline phosphatase, ALT, AST, amylase, cholesterol, glucose, lipase, potassium, triglycerides. May decrease Hgb, lymphocytes, platelets, RBCs; serum albumin, phosphate, magnesium.

AVAILABILITY (Rx)

Tablets: 25 mg, 100 mg.

ADMINISTRATION/HANDLING

PO

• Give without regard to food. • Administer tablets whole; do not break, crush, cut, or divide. Tablets cannot be chewed. Do not give is tablet is broken, cracked, or not intact. • If vomiting occurs after administration, give next dose at regularly scheduled time. • If a dose is missed, administer as soon as possible. • Do not give a missed dose within 4 hrs of next dose.

INDICATIONS/ROUTES/DOSAGE

Non–Small-Cell Lung Cancer

PO: ADULTS, ELDERLY: 100 mg once daily. Continue until disease progression or unacceptable toxicity.

Dose Reduction Schedule

First reduction: 75 mg once daily. **Second reduction:** 50 mg once daily. **Unable to tolerate 50-mg dose:** Permanently discontinue.

Dose Modification

Based on Common Terminology Criteria for Adverse Events (CTCAE).

Atrioventricular (AV) Block

Second-degree AV block: Withhold treatment until PR interval is less than 200 msec, then resume at reduced dose. **First occurrence of complete AV block:** Withhold treatment until PR interval is less than 200 msec or pacemaker is placed. If pacemaker is placed, resume at same dose. If pacemaker is not placed, resume at reduced dose. **Recurrent complete AV block:** Place pacemaker or permanently discontinue.

Central Nervous System (CNS) Effects

Grade 1 CNS effects: Maintain dose or withhold treatment until improved to baseline, then resume at same dose or reduced dose. **Grade 2 or 3 CNS effects:** Withhold treatment until improved to Grade 1 or 0, then resume at reduced dose. **Grade 4 CNS effects:** Permanently discontinue.

Hyperlipidemia

Grade 4 hypercholesterolemia or hypertriglyceridemia: Withhold treatment until improved to Grade 2 or less, then resume at same dose. **Recurrent severe hypercholesterolemia or hypertriglyceridemia:** Resume at reduced dose.

Interstitial Lung Disease (ILD)

Any grade treatment-related ILD: Permanently discontinue.

Other Adverse Reactions

Any Grade 1 or Grade 2 Reaction: Maintain dose or reduce dose.

Any Grade 3 or Grade 4 reaction: Withhold treatment until improved to Grade 2 or less (or baseline), then resume at reduced dose.

Concomitant Use of Strong CYP3A Inhibitors

If strong CYP3A inhibitor cannot be discontinued, reduce dose to 75 mg. If dose was reduced to 75 mg due to adverse reactions and a CYP3A inhibitor is started, reduce dose to 50 mg. If CYP3A inhibitor is discontinued for 3 half-lives, may resume dose prior to starting CYP3A inhibitor.

Concomitant Use of Moderate CYP3A Inducers

Note: Concomitant use of strong CYP3A inducers is contraindicated.

If moderate CYP3A inducer cannot be discontinued, consider discontinuing CYP3A inducer or discontinuing treatment if Grade 2 or higher hepatotoxicity occurs.

Dosage in Renal Impairment

Mild to moderate impairment: No dose adjustment. **Severe impairment:** Not specified; use caution.

Dosage in Hepatic Impairment

Mild impairment: No dose adjustment. **Moderate to severe impairment:** Not specified; use caution.

SIDE EFFECTS

Frequent (57%–18%): Edema (generalized, peripheral), peripheral neuropathy, cognitive effects (amnesia, memory impairment, disorientation), dyspnea, fatigue, asthenia, weight gain, mood effects (aggression, agitation, anxiety, depression, mood swings), arthralgia, diarrhea, headache, cough, nausea. **Occasional (17%–10%):** Myalgia, dizziness, vision disorder, constipation, rash, back pain, extremity pain, vomiting, speech effects (aphasia, dysarthria), pyrexia, sleep effects (abnormal dreams, insomnia, nightmares, sleep talking).

ADVERSE EFFECTS/TOXIC REACTIONS

Anemia, lymphopenia, thrombocytopenia is an expected response to therapy. Concomitant use with moderate CYP3A inducers my increase risk of hepatotoxicity. CNS reactions including hallucinations, seizures, suicidal ideation, and changes in cognitive function, mental status, mood, sleep, speech reported in 54% of pts. Grade 3 or 4 elevations in total cholesterol, triglycerides reported in 18% of pts. AV block and PR internal prolongation reported in 1% of pts. Life-threatening ILD/pneumonitis reported in 2% of pts. Other adverse effects, including pneumonia, pulmonary edema, myocardial infarction, embolism, peripheral artery occlusion, respiratory failure, occur rarely.

NURSING CONSIDERATIONS

BASELINE ASSESSMENT

Obtain CBC, LFT, serum cholesterol, triglycerides, ECG; pregnancy test in female pts of reproductive potential. Confirm compliance of effective contraception. Verify ALK-positive NSCLC status. Discontinue strong CYP3A4 inducers for 3 half-lives prior to initiation. Consider initiating or increasing dose of antihyperlipidemic agents. Screen for active infection. Question history of anxiety, depression, mood disorder, suicidal ideation and behavior; cardiac or pulmonary disease, hepatic impairment. Receive full medication history and screen for interactions/contraindications. Conduct baseline neurologic exam. Offer emotional support.

INTERVENTION/EVALUATION

Monitor CBC, LFT periodically. Monitor serum cholesterol, triglycerides monthly for 2 mos, then periodically thereafter. Monitor ECG periodically (or more frequently if symptoms of AV block occur [dizziness, chest pain, syncope]). If moderate CYP3A inducer cannot be discontinued, monitor LFT 48 hrs after initiation and for at least 3 times during the first week after initiation. Diligently monitor for suicidal ideation and behavior; new-onset or worsening of anxiety, depression, mood disorder. Consider mental health consultation if psychiatric disorder suspected. Conduct regular neurologic exams to rule out CNS effects. Consider ABG, radiologic test if ILD/pneumonitis (excessive cough, dyspnea, hypoxia) is suspected. If treatment related toxicities occur, consider referral to specialist. Assess skin for rash, dermatitis.

PATIENT/FAMILY TEACHING

• Treatment may depress your immune system response and reduce your ability to fight infection. Report symptoms of infection such as body aches, chills, cough, fatigue, fever. Avoid those with active infection. • Seek immediate medical attention if thoughts of suicide, new-onset or worsening of anxiety, depression, or changes in mood occurs. • Neurologic events including altered speech, hallucinations, seizures may occur. • Report symptoms of heart block (dizziness, chest pain, fainting); liver problems (abdominal pain, bruising, clay-colored stool, amber or dark colored urine, yellowing of the skin or eyes); lung inflammation (excessive cough, difficulty breathing, chest pain); skin reactions (rash). • Use effective contraception to avoid pregnancy. Do not breastfeed. • There is a high risk of interactions with other medications. Do not take newly prescribed medications unless approved by prescriber that originally started therapy. • Avoid grapefruit products, herbal supplements (esp. St. John's wort).

losartan

loe-**sar**-tan
(Cozaar)

■ **BLACK BOX ALERT** ■ May cause fetal injury, mortality. Discontinue as soon as possible once pregnancy is detected.

Do not confuse Cozaar with Colace, Coreg, Hyzaar, or Zocor, or losartan with lorcaserin, valsartan.

FIXED-COMBINATION(S)

Hyzaar: losartan/hydroCHLOROthiazide (a diuretic): 50 mg/12.5 mg, 100 mg/12.5 mg, 100 mg/25 mg.

◆CLASSIFICATION

PHARMACOTHERAPEUTIC: Angiotensin II receptor antagonist. **CLINICAL:** Antihypertensive.

USES

Treatment of hypertension in adults and children 6 yrs and older. Used alone or in combination with other antihypertensives. Treatment of diabetic nephropathy with an elevated creatinine and proteinuria (in pts with type 2 diabetes and history of hypertension). **OFF-LABEL:** Slow rate of progression of aortic root dilation in children with Marfan's syndrome. HF in pts intolerant of ACE inhibitors.

PRECAUTIONS

Contraindications: Hypersensitivity to losartan. Concomitant use of aliskiren in pts with diabetes. **Cautions:** Renal/hepatic impairment, unstented renal arterial stenosis, significant aortic/mitral stenosis. Concurrent use of potassium supplements. Pts with history of angioedema.

ACTION

Blocks vasoconstrictor, aldosterone-secreting effects of angiotensin II, inhibiting binding of angiotensin II to AT_1 receptors. **Therapeutic Effect:** Causes vasodilation, decreases peripheral resistance, decreases B/P.

PHARMACOKINETICS

Route	Onset	Peak	Duration
PO	N/A	6 hrs	24 hrs

Well absorbed after PO administration. Protein binding: 98%. Metabolized in liver. Excreted in feces (60%), urine (35%). Not removed by hemodialysis. **Half-life:** 2 hrs; metabolite, 6–9 hrs.

LIFESPAN CONSIDERATIONS

Pregnancy/Lactation: Has caused fetal/neonatal morbidity, mortality. Potential for adverse effects on breastfed infant. Breastfeeding not recommended. **Children:** Safety and efficacy not established. **Elderly:** May be more sensitive to hypotensive effects.

INTERACTIONS

DRUG: **NSAIDs (e.g., ibuprofen, ketorolac, naproxen)** may decrease effects. **Aliskiren** may increase hyperkalemic effect. May increase adverse/toxicity of **ACE inhibitors (e.g., benazepril, lisinopril).** May increase levels/effects of **lithium.** **HERBAL:** **Herbals with hypertensive properties (e.g., licorice, yohimbe) or hypotensive properties (e.g., garlic, ginger, ginkgo biloba)** may alter effects. **FOOD:** None known. **LAB VALUES:** May increase serum bilirubin, ALT, AST, Hgb, Hct. May decrease serum glucose.

AVAILABILITY (Rx)

Tablets: 25 mg, 50 mg, 100 mg.

ADMINISTRATION/HANDLING

PO

- May give without regard to food.

INDICATIONS/ROUTES/DOSAGE

Hypertension

PO: ADULTS, ELDERLY: Initially, 25–50 mg once daily. Evaluate response q4–6 wks. May increase as needed to 100 mg/day in 1–2 divided doses. **CHILDREN 6–16 YRS:** Initially, 0.7 mg/kg (**maximum:** 50 mg) once daily. Adjust dose to BP response. **Maximum:** 1.4 mg/kg or 100 mg/day.

Diabetic Nephropathy

PO: ADULTS, ELDERLY: Initially, 50 mg/day. May increase to 100 mg/day based on B/P response and tolerability.

Dosage in Renal Impairment

Not recommended if glomerular filtration rate (GFR) less than 30 mL/min.

Dosage in Hepatic Impairment

PO: ADULTS, ELDERLY: Initially, 25 mg/day. May increase up to 100 mg/day.

SIDE EFFECTS

Frequent (8%): Upper respiratory tract infection. **Occasional (4%–2%):** Dizziness, diarrhea, cough. **Rare (1% or less):** Insomnia, dyspepsia, heartburn, back/leg pain, muscle cramps, myalgia, nasal congestion, sinusitis, depression.

ADVERSE EFFECTS/TOXIC REACTIONS

Overdosage may manifest as hypotension and tachycardia. Bradycardia occurs less often. Institute supportive measures.

NURSING CONSIDERATIONS

BASELINE ASSESSMENT

Obtain B/P, heart rate immediately before each dose, in addition to regular monitoring (be alert to fluctuations). Question for possibility of pregnancy. Assess medication history (esp. diuretics).

INTERVENTION/EVALUATION

Maintain hydration (offer fluids frequently). Assess for evidence of upper respiratory infection, cough. Monitor B/P, heart rate. Assist with ambulation if dizziness occurs. Monitor daily pattern of bowel activity, stool consistency.

PATIENT/FAMILY TEACHING

• Use effective contraception to avoid pregnancy. • Avoid tasks that require alertness, motor skills until response to drug is established (possible dizziness effect). • Report any sign of infection (sore throat, fever), chest pain. • Do not take OTC cold preparations, nasal decongestants. • Do not stop taking medication. • Limit salt intake.

lovastatin

loe-va-stat-in
(Altoprev)
Do not confuse lovastatin with atorvastatin, Leustatin, Lotensin, nystatin, pitavastatin, or pravastatin.

FIXED-COMBINATION(S)

Advicor: lovastatin/niacin: 20 mg/500 mg, 20 mg/750 mg, 20 mg/1,000 mg.

CLASSIFICATION

PHARMACOTHERAPEUTIC: HMG-CoA reductase inhibitor. **CLINICAL:** Antihyperlipidemic.

USES

Adjunct to diet to decrease elevated serum total and LDL cholesterol in primary hypercholesterolemia; primary prevention of coronary artery disease; reduction of risk of MI, unstable angina, and in coronary revascularization procedures. Slows progression of coronary atherosclerosis in pts with coronary heart disease. Adjunct to diet in adolescent pts (10–17 yrs) with heterozygous familial hypercholesterolemia having LDL greater than 189 mg/dL or LDL greater than 160 mg/dL with positive family history of premature CV disease or LDL greater than 160 mg/dL with presence of at least 2 other CVD risk factors.

PRECAUTIONS

Contraindications: Hypersensitivity to lovastatin. Active hepatic disease, unexplained persistent elevations of serum transaminases. Pregnancy, breastfeeding. Concomitant use of strong CYP3A4 inhibitors. **Cautions:** History of heavy/chronic alcohol use, renal impairment, hepatic disease; concomitant use of amiodarone, cycloSPORINE, fibrates, gemfibrozil, niacin, verapamil (increased risk of myopathy), elderly.

ACTION

Inhibits HMG-CoA reductase, the enzyme that catalyzes the early step in cholesterol synthesis. **Therapeutic Effect:** Decreases LDL, VLDL, triglycerides; increases HDL.

PHARMACOKINETICS

Route	Onset	Peak	Duration
PO (LDL, cholesterol reduction)	3 days	N/A	N/A

Incompletely absorbed from GI tract (increased on empty stomach). Protein binding: 95%. Hydrolyzed in liver. Primarily excreted in feces. Not removed by hemodialysis. **Half-life:** 1.1–1.7 hrs.

LIFESPAN CONSIDERATIONS

Pregnancy/Lactation: Contraindicated in pregnancy (suppression of cholesterol biosynthesis may cause fetal toxicity) and lactation. Unknown if drug is distributed in breast milk. **Children:** Safety and efficacy not established. **Elderly:** No age-related precautions noted.

INTERACTIONS

DRUG: Strong CYP3A4 inhibitors (e.g., clarithromycin, ketoconazole, ritonavir) may increase concentration, risk of myopathy, rhabdomyolysis.

Colchicine, gemfibrozil may increase risk of myopathy. **HERBAL: St. John's wort** may decrease concentration/effect. **FOOD: Grapefruit products** may increase risk of side effects (e.g., myalgia, weakness). **Red yeast rice** may increase concentration (2.4 mg lovastatin/600 mg rice). **LAB VALUES:** May increase serum ALT, AST, creatine kinase (CK).

AVAILABILITY (Rx)

Tablets: 10 mg, 20 mg, 40 mg.

Tablets: ***(Extended-Release [Altoprev]):*** 20 mg, 40 mg, 60 mg.

ADMINISTRATION/HANDLING

PO

• Immediate-release tablet given with evening meal; extended-release at bedtime. • Avoid intake of large quantities of grapefruit juice (greater than 1 quart). • Do not break, crush, dissolve, or divide extended-release tablets.

INDICATIONS/ROUTES/DOSAGE

Hypercholesterolemia, Primary Prevention of CAD

PO: ***(Immediate-Release):*** **ADULTS, ELDERLY:** Initially, 20 mg/day. Adjust at 4-wk intervals. **Maintenance:** 10–80 mg once daily or in 2 divided doses. **Maximum:** 80 mg/day.

PO: ***(Extended-Release):*** **ADULTS, ELDERLY:** Initially, 20–60 mg once daily at bedtime. Adjust at 4-wk intervals. **Maximum:** 60 mg once daily at bedtime.

Heterozygous Familial Hypercholesterolemia

PO: ***(Immediate-Release):*** **CHILDREN 10–17 YRS:** Initially, 10 mg once daily. May increase in 10-mg increments q3mos until target LDL is achieved. Range: 10–40 mg daily. **Maximum:** 80 mg/day.

Dosage With Concurrent Medication

Amiodarone: Maximum: 40 mg/day. **DilTIAZem, dronedarone, verapamil: Maximum:** ***(Immediate-Release):*** 10 mg/day. ***(Extended-Release):*** 20 mg/day. **Lomitapide:** Consider reduction in dose.

Dosage in Renal Impairment

Use caution.

Dosage in Hepatic Impairment

No dose adjustment.

SIDE EFFECTS

Generally well tolerated. Side effects usually mild and transient. **Frequent (9%–5%):** Headache, flatulence, diarrhea, abdominal pain, abdominal cramping, rash, pruritus. **Occasional (4%–3%):** Nausea, vomiting, constipation, dyspepsia. **Rare (2%–1%):** Dizziness, heartburn, myalgia, blurred vision, eye irritation.

ADVERSE EFFECTS/TOXIC REACTIONS

Potential for cataract development. Occasionally produces myopathy manifested as muscle pain, tenderness, weakness with elevated creatine kinase (CK). Severe myopathy may lead to rhabdomyolysis.

NURSING CONSIDERATIONS

BASELINE ASSESSMENT

Obtain LFT, serum cholesterol, triglycerides; pregnancy test in females of reproductive potential. Receive full medication history and screen for interactions. Obtain diet history.

INTERVENTION/EVALUATION

Monitor LFT. Monitor daily pattern of bowel activity, stool consistency. Monitor for headache, dizziness, blurred vision. Assess for rash, pruritus. Monitor serum cholesterol, triglycerides for therapeutic response. Be alert for malaise, muscle cramping/weakness.

PATIENT/FAMILY TEACHING

• Follow special diet (important part of treatment). • Periodic lab tests are essential part of therapy. • Maintain appropriate birth control measures. • Avoid grapefruit juice, alcohol. • Report severe gastric upset, vision changes, myalgia, weakness, changes in color of urine/stool, yellowing of eyes/skin, unusual bruising.

lumateperone

loo-ma-**te**-per-one
(Caplyta)

BLACK BOX ALERT Elderly pts with dementia-related psychosis who are treated with antipsychotic drugs are at increased risk of death. Not approved in pts with dementia-related psychosis.
Do not confuse lumateperone with abiraterone or testosterone, or Caplyta with Kaletra.

CLASSIFICATION

PHARMACOTHERAPEUTIC: Dopamine and serotonin receptor antagonist. **CLINICAL:** Antipsychotic.

USES

Treatment of schizophrenia in adults.

PRECAUTIONS

Contraindications: Hypersensitivity to lumateperone. **Cautions:** Baseline leukopenia, neutropenia; debilitated, diabetes, dyslipidemia, elderly, fall risk, hepatic impairment; pts at risk for orthostatic hypotension, syncope (e.g., dehydration, elderly, hypovolemia, concomitant use of antihypertensives); pts at risk for aspiration, dysphagia (e.g., CVA, myasthenia gravis, Parkinson's disease); conditions that lower seizure threshold (e.g., drug use/withdraw, head trauma, hyponatremia, hyperthermia, history of seizures); conditions predisposing to infection (e.g., diabetes, renal failure, immunocompromised pts, open wounds). Avoid concomitant use of moderate or strong CYP3A inducers, moderate or strong CYP3A inhibitors.

ACTION

Exact mechanism of action unknown. Antagonist of central dopamine D_2 receptors and serotonin 5-HT_{2A} receptors. **Therapeutic Effect:** Diminishes symptoms of psychotic behavior.

PHARMACOKINETICS

Rapidly absorbed and widely distributed. Metabolized in liver. Protein binding: 97.4%. Excreted in urine (58%), feces (29%). Following oral administration, steady state reached in 5 days.

LIFESPAN CONSIDERATIONS

Pregnancy/Lactation: May increase risk of extrapyramidal symptoms, withdrawal syndrome in neonates when given during the third trimester. Unknown if distributed in breast milk. Breastfeeding not recommended. May impair fertility in females and males. **Males:** May have increased risk of dystonia. **Children:** Safety and efficacy not established. **Elderly:** May increase risk of tardive dyskinesia, orthostatic hypotension, syncope. Not indicated in elderly pts with dementia-related psychosis.

INTERACTIONS

DRUG: **Strong CYP3A inhibitors (e.g., clarithromycin, ketoconazole, ritonavir), moderate CYP3A inhibitors (e.g., dilTIAZem, fluconazole, verapamil), UGT inhibitors (e.g., probenecid, valproic acid)** may increase concentration/effect. **Strong CYP3A4 inducers (e.g., carBAMazepine, phenytoin, rifAMPin), moderate CYP3A inducers (e.g., bosentan, nafcillin)** may decrease concentration/effect. **CNS depressants (e.g., lorazepam, morphine, zolpidem)** may increase CNS depression. **HERBAL:** **Herbals with sedative properties (e.g., chamomile, kava kava, valerian)** may increase CNS depression. **FOOD:** **Grapefruit products** may increase concentration/effect. **LAB VALUES:** May increase serum ALT, AST. May decrease leukocytes, neutrophils.

AVAILABILITY (Rx)

Capsules: 42 mg.

ADMINISTRATION/HANDLING

PO

• Give with food. • Administer whole; do not break, crush, cut, or open capsule.

INDICATIONS/ROUTES/DOSAGE

Schizophrenia

PO: ADULTS, ELDERLY: 42 mg once daily.

Dose Modification

Permanently discontinue in pts with neuroleptic malignant syndrome, neutrophil count less than 1000 cells/mm^3. Consider permanent discontinuation in pts with tardive dyskinesia.

Dosage in Renal Impairment

Mild to severe impairment: Not specified; use caution.

L

Dosage in Hepatic Impairment

Mild impairment: No dose adjustment. **Moderate to severe impairment:** Avoid use.

SIDE EFFECTS

Frequent (24%): Somnolence, sedation. **Occasional (9%–6%):** Nausea, dry mouth. **Rare (5%–2%):** Dizziness, fatigue, vomiting, decreased appetite.

ADVERSE EFFECTS/TOXIC REACTIONS

May increase risk of death in elderly pts with dementia-related psychosis. Most deaths appeared to be cardiovascular (e.g., HF, sudden death) or infectious (e.g., pneumonia) in nature. May increase risk of life-threatening neuroleptic malignant syndrome (NMS). Symptoms of NMS may include hyperpyrexia, muscle rigidity, altered mental status, autonomic instability (irregular pulse/blood pressure, tachycardia, diaphoresis, cardiac arrhythmias); elevated CPK, rhabdomyolysis, acute renal failure. Tardive dyskinesia (potentially irreversible, involuntary, dyskinetic movements) has occurred. Metabolic changes including hyperglycemia, ketoacidosis, hyperosmolar coma, diabetes, dyslipidemia may occur. Agranulocytosis, leukopenia, neutropenia was reported. Cognitive and motor impairment reported in 24% of pts. Other effects may include body temperature dysregulation, dysphagia, dystonia, extrapyramidal symptoms, orthostatic hypotension, falls, syncope, seizures.

NURSING CONSIDERATIONS

BASELINE ASSESSMENT

Obtain fasting blood glucose, fasting lipid profile, vital signs; Hgb A1c in pts with diabetes; CBC in pts with baseline leukopenia, neutropenia; pregnancy test in females of reproductive potential. Screen for active infection. Receive full medication history and screen for interactions. Questions history of diabetes, dementia-related psychosis, hepatic impairment, seizures. Assess risk of dysphagia, aspiration. Initiate fall precautions. Assess appearance, behavior, speech pattern, levels of interest. Offer emotional support.

INTERVENTION/EVALUATION

Monitor fasting blood glucose, lipid profile after initiation and periodically thereafter. Monitor CBC, orthostatic vital signs frequently during the first mos of therapy. Monitor for hyperglycemia (blurred vision, confusion, excessive thirst, Kussmaul respirations, polyuria), infections (cough, fatigue, fever), body temperature dysregulation, dysphagia, dystonia, tardive dyskinesia, NMS. Monitor for drug toxicities if discontinuation or dose reduction of concomitant CYP3A inhibitor is unavoidable. Assess for therapeutic response (greater interest in surroundings, improved self-care, increased ability to concentrate, relaxed facial expression).

PATIENT/FAMILY TEACHING

• Treatment may depress your immune system response and reduce your ability to fight infection. Report symptoms of infection such as body aches, chills, cough, fatigue, fever. Avoid those with active infection until response to drug is established. • Report symptoms of high blood sugar levels (e.g., blurred vision, excessive thirst/hunger, headache, frequent urination); nervous system changes (e.g., abnormal, involuntary movements (e.g., lip smacking, puckering, tongue protrusion or chewing, jaw movement, rapid blinking of the eye), difficulty swallowing, seizures, tremor; spasms of the neck, tongue, face). • Treatment may cause NMS (confusion, high fever, muscle rigidity, high or irregular B/P, heart arrhythmias), a life-threatening condition that can be confused with symptoms of severe infection. • Avoid tasks that require alertness, motor skills until response to drug is established. • Go slowly from lying to standing. • There is a high risk of interactions with other medications. Do not take any newly prescribed medications unless approved by prescriber who originally started treatment. Avoid grapefruit products, herbal supplements (esp. St. John's wort). • Do not breastfeed. Treatment may impair fertility. • Avoid overheating and dehydration.

lurasidone

loo-**ras**-i-done
(Latuda)

BLACK BOX ALERT Elderly pts with dementia-related psychosis are at increased risk for mortality due to cardiovascular events, infectious diseases. Increased risk of suicidal thinking/behavior in children, adolescents, young adults.

◆CLASSIFICATION

PHARMACOTHERAPEUTIC: DOPamine, serotonin receptor antagonist. **CLINICAL:** Second-generation (atypical) antipsychotic.

USES

Treatment of schizophrenia in adults and adolescents (13–17 yrs). Treatment of depression associated with bipolar I disorder as monotherapy (children 10 yrs and older, adults) and as adjunctive therapy (adults) with lithium or valproate.

PRECAUTIONS

Contraindications: Hypersensitivity to lurasidone. Concurrent use with strong CYP3A4 inhibitors (e.g., ketoconazole) and inducers (e.g., rifAMPin). **Cautions:** Cardiovascular disease (HF, history of MI, ischemia, conduction abnormalities), cerebrovascular disease (history of CVA in pts with dementia, seizure disorders), diabetes, Parkinson's disease, renal/hepatic impairment, pts at risk for aspiration pneumonia, pts at risk for suicide, disorders where CNS depression is a feature, pts at risk for hypotension, elderly, head trauma, alcoholism, medications that lower seizure threshold.

ACTION

Antagonizes central DOPamine type 2 and serotonin type 2 receptors. **Therapeutic Effect:** Diminishes symptoms of schizophrenia. Reduces incidence of extrapyramidal side effects.

PHARMACOKINETICS

Absorbed in 1–3 hrs. Steady-state concentration occurs in 7 days. Well absorbed from GI tract (unaffected by food). Protein binding: 99%. Metabolized in liver. Excreted in feces (80%), urine (9%). **Half-life:** 18 hrs.

⌛ LIFESPAN CONSIDERATIONS

Pregnancy/Lactation: Unknown if distributed in breast milk. Breastfeeding not recommended. **Children:** Safety and efficacy not established. **Elderly:** More susceptible to postural hypotension. Increased risk of cerebrovascular events (including stroke), mortality, in elderly pts with psychosis.

INTERACTIONS

DRUG: **Alcohol, CNS depressants (e.g., LORazepam, morphine,**

zolpidem) may increase CNS depression. May enhance CNS depressant effect of **azelastine (nasal). Strong CYP3A4 inducers** (e.g., **carBAMazepine, phenytoin, rifAMPin)** decrease concentration/effect. **Strong CYP3A4 inhibitors (e.g., clarithromycin, ketoconazole, ritonavir)** may increase concentration/effect. HERBAL: **Herbals with sedative properties (e.g., chamomile, kava kava, valerian)** may increase CNS depression. **St. John's wort** may decrease concentration/effect. FOOD: **Grapefruit products** may increase concentration/effect. LAB VALUES: May increase prolactin levels.

AVAILABILITY (Rx)

Tablets: 20 mg, 40 mg, 60 mg, 80 mg, 120 mg.

L

ADMINISTRATION/HANDLING

PO

• Give with food. • Tablets may be crushed.

INDICATIONS/ROUTES/DOSAGE

Schizophrenia

PO: ADULTS, ELDERLY: Initially, 40 mg once daily with food. Increase dose based on response and tolerability. **Maximum:** 160 mg once daily with food. **ADOLESCENTS:** Initially, 40 mg once daily with food. **Maximum:** 80 mg once daily with food.

Bipolar Depression

PO: ADULTS, ELDERLY: (Monotherapy or adjunct to lithium or divalproex): Initially, 20 mg once daily, alone or in combination with lithium or divalproex. May increase in 20 mg increments q2–7 days. **Maximum:** 120 mg/day. **CHILDREN 10 YRS AND OLDER: (Monotherapy):** Initially, 20 mg once daily. May increase dose after 1 wk. **Maximum:** 80 mg/day.

Concomitant Use of Moderate CYP3A4 Inhibitors/Inducers

PO: ADULTS, ELDERLY: ***(Inhibitor):*** Initially, 20 mg/day. **Maximum:** 80 mg/day. ***(Inducer):*** May need to increase lurasidone dose if inducer used for 7 or more days.

Moderate to Severe Renal Impairment

CrCl less than 50 mL/min: Initially, 20 mg/day. **Maximum:** 80 mg/day.

Hepatic Impairment

Mild impairment: No dose adjustment. **Moderate impairment:** Initially, 20 mg/day. **Maximum:** 80 mg/day. **Severe impairment:** Initially, 20 mg/day. **Maximum:** 40 mg/day.

SIDE EFFECTS

Frequent (15%–7%): Drowsiness, sedation, insomnia (paradoxical reaction). **Occasional (6%–3%):** Nausea, vomiting, dyspepsia, fatigue, back pain, akathisia, dizziness, agitation, anxiety. **Rare (2%–1%):** Restlessness, salivary hypersecretion, tongue spasm, torticollis, trismus.

ADVERSE EFFECTS/TOXIC REACTIONS

Extrapyramidal disorder (including cogwheel rigidity, drooling, bradykinesia, tardive dyskinesia, tremors) occurs in 5% of pts. Neuroleptic malignant syndrome (fever, muscle rigidity, irregular B/P or pulse, altered mental status, visual changes, dyspnea) occurs rarely.

NURSING CONSIDERATIONS

BASELINE ASSESSMENT

Question history as listed in Precautions. Assess behavior, appearance, emotional status, response to environment, speech pattern, thought content. Renal function, LFT should be obtained before therapy as dose adjustment is required when initiating therapy.

INTERVENTION/EVALUATION

Supervise suicidal risk pt closely during early therapy (as depression lessens, energy level improves, increasing suicide potential). Monitor for potential neuroleptic malignant syndrome. Assess for therapeutic response (greater interest in surroundings, improved self-care, increased ability to concentrate, relaxed facial expression).

PATIENT/FAMILY TEACHING

• Avoid tasks that may require alertness, motor skills until response to drug is established (may cause drowsiness, dizziness). • Avoid alcohol. • Report trembling in fingers, altered gait, unusual muscle/skeletal movements, palpitations, severe dizziness, fainting, visual changes, rash, difficulty breathing. • Report suicidal ideation, unusual changes in behavior.

L

magnesium

HIGH ALERT

mag-**nee**-zee-um

magnesium chloride

(Mag-Delay, Slow-Mag)

magnesium citrate

(Citroma, Citro-Mag 🍁)

magnesium hydroxide

(Milk of Magnesia)

magnesium oxide

(Mag-Ox 400, Uro-Mag)

magnesium sulfate

(Epsom salt, magnesium sulfate injection)

Do not confuse magnesium sulfate with morphine sulfate.

FIXED-COMBINATION(S)

With aluminum and simethicone, an antiflatulent **(Mylanta).**

◆CLASSIFICATION

CLINICAL: Antacid, anticonvulsant, electrolyte, laxative.

USES

Magnesium chloride: Treatment/prevention of hypomagnesemia. Dietary supplement. **Magnesium citrate:** Evacuation of bowel before surgical, diagnostic procedures. Relieves occasional constipation. **Magnesium hydroxide:** Short-term treatment of constipation, symptoms of hyperacidity, laxative. **Magnesium oxide:** Relief of acid indigestion and upset stomach, short-term relief of constipation. Dietary supplement. **Magnesium sulfate:** Treatment/prevention of hypomagnesemia; prevention and treatment of seizures in severe preeclampsia or eclampsia; pediatric acute nephritis, treatment of arrhythmias due to hypomagnesemia (ventricular fibrillation, ventricular tachycardia, or torsades dė pointes). **OFF-LABEL: Magnesium sulfate:** Asthma exacerbation unresponsive to conventional treatment.

PRECAUTIONS

Contraindications: Antacid: Appendicitis, symptoms of appendicitis, ileostomy, intestinal obstruction, severe renal impairment. **Laxative:** Appendicitis, HF, colostomy, hypersensitivity, ileostomy, intestinal obstruction, undiagnosed rectal bleeding. **Systemic:** Heart block, myocardial damage, IV use for pre-eclampsia/eclampsia during the 2 hrs prior to delivery. **Cautions:** Safety in children younger than 6 yrs not known. **Antacids:** Undiagnosed GI/rectal bleeding, ulcerative colitis, colostomy, diverticulitis, chronic diarrhea. **Laxative:** Diabetes, pts on low-salt diet (some products contain sugar, sodium). **Systemic:** Severe renal impairment. Myasthenia gravis or other neuromuscular diseases.

ACTION

Antacid: Acts in stomach to neutralize gastric acid. **Therapeutic Effect:** Increases pH. **Laxative:** Osmotic effect primarily in small intestine, draws water into intestinal lumen. **Therapeutic Effect:** Promotes peristalsis, bowel evacuation. **Systemic (dietary supplement replacement):** Found primarily in intracellular fluids. **Therapeutic Effect:** Essential for enzyme activity, nerve conduction, muscle contraction. Maintains and restores magnesium levels. **Anticonvulsant:** Blocks neuromuscular transmission, amount of acetylcholine released at motor end plate. **Therapeutic Effect:** Produces seizure control.

PHARMACOKINETICS

Antacid, laxative: Minimal absorption through intestine. Absorbed dose primarily excreted in urine. **Systemic:** Widely distributed. Primarily excreted in urine.

LIFESPAN CONSIDERATIONS

Pregnancy/Lactation: Antacid: Unknown if distributed in breast milk. **Parenteral:** Readily crosses placenta. Distributed in breast milk for 24 hrs after magnesium therapy is discontinued. Continuous IV infusion increases risk of magnesium toxicity in neonate. IV administration should not be used 2 hrs preceding delivery. **Children:** No age-related precautions noted. **Elderly:** Increased risk of developing magnesium deficiency (e.g., poor diet, decreased absorption, medications).

INTERACTIONS

DRUG: May decrease absorption of **quinolones (e.g., ciprofloxacin, levoFLOXacin), tetracycline, bisphosphonates.** **HERBAL:** None significant. **FOOD:** None known. **LAB VALUES: Antacid:** May increase gastrin production, pH. **Laxative:** May decrease serum potassium. **Systemic:** None significant.

AVAILABILITY (Rx)

MAGNESIUM CHLORIDE
Tablets: ***(Mag-Delay, Slow-Mag):*** 64 mg.
MAGNESIUM CITRATE
Oral Solution: ***(Citroma):*** 290 mg/5 mL. **Tablets:** 100 mg.
MAGNESIUM HYDROXIDE
Suspension, Oral: ***(Milk of Magnesia):*** 400 mg/5 mL, 1,200 mg/15 mL. **Tablets:** 400 mg.
MAGNESIUM OXIDE
Capsules: ***(Uro-Mag):*** 140 mg. **Tablets:** ***(Mag-Ox 400):*** 400 mg.
MAGNESIUM SULFATE
Infusion Solution: 10 mg/mL, 20 mg/mL, 40 mg/mL, 80 mg/mL. **Injection Solution:** 125 mg/mL, 500 mg/mL.

ADMINISTRATION/HANDLING

IV

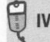

Reconstitution • Must dilute to maximum concentration of 20% for IV infusion. May give IV push, IV piggyback, or continuous infusion.

Rate of administration • For IV push (diluted): Give no faster than 150 mg/min. For IV infusion, maximum rate of infusion is 2 g/hr.

Storage • Store at room temperature.

IM

• For adults, elderly, use 250 mg/mL (25%) or 500 mg/mL (50%) magnesium sulfate concentration. • For infants, children, do not exceed 200 mg/mL (20% diluted solution).

PO (Antacid)

• Shake suspension well before use. • Chewable tablets should be chewed thoroughly before swallowing, followed by full glass of water.

PO (Laxative)

• Drink full glass of liquid (8 oz) with each dose (prevents dehydration). • Flavor may be improved by following with fruit juice, citrus carbonated beverage. • Refrigerate citrate of magnesia (retains potency, palatability).

IV INCOMPATIBILITIES

Amphotericin B complex (Abelcet, AmBisome, Amphotec), cefepime (Maxipime), lansoprazole (Prevacid), pantoprazole (Protonix).

IV COMPATIBILITIES

Amikacin (Amikin), ceFAZolin (Ancef), ciprofloxacin (Cipro), dexmedetomidine (Precedex), DOBUTamine (Dobutrex), enalapril (Vasotec), gentamicin, heparin, HYDROmorphone (Dilaudid), insulin, linezolid (Zyvox), metoclopramide (Reglan), milrinone (Primacor), morphine, piperacillin/tazobactam (Zosyn), potassium chloride, propofol (Diprivan), tobramycin (Nebcin), vancomycin (Vancocin).

INDICATIONS/ROUTES/DOSAGE

MAGNESIUM SULFATE
Hypomagnesemia
Mild to Moderate
IV: ADULTS, ELDERLY: 1–4 g as 1 g/hr. **Maximum:** 12 g/12 hrs.

M

Severe Deficiency

IV: ADULTS, ELDERLY: 4–8 g as 1 g/hr.
IV: CHILDREN: 25–50 mg/kg/dose over 10–20 min. **Maximum single dose:** 2 g.

Usual Dose for Neonates

IM/IV: 25–50 mg/kg/dose q8–12h for 2–3 doses.

Eclampsia/Preeclampsia

IV: ADULTS: 4–6 g loading dose over 20–30 min, then 1–2 g/hr continuous infusion. **Maximum:** 40 g/24 hrs.

MAGNESIUM CHLORIDE

Dietary Supplement

PO: ADULTS, ELDERLY: 2 tablets once daily.

MAGNESIUM CITRATE

Laxative

PO: ADULTS, ELDERLY, CHILDREN 12 YRS AND OLDER: 195–300 mL once or in divided doses. **6–12 YRS:** 100–150 mL once or in divided doses. **2–5 YRS:** 60–90 mL once or in divided doses.

MAGNESIUM HYDROXIDE

Antacid

PO: ADULTS, ELDERLY, CHILDREN 12 YRS AND OLDER: *(400 mg/5 mL):* 5–15 mL as needed up to 4 times/day.

Laxative

PO: ADULTS, ELDERLY, CHILDREN 12 YRS AND OLDER: *(400 mg/5 mL):* 30–60 mL at HS or in divided doses. *(Tablet):* 8 tabs/day in divided doses. **CHILDREN 6–11 YRS:** *(400 mg/5 mL):* 15–30 mL at HS. **CHILDREN 2–5 YRS:** 5–15 mL at HS.

MAGNESIUM OXIDE

Antacid/Dietary Supplement

PO: ADULTS, ELDERLY: 1–2 tablets daily.

Dosage in Renal Impairment

Use caution.

Dosage in Hepatic Impairment

No dose adjustment.

SIDE EFFECTS

Frequent: Antacid: Chalky taste, diarrhea, laxative effect. **Occasional: Antacid:** Nausea, vomiting, stomach cramps. **Antacid, laxative:** Prolonged use or large doses in renal impairment may cause hypermagnesemia (dizziness, palpitations, altered mental status, fatigue, weakness). **Laxative:** Cramping, diarrhea, increased thirst, flatulence. **Systemic (dietary supplement, electrolyte replacement):** Reduced respiratory rate, decreased reflexes, flushing, hypotension, decreased heart rate.

ADVERSE EFFECTS/TOXIC REACTIONS

Magnesium as antacid, laxative has no known adverse reactions. Systemic use may produce prolonged PR interval, widening of QRS interval. Magnesium toxicity may cause loss of deep tendon reflexes, heart block, respiratory paralysis, cardiac arrest. **Antidote:** 10–20 mL 10% calcium gluconate (5–10 mEq of calcium).

NURSING CONSIDERATIONS

BASELINE ASSESSMENT

Assess sensitivity to magnesium. **Antacid:** Assess GI pain (duration, location, quality, time of occurrence, relief with food, causative/exacerbative factors). **Laxative:** Assess for weight loss, nausea, vomiting, history of recent abdominal surgery. **Systemic:** Assess renal function, serum magnesium.

INTERVENTION/EVALUATION

Antacid: Assess for relief of gastric distress. Monitor renal function (esp. if dosing is long term or frequent). **Laxative:** Monitor daily pattern of bowel activity, stool consistency. Maintain adequate fluid intake. **Systemic:** Monitor renal function, magnesium levels, ECG for cardiac function. Test patellar reflexes before giving repeated, rapid parenteral doses (used as indication of CNS depression; suppressed reflexes may be sign of impending respiratory arrest). Patellar reflex must be present, respiratory rate should be 16/min or over before each parenteral dose. Initiate seizure precautions.

PATIENT/FAMILY TEACHING

• **Antacid:** Take at least 2 hrs apart from other medication. • Do not take longer than 2 wks unless directed by physician. • For peptic ulcer, take 1 and 3 hrs after meals and at bedtime for 4–6 wks. • Chew tablets thoroughly, followed by 8 oz of water; shake suspensions well. • Repeat dosing or large doses may have laxative effect. • **Laxative:** Drink full glass (8 oz) liquid to aid stool softening. • Use only for short term. Do not use if abdominal pain, nausea, vomiting is present. • **Systemic:** Report symptoms of hypermagnesemia (altered mental status, difficulty breathing, dizziness, fatigue, palpitations, weakness).

mannitol

man-it-ol
(Osmitrol, Resectisol)
Do not confuse Osmitrol with esmolol.

◆CLASSIFICATION

PHARMACOTHERAPEUTIC: Polyol (sugar alcohol). **CLINICAL:** Osmotic diuretic.

USES

Reduces increased ICP due to cerebral edema, IOP due to acute glaucoma. Promotes urinary excretion of toxic substances. **OFF-LABEL:** Improves renal transplant function. Severe, traumatic brain injury.

PRECAUTIONS

Contraindications: Hypersensitivity to mannitol. Severe dehydration, active intracranial bleeding (except during craniotomy), severe pulmonary edema, congestion, severe renal disease (anuria), progressive HF. **Cautions:** Concurrent nephrotoxic agents, conditions increasing sensitivity to bronchoconstriction (e.g., recent abdominal, thoracic surgery), sepsis, preexisting renal disease, hypernatremia.

ACTION

Increases osmotic pressure of glomerular filtrate, inhibiting tubular reabsorption of water and electrolytes, resulting in increased urine output. Reduces intracranial pressure by decreasing blood viscosity, thereby increasing cerebral blood flow/oxygen transport. **Therapeutic Effect:** Produces diuresis; reduces intraocular pressure (IOP), intracranial pressure (ICP), cerebral edema.

PHARMACOKINETICS

Route	Onset	Peak	Duration
IV (diuresis)	1–3 hrs	N/A	—
IV (reduced ICP)	15–30 min	N/A	1.5–6 hrs

Remains in extracellular fluid. Primarily excreted unchanged in urine. Removed by hemodialysis. **Half-life:** 4.7 hrs.

⌛ LIFESPAN CONSIDERATIONS

Pregnancy/Lactation: Unknown if drug crosses placenta or is distributed in breast milk. **Children:** Safety and efficacy not established in pts younger than 12 yrs. **Elderly:** Age-related renal impairment may require dosage adjustment.

INTERACTIONS

DRUG: May increase nephrotoxic effect of **aminoglycosides (e.g., amikacin, tobramycin).** **HERBAL:** None significant. **FOOD:** None known. **LAB VALUES:** May decrease serum phosphate, potassium. May increase serum sodium, osmolality.

M

AVAILABILITY (Rx)

Injection Solution: ***(Osmitrol):*** 5%, 10%, 15%, 20%, 25%.

ADMINISTRATION/HANDLING

◀ALERT▶ Assess IV site for patency before each dose. Pain, thrombosis noted with extravasation. Use in-line filter (less than 5 microns) for concentrations over 20%. Central venous access is recommended for repeated or scheduled doses.

IV

Rate of administration • Administer test dose for pts with oliguria. • Give IV push over 3–5 min; over 30–60 min for cerebral edema, elevated ICP. Maximum concentration: 25%. • Do not add KCl or NaCl to mannitol 20% or greater. Do not add to whole blood for transfusion.

Storage • Store at room temperature. • If crystals are noted in solution, warm bottle in hot water, shake vigorously at intervals. Cool to body temperature before administration. Do not use if crystals remain after warming procedure.

IV INCOMPATIBILITIES

Cefepime (Maxipime), filgrastim (Neupogen), imipenem-cilastatin (Primaxin).

IV COMPATIBILITIES

CISplatin (Platinol), furosemide (Lasix), linezolid (Zyvox), ondansetron (Zofran), propofol (Diprivan).

INDICATIONS/ROUTES/DOSAGE

USUAL DOSAGE

Elevated Intracranial Pressure

IV: ADULTS, ELDERLY: 0.25–1 g/kg/dose. May repeat q6–8h as needed to maintain serum osmolality <300–325 mOsm/kg. **CHILDREN:** 0.25–1 g/kg/dose; repeat to maintain serum osmolality <300–320 mOsm/kg.

IOP Reduction

IV: ADULTS, ELDERLY: 1.5–2 g/kg over 30–60 min 1–1.5 hrs prior to surgery. **CHILDREN:** 1–2 g/kg over 30–60 min 1–1.5 hrs prior to surgery.

Dosage in Renal Impairment

Contraindicated with severe impairment; caution with underlying renal disease.

Dosage in Hepatic Impairment

No dose adjustment.

SIDE EFFECTS

Frequent: Dry mouth, thirst. **Occasional:** Blurred vision, increased urinary frequency/volume, headache, arm pain, backache, nausea, vomiting, urticaria, dizziness, hypotension, hypertension, tachycardia, fever, angina-like chest pain.

ADVERSE EFFECTS/TOXIC REACTIONS

Fluid, electrolyte imbalance may occur due to rapid administration of large doses or inadequate urine output resulting in overexpansion of extracellular fluid. Circulatory overload may produce pulmonary edema, HF. Excessive diuresis may produce hypokalemia. Fluid loss in excess of electrolyte excretion may produce hypernatremia, hyperkalemia.

NURSING CONSIDERATIONS

BASELINE ASSESSMENT

Obtain serum osmolality, sodium. Obtain baseline B/P, pulse. Assess skin turgor, mucous membranes, mental status, muscle strength. Obtain baseline weight. Assess hydration status.

INTERVENTION/EVALUATION

Monitor urinary output to ascertain therapeutic response. Monitor serum electrolytes, serum osmolality, ICP, renal function, LFT. Assess vital signs, skin turgor, mucous membranes. Weigh daily. Monitor for signs of hypernatremia (confusion, drowsiness, thirst, dry mouth, cold/clammy skin); signs of hypokalemia (changes in muscle strength, tremors, muscle cramps, altered mental status, cardiac arrhythmias). Signs of hyperkalemia include colic, diarrhea, muscle twitching followed by weakness, paralysis, arrhythmias. Inspect IV tubing, in-line filter for crystallization prior to each IV dose.

PATIENT/FAMILY TEACHING

- Expect increased urinary frequency/volume. • May cause dry mouth.

medroxyPROGESTERone

me-**drox**-ee-proe-**jes**-ter-one (Depo-Provera, Depo-SubQ Provera 104, Provera)

■ BLACK BOX ALERT ■ Prolonged use (over 2 yrs) of contraceptive injection form may result in loss of bone mineral density. Limit long-term use (more than 2 yrs). May increase risk of dementia in postmenopausal women. Increased risk of invasive breast cancer in postmenopausal women in combination with conjugated estrogens. **Do not confuse medroxyPROGESTERone with HYDROXYprogesterone, methylPREDNISolone, or methylTESTOSTERone, or Provera with Covera, Femara, Parlodel, or Premarin.**

◆CLASSIFICATION

PHARMACOTHERAPEUTIC: Hormone. **CLINICAL:** Progestin, antineoplastic, contraceptive hormone.

USES

PO: Reduction of endometrial hyperplasia in nonhysterectomized postmenopausal women (concurrently given with estrogen to women with intact uterus), treatment of secondary amenorrhea, abnormal uterine bleeding due to hormonal imbalance. **IM:** Adjunctive therapy, palliative treatment of inoperable, recurrent, metastatic endometrial carcinoma; prevention of pregnancy, endometriosis-associated pain. **OFF-LABEL:** Treatment of paraphilia/hypersexuality.

PRECAUTIONS

Contraindications: Hypersensitivity to medroxyPROGESTERone. Breast cancer (known, suspected, or prior history), history of or active thrombotic disorders (thrombophlebitis, DVT, MI, pulmonary embolism), known or suspected pregnancy, severe hepatic impairment, undiagnosed abnormal vaginal bleeding, cerebrovascular disease. **Cautions:** Conditions aggravated by fluid retention (asthma, seizures, migraine, cardiac/renal dysfunction), diabetes, history of mental depression, preexisting hypercholesterolemia, hypertriglyceridemia.

ACTION

Inhibits secretion of pituitary gonadotropins. **Therapeutic Effect:** Prevents follicular maturation, ovulation. Causes endometrial thinning.

PHARMACOKINETICS

Well absorbed after PO administration. Slowly absorbed after IM administration. Protein binding: 90%. Metabolized in liver. Primarily excreted in urine. **Half-life: PO:** 12–17 hrs. **IM:** 40–50 days.

⌛ LIFESPAN CONSIDERATIONS

Pregnancy/Lactation: Avoid use during pregnancy, esp. first 4 mos (congenital heart, limb reduction defects may occur). Distributed in breast milk. **Children:** Safety and efficacy not established. **Elderly:** No age-related precautions noted.

INTERACTIONS

DRUG: **Strong CYP3A inducers (e.g., carBAMazepine, phenytoin, rifAMPin)** may decrease concentration/effect, resulting in contraceptive failure. May decrease therapeutic effect of **anticoagulants (e.g., warfarin)**. **HERBAL:** **St. John's wort** may decrease effect of progestin contraceptive. **Herbals with progestogenic properties (e.g., bloodroot, chasteberry, yucca)** may increase adverse effects. **FOOD:** None known. **LAB VALUES:** May alter serum thyroid, LFT, PT, HDL, total cholesterol, triglycerides; metapyrone test. May increase LDL.

AVAILABILITY (Rx)

Injection Suspension: ***(Depo-SubQ Provera 104):*** 104 mg/0.65 mL prefilled syringe.

M

(Depo-Provera): 150 mg/mL, 400 mg/mL. **Tablets:** ***(Provera):*** 2.5 mg, 5 mg, 10 mg.

ADMINISTRATION/HANDLING

IM

• Shake vial immediately before administering (ensures complete suspension). • Administer deep IM into gluteal or deltoid muscle. • Shake vigorously prior to administration. • Inject in upper thigh or abdomen (avoid bony areas and umbilicus). • Give over 5–7 sec; do not rub injection area.

PO

• Give with food.

INDICATIONS/ROUTES/DOSAGE

Endometrial Hyperplasia

PO: ADULTS: 5–10 mg/day for 12–14 consecutive days each month starting on day 1 or 16 of cycle.

Secondary Amenorrhea

PO: ADULTS: 5–10 mg/day for 5–10 days, beginning at any time during menstrual cycle.

Abnormal Uterine Bleeding

PO: ADULTS: 5–10 mg/day for 5–10 days, beginning on calculated day 16 or day 21 of menstrual cycle.

Endometrial Carcinoma

IM: ADULTS, ELDERLY: Initially, 400–1,000 mg; repeat at 1-wk intervals.

Pregnancy Prevention

IM: ***(Depo-Provera):*** **ADULTS:** 150 mg q3mos (q13 wks).

SQ: ***(Depo-Subq Provera 104):*** **ADULTS:** 104 mg q3mos (q12–14wks).

Endometriosis

SQ: ***(Depo-SubqProvera 104):*** **ADULTS:** 104 mg q3mos (q12–14 wks).

Dosage in Renal Impairment

No dose adjustment.

Dosage in Hepatic Impairment

Contraindicated with severe impairment.

SIDE EFFECTS

Frequent: Transient menstrual abnormalities (spotting, change in menstrual flow/cervical secretions, amenorrhea) at initiation of therapy. **Occasional:** Edema, weight change, breast tenderness, anxiety, insomnia, fatigue, dizziness. **Rare:** Alopecia, depression, dermatologic changes, headache, fever, nausea.

ADVERSE EFFECTS/TOXIC REACTIONS

Thrombophlebitis, pulmonary/cerebral embolism, retinal thrombosis occur rarely.

NURSING CONSIDERATIONS

BASELINE ASSESSMENT

Obtain usual menstrual history. Question for hypersensitivity to progestins. Obtain baseline weight, B/P, pregnancy test in females of reproductive potential.

INTERVENTION/EVALUATION

Check weight daily; report wkly gain of 5 lb or more. Assess B/P periodically. Assess skin for rash, urticaria. Report development of chest pain, sudden shortness of breath, sudden decrease in vision, migraine headache, pain (esp. with swelling, warmth, redness) in calves, numbness of arm/leg (thrombotic disorders) immediately.

PATIENT/FAMILY TEACHING

• Report sudden loss of vision, severe headache, chest pain, coughing up of blood (hemoptysis), numbness in arm/leg, severe pain/swelling in calf, unusually heavy vaginal bleeding, severe abdominal pain/tenderness. • Depo-Provera Contraceptive injection should be used as long-term birth control method (e.g., longer than 2 yrs) only if other birth control methods are inadequate.

megestrol HIGH ALERT

meh-**jes**-trol
(Megace ES)
Do not confuse megestrol with mesalamine.

◆ CLASSIFICATION

PHARMACOTHERAPEUTIC: Synthetic hormone. **CLINICAL:** Antineoplastic, progestin, appetite stimulant.

USES

Palliative treatment of advanced endometrial or breast carcinoma; treatment of anorexia, cachexia, unexplained significant weight loss in pts with AIDS.

PRECAUTIONS

Contraindications: Hypersensitivity to megestrol. **Suspension:** Known or suspected pregnancy. **Cautions:** History of thrombophlebitis, elderly.

ACTION

Antiestrogenic; interferes with normal estrogen cycle by decreasing release of luteinizing hormone (LH) from anterior pituitary gland by inhibiting pituitary function. Antineoplastic effect may act through an antiluteinizing effect mediated via the pituitary. May increase appetite by antagonizing metabolic effects of catabolic cytokines. **Therapeutic Effect:** Reduces tumor size. Increases appetite.

PHARMACOKINETICS

Well absorbed from GI tract. Metabolized in liver. Excreted in urine. **Half-life:** 13–105 hrs (mean 34 hrs).

LIFESPAN CONSIDERATIONS

Pregnancy/Lactation: If possible, avoid use during pregnancy, esp. first 4 mos. Breastfeeding not recommended. **Children:** Safety and efficacy not established. **Elderly:** Use caution.

INTERACTIONS

DRUG: May decrease therapeutic effect of **anticoagulants (e.g., warfarin).** May increase concentration/effect of **dofetilide. HERBAL:** Avoid **black cohosh, dong quai** in estrogen-dependent tumors. Avoid **herbs with progestogenic properties (e.g., bloodroot, chasteberry, yucca);** may increase adverse effects. **FOOD:** None known. **LAB VALUES:** May alter serum thyroid, LFT, PT, HDL, total cholesterol, triglycerides. May increase LDL.

AVAILABILITY (Rx)

Oral Suspension: ***(Megace ES):*** 40 mg/mL, 625 mg/5 mL. **Tablets:** 20 mg, 40 mg.

ADMINISTRATION/HANDLING

PO

• Store tablets, oral suspension at room temperature. • Shake suspension well before use. • Oral suspension compatible with water, orange juice, apple juice. • Administer without regard to food.

INDICATIONS/ROUTES/DOSAGE

Palliative Treatment of Advanced Breast Cancer

PO: ADULTS, ELDERLY: 40 mg 4 times/day for at least 2 mos.

Palliative Treatment of Advanced Endometrial Carcinoma

PO: ADULTS, ELDERLY: 40–320 mg/day in divided doses for at least 2 mos.

Anorexia, Cachexia, Weight Loss

PO: ADULTS, ELDERLY: Initially, 625 mg (125 mg/mL suspension) or 800 mg (40 mg/mL suspension) daily.

Dosage in Renal Impairment

Use caution.

Dosage in Hepatic Impairment

No dose adjustment.

SIDE EFFECTS

Frequent: Weight gain secondary to increased appetite. **Occasional:** Nausea, breakthrough menstrual bleeding,

M

backache, headache, breast tenderness, carpal tunnel syndrome. **Rare:** Feeling of coldness.

ADVERSE EFFECTS/TOXIC REACTIONS

Thrombophlebitis, pulmonary embolism occur rarely.

NURSING CONSIDERATIONS

BASELINE ASSESSMENT

Obtain pregnancy test in females of reproductive potential. Offer emotional support.

INTERVENTION/EVALUATION

Monitor for tumor response. Monitor pt weight, caloric intake (appetite stimulant).

PATIENT/FAMILY TEACHING

• Contraception is imperative. • Report lower leg (calf) pain, difficulty breathing, vaginal bleeding. • May cause headache, nausea, vomiting, breast tenderness, backache.

M

meloxicam

mel-**ox**-i-kam
(Anjeso, Mobic, Qmiiz ODT, Vivlodex)

■ BLACK BOX ALERT ■ Increased risk of serious cardiovascular thrombotic events, including myocardial infarction, CVA. Increased risk of severe GI reactions, including ulceration, bleeding, GI perforation.

◆CLASSIFICATION

PHARMACOTHERAPEUTIC: NSAID. **CLINICAL:** Anti-inflammatory, analgesic.

USES

Relief of signs/symptoms of osteoarthritis, rheumatoid arthritis (RA). Treatment of juvenile idiopathic arthritis (JIA) in pts 2 yrs of age and older (suspension) and weighing 60 kg or more (tablets).

PRECAUTIONS

Contraindications: Hypersensitivity to meloxicam. Pts with aspirin triad (asthma, rhinitis, aspirin intolerance). History of asthma, urticaria with NSAIDs, perioperative pain in setting of CABG surgery. **Cautions:** Renal/hepatic impairment, asthma, coagulation disorders, hypertension, pts at risk for GI perforation (e.g., Crohn's disease, diverticulitis, GI tract malignancies, peptic ulcers, peritoneal malignancies), history of cardiovascular disease, MI; concurrent use of anticoagulants, fluid retention, HF, dehydration, smoking, alcohol use, elderly, debilitated.

ACTION

Produces analgesic, antipyretic, anti-inflammatory effects by inhibiting prostaglandin synthesis. **Therapeutic Effect:** Reduces inflammatory response, intensity of pain.

PHARMACOKINETICS

Route	Onset	Peak	Duration
PO (Analgesic)	30 min	4–5 hrs	N/A

Well absorbed after PO administration. Protein binding: 99%. Metabolized in liver. Excreted equally in urine, feces. Not removed by hemodialysis. **Half-life:** 15–20 hrs.

⌛ LIFESPAN CONSIDERATIONS

Pregnancy/Lactation: Avoid use at 30 wks gestation or more (may cause premature closure of ductus arteriosus). Distributed in breast milk. May impair fertility in both females and males. **Children:** Safety and efficacy not established in children younger than 2 yrs. **Elderly:** Age-related renal impairment may require dosage adjustment. More susceptible to GI toxicity; lower dosage recommended.

INTERACTIONS

DRUG: May increase anticoagulant effect of **apixaban, dabigatran, edoxaban, rivaroxaban. Bile acid sequestrants (e.g., cholestyramine)** may decrease absorption. May increase nephrotoxic effect of **cycloSPORINE, tacrolimus, tenofovir.** May decrease effect of **loop diuretics**

(e.g., furosemide). May decrease antihypertensive effect of **ACE inhibitors (e.g., enalapril, lisinopril), angiotensin receptor blockers (e.g., losartan, valsartan), beta blockers (e.g., carvedilol, metoprolol).** HERBAL: **Glucosamine, herbals with anticoagulant/antiplatelet properties (e.g., garlic, ginger, ginkgo biloba, ginseng)** may increase concentration/effect. FOOD: None known. LAB VALUES: May increase serum creatinine, ALT, AST.

AVAILABILITY (Rx)

Injection Solution: *(Anjeso):* 30 mg/mL. **Tablets:** *(Mobic):* 7.5 mg, 15 mg. **Capsules:** *(Vivlodex):* 5 mg, 10 mg. **Tablet ODT:** *(Qmiiz):* 7.5 mg, 15 mg.

ADMINISTRATION/HANDLING

IV

• Administer undiluted as an IV bolus over 15 sec.

PO

• Give with food or milk to minimize GI irritation. • **ODT:** Do not remove from blister until ready to administer. Using dry hands, peel backing off the blister; do not push tablet through foil. Remove tablet and place in mouth or on tongue and allow to disintegrate. Swallow with saliva (with or without drinking liquid).

INDICATIONS/ROUTES/DOSAGE

Osteoarthritis, Rheumatoid Arthritis (RA)

PO: *(Mobic):* ADULTS, ELDERLY: Initially, 7.5 mg/day. **Maximum:** 15 mg/day (7.5 mg for pts on dialysis).

Osteoarthritis

PO: *(Vivlodex):* ADULTS, ELDERLY: Initially, 5 mg once daily. May increase to 10 mg once daily.

Pain (Moderate to severe)

IV: ADULTS, ELDERLY: 30 mg once daily.

JIA

PO: CHILDREN, 2 YRS AND OLDER: 0.125 mg/kg once daily. **Maximum:** 7.5 mg.

Dosage in Renal Impairment

Not recommended with severe impairment.

Dosage in Hepatic Impairment

No dose adjustment.

SIDE EFFECTS

Frequent (9%–7%): Dyspepsia, headache, diarrhea, nausea. **Occasional (4%–3%):** Dizziness, insomnia, rash, pruritus, flatulence, constipation, vomiting. **Rare (less than 2%):** Drowsiness, urticaria, photosensitivity, tinnitus.

ADVERSE EFFECTS/TOXIC REACTIONS

May increase risk of severe HF; cardiovascular thrombotic events, including MI. Life-threatening GI effects including inflammation, GI bleeding, ulceration, and perforation of esophagus, small intestines, stomach, and large intestines were reported. Hepatotoxicity reported in 1% of pts. May cause new onset or worsening of hypertension. Hypersensitivity reactions including anaphylaxis may occur. Cutaneous toxicities including Stevens-Johnson syndrome, toxic epidermal necrolysis, exfoliative dermatitis may occur. May mask symptoms of inflammation and fever. Severe renal injury may cause hyperkalemia. In pts treated chronically, peptic ulcer, GI bleeding, gastritis, severe hepatic toxicity (jaundice), nephrotoxicity (hematuria, dysuria, proteinuria), severe hypersensitivity reaction (bronchospasm, angioedema) occur rarely.

NURSING CONSIDERATIONS

BASELINE ASSESSMENT

Assess onset, type, location, duration of pain/inflammation. Inspect appearance of affected joints for immobility, deformities, skin condition. Question history of GI bleeding, gastric or duodenal ulcers, hepatic/renal impairment, asthma.

INTERVENTION/EVALUATION

Monitor CBC, renal function, LFT. Assess for therapeutic response: relief of pain, stiffness, swelling; increased joint mobility; reduced joint tenderness; improved grip strength. Monitor B/P for hypertension. Immediately report abdominal pain, fever, hematemesis, melena; may indicate GI perforation. Monitor for hypersensitivity reactions; symptoms of MI (chest pain, dyspnea, syncope, diaphoresis, arm/jaw pain). Assess skin for cutaneous toxicities. Monitor for symptoms of HF (dyspnea, edema, fatigue, palpitations). Obtain LVEF by echocardiogram if HF is suspected.

PATIENT/FAMILY TEACHING

• Take with food, milk to reduce GI upset. • Treatment may worsen high blood pressure. • Immediately report severe or persistent abdominal pain, bloody stool, fever, vomiting blood; may indicate rupture in GI tract. • Report liver problems (abdominal pain, bruising, clay-colored stool, amber- or dark-colored urine, yellowing of the skin or eyes); kidney problems (decreased urine output, flank pain, darkened urine); toxic skin reactions (rash, skin eruptions); symptoms of heart attack (chest pain, difficulty breathing, jaw pain, nausea, pain that radiates to the left arm, sweating), HF (difficulty breathing, fatigue, palpitations, extremity swelling). Allergic reactions, including anaphylaxis, may occur. • Avoid use after 30 wks gestation.

memantine

TOP 100

me-**man**-teen
(Ebixa ✱, Namenda, Namenda XR)

FIXED-COMBINATION(S)

Namzaric: memantine/donepezil (a cholinesterase inhibitor): 7 mg/10 mg; 14 mg/10 mg; 21 mg/10 mg; 28 mg/10 mg.

◆ CLASSIFICATION

PHARMACOTHERAPEUTIC: NMDA receptor antagonist. **CLINICAL:** Anti-Alzheimer's agent.

USES

Treatment of moderate to severe dementia of Alzheimer's type. **OFF-LABEL:** Treatment of mild to moderate vascular dementia.

PRECAUTIONS

Contraindications: Hypersensitivity to memantine. **Cautions:** Moderate to severe renal impairment, severe hepatic impairment, cardiovascular disease, seizure disorder, GU conditions that raise urine pH level.

ACTION

Decreases effects of glutamate, the principal excitatory neurotransmitter in the brain. Persistent CNS excitation by glutamate is thought to cause symptoms of Alzheimer's disease. **Therapeutic Effect:** May slow clinical deterioration in moderate to severe Alzheimer's disease.

PHARMACOKINETICS

Rapidly, completely absorbed after PO administration. Protein binding: 45%. Undergoes little metabolism; most of dose is excreted unchanged in urine. **Half-life:** 60–80 hrs.

⌛ LIFESPAN CONSIDERATIONS

Pregnancy/Lactation: Unknown if drug crosses placenta or is distributed in breast milk. **Children:** Not prescribed for this pt population. **Elderly:** No age-related precautions noted, but use is not recommended in pts with severe renal impairment (CrCl less than 9 mL/min).

INTERACTIONS

DRUG: Urine alkalinizers (e.g., carbonic anhydrase inhibitors, sodium bicarbonate) may decrease renal elimination. **HERBAL:** None significant. **FOOD:** None known. **LAB VALUES:** None significant.

AVAILABILITY (Rx)

Oral Solution: 10 mg/5 mL. **Tablets:** 5 mg, 10 mg.

Capsules, Extended-Release: ***(Namenda XR):*** 7 mg, 14 mg, 21 mg, 28 mg.

ADMINISTRATION/HANDLING

PO

• Give without regard to food. • Administer oral solution using syringe provided. Do not dilute or mix with other fluids. • Give extended-release capsules whole. Do not crush. May open capsule and sprinkle on applesauce; give immediately.

INDICATIONS/ROUTES/DOSAGE

Alzheimer's Disease

PO: ADULTS, ELDERLY: ***(Immediate-Release):*** Initially, 5 mg once daily. May increase dose at intervals of at least 1 wk in 5-mg increments to 10 mg/day (5 mg twice daily), then 15 mg/day (5 mg and 10 mg as separate doses), then 20 mg/day (10 mg twice daily). Target dose: 20 mg/day. ***(Extended-Release):*** Initially, 7 mg once daily. May increase at intervals of at least 7 days in increments of 7 mg. **Maximum:** 28 mg once daily. Switching from immediate-release to extended-release: Begin the day following last dose of immediate-release.
10 mg twice daily: 28 mg once daily.
5 mg twice daily: 14 mg once daily.

Dosage in Renal Impairment

	Dosage	
Creatinine Clearance	**Immediate-Release**	**Extended-Release**
30 mL/min or greater	No adjustments	No adjustments
5–29 mL/min	5 mg twice daily or 10 mg once daily	14 mg once daily

Dosage in Hepatic Impairment

Mild to moderate impairment: No dose adjustment. **Severe impairment:** Use caution.

SIDE EFFECTS

Occasional (7%–4%): Dizziness, headache, confusion, constipation, hypertension, cough. **Rare (3%–2%):** Back pain, nausea, fatigue, anxiety, peripheral edema, arthralgia, insomnia.

ADVERSE EFFECTS/TOXIC REACTIONS

None known.

NURSING CONSIDERATIONS

BASELINE ASSESSMENT

Assess cognitive, behavioral, functional deficits. Assess renal function. Question history of cardiovascular disease, hepatic/renal impairment, seizure disorder.

INTERVENTION/EVALUATION

Monitor BUN, CrCl, serum creatinine lab values. Monitor cognitive, behavioral, functional status of pt. Monitor urine pH (alterations of urine pH toward the alkaline condition may lead to accumulation of the drug with possible increase in side effects).

PATIENT/FAMILY TEACHING

• Do not reduce or stop medication; do not increase dosage without physician direction. • Ensure adequate fluid intake. • If therapy is interrupted for several days, restart at lowest dose, titrate to current dose at minimum of 1-wk intervals. • Local chapter of Alzheimer's Disease Association can provide a guide to services.

M

meropenem

mer-oh-**pen**-em
(Merrem)
Do not confuse meropenem with doripenem, ertapenem, or imipenem.

◆CLASSIFICATION

PHARMACOTHERAPEUTIC: Carbapenem. **CLINICAL:** Antibiotic.

USES

Treatment of multidrug-resistant infections; meningitis in children 3 mos and older; intra-abdominal infections; complicated skin/skin structure infections caused by susceptible *S. aureus, S. pyogenes, S. agalactiae, S. pneumoniae, H. influenzae, N. meningitidis, M. catarrhalis, E. coli, Klebsiella, Enterobacter, Serratia, P. aeruginosa, B. fragilis*. **OFF-LABEL:** Febrile neutropenia, liver abscess, otitis external, prosthetic joint infection.

PRECAUTIONS

Contraindications: Hypersensitivity to meropenem, anaphylactic reactions to penicillins, cephalosporins, other beta-lactams. **Cautions:** Renal impairment, CNS disorders (particularly with history of seizures, concurrent use with valproic acid).

ACTION

Binds to penicillin-binding proteins. Inhibits bacterial cell wall synthesis. **Therapeutic Effect:** Bactericidal.

PHARMACOKINETICS

Widely distributed into tissues and body fluids, including CSF. Protein binding: 2%. Primarily excreted unchanged in urine. Removed by hemodialysis. **Half-life:** 1 hr.

LIFESPAN CONSIDERATIONS

Pregnancy/Lactation: Unknown if distributed in breast milk. **Children:** Safety and efficacy not established in pts younger than 3 mos. **Elderly:** Age-related renal impairment may require dosage adjustment.

INTERACTIONS

DRUG: May decrease effects of **valproic acid.** **HERBAL:** None significant. **FOOD:** None known. **LAB VALUES:** May increase serum BUN, alkaline phosphatase, LDH, ALT, AST, bilirubin. May decrease Hgb, Hct, WBC.

AVAILABILITY (Rx)

Injection, Powder for Reconstitution: 500 mg, 1 g.

ADMINISTRATION/HANDLING

IV

Reconstitution • Reconstitute each 500 mg with 10 mL Sterile Water for Injection, 0.9% NaCl, or D_5W to provide concentration of 50 mg/mL. • Shake to dissolve until clear. • May further dilute with 0.9% NaCl or D_5W to a concentration of 1–20 mg/mL.

Rate of administration • May give by IV push or IV intermittent infusion (piggyback). • If administering as IV intermittent infusion (piggyback), give over 15–30 min (may also give over 3 hrs); if administered by IV push, give over 3–5 min (at a concentration not greater than 50 mg/mL).

Storage • Store vials at room temperature. • After reconstitution of vials with 0.9% NaCl, stable for 2 hrs at room temperature or 18 hrs if refrigerated (with D_5W, stable for 1 hr at room temperature, 8 hrs if refrigerated). IV infusion with 0.9% NaCl stable for 4 hrs at room temperature or 24 hrs if refrigerated (with D_5W, 1 hr at room temperature or 4 hrs if refrigerated).

IV INCOMPATIBILITIES

Acyclovir (Zovirax), amphotericin B (Fungizone), diazepam (Valium), doxycycline (Vibramycin), metroNIDAZOLE (Flagyl), ondansetron (Zofran).

IV COMPATIBILITIES

Dexamethasone (Decadron), DOBUTamine (Dobutrex), DOPamine (Intropin), furosemide (Lasix), heparin, magnesium, morphine.

INDICATIONS/ROUTES/DOSAGE

Usual Dosage

IV: ADULTS, ELDERLY: 500 mg q6h or 1–2 g q8h. ***(Extended-Infusion):*** 1–2 g over 3 hrs q8h. **CHILDREN, ADOLESCENTS:** 20 mg/kg/dose q8h. **Maximum dose:** 1,000 mg. **NEONATES:** 20–30 mg/kg/dose q8–12h.

Dosage in Renal Impairment

Dosage and frequency are modified based on creatinine clearance.

Creatinine Clearance	Dosage	Interval
26–49 mL/min	Normal dose	q12h
10–25 mL/min	50% of normal dose	q12h
Less than 10 mL/min	50% of normal dose	q24h
Hemodialysis:	500 mg	q24h
Peritoneal dialysis:	Recommended dose (based on indication)	q24h

Continuous Renal Replacement Therapy (CRRT)

	Dosage	Interval
Continuous venovenous hemofiltration	1 gram then 500 mg OR 1 gram	q8h OR q12h
Continuous venovenous hemodialysis/continuous venovenous hemodiafiltration	1 gram then 500 mg OR 1 gram	q6–8h OR q8–12h

Dosage in Hepatic Impairment

No dose adjustment.

SIDE EFFECTS

Frequent (5%–3%): Diarrhea, nausea, vomiting, headache, inflammation at injection site. **Occasional** (2%): Oral candidiasis, rash, pruritus. **Rare** (less than 2%): Constipation, glossitis.

ADVERSE EFFECTS/TOXIC REACTIONS

Antibiotic-associated colitis, other superinfections (abdominal cramps, severe watery diarrhea, fever) may result from altered bacterial balance in GI tract. Anaphylactic reactions have been reported. Seizures may occur in pts with CNS disorders (e.g., brain lesions, history of seizures), bacterial meningitis, renal impairment. Severe cutaneous toxicities including Stevens-Johnson syndrome, toxic epidermal necrolysis, erythema multiforme, acute generalized exanthematous pustulosis, drug reaction with eosinophilia and systemic response (DRESS). DRESS may present with facial swelling, eosinophilia, fever, lymphadenopathy, rash that may be associated with other organ systems, such as hepatitis, hematologic abnormalities, myocarditis, nephritis.

NURSING CONSIDERATIONS

BASELINE ASSESSMENT

Question history of seizures; hypersensitivity, allergic reaction to penicillins, cephalosporins.

INTERVENTION/EVALUATION

Monitor daily pattern of bowel activity, stool consistency. Monitor for nausea, vomiting. Evaluate for inflammation at IV injection site. Monitor skin for cutaneous toxicities. Assess skin for rash. Evaluate hydration status. Monitor I&O, renal function, LFT. Check mental status; be alert to tremors, possible seizures. Assess temperature, B/P twice daily, more often if necessary. Monitor serum electrolytes, esp. potassium.

PATIENT/FAMILY TEACHING

- Report persistent diarrhea, abdominal cramps, fever.

meropenem/vaborbactam

mer-oh-**pen**-em/va-bor-**bak**-tam (Vabomere)

Do not confuse meropenem/vaborbactam with ampicillin/sulbactam, ceftolozane/tazobactam, ceftazidime/avibactam, or piperacillin/tazobactam.

CLASSIFICATION

PHARMACOTHERAPEUTIC: Carbapenem/beta-lactamase inhibitor. **CLINICAL:** Antibacterial.

USES

Treatment of pts 18 yrs and older with complicated urinary tract infections

M

(UTIs), including pyelonephritis, caused by the following susceptible microorganisms: *E. coli, K. pneumoniae, Enterobacter cloacae* species.

PRECAUTIONS

Contraindications: Known hypersensitivity to meropenem, cephalosporins, penicillin; anaphylaxis to beta-lactams. **Cautions:** History of renal impairment, seizure disorder, recent *Clostridioides difficile* infection or antibiotic-associated colitis; prior hypersensitivity to carbapenem, PCN.

ACTION

Meropenem binds to penicillin-binding proteins, inhibiting cell wall synthesis. Vaborbactam protects meropenem from serine beta-lactamase degradation (vaborbactam has no antibacterial activity). **Therapeutic Effect:** Bactericidal.

PHARMACOKINETICS

Widely distributed into tissues and body fluids. Meropenem metabolized by hydrolysis. Vaborbactam does not undergo metabolism. Protein binding: (meropenem): less than 2%; (vaborbactam): 33%. Excreted unchanged in urine. **Half-life:** 1–2 hrs.

LIFESPAN CONSIDERATIONS

Pregnancy/Lactation: Meropenem is secreted in breast milk. Unknown if vaborbactam is distributed in breast milk. **Children:** Safety and efficacy not established. **Elderly:** May have increased risk of adverse effects in pts with renal impairment.

INTERACTIONS

DRUG: **Probenecid** may increase concentration/effect of meropenem. May decrease concentration/effect of **valproic acid, divalproex.** May decrease effect of **BCG (intravesical). HERBAL:** None significant. **FOOD:** None known. **LAB VALUES:** May increase serum ALT, AST. May decrease eosinophils, leukocytes, lymphocytes; serum potassium. May result in positive Coombs' test. May decrease platelets in pts with renal impairment.

AVAILABILITY (Rx)

◀ALERT▶ Meropenem/vaborbactam is a combination product.

Injection, Powder for Reconstitution: meropenem/vaborbactam: 1 g/1 g.

ADMINISTRATION/HANDLING

IV

Reconstitution • Calculate the number of vials needed for dose. • Reconstitute each vial with 20 mL 0.9% NaCl (withdrawn from infusion bag) to a final concentration of 0.05 g/mL of meropenem and 0.05 g/mL of vaborbactam. • Final volume of vial equals 21.3 mL. • Gently mix until powder is fully dissolved. • Visually inspect for particulate matter or discoloration. Solution should appear colorless to slightly yellow in color.

Dilution • **4-g dose (2 vials):** Dilute volume of each vial (21 mL/vial) in 0.9% NaCl bag with a volume of 250 mL (16 mg/mL), or 500 mL (8 mg/mL), or 1,000 mL (4 mg/mL). • **2-g dose (1 vial):** Dilute the volume of vial (21 mL) in 0.9% NaCl bag with a volume of 125 mL (16 mg/mL), or 250 mL (8 mg/mL), or 500 mL (4 mg/mL). • **1-g dose (1 vial):** Dilute half of the volume of vial (10.5 mL) in 0.9% NaCl bag with volume of 70 mL (14.3 mg/mL), or 125 mL (8 mg/mL), or 250 mL (4 mg/mL).

Rate of administration • Infuse over 3 hrs.

Storage • Refrigerate diluted solution for up to 22 hrs or store at room temperature for up to 4 hrs. • Diluted solution must be completely infused within 4 hrs.

IV INCOMPATIBILITIES

Acyclovir (Zovirax), amphotericin B (Fungizone), diazePAM (Valium), doxycycline (Vibramycin), metronidazole (Flagyl), ondansetron (Zofran).

INDICATIONS/ROUTES/DOSAGE

Complicated Urinary Tract Infections Including Pyelonephritis

IV: ADULTS, ELDERLY: 4 g (meropenem 2 g/vaborbactam 2 g) q8h for up to 14 days.

Dosage in Renal Impairment

Note: Infuse after hemodialysis on hemodialysis days. Dosage is modified based on eGFR.

Estimated Glomerular Filtration Rate	Dosage
eGFR 30–49 mL/min	2 g q8h
eGFR 15–29 mL/min	2 g q12h
eGFR less than 15 mL/min	1 g q12h

Dosage in Hepatic Impairment

Mild to severe impairment: No dose adjustment.

SIDE EFFECTS

Occasional (9%–4%): Headache, infusion site reactions (phlebitis, erythema, thrombosis). **Rare (3%–2%):** Diarrhea, pyrexia.

ADVERSE EFFECTS/TOXIC REACTIONS

Hypersensitivity reactions, including anaphylaxis, have been reported in pts treated with beta-lactam antibacterial drugs. Blood and lymphatic disorders such as agranulocytosis, hemolytic anemia, leukopenia, lymphocytosis, neutropenia, thrombocytopenia were reported. Seizures may occur in pts with CNS disorders (e.g., brain lesion, history of seizures, bacterial meningitis), renal impairment. Other CNS reactions may include tremor, paresthesia, lethargy. *Clostridioides difficile*–associated diarrhea, with severity ranging from mild diarrhea to fatal colitis, was reported. *C. difficile* infection may occur more than 2 mos after completion of treatment. May increase risk of development of drug-resistant bacteria when used in the absence of a proven or strongly suspected bacterial infection. Skin and SQ reactions including angioedema, erythema multiforme, pruritus, Stevens-Johnson syndrome, toxic epidermal necrolysis occur rarely. Secondary infections including pharyngitis, oral or vulvovaginal candidiasis may occur.

NURSING CONSIDERATIONS

BASELINE ASSESSMENT

Obtain BUN, serum creatinine, CrCl, GFR in pts with renal impairment. Obtain urine culture and sensitivity. Question history of renal impairment, seizure disorder, recent *C. diff* infection; hypersensitivity reaction to beta-lactams, cephalosporins, PCN. Question pt's usual stool characteristics (color, frequency, consistency).

INTERVENTION/EVALUATION

Periodically monitor WBC. Monitor BUN, serum creatinine, CrCl, GFR, platelet count in pts with renal impairment. Observe daily pattern of bowel activity, stool consistency (increased severity may indicate antibiotic-associated colitis). If frequent diarrhea occurs, obtain *C. difficile* toxin screen and initiate isolation precautions until test result confirmed; manage proper fluid levels/PO intake, electrolyte levels, protein intake. Antibacterial drugs that are not directed against *C. difficile* infection may need to be discontinued. Report any signs of hypersensitivity reaction. Assess skin for toxic skin reactions. Monitor for seizure activity, CNS reactions, IV site reactions.

PATIENT/FAMILY TEACHING

• It is essential to complete drug therapy despite symptom improvement. Early discontinuation may result in antibacterial resistance or may increase risk of recurrent infection. • Report any episodes of diarrhea, esp. the following months after last dose. Frequent loose stool, fever, abdominal pain, blood-streaked stool may indicate infectious diarrhea and may be contagious to oth-

M

ers. • Report abdominal pain, black/tarry stools, bruising, yellowing of skin or eyes; dark urine, decreased urine output; skin problems such as development of sores, rash, skin bubbling/necrosis. • Report any nervous system changes such as anxiety, confusion, hallucinations, muscle jerking, or seizure-like activity. • Severe allergic reactions such as hives, palpitations, shortness of breath, rash, tongue swelling may occur.

mesalamine

me-**sal**-a-meen
(Apriso, Asacol HD, Canasa, Delzicol, Lialda, Mesasal ✱, Pentasa, Rowasa, Salofalk ✱, sfRowasa)
Do not confuse Asacol with Os-Cal, Lialda with Aldara, or mesalamine with megestrol, memantine, or methenamine.

◆CLASSIFICATION

PHARMACOTHERAPEUTIC: Salicylic acid derivative. **CLINICAL:** Anti-inflammatory agent.

USES

PO: Treatment, maintenance of remission of mild to moderate active ulcerative colitis. **Rectal:** Treatment of active mild to moderate distal ulcerative colitis, proctosigmoiditis, or proctitis. **OFF-LABEL:** Crohn's disease.

PRECAUTIONS

Contraindications: Hypersensitivity to mesalamine, salicylates. **Cautions:** Active peptic ulcer, pyloric stenosis, pericarditis, myocarditis, renal/hepatic impairment, elderly.

ACTION

Exact mechanism unknown. May modulate local mediators of inflammation, may inhibit tumor necrosis factor. **Therapeutic Effect:** Decreases inflammation in colon.

PHARMACOKINETICS

Poorly absorbed from colon. Moderately absorbed from GI tract. Metabolized in liver. Unabsorbed portion excreted in feces; absorbed portion excreted in urine. Unknown if removed by hemodialysis. **Half-life:** 0.5–1.5 hrs; metabolite, 5–10 hrs.

LIFESPAN CONSIDERATIONS

Pregnancy/Lactation: Unknown if drug crosses placenta or is distributed in breast milk. **Children:** Safety and efficacy not established. **Elderly:** Age-related renal impairment may require dosage adjustment.

INTERACTIONS

DRUG: **Antacids, histamine H_2-receptor antagonists (e.g., famotidine, ranitidine), proton pump inhibitors (e.g., lansoprazole, pantoprazole)** may decrease therapeutic effect. **HERBAL:** None significant. **FOOD:** None known. **LAB VALUES:** May increase serum alkaline phosphatase, ALT, AST, bilirubin.

AVAILABILITY (Rx)

Rectal Suspension: ***(Rowasa, sfRowasa):*** 4 g/60 mL. **Suppositories:** ***(Canasa):*** 1 g.

Capsules, Controlled-Release: ***(Pentasa):*** 250 mg, 500 mg. **Extended-Release:** ***(Apriso):*** 375 mg. **Capsules, Delayed-Release:** ***(Delzicol):*** 400 mg. **Tablets, Delayed-Release:** ***(Asacol HD):*** 800 mg. ***(Lialda):*** 1.2 g.

ADMINISTRATION/HANDLING

◀ALERT▶ Store rectal suspension, suppository, oral forms at room temperature.

PO

• Have pt swallow whole; do not break outer coating of tablet. • Give without regard to food. • **Apriso:** Do not administer with antacids. • **Lialda:** Administer once daily with meal.

Rectal
• Shake bottle well. • Instruct pt to lie on left side with lower leg extended, upper leg flexed forward. • Knee-chest position may also be used. • Insert applicator tip into rectum, pointing toward umbilicus. • Squeeze bottle steadily until contents are emptied. • Store suppositories at room temperature. Do not refrigerate.

INDICATIONS/ROUTES/DOSAGE

Treatment of Ulcerative Colitis

PO: ***(Capsule [Pentasa]):*** **ADULTS, ELDERLY:** 1 g 4 times daily.

PO: ***(Capsule [Delzicol]):*** **ADULTS, ELDERLY:** 800 mg 3 times daily. **CHILDREN 5 YRS AND OLDER, WEIGHING 54–90 KG:** 1,200 mg in morning and evening. **Maximum:** 2,400 mg/day. **33–53 KG:** 1,200 mg in morning and 800 mg in evening. **Maximum:** 2,000 mg/day. **17–32 KG:** 800 mg in morning and 400 mg in evening. **Maximum:** 1,200 mg/day.

PO: ***(Tablet [Asacol HD]):*** **ADULTS, ELDERLY:** 1.6 g 3 times daily.

PO: ***(Tablet [Lialda]):*** **ADULTS, ELDERLY:** 2.4–4.8 g once daily.

Maintenance of Remission in Ulcerative Colitis

PO: ***(Capsule [Pentasa]):*** **ADULTS, ELDERLY:** 1 g 4 times daily.

PO: ***(Capsule [Delzicol]):*** **ADULTS, ELDERLY:** 1.6 g/day in 2–4 divided doses.

PO: ***(Capsule, Extended-Release [Apriso]):*** **ADULTS, ELDERLY:** 1.5 g once daily in the morning.

PO: ***(Tablet [Lialda]):*** 2.4 g once daily with food.

Distal Ulcerative Colitis, Proctosigmoiditis, Proctitis

Rectal: ***(Retention Enema):*** **ADULTS, ELDERLY:** 60 mL (4 g) at bedtime; retained overnight for approximately 8 hrs for 3–6 wks.

Rectal: ***(1 G Suppository):*** **ADULTS, ELDERLY:** Once daily at bedtime. Continue therapy for 3–6 wks.

◀ALERT▶ Suppository should be retained for 1–3 hrs for maximum benefit.

Dosage of Renal/Hepatic Impairment
Use caution.

SIDE EFFECTS

Mesalamine is generally well tolerated, with only mild, transient effects. **Frequent (greater than 6%): PO:** Abdominal cramps/pain, diarrhea, dizziness, headache, nausea, vomiting, rhinitis, unusual fatigue. **Rectal:** Abdominal/stomach cramps, flatulence, headache, nausea. **Occasional (6%–2%): PO:** Hair loss, decreased appetite, back/joint pain, flatulence, acne. **Rectal:** Alopecia. **Rare (less than 2%): Rectal:** Anal irritation.

ADVERSE EFFECTS/TOXIC REACTIONS

Sulfite sensitivity may occur in susceptible pts, manifested as cramping, headache, diarrhea, fever, rash, urticaria, pruritus, wheezing. Discontinue drug immediately. Hepatitis, pancreatitis, pericarditis occur rarely with oral forms.

NURSING CONSIDERATIONS

BASELINE ASSESSMENT

Obtain BUN, serum creatinine, LFT. Assess for abdominal pain, discomfort.

INTERVENTION/EVALUATION

Encourage adequate fluid intake. Assess bowel sounds for peristalsis. Monitor daily pattern of bowel activity, stool consistency; record time of evacuation. Assess skin for rash, urticaria. Discontinue medication if rash, fever, cramping, or diarrhea occurs.

PATIENT/FAMILY TEACHING

• Report rash, fever, abdominal pain, significant diarrhea. • Avoid tasks that require alertness, motor skills until response to drug is established. • May discolor urine yellow-brown. • Suppositories stain fabrics.

M

metFORMIN

TOP 100 HIGH ALERT

met-**for**-min
(Fortamet, Glucophage, Glucophage XR, Glumetza, Glycon, Riomet)

BLACK BOX ALERT Lactic acidosis occurs very rarely, but mortality rate is 50%. Risk increases with degree of renal impairment, pt's age, those with diabetes, unstable or acute HF.

Do not confuse Glucophage with Glucotrol, or metFORMIN with metroNIDAZOLE.

FIXED-COMBINATION(S)

Actoplus Met: metFORMIN/pioglitazone (an antidiabetic): 500 mg/15 mg, 850 mg/15 mg. **Avandamet:** metFORMIN/rosiglitazone (an antidiabetic): 500 mg/1 mg, 500 mg/2 mg, 500 mg/4 mg, 1,000 mg/2 mg, 1,000 mg/4 mg. **Glucovance:** metFORMIN/glyBURIDE (an antidiabetic): 250 mg/1.25 mg, 500 mg/2.5 mg, 500 mg/5 mg. **Invokamet:** metFORMIN/canagliflozin (an antidiabetic): 500 mg/50 mg, 500 mg/150 mg, 1,000 mg/50 mg, 1,000 mg/150 mg. **Janumet, Janumet XR:** metFORMIN/SITagliptin (an antidiabetic): 500 mg/50 mg, 1,000 mg/50 mg. **Jentadueto, Jentadueto XR:** metFORMIN/linagliptin (an antidiabetic): 500 mg/2.5 mg; 1,000 mg/2.5 mg; 1,000 mg extended-release/2.5 mg; 1,000 mg extended-release/5 mg. **Kazano:** metFORMIN/alogliptin (an antidiabetic): 500 mg/12.5 mg; 1,000 mg/12.5 mg. **Kombiglyze XR:** metFORMIN/SAXagliptin (an antidiabetic): 500 mg/5 mg, 1,000 mg/5 mg, 1,000 mg/2.5 mg. **Metaglip:** metFORMIN/glipiZIDE (an antidiabetic): 250 mg/2.5 mg, 500 mg/2.5 mg, 500 mg/5 mg. **Qternmet XR:** metFORMIN/dapagliflozin (an antidiabetic)/saxagliptin (an antidiabetic): 1,000 mg/2.5 mg/2.5 mg; 1,000 mg/5 mg/2.5 mg; 1,000 mg/5 mg/5 mg; 1,000 mg/10 mg/5 mg. **PrandiMet:** metFORMIN/repaglinide (an antidiabetic): 500 mg/1 mg, 500 mg/2 mg. **Synjardy:** metFORMIN/empagliflozin (an antidiabetic): 500 mg/5 mg, 1,000 mg/5 mg, 500 mg/12.5 mg, 1,000 mg/12.5 mg. **Trijardy XR:** empagliflozin (an antidiabetic)/linagliptin (an antidiabetic)/metFORMIN (an antidiabetic): 10 mg/5 mg/1,000 mg; 25 mg/5 mg/1,000 mg; 5mg/2.5 mg/1,000 mg; 12.5 mg/2.5 mg/1,000 mg.

◆CLASSIFICATION

PHARMACOTHERAPEUTIC: Biguanide antihyperglycemic. **CLINICAL:** Antidiabetic agent.

USES

Management of type 2 diabetes mellitus. **OFF-LABEL:** Polycystic ovarian syndrome, gestational diabetes mellitus. Prevention of type 2 diabetes.

PRECAUTIONS

◀ALERT▶ Lactic acidosis is a rare but potentially severe consequence of metformin therapy. Withhold in pts with conditions that may predispose to lactic acidosis (e.g., hypoxemia, dehydration, hypoperfusion, sepsis).
Contraindications: Hypersensitivity to metformin. Severe renal disease/dysfunction; acute or chronic metabolic acidosis (with or without coma). **Cautions:** HF, hepatic impairment, excessive acute/chronic alcohol intake, elderly. Recommend temporary discontinuation at time of or before iodinated contrast imaging procedures in pts with CrCl of 30–60 mL/min, or with history of hepatic disease, alcoholism, HF.

ACTION

Decreases hepatic production of glucose. Decreases intestinal absorption of glucose, improves insulin sensitivity. **Therapeutic Effect:** Improves glycemic control, stabilizes/decreases body weight, improves lipid profile.

PHARMACOKINETICS

Slowly, incompletely absorbed. Food delays, decreases extent of absorption. Protein binding: Negligible. Primarily distributed to intestinal mucosa, salivary glands. Primarily excreted unchanged in urine. Removed by hemodialysis. **Half-life:** 9–17 hrs.

LIFESPAN CONSIDERATIONS

Pregnancy/Lactation: Insulin is drug of choice during pregnancy. Distributed in breast milk in animals. **Children:** Safety and efficacy not established in children younger than 10 yrs. **Elderly:** Age-related renal impairment or peripheral vascular disease may require dosage adjustment or discontinuation.

INTERACTIONS

DRUG: **Alcohol** may increase adverse effects. **Cimetidine, dolutegravir, ranolazine** may increase concentration/effect. **IV contrast dye** may increase risk of metformin-induced lactic acidosis, acute renal failure (discontinue metFORMIN 24–48 hrs prior to and up to 72 hrs after contrast exposure). **HERBAL:** **Garlic** may cause hypoglycemia. **FOOD:** None known. **LAB VALUES:** May alter cholesterol, LDL, triglycerides, HDL.

AVAILABILITY (Rx)

Oral Solution: ***(Riomet):*** 100 mg/mL. **Tablets:** 500 mg, 850 mg, 1,000 mg. **Oral Suspension:** ***(Riomet ER):*** 500 mg/5 mL.

Tablets, Extended-Release: 500 mg, 750 mg, 1,000 mg.

ADMINISTRATION/HANDLING

PO

• Give extended-release tablets whole. Do not break, crush, dissolve, or divide extended-release tablets. • Give with meals (to decrease GI upset). Give Fortamet with glass of water.

INDICATIONS/ROUTES/DOSAGE

◄ALERT► Allow 1–2 wks between dose titrations.

Diabetes Mellitus

PO: ***(Immediate-Release Tablets, Solution):*** **ADULTS, ELDERLY:** Initially, 500 mg once or twice daily or 850 mg once daily. Titrate in increments of 500 mg or 850 mg q7days. **Usual Maintenance Dose:** 1,000 mg twice daily or 850 mg twice daily. **Maximum:** 2,550 mg/day in 2 or 3 divided doses. **CHILDREN 10–16 YRS:** Initially, 500–1,000 mg once daily or 500 mg twice daily. May increase in 500–1,000 mg increments q1–2wks. **Maximum:** 1,000 mg twice daily or 850 mg 3 times/day.

PO: ***(Extended-Release Tablets):*** **ADULTS, ELDERLY:** Initially, 500–1,000 mg once daily. May increase by 500 mg at 1-wk intervals. **Maximum:** 2,000 mg/day.

Dosage in Renal Impairment

Contraindicated in pts with serum creatinine greater than 1.5 mg/dL (males) or greater than 1.4 mg/dL (females). **Alternative recommendation: CrCl 45–60 mL/min:** Continue use; monitor renal function q3–6 mos. **CrCl 30–44 mL/min:** Use caution. Consider dose reduction; monitor renal function q3mos. **CrCL less than 30 mL/min:** Discontinue use.

Dosage in Hepatic Impairment

Avoid use (risk factor for lactic acidosis).

M

SIDE EFFECTS

Occasional (greater than 3%): GI disturbances (diarrhea, nausea, vomiting, abdominal bloating, flatulence, anorexia) that are transient and resolve spontaneously during therapy. **Rare (3%–1%):** Unpleasant/metallic taste that resolves spontaneously during therapy.

ADVERSE EFFECTS/TOXIC REACTIONS

Lactic acidosis occurs rarely (0.03 cases/1,000 pts) but is a serious and often fatal (50%) complication. Lactic acidosis is characterized by increase in blood lactate levels (greater than 5 mmol/L), decrease in blood pH, electrolyte disturbances. Symptoms include unexplained hyperventilation, myalgia, malaise, drowsiness. May advance to cardiovascular collapse (shock), acute HF, acute MI, prerenal azotemia.

NURSING CONSIDERATIONS

BASELINE ASSESSMENT

Verify pt has not received IV contrast dye within last 48 hrs. Obtain CBC, renal function test, fasting serum glucose, Hgb A1c.

INTERVENTION/EVALUATION

Monitor fasting serum glucose, Hgb A1c, renal function, CBC. Monitor folic acid, renal function tests for evidence of early lactic acidosis. If pt is on concurrent oral sulfonylureas, assess for hypoglycemia (cool/wet skin, tremors, dizziness, anxiety, headache, tachycardia, numbness in mouth, hunger, diplopia). Be alert to conditions that alter glucose requirements: fever, increased activity, stress, surgical procedure. If lactic acidosis occurs, withhold treatment.

PATIENT/FAMILY TEACHING

• Report symptoms of lactic acidosis (unexplained hyperventilation, muscle aches, extreme fatigue, unusual drowsiness). • Prescribed diet is principal part of treatment; do not skip, delay meals. • Diabetes requires lifelong control. • Avoid alcohol. • Report persistent headache, nausea, vomiting, diarrhea or if skin rash, unusual bruising/bleeding, change in color of urine or stool occurs. • Do not take dose for at least 48 hrs after receiving IV contrast dye with radiologic testing.

methadone

meth-a-done
(Dolophine, Metadol ✦, Methadone Intensol, Methadose)

■ BLACK BOX ALERT ■ May prolong QT interval, which may cause serious arrhythmias. May cause serious, life-threatening, or fatal respiratory depression. Monitor for signs of misuse, abuse, addiction. Prolonged maternal use may cause neonatal withdrawal syndrome.

Do not confuse methadone with Mephyton, Metadate CD, Metadate ER, methylphenidate, or morphine.

◆CLASSIFICATION

PHARMACOTHERAPEUTIC: Opioid agonist (Schedule II). **CLINICAL:** Opioid analgesic. Opioid dependency management.

USES

Oral: Moderate to severe pain when a continuous around-the-clock analgesic is needed. Detoxification/maintenance treatment of opioid addiction in conjunction with social/medical services. **Injection:** Management of pain severe enough to require an opioid analgesic when alternate options are inadequate.

PRECAUTIONS

Contraindications: Hypersensitivity to methadone. Severe respiratory depression, acute or severe bronchial asthma (in absence of resuscitative equipment or unmonitored setting), hypercarbia, GI obstruction including paralytic ileus (known or suspected). **Cautions:** Renal/hepatic impairment, elderly/debilitated pts, pts at risk for QTc interval prolongation (congenital long QT syndrome, HF, medications that prolong QTc interval, hypokalemia, hypomagnesemia), cardiovascular disease, pts at high risk for suicidal ideation and behavior; history of drug abuse and misuse, drug-seeking behavior, dependency; respiratory disease, biliary tract dysfunction, acute pancreatitis, hypothyroidism, Addison's disease, head injury, increased intracranial pressure.

ACTION

Binds with opioid receptors within CNS, causing inhibition of ascending pain pathways. **Therapeutic Effect:** Produces generalized CNS depression. Alters processes affecting analgesia, emotional response to pain; reduces withdrawal symptoms from other opioid drugs.

PHARMACOKINETICS

Route	Onset	Peak	Duration
PO	0.5–1 hr	1.5–2 hrs	6–8 hrs
IM	10–20 min	1–2 hrs	4–5 hrs
IV	N/A	15–30 min	3–4 hrs

Well absorbed after IM injection. Protein binding: 85%–90%. Metabolized in liver. Primarily excreted in urine. Not removed by hemodialysis. **Half-life:** 7–59 hrs.

⌛ LIFESPAN CONSIDERATIONS

Pregnancy/Lactation: Crosses placenta. Distributed in breast milk. Respiratory depression may occur in neonate if mother received opiates during labor. Regular use of opiates during pregnancy may produce withdrawal symptoms in neonate (irritability, excessive crying, tremors, hyperactive reflexes, fever, vomiting, diarrhea, yawning, sneezing, seizures). **Children:** Paradoxical excitement may occur. Pts younger than 2 yrs more susceptible to respiratory depressant effects. **Elderly:** More susceptible to respiratory depressant effects. Age-related renal impairment may increase risk of urinary retention.

INTERACTIONS

DRUG: **Alcohol, CNS depressants (e.g., LORazepam, morphine, zolpidem)** may increase CNS effects, respiratory depression, hypotension. **Strong CYP3A4 inducers (e.g., carBAMazepine, phenytoin, rifAMPin)** may decrease concentration/effects. **Strong CYP3A4 inhibitors (e.g., rifAMPin, clarithromycin, ketoconazole, ritonavir)** may increase methadone level. **QT interval–prolonging medications (e.g., amiodarone, azithromycin, ciprofloxacin, haloperidol, sotalol)** may increase risk of QTc interval prolongation. **MAOIs (e.g., phenelzine, selegiline)** may produce serotonin syndrome. **HERBAL:** **Herbals with sedative properties (e.g., chamomile, kava kava, valerian)** may increase CNS depression. **St. John's wort** may decrease concentration/effect. **FOOD:** **Grapefruit products** may alter concentration/effects. **LAB VALUES:** May increase serum amylase, lipase.

AVAILABILITY (Rx)

Injection Solution: 10 mg/mL. **Oral Concentrate:** 10 mg/mL. **Oral Solution:** 5 mg/5 mL, 10 mg/5 mL. **Tablets, Dispersible:** 40 mg. **Tablets:** 5 mg, 10 mg.

ADMINISTRATION/HANDLING

IM, SQ

◀ALERT▶ IM preferred over SQ route (SQ produces pain, local irritation, induration).

• Do not use if solution appears cloudy or contains a precipitate. • Administer slowly. • Those with circulatory impairment experience higher risk of overdosage due to delayed absorption of repeated administration.

PO

• Give without regard to food. • Oral dose for detoxification and maintenance may be given in fruit juice or water. • Dispersible tablet should not be chewed or swallowed; add to liquid, allow to dissolve before swallowing.

INDICATIONS/ROUTES/DOSAGE

Analgesia

PO: ADULTS, ELDERLY: Initially, 2.5 mg q8–12h. May increase by 2.5 mg/dose or 5 mg/day q5–7days.

Dosage in Renal Impairment

CrCl less than 10 mL/min: 50%–75% normal dose. Avoid in severe hepatic disease.

Dosage in Hepatic Impairment

Mild to moderate impairment: No dose adjustment. **Severe Impairment:** Avoid use.

Detoxification

PO: ADULTS, ELDERLY: Initially, dose of 20–30 mg. An additional 5–10 mg may be provided if withdrawal symptoms have not been suppressed or if symptoms reappear after 2–4 hrs. Day 1 dose not to exceed 40 mg. **Maintenance range:** Titrate to a dose that prevents withdrawal symptoms for 24 hrs, reduces craving, reduces euphoria effect of self-administered opioids, while ensuring tolerance to sedative effects of methadone. Usual range: 80–120 mg/day. Dose reduction should be in increments of less than 10% of the maintenance dose every 10–14 days. **Short-term:** Initially, titrate to 40 mg/day in 2 divided doses. Continue 40-mg dose for 2–3 days. After 2–3 days of stabilization at 40 mg, gradually decrease dose to level keeping withdrawal symptoms tolerable.

M

SIDE EFFECTS

Frequent: Sedation, orthostatic hypotension, diaphoresis, facial flushing, constipation, dizziness, nausea, vomiting. **Occasional:** Confusion, urinary retention, palpitations, abdominal cramps, visual changes, dry mouth, headache, decreased appetite, anxiety, insomnia. **Rare:** Allergic reaction (rash, pruritus).

ADVERSE EFFECTS/TOXIC REACTIONS

Overdose results in respiratory depression, skeletal muscle flaccidity, cold/clammy skin, cyanosis, extreme drowsiness progressing to seizures, stupor, coma. Early sign of toxicity presents as increased sedation after being on a stable dose. Cardiac toxicity manifested as QT prolongation, torsades de pointes. Tolerance to analgesic effect, physical dependence may occur with repeated use. **Antidote:** Naloxone (see Appendix J for dosage).

NURSING CONSIDERATIONS

BASELINE ASSESSMENT

Obtain baseline ECG. Assess type, location, intensity of pain. **Detoxification:** Assess pt for opioid withdrawal. Pt should be in recumbent position before drug administration by parenteral route. Obtain vital signs before giving medication. If respirations are 12/min or less (20/min or less in children), withhold medication, contact physician. Assess for potential of abuse/misuse (e.g., drug-seeking behavior, mental health conditions, history of substance abuse).

INTERVENTION/EVALUATION

Monitor vital signs 15–30 min after SQ/IM dose, 5–10 min following IV dose. Oral medication is 50% as potent as parenteral. Assess for adequate voiding. Monitor daily pattern of bowel activity, stool consistency. Assess for clinical improvement, record onset of relief of pain. Provide support to pt in detoxification program; monitor for withdrawal symptoms. Diligently assess for suicidal ideation and behavior; new onset or worsening of anxiety, depression, mood disorder. Screen for drug abuse and misuse, drug-seeking behavior.

PATIENT/FAMILY TEACHING

• Methadone may produce drug dependence, has potential for being abused. • Avoid alcohol. • Do not stop taking abruptly after prolonged use. • May cause dry mouth, drowsiness. • Avoid tasks that require alertness, motor skills until response to drug is established. • Report severe drowsiness, respiratory depression.

methotrexate HIGH ALERT

meth-o-**trex**-ate
(Otrexup, Rasuvo, Trexall, Xatmep)

■ **BLACK BOX ALERT** ■ May cause fetal abnormalities, death. May produce potentially fatal chronic hepatotoxicity, dermatologic reactions, acute renal failure, pneumonitis, myelosuppression, malignant lymphoma, aplastic anemia, GI toxicity. Do not use for psoriasis or rheumatoid arthritis treatment in pregnant women.

Do not confuse methotrexate with metOLazone, methylPREDNISolone, or mitoXANTRONE. MTX is an error-prone abbreviation; do not use as an abbreviation.

◆CLASSIFICATION

PHARMACOTHERAPEUTIC: Antimetabolite. **CLINICAL:** Antineoplastic, antirheumatic disease-modifying, immunosuppressant.

USES

Oncology-related: Treatment of breast, head/neck, non–small-cell lung, small-cell lung carcinomas; trophoblastic tumors, acute lymphocytic, meningeal leukemias; non-Hodgkin's lymphomas (lymphosarcoma, Burkitt's lymphoma), carcinoma of gastrointestinal tract, mycosis fungoides, osteosarcoma. **Non-oncology uses:** Psoriasis, rheumatoid arthritis (including juvenile idiopathic arthritis). **OFF-LABEL:** Treatment of acute myelocytic leukemia, bladder carcinoma, ectopic pregnancy, management of abortion, systemic lupus erythematosus, treatment of and maintenance of remission in Crohn's disease.

PRECAUTIONS

Contraindications: Hypersensitivity to methotrexate. Breastfeeding. **For pts with psoriasis, juvenile idiopathic arthritis or rheumatoid arthritis:** Pregnancy, hepatic disease, alcoholism, immunodeficiency syndrome, preexisting blood dyscrasias. **Cautions:** Peptic ulcer, ulcerative colitis, preexisting myelosuppression, history of chronic hepatic disease, alcohol consumption, obesity, diabetes, hyperlipidemia, use with other hepatotoxic medications, concomitant use of proton pump inhibitors. Use of NSAIDs or aspirin with lower methotrexate doses for rheumatoid arthritis.

ACTION

Irreversibly binds to and inhibits dihydrofolate reductase, inhibiting formation of reduced folates and thymidylate synthetase, which inhibits purine/thymidylic acid synthesis. **Therapeutic Effect:** Interferes with DNA synthesis, repair, and cellular replication.

PHARMACOKINETICS

Variably absorbed from GI tract. Completely absorbed after IM administration. Protein binding: 50%–60%. Widely distributed. Metabolized in liver. Primarily excreted in urine. Removed by hemodialysis but not by peritoneal dialysis. **Half-life:** 3–10 hrs (large doses, 8–15 hrs).

M

LIFESPAN CONSIDERATIONS

Pregnancy/Lactation: Avoid pregnancy during therapy and minimum 3 mos after therapy in males or at least one ovulatory cycle after therapy in females. May cause fetal death, congenital anomalies. Distributed in breast milk. Breastfeeding not recommended. **Children/Elderly:** Renal/hepatic impairment may require dosage adjustment.

INTERACTIONS

DRUG: **Alcohol, hepatotoxic medications (e.g., acetaminophen, acitretin)** may increase risk of hepatotoxicity. **Bone marrow depressants (e.g., cladribine)** may increase myelosuppression. May decrease the therapeutic effect of **vaccines (live).** May increase adverse effects of **natalizumab, vaccines (live). NSAIDs (e.g., ibuprofen, ketorolac, naproxen)** may increase risk of toxicity. **Probenecid, salicylates (e.g., aspirin)** may increase concentration, risk of toxicity. **HERBAL:** **Echinacea** may decrease therapeutic effect. **FOOD:** None known. **LAB VALUES:** May increase serum uric acid, AST.

AVAILABILITY (Rx)

Injection, Powder for Reconstitution: 1 g. **Injection, Autoinjector:** ***(Rasuvo):*** 7.5 mg, 10 mg, 12.5 mg, 15 mg, 17.5 mg, 20 mg, 22.5 mg, 25 mg, 27.5 mg, 30 mg. **Injection Solution:** 25 mg/mL. **Injection, Syringe:** ***(Otrexup):*** 7.5 mg/0.4 mL, 10 mg/0.4 mL, 12.5 mg/0.4 mL, 15 mg/0.4 mL, 17.5 mg/0.4 mL, 20 mg/0.4 mL, 22.5 mg/0.4 mL, 25 mg/0.4 mL. **Solution, Oral:** ***(Xatmep):*** 2.5 mg/mL. **Tablets:** 2.5 mg, 5 mg, 7.5 mg, 10 mg, 15 mg.

ADMINISTRATION/HANDLING

◀ALERT▶ May be carcinogenic, mutagenic, teratogenic. Handle with extreme care during preparation/administration. Wear gloves when preparing solution. If powder or solution comes in contact with skin, wash immediately, thoroughly with soap, water. May give IM, IV, intra-arterially, intrathecally.

IV

Reconstitution • Reconstitute powder with D_5W or 0.9% NaCl to provide concentration of 25 mg/mL or less. • For intrathecal use, dilute with preservative-free 0.9% NaCl to provide a concentration not greater than 2–4 mg/mL.

Rate of administration • Give IV push at rate of 10 mg/min. • Give IV infusion at rate of 4–20 mg/hr (refer to specific protocol).

Storage • Store vials at room temperature. Diluted solutions stable for 24 hrs at room temperature.

IV INCOMPATIBILITIES

Droperidol (Inapsine), gemcitabine (Gemzar), idarubicin (Idamycin), midazolam (Versed), nalbuphine (Nubain).

IV COMPATIBILITIES

CISplatin (Platinol AQ), cyclophosphamide (Cytoxan), DAUNOrubicin (DaunoXome), DOXOrubicin (Adriamycin), etoposide (VePesid), 5-fluorouracil, granisetron (Kytril), leucovorin, mitoMYcin (Mutamycin), ondansetron (Zofran), PACLitaxel (Taxol), vinBLAStine (Velban), vinCRIStine (Oncovin), vinorelbine (Navelbine).

INDICATIONS/ROUTES/DOSAGE

Oncology Uses

◀ALERT▶ Refer to individual specific protocols for optimum dosage, sequence of administration.

Head/Neck Cancer

PO, IV, IM: ADULTS, ELDERLY: 40 mg/m^2 once wkly. Continue until disease progression or unacceptable toxicity.

Breast Cancer

IV: ADULTS, ELDERLY: 40 mg/m^2 days 1 and 8 q4wks in combination with cyclophosphamide and fluorouracil.

Mycosis Fungoides
IM, PO: ADULTS, ELDERLY: 5–50 mg once wkly or 15–37.5 mg twice wkly.

Rheumatoid Arthritis (RA)
PO: ADULTS: Initially, 10–15 mg once wkly. May increase by 5 mg q2–4wks to a maximum dose of 20–30 mg once weekly. **SQ/IM:** Initially, 7.5 mg/wk. Adjust dose gradually to optimal response. **ELDERLY:** Initially, 5–7.5 mg/wk. **Maximum:** 20 mg/wk.

Juvenile Rheumatoid Arthritis (JRA)
PO, IM, SQ: CHILDREN: Initially, 10 mg/m^2 once wkly, then adjust gradually to 20–30 mg/m^2/wk as a single dose. **Usual Maximum Dose:** 25 mg.

Psoriasis
PO: ADULTS, ELDERLY: Initially, 10–25 mg once wkly or 2.5–5 mg q12h for 3 doses once wkly. **IM/SQ:** 10–25 mg once wkly. Adjust dose gradually to optimal response. Titrate to lowest effective dose. Doses greater than 30 mg/wk should usually not be exceeded.

Dosage in Renal Impairment

Creatinine Clearance	Reduce Dose to
61–80 mL/min	75% of normal
51–60 mL/min	70% of normal
10–50 mL/min	30–50% of normal
Less than 10 mL/min	Avoid use

Dosage in Hepatic Impairment
Use caution.

SIDE EFFECTS

Frequent (10%–3%): Nausea, vomiting, stomatitis, burning/erythema at psoriatic site (in pts with psoriasis). **Occasional (3%–1%):** Diarrhea, rash, dermatitis, pruritus, alopecia, dizziness, anorexia, malaise, headache, drowsiness, blurred vision.

ADVERSE EFFECTS/TOXIC REACTIONS

High potential for various severe toxicities. GI toxicity may produce gingivitis, glossitis, pharyngitis, stomatitis, enteritis, hematemesis. Hepatotoxicity more likely to occur with frequent small doses than with large intermittent doses. Pulmonary toxicity characterized by interstitial pneumonitis. Hematologic toxicity, resulting from marked myelosuppression, may manifest as leukopenia, thrombocytopenia, anemia, hemorrhage. Dermatologic toxicity may produce rash, pruritus, urticaria, pigmentation, photosensitivity, petechiae, ecchymosis, pustules. Severe nephrotoxicity produces azotemia, hematuria, renal failure.

NURSING CONSIDERATIONS

BASELINE ASSESSMENT

Obtain pregnancy test in females of reproductive potential. **Rheumatoid arthritis:** Assess pain, range of motion. Obtain baseline CBC, BMP, LFT, rheumatoid factor. **Psoriasis:** Assess skin lesions. Obtain all functional tests before therapy, repeat throughout therapy. Antiemetics may prevent nausea, vomiting.

INTERVENTION/EVALUATION

Monitor CBC, BMP, LFT, urinalysis, chest X-rays, serum uric acid. Monitor for hematologic toxicity (fever, sore throat, signs of local infection, unusual bruising/bleeding from any site), symptoms of anemia (excessive fatigue, weakness). Assess skin for evidence of dermatologic toxicity. Keep pt well hydrated, urine alkaline. Avoid rectal temperatures, traumas that induce bleeding. Apply 5 full min of pressure to IV sites.

PATIENT/FAMILY TEACHING

• Treatment may depress your immune system response and reduce your ability to fight infection. Report symptoms of infection such as body aches, chills, cough, fatigue, fever. Avoid those with active infection. • Report symptoms of lung inflammation (excessive coughing, difficulty breathing, chest pain); liver problems (abdominal pain, bruising, clay-colored stool, amber- or dark-colored urine, yellowing of the skin or eyes), kidney problems (decreased urine output, flank pain, darkened urine); toxic skin reactions

M

(rash, skin eruptions). • Use effective contraception to avoid pregnancy.

methylergonovine

meth-il-er-**goe**-noe-veen
(Methergine)

◆CLASSIFICATION

PHARMACOTHERAPEUTIC: Ergot alkaloid. **CLINICAL:** Oxytocic agent, uterine stimulant.

USES

Management of uterine atony, hemorrhage and subinvolution of uterus following delivery of placenta. Control uterine hemorrhage following delivery of anterior shoulder in second stage of labor.

M

PRECAUTIONS

Contraindications: Hypersensitivity to methylergonovine. Hypertension, pregnancy, toxemia. **Cautions:** Renal/hepatic impairment, coronary artery disease, pts at risk for coronary artery disease (diabetes, obesity, smoking, hypercholesterolemia), concurrent use with CYP3A4 inhibitors, occlusive peripheral vascular disease, sepsis, second stage of labor.

ACTION

Increases tone, rate, amplitude of contraction of uterine smooth muscle. **Therapeutic Effect:** Produces sustained contractions, which shortens third stage of labor, reduces blood loss.

PHARMACOKINETICS

Route	Onset	Peak	Duration
PO	5–10 min	N/A	3 hrs
IV	Immediate	N/A	45 min
IM	2–5 min	N/A	3 hrs

Rapidly absorbed from GI tract after IM administration. Distributed rapidly to plasma, extracellular fluid, tissues. Metabolized in liver. Primarily excreted in urine. **Half-life:** 0.5–2 hrs.

⌛ LIFESPAN CONSIDERATIONS

Pregnancy/Lactation: Contraindicated during pregnancy. Small amounts distributed in breast milk. **Children/Elderly:** No information available.

INTERACTIONS

DRUG: May increase hypertensive effect of **DOPamine, norepinephrine, phenylephrine, vasopressin. Strong CYP3A4 inhibitors (e.g., clarithromycin, ketoconazole, ritonavir)** may increase concentration/effect. **Beta blockers (e.g., carvedilol, labetalol, metoprolol)** may increase vasoconstrictive effect. May decrease vasodilation effect of **nitroglycerin.** May increase vasoconstricting effect of **serotonin 5-HT_{1D} receptor agonists (e.g., SUMAtriptan).** **HERBAL:** None significant. **FOOD:** None known. **LAB VALUES:** May decrease serum prolactin.

AVAILABILITY (Rx)

Injection Solution: 0.2 mg/mL. **Tablets:** 0.2 mg.

ADMINISTRATION/HANDLING

Reconstitution • Dilute with 0.9% NaCl to volume of 5 mL.
Rate of administration • Give over at least 1 min, carefully monitoring B/P.
Storage • Refrigerate ampules.

IV INCOMPATIBILITIES

None known.

IV COMPATIBILITIES

Heparin, potassium.

INDICATIONS/ROUTES/DOSAGE

Prevention/Treatment of Postpartum, Postabortion Hemorrhage
PO: ADULTS: 0.2 mg 3–4 times daily. Continue for up to 7 days.

IV, IM: ADULTS: Initially, 0.2 mg after delivery of anterior shoulder, after delivery of placenta, or during puerperium. May repeat q2–4h as needed.
Note: Initial dose may be given parenterally, followed by oral regimen.
IV use in life-threatening emergencies only.

Dosage in Renal/Hepatic Impairment
Use caution.

SIDE EFFECTS

Frequent: Nausea, uterine cramping, vomiting. **Occasional:** Abdominal pain, diarrhea, dizziness, diaphoresis, tinnitus, bradycardia, chest pain. **Rare:** Allergic reaction (rash, pruritus), dyspnea, severe or sudden hypertension.

ADVERSE EFFECTS/TOXIC REACTIONS

Severe hypertensive episodes may result in CVA, serious arrhythmias, seizures. Hypertensive effects are more frequent with pt susceptibility, rapid IV administration, concurrent use of regional anesthesia, vasoconstrictors. Peripheral ischemia may lead to gangrene.

NURSING CONSIDERATIONS

BASELINE ASSESSMENT

Obtain serum calcium level, B/P, pulse. Assess for any evidence of bleeding before administration.

INTERVENTION/EVALUATION

Monitor uterine tone, bleeding, B/P, pulse q15min until stable (about 1–2 hrs). Assess extremities for color, warmth, movement, pain. Report chest pain promptly. Provide support with ambulation if dizziness occurs.

PATIENT/FAMILY TEACHING

• Avoid smoking: causes increased vasoconstriction. • Report increased cramping, bleeding, foul-smelling lochia. • Report pale, cold hands/feet (possibility of diminished circulation).

methylnaltrexone

meth-il-nal-**trex**-own
(Relistor)
Do not confuse methylnaltrexone with naltrexone.

◆CLASSIFICATION

PHARMACOTHERAPEUTIC: Opioid receptor antagonist. **CLINICAL:** GI agent.

USES

Injection: Treatment of opioid-induced constipation in pts with advanced illness or pain caused by active cancer who require opioid dosage escalation for palliative care. **Injection/Tablets:** Treatment of opioid-induced constipation in pts with chronic pain unrelated to cancer including pts with chronic pain related to prior cancer or its treatment not requiring frequent opioid dosage escalation.

PRECAUTIONS

Contraindications: Hypersensitivity to methylnaltrexone. Known or suspected GI obstruction. Pts at increased risk of recurrent GI obstruction. **Cautions:** Renal impairment, history of GI tract lesions (e.g., peptic ulcer disease, GI tract malignancies).

ACTION

Blocks binding of opioids to peripheral opioid receptors within GI tract. Inhibits opioid-induced decreased GI motility and delay in GI transit time. **Therapeutic Effect:** Decreases constipating effect of opioids.

PHARMACOKINETICS

Absorbed rapidly. Undergoes moderate tissue distribution. Protein binding: 11%–15%. Excreted in urine (50%), feces (35%). **Half-life:** 8 hrs.

LIFESPAN CONSIDERATIONS

Pregnancy/Lactation: Unknown if distributed in breast milk. Breastfeeding not recommended. **Children:** Safety

and efficacy not established. **Elderly:** No age-related precautions noted.

INTERACTIONS

DRUG: May increase adverse/toxic effects of **naloxegol, opioid antagonists.** **HERBAL:** None significant. **FOOD:** None known. **LAB VALUES:** None significant.

AVAILABILITY (Rx)

Injection Solution: 8 mg/0.4 mL, 12 mg/0.6 mL. **Tablets:** 150 mg.

ADMINISTRATION/HANDLING

PO

• Administer with water on an empty stomach at least 30 min before first meal of day.

Preparation • Visually inspect for particulate matter or discoloration. Solution should appear colorless to pale yellow in color. Do not use if solution is cloudy, discolored, or if large particles are observed.

Administration • Insert needle subcutaneously into upper arms, outer thigh, or abdomen, and inject solution. • Do not inject into areas of active skin disease or injury such as sunburns, skin rashes, inflammation, skin infections, or active psoriasis. • Rotate injection sites.

Storage • Once solution is drawn into syringe, may be stored at room temperature. • Administer within 24 hrs.

INDICATIONS/ROUTES/DOSAGE

◀ALERT▶ Usual schedule is once every other day, as needed, but no more frequently than once every 24 hrs.

Constipation (Chronic non-cancer pain)

PO: ADULTS, ELDERLY: 450 mg once daily in the morning. **SQ: ADULTS, ELDERLY:** 12 mg/day. **Note:** Discontinue all laxatives prior to use (if response is not optimal after 3 days, may resume laxative therapy).

Constipation (Advanced illness)

SQ: ADULTS, ELDERLY WEIGHING 38 KG TO LESS THAN 62 KG: 8 mg. **ADULTS, ELDERLY WEIGHING 62–114 KG:** 12 mg. **ADULTS, ELDERLY WHOSE WEIGHT FALLS OUTSIDE THESE RANGES:** Dose at 0.15 mg/kg (round dose up to nearest 0.1 mL of volume).

Dosage in Severe Renal Impairment (CrCl less than 60 mL/min)

SQ: ADULTS, ELDERLY: Administer 50% of recommended dose.

Dosage in Hepatic Impairment

No dose adjustment.

SIDE EFFECTS

Frequent (29%–12%): Abdominal pain, flatulence, nausea. **Occasional (7%–5%):** Diarrhea, dizziness.

ADVERSE EFFECTS/TOXIC REACTIONS

None known.

NURSING CONSIDERATIONS

BASELINE ASSESSMENT

Question characteristics of constipation, frequency of bowel movements. Assess bowel sounds. Question history of GI obstruction, perforation, baseline GI disease; renal impairment. Receive full medication history, including herbal products, and screen for interactions. Assess hydration status.

INTERVENTION/EVALUATION

30% of pts report defecation within 30 min after drug administration. Encourage fluid intake. Assess bowel sounds for peristalsis. Monitor daily pattern of bowel activity, stool consistency. If opioid medication is stopped, drug should be discontinued. Assess for abdominal disturbances.

PATIENT/FAMILY TEACHING

• Laxative effect usually occurs within 30 min but may take up to 24 hrs after medication administration. • Common side effects include transient abdominal pain, nausea, vomiting. • Report persistent or worsening symptoms, or if severe or persistent diarrhea occurs.

methylphenidate

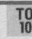

TOP 100

meth-il-**fen**-i-date
(Adhansia XR, Aptensio XR, Concerta, Cotempla XR, Daytrana, Jornay PM, Metadate ER, Methylin, Quillichew ER, Quillivant XR, Relexxii, Ritalin, Ritalin LA)

BLACK BOX ALERT Chronic abuse can lead to marked tolerance, psychological dependence. Abrupt withdrawal from prolonged use may lead to severe depression, psychosis.

Do not confuse Metadate ER with Metadate CD, methylphenidate with methadone, or Ritalin with Rifadin.

CLASSIFICATION

PHARMACOTHERAPEUTIC: CNS stimulant (Schedule II). **CLINICAL:** CNS stimulant.

USES

Treatment of attention-deficit hyperactivity disorder (ADHD). Management of narcolepsy. **OFF-LABEL:** Secondary mental depression (especially elderly pts, medically ill).

PRECAUTIONS

Contraindications: Hypersensitivity to methylphenidate. Use during or within 14 days following MAOI therapy; marked anxiety, tension, agitation, motor tics; family history or diagnosis of Tourette's syndrome, glaucoma. **Metadate:** Severe hypertension, HF, arrhythmia, hyperthyroidism, recent MI or angina. **Cautions:** Hypertension, seizures, acute stress reaction, emotional instability, HF, recent MI, hyperthyroidism or thyrotoxicosis, known structural cardiac abnormality, bipolar disorder, cardiomyopathy, arrhythmias, history of drug abuse and misuse, drug-seeking behavior, dependency.

ACTION

Blocks reuptake of norepinephrine, dopamine into presynaptic neurons. Stimulates cerebral cortex and subcortical structures. **Therapeutic Effect:** Decreases motor restlessness, fatigue. Increases motor activity, attention span, mental alertness. Produces mild euphoria.

PHARMACOKINETICS

Onset	Peak	Duration
Immediate-release	2 hrs	3–6 hrs
Sustained-release	4–7 hrs	8 hrs
Extended-release	N/A	12 hrs
Transdermal	2 hrs	N/A

Slowly, incompletely absorbed from GI tract. Protein binding: 15%. Metabolized in liver. Primarily excreted in urine. Unknown if removed by hemodialysis. **Half-life:** 2–4 hrs.

LIFESPAN CONSIDERATIONS

Pregnancy/Lactation: Unknown if drug crosses placenta or is distributed in breast milk. **Children:** May be more susceptible to developing anorexia, insomnia, stomach pain, decreased weight. Chronic use may inhibit growth. Not approved for children younger than 6 yrs. **Elderly:** No age-related precautions noted.

INTERACTIONS

DRUG: **MAOIs (e.g., phenelzine, selegiline)** may increase hypertensive effects. **Other CNS stimulants (e.g., caffeine, dextroamphetamine, phentermine)** may have additive effect. May inhibit metabolism of **warfarin, anticonvulsants (e.g., carBAMazepine, phenytoin), antidepressants. Alcohol** may increase adverse effects. **HERBAL:** **Ephedra** may cause hypertension, arrhythmias. **Yohimbe** may increase CNS stimulation. **FOOD:** None known. **LAB VALUES:** None significant.

AVAILABILITY (Rx)

Oral Solution: ***(Methylin):*** 5 mg/5 mL, 10 mg/5 mL, 10 mg/1 mL. **Tablets, Chewable:** ***(Methylin):*** 2.5 mg, 5 mg, 10 mg. **Tablets:** ***(Methylin, Ritalin):*** 5 mg, 10 mg, 20 mg. **Topical Patch:** ***(Daytrana):*** 10 mg/9 hrs, 15 mg/9 hrs, 20 mg/9 hrs, 30 mg/9 hrs. **Powder for Suspension, Extended-Release:** ***(Quillivant XR):*** 25 mg/5 mL.

Capsules, Extended-Release: *(Adhansia XR):* 25 mg, 35 mg, 45 mg, 55 mg, 70 mg, 85 mg. *(Aptensio XR):* 10 mg, 15 mg, 20 mg, 30 mg, 40 mg, 50 mg, 60 mg. *(Jornay PM):* 20 mg, 40 mg, 60 mg, 80 mg, 100 mg. *(Ritalin LA):* 10 mg, 20 mg, 30 mg, 40 mg. **Tablets, Extended-Release:** *(Concerta):* 18 mg, 27 mg, 36 mg, 54 mg, 72 mg. *(Relexxii):* 72 mg. *(Metadate ER, Methylin ER):* 10 mg, 20 mg. **Sustained-Release:** *(Ritalin SR):* 20 mg. **Tablets, Extended-Release ODT:** *(Cotempla XR):* 8.6 mg, 17.3 mg, 25.9 mg. **Tablets, Chewable, Extended-Release:** *(Quillichew ER):* 20 mg, 30 mg, 40 mg.

ADMINISTRATION/HANDLING

◀ALERT▶ Sustained-release, extended-release tablets may be given in place of regular tablets once the daily dose is titrated using regular tablets and the titrated dosage corresponds to sustained-release or extended-release tablet strength.

PO

• Do not give in afternoon or evening (may cause insomnia). • Do not crush, break extended-release capsules, extended- or sustained-release tablets. • Immediate-release tablets may be crushed. • Give dose 30–45 min before meals. • **Concerta:** Administer once daily in morning. May take without regard to food but must be taken with water, milk, or juice. • **Methylin Chewable:** Give with at least 8 oz of water or other fluid. • **Metadate CD, Ritalin LA:** • May be opened, sprinkled on applesauce. • Instruct pt to swallow applesauce without chewing. Do not crush or chew capsule contents. • **Quillivant XR:** Administer in morning with or without food. Shake bottle more than 10 sec prior to administration.

Patch

• To be worn daily for 9 hrs. • Replace daily in morning. • Apply to dry, clean area of hip. • Avoid applying to waistline (clothing may cause patch to rub off). • Alternate application site daily. • Press firmly in place for 30 sec to ensure patch is in good contact with skin. • Do not cut patch.

INDICATIONS/ROUTES/DOSAGE

ADHD

PO: ADULTS: *(Immediate-Release):* Initially, 10–20 mg twice daily, before breakfast and lunch. May increase by 5–10 mg/day at wkly intervals. **Maximum:** 60 mg/day in 2–3 divided doses. **CHILDREN 6 YRS AND OLDER:** Initially, 2.5–5 mg before breakfast and lunch. May increase by 5–10 mg/day at wkly intervals. **Usual dose:** 20–30 mg/day in 2–3 divided doses. **Maximum:** 60 mg/day not to exceed 2 mg/kg/day.

PO: *(Concerta):* **CHILDREN 6–12 YRS, ADOLESCENTS 13–17 YRS, ADULTS 18–65 YRS:** Initially, 18 mg once daily; may increase by 18 mg/day at wkly intervals. **Maximum:** 54 mg/day in children 6–12 yrs of age (up to 72 mg/day in adolescents younger than 18 yrs).

PO: *(Metadate CD):* **ADULTS, CHILDREN 6 YRS AND OLDER:** Initially, 20 mg/day. May increase by 10–20 mg/day at wkly intervals. **Maximum:** 60 mg/day.

PO: *(Quillichew ER):* **ADULTS, CHILDREN 6 YRS AND OLDER:** Initially, 20 mg/day. May increase by 10 mg, 15 mg or 20 mg/day at wkly intervals. **Maximum:** 60 mg/day.

PO: *(Quillivant XR):* **ADULTS, CHILDREN 6 YRS AND OLDER:** Initially, 20 mg once daily in the morning. May increase in increments of 10–20 mg/day at wkly increments. **Maximum:** 60 mg/day.

PO: *(Ritalin LA):* **ADULTS, CHILDREN 6 YRS AND OLDER:** Initially, 10–20 mg/day. May increase by 10 mg/day at wkly intervals. **Maximum:** 60 mg/day.

PO: *(Jornay PM):* **ADULTS:** Initially, 20 mg once daily in the evening (between 6:30 PM [1830 hrs] and 9:30 PM [2130 hrs]). May increase by 20 mg/day at wkly intervals. **Maximum:** 100 mg/day.

PO: *(Adhansia XR):* **ADULTS:** Initially, 25 mg in the morning. May increase by 10–15 mg at 5-day intervals or more. **Maximum:** 100 mg/day.

PO: ***(Metadate ER):*** **CHILDREN 6 YRS AND OLDER:** May replace regular tablets after daily dose is titrated and 8-hr dosage corresponds to sustained-release or extended-release tablet strength. **Maximum:** 60 mg/day.
PO: ***(Cotempla XR):*** **CHILDREN, 6–18 YRS:** Initially, 17.3 mg once daily. May increase in wkly intervals in 8.6 to 17.3 mg increments. **Maximum:** 51.8 mg/day.
Patch: ***(Daytrana):*** **ADULTS, ADOLESCENTS, CHILDREN 6–12 YRS:** Initially, 10 mg daily (applied and worn for 9 hrs). Dosage is titrated up to 60 mg/day to desired effect. May increase dose no more frequently than every wk.

Narcolepsy
PO: ADULTS, ELDERLY: ***(Immediate-Release):*** Initially, 10 mg twice daily, before breakfast and lunch. May increase by 5–10 mg/day at wkly intervals. **Maximum:** 60 mg/day in 2–3 divided doses. ***(Extended-Release):*** May be given once the immediate-release dose is titrated and the titrated 8-hr dose corresponds to sustained-release or extended-release tablet strength. **Maximum:** 60 mg/day.

Dosage in Renal/Hepatic Impairment
No dose adjustment.

SIDE EFFECTS

Frequent: Anxiety, insomnia, anorexia. **Occasional:** Dizziness, drowsiness, headache, nausea, abdominal pain, fever, rash, arthralgia, vomiting. **Rare:** Blurred vision, Tourette's syndrome (uncontrolled vocal outbursts, repetitive body movements, tics), palpitations, priapism.

ADVERSE EFFECTS/TOXIC REACTIONS

Prolonged administration to children with ADHD may delay normal weight gain pattern. Overdose may produce tachycardia, palpitations, arrhythmias, chest pain, psychotic episode, seizures, coma. Hypersensitivity reactions, blood dyscrasias occur rarely.

NURSING CONSIDERATIONS

BASELINE ASSESSMENT

ADHD: Assess attention span, impulsivity, interaction with others, distractibility. **Narcolepsy:** Observe/assess frequency of episodes. Question history of seizures. Assess for potential of abuse/misuse (e.g., drug seeking behavior, mental health conditions, history of substance abuse).

INTERVENTION/EVALUATION

Monitor B/P, pulse, changes in ADHD symptoms. CBC with differential should be performed routinely during therapy. If paradoxical return of attention-deficit occurs, dosage should be reduced or discontinued. Monitor growth. Screen for drug abuse and misuse, drug-seeking behavior.

PATIENT/FAMILY TEACHING

• Avoid tasks that require alertness, motor skills until response to drug is established. • Report any increase in seizures. • Take daily dose early in morning to avoid insomnia. • Report anxiety, palpitations, fever, vomiting, skin rash. • Report new or worsened symptoms (e.g., behavior, hostility, concentration ability). • Avoid caffeine. • Do not stop taking abruptly after prolonged use.

methylPREDNISolone

meth-il-pred-**nis**-oh-lone
(Medrol)

methylPREDNISolone acetate

(DEPO-Medrol)

methylPREDNISolone sodium succinate

(SOLU-Medrol)
Do not confuse DEPO-Medrol with SOLU-Medrol, Medrol with

M

Mebaral, or methylPREDNISolone with medroxyPROGESTERone or prednisoLONE.

◆CLASSIFICATION

PHARMACOTHERAPEUTIC: Adrenal corticosteroid. **CLINICAL:** Anti-inflammatory.

USES

Anti-inflammatory or immunosuppressant in the treatment of hematologic, allergic, neoplastic, dermatologic, endocrine, GI, nervous system, ophthalmic, renal, or rheumatic disorders. **OFF-LABEL:** Acute spinal cord injury.

PRECAUTIONS

Contraindications: Hypersensitivity to methylprednisolone. Administration of live or attenuated virus vaccines, systemic fungal infection. **IM:** Idiopathic thrombocytopenia purpura. Intrathecal administration. **Cautions:** Respiratory tuberculosis, untreated systemic infections, hypertension, HF, diabetes, GI disease (e.g., peptic ulcer), myasthenia gravis, renal/hepatic impairment, seizures, cataracts, glaucoma, following acute MI, thyroid disorder, thromboembolic tendencies, cardiovascular disease, elderly, psychiatric conditions, at risk for osteoporosis.

ACTION

Anti-inflammatory: Suppresses migration of polymorphonuclear leukocytes, reverses increased capillary permeability. Exerts effects on modulating carbohydrate, protein, lipid metabolism. Maintains fluid/electrolyte hemostasis. Influences CV, immunologic, endocrine, musculoskeletal, neurologic physiology. **Therapeutic Effect:** Decreases inflammation.

PHARMACOKINETICS

Route	Onset	Peak	Duration
PO	Rapid	1–2 hrs	30–36 hrs
IM	Rapid	4–8 days	1–4 wks
IV	Rapid	N/A	N/A

Well absorbed from GI tract after IM administration. Widely distributed. Metabolized in liver. Excreted in urine. Removed by hemodialysis. **Half-life:** 3.5 hrs.

⌛ LIFESPAN CONSIDERATIONS

Pregnancy/Lactation: Crosses placenta. Distributed in breast milk. May cause cleft palate (chronic use in first trimester). Breastfeeding not recommended. **Children:** Prolonged treatment or high dosages may decrease short-term growth rate, cortisol secretion. **Elderly:** No age-related precautions noted.

INTERACTIONS

DRUG: May increase anticoagulant effects of **warfarin. Strong CYP3A inducers (e.g., carBAMazepine, phenytoin, rifAMPin)** may decrease concentration/effect. **Live virus vaccines** may decrease antibody response to vaccine, increase vaccine side effects, potentiate virus replication. May increase hyponatremic effect of **desmopressin. Strong CYP3A4 inhibitors (e.g., clarithromycin, ketoconazole, ritonavir)** may increase concentration/effect. **HERBAL: Herbals with sedative properties (e.g., chamomile, kava kava, valerian)** may increase CNS depression. **St. John's wort** may decrease concentration/effect. **FOOD:** None known. **LAB VALUES:** May increase serum glucose, cholesterol, lipids, amylase, sodium. May decrease serum calcium, potassium, thyroxine, hypothalamic-pituitary-adrenal (HPA) axis.

AVAILABILITY (Rx)

Injection, Powder for Reconstitution: ***(SOLU):*** 40 mg, 125 mg, 500 mg, 1 g. **Injection, Suspension:** ***(DEPO):*** 20 mg/mL, 40 mg/mL, 80 mg/mL. **Tablets:** ***(Medrol):*** 2 mg, 4 mg, 8 mg, 16 mg, 32 mg. ***(Medrol Dosepak):*** 4 mg (21 tablets).

ADMINISTRATION/HANDLING

◀ALERT▶ Do **not** give methylPREDNIsolone acetate IV.

IV

Reconstitution • For infusion, add to D_5W, 0.9% NaCl.
Rate of administration • Give IV push over 3–15 min. • Give IV piggyback. Dose of 250 mg over 15–30 min; dose of 500–999 mg over at least 30 min; dose of 1 g or greater over 1 hr.
Storage • Store vials at room temperature. Diluted solution is stable for 48 hrs at room temperature or refrigerated.

IM

• MethylPREDNISolone acetate should not be further diluted. • MethylPREDNISolone sodium succinate should be reconstituted with Bacteriostatic Water for Injection. • Give deep IM in gluteus maximus (avoid injection into deltoid muscle).

PO

• Give with food, milk.

IV INCOMPATIBILITIES

Ciprofloxacin (Cipro), dilTIAZem (Cardizem), potassium chloride, propofol (Diprivan).

IV COMPATIBILITIES

Dexmedetomidine (Precedex), DOPamine (Intropin), heparin, midazolam (Versed), theophylline.

INDICATIONS/ROUTES/DOSAGE

Anti-inflammatory, Immunosuppressive

IV: ADULTS, ELDERLY: 40–125 mg/day as a single dose or in divided doses. **CHILDREN:** Initially, 0.11–1.6 mg/kg/day in 3–4 divided doses. Range: 0.5–1.7 mg/kg/day in 2–4 divided doses.

PO: ADULTS, ELDERLY: 16–64 mg/day once daily or in divided doses. **CHILDREN:** 0.5–1.7 mg/kg/day or 5–25 mg/m^2/day in 2–4 divided doses.

IM: *(MethylPREDNISolone Succinate)*: ADULTS, ELDERLY: 40–60 mg as a single dose.

IM: *(Methylprednisolone Acetate)*: ADULTS, ELDERLY: 40–60 mg as a single dose.

Intra-articular, intralesional: ADULTS, ELDERLY: 4–80 mg q1–5wks.

Dosage in Renal/Hepatic Impairment

No dose adjustment.

SIDE EFFECTS

Frequent: Insomnia, heartburn, anxiety, abdominal distention, diaphoresis, acne, mood swings, increased appetite, facial flushing, GI distress, delayed wound healing, increased susceptibility to infection, diarrhea, constipation. **Occasional:** Headache, edema, tachycardia, change in skin color, frequent urination, depression. **Rare:** Psychosis, increased blood coagulability, hallucinations.

ADVERSE EFFECTS/TOXIC REACTIONS

Long-term therapy: Hypocalcemia, hypokalemia, muscle wasting (esp. in arms, legs), osteoporosis, spontaneous fractures, amenorrhea, cataracts, glaucoma, peptic ulcer, HF. **Abrupt withdrawal after long-term therapy:** Anorexia, nausea, fever, headache, severe arthralgia, rebound inflammation, fatigue, weakness, lethargy, dizziness, orthostatic hypotension.

NURSING CONSIDERATIONS

BASELINE ASSESSMENT

Question for hypersensitivity to corticosteroids, components. Obtain height, weight, B/P, serum glucose, electrolytes. Check results of initial tests (tuberculosis [TB] skin test, X-rays, ECG). Question history as listed in Precautions.

INTERVENTION/EVALUATION

Monitor I&O, daily weight; assess for edema. Monitor daily pattern of bowel activity, stool consistency. Check vital signs at least twice daily. Be alert for infection (sore throat, fever, vague symptoms). Monitor serum electrolytes, including B/P, glucose. Monitor for hypocalcemia (muscle twitching, cramps, positive Trousseau's or Chvostek's signs), hy-

M

pokalemia (weakness, muscle cramps, numbness, tingling [esp. lower extremities], nausea/vomiting, irritability, ECG changes). Assess emotional status, ability to sleep.

PATIENT/FAMILY TEACHING

• Take oral dose with food, milk. • Do not change dose/schedule or stop taking drug; must taper off gradually under medical supervision. • Report fever, sore throat, muscle aches, sudden weight gain or loss, edema, loss of appetite, fatigue. • Severe stress (serious infection, surgery, trauma) may require increased dosage. • Follow-up visits, lab tests are necessary. • Children must be assessed for growth retardation. • Inform dentist, other physicians of methylprednisolone therapy now or within past 12 mos.

metoclopramide

met-oh-**kloe**-pra-myde
(Metonia 🍁, Reglan)

BLACK BOX ALERT Prolonged use may cause tardive dyskinesia.
Do not confuse metoclopramide with metOLazone or metoprolol, or Reglan with Renagel.

◆CLASSIFICATION

PHARMACOTHERAPEUTIC: DOPamine, serotonin receptor antagonist. **CLINICAL:** GI agent, antiemetic.

USES

PO: Symptomatic treatment of diabetic gastroparesis, gastroesophageal reflux. **IV/IM:** Symptomatic treatment of diabetic gastroparesis, prevent/treat nausea/vomiting with chemotherapy or after surgery.

PRECAUTIONS

Contraindications: Hypersensitivity to metoclopramide. Concurrent use of medications likely to produce extrapyramidal reactions. Situations in which GI motility may be dangerous (e.g., GI hemorrhage, GI perforation/obstruction), history of seizure disorder, pheochromocytoma. **Cautions:** Renal impairment, HF, cirrhosis, hypertension, depression, Parkinson's disease, elderly.

ACTION

Blocks dopamine/serotonin receptors in chemoreceptor trigger zone of the CNS. Enhances acetylcholine response in upper GI tract, causing increased motility and accelerated gastric emptying without stimulating gastric, biliary, or pancreatic secretions; increases lower esophageal sphincter tone. **Therapeutic Effect:** Accelerates intestinal transit, promotes gastric emptying. Relieves nausea, vomiting.

PHARMACOKINETICS

Route	Onset	Peak	Duration
PO	30–60 min	N/A	1–2 hrs
IV	1–3 min	N/A	1–2 hrs
IM	10–15 min	N/A	1–2 hrs

Well absorbed from GI tract. Metabolized in liver. Protein binding: 30%. Primarily excreted in urine. Not removed by hemodialysis. **Half-life:** 4–6 hrs.

⌛ LIFESPAN CONSIDERATIONS

Pregnancy/Lactation: Crosses placenta. Distributed in breast milk. **Children:** More susceptible to dystonic reactions. **Elderly:** More likely to have parkinsonian dyskinesias after long-term therapy.

INTERACTIONS

DRUG: May increase adverse effects of **antipsychotic (e.g., haloperidol), promethazine, SNRIs (e.g., DULoxetine, venlafaxine), SSRIs (e.g., citalopram, PARoxetine), tramadol, tricyclic antidepressants (e.g., amitriptyline, doxepin). Strong CYP2D6 inhibitors (e.g., FLUoxetine, PARoxetine)** may increase concentration/effect. **HERBAL:** None significant. **FOOD:** None known. **LAB VALUES:** May increase serum aldosterone, prolactin.

AVAILABILITY (Rx)

Injection Solution: 5 mg/mL. **Solution, Oral:** 5 mg/5 mL. **Tablets:** 5 mg, 10 mg.

Tablets, Orally Disintegrating: 5 mg, 10 mg.

ADMINISTRATION/HANDLING

IV

Reconstitution • Dilute doses greater than 10 mg in 50 mL D_5W or 0.9% NaCl.
Rate of administration • Infuse over 15–30 min. • May give undiluted slow IV push at rate of 10 mg over 1–2 min. • Too-rapid IV injection may produce intense feeling of anxiety, restlessness, followed by drowsiness.
Storage • Store vials at room temperature. • After dilution, IV infusion (piggyback) is stable for 24 hrs.

PO

• Give 30 min before meals and at bedtime. • Tablets may be crushed. • Do not cut, divide, break orally disintegrating tablets. Place on tongue, swallow with saliva.

IV INCOMPATIBILITIES

Allopurinol (Aloprim), cefepime (Maxipime), furosemide (Lasix), propofol (Diprivan).

IV COMPATIBILITIES

Dexamethasone, dexmedetomidine (Precedex), dilTIAZem (Cardizem), diphenhy-drAMINE (Benadryl), fentaNYL (Sublimaze), heparin, HYDROmorphone (Dilaudid), morphine, potassium chloride.

INDICATIONS/ROUTES/DOSAGE

Prevention of Chemotherapy-Induced Nausea/Vomiting

PO: ADULTS, ELDERLY: 10 mg q6h prn.

Diabetic Gastroparesis

PO, IV: ADULTS, ELDERLY: 5–10 mg 30 min before meals and at bedtime for up to 12 wks.

Dosage in Renal Impairment

Dosage is modified based on creatinine clearance.

Creatinine Clearance	Dosage
Less than 40 mL/min	50% of normal dose

Dosage in Hepatic Impairment

No dose adjustment.

SIDE EFFECTS

ALERT Doses of 2 mg/kg or greater, or increased length of therapy, may result in a greater incidence of side effects.

Frequent (10%): Drowsiness, restlessness, fatigue, lethargy. **Occasional (3%):** Dizziness, anxiety, headache, insomnia, breast tenderness, altered menstruation, constipation, rash, dry mouth, galactorrhea, gynecomastia. **Rare (less than 3%):** Hypotension, hypertension, tachycardia.

ADVERSE EFFECTS/TOXIC REACTIONS

Extrapyramidal reactions occur most frequently in children, young adults (18–30 yrs) receiving large doses (2 mg/kg) during chemotherapy and usually are limited to akathisia (involuntary limb movement, facial grimacing, motor restlessness). Neuroleptic malignant syndrome (diaphoresis, fever, unstable B/P, muscular rigidity) has been reported.

NURSING CONSIDERATIONS

BASELINE ASSESSMENT

Assess for nausea, vomiting, abdominal distention, bowel sounds. **Antiemetic:** Assess for dehydration (poor skin turgor, dry mucous membranes, longitudinal furrows in tongue).

INTERVENTION/EVALUATION

Monitor renal function, B/P, heart rate. Monitor for anxiety, restlessness, extrapyramidal symptoms (EPS) during IV administration. Monitor daily pattern of bowel activity, stool consistency. Assess skin for rash. Evaluate for therapeutic response from gastroparesis (nausea, vomiting, bloating).

M

PATIENT/FAMILY TEACHING

• Avoid tasks that require alertness, motor skills until response to drug is established. • Report involuntary eye, facial, limb movement (extrapyramidal reaction). • Avoid alcohol.

metOLazone

meh-**toe**-la-zone
(Zaroxolyn ✱)

Do not confuse metOLazone with metaxalone, methotrexate, metoclopramide, or metoprolol, or Zaroxolyn with Zarontin.

◆CLASSIFICATION

PHARMACOTHERAPEUTIC: Thiazide diuretic. **CLINICAL:** Diuretic, antihypertensive.

USES

Treatment of edema due to HF, nephrotic syndrome, or impaired renal function.

PRECAUTIONS

Contraindications: Hypersensitivity to metolazone. Anuria, hepatic coma/precoma. **Cautions:** Hypersensitivity to sulfonamides, thiazide diuretics. Severe renal disease, severe hepatic impairment, gout, prediabetes or diabetes, elevated serum cholesterol, triglycerides.

ACTION

Blocks reabsorption of sodium, potassium, chloride at distal convoluted tubule, increasing excretion of sodium, potassium, water. **Therapeutic Effect:** Reduces B/P, promotes diuresis.

PHARMACOKINETICS

Route	Onset	Peak	Duration
PO (diuretic)	1 hr	—	24 hrs

Incompletely absorbed from GI tract. Protein binding: 95%. Primarily excreted in urine. Not removed by hemodialysis. **Half-life:** 20 hrs.

⌛ LIFESPAN CONSIDERATIONS

Pregnancy/Lactation: Crosses placenta. Small amount distributed in breast milk. Breastfeeding not recommended. **Children:** No age-related precautions noted. **Elderly:** May be more sensitive to hypotensive or electrolyte imbalance. Age-related renal impairment may require dosage adjustment.

INTERACTIONS

DRUG: **Bile acid sequestrants (e.g., cholestyramine)** may decrease absorption. May increase the hypokalemic effect of **topiramate. HERBAL:** **Licorice** may increase the hypokalemic effect. **Herbals with hypotensive properties (e.g., garlic, ginger, ginkgo biloba) or hypertensive properties (e.g., yohimbe)** may alter effects. **FOOD:** None known. **LAB VALUES:** May increase serum glucose, cholesterol, LDL, bilirubin, calcium, creatinine, uric acid, triglycerides. May decrease urinary calcium, serum magnesium, potassium, sodium.

AVAILABILITY (Rx)

Tablets: 2.5 mg, 5 mg, 10 mg.

ADMINISTRATION/HANDLING

PO

• May give with food, milk if GI upset occurs, preferably with breakfast (may prevent nocturia).

INDICATIONS/ROUTES/DOSAGE

Edema

PO: ADULTS: 2.5–10 mg/day. May increase to 20 mg/day.

Dosage in Renal Impairment

Mild to moderate impairment: No dose adjustment. **Severe impairment:** Use caution.

Dosage in Hepatic Impairment

No dose adjustment. Contraindicated with hepatic coma or precoma.

SIDE EFFECTS

Expected: Increased urinary frequency/volume. **Frequent (10%–9%):** Dizziness, light-headedness, headache. **Occasional (6%–4%):** Muscle cramps/spasm, drowsiness, fatigue, lethargy. **Rare (less than 2%):** Asthenia, palpitations, depression, nausea, vomiting, abdominal bloating, constipation, diarrhea, urticaria.

ADVERSE EFFECTS/TOXIC REACTIONS

Vigorous diuresis may lead to profound water loss and electrolyte depletion, resulting in hypokalemia, hyponatremia, dehydration. Acute hypotensive episodes may occur. Hyperglycemia may occur during prolonged therapy. Pancreatitis, paresthesia, blood dyscrasias, pulmonary edema, allergic pneumonitis, dermatologic reactions occur rarely. Overdose can lead to lethargy, coma without changes in electrolytes, hydration.

NURSING CONSIDERATIONS

BASELINE ASSESSMENT

Obtain vital signs, esp. B/P for hypotension. Obtain serum electrolytes. Assess skin turgor, mucous membranes for hydration status. Assess for peripheral edema. Obtain baseline weight. Monitor I&O.

INTERVENTION/EVALUATION

Monitor B/P, vital signs, serum electrolytes, I&O, weight. Note extent of diuresis. Monitor for electrolyte disturbances (hypokalemia may result in weakness, tremors, muscle cramps, nausea, vomiting, altered mental status, tachycardia; hyponatremia may result in confusion, thirst, cold/clammy skin).

PATIENT/FAMILY TEACHING

• Expect increased urinary frequency/volume. • Slowly go from lying to standing to reduce hypotensive effect. • Avoid tasks requiring motor skills, mental alertness until response to drug is established. • Eat foods high in potassium, such as whole grains (cereals), legumes, meat, bananas, apricots, orange juice, potatoes (white, sweet), raisins.

metoprolol

TOP 100 HIGH ALERT

me-**toe**-pro-lol
(Kaspargo, Lopressor, Toprol XL)

BLACK BOX ALERT Abrupt withdrawal can produce acute tachycardia, hypertension, ischemia. Drug should be gradually tapered over 1–2 wks.

Do not confuse metoprolol with atenolol, labetalol, nadolol, or stanozolol, or Toprol XL with TEGretol, TEGretol XR, or Topamax.

FIXED-COMBINATION(S)

Dutoprol: metoprolol/hydroCHLOROthiazide (a diuretic): 25 mg/12.5 mg, 50 mg/12.5 mg, 100 mg/12.5 mg. **Lopressor HCT:** metoprolol/hydrochlorothiazide (a diuretic): 50 mg/25 mg, 100 mg/25 mg, 100 mg/50 mg.

✦CLASSIFICATION

PHARMACOTHERAPEUTIC: Beta$_1$-adrenergic blocker. **CLINICAL:** Antianginal, antihypertensive, MI adjunct.

USES

Treatment of hemodynamically stable acute myocardial infarction (AMI) to reduce CV mortality. Long-term treatment of angina pectoris. Management of hypertension. Treatment of stable symptomatic HF of ischemic, hypertensive, or cardiomyopathic origin to reduce rate of hospitalization in pts receiving ACE inhibitors, diuretics, and/or digoxin. **OFF-LABEL:** Treatment of ventricular arrhythmias, migraine prophylaxis, essential tremor, aggressive behavior, prevent reinfarction post-MI, prevent/treat atrial fibrillation/atrial flutter, hypertrophic cardiomyopathy, thyrotoxicosis.

M

PRECAUTIONS

Contraindications: Hypersensitivity to metoprolol. Second- or third-degree heart block. **Immediate-Release: MI:** Severe sinus bradycardia (HR less than 45 beats/min), systolic B/P less than 100 mm Hg, moderate to severe HF, significant first-degree heart block. **Immediate-Release: HTN/Angina:** Sinus bradycardia, cardiogenic shock, overt HF, sick sinus syndrome (except with pacemaker), severe peripheral arterial disease. **Extended-Release:** Severe bradycardia, cardiogenic shock, decompensated HF, sick sinus syndrome (except with functioning pacemaker). **Cautions:** Arterial obstruction, bronchospastic disease, hepatic impairment, peripheral vascular disease, hyperthyroidism, diabetes mellitus, myasthenia gravis, psychiatric disease, history of severe anaphylaxis to allergens. **Extended-Release***:* Compensated HF.

ACTION

Selectively blocks $beta_1$-adrenergic receptors. **Therapeutic Effect:** Slows heart rate, decreases cardiac output, reduces B/P. Decreases myocardial ischemia severity.

PHARMACOKINETICS

Route	Onset	Peak	Duration
PO	10–15 min	1–2 hrs	N/A
PO (extended-release)	N/A	6–12 hrs	N/A
IV	Immediate	20 min	N/A

Well absorbed from GI tract. Protein binding: 12%. Widely distributed. Metabolized in liver. Primarily excreted in urine. Removed by hemodialysis. **Half-life:** 3–7 hrs.

LIFESPAN CONSIDERATIONS

Pregnancy/Lactation: Crosses placenta; distributed in breast milk. Avoid use during first trimester. May produce bradycardia, apnea, hypoglycemia, hypothermia during delivery, low-birth-weight infants. **Children:** Safety and efficacy not established. **Elderly:** Age-related peripheral vascular disease may increase susceptibility to decreased peripheral circulation.

INTERACTIONS

DRUG: **$Alpha_2$ agonists (e.g., clonidine)** may increase AV-blocking effect. **Strong CYP3A4 inducers (e.g., carBAMazepine, phenytoin, rifAMPin)** may decrease concentration/effect. **Dronedarone, fingolimod, rivastigmine** may increase bradycardic effect. May increase vasoconstriction of **ergot derivatives (e.g., ergotamine).** **HERBAL:** **Herbals with hypertensive properties (e.g., licorice, yohimbe) or hypotensive properties (e.g., garlic, ginger, ginkgo biloba)** may alter effects. **FOOD:** None known. **LAB VALUES:** May increase serum antinuclear antibody titer (ANA), serum BUN, lipoprotein, LDH, alkaline phosphatase, bilirubin, creatinine, potassium, uric acid, ALT, AST, triglycerides.

AVAILABILITY (Rx)

Injection Solution: 5 mg/5 mL. **Tablets, Immediate-Release:** 25 mg, 37.5 mg, 50 mg, 75 mg, 100 mg.

Capsules, Extended-Release Sprinkle: 25 mg, 50 mg, 100 mg, 200 mg. **Tablets, Extended-Release:** 25 mg, 50 mg, 100 mg, 200 mg.

ADMINISTRATION/HANDLING

IV

Rate of administration • May give undiluted. • Administer IV injection over 1 min. • May give by IV piggyback (in 50 mL D_5W or 0.9% NaCl) over 30–60 min. • Monitor ECG, B/P during administration.

Storage • Store at room temperature.

PO

• Tablets may be crushed; do not crush extended-release tablets. • Extended-release tablets may be divided in half. • Give at same time each day. • May be given with or immediately after meals (enhances absorption). • Sprinkle capsules may be given whole or contents may be mixed (1 teaspoonful) on soft food and used within 60 min.

IV INCOMPATIBILITIES

Amphotericin B complex (Abelcet, AmBisome, Amphotec), lidocaine, nitroglycerin.

IV COMPATIBILITIES

Amiodarone, dilTIAZem, furosemide, heparin, morphine.

INDICATIONS/ROUTES/DOSAGE

Hypertension

PO: ***(Immediate-Release):*** **ADULTS, ELDERLY:** Initially, 50 mg twice daily. Increase at wkly (or longer) intervals. Usual range: 100–200 mg/day in 2 divided doses. **Maximum:** 400 mg/day. **CHILDREN:** Initially, 0.5–1 mg/kg/dose. **Maximum Initial Dose:** 25 mg. **Maximum Daily Dose:** 6 mg/kg/day or 200 mg/day, whichever is less.

PO: ***(Extended-Release):*** **ADULTS, ELDERLY:** Initially, 25–100 mg/day as single dose. May increase at least at wkly intervals until optimum B/P attained. Usual range: 50–200 mg once daily. **Maximum:** 400 mg/day. **CHILDREN 6 YRS OR OLDER:** Initially, 1 mg/kg once daily. **Maximum Initial Dose:** 50 mg. May increase to 2 mg/kg/day or 200 mg/day, whichever is less.

Angina Pectoris

PO: ***(Immediate-Release):*** **ADULTS:** Initially, 50 mg twice daily. Increase at wkly (or longer) intervals. Usual range: 50–200 mg twice daily. **Maximum:** 400 mg/day.

PO: ***(Extended-Release):*** **ADULTS:** Initially, 100 mg/day as single dose. May increase by at least at wkly intervals until optimum clinical response achieved. **Maximum:** 400 mg/day.

HF

PO: ***(Extended-Release):*** **ADULTS:** Initially, 12.5–25 mg/day. May titrate gradually by doubling dose q2wks or longer up to target dose of 200 mg/day.

Early Treatment of MI

IV: ADULTS: 5 mg q5min for up to 3 doses, followed by 12.5–50 mg q6–12h in acute setting (begin oral 15–30 min after last IV dose). Transition to metoprolol tartrate twice daily or metoprolol succinate once daily. May increase up to a maximum of 200 mg/day.

Dosage in Renal/Hepatic Impairment

No dose adjustment.

SIDE EFFECTS

Metoprolol is generally well tolerated, with transient and mild side effects. **Frequent:** Diminished sexual function, drowsiness, insomnia, unusual fatigue/weakness. **Occasional:** Anxiety, diarrhea, constipation, nausea, vomiting, nasal congestion, abdominal discomfort, dizziness, difficulty breathing, cold hands/feet. **Rare:** Altered taste, dry eyes, nightmares, paresthesia, allergic reaction (rash, pruritus).

ADVERSE EFFECTS/TOXIC REACTIONS

Overdose may produce profound bradycardia, hypotension, bronchospasm. Abrupt withdrawal may result in diaphoresis, palpitations, headache, tremulousness, exacerbation of angina, MI, ventricular arrhythmias. May precipitate HF, MI in pts with heart disease, thyroid storm in those with thyrotoxicosis, peripheral ischemia in those with existing peripheral vascular disease. Hypoglycemia may occur in pts with previously controlled diabetes (may mask signs of hypoglycemia). **Antidote:** Glucagon (see Appendix J for dosage).

NURSING CONSIDERATIONS

BASELINE ASSESSMENT

Assess B/P, heart rate immediately before drug administration (if pulse is 60/min or less or systolic B/P is less than 90 mm Hg, withhold medication, contact physician). **Antianginal:** Record onset, type (sharp, dull, squeezing), radiation, location, intensity, duration of anginal pain, precipitating factors (exertion, emotional stress).

M

INTERVENTION/EVALUATION

Measure B/P near end of dosing interval (determines whether B/P is controlled throughout day). Monitor B/P for hypotension, respiration for shortness of breath. Assess pulse for quality, rate, rhythm. Assess for evidence of HF: dyspnea (esp. on exertion, lying down), night cough, peripheral edema, distended neck veins. Monitor I&O (increased weight, decreased urinary output may indicate HF). Therapeutic response to hypertension noted in 1–2 wks.

PATIENT/FAMILY TEACHING

• Do not abruptly discontinue medication. • Compliance with therapy regimen is essential to control hypertension, arrhythmias. • Go from lying to standing slowly. • Report excessive fatigue, dizziness. • Avoid tasks that require alertness, motor skills until response to drug is established. • Do not use nasal decongestants, OTC cold preparations (stimulants) without physician approval. • Monitor B/P, pulse before taking medication. • Restrict salt, alcohol intake.

M

metroNIDAZOLE

me-troe-**nye**-da-zole
(Flagyl, MetroCream, MetroGel, NidaGel 🍁, Noritate, Vandazole)
Do not confuse metroNIDAZOLE with meropenem, metFORMIN, methotrexate, or miconazole.

FIXED-COMBINATION(S)

Helidac: metronidazole/bismuth/tetracycline (an anti-infective): 250 mg/262 mg/500 mg. **Pylera:** metroNIDAZOLE/bismuth/tetracycline (an anti-infective): 125 mg/140 mg/125 mg.

◆CLASSIFICATION

PHARMACOTHERAPEUTIC: Nitroimidazole derivative. **CLINICAL:** Antibacterial, antiprotozoal, amebicide.

USES

Systemic: Treatment of anaerobic infections (skin/skin structure, CNS, lower respiratory tract, bone/joints, intra-abdominal, gynecologic, endocarditis, septicemia). Treatment of *H. pylori* (part of multidrug regimen); surgical prophylaxis (colorectal), trichomoniasis, amebiasis. **Topical:** Treatment of acne rosacea or inflammatory lesions. **Vaginal gel:** Treatment of bacterial vaginosis. **OFF-LABEL:** Crohn's disease, urethritis. Antibiotic-associated pseudomembranous colitis (AAPC) caused by *C. difficile*.

PRECAUTIONS

Contraindications: Hypersensitivity to metronidazole. Pregnancy (first trimester with trichomoniasis), use of disulfiram within 2 wks, use of alcohol during therapy or within 3 days of discontinuing metroNIDAZOLE. **Cautions:** Blood dyscrasias, severe hepatic dysfunction, end-stage renal disease, seizure disorder, HF, other sodium-retaining states, elderly.

ACTION

Diffuses into organism, interacting with DNA causing a loss of helical DNA structure and strand breakage, inhibiting protein synthesis. **Therapeutic Effect:** Produces bactericidal, antiprotozoal, amebicidal, trichomonacidal effects. Produces anti-inflammatory, immunosuppressive effects when applied topically.

PHARMACOKINETICS

Well absorbed from GI tract; minimally absorbed after topical application. Protein binding: less than 20%. Widely distributed; crosses blood-brain barrier. Metabolized in liver. Excreted in urine (80%), feces (15%). Removed by hemodialysis. **Half-life:** 8 hrs (increased in cirrhosis, neonates). Active metabolite prolonged in renal failure.

⌛ LIFESPAN CONSIDERATIONS

Pregnancy/Lactation: Readily crosses placenta. Distributed in breast milk. Contraindicated during first trimester in those with trichomoniasis. Topical use during pregnancy, lactation discouraged. **Children:** Safety and efficacy of topical administration not established in pts younger than 21 yrs. **Elderly:** Age-related hepatic impairment may require dosage adjustment.

INTERACTIONS

DRUG: **Alcohol** may cause disulfiram-type reaction (e.g., abdominal cramps, nausea, vomiting, headache, psychotic reactions). **Disulfiram** may increase risk of toxicity. May increase effects of **oral anticoagulants (e.g., warfarin).** **HERBAL:** None significant. **FOOD:** None known. **LAB VALUES:** May increase serum LDH, ALT, AST.

AVAILABILITY (Rx)

Capsules: 375 mg. **Injection, Infusion:** 500 mg/100 mL. **Tablets:** 250 mg, 500 mg. **Topical Cream:** ***(MetroCream):*** 0.75% **(Nuritate):** 1%. **Topical Gel:** ***(MetroGel):*** 0.75%, 1%. **Vaginal Gel:** ***(MetroGel-Vaginal, Vandazole):*** 0.75%.

ADMINISTRATION/HANDLING

IV

Rate of administration • Infuse IV over 30–60 min. Do not give by IV bolus.

Storage • Store at room temperature (ready-to-use infusion bags).

PO

• Give without regard to food. Give with food to decrease GI irritation.

IV INCOMPATIBILITIES

Amphotericin B complex (Abelcet, AmBisome, Amphotec).

IV COMPATIBILITIES

Dexmedetomidine (Precedex), dilTIAZem (Cardizem), DOPamine (Intropin), heparin, HYDROmorphone (Dilaudid), LORazepam (Ativan), magnesium sulfate, midazolam (Versed), morphine.

INDICATIONS/ROUTES/DOSAGE

Amebiasis

PO: ADULTS, ELDERLY: ***(Immediate-Release):*** 500–750 mg q8h for 7–10 days. **CHILDREN:** 35–50 mg/kg/day in divided doses q8h for 7–10 days.

Anaerobic Infections

PO, IV: ADULTS, ELDERLY: 500 mg q6–8h. **PO: CHILDREN, INFANTS:** 30–50 mg/kg/day in divided doses q8h.
IV: CHILDREN, INFANTS: 22.5–40 mg/kg/day in 3 divided doses. **Maximum:** 1,500 mg/day.

Intra-abdominal Infections

IV: ADULTS, ELDERLY: 500 mg q6–8h. **CHILDREN:** 30–40 mg/kg/day in 3 divided doses. **Maximum dose:** 500 mg/dose.

Pseudomembranous Colitis

PO: ADULTS, ELDERLY: 500 mg 3 times/day. **CHILDREN:** 7.5 mg/kg/dose 3–4 times/day for 7–10 days. **Maximum:** 500 mg/dose.

Bacterial Vaginosis

Intravaginal: ADULTS: 0.75% apply 1–2 times/day for 5 days. 1.3% apply once as a single dose. **PO:** 500 mg twice daily for 7 days.

◀ALERT▶ Centers for Disease Control and Prevention (CDC) does not recommend the use of topical agents during pregnancy.

Rosacea

Topical: ADULTS, ELDERLY: (1%): Apply to affected area once daily. **(0.75%):** Apply to affected area twice daily.

Dosage in Renal Impairment

No dose adjustment.

Dosage in Hepatic Impairment

Mild to moderate impairment: Use caution. No dose adjustment. **Severe impairment:** Reduce dose by 50% for

M

immediate-release; not recommended for extended-release.

SIDE EFFECTS

Frequent: Systemic: Anorexia, nausea, dry mouth, metallic taste. **Vaginal:** Symptomatic cervicitis/vaginitis, abdominal cramps, uterine pain. **Occasional: Systemic:** Diarrhea, constipation, vomiting, dizziness, erythematous rash, urticaria, reddish-brown urine. **Topical:** Transient erythema, mild dryness, burning, irritation, stinging, tearing when applied too close to eyes. **Vaginal:** Vaginal, perineal, vulvar itching; vulvar swelling. **Rare:** Mild, transient leukopenia; thrombophlebitis with IV therapy.

ADVERSE EFFECTS/TOXIC REACTIONS

Oral therapy may result in furry tongue, glossitis, cystitis, dysuria, pancreatitis. Peripheral neuropathy (manifested as numbness, tingling of hands/feet) usually is reversible if treatment is stopped immediately upon appearance of neurologic symptoms. Seizures occur occasionally.

NURSING CONSIDERATIONS

BASELINE ASSESSMENT

Obtain baseline CBC, LFT. Question for history of hypersensitivity to metronidazole, other nitroimidazole derivatives (and parabens with topical). Obtain specimens for diagnostic tests, cultures before giving first dose (therapy may begin before results are known).

INTERVENTION/EVALUATION

Monitor daily pattern of bowel activity, stool consistency. Monitor I&O, assess for urinary problems. Be alert to neurologic symptoms (dizziness, paresthesia of extremities). Assess for rash, urticaria. Monitor for onset of superinfection (ulceration/change of oral mucosa, furry tongue, vaginal discharge, genital/anal pruritus).

PATIENT/FAMILY TEACHING

• Urine may be red-brown or dark. • Avoid alcohol, alcohol-containing preparations (cough syrups, elixirs) for at least 48 hrs after last dose. • If taking metroNIDAZOLE for trichomoniasis, refrain from sexual intercourse until full treatment is completed. • For amebiasis, frequent stool specimen checks will be necessary. • **Topical:** Avoid contact with eyes. • May apply cosmetics after application. • Metronidazole acts on erythema, papules, pustules but has no effect on rhinophyma (hypertrophy of nose), telangiectasia, ocular problems (conjunctivitis, keratitis, blepharitis). • Other recommendations for rosacea include avoidance of hot/spicy foods, alcohol, extremes of hot/cold temperatures, excessive sunlight.

micafungin

mye-ka-**fun**-jin
(Mycamine)

◆CLASSIFICATION

PHARMACOTHERAPEUTIC: Echinocandin antifungal. **CLINICAL:** Antifungal.

USES

Treatment of esophageal candidiasis, candidemia, candida peritonitis, abscesses, acute disseminated candidiasis, prophylaxis of *Candida* infection in pts undergoing hematopoietic stem cell transplant. **OFF-LABEL:** Treatment of infections due to *Aspergillus* spp.

PRECAUTIONS

Contraindications: Hypersensitivity to micafungin. **Cautions:** Hepatic/renal impairment, concomitant hepatotoxic medications.

ACTION

Inhibits synthesis of glucan (vital component of fungal cell formation), damaging fungal cell membrane. **Therapeutic Effect:** Decreased glucan content leads to cellular lysis.

PHARMACOKINETICS

Slowly metabolized in liver. Protein binding: greater than 99%. Primarily excreted in feces. Not removed by hemodialysis. **Half-life:** 11–21 hrs.

LIFESPAN CONSIDERATIONS

Pregnancy/Lactation: May reduce sperm count. May be embryotoxic. Unknown if distributed in breast milk. **Children:** Safety and efficacy not established. **Elderly:** No age-related precautions noted.

INTERACTIONS

DRUG: May decrease therapeutic effect of ***Saccharomyces boulardii.*** May increase concentration/effect of **sirolimus. HERBAL:** None significant. **FOOD:** None known. **LAB VALUES:** May increase serum creatinine, alkaline phosphatase, LDH, ALT, AST.

AVAILABILITY (Rx)

Injection, Powder for Reconstitution: 50 mg, 100 mg.

ADMINISTRATION/HANDLING

IV

Reconstitution • Add 5 mL 0.9% NaCl (without bacteriostatic agent) to each 50-mg vial (10 mL to 100-mg vial) to yield micafungin 10 mg/mL. • Gently swirl to dissolve; do not shake. • Further dilute in 0.9% NaCl or D_5W to final concentration of 0.5–1.5 mg/mL. • Alternatively, D_5W may be used for reconstitution and dilution. • Flush existing IV line with 0.9% NaCl or D_5W before infusion.

Rate of administration • Infuse over 60 min.

Storage • Reconstituted solution is stable for 24 hrs at room temperature. • Discard if precipitate is present.

IV INCOMPATIBILITIES

Amiodarone, nicardipine.

IV COMPATIBILITIES

Bumetanide (Bumex), calcium gluconate, heparin.

INDICATIONS/ROUTES/DOSAGE

Esophageal Candidiasis

IV: ADULTS, ELDERLY: 150 mg/day for 10–30 days. **CHILDREN 4 MOS OR OLDER WEIGHING MORE THAN 30 KG:** 2.5 mg/kg/day. **Maximum:** 150 mg daily. **30 KG OR LESS:** 3 mg/kg/day.

Candida Prophylaxis in Stem Cell Pts

IV: ADULTS, ELDERLY: 50 mg/day. **CHILDREN 4 MOS OR OLDER:** 1 mg/kg/day. **Maximum:** 50 mg/day.

Candidemia, Disseminated Candidiasis, Peritonitis, Abscesses

IV: ADULTS, ELDERLY: 100 mg/day for 15 days. **CHILDREN 4 MOS OR OLDER:** 2 mg/kg/day. **Maximum:** 100 mg daily.

Dosage in Renal/Hepatic Impairment

No dose adjustment.

SIDE EFFECTS

Occasional (3%–2%): Nausea, headache, diarrhea, vomiting, fever. **Rare (1%):** Dizziness, drowsiness, pruritus, abdominal pain, dyspepsia.

ADVERSE EFFECTS/TOXIC REACTIONS

Hypersensitivity reaction characterized by rash, pruritus, facial edema occurs rarely. Anaphylaxis, hemoglobinuria, hemolytic anemia have been reported.

NURSING CONSIDERATIONS

BASELINE ASSESSMENT

Obtain renal function, LFT.

INTERVENTION/EVALUATION

Monitor BUN, serum creatinine, CrCl, LFT. Monitor for hepatotoxicity.

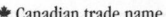

M

PATIENT/FAMILY TEACHING

• Report liver problems such as bruising, confusion; dark amber or orange-colored urine; right upper abdominal pain; yellowing of the skin or eyes. • Report decreased urine output; dark, amber urine; swelling of the hands or feet. • Do not take OTC medications that are toxic to the liver (e.g., acetaminophen).

midazolam HIGH ALERT

mye-**da**-zoe-lam
(Nayzilam)

BLACK BOX ALERT May cause severe respiratory depression, respiratory arrest, apnea. Initial doses in elderly should be conservative. Do not administer by rapid IV injection in neonates (may cause severe hypotension/seizures). Use with opioids may cause profound sedation, respiratory depression, coma, or death.

Do not confuse midazolam with, ALPRAZolam or LORazepam.

◆CLASSIFICATION

PHARMACOTHERAPEUTIC: Benzodiazepine (Schedule IV). **CLINICAL:** Sedative, anxiolytic.

USES

Sedation, anxiolytic, amnesia before procedure or induction of anesthesia, conscious sedation before diagnostic/radiographic procedure, continuous IV sedation of intubated or mechanically ventilated pts. **Nasal:** Acute treatment of seizure clusters. **OFF-LABEL:** Anxiety, status epilepticus, conscious sedation (intranasal route).

PRECAUTIONS

Contraindications: Hypersensitivity to midazolam. Acute narrow-angle glaucoma, concurrent use of protease inhibitors (e.g., atazanavir, darunavir). **Cautions:** Renal/hepatic/pulmonary impairment, impaired gag reflex, HF, treated open-angle glaucoma, concurrent CNS depressants, obesity, elderly, debilitated.

ACTION

Enhances action of gamma-aminobutyric acid (GABA), one of the major inhibitory neurotransmitters in the brain. **Therapeutic Effect:** Produces anxiolytic, hypnotic, anticonvulsant, muscle relaxant, amnestic effects.

PHARMACOKINETICS

Route	Onset	Peak	Duration
PO	10–20 min	N/A	N/A
IV	1–5 min	5–7 min	20–30 min
IM	5–15 min	30–60 min	2–6 hrs

Well absorbed after IM administration. Protein binding: 97%. Metabolized in liver. Primarily excreted in urine. Not removed by hemodialysis. **Half-life:** 1–5 hrs.

⌛ LIFESPAN CONSIDERATIONS

Pregnancy/Lactation: Crosses placenta. Unknown if distributed in breast milk. **Children:** Neonates more likely to have respiratory depression. **Elderly:** Age-related renal impairment may require dosage adjustment.

INTERACTIONS

DRUG: **Alcohol, other CNS depressants (e.g., LORazepam, morphine, zolpidem)** may increase CNS effects, respiratory depression, hypotensive effect. **Strong CYP3A4 inhibitors (e.g., clarithromycin, ketoconazole, ritonavir)** may increase concentration/effect. **Strong CYP3A4 inducers (e.g., carBAMazepine, phenytoin, rifAMPin)** may decrease concentration/effect. **HERBAL:** **Herbals with sedative properties (e.g., chamomile, kava kava, valerian)** may increase CNS depression. **St. John's wort** may decrease concentration. **FOOD:** **Grapefruit products** increase oral absorption, systemic availability. **LAB VALUES:** None significant.

AVAILABILITY (Rx)

Injection Solution: 1 mg/mL, 5 mg/mL. **Nasal Spray:** 5 mg/0.1 ml. **Syrup:** 2 mg/mL.

ADMINISTRATION/HANDLING

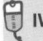

IV

Rate of administration
• May give undiluted or as infusion. • Resuscitative equipment, O_2 must be readily available before IV administration. • Administer by slow IV injection over at least 2–5 min at concentration of 1–5 mg/mL. • Reduce IV rate in those older than 60 yrs, debilitated pts with chronic disease states, pulmonary impairment. • Too-rapid IV rate, excessive doses, or single large dose increases risk of respiratory depression/arrest.
Storage • Store vials at room temperature.

IM
• Give deep IM into large muscle mass. **Maximum concentration:** 1 mg/mL.

PO
• Do not mix with grapefruit juice.

IV INCOMPATIBILITIES

Albumin, amphotericin B complex (Abelcet, AmBisome, Amphotec), ampicillin (Polycillin), ampicillin and sulbactam (Unasyn), bumetanide (Bumex), co-trimoxazole (Bactrim), dexamethasone (Decadron), fosphenytoin (Cerebyx), furosemide (Lasix), hydrocortisone (Solu-Cortef), methotrexate, nafcillin (Nafcil), sodium bicarbonate.

IV COMPATIBILITIES

Amiodarone (Cordarone), atropine, calcium gluconate, dexmedetomidine (Precedex), dilTIAZem (Cardizem), diphenhydrAMINE (Benadryl), DOBUTamine (Dobutrex), DOPamine (Intropin), etomidate (Amidate), fentaNYL (Sublimaze), glycopyrrolate (Robinul), heparin, HYDROmorphone (Dilaudid), hydrOXYzine (Vistaril), insulin, LORazepam (Ativan), milrinone (Primacor), morphine, nitroglycerin, norepinephrine (Levophed), potassium chloride, propofol (Diprivan).

INDICATIONS/ROUTES/DOSAGE

Continuous Sedation During Mechanical Ventilation
IV: ADULTS, ELDERLY: Initially, 0.01–0.05mg/kg (1–5 mg in 70-kg adult). May repeat at 5- to 15-min intervals until adequate sedation achieved or continuous infusion rate of 0.02–0.1 mg/kg/hr and titrated to desired effect. **CHILDREN:** Initially, 0.05–0.2 mg/kg followed by continuous infusion of 0.06–0.12 mg/kg/hr (1–2 mcg/kg/min) titrated to desired effect. Usual range: 0.4–6 mcg/kg/min.

Seizure Clusters
Nasal: ADULTS, CHILDREN 12 YRS AND OLDER: Initially, one spray (5-mg dose) into one nostril. One additional spray (5-mg dose) into the opposite nostril may be administered after 10 min. **Maximum dose:** 10 mg (2 sprays) per episode. **Maximum frequency:** 1 episode q3days; 5 episodes/mos.

Dosage in Renal Impairment
No dose adjustment.

Dosage in Hepatic Impairment
Use caution.

SIDE EFFECTS

Frequent (10%–4%): Decreased respiratory rate, tenderness at IM or IV injection site, pain during injection, oxygen desaturation, hiccups. **Occasional (3%–2%):** Hypotension, paradoxical CNS reaction. **Rare (less than 2%):** Nausea, vomiting, headache, coughing.

ADVERSE EFFECTS/TOXIC REACTIONS

Inadequate or excessive dosage, improper administration may result in cerebral hypoxia, agitation, involuntary movements, hyperactivity, combativeness. Too-rapid IV rate, excessive doses, or single large dose increases risk of respiratory depression/arrest. Respiratory depression/apnea may produce hypoxia, cardiac arrest.

M

NURSING CONSIDERATIONS

BASELINE ASSESSMENT

Resuscitative equipment, oxygen must be available. Obtain vital signs before administration. Assess level of consciousness.

INTERVENTION/EVALUATION

Monitor respiratory rate, oxygen saturation continuously during administration for underventilation, apnea. Monitor vital signs, level of sedation q3–5min during recovery period. Assess level of consciousness for effectiveness.

midodrine

mye-doe-dreen
(Amatine ✱, Apo-Midodrine ✱)

■ BLACK BOX ALERT ■ Can cause marked rise in supine blood pressure; use in pts for whom orthostatic hypotension significantly impairs daily life.

Do not confuse Amatine with amantadine or protamine, or midodrine with Midrin.

◆CLASSIFICATION

PHARMACOTHERAPEUTIC: Alpha$_1$ agonist. **CLINICAL:** Vasopressor.

USES

Treatment of symptomatic orthostatic hypotension. **OFF-LABEL:** Vasovagal syncope, prevention of dialysis-induced hypotension.

PRECAUTIONS

Contraindications: Hypersensitivity to midodrine. Acute renal failure, persistent supine hypertension, pheochromocytoma, severe cardiac disease, thyrotoxicosis, urinary retention. **Cautions:** Renal/hepatic impairment, history of visual problems, diabetes, immobility, pts who are unable to stand. Concurrent administration with digoxin, beta blockers (e.g., metoprolol), vasoconstrictors (e.g., norepinephrine).

ACTION

Forms active metabolite desglymidodrine, an alpha$_1$ agonist, increasing arteriolar and venous tone. **Therapeutic Effect:** Increases standing, sitting, and supine systolic B/P in pts with orthostatic hypotension.

PHARMACOKINETICS

Route	Onset	Peak	Duration
PO	1 hr	—	2–3 hrs

Rapid absorption from GI tract following PO administration. Protein binding: Low. Undergoes enzymatic hydrolysis in systemic circulation. Excreted in urine. **Half-life:** 0.5 hr.

⌛ LIFESPAN CONSIDERATIONS

Pregnancy/Lactation: Unknown if drug crosses placenta or is distributed in breast milk. **Children:** Safety and efficacy not established. **Elderly:** Age-related renal impairment may require dosage adjustment.

INTERACTIONS

DRUG: Ergot derivatives (e.g., ergotamine), linezolid, MAOIs (e.g., phenelzine, selegiline) may increase hypertensive effects. May increase bradycardic effect of **beta blockers (e.g., metoprolol), digoxin. HERBAL:** None significant. **FOOD:** None known. **LAB VALUES:** None significant.

AVAILABILITY (Rx)

Tablets: 2.5 mg, 5 mg, 10 mg.

ADMINISTRATION/HANDLING

• Give without regard to food. • Last dose of day should be given 3–4 hrs before bedtime.

INDICATIONS/ROUTES/DOSAGE

Orthostatic Hypotension

PO: ADULTS, ELDERLY: 2.5–10 mg 3 times/day (q3–4hrs). Give during the day when pt is upright, such as upon arising, midday, and late afternoon. Do not give less than 4h before bedtime. **Maximum:** 40 mg/day.

Dosage in Renal Impairment

2.5 mg 3 times/day; increase gradually, as tolerated. **Hemodialysis:** Dose after HD unless used to prevent HD-induced hypotension.

Dosage in Hepatic Impairment

Use caution.

SIDE EFFECTS

Frequent (20%–7%): Paresthesia, piloerection, pruritus, dysuria, supine hypertension. **Occasional (6%–1%):** Pain, rash, chills, headache, facial flushing, confusion, dry mouth, anxiety.

ADVERSE EFFECTS/TOXIC REACTIONS

May cause marked increase of supine systolic BP (supine hypertension). May cause bradycardia due to vagal reflex.

NURSING CONSIDERATIONS

BASELINE ASSESSMENT

Obtain B/P, heart rate. Assess sensitivity to midodrine, other medications (esp. digoxin, sodium-retaining vasoconstrictors). Assess medical history, esp. for renal impairment, severe hypertension, cardiac disease.

INTERVENTION/EVALUATION

Monitor B/P, heart rate; renal, hepatic, cardiac function.

PATIENT/FAMILY TEACHING

• Do not take last dose of the day after evening meal or less than 4 hrs before bedtime. • Do not give if pt will be supine. • Use caution with OTC medications that may affect B/P (e.g., cough and cold, diet medications).

midostaurin

mye-doe-**staw**-rim
(Rydapt)

Do not confuse midostaurin with midodrine.

◆CLASSIFICATION

PHARMACOTHERAPEUTIC: FLT inhibitor. Tyrosine kinase inhibitor. **CLINICAL:** Antineoplastic.

USES

Treatment of adult pts with newly diagnosed acute myeloid leukemia (AML) who are FLT3 mutation–positive, as detected by an FDA-approved test (in combination with standard cytarabine and daunorubicin induction and cytarabine consolidation chemotherapy). Treatment of adult pts with aggressive systemic mastocytosis (ASM), systemic mastocytosis with associated hematologic neoplasm (SM-AHN), or mast cell leukemia (MCL).

PRECAUTIONS

Contraindications: Hypersensitivity to midostaurin. **Cautions:** Baseline cytopenias; concomitant use of strong CYP3A inhibitors, strong CYP3A inducers; pts at risk for hemorrhage (e.g., history of GI bleeding, coagulation disorders, recent trauma; concomitant use of anticoagulants, NSAIDs, antiplatelet medication).

ACTION

Inhibits multiple receptors including FLT3 receptor signaling, and cell proliferation. **Therapeutic Effect:** Induces apoptosis in ITD and ITD mutant expressing leukemic cells.

PHARMACOKINETICS

Widely distributed. Metabolized in liver. Protein binding: 99.8%. Peak plasma concentration: 1–3 hrs. Steady state reached in 28 days. Excreted in feces (95%), urine (5%). **Half-life:** 21 hrs.

⌛ LIFESPAN CONSIDERATIONS

Pregnancy/Lactation: Avoid pregnancy; may cause fetal harm. Females and males with female partners of reproductive

M

potential should use effective contraception during treatment and for at least 4 mos after discontinuation. Unknown if distributed in breast milk. Breastfeeding not recommended. May impair fertility in both females and males. **Children:** Safety and efficacy not established. **Elderly:** No age-related precautions noted.

INTERACTIONS

DRUG: **Moderate CYP3A4 inhibitors (e.g., ciprofloxacin, fluconazole, verapamil), strong CYP3A4 inhibitors (e.g., clarithromycin, ketoconazole, ritonavir)** may increase concentration/effect. **Strong CYP3A4 inducers (e.g., carBAMazepine, phenytoin, rifAMPin)** may decrease concentration/effect. **QT-prolonging agents (e.g., amiodarone, haloperidol, moxifloxacin, sotalol)** may enhance QT-prolonging effect. May decrease therapeutic effect of BCG. **HERBAL:** **St. John's wort** may decrease concentration/effect. **FOOD:** **Grapefruit products** may increase concentration/effect. **LAB VALUES:** May increase serum alkaline phosphatase, ALT, AST, bilirubin, creatinine, GGT, glucose, lipase, sodium, uric acid. May decrease Hgb, Hct, lymphocytes, leukocytes, neutrophils, platelets, RBCs; serum albumin, magnesium, phosphate, potassium. May increase or decrease serum calcium or sodium. May prolong aPTT.

AVAILABILITY (Rx)

Capsules: 25 mg.

ADMINISTRATION/HANDLING

PO

• Give with food. • Administer whole; do not cut, crush, open capsules.

INDICATIONS/ROUTES/DOSAGE

Acute Myeloid Leukemia (FLT positive)

PO: ADULTS, ELDERLY: 50 mg twice daily (at 12-hr intervals) on days 8–21 of each induction in combination with cytarabine and daunorubicin, and on days 8–21 of each cycle of consolidation with high-dose in combination with cytarabine.

Systemic Mastocytosis, Mast Cell Leukemia

PO: ADULTS, ELDERLY: 100 mg twice daily. Continue until disease progression or unacceptable toxicity.

DOSE MODIFICATION FOR SYSTEMIC MASTOCYTOSIS

Neutropenia

ANC less than 1,000 cells/mm^3 in pts without MCL; ANC less than 500 cells/mm^3 in pts with baseline ANC 500–1,500 cells/mm^3: Withhold treatment until ANC greater than or equal to 1,000 cells/mm^3, then resume at 50-mg twice daily. May increase to 100 mg twice daily if 50 mg dose is tolerated. If neutropenia persists for more than 21 days, permanently discontinue.

Thrombocytopenia

Platelet count less than 50,000 cells/mm^3 in pts without MCL; platelet count less than 25,000 cells/mm^3 in pts with baseline platelet count 25,000–75,000 cells/mm^3: Withhold treatment until platelet count greater than or equal to 50,000 cells/mm^3, then resume at 50 mg twice daily. May increase to 100 mg twice daily if 50-mg dose is tolerated. If thrombocytopenia persists for more than 21 days, permanently discontinue.

Anemia

Hgb less than 8 g/dL in pts without MCL; life-threatening anemia with baseline Hgb 8–10 g/dL: Withhold treatment until Hgb greater than or equal to 8 g/dL, then resume at 50 mg twice daily. May increase to 100 mg twice daily if 50-mg dose is tolerated. If treatment-induced anemia persists for more than 21 days, permanently discontinue.

Nausea, Vomiting

Grade 3 or 4 nausea, vomiting despite antiemetic therapy: Withhold treatment for 3 days (6 doses), then resume at 50 mg twice daily. May increase to 100 mg twice daily if 50-mg dose is tolerated.

Nonhematologic Toxicities

Any other grade toxicities: Withhold treatment until resolved to Grade 2 or less, then resume at 50 mg twice daily. May increase to 100 mg twice daily if 50-mg dose is tolerated.

Dosage in Rena/Hepatic Impairment

Not specified; use caution.

SIDE EFFECTS

AML: Frequent (83%–24%): Nausea, mucositis, stomatitis, laryngeal pain, vomiting, headache, petechiae, musculoskeletal pain. **Occasional (20%–7%):** Hyperglycemia, hemorrhoids, arthralgia, hyperhidrosis, insomnia, hypertension, dry skin, increased weight. **Rare (4%–3%):** Tremor, eyelid edema. **Systemic mastocytosis: Frequent (82%–23%):** Nausea, vomiting, diarrhea, edema, peripheral edema, fatigue, asthenia, musculoskeletal pain, back pain, extremity pain, abdominal pain, constipation, pyrexia, headache, dyspnea, bronchospasm. **Occasional (19%–6%):** Arthralgia, cough, rash, dizziness, insomnia, hypotension, dyspepsia. **Rare (5%–4%):** Vertigo, chills, mental status change.

ADVERSE EFFECTS/TOXIC REACTIONS

Myelosuppression (anemia, leukopenia, lymphopenia, neutropenia, thrombocytopenia) is an expected response to therapy. Hypersensitivity reactions including anaphylaxis, angioedema, dyspnea, itching, flushing may occur. Infections including bronchitis, bronchopulmonary aspergillosis, colitis, cellulitis, device-related infection, erysipelas, fungal pneumonia, gastroenteritis, hepatic candidiasis, herpes zoster, nasopharyngitis, oral herpes, pneumonia, sepsis, sinusitis, splenic fungal infection, upper respiratory tract infection, UTI have occurred. Renal failure, acute kidney injury may occur. Other adverse effects including angina pectoris, cardiac failure, contusion, duodenal ulcer hemorrhage, epistaxis, gastritis, febrile neutropenia, GI bleeding, hematoma, interstitial lung disease, myocardial infarction, myocardial ischemia, pericardial effusion, pneumonitis, pulmonary congestion, pulmonary edema, thrombosis were reported. May prolong QT interval.

NURSING CONSIDERATIONS

BASELINE ASSESSMENT

Obtain ANC, CBC, BMP, LFT; serum magnesium; vital signs. Ensure electrolytes are corrected prior to initiation. In females of reproductive potential, obtain pregnancy test within 7 days of initiation. Screen for active infection. To reduce risk of nausea/vomiting, administer antiemetic before treatment. Obtain ECG in pts taking QT interval–prolonging medications. Receive full medication history and screen for interactions. Question history as listed in Precautions. Confirm compliance of effective contraception. Offer emotional support.

INTERVENTION/EVALUATION

Monitor ANC, CBC for myelosuppression. Monitor BMP for renal insufficiency, electrolyte imbalance (esp. in pts with diarrhea, vomiting, malnutrition); LFT for transaminitis, hepatotoxicity. Diligently screen for infections, sepsis; provide appropriate antimicrobial therapy if indicated. Obtain ABG, radiologic test if interstitial lung disease or pneumonitis suspected. Monitor for toxicities at least wkly for 4 wks, then every other wk for 8 wks, then monthly thereafter. If treatment-related toxicities occur, consider referral to specialist. Monitor for hemorrhage, melena, hematuria; hypersensitivity reactions; myocardial infarction, pulmonary disease, thrombosis. Monitor I&O.

PATIENT/FAMILY TEACHING

• Treatment may depress your immune system and reduce your ability to fight infection. Report symptoms of infection

M

such as body aches, burning with urination, chills, cough, fatigue, fever. Avoid those with active infection. • Report symptoms of kidney failure (decreased urination, amber-colored urine, flank pain, fatigue, swelling of the hands or feet); liver problems (bruising, confusion; amber, dark, orange-colored urine; right upper abdominal pain, yellowing of the skin or eyes); lung problems (severe cough, difficulty breathing, lung pain, shortness of breath). • Use effective contraception to avoid pregnancy. • Avoid grapefruit products, Seville oranges, starfruit, herbal supplements. • Do not take newly prescribed medications unless approved by the prescriber who originally started treatment. • Heart attacks have occurred; immediately report chest pain, sweating, fainting, palpitations, jaw pain, pain that radiates to the left arm. • Report bleeding of any kind, esp. nosebleeds, blood in stool or urine. • Allergic reactions such as anaphylaxis, difficulty breathing, itching, flushing, rash may occur.

M

milnacipran

mil-**nay**-sip-ran
(Savella)

BLACK BOX ALERT Increased risk of suicidal ideation and behavior in children, adolescents, and young adults 18–24 yrs with major depressive disorder, other psychiatric disorders. Not approved for use in children.

Do not confuse Savella with cevimeline or sevelamer.

CLASSIFICATION

PHARMACOTHERAPEUTIC: Serotonin, norepinephrine reuptake inhibitor. **CLINICAL:** Fibromyalgia agent.

USES

Management of fibromyalgia.

PRECAUTIONS

Contraindications: Hypersensitivity to milnacipran. Concomitant use of MAOIs to treat psychiatric disorders (concurrently or within 5 days of discontinuing milnacipran or within 2 wks of discontinuing MAOI), initiation of milnacipran in pts receiving linezolid or IV methylene blue. **Cautions:** Depression, pts at increased risk of suicide, other psychiatric disorders; elevated B/P or heart rate, seizure disorder, pts with substantial alcohol use or chronic hepatic disease, pts with history of dysuria (e.g., prostatic hypertrophy, prostatitis), controlled narrow-angle glaucoma, renal impairment, cardiovascular disease, elderly.

ACTION

Inhibits serotonin and norepinephrine reuptake at CNS neuronal presynaptic membranes. **Therapeutic Effect:** Reduces chronic pain, fatigue, depression, sleep disorders associated with fibromyalgia syndrome; improves physical function.

PHARMACOKINETICS

Well absorbed following PO administration. Protein binding: 13%. Excreted unchanged in urine. Steady state reached in 36–48 hrs. **Half-life:** 6–8 hrs.

LIFESPAN CONSIDERATIONS

Pregnancy/Lactation: Increased risk of fetal complications, including need for respiratory support, if given during third trimester. Unknown if distributed in breast milk. **Children:** Safety and efficacy not established. **Elderly:** Severe renal impairment requires dosage adjustment.

INTERACTIONS

DRUG: **Alcohol, clomipramine, metoclopramide** may increase adverse effects. May increase adverse effects of **digoxin. Linezolid, MAOIs (e.g. phenelzine, selegiline)** may increase serotonergic effect. **EPINEPHrine, norepinephrine** may produce paroxysmal hypertension, arrhythmias. May inhibit antihypertensive effect of **cloNIDine**. **HERBAL**: **Glucosamine, herbals with anticoagulant/antiplatelet activity (e.g., garlic, ginger, ginkgo biloba)** may increase adverse effects. **FOOD**: None known. **LAB VALUES**: May decrease serum sodium.

AVAILABILITY (Rx)

Tablets, Film-Coated: 12.5 mg, 25 mg, 50 mg, 100 mg.

ADMINISTRATION/HANDLING

• Give without regard to food. • Do not break, crush, dissolve, or divide film-coated tablets.

INDICATIONS/ROUTES/DOSAGE

Fibromyalgia

PO: ADULTS, ELDERLY: Day 1: 12.5 mg once. **Days 2–3:** 25 mg/day (12.5 mg twice daily). **Days 4–7:** 50 mg/day (25 mg twice daily). **After Day 7:** 100 mg/day (50 mg twice daily thereafter). Dose may be increased to 200 mg/day (100 mg twice daily).

Dosage in Renal Impairment

Mild impairment: No dose adjustment. **Moderate impairment:** Use caution. **Severe impairment:** Reduce maintenance dose by 50% to 50 mg/day (25 mg twice daily). Based on pt response, dose may be increased to 100 mg/day (50 mg twice daily). Not recommended in end-stage renal disease.

Dosage in Hepatic Impairment

Mild to moderate impairment: No dose adjustment. **Severe impairment:** Use caution.

SIDE EFFECTS

Frequent (37%–18%): Nausea, headache. **Occasional (16%–5%):** Constipation, insomnia, hot flashes, dizziness, hyperhidrosis, palpitations, vomiting, URI. **Rare (less than 5%):** Dry mouth, increased B/P, anxiety, skin flushing, rash, blurred vision, abdominal pain, chest pain, chills, pruritus, paresthesia, tachycardia.

ADVERSE EFFECTS/TOXIC REACTIONS

Abrupt discontinuation may present withdrawal symptoms (dysphoria, irritability, agitation, dizziness, paresthesia, anxiety, confusion, headache, lethargy, emotional lability, tinnitus, seizures). Serotonin syndrome symptoms may include mental status changes (agitation, hallucinations), hyperreflexia, incoordination. May increase risk of bleeding events (e.g., ecchymoses, hematomas, epistaxis).

NURSING CONSIDERATIONS

BASELINE ASSESSMENT

Obtain pain intensity, location(s) of pain, tenderness. Obtain baseline B/P, heart rate. Question for history of changes in day-to-day pain intensity.

INTERVENTION/EVALUATION

Monitor for increase in B/P, pulse. Question for changes in visual acuity. Assess for clinical improvement and record onset of pain control, decreased fatigue, lessening of depressive symptoms, improvement in sleep pattern. Monitor for suicidal ideation.

PATIENT/FAMILY TEACHING

• Avoid tasks that require alertness, motor skills until response to drug is established. • Do not abruptly discontinue medication. • Increase fluids, bulk to prevent constipation. • Report unusual changes in behavior, suicidal ideation; hot flushing that becomes intolerant, excessive sweating. • Caution about risk of bleeding associated with concomitant use of NSAIDs, aspirin.

milrinone

HIGH ALERT

mil-ri-none

◆CLASSIFICATION

PHARMACOTHERAPEUTIC: Cardiac inotropic agent. **CLINICAL:** Vasodilator.

M

USES

Short-term management of decompensated HF. **OFF-LABEL:** Inotropic therapy for pts unresponsive to other therapy, outpatient inotropic therapy for heart transplant candidates, palliation of symptoms in end-stage HF.

PRECAUTIONS

Contraindications: Hypersensitivity to milrinone. **Cautions:** Severe obstructive aortic or pulmonic valvular disease, history of ventricular arrhythmias, atrial fibrillation/flutter, renal impairment. Not recommended in pts with acute MI.

ACTION

Inhibits phosphodiesterase in cardiac and vascular tissue, which increases cyclic adenosine monophosphate (cAMP), potentiating delivery of calcium to myocardial contractile systems. **Therapeutic Effect:** Relaxes vascular muscle, causing vasodilation. Increases cardiac output, decreases pulmonary capillary wedge pressure, vascular resistance.

PHARMACOKINETICS

Route	Onset	Peak	Duration
IV	5–15 min	N/A	N/A

Protein binding: 70%. Metabolized in liver. Primarily excreted in urine. **Half-life:** 1.7–2.7 hrs.

LIFESPAN CONSIDERATIONS

Pregnancy/Lactation: Unknown if drug crosses placenta or is distributed in breast milk. **Children:** Safety and efficacy not established. **Elderly:** Age-related renal impairment may require dosage adjustment.

INTERACTIONS

DRUG: None significant. **HERBAL:** None significant. **FOOD:** None known. **LAB VALUES:** None significant.

AVAILABILITY (Rx)

Injection Solution: ***(Primacor):*** 1 mg/mL, 10-mL vial. **Injection Solution, Premix:** ***(Primacor):*** 200 mcg/mL (100 mL, 200 mL).

ADMINISTRATION/HANDLING

IV

Reconstitution • For IV infusion, dilute 20-mg (20-mL) vial with 80 mL 0.9% NaCl or D_5W to provide concentration of 0.2 mg/mL (200 mcg/mL).

Rate of administration • For IV injection (loading dose), administer undiluted slowly over 10 min. • Monitor for arrhythmias, hypotension during IV therapy; reduce or temporarily discontinue infusion until condition stabilizes. Infuse via infusion pump.

Storage • Diluted solutions stable for 72 hrs at room temperature.

IV INCOMPATIBILITIES

Furosemide (Lasix), imipenem-cilastatin (Primaxin), procainamide (Pronestyl).

IV COMPATIBILITIES

Calcium gluconate, dexamethasone (Decadron), dexmedetomidine (Precedex), digoxin (Lanoxin), dilTIAZem (Cardizem), DOBUTamine (Dobutrex), DOPamine (Intropin), heparin, HYDROmorphone (Dilaudid), lidocaine, magnesium, midazolam (Versed), morphine, nitroglycerin, potassium, propofol (Diprivan).

INDICATIONS/ROUTES/DOSAGE

Management of HF

IV: ADULTS: Initially, 50 mcg/kg over 10 min. Continue with maintenance infusion rate of 0.125–0.75 mcg/kg/min based on hemodynamic and clinical response.

Dosage in Renal Impairment

Creatinine Clearance	Dosage
50 mL/min	0.43 mcg/kg/min
40 mL/min	0.38 mcg/kg/min
30 mL/min	0.33 mcg/kg/min
20 mL/min	0.28 mcg/kg/min
10 mL/min	0.23 mcg/kg/min
5 mL/min	0.2 mcg/kg/min

Dosage in Hepatic Impairment
No dose adjustment.

SIDE EFFECTS

Occasional (3%–1%): Headache, hypotension. **Rare (less than 1%):** Angina, chest pain.

ADVERSE EFFECTS/TOXIC REACTIONS

Supraventricular/ventricular arrhythmias, nonsustained ventricular tachycardia, sustained ventricular tachycardia may occur. Ventricular fibrillation (0.2% of pts) has been documented.

NURSING CONSIDERATIONS

BASELINE ASSESSMENT

Obtain BN peptide. Assess B/P, heart rate before treatment begins and during IV therapy. Assess lung sounds; observe for edema.

INTERVENTION/EVALUATION

Monitor B/P, heart rate, cardiac output, ECG, serum potassium, renal function, signs/symptoms of HF.

mirabegron

mir-a-**beg**-ron
(Myrbetriq)

◆CLASSIFICATION

PHARMACOTHERAPEUTIC: Beta$_3$-adrenergic agonist. **CLINICAL:** Smooth muscle relaxant.

USES

Treatment of overactive bladder with symptoms of urinary incontinence, urgency, frequency as monotherapy or in combination with solifenacin.

PRECAUTIONS

Contraindications: Hypersensitivity to mirabegron. **Cautions:** Bladder outlet obstruction, pts taking antimuscarinic medications (increases urinary retention), mild to moderate hepatic/renal impairment, pts at risk for QTc interval prolongation (congenital long QT syndrome, HF, medications that prolong QTc interval, hypokalemia, hypomagnesemia). Not recommended in pts with severe uncontrolled hypertension (SBP equal to or greater than 180 mm Hg and/or DBP equal to or greater than 110 mm Hg).

ACTION

Relaxes detrusor smooth muscle of bladder through beta$_3$ stimulation during storage phase of urinary bladder fill–void cycle. **Therapeutic Effect:** Increases bladder capacity, reduces symptoms of urinary urgency, increased voiding frequency, urge incontinence, nocturia.

PHARMACOKINETICS

Widely distributed. Protein binding: 71%. Eliminated in urine (55%), feces (35%). **Half-life:** 50 hrs.

LIFESPAN CONSIDERATIONS

Pregnancy/Lactation: Unknown if distributed in breast milk. **Children:** Safety and efficacy not established. **Elderly:** No age-related precautions noted.

INTERACTIONS

DRUG: May increase concentration/effects of **desipramine, digoxin, thioridazine, flecainide, propafenone.** May decrease concentration/effect of **tamoxifen.** **HERBAL:** None significant. **FOOD:** None known. **LAB VALUES:** May increase GGT, LDH; temporarily increase ALT, AST.

AVAILABILITY (Rx)

Tablets, Extended-Release: 25 mg, 50 mg.

ADMINISTRATION/HANDLING

PO

• Give without regard to food. • Administer with water. • Do not break, crush, dissolve, or divide film-coated tablets.

INDICATIONS/ROUTES/DOSAGE

Overactive Bladder

PO: ADULTS, ELDERLY: (Monotherapy): Initially, 25 mg once daily. Efficacy seen within 8 wks for 25-mg dose. May increase to 50 mg once daily. **(Combination with solifenacin):** Initially, 25 mg once daily with solifenacin 5 mg once daily. May increase mirabegron to 50 mg once daily after 4–8 wks.

Dosage in Renal Impairment

Mild to moderate impairment: No dosage adjustment. **Severe impairment:** Do not exceed 25 mg once daily.

Dosage in Hepatic Impairment

Mild impairment: No dosage adjustment. **Moderate impairment:** Do not exceed 25 mg once daily. **Severe impairment:** Not recommended.

M

SIDE EFFECTS

Occasional (9%–4%): Hypertension, headache, nasopharyngitis. **Rare (2%–1%):** Constipation, arthralgia, diarrhea, tachycardia, fatigue.

ADVERSE EFFECTS/TOXIC REACTIONS

Worsening of preexisting hypertension reported infrequently. UTI occurred in 6% of pts, influenza in 3%, and upper respiratory infection in 1.5%.

NURSING CONSIDERATIONS

BASELINE ASSESSMENT

Obtain B/P. Receive full medication history, and screen for possible drug interactions. Monitor I&O (particularly in pts with history of urinary retention).

INTERVENTION/EVALUATION

Palpate bladder for urinary retention. Measure B/P near end of dosing interval (determines whether B/P is controlled throughout day). Monitor B/P periodically especially in hypertensive pts. For pts taking digoxin, monitor digoxin serum level for therapeutic effect (very narrow line between therapeutic and toxic level). Assess pulse for quality, irregular rate, bradycardia. Question for evidence of headache.

PATIENT/FAMILY TEACHING

• Report urinary retention. • Do not use nasal decongestants, over-the-counter cold preparations without doctor approval. Restrict salt, alcohol intake.

mirtazapine

mir-**taz**-a-peen
(Remeron, Remeron Soltab)

BLACK BOX ALERT Increased risk of suicidal thinking and behavior in children, adolescents, young adults 18–24 yrs with major depressive disorder, other psychiatric disorders.

Do not confuse Remeron with Premarin, Rozerem, or Zemuron.

CLASSIFICATION

PHARMACOTHERAPEUTIC: Alpha 2-antagonist. **CLINICAL:** Antidepressant.

USES

Treatment of major depressive disorder (MDD).

PRECAUTIONS

Contraindications: Hypersensitivity to mirtazapine. Use of MAOIs to treat psychiatric disorders (concurrently or within 14 days of discontinuing either MAOI or mirtazapine), initiation of mirtazapine in pts receiving linezolid or IV methylene blue. **Cautions:** Renal/hepatic impairment, elderly, seizure disorder, suicidal ideation or behavior, alcoholism, concurrent medications that lower seizure threshold, cardiovascular disease, pts at risk for QTc interval prolongation (congenital long QT syndrome, HF, medications that prolong QTc interval, hypokalemia, hypomagnesemia).

ACTION

Acts as antagonist at presynaptic $alpha_2$-adrenergic receptors, increasing norepinephrine, serotonin neurotransmission. Has low anticholinergic activity. **Therapeutic Effect:** Relieves depression.

PHARMACOKINETICS

Rapidly absorbed and widely distributed. Protein binding: 85%. Metabolized in liver. Primarily excreted in urine. Unknown if removed by hemodialysis. **Half-life:** 20–40 hrs (longer in males [37 hrs] than females [26 hrs]).

LIFESPAN CONSIDERATIONS

Pregnancy/Lactation: Unknown if distributed in breast milk. **Children:** Safety and efficacy not established. **Elderly:** Age-related renal impairment may require dosage adjustment.

INTERACTIONS

DRUG: **Alcohol, CNS depressant medications (e.g., LORazepam, morphine, zolpidem)** may increase impairment of cognition, motor skills. **Serotonergic drugs (e.g., venlafaxine)** may increase risk of serotonin syndrome. **Strong CYP3A4 inducers (e.g., carBAMazepine, phenytoin, rifAMPin)** may decrease concentration/effect. **Strong CYP3A4 inhibitors (e.g., clarithromycin, ketoconazole, ritonavir)** may increase concentration/effect. **MAOIs (e.g., phenelzine, selegiline)** may increase risk of neuroleptic malignant syndrome, hypertensive crisis, severe seizures. **QT interval–prolonging medications (e.g., amiodarone, azithromycin, ciprofloxacin, haloperidol, methadone, sotalol)** may increase risk of QTc interval prolongation. **HERBAL:** **Herbals with sedative properties (e.g., chamomile, kava kava, valerian)** may increase CNS depression. **St. John's wort** may decrease concentration/effects, may increase risk of serotonin syndrome. **FOOD:** None known. **LAB VALUES:** May increase serum cholesterol, triglycerides, ALT.

AVAILABILITY (Rx)

Tablets: 7.5 mg, 15 mg, 30 mg, 45 mg. **Tablets, Orally Disintegrating:** 15 mg, 30 mg, 45 mg.

ADMINISTRATION/HANDLING

PO

• Give without regard to food. • May crush/break scored tablets.

Orally Disintegrating Tablets

• Give without regard to food. • Do not split tablet. • Place on tongue; dissolves without water.

INDICATIONS/ROUTES/DOSAGE

Depression

Note: When discontinuing, gradually taper dose to minimize withdrawal symptoms and to allow detection of re-emerging symptoms. **PO: ADULTS:** Initially, 15 mg at bedtime. May increase by 15 mg/day q1–2wks. **Maximum:** 45 mg/day. **ELDERLY:** Initially, 7.5 mg at bedtime. May increase by 7.5–15 mg/day q1–2wks. **Maximum:** 45 mg/day.

Dosage in Renal/Hepatic Impairment

Use caution.

SIDE EFFECTS

Frequent (54%–12%): Drowsiness, dry mouth, increased appetite, constipation, weight gain. **Occasional (89%–4%):** Asthenia, dizziness, flu-like symptoms, abnormal dreams. **Rare:** Abdominal discomfort, vasodilation, paresthesia, acne, dry skin, thirst, arthralgia.

ADVERSE EFFECTS/TOXIC REACTIONS

Higher incidence of seizures than with tricyclic antidepressants (esp. in pts with no history of seizures). Overdose may produce cardiovascular effects (severe orthostatic hypotension, dizziness, tachycardia, palpitations, arrhythmias). Abrupt discontinuation from prolonged therapy may produce headache, malaise, nausea, vomiting, vivid dreams. Agranulocytosis occurs rarely.

NURSING CONSIDERATIONS

BASELINE ASSESSMENT

Assess mental status, appearance, behavior, speech pattern, level of interest, mood. Obtain baseline weight.

INTERVENTION/EVALUATION

For pts on long-term therapy, renal function, LFT, CBC should be performed periodically. Supervise suicidal-risk pt closely during early therapy (as depression lessens, energy level improves, increasing suicide potential). Children, adolescents are at increased risk for suicidal thoughts/behavior and worsening of depression, esp. during first few mos of therapy. Assess appearance, behavior, speech pattern, level of interest, mood. Monitor for hypotension, arrhythmias.

PATIENT/FAMILY TEACHING

• Take as single bedtime dose. • Avoid alcohol, depressant/sedating medications. • Avoid tasks requiring alertness, motor skills until response to drug established. • Report worsening depression, suicidal ideation, unusual changes in behavior.

miSOPROStol

mis-oh-**pros**-tol
(Cytotec)

■ **BLACK BOX ALERT** ■ Use during pregnancy can cause abortion, premature birth, birth defects. Not recommended in women of childbearing potential unless pt is capable of complying with effective contraception.

Do not confuse Cytotec with Cytoxan, or miSOPROStol with metoprolol or miFEPRIStone.

FIXED-COMBINATION(S)

Arthrotec: miSOPROStol/diclofenac (an NSAID): 200 mcg/50 mg, 200 mcg/75 mg.

◆CLASSIFICATION

PHARMACOTHERAPEUTIC: Prostaglandin. **CLINICAL:** Antisecretory, gastric protectant.

USES

Prevention of NSAID-induced gastric ulcers and in pts at high risk for developing gastric ulcer/gastric ulcer complications. Medical termination of intrauterine pregnancy through 70 days' gestation (in conjunction with miFEPRIStone). **OFF-LABEL:** Cervical ripening, labor induction, treatment/prevention of postpartum hemorrhage, treatment of incomplete or missed abortion.

PRECAUTIONS

Contraindications: Hypersensitivity to misoprostol, other prostaglandins; pregnancy. **Cautions:** Renal impairment, cardiovascular disease, elderly.

ACTION

Replaces protective prostaglandins consumed with prostaglandin-inhibiting therapies (e.g., NSAIDs). Induces uterine contractions. **Therapeutic Effect:** Reduces acid secretion from gastric parietal cells, stimulates bicarbonate production from gastric/duodenal mucosa.

PHARMACOKINETICS

Route	Onset	Peak	Duration
PO	30 min	1–1.5 hrs	3–6 hrs

Rapidly absorbed from GI tract. Protein binding: 80%–90%. Primarily excreted in urine. Unknown if removed by hemodialysis. **Half-life:** 20–40 min.

⌛ LIFESPAN CONSIDERATIONS

Pregnancy/Lactation: Unknown if distributed in breast milk. Produces uterine contractions, uterine bleeding, expulsion of products of conception (abortifacient property). **Children:** Safety and efficacy not established. **Elderly:** No age-related precautions noted.

INTERACTIONS

DRUG: **Antacids** may increase concentration. May increase adverse effects of **oxytocin.** **HERBAL:** None significant. **FOOD:** None known. **LAB VALUES:** None significant.

AVAILABILITY (Rx)

Tablets: 100 mcg, 200 mcg.

ADMINISTRATION/HANDLING

PO

• Give with or after meals (minimizes diarrhea).

INDICATIONS/ROUTES/DOSAGE

Prevention of NSAID-Induced Gastric Ulcer

PO: ADULTS, ELDERLY: 200 mcg 4 times/day with food (last dose at bedtime). Continue for duration of NSAID therapy. May reduce dosage to 100 mcg 4 times/day.

Termination of Intrauterine Pregnancy

See manufacturer guidelines for miFEPRIstne.

Early Pregnancy Loss

Intravaginal: 800 mcg once; may repeat 3 or more hrs after first dose and within 7 days of no response to initial dose.

Incomplete Abortion, Postpartum Hemorrhage

PO: 600 mcg as a single dose.

Labor Induction or Cervical Ripening

Intravaginal: 25 mcg q2h.

Postpartum Hemorrhage (Prevention)

PO: ADULTS: 600 mcg as a single dose given immediately after delivery.

Postpartum Hemorrhage (Treatment)

PO/Rectal: ADULTS: 600–1,000 mcg as a single dose.

Dosage in Renal/Hepatic Impairment

No dose adjustment.

SIDE EFFECTS

Frequent (40%–20%): Abdominal pain, diarrhea. **Occasional (3%–2%):** Nausea, flatulence, dyspepsia, headache. **Rare (1%):** Vomiting, constipation.

ADVERSE EFFECTS/TOXIC REACTIONS

Overdosage may produce sedation, tremor, seizures, dyspnea, palpitations, hypotension, bradycardia.

NURSING CONSIDERATIONS

BASELINE ASSESSMENT

Question for possibility of pregnancy before initiating therapy.

PATIENT/FAMILY TEACHING

• Avoid magnesium-containing antacids (minimizes potential for diarrhea). • Women of childbearing potential must not be pregnant before or during medication therapy (may result in hospitalization, surgery, infertility, fetal death). • Take with food to reduce diarrhea.

M

mitoMYcin

HIGH ALERT

mye-toe-**mye**-sin
(Mutamycin)

BLACK BOX ALERT Potent vesicant. Marked myelosuppression. Infiltration produces ulceration, necrosis, cellulitis, tissue sloughing. Hemolytic-uremic syndrome reported. Must be administered by certified chemotherapy personnel.

Do not confuse mitoMYcin with mithramycin or mitoXANTRONE.

CLASSIFICATION

PHARMACOTHERAPEUTIC: Antibiotic. **CLINICAL:** Antineoplastic.

USES

Treatment of disseminated adenocarcinoma of stomach, pancreas (in combination with other chemotherapy agents and as palliative treatment when other modalities have failed). OFF-LABEL: Treatment of bladder cancer, anal carcinoma; cervical, esophageal, gastric, non–small-cell lung cancer.

PRECAUTIONS

Contraindications: Hypersensitivity to mitomycin. Coagulation disorders, other increased bleeding tendencies, thrombocytopenia. **Cautions:** Myelosuppression, renal (serum creatinine greater than 1.7 mg/dL)/hepatic impairment, pregnancy, prior radiation treatment.

ACTION

Alkylating agent, produces DNA cross-linking. **Therapeutic Effect:** Inhibits DNA, RNA synthesis.

PHARMACOKINETICS

Widely distributed. Does not cross blood-brain barrier. Metabolized in liver. Excreted in urine. **Half-life:** 50 min.

LIFESPAN CONSIDERATIONS

Pregnancy/Lactation: If possible, avoid use during pregnancy, esp. first trimester. Breastfeeding not recommended. **Children:** Safety and efficacy not established. **Elderly:** Age-related renal impairment may require dosage adjustment.

INTERACTIONS

DRUG: **Bone marrow depressants (e.g., cladribine)** may increase myelosuppression. **Live virus vaccines** may potentiate virus replication, increase vaccine side effects, decrease pt's antibody response to vaccine. **HERBAL:** **Echinacea** may decrease the therapeutic effect. **FOOD:** None known. **LAB VALUES:** May increase serum BUN, creatinine.

AVAILABILITY (Rx)

Injection, Powder for Reconstitution: 5 mg, 20 mg, 40 mg.

ADMINISTRATION/HANDLING

◀ALERT▶ May be carcinogenic, mutagenic, teratogenic. Handle with extreme care during preparation/administration. Give via IV push, IV infusion. Extremely irritating to vein. Injection may produce pain with induration, thrombophlebitis, paresthesia.

IV

Reconstitution • Reconstitute with Sterile Water for Injection to provide solution containing 0.5–1 mg/mL. • Do not shake vial to dissolve. • Allow vial to stand at room temperature until complete dissolution occurs. • For IV infusion, further dilute with 50–100 mL D_5W or 0.9% NaCl (concentration 20–40 mcg/mL).

Rate of administration • Give slow IV push or by IV infusion over 15–30 min. • Extravasation may produce cellulitis, ulceration, tissue sloughing. Terminate administration immediately, inject ordered antidote. Apply ice intermittently for up to 72 hrs; keep area elevated.

Storage • Use only clear, blue-gray solutions. • Concentration of 0.5 mg/mL (reconstituted vial or syringe) is stable for 7 days at room temperature or 2 wks if refrigerated. Further diluted solution with D_5W is stable for 3 hrs, 12 hrs if diluted with 0.9% NaCl at room temperature.

IV INCOMPATIBILITIES

Aztreonam (Azactam), bleomycin (Blenoxane), cefepime (Maxipime), filgrastim (Neupogen), heparin, piperacillin/tazobactam (Zosyn), sargramostim (Leukine), vinorelbine (Navelbine).

IV COMPATIBILITIES

Cisplatin (Platinol AQ), cyclophosphamide (Cytoxan), DOXOrubicin (Adriamycin), 5-fluorouracil, granisetron (Kytril), leucovorin, methotrexate, ondansetron (Zofran), vinBLAStine (Velban), vinCRIStine (Oncovin).

INDICATIONS/ROUTES/DOSAGE

Stomach, Pancreatic Cancer

IV: **ADULTS, ELDERLY, CHILDREN:** 20 mg/m^2 as single dose. Repeat q6–8wks.

Bladder Cancer (Non–muscle invasive)
Intravesicular Instillation: ADULTS, ELDERLY: Low risk of recurrence: 40 mg as single dose postoperatively (retain in bladder for 1–2 hrs). High risk of recurrence: 20 mg/wk for 6 wks, then 20 mg qmo for 3 yrs (retain in bladder for 1–2 hrs).

Dose Modification for Toxicity

Leukocytes 2,000 to less than 3,000 cells/mm^3	Hold therapy until leukocytes 4,000 or more cells/mm^3; reduce dose to 70% or more in subsequent cycles
Leukocytes less than 2,000 cells/mm^3	Hold therapy until leukocytes 4,000 or more cells/mm^3; reduce dose to 50% in subsequent cycles
Platelets 25,000 to less than 75,000 cells/mm^3	Hold therapy until platelets 100,000 or more cells/mm^3; reduce dose to 70% in subsequent cycles
Platelets less than 25,000 cells/mm^3	Hold therapy until platelets 100,000 or more cells/mm^3; reduce dose to 50% in subsequent cycles

Dosage in Renal Impairment
CrCl less than 10 mL/min: Give 75% of normal dose.

Dosage in Hepatic Impairment
No dose adjustment.

SIDE EFFECTS

Frequent (greater than 10%): Fever, anorexia, nausea, vomiting. **Occasional (10%–2%):** Stomatitis, paresthesia, purple colored bands on nails, rash, alopecia, unusual fatigue. **Rare (less than 1%):** Thrombophlebitis, cellulitis with extravasation.

ADVERSE EFFECTS/TOXIC REACTIONS

Marked myelosuppression results in hematologic toxicity manifested as leukopenia, thrombocytopenia, and, to a lesser extent, anemia (generally occurs within 2–4 wks after initial therapy). Renal toxicity may be evidenced by increased serum BUN, creatinine levels. Pulmonary toxicity manifested as dyspnea, cough, hemoptysis, pneumonia. Long-term therapy may produce hemolytic uremic syndrome, characterized by hemolytic anemia, thrombocytopenia, renal failure, hypertension.

NURSING CONSIDERATIONS

BASELINE ASSESSMENT

Obtain CBC with differential, PT, bleeding time, before and periodically during therapy. Antiemetics before and during therapy may alleviate nausea/vomiting. Offer emotional support.

INTERVENTION/EVALUATION

Monitor hematologic status, renal function studies. Assess IV site for phlebitis, extravasation. Monitor for hematologic toxicity (fever, sore throat, signs of local infection, unusual bruising/bleeding from any site), symptoms of anemia (excessive fatigue, weakness). Assess for renal toxicity (foul odor from urine, elevated serum BUN, creatinine).

PATIENT/FAMILY TEACHING

• Treatment may depress your immune system and reduce your ability to fight infection. Report symptoms of infection such as body aches, chills, cough, fatigue, fever. Avoid those with active infection. • Maintain strict oral hygiene. • Immediately report stinging, burning, pain at injection site. • Do not have immunizations without physician's approval (drug lowers resistance to infection). • Report nausea/vomiting, fever, sore throat, bruising, bleeding, shortness of breath, painful urination.

modafinil

TOP 100

moe-**daf**-i-nil
(Alertec ✤, Provigil)

◆CLASSIFICATION

PHARMACOTHERAPEUTIC: Alpha$_1$-agonist, CNS stimulant (Schedule IV). **CLINICAL:** Wakefulness-promoting agent, antinarcoleptic.

USES

Treatment of excessive daytime sleepiness associated with narcolepsy, shift work sleep disorder, adjunct therapy for obstructive sleep apnea/hypopnea syndrome. **OFF-LABEL:** Treatment of ADHD, multiple sclerosis–related fatigue.

PRECAUTIONS

Contraindications: Hypersensitivity to modafinil, armodafinil. **Cautions:** History of clinically significant mitral valve prolapse, left ventricular hypertrophy, renal/hepatic impairment, angina, cardiac disease, myocardial ischemia, recent MI, preexisting psychosis or bipolar disorder, Tourette's syndrome.

ACTION

Exact mechanism unknown. Increases dopamine in brain. Increases alpha activity, decreasing delta, theta, brain wave activity. **Therapeutic Effect:** Reduces number of sleep episodes, total daytime sleep. Increases mental alertness.

PHARMACOKINETICS

Widely distributed. Protein binding: 60%. Widely distributed. Metabolized in liver. Excreted by kidneys. Unknown if removed by hemodialysis. **Half-life:** 15 hrs.

⌛ LIFESPAN CONSIDERATIONS

Pregnancy/Lactation: Unknown if excreted in breast milk. Use caution if given to pregnant women. **Children:** Safety and efficacy not established in pts younger than 16 yrs. **Elderly:** Age-related renal/hepatic impairment may require decreased dosage.

INTERACTIONS

DRUG: May decrease concentration/effect of **cycloSPORINE, oral contraceptives. Alcohol** may decrease therapeutic effect. **Strong CYP3A4 inducers (e.g., carBAMazepine, phenytoin, rifAMPin)** may decrease concentration/effect. **HERBAL: St. John's wort** may decrease concentration/effect. **FOOD:** None known. **LAB VALUES:** None significant.

AVAILABILITY (Rx)

Tablets: ***(Provigil):*** 100 mg, 200 mg.

ADMINISTRATION/HANDLING

PO

- Give without regard to food.

INDICATIONS/ROUTES/DOSAGE

Narcolepsy, Obstructive Sleep Apnea/ Hypopnea Syndrome

PO: ADULTS: 200 mg/day in the morning. **ELDERLY:** 100 mg/day in the morning.

Shift Work Sleep Disorder

PO: ADULTS: 200 mg about 1 hr before start of work shift.

Dosage in Renal Impairment

No dose adjustment.

Dosage in Hepatic Impairment

Mild to moderate impairment: No dose adjustment. Reduce dose 50% with severe impairment.

SIDE EFFECTS

Generally well tolerated. **Occasional (5%):** Headache, nausea, dizziness, insomnia, palpitations, diarrhea.

ADVERSE EFFECTS/TOXIC REACTIONS

Agitation, excitation, increased B/P, insomnia may occur. Psychiatric disturbances (anxiety, hallucinations, suicidal ideation), serious allergic reactions (angioedema, Stevens-Johnson syndrome) have been noted.

NURSING CONSIDERATIONS

BASELINE ASSESSMENT

Obtain baseline evidence of narcolepsy or other sleep disorders, including pattern, environmental situations, length of sleep episodes. Question for sudden loss of muscle tone (cataplexy) precipitated by strong emotional responses before sleep episode. Assess frequency/severity of sleep episodes before drug therapy.

INTERVENTION/EVALUATION

Monitor sleep pattern, evidence of restlessness during sleep, length of insomnia episodes at night. Assess for dizziness, anxiety; initiate fall precautions.

PATIENT/FAMILY TEACHING

• Avoid alcohol. • Do not increase dose without physician approval. • Use alternative contraceptives during therapy and 1 mo after discontinuing modafinil (reduces effectiveness of oral contraceptives).

mometasone

TOP 100

moe-**met**-a-sone
(Asmanex, Asmanex HFA, Elocon, Nasonex, Apo-Mometasone ✱)

FIXED-COMBINATION(S)

Dulera: mometasone/formoterol (beta-adrenergic agonist): 100 mcg/5 mcg, 200 mcg/5 mcg.

◆CLASSIFICATION

PHARMACOTHERAPEUTIC: Adrenocorticosteroid. **CLINICAL:** Anti-inflammatory.

USES

Nasal: Treatment of nasal symptoms of seasonal/perennial allergic rhinitis in adults, children 2 yrs and older. Relief of nasal symptoms of seasonal allergic rhinitis in adults, children 2 yrs and older. Treatment of nasal polyps in adults. **Inhalation:** Maintenance treatment of asthma as prophylactic therapy in adults and children 4 yrs and older. **Topical:** Relief of inflammatory, pruritic manifestations of steroid-responsive dermatoses.

PRECAUTIONS

Contraindications: Hypersensitivity to mometasone, milk proteins. **Asmanex:** Primary treatment of status asthmaticus or acute bronchospasm. **Cautions:** Thyroid/hepatic/renal impairment, elderly, diabetes, cardiovascular disease, glaucoma, cataracts, myasthenia gravis, pts at risk for osteoporosis, seizures, GI disease (e.g., ulcer, colitis); following MI. Untreated systemic fungal, viral, bacterial infections.

ACTION

Inhibits formation, release, and activity of mediators of inflammation (e.g., histamine, kinins). Reverses the dilation and increased nasal permeability of inflammation. **Therapeutic Effect:** Improves symptoms of asthma, rhinitis.

PHARMACOKINETICS

Undetectable in plasma. Protein binding: 98%–99%. Swallowed portion undergoes extensive metabolism. Excreted in bile (74%), urine (8%). **Half-life:** 5 hrs.

⌛ LIFESPAN CONSIDERATIONS

Pregnancy/Lactation: Unknown if drug crosses placenta or is distributed in breast milk. **Children:** Prolonged treatment/high doses may decrease short-term growth rate, cortisol secretion. **Elderly:** No age-related precautions noted.

INTERACTIONS

DRUG: May increase hyponatremic effect of **desmopressin.** May increase antineoplastic effect of **aldesleukin.** **HERBAL:** None significant. **FOOD:** None known. **LAB VALUES:** None significant.

AVAILABILITY (Rx)

Cream: ***(Elocon):*** 0.1%. **Lotion:** ***(Elocon):*** 0.1%. **Nasal Spray:** ***(Nasonex):*** 50 mcg/spray. **Ointment:** ***(Elocon):*** 0.1%. **Powder for Oral Inhaler:** ***(Asmanex):*** 110 mcg (delivers 100 mcg/actuation), 220 mcg (delivers 200 mcg/actuation). ***(Asmanex HFA):*** 100 mcg/actuation, 200 mcg/actuation.

ADMINISTRATION/HANDLING

Inhalation

• Do not shake or prime. • Hold twisthaler straight up with pink portion (base) on bottom, remove cap. • Exhale fully. • Firmly close lips around mouthpiece and inhale a fast, deep breath. • Hold breath for 10 sec.

Intranasal

• Instruct pt to clear nasal passages as much as possible before use. • Tilt head slightly forward. • Insert spray tip into nostril, pointing toward nasal passages, away from nasal septum. • Spray into one nostril while pt holds other nostril closed, concurrently inspiring through nose to permit medication as high into nasal passages as possible.

M

Topical

• Apply thin layer of cream, lotion, ointment to cover affected area. Rub in gently. • Do not cover area with occlusive dressing.

INDICATIONS/ROUTES/DOSAGE

Allergic Rhinitis

Nasal Spray: **ADULTS, ELDERLY, CHILDREN 12 YRS AND OLDER:** 2 sprays (100 mcg) in each nostril once daily. Total daily dose: 200 mcg. When used to prevent nasal rhinitis, begin 2–4 wks before start of pollen season. **CHILDREN 2–11 YRS:** 1 spray (50 mcg) in each nostril once daily. Total daily dose: 100 mcg.

Asthma

Inhalation: **ADULTS, ELDERLY, CHILDREN 12 YRS AND OLDER (Previous therapy with bronchodilators):** ***(Asmanex):*** Initially, inhale 220 mcg (1 puff) once daily. **Maximum:** 440 mcg/day as single or 2 divided doses. **(Previous therapy with inhaled corticosteroids):** ***(Asmanex HFA):*** Initially, 200 mcg twice daily. **Maximum:** 400 mcg twice daily. **(Previous therapy with oral corticosteroids):** ***(Asmanex):*** 440 mcg (2 puffs) twice daily. ***(Asmanex HFA):*** 400 mcg twice daily. Reduce predniSONE no faster than 2.5 mg/day beginning after at least 1 wk of mometasone. **CHILDREN 4–11 YRS:** ***(Asmanex):*** 110 mcg once daily in evening.

Skin Disease

Topical: **ADULTS, ELDERLY, CHILDREN 12 YRS AND OLDER:** Apply cream, lotion, or ointment sparingly to affected area once daily.

Nasal Polyp

Nasal Spray: **ADULTS, ELDERLY:** 2 sprays (100 mcg) in each nostril once or twice daily. Total daily dose: 400 mcg.

Dosage in Renal/Hepatic Impairment

No dose adjustment.

SIDE EFFECTS

Occasional: **Inhalation:** Headache, allergic rhinitis, upper respiratory infection, muscle pain, fatigue. **Nasal:** Nasal irritation, stinging. **Topical:** Burning. **Rare:** **Inhalation:** Abdominal pain, dyspepsia, nausea. **Nasal:** Nasal/pharyngeal candidiasis. **Topical:** Pruritus.

ADVERSE EFFECTS/TOXIC REACTIONS

Acute hypersensitivity reaction (urticaria, angioedema, severe bronchospasm) occurs rarely. Transfer from systemic to local steroid therapy may unmask previously suppressed bronchial asthma condition.

NURSING CONSIDERATIONS

BASELINE ASSESSMENT

Question for hypersensitivity to any corticosteroids. Auscultate lung sounds. Teach proper use of nasal spray, oral inhaler.

INTERVENTION/EVALUATION

Monitor for relief of rhinitis, asthma symptoms. Assess lung sounds for wheezing, rales.

PATIENT/FAMILY TEACHING

• Do not change dose schedule or stop taking drug; must taper off gradually under medical supervision. **Nasal:** Report if symptoms do not improve; report if sneezing, nasal irritation occur. • Clear nasal passages prior to use. **Inhalation:** Inhale rapidly, deeply; rinse mouth after inhalation. • Not indicated for acute asthma attacks. **Topical:** Do not cover affected area with bandage, dressing.

montelukast

mon-**tee**-loo-kast
(Singulair)
Do not confuse Singulair with SINEquan.

◆CLASSIFICATION

PHARMACOTHERAPEUTIC: Leukotriene receptor inhibitor. **CLINICAL:** Antiasthmatic.

USES

Prophylaxis, chronic treatment of asthma. Prevention of exercise-induced bronchoconstriction. Relief of symptoms of seasonal allergic rhinitis (hay fever), perennial allergic rhinitis. **OFF-LABEL:** Urticaria.

PRECAUTIONS

Contraindications: Hypersensitivity to montelukast. **Cautions:** Systemic corticosteroid treatment reduction during montelukast therapy. Concomitant use of CYP3A4 inducers. Not for use in acute asthma attacks.

ACTION

Binds to cysteinyl leukotriene receptors, inhibiting effects of leukotrienes on bronchial smooth muscle. **Therapeutic Effect:** Decreases bronchoconstriction, vascular permeability, mucosal edema, mucus production.

PHARMACOKINETICS

Route	Onset	Peak	Duration
PO	N/A	N/A	24 hrs
PO (chewable)	N/A	N/A	24 hrs

Rapidly absorbed. Protein binding: 99%. Extensively metabolized in liver. Excreted almost exclusively in feces. **Half-life:** 2.7–5.5 hrs (slightly longer in elderly).

LIFESPAN CONSIDERATIONS

Pregnancy/Lactation: Unknown if distributed in breast milk. **Children/Elderly:** No age-related precautions noted in pts older than 6 yrs or the elderly.

INTERACTIONS

DRUG: None significant. **HERBAL:** None significant. **FOOD:** None known. **LAB VALUES:** May increase serum ALT, AST, eosinophils.

AVAILABILITY (Rx)

Oral Granules: 4 mg per packet. **Tablets:** 10 mg. **Tablets, Chewable:** 4 mg, 5 mg.

ADMINISTRATION/HANDLING

PO

• May take without regard to food. When treating asthma, administer in evening. • When treating allergic rhinitis, may individualize administration times. • Granules may be given directly in mouth or mixed with carrots, rice, applesauce, ice cream, baby formula, or breast milk (do not add to any other liquid or food). • Give within 15 min of opening packet.

INDICATIONS/ROUTES/DOSAGE

Bronchial Asthma

PO: ADULTS, ELDERLY, CHILDREN 15 YRS AND OLDER: 10-mg tablet daily, taken in the evening. **CHILDREN 6–14 YRS:** 5-mg chewable tablet daily, taken in the evening. **CHILDREN 1–5 YRS:** 4-mg chewable tablet or oral granules daily, taken in the evening.

Seasonal Allergic Rhinitis

PO: ADULTS, ELDERLY, CHILDREN 15 YRS AND OLDER: 10-mg tablet, taken in the evening. **CHILDREN 6–14 YRS:** 5-mg chewable tablet, taken in the evening. **CHILDREN 2–5 YRS:** 4-mg chewable tablet, or oral granules taken in the evening.

Perennial Allergic Rhinitis

PO: ADULTS, ELDERLY, CHILDREN 15 YRS AND OLDER: 10-mg tablet, taken in the evening. **CHILDREN 6–14 YRS:** 5-mg chewable tablet, taken in the evening. **CHILDREN 2–5 YRS:** 4-mg chewable tablet or oral granules, taken in the evening. **CHILDREN 6–23 MOS:** 4 mg oral granules, taken in the evening.

Exercise-Induced Bronchoconstriction Prevention

PO: ADULTS, ELDERLY, CHILDREN 15 YRS AND OLDER: 10 mg 2 or more hrs before exercise. No additional doses within 24 hrs. **CHILDREN 6–14 YRS:** 5 mg (chew tab) 2 or more hrs prior to exercise. No additional doses within 24 hrs.

Dosage in Renal/Hepatic Impairment

No dose adjustment.

M

SIDE EFFECTS

ADULTS, CHILDREN 15 YRS AND OLDER: Frequent (18%): Headache. **Occasional (4%):** Influenza. **Rare (3%–2%):** Abdominal pain, cough, dyspepsia, dizziness, fatigue, dental pain. **CHILDREN 6–14 YRS: Rare (less than 2%):** Diarrhea, laryngitis, pharyngitis, nausea, otitis media, sinusitis, viral infection.

ADVERSE EFFECTS/TOXIC REACTIONS

Suicidal ideation and behavior, depression have been noted.

NURSING CONSIDERATIONS

BASELINE ASSESSMENT

Chewable tablet contains phenylalanine (component of aspartame); parents of phenylketonuric pts should be informed. Assess lung sounds for wheezing. Assess for allergy symptoms. Question history of depression, suicidal ideation.

INTERVENTION/EVALUATION

Monitor rate, depth, rhythm, type of respirations; quality/rate of pulse. Assess lung sounds for wheezing. Monitor for change in mood, behavior.

PATIENT/FAMILY TEACHING

• Increase fluid intake (decreases lung secretion viscosity). • Take as prescribed, even during symptom-free periods as well as during exacerbations of asthma. • Drug is not for treatment of acute asthma attacks. • Report increased use or frequency of short-acting bronchodilators, changes in behavior, suicidal ideation.

morphine

TOP 100 HIGH ALERT

mor-feen

(Arymo ER, Duramorph, Infumorph, Kadian, M-Eslon ✦, Mitigo, MS Contin, MS-IR ✦)

■ BLACK BOX ALERT ■ Risk of severe adverse effects when epidural route of administration is used. Ingestion of alcohol with morphine ER may increase risk of overdose. Risk of opioid addiction, abuse, and misuse. Serious, life-threatening, or fatal respiratory depression may occur. Prolonged use during pregnancy may result in neonatal opioid withdrawal syndrome. Accidental ingestion of even one dose may result in a fatal overdose. Concomitant use with benzodiazepines, other CNS depressants may result in profound sedation, respiratory depression, coma, or death.

Do not confuse morphine with HYDROmorphone, or morphine sulfate with magnesium sulfate, MS Contin with OxyCONTIN. MSO_4 and MS are error-prone abbreviations.

FIXED-COMBINATION(S)

Embeda: morphine/naloxone (an opioid antagonist): 20 mg/0.8 mg, 30 mg/1.2 mg, 50 mg/2 mg, 60 mg/2.4 mg, 80 mg/3.2 mg, 100 mg/4 mg.

◆CLASSIFICATION

PHARMACOTHERAPEUTIC: Opioid agonist (Schedule II). **CLINICAL:** Opioid analgesic.

USES

Relief of moderate to severe, acute, or chronic pain; analgesia during labor, pain due to MI, dyspnea from pulmonary edema not resulting from chemical respiratory irritant. **Infumorph:** Use in devices for managing intractable chronic pain. **Extended-Release:** Use only when repeated doses for extended periods of time are required around the clock.

PRECAUTIONS

Contraindications: Hypersensitivity to morphine. Acute or severe asthma, GI obstruction, known or suspected paralytic ileus, concurrent use of MAOIs or use of MAOIs within 14 days, severe respiratory depression. **Extreme Caution:** COPD, cor pulmonale, hypoxia, hypercapnia, preexisting respiratory depression, head injury, increased ICP, severe hypotension. **Cautions:** Biliary tract disease, pancreatitis, Addison's disease, cardiovascular disease, morbid obesity, adrenal insufficiency, elderly, hypothyroidism, urethral stricture, prostatic hyperplasia, debilitated pts, pts with CNS depression, toxic psychosis, seizure disorders, history of drug abuse and misuse, drug-seeking behavior, dependency.

ACTION

Binds with opioid receptors within CNS, inhibiting ascending pain pathways. **Therapeutic Effect:** Alters pain perception, emotional response to pain.

PHARMACOKINETICS

Route	Onset	Peak	Duration
Oral solution	30 min	1 hr	3–5 hrs
Tablets	30 min	1 hr	3–5 hrs
Tablets (extended-release)	N/A	3–4 hrs	8–12 hrs
IV	Rapid	0.3 hr	3–5 hrs
IM	5–30 min	0.5–1 hr	3–5 hrs
Epidural	15–60 min	1 hr	12–20 hrs
SQ	10–30 min	1.1–5 hrs	3–5 hrs
Rectal	20–60 min	0.5–1 hr	3–7 hrs

Variably absorbed from GI tract. Readily absorbed after IM, SQ administration. Protein binding: 20%–35%. Widely distributed. Metabolized in liver. Primarily excreted in urine. Removed by hemodialysis. **Half-life:** 2–4 hrs (increased in hepatic disease).

LIFESPAN CONSIDERATIONS

Pregnancy/Lactation: Crosses placenta. Distributed in breast milk. May prolong labor if administered in latent phase of first stage of labor or before cervical dilation of 4–5 cm has occurred. Respiratory depression may occur in neonate if mother received opiates during labor. Regular use of opiates during pregnancy may produce withdrawal symptoms in neonate (irritability, excessive crying, tremors, hyperactive reflexes, fever, vomiting, diarrhea, yawning, sneezing, seizures). **Children:** Paradoxical excitement may occur; those younger than 2 yrs are more susceptible to respiratory depressant effects. **Elderly:** Paradoxical excitement may occur. Age-related renal impairment may increase risk of urinary retention.

INTERACTIONS

DRUG: **Alcohol, other CNS depressants (e.g., LORazepam, gabapentin, zolpidem)** may increase CNS effects, respiratory depression, hypotension. **MAOIs (e.g., phenelzine, selegiline)** may produce serotonin syndrome. (Reduce dosage to one-fourth of usual morphine dose.) **HERBAL:** **Herbals with sedative properties (e.g., chamomile, kava kava, valerian)** may increase CNS depression. **FOOD:** None known. **LAB VALUES:** May increase serum amylase, lipase.

AVAILABILITY (Rx)

Injection Solution: 2 mg/mL, 4 mg/mL, 5 mg/mL, 10 mg/mL. **Injection Solution (Epidural, Intrathecal, IV Infusion):** ***(Duramorph):*** 0.5 mg/mL, 1 mg/mL. **Injection Solution, Epidural or Intrathecal:** ***(Infumorph):*** 10 mg/mL, 25 mg/mL. **Injection Solution:** ***(Mitigo):*** 10 mg/mL, 25 mg/mL. **Injection Solution, Patient-Controlled**

M

Analgesia (PCA) Pump: 1 mg/mL. **Solution, Oral:** 10 mg/5 mL, 20 mg/5 mL, 20 mg/mL. **Suppository:** 5 mg, 10 mg, 20 mg, 30 mg. **Tablets:** 15 mg, 30 mg.

Capsules, Extended-Release: 45 mg, 75 mg, 90 mg, 120 mg. **Capsules, Sustained-Release:** 10 mg, 20 mg, 30 mg, 50 mg, 60 mg, 80 mg, 100 mg. **Tablets, Extended-Release:** 15 mg, 30 mg, 60 mg, 100 mg, 200 mg. **Tablets, Extended-Release (Abuse Deterrent):** 15 mg, 30 mg, 60 mg.

ADMINISTRATION/HANDLING

IV

Reconstitution • May give undiluted. • For IV injection, may dilute in Sterile Water for Injection or 0.9% NaCl to final concentration of 1–2 mg/mL. • For continuous IV infusion, dilute to concentration of 0.1–1 mg/mL in D_5W and give through controlled infusion device.

Rate of administration • Always administer very slowly. Rapid IV increases risk of severe adverse reactions (apnea, chest wall rigidity, peripheral circulatory collapse, cardiac arrest, anaphylactoid effects).

Storage • Store at room temperature.

IM, SQ

• Administer slowly, rotating injection sites. • Pts with circulatory impairment experience higher risk of overdosage due to delayed absorption of repeated administration.

PO

• May give without regard to food. • Mix liquid form with fruit juice to improve taste. • Do not break, crush, dissolve, or divide extended-release capsule, tablets. • **Avinza, Kadian:** May mix with applesauce immediately prior to administration.

Rectal

• If suppository is too soft, chill for 30 min in refrigerator or run cold water over foil wrapper. • Moisten suppository with cold water before inserting well into rectum.

IV INCOMPATIBILITIES

Amphotericin B complex (Abelcet, AmBisome, Amphotec), cefepime (Maxipime), doxorubicin (Doxil), phenytoin (Dilantin).

IV COMPATIBILITIES

Amiodarone (Cordarone), atropine, bumetanide (Bumex), bupivacaine (Marcaine, Sensorcaine), dexmedetomidine (Precedex), dilTIAZem (Cardizem), diphenhydrAMINE (Benadryl), DOBUTamine (Dobutrex), DOPamine (Intropin), glycopyrrolate (Robinul), heparin, hydrOXYzine (Vistaril), lidocaine, LORazepam (Ativan), magnesium, midazolam (Versed), milrinone (Primacor), nitroglycerin, potassium, propofol (Diprivan).

INDICATIONS/ROUTES/DOSAGE

◄ALERT► Dosage should be titrated to desired effect.

Analgesia

PO: ***(Immediate-Release):*** **ADULTS, ELDERLY:** 10–30 mg q4h as needed. **CHILDREN 6 MOS AND OLDER WEIGHING 50 KG OR MORE:** 15–20 mg q3–4h as needed. **CHILDREN 6 MOS AND OLDER WEIGHING LESS THAN 50 KG:** 0.2–0.5 mg/kg q3–4h as needed. **CHILDREN YOUNGER THAN 6 MOS:** ***(Oral Solution):*** 0.08–0.1 mg/kg q3–4h as needed.

◄ALERT► For the Avinza dosage below, be aware that this drug is to be administered once daily only.

◄ALERT► For the Kadian dosage information below, be aware that this drug is to be administered q12h or once daily.

◄ALERT► Be aware that pediatric dosages of extended-release preparations of Kadian and AVINza have not been established.

◄ALERT► For the MS Contin dosage information below, be aware that the daily dosage is divided and given q8h or q12h.

PO: ***(Extended-Release [Avinza]):*** **ADULTS, ELDERLY:** Dosage requirement should be established using prompt-release formulations and is based on total daily dose. AVINza is given once daily only.
PO: ***(Extended-Release [Kadian]):*** **ADULTS, ELDERLY:** Dosage requirement should be established using prompt-release formulations and is based on total daily dose. Dose is given once daily or divided and given q12h.
PO: ***(Extended-Release [MS Contin]):*** **ADULTS, ELDERLY:** Dosage requirement should be established using prompt-release formulations and is based on total daily dose. Daily dose is divided and given q8h or q12h.
IV: ADULTS, ELDERLY: 2.5–5 mg q3–4h as needed. **Note:** Repeated doses (e.g., 1–2 mg) may be given more frequently (e.g., every hr) if needed. **CHILDREN WEIGHING 50 KG OR MORE:** Initially, 2–5 mg q2–4h as needed. **CHILDREN WEIGHING LESS THAN 50 KG:** Initially, 0.05 mg/kg. Range: 0.1–0.2 mg/kg q2–4h as needed. **NEONATES:** Initially, 0.05–0.1 mg/kg/dose q4–6h as needed.
IV continuous infusion: ADULTS, ELDERLY: 0.8–10 mg/hr. Range: 20–50 mg/hr. **CHILDREN WEIGHING 50 KG OR MORE:** 1.5 mg/hr. **CHILDREN WEIGHING LESS THAN 50 KG:** Initially, 0.01 mg/kg/hr. Range: 0.01–0.04 mg/kg/hr (10–40 mcg/kg/hr). **NEONATES:** Initially, 0.01 mg/kg/hr (10 mcg/kg/hr). **Maximum:** 0.015–0.02 mg/kg/hr.

Patient-Controlled Analgesia (PCA)
IV: ADULTS, ELDERLY: Usual concentration: 1 mg/mL. **Demand dose:** 1 mg (range: 0.5–2.5 mg). **Lockout interval:** 5–10 min.

Dosage in Renal Impairment

Creatinine Clearance	Dose
10–50 mL/min, CRRT	75% of normal dose
Less than 10 mL/min, HD, PD	50% of normal dose

Dosage in Hepatic Impairment
No dose adjustment.

SIDE EFFECTS

◀ALERT▶ Ambulatory pts, pts not in severe pain may experience nausea, vomiting more frequently than pts in supine position or who have severe pain. **Frequent:** Sedation, decreased B/P (including orthostatic hypotension), diaphoresis, facial flushing, constipation, dizziness, drowsiness, nausea, vomiting. **Occasional:** Allergic reaction (rash, pruritus), dyspnea, confusion, palpitations, tremors, urinary retention, abdominal cramps, vision changes, dry mouth, headache, decreased appetite, pain/burning at injection site. **Rare:** Paralytic ileus.

ADVERSE EFFECTS/TOXIC REACTIONS

Overdose results in respiratory depression, skeletal muscle flaccidity, cold/clammy skin, cyanosis, extreme drowsiness progressing to seizures, stupor, coma. Tolerance to analgesic effect, physical dependence may occur with repeated use. Prolonged duration of action, cumulative effect may occur in those with hepatic/renal impairment. **Antidote:** Naloxone (see Appendix J for dosage).

NURSING CONSIDERATIONS

BASELINE ASSESSMENT

Assess onset, type, location, duration of pain. Obtain vital signs before giving medication. If respirations are 12/min or less (20/min or less in children), withhold medication, contact physician. Effect of medication is reduced if full pain recurs before next dose. Assess for potential of abuse/misuse (e.g., drug-seeking behavior, mental health conditions, history of substance abuse).

M

INTERVENTION/EVALUATION

Monitor vital signs 5–10 min after IV administration, 15–30 min after SQ, IM. Be alert for decreased respirations, B/P. Check for adequate voiding. Monitor daily pattern of bowel activity, stool consistency; avoid constipation. Initiate deep breathing, coughing exercises, particularly in those with pulmonary impairment. Assess for clinical improvement; record onset of pain relief. Screen for drug abuse and misuse, drug-seeking behavior.

PATIENT/FAMILY TEACHING

• Change positions slowly to avoid orthostatic hypotension. • Avoid tasks that require alertness, motor skills until response to drug is established. • Avoid alcohol, CNS depressants. • Tolerance, dependence may occur with prolonged use of high doses. • Report ineffective pain control, constipation, urinary retention.

M

mycophenolate

mye-koe-**fen**-o-late
(CellCept, Myfortic)

BLACK BOX ALERT Increased risk of congenital malformation, spontaneous abortion. Increased risk for development of lymphoma, skin malignancy. Increased susceptibility to infections. Administer under supervision of physician experienced in immunosuppressive therapy.

◆CLASSIFICATION

PHARMACOTHERAPEUTIC: Immunologic agent. **CLINICAL:** Immunosuppressant.

USES

Should be used concurrently with other immunosuppressants **CellCept:** Prophylaxis of organ rejection in pts receiving allogeneic hepatic/renal/cardiac transplant. **Myfortic:** Renal transplants. **OFF-LABEL:** Treatment of hepatic transplant rejection in pts unable to tolerate tacrolimus or cycloSPORINE due to toxicity, mild heart transplant rejection, moderate to severe psoriasis, proliferative lupus nephritis, myasthenia gravis, graft-vs-host disease. Treatment of autoimmune hepatitis (refractory).

PRECAUTIONS

Contraindications: Hypersensitivity to mycophenolate, mycophenolic acid or polysorbate 80 (IV formulation). **Cautions:** Active severe GI disease, renal impairment, neutropenia, women of childbearing potential (use caution when handling).

ACTION

Suppresses immunologically mediated inflammatory response by inhibiting inosine monophosphate dehydrogenase, an enzyme that deprives lymphocytes of nucleotides necessary for DNA, RNA synthesis, thus inhibiting proliferation of T and B lymphocytes. **Therapeutic Effect:** Prevents transplant rejection.

PHARMACOKINETICS

Widely distributed. Protein binding: 97%. Completely hydrolyzed to active metabolite mycophenolic acid. Primarily excreted in urine. Not removed by hemodialysis. **Half-life:** 17.9 hrs.

⌛ LIFESPAN CONSIDERATIONS

Pregnancy/Lactation: Avoid use; may cause fetal harm. Females of reproductive potential should use effective contraception during treatment and for at least 6 wks after discontinuation. Breastfeeding not recommended. **Children:** Safety and efficacy not established in children younger than 3 mos. **Elderly:** Age-related renal impairment may require dosage adjustment.

INTERACTIONS

DRUG: May increase concentration/effects of **acyclovir, ganciclovir. Antacids (aluminum- and magnesium-containing), cholestyramine**

may decrease absorption. **Live virus vaccines** may potentiate virus replication, increase vaccine side effects, decrease pt's antibody response to vaccine. **Rifampin** may decrease concentration/effect. May decrease therapeutic effect of **oral contraceptives.** HERBAL: **Echinacea** may decrease therapeutic effect. FOOD: **All foods** may decrease concentration. LAB VALUES: May increase serum cholesterol, alkaline phosphatase, creatinine, ALT, AST. May alter serum glucose, lipids, calcium, potassium, phosphate, uric acid.

AVAILABILITY (Rx)

Capsules: *(CellCept):* 250 mg. **Injection, Powder for Reconstitution:** *(CellCept):* 500 mg. **Oral Suspension:** *(CellCept):* 200 mg/mL. **Tablets:** *(CellCept):* 500 mg.

Tablets, Delayed-Release: *(Myfortic):* 180 mg, 360 mg.

ADMINISTRATION/HANDLING

IV

Reconstitution • Reconstitute each 500-mg vial with 14 mL D_5W. Gently agitate. • For 1-g dose, further dilute with 140 mL D_5W; for 1.5-g dose, further dilute with 210 mL D_5W, providing a concentration of 6 mg/mL.

Rate of administration • Infuse over at least 2 hrs. • Begin infusion within 4 hrs of reconstitution.

Storage • Store at room temperature.

PO

• Give on empty stomach (1 hr before or 2 hrs after food). • Do not break, crush, or open capsules or break, crush, dissolve, or divide delayed-release tablets. Avoid inhalation of powder in capsules, direct contact of powder on skin/mucous membranes. If contact occurs, wash thoroughly, with soap, water. Rinse eyes profusely with plain water. • May store reconstituted suspension in refrigerator or at room temperature. • Suspension is stable for 60 days after reconstitution. • Suspension can be administered orally or via an NG tube (minimum size 8 French).

IV INCOMPATIBILITIES

Mycophenolate is compatible only with D_5W. Do not infuse concurrently with other drugs or IV solutions.

INDICATIONS/ROUTES/DOSAGE

Prevention of Renal Transplant Rejection

PO, IV: *(CellCept):* **ADULTS, ELDERLY:** 1 g twice daily. **PO: CHILDREN 3 MONTHS AND OLDER:** *(CellCept Suspension):* 600 mg/m^2/dose twice daily. **Maximum:** 1 g twice daily. *(Tablets, Capsules):* **BSA greater than or equal to 1.5 m^2:** 1,000 mg twice daily. **BSA 1.25–1.5 m^2:** 750 mg twice daily. **PO:** *(Myfortic):* **ADULTS, ELDERLY:** 720 mg twice daily. **CHILDREN 5–16 YRS:** 400 mg/m^2 twice daily. **Maximum:** 720 mg twice daily. **BSA greater than 1.58 m^2:** 720 mg twice daily. **BSA 1.19–1.58 m^2:** 540 mg twice daily.

Prevention of Heart Transplant Rejection

PO, IV: *(CellCept):* **ADULTS, ELDERLY:** 1.5 g twice daily in combination with cyclosporine and initially with corticosteroids; or 1 g twice daily in combination with other immunosuppressants (e.g., tacrolimus, everolimus, or sirolimus).

Prevention of Hepatic Transplant Rejection

PO, IV: *(CellCept):* **ADULTS, ELDERLY:** 1.5 g twice daily in combination with cyclosporine and initially with corticosteroids; or 1 g twice daily in combination with other immunosuppressants (e.g., tacrolimus, everolimus, or sirolimus).

Dosage in Renal/Hepatic Impairment

No dose adjustment.

SIDE EFFECTS

Frequent (37%–20%): UTI, hypertension, peripheral edema, diarrhea, constipation, fever, headache, nausea. **Occasional (18%–10%):** Dyspepsia, dyspnea, cough, hematuria, asthenia, vomiting, edema, tremors, oral candidiasis, acne;

M

abdominal, chest, back pain. **Rare (9%–6%):** Insomnia, respiratory tract infection, rash, dizziness.

ADVERSE EFFECTS/TOXIC REACTIONS

Significant anemia, leukopenia, thrombocytopenia, neutropenia, leukocytosis may occur, particularly in pts undergoing renal transplant rejection. Sepsis, infection occur occasionally. GI tract hemorrhage occurs rarely. May increase risk of new malignancies. Immunosuppression results in increased susceptibility to infection.

NURSING CONSIDERATIONS

BASELINE ASSESSMENT

Obtain pregnancy test in females of reproductive potential. Assess medical history, esp. renal function, existence of active digestive system disease, drug history, esp. other immunosuppressants.

INTERVENTION/EVALUATION

CBC should be performed wkly during first mo of therapy, twice monthly during second and third mos of treatment, then monthly throughout the first yr. If rapid fall in WBC occurs, dosage should be reduced or discontinued. Assess for delayed bone marrow suppression. Monitor for infections (cough, fatigue, fever).

PATIENT/FAMILY TEACHING

• Treatment may depress your immune system and reduce your ability to fight infection. Report symptoms of infection such as body aches, chills, cough, fatigue, fever. Avoid those with active infection. • Report unusual bleeding/bruising, sore throat, mouth sores, abdominal pain, fever. • May cause new cancers. • Use effective contraception to avoid pregnancy. Laboratory follow-up while taking medication is important part of therapy.

nafcillin

naf-**sil**-in

◆CLASSIFICATION

PHARMACOTHERAPEUTIC: Penicillin. **CLINICAL:** Antibiotic.

USES

Treatment of respiratory tract, skin/skin structure infections, osteomyelitis, endocarditis, meningitis; perioperatively, esp. in cardiovascular, orthopedic procedures. Predominant treatment of infections caused by susceptible strains of staphylococci.

PRECAUTIONS

Contraindications: Hypersensitivity to nafcillin, other penicillins. **Cautions:** History of allergies, particularly cephalosporins; severe renal/hepatic impairment, asthma, HF.

ACTION

Binds to bacterial membranes. **Therapeutic Effect:** Inhibits cell wall synthesis. Bactericidal.

LIFESPAN CONSIDERATIONS

Pregnancy/Lactation: Readily crosses placenta; appears in cord blood, amniotic fluid. Distributed in breast milk. May lead to rash, diarrhea, candidiasis in neonate, infant. **Children:** Immature renal function in neonates may delay renal excretion. **Elderly:** Age-related renal impairment may require dosage adjustment.

INTERACTIONS

DRUG: High doses (2 g q4h) may decrease effects of **warfarin.** May decrease effects of **BCG (intravesical), axitinib, bosutinib, cobimetinib, elbasvir, grazoprevir, neratinib, olaparib, ranolazine, sonidegib. HERBAL:** None significant. **FOOD:** None known. **LAB VALUES:** May cause false-positive Coombs' test.

AVAILABILITY (Rx)

Injection, Powder for Reconstitution: 1 g, 2 g. **Infusion, Premix:** 1 g/50 mL, 2g/100 mL.

ADMINISTRATION/HANDLING

◀ALERT▶ Space doses evenly around the clock.

IV

Reconstitution • Reconstitute each vial with 10 mL Sterile Water for Injection or 0.9% NaCl. • For intermittent IV infusion (piggyback), further dilute with 50–100 mL 0.9% NaCl or D_5W.

Rate of administration • Infuse over 30–60 min. • Stop infusion if pt complains of pain at IV site.

Storage • Refrigerate diluted solution for up to 7 days or store at room temperature for up to 24 hrs. • Discard if precipitate forms.

IM

• Reconstitute each 500 mg with 1.7 mL Sterile Water for Injection or 0.9% NaCl to provide concentration of 250 mg/mL. • Inject IM into large muscle mass.

IV INCOMPATIBILITIES

Aztreonam (Azactam), dilTIAZem (Cardizem), droperidol (Inapsine), fentaNYL, gentamicin, insulin, labetalol (Normodyne, Trandate), methylPREDNISolone (Solu-Medrol), midazolam (Versed), nalbuphine (Nubain), vancomycin (Vancocin), verapamil (Isoptin).

IV COMPATIBILITIES

Acyclovir, famotidine (Pepcid), fluconazole (Diflucan), heparin, HYDROmorphone (Dilaudid), lidocaine, lipids, magnesium, morphine, potassium chloride, propofol (Diprivan).

INDICATIONS/ROUTES/DOSAGE

Usual Dosage

IV: ADULTS, ELDERLY: 1–2 g q4–6h. **CHILDREN: Mild to moderate infections:** 100–150 mg/kg/day in divided doses q6h. **Maximum:** 4 g/day. **Severe infections:** 150–200 mg/kg/day in divided doses q4–6h. **Maximum:** 12 g/day. **NEONATES:** 25 mg/kg/dose in divided doses q6–12h. Dose based on body weight and postnatal age.

Dosage in Renal/Hepatic Impairment

No dose adjustment.

SIDE EFFECTS

Frequent: Mild hypersensitivity reaction (fever, rash, pruritus), GI effects (nausea, vomiting, diarrhea). **Occasional:** Hypokalemia with high IV dosages, phlebitis, thrombophlebitis (common in elderly). **Rare:** Extravasation with IV administration.

N

ADVERSE EFFECTS/TOXIC REACTIONS

Potentially fatal antibiotic-associated colitis, superinfections (abdominal cramps, severe watery diarrhea, fever) may result from altered bacterial balance in GI tract. Hematologic effects (esp. involving platelets, WBCs), severe hypersensitivity reactions, anaphylaxis occur rarely.

NURSING CONSIDERATIONS

BASELINE ASSESSMENT

Question for history of allergies, esp. penicillins, cephalosporins.

INTERVENTION/EVALUATION

Hold medication, promptly report rash (possible hypersensitivity), diarrhea (fever, abdominal pain, mucus/blood in stool may indicate antibiotic-associated colitis). Evaluate IV site frequently for phlebitis (heat, pain, red streaking over vein), infiltration (potential extravasation). Be alert for superinfection: fever, vomiting, diarrhea, anal/genital pruritus, oral mucosal changes (ulceration, pain, erythema).

PATIENT/FAMILY TEACHING

• Continue antibiotic for full length of treatment. • Doses should be evenly spaced. • Discomfort may occur with IM injection. • Report IV discomfort immediately. • Report diarrhea, rash, other new symptoms.

naldemedine

nal-**dem**-e-deen
(Symproic)

◆CLASSIFICATION

PHARMACOTHERAPEUTIC: Opioid receptor antagonist (peripheral acting) **(Schedule II)**. **CLINICAL:** GI agent.

USES

Treatment of opioid-induced constipation (OIC) in adult pts with chronic noncancer pain, including pts with chronic pain related to prior cancer or its treatment, who do not require frequent (e.g., weekly) opioid dosage escalation.

PRECAUTIONS

Contraindications: Hypersensitivity to naldemedine. Known or suspected mechanical GI obstruction. Pts at risk of recurrent GI obstruction. **Cautions:** Severe hepatic impairment, advanced illness associated with impaired structural integrity of the GI wall or conditions that may impair integrity of GI wall (e.g., Crohn's disease, diverticulitis, GI tract malignancies, intestinal adhesions, Ogilvie's syndrome, peptic ulcers, peritoneal malignancies). Concomitant use of strong CYP3A inducers, other opioid antagonists. Pts with disruption to the blood-brain barrier (may precipitate symptoms of opioid withdrawal).

ACTION

Blocks opioid binding at the peripheral mu, delta, and kappa opioid receptors in GI tract. Inhibits the delay in GI transit times. **Therapeutic Effect:** Decreases constipating effects of opioids.

PHARMACOKINETICS

Widely distributed. Metabolized in liver. Protein binding: 93%–94%. Peak plasma concentration: 45 min (with food: 2.5 hrs). Excreted in urine (57%), feces (35%). Not removed by dialysis. **Half-life:** 11 hrs.

⌛ LIFESPAN CONSIDERATIONS

Pregnancy/Lactation: May cross the placenta and cause fetal opiate withdrawal due to immature blood-brain barrier. Due to risk of opiate withdrawal in nursing infants, breastfeeding not recommended during treatment and for at least 3 days after discontinuation. **Children:** Safety and efficacy not established. **Elderly:** No age-related precautions noted.

INTERACTIONS

DRUG: P-gp/ABCB1 inhibitors (e.g., amiodarone), dilTIAZem, proton pump inhibitors (e.g., omeprazole, pantoprazole), strong CYP3A inhibitors (e.g., clarithromycin, ketoconazole, ritonavir) may increase concentration/effect. **Strong CYP3A inducers (e.g., carBAMazepine, phenytoin, rifAMPin)** may decrease concentration/effect. **Methylnaltrexone, opioid antagonists** may increase adverse/toxic effects. **HERBAL: St. John's wort** may decrease concentration/effect. **FOOD:** None known. **LAB VALUES:** None known.

AVAILABILITY (Rx)

Tablets: 0.2 mg.

ADMINISTRATION/HANDLING

PO

- Give with or without food.

INDICATIONS/ROUTES/DOSAGE

Opioid-Induced Constipation

PO: ADULTS, ELDERLY: 0.2 mg once daily. (Discontinue if opioid pain medication is discontinued.)

Dosage in Renal Impairment

No dose adjustment.

Dosage in Hepatic Impairment

Mild to moderate impairment: No dose adjustment. **Severe impairment:** Not recommended.

SIDE EFFECTS

Frequent (21%–12%): Abdominal pain. **Occasional (9%–3%):** Diarrhea, nausea, flatulence, vomiting, headache, hyperhidrosis.

ADVERSE EFFECTS/TOXIC REACTIONS

Severe abdominal pain, diarrhea requiring hospitalization may occur. GI perforation was reported in pts with baseline GI disease (Crohn's disease, diverticulitis, GI tract malignancies, peptic ulcers, Ogilvie's syndrome, peritoneal malignancies). Symptoms of opiate withdrawal including abdominal pain, anxiety, chills, diarrhea, feeling cold, flushing, hyperhidrosis, increased lacrimation, irritability, nausea were reported, esp. in pts taking methadone or with disruptions to the blood-brain barrier. May increase risk of adverse effects in pts with renal impairment.

NURSING CONSIDERATIONS

BASELINE ASSESSMENT

Discontinue all maintenance laxative therapy prior to initiation. Laxatives may be restarted if therapy has been ineffective for 3 days. Changes to analgesic dosage prior to initiation is not required. Question characteristics of constipation, frequency of bowel movements. Assess bowel sounds. Question history of GI obstruction, GI perforation, or baseline GI disease. Receive full medication history, including herbal products, and screen for interactions. Assess hydration status.

INTERVENTION/EVALUATION

Pts may be less responsive to therapy if taking opioids for less than 4 wks. Monitor for opioid withdrawal symptoms, esp. in pts taking methadone or with disruptions to blood-brain barrier. Monitor for severe, persistent, or worsening of abdominal pain; may indicate GI tract obstruction or perforation. Encourage fluid intake. Monitor daily pattern of bowel activity, stool consistency. Discontinue treatment if opioid pain medication is also discontinued. If dose is increased to 25 mg/day in pts with renal impairment, monitor for adverse effects.

PATIENT/FAMILY TEACHING

• Do not take laxatives unless approved by prescriber. • Notify prescriber if opioid pain medication is discontinued. • Immediately report severe, persistent abdominal pain; may indicate rupture or blockage in GI tract. • Do not ingest grapefruit products or take herbal supplements. • Opioid withdrawal may occur in a fetus of pregnant females due to undeveloped fetal blood-brain barrier. • Do not take newly prescribed medication unless approved by prescriber who originally started treatment.

naloxegol

nal-**ox**-ee-gol
(Movantik)

Do not confuse naloxegol with naloxone.

◆CLASSIFICATION

PHARMACOTHERAPEUTIC: Mu-opioid receptor antagonist (Peripherally acting). **CLINICAL:** GI agent.

USES

Treatment of opioid-induced constipation (OIC) in adult pts with chronic noncancer pain, including pts with chronic pain related to prior cancer or its treatment who do not require frequent (e.g., weekly) opioid dosage escalation.

PRECAUTIONS

Contraindications: Hypersensitivity to naloxegol. Known or suspected mechanical GI obstruction, pts at risk for recurrent GI obstruction. Concomitant use of strong CYP3A inhibitors. **Cautions:** Moderate to severe renal impairment, end-stage renal disease, severe hepatic impairment; pts with risk or reduction of structural wall integrity of GI tract (e.g., Crohn's disease, diverticulitis, GI tract malignancies, peptic ulcers, Ogilvie's syndrome, peritoneal metastases). Pts with disruptions to the blood-brain barrier. Concomitant use of moderate CYP3A inhibitors, P-glycoprotein (P-gp) inhibitors. Avoid concomitant use of strong CYP3A inducers, other opioid antagonists.

ACTION

Blocks opioid binding at peripheral mu-opioid receptors in GI tract. **Therapeutic Effect:** Decreases constipating effects of opioids.

PHARMACOKINETICS

Rapidly absorbed. Widely distributed. Metabolized in liver. Protein binding: 4.2%. Peak plasma concentration: less than 2 hrs. Excreted in feces (68%), urine (16%). **Half-life:** 6–11 hrs.

⌛ LIFESPAN CONSIDERATIONS

Pregnancy/Lactation: Known to cross the placenta. Use during pregnancy may induce fetal opiate withdrawal due to immature blood-brain barrier. Unknown if excreted in breast milk. Breastfeeding not recommended due to risk of opiate withdrawal in nursing infants. **Children:** Safety and efficacy not established. **Elderly:** No age-related precautions noted.

INTERACTIONS

DRUG: P-gp/ABCB1 inhibitors (e.g., amiodarone, cycloSPORINE), dilTIAZem, PPIs (e.g., pantoprazole), moderate CYP3A inhibitors (e.g., erythromycin, fluconazole, verapamil), strong CYP3A inhibitors (e.g.,

clarithromycin, ketoconazole, ritonavir) may increase concentration/effect; may increase risk of opiate withdrawal. **Strong CYP3A inducers (e.g., carBAMazepine, phenytoin, rifAMPin)** may decrease concentration/effect. **Methylnaltrexone, opioid antagonists** may increase adverse/toxic effects. **HERBAL: St John's wort** may decrease concentration/effect. **FOOD: Grapefruit products** may increase concentration/effect. **LAB VALUES:** None known.

AVAILABILITY (Rx)

Tablets: 12.5 mg, 25 mg.

ADMINISTRATION/HANDLING

PO

• Give on empty stomach at least 1 hr prior to first meal or 2 hrs after first meal. • Administer whole; do not chew. For pts unable to swallow tablet whole, tablets may be crushed and mixed with 120 mL water for oral administration or mixed with 60 mL for NG tube administration. After administration of crushed tablet, refill container with 120 mL (oral) or 60 mL (NG tube) of water, stir well, and give remaining contents. • Do not give with grapefruit products.

INDICATIONS/ROUTES/DOSAGE

Note: Discontinue all maintenance laxative therapy prior to use. May reintroduce laxatives if suboptimal response to naloxegol after 3 days.

Opioid-Induced Constipation

PO: ADULTS, ELDERLY: 25 mg once daily in the morning. May reduce dose to 12.5 mg once daily if 25-mg dose is not tolerated.

Dose Modification

Concomitant use of moderate CYP3A inhibitors: 12.5 mg daily in the morning. **Strong CYP3A inhibitors:** Contraindicated.

Dosage in Renal Impairment

Mild impairment: No dose adjustment. **Moderate to severe impairment: ESRD:** Reduce dose to 12.5 mg once daily in the morning. If tolerated, may increase to 25 mg once daily in the morning.

Dosage in Hepatic Impairment

Mild to moderate impairment: No dose adjustment. **Severe impairment:** Not recommended; avoid use.

SIDE EFFECTS

Frequent (21%–12%): Abdominal pain. **Occasional (9%–3%):** Diarrhea, nausea, flatulence, vomiting, headache, hyperhidrosis.

ADVERSE EFFECTS/TOXIC REACTIONS

Severe abdominal pain, diarrhea requiring hospitalization have occurred. GI perforation was reported in pts with baseline GI disease (Crohn's disease, diverticulitis, GI tract malignancies, peptic ulcers, Ogilvie's syndrome, peritoneal malignancies). Symptoms of opiate withdrawal, including abdominal pain, anxiety, chills, diarrhea, hyperhidrosis, irritability, yawning, were reported, esp. in pts taking methadone or with disruptions to the blood-brain barrier. May increase risk of adverse effects in pts with renal impairment who have increased dose to 25 mg/day.

NURSING CONSIDERATIONS

BASELINE ASSESSMENT

Discontinue all maintenance laxative therapy prior to initiation. Laxatives may be restarted if therapy has been ineffective for 3 days. Changes to analgesic dosage prior to initiation are not required. Question characteristics of constipation, frequency of bowel movements. Assess bowel sounds. Question history of GI obstruction, perforation, baseline GI disease. Receive full medication history including herbal products and screen for interactions. Assess hydration status.

INTERVENTION/EVALUATION

Pts may be less responsive to therapy if taking opioids for less than 4 wks. Monitor for opioid withdrawal symptoms, esp. in pts taking methadone or with disruptions to blood-brain barrier. Monitor for severe, persistent, worsening of abdominal pain; may indicate GI tract obstruction, perforation. Encourage fluid intake. Monitor daily pattern of bowel activity, stool consistency. Discontinue treatment if opioid pain medication is also discontinued. If dose is increased to 25 mg/day in pts with renal impairment, monitor for increased adverse effects.

PATIENT/FAMILY TEACHING

• Do not take laxatives unless approved by prescriber. • Tablets may be taken whole or crushed and mixed in water. • Notify prescriber if opioid pain medication is discontinued. • Immediately report severe, persistent abdominal pain; may indicate rupture or blockage in GI tract. • Do not ingest grapefruit products or take herbal supplements. • Opioid withdrawal may occur in a fetus of pregnant females due to undeveloped fetal blood-brain barrier. • Do not breastfeed.

N

naloxone

nal-**ox**-own
(Evzio, Narcan, Narcan Nasal Spray)
Do not confuse naloxone with Lanoxin or naltrexone.

FIXED-COMBINATION(S)

Embeda: naloxone/morphine (an opioid agonist): 0.8 mg/20 mg, 1.2 mg/30 mg, 2 mg/50 mg, 2.4 mg/60 mg, 3.2 mg/80 mg, 4 mg/100 mg. **Suboxone (sublingual film):** naloxone/buprenorphine (an analgesic): 0.5 mg/2 mg, 1 mg/4 mg, 2 mg/8 mg, 3 mg/12 mg. **Zubsolv:** naloxone/buprenorphine: 0.36 mg/1.4 mg, 1.4 mg/ 5.7 mg.

◆CLASSIFICATION

PHARMACOTHERAPEUTIC: Opioid antagonist. **CLINICAL:** Antidote.

USES

Narcan: Complete or partial reversal of opioid depression including respiratory depression. Diagnosis of suspected opioid tolerance or acute opioid overdose. **Evzio, Narcan Nasal Spray:** Emergency treatment of known or suspected opioid overdose. **OFF-LABEL:** Opioid-induced pruritus.

PRECAUTIONS

Contraindications: Hypersensitivity to naloxone. **Cautions:** Cardiac/pulmonary disease. Medications with potential for adverse cardiovascular effects (e.g., hypotension, arrhythmias).

ACTION

Displaces opioids at opioid-occupied receptor sites in CNS. **Therapeutic Effect:** Reverses opioid-induced sleep/sedation, increases respiratory rate, raises B/P to normal range.

PHARMACOKINETICS

Route	Onset	Peak	Duration
IV	1–2 min	N/A	20–60 min
IM	2–5 min	N/A	20–60 min
SQ	2–5 min	N/A	20–60 min

Well absorbed after IM, SQ administration. Metabolized in liver. Primarily excreted in urine. **Half-life:** 60–100 min.

⌛ LIFESPAN CONSIDERATIONS

Pregnancy/Lactation: Unknown if drug crosses placenta or is distributed in breast milk. **Children/Elderly:** No age-related precautions noted.

INTERACTIONS

DRUG: **Methylnaltrexone** may increase adverse/toxic effects. May increase adverse/toxic effects of **naldemedine, naloxegol.** **HERBAL:** None significant. **FOOD:** None known. **LAB VALUES:** None significant.

AVAILABILITY (Rx)

Injection, Autoinjector: ***(Evzio):*** 2 mg/0.4 mL. **Injection Solution:** 0.4 mg/mL, 1 mg/mL. **Narcan Nasal Spray:** 4 mg/0.1 mL.

ADMINISTRATION/HANDLING

IV

Reconstitution • For IV push, may give undiluted (0.4 mg/mL or diluted with 9 mL 0.9% NaCl to concentration of 0.04 mg/mL). • For continuous IV infusion, dilute each 2 mg of naloxone with 500 mL of D_5W or 0.9% NaCl, producing solution containing 0.004 mg/mL (4 mcg/mL).
Rate of administration • May give IV push over 30 sec.
Storage • Store parenteral form at room temperature. • Use mixture within 24 hrs; discard unused solution. • Protect from light. • Stable in D_5W or 0.9% NaCl at 4 mcg/mL for 24 hrs.

IM

- Give deep IM in large muscle mass.

IV INCOMPATIBILITIES

Amphotericin B complex (Abelcet, AmBisome, Amphotec).

IV COMPATIBILITIES

Heparin, ondansetron (Zofran), propofol (Diprivan).

INDICATIONS/ROUTES/DOSAGE

Note: If no response seen after a total of 10 mg, consider other causes of respiratory depression.

Opioid Overdose

IV, IM, SQ: ADULTS, ELDERLY: 0.4–2 mg q2–3min as needed. After reversal, additional doses may be required at later intervals (e.g., 20–60 min) depending on type/duration of opioid. **CHILDREN 5 YRS AND OLDER, WEIGHING 20 KG OR MORE:** 2 mg/dose; if no response, may repeat q2–3min. May need to repeat doses q20–60min. **CHILDREN YOUNGER THAN 5 YRS, WEIGHING LESS THAN 20 KG:** 0.1 mg/kg (**Maximum:** 2 mg); if no response, repeat q2–3min. May need to repeat doses q20–60min. ***(Narcan Nasal Spray):*** **ADULTS, ELDERLY, CHILDREN:** Single spray (4 mg) into one nostril. May give q2–3min until emergency medical assistance arrives. ***(Evzio):*** **IM: ADULTS, ELDERLY, CHILDREN:** 2 mg (contents of 1 auto-injector) as a single dose; may repeat q2–3min until emergency medical assistance becomes available.

Reversal of Respiratory Depression With Therapeutic Opioid Dosing

IV, IM, SQ: ADULTS, ELDERLY: Initially, 0.02–0.2 mg. Titrate to avoid profound withdrawal, seizures, arrhythmias, or severe pain. **CHILDREN:** 0.001–0.015 mg/kg. Titrate to desired effect. If administered IM or SQ, dose is to be given in divided doses.

Dosage in Renal/Hepatic Impairment

No dose adjustment.

SIDE EFFECTS

None known; little or no pharmacologic effect in absence of narcotics.

ADVERSE EFFECTS/TOXIC REACTIONS

Too-rapid reversal of narcotic-induced respiratory depression may result in agitation, nausea, vomiting, tremors, increased B/P, tachycardia, seizures. Excessive dosage in postoperative pts may produce significant reversal of analgesia, agitation, tremors. Hypotension or hypertension, ventricular tachycardia/fibrillation, pulmonary edema may occur in pts with cardiovascular disease.

NURSING CONSIDERATIONS

BASELINE ASSESSMENT

Maintain patent airway. Obtain weight of children to calculate drug dosage.

INTERVENTION/EVALUATION

Monitor vital signs, esp. rate, depth, rhythm of respiration, during and frequently following administration. Carefully observe pt after satisfactory response (duration of opiate may exceed duration of naloxone, resulting in recurrence of respiratory depression). Assess for increased pain, seizure activity with reversal of opiate.

N

naproxen

na-**prox**-en
(Aleve, EC-Naprosyn, Naprelan, Naprosyn)

■ BLACK BOX ALERT ■
Increased risk of serious cardiovascular thrombotic events, including myocardial infarction, CVA. Increased risk of severe GI reactions, including ulceration, bleeding, perforation of stomach, intestines.

Do not confuse Aleve with Alesse, or Anaprox with Anaspaz or Avapro.

FIXED-COMBINATION(S)

Prevacid NapraPac: naproxen/lansoprazole (proton pump inhibitor): 375 mg/15 mg, 500 mg/15 mg. **Treximet:** naproxen/SUMAtriptan (an antimigraine): 60 mg/10 mg; 500 mg/85 mg. **Vimovo:** naproxen/esomeprazole (proton pump inhibitor): 375 mg/20 mg, 500 mg/20 mg.

◆CLASSIFICATION

PHARMACOTHERAPEUTIC: NSAID. **CLINICAL:** Analgesic, nonopioid.

N

USES

Treatment of acute or long-term mild to moderate pain, primary dysmenorrhea, rheumatoid arthritis (RA), juvenile rheumatoid arthritis (JRA), osteoarthritis, ankylosing spondylitis, acute gouty arthritis, bursitis, tendonitis, fever. **OFF-LABEL:** Migraine prophylaxis.

PRECAUTIONS

Contraindications: History of asthma, urticaria; hypersensitivity to naproxen, other NSAIDs. Perioperative pain in setting of CABG surgery. **Cautions:** GI disease (bleeding, ulcers), fluid retention, renal/hepatic impairment, asthma, HF, concurrent use of anticoagulants, smoking, use of alcohol, elderly pts, debilitated pts.

ACTION

Reversibly inhibits COX-1 and COX-2 enzymes, resulting in decreased formation of prostaglandin precursors. **Therapeutic Effect:** Reduces inflammatory response, fever, intensity of pain.

PHARMACOKINETICS

Route	Onset	Peak	Duration
PO (analgesic)	1 hr	2–4 hrs	7 hrs or less
PO (anti-inflammatory)	2 wks	2–4 wks	12 hrs

Completely absorbed from GI tract. Protein binding: 99%. Metabolized in liver. Primarily excreted in urine. Not removed by hemodialysis. **Half-life:** 13 hrs.

⧗ LIFESPAN CONSIDERATIONS

Pregnancy/Lactation: Crosses placenta. Distributed in breast milk. Avoid use during third trimester (may adversely affect fetal cardiovascular system: premature closing of ductus arteriosus). **Children:** Safety and efficacy not established in pts younger than 2 yrs. Children older than 2 yrs at increased risk for skin rash. **Elderly:** Age-related renal impairment may increase risk of hepatic/renal toxicity; reduced dosage recommended. More likely to have serious adverse effects with GI bleeding/ulceration.

INTERACTIONS

DRUG: May increase effect of **apixaban, dabigatran, edoxaban, rivaroxaban. Bile acid sequestrants (e.g., cholestyramine)** may decrease absorption. May increase nephrotoxic effect of **aliskiren, cyclosporine**. **HERBAL: Glucosamine, herbals with anticoagulant/antiplatelet properties (e.g., garlic, ginger, ginseng, ginkgo biloba)** may increase concentration/effect. **FOOD:** None known. **LAB VALUES:** May prolong bleeding time. May increase serum BUN, creatinine, ALT, AST, alkaline phosphatase. May decrease Hgb, Hct, leukocytes, platelets, uric acid.

AVAILABILITY (Rx)

Capsule: 220 mg. **Oral Suspension:** 125 mg/5 mL naproxen. **Tablets:** 220 mg, 250 mg, 275 mg, 375 mg, 500 mg, 550 mg.

Tablets, Delayed-Release: 375 mg, 500 mg. **Extended-Release:** 375 mg, 500 mg, 750 mg.

ADMINISTRATION/HANDLING

PO

• Give controlled-release form whole. Do not break, crush, dissolve, or divide. • Best taken with food or milk (decreases GI irritation). • Shake suspension well.

INDICATIONS/ROUTES/DOSAGE

Note: Dosage expressed as naproxen base (200 mg naproxen base equivalent to 220 mg naproxen sodium).

Rheumatoid Arthritis (RA), Osteoarthritis, Ankylosing Spondylitis

PO: ADULTS, ELDERLY: ***(Immediate-Release):*** 500–1,000 mg/day in 2 divided doses. May increase to 1,500 mg/day for limited time (less than 6 mos). ***(Extended-Release):*** Initially, 750–1,000 mg once daily. May increase temporarily to 1,500 mg once daily.

Acute Gouty Arthritis

PO: ADULTS, ELDERLY: 500 mg twice daily (start within 24–48 hrs of flare-up). Discontinue 2–3 days after clinical signs resolve. (Usual duration: 5–7 days.)

Mild to Moderate Pain, Dysmenorrhea, Bursitis, Tendonitis

PO: ADULTS, ELDERLY: ***(Immediate-Release)***: Initially, 500 mg, then 500 mg q12h or 250 mg q6–8h as needed. **Maximum:** 1,250 mg on day 1, then 1,000 mg once daily. ***(Extended-Release):*** Initially, 1,000 mg once daily. May temporarily increase to 1,500 mg once daily, then reduce to 1,000 mg once daily.

Juvenile Idiopathic Arthritis (JIA)

PO: ***(Oral Suspension Recommended):*** **CHILDREN OLDER THAN 2 YRS:** 10–15 mg/kg/day in 2 divided doses. **Maximum:** 1,000 mg/day.

OTC Uses (Pain, fever)

PO: ADULTS 65 YRS AND YOUNGER, CHILDREN 12 YRS AND OLDER: Initially, 400 mg once, then 200 mg q8–12h. **Maximum:** 400 mg in any 8- to12-hr period or 600 mg/day. **ELDERLY:** Use with caution (consider a lower dose).

Dosage in Renal Impairment

Not recommended with CrCl less than 30 mL/min.

Dosage in Hepatic Impairment

Use caution.

SIDE EFFECTS

Frequent (9%–4%): Nausea, constipation, abdominal cramps/pain, heartburn, dizziness, headache, drowsiness. **Occasional (3%–1%):** Stomatitis, diarrhea, indigestion. **Rare (less than 1%):** Vomiting, confusion.

ADVERSE EFFECTS/TOXIC REACTIONS

Rare reactions with long-term use include peptic ulcer, GI bleeding, gastritis, severe hepatic reactions (cholestasis, jaundice), nephrotoxicity (dysuria, hematuria, proteinuria, nephrotic syndrome), and severe hypersensitivity reaction (fever, chills, bronchospasm).

NURSING CONSIDERATIONS

BASELINE ASSESSMENT

Assess onset, type, location, duration of pain/inflammation. Inspect appearance of affected joints for immobility, deformities, skin condition. Question history of GI bleeding, gastric or duodenal ulcers, hypertension.

INTERVENTION/EVALUATION

Periodically monitor renal function test during chronic use. Monitor daily pattern of bowel activity, stool consistency. Evaluate for therapeutic response: relief of pain, stiffness, swelling; increased joint mobility, reduced joint tenderness, improved grip strength.

PATIENT/FAMILY TEACHING

• Take with food, milk. • Avoid aspirin, alcohol during therapy (increases risk of GI bleeding). • Report headache, rash, visual disturbances, weight gain, black or tarry stools, bleeding, persistent headache.

naratriptan

nar-a-**trip**-tan
(Amerge)

Do not confuse naratriptan with eletriptan or almotriptan, or Amerge with Altace or Amaryl.

◆CLASSIFICATION

PHARMACOTHERAPEUTIC: Serotonin receptor agonist. **CLINICAL:** Antimigraine.

USES

Treatment of acute migraine headache with or without aura in adults.

PRECAUTIONS

Contraindications: Hypersensitivity to naratriptan. Basilar/hemiplegic migraine, cerebrovascular disease, peripheral vascular disease, coronary artery disease, ischemic heart disease (including angina pectoris, history of MI, silent ischemia, Prinzmetal's angina), severe hepatic impairment (Child-Pugh Grade C), severe renal impairment (CrCl less than 15 mL/min), uncontrolled hypertension, use within 24 hrs of ergotamine-containing preparations or another serotonin receptor agonist, 5-HT agonist (e.g., SUMAtriptan), MAOI use within 14 days. **Cautions:** Mild to moderate renal/hepatic impairment, elderly.

ACTION

Binds selectively to serotonin receptors, producing vasoconstrictive effect on cranial blood vessels. **Therapeutic Effect:** Relieves migraine headache.

PHARMACOKINETICS

Widely distributed. Protein binding: 28%–31%. Metabolized in liver. Eliminated primarily in urine. **Half-life:** 6 hrs (increased in hepatic/renal impairment).

LIFESPAN CONSIDERATIONS

Pregnancy/Lactation: Unknown if drug is distributed in breast milk. **Children:** Safety and efficacy not established. **Elderly:** Not recommended in the elderly.

INTERACTIONS

DRUG: **Ergotamine-containing medications** may produce vasospastic reaction. **SSRIs (e.g., escitalopram, paroxetine, sertraline), SNRIs (e.g., duloxetine, venlafaxine)** may produce serotonin syndrome. **HERBAL:** None significant. **FOOD:** None known. **LAB VALUES:** None significant.

AVAILABILITY (Rx)

Tablets: 1 mg, 2.5 mg.

ADMINISTRATION/HANDLING

PO

• Give without regard to food. • Do not break, crush, dissolve, or divide tablets. Administer whole with water.

INDICATIONS/ROUTES/DOSAGE

Acute Migraine Attack

PO: ADULTS: 1–2.5 mg. If headache improves but then returns, dose may be repeated after 4 hrs. **Maximum:** 5 mg/24 hrs.

Dosage in Renal/Hepatic Impairment

Hepatic Failure	Creatinine Clearance	Dosage
Mild to moderate	15–39 mL/min	Initial, 1 mg; Max: 2.5 mg/24 hrs
Severe	Less than 15 mL/min	Contraindicated

SIDE EFFECTS

Occasional (5%): Nausea. **Rare (2%):** Paresthesia, dizziness, fatigue, drowsiness, feeling of pressure in throat, neck, jaw.

ADVERSE EFFECTS/TOXIC REACTIONS

Corneal opacities, other ocular defects may occur. Cardiac events (ischemia, coronary artery vasospasm, MI), noncardiac vasospasm-related reactions (hemorrhage, cerebrovascular accident [CVA]) occur rarely, particularly in pts with hypertension, diabetes, strong family history of coronary artery disease, obesity, smokers, males older than 40 yrs, postmenopausal women.

NURSING CONSIDERATIONS

BASELINE ASSESSMENT

Question medical history as listed in Precautions. Question characteristics of migraine headaches (onset, location, duration, possible precipitating symptoms).

INTERVENTION/EVALUATION

Evaluate for relief of migraine headaches (photophobia, phonophobia, nausea, vomiting, pain, dizziness, fogginess).

PATIENT/FAMILY TEACHING

• May cause dizziness, fatigue, drowsiness. • Avoid tasks that require alertness, motor skills until response to drug is established. • Report any chest pain, palpitations, tightness in throat, rash, hallucinations, anxiety, panic.

necitumumab

ne-si-**toom**-oo-mab
(Portrazza)

BLACK BOX ALERT Cardiopulmonary arrest and/or sudden death may occur (when treated in combination with gemcitabine and cisplatin). Closely monitor serum electrolytes, esp. serum calcium, magnesium, potassium, and aggressively replace as appropriate. Hypomagnesemia occurred in 83% of pts and was severe in 20%. Monitor for hypomagnesemia, hypocalcemia, hypokalemia prior to each dose, during treatment, and up to 8 wks after discontinuation. Withhold treatment for CTCAE Grade 3 or 4 electrolyte abnormality.

Do not confuse necitumumab with adalimumab, belimumab, daratumumab, ipilimumab, nivolumab, ofatumumab, or panitumumab.

◆CLASSIFICATION

PHARMACOTHERAPEUTIC: Epidermal growth factor receptor (EGFR) inhibitor. Monoclonal antibody. **CLINICAL:** Antineoplastic.

USES

First-line treatment (in combination with gemcitabine and CISplatin) of metastatic squamous non–small-cell lung cancer (NSCLC).

PRECAUTIONS

Contraindications: Severe hypersensitivity to necitumumab. **Cautions:** COPD, chronic arrhythmias, coronary artery disease, HF, recent MI (within 6 mos), pts at risk for electrolyte imbalance (e.g., adrenal insufficiency, alcoholism, renal failure, thyroid disorders, malnutrition, chronic diarrhea; concomitant use of medication known to cause electrolyte abnormalities); history of venous or arterial thrombosis (e.g., CVA, DVT, MI, pulmonary embolism). Not indicated for treatment of nonsquamous non–small-cell lung cancer.

ACTION

Binds to ligand-binding site of EGFR and prevents activation, expression, signaling of EGFR. **Therapeutic Effect:** Inhibits tumor cell growth and metastasis.

PHARMACOKINETICS

Widely distributed. Metabolism not specified. Elimination not specified. **Half-life:** 14 days.

N

LIFESPAN CONSIDERATIONS

Pregnancy/Lactation: Avoid pregnancy; may cause fetal harm. Females of reproductive potential should use effective contraception during treatment and for at least 3 mos after discontinuation. Unknown if distributed in breast milk. Breastfeeding not recommended during treatment and up to 3 mos after discontinuation. **Children:** Safety and efficacy not established. **Elderly:** May have increased risk of venous thromboembolism (including pulmonary embolism).

INTERACTIONS

DRUG: None known. **HERBAL:** None known. **FOOD:** None known. **LAB VALUES:** May decrease serum calcium, magnesium, potassium.

AVAILABILITY (Rx)

Injection Solution: 800 mg/50 mL (16 mg/mL).

ADMINISTRATION/HANDLING

IV

Preparation • Visually inspect for particulate matter or discoloration. • Solution should appear clear to slightly opalescent, colorless to slightly yellow in color. Discard if solution is cloudy or particulate matter is observed. • Dilute in 250 mL 0.9% NaCl bag. • Do not use solutions containing dextrose. • Gently invert to mix. Do not shake or agitate.

Infusion guidelines • For pts with prior Grade 1 or 2 infusion reaction, premedicate with diphenhydrAMINE (or equivalent) before each subsequent infusion. • For pts with recurrent Grade 1 or 2 infusion reaction (despite administration of diphenhydrAMINE), premedicate with dexamethasone (or equivalent), acetaminophen, diphenhydrAMINE (or equivalent) before each subsequent infusion. • Once infusion is complete, flush IV line with 0.9% NaCl only.

Rate of administration • Infuse over 60 min via dedicated line.

Storage • Refrigerate unused vials in original carton until time of use. • Protect from light. • May refrigerate diluted solution up to 24 hours or at room temperature up to 4 hrs.

IV INCOMPATIBILITIES

Do not mix with dextrose-containing solutions. Do not infuse with other medications or electrolytes.

INDICATIONS/ROUTES/DOSAGE

Non–Small-Cell Lung Cancer

IV: ADULTS, ELDERLY: 800 mg on days 1 and 8 of each 3-wk cycle (in combination with gemcitabine and CISplatin). Continue until disease progression or unacceptable toxicity.

Dose Modification

Based on Common Terminology Criteria for Adverse Events (CTCAE).

Infusion Reactions

Any Grade 1 reaction: Decrease rate by 50%. **Grade 2 reaction:** Interrupt infusion until resolved to Grade 1 or 0, then resume with rate reduced by 50% for all subsequent infusions. **Grade 3 reaction:** Permanently discontinue.

Dermatological Toxicity

Grade 3 rash or acneiform rash: Withhold treatment until resolved to Grade 2 or better, then reduce dose to 400 mg for at least 1 treatment cycle. If tolerated, may increase dose to 600 mg and 800 mg for subsequent cycles.

Permanent discontinuation: Grade 3 rash or acneiform rash that does not resolve to Grade 2 or better within 6 wks; worsening of skin reaction or intolerance at 400 mg dose; Grade 3 skin induration or fibrosis; Grade 4 dermatologic toxicity.

Electrolyte Imbalance

Withhold treatment for any Grade 3 or 4 electrolyte abnormalities. Resume once abnormalities resolve to Grade 2 or less.

Venous/Arterial Thrombosis
Any occurrence: Permanently discontinue.

Dosage in Renal Impairment
No dose adjustment.

Dosage in Hepatic Impairment
Mild to moderate impairment: No dose adjustment. **Severe impairment:** Not specified; use caution.

SIDE EFFECTS

Frequent (44%–29%): Rash, vomiting. **Occasional (16%–5%):** Diarrhea, dermatitis acneiform, decreased weight, stomatitis, headache, acne, pruritus, dry skin, paronychia, conjunctivitis, blurry vision, dry eye, reduced visual acuity, blepharitis, eye pain, increased lacrimation, ocular hyperemia, visual impairment, eye pruritus, skin fissures. **Rare (3%–1%):** Dysphagia, muscle spasm, oropharyngeal pain.

ADVERSE EFFECTS/TOXIC REACTIONS

All cases were reported in combination with gemcitabine and CISplatin. Pts with severe hypomagnesemia, hypokalemia, hypocalcemia are at an increased risk for cardiac arrhythmias or sudden death. Cardiopulmonary arrest and/or sudden death occurred in 3% of pts. Most cases of cardiopulmonary arrest occurred within 30 days of the last dose and involved comorbidities including COPD, coronary artery disease, hypomagnesemia, hypertension. Hypomagnesemia reported in 83% of pts with median onset of approx. 6 wks. Severe hypomagnesemia (Grade 3 or 4) reported in 20% of pts. Infusion reaction (any grade) reported in 1.5% of pts. Life-threatening venous and arterial thromboembolic events including pulmonary embolism (5% of pts), DVT (2% of pts), CVA (2% of pts), MI (1% of pts); thrombosis of mesenteric veins, pulmonary artery/vein, axillary vein, vena cava, subclavian vein; thrombophlebitis may occur. Hemoptysis reported in 10% of pts. Ocular toxicities including conjunctivitis, conjunctival hemorrhage, eye infections were reported. Severe skin toxicities occurred in 8% of pts. Immunogenicity (auto-necitumumab antibodies) occurred in 4% of pts.

NURSING CONSIDERATIONS

BASELINE ASSESSMENT

Obtain baseline BMP, serum magnesium, ionized calcium; vital signs prior to each dose. Obtain pregnancy test in female pts of reproductive potential. Receive full medication history and screen for drugs known to cause electrolyte imbalance. Assess nutritional status. Question history of CVA, DVT, pulmonary embolism, cardiac disease, recent MI; conditions known to cause electrolyte imbalance; prior hypersensitivity reaction to any drug in treatment regimen; prior infusion reaction. Offer emotional support. Conduct full dermatological exam.

INTERVENTION/EVALUATION

Diligently monitor serum electrolytes, esp. serum magnesium, potassium, calcium, ionized calcium, during therapy and up to 8 wks after discontinuation. Monitor for symptoms of hypocalcemia, hypokalemia, hypomagnesemia. Obtain ECG, vital signs if arrhythmia, chest pain, palpitations, syncope occurs. Aggressively replace electrolytes as appropriate. Pts with sudden chest pain, dyspnea, hypoxia, tachycardia should be evaluated for pulmonary embolism. Monitor for symptoms of DVT (leg or arm pain/swelling), CVA (aphasia, altered LOC, hemiplegia, vision loss, headache, homonymous hemianopsia [vision loss on the same side of both eyes]), MI (chest pain, dyspnea, syncope, diaphoresis, left arm pain, jaw pain). Monitor for hemoptysis. Assess skin for rash, hypersensitivity reaction; eyes for infection, subconjunctival hemorrhage.

PATIENT/FAMILY TEACHING

• Therapy may cause low levels of potassium, magnesium, calcium in the

N

blood and may be life-threatening. Replace electrolytes exactly as instructed. • Report symptoms of electrolyte imbalance such as fainting, fatigue, muscle cramps, palpations, paralysis, numbness or tingling, seizures, weakness. • Use effective contraception to avoid pregnancy. Do not breastfeed. • Treatment may cause blood clots in the arms, legs, lungs, brain, heart, or abdomen. Immediately report symptoms of stroke (difficulty speaking, confusion, paralysis, vision loss), heart attack (chest pain, shortness of breath, fainting, dizziness, profuse sweating, left arm or jaw pain), lung embolism (difficulty breathing, fast heart rate, chest pain), or blood clots in the arms or legs (pain/swelling). • Report skin rashes, allergic reactions, coughing up blood; eye problems such as infection, vision impairment, collection of blood in the whites of the eyes. • Avoid sunlight, tanning beds. Wear protective clothing, high SPF sunscreen, and lip balm when outdoors.

N

neratinib

ne-**ra**-ti-nib
(Nerlynx)
Do not confuse neratinib with afatinib, axitinib, bosutinib, cabozantinib, dasatinib, gefitinib, imatinib, ponatinib, tofacitinib.

CLASSIFICATION

PHARMACOTHERAPEUTIC: Epidermal growth factor receptor (EGFR) inhibitor. Tyrosine kinase inhibitor. **CLINICAL:** Antineoplastic.

USES

Extended adjuvant treatment of adult pts with early stage HER2-overexpressed/amplified breast cancer, to follow adjuvant trastuzumab-based therapy. Treatment of advanced or metastatic HER2-positive breast cancer (in combination with capecitabine) in pts who have received 2 or more prior anti–HER2-based regimens in the metastatic setting.

PRECAUTIONS

Contraindications: Hypersensitivity to neratinib. **Cautions:** Dehydration, electrolyte imbalance, hepatic impairment, irritable bowel syndrome with diarrhea. Avoid concomitant use of strong or moderate CYP3A inhibitors, CYP3A inducers; proton pump inhibitors, H_2 receptor antagonists, antacids.

ACTION

Irreversibly binds to epidermal growth factor receptor (EGFR), human epidermal growth factor receptor 2 (HER2), HER4, reducing autophosphorylation and signaling of EGFR and HER2. **Therapeutic Effect:** Exhibits antitumor activity in EGFR and/or HER2 expressing cancer cell lines.

PHARMACOKINETICS

Widely distributed. Metabolized in liver. Protein binding: 99%. Peak plasma concentration: 2–8 hrs. Excreted in feces (97%), urine (1%). **Half-life:** 7–17 hrs.

LIFESPAN CONSIDERATIONS

Pregnancy/Lactation: Avoid pregnancy; may cause fetal harm/malformations. Unknown if distributed in breast milk. Breastfeeding not recommended during treatment and for at least 1 month after last dose. Females of reproductive potential should use effective contraception during treatment and for at least 1 mo after discontinuation. **Males:** Males with female partners of reproductive potential should use effective contraception during treatment and up to 3 mos after discontinuation. **Children:** Safety and efficacy not established. **Elderly:** May have increased risk of adverse reactions/toxic effects. Use caution.

INTERACTIONS

DRUG: **Aluminum-, magnesium-, calcium-containing antacids, H_2 receptor antagonists (e.g., famotidine), proton pump inhibitors (e.g., omeprazole, pantoprazole)** may decrease concentration/effect. **Strong CYP3A4 inhibitors (e.g., clarithromycin, ketoconazole, ritonavir), moderate CYP3A inhibitors (e.g., erythromycin, ciprofloxacin, dilTIAZem, dronedarone, fluconazole, verapamil)** may increase concentration/effect. **CYP3A4 inducers (e.g., carBAMazepine, phenytoin, rifAMPin)** may decrease concentration/effect. May increase concentration of **pazopanib, topotecan. HERBAL**: None significant. **FOOD**: **Grapefruit products** may increase concentration/effect. **LAB VALUES**: May increase serum ALT, AST, bilirubin.

AVAILABILITY (Rx)

Tablets: 40 mg.

ADMINISTRATION/HANDLING

PO

• Give with food. • Administer whole; do not break, cut, crush, or divide tablets. • If a dose is missed or vomiting occurs after administration, do not give extra dose. Administer next dose at regularly scheduled time. • Take 3 hours after aluminum-, magnesium-, or calcium-containing antacids are given.

INDICATIONS/ROUTES/DOSAGE

Note: Recommend antidiarrheal prophylaxis during first 2 cycles (56 days) of therapy.

Breast Cancer (extended adjuvant therapy)

PO: ADULTS, ELDERLY: 240 mg (6 tablets) once daily for 1 yr.

Breast Cancer (HER2-positive; advanced or metastatic)

PO: ADULTS, ELDERLY: 240 mg once daily on days 1–21 of a 21-day cycle (in combination with capecitabine on days 1–14). Continue until disease progression or unacceptable toxicity.

Loperamide (Antidiarrheal) Prophylaxis

Wks 1–2 (days 1–14): 4 mg three times/day. **Wks 3–8 (days 15–56):** 4 mg twice daily. **Wks 9–52 (days 57–365):** 4 mg as needed (do not exceed 16 mg/day).

Dose Reduction Schedule (Neratinib)

First dose reduction: 200 mg daily. **Second dose reduction:** 160 mg daily. **Third dose reduction:** 120 mg daily.

Dose Modification

Based on Common Terminology Criteria for Adverse Events (CTCAE).

Diarrhea

Grade 1 diarrhea; Grade 2 diarrhea lasting more than 5 days; Grade 3 diarrhea lasting more than 2 days: Adjust antidiarrheal therapy, diet. Maintain fluid intake (approx. 2 L/day). Once improved to Grade 1 or 0, start loperamide 4 mg with each administration. **Any grade diarrhea with complications (fever, hypotension, renal failure, or Grade 3 or 4 neutropenia):** Withhold treatment and adjust antidiarrheal therapy, diet. Maintain fluid intake (approx. 2 L/day). If diarrhea improves to Grade 1 or 0 within 7 days, resume treatment at same dose level. If diarrhea improves to Grade 1 or 0 for more than 7 days, resume treatment at the next reduced dose level. Once improved to Grade 1 or 0, start loperamide 4 mg with each administration. **Grade 4 diarrhea; recurrent Grade 2 diarrhea (or higher) at 120 mg dose:** Permanently discontinue.

Hepatotoxicity

Grade 3 serum ALT elevation; Grade 3 serum bilirubin elevation: Withhold treatment until improved to Grade 1 or 0 and investigate cause. If serum ALT elevation improves to Grade 1 or 0 within 3 wks, resume treatment at reduced dose level.

N

Grade 4 serum ALT elevation; Grade 4 serum bilirubin elevation: Permanently discontinue and investigate cause.

Other Toxicities

Any other Grade 3 toxicity: Withhold treatment until improved to Grade 1 or 0 (or baseline), then resume at reduced dose level. **Any other Grade 4 toxicity:** Permanently discontinue.

Dosage in Renal Impairment

Not specified; use caution.

Dosage in Hepatic Impairment

Mild to moderate impairment: No dose adjustment. **Severe impairment:** Reduce starting dose to 80 mg.

SIDE EFFECTS

Frequent (95%–26%): Diarrhea, nausea, abdominal pain, vomiting. **Occasional (18%–4%):** Rash (erythematous, follicular, generalized, pruritic, pustular, maculopapular, papular, dermatitis, dermatitis acneiform, toxic skin eruption), stomatitis, mouth ulceration, oral mucosal blistering, mucosal inflammation, oropharyngeal pain, oral pain, glossodynia, glossitis, cheilitis, decreased appetite, muscle spasm, dyspepsia, nail disorder (paronychia, onychoclasis, nail discoloration, nail toxicity, abnormal nail growth, nail dystrophy), dry skin, abdominal distention, decreased weight, dehydration. **Rare (3%):** Dry mouth.

N

ADVERSE EFFECTS/TOXIC REACTIONS

Diarrhea reported in 95% of pts. Grade 3 diarrhea reported in 40% of pts. Grade 4 diarrhea reported in less than 1% of pts. Median time of onset of diarrhea was days to wks. Severe diarrhea, dehydration, hypotension, renal failure may occur. Hepatotoxicity reported in 5%–10% of pts.

NURSING CONSIDERATIONS

BASELINE ASSESSMENT

Obtain LFT, vital signs. Obtain BMP and screen for electrolyte imbalance. Confirm HER2-positive status. Obtain pregnancy test prior to initiation. Stress the importance of antidiarrheal therapy. Question history of IBS with chronic diarrhea, hepatic impairment. Assess hydration status. Question usual bowel movement patterns, stool characteristics. Receive full medication history and screen for interactions. Offer emotional support.

INTERVENTION/EVALUATION

Monitor LFT monthly for the first 3 mos, then q3mos thereafter. Monitor for hepatotoxicity (abdominal pain, ascites, confusion, dark-colored urine, jaundice). Obtain BMP (note electrolytes) if severe diarrhea occurs. Ensure compliance of antidiarrheal therapy. Additional antidiarrheal medication may be needed to manage diarrhea despite treatment with loperamide. Monitor daily pattern of bowel activity, stool consistency. If treatment-related toxicities occur, consider referral to specialist. Monitor I&O. Assess skin, nails, oral mucosa for toxic reactions.

PATIENT/FAMILY TEACHING

• Treatment may cause severe diarrhea, which may lead to life-threatening dehydration or hospitalization. Take antidiarrheal medication exactly as prescribed (goal is 1–2 bowel movements/day). Report worsening of diarrhea or dehydration. • Drink plenty of fluids (at least 2 L/day if severe diarrhea occurs). • Report liver problems such as bruising; confusion; amber, dark, orange-colored urine; right upper abdominal pain; yellowing of the skin or eyes. • Use effective contraception to avoid pregnancy. Do not breastfeed. • Avoid grapefruit products, Seville oranges, starfruit, herbal supplements. • Acid-reducing medications may interfere with absorption; avoid use. Do not take aluminum-, magnesium-, calcium-containing antacids 3 hrs before or 3 hrs after dose. • Do not take newly prescribed medications unless approved by the prescriber who originally started treatment.

niCARdipine

nye-**kar**-di-peen
(Cardene IV)
Do not confuse Cardene SR with Cardizem SR or codeine, or niCARdipine with NIFEdipine or niMODipine.

◆CLASSIFICATION

PHARMACOTHERAPEUTIC: Calcium channel blocker. Dihydropyridine. **CLINICAL:** Antianginal, antihypertensive.

USES

PO: Immediate-Release: Treatment of chronic stable (effort-associated) angina, hypertension. **Sustained-Release:** Treatment of hypertension. **Parenteral:** Short-term treatment of hypertension when oral therapy not feasible or desirable. **OFF-LABEL:** Blood pressure control in acute ischemic stroke and intracranial hemorrhage.

PRECAUTIONS

Contraindications: Hypersensitivity to niCARdipine. Advanced aortic stenosis. **Cautions:** Cardiac/renal/hepatic dysfunction, HF, hypertrophic cardiomyopathy with outflow tract obstruction, aortic stenosis, coronary artery disease, portal hypertension.

ACTION

Inhibits calcium ion movement across cell membranes of cardiac, vascular smooth muscle. **Therapeutic Effect:** Relaxes coronary vascular smooth muscle. Causes coronary vasodilation, increasing myocardial oxygen delivery in angina.

PHARMACOKINETICS

Route	Onset	Peak	Duration
PO	0.5–2 hrs	—	8 hrs
IV	10 min	—	8 hrs or less

Rapidly, completely absorbed from GI tract. Protein binding: 95%. Metabolized in liver. Primarily excreted in urine. Not removed by hemodialysis. **Half-life:** 2–4 hrs.

⌛ LIFESPAN CONSIDERATIONS

Pregnancy/Lactation: Unknown if distributed in breast milk. **Children:** Safety and efficacy not established. **Elderly:** Age-related renal impairment may require dosage adjustment.

INTERACTIONS

DRUG: May increase concentration/effects of **cycloSPORINE, fosphenytoin, phenytoin. Azole antifungals (e.g., ketoconazole, itraconazole)** may increase adverse effects. **Strong CYP3A4 inhibitors (e.g., clarithromycin, ketoconazole, ritonavir)** may increase concentration/effect. **Strong CYP3A4 inducers (e.g., carbamazepine, phenytoin, rifampin)** may decrease concentration/effect. **HERBAL: Herbals with hypertensive properties (e.g., licorice, yohimbe) or hypotensive properties (e.g., garlic, ginger, ginkgo biloba)** may alter effects. **St. John's wort** may decrease concentration/effect. **FOOD: Grapefruit products** may decrease concentration/effect. **LAB VALUES:** None significant.

AVAILABILITY (Rx)

Capsules, Sustained-Release: 30 mg. **Infusion, Ready to Use:** 20 mg/200 mL, 40 mg/200 mL. **Injection Solution:** 2.5 mg/mL (10-mL vial).

ADMINISTRATION/HANDLING

IV

Reconstitution • Dilute in 240 mL D_5W, 0.45% NaCl, or 0.9% NaCl to provide concentration of 0.1 mg/mL.

Rate of administration • Titrate to desired effect. • Change IV site q12h if administered peripherally.

Storage • Store at room temperature. • Diluted IV solution is stable for 24 hrs at room temperature.

PO

• Give without regard to food. • Do not break, crush, or open capsules. Give whole.

IV INCOMPATIBILITIES

Ampicillin (Principen), ampicillin/sulbactam (Unasyn), cefepime (Maxipime), cefTAZidime (Fortaz), furosemide (Lasix), heparin, sodium bicarbonate.

IV COMPATIBILITIES

DilTIAZem (Cardizem), DOBUTamine (Dobutrex), DOPamine (Intropin), EPINEPHrine, HYDROmorphone (Dilaudid), labetalol (Trandate), LORazepam (Ativan), midazolam (Versed), milrinone (Primacor), morphine, nitroglycerin, norepinephrine (Levophed), potassium chloride.

INDICATIONS/ROUTES/DOSAGE

Chronic Stable Angina

PO: ADULTS, ELDERLY: Initially, 20 mg 3 times/day. Range: 20–40 mg 3 times/day (allow at least 3 days between dosage increases).

Hypertension

PO: ADULTS, ELDERLY *(Sustained-Release):* Initially, 30 mg twice daily. Usual dosage: 30–60 mg twice daily.

Acute Hypertension

IV: ADULTS, ELDERLY (GRADUAL B/P DECREASE): Initially, 5 mg/hr. May increase by 2.5 mg/hr q5–15min. **Maximum:** 15 mg/hr. After B/P goal is achieved, adjust dose to maintain desired BP.

Dosage in Renal Impairment

ADULTS, ELDERLY: PO: Initially, give 20 mg q8h (30 mg twice daily [sustained-release capsules]), then titrate. **IV:** No dose adjustment.

Dosage in Hepatic Impairment

ADULTS, ELDERLY: PO: Initially, give 20 mg twice daily, then titrate. **IV:** No dose adjustment.

SIDE EFFECTS

Frequent (10%–7%): Headache, facial flushing, peripheral edema, light-headedness, dizziness. **Occasional (6%–3%):** Asthenia, palpitations, angina, tachycardia. **Rare (less than 2%):** Nausea, abdominal cramps, dyspepsia, dry mouth, rash.

ADVERSE EFFECTS/TOXIC REACTIONS

Overdose produces confusion, slurred speech, drowsiness, marked hypotension, bradycardia.

NURSING CONSIDERATIONS

BASELINE ASSESSMENT

Concurrent therapy with sublingual nitroglycerin may be used for relief of anginal pain. Record onset, type (sharp, dull, squeezing), radiation, location, intensity, duration of anginal pain, precipitating factors (exertion, emotional stress).

INTERVENTION/EVALUATION

Monitor B/P, heart rate during and following IV infusion. Assess for peripheral edema, thrombophlebitis. Assess skin for facial flushing, dermatitis, rash. Question for asthenia, headache. Monitor LFT results. Assess ECG, pulse for tachycardia. Rotate infusion sites to decrease occurrence of thrombophlebitis.

PATIENT/FAMILY TEACHING

• Sustained-release capsule taken whole; do not break, chew, crush, or open. • Avoid alcohol, grapefruit products; limit caffeine. • Report if anginal pain not relieved or if palpitations, shortness of breath, swelling, dizziness, constipation, nausea, hypotension occurs. • Avoid tasks requiring motor skills, alertness until response to drug is established.

nicotine

nik-o-teen
(Good Sense Nicotine, NicoDerm CQ, Nicorette, Nicotrol, Nicotrol NS, Thrive)

Do not confuse NicoDerm with Nitroderm.

◆CLASSIFICATION

PHARMACOTHERAPEUTIC: Cholinergic-receptor agonist. **CLINICAL:** Smoking deterrent.

USES

Treatment to aid smoking cessation for relief of nicotine withdrawal symptoms (including nicotine craving). **OFF-LABEL: Transdermal:** Management of ulcerative colitis.

PRECAUTIONS

Contraindications: Hypersensitivity to nicotine. **Cautions:** Smoking post-MI period, severe or worsening angina, active temporomandibular joint disease (gum), pregnancy, hyperthyroidism, pheochromocytoma, insulin-dependent diabetes, severe renal impairment, eczematous dermatitis, oropharyngeal inflammation, esophagitis, peptic ulcer (delays healing in peptic ulcer disease), coronary artery disease, recent MI, serious cardiac arrhythmias, vasospastic disease, angina, hypertension, hepatic impairment, use of oral inhaler/nasal spray with bronchospastic disease.

ACTION

Binds to nicotinic-cholinergic receptors at the autonomic ganglia, in the adrenal medulla, at neuromuscular junction, and in the brain, producing stimulating effect in the cortex and a rewards effect in the limbic system. **Therapeutic Effect:** Provides source of nicotine during nicotine withdrawal, reduces withdrawal symptoms.

PHARMACOKINETICS

Absorbed slowly after transdermal administration. Protein binding: 5%. Metabolized in liver. Excreted primarily in urine. **Half-life:** 4 hrs.

⌛ LIFESPAN CONSIDERATIONS

Pregnancy/Lactation: Distributed in breast milk. Use of cigarettes, nicotine gum associated with decrease in fetal breathing movements. **Children:** Not recommended in this pt population. **Elderly:** Age-related decrease in cardiac function may require dosage adjustment.

INTERACTIONS

DRUG: None significant. **HERBAL:** None significant. **FOOD:** None known. **LAB VALUES:** None significant.

AVAILABILITY (OTC)

Chewing Gum: 2 mg, 4 mg. **Inhalation (Nicotrol Inhaler):** 10-mg cartridge. **Lozenges:** 2 mg, 4 mg. **Nasal Spray (Nicotrol NS):** 0.5 mg/spray. **Transdermal Patch:** 7 mg/24 hrs, 14 mg/24 hrs, 21 mg/24 hrs.

ADMINISTRATION/HANDLING

Gum

• Do not swallow. • Chew 1 piece when urge to smoke present. • Chew slowly and intermittently for 30 min. • Chew until distinctive nicotine taste (peppery) or slight tingling in mouth perceived, then stop; when tingling almost gone (about 1 min), repeat chewing procedure (this allows constant slow buccal absorption). • Too-rapid chewing may cause excessive release of nicotine, resulting in adverse effects similar to oversmoking (e.g., nausea, throat irritation).

Inhaler

• Insert cartridge into mouthpiece. • Puff on nicotine cartridge mouthpiece for 20 min.

Lozenge

• Do not chew or swallow. • Allow to dissolve slowly (20–30 min).

Transdermal

• Apply promptly upon removal from protective pouch (prevents evaporation, loss of nicotine). • Use only intact pouch. Do not cut patch. • Apply only once daily to hairless, clean, dry skin on upper body, outer arm. • Replace daily; rotate sites; do not use same site within 7 days; do not use same patch longer than 24 hrs. • Normal exposure to water (e.g., bathing, swimming) should not affect patch. • Wash hands with water alone after applying patch (soap may increase nicotine absorption). • Discard used patch by folding patch in half (sticky side together), placing in pouch of new patch, and throwing away in such a way as to prevent child or pet accessibility. • Patch may contain conducting metal; remove prior to MRI.

INDICATIONS/ROUTES/DOSAGE

Smoking Cessation Aid to Relieve Nicotine Withdrawal Symptoms

PO: ***(Chewing Gum):*** **ADULTS, ELDERLY:** 2 mg. Use 4 mg in pts who smoke first cigarette within 30 min of waking. Chew 1 piece of gum when urge to smoke, up to 24/day. Use following schedule: wks 1–6: q1–2h (at least 9 pieces/day); wks 7–9: q2–4h; wks 10–12: q4–8h.

N

PO: ***(Lozenge):***

◀ALERT▶ For pts who smoke the first cigarette within 30 min of waking, administer the 4-mg lozenge; otherwise, administer the 2-mg lozenge.

ADULTS, ELDERLY: One 4-mg or 2-mg lozenge q1–2h for the first 6 wks (use at least 9 lozenges/day first 6 wks); 1 lozenge q2–4h for wks 7–9; and 1 lozenge q4–8h for wks 10–12. **Maximum:** 1 lozenge at a time, 5 lozenges/6 hrs, 20 lozenges/day.

Transdermal:

◀ALERT▶ Apply 1 new patch q24h. **ADULTS, ELDERLY WHO SMOKE 10 CIGARETTES OR MORE PER DAY:** Follow the guidelines below. **Step 1:** 21 mg/day for 6 wks. **Step 2:** 14 mg/day for 2 wks. **Step 3:** 7 mg/day for 2 wks. **ADULTS, ELDERLY WHO SMOKE LESS THAN 10 CIGARETTES PER DAY:** Follow the guidelines below. **Step 1:** 14 mg/day for 6 wks. **Step 2:** 7 mg/day for 2 wks.

Nasal: ADULTS, ELDERLY: Each dose (2 sprays, 1 spray in each nostril) = 1 mg nicotine. Initially, 1–2 doses/hr. **Maximum:** 5 doses/hr (10 sprays), 40 doses/day (80 sprays). For best results, take at least 8 doses/day (16 sprays). Use beyond 6 mos not recommended.

Inhaler: ***(Nicotrol):*** **ADULTS, ELDERLY:** Initially, 6–16 cartridges per day. Puff on nicotine cartridge mouthpiece for about 20 min as needed. **Maximum:** 16 cartridges/day. Use beyond 6 mos not recommended.

Dosage in Renal/Hepatic Impairment

No dose adjustment.

SIDE EFFECTS

Frequent: All forms: Hiccups, nausea. **Gum:** Mouth/throat soreness. **Transdermal:** Erythema, pruritus, burning at application site. **Occasional: All forms:** Eructation, GI upset, dry mouth, insomnia, diaphoresis, irritability. **Gum:** Hoarseness. **Inhaler:** Mouth/throat irritation, cough. **Rare: All forms:** Dizziness, myalgia, arthralgia.

ADVERSE EFFECTS/TOXIC REACTIONS

Overdose produces palpitations, tachyarrhythmias, seizures, depression, confusion, diaphoresis, hypotension, rapid/weak pulse, dyspnea. Lethal dose for adults is 40–60 mg. Death results from respiratory paralysis.

NURSING CONSIDERATIONS

BASELINE ASSESSMENT

Screen, evaluate those with coronary heart disease (history of MI, angina pectoris), serious cardiac arrhythmias, Buerger's disease, Prinzmetal's variant angina.

INTERVENTION/EVALUATION

Monitor smoking habits, B/P, pulse, sleep pattern, skin for erythema, pruritus, burning at application site if transdermal system used.

PATIENT/FAMILY TEACHING

• Follow guidelines for proper application of transdermal system. • Chew gum slowly to avoid jaw ache, maximize benefit. • Report persistent rash, pruritus that occurs with patch. • Do not smoke while wearing patch.

NIFEdipine

nye-**fed**-i-peen
(Adalat CC, Adalat XL ✦, Procardia, Procardia XL)
Do not confuse NIFEdipine with niCARdipine or niMODipine, or Procardia XL with Cartia XT.

◆CLASSIFICATION

PHARMACOTHERAPEUTIC: Calcium channel blocker, dihydropyridine. **CLINICAL:** Antianginal, antihypertensive.

USES

Immediate-/Extended-Release: Treatment of angina due to coronary artery spasm (Prinzmetal's variant angina), chronic stable angina (effort-associated angina). **Extended-Release:** Treatment of hypertension. **OFF-LABEL:** Treatment of Raynaud's phenomenon, pulmonary hypertension, preterm labor, prevention/treatment of high-altitude pulmonary edema.

PRECAUTIONS

Contraindications: Hypersensitivity to NIFEdipine. ST elevation myocardial infarction (STEMI). **Cautions:** Renal/hepatic impairment, obstructive coronary disease, HF, severe aortic stenosis, edema, severe left ventricular dysfunction, hypertrophic cardiomyopathy, before major surgery, bradycardia, concurrent use with beta blockers or digoxin, CYP3A4 inhibitors/inducers.

ACTION

Inhibits calcium ion movement across cell membranes of vascular smooth muscle and myocardium during depolarization. **Therapeutic Effect:** Relaxes coronary vascular smooth muscle and coronary vasodilation, increases myocardial oxygen delivery (angina), reduces peripheral vascular resistance, reduces arterial B/P.

PHARMACOKINETICS

Rapidly, completely absorbed from GI tract. Protein binding: 92%–98%. Metabolized in liver. Primarily excreted in urine. Not removed by hemodialysis. **Half-life:** 2–5 hrs.

LIFESPAN CONSIDERATIONS

Pregnancy/Lactation: Insignificant amount distributed in breast milk. **Children:** Safety and efficacy not established. **Elderly:** Age-related renal impairment may require dosage adjustment. Use lower initial doses and titrate to response.

INTERACTIONS

DRUG: **Strong CYP3A4 inducers (e.g., rifAMPin, PHENobarbital, phenytoin, carBAMazepine)** may decrease concentration/effect. **CYP3A4 inhibitors (e.g., clarithromycin, ketoconazole)** may increase concentration/effect. **Beta blockers (e.g., carvedilol, metoprolol)** may have additive effect. May increase **digoxin** concentration, risk of toxicity. **Hypokalemia-producing agents (e.g., furosemide, other diuretics)** may increase risk of arrhythmias. **HERBAL:** **Herbals with hypertensive properties (e.g., licorice, yohimbe) or hypotensive properties (e.g., garlic, ginger, ginkgo biloba)** may alter effects. **St. John's wort** may decrease concentration/effect. **FOOD:** **Grapefruit products** may increase risk for flushing, headache, tachycardia, hypotension. **LAB VALUES:** May cause positive ANA, direct Coombs' test.

AVAILABILITY (Rx)

Capsules: 10 mg, 20 mg.

Tablets, Extended-Release: 30 mg, 60 mg, 90 mg.

ADMINISTRATION/HANDLING

PO

• Do not break, crush, dissolve, or divide extended-release tablets. • Give without regard to food (Adalat CC, Nifediac CC should be taken on an empty stomach).

N

Sublingual
• Capsules must be punctured, chewed, and/or squeezed to express liquid into mouth.

INDICATIONS/ROUTES/DOSAGE

Prinzmetal's Variant Angina, Chronic Stable (Effort-associated) Angina

PO: *(Extended-Release):* ADULTS, ELDERLY: Initially, 30–60 mg/day. May increase at 7- to 14-day intervals. **Maximum:** 120 mg/day.

Hypertension

PO: *(Extended-Release):* ADULTS, ELDERLY: Initially, 30–60 mg once daily. May increase at 7- to 14-day intervals. **Usual range:** 30–90 mg once daily. **Maximum:** 90–120 mg/day. CHILDREN 1–17 YRS: Initially, 0.25–5 mg/kg/day. **Maximum:** 3 mg/kg/day or 120 mg/day.

Dosage in Renal/Hepatic Impairment
No dose adjustment.

SIDE EFFECTS

Frequent (30%–11%): Peripheral edema, headache, flushed skin, dizziness. **Occasional (12%–6%):** Nausea, shakiness, muscle cramps/pain, drowsiness, palpitations, nasal congestion, cough, dyspnea, wheezing. **Rare (5%–3%):** Hypotension, rash, pruritus, urticaria, constipation, abdominal discomfort, flatulence, sexual dysfunction.

ADVERSE EFFECTS/TOXIC REACTIONS

May precipitate HF, MI in pts with cardiac disease, peripheral ischemia. Overdose produces nausea, drowsiness, confusion, slurred speech. **Antidote:** Glucagon (see Appendix J for dosage).

NURSING CONSIDERATIONS

BASELINE ASSESSMENT
Concurrent therapy with sublingual nitroglycerin may be used for relief of anginal pain. Record onset, type (sharp, dull, squeezing), radiation, location, intensity, duration of anginal pain; precipitating factors (exertion, emotional stress). Check B/P for hypotension immediately before giving medication.

INTERVENTION/EVALUATION
Monitor B/P. Assist with ambulation if light-headedness, dizziness occurs. Assess for peripheral edema. Assess skin for flushing. Monitor LFT. Observe for signs/symptoms of HF.

PATIENT/FAMILY TEACHING
• Go from lying to standing slowly. • Report palpitations, shortness of breath, pronounced dizziness, nausea, exacerbations of angina. • Avoid alcohol; concomitant grapefruit product use.

niMODipine

nye-**mode**-i-peen
(Nimotop ✱, Nymalize)

■ BLACK BOX ALERT ■ Severe cardiovascular events, including fatalities, have resulted when capsule contents have been withdrawn by syringe and administered by IV injection rather than orally or via nasogastric tube.

Do not confuse niMODipine with niCARdipine or NIFEdipine.

◆CLASSIFICATION

PHARMACOTHERAPEUTIC: Calcium channel blocker, dihydropyridine. **CLINICAL:** Cerebral vasospasm agent.

USES

Improvement of neurologic deficits due to cerebral vasospasm following subarachnoid hemorrhage from ruptured intracranial aneurysms.

PRECAUTIONS

Contraindications: Hypersensitivity to niMODipine. Concurrent use with strong CYP3A4 inhibitors (e.g., clarithromycin, voriconazole). **Cautions:** Pts with cirrhosis, baseline hypotension, bradycardia.

LIFESPAN CONSIDERATIONS

Pregnancy/Lactation: Unknown if drug crosses placenta or is distributed in breast milk. **Children:** Safety and efficacy not established. **Elderly:** Age-related renal impairment may require dosage adjustment. May experience greater hypotensive response, constipation.

ACTION

Inhibits movement of calcium ions across vascular smooth muscle cell membranes. Exerts greatest effect on cerebral arteries. **Therapeutic Effect:** Produces favorable effect on severity of neurologic deficits due to cerebral vasospasm. May prevent cerebral vasospasm.

PHARMACOKINETICS

Rapidly absorbed from GI tract. Protein binding: 95%. Metabolized in liver. Excreted in bile (80%), urine (20%). Not removed by hemodialysis. **Half-life:** 1–2 hrs.

INTERACTIONS

DRUG: **Beta blockers (e.g., carvedilol, metoprolol)** may have additive effect, increase depression of cardiac SA/AV conduction. **CYP3A4 inhibitors (e.g., clarithromycin, ketoconazole, ritonavir)** increase concentration/effect. **CYP3A4 inducers (e.g., carBAMazepine, phenytoin, rifAMPin)** may decrease concentration/effect. **HERBAL:** **Herbals with hypertensive properties (e.g., licorice, yohimbe) or hypotensive properties (e.g., garlic, ginger, ginkgo biloba)** may alter effects. **St. John's wort** may decrease concentration/effect. **FOOD:** **Grapefruit products** may increase concentration, risk of toxicity. **LAB VALUES:** None significant.

AVAILABILITY (Rx)

Solution, Oral: ***(Nymalize)*:** 60 mg/20 mL.

Capsules: 30 mg.

ADMINISTRATION/HANDLING

PO

• Administer 1 hr before or 2 hrs after meals. • If pt unable to swallow, place hole in both ends of capsule with 18-gauge needle to extract contents into syringe. Empty into NG tube; flush tube with 30 mL water.

INDICATIONS/ROUTES/DOSAGE

Subarachnoid Hemorrhage

PO: ADULTS, ELDERLY: 60 mg q4h for 21 days. Begin within 96 hrs of subarachnoid hemorrhage.

Dosage in Renal Impairment

No dose adjustment.

Dosage in Hepatic Impairment

PO: ADULTS, ELDERLY: Reduce dose to 30 mg q4h in pts with cirrhosis.

SIDE EFFECTS

Occasional (6%–2%): Hypotension, peripheral edema, diarrhea, headache. **Rare (less than 2%):** Allergic reaction (rash, urticaria), tachycardia, flushing of skin.

ADVERSE EFFECTS/TOXIC REACTIONS

Overdose produces nausea, weakness, dizziness, drowsiness, confusion, slurred speech.

NURSING CONSIDERATIONS

BASELINE ASSESSMENT

Assess level of consciousness, neurologic response, initially and throughout therapy. Assess B/P, heart rate immediately before drug administration. Assess hydration status.

INTERVENTION/EVALUATION

The benefit of giving nimodipine for prevention of cerebral vasospasm must be considered if manageable bradycardia or hypotension occurs. Consider administering 30-mg dose q2h if bradycardia; hypotension is a concern in the acute care setting. Monitor CNS response, heart rate, B/P for evidence of hypoten-

N

sion, bradycardia. Monitor transcranial Doppler results for evidence of vasospasm.

PATIENT/FAMILY TEACHING

• Report palpitations, shortness of breath, swelling, constipation, nausea, dizziness. Immediately report headache, blurry vision, confusion (may indicate vasospasm). Drink plenty of fluids to maintain hydration.

niraparib

nye-**rap**-a-rib
(Zejula)
Do not confuse niraparib with olaparib, neratinib, or rucaparib.

◆CLASSIFICATION

PHARMACOTHERAPEUTIC: Poly(ADP-ribose) polymerase (PARP) inhibitor. **CLINICAL:** Antineoplastic.

N

USES

Maintenance treatment of adult pts with recurrent epithelial ovarian, fallopian tube, or primary peritoneal cancer who are in a complete or partial response to platinum-based chemotherapy. Treatment of adults with advanced ovarian, fallopian tube, or primary peritoneal cancer who have been treated with 3 or more prior chemotherapy regimens and whose cancer is associated with homologous recombination deficiency (HRD)–positive status. Maintenance treatment of adults with advanced epithelial ovarian, fallopian tube, or primary peritoneal cancer who are in a complete or partial response to first-line platinum-based chemotherapy.

PRECAUTIONS

Contraindications: Hypersensitivity to niraparib. **Cautions:** Baseline cytopenias; history of hypertension, cardiac disease; pts at risk for hemorrhage (e.g., history of GI bleeding, coagulation disorders, recent trauma; conditions predisposing to infection (e.g., diabetes, renal failure, immunocompromised pts, open wounds); concomitant use of anticoagulants, antiplatelet medication, NSAIDs).

ACTION

Inhibits poly(ADP-ribose) polymerase (PARP) enzymatic activity, resulting in DNA damage, apoptosis, and cellular death. **Therapeutic Effect:** Induces cytotoxicity in tumor cell lines with and without BRCA deficiencies.

PHARMACOKINETICS

Well absorbed. Widely distributed. Metabolized by carboxylesterase to inactive metabolite. Protein binding: 83%. Peak plasma concentration: 3 hrs. Excreted in urine (48%), feces (39%). **Half-Life:** 36 hrs.

⌛ LIFESPAN CONSIDERATIONS

Pregnancy/Lactation: Avoid pregnancy; may cause fetal harm/malformations. Females of reproductive potential should use effective contraception during treatment and for at least 6 mos after discontinuation. Unknown if distributed in breast milk. Breastfeeding not recommended during treatment and up to 1 mo after discontinuation. May impair fertility in males. **Children:** Safety and efficacy not established. **Elderly:** No age-related precautions noted.

INTERACTIONS

DRUG: May decrease therapeutic effect of **BCG (intravesical)**. **HERBAL:** None significant. **FOOD:** None known. **LAB VALUES:** May increase serum alkaline phosphatase, ALT, AST, creatinine, GGT. May decrease ANC, Hgb, Hct, leukocytes, neutrophils, RBCs; serum potassium.

AVAILABILITY (Rx)

Capsules: 100 mg.

ADMINISTRATION/HANDLING

PO

• Give with or without food. • Administer whole; do not break, cut, crush, or open capsules. • If a dose is missed or vomiting occurs after administration, do not give extra dose. Administer next dose at regularly scheduled time. • Administration at bedtime may decrease occurrence of nausea.

INDICATIONS/ROUTES/DOSAGE

Recurrent Epithelial Ovarian, Fallopian Tube, Peritoneal Cancer

PO: ADULTS, ELDERLY: 300 mg once daily, initiated no later than 8 wks after most recent platinum-containing regimen. Continue until disease progression or unacceptable toxicity.

Advanced Epithelial Ovarian, Fallopian Tube, Peritoneal Cancer

PO: ADULTS, ELDERLY: 200 mg once daily (if weight less than 77 kg or platelet count is less than 150,000 cells/mm^3) or 300 mg once daily (if weight greater than or equal to 77 kg and platelet count greater than or equal to 150,000 cells/mm^3).

Dose Reduction Schedule

First dose reduction: 200 mg daily. **Second dose reduction:** 100 mg daily.

Dose Modification

Based on Common Terminology Criteria for Adverse Events (CTCAE).

Note: If acute myeloid leukemia or myelodysplastic syndrome is confirmed, permanently discontinue.

Anemia, Neutropenia

ANC less than 1,000 cells/mm^3, Hgb less than 8 g/dL: Withhold treatment for maximum of 28 days until ANC improves to greater than or equal to 1,500 cells/mm^3 or Hgb level improves to 9 g/dL or greater, then resume at reduced dose level. If ANC or Hgb level does not improve to an acceptable level within 28 days or if dose is already reduced to 100 mg/day, permanently discontinue.

Hematologic Toxicity Requiring Transfusion

Platelet count less than or equal to 10,000 cells/mm^3: Consider transfusion, then resume at reduced dose level.

Nonhematologic Toxicity

Any nonhematologic Grade 3 or 4 toxicity when prophylactic treatment is not possible or toxicity persists despite treatment: Withhold treatment for maximum of 28 days until resolved, then resume at next lower dose level.

Any nonhematologic Grade 3 or 4 toxicity lasting more than 28 days with 100 mg/day regimen: Permanently discontinue.

Thrombocytopenia

Platelet count less than 100,000 cells/mm^3: First occurrence: Withhold treatment for maximum of 28 days until improved to greater than or equal to 100,000 cells/mm^3, then resume at same dose or reduced dose level. If platelet count is less than 75,000 cells/mm^3, resume at reduced dose level. **Second occurrence:** Withhold treatment for maximum of 28 days until improved to greater than or equal to 100,000 cells/mm^3, then resume at reduced dose level. If platelet count does not improve to an acceptable level within 28 days or if dose is already reduced to 100 mg/day, permanently discontinue.

Dosage in Renal Impairment

Mild to moderate impairment: No dose adjustment. **Severe impairment, ESRD:** Not specified; use caution.

Dosage in Hepatic Impairment

Mild impairment: No dose adjustment. **Moderate to severe impairment:** Not specified; use caution.

SIDE EFFECTS

Frequent (74%–20%): Nausea, fatigue, asthenia, constipation, vomiting, abdominal pain/distention, insomnia, headache, decreased appetite, rash, mucositis, stomatitis, hypertension, dyspnea. **Occasional (19%–10%):** Myalgia, back pain, dizziness, dyspepsia, cough, arthralgia, anxiety, dysgeusia, dry mouth, palpitations, tachycardia, peripheral edema, decreased weight, depression.

N

ADVERSE EFFECTS/TOXIC REACTIONS

Myelosuppression (anemia neutropenia, leukopenia, thrombocytopenia) is an expected response to therapy, but more severe reactions including bone marrow failure may result in life-threatening event. Fatal cases of acute myeloid leukemia, myelodysplastic syndrome reported in 1% of pts. Hypertension, hypertensive crisis reported in 9% of pts. Infections including bronchitis, conjunctivitis, nasopharyngitis (23% of pts), UTI (13% of pts) may occur. Epistaxis may occur, esp. in pts with treatment-induced thrombocytopenia.

NURSING CONSIDERATIONS

BASELINE ASSESSMENT

Obtain ANC, CBC, BMP, LFT; vital signs. Obtain pregnancy test in females of reproductive potential. Confirm compliance of effective contraception. Question history of cardiac disease, hypertension. Assess hydration status. Screen for active infection. Offer emotional support.

INTERVENTION/EVALUATION

Monitor ANC, CBC for myelosuppression wkly for first 4 wks, then monthly for 11 mos, then periodically thereafter. In pts with platelet count less than 10,000 cells/mm^3, consider withholding anticoagulant, antiplatelet drugs or proceed with transfusion (if applicable). Monitor for acute myeloid leukemia, myelodysplastic syndrome (bleeding or bruising easily, fatigue, frequent infections, pyrexia, hematuria, melena, weakness, weight loss, cytopenias, increased requirements for blood transfusion). Diligently screen for infections (cough, fatigue, fever). Monitor vital signs for arrhythmia, hypertension, tachycardia. Offer antiemetic if nausea, vomiting occurs. Assess skin for rash, toxic reactions. Encourage nutritional intake.

PATIENT/FAMILY TEACHING

• Treatment may depress your immune system and reduce your ability to fight infection. Report symptoms of infection such as body aches, burning with urination, chills, cough, fatigue, fever. Avoid those with active infection. • Treatment may cause severe bone marrow depression or new-onset myeloid leukemia; report bruising, fatigue, fever, frequent infections, shortness of breath, weight loss, bleeding easily, blood in urine or stool. • Use effective contraception to avoid pregnancy. Do not breastfeed. • Dose administration at bedtime may decrease occurrence of nausea.

nitrofurantoin

nye-troe-fue-**ran**-toyn
(Macrobid, Macrodantin)
Do not confuse Macrobid with MicroK or Nitro-Bid, or nitrofurantoin with Neurontin or nitroglycerin.

◆CLASSIFICATION

PHARMACOTHERAPEUTIC: Antibacterial. **CLINICAL:** Antibiotic, UTI prophylaxis.

USES

Prevention/treatment of UTI caused by susceptible gram-negative, gram-positive organisms, including *E. coli, S. aureus, Enterococcus, Klebsiella, Enterobacter.*

PRECAUTIONS

Contraindications: Hypersensitivity to nitrofurantoin. Anuria, oliguria, renal impairment (CrCl less than 60 mL/min), infants younger than 1 mo due to risk of hemolytic anemia. Pregnancy at term, during labor, or delivery, or when onset of labor is imminent. History of cholestatic jaundice or hepatic impairment with previous nitrofurantoin therapy. **Cautions:** Renal impairment, diabetes, electrolyte imbalance, anemia, vitamin B deficiency, debilitated (greater risk of peripheral neuropathy), G6PD deficiency (greater risk of hemolytic anemia), elderly, prolonged therapy (may cause pulmonary toxicity).

ACTION

Inhibits bacterial enzyme systems, interfering with protein synthesis, anaerobic energy metabolism, DNA, RNA, and cell wall synthesis. **Therapeutic Effect:** Bactericidal at therapeutic doses.

PHARMACOKINETICS

Microcrystalline form rapidly, completely absorbed; macrocrystalline form more slowly absorbed. Food increases absorption. Protein binding: 60%. Primarily concentrated in urine, kidneys. Metabolized in most body tissues. Primarily excreted in urine. Removed by hemodialysis. **Half-life:** 20–60 min.

LIFESPAN CONSIDERATIONS

Pregnancy/Lactation: Readily crosses placenta. Distributed in breast milk. Contraindicated at term and during lactation when infant suspected of having G6PD deficiency. **Children:** No age-related precautions noted in pts older than 1 mo. **Elderly:** Avoid use. More likely to develop acute pneumonitis, peripheral neuropathy. Age-related renal impairment may require dosage adjustment.

INTERACTIONS

DRUG: **Antacids containing magnesium trisilicate** may decrease absorption. **Probenecid** may increase concentration, risk of toxicity. May decrease effect of **norfloxacin**. **HERBAL:** None significant. **FOOD:** None known. **LAB VALUES:** May increase serum ALT, AST, phosphorus. May decrease Hgb.

AVAILABILITY (Rx)

Capsules: ***(Macrocrystalline [Macrobid]):*** 100 mg. **Capsules:** ***(Macrocrystalline [Macrodantin]):*** 25 mg, 50 mg, 100 mg. **Oral Suspension:** ***(Microcrystalline):*** 25 mg/5 mL.

ADMINISTRATION/HANDLING

PO

• Give with food, milk to enhance absorption, reduce GI upset. • May mix suspension with water, milk, fruit juice; shake well.

INDICATIONS/ROUTES/DOSAGE

UTI

PO: ***(Macrodantin):*** **ADULTS, ELDERLY:** 50–100 mg q6h; treat males for 7 days or females for 5 days. **Maximum:** 400 mg/day. **CHILDREN, ADOLESCENTS:** 5–7 mg/kg/day in divided doses q6h for 7 days or at least 3 days after obtaining sterile urine. **Maximum:** 400 mg/day (100 mg/dose).

PO: ***(Macrobid):*** **ADULTS, ELDERLY, ADOLESCENTS:** 100 mg twice daily; treat males for 7 days or females for 5 days.

Long-Term Prevention of UTI

PO: **ADULTS, ELDERLY:** 50–100 mg at bedtime. **CHILDREN OLDER THAN 1 MONTH:** 1–2 mg/kg/day in 2 divided doses. **Maximum:** 100 mg/day.

Dosage in Renal Impairment

Contraindicated in pts with CrCl less than 60 mL/min.

Dosage in Hepatic Impairment

No dose adjustment.

SIDE EFFECTS

Frequent: Anorexia, nausea, vomiting, dark urine. **Occasional:** Abdominal pain, diarrhea, rash, pruritus, urticaria, hypertension, headache, dizziness, drowsiness. **Rare:** Photosensitivity, transient alopecia, asthmatic exacerbation in those with history of asthma.

ADVERSE EFFECTS/TOXIC REACTIONS

Superinfection, hepatotoxicity, peripheral neuropathy (may be irreversible), Stevens-Johnson syndrome, permanent pulmonary impairment, anaphylaxis occur rarely.

NURSING CONSIDERATIONS

BASELINE ASSESSMENT

Question for history of asthma. Evaluate baseline renal function, LFT. Question medical history as listed in Precautions, and screen for contraindications.

INTERVENTION/EVALUATION

Monitor CBC, BMP, LFT; I&O. Monitor daily pattern of bowel activity, stool consistency. Assess skin for rash, urticaria. Be alert for numbness/tingling, esp. of lower extremities (may signal onset of peripheral neuropathy). Observe for signs of hepatotoxicity (fever, rash, arthralgia, hepatomegaly). Monitor respiratory status, esp. in pts with asthma.

PATIENT/ FAMILY TEACHING

• Urine may become dark yellow/brown. • Take with food, milk for best results, to reduce GI upset. • Complete full course of therapy. • Avoid sun, ultraviolet light; use sunscreen, wear protective clothing. • Report cough, fever, chest pain, difficulty breathing, numbness/tingling of fingers, toes. • Rare occurrence of alopecia is transient.

N

nitroglycerin

nye-troe-**glis**-er-in
(GoNitro, Minitran, Nitro-Bid, Nitro-Dur, Nitrolingual, NitroMist, Nitrostat, Rectiv, Trinipatch ✱)
Do not confuse Nitro-Bid with Macrobid or Nicobid, Nitro-Dur with Nicoderm, nitroglycerin with nitrofurantoin or nitroprusside, or Nitrostat with Nilstat or Nystatin.

◆CLASSIFICATION

PHARMACOTHERAPEUTIC: Nitrate. **CLINICAL:** Antianginal, antihypertensive, coronary vasodilator.

USES

Treatment/prevention of angina pectoris. Extended-release, topical forms used for prophylaxis, long-term angina management. IV form used in treatment of HF, acute MI, perioperative hypertension, induction of intraoperative hypotension. **Rectiv:** Treatment of moderate to severe pain associated with chronic anal fissure. **OFF-LABEL:** Short-term management of pulmonary hypertension, esophageal spastic disorders, uterine relaxation, treatment of sympathomimetic vasopressor extravasation.

PRECAUTIONS

Contraindications: Hypersensitivity to nitroglycerin. Allergy to adhesives (transdermal); concurrent use of sildenafil, tadalafil, vardenafil (PDE5 inhibitors). Concurrent use with riociguat. **IV:** Restrictive cardiomyopathy, pericardial tamponade, constrictive pericarditis, increased ICP, uncorrected hypovolemia. **Sublingual, Rectal:** Increased intracranial pressure, severe anemia. **Sublingual:** Acute circulatory failure or shock, early MI. **Cautions:** Blood volume depletion, severe hypotension (systolic B/P less than 90 mm Hg), bradycardia (less than 50 beats/min), inferior wall MI and suspected right ventricular involvement.

ACTION

Forms nitric oxide, which increases cGMP, causing dephosphorylation of myosin light chains and smooth muscle relaxation. Produces vasodilation on peripheral veins and arteries (more prominent effect on veins). **Therapeutic Effect:** Decreases myocardial oxygen demand by decreasing preload (LVDP). Improves collateral flow to ischemic areas. **Rectal:** Decreases sphincter tone and intra-anal pressure.

PHARMACOKINETICS

Route	Onset	Peak	Duration
Sublingual	1–3 min	4–8 min	30–60 min
Translingual spray	2 min	4–10 min	30–60 min
Buccal tablet	2–5 min	4–10 min	2 hrs
PO (extended-release)	20–45 min	45–120 min	4–8 hrs

Route	Onset	Peak	Duration
Topical	15–60 min	30–120 min	2–12 hrs
Transdermal patch	40–60 min	60–180 min	18–24 hrs
IV	1–2 min	Immediate	3–5 min

Well absorbed after PO, sublingual, topical administration. Metabolized in liver, by enzymes in bloodstream. Protein binding: 60%. Excreted in urine. Not removed by hemodialysis. **Half-life:** 1–4 min.

LIFESPAN CONSIDERATIONS

Pregnancy/Lactation: Unknown if drug crosses placenta or is distributed in breast milk. **Children:** Safety and efficacy not established. **Elderly:** More susceptible to hypotensive effects. Age-related renal impairment may require dosage adjustment.

INTERACTIONS

DRUG: **Alcohol, other antihypertensives (e.g., amLODIPine, lisinopril, valsartan), vasodilators** may increase risk of orthostatic hypotension. Concurrent use of **sildenafil, tadalafil, vardenafil** (PDE5 inhibitors) produces significant hypotension. **Ergot derivatives (e.g., ergotamine)** may decrease effect of vasodilation. May increase hypotensive effect of **riociguat**. **HERBAL:** **Herbals with hypertensive properties (e.g., licorice, yohimbe) or hypotensive properties (e.g., garlic, ginger, ginkgo biloba)** may alter effects. **FOOD:** None known. **LAB VALUES:** May increase serum methemoglobin, urine catecholamine concentrations.

AVAILABILITY (Rx)

Infusion, Premix: 25 mg/250 mL, 50 mg/250 mL, 100 mg/250 mL. **Injection Solution:** 5 mg/mL. **Ointment:** *(Nitro-Bid):* 2%. **Ointment, Rectal** *(Rectiv):* 0.4%. **Translingual Spray:** 0.4 mg/spray. **Transdermal Patch:** 0.1 mg/hr, 0.2 mg/hr, 0.4 mg/hr, 0.6 mg/hr.

Capsules, Extended-Release: 2.5 mg, 6.5 mg, 9 mg. **Tablets, Sublingual:** 0.3 mg, 0.4 mg, 0.6 mg.

ADMINISTRATION/HANDLING

◀ALERT▶ Cardioverter/defibrillator must not be discharged through paddle electrode overlying nitroglycerin (transdermal, ointment) application. May cause burns to pt or damage to paddle via arcing.

IV

Reconstitution • Available in ready-to-use injectable containers. • Dilute vials in D_5W or 0.9% NaCl. **Maximum concentration:** 400 mcg/mL. • Use glass bottles.

Rate of administration • Use microdrop or infusion pump.

Storage • Store at room temperature. • Reconstituted solutions stable for 48 hrs at room temperature or 7 days if refrigerated.

PO

• Do not break, crush, or open extended-release capsules. • Do not shake oral aerosol canister before lingual spraying.

Sublingual

• Instruct pt to not swallow. • Dissolve under tongue. • Administer while seated. • Slight burning sensation under tongue may be lessened by placing tablet in buccal pouch. • Keep sublingual tablets in original container.

Topical

• Spread thin layer on clean, dry, hairless skin of upper arm or body (not below knee or elbow), using applicator or dose-measuring papers. Do not use fingers; do not rub/massage into skin.

Transdermal

• Apply patch on clean, dry, hairless skin of upper arm or body (not below

N

knee or elbow). • May keep patch on when bathing/showering. • Do not cut/trim to adjust dose.

IV INCOMPATIBILITIES

Alteplase (Activase), phenytoin (Dilantin).

IV COMPATIBILITIES

Amiodarone (Cordarone), dexmedetomidine (Precedex), dilTIAZem (Cardizem), DOBUTamine (Dobutrex), DOPamine (Intropin), EPINEPHrine, famotidine (Pepcid), fentaNYL (Sublimaze), furosemide (Lasix), heparin, HYDROmorphone (Dilaudid), insulin, labetalol (Trandate), lidocaine, lipids, LORazepam (Ativan), midazolam (Versed), milrinone (Primacor), morphine, niCARdipine (Cardene), nitroprusside (Nipride), norepinephrine (Levophed), propofol (Diprivan).

INDICATIONS/ROUTES/DOSAGE

Angina, CAD

Translingual spray: ADULTS, ELDERLY: 1 spray (0.4 mg) q5min up to 3 doses in response to chest pain. If chest pain fails to improve or worsens in 3–5 min after 1 dose, call 911.

Sublingual: ADULTS, ELDERLY: One tablet (0.3–0.4 mg) under tongue. If chest pain fails to improve or worsens in 3–5 min, call 911. After the call, may take additional tablet. A third tablet may be taken 5 min after second dose (maximum of 3 tablets).

PO: ***(Extended-Release):*** **ADULTS, ELDERLY:** 2.5–6.5 mg 3–4 times/day. **Maximum:** 26 mg 4 times/day.

Topical: ADULTS, ELDERLY: Initially, 1/2 inch upon waking and 1/2 inch 6 hrs later. May double dose to 1 inch and double again to 2 inches. **Maximum:** 2 doses/day including nitrate-free interval of 10–12 hrs.

Transdermal patch: ADULTS, ELDERLY: Initially, 0.2–0.4 mg/hr. **Maintenance:** 0.4–0.8 mg/hr. Consider patch on for 12–14 hrs, patch off for 10–12 hrs (prevents tolerance).

HF, Acute MI

IV: ADULTS, ELDERLY: Initially, 10 mcg/min via infusion pump. Increase in 5-mcg/min increments at 3- to 5-min intervals until B/P response is noted or until dosage reaches 20 mcg/min, then increase by 10–20 mcg/min q3–5min. Dosage may be further titrated according to clinical, therapeutic response up to 400 mcg/min.

Anal Fissure

Rectal: ADULTS, ELDERLY: One inch (1.5 mg) q12h for up to 3 wks.

Dosage in Renal/Hepatic Impairment

No dose adjustment.

SIDE EFFECTS

Frequent: Headache (possibly severe; occurs mostly in early therapy, diminishes rapidly in intensity, usually disappears during continued treatment), transient flushing of face/neck, dizziness (esp. if pt is standing immobile or is in a warm environment), weakness, orthostatic hypotension. **Sublingual:** Burning, tingling sensation at oral point of dissolution. **Ointment:** Erythema, pruritus. **Occasional:** GI upset. **Transdermal:** Contact dermatitis.

ADVERSE EFFECTS/TOXIC REACTIONS

Discontinue drug if blurred vision, dry mouth occurs. Severe orthostatic hypotension may occur, manifested by syncope, pulselessness, cold/clammy skin, diaphoresis. Tolerance may occur with repeated, prolonged therapy; minor tolerance may occur with intermittent use of sublingual tablets. High doses tend to produce severe headache.

NURSING CONSIDERATIONS

BASELINE ASSESSMENT

Record onset, type (sharp, dull, squeezing), radiation, location, intensity, duration of anginal pain; precipitating factors (exertion, emotional stress). Assess B/P, apical pulse before administration and periodically following dose. Pt must have continuous

ECG monitoring for IV administration. Rule out right-sided MI, if applicable (may precipitate life-threatening hypotension). Receive full medication history, and screen for interactions, esp. use of PDE5 inhibitors. Question medical history and screen for contraindications.

INTERVENTION/EVALUATION

Monitor B/P, heart rate. Assess for facial, neck flushing. Cardioverter/defibrillator must not be discharged through paddle electrode overlying nitroglycerin (transdermal, ointment) system (may cause burns to pt or damage to paddle via electrical arcing). Consider NS boluses for hypotension.

PATIENT/FAMILY TEACHING

• Go from lying to standing slowly. • Take oral form on empty stomach (however, if headache occurs during therapy, take medication with meals). • Use spray only when lying down. • Dissolve sublingual tablet under tongue; do not swallow. • Take at first sign of angina. • May take additional dose q5min if needed up to a total of 3 doses. • If not relieved within 5 min, contact physician or immediately go to emergency room. • Do not inhale lingual aerosol but spray onto or under tongue (avoid swallowing after spray is administered). • Expel from mouth any remaining lingual, sublingual, intrabuccal tablet after pain is completely relieved. • Place transmucosal tablets under upper lip or buccal pouch (between cheek and gum); do not chew/swallow tablet. • Avoid alcohol (intensifies hypotensive effect). If alcohol is ingested soon after taking nitroglycerin, possible acute hypotensive episode (marked drop in B/P, vertigo, diaphoresis, pallor) may occur. • Do not use within 48 hrs of sildenafil, tadalafil, vardenafil (PDE5 inhibitors); may cause acute hypotensive episode.

nivolumab

nye-**vol**-ue-mab
(Opdivo)
Do not confuse nivolumab with denosumab, adalimumab, or palivizumab.

CLASSIFICATION

PHARMACOTHERAPEUTIC: Anti-PD-1 monoclonal antibody. Immune checkpoint inhibitor. **CLINICAL:** Antineoplastic.

USES

Treatment of BRAF V600 wild-type unresectable or metastatic melanoma, as a single agent; BRAF V600 mutation-positive unresectable melanoma, as a single agent; unresectable or metastatic melanoma, in combination with ipilimumab. Adjuvant treatment of melanoma with involvement of lymph nodes or metastatic disease following complete resection. Treatment of metastatic non–small-cell lung cancer (NSCLC) with progression on or after platinum-based chemotherapy. Treatment of metastatic small-cell lung cancer (SCLC) in pts with progression following platinum-based chemotherapy and at least one other line of therapy. Treatment of advanced renal cell cancer (RCC) in pts receiving prior antiangiogenic therapy. First-line treatment of advanced previously untreated RCC (in combination with ipilimumab). Treatment of classical Hodgkin lymphoma (cHL) that relapsed or progressed following autologous hematopoietic stem cell transplant (HSCT) and post-brentuximab, or 3 or more lines of systemic therapy that includes autologous HSCT. Treatment of recurrent or metastatic squamous cell carcinoma of the head and neck. Treatment of locally advanced or metastatic urothelial carcinoma with disease progression during or following platinum-containing chemotherapy; or within 12 mos of neoadjuvant or adjuvant

N

treatment with platinum-containing chemotherapy. Treatment (as a single agent or in combination with ipilimumab) of microsatellite instability-high (MSI-H) or mismatch repair deficient (dMMR) metastatic colorectal cancer in adults and children 12 yrs of age and older that has progressed following treatment with fluoropyrimidine, oxaliplatin, and irinotecan. Treatment of hepatocellular carcinoma in pts previously treated with sorafenib. Treatment of unresectable advanced, recurrent, or metastatic esophageal squamous cell carcinoma after prior fluoropyrimidine- and platinum-based chemotherapy. First-line treatment of metastatic non–small-cell lung cancer (NSCLC) (in combination with ipilimumab) in adults whose tumors express PD-L1 (greater than or equal to1%) and with no epidermal growth factor receptor (EGFR) or anaplastic lymphoma kinase (ALK) genomic tumor aberrations. First-line treatment of metastatic or recurrent NSCLC (in combination with ipilimumab and 2 cycles of platinum doublet chemotherapy) in adults with no EGFR or ALK genomic tumor aberrations. First-line treatment in adults (in combination with ipilimumab) of unresectable malignant pleural mesothelioma.

PRECAUTIONS

Contraindications: Hypersensitivity to nivolumab. **Cautions:** Thyroid/pituitary disease, hepatic/renal impairment, interstitial lung disease, electrolyte imbalance.

ACTION

Binds PD-1 ligands to PD-1 receptor found on T cells, blocking its interaction with the ligands (PD-L1 and PD-L2). Releases PD-1 pathway–mediated inhibition of immune response (including antitumor immune response). **Therapeutic Effect:** Inhibits T-cell proliferation and cytokine production. Inhibits tumor cell growth and metastasis.

PHARMACOKINETICS

Information on metabolism and elimination is not available. Steady-state concentration reached in 12 wks. **Half-life:** 26.7 days.

LIFESPAN CONSIDERATIONS

Pregnancy/Lactation: Avoid pregnancy; may cause fetal harm. Unknown if distributed in breast milk. Females of reproductive potential should use effective contraception during treatment and up to 5 mos after discontinuation. **Children:** Safety and efficacy not established. **Elderly:** May have increased risk of endocrine/hepatic/pulmonary/optic/renal injury due to age-related diseases.

INTERACTIONS

DRUG: May enhance adverse/toxic effects of **belimumab**. **HERBAL:** None significant. **FOOD:** None known. **LAB VALUES:** **Single Therapy:** May increase serum alkaline phosphatase, ALT, AST, potassium. May decrease serum sodium. **Combo Therapy:** May increase serum alkaline phosphatase, ALT, AST, amylase, creatinine, lipase. May decrease RBC, Hct, Hgb, lymphocytes, neutrophils, platelets; serum calcium, sodium, magnesium. May increase or decrease serum calcium, potassium.

AVAILABILITY (Rx)

Injection Solution: 40 mg/4 mL, 100 mg/10 mL, 240 mg/24 mL vials.

ADMINISTRATION/HANDLING

IV

Preparation • Visually inspect solution for particulate matter or discoloration. Solution should appear opalescent, colorless to pale yellow. Discard if solution is cloudy or contains particulate matter other than a few translucent to white proteinaceous particles. • Do not shake vial. • Withdraw required dose volume and dilute in 0.9% NaCl or D_5W. Final concentration will equal 1–10 mg/mL based on volume of diluent. • Mix by gentle inversion. • Do not shake. • Discard partially used or empty vials.

Rate of administration • Infuse over 60 min using sterile, nonpyrogenic, low protein-binding, 0.2- to 1.2-micron in-line filter. • Flush IV line upon completion.

Storage • Refrigerate diluted solution up to 24 hrs or store at room temperature for no more than 4 hrs (includes time of preparation and infusion). • Do not freeze.

IV INCOMPATIBILITIES

Do not infuse with other medications.

INDICATIONS/ROUTES/DOSAGE

Melanoma

IV: ADULTS, ELDERLY: (Single Agent): 240 mg q2wks or 480 mg q4wks until disease progression or unacceptable toxicity. **(In combination with ipilimumab):** 1 mg/kg, followed by ipilimumab on the same day, q3wks for 4 doses. Subsequent single-agent therapy dose is 240 mg q2wks or 480 mg q4wks until disease progression or unacceptable toxicity.

Metastatic Non–Small-Cell Lung Cancer (NSCLC)

IV: ADULTS, ELDERLY: 240 mg q2wks until disease progression or unacceptable toxicity.

Advanced Renal Cell Carcinoma (Previously treated), Urothelial Carcinoma, Hepatocellular Carcinoma, Melanoma (Adjuvant treatment)

IV: ADULTS, ELDERLY: 240 mg q2wks or 480 mg q4wks until disease progression or unacceptable toxicity.

cHL (Recurrent or metastatic), Esophageal Carcinoma, Squamous Cell Carcinoma (Unresectable advanced, recurrent, or metastatic)

IV: ADULTS, ELDERLY: 240 mg once q2wks or 480 mg once q4wks until disease progression or unacceptable toxicity.

Colorectal Cancer, Metastatic (Single agent)

IV: ADULTS, ELDERLY: 240 mg q2wks or 480 mg once q4wks until disease progression or unacceptable toxicity.

Colorectal Cancer, Metastatic (Combination therapy)

IV: ADULTS, ELDERLY: (In combination with ipilimumab): 3 mg/kg, in combination with ipilimumab, q3wks for 4 doses. Subsequent single-agent therapy dose is 240 mg q2wks or 480 mg once q4wks until disease progression or unacceptable toxicity.

Metastatic SCLC

IV: ADULTS, ELDERLY: (Single Agent): 3 mg/kg once q2wks until disease progression or unacceptable toxicity. **(In combination with ipilimumab):** 1 mg/kg once q3wks for 4 combination doses, then 3 mg/kg once q2wks as single agent until disease progression or unacceptable toxicity.

RCC Combination Therapy (Previously untreated)

IV: ADULTS, ELDERLY: (In combination with ipilimumab): 3 mg/kg, in combination with ipilimumab, q3wks for 4 doses. Subsequent single-agent therapy dose is 240 mg q2wks or 480 mg q4wks until disease progression or unacceptable toxicity.

Head and Neck Carcinoma

IV: ADULTS, ELDERLY: 240 mg once q2wks or 480 mg once q4wks until disease progression or unacceptable toxicity.

NSCLC (Metastatic, PD-L1–expressing)

IV: ADULTS, ELDERLY: 3 mg/kg q2wks (with ipilimumab). Continue until disease progression or unacceptable toxicity or for up to 2 yrs in pts without disease progression.

NSCLC (Metastatic or recurrent)

IV: ADULTS, ELDERLY: 360 mg q3wks (in combination with ipilimumab and 2 cycles of histology-based platinum-doublet chemotherapy). Continue until disease progression or unacceptable toxicity or for up to 2 yrs in pts without disease progression.

Malignant Pleural Mesothelioma

IV: ADULTS, ELDERLY: 360 mg q3wks (in combination with ipilimumab). Continue until disease progression or unacceptable toxicity or for up to 2 yrs in pts without disease progression.

Dose Modification

Based on Common Terminology Criteria for Adverse Events (CTCAE).

N

Withhold Treatment for Any of the Following Adverse Events

Grade 2 or 3 diarrhea or colitis; single-agent therapy–associated colitis; Grade 2 pneumonitis; serum AST or ALT greater than 3–5 times upper limit of normal (ULN) or serum bilirubin 1.5–3 times ULN; Grade 2 or 3 hypophysitis; Grade 2 adrenal insufficiency; serum creatinine greater than 1.5–6 times ULN; Grade 3 rash; first occurrence of any other Grade 3 adverse reaction. When nivolumab is administered in combination with ipilimumab and nivolumab is withheld, then ipilimumab should also be withheld.

Restarting Therapy

Resume when adverse reactions return to Grade 0 or 1.

Permanently Discontinue for Any of the Following Adverse Events

Combo-agent therapy (ipilimumab)–associated colitis; Grade 3 or 4 pneumonitis; serum AST or ALT greater than 5 times ULN or serum bilirubin 3 times ULN; pts with liver metastasis who begin treatment with baseline Grade 2 serum ALT or AST elevation who experience serum ALT or AST elevation greater than or equal to 50% from baseline that persists for at least 1 wk; Grade 4 hypophysitis; Grade 3 or 4 adrenal insufficiency; serum creatinine greater than 6 times ULN; Grade 4 rash; recurrence of any other Grade 3 adverse reaction; any life-threatening or Grade 4 adverse reaction; requirement for predniSONE 10 mg/day or greater (or equivalent) for more than 12 wks; persistent Grade 2 or 3 adverse reaction lasting longer than 12 wks.

Dosage in Renal Impairment

No dose adjustment.

Dosage in Hepatic Impairment

Mild to moderate impairment: No dose adjustment. **Severe impairment:** Not specified; use caution.

SIDE EFFECTS

Note: Percentage of side effects may vary depending on the use of single or combination therapy. **Frequent (50%–24%):** Fatigue, dyspnea, musculoskeletal pain, decreased appetite, cough, nausea, headache, constipation. **Occasional (19%–10%):** Vomiting, asthenia, diarrhea, edema, pyrexia, cough, dehydration, rash, abdominal pain, chest pain, arthralgia, decreased weight, blurred vision, pruritus, peripheral edema, generalized pain.

ADVERSE EFFECTS/TOXIC REACTIONS

Anemia, lymphopenia, neutropenia, thrombocytopenia is an expected response to therapy. May cause severe immune-mediated events including interstitial lung disease or pneumonitis (3%–10% of pts), colitis (21%–57% of pts), hepatitis (15%–28% of pts), hypophysitis (13% of pts), renal failure or nephritis (1%–2% of pts), hyperthyroidism (1% of pts), hypothyroidism (3%–19% of pts), rash (up to 37% of pts). Other adverse events including autoimmune nephropathy, demyelination, diabetic ketoacidosis, duodenitis, erythema multiforme, exfoliative dermatitis, facial and abducens nerve paresis, gastritis, iridocyclitis, motor dysfunction, pancreatitis, psoriasis, sarcoidosis, uveitis, vasculitis, ventricular arrhythmia, vitiligo reported in less than 2% of pts. Severe infusion-related reactions reported in less than 1% of pts. Occurrence of events is dependent on use of single or combination therapy. Upper respiratory tract infections including nasopharyngitis, pharyngitis, rhinitis reported in 11% of pts. Immunogenicity (auto-nivolumab antibodies) occurred in 8.5% of pts.

NURSING CONSIDERATIONS

BASELINE ASSESSMENT

Obtain CBC, BMP, LFT, TSH; vital signs; urine pregnancy. Record weight in kg. Screen for history of arrhythmias, pituitary/pulmonary/thyroid disease, autoimmune disorders, diabetes, hepatic/renal impairment; allergy to predniSONE. Along with routine assessment, conduct full dermatologic exam, ophthalmologic exam/visual acuity. Receive full medication history and screen for interactions.

INTERVENTION/EVALUATION

Monitor CBC, LFT, serum electrolytes; thyroid panel if applicable. Diligently monitor for immune-mediated adverse events as listed in Adverse Effects/Toxic Reactions. Notify physician if any toxicities occur (see Appendix M) and initiate proper treatment. Obtain chest X-ray if interstitial lung disease, pneumonitis suspected. Screen for tumor lysis syndrome in pts with high tumor burden. Monitor I&O, daily weight. If predniSONE therapy is initiated for immune-mediated events, monitor capillary blood glucose and screen for corticosteroid side effects.

PATIENT/FAMILY TEACHING

• Serious adverse reactions may affect lungs, GI tract, kidneys, or hormonal glands; anti-inflammatory medication may need to be started. • Immediately contact physician if serious or life-threatening inflammatory reactions occur in the following body systems: colon (severe abdominal pain or diarrhea); kidney (decreased or dark-colored urine, flank pain); lung (chest pain, cough, shortness of breath); liver (bruising easily, dark-colored urine, clay-colored/tarry stools, yellowing of skin or eyes); pituitary (persistent or unusual headache, dizziness, extreme weakness, fainting, vision changes); thyroid (trouble sleeping, high blood pressure, fast heart rate [overactive thyroid]), (fatigue, goiter, weight gain [underactive thyroid]). • Use effective contraction to avoid pregnancy. Do not breastfeed.

norepinephrine HIGH ALERT

nor-ep-i-**nef**-rin
(Levophed)

■ **BLACK BOX ALERT** ■
Extravasation may produce severe tissue necrosis, sloughing. Using fine hypodermic needle, liberally infiltrate area with 10–15 mL saline solution containing 5–10 mg phentolamine.

Do not confuse Levophed with Levaquin or levoFLOXacin, or norepinephrine with EPINEPHrine.

◆CLASSIFICATION

PHARMACOTHERAPEUTIC: Alpha, beta agonist. **CLINICAL:** Vasopressor.

USES

Severe hypotension, treatment of shock persisting after adequate fluid volume replacement.

PRECAUTIONS

Contraindications: Hypersensitivity to norepinephrine. Hypotension related to hypovolemia (except in emergency to maintain coronary/cerebral perfusion until volume replaced), mesenteric/peripheral vascular thrombosis (unless it is lifesaving procedure). **Cautions:** Concurrent use of MAOIs.

ACTION

Stimulates $beta_1$-adrenergic receptors, alpha-adrenergic receptors, increasing contractility, heart rate and producing vasoconstriction. **Therapeutic Effect:** Increases systemic B/P, coronary blood flow.

PHARMACOKINETICS

Route	Onset	Peak	Duration
IV	Rapid	1–2 min	N/A

Localized in sympathetic tissue. Metabolized in liver. Primarily excreted in urine.

⌛ LIFESPAN CONSIDERATIONS

Pregnancy/Lactation: Readily crosses placenta. May produce fetal anoxia due to uterine contraction, constriction of uterine blood vessels. **Children/Elderly:** No age-related precautions noted.

INTERACTIONS

DRUG: MAOIs (e.g., phenelzine, selegiline), antidepressants (tricyclic) may prolong hypertension.

N

SNRIs (e.g., duloxetine), tramadol may increase tachycardic effect. **HERBAL:** None significant. **FOOD:** None known. **LAB VALUES:** None significant.

AVAILABILITY (Rx)

Injection Solution: 1 mg/mL.

ADMINISTRATION/HANDLING

IV

Reconstitution • Add 4 mL (4 mg) to 250 mL D_5W (16 mcg/mL). **Maximum concentration:** 32 mL (32 mg) to 250 mL (128 mcg/mL).

Rate of administration • Closely monitor IV infusion flow rate (use infusion pump). • Monitor B/P q2min during IV infusion until desired therapeutic response is achieved, then q5min during remaining IV infusion. • Never leave pt unattended. • Maintain B/P at 90–100 mm Hg in previously normotensive pts, and 30–40 mm Hg below preexisting B/P in previously hypertensive pts. • Reduce IV infusion gradually. Avoid abrupt withdrawal. • If using peripherally inserted catheter, it is imperative to check the IV site frequently for free flow and infused vein for blanching, hardness to vein, coldness, pallor to extremity. • If extravasation occurs, area should be infiltrated with 10–15 mL sterile saline containing 5–10 mg phentolamine (does not alter pressor effects of norepinephrine).

Storage • Do not use if solution is brown or contains precipitate. • Store at room temperature. Diluted solution stable for 24 hrs at room temperature.

IV INCOMPATIBILITIES

Pantoprazole (Protonix), regular insulin.

IV COMPATIBILITIES

Amiodarone (Cordarone), calcium gluconate, dexmedetomidine (Precedex), dilTIAZem (Cardizem), DOBUTamine (Dobutrex), DOPamine (Intropin), EPINEPHrine, esmolol (Brevibloc), fentaNYL (Sublimaze), furosemide (Lasix), haloperidol (Haldol), heparin, HYDROmorphone (Dilaudid), labetalol (Trandate), lipids, LORazepam (Ativan), magnesium, midazolam (Versed), milrinone (Primacor), morphine, niCARdipine (Cardene), nitroglycerin, potassium chloride, propofol (Diprivan).

INDICATIONS/ROUTES/DOSAGE

◀ **ALERT** ▶ If possible, blood, fluid volume depletion should be corrected before drug is administered. Recommend infusion via central venous access.

Acute Hypotension Unresponsive to Fluid Volume Replacement

IV infusion: ADULTS, ELDERLY: Initially, administer at 8–12 mcg/min. Adjust rate of flow to desired response. Average maintenance range: 2–4 mcg/min (varies greatly based on clinical situation). **CHILDREN:** Initially, 0.05–0.1 mcg/kg/min; titrate to desired effect. **Maximum:** 2 mcg/kg/min.

Dosage in Renal/Hepatic Impairment

No dose adjustment.

SIDE EFFECTS

Norepinephrine produces less pronounced, less frequent side effects than EPINEPHrine. **Occasional (5%–3%):** Anxiety, bradycardia, palpitations. **Rare (2%–1%):** Nausea, anginal pain, shortness of breath, fever.

ADVERSE EFFECTS/TOXIC REACTIONS

Extravasation may produce tissue necrosis, sloughing. Overdose manifested as severe hypertension with violent headache (may be first clinical sign of overdose), arrhythmias, photophobia, retrosternal or pharyngeal pain, pallor, diaphoresis, vomiting. Prolonged therapy may result in plasma volume depletion. Hypotension may recur if plasma volume is not maintained.

NURSING CONSIDERATIONS

BASELINE ASSESSMENT

Assess ECG, B/P continuously (be alert to precipitous B/P drop). Be alert to pt complaint of headache.

INTERVENTION/EVALUATION

Monitor IV flow rate diligently. Assess for extravasation characterized by blanching of skin over vein, coolness (results from local vasoconstriction); color, temperature of IV site extremity (pallor, cyanosis, mottling). Assess nailbed capillary refill. Monitor I&O; measure output hourly, report urine output less than 30 mL/hr. Once B/P parameter has been reached, IV infusion should not be restarted unless systolic B/P falls below 90 mm Hg.

obinutuzumab

oh-bi-nue-**tooz**-ue-mab
(Gazyva)

■ **BLACK BOX ALERT** ■ Hepatitis B virus reactivation, resulting in hepatic failure, fulminant hepatitis, and death have occurred. Screen all pts for hepatitis B virus infection before initiating treatment. Progressive multifocal leukoencephalopathy (PML) including fatal PML reported.

◆CLASSIFICATION

PHARMACOTHERAPEUTIC: Anti-CD20 monoclonal antibody. **CLINICAL:** Antineoplastic.

USES

Treatment of previously untreated chronic lymphocytic leukemia (CLL), in combination with chlorambucil. Treatment of follicular lymphoma (in combination with bendamustine) in pts who relapsed after, or are refractory to, a riTUXimab-containing regimen. Treatment of previously untreated stage II bulky, stage III, or stage IV follicular lymphoma in combination with chemotherapy and followed by obinutuzumab monotherapy.

PRECAUTIONS

Contraindications: Hypersensitivity to obinutuzumab. **Cautions:** Baseline cytopenias, HBV infection, preexisting cardiac/pulmonary impairment; hematologic abnormalities (e.g., leukopenia, thrombocytopenia); electrolyte imbalance; conditions predisposing to infection (e.g., diabetes, renal failure, immunocompromised pts, open wounds).

ACTION

Targets CD20 antigen expressed on surface of B lymphocytes. Mediates B-cell lysis by activating complement-dependent cytotoxicity, antibody-dependent cellular cytotoxicity. **Therapeutic Effect:** Inhibits tumor cell growth and proliferation in CLL.

PHARMACOKINETICS

Metabolism and elimination not specified. **Half-life:** 28 days.

⌛ LIFESPAN CONSIDERATIONS

Pregnancy/Lactation: Unknown if distributed in breast milk. Monoclonal antibodies are known to cross placenta. Effective contraception, discontinuation of breastfeeding recommended during therapy and for at least 18 mos after discontinuation. **Children:** Safety and efficacy not established. **Elderly:** May have increased risk of adverse reactions.

INTERACTIONS

DRUG: May increase hypotensive effect of **ACE inhibitors (e.g., enalapril, lisinopril), angiotensin receptor blockers (e.g., losartan), beta blockers (e.g., metoprolol).** May decrease the therapeutic effect of **BCG (intravesical), vaccines (live)**. May increase adverse effects of **belimumab, natalizumab, vaccines (live). HERBAL: Echinacea** may diminish the therapeutic effect. **FOOD:** None known. **LAB VALUES:** May increase serum alkaline phosphatase, ALT, AST, bilirubin, creatinine, uric acid. May decrease albumin, Hgb, Hct, lymphocytes, neutrophils, platelets; serum potassium, sodium.

AVAILABILITY (Rx)

Injection Solution: 1,000 mg/40 mL (25 mg/mL) single-use vial.

ADMINISTRATION/HANDLING

◀ALERT▶ Administer via dedicated line. Do not administer IV push or bolus. Withhold hypertensive medications at least 12 hrs before and 1 hr after administration. Do not mix with dextrose-containing fluids.

IV

Reconstitution • Visually inspect for particulate matter or discoloration. • For 100-mg dose: withdraw 40 mL solution from vial and dilute only 4 mL (100 mg) in 100 mL 0.9% NaCl for immediate administration. Dilute remaining 36 mL (900 mg) into 250 mL 0.9% NaCl at same time and refrigerate for up to 24 hrs for cycle 1: day 2. For remaining infusions (day 8 and day 15 of cycle 1 and day 1 of cycles 2–6), dilute 40 mL (1,000 mg) solution in 250 mL NaCl infusion bag. • Gently mix by inversion. • Do not shake.

Rate of administration • **Day 1 of cycle 1 (100 mg):** Infuse over 4 hrs (25 mg/hr). • Do not increase infusion rate. • **Day 2 of cycle 1 (900 mg):** Infuse at 50 mg/hr. • May increase by 50 mg/hr every 30 min to maximum rate of 400 mg/hr. • Increase rate based on tolerability.

Storage • Solution should appear clear, colorless to slightly brown. • May refrigerate diluted solution up to 24 hrs.

INDICATIONS/ROUTES/DOSAGE

Chronic Lymphocytic Leukemia (CLL)

◀ALERT▶ Premedicate with glucocorticoid, acetaminophen, and antihistamine to decrease severity of infusion reaction. Consider premedication with antihyperuricemics (allopurinol) 12–24 hrs for pts with high tumor burden or high circulating absolute lymphocyte count greater than 25 × 10^9/L. Recommend antimicrobial prophylaxis throughout treatment for pts with neutropenia.

IV: ADULTS/ELDERLY: Six treatment cycles of 28-day cycle. **Day 1 of cycle 1:** 100 mg. **Day 2 of cycle 1:** 900 mg. **Day 8 and Day 15 of cycle 1:** 1000 mg. **Cycles 2–6:** 1000 mg on day 1 of each subsequent 28-day cycle for 5 doses. Discontinue treatment if any severe to life-threatening infusion reactions occur.

Follicular Lymphoma (Relapsed/refractory)

IV: ADULTS, ELDERLY: Six treatment cycles of 28 days (in combination with bendamustine). **Cycle 1:** 1,000 mg on days 1, 8, 15. **Cycles 2–6:** 1,000 mg on day 1 of each subsequent 28-day cycle for 5 doses. If achieves stable disease, complete or partial response, continue obinutuzumab (as monotherapy) 1,000 mg q2mos for 2 yrs.

Follicular Lymphoma (Previously untreated)

IV: ADULTS, ELDERLY: Cycle 1 (either in combination with bendamustine or with CHOP or CVP chemotherapy): 1,000 mg wkly on days 1, 8, and 15. **Cycles 2–6 (in combination with bendamustine):** 1,000 mg on day 1 q28days for 5 doses. **Cycles 2–8 (in combination with CHOP):** 1,000 mg on day1 q21days for 5 doses (with CHOP), then 1,000 mg on day 1 q21 days for 2 doses (as monotherapy). **Cycles 2–8 (in combination with CVP):** 1,000 mg on day 1 q21days for 7 doses. **Then as monotherapy:** 1,000 mg q2mos for up to 2 yrs beginning approximately 2 mos after last induction phase.

Dosage in Renal/Hepatic Impairment

No dose adjustment.

SIDE EFFECTS

Frequent (69%): Infusion reactions (pruritus, flushing, urticaria). **Occasional (10%):** Pyrexia, cough.

ADVERSE EFFECTS/TOXIC REACTIONS

Myelosuppression (leukopenia, lymphopenia, neutropenia, thrombocytopenia) is an expected response to therapy, but more severe reactions including bone marrow failure, febrile neutropenia, opportunistic infection may result in life-threatening events. Hepatitis B virus reactivation may occur. Infusion reactions including hypotension, tachycardia, dyspnea, bronchospasm, wheezing, laryngeal edema, nausea, vomiting, flushing, pyrexia may occur during infusion. Tumor lysis syndrome may present as acute renal failure, hypocalcemia, hyperuricemia, hyperphosphatemia within 12–24 hrs of infusion. Immunogenicity (autoantibodies) occurred in 13% of pts. Progressive multifocal leukoencephalopathy (PML) occurred rarely and may include weakness, paralysis, vision loss, aphasia, cognition impairment.

NURSING CONSIDERATIONS

BASELINE ASSESSMENT

Obtain CBC, BMP, uric acid; pregnancy test in females of reproductive potential. Screen for history of anemia, asthma, arrhythmias, COPD, diabetes, GI bleeding, hypertension, hepatitis B virus infection, hepatic/renal impairment, peripheral edema. Receive full medication history, esp. hypertension, anticoagulant medications. Perform baseline visual acuity. Offer emotional support.

INTERVENTION/EVALUATION

Monitor CBC, serum electrolytes, LFT, vital signs. Monitor for cardiovascular alterations, respiratory distress. If respiratory reactions occur, consider administration of oxygen, EPINEPHrine, albuterol treatments. Locate rapid-sequence intubation kit if respiratory compromise occurs. Monitor strict I&O, hydration status. If PML suspected, consult neurologist for proper management. Obtain ECG for palpitations, severe hypokalemia, hyponatremia. Monitor for infection (cough, fatigue, fever).

PATIENT/FAMILY TEACHING

• Treatment may depress your immune system and reduce your ability to fight infection. Report symptoms of infection such as body aches, chills, cough, fatigue, fever. Avoid those with active infection. • Avoid alcohol. • Immediately report difficult breathing, severe coughing, chest tightness, wheezing. • Paralysis, vision changes, impaired speech, altered mental status may indicate life-threatening neurologic event. • Use effective contraception to avoid pregnancy.

ocrelizumab

ok-re-**liz**-ue-mab
(Ocrevus)
Do not confuse ocrelizumab with certolizumab, daclizumab, efalizumab, mepolizumab, natalizumab, or omalizumab.

◆CLASSIFICATION

PHARMACOTHERAPEUTIC: Anti-CD20 monoclonal antibody. **CLINICAL:** Multiple sclerosis agent.

USES

Treatment of adult pts with relapsing or primary progressive forms of multiple sclerosis (MS).

PRECAUTIONS

Contraindications: Life-threatening infusion reaction to ocrelizumab. Active hepatitis B virus (HBV) infection confirmed by positive results for hepatitis B surface antigen (HBsAg) and anti-HBV tests. **Cautions:** History of chronic opportunistic infections (esp. bacterial, invasive fungal, mycobacterial, protozoal, viral, tuberculosis); active infection, conditions predisposing to infection (e.g., diabetes, immunocompromised pts, renal failure, open wounds); intolerance to corticosteroids; history of depression, malignancies, breast cancer. Avoid administration of live or live attenuated vaccines during treatment and after discontinuation until B cells are no longer depleted.

ACTION

Monoclonal antibody that is directed against B cells, which express the cell surface antigen CD20 (thought to influence the course of MS through antigen presentation, autoantibody production, cytokine regulation, and formation of ectopic lymphoid aggregates in meninges). Binds to the cell surface to deplete CD20-expressing B cells. **Therapeutic Effect:** Reduces progression of MS.

PHARMACOKINETICS

Onset of action: serum CD-19+ B-cell count reduced within 14 days. Duration of action: 72 wks (Range: 27–175 wks). Antibodies are primarily cleared by catabolism. **Half-life:** 26 days.

LIFESPAN CONSIDERATIONS

Pregnancy/Lactation: May cause transient peripheral B-cell depletion and lymphocytopenia in neonates when used during pregnancy. Immunoglobulins are known to cross the placenta. Females of reproductive potential must use effective contraception during treatment and up to 6 mos after discontinuation. Unknown if distributed in breast milk; however, immunoglobulin G (IgG) is present in breast milk. Breastfeeding not recommended. **Children:** Safety and efficacy not established. **Elderly:** No age-related precautions noted.

INTERACTIONS

DRUG: May decrease effect of **BCG, vaccines (live).** May increase adverse effects/toxicity of **belimumab, natalizumab, tacrolimus.** **HERBAL:** **Echinacea** may diminish therapeutic effect. **FOOD:** None known. **LAB VALUES:** May decrease immunoglobulin A (IgA), immunoglobulin M (IgM), immunoglobulin G (IgG), neutrophils.

AVAILABILITY (Rx)

Injection Solution: 300 mg/10 mL (30 mg/mL).

ADMINISTRATION/HANDLING

IV

Preparation • Visually inspect for particulate matter or discoloration. Solution should appear clear to slightly opalescent, colorless to pale brown in color. • Do not use if solution is cloudy, discolored, or if visible particles are observed. • Withdraw proper dose from vial (10 mL for 300-mg dose; 20 mL for 600-mg dose) and dilute into 0.9% NaCl bag to a final concentration of approx. 1.2 mg/mL (300-mg dose in 250 mL 0.9% NaCl; 600-mg dose in 500 mL 0.9% NaCl). • Mix by gentle inversion. • Do not shake or agitate.

Rate of administration • **First and Second Infusion:** Start at 30 mL/hr via dedicated line using 0.2- or 0.22-micron in-line filter. If tolerated, increase rate by 30 mL/hr q30min to a maximum rate of 180 mL/hr for a duration of 2.5 hrs or longer. • **Subsequent Infusions:** Start at 40 mL/hr via dedicated line using 0.2- or 0.22-micron in-line filter. If tolerated, increase rate by 40 mL/hr q30min to a maximum rate of 200 mL/hr for a duration of 3.5 hrs or longer. • **Mild Infusion Reactions:** Decrease rate by 50% and continue reduced rate for at least 30 min. If tolerated, may increase infusion rate as described above. • **Severe Infusion Reactions:** Interrupt infusion until symptoms resolve, then resume infusion at 50% of the initial infusion rate. • **Life-threatening Infusion Reaction:** Immediately stop infusion and permanently discontinue; do not restart.

Storage • May refrigerate diluted solution up to 24 hrs or store at room temperature for up to 8 hrs (includes infusion time). • If diluted solution is refrigerated, allow to warm to room temperature before administration. • Discard solution if not administered within required time frame.

IV INCOMPATIBILITIES

Do not dilute with other IV solutions. Do not mix or infuse with other medications.

INDICATIONS/ROUTES/DOSAGE

◀ALERT▶ Must be administered under the direct supervision of health care professionals with access to emergency medical supplies and who are trained to manage severe infusion reactions. If a dose is missed, administer as soon as possible; do not wait until the next regularly scheduled dose. Reset administration schedule so that the next subsequent infusion is 6 mos after the most recent dose. Subsequent doses must be separated by at least 5 mos.

Premedication

• To reduce severity and frequency of infusion reaction, premedicate with methylprednisolone 100 mg (or equivalent) approx. 30 min prior to infusion and an antihistamine (e.g., diphenhydramine) approx. 30–60 min prior to infusion. • Consider an antipyretic (e.g., acetaminophen) based on previous infusion reactions.

Multiple Sclerosis

IV: ADULTS, ELDERLY: 300 mg once at wk 0 and wk 2, then 600 mg q6mos (beginning 6 mos after the first 300-mg dose). Observe pt for at least 1 hr after completion of infusion.

Dosage in Renal/Hepatic Impairment

Mild impairment: No dose adjustment. **Moderate to severe impairment:** Not specified; use caution.

SIDE EFFECTS

Occasional (8%–5%): Back pain, cough, diarrhea, peripheral edema, extremity pain.

ADVERSE EFFECTS/TOXIC REACTIONS

Infusion-related reactions including bronchospasm, dizziness, dyspnea, erythema, fatigue, flushing, headache, hypotension, nausea, oropharyngeal pain, pharyngeal/laryngeal edema, pruritus, pyrexia, rash, tachycardia, throat irritation, urticaria was reported in 34%–40% of pts. Serious infusion reactions requiring hospitalization occurred in less than 1% of pts. Infections including upper respiratory tract infections (40%–49% of pts), lower respiratory tract infections (10% of pts), skin infections (16% of pts), herpes infection (6% of pts) may occur. Progressive multifocal leukoencephalopathy (PML), an opportunistic viral infection of the brain caused by the JC virus, has occurred in pts treated with other anti-CD20 antibodies; may result in progressive permanent disability and death. Symptoms of PML include altered mental status, aphasia, paralysis, vision loss, weakness. HBV reactivation was reported in pts treated with other anti-CD20 antibodies; may result in fulminant hepatitis, hepatic failure, death. May increase risk of malignancies including breast cancer. Immunogenicity (auto anti-ocrelizumab antibodies) reported in 1% of pts. Depression reported in 8% of pts.

NURSING CONSIDERATIONS

BASELINE ASSESSMENT

Assess baseline symptoms of MS (e.g., bladder/bowel dysfunction, cognitive impairment, depression, dysphagia, fatigue, gait disorder, numbness/tingling, pain, seizures, spasticity, tremors, weakness). Obtain vital signs. Question history of hypersensitivity reactions, infusion-related reactions. Ensure that proper resuscitative equipment, medical supplies are readily available (e.g., albuterol, antipyretics, antihistamines, epinephrine, isotonic IV fluids, bag-valve mask, oxygen, rapid sequence intubation kit). Screen for active HBV. Pts who test negative for HBsAg and positive for anti-HBcAb+ should be referred to a hepatic specialist. If applicable, immunizations should be up-to-date according to guidelines at least 6 wks prior to initiation. Question history of chronic infections, herpes infection, depression, malignancies, breast cancer. Screen for active infection. Verify use of effective contraception in females of reproductive potential.

INTERVENTION/EVALUATION

Monitor vital signs. Diligently monitor for infusion-related reactions during infusion and for at least 1 hr after completion (esp. during initial infusions). If severe or life-threatening reactions occur, immediately stop infusion and provide appropriate medical support. Due to risk of respiratory compromise, pts with bronchospasm, dyspnea, hypoxia should be given immediate supplemental oxygen, hypersensitivity medications, hemodynamic support. If laryngeal or pharyngeal edema occurs, airway protection or possible intubation may be required. Mild to moderate infusion reactions may require interruption of infusion, decrease of infusion rate, symp-

O

tom management. Closely monitor for HBV reactivation, symptoms of PML, new malignancies including breast cancer, infections. Conduct neurologic assessment. Assess for symptom improvement of MS.

PATIENT/FAMILY TEACHING

• Life-threatening infusion reactions, allergic reactions may occur during infusion and up to 24 hrs after completion of infusion. Immediately report difficulty breathing, chest pain, chest tightness, chills, dizziness, fast heart rate, fever, flushing, headache, hives, itching, low blood pressure, nausea, throat pain or swelling, rash. • If applicable, vaccinations should be up to date at least 6 wks before starting treatment. Do not receive live vaccines. • Treatment may depress your immune system and reduce your ability to fight infection. Report symptoms of infection such as body aches, burning with urination, chills, cough, fatigue, fever. Avoid those with active infection. • Use effective contraception to avoid pregnancy. Do not breastfeed. • Due to pretreatment with a corticosteroid, pts with diabetes may experience a transient rise in blood sugar levels. • PML, an opportunistic viral infection of the brain, may cause progressive, permanent disabilities and death. Report symptoms of PML such as confusion, memory loss, paralysis, trouble speaking, vision loss, seizures, weakness. • Treatment may cause reactivation of HBV, depression, new cancers including breast cancer. • Notify physician if symptoms of MS do not improve.

octreotide

ock-**tree**-oh-tide
(SandoSTATIN, SandoSTATIN LAR Depot)

Do not confuse SandoSTATIN with SandIMMUNE, SandoSTATIN LAR, sargramostim, or simvastatin.

◆CLASSIFICATION

PHARMACOTHERAPEUTIC: Somatostatin analogue. **CLINICAL:** Secretory inhibitory, growth hormone suppressant; antidiarrheal.

USES

Control of diarrhea and flushing in pts with metastatic carcinoid tumors, treatment of watery diarrhea associated with vasoactive intestinal peptic-secreting tumors (VIPomas), acromegaly (to reduce blood levels of growth hormone and insulin-like growth factor). **OFF-LABEL:** Control of bleeding esophageal varices, treatment of AIDS-associated secretory diarrhea, diarrhea, diarrhea associated with graft-vs-host disease, chemotherapy-induced diarrhea, insulinomas, small-bowel fistulas, Zollinger-Ellison syndrome, Cushing's syndrome, hypothalamic obesity, malignant bowel obstruction, postgastrectomy dumping syndrome, islet cell tumors, sulfonylurea-induced hypoglycemia.

PRECAUTIONS

Contraindications: Hypersensitivity to octreotide. **Cautions:** Diabetic pts with gastroparesis, renal failure, hepatic impairment, HF, concomitant medications altering heart rate or rhythm. Concurrent use of medications that prolong QT interval, elderly.

ACTION

Suppresses secretion of serotonin, gastrin, VIP, insulin, glucagon, secretin, pancreatic polypeptide. **Therapeutic Effect:** Prolongs intestinal transit time. Decreases growth hormone in acromegaly.

PHARMACOKINETICS

Route	Onset	Peak	Duration
SQ	N/A	N/A	Up to 12 hrs

Rapidly, completely absorbed from injection site. Protein binding: 65%. Metabolized in liver. Excreted in urine. Removed by hemodialysis. **Half-life:** 1.7–1.9 hrs.

O

LIFESPAN CONSIDERATIONS

Pregnancy/Lactation: Unknown if distributed in breast milk. **Children:** Safety and efficacy not established. **Elderly:** No age-related precautions noted.

INTERACTIONS

DRUG: May decrease effectiveness of **cycloSPORINE. Glucagon, growth hormone, insulin, oral antidiabetics (e.g., glipiZIDE, metFORMIN)** may alter glucose concentrations. **HERBAL: Herbals with hypoglycemic properties (e.g., fenugreek)** may increase hypoglycemic effect. **FOOD:** None known. **LAB VALUES:** May decrease serum thyroxine (T_4). May increase serum alkaline phosphatase, ALT, AST, GGT.

AVAILABILITY (Rx)

Injection Solution: ***(SandoSTATIN):*** 50 mcg/mL, 100 mcg/mL, 200 mcg/mL, 500 mcg/mL, 1,000 mcg/mL. **Injection Suspension:** ***(SandoSTATIN LAR):*** 10-mg, 20-mg, 30-mg vials.

O

ADMINISTRATION/HANDLING

◀ALERT▶ SandoSTATIN may be given IV, IM, SQ. SandoSTATIN LAR Depot may be given only IM. Refrigerate.

IM

• Give immediately after mixing. • Administer deep IM in large muscle mass at 4-wk intervals. • Avoid deltoid injections.

SQ

• Do not use if discolored or particulates form. • Avoid multiple injections at same site within short periods.

IV

• Dilute in 50–100 mL 0.9% NaCl or D_5W and infuse over 15–30 min. In emergency, may give IV push over 3 min. Following dilution, stable for 96 hrs at room temperature when diluted with 0.9% NaCl (24 hrs with D_5W). Infuse over 15–30 min.

INDICATIONS/ROUTES/DOSAGE

Note: Schedule injections between meals (to decrease GI effects).

Carcinoid Tumor

IV, SQ: ***(Sandostatin):*** **ADULTS, ELDERLY:** Initial 2 wks, 100–600 mcg/day in 2–4 divided doses. Range: 50–750 mcg.
IM: ***(Sandostatin Lar):*** **ADULTS, ELDERLY:** Must be stabilized on SQ octreotide for at least 2 wks; 20 mg q4wks for 2 mos, then modify based on response. **Maximum:** 30 mg q4wks.

Vasoactive Intestinal Peptic-Secreting Tumor (VIPoma)

IV, SQ: ***(Sandostatin):*** **ADULTS, ELDERLY:** Initial 2 wks, 200–300 mcg/day in 2–4 divided doses. Titrate dose based on response/tolerance. Range: 150–750 mcg.
IM: ***(Sandostatin Lar):*** **ADULTS, ELDERLY:** Must be stabilized on SQ octreotide for at least 2 wks; 20 mg q4wks for 2 mos, then modify based on response. **Maximum:** 30 mg q4wks.

Acromegaly

IV, SQ: ***(Sandostatin):*** **ADULTS, ELDERLY:** Initially, 50 mcg 3 times/day. Increase as needed. Range: 300–1,500 mcg/day. Usual effective dose: 100 mcg 3 times/day.
IM: ***(Sandostatin Lar):*** **ADULTS, ELDERLY:** Must be stabilized on SQ octreotide for at least 2 wks. 20 mg q4wks for 3 mos, then modify based on response. **Maximum:** 40 mg q4wks.

Dosage in Renal/Hepatic Impairment

No dose adjustment.

SIDE EFFECTS

Frequent (10%–6%; 58%–30% in acromegaly pts): Diarrhea, nausea, abdominal discomfort, headache, injection site pain. **Occasional (5%–1%):** Vomiting, flatulence, constipation, alopecia, facial flushing, pruritus, dizziness, fatigue, arrhythmias, ecchymosis, blurred vision. **Rare (less than 1%):** Depression, diminished libido, vertigo, palpitations, dyspnea.

ADVERSE EFFECTS/TOXIC REACTIONS

Increased risk of cholelithiasis. Prolonged high-dose therapy may produce hypothyroidism. GI bleeding, hepatitis, seizures occur rarely.

NURSING CONSIDERATIONS

BASELINE ASSESSMENT

Establish baseline B/P, weight, thyroid function, serum glucose, electrolytes.

INTERVENTION/EVALUATION

Monitor serum glucose, electrolytes, thyroid function. In acromegaly, monitor growth hormone levels. Weigh every 2–3 days, report over 5-lb gain per wk. Monitor B/P, pulse, respirations periodically during treatment. Be alert for decreased urinary output, peripheral edema. Monitor daily pattern of bowel activity, stool consistency.

PATIENT/FAMILY TEACHING

- Therapy should provide significant improvement of severe, watery diarrhea.

ofatumumab

oh-fa-**tue**-mue-mab
(Arzerra)

BLACK BOX ALERT Hepatitis B virus (HBV) reactivation may occur, resulting in hepatitis, hepatic failure, death. Progressive multifocal leukoencephalopathy (PML) resulting in death may occur.

Do not confuse ofatumumab with omalizumab.

CLASSIFICATION

PHARMACOTHERAPEUTIC: Anti-CD20 monoclonal antibody. **CLINICAL:** Antineoplastic.

USES

Treatment of chronic lymphocytic leukemia (CLL) in pts previously untreated, relapsed, or who require extended therapy. Treatment of CLL refractory to fludarabine and alemtuzumab.

PRECAUTIONS

Contraindications: Hypersensitivity to ofatumumab. **Cautions:** Hepatitis B virus infection, conditions predisposing to infection (e.g., diabetes, renal failure, immunocompromised pts, open wounds).

ACTION

Binds to CD20 molecule, the antigen on surface of B-cell lymphocytes; inhibits early-stage B-lymphocyte activation. **Therapeutic Effect:** Controls tumor growth, triggers cell death.

PHARMACOKINETICS

Eliminated through both a target-independent route and a B-cell–mediated route. Due to depletion of B cells, clearance is decreased substantially after subsequent infusions compared with first infusion. **Half-life:** 12–16 days.

LIFESPAN CONSIDERATIONS

Pregnancy/Lactation: Unknown if distributed in breast milk. **Children:** Safety and efficacy not established. **Elderly:** No age-related precautions noted.

INTERACTIONS

DRUG: **Bone marrow depressants (e.g., cladribine)** may increase myelosuppression. **Live virus vaccines** may potentiate virus replication, increase vaccine side effects, decrease pt's antibody response to vaccine. **HERBAL:** **Echinacea** may decrease concentration/effects. **FOOD:** None known. **LAB VALUES:** May decrease neutrophils, platelets.

AVAILABILITY (Rx)

Injection Solution: 100 mg/5 mL, 1000 mg/50 mL.

ADMINISTRATION/HANDLING

IV

ALERT Do not give by IV push or bolus. Use in-line filter supplied with product.

O

Reconstitution • **300-mg dose:** Withdraw and discard 15 mL from 1,000 mL 0.9% NaCl bag. • Withdraw 5 mL from each of 3 single-use 100-mg vials and add to bag. • Gently invert. • **1,000-mg dose:** Withdraw and discard 50 mL from 1,000 mL NaCl bag. Withdraw 50 mL from 1 single-use 1,000-mg vial and add to bag. • Gently invert to mix. **2,000-mg dose:** Withdraw and discard 100 mL from 1,000 mL NaCl bag. Withdraw 50 mL from 2 single-use 1,000-mg vials and add to bag. • Gently invert to mix.

Rate of administration • **Dose 1:** Initiate infusion at rate of 3.6 mg/hr (12 mL/hr). • **Dose 2:** Initiate infusion at rate of 24 mg/hr (12 mL/hr). • **Dose 3–12:** Initiate infusion at rate of 50 mg/hr (25 mL/hr). • If no infusion toxicity, rate of infusion may be increased every 30 min, using following table:

Interval After Start of Infusion (min)	Dose 1 (mL/hr)	Dose 2 (mL/hr)	Doses 3–12 (mL/hr)
0–30	12	12	25
31–60	25	25	50
61–90	50	50	100
91–120	100	100	200
Over 120	200	200	400

Storage • Refrigerate vials. • Diluted solution should be used within first 12 hrs; discard preparation after 24 hrs. • Discard if discoloration is present, but solution may contain visible, translucent-to-white particulates (will be removed by in-line filter).

IV COMPATIBILITIES

Prepare all doses with 0.9% NaCl. Do not mix with dextrose solutions or any other medications.

INDICATIONS/ROUTES/DOSAGE

◀ALERT▶ Premedicate 30 min to 2 hrs before each infusion with acetaminophen, an antihistamine, and a corticosteroid as prophylaxis for infusion reaction. Flush IV line with 0.9% NaCl before and after each dose. Interrupt infusion if infusion reaction of any severity occurs (do not resume for Grade 4 reaction).

CLL (untreated)

IV infusion: ADULTS, ELDERLY: Cycle 1: 300 mg, then 1,000 mg on day 8. Subsequent cycles: 1,000 mg on day 1 q28days. Continue for at least 3 cycles or a maximum of 12 cycles (in combination with chlorambucil).

CLL (refractory)

IV infusion: ADULTS, ELDERLY: Recommended dosage is 12 doses given on the following schedule: 300 mg initial dose (dose 1), followed 1 wk later by 2,000 mg wkly for 7 doses (doses 2–8), followed 4 wks later by 2,000 mg every 4 wks for 4 doses (doses 9–12).

CLL (relapsed)

IV infusion: ADULTS, ELDERLY: 300 mg once on day 1, then 1,000 mg on day 8, then 1,000 mg on day 1 of subsequent 28-day cycles for a maximum of 6 cycles (in combination with fludarabine and cyclophosphamide).

Extended Treatment of CLL

IV infusion: ADULTS, ELDERLY: 300 mg once on day 1, then 1,000 mg on day 8, then 1,000 mg 7 wks later and q8wks thereafter up to a maximum of 2 yrs.

Dosage in Renal/Hepatic Impairment

No dose adjustment.

SIDE EFFECTS

Frequent (20%–14%): Fever, cough, diarrhea, fatigue, rash. **Occasional (13%–5%):** Nausea, bronchitis, peripheral edema, nasopharyngitis, urticaria, insomnia, headache, sinusitis, muscle spasm, hypertension.

ADVERSE EFFECTS/TOXIC REACTIONS

Most common serious adverse reactions were bacterial, viral, fungal infections (including pneumonia and sepsis), septic shock, neutropenia, thrombocytopenia. Infusion reactions occur more frequently with first 2 infusions. Severe infusion reactions manifested as angioedema, bronchospasm, dyspnea, fever, chills, back pain, hypotension. Progressive multifocal leukoencephalopathy may occur. Small bowel obstruction has been noted.

NURSING CONSIDERATIONS

BASELINE ASSESSMENT

Obtain CBC; pregnancy test in females of reproductive potential. Test for hepatitis B virus infection. Screen for active infection. Screen pts at high risk of hepatitis B virus. Assess baseline CBC prior to therapy. Offer emotional support.

INTERVENTION/EVALUATION

Monitor renal function, electrolytes. Monitor CBC for evidence of myelosuppression during therapy, and increase frequency of monitoring in pts who develop Grade 3 or 4 cytopenia. Monitor for blood dyscrasias (fever, sore throat, signs of local infection, unusual bruising/bleeding from any site), symptoms of anemia (excessive fatigue, weakness). Closely monitor for infusion reactions.

PATIENT/FAMILY TEACHING

• Treatment may depress your immune system and reduce your ability to fight infection. Report symptoms of infection such as body aches, chills, cough, fatigue, fever. Avoid those with active infection. • Report symptoms of infusion reactions (e.g., fever, chills, breathing problems, rash); bleeding, bruising, petechiae, worsening weakness or fatigue; new neurologic symptoms (e.g., confusion, loss of balance, vision problems); symptoms of hepatitis (e.g., fatigue, yellow discoloration of skin/eyes); worsening abdominal pain, nausea.

OLANZapine

oh-**lan**-za-peen
(Apo-OLANZapine ✦, ZyPREXA, ZyPREXA Relprevv, ZyPREXA Zydis)

BLACK BOX ALERT
Elderly pts with dementia-related psychosis are at increased risk for mortality due to cerebrovascular events. Sedation (including coma), delirium reported following use of ZyPREXA Relprevv.
Do not confuse OLANZapine with olsalazine or QUEtiapine, or ZyPREXA with CeleXA or ZyrTEC.

FIXED-COMBINATION(S)

Symbyax: OLANZapine/FLUoxetine (an antidepressant): 6 mg/25 mg, 6 mg/50 mg, 12 mg/25 mg, 12 mg/50 mg.

◆CLASSIFICATION

PHARMACOTHERAPEUTIC: Second-generation (atypical) antipsychotic. **CLINICAL:** Antipsychotic.

USES

PO: Management of manifestations of schizophrenia. Treatment of acute mania associated with bipolar I disorder as monotherapy or in combination with lithium or valproate. In combination with FLUoxetine: treatment of depressive episodes associated with bipolar I disorder and treatment of treatment-resistant bipolar depression. Maintenance treatment of bipolar I disorder. **IM: ZyPREXA Intramuscular:** Controls acute agitation in schizophrenia and bipolar mania. **Relprevv:** Long-acting antipsychotic for IM injection for treatment of schizophrenia. **OFF-LABEL:** Prevention of chemotherapy-induced nausea/vomiting. Acute treatment of delirium. Treatment of anorexia nervosa, Tourette's syndrome, tic disorder.

PRECAUTIONS

Contraindications: Hypersensitivity to OLANZapine. **Cautions:** Disorders in which CNS depression is prominent; cardiac disease, hemodynamic instability, prior MI, ischemic heart disease; hyperlipidemia, pts at risk for aspiration pneumonia, decreased GI motility, urinary

O

retention, BPH, narrow-angle glaucoma, diabetes, elderly, pts at risk for suicide, Parkinson's disease, severe renal/hepatic impairment, predisposition to seizures.

ACTION

Antagonizes alpha$_1$-adrenergic, DOPamine, histamine, muscarinic, serotonin receptors. Produces anticholinergic, histaminic, CNS depressant effects. **Therapeutic Effect:** Diminishes psychotic symptoms through combined antagonism of dopamine and serotonin receptors.

PHARMACOKINETICS

Well absorbed after PO administration. Rapid absorption following IM administration. Protein binding: 93%. Widely distributed. Excreted in urine (57%), feces (30%). Not removed by dialysis. **Half-life:** 21–54 hrs.

⌛ LIFESPAN CONSIDERATIONS

Pregnancy/Lactation: Unknown if drug crosses placenta or is distributed in breast milk. **Children:** Safety and efficacy not established. **Elderly:** Use caution. Consider lower starting doses.

O

INTERACTIONS

DRUG: **Alcohol, CNS depressants (e.g., LORazepam, morphine, zolpidem)** may increase CNS depressant effects. **Anticholinergics (e.g., aclidinium, ipratropium, tiotropium, umeclidinium)** may increase anticholinergic effect. **QT-prolonging agents (e.g., amiodarone, haloperidol, moxifloxacin, sotalol)** may cause QT interval prolongation. **HERBAL:** **Herbals with sedative properties (e.g., chamomile, kava kava, valerian)** may increase CNS depression. **FOOD:** None known. **LAB VALUES:** May increase serum GGT, cholesterol, prolactin, ALT, AST.

AVAILABILITY (Rx)

Injection, Powder for Reconstitution: *(ZyPREXA):* 10 mg. **Suspension for IM Injection:** *(Relprevv):* 210 mg, 300 mg, 405 mg. **Tablets:** *(ZyPREXA):* 2.5 mg, 5 mg, 7.5 mg, 10 mg, 15 mg, 20 mg. **Tablets, Orally Disintegrating:** *(ZyPREXA Zydis):* 5 mg, 10 mg, 15 mg, 20 mg.

ADMINISTRATION/HANDLING

PO

• Give without regard to food.

Orally Disintegrating

• Remove by peeling back foil (do not push through foil). • Place in mouth immediately. • Tablet dissolves rapidly with saliva and may be swallowed with or without liquid.

IM (ZyPREXA Intramuscular)

• Reconstitute 10-mg vial with 2.1 mL Sterile Water for Injection to provide concentration of 5 mg/mL. • Use within 1 hr following reconstitution. • Discard unused portion.

IM (Relprevv)

• Dilute to final concentration of 150 mg/mL. • Shake vigorously to mix. • Store at room temperature for up to 24 hrs.

INDICATIONS/ROUTES/DOSAGE

Schizophrenia

Note: Discontinue gradually to avoid withdrawal symptoms and reduce relapse.

PO: **ADULTS, ELDERLY:** Initially, 5–10 mg once daily. May increase to 10 mg/day within 5–7 days. If further adjustments are indicated, may increase by 5 mg/day at 7-day intervals. **Maintenance:** 10–20 mg/day. **Maximum:** 20 mg/day. **CHILDREN 13 YRS AND OLDER:** Initially, 2.5–5 mg/day. Titrate in 2.5- or 5-mg increments at wkly intervals. Target dose: 10 mg. **Maximum:** 20 mg/day.

IM: ***(Long-Acting [Relprevv]):*** **ADULTS, ESTABLISHED ON 10 MG/DAY ORALLY:** 210 mg q2wks for 4 doses or 405 mg q4wks for 2 doses. **Maintenance:** 150 mg q2wks or 300 mg q4wks. **ESTABLISHED ON 15 MG/DAY ORALLY:** 300 mg q2wks for 4 doses. **Maintenance:** 210 mg q2wks or 405 mg q4wks. **ESTABLISHED ON 20 MG/DAY ORALLY:** 300 mg q2wks.

Depression Associated With Bipolar Disorder (with FLUoxetine)

PO: ADULTS, ELDERLY: Initially, 5 mg in evening. May increase dose in 5 mg increments at intervals of q1–7 days based on response and tolerability up to 15 mg/day (adjunctive therapy) or up to 20 mg/day (monotherapy). **CHILDREN 10–17 yrs:** Initially, 2.5 mg once daily in evening. Adjust dose as tolerated.

Treatment-Resistant Depression (with FLUoxetine)

PO: ADULTS, ELDERLY: Initially, 5 mg in evening. May gradually increase dose based on response and tolerability up to 20 mg/day. Range: 5–20 mg/day.

Bipolar Mania

PO: ADULTS, ELDERLY: ***(Monotherapy):*** Initially, 10–15 mg/day. May increase by 5 mg/day at intervals of at least 24 hrs. Range: 5–20 mg/day. **Maximum:** 20 mg/day. ***(In Combination With Lithium or Valproate):*** Initially, 10 mg/day. Range: 5–20 mg/day. **CHILDREN 13 YRS OF AGE AND OLDER:** Initially, 2.5–5 mg/day. Adjust dose by 2.5–5 mg daily to target dose of 10 mg/day. Range: 2.5–20 mg/day.

Dosage for Elderly, Debilitated Pts, Pts Predisposed to Hypotensive Reactions

Initial dosage: 5 mg/day.

Control of Agitation

IM: ADULTS, ELDERLY: ***(Short-Acting):*** Initially, 5–10 mg. Additional doses (up to 10 mg) may be considered. However, allow at least 2 hrs (after initial dose) or 4 hrs (after second dose) to evaluate response. **Maximum:** 30 mg/day.

Dosage in Renal/Hepatic Impairment

No dose adjustment.

SIDE EFFECTS

Frequent (26%–10%): Drowsiness, agitation, insomnia, headache, nervousness, hostility, dizziness, rhinitis. **Occasional (9%–5%):** Anxiety, constipation, nonaggressive atypical behavior, dry mouth, weight gain, orthostatic hypotension, fever, arthralgia, restlessness, cough, pharyngitis, visual changes (dim vision). **Rare:** Tachycardia; back, chest, abdominal, or extremity pain; tremor.

ADVERSE EFFECTS/TOXIC REACTIONS

Rare reactions include seizures, neuroleptic malignant syndrome, a potentially fatal syndrome characterized by hyperpyrexia, muscle rigidity, irregular pulse or B/P, tachycardia, diaphoresis, cardiac arrhythmias. Extrapyramidal symptoms (EPS), dysphagia may occur. Overdose (300 mg) produces drowsiness, slurred speech.

NURSING CONSIDERATIONS

BASELINE ASSESSMENT

Obtain LFT, serum glucose, weight, lipid profile before initiating treatment. Assess behavior, appearance, emotional status, response to environment, speech pattern, thought content. Question history of suicidal ideation and behavior.

INTERVENTION/EVALUATION

Monitor B/P, serum glucose, lipids, LFT. Assess for tremors, changes in gait, abnormal muscular movements, behavior. Supervise suicidal-risk pt closely during early therapy (as depression lessens, energy level improves, increasing suicide potential). Assess for therapeutic response (interest in surroundings, improvement in self-care, increased ability to concentrate, relaxed facial expression). Assist with ambulation if dizziness occurs. Assess sleep pattern. Notify physician if extrapyramidal symptoms (EPS) occur.

PATIENT/FAMILY TEACHING

• Avoid dehydration, particularly during exercise, exposure to extreme heat, concurrent use of medication causing dry mouth, other drying effects. • Take medication as prescribed; do not stop taking or increase dosage. • Slowly go from lying to standing. • Avoid alcohol. • Avoid tasks that require alertness, motor skills until response to drug is established.

O

olaparib

oh-**lap**-a-rib
(Lynparza)

◆CLASSIFICATION

PHARMACOTHERAPEUTIC: PARP inhibitor. **CLINICAL:** Antineoplastic.

USES

Treatment of deleterious or suspected deleterious germline BRCA-mutated advanced ovarian cancer in pts who have been treated with three or more prior lines of chemotherapy. First-line maintenance treatment (in combination with bevacizumab) of advanced epithelial ovarian, fallopian tube, or primary peritoneal cancer in adults who are in complete or partial response to first-line, platinum-based chemotherapy and whose cancer is associated with homologous recombination deficiency (HRD)–positive status. Maintenance treatment of recurrent epithelial ovarian, fallopian tube, or primary peritoneal cancer in adults who are in complete or partial response to platinum-based chemotherapy. Maintenance treatment of adults with recurrent epithelial ovarian, fallopian tube, or primary peritoneal cancer who are in complete or partial response to platinum-based chemotherapy. Treatment of germline BRCA-mutated, HER2-negative metastatic breast cancer in pts who have been treated with chemotherapy. First-line treatment of germline BRCA-mutated metastatic pancreatic cancer in pts whose disease has not progressed on at least 16 wks of first-line, platinum-based chemotherapy. Treatment of deleterious or suspected deleterious germline or somatic homologous recombination repair (HRR) gene–mutated metastatic castration-resistant prostate cancer in adults who have progressed following prior enzalutamide or abiraterone treatment.

PRECAUTIONS

Contraindications: Hypersensitivity to olaparib. **Cautions:** Baseline cytopenias, conditions predisposing to infection (e.g., diabetes, renal failure, immunocompromised pts, open wounds). History of pulmonary disease. Avoid concomitant use of strong or moderate CYP3A inhibitors, strong or moderate CYP3A inducers.

ACTION

Inhibits poly(ADP-ribose) polymerase (PARP) enzymes, involved in normal cellular hemostasis (e.g., DNA transcription, cell cycle regulation, and DNA repair). Disrupts cellular homeostasis, resulting in cell death. **Therapeutic Effect:** Inhibits tumor cell growth and metastasis.

PHARMACOKINETICS

Rapidly absorbed. Metabolized in liver. Protein binding: 82%. Peak plasma concentration: 1–3 hrs. Steady-state concentration: 3–4 days. Excreted in urine (44%), feces (42%). **Half-life:** 11.9 hrs.

⌛ LIFESPAN CONSIDERATIONS

Pregnancy/Lactation: Avoid pregnancy; may cause fetal harm. Females of reproductive potential should use effective contraception during treatment and for at least 6 mos after discontinuation. Unknown if distributed in breast milk. **Children:** Safety and efficacy not established. **Elderly:** No age-related precautions noted.

INTERACTIONS

DRUG: Strong CYP3A inhibitors (e.g., clarithromycin, ketoconazole, ritonavir), moderate CYP3A inhibitors (e.g., atazanavir, ciprofloxacin) may increase concentration/effect. **Strong CYP3A inducers (e.g., carBAMazepine), moderate CYP3A inducers (e.g., nafcillin)** may decrease concentration/effect. **HERBAL: Bitter orange** may increase concentration/effect. **FOOD: Grapefruit products,**

Seville oranges may increase concentration/effect. **High-fat food** may delay absorption. **LAB VALUES:** May increase mean corpuscular volume, serum creatinine. May decrease Hct, Hgb, lymphocytes, neutrophils, RBC.

AVAILABILITY (Rx)

Tablets: 100 mg, 150 mg.

ADMINISTRATION/HANDLING

PO

Capsules: • Give without regard to food. • Administer capsules whole; do not break, cut, crush, or open. **Tablets:** May give with or without food. Administer tablet whole; do not break, cut, crush, or divide.

INDICATIONS/ROUTES/DOSAGE

Note: Do not substitute tablets with capsules on a mg to mg basis.

Ovarian Cancer (Advanced, germline or somatic BRCA-mutated), first-line maintenance therapy (monotherapy)

PO: ADULTS, ELDERLY: 300 mg twice daily until disease progression, unacceptable toxicity, or completion of 2 yrs of therapy. Pts with complete response at 2 yrs should discontinue treatment. Pts with evidence of disease at 2 yrs may continue treatment beyond 2 yrs.

Ovarian Cancer (Advanced, recurrent)

PO: ADULTS, ELDERLY: 300 mg twice daily until disease progression or unacceptable toxicity.

Ovarian Cancer (Advanced HRD-positive), First-line Maintenance Therapy (Combination therapy)

PO: ADULTS, ELDERLY: 300 mg twice daily (in combination with bevacizumab). Continue until disease progression, unacceptable toxicity, or completion of 2 yrs of therapy. Pts with a complete response at 2 yrs should discontinue olaparib. Pts with evidence of disease at 2 yrs may continue treatment (beyond 2 years). Bevacizumab duration is for a total of 15 mos.

Breast Cancer (Metastatic, HER2-negative, BRCA-mutated)

PO: ADULTS, ELDERLY: ***(Tablet):*** 300 mg (2 × 150 mg) twice daily. Continue until disease progression or unacceptable toxicity.

Pancreatic Cancer

PO: ADULTS, ELDERLY: 300 mg twice daily until disease progression or unacceptable toxicity.

Dose Modification

Dose Reduction for Adverse Reactions

PO: ADULTS, ELDERLY: Interrupt treatment until resolved. Then decrease to 200 mg twice daily. If further dose reduction is indicated, decrease to 100 mg twice daily.

Concomitant Use of Strong CYP3A Inhibitors

PO: ADULTS, ELDERLY: 150 mg twice daily.

Concomitant Use of Moderate CYP3A Inhibitors

PO: ADULTS, ELDERLY: 200 mg twice daily.

Dosage in Renal Impairment

Mild impairment: No dose adjustment. **Moderate to severe impairment:** Not specified; use caution.

Dosage in Hepatic Impairment

Not specified; use caution.

SIDE EFFECTS

Frequent (66%–21%): Fatigue, asthenia, nausea, vomiting, abdominal pain, diarrhea, dyspepsia, decreased appetite, headache, back pain, rash, myalgia, arthralgia, musculoskeletal pain, dysgeusia, cough.

ADVERSE EFFECTS/TOXIC REACTIONS

Myelodysplastic syndrome/acute myeloid leukemia reported in 2% of pts. Pneumonitis, including fatal cases, occurred in less than 1% of pts. Respiratory tract infections including nasopharyngitis, pharyngitis, upper respiratory tract infection occurred in 43% of pts.

O

NURSING CONSIDERATIONS

BASELINE ASSESSMENT

Obtain CBC. Do not initiate therapy until pts have recovered from hematologic toxicities caused by previous chemotherapy. Question history of pulmonary disease. Receive full medication history and screen for interactions. Offer emotional support.

INTERVENTION/EVALUATION

Monitor CBC monthly. For prolonged hematologic toxicities, interrupt treatment and monitor CBC wkly until recovery. If hematologic levels have not recovered to CTCAE Grade 1 or 0 after 4 wks of treatment interruption, consider hematology consultation for further investigations such as bone marrow analysis and blood sample for cytogenetics. Monitor for myelodysplastic syndrome/acute myeloid leukemia, pneumonitis. Monitor for infections (cough, fatigue, fever).

PATIENT/FAMILY TEACHING

• Treatment may depress your immune system and reduce your ability to fight infection. Report symptoms of infection such as body aches, burning with urination, chills, cough, fatigue, fever. Avoid those with active infection. • Report symptoms of bone marrow depression such as bruising, fatigue, fever, shortness of breath, weight loss; bleeding easily, bloody urine or stool. • Report new or worsening respiratory symptoms such as cough, difficulty breathing, fever, wheezing; may indicate severe lung inflammation. • Do not ingest grapefruit product, Seville oranges. • Do not take herbal products. • Use effective contraception to avoid pregnancy. Do not breastfeed.

olmesartan

TOP 100

ol-me-**sar**-tan
(Benicar, Olmetec ✱)

BLACK BOX ALERT May cause fetal injury, mortality. Discontinue as soon as possible once pregnancy is detected.

Do not confuse Benicar with Mevacor.

FIXED-COMBINATION(S)

Azor: olmesartan/amLODIPine (calcium channel blocker): 20 mg/5 mg, 40 mg/5 mg, 20 mg/10 mg, 40 mg/10 mg. **Benicar HCT:** olmesartan/hydroCHLOROthiazide (a diuretic): 20 mg/12.5 mg, 40 mg/12.5 mg, 40 mg/25 mg. **Tribenzor:** olmesartan/hydroCHLOROthiazide/amLODIPine: 20 mg/12.5 mg/5 mg, 40 mg/12.5 mg/5 mg, 40 mg/25 mg/5 mg, 40 mg/12.5 mg/10 mg, 40 mg/25 mg/10 mg.

◆CLASSIFICATION

PHARMACOTHERAPEUTIC: Angiotensin II receptor antagonist. **CLINICAL:** Antihypertensive.

USES

Treatment of hypertension alone or in combination with other antihypertensives.

PRECAUTIONS

Contraindications: Hypersensitivity to olmesartan. Concomitant use with aliskiren in pts with diabetes. **Cautions:** Renal impairment, unstented unilateral or bilateral renal arterial stenosis, significant aortic/mitral stenosis. Concurrent potassium supplements; pts who are volume depleted.

ACTION

Blocks vasoconstrictor, aldosterone-secreting effects of angiotensin II by inhibiting binding of angiotensin II to AT_1 receptors in vascular smooth muscle. **Therapeutic Effect:** Causes vasodilation, decreases peripheral resistance, decreases B/P.

PHARMACOKINETICS

Moderately absorbed after PO administration. Hydrolyzed in GI tract to olmesartan. Protein binding: 99%. Excreted in urine (35%–50%), remainder in feces. Not removed by hemodialysis. **Half-life:** 13 hrs.

LIFESPAN CONSIDERATIONS

Pregnancy/Lactation: Unknown if distributed in breast milk. **Children:** Safety and efficacy not established in children younger than 6 yrs of age. **Elderly:** No age-related precautions noted.

INTERACTIONS

DRUG: **NSAIDs (e.g., ibuprofen, naproxen)** may decrease antihypertensive effect. **Aliskiren** may increase hyperkalemic effect. May increase adverse effects of **ACE inhibitors (e.g., benazepril, lisinopril).** **HERBAL:** **Herbals with hypertensive properties (e.g., licorice, yohimbe) or hypotensive properties (e.g., garlic, ginger, ginkgo biloba)** may alter effects. **FOOD:** None known. **LAB VALUES:** May slightly decrease Hgb, Hct. May increase serum BUN, creatinine, bilirubin, ALT, AST.

AVAILABILITY (Rx)

Tablets: 5 mg, 20 mg, 40 mg.

ADMINISTRATION/HANDLING

PO

- Give without regard to food.

INDICATIONS/ROUTES/DOSAGE

Hypertension

PO: ADULTS, ELDERLY: Initially, 20 mg/day. May increase to 40 mg/day after 2 wks. Lower initial dose may be necessary in pts receiving volume-depleting medications (e.g., diuretics). **CHILDREN 6–16 YRS, WEIGHING 20 TO LESS THAN 35 KG:** Initially, 10 mg once daily. Range: 10–20 mg once daily. **WEIGHING 35 KG OR MORE:** Initially, 20 mg once daily. Range: 20–40 mg once daily. Use with caution.

Dosage in Renal/Hepatic Impairment

Use caution.

SIDE EFFECTS

Occasional (3%): Dizziness. **Rare (less than 2%):** Headache, diarrhea, upper respiratory tract infection.

ADVERSE EFFECTS/TOXIC REACTIONS

Overdosage may manifest as hypotension, tachycardia. Bradycardia occurs less often. Rare cases of rhabdomyolysis have been reported.

NURSING CONSIDERATIONS

BASELINE ASSESSMENT

Obtain B/P immediately before each dose in addition to regular monitoring (be alert to fluctuations). If excessive reduction in B/P occurs, place pt in supine position, feet slightly elevated. Question for possibility of pregnancy. Assess medication history (esp. diuretics).

INTERVENTION/EVALUATION

Assess B/P for hypertension, hypotension. Maintain hydration. Assess for upper respiratory infection. Assist with ambulation if dizziness occurs. Monitor serum potassium level.

PATIENT/FAMILY TEACHING

• Maintain adequate hydration. • Avoid pregnancy. • Avoid tasks that require alertness, motor skills until response to drug is established (possible dizziness effect). • Report symptoms of infection (sore throat, fever). • Therapy requires lifelong control, diet, exercise.

olodaterol

oh-loe-**da**-ter-ol

(Striverdi Respimat)

BLACK BOX ALERT Long-acting $beta_2$-adrenergic agonists (LABA) increase risk of asthma-related deaths. Not indicated for treatment of asthma.

Do not confuse olodaterol with albuterol, indacaterol, formoterol, or salmeterol.

FIXED-COMBINATION(S)

Stiolto Respimat: olodaterol/tiotropium (bronchodilator): 2.5 mcg/2.5 mcg.

O

◆CLASSIFICATION

PHARMACOTHERAPEUTIC: Sympathomimetic (beta$_2$-adrenergic agonist). **CLINICAL:** Bronchodilator.

USES

Long-term, once-daily maintenance bronchodilator treatment of airflow obstruction in pts with chronic obstructive pulmonary disease (COPD), including chronic bronchitis and emphysema. Not indicated in asthma, acute deterioration of COPD.

PRECAUTIONS

Contraindications: Hypersensitivity to olodaterol. Asthma without use of long-term asthma control medication, history of hypersensitivity to sympathomimetics. **Cautions:** Diabetes, cardiovascular disorders (e.g., coronary insufficiency, arrhythmias, hypertension, hypertrophic obstructive cardiomyopathy), seizure disorder, hyperthyroidism; history of severe bronchospasm, pts at risk for QTc interval prolongation (congenital long QT syndrome, HF, medications that prolong QTc interval, hypokalemia, hypomagnesemia), electrolyte imbalance.

ACTION

Stimulates beta$_2$-adrenergic receptors in lungs, resulting in relaxation of bronchial smooth muscle. **Therapeutic Effect:** Relieves bronchospasm, reduces airway resistance, improves bronchodilation.

PHARMACOKINETICS

Rapidly absorbed following inhalation. Extensively distributed in tissue. Metabolized in liver. Protein binding: 60%. Peak plasma concentration: 10–20 min. Excreted in urine. **Half-life:** 45 hrs.

⌛ LIFESPAN CONSIDERATIONS

Pregnancy/Lactation: Excretion into breast milk is probable. Breastfeeding not recommended. May interfere with uterine contractility. **Children:** Safety and efficacy not established. **Elderly:** No age-related precaution noted.

INTERACTIONS

DRUG: **Beta blockers (e.g., metoprolol)** may decrease therapeutic effect, cause bronchospasms. **Beta$_2$-adrenergic agonists (e.g., salmeterol)** may potentiate sympathomimetic effects. **Linezolid** may increase hypertensive effect. **HERBAL:** None significant. **FOOD:** None known. **LAB VALUES:** May increase serum glucose. May decrease serum potassium.

AVAILABILITY (Rx)

Inhalation Spray (2.5 mcg/actuation): 28 metered actuations/cartridge with inhaler, 60 metered actuations/cartridge with inhaler.

ADMINISTRATION/HANDLING

Inhalation

• While taking slow, deep breath through the mouth, press and release button and continue slow inhalation as long as possible. (See manufacturer guidelines for priming instructions and further information.)

INDICATIONS/ROUTES/DOSAGE

COPD

Inhalation: ADULTS, ELDERLY: Two inhalations (2.5 mcg per inhalation for total of 5 mcg) once daily, at same time each day. **Maximum:** 5 mcg within 24-hr period.

Dosage in Renal Impairment

No dose adjustment.

Dosage in Hepatic Impairment

Mild to moderate impairment: No dose adjustment. **Severe impairment:** Use caution.

SIDE EFFECTS

Occasional (11%–4%): Nasopharyngitis, upper respiratory tract infection, bronchitis, cough, back pain. **Rare (3%–2%):** Dizziness, insomnia, dry mouth, arthralgia, urinary retention.

ADVERSE EFFECTS/TOXIC REACTIONS

Life-threatening asthma-related events, bronchospasm, or worsening of

O

COPD-related symptoms have been reported. Serious cardiovascular events including arrhythmias, angina pectoris, cardiac arrest, hypertension, tachycardia; flattening of T wave, prolongation of QTc interval, ST segment depression have occurred. All beta-adrenergic agonists carry risk of hyperglycemia or significant hypokalemia. Pts with severe COPD or hypokalemia have additional increased risk of adverse effects related to hypoxia and concomitant medications.

NURSING CONSIDERATIONS

BASELINE ASSESSMENT

Obtain ABG, capillary glucose, O_2 saturation, serum potassium level, vital signs; ECG, pulmonary function test if applicable. Assess respiratory rate, depth, rhythm. Assess lung sounds for wheezing, rales. Receive full medication history and screen for drug interactions. Question history of asthma, cardiovascular disease, diabetes, long QT syndrome, seizure disorder. Teach proper inhaler priming and administration techniques.

INTERVENTION/EVALUATION

Routinely monitor capillary glucose, O_2 saturation, serum potassium level, vital signs. Auscultate lung sounds. Obtain ECG for palpitation, tachycardia; symptomatic hypokalemia. Recommend discontinuation of short-acting beta$_2$-agonists (use only for symptomatic relief of acute respiratory symptoms). Monitor for hypoglycemia.

PATIENT/FAMILY TEACHING

• Refill prescription when dose indicator on left of inhaler reaches red area of scale. • Follow manufacturer guidelines for proper use of inhaler. • Drink plenty of fluids (decreases lung secretion viscosity). • Rinse mouth with water after inhalation to decrease mouth/throat irritation. • Avoid excessive use of caffeine derivatives (chocolate, coffee, tea, cola). • Report fever, productive cough, body aches, difficulty breathing; may indicate lung infection or worsening of COPD.

omacetaxine

oh-ma-se-**tax**-een
(Synribo)

◆CLASSIFICATION

PHARMACOTHERAPEUTIC: Protein synthesis inhibitor. **CLINICAL:** Antineoplastic.

USES

Treatment of adult pts with chronic or accelerated phase chronic myeloid leukemia (CML) with resistance and/or intolerance to two or more tyrosine kinase inhibitors.

PRECAUTIONS

Contraindications: Hypersensitivity to omacetaxine. **Cautions:** Glucose intolerance, poorly controlled diabetes, elderly, recent GI bleeding. Avoid all use of anticoagulants, aspirin, NSAIDs; all pts with baseline platelets less than 50,000 cells/mm^3.

ACTION

Binds to A-site cleft of ribosomal unit. Interferes with chain elongation and inhibits protein synthesis. **Therapeutic Effect:** Inhibits tumor proliferation and growth during accelerated and chronic stages of CML.

PHARMACOKINETICS

Rapidly absorbed following SQ administration. **Maximum concentration:** 30 min. Protein binding: Less than 50%. Hydrolyzed via plasma esterases. **Half-life:** 6 hrs.

⌛ LIFESPAN CONSIDERATIONS

Pregnancy/Lactation: May cause fetal harm. Not recommended in nursing mothers. Unknown if distributed in breast milk. **Children:** Safety and efficacy not established. **Elderly:** Increased risk for toxicity (e.g., hematologic).

INTERACTIONS

DRUG: **NSAIDs (e.g., ibuprofen, ketorolac, naproxen), anticoagulants**

O

(e.g., heparin, warfarin), aspirin, antiplatelets (e.g., clopidogrel) may increase risk for bleeding. **HERBAL: Echinacea** may decrease levels/effects. **FOOD:** None known. **LAB VALUES:** May decrease platelets, Hgb, Hct, leukocytes, lymphocytes. May increase serum ALT.

AVAILABILITY (Rx)

Injection, Powder for Reconstitution: 3.5-mg vial.

ADMINISTRATION/HANDLING

◀ALERT▶ Must be administered by health care workers trained in proper chemotherapy handling and disposal procedures.

SQ

Reconstitution • Reconstitute with 1 mL 0.9% NaCl. • Gently swirl until powder is completely dissolved. • Inspect vial for particular matter or discoloration. • Reconstituted vial will provide a concentration of 3.5 mg/mL. • Avoid contact with skin.

Storage • Solution should appear clear. • May store solution at room temperature for up to 12 hrs or may refrigerate up to 24 hrs. • Discard unused solution.

INDICATIONS/ROUTES/DOSAGE

Note: If dose is missed, skip dose and resume next regularly scheduled dose.

Chronic or Accelerated Myeloid Leukemia

SQ: ADULTS, ELDERLY: Induction dose: 1.25 mg/m^2 twice daily for 14 consecutive days every 28 days, over 28-day cycle. Continue induction dose until hematologic response achieved. **Maintenance dose:** 1.25 mg/m^2 twice daily for 7 consecutive days every 28 days of a 28-day cycle. Continue until no longer achieving clinical treatment benefit.

Dose Modification

Hematologic toxicity: If neutrophils less than 500 cells/mm^3 or platelets less than 50,000 cells/mm^3, interrupt therapy. Restart when neutrophil count greater than or equal to 1000 cells/mm^3 or platelet count greater than or equal to 50,000 cells/mm^3 and reduce number of dosing days by 2. **Nonhematologic toxicity:** Interrupt therapy until toxicity/adverse effects resolved. Continue indefinitely until pt no longer benefits from therapy.

Dosage in Renal/Hepatic Impairment

No dose adjustment.

SIDE EFFECTS

Chronic Phase

Frequent (45%–25%): Diarrhea, nausea, fatigue, pyrexia, asthenia. **Occasional (20%–11%):** Headache, arthralgia, cough, epistaxis, alopecia, constipation, abdominal pain, peripheral edema, vomiting, back pain, insomnia, rash.

Accelerated Phase

Occasional (19%–7%): Diarrhea, nausea, fatigue, pyrexia, asthenia, vomiting, cough, abdominal pain, chills, anorexia, headache. **Rare (7% or less):** Dyspnea, epistaxis.

ADVERSE EFFECTS/TOXIC REACTIONS

Myelosuppression (leukopenia, lymphopenia neutropenia, thrombocytopenia) is an expected response to therapy, but more severe reactions including bone marrow failure, febrile neutropenia may result in life-threatening events. Pts with neutropenia are at increased risk for infection. Thrombocytopenia may increase risk for intracranial hemorrhage, GI bleeding. Hyperglycemic events including hyperglycemic hyperosmolar nonketotic syndrome (HHNK) may occur. Pts with uncontrolled diabetes are at increased risk for hyperglycemic emergency.

NURSING CONSIDERATIONS

BASELINE ASSESSMENT

Obtain CBC; pregnancy test in females of reproductive potential. Obtain full medication history including herbal products, anticoagulants. Question for history of diabetes, GI bleeding. Offer emotional support.

O

INTERVENTION/EVALUATION

Monitor CBC wkly, then q2wks during maintenance phase. Obtain frequent blood glucose levels, especially in diabetic pts. Monitor LFT if hepatic impairment suspected. If drug exposure occurs, immediately wash affected area with soap and water. Consider isolation protocol if pt develops neutropenia.

PATIENT/FAMILY TEACHING

• Use effective contraception to avoid pregnancy. Do not breastfeed. • Immediately report yellowing of skin or eyes, abdominal pain, bruising, black/tarry stools, dark urine, dehydration, GI bleeding, nausea, vomiting, rash. • Report fever, cough, night sweats, flu-like symptoms, skin changes. • Shortness of breath, pale skin, weakness may indicate bleeding or severe myelosuppression. • Avoid tasks that require alertness, motor skills until response to drug is established.

omalizumab

TOP 100

oh-ma-**liz**-ue-mab
(Xolair)

■ BLACK BOX ALERT ■ Anaphylaxis (severe bronchospasm, hypotension, angioedema, syncope, urticaria) has occurred after first dose and in some cases after 1 yr of regular treatment.

Do not confuse omalizumab with ofatumumab.

CLASSIFICATION

PHARMACOTHERAPEUTIC: Monoclonal antibody. **CLINICAL:** Antiasthmatic.

USES

Treatment of moderate to severe persistent asthma in adults and children 6 yrs of age and older reactive to perennial allergens and with symptoms inadequately controlled with inhaled corticosteroids. Chronic idiopathic urticaria in adults and children 12 yrs and older.

PRECAUTIONS

Contraindications: Hypersensitivity to omalizumab. Do not use to treat acute bronchospasm, status asthmaticus. **Cautions:** Pts at risk for parasitic infections.

ACTION

Selectively binds to human immunoglobulin E (IgE). Inhibits binding of IgE on surface of mast cells, basophils. **Therapeutic Effect:** Prevents/reduces number of asthmatic attacks and corticosteroid use.

PHARMACOKINETICS

Absorbed slowly after SQ administration, with peak concentration in 7–8 days. Excreted primarily via hepatic degradation. **Half-life:** 26 days.

LIFESPAN CONSIDERATIONS

Pregnancy/Lactation: Because IgE is present in breast milk, omalizumab is expected to be present in breast milk. Use only if clearly needed. **Children:** Safety and efficacy not established in pts younger than 6 yrs. **Elderly:** No age-related precautions noted.

INTERACTIONS

DRUG: May enhance the adverse/toxic effects of **belimumab, loxapine. HERBAL: Echinacea** may decrease therapeutic effect. **FOOD:** None known. **LAB VALUES:** May increase serum IgE levels.

AVAILABILITY (Rx)

Injection, Prefilled Syringe: 75 mg/0.5 mL, 150 mg/mL. **Injection, Powder for Reconstitution:** 150 mg/1.2 mL after reconstitution.

ADMINISTRATION/HANDLING

SQ

Reconstitution • Use only Sterile Water for Injection to prepare for SQ administration. • Medication takes 15–20 min to

O

dissolve. • Draw 1.4 mL Sterile Water for Injection into 3-mL syringe with 1-inch, 18-gauge needle; inject contents into powdered vial. • Swirl vial for approximately 1 min (do not shake) and again swirl vial for 5–10 sec every 5 min until no gel-like particles appear in the solution. • Do not use if contents do not dissolve completely within 40 min. • Invert vial for 15 sec (allows solution to drain toward the stopper). • Using new 3-mL syringe with 1-inch 18-gauge needle, obtain required 1.2-mL dose, replace 18-gauge needle with 25-gauge needle for SQ administration.

Rate of administration • SQ administration may take 5–10 sec to administer due to its viscosity.

Storage • Use only clear or slightly opalescent solution; solution is slightly viscous. • Refrigerate. • Reconstituted solution is stable for 8 hrs if refrigerated or within 4 hrs of reconstitution when stored at room temperature.

INDICATIONS/ROUTES/DOSAGE

◀ALERT▶ Give only under direct medical supervision. Should be administered in health care setting by health professionals. Dosage and frequency of administration are based upon total IgE levels and body weight (see table). IgE levels should be measured prior to initiating treatment and not during treatment. Pts should be observed a minimum of 2 hrs following each omalizumab treatment.

Asthma

SQ: ADULTS, ELDERLY, CHILDREN 6 YRS AND OLDER: 75–375 mg every 2 or 4 wks; dose and dosing frequency are individualized based on body weight and pretreatment IgE level (as shown in table). (Consult specific product labeling.)

Chronic Idiopathic Urticaria

SQ: ADULTS, CHILDREN 12 YRS AND OLDER: 150 mg or 300 mg q4wks. Dosing not dependent on IgE level or body weight.

Dosage in Renal/Hepatic Impairment

No dose adjustment.

4-Wk Dosing Table

Pretreatment Serum IgE Levels (units/mL)	Weight 30–60 kg	Weight 61–70 kg	Weight 71–90 kg	Weight 91–150 kg
30–100	150 mg	150 mg	150 mg	300 mg
101–200	300 mg	300 mg	300 mg	See next table
201–300	300 mg	See next table	See next table	See next table

2-Wk Dosing Table

Pretreatment Serum IgE Levels (units/mL)	Weight 30–60 kg	Weight 61–70 kg	Weight 71–90 kg	Weight 91–150 kg
101–200	See preceding table	See preceding table	See preceding table	225 mg
201–300	See preceding table	225 mg	225 mg	300 mg
301–400	225 mg	225 mg	300 mg	Do not dose
401–500	300 mg	300 mg	375 mg	Do not dose
501–600	300 mg	375 mg	Do not dose	Do not dose
601–700	375 mg	Do not dose	Do not dose	Do not dose

SIDE EFFECTS

Frequent (45%–11%): Injection site ecchymosis, redness, warmth, stinging, urticaria, viral infection, sinusitis, headache, pharyngitis. **Occasional (8%–3%):** Arthralgia, leg pain, fatigue, dizziness. **Rare (2%):** Arm pain, earache, dermatitis, pruritus.

ADVERSE EFFECTS/TOXIC REACTIONS

Anaphylaxis, occurring within 2 hrs of first dose or subsequent doses, occurs in 0.1% of pts. Malignant neoplasms occur in 0.5% of pts.

NURSING CONSIDERATIONS

BASELINE ASSESSMENT

Obtain baseline serum total IgE level before initiation of treatment (dosage is based on pretreatment levels). Drug is not for treatment of acute exacerbations of asthma, acute bronchospasm, status asthmaticus.

INTERVENTION/EVALUATION

Monitor rate, depth, rhythm, type of respirations, quality/rate of pulse. Assess lung sounds for rhonchi, wheezing, rales. Observe lips, fingernails for cyanosis.

PATIENT/FAMILY TEACHING

• Increase fluid intake (decreases viscosity of pulmonary secretions). • Do not alter/stop other asthma medications. • Report allergic reactions (e.g., breathing difficulty, swelling of throat/tongue).

ombitasvir/ paritaprevir/ ritonavir/dasabuvir

om-**bit**-as-vir/**par**-i-**ta**-pre-vir/rit-**oh**-na-vir/da-**sa**-bue-vir
(Viekira Pak, Holkira PAK ✱, Viekira XR)

Test all pts for hepatitis B virus (HBV) infection prior to initiation. HBV reactivation was reported in HBV/HCV coinfected pts who were undergoing or had completed treatment with hepatitis C virus (HCV) direct-acting antivirals and were not receiving HBV antiviral therapy. HBV reactivation may cause fulminant hepatitis, hepatic failure, and death. Monitor HCV/HBV coinfected pts for hepatitis flare or HBV reactivation during HCV infection and as clinically indicated.

Do not confuse ombitasvir with daclatasvir, or paritaprevir with boceprevir or simeprevir, or ritonavir with Retrovir, lopinavir, darunavir, or saquinavir, or dasabuvir with sofosbuvir.

◆ CLASSIFICATION

PHARMACOTHERAPEUTIC: NS5A inhibitor, protease inhibitor, CYP3A inhibitor, nonnucleoside inhibitor. **CLINICAL:** Antihepaciviral.

USES

Treatment of adults with chronic hepatitis C virus (HCV) infection genotype 1a without cirrhosis or with compensated cirrhosis (in combination with ribavirin), and genotype 1b without cirrhosis or with compensated cirrhosis.

PRECAUTIONS

Contraindications: Hypersensitivity to any component. Moderate to severe hepatic impairment; decompensated hepatic cirrhosis; contraindication or known hypersensitivity to ribavirin; concomitant use of strong CYP3A inducers, strong CYP2C8 inducers or strong CYP2C8 inhibitors; drugs highly dependent on CYP3A for clearance and for which elevated plasma concentrations are associated with serious and/or life-threatening events. Concurrent use of alfuzosin, carBAMazepine, colchicine, dronedarone, efavirenz, ergotamine, dihydroergotamine, ethinyl estradiol–containing drugs including combined oral contraceptives, gemfibrozil, lovastatin, lurasidone, midazolam

O

(oral), phenytoin, PHENobarbital, pimozide, ranolazine, rifAMPin, sildenafil (when used for pulmonary arterial hypertension), simvastatin, St. John's wort, triazolam. **Cautions:** History of anemia, hepatitis B virus infection, HIV infection.

ACTION

Ombitasvir inhibits HCV NS5A needed for essential RNA replication and virion assembly. Paritaprevir inhibits HCV protease needed for cleavage of HCV-encoded polyproteins and viral replication. Ritonavir inhibits CYP3A clearance; increases plasma concentrations of paritaprevir. Dasabuvir inhibits HCV RNA-dependent RNA polymerase needed for replication of viral genome. **Therapeutic Effect:** Inhibits viral replication of hepatitis C virus.

PHARMACOKINETICS

Readily absorbed. Paritaprevir, ritonavir, dasabuvir metabolized in liver. Ombitasvir metabolized by amide hydrolysis. Protein binding: ombitasvir: greater than 99%, paritaprevir: 97%–99%, ritonavir: 99%, dasabuvir: 99%. Peak plasma concentration: 4–5 hrs. Steady-state concentration: 12 days. Elimination: ombitasvir: feces (92%), urine (2%); paritaprevir: feces (88%), urine (9%); ritonavir: feces (86%), urine (11%); dasabuvir: feces (94%), urine (2%). **Half-life:** Ombitasvir: 21–25 hrs; paritaprevir: 5.5 hrs; ritonavir: 4 hrs; dasabuvir: 5.5–6 hrs.

O

LIFESPAN CONSIDERATIONS

Pregnancy/Lactation: Avoid pregnancy; may cause fetal harm. When administered with ribavirin, therapy is contraindicated in pregnant women and in men whose female partners are pregnant. Unknown if distributed in breast milk. Concomitant use of ethinyl estradiol–containing drugs is contraindicated. Alternative contraception methods including progestin-only drugs, barrier methods, abstinence are recommended. **Children:** Safety and efficacy not established. **Elderly:** No age-related precautions noted.

INTERACTIONS

DRUG: May increase concentration/effects of **antiarrhythmics (e.g., amiodarone), antifungals (e.g., itraconazole), calcium channel blockers (e.g., amLODIPine, NIFEdipine), corticosteroids (e.g., fluticasone), immunosuppressants (e.g., cycloSPORINE), digoxin, HIV antiretrovirals (e.g., paritaprevir, rilpivirine), phosphodiesterase-5 inhibitors (e.g., sildenafil), sedative/hypnotics (e.g., temazepam), statins (e.g., atorvastatin, simvastatin), sirolimus, tacrolimus. Anticonvulsants (e.g., carBAMazepine, phenytoin), dexamethasone, efavirenz, omeprazole, rifAMPin** may decrease concentration/effect. **HERBAL: St. John's wort** may decrease concentration/effect. **Kava kava** may increase risk of hepatotoxicity. **Red yeast** may increase risk of myopathy, rhabdomyolysis. **Meals** increase absorption. **FOOD: Grapefruit products, Seville oranges** may increase concentration/effect. **LAB VALUES:** May increase serum alkaline phosphatase, ALT, INR. May decrease Hct, Hgb.

AVAILABILITY (Rx)

Fixed-Dose Combination Tablets (Co-packaged with dasabuvir tablets): ***(Viekira Pak):*** Ombitasvir 12.5 mg/paritaprevir 75 mg/ritonavir 50 mg; dasabuvir 250 mg. ***(Viekira XR):*** Ombitasvir 8.33 mg/paritaprevir 50 mg/ritonavir 33.3 mg/dasabuvir 200 mg.

ADMINISTRATION/HANDLING

PO

• Give with food. Do not cut, crush, break, or divide XR tablets.

INDICATIONS/ROUTES/DOSAGE

Hepatitis C Virus Infection

PO: ADULTS, ELDERLY: ***(Viekira Pak):*** 2 tablets of ombitasvir, paritaprevir, ritonavir once daily, plus 1 tablet of dasabuvir twice daily with or without ribavirin. ***(Viekira XR):*** 3 tablets once daily.

Treatment Regimen and Duration

Genotype 1a, without cirrhosis (in combination with ribavirin); genotype 1b without cirrhosis or compensated cirrhosis: Fixed-combination regimen with ribavirin for 12 wks. **Recommended dose of ribavirin based on weight in kg: LESS THAN 75 KG:** 1,000 mg/day in 2 divided doses. **75 KG OR GREATER:** 1,200 mg/day in 2 divided doses. For ribavirin dose modifications, refer to prescribing information.

Dose Modification

Liver Transplant Recipients

PO: ADULTS, ELDERLY: 2 tablets of ombitasvir, paritaprevir, ritonavir once daily, plus 1 tablet of dasabuvir twice daily with ribavirin for 24 wks, irrespective of HCV genotype 1 subtype in pts with normal hepatic function and mild fibrosis.

HCV/HIV-1 Coinfection

Follow dose recommendations as listed in Treatment Regimen and Duration. Consider suppressive antiretroviral drug therapy during treatment.

Dosage in Renal Impairment

No dose adjustment.

Dosage in Hepatic Impairment

Mild impairment: No dose adjustment. **Moderate impairment:** Treatment not recommended. **Severe impairment:** Treatment contraindicated.

SIDE EFFECTS

Frequent (34%–22%): Fatigue, nausea. **Occasional (18%–14%):** Pruritus, rash, erythema, eczema, allergic dermatitis, skin exfoliation, urticaria, photosensitivity reaction, skin ulcer, insomnia, asthenia.

ADVERSE EFFECTS/TOXIC REACTIONS

HBV reactivation was reported in pts coinfected with HBV/HVC; may result in fulminant hepatitis, hepatic failure, death. Serum ALT greater than 5 times upper limit of normal (ULN) reported in 1% of pts (usually occurred during the first 4 wks of treatment). Elevations of serum ALT were significantly higher in female pts using ethinyl estradiol–containing drugs such as contraceptive patches, combined oral contraceptives, vaginal rings. May increase risk of drug resistance in HCV/HIV-1 coinfected pts using HIV-1 protease inhibitors. Hypersensitivity reaction including angioedema may occur.

NURSING CONSIDERATIONS

BASELINE ASSESSMENT

Obtain CBC, LFT, HCV-RNA level, pregnancy test in females of reproductive potential. Confirm HCV genotype. Test for hepatitis B virus (HBV) infection prior to initiation. Receive full medication history and screen for contraindications/interactions. Ethinyl estradiol–containing contraceptive drugs should be discontinued prior to initiation. Question history as listed in Precautions. To reduce risk of HIV-1 protease inhibitor drug resistance, consider suppressive antiretroviral drug therapy upon initiation.

INTERVENTION/EVALUATION

Monitor LFT periodically during the first 4 wks of treatment, then as clinically indicated thereafter. Discontinue treatment for serum ALT persistently greater than 10 times ULN; serum ALT elevation associated with increase in serum alkaline phosphatase, bilirubin, or INR; hepatic injury. Periodically monitor CBC for anemia, HCV-RNA level for treatment effectiveness. Monitor for abdominal pain, bruising, jaundice, nausea, vomiting; may indicate hepatic injury. Ethinyl estradiol–containing contraceptives may be restarted approx. 2 wks after discontinuation.

PATIENT/FAMILY TEACHING

• Treatment must be used in combination with ribavirin. • Take with meals. • Inform pt of contraindications/adverse effects of therapy. • Do not take newly prescribed medication unless approved by doctor who originally started treatment. Do not take herbal products. • Pregnancy should be avoided when combination regimen is

O

given with ribavirin. Use effective contraception to avoid pregnancy. Do not breastfeed. • Report abdominal pain, bruising easily, dark-colored urine, fatigue, yellowing of the skin or eyes. • Avoid alcohol. • Report skin changes such as rash, peeling, ulcers; allergic reactions such as difficulty breathing, itching, hives, tongue swelling.

omega-3 acid-ethyl esters

TOP 100

oh-**may**-ga 3 **as**-id **eth**-il **es**-ters
(Lovaza, Vascepa)
Do not confuse Lovaza with LORazepam.

CLASSIFICATION

PHARMACOTHERAPEUTIC: Omega-3 fatty acid. **CLINICAL:** Antilipemic agent.

O

USES

Adjunct to diet to reduce very high (500 mg/dL or higher) serum triglyceride levels in adult pts. Dietary supplement for pts with early risk of CAD. **(Vascepa)**: Cardiovascular risk reduction with mild hypertriglyceridemia. **OFF-LABEL:** Treatment of IgA nephropathy.

PRECAUTIONS

Contraindications: Hypersensitivity to omega-3 fatty acids. **Cautions:** Known sensitivity, allergy to fish.

ACTION

Reduces hepatic production of triglyceride-rich very low density lipoproteins (VLDL). **Therapeutic Effect:** Reduces serum triglyceride levels.

PHARMACOKINETICS

Well absorbed following PO administration. Incorporated into phospholipids. **Half-life:** N/A.

LIFESPAN CONSIDERATIONS

Pregnancy/Lactation: Unknown if distributed in breast milk. **Children:** Safety and efficacy not established in pts younger than 18 yrs. **Elderly:** No age-related precautions noted.

INTERACTIONS

DRUG: May increase antiplatelet effect of **antiplatelets (e.g., aspirin, clopidogrel).** May increase anticoagulant effect of **anticoagulants (e.g., warfarin).** **HERBAL:** None significant. **FOOD:** None known. **LAB VALUES:** May increase serum ALT, LDL.

AVAILABILITY (Rx)

Capsules: 500 mg, 1,000 mg.

ADMINISTRATION/HANDLING

PO

• Give without regard to food.

INDICATIONS/ROUTES/DOSAGE

◀ALERT▶ Before initiating therapy, pt should be on standard cholesterol-lowering diet for minimum of 3–6 mos. Continue diet throughout therapy.

Usual Dosage

PO: ADULTS, ELDERLY: (Lovaza): 4 g (4 capsules) once daily or 2 g (2 capsules) twice daily. **(Vascepa):** 2 g (2 [1 gram] capsules or 4 [0.5 g] capsules) twice daily with meals. 4 g/day, given as a single daily dose or twice daily.

Dosage in Renal/Hepatic Impairment

No dose adjustment.

SIDE EFFECTS

Occasional (5%–3%): Eructation, altered taste, dyspepsia. **Rare (2%–1%):** Rash, back pain.

ADVERSE EFFECTS/TOXIC REACTIONS

None known.

NURSING CONSIDERATIONS

BASELINE ASSESSMENT

Assess serum triglyceride level, LFT. Obtain diet history, esp. fat consumption.

INTERVENTION/EVALUATION

Monitor serum triglyceride levels for therapeutic response. Monitor serum ALT, LDL periodically during therapy. Discontinue therapy if no response after 2 mos of treatment.

PATIENT/FAMILY TEACHING

• Continue to adhere to lipid-lowering diet (important part of treatment). • Periodic lab tests are essential part of therapy to determine drug effectiveness.

omeprazole

TOP 100

oh-**mep**-ra-zole
(Losec ✱, PriLOSEC, PriLOSEC OTC)
Do not confuse omeprazole with ARIPiprazole, pantoprazole, or esomeprazole, or PriLOSEC with Plendil, Prevacid, Prinivil, or PROzac.

FIXED-COMBINATION(S)

Yosprala: omeprazole/aspirin (a platelet aggregation inhibitor): 40 mg/81 mg, 40 mg/325 mg. **Zegerid:** omeprazole/sodium bicarbonate (an antacid): 20 mg/1,100 mg, 40 mg/1,100 mg. **Zegerid Powder:** 20 mg/1,680 mg, 40 mg/1,680 mg.

◆CLASSIFICATION

PHARMACOTHERAPEUTIC: Benzimidazole. **CLINICAL:** Proton pump inhibitor.

USES

Short-term treatment (4–8 wks) of erosive esophagitis (diagnosed by endoscopy), symptomatic gastroesophageal reflux disease (GERD) poorly responsive to other treatment. *H. pylori*–associated duodenal ulcer (with amoxicillin and clarithromycin). Long-term treatment of pathologic hypersecretory conditions, treatment of active duodenal ulcer or active benign gastric ulcer. Maintenance healing of erosive esophagitis. **OTC, short-term:** Treatment of frequent, uncomplicated heartburn occurring 2 or more days/wk. **OFF-LABEL:** Prevention/treatment of NSAID-induced ulcers, stress ulcer prophylaxis in critically ill pts.

PRECAUTIONS

Contraindications: Hypersensitivity to omeprazole, other proton pump inhibitors. Concomitant use with products containing rilpivirine. **Cautions:** May increase risk of fractures, gastrointestinal infections. Hepatic impairment, pts of Asian descent.

ACTION

Inhibits hydrogen-potassium adenosine triphosphatase (H^+/K^+ ATP pump), an enzyme on the surface of gastric parietal cells. **Therapeutic Effect:** Increases gastric pH, reduces gastric acid production.

PHARMACOKINETICS

Route	Onset	Peak	Duration
PO	1 hr	2 hrs	72 hrs

Rapidly absorbed from GI tract. Protein binding: 95%. Primarily distributed into gastric parietal cells. Metabolized in liver. Primarily excreted in urine. Unknown if removed by hemodialysis. **Half-life:** 0.5–1 hr (increased in hepatic impairment).

⌛ LIFESPAN CONSIDERATIONS

Pregnancy/Lactation: Unknown if drug crosses placenta or is distributed in breast milk. **Children:** Safety and efficacy not established. **Elderly:** Use caution (bioavailability may be increased).

INTERACTIONS

DRUG: May decrease concentration/effects of **acalabrutinib, atazanavir, bosutinib, cefuroxime, clopidogrel, dasatinib, neratinib.** May increase concentration/effects of **escitalopram,**

O

voriconazole, oral anticoagulants (e.g., warfarin), phenytoin. **HERBAL:** **St. John's wort** may decrease concentration/effects. **FOOD:** None known. **LAB VALUES:** May increase serum alkaline phosphatase, ALT, AST.

AVAILABILITY (Rx)

Oral Suspension: 2.5 mg/packet, 10 mg/packet.

Capsules, Delayed-Release: ***(PriLOSEC):*** 10 mg, 20 mg, 40 mg. **Tablets, Delayed-Release:** ***(PriLOSEC OTC):*** 20 mg.

ADMINISTRATION/HANDLING

PO

• Give before meals (breakfast preferred). • Give whole. Do not break, crush, dissolve, or divide delayed-release forms. • May open capsule, mix with applesauce, and give immediately.

PO (Suspension)

• Following reconstitution, allow to thicken (2–3 min). • Administer within 30 min.

INDICATIONS/ROUTES/DOSAGE

Active Duodenal Ulcer

PO: ADULTS, ELDERLY: 20–40 mg once daily for 4 wks.

Symptomatic GERD

PO: ADULTS, ELDERLY, CHILDREN WEIGHING 20 KG OR MORE: 10 mg once daily. May increase to 20 mg once daily after 4–8 wks if necessary. Discontinue once asymptomatic for 8 wks. **10–19 KG:** 10 mg/day for up to 4 wks. **5–9 KG:** 5 mg/day for up to 4 wks.

Erosive Esophagitis

PO: ADULTS, ELDERLY, CHILDREN WEIGHING 20 KG OR MORE: Treatment: 20–40 mg once daily. Once symptoms are controlled, continue for at least 8 wks. **CHILDREN 1–16 YRS WEIGHING 10–19 KG:** 10 mg/day. **WEIGHING 5–9 KG:** 5 mg/day. **CHILDREN 1–11 MOS WEIGHING 10 KG OR MORE:** 10 mg/day. **WEIGHING 5–9 KG:** 5 mg/day. **WEIGHING 3–4 KG:** 2.5 mg/day. **Maintenance: ADULTS, ELDERLY, CHILDREN WEIGHING 20 KG OR MORE:** 20 mg/day for up to 12 mos (including treatment period). **ASIAN PTS, CHILDREN WEIGHING 10–19 KG:** 10 mg/day. **WEIGHING 5–9 KG:** 5 mg/day.

Pathologic Hypersecretory Conditions

Note: Doses more than 80 mg in divided doses. **PO: ADULTS, ELDERLY:** Initially, 40 mg twice daily. May titrate up to 180 mg/day.

***H. pylori* Duodenal Ulcer**

PO: ADULTS, ELDERLY: 20 mg or 40 mg twice daily as part of an appropriate combination regimen with antibiotics (dose depends on the selected regimen).

Gastric Ulcer

PO: ADULTS, ELDERLY: 20–40 mg once daily for 8 wks.

OTC Use (Frequent heartburn)

PO: ADULTS, ELDERLY: 20 mg/day for 14 days. May repeat after 4 mos if needed.

Dosage in Renal/Hepatic Impairment

No dose adjustment.

SIDE EFFECTS

Frequent (7%): Headache. **Occasional (3%–2%):** Diarrhea, abdominal pain, nausea. **Rare (2%):** Dizziness, asthenia, vomiting, constipation, upper respiratory tract infection, back pain, rash, cough.

ADVERSE EFFECTS/TOXIC REACTIONS

Pancreatitis, hepatotoxicity, interstitial nephritis occur rarely. May increase risk of *C. difficile* infection.

NURSING CONSIDERATIONS

INTERVENTION/EVALUATION

Evaluate for therapeutic response (relief of GI symptoms). Question if GI discomfort, nausea, diarrhea occurs.

PATIENT/FAMILY TEACHING

• Report headache, onset of black, tarry stools, diarrhea, abdominal pain. • Avoid alcohol. • Swallow capsules whole; do not chew, crush, dissolve, or divide. • Take before eating.

ondansetron

on-**dan**-se-tron
(Zofran)
Do not confuse ondansetron with dolasetron, granisetron, or palonosetron, or Zofran with Zantac or Zosyn.

CLASSIFICATION

PHARMACOTHERAPEUTIC: Selective 5-HT_3 receptor antagonist. **CLINICAL:** Antinausea, antiemetic.

USES

Prevention/treatment of nausea/vomiting due to cancer chemotherapy (including high-dose CISplatin). Prevention and treatment of postop nausea, vomiting. Prevention of radiation-induced nausea, vomiting. **OFF-LABEL:** Breakthrough treatment of nausea and vomiting associated with chemotherapy, hyperemesis gravidarum.

PRECAUTIONS

Contraindications: Hypersensitivity to ondansetron, other HT_3 antagonists. Concomitant use of apomorphine. **Cautions:** Mild to moderate hepatic impairment, pts at risk for QT prolongation or ventricular arrhythmia (congenital long QT prolongation, medications prolonging QT interval, hypokalemia, hypomagnesemia).

ACTION

Blocks serotonin, both peripherally on vagal nerve terminals and centrally in chemoreceptor trigger zone. **Therapeutic Effect:** Prevents nausea/vomiting.

PHARMACOKINETICS

Readily absorbed from GI tract. Protein binding: 70%–76%. Metabolized in liver. Primarily excreted in urine. Unknown if removed by hemodialysis. **Half-life:** 3–6 hrs (increased in hepatic impairment).

LIFESPAN CONSIDERATIONS

Pregnancy/Lactation: Unknown if drug crosses placenta or is distributed in breast milk. **Children:** Safety and efficacy not established in children younger than 1 mo. **Elderly:** No age-related precautions noted.

INTERACTIONS

DRUG: **Apomorphine** may cause profound hypotension, altered LOC. **QT interval–prolonging medications (e.g., amiodarone, azithromycin, ciprofloxacin, haloperidol)** may increase risk of QT interval prolongation, torsades de pointes. **HERBAL:** **St. John's wort** may decrease concentration. **FOOD:** None known. **LAB VALUES:** May transiently increase serum bilirubin, ALT, AST.

AVAILABILITY (Rx)

Injection Solution: ***(Zofran):*** 2 mg/mL. **Oral Solution:** 4 mg/5 mL. **Tablets:** ***(Zofran):*** 4 mg, 8 mg, 24 mg. **Tablets, Orally Disintegrating:** 4 mg, 8 mg.

ADMINISTRATION/HANDLING

IV

Reconstitution • May give undiluted. • For IV infusion, dilute with 50 mL D_5W or 0.9% NaCl before administration.
Rate of administration • Give IV push over 2–5 min. • Give IV infusion over 15–30 min.
Storage • Store at room temperature. • Stable for 48 hrs at room temperature following dilution.

IM

• Inject undiluted into large muscle mass.

PO

• Give without regard to food.

Orally Disintegrating Tablets

• Do not remove from blister pack until needed. • Peel backing off; do not push through. • Place tablet on tongue; allow to dissolve. • Swallow with saliva.

O

Oral Soluble Film

• Keep film in pouch until ready to use. • Remove film strip from pouch and place on top of tongue; allow to dissolve. • Swallow after film dissolves. Do not chew or swallow film whole. • If using more than one, each should be allowed to dissolve before administering the next one.

IV INCOMPATIBILITIES

Acyclovir (Zovirax), allopurinol (Aloprim), amphotericin B (Fungizone), amphotericin B complex (Abelcet, AmBisome, Amphotec), ampicillin (Polycillin), ampicillin and sulbactam (Unasyn), cefepime (Maxipime), 5-fluorouracil, LORazepam (Ativan), meropenem (Merrem IV), methylPREDNISolone (SOLU-Medrol).

IV COMPATIBILITIES

CARBOplatin (Paraplatin), CISplatin (Platinol), cyclophosphamide (Cytoxan), cytarabine (Cytosar), dacarbazine (DTIC-Dome), DAUNOrubicin (Cerubidine), dexmedetomidine (Precedex), dexamethasone (Decadron), diphenhydrAMINE (Benadryl), DOCEtaxel (Taxotere), DOPamine (Intropin), etoposide (VePesid), gemcitabine (Gemzar), heparin, HYDROmorphone (Dilaudid), ifosfamide (Ifex), magnesium, mannitol, mesna (Mesnex), methotrexate, metoclopramide (Reglan), mitoMYcin (Mutamycin), mitoXANTRONE (Novantrone), morphine, PACLitaxel (Taxol), potassium chloride, teniposide (Vumon), topotecan (Hycamtin), vinBLAStine (Velban), vinCRIStine (Oncovin), vinorelbine (Navelbine).

INDICATIONS/ROUTES/DOSAGE

Chemotherapy-Induced Nausea/Vomiting

IV: ADULTS, ELDERLY, CHILDREN 6 MOS AND OLDER: 0.15 mg/kg (**Maximum:** 16 mg/dose).

PO: ADULTS, ELDERLY: 8 mg twice daily with first dose administered prior to chemotherapy.

Prevention of Postop Nausea/Vomiting

IV, IM: ADULTS, ELDERLY, CHILDREN OLDER THAN 12 YRS: 4 mg as a single dose. **CHILDREN 1 MO–12 YRS WEIGHING MORE THAN 40 KG:** 4 mg as a single dose. **CHILDREN 1 MO–12 YRS WEIGHING 40 KG OR LESS:** 0.1 mg/kg as a single dose.

PO: ADULTS, ELDERLY: 8 mg 1 hr before induction of anesthesia.

Prevention of Radiation-Induced Nausea/Vomiting

IV: ADULTS, ELDERLY: 8 mg or 0.15 mg/kg (maximum: 16 mg) once or twice daily 1–2 hrs prior to each fraction of radiation (give with dexamethasone).

PO: 8 mg once or twice daily 1–2 hrs prior to each fraction of radiation (give with dexamethasone).

Dosage in Renal Impairment

No dose adjustment.

Dosage in Hepatic Impairment

Mild to moderate impairment: No dose adjustment. **Severe impairment: Maximum daily dose:** 8 mg.

SIDE EFFECTS

Frequent (13%–5%): Anxiety, dizziness, drowsiness, headache, fatigue, constipation, diarrhea, hypoxia, urinary retention. **Occasional (4%–2%):** Abdominal pain, xerostomia, fever, feeling of cold, redness/pain at injection site, paresthesia, asthenia (loss of strength, energy). **Rare (1%):** Hypersensitivity reaction (rash, pruritus), blurred vision.

ADVERSE EFFECTS/TOXIC REACTIONS

Hypertension, acute renal failure, GI bleeding, respiratory depression, coma, extrapyramidal effects occur rarely. QT interval prolongation, torsades de pointes may occur.

NURSING CONSIDERATIONS

BASELINE ASSESSMENT

Assess degree of nausea, vomiting. Assess for dehydration if excessive vomiting occurs (poor skin turgor, dry mucous membranes, longitudinal furrows in tongue). Provide emotional support.

INTERVENTION/EVALUATION

Monitor ECG in pts with electrolyte abnormalities (e.g., hypokalemia, hypomagnesemia), HF, bradyarrhythmias, concurrent use of other medications that may cause QT prolongation, pts receiving high doses or frequent doses. Provide supportive measures. Assess mental status. Assess bowel sounds for peristalsis. Monitor daily pattern of bowel activity, stool consistency. Record time of evacuation.

PATIENT/FAMILY TEACHING

• Relief from nausea/vomiting generally occurs shortly after drug administration. • Avoid alcohol, barbiturates. • Report persistent vomiting. • Avoid tasks that require alertness, motor skills until response to drug is established (may cause drowsiness, dizziness).

oseltamivir

TOP 100

oh-sel-**tam**-i-veer
(Tamiflu)
Do not confuse Tamiflu with Thera-flu.

CLASSIFICATION

PHARMACOTHERAPEUTIC: Neuraminidase inhibitor. **CLINICAL:** Antiviral.

USES

Symptomatic treatment of uncomplicated acute illness caused by influenza A or B virus in adults and children 2 wks of age and older who are symptomatic no longer than 2 days. Prevention of influenza in adults, children.

PRECAUTIONS

Contraindications: Hypersensitivity to oseltamivir. **Cautions:** Renal impairment.

ACTION

Selective inhibitor of influenza virus neuraminidase, an enzyme essential for viral replication. Acts against influenza A and B viruses. **Therapeutic Effect:** Suppresses spread of infection within respiratory system, reduces duration of clinical symptoms.

PHARMACOKINETICS

Readily absorbed after PO administration. Protein binding: 3%. Metabolized in liver. Primarily excreted in urine. **Half-life:** 6–10 hrs.

LIFESPAN CONSIDERATIONS

Pregnancy/Lactation: Unknown if distributed in breast milk. **Children:** Safety and efficacy not established in pts younger than 2 wks. **Elderly:** No age-related precautions noted.

INTERACTIONS

DRUG: **Live attenuated influenza virus vaccine intranasal** may interfere with effect. **HERBAL:** None significant. **FOOD:** None known. **LAB VALUES:** None significant.

AVAILABILITY (Rx)

Capsules: 30 mg, 45 mg, 75 mg. **Powder for Oral Suspension:** 6 mg/mL.

ADMINISTRATION/HANDLING

PO

• Give without regard to food. • May open capsules and mix with sweetened liquid. • Oral suspension stable for 10 days (room temperature) or 17 days (refrigerated) following reconstitution.

INDICATIONS/ROUTES/DOSAGE

Treatment of Influenza

Note: Hospitalized pts may require longer treatment course. Initiate within 48 hrs of onset of symptoms. Consider duration longer than 5 days in pts with severe or complicated influenza.

PO: ADULTS, ELDERLY, CHILDREN 13 YRS AND OLDER: 75 mg twice daily for 5 days. **CHILDREN 1–12 YRS, WEIGHING MORE THAN 40 KG:** 75 mg twice daily for 5 days. **WEIGHING 24–40 KG:** 60 mg twice daily for 5 days. **WEIGHING 16–23 KG:** 45 mg twice daily for 5 days. **WEIGHING 15 KG OR LESS:** 30 mg twice daily for 5

O

days. **NEONATES, INFANTS AGES 2 WKS TO YOUNGER THAN 1 YR:** 3 mg/kg twice daily for 5 days.

Prevention of Influenza

Note: Initiate within 48 hrs of contact with an infected individual. Duration: 7–10 days (longer during community outbreaks).

PO: ADULTS, ELDERLY, CHILDREN 13 YRS AND OLDER: 75 mg once daily. **CHILDREN 1–12 YRS, WEIGHING MORE THAN 40 KG:** 75 mg once daily. **WEIGHING 24–40 KG:** 60 mg once daily. **WEIGHING 15–23 KG:** 45 mg once daily. **WEIGHING LESS THAN 15 KG:** 30 mg once daily. **INFANTS 9–11 MOS:** 3.5 mg/kg/dose. **INFANTS 3–8 MOS:** 3 mg/kg/dose.

Dosage in Renal Impairment

CrCl 31–60 mL/min: Treatment: 30 mg twice daily. Prevention: 30 mg once daily. **CrCl 11–30 mL/min:** Treatment: 30 mg once daily. Prevention: 30 mg every other day. **End-stage renal disease:** Not recommended.

Dosage in Hepatic Impairment

No dose adjustment.

SIDE EFFECTS

Frequent (10%–7%): Nausea, vomiting, diarrhea. **Rare (2%–1%):** Abdominal pain, bronchitis, dizziness, headache, cough, insomnia, fatigue, vertigo.

ADVERSE EFFECTS/TOXIC REACTIONS

Colitis, pneumonia, tympanic membrane disorder, fever occur rarely.

NURSING CONSIDERATIONS

BASELINE ASSESSMENT

Confirm presence of influenza A or B virus.

INTERVENTION/EVALUATION

Monitor for improvement of flu-like symptoms.

PATIENT/FAMILY TEACHING

• Begin as soon as possible from first appearance of flu symptoms (recommended within 2 days from symptom onset). • Avoid contact with those who are at high risk for influenza. • Not a substitute for flu shot.

osimertinib

oh-sim-**er**-ti-nib
(Tagrisso)

Do not confuse osimertinib with afatinib, dasatinib, erlotinib, ibrutinib, imatinib, olaparib, or ospemifene, or Tagrisso with Targretin or Tasigna.

CLASSIFICATION

PHARMACOTHERAPEUTIC: Epidermal growth factor receptor (EGFR) inhibitor. Tyrosine kinase inhibitor. **CLINICAL:** Antineoplastic.

USES

Treatment of pts with metastatic epidermal growth factor receptor (EGFR) T790M mutation-positive non–small-cell lung cancer (NSCLC), as detected by FDA-approved test, who have progressed on or after EGFR therapy. First-line treatment of metastatic NSCLC in pts with EGFR exon 19 deletions or exon 21 L858R mutations.

PRECAUTIONS

Contraindications: Hypersensitivity to osimertinib. **Cautions:** Baseline cytopenias, COPD, heart disease (bradycardia, cardiomyopathy, heart block, HF, recent MI), conditions predisposing to infection (e.g., diabetes, renal failure, immunocompromised pts, open wounds), pts at risk for QTc interval prolongation or ventricular arrhythmia (congenital long QT syndrome, history for QT prolongation, medications that prolong QT interval, hypokalemia, hypomagnesemia); history of CVA, pulmonary embolism. Concomitant use of CYP3A inducers.

ACTION

Exhibits antitumor activity by irreversibly binding to mutant forms of EGFR.

Therapeutic Effect: Inhibits tumor cell growth and metastasis.

PHARMACOKINETICS

Widely distributed. Metabolized in liver. Protein binding: Likely high. Peak plasma concentration: 3–24 hrs (median: 6 hrs). Steady state reached in 15 days. Excreted in feces (68%), urine (14%). **Half-life:** 48 hrs.

LIFESPAN CONSIDERATIONS

Pregnancy/Lactation: Avoid pregnancy; may cause fetal harm. Females of reproductive potential should use effective contraception during treatment and for at least 6 wks after discontinuation. Males with female partners of reproductive potential must use effective barrier methods during treatment and at least 4 mos after discontinuation. Unknown if distributed in breast milk. Breastfeeding not recommended during treatment and for up to 2 wks after discontinuation. May impair fertility in both females and males. **Children:** Safety and efficacy not established. **Elderly:** May have increased risk of Grade 3 or 4 adverse events. May require more frequent dose modifications.

INTERACTIONS

DRUG: **QTc interval–prolonging medications (e.g., amiodarone, FLUoxetine, haloperidol, sotalol)** may increase risk of QTc prolongation. **Strong CYP3A inducers (e.g., carBAMazepine, phenytoin, rifAMPin)** may decrease concentration/effect. **Strong CYP3A inhibitors (e.g., clarithromycin, ketoconazole, ritonavir)** may increase concentration/risk of adverse effects. May decrease the therapeutic effect of **BCG (intravesical), vaccines (live)**. May increase adverse/toxic effects of **belimumab, natalizumab, vaccines (live)**. **HERBAL:** **St. John's wort** may decrease concentration/effect. **Echinacea** may diminish therapeutic effect. **FOOD:** None known. **LAB VALUES:** May decrease serum sodium, magnesium; Hgb, Hct, lymphocytes, neutrophils, platelets, RBCs. May decrease diagnostic effect of *Coccidioides immitis* skin test.

AVAILABILITY (Rx)

Tablets: 40 mg, 80 mg.

ADMINISTRATION/HANDLING

PO

• Tablets are hazardous; use cytotoxic precautions during handling and disposal. Recommend single gloving when handling intact tablets; double gloving, protective gown when handling liquid preparations. • Do not divide, crush, cut, or ultrasonicate tablets. • Give without regard to food. • If a dose is missed, skip missed dose and administer the next dose on schedule. • **Pts with dysphagia:** Disperse tablet in 60 mL of water (noncarbonated) only. • Stir until dissipated into small pieces (does not completely dissolve). • Deliver orally or via gastric tube. • Rinse container with 120–240 mL of water and administer any remaining drug residue. After oral administration of residue, instruct pt to thoroughly rinse mouth with water and swallow.

O

INDICATIONS/ROUTES/DOSAGE

Non–Small-Cell Lung Cancer

PO: **ADULTS, ELDERLY:** 80 mg once daily. Continue until disease progression or unacceptable toxicity.

Dose Modification

Based on Common Terminology Criteria for Adverse Events (CTCAE).

Cardiac Toxicity

QTc interval greater than 500 msec on at least two separate ECGs: Withhold treatment until QTc interval is less than 481 msec or recovers to baseline. Once resolved, resume at 40 mg once daily. **QTc interval prolongation with symptoms of life-threatening arrhythmia:** Permanently discontinue. **Asymptomatic, absolute decrease in left ventricular ejection fraction (LVEF) of 10% from baseline and below 50%:** Withhold treatment for up to 4 wks. Resume treatment if improved to baseline. If not improved to baseline, permanently discontinue.

Pulmonary Toxicity
Interstitial lung disease/pneumonitis: Permanently discontinue.

Other Toxicities
Any Grade 3 or higher reaction: Withhold treatment for up to 3 wks. Resume treatment at 80 mg once daily or 40 mg once daily if improved to Grade 2 or lower within 3 wks. If not improved within 3 wks, permanently discontinue. **Concomitant use of strong CYP3A4 inducers:** Start dose at 160 mg once daily. May decrease dose to 80 mg once daily if strong CYP3A4 inducer has been discontinued for at least 3 wks.

Dosage in Renal/Hepatic Impairment
Mild to moderate impairment: No dose adjustment. **Severe impairment:** Not specified; use caution.

O

SIDE EFFECTS

Frequent (42%–17%): Diarrhea, rash (generalized, erythematous, macular, maculopapular, papular, pustular), erythema, folliculitis, acne, dermatitis, acneiform dermatitis, dry skin, eczema, skin fissures, xerosis, nail disorders (inflammation, tenderness, discoloration, dystrophy, infection, ridging, onychoclasis, onycholysis, onychomadesis, paronychia), dry eye, blurry vision, keratitis, cataract, eye irritation, blepharitis, eye pain, increased lacrimation, vitreous floaters, nausea. **Occasional (16%–10%):** Decreased appetite, constipation, pruritus, cough, fatigue, back pain, stomatitis, headache.

ADVERSE EFFECTS/TOXIC REACTIONS

Myelosuppression (anemia, leukopenia, neutropenia, thrombocytopenia) is an expected response to therapy. Interstitial lung disease/pneumonitis reported in 3% of pts. May cause QTc interval prolongation (up to 3% of pts); cardiac toxicities including cardiomyopathy (1% of pts), decreased LVEF (2% of pts); other adverse effects including CVA, intracranial hemorrhage; pneumonia (4% of pts); venous thromboembolism including pulmonary embolism, jugular venous thrombosis, DVT (7% of pts).

NURSING CONSIDERATIONS

BASELINE ASSESSMENT

Obtain CBC, BMP, serum magnesium; vital signs; ECG. Confirm presence of T790M mutation in tumor specimen prior to initiation. Obtain pregnancy test in females of reproductive potential. Receive full medication history and screen for interactions. Question history of CVA, DVT, pulmonary embolism, pulmonary disease, cardiac disease. Obtain baseline echocardiogram to assess LVEF. Obtain visual acuity. Screen for active infection. Offer emotional support.

INTERVENTION/EVALUATION

Monitor CBC for cytopenias; BMP, serum magnesium for electrolyte abnormalities. Pts with cough, dyspnea, fever, worsening of respiratory status should be investigated for interstitial lung disease/pneumonitis. Pts with sudden chest pain, dyspnea, hypoxia, tachycardia should be evaluated for pulmonary embolism. Monitor for symptoms of DVT (leg or arm pain/swelling); CVA, intracranial hemorrhage (aphasia, altered LOC, facial droop, headache, hemiplegia, seizures). Assess LVEF by echocardiogram q3mos during therapy or more frequently in pts suspected of HF, congestive HF. Assess for eye pain, visual changes. Monitor for skin rash/toxicities, hypersensitivity reaction. Diligently monitor for infection. Monitor daily stool pattern, consistency.

PATIENT/FAMILY TEACHING

• Treatment may depress your immune system and reduce your ability to fight infection. Report symptoms of infection such as body aches, burning with urination, chills, cough, fatigue, fever. Avoid those with active infection. • Report symptoms of bone marrow depression such as bruising, fatigue, fever, shortness of breath, weight loss; bleeding easily, bloody urine or stool. • Report symptoms of abnormal heartbeats (dizziness, fainting, light-headedness, palpitations), heart failure (shortness of breath, fast or slow heart rate, exercise intolerance, swelling of the ankles or legs), severe lung inflammation (difficulty breathing, cough with fever, lung pain). • Use effective contraception to avoid pregnancy. Do not breastfeed. • Treatment may cause blood clots in the arms, legs, lungs, or brain. Immediately report symptoms of stroke (difficulty speaking, confusion, paralysis, vision loss), lung embolism (difficulty breathing, fast heart rate, chest pain), blood clots in the arms or legs (pain/swelling). • Do not take any newly prescribed medications unless approved by doctor who originally started treatment. • Do not take herbal supplements.

oxaliplatin HIGH ALERT

ox-**al**-i-**pla**-tin

BLACK BOX ALERT
Anaphylactic-like reaction may occur within minutes of administration; may be controlled with EPINEPHrine, corticosteroids, antihistamines.

Do not confuse oxaliplatin with Aloxi, CARBOplatin, or CISplatin.

◆CLASSIFICATION

PHARMACOTHERAPEUTIC: Platinum-containing complex. Alkylating agent. **CLINICAL:** Antineoplastic.

USES

Treatment of stage III colon cancer after complete resection of primary tumor (in combination with infusional 5-fluorouracil and leucovorin); treatment of advanced colon cancer (in combination with infusional 5-fluorouracil and leucovorin). **OFF-LABEL:** Treatment of ovarian cancer, pancreatic cancer, hepatobiliary cancer, testicular cancer, esophageal cancer, gastric cancer, non-Hodgkin's lymphoma, chronic lymphocytic leukemia.

PRECAUTIONS

Contraindications: History of allergy to oxaliplatin, other platinum compounds. **Cautions:** Previous therapy with other antineoplastic agents; radiation, renal impairment, pregnancy, immunosuppression, presence or history of peripheral neuropathy, elderly pts.

ACTION

Inhibits DNA replication and transcription by cross-linking with DNA strands. Cell cycle–phase nonspecific. **Therapeutic Effect:** Causes cellular death (apoptosis).

PHARMACOKINETICS

Rapidly distributed. Protein binding: 90%. Undergoes rapid, extensive nonenzymatic biotransformation. Excreted in urine. **Half-life:** 391 hrs.

LIFESPAN CONSIDERATIONS

Pregnancy/Lactation: If possible, avoid use during pregnancy, esp. first trimester. May cause fetal harm. Breastfeeding not recommended. **Children:** Safety and efficacy not established. **Elderly:** Increased incidence of diarrhea, dehydration, hypokalemia, fatigue.

INTERACTIONS

DRUG: Bone marrow depressants (e.g., cladribine) may increase myelosuppression, GI effects. **Live virus vaccines** may potentiate virus replication, increase vaccine side effects, decrease pt's antibody response to vaccine. **HERBAL: Echinacea** may decrease effects. **FOOD:** None known. **LAB VALUES:** May increase serum creatinine,

O

bilirubin, ALT, AST, INR. May prolong prothrombin time.

AVAILABILITY (Rx)

Injection Solution: 5 mg/mL (10-mL, 20-mL vials).

ADMINISTRATION/HANDLING

◀ALERT▶ Wear protective gloves during handling of oxaliplatin. If solution comes in contact with skin, wash skin immediately with soap, water. Do not use aluminum needles or administration sets that may come in contact with drug; may cause degradation of platinum compounds.

◀ALERT▶ Pt should avoid ice, drinking cold beverages, touching cold objects during infusion and for 5 days thereafter (can exacerbate acute neuropathy).

IV

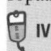

Reconstitution • Dilute with 250–500 mL D_5W (never dilute with sodium chloride solution or other chloride-containing solutions) to final concentration of 0.2–0.6 mg/mL.

Rate of administration • Infuse over 2–6 hrs.

Storage • Do not freeze. • Protect from light. • Store vials at room temperature. • After dilution, solution is stable for 6 hrs at room temperature, 24 hrs if refrigerated.

IV INCOMPATIBILITIES

Do not infuse oxaliplatin with alkaline medications.

IV COMPATIBILITIES

Dexamethasone, diphenhydrAMINE (Benadryl), granisetron (Kytril), ondansetron (Zofran), palonosetron (Aloxi).

INDICATIONS/ROUTES/DOSAGE

Refer to individual protocols.

◀ALERT▶ Pretreat pt with antiemetics. Repeat courses should not be given more frequently than every 2 wks.

Colon Cancer, Advanced

IV: ADULTS: 85 mg/m² q2wks until disease progression or unacceptable toxicity (in combination with fluorouracil/leucovorin).

Colon Cancer, Stage III (adjuvant therapy)

IV: ADULTS: 85 mg/m² q2wks for total of 6 months (in combination with fluorouracil/leucovorin).

Dosage in Renal Impairment

CrCl less than 30 mL/min: Reduce dose to 65 mg/m².

Dosage in Hepatic Impairment

No dose adjustment.

SIDE EFFECTS

Frequent (76%–20%): Peripheral/sensory neuropathy (usually occurs in hands, feet, perioral area, throat but may present as: jaw spasm, abnormal tongue sensation, eye pain, chest pressure, difficulty walking, swallowing, writing), nausea, fatigue, diarrhea, vomiting, constipation, abdominal pain, fever, anorexia. **Occasional (14%–10%):** Stomatitis, earache, insomnia, cough, difficulty breathing, backache, edema. **Rare (7%–3%):** Dyspepsia, dizziness, rhinitis, flushing, alopecia.

ADVERSE EFFECTS/TOXIC REACTIONS

Peripheral/sensory neuropathy can occur without any prior event by drinking or holding a glass of cold liquid during IV infusion. Pulmonary fibrosis (characterized as nonproductive cough, dyspnea, crackles, radiologic pulmonary infiltrates) may warrant drug discontinuation. Hypersensitivity reaction (rash, urticaria, pruritus) occurs rarely.

NURSING CONSIDERATIONS

BASELINE ASSESSMENT

Obtain CBC, renal function test. Question medical history as listed in Precautions. Offer emotional support.

INTERVENTION/EVALUATION

Monitor for decrease in WBC, platelets (myelosuppression is minimal). Monitor daily pattern of bowel activity, stool consistency. Monitor for diarrhea, GI bleeding (bright red, black tarry stool), neuropathy. Pt should avoid ice or drinking, holding glass of cold liquid during IV infusion and for 5 days following completion of infusion; may precipitate/exacerbate neuropathy (occurs within hrs or 1–2 days of dosing, lasts up to 14 days). Maintain strict I&O. Assess oral mucosa for stomatitis.

PATIENT/FAMILY TEACHING

• Promptly report fever, sore throat, signs of local infection, unusual bruising/bleeding from any site, persistent diarrhea, difficulty breathing. • Do not have immunizations without physician's approval (drug lowers resistance). • Avoid contact with those who have recently taken oral polio vaccine. • Avoid cold drinks, ice, cold objects (may produce neuropathy).

OXcarbazepine

ox-kar-**baz**-e-peen
(Oxtellar XR, Trileptal)
Do not confuse OXcarbazepine with carBAMazepine, or Trileptal with TriLipix.

◆CLASSIFICATION

PHARMACOTHERAPEUTIC: Carboxamide derivative, anticonvulsant. **CLINICAL:** Anticonvulsant.

USES

Immediate-Release: Monotherapy, adjunctive therapy in treatment of partial seizures in adults. Monotherapy in children 4 yrs and older, adjunctive therapy in children 2 yrs and older. **Extended-Release:** Treatment of partial seizures in adults and children 6 yrs and older. **OFF-LABEL:** Treatment of neuropathic pain, bipolar disorder.

PRECAUTIONS

Contraindications: Hypersensitivity to OXcarbazepine. **Cautions:** Renal impairment, sensitivity to carBAMazepine, pts at increased risk for suicide.

ACTION

Blocks sodium channels, stabilizing hyperexcited neural membranes, inhibiting repetitive neuronal firing, diminishing synaptic impulses. **Therapeutic Effect:** Prevents seizures.

PHARMACOKINETICS

Completely absorbed from GI tract. Metabolized in liver. Protein binding: 40%. Primarily excreted in urine. **Half-life:** 2 hrs; metabolite, 6–10 hrs.

LIFESPAN CONSIDERATIONS

Pregnancy/Lactation: Crosses placenta. Distributed in breast milk. **Children:** Safety and efficacy not established in children younger than 2 yrs. **Elderly:** Age-related renal impairment may require dosage adjustment.

INTERACTIONS

DRUG: **Alcohol, CNS depressants (e.g., LORazepam, morphine, zolpidem)** may have additive sedative effect. May decrease effectiveness of **oral contraceptives, dolutegravir, doravirine, elvitegravir, rilpivirine, simeprevir, sofosbuvir, tenofovir alafenamide.** May increase serotonergic effect of **selegiline.** May increase concentration, risk of toxicity of **PHENobarbital, phenytoin.** **HERBAL:** None significant. **FOOD:** None known. **LAB VALUES:** May increase serum alkaline phosphatase, ALT, AST. May decrease serum sodium.

AVAILABILITY (Rx)

Oral Suspension: 300 mg/5 mL. **Tablets:** 150 mg, 300 mg, 600 mg.

Tablets, Extended-Release: 150 mg, 300 mg, 600 mg.

ADMINISTRATION/HANDLING

PO

- Give without regard to food. Do not break, crush, dissolve, or divide extended-release tablets. Swallow whole.

INDICATIONS/ROUTES/DOSAGE

Adjunctive Treatment of Seizures

PO: ADULTS, ELDERLY: ***(Immediate-Release):*** Initially, 600 mg/day in 2 divided doses. May increase by up to 600 mg/day at wkly intervals. **Maximum:** 1,200 mg/day. **Usual maintenance dose:** 600 mg twice daily. **ADOLESCENTS:** Initially, 300 mg twice daily. May increase in increments up to 600 mg/day at wkly intervals. **CHILDREN 4–16 YRS:** Initially, 8–10 mg/kg in 2 divided doses. **Maximum:** 600 mg/day. Increase dose slowly over 2 wks. **Maintenance (based on weight): CHILDREN WEIGHING MORE THAN 39 KG:** 1,800 mg/day in 2 divided doses; **CHILDREN WEIGHING 29.1–39 KG:** 1,200 mg/day in 2 divided doses; **CHILDREN WEIGHING 20–29 KG:** 900 mg/day in 2 divided doses. **CHILDREN 2–3 YRS:** Initially, 8–10 mg/kg/day in 2 divided doses. **Maximum:** 600 mg/day in 2 divided doses. Increase dose slowly over 2–4 wks up to a **maximum** of 60 mg/kg/day in 2 divided doses. ***(Extended-Release):*** **ADULTS:** Initially, 600 mg once daily. May increase by 600 mg/day at wkly intervals. Range: 1,200–2,400 mg/day. **ELDERLY:** Initially, 300–450 mg/day. May increase by 300–450 mg/day at wkly intervals to desired clinical response. Range: Up to 2,400 mg/day.

Conversion to Monotherapy

PO: ADULTS, ELDERLY: ***(Immediate-Release):*** 600 mg/day in 2 divided doses (while decreasing concomitant anticonvulsant over 3–6 wks). May increase by 600 mg/day at wkly intervals up to 2,400 mg/day. **CHILDREN 4–16 YRS:** Initially, 8–10 mg/kg/day in 2 divided doses with simultaneous initial reduction of dose of concomitant antiepileptic over 3–6 wks. May increase by maximum of 10 mg/kg/day at wkly intervals (see below for recommended daily dose by weight).

Initiation of Monotherapy

PO: ADULTS, ELDERLY: ***(Immediate-Release):*** 600 mg/day in 2 divided doses. May increase by 300 mg/day every 3 days up to 1,200 mg/day. ***(Extended-Release):*** Initially, 600 mg once daily. May increase by 600 mg/day at wkly intervals up to 1,200–2,400 mg once daily. **CHILDREN 4–16 YRS:** ***(Immediate-Release):*** Initially, 8–10 mg/kg/day in 2 divided doses. Increase at 3-day intervals by 5 mg/kg/day to achieve maintenance dose by weight as follows:

Weight	Dosage
70+ kg	1,500–2,100 mg/day
60–69 kg	1,200–2,100 mg/day
50–59 kg	1,200–1,800 mg/day
41–49 kg	1,200–1,500 mg/day
35–40 kg	900–1,500 mg/day
25–34 kg	900–1,200 mg/day
20–24 kg	600–900 mg/day

Dosage in Renal Impairment

Mild to moderate impairment: No dose adjustment. **CrCl less than 30 mL/min:** Give 50% of normal starting dose, then titrate slowly to desired dose.

Dosage in Hepatic Impairment

Mild to moderate impairment: No dose adjustment. **Severe impairment:** Use caution with immediate-release; not recommended with extended-release.

SIDE EFFECTS

Frequent (22%–13%): Dizziness, nausea, headache. **Occasional (7%–5%):** Vomiting, diarrhea, ataxia (muscular incoordination), nervousness, dyspepsia, constipation. **Rare (4%):** Tremor, rash, back pain, epistaxis, sinusitis, diplopia.

ADVERSE EFFECTS/TOXIC REACTIONS

Clinically significant hyponatremia may occur, manifested as leg cramping, hypotension, cold/clammy skin, increased pulse rate, headache, nausea, vomiting, diarrhea. Suicidal ideation occurs rarely.

NURSING CONSIDERATIONS

BASELINE ASSESSMENT

Review history of seizure disorder (type, onset, intensity, frequency, duration, LOC), drug history (esp. other anticonvulsants). Provide safety precautions; quiet, dark environment.

INTERVENTION/EVALUATION

Assist with ambulation if dizziness, ataxia occur. Assess for visual abnormalities, headache. Monitor serum sodium. Assess for signs of hyponatremia (nausea, malaise, headache, lethargy, confusion). Assess for clinical improvement (decrease in intensity, frequency of seizures). Monitor for worsening depression, suicidal ideation.

PATIENT/FAMILY TEACHING

• Do not abruptly stop taking medication (may increase seizure activity). • Report if rash, nausea, headache, dizziness occurs. • May need periodic blood tests. • Avoid tasks that require alertness, motor skills until response to drug is established. • Avoid alcohol. • May decrease effectiveness of oral contraceptives. • Seek immediate medical attention if thoughts of suicide, new onset or worsening of anxiety, depression, or changes in mood occur.

oxybutynin

ox-i-**bue**-ti-nin
(Ditropan XL, Gelnique, Oxytrol for Women)
Do not confuse oxybutynin with OxyContin.

◆CLASSIFICATION

PHARMACOTHERAPEUTIC: Anticholinergic. **CLINICAL:** Urinary antispasmodic.

USES

Relief of symptoms (urgency, incontinence, frequency, nocturia, urge incontinence) associated with uninhibited neurogenic bladder, reflex neurogenic bladder. **Extended-Release (additional):** Treatment of symptoms associated with detrusor overactivity due to neurologic disorder (e.g., spina bifida).

PRECAUTIONS

Contraindications: Hypersensitivity to oxybutynin. Uncontrolled narrow-angle glaucoma, urinary retention, gastric retention, or conditions with severely decreased GI motility. **Cautions:** Renal/hepatic impairment, bladder outflow obstruction, treated narrow-angle glaucoma, hyperthyroidism, coronary artery disease, HF, hypertension, arrhythmias, prostatic hyperplasia, myasthenia gravis, reduced GI motility, GI obstructive disorder, gastroesophageal reflux.

ACTION

Direct antispasmodic effect on smooth muscle; inhibits action of acetylcholine on smooth muscle. **Therapeutic Effect:** Increases bladder capacity, delays desire to void. Decreases urgency and frequency.

PHARMACOKINETICS

Route	Onset	Peak	Duration
PO	0.5–1 hr	3–6 hrs	6–10 hrs

Rapidly, well absorbed from GI tract. Metabolized in liver. Primarily excreted in urine. Unknown if removed by hemodialysis. **Half-life:** 1–2.3 hrs; metabolite, 7–8 hrs.

⌛ LIFESPAN CONSIDERATIONS

Pregnancy/Lactation: Unknown if drug crosses placenta or is distributed in breast milk. **Children:** No age-related precautions noted in pts older than 5 yrs. **Elderly:** May be more sensitive to anticholinergic effects (e.g., dry mouth, urinary retention).

INTERACTIONS

DRUG: **Medications with anticholinergic action (e.g., aclidinium, ipratropium, tiotropium, umeclidinium)** may increase anticholinergic effects. **HERBAL:** None significant. **FOOD:** None known. **LAB VALUES:** None significant.

AVAILABILITY (Rx)

Syrup: 5 mg/5 mL. **Tablets:** 5 mg. **Topical Gel (10%):** ***(Gelnique):*** 100 mg/unit dose sachet. **Transdermal:** ***(Oxytrol for Women):*** 3.9 mg/24 hrs.

Tablets, Extended-Release: 5 mg, 10 mg, 15 mg.

ADMINISTRATION/HANDLING

PO

• Give without regard to food. • Extended-release tablet must be swallowed whole; do not break, crush, dissolve, or divide.

Transdermal

• Apply patch to dry, intact skin on abdomen, hip, buttock. • Use new application site for each new patch; avoid reapplication to same site within 7 days. • Normal exposure to water (e.g., bathing, swimming) should not affect patch.

Topical Gel

• **Gelnique:** Apply contents of 1 sachet once daily to dry, intact skin on abdomen, upper arms/shoulders, or thighs. • Do not bathe/shower until 1 hr after gel is applied.

INDICATIONS/ROUTES/DOSAGE

Neurogenic Bladder

PO: ***(Immediate-Release):*** **ADULTS:** 5 mg 2–3 times/day. May increase to 5 mg 4 times/day. **ELDERLY:** 2.5–5 mg 2–3 times/day. **CHILDREN OLDER THAN 5 YRS:** 5 mg twice daily. May increase to 5 mg 3 times/day. **Maximum:** 5 mg 4 times/day.

PO: ***(Extended-Release):*** **ADULTS, ELDERLY:** 5–10 mg/day. May increase by 5-mg increments at wkly intervals. **Maximum:** 30 mg/day. **CHILDREN 6 YRS AND OLDER:** Initially, 5–10 mg once daily. May increase in 5 mg increments at wkly intervals. **Maximum:** 20 mg/day.

Transdermal: **ADULTS:** 3.9 mg applied twice wkly. Apply every 3–4 days.

Topical gel: **ADULTS, ELDERLY:** (10%) 100 mg once daily.

Dosage in Renal/Hepatic Impairment

No dose adjustment.

SIDE EFFECTS

Frequent: Constipation, dry mouth, drowsiness, decreased perspiration. **Occasional:** Decreased lacrimation/salivation, impotence, urinary hesitancy/retention, suppressed lactation, blurred vision, mydriasis, nausea/vomiting, insomnia.

ADVERSE EFFECTS/TOXIC REACTIONS

Overdose produces CNS excitation (nervousness, restlessness, hallucinations, irritability), hypotension/hypertension, confusion, tachycardia, facial flushing, respiratory depression.

NURSING CONSIDERATIONS

BASELINE ASSESSMENT

Assess degree of dysuria, urgency, frequency, incontinence. Question medical history as listed in Precautions.

INTERVENTION/EVALUATION

Monitor for symptomatic relief. Monitor I&O; palpate bladder for urine retention. Monitor daily pattern of bowel activity, stool consistency.

PATIENT/FAMILY TEACHING

• Avoid alcohol. • May cause dry mouth (sugarless candy/gum may reduce effect). • Avoid tasks that require alertness, motor skills until response to drug is established (may cause drowsiness). • Avoid strenuous activity in warm environment.

oxyCODONE

TOP 100 HIGH ALERT

ox-ee-**koe**-done
(Oxaydo, Oxy CONTIN, OxyIR ✱, Roxicodone, Supeudol ✱, Xtampza ER)

BLACK BOX ALERT **OxyContin (controlled-release):** Not intended as an "as needed" analgesic or for immediate postop pain control. Extended-release should not be crushed, broken, or chewed (otherwise leads to rapid release and absorption of potentially fatal dose). Be alert to signs of abuse, misuse, and diversion. May cause potentially life-threatening respiratory depression. Prolonged use during pregnancy can cause neonatal withdrawal syndrome. Use of CYP3A4 inhibitors may increase effects/cause fatal respiratory depression.

Do not confuse oxyCODONE with HYDROcodone, oxybutynin, or oxyMORphone, OxyCONTIN with MS Contin or oxybutynin, or Roxicodone with Roxanol.

FIXED-COMBINATION(S)

Combunox: oxyCODONE/ibuprofen (an NSAID): 5 mg/400 mg. **Endocet:** oxyCODONE/acetaminophen (a nonnarcotic analgesic): 5 mg/325 mg, 7.5 mg/325 mg, 7.5 mg/500 mg, 10 mg/325 mg, 10 mg/650 mg. **Magnacet:** oxyCODONE/acetaminophen (a nonnarcotic analgesic): 2.5 mg/400 mg, 7.5 mg/400 mg, 10 mg/400 mg. **Percocet:** oxyCODONE/acetaminophen: 2.5 mg/325 mg, 5 mg/325 mg, 5 mg/500 mg, 7.5 mg/325 mg, 7.5 mg/500 mg, 10 mg/325 mg, 10 mg/650 mg. **Percocet, Roxicet, Tylox:** oxyCODONE/acetaminophen (a nonnarcotic analgesic): 5 mg/500 mg. **Percodan:** oxyCODONE/aspirin (a nonnarcotic analgesic): 2.25 mg/325 mg, 4.5 mg/325 mg. **Targiniq ER:** oxyCODONE/naloxone (opioid antagonist): 10 mg/5 mg, 20 mg/10 mg, 40 mg/20 mg. **Troxyca ER:** oxyCODONE/naltrexone (an opioid antagonist): 10 mg/1.2 mg, 20 mg/2.4 mg, 30 mg/3.6 mg, 40 mg/4.8 mg, 60 mg/7.2 mg, 9.6 mg/80 mg. **Xartemis XR:** oxyCODONE/acetaminophen (nonnarcotic analgesic): 7.5 mg/325 mg.

◆CLASSIFICATION

PHARMACOTHERAPEUTIC: Opioid agonist (Schedule II). **CLINICAL:** Analgesic.

USES

Immediate-Release: Relief of acute or chronic, moderate to severe pain (usually in combination with nonopioid analgesics). **Extended-Release:** Around-the-clock management of moderate to severe pain when continuous analgesic is needed.

PRECAUTIONS

Contraindications: Hypersensitivity to oxyCODONE. Acute or severe bronchial asthma, hypercarbia, paralytic ileus (known or suspected), GI obstruction, significant respiratory depression. **Extreme Caution:** CNS depression, anoxia, hypercapnia, respiratory depression, seizures, acute alcoholism, shock, untreated myxedema, respiratory dysfunction. **Cautions:** Elevated ICP, hepatic/renal impairment, coma, debilitated pts, head injury, biliary tract disease, toxic psychosis, acute abdominal conditions, hypothyroidism, prostatic hypertrophy, Addison's disease, urethral stricture, COPD, elderly, history of drug abuse and misuse, drug-seeking behavior, dependency.

ACTION

Binds with opioid receptors within CNS, causing inhibition of ascending pain pathway. **Therapeutic Effect:** Alters perception of and emotional response to pain.

PHARMACOKINETICS

Route	Onset	Peak	Duration
PO (immediate-release)	10–15 min	0.5–1 hr	3–6 hrs

O

Route	Onset	Peak	Duration
PO (controlled-release)	10–15 min	0.5–1 hr	Up to 12 hrs

Moderately absorbed from GI tract. Protein binding: 38%–45%. Widely distributed. Metabolized in liver. Excreted in urine. Unknown if removed by hemodialysis. **Half-life:** 2–3 hrs (5 hrs controlled-release).

LIFESPAN CONSIDERATIONS

Pregnancy/Lactation: Readily crosses placenta. Distributed in breast milk. Respiratory depression may occur in neonate if mother received opiates during labor. Regular use of opiates during pregnancy may produce withdrawal symptoms in neonate (irritability, excessive crying, tremors, hyperactive reflexes, fever, vomiting, diarrhea, yawning, sneezing, seizures). **Children:** Paradoxical excitement may occur. Pts younger than 2 yrs are more susceptible to respiratory depressant effects. **Elderly:** Age-related renal impairment may increase risk of urinary retention. May be more susceptible to respiratory depressant effects.

INTERACTIONS

DRUG: **Alcohol, other CNS depressants (e.g., LORazepam, gabapentin, zolpidem)** may increase CNS effects, respiratory depression, hypotension. **Strong CYP3A4 inhibitors (clarithromycin, ketoconazole, ritonavir)** may increase concentration, toxicity. **Strong CYP3A4 inducers (carBAMazepine, phenytoin, rifAMPin)** may decrease concentration/effect. **MAOIs** may produce serotonin syndrome, a severe, sometimes fatal reaction. **HERBAL:** **Herbals with sedative properties (e.g., chamomile, kava kava, valerian)** may increase CNS depression. **St. John's wort** may decrease concentration/effect. **FOOD:** **Grapefruit products** may increase potential for respiratory depression. **LAB VALUES:** May increase serum amylase, lipase.

AVAILABILITY (Rx)

◀ALERT▶ New formulation of controlled-release is intended to prevent medication from being cut, broken, chewed, crushed, or dissolved to reduce risk of overdose due to tampering, snorting, or injection.

Capsules: 5 mg. **Oral Concentrate:** 20 mg/mL. **Oral Solution:** 5 mg/5 mL. **Tablets:** 5 mg, 10 mg, 15 mg, 20 mg, 30 mg. **Tablets, Abuse Deterrent:** ***(Oxaydo):*** 5 mg, 7.5 mg.

Capsules, Extended-Release: ***(Xtampza):*** 9 mg, 13.5 mg, 18 mg, 27 mg, 36 mg. **Tablets, Controlled-Release 12-Hour Abuse Deterrent:** ***(OxyCONTIN):*** 10 mg, 15 mg, 20 mg, 30 mg, 40 mg, 60 mg, 80 mg.

ADMINISTRATION/HANDLING

PO

- Give without regard to food.
- **Controlled-release:** Swallow whole; do not break, crush, dissolve, or divide.

INDICATIONS/ROUTES/DOSAGE

Note: All doses should be titrated to desired effect. Do not abruptly discontinue in physically dependent pts. **Discontinuation:** ***(Immediate-Release):*** Reduce dose by 25%–50% q2–4 days while monitoring for withdrawal; ***(Extended-Release):*** Gradually titrate downward.

Analgesia

PO: ***(Immediate-Release):*** **ADULTS, ELDERLY:** Initially, 5–15 mg q4–6h as needed. Range: 5–20 mg/dose. **CHILDREN (GREATER THAN 6 MOS) 50 KG OR GREATER:** Initially, 5–10 mg q4–6h. **Maximum:** 20 mg/dose. **LESS THAN 50 KG:** 0.1–0.2 mg/kg/dose q4–6h. **Maximum dose range:** 5–10 mg.

Opioid Naive

PO: ***(Controlled-Release):*** **ADULTS, ELDERLY:** ***(Tablets):*** Initially, 10 mg q12h. ***(Capsules):*** Initially, 9 mg q12h.

◀ALERT▶ To convert from other opioids or nonopioid analgesics to oxyCODONE controlled-release, refer to OxyCONTIN package insert. Dosages are reduced in pts with severe hepatic disease.

Dosage in Renal/Hepatic Impairment

Use caution. Titrate carefully.

SIDE EFFECTS

◀ALERT▶ Effects are dependent on dosage amount. Ambulatory pts, pts not in severe pain may experience dizziness, nausea, vomiting, hypotension more frequently than those in supine position or having severe pain. **Frequent:** Drowsiness, dizziness, hypotension (including orthostatic hypotension), anorexia. **Occasional:** Confusion, diaphoresis, facial flushing, urinary retention, constipation, dry mouth, nausea, vomiting, headache. **Rare:** Allergic reaction, depression, paradoxical CNS hyperactivity, nervousness in children, paradoxical excitement, restlessness in elderly, debilitated pts.

ADVERSE EFFECTS/TOXIC REACTIONS

Overdose results in respiratory depression, skeletal muscle flaccidity, cold/clammy skin, cyanosis, extreme drowsiness progressing to seizures, stupor, coma. Hepatotoxicity may occur with overdose of acetaminophen component of fixed-combination product. Tolerance to analgesic effect, physical dependence may occur with repeated use. **Antidote:** Naloxone (see Appendix J for dosage).

NURSING CONSIDERATIONS

BASELINE ASSESSMENT

Assess onset, type, location, duration of pain. Effect of medication is reduced if full pain recurs before next dose. Obtain vital signs before giving medication. If respirations are 12/min or less (20/min or less in children), withhold medication, contact physician. Assess for potential of abuse/misuse (e.g., drug-seeking behavior, mental health conditions, history of substance abuse).

INTERVENTION/EVALUATION

Palpate bladder for urinary retention. Monitor daily pattern of bowel activity, stool consistency. Initiate deep breathing, coughing exercises, esp. in pts with pulmonary impairment. Monitor pain relief, respiratory rate, mental status, B/P, level of consciousness. Screen for drug abuse and misuse, drug-seeking behavior

PATIENT/FAMILY TEACHING

• May cause dry mouth, drowsiness. • Avoid tasks that require alertness, motor skills until response to drug is established. • Avoid alcohol. • May be habit forming. • Do not chew, crush, dissolve, or divide controlled-release tablets. • Report severe constipation, absence of pain relief.

oxytocin HIGH ALERT

ox-ee-**toe**-sin

(Pitocin)

■ BLACK BOX ALERT ■ Not to be given for elective labor induction, but can be used when there is a clear medical indication for induction.

Do not confuse Pitocin with Pitressin.

◆CLASSIFICATION

PHARMACOTHERAPEUTIC: Uterine smooth muscle stimulant. **CLINICAL:** Oxytocic agent.

USES

Antepartum: Induction of labor in pts with medical indication (e.g., at or near term), to stimulate reinforcement of labor, as adjunct in managing incomplete or inevitable abortion. **Postpartum:** To produce uterine contractions during third stage of labor and to control postpartum bleeding/hemorrhage.

PRECAUTIONS

Contraindications: Hypersensitivity to oxytocin. Adequate uterine activity that fails to progress, cephalopelvic disproportion, fetal distress without imminent delivery, grand multiparity, hyperactive or hypertonic uterus, obstetric emergencies

O

that favor surgical intervention, prematurity, unengaged fetal head, unfavorable fetal position/presentation, when vaginal delivery is contraindicated (e.g., active genital herpes infection, invasive cervical cancer, placenta previa, cord presentation). **Cautions:** Induction of labor should be for medical, not elective, reasons. Generally not recommended in fetal distress, hydramnios, partial placental previa, predisposition to uterine rupture.

ACTION

Activates receptors that trigger increase in intracellular calcium levels in uterine myofibrils; increases prostaglandin production. **Therapeutic Effect:** Stimulates uterine contractions.

PHARMACOKINETICS

Route	Onset	Peak	Duration
IV	Immediate	N/A	1 hr
IM	3–5 min	N/A	2–3 hrs

Rapidly absorbed through nasal mucous membranes. Protein binding: 30%. Distributed in extracellular fluid. Metabolized in liver, kidney. Primarily excreted in urine. **Half-life:** 1–6 min.

LIFESPAN CONSIDERATIONS

Pregnancy/Lactation: Used as indicated, not expected to present risk of fetal abnormalities. Small amounts in breast milk. Breastfeeding not recommended. **Children/Elderly:** Not used in these pt populations.

INTERACTIONS

DRUG: **Dinoprostone, misoprostol** may increase adverse effects. **HERBAL:** None significant. **FOOD:** None known. **LAB VALUES:** None significant.

AVAILABILITY (Rx)

Injection: ***(Pitocin):*** 10 units/mL. **Injection Solution:** 30 units/500 mL.

ADMINISTRATION/HANDLING

IV

Reconstitution • Dilute 10–40 units (1–4 mL) in 1,000 mL of 0.9% NaCl, lactated Ringer's, or D_5W to provide concentration of 10–40 milliunits/mL solution.

Rate of administration • Give by IV infusion (use infusion device to carefully control rate of flow as ordered by physician).

Storage • Store at room temperature.

IV INCOMPATIBILITIES

No known incompatibilities via Y-site administration.

IV COMPATIBILITIES

Heparin, insulin (regular), multivitamins, potassium chloride, zidovudine.

INDICATIONS/ROUTES/DOSAGE

Induction or Stimulation of Labor

IV: ADULTS: 0.5–1 milliunit/min. May gradually increase in increments of 1–2 milliunits/min q30–60 minutes until desired contraction pattern is established. Rates greater than 9–10 milliunits/min are rarely required.

Abortion

IV: ADULTS: (Midterm elective abortion): 10–20 milliunits/min. **Maximum:** 30 units/12-hr dose. **(Incomplete, inevitable, or elective abortion):** 10 units as IV infusion after suction or a sharp curettage.

Control of Postpartum Bleeding

IV infusion: ADULTS: 5–10 units may be given initially and can be followed by a maintenance infusion of 10–40 units in 1,000 mL IV fluid at rate sufficient to sustain uterine contractions and control uterine atony.

IM: ADULTS: 10 units (total dose) after delivery.

O

Dosage in Renal/Hepatic Impairment
No dose adjustment.

SIDE EFFECTS

Occasional: Tachycardia, premature ventricular contractions, hypotension, nausea, vomiting. **Rare: Nasal:** Lacrimation/tearing, nasal irritation, rhinorrhea, unexpected uterine bleeding/contractions.

ADVERSE EFFECTS/TOXIC REACTIONS

Hypertonicity may occur with tearing of uterus, increased bleeding, abruptio placentae (i.e., placental abruption), cervical/vaginal lacerations. **Fetal:** Bradycardia, CNS/brain damage, trauma due to rapid propulsion, low Apgar score at 5 min, retinal hemorrhage occur rarely. Prolonged IV infusion of oxytocin with excessive fluid volume has caused severe water intoxication with seizures, coma, death.

NURSING CONSIDERATIONS

BASELINE ASSESSMENT

Assess baselines for vital signs, B/P, fetal heart rate. Determine frequency, duration, strength of contractions.

INTERVENTION/EVALUATION

Monitor B/P, pulse, respirations, fetal heart rate, intrauterine pressure, contractions (duration, strength, frequency) q15min. Notify physician of contractions that last longer than 1 min, occur more frequently than every 2 min, or stop. Maintain careful I&O; be alert to potential water intoxication. Check for blood loss.

PATIENT/FAMILY TEACHING

- Keep pt, family informed of labor progress.

ozanimod

oh-zan-i-mod
(Zeposia)
Do not confuse ozanimod with fingolimod, or siponimod.

◆CLASSIFICATION

PHARMACOTHERAPEUTIC: Sphingosine 1-phosphate (S1P) receptor modulator. **CLINICAL:** Multiple sclerosis agent.

USES

Treatment of relapsing forms of multiple sclerosis (MS) in adults, including clinically isolated syndrome, relapsing-remitting disease, and active secondary progressive disease.

PRECAUTIONS

Contraindications: Hypersensitivity to ozanimod; recent (within 6 mos) MI; unstable angina; CVA; TIA; decompensated HF requiring hospitalization; NYHA class III/IV HF; sick sinus syndrome; Mobitz type II second- or third-degree AV block (unless pt has functioning pacemaker); severe, untreated sleep apnea; concomitant use of MAOIs. **Cautions:** Baseline lymphopenia; conditions predisposing to infection (e.g., diabetes, immunocompromised pts, renal failure, open wounds); baseline sinus bradycardia; hypertension; altered pulmonary function; pts at risk for developing AV block (congenital heart disease, ischemic heart disease, HF); pts at risk for macular edema (e.g., diabetes, history of uveitis); concomitant use of antiarrhythmics, beta blockers, calcium channel blockers. Not recommended with concomitant QT interval-prolonging medications, strong CYP2C8 inhibitors or inducers, breast cancer resistance protein (BCRP) inhibitors, adrenergic and serotonergic drugs (e.g., SSRI, SNRI, opioids), foods containing high amounts of tyramine. Not recommended in pts with severe active infection, history of cardiac arrest, hepatic impairment, cerebrovascular disease, uncontrolled hypertension.

ACTION

Exact mechanism of action unknown. Binds to S1P receptors 1 and 5, blocking capacity of lymphocytes to move out from lymph nodes, reducing the number of lymphocytes available to the CNS. **Therapeutic Effect:** May involve reduction of lymphocyte migration into the CNS, reducing inflammation.

PHARMACOKINETICS

Widely distributed. Metabolized in liver. Protein binding: 98%. Peak plasma concentration: 6–8 hrs. Excreted in feces (37%), urine (26%). **Half-life:** 21 hrs.

LIFESPAN CONSIDERATIONS

Pregnancy/Lactation: Avoid pregnancy; may cause fetal harm. Females of reproductive potential should use effective contraception during treatment and for at least 3 mos after discontinuation. Unknown if distributed in breast milk. **Children:** Safety and efficacy not established. **Elderly:** Not specified; use caution.

INTERACTIONS

DRUG: **Beta-blockers (e.g., carvedilol, metoprolol), calcium channel blockers (e.g., diltiazem, verapamil), certinib, lacosamide** may increase risk of AV block, bradycardia. **Class III antiarrhythmics (e.g., amiodarone, sotolol)** may increase risk of Torsades de Pointes in pts with baseline sinus bradycardia. **QT-interval prolonging agents (e.g., amiodarone, azithromycin, ciprofloxacin, haloperidol)** may enhance QT prolongation. May decrease therapeutic effect of **BCG (intravesical), vaccines (live) varicella vaccines**. **Strong CYP2C8 inhibitors (e.g., gemfibrozil)** may increase concentration/effect. **Strong CYP2C8 inducers (e.g., rifampin)** may decrease concentration/effect. **MAOIs (e.g., phenelzine, selegiline), SSRIs (e.g., escitalopram, sertraline), SNRIs (e.g., duloxetine, venlafaxine)** may increase risk of hypertensive crisis. **Alemtuzumab** may enhance immunosuppressive effect. May increase adverse/toxic effects of **natalizumab.** HERBAL: **Echinacea** may decrease concentration/effect. FOOD: **Foods or beverages containing high amounts of tyramine (e.g., aged cheese, pickled herring, red wine)** may cause release of norepinephrine, resulting hypertension. LAB VALUES: May increase serum ALT, AST, bilirubin. Expected to cause a dose-dependent reduction in peripheral lymphocyte count to 45% of baseline values.

AVAILABILITY (Rx)

Capsules: 0.23 mg, 0.46 mg, 0.92 mg.

ADMINISTRATION/HANDLING

PO

- Give without regard to meals. Administer capsule whole; do not break, cut, or crush.
- If a dose is missed during the first 2 wks of therapy, reinitiate treatment starting with day 1 of titration regimen. If a dose is missed after the first 2 wks of therapy, continue maintenance regimen.

INDICATIONS/ROUTES/DOSAGE

Multiple Sclerosis

PO: ADULTS: Titration: 0.23 mg once daily on days 1–4, then increase to 0.46 mg once daily on days 5–7, then increase to 0.92 mg once daily on day 8. **Maintenance:** 0.92 mg once daily.

Dosage in Renal Impairment

Mild to severe impairment: No dose adjustment.

Dosage in Hepatic Impairment

Mild to severe impairment: Not recommended.

SIDE EFFECTS

Rare (4%–2%): Orthostatic hypotension, back pain, hypertension, abdominal pain.

ADVERSE EFFECTS/TOXIC REACTIONS

Life-threatening infections (bronchitis, laryngitis, pharyngitis, upper respiratory tract infection, UTI) may occur. Fatal cases of cryptococcal meningitis, disseminated cryptococcal infections were reported. Herpes zoster infections reported in less than 1% of pts. Reactivation of herpes zoster infection may cause varicella zoster meningitis. Progressive multifocal leukoencephalopathy (PML), an opportunistic viral infection of the brain caused by the JC virus, may result in progressive permanent disability and death. Posterior reversible encephalopathy syndrome, a dysfunction of the brain that may evolve into an ischemic CVA or cerebral hemorrhage, may occur. Macular edema reported in less than 1% of pts. Pts with diabetes or history of uveitis are at an increased risk for developing macular edema. May result in transient bradycardia, AV conduction delays. Dose-dependent reductions of pulmonary function (absolute forced expiratory volume over 1 second) were reported. Hepatic injury (transaminitis) reported in 3–5% of pts. Severe exacerbation of disability, including rebound disease, may occur after discontinuation. Malignancies including basal cell carcinoma, breast cancer, melanoma, seminoma may occur. Hypersensitivity reactions including rash, urticaria were reported.

NURSING CONSIDERATIONS

BASELINE ASSESSMENT

Obtain CBC, LFT, ECG. Assess baseline symptoms of MS (e.g., bladder/bowel dysfunction, cognitive impairment, depression, dysphagia, fatigue, gait disorder, numbness/tingling, pain, seizures, spasticity, tremors, weakness). Consultation with a cardiologist is advised in pts with QT interval prolongation greater than 450 msec in males or greater than 470 in females; arrhythmias requiring treatment with Class Ia or Class III antiarrhythmics; ischemic heart disease, HF, recent MI; history of Mobitz type II second- or third-degree AV block, sick sinus syndrome, sino-atrial heart block, cerebrovascular disease, uncontrolled hypertension. Pts without a documented history of vaccination against varicella zoster or a confirmed history of varicella infection (chickenpox) should be tested for antibodies prior to initiation. A full vaccination course for varicella in antibody-negative pts is recommended prior to initiation. If live attenuated vaccine immunization is required, give at least 1 mo prior to initiation. Receive full medication history and screen for interaction. Question history as listed in PRECAUTIONS. Conduct ophthalmologic evaluation of the fundus (including the macula) prior to initiation. Withhold treatment in pts with active infection until resolved.

INTERVENTION/EVALUATION

Obtain LFT if hepatotoxicity (abdominal pain, clay-colored stool, amber or dark colored urine, jaundice, nausea) is suspected. During initiation, bradycardia and AV conduction delay is transient (initial effects lessened by titration). Conduct ophthalmic examination with any change of vision (or at regular intervals in pts with diabetes or history of uveitis). Pts with altered mental status, seizures, visual disturbances, unilateral weakness should be evaluated for cryptococcal meningitis, varicella zoster meningitis, posterior reversible encephalopathy syndrome, PML. Closely monitor for infections (body aches, cough, fever) during treatment and for at least 3 mos after discontinuation. If herpes zoster infection or other serious infection occurs, consider withholding treatment and initiate antimicrobial therapy. Closely monitor for adverse effects if other immunosuppresants are initiated within 3 mos after discontinuation. Monitor B/P for hypertension. Monitor for hypersensitivity reactions,

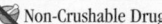

O

new malignancies. Conduct neurological assessment. Assess for symptoms improvement of MS.

PATIENT/FAMILY TEACHING

• Treatment may depress your immune system and reduce your ability to fight infection. Report symptoms of infection such as body aches, burning with urination, chills, cough, fatigue, fever. Avoid those with active infection. Report travel plans to possible endemic areas. • Any changes of vision will require an immediate eye examination. • PML, an opportunistic viral infection of the brain, may cause progressive, permanent disabilities or death. Report symptoms of PML such as confusion, memory loss, paralysis, trouble speaking, loss of vision, seizures, weakness. • Posterior reversible encephalopathy syndrome, a condition resulting in brain swelling and narrowing of blood vessels, may lead to stroke; report confusion, severe headache, loss of vision, seizures, weakness. • Treatment may worsen high blood pressure or cause new cancers. • Report liver problems (abdominal pain, bruising, clay-colored stool, amber or dark colored urine, yellowing of the skin or eyes), lung problems (reduced lung function, shortness of breath), heart arrhythmias (chest pain, dizziness, fainting, palpitations, slow or rapid heart rate, irregular heart rate). • There is a high risk of interactions with other medications. Do not take newly prescribed medications unless approved by prescriber who originally started treatment. • Severe worsening of MS symptoms may occur after stopping treatment. • Avoid foods high in tyramine (aged, cured, fermented, pickled, smoked food).

PACLitaxel

HIGH ALERT

pak-li-**tax**-el
(Abraxane, Apo-**Pacl**itaxel ✱)

■ BLACK BOX ALERT ■ Myelosuppression is a major dose-limiting toxicity. Must be administered by certified chemotherapy personnel. Severe hypersensitivity reactions reported.

Do not confuse PACLitaxel with DOCEtaxel, PARoxetine, or Paxil.

◆CLASSIFICATION

PHARMACOTHERAPEUTIC: Taxane derivative, antimitotic agent. **CLINICAL:** Antineoplastic.

USES

Conventional: Treatment of node-positive breast cancer, metastatic breast cancer after failure of combination therapy or relapse within 6 mos of adjuvant therapy; subsequent therapy for advanced ovarian cancer or as first-line therapy (in combination with CISplatin). Treatment of AIDS-related Kaposi's sarcoma; non–small-cell lung cancer (NSCLC) as first-line therapy (in combination with CISplatin). **Abraxane:** Treatment of breast cancer after failure of combination chemotherapy or relapse within 6 mos of adjuvant chemotherapy. First-line treatment of metastatic adenocarcinoma of pancreas. Treatment of locally advanced or metastatic NSCLC. **OFF-LABEL:** Bladder, cervical, small-cell lung, head and neck cancers. Treatment of adenocarcinoma. **Abraxane:** Recurrent/persistent ovarian, fallopian tube, primary peritoneal cancers.

PRECAUTIONS

Contraindications: Hypersensitivity to PACLitaxel. Hypersensitivity to drugs developed with Cremophor EL (polyoxyethylated castor oil). Treatment of solid tumors with baseline neutrophil count less than 1,500 cells/mm^3; treatment of Kaposi's sarcoma with baseline neutrophil count less than 1,000 cells/mm^3. **Cautions:** Baseline cytopenias, cardiovascular disease, pulmonary disease, conditions predisposing to infection (e.g., diabetes, renal failure, immunocompromised pts, open wounds), hepatic impairment, concomitant use of strong CYP3A inhibitors, strong CYP3A inducers.

ACTION

Promotes microtubule assembly by enhancing action of tubulin dimers; stabilizes existing microtubules; inhibits their disassembly; interferes with late G_2 mitotic phase and inhibits cell lication. **Therapeutic Effect:** Inhibits cellular mitosis; suppresses cell proliferation, and modulates immune response.

PHARMACOKINETICS

Does not readily cross blood-brain barrier. Protein binding: 89%–98%. Metabolized in liver. Excreted in feces (71%), urine (14%). Not removed by hemodialysis. **Half-life:** 3-hr infusion: 13.1–20.2 hrs; 24 hr infusion. 15.7–52.7 hrs.

⌛ LIFESPAN CONSIDERATIONS

Pregnancy/Lactation: Avoid pregnancy; may cause fetal harm. Females of reproductive potential must use effective contraception during treatment and for at least 6 mos after discontinuation. Breastfeeding not recommended during treatment and for at least 2 wks after discontinuation. May impair fertility in both females and males. **Males:** Males with female partners of reproductive potential must use effective contraception during treatment and for at least 3 mos after discontinuation. **Children:** Safety and efficacy not established. **Elderly:** May have increased risk of adverse effects.

INTERACTIONS

DRUG: **Strong CYP3A4 inhibitors (e.g., clarithromycin, ketoconazole, ritonavir)** may increase concentration/effect. **Strong CYP3A4 inducers (e.g., carBAMazepine, phenytoin, rifAMPin)** may decrease effect. **Bone marrow depressants (e.g., cladribine)** may increase myelosuppression. **Strong CYP2C8**

P

inhibitors (e.g., gemfibrozil) may increase concentration/effect. **Live virus vaccines** may potentiate virus replication, increase vaccine side effects, decrease pt's antibody response to vaccine. HERBAL: **Herbals with hypotensive properties (e.g., garlic, ginger, gingko biloba)** may increase effect. **Echinacea** may decrease therapeutic effect. **St. John's wort** may decrease concentration/effect. FOOD: None known. LAB VALUES: May increase serum alkaline phosphatase, bilirubin, ALT, AST, triglycerides.

AVAILABILITY (Rx)

Injection, Powder for Reconstitution (Abraxane): 100-mg vial. **Injection Solution:** 6 mg/mL (5-mL, 16.7-mL, 25-mL, 50-mL vials).

ADMINISTRATION/HANDLING

IV

◄ALERT► Wear gloves during handling; if contact with skin occurs, wash hands thoroughly with soap, water. If contact with mucous membranes occurs, flush with water.

P

PACLitaxel

Reconstitution • Dilute with 250–1,000 mL 0.9% NaCl, D_5W to final concentration of 0.3–1.2 mg/mL.

Rate of administration • Administer at rate per protocol (range: 1–96 hrs) through in-line filter not greater than 0.22 microns. • Monitor vital signs during infusion, esp. during first hour. • Discontinue administration if severe hypersensitivity reaction occurs.

Storage • Store unopened vials at room temperature. • Reconstituted solution is stable at room temperature for 72 hrs. • Store diluted solutions in bottles or plastic bags. Administer through polyethylene-lined administration sets (avoid plasticized PVC equipment or devices).

Abraxane (PACLitaxel—protein bound)

Reconstitution • Reconstitute each vial with 20 mL 0.9% NaCl to provide concentration of 5 mg/mL. • Slowly inject onto inside wall of vial; gently swirl over 2 min to avoid foaming. • Inject appropriate amount into empty PVC-type bag.

Rate of administration • Infuse over 30 min. Do not use in-line filter.

Storage • Store unopened vials at room temperature. • Once reconstituted, use immediately but may refrigerate for up to 8 hrs.

IV INCOMPATIBILITIES

◄ALERT► Data for Abraxane not known; avoid mixing with other medication.

Amphotericin B complex (Abelcet, AmBisome, Amphotec), DOXOrubicin liposomal (Doxil), hydrOXYzine (Vistaril), methylPREDNISolone (SOLU-Medrol), mitoXANTRONE (Novantrone).

IV COMPATIBILITIES

CARBOplatin (Paraplatin), CISplatin (Platinol AQ), cyclophosphamide (Cytoxan), cytarabine (Cytosar), dacarbazine (DTIC-Dome), dexamethasone (Decadron), diphenhydrAMINE (Benadryl), DOXOrubicin (Adriamycin), etoposide (VePesid), gemcitabine (Gemzar), granisetron (Kytril), HYDROmorphone (Dilaudid), lipids, magnesium sulfate, mannitol, methotrexate, morphine, ondansetron (Zofran), potassium chloride, vinBLAStine (Velban), vinCRIStine (Oncovin).

INDICATIONS/ROUTES/DOSAGE

Note: Premedication with dexamethasone, diphenhydrAMINE, and cimetidine, famotidine, or raNITIdine recommended. Refer to individual protocols.

PACLitaxel (Conventional)

Ovarian Cancer

IV: ADULTS, ELDERLY: (Previously treated): 135–175 mg/m²/dose over 3 hrs q3wks. **(Previously untreated):** 175 mg/m² over 3 hrs q3wks (in combination with CISplatin) or 135 mg/m² over 24 hrs q3wks (in combination with CISplatin).

Breast Cancer (Adjuvant)
IV: ADULTS, ELDERLY: 175 mg/m^2 over 3 hrs q3wks for 4 cycles (give sequentially following anthracycline-containing regimen).

Breast Cancer (Metastatic/relapsed)
IV: ADULTS, ELDERLY: 175 mg/m^2 over 3 hrs q3wks.

Non–Small-Cell Lung Cancer
IV: ADULTS, ELDERLY: 135 mg/m^2 over 24 hrs q3wks (in combination with CISplatin) **or** 200 mg/m^2 q3wks for 4 cycles (in combination with pembrolizumab and carboplatin), followed by pembrolizumab maintenance therapy **or** 200 mg/m^2 (175 mg/m^2 for Asian pts) q3wks for 4–6 cycles (in combination with atezolizumab, bevacizumab, and CARBOplatin), followed by atezolizumab/bevacizumab maintenance therapy.

Kaposi's Sarcoma (AIDS-related)
IV: ADULTS, ELDERLY: 135 mg/m^2/dose over 3 hrs q3wks or 100 mg/m^2/dose over 3 hrs q2wks.

Dosage in Renal Impairment
No dose adjustment.

Dosage in Hepatic Impairment

Transaminase Level	Bilirubin	Dose
24-HR INFUSION		
Less than 2 times ULN	1.5 mg/dL or less	135 mg/m^2
2 to less than 10 times ULN	1.5 mg/dL or less	100 mg/m^2
Less than 10 times ULN	1.6–7.5 mg/dL or less	50 mg/m^2
3-HR INFUSION		
Less than 10 times ULN	1.25 mg/dL or less	175 mg/m^2
Less than 10 times ULN	1.26–2 times ULN	135 mg/m^2
Less than 10 times ULN	2.01–5 times ULN	90 mg/m^2
10 times ULN or greater	Greater than 5 times ULN	Avoid use

ULN: upper limit of normal

Dose Modification
Courses of PACLitaxel should be withheld until neutrophil count is 1,500 cells/mm^3 or more, and platelet count is 100,000 cells/mm^3 or more.

Abraxane (Protein bound)
Breast Cancer (metastatic)
IV infusion: ADULTS, ELDERLY: 260 mg/m^2 q3wks **or** 100 mg/m^2 on days 1, 8, 15 of a 28-day cycle (in combination with atezolizumab). Continue until disease progression or unacceptable toxicity.

Dose Modification
Severe neutropenia (ANC less than 500 cells/mm^3 for 1 wk or longer); severe sensory neuropathy: Reduce dose to 220 mg/m^2 for subsequent courses. **Recurrence of severe neutropenia, severe neuropathy:** Reduce dose to 180 mg/m^2 q3wks for subsequent courses. **CTCAE Grade 3 sensory neuropathy:** Hold until resolved to Grade 2 or 1, then reduce dose for subsequent courses. **Dosage of Abraxane for serum bilirubin greater than 1.5 mg/dL:** Dose unknown.

NSCLC (Locally advanced or metastatic)
IV: ADULTS, ELDERLY: 100 mg/m^2 on days 1, 8, 15 of each 21-day cycle (in combination with CARBOplatin) **or** 100 mg/m^2 on days 1, 8, 15 of a 28-day cycle (in combination with atezolizumab and CARBOplatin) for 4–6 cycles, followed by atezolizumab maintenance therapy **or** 100 mg/m^2 on days 1, 8, 15 of a 28-day cycle (in combination with pembrolizumab and CARBOplatin) for 4 cycles, followed by pembrolizumab maintenance therapy.

Adenocarcinoma of Pancreas (Metastatic) (in combination with gemcitabine)
IV: ADULTS, ELDERLY: 125 mg/m^2 on days 1, 8, 15 of each 28-day cycle (in combination with gemcitabine).

Dosage in Renal Impairment
No dose adjustment.

Dosage in Hepatic Impairment

	Mild Impairment (AST less than 10 times upper limit of normal [ULN], bilirubin 1.25 times ULN or less)	Moderate Impairment (AST less than 10 times ULN, bilirubin 1.26–2 times ULN)	Severe Impairment (AST less than 10 times ULN, bilirubin 2.01–5 times ULN)	Severe Impairment (AST more than 10 times ULN or bilirubin > 5 times ULN)
Breast cancer	No adjustment	Reduce dose to 200 mg/m²	Reduce dose to 130 mg/m² (may increase to 200 mg/m² in subsequent cycles)	Not recommended
NSCLC	No adjustment	Reduce dose to 75 mg/m²	Reduce dose to 50 mg/m² (may increase to 75 mg/m² in subsequent cycles)	Not recommended
Pancreatic	No adjustment	Not recommended	Not recommended	Not recommended

SIDE EFFECTS

Expected (90%–70%): Diarrhea, alopecia, nausea, vomiting. **Frequent (48%–46%):** Myalgia, arthralgia, peripheral neuropathy. **Occasional (20%–13%):** Mucositis, hypotension during infusion, pain/redness at injection site. **Rare (3%):** Bradycardia.

ADVERSE EFFECTS/TOXIC REACTIONS

Myelosuppression (anemia, neutropenia, thrombocytopenia) is an expected response to therapy, but more severe reactions including febrile neutropenia, sepsis may occur. Infections (candidiasis, respiratory tract infections, pneumonia) reported in 24% of pts. Pts with hepatic impairment may have increased risk of myelosuppression. Severe neuropathy was reported. Ocular toxicities (blurry vision, keratitis) reported in 10% of pts. Fatal interstitial lung disease (ILD), pneumonitis reported in 4% of pts. Severe hypersensitivity reactions, including anaphylaxis, may occur. Severe cardiovascular events (cardiac ischemia/infarction, chest pain, cardiac arrest, CVA, edema, hypertension, pulmonary embolism, SVT, transient ischemic attack, thrombosis) were reported.

NURSING CONSIDERATIONS

BASELINE ASSESSMENT

Obtain CBC, LFT prior to each course; pregnancy test in females of reproductive potential. Confirm compliance of effective contraception. Screen for active infection. Question history of cardiovascular disease, pulmonary disease, hepatic impairment. Receive full medication history and screen for interactions. Assess hydration status. Offer emotional support.

INTERVENTION/EVALUATION

Monitor CBC for myelosuppression; LFT for hepatotoxicity. Monitor for symptoms of hepatotoxicity (abdominal pain, jaundice, nausea, vomiting, weight loss) esp. in pts with hepatic impairment. Consider ABG, radiologic test if ILD/pneumonitis (excessive cough, dyspnea, fever, hypoxia) is suspected. Consider treatment with corticosteroids if ILD/pneumonitis is confirmed. Monitor for infections (cough, fatigue, fever). Monitor daily pattern of bowel activity, stool consistency. Monitor for ocular toxicities, hypersensitivity reactions. Monitor for symptoms of DVT (leg or arm pain/swelling), CVA (aphasia, altered mental status, headache, hemiplegia, vision loss); MI (chest pain, dyspnea, syncope, diaphoresis, arm/jaw pain), PE (chest pain, dyspnea, tachycardia).

PATIENT/FAMILY TEACHING

• Treatment may depress your immune system response and reduce your ability to fight infection. Report symptoms of infection such as body aches, chills, cough, fatigue, fever. Avoid those with active infection. • Report symptoms of bone marrow depression (e.g., bruising, fatigue, fever, shortness of breath, weight loss; bleeding easily, bloody urine or stool). • Report symptoms of lung inflammation (excessive coughing, difficulty breathing, chest pain); liver problems (abdominal pain, bruising, clay-colored stool, amber- or dark-colored urine, yellowing of the skin or eyes). • Life-threatening blood clots may occur; report symptoms of DVT (swelling, pain, hot feeling in the arms or legs; discoloration of extremity), lung embolism (difficulty breathing, chest pain, rapid heart rate), stroke (confusion, one-sided weakness or paralysis, difficulty speaking), heart attack (chest pain, difficulty breathing, jaw pain, nausea, pain that radiates to the arm or jaw, sweating). • Use effective contraception to avoid pregnancy. Do not breastfeed. • Report any vision changes, eye redness. • Maintain proper hydration and nutrition. • Do not take newly prescribed medications unless approved by prescriber who originally started treatment. • Report allergic reactions of any kind.

palbociclib

pal-boe-**sye**-klib
(Ibrance)

◆CLASSIFICATION

PHARMACOTHERAPEUTIC: Cyclin-dependent kinase inhibitor. **CLINICAL:** Antineoplastic.

USES

Used in combination with an aromatase inhibitor (e.g., letrozole) for treatment of postmenopausal women and adult men with estrogen receptor–positive, human epidermal growth factor receptor 2 *(HER2)*–negative advanced breast cancer as initial endocrine-based therapy for metastatic disease or in combination with fulvestrant in women with disease progression following endocrine therapy.

PRECAUTIONS

Contraindications: Hypersensitivity to palbociclib. **Cautions:** Baseline cytopenias. History of pulmonary embolism. Avoid concomitant use of strong or moderate CYP3A inhibitors, strong or moderate CYP3A inducers.

ACTION

Reduces proliferation of breast cancer cell lines by preventing cellular progression from G1 into S phase of cell cycle. Combination with an aromatase inhibitor provides increased inhibition. **Therapeutic Effect:** Inhibits tumor cell growth and survival.

PHARMACOKINETICS

Readily absorbed. Widely distributed. Metabolized in liver. Protein binding: 85%. Peak plasma concentration: 6–12 hrs. Steady state reached in 8 days. Excreted in feces (74%), urine (18%). **Half-life:** 29 hrs.

LIFESPAN CONSIDERATIONS

Pregnancy/Lactation: Treatment is indicated for postmenopausal women. However, treatment may cause fetal harm when administered during pregnancy. Females of reproductive potential should use effective contraception during treatment and up to 2 wks after discontinuation. Unknown if distributed in breast milk. **Children:** Safety and efficacy not established. Not indicated for this pt population. **Elderly:** No age-related precautions noted.

INTERACTIONS

DRUG: Strong CYP3A inhibitors (e.g., clarithromycin, ketoconazole, ritonavir), moderate CYP3A inhibitors (e.g.,

dilTIAZem, fluconazole, verapamil) may increase concentration/effect. **Strong CYP3A inducers (e.g., carBAMazepine, rifAMPin), moderate CYP3A inducers (e.g., nafcillin)** may decrease concentration/effect. May decrease the therapeutic effect of **vaccines (live)**. May increase adverse/toxic effects of **natalizumab, vaccines (live)**. **HERBAL: St. John's wort** may decrease concentration/effect. **Echinacea** may decrease therapeutic effect. **FOOD: Grapefruit products** may increase concentration/effect. **LAB VALUES:** May decrease Hgb, lymphocytes, neutrophils, platelets, WBC.

AVAILABILITY (Rx)

Capsules: 75 mg, 100 mg, 125 mg.

ADMINISTRATION/HANDLING

PO

• Give with food. • Administer whole; do not break, crush, cut, or open capsule. • If vomiting occurs after dosing, do not readminister dose; give next dose at next scheduled time.

P

INDICATIONS/ROUTES/DOSAGE

Breast Cancer (Initial endocrine-based therapy)

PO: ADULTS, ELDERLY: 125 mg once daily for 21 days, followed by a 7-day rest period to complete a 28-day cycle. Use in combination with an aromatase inhibitor (e.g., letrozole) once daily throughout 28-day cycle. Continue until disease progression or unacceptable toxicity.

Breast Cancer (Disease progression)

PO: ADULTS, ELDERLY: 125 mg once daily for 21 days, then 7 days off. Repeat q28 days (in combination with fulvestrant [and an LHRH agonist (e.g., goserelin) if pre- or perimenopausal]). Continue until disease progression or unacceptable toxicity.

Dose Reduction for Adverse Events

Dose Level	Dose
Recommended starting dose	125 mg/day
First dose reduction	100 mg/day
Second dose reduction	75 mg/day
Unable to tolerate 75 mg/day	Permanently discontinue

Dose Modification

Based on Common Terminology Criteria for Adverse Events (CTCAE).

Hematologic Toxicities

Grade 1 or 2: No dose adjustment. **Grade 3 (except lymphopenia unless associated with clinical events [e.g., opportunistic infection]):** No dose adjustment. Withhold treatment until recovery to less than Grade 2. **Grade 3, ANC 500–1000 cells/mm^3 plus fever that is greater than or equal to 38.5°C and/or active infection:** Interrupt treatment (and initiation of the next cycle) until recovery to Grade 2 or less. Resume at reduced dose upon starting.

Nonhematologic Toxicities

Grade 1 or 2: No dose adjustment. **Grade 3 or greater (if persistent despite optimal medical management):** Interrupt treatment until resolved to Grade 1 or less; Grade 2 or less if the event is not considered a serious medical risk. Resume at reduced dose upon starting.

Concomitant Use of Strong CYP3A Inhibitors

PO: ADULTS, ELDERLY: 75 mg once daily if unable to use alternative drug with minimal CYP3A inhibition. If CYP3A inhibitor is discontinued, increase palbociclib dose (after 3–5 half-lives of CYP3A inhibitor have elapsed) to the dose used prior to initiating strong CYP3A inhibitor.

Dosage in Renal Impairment

Mild to moderate impairment: No dose adjustment. **Severe impairment:** Not studied; use caution.

Dosage in Hepatic Impairment

Mild impairment: No dose adjustment. **Moderate to severe impairment:** Not studied; use caution.

SIDE EFFECTS

Frequent (41%–21%): Fatigue, nausea, alopecia, diarrhea. **Occasional (16%–**

13%): Decreased appetite, vomiting, asthenia.

ADVERSE EFFECTS/TOXIC REACTIONS

Anemia, leukopenia, neutropenia, thrombocytopenia are expected responses to therapy. Grade 3 neutropenia reported in 57% of pts. The median onset of neutropenia was 15 days. Pulmonary embolism (5% of pts); upper respiratory tract infections including influenza, laryngitis, nasopharyngitis, pharyngitis, rhinitis, sinusitis (31% of pts); peripheral neuropathy (31% of pts); cheilitis, glossitis, glossodynia, mouth ulceration, stomatitis (25% of pts); epistaxis (11% of pts) were reported.

NURSING CONSIDERATIONS

BASELINE ASSESSMENT

Obtain ANC, CBC; pregnancy test in females of reproductive potential. Confirm estrogen receptor–positive, *HER2*-negative status. Screen for history of pulmonary embolism. Receive full medication history and screen for interactions. Assess hydration status. Screen for active infection. Offer emotional support.

INTERVENTION/EVALUATION

Monitor ANC, CBC at start of each cycle and on day 14 on the first two cycles. If any Grade 3 or 4 hematologic toxicity occurs, repeat CBC 7 days after interruption of therapy and at start of next cycle. If neutropenia occurs specifically, recommend treatment interruption, dose reduction, or delay in starting treatment for next cycle. Monitor for neurotoxicity (peripheral neuropathy), epistaxis. If chest pain, dyspnea, tachycardia occurs, provide supplemental O_2 and obtain radiologic testing to rule out pulmonary embolism.

PATIENT/FAMILY TEACHING

• Treatment may depress your immune system response and reduce your ability to fight infection. Report symptoms of infection such as body aches, chills, cough, fatigue, fever. Avoid those with active infection. • Report symptoms of bone marrow depression (e.g., bruising, fatigue, fever, shortness of breath, weight loss; bleeding easily, bloody urine or stool). • Immediately report chest pain, difficult breathing, fast heart rate, rapid breathing; may indicate life-threatening blood clot in the lungs. • Use effective contraception to avoid pregnancy. Do not breastfeed. • Drink plenty of fluids. • Do not ingest grapefruit products or herbal supplements.

paliperidone

TOP 100

pal-ee-**per**-i-done
(Invega, Invega Sustenna, Invega Trinza)

Do not confuse Invega with Intuniv.

BLACK BOX ALERT Elderly pts with dementia-related psychosis are at increased risk for mortality due to cerebrovascular events.

◆CLASSIFICATION

PHARMACOTHERAPEUTIC: Benzisoxazole derivative. **CLINICAL:** Second-generation (atypical) antipsychotic.

USES

PO: Treatment of schizophrenia. **PO, IM:** Treatment of schizoaffective disorder. **OFF-LABEL:** Treatment of irritability associated with autistic disorder.

PRECAUTIONS

Contraindications: Sensitivity to paliperidone, risperiDONE. **Cautions:** History of cardiac arrhythmias, mild renal impairment (not recommended in moderate to severe impairment), HF, active seizures or predisposition to seizures, history of seizures, cardiovascular disease, pts at risk for QTc interval prolongation (congenital long QT syndrome, HF, medications that prolong QTc interval, hypokalemia, hypomagnesemia), pts at risk for aspiration pneumonia. May increase risk of stroke in pts with

P

dementia-related psychosis. CNS depression, concomitant use of antihypertensives, hypovolemia or dehydration, high risk for suicide. Pts with breast cancer, other prolactin-dependent tumors; children, adolescents.

ACTION

Exact mechanism unknown. May be a result of mixed central DOPamine and serotonin antagonism. **Therapeutic Effect:** Improves negative symptoms of psychosis; reduces incidence of extrapyramidal side effects.

PHARMACOKINETICS

Absorbed from GI tract. Metabolized in liver. Primarily excreted in urine. **Half-life:** 23 hrs.

LIFESPAN CONSIDERATIONS

Pregnancy/Lactation: Unknown if drug crosses placenta or is distributed in breast milk. **Children:** Safety and efficacy not established. **Elderly:** Potential for orthostatic hypotension. Age-related renal impairment may require dosage adjustment.

P

INTERACTIONS

DRUG: May decrease effects of **DOPamine agonists, levodopa. Alcohol, CNS depressants (e.g., LORazepam, morphine, zolpidem)** may increase CNS depression. **Strong CYP3A4 inducers (e.g., carBAMazepine, phenytoin, rifAMPin)** may decrease concentration/effect. **QT interval–prolonging medications (e.g., amiodarone, azithromycin, ciprofloxacin, haloperidol, methadone, sotalol)** may increase risk of QTc interval prolongation. **HERBAL:** **St. John's wort** may decrease concentration/effect. **Herbals with sedative properties (e.g., chamomile, kava kava, valerian)** may increase CNS depression. **FOOD:** None known. **LAB VALUES:** May increase serum creatine phosphatase, uric acid, triglycerides, ALT, AST, prolactin. May decrease serum potassium, sodium, protein, glucose.

AVAILABILITY (Rx)

Injection Suspension: ***(Invega Sustenna):*** 39 mg/0.25 mL, 78 mg/0.5 mL, 117 mg/0.75 mL, 156 mg/mL, 234 mg/1.5 mL. ***(Invega Trinza):*** 273 mg, 410 mg, 546 mg, 819 mg.

Tablets, Extended-Release: 1.5 mg, 3 mg, 6 mg, 9 mg.

ADMINISTRATION/HANDLING

PO

• May give without regard to food. • Do not break, crush, dissolve, or divide extended-release tablets.

IM

• Administer both initial injections (first injection on day 1 and the second injection 1 wk later) into deltoid muscle (helps attain therapeutic concentration rapidly). • Maintenance doses may be given in gluteal or deltoid muscle.

INDICATIONS/ROUTES/DOSAGE

Schizophrenia

PO: **ADULTS, ELDERLY:** Initially, 6 mg once daily in the morning. May increase dose in increments of 3 mg/day at intervals of more than 5 days. Range: 3–12 mg/day. **ADOLESCENTS 12–17 YRS: 51 KG OR MORE:** Initially, 3 mg once daily. Range: 3–12 mg/day. **50 KG OR LESS:** Initially, 3 mg once daily. Range: 3–6 mg/day.

IM: ***(Invega Sustenna):*** **ADULTS, ELDERLY:** Initially, 234 mg on day 1 followed by 156 mg 1 wk later (second dose may be given 4 days before or after the wkly time point). **Maintenance:** Following the 1-wk initiation regimen, begin 117 mg monthly. Range: 39–234 mg (based on response and tolerability). Monthly maintenance dose may be given 7 days before or after the monthly time point. ***(Invega Trinza):*** 273 mg to 819 mg q3mos (based on last dose of Invega Sustenna). Three-month IM used only after monthly IM dose established for at least 4 mos. The last 2 mos of monthly IM should be the same dosage strength before starting 3-mo injections.

Schizoaffective Disorder

PO: ADULTS, ELDERLY: 6 mg once daily in the morning. May increase in increments of 3 mg/day at intervals of more than 4 days. Range: 3–12 mg/day. **IM: ADULTS, ELDERLY:** Initially, 234 mg, then 156 mg 1 wk later. **Maintenance range:** 39–234 mg monthly (based on response and tolerability). May be given 7 days before or after the monthly time point.

Dosage in Renal Impairment

Creatinine Clearance	Oral Dosage	IM Dosage
50–79 mL/min	Initially, 3 mg/d Maximum: 6 mg/d	Initially, 156 mg, then 117 mg 1 wk later, then 78 mg monthly
10–49 mL/min	Initially, 1.5 mg/d Maximum: 3 mg/d	Not recommended
Less than 10 mL/min	Not recommended	Not recommended

Dosage in Hepatic Impairment

No dose adjustment.

SIDE EFFECTS

Occasional (14%–4%): Tachycardia, headache, drowsiness, akathisia, anxiety, dizziness, dyspepsia, nausea.

ADVERSE EFFECTS/TOXIC REACTIONS

Neuroleptic malignant syndrome (NMS), hyperpyrexia, muscle rigidity, change in mental status, unstable pulse or B/P, tachycardia, diaphoresis, cardiac arrhythmias, rhabdomyolysis, acute renal failure, tardive dyskinesia (protrusion of tongue, puffing of cheeks, chewing/puckering of mouth) may occur rarely. May prolong QT interval.

NURSING CONSIDERATIONS

BASELINE ASSESSMENT

Obtain renal function tests. Assess behavior, appearance, emotional status, response to environment, speech pattern, thought content. Screen for comorbidities as listed in Precautions.

INTERVENTION/EVALUATION

Monitor B/P, heart rate, weight, renal function tests, ECG. Monitor for fine tongue movement (may be first sign of tardive dyskinesia). Supervise suicidal-risk pt closely during early therapy (as depression lessens, energy level improves, increasing suicide potential). Assess for therapeutic response (greater interest in surroundings, improved self-care, increased ability to concentrate, relaxed facial expression). Monitor for potential neuroleptic malignant syndrome (fever, muscle rigidity, unstable B/P or pulse, altered mental status).

PATIENT/FAMILY TEACHING

• Avoid tasks that may require alertness, motor skills until response to drug is established. • Use caution when changing position from lying or sitting to standing. • Report trembling in fingers, altered gait, unusual muscle/skeletal movements, palpitations, severe dizziness, fainting, swelling/pain in breasts, visual changes, rash, difficulty in breathing.

P

palonosetron

pal-oh-**noe**-se-tron

(Aloxi)

Do not confuse Aloxi with Eloxatin or oxaliplatin, or palonosetron with dolasetron, granisetron, or ondansetron.

FIXED-COMBINATION(S)

Akynzeo: palonosetron/netupitant (a substance P/neurokinin receptor antagonist): 0.5 mg/300 mg.

◆CLASSIFICATION

PHARMACOTHERAPEUTIC: Selective 5-HT_3 receptor antagonist. **CLINICAL:** Antiemetic.

USES

Prevention of acute and delayed nausea/vomiting associated with initial/repeated courses of moderately or highly emetogenic chemotherapy. Prevention of postop nausea/vomiting for up to 24 hrs following surgery.

PRECAUTIONS

Contraindications: Hypersensitivity to palonosetron. **Cautions:** History of cardiovascular disease; pts at risk for QTc interval prolongation (congenital long QT syndrome, HF, medications that prolong QTc interval, hypokalemia, hypomagnesemia), pts at risk for ventricular arrhythmias.

ACTION

Antagonizes 5-HT_3 receptors, blocking serotonin on both peripheral and vagal nerve terminals in chemoreceptor trigger zone. **Therapeutic Effect:** Decreases episodes of nausea/vomiting associated with chemotherapy or postoperative recovery.

PHARMACOKINETICS

Protein binding: 52%. Metabolized in liver. Excreted in urine. **Half-life:** 40 hrs.

LIFESPAN CONSIDERATIONS

Pregnancy/Lactation: Unknown if distributed in breast milk. **Children:** Safety and efficacy not established. **Elderly:** No age-related precautions noted.

INTERACTIONS

DRUG: **FentaNYL, lithium, MAOIs (e.g., phenelzine, selegiline), SNRIs (e.g., DULoxetine, venlafaxine), SSRIs (e.g., citalopram, FLUoxetine, sertraline), tricyclic antidepressants (e.g., amitriptyline, doxepin)** may increase risk of serotonin syndrome. **QT interval–prolonging medications (e.g., amiodarone, azithromycin, ciprofloxacin, haloperidol, methadone, sotalol)** may increase risk of QTc interval prolongation. **HERBAL:** None significant. **FOOD:** None known. **LAB VALUES:** May transiently increase serum bilirubin, ALT, AST.

AVAILABILITY (Rx)

Injection Solution: 0.25 mg/5 mL.

ADMINISTRATION/HANDLING

IV

Reconstitution • Give undiluted as IV push.

Rate of administration • Give IV push over 30 sec. Children: Infuse over 15 min. • Flush IV line with 0.9% NaCl before and following administration.

Storage • Store at room temperature. Solution should appear colorless, clear. Discard if cloudy precipitate forms.

IV COMPATIBILITIES

Famotidine (Pepcid), LORazepam (Ativan), midazolam (Versed), potassium chloride.

INDICATIONS/ROUTES/DOSAGE

Chemotherapy-Induced Nausea/Vomiting

IV: ADULTS, ELDERLY: 0.25 mg as single dose 30 min before starting chemotherapy. **CHILDREN 1 MO TO YOUNGER THAN 17 YRS:** 20 mcg/kg as single dose 30 min before starting chemotherapy. **Maximum:** 1.5 mg.

Postop Nausea/Vomiting

IV: ADULTS, ELDERLY: 0.075 mg over 10 sec immediately before induction of anesthesia.

Dosage in Renal/Hepatic Impairment

No dose adjustment.

SIDE EFFECTS

Occasional (9%–5%): Headache, constipation. **Rare (less than 1%):** Diarrhea, dizziness, fatigue, abdominal pain, insomnia.

ADVERSE EFFECTS/TOXIC REACTIONS

Overdose may produce combination of CNS stimulation, depressant effects. May prolong QT interval. 5-HT_3 receptor antagonists are known to potentiate serotonin syndrome, esp. in pts taking serotonergic medications.

NURSING CONSIDERATIONS

BASELINE ASSESSMENT

Obtain BMP, serum magnesium in pts at risk for hypokalemia, hypomagnesemia, QT interval prolongation. Assess for signs of dehydration due to excessive vomiting (poor skin turgor, dry mucous membranes). Question history of cardiac disease, long QT syndrome, cardiac arrhythmias. Screen for concomitant home medications that prolong QT interval, increase risk of serotonin syndrome.

INTERVENTION/EVALUATION

Monitor BMP, serum magnesium; ECG in pts suspected of arrhythmia, QT interval prolongation. Monitor for nausea/vomiting. Assess for symptoms of serotonin syndrome (e.g., altered mental status, tachycardia, labile B/P, diaphoresis, hyperthermia, tremor, hyperreflexia, diarrhea, seizures). Monitor for hypersensitivity reaction.

PATIENT/FAMILY TEACHING

• Relief from nausea/vomiting generally occurs shortly after drug administration. • Report symptoms of serotonin overproduction such as confusion, excessive talking, fever, hallucinations, headache, hyperactivity, insomnia, racing thoughts, seizure activity, sexual dysfunction, tremors. • Report persistent vomiting. • Report palpitations, light-headedness, fainting; allergic reactions of any kind.

pamidronate

pam-id-**roe**-nate
(Aredia ✦)
Do not confuse Aredia with Adriamycin, or pamidronate with alendronate, ibandronate, or risedronate.

◆CLASSIFICATION

PHARMACOTHERAPEUTIC: Bisphosphonate. **CLINICAL:** Hypocalcemic.

USES

Treatment of moderate to severe hypercalcemia associated with malignancy (with/without bone metastases). Treatment of moderate to severe Paget's disease. Treatment of osteolytic bone lesions of multiple myeloma or bone metastases of breast cancer. **OFF-LABEL:** Inhibition of bone resorption in osteogenesis imperfecta. Treatment of bone metastases of thyroid cancer. Prevention of bone loss associated with androgen deprivation treatment in prostate cancer.

PRECAUTIONS

Contraindications: Hypersensitivity to pamidronate, other bisphosphonates (e.g., risedronate, alendronate). **Cautions:** Baseline cytopenias, renal impairment, concurrent use with other nephrotoxic medications, history of thyroid surgery.

ACTION

Inhibits bone resorption, decreases mineralization by disrupting activity of osteoclasts. **Therapeutic Effect:** Lowers serum calcium concentration.

PHARMACOKINETICS

Route	Onset	Peak	Duration
IV	24–48 hrs	3–7 days	N/A

Rapidly absorbed by bone. Excreted in urine. Unknown if removed by hemodialysis. **Half-life:** 21–35 hrs.

LIFESPAN CONSIDERATIONS

Pregnancy/Lactation: Unknown if crosses placenta. Recommend discontinuation of drug as early as possible before a planned pregnancy. Unknown if fetal harm can occur. Unknown if distributed in breast milk. **Children:** Safety and efficacy not established. **Elderly:** May become overhydrated. Careful monitoring of fluid and electrolytes indicated; recommend dilution in smaller volume.

INTERACTIONS

DRUG: **NSAIDs (e.g., diclofenac, meloxicam, naproxen)** may increase adverse/

toxic effects (e.g., increased risk of ulcer). **Proton pump inhibitors (e.g., omeprazole, pantoprazole)** may decrease effect. **Aminoglycosides (e.g., gentamicin)** may increase risk of hypokalemia. **HERBAL:** None significant. **FOOD:** None known. **LAB VALUES:** None significant.

AVAILABILITY (Rx)

Injection, Powder for Reconstitution: 30 mg, 90 mg. **Injection Solution:** 3 mg/mL, 6 mg/mL, 9 mg/mL.

ADMINISTRATION/HANDLING

IV

Reconstitution • Reconstitute each vial with 10 mL Sterile Water for Injection to provide concentration of 3 mg/mL or 9 mg/mL. • Allow drug to dissolve before withdrawing. • Dilute in 250–1,000 mL bag containing 0.45% or 0.9% NaCl or D_5W (1,000 mL for hypercalcemia of malignancy, 500 mL for Paget's disease, multiple myeloma, 250 mL for breast cancer).

Rate of administration • Adequate hydration is essential in conjunction with pamidronate therapy (avoid overhydration in pts with potential for HF). • Administer as IV infusion over 2–24 hrs for treatment of hypercalcemia; over 2 hrs for breast cancer; over 4 hrs for Paget's disease or multiple myeloma.

Storage • Store at room temperature. • Reconstituted vial is stable for 24 hrs if refrigerated; IV solution is stable for 24 hrs after dilution.

P

IV INCOMPATIBILITIES

Calcium-containing IV fluids.

INDICATIONS/ROUTES/DOSAGE

Hypercalcemia of Malignancy

IV infusion: ADULTS, ELDERLY: Moderate hypercalcemia (corrected serum calcium level 12–13.5 mg/dL): 60–90 mg as a single dose over 2–24 hrs. **Severe hypercalcemia (corrected serum calcium level greater than 13.5 mg/dL):** 90 mg as a single dose over 2–24 hrs.

Paget's Disease

IV infusion: ADULTS, ELDERLY: 30 mg/day over 4 hrs for 3 consecutive days. May retreat if clinically indicated.

Osteolytic Bone Lesion (Multiple myeloma)

IV infusion: ADULTS, ELDERLY: 90 mg over 4 hrs once monthly.

Osteolytic Bone Metastases (Breast cancer)

IV infusion: ADULTS, ELDERLY: 90 mg over 2 hrs q3–4wks.

Dosage in Renal Impairment

Not recommended.

Dosage in Hepatic Impairment

No dose adjustment.

SIDE EFFECTS

Frequent (27%–18%): Temperature elevation (at least 1°C) 24–48 hrs after administration; erythema, swelling, induration, pain at catheter site in pts receiving 90 mg; anorexia, nausea, fatigue. **Occasional (10%–1%):** Constipation, rhinitis.

ADVERSE EFFECTS/TOXIC REACTIONS

Hypophosphatemia, hypokalemia, hypomagnesemia, hypocalcemia occur more frequently with higher dosages. Anemia, hypertension, tachycardia, atrial fibrillation, drowsiness occur more frequently with 90-mg doses. GI hemorrhage occurs rarely.

NURSING CONSIDERATIONS

BASELINE ASSESSMENT

Obtain CBC, serum calcium, ionized calcium, magnesium, phosphate; renal function test level prior to therapy. Assess hydration status.

INTERVENTION/EVALUATION

Monitor serum calcium, ionized calcium, potassium, magnesium, creatinine, CBC. Provide adequate hydration; assess overhydration. Monitor I&O; assess lungs for crackles, dependent body parts for edema.

Monitor B/P, temperature, pulse. Assess catheter site for redness, swelling, pain. Monitor food intake, daily pattern of bowel activity, stool consistency. Monitor for potential GI hemorrhage with 90-mg dosage.

PATIENT/FAMILY TEACHING

• Report symptoms of low blood calcium levels, including confusion, muscle twitching/cramps, numbness, seizures, tingling, jaw pain. • Immediately report GI bleeding.

panitumumab

pan-i-**toom**-ue-mab
(Vectibix)

BLACK BOX ALERT 90% of pts experience dermatologic toxicities (dermatitis acneiform, pruritus, erythema, rash, skin exfoliation, skin fissures, abscess). Severe infusion reactions (anaphylaxis, bronchospasm, fever, chills, hypotension), fatal reactions have occurred.

Do not confuse panitumumab with daratumumab, necitumumab, ofatumumab.

◆CLASSIFICATION

PHARMACOTHERAPEUTIC: Epidermal growth factor receptor (EGFR) inhibitor, monoclonal antibody. **CLINICAL:** Antineoplastic.

USES

Treatment of wild-type RAS metastatic colorectal cancer either as first-line therapy in combination with FOLFOX or as monotherapy following disease progression after prior treatment with fluoropyrimidine-, oxaliplatin-, or irinotecan-based regimens.

PRECAUTIONS

Contraindications: Hypersensitivity to panitumumab. **Cautions:** Baseline electrolyte imbalance (esp. hypomagnesemia, hypokalemia), pulmonary disease, ocular disease, dehydration, skin disease (e.g., poorly healed wounds, skin fissures), elderly. Not indicated in pts with *RAS*-mutant metastatic colorectal cancer or for whom *RAS* mutation status is unknown.

ACTION

Binds specifically to epidermal growth factor receptor (EGFR) and competitively inhibits binding of epidermal growth factor. Blocks activation of intracellular tyrosine kinase. **Therapeutic Effect:** Inhibits tumor cell growth, survival, and proliferation.

PHARMACOKINETICS

Clearance varies by body weight, gender, tumor burden. **Half-life:** 3–10 days.

LIFESPAN CONSIDERATIONS

Pregnancy/Lactation: Avoid pregnancy; may cause fetal harm. Females of reproductive potential must use effective contraception during treatment and for at least 2 mos after discontinuation. Breastfeeding not recommended during treatment and for at least 2 mos after discontinuation. May impair fertility. **Children:** Safety and efficacy not established. **Elderly:** May have increased risk of adverse effects, severe diarrhea.

INTERACTIONS

DRUG: None significant. **HERBAL:** None significant. **FOOD:** None known. **LAB VALUES:** May decrease serum magnesium, calcium.

AVAILABILITY (Rx)

Injection Solution: 20 mg/mL vial (5-mL, 20-mL vials).

ADMINISTRATION/HANDLING

IV

◀ALERT▶ Do not give by IV push or bolus. Use low protein-binding 0.2- or 0.22-micron in-line filter. Flush IV line before and after chemotherapy administration with 0.9% NaCl.

Reconstitution • Dilute in 100–150 mL 0.9% NaCl to provide concentration of 10 mg/mL or less. • Do not shake

P

solution. Invert gently to mix. • Discard any unused portion.

Rate of administration • Give as IV infusion over 60 min. • Infuse doses greater than 1,000 mg over 90 min.

Storage • Refrigerate vials. • After dilution, solution may be stored for up to 6 hrs at room temperature, up to 24 hrs if refrigerated. • Discard if discolored, but solution may contain visible, translucent-to-white particulates (will be removed by in-line filter).

IV INCOMPATIBILITIES

Do not mix with dextrose solutions or any other medications.

INDICATIONS/ROUTES/DOSAGE

◀ALERT▶ Stop infusion immediately in pts experiencing severe infusion reactions.

Metastatic Colorectal Cancer

IV infusion: ADULTS, ELDERLY: 6 mg/kg once q14 days as a single agent or in combination with FOLFOX (fluorouracil, leucovorin, and oxaliplatin). Continue until disease progression or unacceptable toxicity.

P

Dose Modification

Infusion Reactions

Mild to moderate reactions: Reduce infusion rate by 50% for remainder of infusion. **Severe reactions:** Discontinue infusion. Depending on severity, consider permanent discontinuation.

Skin Toxicity

For all CTCAE Grade 3 skin toxicities, withhold treatment for 1–2 doses until improved to Grade 2 or less, then reduce dose as follows: **First occurrence of CTCAE Grade 3:** Resume at same dose. **Second occurrence of CTCAE Grade 3:** Reduce dose to 80% of initial dose. **Third occurrence of CTCAE Grade 3:** Reduce dose to 60% of initial dose. **Fourth occurrence of CTCAE Grade 3:** Permanently discontinue.

Dosage in Renal/Hepatic Impairment

No dose adjustment.

SIDE EFFECTS

Frequent (66%–17%): Erythema, pruritus, fatigue, nausea, rash, diarrhea, vomiting, dyspnea, pyrexia. **Occasional (15%–6%):** Cough, acne, dry skin, stomatitis, mucosal inflammation, growth of eyelashes.

ADVERSE EFFECTS/TOXIC REACTIONS

Dermatologic toxicities (acneiform dermatitis, erythema, paronychia, pruritus, rash, skin exfoliation, fissures) reported in 90% of pts. Fatal cutaneous or soft issue toxicities including abscesses, bullous mucocutaneous disease, necrotizing fasciitis, sepsis may occur. Sunlight/UV exposure may worsen dermatologic toxicities. May cause electrolyte depletion (hypomagnesemia, hypokalemia). Grade 3 or 4 infusion reactions (bronchospasm, chills, dyspnea, hypotension) reported in 4% of pts. Severe diarrhea may lead to dehydration, acute renal failure. Fatal interstitial lung disease (ILD), pneumonitis reported in 1% of pts. Ocular toxicities (keratitis, ulcerative keratitis, corneal perforation) may occur. Increased mortality/toxicity was reported when therapy used in combination with bevacizumab and chemotherapy. Immunogenicity (auto-panitumumab antibodies) reported in less than 1% of pts.

NURSING CONSIDERATIONS

BASELINE ASSESSMENT

Obtain serum magnesium, potassium; pregnancy test in females of reproductive potential. Screen for active infection. Question history of pulmonary/ocular/skin disease. Conduct dermatologic exam. Review occurrence of prior infusion reactions prior to each dose. Assess usual bowel movement patterns, stool characteristics. Assess and correct hydration status. Offer emotional support. Assess *KRAS* mutational status in colorectal tumors and confirm the absence of a *RAS* mutation.

INTERVENTION/EVALUATION

Monitor serum magnesium, potassium periodically and for 8 wks after discontinuation. Monitor serum electrolytes if severe diarrhea occurs. Replete electrolytes as clinically indicated. Consider ABG, radiologic test if ILD/pneumonitis (excessive cough, dyspnea, fever, hypoxia) is suspected. Monitor daily pattern of bowel activity, stool consistency. Diarrhea must be treated promptly to reduce occurrence of severe dehydration, acute renal failure. Diligently assess for ocular toxicities (redness, pain of eye; dry eye, change of vision); skin for cutaneous and soft tissue toxicities.

PATIENT/FAMILY TEACHING

• Severe infusion reaction may occur; report chills, difficulty breathing, dizziness, fever. • Diarrhea may cause dehydration, electrolyte imbalance, low blood pressure, kidney injury, and may be life-threatening. Drink plenty of fluids. Report diarrhea or dehydration that does not improve with medical management. • Report toxic skin reactions (abscess, itching, peeling, rash, redness, sloughing, swelling); kidney problems (decreased urine output, flank pain, darkened urine), symptoms of lung inflammation (excessive coughing, difficulty breathing, chest pain); eye problems (redness, pain of eye; dry eye, change of vision). • Limit sunlight, UV exposure. Wear protective sunscreen, hats, clothing when outdoors. • Use effective contraception to avoid pregnancy. Do not breastfeed.

panobinostat

pan-oh-**bin**-oh-stat
(Farydak)

BLACK BOX ALERT Severe diarrhea reported in 25% of pts. If diarrhea occurs, interrupt treatment, initiate antidiarrheal therapy, then reduce or discontinue treatment. Severe and/or fatal cardiac arrhythmias, cardiac ischemic events, ECG changes may occur. Electrolyte abnormalities may increase risk of arrhythmias. Obtain ECG, serum electrolytes at baseline and monitor during treatment.

Do not confuse panobinostat with febuxostat or pentostatin.

◆CLASSIFICATION

PHARMACOTHERAPEUTIC: Histone deacetylase (HDAC) inhibitor. **CLINICAL:** Antineoplastic.

USES

Used in combination with bortezomib and dexamethasone for treatment of pts with multiple myeloma who have received at least 2 prior regimens, including bortezomib and an immunomodulatory agent.

PRECAUTIONS

Contraindications: Hypersensitivity to panobinostat. **Cautions:** Baseline cytopenias, conditions predisposing to infection (e.g., diabetes, renal failure, immunocompromised pts, open wounds), pts at risk for QTc interval prolongation (congenital long QT syndrome, HF, medications that prolong QTc interval, hypokalemia, hypomagnesemia). Not recommended in pts with recent MI or unstable angina, severe hepatic impairment. Concurrent use of strong CYP3A inhibitors and/or CYP3A inducers, CYP2D6 substrates not recommended. Avoid use in pts with active infection.

ACTION

Inhibits enzymatic activity of histone deacetylase. Increases acetylation of histone proteins, resulting in cell cycle arrest and/or cellular death (apoptosis). **Therapeutic Effect:** Inhibits tumor growth and survival.

PHARMACOKINETICS

Widely distributed. Extensively metabolized. Protein binding: 90%. Peak plasma concentration: 2 hrs. Excreted in feces (44%–77%), urine (29%–51%). **Half-life:** 37 hrs.

LIFESPAN CONSIDERATIONS

Pregnancy/Lactation: Avoid pregnancy; may cause fetal harm/malformations.

P

Females of reproductive potential should use effective contraception during treatment and up to 1 mo after discontinuation. Unknown if distributed in breast milk. **Males:** Males should use condoms during sexual activity during treatment and up to 3 mos after discontinuation. **Children:** Safety and efficacy not established. **Elderly:** May have increased risk of adverse effects (e.g., cardiac/GI/hematologic toxicities).

INTERACTIONS

DRUG: **Strong CYP3A inhibitors (e.g., clarithromycin, ketoconazole, ritonavir)** may increase concentration/effect. **Strong CYP3A inducers (e.g., carBAMazepine, rifAMPin)** may decrease concentration/effect. May increase concentration/effects of **CYP2D6 substrates (e.g., metoprolol, venlafaxine). QT interval–prolonging medications (e.g., amiodarone, azithromycin, ciprofloxacin, haloperidol, methadone, sotalol)** may increase risk of QTc interval prolongation. May decrease the therapeutic effect; increase adverse effects of **vaccines (live)**. **HERBAL:** **St. John's wort** may decrease concentration/effect. **FOOD:** **Grapefruit products, star fruit** may increase concentration/effect. **LAB VALUES:** May decrease Hct, Hgb, leukocytes, lymphocytes, neutrophils, platelets; serum albumin, calcium, potassium, sodium. May increase serum bilirubin, creatinine, magnesium. May increase or decrease phosphate.

AVAILABILITY (Rx)

Capsules: 10 mg, 15 mg, 20 mg.

ADMINISTRATION/HANDLING

PO

• May give without regard to food; avoid grapefruit products (dexamethasone should be given with food to decrease GI upset). • Administer capsule whole; do not break, cut, crush, or open. • If vomiting occurs after dosing, do not readminister dose; give dose at next scheduled time.

INDICATIONS/ROUTES/DOSAGE

Multiple Myeloma

PO: ADULTS, ELDERLY: 20 mg once every other day for 3 doses/wk during wk 1 and 2 of each 21-day cycle for up to 8 cycles, in combination with bortezomib and dexamethasone. Consider continuing treatment for additional 8 cycles based on tolerability. **Total duration:** Up to 16 cycles (48 wks). **Recommended dose of bortezomib:** 1.3 mg/m^2 as injection/day per dosing schedule. **Recommended dose of dexamethasone:** 20 mg orally/day on a full stomach per dosing schedule.

Dosing Schedule for Cycles 1–8 of 21-Day Cycle

Wk 1: Panobinostat: days 1, 3, 5. Bortezomib: days 1, 4. Dexamethasone: days 1, 2, 4, 5. **Wk 2:** Panobinostat: days 8, 10, 12. Bortezomib: days 8, 11. Dexamethasone: days 8, 9, 11, 12. **Wk 3:** Rest period (all 3 drugs).

Dosing Schedule for Cycles 9–16 of 21-Day Cycle

Wk 1: Panobinostat: days 1, 3, 5. Bortezomib: day 1 only. Dexamethasone: days 1, 2. **Wk 2:** Panobinostat: days 8, 10, 12. Bortezomib: day 8 only. Dexamethasone: days 8, 9. **Wk 3:** Rest period (all 3 drugs).

Dose Reduction for Adverse Events

If reduction required, reduce panobinostat in increments of 5 mg. If the reduced dose is less than 10 mg 3 times/wk, discontinue treatment. Keep same schedule (21-day cycle) when dose reduced.

Dose Modification for Clinical Toxicities

Based on Common Terminology Criteria for Adverse Events (CTCAE).

Thrombocytopenia

Grade 3: No dose adjustment. ***(Bortezomib):*** No dose adjustment. **Grade 3 with bleeding/Grade 4:** Interrupt treatment until platelet count 50,000 cells/mm^3 or greater, then resume at reduced dose. ***(Bortezomib):*** Interrupt bortezomib until platelet count 75,000 cells/mm^3 or greater. If only 1 dose was held prior to resolution of platelet count, resume bortezomib at same dose. If more than 2 doses were held consecutively, resume bortezomib at reduced dose.

Neutropenia

Grade 3: No dose adjustment. ***(Bortezomib):*** No dose adjustment. **Two or more occurrences of Grade 3:** Withhold treatment until ANC 1,000 cells/mm^3 or greater, then resume at same dose. ***(Bortezomib):*** No dose adjustment. **Grade 3 with febrile neutropenia/Grade 4:** Withhold treatment until febrile neutropenia resolves and ANC is 1,000 cells/mm^3 or greater, then resume at reduced dose. ***(Bortezomib):*** Withhold bortezomib until febrile neutropenia resolves and ANC is 1,000 cells/mm^3 or greater. If only 1 dose was held prior resolution of platelet count, resume bortezomib at same dose. If more than 2 doses were held consecutively, resume bortezomib at reduced dose.

Anemia

Grade 3: Withhold panobinostat until Hgb greater than or equal to 10 g/dL, then resume at reduced dose. ***(Bortezomib):*** Not specified.

Diarrhea

Grade 2: Withhold treatment until resolved, then resume at same dose. ***(Bortezomib):*** Consider interruption of bortezomib until resolved, then resume at same dose. **Grade 3 or hospitalization/administration of IV fluids:** Interrupt until resolved, then resume at reduced dose. ***(Bortezomib):*** Withhold until resolved, then resume bortezomib at reduced dose. **Grade 4:** Permanently discontinue panobinostat and bortezomib.

Nausea/Vomiting

Grade 3 or 4: Withhold until resolved, then resume at reduced dose. ***(Bortezomib):*** Not specified.

Other Toxicities (Other CTCAE grades)

Any Grade 2 recurrence, any other Grade 3 or 4: Withhold until resolved to Grade 1 or 0, then resume at reduced dose. ***(Bortezomib):*** Not specified. **Any other Grade 3 or 4 recurrence:** Consider further dose reduction once resolved to Grade 1 or 0.

Concomitant Use of Strong CYP3A Inhibitors

PO: ADULTS, ELDERLY: 10 mg per dosing schedule.

Dosage in Renal Impairment

No dose adjustment.

Dosage in Hepatic Impairment

PO: ADULTS, ELDERLY: Mild impairment: 15 mg per dosing schedule. **Moderate impairment:** 10 mg per dosing schedule. **Severe impairment:** Treatment not recommended.

SIDE EFFECTS

Frequent (60%–2%): Fatigue, asthenia, lethargy, diarrhea, nausea, peripheral edema, decreased appetite, vomiting, pyrexia. **Occasional (12%):** Decreased weight.

ADVERSE EFFECTS/TOXIC REACTIONS

Myelosuppression (anemia, leukopenia, neutropenia, thrombocytopenia) is an expected response to therapy. Diarrhea occurred in 68% of pts. Severe cases of diarrhea occurred in 25% of pts. Cardiac toxicities such as cardiac ischemic events, ST-segment depression, T-wave abnormalities were reported. Cardiac arrhythmias including atrial fibrillation, atrial flutter, bradycardia, SVT, atrial/ventricular/sinus tachycardia occurred in 12% of pts. Severe thrombocytopenia may increase risk of fatal hemorrhage. Infectious processes such as bacterial infections, invasive fungal infections, pneumonia, sepsis, viral infections were reported. Severe and/or fatal infections occurred in 31% of pts.

P

NURSING CONSIDERATIONS

BASELINE ASSESSMENT

Obtain ANC, CBC, BMP, LFT; serum magnesium, phosphate; ECG, pregnancy test in females of reproductive potential. Correct electrolyte imbalances prior to each cycle. Verify platelet count is at least 100,000 cells/mm^3, ANC is 1,500 cells/mm^3, QTc interval is less than 450 msec on ECG prior to each cycle. Verify pregnancy status. Assess hydration status, usual stool characteristics. Question history if acute MI, unstable angina, arrhythmia. Screen for active infection.

INTERVENTION/EVALUATION

Monitor CBC, BMP; serum magnesium, phosphate wkly; LFT as indicated; vital signs. Monitor ECG periodically. If QTc interval increases to greater than 480 msec on ECG, interrupt treatment and correct any electrolyte abnormalities. If QT prolongation does not resolve, permanently discontinue treatment. Initiate medical management for nausea, vomiting, diarrhea prior to any interruption or dose reduction. Consider blood transfusion in pts with severe anemia, thrombocytopenia. Diligently monitor daily pattern bowel activity, stool consistency. Start antidiarrheal therapy at first sign of loose stool/diarrhea. Obtain 2D cardiac echocardiogram, ECG if cardiac decompensation is suspected. Monitor for infection.

PATIENT/FAMILY TEACHING

• Treatment may depress your immune system response and reduce your ability to fight infection. Report symptoms of infection such as body aches, chills, cough, fatigue, fever. Avoid those with active infection. • Report symptoms of bone marrow depression (e.g., bruising, fatigue, fever, shortness of breath, weight loss; bleeding easily, bloody urine or stool). • Report liver problems (abdominal pain, bruising, clay-colored stool, amber- or dark-colored urine, yellowing of the skin or eyes); heart problems (chest tightness, dizziness, fainting, palpitations, shortness of breath); kidney problems (dark-colored urine, decreased urine output, extremity swelling, flank pain), skin problems (redness, rash); mouth ulceration. • Use effective contraception to avoid pregnancy. Do not breastfeed. • Report bleeding of any kind.

P

pantoprazole

TOP 100

pan-**toe**-pra-zole
(Protonix, Tecta ✱)
Do not confuse pantoprazole with ARIPiprazole.

◆CLASSIFICATION

PHARMACOTHERAPEUTIC: Benzimidazole. **CLINICAL:** Proton pump inhibitor.

USES

PO: Treatment, maintenance of healing of erosive esophagitis associated with gastroesophageal reflux disease (GERD) and reduction of relapse rate of heartburn symptoms in GERD. Treatment of hypersecretory conditions including Zollinger-Ellison syndrome. **IV:** Short-term treatment of erosive esophagitis associated with GERD, treatment of hypersecretory conditions. **OFF-LABEL:** Peptic ulcer disease, active ulcer bleeding (injection), adjunct in treatment of *H. pylori,* stress ulcer prophylaxis in critically ill pts.

PRECAUTIONS

Contraindications: Hypersensitivity to pantoprazole, other proton pump inhibitors (e.g., omeprazole). **Cautions:** May increase risk of fractures, GI infections.

ACTION

Irreversibly binds to, inhibits hydrogen-potassium adenosine triphosphate, an enzyme on surface of gastric parietal cells. Inhibits hydrogen ion transport into gastric lumen. **Therapeutic Effect:** Increases gastric pH, reduces gastric acid production.

PHARMACOKINETICS

Route	Onset	Peak	Duration
PO	N/A	N/A	24 hrs

Primarily distributed into gastric parietal cells. Metabolized in liver. Protein binding: 98%. Primarily excreted in urine. Not removed by hemodialysis. **Half-life:** 1 hr.

LIFESPAN CONSIDERATIONS

Pregnancy/Lactation: Unknown if drug crosses placenta or is distributed in breast milk. **Children:** Safety and efficacy not established. **Elderly:** No age-related precautions noted.

INTERACTIONS

DRUG: May decrease concentration/effects of **acalabrutinib, cefuroxime, erlotinib, neratinib, pazopanib. Strong CYP2C19 inducers (e.g., FLUoxetine), strong CYP3A4 inducers (e.g., carBAMazepine, phenytoin, rifAMPin)** may decrease concentration/effect. **HERBAL:** None significant. **FOOD:** None known. **LAB VALUES:** May increase serum creatinine, cholesterol, uric acid, glucose, lipoprotein, ALT.

AVAILABILITY (Rx)

Granules for Suspension: 40 mg/packet. **Injection, Powder for Reconstitution:** ***(Protonix):*** 40 mg.

Tablets, Delayed-Release: ***(Protonix):*** 20 mg, 40 mg.

ADMINISTRATION/HANDLING

IV

Reconstitution • Mix 40-mg vial with 10 mL 0.9% NaCl injection. • May be further diluted with 100 mL D_5W, 0.9% NaCl.

Rate of administration • Infuse 10 mL solution over at least 2 min. • Infuse 100 mL solution over at least 15 min. or as continuous infusion. • Flush IV line after administration.

Storage • Store vials at room temperature. • Once diluted with 10 mL 0.9% NaCl, stable for 96 hrs at room temperature; when further diluted with 100 mL, stable for 96 hrs at room temperature.

PO

• Give without regard to food. Best given before breakfast. • Do not break, crush, dissolve, or divide tablets; give whole. • Administer oral suspension only in apple juice or applesauce. Best taken 30 min before a meal.

IV INCOMPATIBILITIES

DOBUTamine.

IV COMPATIBILITIES

DOPamine, EPINEPHrine, furosemide (Lasix), insulin (regular), potassium chloride, vasopressin.

INDICATIONS/ROUTES/DOSAGE

Erosive Esophagitis (Treatment)

PO: ADULTS, ELDERLY: 40 mg/day for up to 8 wks. If not healed after 8 wks, may continue an additional 8 wks. **CHILDREN 5 YRS AND OLDER (WEIGHING 40 KG OR MORE):** 40 mg/day for up to 8 wks. **(WEIGHING 15–39 KG):** 20 mg/day for up to 8 wks.

IV: ADULTS, ELDERLY: 40 mg/day for 7–10 days.

Maintenance of Healing of Erosive Esophagitis

PO: ADULTS, ELDERLY: 40 mg once daily.

Hypersecretory Conditions

PO: ADULTS, ELDERLY: Initially, 80 mg twice daily. May titrate upward early in therapy. **Maximum:** 240 mg/day (as either 80 mg three times daily or 120 mg twice daily).

IV: ADULTS, ELDERLY: 80 mg twice daily. May increase to 80 mg q8h.

Prevention of Rebleeding in Peptic Ulcer Bleed (Unlabeled)

IV: ADULTS, ELDERLY: 80 mg followed by 8 mg/hr infusion for 72 hrs or 80 mg then 40 mg q12h for 72 hrs.

Dosage in Renal/Hepatic Impairment

No dose adjustment.

SIDE EFFECTS

Rare (less than 2%): Diarrhea, headache, dizziness, pruritus, rash.

ADVERSE EFFECTS/TOXIC REACTIONS

Hyperglycemia occurs rarely. May increase risk of *Clostridioides difficile*–associated diarrhea.

NURSING CONSIDERATIONS

BASELINE ASSESSMENT

Question history of GI disease, ulcers, GERD.

INTERVENTION/EVALUATION

Evaluate for therapeutic response (relief of GI symptoms). Monitor for symptoms of *C. difficile* (abdominal pain, diarrhea, fever).

PATIENT/FAMILY TEACHING

• Best if taken before breakfast. • Frequent, loose stool; fever, abdominal pain, blood-streaked stool may indicate infectious diarrhea and may be contagious to others.

P

PARoxetine

par-**ox**-e-teen
(Brisdelle, Paxil, Paxil CR, Pexeva)

BLACK BOX ALERT Increased risk of suicidal thinking and behavior in children, adolescents, young adults 18–24 yrs with major depressive disorder, other psychiatric disorders.

Do not confuse PARoxetine with DULoxetine, FLUoxetine, piroxicam, pyridoxine, or vortioxetine, or Paxil with Doxil, Plavix, PROzac, or Taxol.

◆CLASSIFICATION

PHARMACOTHERAPEUTIC: Selective serotonin reuptake inhibitor (SSRI). **CLINICAL:** Antidepressant, antiobsessive-compulsive, antianxiety.

USES

Treatment of major depressive disorder (MDD). Treatment of panic disorder, obsessive-compulsive disorder (OCD). Treatment of social anxiety disorder (SAD), generalized anxiety disorder (GAD), premenstrual dysphoric disorder (PMDD), posttraumatic stress disorder (PTSD). **Brisdelle:** Treatment of moderate to severe vasomotor symptoms associated with menopause. **OFF-LABEL:** Social anxiety disorder in children, self-injurious behavior, treatment of depression and OCD in children.

PRECAUTIONS

Contraindications: Hypersensitivity to PARoxetine. Concurrent use of MAOIs with or within 14 days of MAOIs intended to treat psychiatric disorders, initiation in pts treated with linezolid or methylene blue; concomitant use with thioridazine, pimozide. **Brisdelle:** Pregnancy. **Cautions:** History of suicidal ideation and behavior; seizure disorder, hepatic/renal impairment, elderly, narrow-angle glaucoma, alcohol use. Avoid use in first trimester of pregnancy, alcohol use.

ACTION

Selectively blocks uptake of neurotransmitter serotonin at CNS neuronal presynaptic membranes, increasing its availability at postsynaptic receptor sites. **Therapeutic Effect:** Relieves depression, reduces obsessive-compulsive behavior, decreases anxiety.

PHARMACOKINETICS

Widely distributed. Metabolized in liver. Protein binding: 95%. Excreted in urine. Not removed by hemodialysis. **Half-life:** 24 hrs.

⌛ LIFESPAN CONSIDERATIONS

Pregnancy/Lactation: May impair reproductive function. Not distributed in breast milk. May increase risk of congenital malformations. **Children:** Safety and efficacy not established. **Elderly:** Age-related renal impairment may require dosage adjustment. Use caution.

INTERACTIONS

DRUG: **Alcohol** may increase adverse effects. **Lithium, MAOIs (e.g., phenelzine, selegiline)** may increase the serotonergic effect. May increase antiplatelet effect of **NSAIDs (e.g., diclofenac, meloxicam, naproxen).** May decrease concentration/effect of **tamoxifen**. May increase adverse effects of **tricyclic antidepressants (e.g., amitriptyline)**. **HERBAL: Glucosamine, herbals with anticoagulant/antiplatelet properties (e.g., garlic, ginger, ginkgo biloba)** may increase effect. **FOOD:** None known. **LAB VALUES:** May decrease Hgb, Hct, WBC count.

AVAILABILITY (Rx)

Capsules: ***(Brisdelle):*** 7.5 mg. **Oral Suspension:** ***(Paxil):*** 10 mg/5 mL. **Tablets:** ***(Paxil, Pexeva):*** 10 mg, 20 mg, 30 mg, 40 mg.

Tablets, Controlled-Release: ***(Paxil CR):*** 12.5 mg, 25 mg, 37.5 mg.

ADMINISTRATION/HANDLING

PO

• Give without regard to food. • Give with food, milk if GI distress occurs. • Scored tablet may be crushed. • Do not crush, break, dissolve, or divide controlled-release tablets.

INDICATIONS/ROUTES/DOSAGE

Depression

PO: ***(Immediate-Release):*** **ADULTS:** Initially, 10–20 mg/day. May increase by 10–20 mg/day at intervals of more than 1 wk. **Maximum:** 50 mg/day.

PO: ***(Controlled-Release):*** **ADULTS:** Initially, 25 mg/day. May increase by 12.5 mg/day at intervals of more than 1 wk. **Maximum:** 62.5 mg/day.

Generalized Anxiety Disorder (GAD)

PO: ***(Immediate-Release):*** **ADULTS:** Initially, 10 mg/day. May increase by 10 mg/day at intervals of more than 1 wk. Range: 20–50 mg/day.

Obsessive-Compulsive Disorder (OCD)

PO: ***(Immediate-Release):*** **ADULTS:** Initially, 20 mg/day. May increase by 10 mg/day at intervals of more than 1 wk. Recommended dose: 40–60 mg/day.

Panic Disorder

PO: ***(Immediate-Release):*** **ADULTS:** Initially, 10 mg/day. May increase by 10 mg/day at intervals of more than 1 wk. Usual dose: 20–40 mg/day. **Maximum:** 60 mg/day.

PO: ***(Controlled-Release):*** **ADULTS, ELDERLY:** Initially, 12.5 mg once daily. May increase by 12.5 mg/day at wkly intervals. **Maximum:** 75 mg/day.

Social Anxiety Disorder (SAD)

PO: ***(Immediate-Release):*** **ADULTS:** Initially, 10 mg/day. May increase by 10 mg/day at intervals of more than 1 wk. **Maximum:** 60 mg/day.

PO: ***(Controlled-Release):*** **ADULTS, ELDERLY:** Initially, 12.5 mg once daily. May increase by 12.5 mg/day at wkly intervals. **Maximum:** 37.5 mg/day.

Posttraumatic Stress Disorder (PTSD)

PO: ***(Immediate-Release):*** **ADULTS:** Initially, 20 mg/day. May increase by 10–20 mg/day at intervals of more than 1 wk. **Maximum:** 60 mg/day.

Premenstrual Dysphoric Disorder (PMDD)

PO: ***(Controlled-Release):*** **ADULTS:** Initially, 12.5 mg/day. May increase by 12.5 mg at wkly intervals. **Maximum:** 50 mg/day.

Vasomotor Symptoms

PO: **ADULTS:** ***(Brisdelle):*** 7.5 mg once daily at bedtime.

Usual Elderly Dosage

PO: Initially, 10 mg/day. May increase by 10 mg/day at intervals of more than 1 wk. **Maximum:** 40 mg/day.

PO: ***(Controlled-Release):*** Initially, 12.5 mg/day. May increase by 12.5 mg/day at intervals of more than 1 wk. **Maximum:** 50 mg/day (37.5 mg for SAD).

Dosage Renal/Hepatic Impairment

CrCl less than 30 mL/min, severe hepatic impairment: ***(Immediate-Release):*** Initially, 10 mg/day. May increase by 10 mg/dose at wkly intervals. **Maximum:** 40 mg/day. ***(Extended-***

P

Release): Initially, 12.5 mg/day. May increase by 12.5 mg/day at wkly intervals. **Maximum:** 50 mg/day. ***(Brisdelle):*** No dosage adjustment.

SIDE EFFECTS

Frequent (26%–8%): Nausea, drowsiness, headache, dry mouth, asthenia, constipation, dizziness, insomnia, diarrhea, diaphoresis, tremor. **Occasional (6%–3%):** Decreased appetite, respiratory disturbance (e.g., increased cough), anxiety, flatulence, paresthesia, yawning, decreased libido, sexual dysfunction, abdominal discomfort. **Rare:** Palpitations, vomiting, blurred vision, altered taste, confusion.

ADVERSE EFFECTS/TOXIC REACTIONS

Hyponatremia, seizures have been reported. Serotonin syndrome (agitation, confusion, diaphoresis, hallucinations, hyperreflexia) occurs rarely.

NURSING CONSIDERATIONS

BASELINE ASSESSMENT

Obtain LFT. Assess appearance, behavior, speech pattern, level of interest, mood. Question history of suicidal ideation and behavior.

INTERVENTION/EVALUATION

For pts on long-term therapy, CBC, LFT, renal function test should be performed periodically. Assess mental status for depression, suicidal ideation (esp. at beginning of therapy or change in dosage), anxiety, social functioning, panic attacks. Assess appearance, behavior, speech pattern, level of interest, mood.

PATIENT/FAMILY TEACHING

• Avoid alcohol, St. John's wort. • Therapeutic effect may be noted within 1–4 wks. • Do not abruptly discontinue medication. • Avoid tasks that require alertness, motor skills until response to drug is established. • Seek immediate medical attention if thoughts of suicide, new onset or worsening of anxiety, depression, or changes in mood occur.

P

PAZOPanib

paz-**oh**-pa-nib
(Votrient)

■ BLACK BOX ALERT ■ Severe, fatal hepatotoxicity has been observed.

Do not confuse PAZOPanib with nintedanib, pegaptanib, tivozanib, or vandetanib.

◆CLASSIFICATION

PHARMACOTHERAPEUTIC: Vascular endothelial growth factor (VEGF) inhibitor. Tyrosine kinase inhibitor. **CLINICAL:** Antineoplastic.

USES

Treatment of advanced renal cell carcinoma (RCC), advanced soft-tissue sarcoma (STS) (in pts previously treated with chemotherapy). **OFF-LABEL:** Advanced thyroid cancer.

PRECAUTIONS

Contraindications: Hypersensitivity to PAZOPanib. **Cautions:** Baseline cytopenias, hepatic impairment, hypertension, cardiac disease (cardiomyopathy, HF), pulmonary disease, hypothyroidism, ocular disease, poorly healed wound, conditions predisposing to infection (e.g., diabetes, immunocompromised pts, renal failure, open wounds); history of thromboembolic events (CVA, DVT, MI, pulmonary embolism (PE). Pts at risk for: GI perforation (e.g., Crohn's disease, diverticulitis, GI tract malignancies, peptic ulcers, peritoneal malignancies), tumor lysis syndrome (high tumor burden, dehydration), QTc interval prolongation, cardiac arrhythmias (congenital long QT syndrome, HF, QT interval–prolonging medications, hypokalemia, hypomagnesemia), bleeding (e.g., history of intracranial/GI/GU bleeding, coagulation disorders, recent trauma; concomitant use of anticoagulants, NSAIDs, antiplatelets). Do not initiate in pts with uncontrolled hypertension. Avoid use concomitant use of strong CYP3A4 inhibitors or inducers, gastric acid–reducing agents, QT interval–prolonging medications.

ACTION

Inhibits cell surface vascular endothelial growth factor (VEGF) receptors. **Therapeutic Effect:** Inhibits angiogenesis, blocks tumor growth.

PHARMACOKINETICS

Widely distributed. Metabolized in liver. Protein binding: greater than 99%. Peak plasma concentration: 2–4 hrs. Excreted primarily in feces, urine (4%). **Half-life:** 31 hrs.

LIFESPAN CONSIDERATIONS

Pregnancy/Lactation: Avoid pregnancy; may cause fetal harm. Females and males with female partners of reproductive potential must use effective contraception during treatment and for at least 2 wks after discontinuation. Breastfeeding not recommended during treatment and for at least 2 wks after discontinuation. May impair fertility in both female and males. **Children:** Safety and efficacy not established. **Elderly:** May have increased risk of adverse effects.

INTERACTIONS

DRUG: **H_2 antagonists (e.g., famotidine, ranitidine), proton pump inhibitors (e.g., omeprazole, pantoprazole)** may decrease concentration/effect. **QT interval–prolonging medications (e.g., amiodarone, azithromycin, ciprofloxacin, haloperidol, methadone, sotalol)** may increase risk of QTc interval prolongation. **CYP3A4 inhibitors (e.g., clarithromycin, ketoconazole, ritonavir)** may increase concentration/effect. **CYP3A4 inducers (e.g., carBAMazepine, phenytoin, rifAMPin)** may decrease concentration/effect. May decrease the therapeutic effect; increase adverse effects of **vaccines (live)**. **HERBAL:** **St. John's wort** decreases concentration/effect. **FOOD:** **Food** may increase concentration/effect. **Grapefruit products** may increase concentration, potential for torsades de pointes, myelotoxicity. **LAB VALUES:** May increase serum ALT, AST, bilirubin. May decrease serum magnesium, phosphate, potassium, sodium; leukocytes, lymphocytes, neutrophils, platelets. May increase or decrease serum glucose.

AVAILABILITY (Rx)

Tablets: 200 mg.

ADMINISTRATION/HANDLING

PO

• Give at least 1 hr before or 2 hrs after ingestion of food. • Give tablets whole; do not break, crush, dissolve, or divide.

INDICATIONS/ROUTES/DOSAGE

Renal Cell Carcinoma, Soft-Tissue Sarcoma

PO: ADULTS, ELDERLY: 800 mg once daily. If concomitant CYP3A4 inhibitor cannot be discontinued, reduce initial dose to 400 mg/day.

Dose Reduction Schedule

(Renal cell carcinoma): First reduction: 400 mg once daily. **Second reduction:** 200 mg once daily. **(Soft tissue carcinoma): First reduction:** 600 mg once daily. **Second reduction:** 400 mg once daily.

Dose Modification

Based on Common Terminology for Adverse Events.

Cardiac Toxicity

Symptomatic or Grade 3 left ventricular systolic dysfunction: Withhold treatment until improved to less than Grade 3, then resume if benefit outweighs risk. **Grade 4:** Permanently discontinue.

GI Fistula

Grade 2 or 3 GI fistula: Withhold treatment until improved, then resume if benefit outweighs risk. **Grade 4 GI fistula:** Permanently discontinue.

Hemorrhagic Events

Grade 2 hemorrhage: Withhold treatment until improved to Grade 1 or 0, then resume at reduced dose. **Grade 3 or 4**

hemorrhage; recurrence of Grade 2 hemorrhage: Permanently discontinue.

Hepatotoxicity

Serum ALT 3–8 times ULN: Continue same dose and monitor LFT wkly until improved to Grade 1 or baseline. **Serum ALT greater than 8 times ULN:** Withhold treatment until improved to Grade 1 or baseline, then resume at no more than 400 mg daily if benefit outweighs risk. Continue to monitor LFT wkly for 8 wks. **Serum ALT greater than 3 times ULN with serum bilirubin greater than 2 times ULN; recurrence of serum ALT greater than 3 times ULN despite dose reduction:** Permanently discontinue.

Hypertension

Grade 2 or 3 hypertension: Reduce dose and start antihypertensive therapy. Permanently discontinue if Grade 3 hypertension persists despite dose reduction and antihypertensive therapy. **Grade 4 hypertension:** Permanently discontinue.

Proteinuria

24-hr urine protein 3 grams or greater: Withhold treatment until improved to Grade 1 or 0, then resume at reduced dose. Permanently discontinue if 24-hr urine protein does not improve or recurs. **Confirmed nephrotic syndrome:** Permanently discontinue.

Venous Thrombosis

Grade 3 venous thrombosis: Withhold treatment and manage for at least 1 wk, then resume at same dose. **Grade 4 venous thrombosis:** Permanently discontinue.

Other Events Requiring Permanent Discontinuation

Permanently discontinue if arterial thrombosis, thrombotic microangiopathy, GI perforation, ILD/pneumonitis, posterior reversible encephalopathy syndrome occurs.

Concomitant Use of Strong CYP3A4 Inhibitors, Gastric Acid Reducers

If strong CYP3A4 inhibitor cannot be discontinued, reduced PAZOPanib dose to 400 mg. If gastric acid–reducing agents cannot be discontinued, consider short-acting antacid instead of proton pump inhibitor, H_2-receptor antagonist.

Dosage in Renal Impairment

No dose adjustment.

Dosage in Hepatic Impairment

Mild impairment: No dose adjustment. **Moderate impairment:** Reduce dose to 200 mg/day. **Severe impairment:** Not recommended.

SIDE EFFECTS

Note: Frequency and occurrence of side effects may vary depending on indicated treatment.

Frequent (69%–20%): Fatigue, diarrhea, nausea, decreased weight, hypertension, decreased appetite, change of hair color, vomiting, tumor pain, dysgeusia, headache, musculoskeletal pain, myalgia, abdominal pain, dyspnea. **Occasional (18%–5%):** Rash, cough, edema, mucositis, alopecia, dizziness, skin disorder, skin hypopigmentation, stomatitis, chest pain, insomnia, dysphonia, dyspepsia, dry skin, chills, vision blurred, nail disorder.

ADVERSE EFFECTS/TOXIC REACTIONS

Fatal hepatotoxicity may occur. Cardiac toxicities including QT interval prolongation, torsades de pointes; cardiac dysfunction (decreased left ventricular ejection fraction, HF) were reported. Fatal hemorrhagic events including epistaxis (8% of pts), mouth hemorrhage (3% of pts), rectal hemorrhage (2% of pts), Grade 4 hemorrhage (intracranial/subarachnoid/peritoneal hemorrhage), hemoptysis may occur. Fatal thromboembolism including CVA, DVT, MI, pulmonary embolism, transient ischemic attack was reported. Thrombotic microangiopathy including thrombotic thrombocytopenic purpura (TTP), hemolytic uremic syndrome reported in 1%–5% of pts. GI perforation or fistula reported in 1% of pts. Fatal interstitial lung disease (ILD), pneumonitis reported in less than 1% of pts. Posterior reversible encephalopathy syndrome, a dysfunction of the brain that may evolve into an ischemic CVA or cerebral hemorrhage, may occur. Grade 3 hypertension reported in 1%–3% of pts. May impair healing of wounds. Tumor lysis syndrome may present as acute renal failure, hypocalcemia, hyperuricemia, hyperphosphatemia. Vascular disorders including arterial aneurysm, dissection, rupture may occur. Other reactions may include retinal changes/detachment, hypothyroidism, pancreatitis, pneumothorax, nephrotic syndrome.

NURSING CONSIDERATIONS

BASELINE ASSESSMENT

Obtain CBC, LFT; ECG; pregnancy test in females of reproductive potential. Confirm compliance of effective contraception. Assess LVEF by echocardiogram in pts with cardiomyopathy. Screen for active infection. Assess risk for bleeding. Assess usual bowel movement patterns, stool characteristics. Receive full medication history and screen for interactions. Assess skin for open wounds, surgical incisions. Assess adequate hydration prior to initiation due to increased risk of tumor lysis syndrome, diarrhea, vomiting. Question history as listed in Precautions. Offer emotional support.

INTERVENTION/EVALUATION

Monitor CBC for myelosuppression; LFT for hepatotoxicity; ECG for QT interval prolongation; urine protein level. Monitor for symptoms of hepatotoxicity (abdominal pain, jaundice, nausea, vomiting, weight loss) esp. in pts with hepatic impairment. Monitor B/P for hypertension. Consider ABG, radiologic test if ILD/pneumonitis (excessive cough, dyspnea, fever, hypoxia) is suspected. Consider treatment with corticosteroids if ILD/pneumonitis is confirmed. Assess LVEF by echocardiogram periodically if cardiomyopathy (dyspnea, extremity swelling, palpitations) is suspected. Monitor for infections (cough, fatigue, fever). Monitor daily pattern of bowel activity, stool consistency. Ensure adequate hydration/nutrition. Monitor for ocular toxicities; symptoms of DVT (leg or arm pain/swelling); CVA, intracranial hemorrhage (aphasia, altered mental status, facial droop, hemiplegia, vision loss); MI (chest pain, diaphoresis, left arm/jaw pain, increased serum troponin, ST segment elevation), PE (chest pain, dyspnea, tachycardia). Bleeding of any kind can be life-threatening and must be treated promptly.

Monitor serum uric acid level if tumor lysis syndrome (acute renal failure, electrolyte imbalance, cardiac arrhythmias, seizures) is suspected. Conduct neurological assessment. Pts with altered mental status, seizures, visual disturbances, unilateral weakness should be evaluated for posterior reversible encephalopathy syndrome. Assess for skin toxicities, poorly healed wounds.

PATIENT/FAMILY TEACHING

• Treatment may depress your immune system response and reduce your ability to fight infection. Report symptoms of infection such as body aches, chills, cough, fatigue, fever. Avoid those with active infection. • Report symptoms of bone marrow depression (e.g., bruising, fatigue, fever, shortness of breath, weight loss; bleeding easily, bloody urine or stool). • Report symptoms of lung inflammation (excessive coughing, difficulty breathing, chest pain); liver problems (abdominal pain, bruising, clay-colored stool, amber- or dark-colored urine, yellowing of the skin or eyes), eye problems (eye pain, change of vision), toxic skin reactions (rash, redness, sloughing, swelling). • Life-threatening blood clots may occur; report symptoms of DVT (swelling, pain, hot feeling in the arms or legs; discoloration of extremity), lung embolism (difficulty breathing, chest pain, rapid heart rate), stroke (confusion, one-sided weakness or paralysis, difficulty speaking), heart attack (chest pain, difficulty breathing, jaw pain, nausea, pain that radiates to the arm or jaw, sweating). • Life-threatening tumor lysis syndrome (a condition

P

caused by the rapid breakdown of cancer cells), which can cause kidney failure, may occur. Report decreased urination, amber-colored urine; confusion, difficulty breathing, fatigue, fever, muscle or joint pain, palpitations, seizures, vomiting. • Bleeding of any kind can be life-threatening. • Use effective contraception to avoid pregnancy. Do not breastfeed. • Drink plenty of fluids. • Do not take newly prescribed medications unless approved by prescriber who originally started treatment. • Treatment may affect the heart's ability to pump blood or alter the electrical conduction of the heart; report chest pain, difficulty breathing, dizziness, swelling of extremities, fainting, palpitations. • Take on empty stomach. • Treatment may worsen high blood pressure. • Immediately report severe or persistent abdominal pain, bloody stool, fever, vomiting blood; may indicate rupture in GI tract.

pegfilgrastim

TOP 100

peg-fil-**gras**-tim
(Neulasta, Neulasta Onpro, Fulphila, Udenyca, Ziextenzo)
Do not confuse Neulasta with Lunesta, Neumega, or Neupogen, or pegfilgrastim with filgrastim.

CLASSIFICATION

PHARMACOTHERAPEUTIC: Colony-stimulating factor. **CLINICAL:** Hematopoietic agent.

USES

Decreases incidence of infection (as manifested by febrile neutropenia) in cancer pts receiving myelosuppressive chemotherapy associated with febrile neutropenia. To increase survival in pts acutely exposed to myelosuppressive doses of radiation.

PRECAUTIONS

Contraindications: Hypersensitivity to pegfilgrastim, filgrastim. **Cautions:** Any malignancy with myeloid characteristics, sickle cell disease. The 6-mg fixed dose should not be used in infants, children, or adolescents weighing less than 45 kg. Do not administer within 14 days before and 24 hrs after cytotoxic chemotherapy.

ACTION

Stimulates production, maturation, and activation of neutrophils within bone marrow. **Therapeutic Effect:** Increases phagocytic ability, antibody-dependent destruction; decreases incidence of infection.

PHARMACOKINETICS

Readily absorbed after SQ administration. **Half-life:** 15–80 hrs.

LIFESPAN CONSIDERATIONS

Pregnancy/Lactation: Unknown if drug crosses placenta or is distributed in breast milk. **Children:** Safety and efficacy not established in children younger than 12 yrs. **Elderly:** No age-related precautions noted.

INTERACTIONS

DRUG: **Pegloticase** may decrease effect. **HERBAL:** None significant. **FOOD:** None known. **LAB VALUES:** May increase serum LDH, alkaline phosphatase, uric acid.

AVAILABILITY (Rx)

Injection Solution: ***(Neulasta):*** 6 mg/0.6 mL syringe. **Prefilled Syringe Kit:** ***(Neulasta Onpro):*** 6 mg/0.6 mL; dose delivers over 45 min time period about 27 hrs after application. **Prefilled Syringe:** ***(Fulphila, Udenyca, Ziextenzo):*** 6 mg/0.6 mL.

ADMINISTRATION/HANDLING

SQ

Preparation • Remove syringe from refrigerator and allow solution to warm to room temperature. • Visually inspect for particulate matter or discoloration. Do not use if solution is cloudy, discolored, or visible particles are observed.
Administration • Insert needle subcutaneously into outer abdomen, upper arm, or outer thigh and inject solution. • Do not inject into areas of active skin

disease or injury such as sunburns, skin rashes, inflammation, skin infections, or active psoriasis. • Rotate injection sites. • Do not administer IV or intramuscularly. **Storage** • Refrigerate in original carton until time of use. • Protect from light. • Do not shake. • Discard if left at room temperature for more than 48 hrs. • May store syringe at room temperature for up to 4 hrs. • Avoid freezing. If accidentally frozen, may thaw in refrigerator. Discard if frozen more than once.

On Body Injector (Onpro)

A health care provider must fill the injector prior to applying to pt's skin. Apply to intact, nonirritated skin on back of arms or abdomen. • Delivers pegfilgrastim over 45 min time period about 27 hrs after application. • May apply on same day as chemotherapy. Keep injector at least 4 inches away from electrical equipment. **Storage** • Store in refrigerator until 30 min prior to use. • Kit should not be at room temperature for more than 12 hrs (including injecting time). Discard if at room temperature for more than 12 hrs.

INDICATIONS/ROUTES/DOSAGE

Neutropenia (Chemotherapy-Induced)

SQ: ADULTS, ELDERLY, CHILDREN 12–17 YRS, WEIGHING MORE THAN 45 KG: Give as single 6-mg injection once per chemotherapy cycle beginning at least 24 hrs after completion of chemotherapy.

◀ALERT▶ Do not administer between 14 days before and 24 hrs after cytotoxic chemotherapy. Manufacturer Recommendation: Do not use in infants, children, adolescents weighing less than 45 kg (dose less than 6 mg).

Radiation Injury Syndrome

Note: Prefilled syringe not designed to give doses less than 6 mg. Not recommended; use caution to avoid dosing errors.

SQ: ADULTS, ELDERLY, CHILDREN WEIGHING 45 KG OR MORE: 6 mg once wkly for 2 doses. **31–44 KG:** 4 mg once wkly for 2 doses. **21–30 KG:** 2.5 mg once wkly for 2 doses. **10–20 KG:** 1.5 mg once wkly for 2 doses. **LESS THAN 10 KG:** 0.1 mg/kg once wkly for 2 doses.

Dosage in Renal/Hepatic Impairment

No dose adjustment.

SIDE EFFECTS

Frequent (72%–15%): Bone pain, nausea, fatigue, alopecia, diarrhea, vomiting, constipation, anorexia, abdominal pain, arthralgia, generalized weakness, peripheral edema, dizziness, stomatitis, mucositis, neutropenic fever.

ADVERSE EFFECTS/TOXIC REACTIONS

Capillary leak syndrome (hypoalbuminemia, hypotension, fluid overload, leukocytosis, hemoconcentration), glomerulonephritis, fatal splenic rupture may occur. Acute respiratory distress syndrome (ARDS) may occur in pts with sepsis. Serious hypersensitivity reactions including anaphylaxis, skin rash, urticaria, erythema, flushing may occur. Fatal sickle cell crisis may occur in pts with sickle cell disease. May act as growth factor stimulator for tumors of any type. Potential device failures of Neulasta Onpro may cause partial delivery of medication, increasing risk of neutropenia, febrile neutropenia. Abdominal pain, malaise, back pain, increased inflammatory markers (C-reactive protein, WBC) may indicate aortitis. Other reactions including Sweet syndrome (acute febrile neutropenic dermatosis), contact dermatitis, and local skin reactions may occur. Immunogenicity (auto-pegfilgrastim antibodies) reported in 6% of pts.

NURSING CONSIDERATIONS

BASELINE ASSESSMENT

Obtain CBC prior to initiation and routinely thereafter. Question history of sickle cell disease, glomerulonephritis, splenic disease, hypersensitivity reaction to acrylic adhesive on body (injector uses acrylic adhesive).

INTERVENTION/EVALUATION

Monitor neutrophil count for treatment effectiveness. Monitor for hypersensitivity reactions. Assess for hypoalbuminemia,

P

peripheral edema, respiratory symptoms (cough, dyspnea) if weight has increased by 5% (or greater) and pt is hypotensive; may indicate capillary leak syndrome. Severe capillary leak syndrome should be treated with supportive measures (corticosteroids; monitoring of weight, B/P, albumins levels) until resolution. Monitor Neulasta Onpro for device failures. Septic pts should be monitored for ARDS.

PATIENT/FAMILY TEACHING

• Drink plenty of fluids to maintain hydration. • Immediately report symptoms of capillary leak syndrome (dizziness, fatigue, sudden weight gain, shortness of breath, swelling of face or extremities). A delay in reporting symptoms may be life-threatening. • Fatal rupturing of the spleen can occur; report sudden abdominal pain or swelling, low blood pressure, fast heart rate. • Report chest pain, fever, palpitations, severe bone pain.

P

pembrolizumab

pem-broe-**liz**-ue-mab
(Keytruda)
Do not confuse pembrolizumab with atezolizumab, durvalumab, necitumumab, nivolumab, palivizumab, or panitumumab.

◆CLASSIFICATION

PHARMACOTHERAPEUTIC: Anti PD-1 monoclonal antibody. **CLINICAL:** Antineoplastic.

USES

Treatment of unresectable or metastatic melanoma. Treatment of metastatic head and neck squamous cell carcinoma (HNSCC) (recurrent or metastatic) with disease progression on or after platinum-containing chemotherapy. Treatment of metastatic non–small-cell lung cancer (NSCLC) in pts with PD-L1–expressing tumors as a single agent for first-line tx, with disease progression on or after platinum-containing chemotherapy; or in combination with pemetrexed and carboplatin, as first-line tx of metastatic nonsquamous NSCLC or as first-line single-agent treatment of metastatic NSCLC in pts with tumors with PD-L1 expression and with no EGFR or ALK genomic tumor aberrations. Treatment of refractory classical Hodgkin lymphoma (cHL) or relapse after 3 or more lines of therapy. Treatment of locally advanced or metastatic urothelial carcinoma not eligible for cisplatin-containing chemotherapy or who have disease progression during or following platinum-containing chemotherapy; or with 12 mos of neoadjuvant or adjuvant tx with platinum-containing chemotherapy. Treatment of unresectable or metastatic microsatellite instability high (MSI-H) or mismatch repair deficient solid tumors or colorectal cancer. Treatment of gastric cancer (advanced or metastatic) or gastroesophageal junction adenocarcinoma in pts with tumors with PD-L1 expression and with disease progression on or after 2 or more lines of therapy. Treatment of recurrent or metastatic cervical cancer in pts with tumors with PD-L1 expression and with disease progression on or after chemotherapy. Treatment of primary mediastinal large B-cell lymphoma (PMBCL) in adult and pediatric pts with refractory disease or relapsed after 2 or more lines of therapy. Treatment of hepatocellular carcinoma in pts previously treated with sorafenib. Adjuvant treatment of melanoma with lymph node involvement following complete resection. Treatment of recurrent locally advanced or metastatic Merkel cell carcinoma. Treatment of advanced renal cell carcinoma (in combination with axitinib). Treatment of metastatic small-cell lung cancer (SCLC) in pts with disease progression on or after platinum-based chemotherapy and at least one other prior line of therapy. Treatment of HNSCC. Treatment of metastatic squamous cell carcinoma of esophagus. Treatment of advanced endometrial carcinoma (in combination with lenvatinib) that is not MSI-H or dMMR, having disease progression following prior systemic therapy, and who are not candidates for curative surgery or radiation. Treatment of recurrent or metastatic cutaneous squamous cell carcinoma (cSCC) not curable by surgery or radiation. Treatment of classical Hodgkin lymphoma (relapsed or refractory) in adults and pediatric pts who have relapsed after 3 or more prior lines of therapy. Treatment of locally recurrent unresectable or metastatic triple- negative breast cancer (TNBC) in combination with chemotherapy.

PRECAUTIONS

Contraindications: Hypersensitivity to pembrolizumab. **Cautions:** Thyroid disease, hepatic/renal impairment, interstitial lung disease, electrolyte imbalance, hypertriglyceridemia.

ACTION

Inhibits programmed cell death-1 (PD-1) activity by binding to PD-1 receptors on T cell, blocking PD-1 ligands from binding, which inhibits the negative immune regulation caused by PD-1 signaling. **Therapeutic Effect:** Inhibits T-cell proliferation and cytokine production. Induces antitumor responses.

PHARMACOKINETICS

Metabolism not specified. Elimination not specified. Steady-state concentration: 18 wks. **Half-life:** 26 days.

LIFESPAN CONSIDERATIONS

Pregnancy/Lactation: Avoid pregnancy; may cause fetal harm. Unknown if distributed in breast milk. Females of reproductive potential must use effective contraception during treatment and up to 4 mos after discontinuation. **Children:** Safety and efficacy not established. **Elderly:** No age-related precautions noted.

INTERACTIONS

DRUG: None known. **HERBAL:** None significant. **FOOD:** None known. **LAB VALUES:** May increase serum AST, glucose, triglycerides. May decrease albumin, serum calcium, sodium.

AVAILABILITY (Rx)

Injection Solution: 100 mg/4 mL.

ADMINISTRATION/HANDLING

IV

◀ALERT▶ Use 0.2–0.5-micron in-line filter.

Reconstitution • Withdraw required dose and mix into 0.9% NaCl infusion bag (diluent volume depends on dose required). • Final concentration of diluent bag should equal 1–10 mg/mL. • Allow refrigerated solution to warm to room temperature before infusing.

Rate of administration • Infuse via dedicated line over 30 min using a 0.2–0.5-micron filter.

Storage • Diluted solution up to 24 hrs, or at room temperature up to 4 hrs. Store time should not exceed total combined time of reconstitution, dilution, storage, and infusion.

INDICATIONS/ROUTES/DOSAGE

cHL, MSI-H Cancer, Merkel Cell Carcinoma, cSCC

IV: ADULTS, ELDERLY: 200 mg q3wks (or 400 mg q6wks) until disease progression or unacceptable toxicity for up to 2 mos. **CHILDREN:** 2 mg/kg (up to 200 mg) q3wks until disease progression or unacceptable toxicity for up to 2 mos.

Cervical Cancer, Gastric Cancer, HNSCC, NSCLC (Single-agent therapy), Primary Mediastinal Large B-Cell Lymphoma, Melanoma, Urothelial Cancer, Hepatocellular Carcinoma, Head and Neck Squamous Cell, Melanoma (Adjuvant treatment), Renal Cell Carcinoma, SCLC, Squamous Cell Carcinoma of Esophagus, Endometrial Carcinoma

IV: ADULTS, ELDERLY: 200 mg q3wks (or 400 mg q6wks. Continue until disease progression or unacceptable toxicity, or in pts without disease progression.

NSCLC (Combination therapy)

IV: ADULTS, ELDERLY: 200 mg q3wks (in combination with pemetrexed and carboplatin) for 4 cycles, then 200 mg q3wks (with or without optional indefinite pemetrexed maintenance therapy). Continue until disease progression or unacceptable toxicity, or in pts without disease progression for up to 24 months.

TNBC

IV: ADULTS, ELDERLY: 200 mg q3wks or 400 mg q6wks. Continue until disease progression, unacceptable toxicity or (pts without disease progression) for up to 24 mos.

Dose Modification

Based on Common Terminology Criteria for Adverse Events (CTCAE).

Withhold treatment for any of the following adverse events: ALT or AST greater than 3–5 times upper limit of normal (ULN) or bilirubin 1.5–3 times ULN, Grade 2 or 3 colitis, Grade 3 hyperthyroidism, Grade 2 nephritis, Grade 2 pneumonitis, symptomatic hypophysitis; any Grade 3 treatment-related adverse reaction. **Permanently discontinue for any of the following adverse events:** ALT or AST greater than 5 times ULN or bilirubin 3 times ULN (or pts with liver metastasis who begin treatment with Grade 2 ALT, AST, if ALT or AST increases greater than or equal to 50% from baseline and lasts for at least 1 wk), Grade 3 or 4 infusion-related reaction, Grade 3 or 4 nephritis, Grade 3 or 4 pneumonitis; inability to reduce corticosteroid dose to 10 mg/day or less (or predniSONE equivalent) after last dose; persistent Grade 2 or 3 adverse reaction that does not recover to Grade 0–1 within 12 wks after last dose; any severe or Grade 3 treatment-related adverse reaction that reoccurs.

Dosage in Renal Impairment

No dose adjustment.

Dosage in Hepatic Impairment

Mild impairment: No dose adjustment. **Moderate to severe impairment:** Not studied, use caution.

SIDE EFFECTS

Frequent (47%–20%): Fatigue, nausea, cough, pruritus, rash, decreased appetite, constipation, diarrhea, arthralgia. **Occasional (18%–11%):** Dyspnea, extremity pain, peripheral edema, vomiting, headache, chills, insomnia, myalgia, abdominal pain, back pain, pyrexia, vitiligo, dizziness, upper respiratory tract infection.

ADVERSE EFFECTS/TOXIC REACTIONS

May cause severe immune-mediated events such as pneumonitis (2.9% of pts), colitis (1% of pts), hepatitis (0.5% of pts), hypophysitis (0.5% of pts), renal failure or nephritis (0.7% of pts), hyperthyroidism (1.2% of pts), hypothyroidism (8.3% of pts). Other reported events include adrenal insufficiency, arthritis, cellulitis, exfoliative dermatitis, hemolytic anemia, myositis, myasthenic syndrome, pancreatitis, partial seizures, pneumonia, optic neuritis, rhabdomyolysis, sepsis. Immunogenicity (anti-pembrolizumab antibody formation) may occur.

NURSING CONSIDERATIONS

BASELINE ASSESSMENT

Obtain CBC, BMP, LFT, TSH; pregnancy test in females of reproductive potential. Obtain weight in kg. Question history of adrenal/pituitary/pulmonary/thyroid disease, autoimmune disorders, hepatic/renal impairment, allergy to predniSONE. Conduct dermatologic exam, visual acuity. Offer emotional support.

INTERVENTION/EVALUATION

Monitor CBC, LFT, serum electrolytes; thyroid panel if applicable. Monitor for immune-mediated adverse events. Notify physician if any CTCAE toxicities occur (see Appendix M) and initiate proper treatment. Obtain chest X-ray if pneumonitis suspected. Screen for tumor lysis syndrome in pts with high tumor burden. Offer antiemetics if nausea, vomiting occurs. Monitor I&O, daily weight.

PATIENT/FAMILY TEACHING

• Serious adverse reactions may affect lungs, GI tract, kidneys, or hormonal glands, and predniSONE therapy may need to be started. • Immediately contact physician if serious or life-threatening inflammatory reactions occur in the following body systems: lung (chest pain, cough, shortness of

P

breath); colon (severe abdominal pain or diarrhea); liver (bruising, clay-colored/tarry stools, yellowing of skin or eyes); pituitary (persistent or unusual headache, dizziness, extreme weakness, fainting, vision changes); kidney (decreased or dark-colored urine, flank pain); thyroid (insomnia, hypertension, tachycardia [overactive thyroid]), (fatigue, goiter, weight gain [underactive thyroid]). • Use effective contraception to avoid pregnancy. Do not breastfeed.

PEMEtrexed

TOP 100 HIGH ALERT

pem-e-**trex**-ed
(Alimta)

CLASSIFICATION

PHARMACOTHERAPEUTIC: Folate analog metabolic inhibitor. Antimetabolite. **CLINICAL:** Antineoplastic.

Do not confuse PEMEtrexed with methotrexate or PRALAtrexate.

USES

Treatment of unresectable malignant pleural mesothelioma in combination with CISplatin. Initial treatment of locally advanced or metastatic nonsquamous non–small-cell lung cancer (NSCLC) in combination with CISplatin. Single-agent maintenance treatment of NSCLC in pts whose disease has not progressed following 4 cycles of platinum-based first-line chemotherapy. **OFF-LABEL:** Treatment of bladder, cervical, ovarian, thymic malignancies; malignant pleural mesothelioma.

PRECAUTIONS

Contraindications: Severe hypersensitivity to PEMEtrexed. **Cautions:** Hepatic/renal impairment, concurrent use of nephrotoxic medications, preexisting myelosuppression. Not indicated for squamous cell NSCLC.

ACTION

Inhibits biosynthesis of purine and thymidine nucleotides. Inhibits protein synthesis. **Therapeutic Effect:** Disrupts folate-dependent enzymes essential for cell replication.

PHARMACOKINETICS

Protein binding: 81%. Not metabolized. Excreted in urine. **Half-life:** 3.5 hrs.

LIFESPAN CONSIDERATIONS

Pregnancy/Lactation: Avoid pregnancy; may cause fetal harm. Females of reproductive potential must use effective contraception during treatment and for at least 6 mos after discontinuation. Unknown if distributed in breast milk. Breastfeeding not recommended during treatment and for at least 7 days after discontinuation. Males must use effective contraception during treatment and for at least 3 mos after discontinuation. **Children:** Safety and efficacy not established in pts younger than 18 yrs. **Elderly:** Higher incidence of fatigue, leukopenia, neutropenia, thrombocytopenia in pts 65 yrs and older.

INTERACTIONS

DRUG: **Ibuprofen** may increase concentration/adverse effects. **Bone marrow depressants (e.g., cladribine)** may increase risk of myelosuppression. **Live virus vaccines** may potentiate virus replication, increase vaccine side effects, decrease pt's antibody response to vaccine. **HERBAL:** **Echinacea** may decrease therapeutic effect. **FOOD:** None known. **LAB VALUES:** May increase serum ALT, AST, creatinine.

AVAILABILITY (Rx)

Injection, Powder for Reconstitution: 100 mg; 500 mg.

ADMINISTRATION/HANDLING

IV Infusion

Reconstitution • Dilute 500-mg vial with 20 mL (4.2 mL to 100-mg vial) 0.9% NaCl to provide concentration of 25 mg/mL. • Gently swirl each vial until powder is completely dissolved. • Solution appears clear and ranges in color from colorless to yellow or green-yellow. • Dilute in 100 mL 0.9% NaCl.

Rate of administration • Infuse over 10 min.
Storage • Store at room temperature. • Diluted solution is stable for up to 24 hrs at room temperature or if refrigerated.

IV INCOMPATIBILITIES

Use only 0.9% NaCl to reconstitute; flush line prior to and following infusion. Do not add any other medications to IV line.

INDICATIONS/ROUTES/DOSAGE

◄ALERT► Pretreatment with dexamethasone (or equivalent) will reduce risk, severity of cutaneous reaction; treatment with folic acid and vitamin B_{12} beginning 1 wk before treatment and continuing for 21 days after last PEMEtrexed dose will reduce risk of side effects. Do not begin new treatment cycles unless ANC 1,500 cells/mm^3 or greater, platelets 100,000 cells/mm^3 or greater, and CrCl 45 mL/min or greater.

Malignant Pleural Mesothelioma

IV: ADULTS, ELDERLY: 500 mg/m^2 on day 1 of each 21-day cycle in combination with CISplatin. Continue until disease progression or unacceptable toxicity.

Nonsquamous Non–Small-Cell Lung Cancer (NSCLC)

IV: ADULTS, ELDERLY: Initial treatment 500 mg/m^2 on day 1 of each 21-day cycle (in combination with CISplatin) for up to 6 cycles or until disease progression or unacceptable toxicity. **Maintenance or second-line treatment:** 500 mg/m^2 on day 1 of each 21-day cycle (as single agent). Continue until disease progression or unacceptable toxicity.

Dose Modification for Hematologic Toxicity

ANC less than 500 cells/mm^3 and platelets 50,000 cells/mm^3 or more: Reduce dose to 75% of previous dose. **Platelets less than 50,000 cells/mm^3 without bleeding:** Reduce dose to 75% of previous dose. **Platelets less than 50,000 cells/mm^3 with bleeding:** Reduce dose to 50% of previous dose. **Nonhematologic toxicity Grade 3 or greater (excluding neurotoxicity):** Reduce dose to 75% of previous dose (excluding mucositis). **Grade 3 or 4 mucositis:** Reduce dose to 50% of previous dose.

Dosage in Renal Impairment

Not recommended with CrCl less than 45 mL/min.

Dosage in Hepatic Impairment

Grade 3 or 4 hepatic impairment: 75% of previous dose.

SIDE EFFECTS

Frequent (12%–10%): Fatigue, nausea, vomiting, rash, desquamation. **Occasional (8%–4%):** Stomatitis, pharyngitis, diarrhea, anorexia, hypertension, chest pain. **Rare (less than 3%):** Constipation, depression, dysphagia.

ADVERSE EFFECTS/TOXIC REACTIONS

Myelosuppression (anemia, neutropenia, thrombocytopenia) is an expected response to therapy. Severe, sometimes fatal renal toxicity may occur. Serious cutaneous events including bullous, blistering, and exfoliative skin toxicities, Stevens-Johnson syndrome, epidermal necrolysis may occur. Fatal cases of interstitial pneumonitis were reported. Radiation recall may occur in pts who have received radiation wks to yrs previously.

NURSING CONSIDERATIONS

BASELINE ASSESSMENT

Obtain CBC, BMP, LFT; pregnancy test in females of reproductive potential. Question history of hepatic/renal impairment. Receive full medication history and screen for interactions (esp. use of NSAIDs). Assess hydration status. Offer emotional support.

INTERVENTION/EVALUATION

Monitor CBC as clinically indicated; BMP, LFT periodically. Monitor for hematologic toxicity (fever, sore throat, signs of local infection, unusual bruising/bleeding from any site), symptoms of anemia (excessive fatigue, weakness), renal toxicity. Assess skin for rash, lesions, dermatological toxicities. Obtain CXR if interstitial lung disease, pneumonitis suspected. Ensure adequate hydration.

PATIENT/FAMILY TEACHING

• Treatment may depress your immune system response and reduce your ability to fight infection. Report symptoms of infection such as body aches, chills, cough, fatigue, fever. Avoid those with active infection. • Use effective contraception to avoid pregnancy. Do not breastfeed. • Report unusual bruising or bleeding of any kind. • Treatment may cause severe lung inflammation; report cough, difficulty breathing, fever. • Report skin toxicities such as blistering, bubbling, sloughing of the skin; liver problems (bruising, confusion, amber- or orange-colored urine, abdominal pain, yellowing of the skin or eyes); kidney problems (decreased urine output, dark-colored urine, flank pain).

penicillin G potassium

pen-i-**sil**-in G po-**tas**-ee-um
(Pfizerpen-G)
Do not confuse penicillin with penicillAMINE.

◆CLASSIFICATION

PHARMACOTHERAPEUTIC: Penicillin. **CLINICAL:** Antibiotic.

USES

Treatment of susceptible infections including sepsis, meningitis, endocarditis, pneumonia. Active against gram-positive organisms (except *S. aureus*), some gram-negative organisms (e.g., *N. gonorrhoeae*), and some anaerobes and spirochetes.

PRECAUTIONS

Contraindications: Hypersensitivity to any penicillin. **Cautions:** Renal/hepatic impairment, seizure disorder, hypersensitivity to cephalosporins, asthma.

ACTION

Inhibits bacterial cell wall synthesis by binding to one or more of the penicillin-binding proteins of bacteria. **Therapeutic Effect:** Bactericidal.

PHARMACOKINETICS

Protein binding: 60%. Widely distributed (poor CNS penetration). Metabolized in liver. Primarily excreted in urine. **Half-life:** 0.5–1 hr (increased in renal impairment).

LIFESPAN CONSIDERATIONS

Pregnancy/Lactation: Readily crosses placenta; distributed in breast milk. **Children:** May delay renal excretion in neonates, young infants. **Elderly:** Age-related renal impairment may require dosage adjustment.

INTERACTIONS

DRUG: **Probenecid** may increase concentration/effect. **HERBAL:** None significant. **FOOD:** None significant. **LAB VALUES:** May cause positive Coombs' test. May increase serum ALT, AST, alkaline phosphatase, LDH. May decrease WBC count.

AVAILABILITY (Rx)

Injection, Powder for Reconstitution: 5 million units.

ADMINISTRATION/HANDLING

IV

Reconstitution • After reconstitution, further dilute with 50–100 mL D_5W or 0.9% NaCl for final concentration of 100,000–500,000 units/mL (50,000 units/mL for infants, neonates).
Rate of administration • Infuse over 15–30 min.
Storage • Reconstituted solution is stable for 7 days if refrigerated.

IV INCOMPATIBILITIES

DOPamine (Intropin), sodium bicarbonate.

IV COMPATIBILITIES

Amiodarone (Cordarone), calcium gluconate, dilTIAZem (Cardizem), heparin, magnesium sulfate, potassium chloride.

INDICATIONS/ROUTES/DOSAGE

Usual Dosage

IV: ADULTS, ELDERLY: 12–24 million units/day in divided doses q4–6h. **CHILDREN: Mild to moderate infection:** 100,000–150,000 units/kg/day in divided doses q6h. **Maximum:** 8 million units/day. **Severe infections:** 200,000–300,000 units/kg/day in divided doses q4–6h. **Maximum:** 24 million units/day. **NEONATES:** 25,000–50,000 units/kg/dose q8–12h.

Dosage in Renal Impairment

Dosage interval is modified based on creatinine clearance.

Creatinine Clearance	Dosage
Greater than 50 mL/min	No dose adjustment
10–50 mL/min	75% normal dose
Less than 10 mL/min	20%–50% normal dose
Hemodialysis	50%–100% normal dose q8–12h
Continuous renal replacement therapy	
Continuous venovenous hemofiltration	Loading dose 4 million units, then 2 million units q4–6h
Continuous venovenous hemodialysis	Loading dose 4 million units, then 2–3 million units q4–6h
Continuous venovenous hemodiafiltration	Loading dose 4 million units, then 2–4 million units q4–6h

Dosage in Hepatic Impairment

No dose adjustment.

SIDE EFFECTS

Occasional: Lethargy, fever, dizziness, rash, electrolyte imbalance, diarrhea, thrombophlebitis. **Rare:** Seizures, interstitial nephritis.

ADVERSE EFFECTS/TOXIC REACTIONS

Hypersensitivity reactions ranging from rash, fever, chills to anaphylaxis occur occasionally.

NURSING CONSIDERATIONS

BASELINE ASSESSMENT

Question for history of allergies, particularly penicillins, cephalosporins.

INTERVENTION/EVALUATION

Promptly report rash (hypersensitivity), diarrhea (with fever, abdominal pain, mucus, or blood in stool, may indicate antibiotic-associated colitis). Monitor I&O, urinalysis, electrolytes, renal function tests for nephrotoxicity.

penicillin V potassium

pen-i-**sil**-in V po-**tas**-ee-um (Apo-Pen-VK ✦, Novo-Pen-VK ✦, NuPen VK ✦)

◆CLASSIFICATION

PHARMACOTHERAPEUTIC: Penicillin. **CLINICAL:** Antibiotic.

USES

Treatment of infections of respiratory tract, skin/skin structure, otitis media, necrotizing ulcerative gingivitis; prophylaxis for rheumatic fever, dental procedures. **OFF-LABEL:** Prosthetic joint infection.

PRECAUTIONS

Contraindications: Hypersensitivity to any penicillin. **Cautions:** Severe renal impairment, history of allergies (particularly cephalosporins), seizure disorder, asthma.

ACTION

Inhibits cell wall synthesis by binding to bacterial cell membranes. **Therapeutic Effect:** Bactericidal.

PHARMACOKINETICS

Moderately absorbed from GI tract. Protein binding: 80%. Widely distributed. Metabolized in liver. Primarily excreted in urine. **Half-life:** 1 hr (increased in renal impairment).

⌛ LIFESPAN CONSIDERATIONS

Pregnancy/Lactation: Readily crosses placenta; appears in cord blood, amniotic fluid. Distributed in breast milk in low concentrations. May lead to allergic sensitization, diarrhea, candidiasis, skin rash in infant. **Children:** Use caution in neonates and young infants (may delay renal elimination). **Elderly:** Age-related renal impairment may require dosage adjustment.

INTERACTIONS

DRUG: May increase concentration/effect of **methotrexate. Probenecid** may increase concentration/effect. **Tetracycline** may decrease concentration/effect. **HERBAL:** None significant. **FOOD:** None known. **LAB VALUES:** May cause positive Coombs' test. May increase serum ALT, AST, alkaline phosphatase, LDH. May decrease WBC count.

AVAILABILITY (Rx)

Powder for Oral Solution: 125 mg/5 mL, 250 mg/5 mL. **Tablets:** 250 mg, 500 mg.

ADMINISTRATION/HANDLING

PO

• Give on empty stomach 1 hr before or 2 hrs after meals (increases absorption). • After reconstitution, oral solution is stable for 14 days if refrigerated. • Space doses evenly around the clock.

INDICATIONS/ROUTES/DOSAGE

Usual Dosage

PO: ADULTS, ELDERLY, CHILDREN 12 YRS AND OLDER: 125–500 mg q6–8h. **CHILDREN YOUNGER THAN 12 YRS:** 25–75 mg/kg/day in divided doses q6–8h. **Maximum:** 2,000 mg/day.

Dosage in Renal/Hepatic Impairment

No dose adjustment.

SIDE EFFECTS

Frequent: Mild hypersensitivity reaction (chills, fever, rash), nausea, vomiting, diarrhea. **Rare:** Bleeding, allergic reaction.

ADVERSE EFFECTS/TOXIC REACTIONS

Severe hypersensitivity reactions, including anaphylaxis, may occur. Nephrotoxicity, antibiotic-associated colitis, other superinfections (abdominal cramps, severe watery diarrhea, fever) may result from high dosages, prolonged therapy.

NURSING CONSIDERATIONS

BASELINE ASSESSMENT

Question for history of allergies, particularly penicillins, cephalosporins.

INTERVENTION/EVALUATION

Monitor for rash (hypersensitivity), diarrhea (with fever, abdominal pain, mucus or blood in stool may indicate antibiotic-associated colitis). Be alert for superinfection: fever, vomiting, diarrhea, anal/genital pruritus, oral mucosal change (ulceration, pain, erythema). Monitor I&O, urinalysis, renal function tests for nephrotoxicity.

PATIENT/FAMILY TEACHING

• Continue antibiotic for full length of treatment. • Space doses evenly. • Report immediately if rash, diarrhea, bleeding, bruising, other new symptoms occur.

P

pertuzumab

per-**tue**-zue-mab
(Perjeta)

■ BLACK BOX ALERT ■ Can result in embryo-fetal death, birth defects. Pts must be made aware of danger to fetus, need for effective contraception. May result in cardiac failure. Assess left ventricular ejection fraction.

◆CLASSIFICATION

PHARMACOTHERAPEUTIC: *HER2* receptor antagonist. Monoclonal antibody. **CLINICAL:** Antineoplastic.

USES

Treatment of *HER2*-positive metastatic breast cancer in pts who have not received prior anti-*HER2* therapy or chemotherapy for metastatic disease in combination with trastuzumab and DOCEtaxel. Neoadjuvant treatment of pts with *HER2*-positive, locally advanced inflammatory, or early-stage breast cancer in combination with trastuzumab and DOCEtaxel. Adjuvant treatment of *HER2*-positive early breast cancer at high risk of recurrence (in combination with trastuzumab and chemotherapy).

PRECAUTIONS

Contraindications: Hypersensitivity to pertuzumab. **Cautions:** Cardiomyopathy, HF, history of infusion-related reaction. Prior anthracycline therapy or irradiation. Conditions predisposing to infection (e.g., diabetes, immunocompromised pts, renal failure, open wounds), pts at risk for tumor lysis syndrome (high tumor burden).

ACTION

Targets human epidermal growth factor 2 (*HER2*), blocking ligand-initiated intercellular signaling, which can result in cell growth arrest and cell death. **Therapeutic Effect:** Inhibits cell growth and metastasis.

PHARMACOKINETICS

Peak plasma concentration reached after first maintenance dose. **Half-life:** 18 days.

LIFESPAN CONSIDERATIONS

Pregnancy/Lactation: Avoid pregnancy; may cause fetal harm. Females of reproductive potential must use effective contraception during treatment and for at least 7 mos after discontinuation. Unknown if distributed in breast milk. However, human immunoglobulin G (IgG) is present in breast milk and is known to cross the placenta. **Children:** Safety and efficacy not established. **Elderly:** No age-related precautions noted.

INTERACTIONS

DRUG: May increase concentration/effect of **belimumab**. **HERBAL:** None significant. **FOOD:** None known. **LAB VALUES:** May decrease Hgb, Hct, leukocytes, neutrophils.

AVAILABILITY (Rx)

Injection Solution: 420 mg/14 mL (30 mg/mL) vial.

ADMINISTRATION/HANDLING

IV

Reconstitution • Visually inspect for particulate matter or discoloration. Do not use if solution is cloudy, discolored, or if visible particles are observed. • Dilute in 250 mL 0.9% NaCl only (do not use D_5W). • Mix by gentle inversion. • Do not shake.

Rate of administration • Initial dose to be infused over 60 min. • Subsequent doses may be infused over 30–60 min.

Storage • Refrigerate unused vials. Store vials in outside cartons (protects from light). • May refrigerate diluted solution for up to 24 hrs. • Do not freeze.

IV INCOMPATIBILITIES

Do not mix with any other medications.

INDICATIONS/ROUTES/DOSAGE

◀ALERT▶ Give as an IV infusion only. Do not give by IV push or bolus.

Breast Cancer (Metastatic)

IV infusion: ADULTS/ELDERLY: Initially, 840, followed by maintenance dose of 420 mg given over q3wks until disease progression or unacceptable toxicity (in combination with trastuzumab and DOCEtaxel).

Breast Cancer (Adjuvant)

IV infusion: ADULTS, ELDERLY: 840 mg, followed by maintenance dose of 420 mg q3wks for a total of 1 yr (up to 18 cycles) or until disease progression or unacceptable toxicity (as part of combination regimen containing trastuzumab and standard anthracycline- and/or taxane-based therapy). Pertuzumab and trastuzumab should begin on day 1 of the first taxane-containing cycle.

Breast Cancer (Neoadjuvant)

IV infusion: ADULTS, ELDERLY: 840 mg once, followed by 420 mg q3wks for 3–6 cycles. May be administered as one of the following regimens: 4 preoperative cycles of pertuzumab, trastuzumab, DOCEtaxel, then 3 postoperative cycles of 5-fluorouracil, epiRUBicin, and cyclophosphamide (FEC) **or** 3 or 4 preoperative cycles of FEC alone, then 3 or 4 preoperative cycles of pertuzumab, trastuzumab, DOCEtaxel **or** 6 preoperative cycles of pertuzumab, trastuzumab, DOCEtaxel, and CARBOplatin **or** 4 preoperative cycles of dose-dense DOXOrubicin and cyclophosphamide alone, then 4 preoperative cycles of pertuzumab, trastuzumab, and PACLitaxel. **Note:** Continue trastuzumab postoperatively to complete 1 yr of treatment.

Dosage in Renal/Hepatic Impairment

No dose adjustment.

SIDE EFFECTS

Frequent (67%–21%): Diarrhea, alopecia, nausea, fatigue, rash, peripheral neuropathy, anorexia, asthenia, mucosal inflammation, vomiting, peripheral edema, myalgia, nail disorder, headache. **Occasional (19%–12%):** Stomatitis, pyrexia, dysgeusia, arthralgia, constipation, increased lacrimation, pruritus, insomnia, dizziness. **Rare (10%–7%):** Nasopharyngitis, dry skin, paronychia.

ADVERSE EFFECTS/TOXIC REACTIONS

Myelosuppression (anemia, leukopenia, neutropenia) is an expected response to therapy, but more severe reactions including febrile neutropenia may be life-threatening. Upper respiratory tract infection occurs in 17% of pts. Pleural effusion occurred in 5% of pts. Tumor lysis syndrome may present as acute renal failure, hypocalcemia, hyperuricemia, hyperphosphatemia. Immunogenicity (auto-pertuzumab antibodies) reported in 3% of pts. Decreases in LVEF occurred in 4% of pts. Prior treatment with anthracyclines, chest radiotherapy may further increase risk of decreased LVEF.

NURSING CONSIDERATIONS

BASELINE ASSESSMENT

Obtain CBC. Assess left ventricular ejection fraction (LVEF) by echocardiogram. Negative pregnancy test must be confirmed before initiating treatment. Obtain *HER2* testing by an FDA-approved laboratory. Screen for active infection. Offer emotional support.

INTERVENTION/EVALUATION

Monitor ANC, CBC periodically. Assess LVEF at regular intervals. Monitor for symptoms of left ventricular dysfunction (arrhythmia, cough, dyspnea, peripheral edema). Monitor for infusion reactions, hypersensitivity reactions, anaphylaxis. If a significant infusion reaction occurs, slow or interrupt infusion and administer appropriate medical treatment. Observe pt closely for 60 min after the first infusion and for 30 min after subsequent infusions. Monitor for symptoms of tumor

P

lysis syndrome (acute renal failure, hypocalcemia, hyperuricemia, hyperphosphatemia).

PATIENT/FAMILY TEACHING

• Treatment may depress your immune system response and reduce your ability to fight infection. Report symptoms of infection such as body aches, chills, cough, fatigue, fever. Avoid those with active infection. • Report symptoms of bone marrow depression such as bruising, fatigue, fever, shortness of breath, weight loss; bleeding easily, bloody urine or stool. • New-onset left heart dysfunction may occur; report shortness of breath, cough, swelling of ankles or feet, palpitations. • Therapy may cause life-threatening tumor lysis syndrome (a condition caused by the rapid breakdown of cancer cells), which can cause kidney failure. Report decreased urination, amber-colored urine; confusion, difficulty breathing, fatigue, fever, muscle or joint pain, palpitations, seizures, vomiting. • Use effective contraception to avoid pregnancy. Do not breastfeed.

P

PHENobarbital

fee-noe-**bar**-bi-tal
Do not confuse PHENobarbital with Phenergan, or phenytoin.

FIXED-COMBINATION(S)

Donnatal: PHENobarbital/atropine (an anticholinergic)/hyoscyamine (an anticholinergic)/scopolamine (an anticholinergic): 16.2 mg/0.0194 mg/0.1037 mg/0.0065 mg.

◆CLASSIFICATION

PHARMACOTHERAPEUTIC: Barbiturate (Schedule IV). **CLINICAL:** Anticonvulsant.

USES

Management of generalized tonic-clonic (grand mal) seizures, partial seizures, control of acute seizure episodes (status epilepticus). **OFF-LABEL:** Treatment of alcohol withdrawal, sedative/hypnotic withdrawal.

PRECAUTIONS

Contraindications: Hypersensitivity to PHENobarbital, other barbiturates, porphyria, dyspnea or airway obstruction, use in nephritic pts (large doses), severe hepatic impairment. History of sedative/hypnotic addiction. Intra-arterial or SQ administration. **Cautions:** Renal/hepatic impairment, acute/chronic pain, depression, suicidal tendencies, history of drug abuse, elderly, debilitated, children, hemodynamically unstable pts, hypoadrenalism, respiratory disease.

ACTION

Depresses sensory cortex, decreases motor activity, alters cerebellar function. **Therapeutic Effect:** Induces drowsiness, sedation, anticonvulsant activity.

PHARMACOKINETICS

Route	Onset	Peak	Duration
PO	20–60 min	N/A	6–10 hrs
IV	5 min	30 min	4–10 hrs

Widely distributed. Protein binding: 20%–45%. Metabolized in liver. Primarily excreted in urine. Removed by hemodialysis. **Half-life:** 53–140 hrs.

⌛ LIFESPAN CONSIDERATIONS

Pregnancy/Lactation: Readily crosses placenta. Distributed in breast milk. Produces respiratory depression in neonates during labor. May cause postpartum hemorrhage, hemorrhagic disease in newborn. Withdrawal symptoms may appear in neonates born to women receiving barbiturates during last trimester of pregnancy. Lowers serum bilirubin in neonates. **Children:** May cause paradoxical excitement. **Elderly:** May exhibit excitement, confusion, mental depression. Use caution.

INTERACTIONS

DRUG: **Alcohol, CNS depressants (e.g., LORazepam, morphine)** may increase CNS depression. May decrease effects of **warfarin, oral contraceptives. Valproic acid** may increase concentration, risk of toxicity. **Strong CYP2C19 inducers (e.g., carBAMazepine, rifAMPin)** may decrease concentration/effect. **Strong CYP2C19 inhibitors (e.g., FLUoxetine, fluvoxaMINE)** may increase concentration/effect. May decrease concentration/effect of **dolutegravir, tenofovir, voriconazole. HERBAL: Herbals with sedative properties (e.g., chamomile, kava kava, valerian)** may increase CNS depression. **FOOD:** None known. **LAB VALUES:** May decrease serum bilirubin. **Therapeutic serum level:** 10–40 mcg/mL; **toxic serum level:** greater than 40 mcg/mL.

AVAILABILITY (Rx)

Elixir: 20 mg/5 mL. **Oral Solution:** 20 mg/5 mL. **Injection Solution:** 65 mg/mL, 130 mg/mL. **Tablets:** 15 mg, 30 mg, 60 mg, 100 mg.

ADMINISTRATION/HANDLING

IV

Reconstitution • May give undiluted or may dilute with NaCl.

Rate of administration • Adequately hydrate before and immediately after drug therapy (decreases risk of adverse renal effects). • Do not inject IV faster than 30 mg/min for children and 60 mg/min for adults. Too-rapid IV may produce severe hypotension, marked respiratory depression. • Inadvertent intra-arterial injection may result in arterial spasm with severe pain, tissue necrosis. Extravasation in SQ tissue may produce redness, tenderness, tissue necrosis.

Storage • Store vials at room temperature.

IM

• Do not inject more than 5 mL in any one IM injection site (produces tissue irritation). • Inject deep IM into large muscle mass.

PO

• Give without regard to food. • Tablets may be crushed. • Elixir may be mixed with water, milk, fruit juice.

IV INCOMPATIBILITIES

Amphotericin B complex (Abelcet, AmBisome, Amphotec).

IV COMPATIBILITIES

Calcium gluconate, enalapril (Vasotec), fosphenytoin (Cerebyx), propofol (Diprivan).

INDICATIONS/ROUTES/DOSAGE

Status Epilepticus

IV: ADULTS, ELDERLY, CHILDREN: 15 mg/kg as a single dose. **CHILDREN:** 15–20 mg/kg (**Maximum:** 1,000 mg) over 10 min; may repeat after 15 min (**Maximum:** 40 mg/kg).

Seizure Control (Maintenance)

Note: Maintenance dose usually starts 12 hrs after loading dose.

PO, IV: ADULTS, ELDERLY: 2 mg/kg/day in divided doses. **ADOLESCENTS:** 1–3 mg/kg/day in 1–2 divided doses. **CHILDREN 5–12 YRS:** 4–6 mg/kg/day in divided doses. **CHILDREN 1–5 YRS:** 6–8 mg/kg/day in divided doses. **CHILDREN YOUNGER THAN 1 YR:** 5–6 mg/kg/day in 1–2 divided doses. **NEONATES:** 3–4 mg/kg/day given once daily.

Dosage in Renal/Hepatic Impairment

No dose adjustment.

SIDE EFFECTS

Occasional (3%–1%): Drowsiness. **Rare (less than 1%):** Confusion, paradoxical

CNS reactions (hyperactivity, anxiety in children; excitement, restlessness in elderly, generally noted during first 2 wks of therapy, particularly in presence of uncontrolled pain).

ADVERSE EFFECTS/TOXIC REACTIONS

Abrupt withdrawal after prolonged therapy may produce increased dreaming, nightmares, insomnia, tremor, diaphoresis, vomiting, hallucinations, delirium, seizures, status epilepticus. Skin eruptions appear as hypersensitivity reaction. Blood dyscrasias, hepatic disease, hypocalcemia occur rarely. Overdose produces cold/clammy skin, hypothermia, severe CNS depression, cyanosis, tachycardia, Cheyne-Stokes respirations. Toxicity may result in severe renal impairment.

NURSING CONSIDERATIONS

BASELINE ASSESSMENT

Assess B/P, heart rate, respirations immediately before administration. **Hypnotic:** Raise bed rails, provide environment conducive to sleep (back rub, quiet environment, low lighting). **Seizures:** Review history of seizure disorder (length, presence of auras, LOC). Observe for recurrence of seizure activity. Initiate seizure precautions.

INTERVENTION/EVALUATION

Monitor CNS status, seizure activity, hepatic/renal function, respiratory rate, heart rate, B/P. Monitor for therapeutic serum level. Neurologic assessments may be inaccurate until drug has properly cleared the body. **Therapeutic serum level:** 10–40 mcg/mL; **toxic serum level:** greater than 40 mcg/mL.

PATIENT/FAMILY TEACHING

• Avoid alcohol, limit caffeine. • May be habit-forming. • Do not discontinue abruptly. • May cause dizziness/drowsiness; avoid tasks that require alertness, motor skills until response to drug is established.

P

phenylephrine HIGH ALERT

fen-il-**ef**-rin
(AK-Dilate, Mydfrin, Neo-Synephrine, Sudafed PE)

BLACK BOX ALERT Intravenous use should be administered by adequately trained individuals familiar with its use.

Do not confuse Mydfrin with Midrin, or Sudafed PE with Sudafed.

CLASSIFICATION

PHARMACOTHERAPEUTIC: Alpha-adrenergic agonist. **CLINICAL:** Nasal decongestant, mydriatic, vasopressor.

USES

Nasal decongestant: Topical application to nasal mucosa reduces nasal secretion, promoting drainage of sinus secretions. **Parenteral:** Vascular failure in shock, supraventricular tachycardia, hypotension.

PRECAUTIONS

Contraindications: Hypersensitivity to phenylephrine. **Injection:** Severe hypertension, ventricular tachycardia. **Oral:** Use within 14 days of MAOI therapy. **Cautions: Injection:** Elderly, hyperthyroidism, bradycardia, partial heart block, cardiac disease, HF, cardiogenic shock, hypertension. **Oral:** Asthma, bowel obstruction, cardiac disease, ischemic heart disease, hypertension, increased intraocular pressure, elderly, prostatic hyperplasia.

ACTION

Acts on alpha-adrenergic receptors of vascular smooth muscle. Causes vasoconstriction of arterioles of nasal mucosa/conjunctiva; produces systemic arterial vasoconstriction. **Therapeutic Effect:** Decreases mucosal blood flow, relieves congestion. Increases B/P. Reduces heart rate due to decrease in cardiac output.

PHARMACOKINETICS

Route	Onset	Peak	Duration
IV	Immediate	N/A	15–20 min
IM	10–15 min	N/A	0.5–2 hrs
SQ	10–15 min	N/A	1 hr

Minimal absorption after intranasal, ophthalmic administration. Metabolized in liver, GI tract. Primarily excreted in urine. **Half-life:** 2.5 hrs.

LIFESPAN CONSIDERATIONS

Pregnancy/Lactation: Crosses placenta. Distributed in breast milk. **Children:** May exhibit increased absorption, toxicity with nasal preparation. No age-related precautions noted with systemic use. **Elderly:** More likely to experience adverse effects.

INTERACTIONS

DRUG: **Linezolid, MAOIs (e.g., phenelzine, selegiline)** may increase vasopressor effects. **Tricyclic antidepressants (e.g., amitriptyline, doxepin)** may increase vasopressor effect. **Ergot derivatives (e.g., ergotamine)** may increase hypertensive effect. **HERBAL:** None significant. **FOOD:** None known. **LAB VALUES:** None significant.

AVAILABILITY (OTC)

Injection, Solution: 10 mg/mL. **Solution, Nasal Drops (Neo-Synephrine):** 0.125%, 0.25%. **Solution, Nasal Spray (Neo-Synephrine):** 0.25%, 0.5%. **Solution, Oral:** 2.5 mg/5 mL. **Tablets (Sudafed PE):** 10 mg.

ADMINISTRATION/HANDLING

IV

Reconstitution • For IV push, dilute with NS to a concentration of 0.1–1 mg/mL. • For IV infusion, dilute 10–100 mg with 500 mL 0.9% NaCl or D_5W.

Rate of administration • For IV push, give over 20–30 sec. • For IV infusion, titrate dose to maintain systolic B/P greater than 90 mm Hg.

Storage • Store vials at room temperature.

Nasal

• Instruct pt to blow nose prior to administering medication. • With head tilted back, apply drops in 1 nostril. Wait 5 min before applying drops in other nostril. • Sprays should be administered into each nostril with head erect. • Pt should sniff briskly while squeezing container, then wait 3–5 min before blowing nose gently. • Rinse tip of spray bottle.

IV INCOMPATIBILITIES

Furosemide (Lasix).

IV COMPATIBILITIES

Amiodarone (Cordarone), dexmedetomidine (Precedex), DOBUTamine (Dobutrex), lidocaine, potassium chloride, propofol (Diprivan), vasopressin.

INDICATIONS/ROUTES/DOSAGE

Nasal Decongestant

◀ALERT▶ Do not use for more than 3 days.

Intranasal: ADULTS, ELDERLY, CHILDREN 12 YRS AND OLDER: 2–3 drops or 2–3 sprays of 0.25%–0.5% solution into each nostril q4h as needed. **CHILDREN 6–11 YRS:** 2–3 drops or 2–3 sprays of 0.25% solution into each nostril q4h as needed. **CHILDREN 2–5 YRS:** 1 drop of 0.125% solution (dilute 0.5% solution with 0.9% NaCl to achieve 0.125%) in each nostril. Repeat q2–4h as needed.

PO: ADULTS, ELDERLY, CHILDREN 13 YRS AND OLDER: 10 mg q4h as needed for up to 7 days. **Maximum:** 60 mg/day. **CHILDREN 6–11 YRS:** 5 mg q4h as needed for up to 7 days. **Maximum:** 30 mg/day. **CHILDREN 4–5 YRS:** 2.5 mg q4h as needed for up to 7 days. **Maximum:** 15 mg/day.

Hypotension, Shock

IV infusion: ADULTS, ELDERLY: 0.5–6 mcg/kg/min. Titrate to desired response. **CHILDREN:** Initially, 0.1–0.5 mcg/kg/min. Titrate to desired effect.

P

SIDE EFFECTS

Frequent: Nasal: Rebound nasal congestion due to overuse, esp. when used longer than 3 days. **Occasional:** Mild CNS stimulation (restlessness, nervousness, tremors, headache, insomnia, particularly in those hypersensitive to sympathomimetics, such as elderly pts). **Nasal:** Stinging, burning, drying of nasal mucosa.

ADVERSE EFFECTS/TOXIC REACTIONS

Large doses may produce tachycardia, palpitations (particularly in pts with cardiac disease), dizziness, nausea, vomiting. Overdose in pts older than 60 yrs may result in hallucinations, CNS depression, seizures. Prolonged nasal use may produce chronic swelling of nasal mucosa, rhinitis. If phenylephrine 10% ophthalmic is instilled into denuded/damaged corneal epithelium, corneal clouding may result.

NURSING CONSIDERATIONS

P

BASELINE ASSESSMENT

Obtain baseline symptomology, vital signs. Question history of hypertension, cardiac disease, asthma, recent use of MAOI therapy.

INTERVENTION/EVALUATION

Monitor B/P, heart rate. For severe hypotension or shock states, monitor central venous pressure noninvasive hemodynamic monitoring systems.

PATIENT/FAMILY TEACHING

• Discontinue if adverse reactions occur. • Do not use for nasal decongestion for longer than 3 days (rebound congestion). • Discontinue if insomnia, dizziness, weakness, tremor, palpitations occur. • **Nasal:** Stinging/burning of nasal mucosa may occur. • **Ophthalmic:** Blurring of vision with eye instillation generally subsides with continued therapy. • Discontinue medication if redness/swelling of eyelids, itching occurs.

phenytoin

fen-i-toyn
(Dilantin, Phenytek)

■ BLACK BOX ALERT ■ Do not exceed IV rate of 50 mg/min in adults and 1–3 mg/kg/min in pediatric pts.
Do not confuse Dilantin with Dilaudid or dilTIAZem, or phenytoin with phenelzine or fosphenytoin.

◆CLASSIFICATION

PHARMACOTHERAPEUTIC: Hydantoin. **CLINICAL:** Anticonvulsant.

USES

Management of generalized tonic-clonic seizures (grand mal), complex partial seizures, status epilepticus. Prevention of seizures following head trauma/neurosurgery. **OFF-LABEL:** Prevention of early posttraumatic seizures following traumatic brain injury.

PRECAUTIONS

Contraindications: Hypersensitivity to phenytoin, other hydantoins. Concurrent use of delavirdine. History of acute phenytoin therapy–induced hepatotoxicity. **IV (additional):** Second- and third-degree AV block, sinoatrial block, sinus bradycardia, Adams-Stokes syndrome. **Cautions:** Porphyria, diabetes, renal/hepatic impairment, pts at increased risk of suicidal behavior/thoughts, elderly, debilitated, hypoalbuminemia, cardiac disease, hypothyroidism, pts of Asian descent.

ACTION

Stabilizes neuronal membranes in motor cortex. Decreases influx of sodium during generation of nerve impulses. **Therapeutic Effect:** Decreases seizure activity.

PHARMACOKINETICS

Widely distributed. Protein binding: 90%–95%. Metabolized in liver. Primarily excreted in urine. Not removed by hemodialysis. **Half-life:** 7–42 hrs.

LIFESPAN CONSIDERATIONS

Pregnancy/Lactation: Crosses placenta; distributed in small amount in breast milk. Fetal hydantoin syndrome (craniofacial abnormalities, nail/digital hypoplasia, prenatal growth deficiency) has been reported. Increased frequency of seizures in pregnant women due to altered absorption of metabolism of phenytoin. May increase risk of hemorrhage in neonate, maternal bleeding during delivery. **Children:** More susceptible to gingival hyperplasia, coarsening of facial features; excess body hair. **Elderly:** No age-related precautions noted but lower dosages recommended.

INTERACTIONS

DRUG: **Alcohol, CNS depressants (e.g., LORazepam, morphine, zolpidem)** may increase CNS depression. **Amiodarone, cimetidine, disulfiram, FLUoxetine, isoniazid, sulfonamides** may increase concentration/effect, risk of toxicity. May decrease effects of **glucocorticoids (e.g., dexamethasone, predniSONE), oral contraceptives. Lidocaine, propranolol** may increase cardiac depressant effect. **Valproic acid** may decrease metabolism, increase concentration/effect. May decrease concentration/effects of **apixaban, axitinib, dabigatran, dronedarone, itraconazole, ivabradine, niMODipine, rivaroxaban.** HERBAL: **Herbals with sedative properties (e.g., chamomile, kava kava, valerian)** may increase CNS depression. FOOD: None known. LAB VALUES: May increase serum glucose, GGT, alkaline phosphatase. **Therapeutic serum level:** 10–20 mcg/mL; **toxic serum level:** greater than 20 mcg/mL.

AVAILABILITY (Rx)

Capsules, Extended-Release: 30 mg, 100 mg, 200 mg, 300 mg. **Injection Solution:** 50 mg/mL. **Suspension, Oral:** 125 mg/5 mL. **Tablets, Chewable:** 50 mg.

ADMINISTRATION/HANDLING

IV

◄ALERT► Give by IV push or IV piggyback. IV push can be painful (chemical irritation of vein due to alkalinity of solution). To minimize effect of irritation, flush IV with sterile saline after dose is administered.

Reconstitution • May give undiluted or may dilute with 0.9% NaCl to a concentration of 5 mg/mL or more.

Rate of administration • Administer at rate not exceeding 50 mg/min in adults, 20 mg/min in elderly, pts with preexisting cardiovascular conditions. In neonates, administer at rate not exceeding 1–3 mg/kg/min. • Infuse diluted solutions using an in-line filter. • Severe hypotension, cardiovascular collapse occur if rate of IV injection exceeds 50 mg/min for adults. • IV toxicity characterized by CNS depression, cardiovascular collapse.

Storage • Precipitate may form if parenteral form is refrigerated. • Slight yellow discoloration of parenteral form does not affect potency, but do not use if solution is cloudy or precipitate forms. Discard if not used within 4 hrs of preparation.

PO

- Give with food if GI distress occurs.
- Tablets may be chewed. • Shake oral suspension well before using. • Separate administration of phenytoin with antacids or tube feeding by 2 hrs.

IV INCOMPATIBILITIES

DilTIAZem (Cardizem), DOBUTamine (Dobutrex), enalapril (Vasotec), heparin, HYDROmorphone (Dilaudid), insulin, lidocaine, morphine, nitroglycerin, norepinephrine (Levophed), potassium chloride, propofol (Diprivan).

INDICATIONS/ROUTES/DOSAGE

Status Epilepticus

IV: ADULTS, ELDERLY, ADOLESCENTS: **Loading dose:** 20 mg/kg at maximum

P

rate of 25–50 mg/min. May repeat in 10 min after loading dose with dose of 5–10 mg/kg. INFANTS, CHILDREN: **Loading dose:** 20 mg/kg at maximum rate of 1 mg/kg/min. May give additional dose of 5–10 mg/kg after loading dose.

Seizure Control (Maintenance)

Note: Loading dose not used in pts with history of renal/hepatic disease.

PO: ADULTS, ELDERLY: **Loading Dose:** 1 g divided into 3 doses given at 2-hr intervals. **Maintenance** (begins 24 hrs after loading dose): Initially 100 mg 3 times/day; adjust at no less than 7–10-day intervals. Usual dose: 100 mg 3–4 times/day up to 200 mg 3 times/day (may consider 300 mg once daily in pts established on 100 mg 3 times/day). CHILDREN: Initially, 5 mg/kg/day in 2–3 divided doses. Adjust dose at 7- to 10-day intervals. **Maintenance:** 4–8 mg/kg/day. **Maximum:** 300 mg/day.

Dosage in Renal/Hepatic Impairment

No dose adjustment.

P

SIDE EFFECTS

Frequent: Drowsiness, lethargy, confusion, slurred speech, irritability, gingival hyperplasia, hypersensitivity reaction (fever, rash, lymphadenopathy), constipation, dizziness, nausea. **Occasional:** Headache, hirsutism, coarsening of facial features, insomnia, muscle twitching.

ADVERSE EFFECTS/TOXIC REACTIONS

Abrupt withdrawal may precipitate status epilepticus. Blood dyscrasias, osteomalacia (due to interference of vitamin D metabolism) may occur. Toxic phenytoin blood concentration (25 mcg/mL or more) may produce ataxia, nystagmus, diplopia. As level increases, extreme lethargy to comatose state occurs. May increase risk of suicidal thoughts and behavior. Severe cutaneous reactions including toxic epidermal necrolysis, Stevens-Johnson syndrome may occur. Life-threatening drug reaction with eosinophilia and systemic symptoms (DRESS) (multi-organ hypersensitivity) may present as lymphadenopathy, fever, facial swelling, hepatitis, nephritis, myocarditis, myositis. Hepatotoxicity, acute hepatic failure were reported.

NURSING CONSIDERATIONS

BASELINE ASSESSMENT

Anticonvulsant: Review history of seizure disorder (intensity, frequency, duration, LOC). Initiate seizure precautions. LFT, CBC should be performed before beginning therapy and periodically during therapy.

INTERVENTION/EVALUATION

Repeat CBC 2 wks following initiation of therapy and 2 wks following administration of maintenance dose. Observe frequently for recurrence of seizure activity. Monitor ECG for cardiac arrhythmia. Assess for clinical improvement (decrease in intensity/frequency of seizures). Monitor for depression, suicidal tendencies, unusual behavior. Monitor CBC with differential, renal function, LFT, B/P (with IV use). Assist with ambulation if drowsiness, lethargy occurs. Monitor for therapeutic serum level (10–20 mcg/mL). **Therapeutic serum level:** 10–20 mcg/mL; **toxic serum level:** greater than 20 mcg/mL. **Free unbound levels: Therapeutic:** 1–2 mcg/mL; **toxic:** more than 2 mcg/mL.

PATIENT/FAMILY TEACHING

• Pain may occur with IV injection. • To prevent gingival hyperplasia (bleeding, tenderness, swelling of gums), maintain good oral hygiene, gum massage, regular dental visits. • Report sore throat, fever, glandular swelling, skin reaction (hematologic toxicity). • Drowsiness usually diminishes with continued therapy. • Avoid tasks that require alertness, motor skills until response to drug is established. • Do not abruptly withdraw medication after long-term use (may precipitate seizures). • Strict maintenance of drug therapy is essential for seizure control, arrhythmias. • Avoid alcohol. • Report changes in behavior, thoughts of suicide.

phosphates potassium sodium

fos-fates

◆CLASSIFICATION

PHARMACOTHERAPEUTIC: Electrolyte supplement. **CLINICAL:** Mineral.

USES

Prevention and treatment of hypophosphatemia.

PRECAUTIONS

Contraindications: K-phosphate: Hyperkalemia, hyperphosphatemia, hypocalcemia. **Na-phosphate:** Hypocalcemia, hypernatremia, hyperphosphatemia. **Cautions:** Renal impairment, concomitant use of potassium-sparing drugs, acid-base alteration, digitalized pts, cardiac disease, metabolic alkalosis.

ACTION

Active in bone deposition, calcium metabolism, utilization of B complex vitamins. Act as buffers in maintaining acid-base balance. Exert osmotic effect in small intestine. **Therapeutic Effect:** Correct hypophosphatemia, acidify urine, prevent calcium deposits in urinary tract, promote peristalsis in GI tract.

PHARMACOKINETICS

Poorly absorbed after PO administration. PO form excreted in feces; IV form excreted in urine.

LIFESPAN CONSIDERATIONS

Pregnancy/Lactation: Use caution in pregnant women with other medical conditions (e.g., preeclampsia). **Children:** Increased risk of dehydration in pts younger than 12 yrs. **Elderly:** No age-related precautions noted.

INTERACTIONS

DRUG: ACE inhibitors (e.g., enalapril, lisinopril), eplerenone, iron salts, magnesium salts, potassium-containing medications, potassium-sparing diuretics (e.g., spironolactone), salt substitutes containing potassium phosphate may increase serum potassium. **Antacids, sucralfate** may decrease absorption. **Calcium-containing medications** may increase risk of calcium deposition in soft tissues, decrease phosphate absorption. **HERBAL:** None significant. **FOOD:** None known. **LAB VALUES:** None significant.

AVAILABILITY (Rx)

Injection Solution (Potassium Phosphate): 3 mmol phosphate and 4.4 mEq potassium per mL. **Injection Solution (Sodium Phosphate):** 3 mmol phosphate and 4 mEq sodium per mL.

ADMINISTRATION/HANDLING

IV

Reconstitution • Must be diluted. Soluble in all commonly used IV solutions.

Rate of administration • Infuse over minimum of 4 hrs (usually over 6 hrs). **Maximum rate:** 0.06 mmol/kg/hr.

Storage • Store at room temperature.

IV INCOMPATIBILITIES

Amiodarone, DOBUTamine (Dobutrex), pantoprazole (Protonix).

IV COMPATIBILITIES

DilTIAZem (Cardizem), enalapril (Vasotec), famotidine (Pepcid), metoclopramide (Reglan), niCARdipine (Cardene).

P

INDICATIONS/ROUTES/DOSAGE

Note: ***(K-Phosphate):*** For each mmol of phosphate, 1.5 mEq of K will be given. ***(Na-Phosphate):*** For each mmol of phosphate, 1.3 mEq of Na will be given.

Hypophosphatemia

(Potassium/Sodium Phosphate): **Phosphate level 2.3–3 mg/dL:** 0.16–0.32 mmol/kg over 4–6 hr. **Phosphate level 1.6–2.2 mg/dL:** 0.32–0.64 mmol/kg over 4–6 hr. **Phosphate level less than 1.5 mg/dL:** 0.64–1 mmol/kg over 8–12 hr.

SIDE EFFECTS

Frequent: Mild laxative effect (in first few days of therapy). **Occasional:** Diarrhea, nausea, abdominal pain, vomiting. **Rare:** Headache, dizziness, confusion, heaviness of lower extremities, fatigue, muscle cramps, paresthesia, peripheral edema, arrhythmias, weight gain, thirst.

ADVERSE EFFECTS/TOXIC REACTIONS

Hyperphosphatemia may produce extraskeletal calcification.

P

NURSING CONSIDERATIONS

BASELINE ASSESSMENT

Obtain BMP, serum phosphate, ionized calcium. Question history of renal impairment, cardiac disease. Assess hydration status.

INTERVENTION/EVALUATION

Monitor serum phosphate, potassium, calcium.

PATIENT/FAMILY TEACHING

- Report diarrhea, nausea, vomiting.

piperacillin/ tazobactam

pye-per-a-**sil**-in/tay-zoe-**bak**-tam (Zosyn)
Do not confuse Zosyn with Zofran or Zyvox.

◆CLASSIFICATION

PHARMACOTHERAPEUTIC: Penicillin. **CLINICAL:** Antibiotic.

USES

Treatment of moderate to severe bacterial infections, including community-acquired/nosocomial pneumonia, intra-abdominal, pelvic, skin, and skin structure infections. Tazobactam expands piperacillin activity to include beta-lactamase–producing strains of *S. aureus, H. influenzae, Bacteroides, PsAg, Acinetobacter, Klebsiella pneumoniae, E. coli.* **OFF-LABEL:** Surgical prophylaxis, complicated intra-abdominal infections.

PRECAUTIONS

Contraindications: Hypersensitivity to piperacillin/tazobactam, any penicillin. **Cautions:** History of allergies (esp. cephalosporins, beta-lactamase inhibitors), renal impairment, seizure disorder.

ACTION

Piperacillin: Inhibits bacterial cell wall synthesis by binding to PCN-binding proteins, which inhibit the final step of peptidoglycan synthesis. **Therapeutic Effect:** Bactericidal. **Tazobactam:** Inactivates bacterial beta-lactamase. **Therapeutic Effect:** Protects piperacillin from enzymatic degradation, extends its spectrum of activity, prevents bacterial overgrowth.

PHARMACOKINETICS

Widely distributed. Protein binding: 16%–30%. Primarily excreted unchanged in urine. Removed by hemodialysis. **Half-life:** 0.7–1.2 hrs (increased in hepatic cirrhosis, renal impairment).

⌛ LIFESPAN CONSIDERATIONS

Pregnancy/Lactation: Readily crosses placenta; appears in cord blood, amniotic fluid. Distributed in breast milk in low concentrations. May lead to allergic sensitization, diarrhea, candidiasis, skin rash in infant. **Children:** Dosage not established for pts younger than 12 yrs. **Elderly:** Age-related renal impairment may require dosage adjustment.

INTERACTIONS

DRUG: May decrease concentration/effects of **aminoglycosides (e.g., gentamicin, tobramycin)**. May increase concentration, toxicity of **methotrexate. Probenecid** may increase concentration, risk of toxicity. **HERBAL:** None significant. **FOOD:** None known. **LAB VALUES:** May increase serum sodium, alkaline phosphatase, bilirubin, LDH, ALT, AST, BUN, creatinine, PT, PTT. May decrease serum potassium. May cause positive Coombs' test.

AVAILABILITY (Rx)

◀ALERT▶ Piperacillin/tazobactam is a combination product in an 8:1 ratio of piperacillin to tazobactam. **Injection Powder:** 2.25 g, 3.375 g, 4.5 g. **Premix Ready to Use:** 2.25 g (50 mL), 3.375 g (50 mL), 4.5 g (100 mL).

ADMINISTRATION/HANDLING

IV

Reconstitution • Reconstitute each 1 g with 5 mL D_5W or 0.9% NaCl. Shake vigorously to dissolve. • Further dilute with at least 50 mL D_5W or 0.9% NaCl.

Rate of administration • Infuse over 30 min. Expanded infusion over 3–4 hrs.

Storage • Reconstituted vial is stable for 24 hrs at room temperature or 48 hrs if refrigerated. • After further dilution, stable for 24 hrs at room temperature or 7 days if refrigerated.

IV INCOMPATIBILITIES

Amphotericin B (Fungizone), amphotericin B complex (Abelcet, AmBisome, Amphotec), famotidine (Pepcid), haloperidol (Haldol), hydrOXYzine (Vistaril), vancomycin (Vancocin).

IV COMPATIBILITIES

Bumetanide (Bumex), calcium gluconate, dexmedetomidine (Precedex), diphenhydrAMINE (Benadryl), DOPamine (Intropin), enalapril (Vasotec), furosemide (Lasix), granisetron (Kytril), heparin, hydrocortisone (Solu-CORTEF), HYDROmorphone (Dilaudid), LORazepam (Ativan), magnesium sulfate, methylPREDNISolone (SOLU-Medrol), metoclopramide (Reglan), morphine, ondansetron (Zofran), potassium chloride.

INDICATIONS/ROUTES/DOSAGE

Note: Extended Infusion: ADULTS, ELDERLY: 3.375–4.5 g over 4 hrs q8h.

Usual Dosage

IV: ADULTS, ELDERLY: 4.5 g q6–8h or 3.375 g q6h. **Maximum:** 18 g daily. **ADOLESCENTS, CHILDREN, INFANTS OLDER THAN 9 MOS:** 100 mg piperacillin component/kg/dose q8h. **Maximum:** 16 g piperacillin/day. **2–9 MOS:** 80 mg piperacillin component/kg/dose q8h. **LESS THAN 2 MOS:** 80 mg piperacillin component/kg/dose q6h. **NEONATES:** 80–100 mg piperacillin component/kg/dose q6–8h.

Creatinine Clearance	Dosage
20–40 mL/min	2.25 g q6h (if usual dose is 3.375g q6h) or 4.5 g q8h or 3.375g q6h (if usual dose is 4.5 g q6h). Extended infusion over 4h (3.375g q8-12h).
Less than 20 mL/min	2.25 g q8h (if usual dose is 3.375g q6h) or 4.5 g q12h or 2.25 g q6h (if usual dose is 4.5 g q6h). Extended infusion over 4h (3.375g q12h).

Dosage for Hemodialysis

IV: ADULTS, ELDERLY: 2.25 g q12 with additional dose of 0.75 g after each dialysis session.

Dosage for CRRT

CVVH	2.25–3.375 g q6–8h
CVVHD	2.25–3.375 g q6h
CVVHDF	3.375 g q6h

Dosage in Renal Impairment

Dosage and frequency are modified based on creatinine clearance.

P

Dosage in Hepatic Impairment
No dose adjustment.

SIDE EFFECTS

Frequent: Diarrhea, headache, constipation, nausea, insomnia, rash. **Occasional:** Vomiting, dyspepsia, pruritus, fever, agitation, candidiasis, dizziness, abdominal pain, edema, anxiety, dyspnea, rhinitis.

ADVERSE EFFECTS/TOXIC REACTIONS

Antibiotic-associated colitis, other superinfections (abdominal cramps, severe watery diarrhea, fever) may result from altered bacterial balance in GI tract. Overdose, more often with renal impairment, may produce seizures, neurologic reactions. Severe hypersensitivity reactions, including anaphylaxis, occur rarely.

NURSING CONSIDERATIONS

BASELINE ASSESSMENT

Question for history of allergies, esp. to penicillins, cephalosporins. Obtain CBC; LFT in pts with hepatic impairment.

P

INTERVENTION/EVALUATION

Monitor daily pattern of bowel activity, stool consistency; mild GI effects may be tolerable, but increasing severity may indicate onset of antibiotic-associated colitis. Be alert for superinfection: fever, vomiting, diarrhea, anal/genital pruritus, oral mucosal changes (ulceration, pain, erythema). Monitor I&O, urinalysis. Monitor serum electrolytes, esp. potassium, renal function tests.

plecanatide

ple-**kan**-a-tide
(Trulance)

■ **BLACK BOX ALERT** ■ Contraindicated in pts younger than 6 yrs due to risk of life-threatening dehydration and death. Safety and efficacy not established in pts younger than 18 yrs; avoid use.

Do not confuse plecanatide with exenatide, lixisenatide, pramlintide or Trulance with Truvada.

◆CLASSIFICATION

PHARMACOTHERAPEUTIC: Guanylate cyclase-C agonist. **CLINICAL:** GI agent.

USES

Treatment of adults with chronic idiopathic constipation or irritable bowel syndrome with constipation.

PRECAUTIONS

Contraindications: Hypersensitivity to plecanatide. Pts younger than 6 yrs of age, mechanical GI obstruction (known or suspected). **Cautions:** Dehydration. Avoid use in pts younger than 18 yrs of age.

ACTION

Binds and agonizes guanylate cyclase-C on luminal surface of intestinal epithelium, increasing cyclic guanosine monophosphate (cGMP), resulting in chloride and bicarbonate secretion into the intestinal lumen. **Therapeutic Effect:** Increases intestinal fluid and accelerates GI transit time.

PHARMACOKINETICS

Minimal absorption systemically; mainly confined to GI tract. Metabolized within GI tract to active metabolite. Undergoes proteolytic degradation within intestinal lumen to smaller peptides and amino acids. **Half-life:** Not specified.

⌛ LIFESPAN CONSIDERATIONS

Pregnancy/Lactation: Unknown if distributed in breast milk. **Children:** Contraindicated in pts younger than 6 yrs. Safety and efficacy not established in pts aged 6 to less than 18 yrs. Severe, possibly fatal, dehydration may occur in pediatric pts younger than 18 yrs due to increased intestinal fluid secretion; avoid use. **Elderly:** No age-related precautions noted.

INTERACTIONS

DRUG: None known. **HERBAL:** None significant. **FOOD:** None known. **LAB VALUES:** May increase serum ALT, AST.

AVAILABILITY (Rx)

Tablets: 3 mg.

ADMINISTRATION/HANDLING

PO

• Give without regard to food. • If a dose is missed, skip the dose and give at next regularly scheduled time; do not double dose. • Give tablet whole; do not break, cut, or divide. • For pts with dysphagia, tablet may be crushed and mixed in applesauce, or dispersed in 30 mL of water and given orally or via NG tube. After administration of dispersed tablet, refill container with additional 30 mL of water and give remaining contents. Flush NG tube with additional 10 mL of water.

INDICATIONS/ROUTES/DOSAGE

Chronic Idiopathic Constipation, Irritable Bowel Syndrome

PO: ADULTS, ELDERLY: 3 mg once daily.

Dosage in Renal/Hepatic Impairment

Not specified; use caution.

SIDE EFFECTS

Occasional (5%): Diarrhea. **Rare (less than 2%):** Abdominal pain/tenderness, flatulence.

ADVERSE EFFECTS/TOXIC REACTIONS

Severe diarrhea reported in less than 1% of pts; usually occurred within the first 3 days.

NURSING CONSIDERATIONS

BASELINE ASSESSMENT

Question characteristics of constipation, frequency of bowel movements. Assess bowel sounds. Assess hydration status.

INTERVENTION/EVALUATION

Encourage fluid intake. Monitor daily pattern of bowel activity, stool consistency. Monitor for abdominal pain, dehydration.

PATIENT/FAMILY TEACHING

• Report severe diarrhea. • Drink plenty of fluids. • Do not take laxatives unless approved by prescriber. • Tablets may be taken whole, dispersed in water, or crushed and mixed in applesauce. • Securely store tablets away from children; life-threating dehydration may occur if accidentally ingested by children younger than 6 yrs.

polatuzumab vedotin-piiq

pol-a-**tooz**-ue-mab ve-**doe**-tin
(Polivy)

Do not confuse polatuzumab vedotin-piiq with brentuximab vedotin, panitumumab, pembrolizumab, pertuzumab, or riTUXimab.

◆CLASSIFICATION

PHARMACOTHERAPEUTIC: CD79b-directed antibody-drug conjugate (ADC), monoclonal antibody. **CLINICAL:** Antineoplastic.

USES

Treatment of adults with relapsed or refractory diffuse large B-cell lymphoma (in combination with bendamustine and a riTUXimab product), not otherwise specified, after at least two prior therapies.

PRECAUTIONS

Contraindications: Hypersensitivity to polatuzumab vedotin-piiq. **Cautions:** Baseline cytopenias, hepatic impairment, pts at high risk for tumor lysis syndrome (high tumor burden); conditions predisposing to infection (e.g., diabetes, renal failure, immunocompromised pts, open wounds); chronic opportunistic

P

infections (e.g., herpesvirus infection, fungal infections).

ACTION

An antibody drug conjugate consisting of three components: a protease-cleavable linker, a microtubule-disrupting agent (monomethyl auristatin E [MMAE]), and humanized immunoglobulin G1 (IgG1) monoclonal antibody. Binds to CD79b (B-cell–specific cell surface protein) commonly expressed in B-cell lymphoma. Forms a complex that disrupts microtubule network. **Therapeutic Effect:** Induces cell cycle arrest and apoptosis.

PHARMACOKINETICS

Widely distributed. Metabolized via catabolism into small peptides, amino acids, unconjugated MMAE, catabolites. Protein binding: 71%–77%. Excretion not specified. **Half-life:** (antibody-conjugated MMAE): 12 days; (unconjugated MMAE): 4 days.

LIFESPAN CONSIDERATIONS

Pregnancy/Lactation: Avoid pregnancy; may cause fetal harm. Females of reproductive potential must use effective contraception during treatment and for at least 3 mos after discontinuation. Unknown if distributed in breast milk. Breastfeeding not recommended during treatment and for at least 2 mos after discontinuation. **Males:** Males with female partners of reproductive potential must use effective contraception during treatment and for at least 5 mos after discontinuation. May impair fertility. **Children:** Safety and efficacy not established. **Elderly:** May have increased risk of adverse reactions/toxic effects.

INTERACTIONS

DRUG: May decrease therapeutic effect of **BCG (intravesical).** May decrease therapeutic effect; increase adverse effects of **live vaccines.** May increase adverse/toxic effects of **natalizumab. Pimecrolimus, tacrolimus (topical)** may increase adverse/toxic effects. **HERBAL:** Echinacea may decrease therapeutic effect. **FOOD: Grapefruit products** may increase concentration/effect. **LAB VALUES:** May increase serum amylase, ALT, AST, creatinine, lipase. May decrease serum calcium, phosphate, potassium; Hgb, lymphocytes, neutrophils, platelets, RBCs.

AVAILABILITY (Rx)

Injection, Powder for Reconstitution: 140 mg.

ADMINISTRATION/HANDLING

IV

Premedication • Premedicate with an antipyretic and an antihistamine 30–60 min prior to each dose.

Infusion Guidelines • Infuse via dedicated IV line using a sterile, nonpyrogenic, low-protein-binding 0.2 or 0.22 micron in-line filter. • Do not administer as IV push or bolus. If a dose is missed, give as soon as possible and adjust schedule to maintain treatment interval.

Reconstitution • Must be prepared by personal trained in aseptic manipulations and admixing of cytotoxic drugs. • Calculate the number of vials needed for reconstitution based on weight in kg. • While directing stream toward glass wall of vial, reconstitute each vial with 7.2 mL of Sterile Water for Injection to a final concentration of 20 mg/mL. • Swirl vial gently until powder is completely dissolved. Do not shake or agitate. • Visually inspect for particulate matter or discoloration. Solution should appear slightly opalescent and colorless to slightly brown in color. Do not use if solution is cloudy or discolored or if visible particles are observed. • Dilute in an infusion bag with a minimum of 50 mL containing 0.9% NaCl, 0.45% NaCl, or D_5W to a final concentration of 0.72–2.7 mg/mL. • Mix by gentle inversion. • Do not shake or agitate. • Discard used portions of vial.

Rate of administration • **Initial infusion:** Infuse over 90 min.

• **Subsequent Infusions:** Infuse over 30 min if previous infusion was tolerated.

Infusion Reactions • If grade 1–3 infusion-related reactions occur, interrupt infusion and treat symptoms. If symptoms resolve, resume infusion at 50% of the infusion rate prior to interruption. If symptoms do not recur, may increase infusion rate in increments of 50 mL/hr q30min. • For next cycle, may infuse over 90 min. If no infusion-related reactions occur, subsequent infusion may be infused over 30 min. If grade 4 infusion-related reactions occur, discontinue infusion and treat symptoms.

Storage • Refrigerate unused vials in original carton. • May refrigerate reconstituted vials for up to 48 hrs or store at room temperature for up to 8 hrs. Diluted solutions containing 0.9% NaCl may be refrigerated for up to 24 hrs or stored at room temperature for up to 4 hrs. Diluted solutions containing 0.45% NaCl may be refrigerated for up to 18 hrs or stored at room temperature for up to 4 hrs. Diluted solutions containing D_5W may be refrigerated for up to 36 hrs or stored at room temperature for up to 6 hrs. Limit transportation of refrigerated, diluted solutions to 12 hrs or room temperature solutions to 30 min. The total storage time plus transportation of diluted solution should not exceed the storage duration.

IV INCOMPATABILITIES

Do not mix or infuse with other solutions or medications.

INDICATIONS/ROUTES/DOSAGE

Diffuse Large B-Cell Lymphoma (relapsed or refractory)

IV: ADULTS: 1.8 mg/kg q21days for 6 cycles (in combination with bendamustine 90 mg/m²/day on day 1 and 2 of each cycle, and rituximab 375 mg/m² on day 1 of each cycle).

Dose Modification

Based on Common Terminology Criteria for Adverse Events (CTCAE).

Peripheral Neuropathy

Grade 2 or 3 peripheral neuropathy: Withhold treatment until improved to grade 1 or 0. If recovered to grade 1 or 0 before day 14, resume at permanently reduced dose of 1.4 mg/kg. **Permanent discontinuation:** Permanently discontinue if unable to tolerate 1.4 mg/kg dose; if not recovered to grade 1 or 0 by day 14; if grade 4 peripheral neuropathy occurs.

Neutropenia

Grade 3 or 4 neutropenia: Withhold treatment until absolute neutrophil count (ANC) greater than 1,000 cells/mm³. **ANC improved to greater than 1,000 cells/mm3 on or before day 7:** Resume all treatments at same dose and consider granulocyte colony-stimulating factor prophylaxis for subsequent cycles (if not previously given). **ANC improved to greater than 1,000 cells/mm3 after day 7:** Resume all treatments at same dose and consider granulocyte colony-stimulating factor prophylaxis for subsequent cycles (if not previously given). Consider dose reduction of bendamustine if granulocyte colony-stimulating factor prophylaxis was given. If bendamustine dose was already reduced, then reduce polatuzumab vedotin-piiq dose to 1.4 mg/kg.

Thrombocytopenia

Grade 3 or 4 thrombocytopenia: Withhold treatment until platelet count improves to greater than 75,000 cells/mm³. **Platelet count improved to greater than 75,000 cells/mm³ on or before day 7:** Resume all treatments at same dose. **Platelet count improved to greater than 75,000 cells/mm³ after day 7:** Resume all treatments and reduce dose of bendamustine. If bendamustine dose was already reduced, then reduce polatuzumab vedotin-piiq dose to 1.4 mg/kg.

Infusion-Related Reactions

Permanently discontinue in pts with first occurrence of grade 3 bronchospasm,

P

generalized urticaria, wheezing; recurrent grade 2 wheezing, urticaria; recurrence of any grade 3 symptoms; any grade 4 symptoms.

Dosage in Renal Impairment.

Mild to severe impairment: Not specified; use caution.

Dosage in Hepatic Impairment.

Mild impairment: No dose adjustment. Moderate to severe impairment: Not recommended.

SIDE EFFECTS

Frequent (38%–18%): Diarrhea, pyrexia, decreased appetite, vomiting. **Occasional (16%–7%):** Decreased weight, dizziness, arthralgia. **Rare (1%):** Blurred vision.

ADVERSE EFFECTS/TOXIC REACTIONS

Myelosuppression (anemia, lymphopenia, neutropenia, thrombocytopenia) is an expected response to therapy but more severe reactions including severe neutropenia, febrile neutropenia may be life threatening. Peripheral neuropathy including hypoesthesia, hyperesthesia, gait disturbance, muscular weakness, paresthesia, peripheral motor/sensorimotor neuropathy, neuropathic pain reported in 40% of pts. Infusion reactions including chills, dyspnea, fever, flushing, hypotension, urticaria reported in 7% of pts. Fatal infections, including opportunistic infections, such as cytomegalovirus infection, herpes virus infection, pneumonia (*Pneumocystis jiroveci* and fungal pneumonia), sepsis have occurred. Grade 3 or higher infections reported in 32% of pts. Progressive multifocal leukoencephalopathy (PML), an opportunistic viral infection of the brain caused by the JC virus, may result in progressive, permanent disability and death. Tumor lysis syndrome may present as acute renal failure, hypocalcemia, hyperuricemia, hyperphosphatemia. Hepatotoxicity reported in 2% of pts. Pneumonitis reported in 4% of pts. Immunogenicity (auto-polatuzumab vedotin-piiq antibodies) reported in 6% of pts.

P

NURSING CONSIDERATIONS

BASELINE ASSESSMENT

Obtain ANC, CBC, LFT; pregnancy test in females of reproductive potential. Verify use of effective contraception. Recommend prophylactic treatment of *Pneumocystis jiroveci* pneumonia and herpes zoster throughout therapy. Question occurrence of infusion-related reactions prior to each treatment. Due to increased risk of tumor lysis syndrome, assess hydration status prior to each treatment. Screen for active infection. Question history of hepatic impairment, herpesvirus infection, chronic opportunistic infections. Receive full medication history and screen for interactions. Offer emotional support.

INTERVENTION/EVALUATION

Monitor ANC, CBC throughout treatment. Monitor LFT for hepatotoxicity (bruising, hematuria, jaundice, right upper abdominal pain, nausea, vomiting, weight loss) periodically. Monitor for infusion reactions during each infusion. If infusion reactions occur, interrupt infusion and manage symptoms. Consider ABG, radiologic test if pneumonitis (excessive cough, dyspnea, fever, hypoxia) is suspected. Consider treatment with corticosteroids if pneumonitis is confirmed. Pts with altered mental status, seizures, visual disturbances, generalized or unilateral weakness should be evaluated for PML. Diligently monitor for infections (cough, fatigue, fever). If serious infection occurs, initiate appropriate antimicrobial therapy. Offer antiemetics if nausea occurs; antidiarrheal agent if diarrhea occurs. Monitor daily pattern of bowel activity, stool consistency.

PATIENT/FAMILY TEACHING

• Treatment may depress your immune system response and reduce your ability to fight infection. Report symptoms of infection such as body aches, chills, cough, fatigue, fever. Avoid those with active infection. • Report symptoms of bone marrow depression such as bruising, fatigue, fever, shortness of breath, weight loss; bleeding easily, bloody urine or stool. • Report liver problems (abdominal pain, bruising, clay-colored stool, dark or amber-colored urine, yellowing of the skin or eyes), inflammation of the lung (excessive cough, difficulty breathing, chest pain), nervous system changes (gait disturbance, pain, numbness, trouble walking). • PML, an opportunistic viral infection of the brain, may cause progressive, permanent disabilities or death. Report symptoms of PML brain such as confusion, memory loss, paralysis, trouble speaking, vision loss, seizures, weakness. • Therapy may cause tumor lysis syndrome (a condition caused by the rapid breakdown of cancer cells), which can cause kidney failure, and can be fatal. Report decreased urination, amber-colored urine; confusion, difficulty breathing, fatigue, fever, muscle or joint pain, palpitations, seizures, vomiting. • Use effective contraception to avoid pregnancy. Do not breastfeed. • Allergic reactions such as chills, difficulty breathing, fever, flushing, itching, low blood pressure can happen at any time during infusion. If allergic reaction occurs, seek immediate medical attention.

polyethylene glycol

polyethylene glycol–electrolyte solution

pol-ee-**eth**-il-een-**glye**-kol
(CoLyte, GoLYTELY, Klean-Prep ✱, MiraLax, NuLytely, Peglyte ✱, TriLyte)
Do not confuse MiraLax with Mirapex.

◆CLASSIFICATION

PHARMACOTHERAPEUTIC: Osmotic. **CLINICAL:** Bowel evacuant, laxative.

USES

Polyethylene glycol-electrolyte solution: Bowel cleansing before GI examination, colon surgery. **Polyethylene glycol:** Treatment of occasional constipation.

PRECAUTIONS

Contraindications: Hypersensitivity to polyethylene glycol. Bowel perforation, gastric retention, GI obstruction, megacolon, toxic colitis, toxic ileus. **Cautions: Propylene glycol:** Renal impairment. **Propylene glycol–electrolyte solution:** Ulcerative colitis, dehydration, medications altering electrolytes, hyponatremia, cardiac arrhythmias, impaired gag reflex, seizure disorder, elderly.

ACTION

Induces catharsis by osmotic effect. **Therapeutic Effect:** Alleviates constipation, cleanses bowel without depleting electrolytes.

PHARMACOKINETICS

Route	Onset	Peak	Duration
PO (bowel cleansing)	1–2 hrs	N/A	N/A
PO (constipation)	2–4 days	N/A	N/A

⌛ LIFESPAN CONSIDERATIONS

Pregnancy/Lactation: Unknown if drug crosses placenta or is distributed in breast milk. **Children/Elderly:** No age-related precautions noted.

INTERACTIONS

DRUG: None significant. **HERBAL:** None significant. **FOOD:** None known. **LAB VALUES:** None significant.

AVAILABILITY (Rx)

Powder for Oral Solution: Propylene glycol: *(MiraLax):* 17 g/dose. **Propylene glycol–electrolyte solution:** *(CoLyte, GoLYTELY):* See individual product for specific ingredients.

ADMINISTRATION/HANDLING

PO

Polyethylene glycol–electrolyte solution: • Refrigerate reconstituted solutions; use within 48 hrs. • May use tap water to prepare solution. Shake vigorously for several min to ensure complete dissolution of powder. • Fasting should occur for more than 3 hrs prior to ingestion of solution (always avoid solid food less than 2 hrs prior to administration). • Only clear liquids permitted after administration. • May give via NG tube. • Rapid drinking preferred. Chilled solution is more palatable.

Polyethylene glycol: • Add to 4- to 8-oz beverage.

INDICATIONS/ROUTES/DOSAGE

Bowel Evacuant

PO: ADULTS, ELDERLY: Before GI examination: 240 mL (8 oz) q10min until 4 L consumed or rectal effluent clear. NG tube: 20–30 mL/min until 4 L given.

Constipation

PO: ***(MiraLax):*** **ADULTS:** 17 g or 1 heaping tbsp/day. **CHILDREN 6 MOS AND OLDER:** 0.2–0.8 g/kg/day. **Maximum:** 17 g/day.

Dosage in Renal/Hepatic Impairment

No dose adjustment.

SIDE EFFECTS

Frequent (50%): Some degree of abdominal fullness, nausea, bloating. **Occasional (10%–1%):** Abdominal cramping, vomiting, anal irritation. **Rare (less than 1%):** Urticaria, rhinorrhea, dermatitis.

ADVERSE EFFECTS/TOXIC REACTIONS

None known.

NURSING CONSIDERATIONS

BASELINE ASSESSMENT

Do not give oral medication within 1 hr of start of therapy (may not adequately be absorbed before GI cleansing).

INTERVENTION/EVALUATION

Assess bowel sounds for peristalsis. Monitor daily pattern of bowel activity, stool consistency. Assess for abdominal disturbances.

PATIENT/FAMILY TEACHING

• May take 2–4 days to produce a bowel movement. • Report unusual cramps, bloating, diarrhea.

pomalidomide

poe-ma-**lid**-oh-mide
(Pomalyst)

BLACK BOX ALERT May cause life-threatening birth defects. Pregnancy contraindicated. Exclude pregnancy before initiating treatment. Females of reproductive potential must use two reliable forms of contraception or continuously abstain during treatment and for 4 wks after treatment. Deep vein thrombosis and pulmonary embolism may occur. Consider venous thromboembolism (VTE) prophylaxis during treatment.

◆CLASSIFICATION

PHARMACOTHERAPEUTIC: Thalidomide analogue. **CLINICAL:** Antineoplastic.

USES

Treatment of multiple myeloma in pts who have received at least two prior therapies including lenalidomide and bortezomib and who have demonstrated disease progression on or within 60 days of completion of the last therapy.

Treatment of adults with AIDS-related Kaposi sarcoma (KS) after failure of highly active antiretroviral therapy (HAART) or in pts with KS who are HIV negative.

PRECAUTIONS

◀ALERT▶ Do not donate blood products during therapy and for 1 month after therapy discontinuation; male pts must not donate sperm.

Contraindications: Hypersensitivity to pomalidomide. Pregnancy. **Cautions:** Anemia, HF, hepatic/renal impairment, smoking, breastfeeding, or prior history of CVA, MI, DVT, PE.

ACTION

Inhibits tumor cell proliferation and induces apoptosis (cell death) of hematopoietic cells. Enhances T-cell– and natural killer (NK) cell–mediated immunity. Inhibits proinflammatory cytokines. **Therapeutic Effect:** Inhibits tumor cell growth and metastasis.

PHARMACOKINETICS

Widely distributed. Metabolized in liver. Protein binding: 12%–44%. Peak plasma concentration: 2–3 hrs. Excreted in urine (73%), feces (15%). **Half-life:** 8–10 hrs.

LIFESPAN CONSIDERATIONS

Pregnancy/Lactation: Pregnancy/breastfeeding contraindicated. May cause fetal harm. Unknown if distributed in breast milk. Do not breastfeed. Must verify negative pregnancy status before initiation. Must use two reliable forms of birth control (intrauterine device [IUD], tubal ligation) plus barrier methods. Avoid pregnancy for at least 4 wks after discontinuation. **Males:** Must use condoms during treatment and up to 1 mo after treatment, despite prior history of vasectomy. Do not donate sperm. **Children:** Safety and efficacy not established. **Elderly:** May have increased risk of serious adverse effects, renal failure, electrolyte imbalance.

INTERACTIONS

DRUG: May decrease the therapeutic effect; increase adverse effects of **vaccines (live). CNS depressants (e.g., alcohol, morphine, zolpidem)** may increase CNS depression. **HERBAL: Herbals with sedative properties (e.g., chamomile, kava kava, valerian)** may increase CNS depression. **Echinacea** may decrease therapeutic effect. **FOOD:** None significant. **LAB VALUES:** May decrease Hgb, Hct, neutrophils, platelets, leukocytes, lymphocytes, serum calcium, potassium, sodium. May increase serum calcium, creatinine, glucose.

AVAILABILITY (Rx)

Capsules: 1 mg, 2 mg, 3 mg, 4 mg.

ADMINISTRATION/HANDLING

PO

• Do not break, crush, or open capsule. • Give on empty stomach; must administer at least 2 hrs before or 2 hrs after meal.

INDICATIONS/ROUTES/DOSAGE

Note: Absolute neutrophil count (ANC) should be 500 cells/mm^3 or greater and platelet count 50,000 cells/mm^3 or greater prior to starting new cycles of therapy.

Multiple Myeloma

PO: ADULTS/ELDERLY: 4 mg once daily on days 1–21 of 28-day cycle (in combination with dexamethasone; or dexamethasone and elotuzumab; or dexamethasone and daratumumab). Continue until disease progression or unacceptable toxicity.

Dose Modification

Neutropenia

ANC less than 500 cells/mm^3 or febrile neutropenia: Withhold treatment until ANC is greater than 500 cells/mm^3, then reduce dose to 3 mg once daily. **Any subsequent drop of ANC less than 500 cells/mm^3 after prior reduction:** Withhold treatment until ANC is greater than 500 cells/mm^3, then reduce dose by 1 mg less than previous dose. Discontinue if 1-mg dose is intolerable.

Thrombocytopenia

Platelet count less than 25,000 cells/mm³: Withhold treatment until platelet count greater than 50,000 cells/mm³, then reduce dose to 3 mg once daily. **Any subsequent platelet drop to less than 25,000 cells/mm³:** Withhold treatment until platelet count greater than 50,000 cells/mm³, then reduce dose by 1 mg less than previous dose. Discontinue if 1-mg dose is intolerable.

Kaposi Sarcoma

PO: ADULTS: 5 mg once daily on days 1–21 of a 28-day cycle. Continue until disease progression or unacceptable toxicity. Continue HAART as HIV treatment in pts with AIDS-related Kaposi sarcoma.

Dosage in Renal Impairment

Avoid use in pts with serum creatinine more than 3 mg/dL or CrCl less than 45 mL/min.

Dosage in Hepatic Impairment

Avoid use in pts with serum bilirubin more than 2 mg/dL and ALT, AST more than 3 times upper limit of normal (ULN).

SIDE EFFECTS

Frequent (55%–22%): Fatigue, constipation, nausea, diarrhea, dyspnea, back pain, peripheral edema, musculoskeletal chest pain, anorexia, rash. **Occasional (20%–7%):** Dizziness, pyrexia, muscle spasms, arthralgia, pruritus, vomiting, cough, weight loss, headache, bone pain, muscular weakness, anxiety, musculoskeletal pain, peripheral neuropathy, chills, dry skin, tremor, insomnia. **Rare (6%–1%):** Hyperhidrosis, extremity pain, back pain, night sweats, constipation.

ADVERSE EFFECTS/TOXIC REACTIONS

Myelosuppression (neutropenia, leukopenia, thrombocytopenia) is an expected outcome of therapy; may increase risk of infection such as pneumonia, upper respiratory tract infection, UTI. Neurologic events such as acute confusion, dizziness reported. Peripheral neuropathy occurred in 18% of pts. Venous thromboembolism including DVT, PE occurred in 3% of pts. Epistaxis occurred in 15% of pts. Increased risk of secondary malignancies reported. Acute renal failure reported in 16% of pts. Additional adverse events may include interstitial lung disease (ILD), neutropenic sepsis, *Pneumocystis jiroveci* pneumonia, respiratory syncytial virus infection, urinary retention, vertigo.

NURSING CONSIDERATIONS

BASELINE ASSESSMENT

Obtain CBC, BMP; pregnancy test in females of reproductive potential. Receive full medication history. Obtain baseline neurologic exam. Question history of diabetes mellitus, electrolyte imbalance, hepatic/renal impairment, pulmonary disease, thromboembolism, smoking.

INTERVENTION/EVALUATION

Monitor CBC, BMP. Obtain ECG for palpitations, chest pain, hypokalemia, hyperkalemia, hypocalcemia, bradycardia, ventricular arrhythmias. Immediately report dyspnea, chest pain, hypoxia, unilateral peripheral edema/pain (may indicate thromboembolic event). Perform routine neurologic assessments to screen for confusion, delirium. Monitor urine output, frequency.

PATIENT/FAMILY TEACHING

• Treatment may depress your immune system response and reduce your ability to fight infection. Report symptoms of infection such as body aches, chills, cough, fatigue, fever. Avoid those with active infection. • Report symptoms of bone marrow depression (e.g., bruising, fatigue, fever, shortness of breath, weight loss; bleeding easily, bloody urine or stool). • Do not donate blood. • Use effective contraception to avoid pregnancy. Do not breastfeed. • Go from lying to standing slowly (prevents postural hypotension, dizziness). Avoid tasks that require alertness, motor skills until response to drug is established. • Do not smoke. • Do not eat 2 hrs before or 2 hrs after dose. • Avoid alcohol. • Report difficulty breathing, chest pain, extremity pain or swelling, dizziness, confusion.

ponatinib

poe-**na**-ti-nib
(Iclusig)

■ **BLACK BOX ALERT** ■ Arterial occlusions have occurred, including CVA, fatal MI, large arterial vessel stenosis of the brain, severe peripheral vascular disease requiring revascularization. Events may occur in pts with or without cardiovascular risks, including pts younger than 50 yrs of age. Venous thromboembolism, serious HF, or left ventricular dysfunction were reported. Hepatotoxicity, including fatal hepatic failure, may occur.

Do not confuse ponatinib with afatinib, alectinib, dasatinib, bosutinib, gefitinib, imatinib, lapatinib, lenvatinib, neratinib, or tofacitinib.

◆CLASSIFICATION

PHARMACOTHERAPEUTIC: BCR-ABL tyrosine kinase inhibitor. **CLINICAL:** Antineoplastic.

USES

Treatment of pts with chronic, accelerated, or blast phase chronic myeloid leukemia (CML) or Philadelphia chromosome (Ph+) acute lymphoblastic leukemia (ALL) for whom no other kinase inhibitor therapy is indicated. Treatment of adults with T315I-positive CML (chronic, accelerated, or blast phase) or T315I-positive ALL (Ph+ ALL). Not indicated for treatment of newly diagnosed chronic phase CML.

PRECAUTIONS

Contraindications: Hypersensitivity to ponatinib. **Cautions:** Baseline hematologic cytopenias; conditions predisposing to infection (e.g., diabetes, immunocompromised pts, open wounds), history of arterial/venous thrombosis (e.g., CVA, DVT, MI, PE), cardiac disease, cardiac conduction disorders, HF, hypertension; diabetes, electrolyte imbalance, glaucoma, hepatic impairment, hyperlipidemia, GI perforation, neuropathy (peripheral or cranial), ocular disorders, pancreatitis or alcohol abuse, history of ischemia, vascular stenosis; pts with high tumor burden; pts at risk for hemorrhage (e.g., history of intracranial/GI bleeding, coagulation disorders, recent trauma; concomitant use of anticoagulants, antiplatelets, NSAIDs).

ACTION

Inhibits viability of cells expressing native or mutant BCR-ABL tyrosine kinase, including T315I mutation, created by the Philadelphia chromosome abnormality. **Therapeutic Effect:** Inhibits tumor cell growth and metastasis.

PHARMACOKINETICS

Widely distributed. Metabolized in liver. Protein binding: greater than 99%. Peak plasma concentration: 6 hrs or less. Excreted in feces (87%), urine (5%). **Half-life:** 24 hrs (Range: 12–66 hrs).

⌛ LIFESPAN CONSIDERATIONS

Pregnancy/Lactation: Avoid pregnancy; may cause fetal harm/malformations. Unknown if distributed in breast milk. Breastfeeding not recommended during treatment and for at least 6 days after discontinuation. Females of reproductive potential and males with female partners of reproductive potential should use effective contraception during treatment and for at least 3 wks after discontinuation. May impair fertility in females. **Children:** Safety and efficacy not established. **Elderly:** May have increased risk of adverse reactions/toxic effects. Use caution.

INTERACTIONS

DRUG: Strong CYP3A4 inhibitors (e.g., clarithromycin, ketoconazole, ritonavir) may increase concentration/

effect. **Strong CYP3A4 inducers (e.g., carBAMazepine, phenytoin, rifAMPin)** may decrease concentration/effect. May decrease therapeutic effect of **BCG (intravesical)**. **HERBAL: St. John's wort** may decrease concentration/effect. **FOOD: Grapefruit products** may increase concentration/effect. **LAB VALUES:** May increase serum alkaline phosphatase, amylase, ALT, AST, bilirubin, creatinine, lipase, triglycerides, uric acid. May decrease Hgb, Hct, leukocytes, lymphocytes, neutrophils, platelets; serum albumin, bicarbonate, phosphate. May increase or decrease serum calcium, glucose, potassium, sodium.

AVAILABILITY (Rx)

Tablets: 15 mg, 45 mg.

ADMINISTRATION/HANDLING

PO

• Give without regard to food. • Administer tablets whole; do not break, cut, crush, or divide.

INDICATIONS/ROUTES/DOSAGE

CML, Ph+ ALL

PO: ADULTS, ELDERLY: 45 mg once daily. Consider dose reduction in pts with chronic or accelerated phase CML who have achieved a major cytogenetic response. If an adequate response has been not achieved within 90 days, consider discontinuation.

Dose Modification

Based on Common Terminology for Adverse Events (CTCAE).

Hepatotoxicity

Grade 2 or greater serum ALT/AST elevation: Withhold treatment until improved to Grade 1 or 0, then resume dose based on occurrence. **Occurrence at 45-mg dose:** Resume treatment at 30-mg dose. **Occurrence at 30-mg dose:** Resume treatment at 15-mg dose. **Occurrence at 15-mg dose:** Permanently discontinue. **Serum ALT/AST elevation greater than or equal to 3 times ULN with concurrent serum bilirubin elevation greater than 2 times ULN and serum alkaline phosphatase less than 2 times ULN:** Permanently discontinue.

Neutropenia/Thrombocytopenia

ANC less than 1000 cells/mm^3; platelet count less than 50,000 cells/mm^3: Withhold treatment until ANC greater than or equal to 1500 cells/mm^3; or platelet count greater than or equal to 75,000 cells/mm^3, then resume dose based on occurrence. **First occurrence:** Resume treatment at 45-mg dose. **Second occurrence:** Resume treatment at 30-mg dose. **Third occurrence:** Resume treatment at 15-mg dose.

Pancreatitis/Elevated Lipase

Asymptomatic Grade 1 or 2 serum lipase elevation: Consider withholding treatment or reducing dose. **Asymptomatic Grade 3 or 4 serum lipase elevation; asymptomatic radiologic pancreatitis (Grade 2 pancreatitis):** Withhold treatment until improved to Grade 1 or 0, then resume dose based on occurrence. **Occurrence at 45-mg dose:** Resume treatment at 30-mg dose. **Occurrence at 30-mg dose:** Resume treatment at 15-mg dose. **Occurrence at 15-mg dose:** Permanently discontinue. **Grade 4 pancreatitis:** Permanently discontinue.

Concomitant Use of Strong CYP3A4 Inhibitors

Reduce initial dose to 30 mg.

Dosage in Renal Impairment

Not specified; use caution.

Dosage in Hepatic Impairment

Mild, moderate, severe impairment: Reduce initial dose to 30 mg.

SIDE EFFECTS

Note: Percentages of side effects of chronic phase, accelerated phase, blast phase CML; Ph+ ALL may vary.

Frequent (69%–18%): Hypertension, abdominal pain, fatigue, asthenia, headache, dry skin, constipation, arthralgia, nausea, pyrexia, burning sensation, hyperesthesia, hypoesthesia, neuralgia, paresthesia, dysgeusia, muscular weakness, gait disturbance, areflexia, hypotonia, restless legs syndrome, myalgia, extremity pain, back pain, diarrhea, vomiting. **Occasional (17%–2%):** Dyspnea, dizziness, peripheral edema, cough, bone pain, musculoskeletal pain, mucositis, aphthous stomatitis, lip blister, mouth ulceration, mucosal eruption, oral pain, oropharyngeal pain, stomatitis, tongue ulceration, muscle spasm, conjunctival irritation, corneal abrasion/erosion, dry eye, hyperemia, eye pain, pruritus, decreased appetite, insomnia, decreased weight, generalized pain, erythema, alopecia, chills, blurry vision, tachycardia.

ADVERSE EFFECTS/TOXIC REACTIONS

Myelosuppression (anemia, leukopenia, neutropenia, thrombocytopenia) is an expected response to therapy, but more severe reactions including bone marrow failure, febrile neutropenia may be life-threatening. Fatal arterial occlusions including CVA, MI, stenosis of large arterial vessel of the brain, severe peripheral vascular disease requiring revascularization reported in 35% of pts; may occur within 2 wks of initiation (even at reduced doses of 15 mg/day). Coronary artery occlusion, MI occurred in 21% of pts. Venous thromboembolism (DVT, PE, superficial thrombophlebitis) occurred in 5–9% of pts. Life-threatening events including cardiac bradyarrhythmias (requiring pacemaker implantation), complete heart block, sick sinus syndrome, atrial fibrillation with bradycardic pauses, atrial fibrillation, SVT, ventricular tachycardia; emergent hypertension (68% of pts), GI/intracranial hemorrhage (28% of pts), hepatotoxicity (54% of pts), pancreatitis (6%), HF, left ventricular dysfunction (6% of pts); infections including cellulitis, nasopharyngitis, pneumonia, sepsis, upper respiratory tract infection, UTI; ocular toxicities including blindness, conjunctival hemorrhage, cataracts, periorbital edema, ocular hyperemia, iritis, iridocyclitis, ulcerative keratinitis; peripheral edema (31% of pts), pleural effusion (2% of pts), pericardial effusion (1% of pts); peripheral neuropathy, polyneuropathy, nerve compression (20% of pts) may occur. Tumor lysis syndrome may present as acute renal failure, hypocalcemia, hyperuricemia, hyperphosphatemia. Reversible posterior leukoencephalopathy may include aphasia, cognition impairment, paralysis, vision loss, weakness. Pts with newly diagnosed CML have an increased risk of severe toxicities. Improper wound healing, GI perforation may occur.

NURSING CONSIDERATIONS

BASELINE ASSESSMENT

Obtain CBC, BMP, LFT, serum ionized calcium, phosphate, uric acid; vital signs; weight. Obtain pregnancy test in females of reproductive potential. Receive full medication history including herbal products and screen for interactions. Question history as listed in Precautions. Screen for active infection. Conduct ophthalmologic, neurologic exam. Due to increased risk of tumor lysis syndrome, assess adequate hydration prior to initiation. Consider correcting electrolyte abnormalities prior to initiation. Obtain dietary consult. Screen for risk of bleeding; active infection. Assess skin for rash, lesions. Offer emotional support.

INTERVENTION/EVALUATION

Obtain ANC, CBC for myelosuppression q2wks for 3 mos, then monthly thereafter. Monitor serum lipase monthly; BMP, LFT, serum ionized calcium, phosphate, uric acid as indicated. Monitor ECG for cardiac arrhythmias. Due to extremely high risk for arterial occlusions, be vigilant when screening for CVA (aphasia, confusion, paresthesia, hemiparesis, seizures), MI (chest pain, diaphoresis, left arm/jaw pain, increased serum troponin, ST segment elevation), vascular compromise. Be alert for serious infection, opportunistic

P

infection, sepsis. Monitor for GI perforation, hepatotoxicity, ocular disease, pancreatitis; symptoms of thromboembolism (arm/leg pain, swelling; chest pain, dyspnea, hypoxia, tachycardia), reversible posterior leukoencephalopathy, tumor lysis syndrome; other toxicities as listed in Adverse Reactions/Toxic Effects. Monitor daily pattern of bowel activity, stool consistency. Ensure adequate hydration, nutrition. Monitor weight, I&O.

PATIENT/FAMILY TEACHING

• Treatment may depress your immune system response and reduce your ability to fight infection. Report symptoms of infection such as body aches, chills, cough, fatigue, fever. Avoid those with active infection. • Report symptoms of bone marrow depression (e.g., bruising, fatigue, fever, shortness of breath, weight loss; bleeding easily, bloody urine or stool). • Life-threatening arterial blood clots may occur; report symptoms of heart attack (chest pain, difficulty breathing, jaw pain, nausea, pain that radiates to the left arm, sweating), stroke (blindness, confusion, one-sided weakness, loss of consciousness, trouble speaking, seizures). • Report symptoms of DVT (swelling, pain, hot feeling in the arms or legs), lung embolism (difficulty breathing, chest pain, rapid heart rate); liver problems (abdominal pain, bruising, clay-colored stool, amber or dark-colored urine, yellowing of the skin or eyes); HF (difficulty breathing, extremity swelling, sudden loss of breath, palpitations); inflammation of the pancreas (abdominal bruising; persistent, severe abdominal pain that radiates to the back [with or without vomiting]); eye problems (blindness, blurred vision, eye inflammation or bleeding, severe eye or head pain); heart arrhythmias (chest pain, dizziness, fainting, palpitations, slow or rapid heart rate, irregular heart rate); intestinal perforation (severe abdominal pain, fever, nausea). • Use effective contraception to avoid pregnancy. Do not breastfeed. • Report planned surgical/dental procedures. • Immediately report bleeding of any kind. • Do not ingest grapefruit products, herbal supplements. • Do not take newly prescribed medications unless approved by the prescriber who originally started treatment.

potassium acetate

HIGH ALERT

potassium bicarbonate/citrate

(Effer-K, Klor-Con EF)

potassium chloride

(Kaon-Cl, Klor-Con, Klor-Con M10, Klor-Con M20, Micro-K)

Do not confuse Micro-K with Macrobid or Micronase.

◆CLASSIFICATION

PHARMACOTHERAPEUTIC: Electrolyte. **CLINICAL:** Potassium replenisher.

USES

Potassium acetate, potassium bicarbonate/citrate: Treatment, prevention of hypokalemia when necessary to avoid chloride or acid/base imbalance (requires bicarbonate). **Potassium chloride:** Treatment, prevention of hypokalemia.

PRECAUTIONS

Contraindications: Acetate: Severe renal impairment, adrenal insufficiency, hyperkalemia. **Chloride:** Renal failure, hyperkalemia, conditions in which potassium retention is present. Solid oral dosage form in pts in whom there is structural, pathologic cause for delay in passage through

P

GI tract. **Cautions:** Cardiac disease, acid-base disorders, potassium-altering disorders, digitalized pts, concomitant therapy that increases serum potassium (e.g., ACE inhibitors), renal impairment. Do not administer IV undiluted.

ACTION

Necessary for multiple cellular metabolic processes. Primary action is intracellular. **Therapeutic Effect:** Required for nerve impulse conduction, contraction of cardiac, skeletal, smooth muscle; maintains normal renal function, acid-base balance.

PHARMACOKINETICS

Well absorbed from GI tract. Enters cells by active transport from extracellular fluid. Primarily excreted in urine.

LIFESPAN CONSIDERATIONS

Pregnancy/Lactation: Unknown if drug crosses placenta or is distributed in breast milk. **Children:** No age-related precautions noted. **Elderly:** May be at increased risk for hyperkalemia. Age-related ability to excrete potassium is reduced.

INTERACTIONS

DRUG: **ACE inhibitors (e.g., enalapril, lisinopril), eplerenone, potassium-containing medications, potassium-sparing diuretics (e.g., spironolactone, triamterene), salt substitutes** may increase serum potassium concentration. **HERBAL:** None significant. **FOOD:** None known. **LAB VALUES:** None known.

AVAILABILITY (Rx)

Potassium Acetate
Injection Solution: 2 mEq/mL.
Potassium Bicarbonate and Potassium Citrate
Tablets for Solution: *(Effer-K):* 10 mEq, 20 mEq, 25 mEq. *(Klor-Con EF):* 25 mEq.
Potassium Chloride
Injection Solution: 2 mEq/mL. **Oral Solution:** 20 mEq/15 mL, 40 mEq/15 mL. **Powder for Oral Solution:** 20 mEq/packet, 25 mEq/packet.
Capsules, Extended-Release: *(Micro-K):* 8 mEq, 10 mEq. **Tablets, Extended-Release:** 8 mEq, 10 mEq, 15 mEq, 20 mEq.

ADMINISTRATION/HANDLING

IV

Reconstitution • For IV infusion only, must dilute before administration, mix well, infuse slowly. • Avoid adding potassium to hanging IV.

Rate of administration • Routinely, give at concentration of no more than 40 mEq/L, no faster than 10 mEq/hr for peripheral infusion, 20–40 mEq/hr for central infusion.

Storage • Store at room temperature. Use admixtures within 24 hrs.

PO

• Take with or after meals, with full glass of water (decreases GI upset). • Liquids, powder, effervescent tablets: Mix, dissolve with juice, water before administering. • Do not break, crush, dissolve, or divide tablets; give whole.

IV INCOMPATIBILITIES

Amphotericin B complex (Abelcet, AmBisome, Amphotec), phenytoin (Dilantin).

IV COMPATIBILITIES

Amiodarone (Cordarone), atropine, aztreonam (Azactam), calcium gluconate, cefepime (Maxipime), ciprofloxacin (Cipro), clindamycin (Cleocin), dexamethasone (Decadron), dexmedetomidine (Precedex), digoxin (Lanoxin), dilTIAZem (Cardizem), diphenhydrAMINE (Benadryl), DOBUTamine (Dobutrex), DOPamine (Intropin), enalapril (Vasotec), famotidine (Pepcid), fluconazole (Diflucan), furosemide (Lasix), granisetron (Kytril), heparin, hydrocortisone (Solu-CORTEF), insulin, lidocaine, LORazepam (Ativan), magnesium sulfate, methylPREDNISolone (SOLU-Medrol), metoclopramide (Reglan), midazolam (Versed), milrinone (Primacor), morphine, norepinephrine (Levophed), ondansetron (Zofran), oxytocin (Pitocin),

P

piperacillin and tazobactam (Zosyn), procainamide (Pronestyl), propofol (Diprivan), propranolol (Inderal).

INDICATIONS/ROUTES/DOSAGE

Treatment of Hypokalemia

Potassium Acetate

IV: ADULTS, ELDERLY: 5–10 mEq/dose (**Maximum:** 40 mEq/dose) to infuse over 2–3 hrs. **Usual Range:** 40–100 mEq/day.

Dose/Rate Guidelines

Serum potassium	Greater than 2.5–3.5 mEq/L	2.5 mEq/L or less
Maximum infusion rate	10 mEq/hr	40 mEq/hr
Maximum 24-hr dose	200 mEq	400 mEq

Potassium Chloride

PO: ADULTS, ELDERLY: Mild to moderate: Initially, 10–20 mEq given 2–4 times/day. **Severe:** Initially, 40 mEq given 3–4 times/day. (May also give 20 mEq q2–3h in conjunction with careful monitoring.) **CHILDREN:** Initially, 1–2 mEq/kg, then as needed based on lab values.

IV: ADULTS, ELDERLY: 10 mEq/hr (or less); repeat as needed based on lab values. **CHILDREN:** 0.5–1 mEq/kg/dose (**Maximum:** 40 mEq); repeat as needed based on lab values.

Dosage in Renal/Hepatic Impairment

No dose adjustment. Use caution with potassium acetate (may increase serum aluminum and/or potassium).

SIDE EFFECTS

Occasional: Nausea, vomiting, diarrhea, flatulence, abdominal discomfort with distention, phlebitis with IV administration (particularly when potassium concentration of greater than 40 mEq/L is infused). **Rare:** Rash.

ADVERSE EFFECTS/TOXIC REACTIONS

Hyperkalemia (more common in elderly, pts with renal impairment) manifested as paresthesia, motor weakness, cold skin, hypotension, confusion, irritability, paralysis, cardiac arrhythmias. Too-rapid infusion may cause cardiac arrhythmia, ventricular fibrillation, cardiac arrest.

NURSING CONSIDERATIONS

BASELINE ASSESSMENT

Assess for hypokalemia (weakness, fatigue, polyuria, polydipsia). PO form should be given with food or after meals with full glass of water, fruit juice (minimizes GI irritation).

INTERVENTION/EVALUATION

Monitor serum potassium, calcium, phosphate. If GI disturbance occurs, dilute preparation further or give with meals. Monitor for decreased urinary output (may be indication of renal insufficiency). Check IV site closely during infusion for evidence of phlebitis (heat, pain, red streaking of skin over vein, hardening of vein), extravasation (swelling, pain). Be alert to evidence of hyperkalemia (skin pallor/coldness, paresthesia, feeling of heaviness of lower extremities).

PATIENT/FAMILY TEACHING

- Report symptoms of high potassium levels (irregular heartbeat, muscle weakness, nausea, numbness, tingling).

PRALAtrexate

pral-a-**trex**-ate
(Folotyn)
Do not confuse Folotyn with Focalin, or PRALAtrexate with methotrexate or PEMEtrexed.

◆CLASSIFICATION

PHARMACOTHERAPEUTIC: Antimetabolite. **CLINICAL:** Antineoplastic.

USES

Treatment of relapsed or refractory peripheral T-cell lymphoma (PTCL). **OFF-LABEL:** Treatment of relapsed/refractory cutaneous T-cell lymphoma.

PRECAUTIONS

Contraindications: Hypersensitivity to PRALAtrexate. **Cautions:** Baseline cytopenias, mouth ulcers; conditions predisposing to infection (e.g., diabetes, renal failure, immunocompromised pts, open wounds), hepatic impairment, severe renal impairment, pts at risk for tumor lysis syndrome (high tumor burden). Avoid use in pts with end-stage renal disease (ESRD).

ACTION

Folate analogue metabolic inhibitor that competes with enzymes necessary for tumor cell reproduction. Inhibits DNA, RNA, protein synthesis. **Therapeutic Effect:** Inhibits tumor growth.

PHARMACOKINETICS

Protein binding: 67%. Partially excreted in urine. **Half-life:** 12–18 hrs.

LIFESPAN CONSIDERATIONS

Pregnancy/Lactation: Avoid pregnancy; may cause fetal harm. Females of reproductive potential must use effective contraception during treatment and for at least 6 mos after discontinuation. Breastfeeding not recommended during treatment and for at least 1 wk after discontinuation. **Males:** Males with female partners of reproductive potential must use effective contraception during treatment and for at least 3 mos after discontinuation. **Children:** Safety and efficacy not established. **Elderly:** No age-related precautions noted.

INTERACTIONS

DRUG: NSAIDs (e.g., diclofenac, meloxicam, naproxen), probenecid, salicylates (e.g., aspirin), trimethoprim/sulfamethoxazole may delay clearance, increase concentration. May decrease the therapeutic effect; increase adverse effects of **vaccines (live)**. **HERBAL: Echinacea** may decrease therapeutic effect. **FOOD:** None known. **LAB VALUES:** May decrease RBC, WBC, Hgb, Hct, platelet count, serum potassium. May increase serum ALT, AST.

AVAILABILITY (Rx)

Injection Solution: 20 mg/mL.

ADMINISTRATION/HANDLING

◀ALERT▶ May be carcinogenic, mutagenic, teratogenic. Handle with extreme care during preparation/administration. Wear gloves when preparing solution. If powder or solution comes in contact with skin, wash immediately, thoroughly with soap, water.

IV

Reconstitution • Withdraw calculated dose into syringe for immediate use. • Intended for single use only. • Do not dilute.

Rate of administration • Administer as IV push over 3–5 min into IV infusion of 0.9% NaCl.

Storage • Refrigerate vials until use, protect from light. Stable at room temperature for 72 hrs. • Discard vial if solution is discolored (solution should appear clear to yellow) or particulate matter is present.

IV INCOMPATIBILITIES

Do not mix with any other medication.

INDICATIONS/ROUTES/DOSAGE

◀ALERT▶ Prior to any dose, mucositis should be no higher than CTCAE Grade 1, platelets 100,000 cells/mm^3 or greater for first dose and 50,000 cells/mm^3 or greater for subsequent doses, and absolute neutrophil count (ANC) 1,000 cells/mm^3 or greater. Pt should begin taking oral folic acid (1 mg) daily starting 10 days prior to first IV PRALAtrexate dose and continue for 30 days after last dose.

P

Pt should also receive vitamin B_{12} (1 mg) IM injection no more than 10 wks prior to first IV PRALAtrexate dose and every 8–10 wks thereafter.

Refractory/Relapsed Peripheral T-Cell Lymphoma

IV: ADULTS, ELDERLY: 30 mg/m^2 administered once wkly for 6 wks in 7-wk cycles. Dose may be decreased to 20 mg/m^2 to manage adverse reactions. Continue until disease progression or unacceptable toxicity.

Dosage in Renal Impairment

Note: Further dose modifications may be required based on tolerability and history of renal impairment.

Mild to moderate impairment: No dose adjustment. **Severe impairment:** Reduce dose to 15 mg/m^2. **ESRD:** Avoid use.

Dosage in Hepatic Impairment

CTCAE Grade 3: Withhold dose; decrease to 20 mg/m^2 when Grade 2 or less. **CTCAE Grade 4:** Discontinue.

SIDE EFFECTS

Common (70%–36%): Mucositis, nausea, fatigue. **Frequent (34%–10%):** Constipation/diarrhea, pyrexia, edema, cough, epistaxis, vomiting, dyspnea, anorexia, rash, throat/abdominal/back pain, night sweats, asthenia, tachycardia.

ADVERSE EFFECTS/TOXIC REACTIONS

Myelosuppression (anemia, leukopenia, neutropenia) is an expected response to therapy, but more severe reactions including febrile neutropenia, sepsis may occur. Mucositis reported in 70% of pts. Mucositis is less severe when folic acid, vitamin B_{12} therapy is ongoing. Cutaneous toxicities, including toxic epidermal necrolysis, may occur. Tumor lysis syndrome may present as acute renal failure, hypocalcemia, hyperuricemia, hyperphosphatemia. May cause hepatotoxicity. Pts with renal impairment have an increased risk of toxicity. Epistaxis reported in 26% of pts. Upper respiratory tract infections reported in 10% of pts. Overdosage requires general supportive care. Prompt administration of leucovorin should be considered in case of overdose, based on mechanism of action of PRALAtrexate.

NURSING CONSIDERATIONS

BASELINE ASSESSMENT

Obtain CBC, renal function, LFT; pregnancy test in females of reproductive potential. Initiate folic acid, vitamin B_{12} therapy prior to and throughout therapy. Assess risk of tumor lysis syndrome. Ensure adequate hydration. Screen for active infection. Ensure proper parameters prior to each dose: mucositis Grade 1 or 0; platelet count 100,000 cells/mm^3 or greater (first dose) or 50,000 cells/mm^3 or greater (subsequent doses); ANC 1000 cells/mm^3 or greater. Verify compliance of folic acid, vitamin B_{12} therapy prior to initiation and during treatment. Receive full medication history and screen for interactions. Question history of hepatic/renal disease.

INTERVENTION/EVALUATION

Monitor CBC for myelosuppression; LFT for hepatotoxicity (bruising, hematuria, jaundice, right upper abdominal pain, nausea, vomiting, weight loss); renal function. An increase of serum creatinine greater than 0.4 mg/dL from baseline may indicate renal impairment. Monitor serum uric acid level if tumor lysis syndrome (acute renal failure, electrolyte imbalance, cardiac arrhythmias, seizures) is suspected. Diligently monitor for infection (cough, fatigue, fever). Assess for mucositis (oropharyngeal ulcers, oral/throat pain, local infection). Monitor skin for cutaneous toxicities. Monitor daily pattern of bowel activity, stool consistency.

PATIENT/FAMILY TEACHING

- Treatment may depress your immune system response and reduce your ability to fight infection. Report symptoms of infection such as body aches, chills, cough, fatigue, fever. Avoid those with active infection. • Report symptoms of bone marrow depression such as bruising, fatigue, fever, shortness of breath, weight loss; bleeding easily, bloody urine or stool. • Folic acid, vitamin B_{12} therapy is essential to reduce adverse effects. • Therapy may cause life-threatening tumor lysis syndrome (a condition caused by the rapid breakdown of cancer cells), which can cause kidney failure. Report decreased urination, amber-colored urine; confusion, difficulty breathing, fatigue, fever, muscle or joint pain, palpitations, seizures, vomiting. Report liver problems (abdominal pain, bruising, clay-colored stool, amber- or dark-colored urine, yellowing of the skin or eyes), toxic skin reactions (rash, redness, sloughing, swelling); symptoms of mucositis (oral/throat pain or ulcers, local infection). • Maintain strict oral hygiene. Use effective contraception to avoid pregnancy. Do not breastfeed.

pramipexole

pram-i-**pex**-ole
(Apo-Pramipexole ✤, Mirapex, Mirapex ER)
Do not confuse Mirapex with Mifeprex or MiraLax.

CLASSIFICATION

PHARMACOTHERAPEUTIC: DOPamine receptor agonist. **CLINICAL:** Antiparkinson agent.

USES

Mirapex: Treatment of Parkinson's disease, moderate to severe primary restless legs syndrome. **Mirapex ER:** Treatment of Parkinson's disease. **OFF-LABEL: Immediate-Release:** Depression (due to bipolar disorder), fibromyalgia.

PRECAUTIONS

Contraindications: Hypersensitivity to pramipexole. **Cautions:** History of orthostatic hypotension, pts at risk for hypotension, syncope, hallucinations, renal impairment (extended-release not recommended with CrCl less than 30 mL/min), concomitant use of CNS depressants, preexisting dyskinesia, elderly pts.

ACTION

Stimulates DOPamine receptors in striatum and substantia nigra. **Therapeutic Effect:** Relieves signs/symptoms of Parkinson's disease. Improves motor function.

PHARMACOKINETICS

Widely distributed. Protein binding: 15%. Steady-state concentrations achieved within 2 days. Primarily excreted in urine. Not removed by hemodialysis. **Half-life:** 8 hrs (12 hrs in pts older than 65 yrs).

LIFESPAN CONSIDERATIONS

Pregnancy/Lactation: Unknown if drug is distributed in breast milk. **Children:** Safety and efficacy not established. **Elderly:** Increased risk of hallucinations.

INTERACTIONS

DRUG: Antipsychotic agents (e.g., haloperidol) may decrease therapeutic effect. **Levodopa-containing products** may increase the hypotensive effect. **HERBAL: Herbals with hypotensive properties (e.g., garlic, ginger, gingko biloba)** may increase hypotensive effect. **FOOD: All foods** delay peak drug plasma levels by 1 hr (extent of absorption not affected). **LAB VALUES:** None significant.

AVAILABILITY (Rx)

Tablets: 0.125 mg, 0.25 mg, 0.5 mg, 0.75 mg, 1 mg, 1.5 mg.

Tablets, Extended-Release: *(Mirapex ER):* 0.375 mg, 0.75 mg, 1.5 mg, 2.25 mg, 3 mg, 3.75 mg, 4.5 mg.

P

ADMINISTRATION/HANDLING

PO

Mirapex: • Give without regard to food. **Mirapex ER:** • Give once daily, without regard to food. • Give whole; do not break, crush, dissolve, or divide tablets.

INDICATIONS/ROUTES/DOSAGE

Parkinson's Disease

Note: When discontinuing, reduce dose by 0.75 mg/day until daily dose is 0.75 mg once daily, then reduce by 0.375 mg/day thereafter.

PO: ***(Immediate-Release):*** **ADULTS, ELDERLY:** Initially, 0.125 mg 3 times/day. Increase no more frequently than every 5–7 days. **Maintenance:** 0.5–1.5 mg 3 times/day. ***(Extended-Release):*** Initially, 0.375 mg once daily. May increase to 0.75 mg, then by 0.75-mg increments no more frequently than 5–7 days. **Maximum:** 4.5 mg once daily. **Note:** May switch overnight from immediate-release to extended-release at same daily dose.

P

Restless Legs Syndrome

Note: When discontinuing, gradually reduce dose q4–7 days.

PO: ADULTS, ELDERLY: ***(Immediate-Release):*** Initially, 0.125 mg once daily 2–3 hrs before bedtime. May increase to 0.25 mg after 4–7 days, then to 0.5 mg after 4–7 days (interval is 14 days in pts with renal impairment). **Maximum:** 0.75 mg/day.

Dosage in Renal Impairment

Dosage and frequency are modified based on creatinine clearance.

Parkinson's Disease

Immediate-Release

Creatinine Clearance	Initial Dosage	Maximum Dosage
30–50 mL/min	0.125 mg twice daily	0.75 mg 3 times/day
15–29 mL/min	0.125 mg once daily	1.5 mg once daily

Extended-Release

CrCl 30–50 mL/min: Initially, 0.375 mg every other day. May increase by 0.375 mg/day in 7 days or longer. **Maximum:** 2.25 mg once daily. **CrCl less than 30 mL/min:** Not recommended.

Restless Legs Syndrome

No dose adjustment.

Dosage in Hepatic Impairment

No dose adjustment.

SIDE EFFECTS

Frequent: Early Parkinson's disease (28%–10%): Nausea, asthenia, dizziness, drowsiness, insomnia, constipation. **Advanced Parkinson's disease (53%–17%):** Orthostatic hypotension, extrapyramidal reactions, insomnia, dizziness, hallucinations. **Occasional: Early Parkinson's disease (5%–2%):** Edema, malaise, confusion, amnesia, akathisia, anorexia, dysphagia, peripheral edema, vision changes, impotence. **Advanced Parkinson's disease (10%–7%):** Asthenia, drowsiness, confusion, constipation, abnormal gait, dry mouth. **Rare: Advanced Parkinson's disease (6%–2%):** General edema, malaise, angina, amnesia, tremor, urinary frequency/incontinence, dyspnea, rhinitis, vision changes. **Restless legs syndrome: Frequent (16%):** Headache, nausea. **Occasional (13%–9%):** Insomnia, fatigue. **Rare (6%–3%):** Drowsiness, constipation, diarrhea, dry mouth.

ADVERSE EFFECTS/TOXIC REACTIONS

Vascular disease, atrial fibrillation, arrhythmias, pulmonary embolism, impulsive/compulsive behavior (pathological gambling, hypersexuality, binge eating) have been reported.

NURSING CONSIDERATIONS

BASELINE ASSESSMENT

Parkinson's disease: Assess for tremor, muscle weakness and rigidity, ataxia. **Restless legs syndrome:** Assess frequency of symptoms, sleep pattern.

INTERVENTION/EVALUATION

Assess for clinical improvement. Assist with ambulation if dizziness occurs. Assess for constipation; encourage fiber, fluids, exercise.

PATIENT/FAMILY TEACHING

• Hallucinations may occur, esp. in the elderly. • Go from lying to standing slowly. • Avoid tasks that require alertness, motor skills until response to drug is established. • If nausea occurs, take medication with food. • Avoid abrupt withdrawal. • Avoid alcohol. • Report new or increased impulsive/compulsive behaviors (e.g., gambling, sexual urges, compulsive eating or buying).

pravastatin

TOP 100

pra-va-sta-tin
(Pravachol)

Do not confuse pravastatin with atorvastatin, lovastatin, nystatin, pitavastatin, or simvastatin, or Pravachol with Prevacid, Prinivil, or propranolol.

FIXED-COMBINATION(S)

Pravigard: pravastatin/aspirin (anticoagulant): 20 mg/81 mg, 40 mg/81 mg, 80 mg/81 mg, 20 mg/325 mg, 40 mg/325 mg, 80 mg/325 mg.

◆CLASSIFICATION

PHARMACOTHERAPEUTIC: Hydroxymethylglutaryl CoA (HMG-CoA) reductase inhibitor. **CLINICAL:** Antihyperlipidemic.

USES

Adjunct to diet in the treatment of primary hyperlipidemias and mixed dyslipidemias to reduce total cholesterol, LDL cholesterol, apolipoprotein B, triglycerides; increase HDL cholesterol. Reduces risk of MI, revascularization, and mortality in hypercholesterolemia without clinically evident CHD. Reduces mortality risk in pts with CHD. Reduces elevated triglycerides in hypertriglyceridemia. Treatment of heterozygous familial hypercholesterolemia in pediatric pts 8–18 yrs.

PRECAUTIONS

Contraindications: Hypersensitivity to pravastatin. Active hepatic disease or unexplained, persistent elevations of LFT results. Pregnancy, breastfeeding. **Cautions:** Hepatic impairment, substantial alcohol consumption. Withholding/discontinuing pravastatin may be necessary when pt is at risk for renal failure secondary to rhabdomyolysis, elderly.

ACTION

Interferes with cholesterol biosynthesis by preventing conversion of HMG-CoA reductase to mevalonate, a precursor to cholesterol. **Therapeutic Effect:** Lowers LDL, VLDL cholesterol, plasma triglycerides; increases HDL.

PHARMACOKINETICS

Widely distributed. Protein binding: 50%. Metabolized in liver. Primarily excreted in feces. Not removed by hemodialysis. **Half-life:** 2–3 hrs. (Half-life including all metabolites: 77 hrs.)

LIFESPAN CONSIDERATIONS

Pregnancy/Lactation: Contraindicated in pregnancy (suppression of cholesterol biosynthesis may cause fetal toxicity) and lactation. Small amount is distributed in breast milk, but there is risk of serious adverse reactions in breastfeeding infants. Breastfeeding not recommended. **Children/Elderly:** No age-related precautions noted.

INTERACTIONS

DRUG: **CycloSPORINE, clarithromycin, colchicine, erythromycin, gemfibrozil, niacin** increase risk of myopathy, rhabdomyolysis. **Bile acid sequestrants (e.g., cholestyramine)** may decrease absorption. **HERBAL:** None

P

significant. **FOOD:** **Red yeast rice** contains 2.4 mg **lovastatin** per 600 mg rice (may increase adverse effects). **LAB VALUES:** May increase serum creatine kinase (CK), transaminase.

AVAILABILITY (Rx)

Tablets: 10 mg, 20 mg, 40 mg, 80 mg.

ADMINISTRATION/HANDLING

PO

- Give without regard to food.

INDICATIONS/ROUTES/DOSAGE

◀ALERT▶ Prior to initiating therapy, pt should be on standard cholesterol-lowering diet for 3–6 mos. Low-cholesterol diet should be continued throughout pravastatin therapy.

Hyperlipidemia, Prevention of Coronary/Cardiovascular Events

PO: ADULTS, ELDERLY: Initially, 40 mg/day. Titrate to desired response. Range: 10–80 mg/day.

Heterozygous Familial Hypercholesterolemia

PO: CHILDREN 14–18 YRS: 40 mg/day. **CHILDREN 8–13 YRS:** 20 mg/day. Range: 5–20 mg/day.

Dosage with Clarithromycin

Maximum: 40 mg/day.

Dosage with CycloSPORINE

ADULTS, ELDERLY: Initially, 10 mg/day. **Maximum:** 20 mg/day.

Dosage in Renal Impairment

For adults, give 10 mg/day initially. Titrate to desired response.

Dosage in Hepatic Impairment

See contraindications.

SIDE EFFECTS

Occasional (7%–4%): Nausea, vomiting, diarrhea, constipation, abdominal pain, headache, rhinitis, rash, pruritus. **Rare (3%–2%):** Heartburn, myalgia, dizziness, cough, fatigue, flu-like symptoms, depression, photosensitivity.

ADVERSE EFFECTS/TOXIC REACTIONS

Potential for malignancy, cataracts. Hypersensitivity, myopathy occur rarely. Rhabdomyolysis has been reported.

NURSING CONSIDERATIONS

BASELINE ASSESSMENT

Obtain lipid panel, LFT; pregnancy test in females of reproductive potential. Obtain dietary history, esp. fat consumption.

INTERVENTION/EVALUATION

Monitor serum cholesterol, triglycerides for therapeutic response. Monitor LFT. Monitor daily pattern of bowel activity, stool consistency. Assess for rash, pruritus. Be alert for malaise, muscle cramping/weakness; if accompanied by fever, may require discontinuation of medication.

PATIENT/FAMILY TEACHING

• Follow special diet (important part of treatment). • Report promptly any muscle pain/weakness, esp. if accompanied by fever, malaise. • Use nonhormonal contraception. • Avoid direct exposure to sunlight.

prednisoLONE

pred-**niss**-oh-lone
(Millipred, Orapred ODT, Pred Forte, Pred Mild, Veripred)
Do not confuse Pediapred with Pediazole, prednisoLONE with predniSONE or primidone, or Prelone with PROzac.

FIXED-COMBINATION(S)

Blephamide: prednisoLONE/sulfacetamide (an anti-infective): 0.2%/10%. **Vasocidin:** prednisoLONE/sulfacetamide: 0.25%/10%.

◆CLASSIFICATION

PHARMACOTHERAPEUTIC: Adrenal corticosteroid. **CLINICAL:** Anti-inflammatory, immunosuppressant.

USES

Systemic: Endocrine, rheumatic, hematologic disorders; collagen, respiratory, neoplastic, GI diseases; allergic states; acute or chronic solid organ rejection. **Ophthalmic:** Treatment of conjunctivitis, corneal injury (from chemical/thermal burns, foreign body).

PRECAUTIONS

Contraindications: Hypersensitivity to prednisoLONE. Acute superficial herpes simplex keratitis, systemic fungal infections, varicella, live or attenuated virus vaccines. **Cautions:** Hyperthyroidism, cirrhosis, ocular herpes simplex, respiratory tuberculosis, untreated systemic infections, renal/hepatic impairment, diabetes, cataracts, glaucoma, seizure disorder, peptic ulcer disease, osteoporosis, myasthenia gravis, hypertension, HF, ulcerative colitis, thromboembolic disorders, elderly.

ACTION

Inhibits accumulation of inflammatory cells at inflammation sites, phagocytosis, lysosomal enzyme release/synthesis, release of mediators of inflammation. **Therapeutic Effect:** Prevents/suppresses cell-mediated immune reactions. Decreases/prevents tissue response to inflammatory process.

PHARMACOKINETICS

Protein binding: 65%–91%. Metabolized in liver. Excreted in urine. **Half-life:** 3.6 hrs.

LIFESPAN CONSIDERATIONS

Pregnancy/Lactation: Crosses placenta. Distributed in breast milk. Fetal cleft palate often occurs with chronic, first-trimester use. Breastfeeding not recommended. **Children:** Prolonged treatment or high dosages may decrease short-term growth rate, cortisol secretion. **Elderly:** May be more susceptible to developing hypertension or osteoporosis.

INTERACTIONS

DRUG: CYP3A4 inducers (e.g., carBAMazepine, phenytoin, rifAMPin) may decrease effects. **Live virus vaccines** increase vaccine side effects, potentiate virus replication, decrease pt's antibody response to vaccine. May increase effect of **warfarin**. May decrease therapeutic effect of **aldesleukin**. May increase hyponatremic effect of **desmopressin**. **HERBAL: Echinacea** may decrease therapeutic effect. **FOOD:** None known. **LAB VALUES:** May increase serum glucose, lipids, sodium, uric acid. May decrease serum calcium, WBC, hypothalamic pituitary adrenal (HPA) axis function, potassium.

AVAILABILITY (Rx)

Solution, Ophthalmic: 1%. **Solution, Oral:** 15 mg/5 mL, 5 mg/5 mL, 10 mg/5 mL, 20 mg/5 mL, 25 mg/5 mL. **Suspension, Ophthalmic:** 1%, 0.12%. **Tablets:** 5 mg.

Tablets, Orally Disintegrating: 10 mg, 15 mg, 30 mg.

ADMINISTRATION/HANDLING

PO

• Give with food or fluids to decrease GI side effects.

Orally Disintegrating Tablets

• Do not break, crush, or divide tablets. • Remove from blister just prior to giving; place on tongue. • Pt may swallow whole or allow to dissolve in mouth with/without water.

Ophthalmic

• For ophthalmic solution, shake well before using. • Instill drops into conjunctival sac, as prescribed. • Avoid touching applicator tip to conjunctiva to avoid contamination.

INDICATIONS/ROUTES/DOSAGE

Usual Dosage

PO: ADULTS, ELDERLY: 5–60 mg/day in divided doses. **CHILDREN:** 0.1–2 mg/kg/day in 3–4 divided doses.

P

Treatment of Conjunctivitis, Corneal Injury
Ophthalmic: ADULTS, ELDERLY, CHILDREN: 1–2 drops every hr during day and q2h during night. After response, decrease dosage to 1 drop q4h, then 1 drop 3–4 times/day.

Dosage in Renal/Hepatic Impairment
No dose adjustment.

SIDE EFFECTS

Frequent: Insomnia, heartburn, nervousness, abdominal distention, diaphoresis, acne, mood swings, increased appetite, facial flushing, delayed wound healing, increased susceptibility to infection, diarrhea, constipation. **Occasional:** Headache, edema, change in skin color, frequent urination. **Rare:** Tachycardia, allergic reaction (rash, urticaria), psychological changes, hallucinations, depression. **Ophthalmic:** Stinging/burning, posterior subcapsular cataracts.

ADVERSE EFFECTS/TOXIC REACTIONS

Long-term therapy: Hypocalcemia, hypokalemia, muscle wasting (esp. arms, legs), osteoporosis, spontaneous fractures, amenorrhea, cataracts, glaucoma, peptic ulcer, HF, immunosuppression. **Abrupt withdrawal following long-term therapy:** Anorexia, nausea, fever, headache, severe/sudden joint pain, rebound inflammation, fatigue, weakness, lethargy, dizziness, orthostatic hypotension. Sudden discontinuance may be fatal.

NURSING CONSIDERATIONS

BASELINE ASSESSMENT

Question medical history as listed in Precautions. Obtain height, weight, B/P, serum glucose, electrolytes. Check results of initial tests (tuberculosis [TB] skin test, X-rays, ECG).

INTERVENTION/EVALUATION

Monitor B/P, weight, serum electrolytes, glucose, results of bone mineral density test, height, weight in children. Be alert to infection (sore throat, fever, vague symptoms); assess oral cavity daily for signs of *Candida* infection. Monitor for symptoms of adrenal insufficiency, immunosuppression.

PATIENT/FAMILY TEACHING

• Report fever, sore throat, muscle aches, sudden weight gain, swelling, loss of appetite, fatigue. • Avoid alcohol, limit caffeine. • Do not abruptly discontinue without physician's approval. • Avoid exposure to chickenpox, measles. • Long-term use may significantly increase risk of serious infections.

predniSONE

pred-ni-sone
(Apo-PredniSONE ✦, PredniSONE Intensol, Rayos, Winpred ✦)
Do not confuse predniSONE with methylPREDNISolone, prazosin, prednisoLONE, PriLOSEC, primidone, or promethazine.

◆CLASSIFICATION

PHARMACOTHERAPEUTIC: Adrenal corticosteroid. **CLINICAL:** Anti-inflammatory, immunosuppressant.

USES

Substitution therapy in deficiency states: Acute or chronic adrenal insufficiency, congenital adrenal hyperplasia, adrenal insufficiency secondary to pituitary insufficiency. **Nonendocrine disorders:** Arthritis, rheumatic carditis; allergic, collagen, intestinal tract, multiple sclerosis exacerbations; liver, ocular, renal, skin diseases; bronchial asthma, cerebral edema, malignancies. **OFF-LABEL:** Prevention of postherpetic neuralgia, relief of acute pain in pts with herpes zoster, autoimmune hepatitis.

PRECAUTIONS

Contraindications: Hypersensitivity to predniSONE. Acute superficial herpes simplex keratitis, systemic fungal infections, varicella, administration of live or attenuated virus vaccines. **Cautions:** Hyperthyroidism, cirrhosis, ocular herpes simplex, respiratory tuberculosis, untreated systemic infections, renal/hepatic impairment, following acute MI, cataracts, glaucoma, seizure disorder, peptic ulcer disease, osteoporosis, myasthenia gravis, hypertension, HF, ulcerative colitis, thromboembolic disorders, elderly, pts at risk for hyperglycemia (e.g., diabetes, recent surgery).

ACTION

Inhibits accumulation of inflammatory cells at inflammation sites, phagocytosis, lysosomal enzyme release/synthesis, release of mediators of inflammation. **Therapeutic Effect:** Prevents/suppresses cell-mediated immune reactions. Decreases/prevents tissue response to inflammatory process.

PHARMACOKINETICS

Well absorbed from GI tract. Protein binding: 70%–90%. Widely distributed. Metabolized in liver, converted to prednisoLONE. Primarily excreted in urine. Not removed by hemodialysis. **Half-life:** 2.5–3.5 hrs.

LIFESPAN CONSIDERATIONS

Pregnancy/Lactation: Crosses placenta. Distributed in breast milk. Fetal cleft palate often occurs with chronic, first trimester use. Breastfeeding not recommended. **Children:** Prolonged treatment or high dosages may decrease short-term growth rate, cortisol secretion. **Elderly:** May be more susceptible to developing hypertension or osteoporosis.

INTERACTIONS

DRUG: **CYP3A4 inducers (e.g., carBAMazepine, phenytoin, rifAMPin)** may decrease effects. **Live virus vaccines** may increase vaccine side effects, potentiate virus replication, decrease pt's antibody response to vaccine. May increase effect of **warfarin**. May decrease therapeutic effect of **aldesleukin**. May increase hyponatremic effect of **desmopressin**. **HERBAL:** **Echinacea** may decrease therapeutic effect. **FOOD:** None known. **LAB VALUES:** May increase serum glucose, lipids, sodium, uric acid. May decrease serum calcium, potassium, WBC, hypothalamic pituitary adrenal (HPA) axis function.

AVAILABILITY (Rx)

Solution, Oral: 1 mg/mL. **Solution, Oral Concentrate:** ***(Prednisone Intensol):*** 5 mg/mL. **Tablets:** 1 mg, 2.5 mg, 5 mg, 10 mg, 20 mg, 50 mg.

Tablet, Delayed-Release: ***(Rayos)***: 1 mg, 2 mg, 5 mg.

ADMINISTRATION/HANDLING

PO

• Give with food or fluids to decrease GI side effects. • Give single doses before 9 AM, multiple doses at evenly spaced intervals. • Give delayed-release tablet whole; do not break, crush, dissolve, or divide.

INDICATIONS/ROUTES/DOSAGE

Note: Dose dependent upon condition treated, pt response rather than by rigid adherence to age, weight, or body surface area.

Usual Dosage

PO: **ADULTS, ELDERLY:** 10–60 mg/day in divided doses. **Range:** 2.5–100 mg/day. **CHILDREN:** 0.05–2 mg/kg/day in 1–4 divided doses.

Dosage in Renal/Hepatic Impairment

No dose adjustment.

SIDE EFFECTS

Frequent: Insomnia, heartburn, nervousness, abdominal distention, diaphoresis, acne, mood swings, increased appetite, facial flushing, delayed wound healing, increased susceptibility to infection, diarrhea, constipation. **Occasional:** Headache, edema, change in skin color, frequent urination. **Rare:** Tachycardia, allergic reaction (rash, urticaria), psychological changes, hallucinations, depression.

ADVERSE EFFECTS/TOXIC REACTIONS

Long-term therapy: Muscle wasting (esp. in arms, legs), osteoporosis, spontaneous fractures, amenorrhea, cataracts, glaucoma, peptic ulcer, HF. **Abrupt withdrawal following long-term therapy:** Anorexia, nausea, fever, headache, rebound inflammation, fatigue, weakness, lethargy, dizziness, orthostatic hypotension. Sudden discontinuance may be fatal.

NURSING CONSIDERATIONS

BASELINE ASSESSMENT

Question medical history as listed in Precautions. Obtain height, weight, B/P, serum glucose, electrolytes. Check results of initial tests (tuberculosis [TB] skin test, X-rays, ECG).

INTERVENTION/EVALUATION

Monitor B/P, serum electrolytes, glucose, results of bone mineral density test, height, weight in children. Be alert to infection (sore throat, fever, vague symptoms); assess oral cavity daily for signs of *Candida* infection. Monitor for symptoms of adrenal insufficiency, immunosuppression.

PATIENT/FAMILY TEACHING

• Report fever, sore throat, muscle aches, sudden weight gain, swelling, loss of appetite, or fatigue. • Avoid alcohol, minimize use of caffeine. • Report symptoms of elevated blood sugar levels (blurred vision, headache, increased thirst, frequent urination). • Do not abruptly discontinue without physician's approval. • Avoid exposure to chickenpox, measles. • Long-term use may significantly increase risk of serious infections.

pregabalin

TOP 100

pre-**gab**-a-lin
(Lyrica, Lyrica CR)

◆CLASSIFICATION

PHARMACOTHERAPEUTIC: GABA analogue. **CLINICAL:** Anticonvulsant, antineuralgic, analgesic (Schedule V).

USES

Lyrica: Adjunctive therapy in treatment of partial-onset seizures. Management of neuropathic pain associated with diabetic peripheral neuropathy or spinal cord injury. Management of postherpetic neuralgia. Management of fibromyalgia. **Lyrica CR:** Management of neuropathic pain associated with diabetic peripheral neuropathy, postherpetic neuralgia.

PRECAUTIONS

Contraindications: Hypersensitivity to pregabalin. **Cautions:** HF, renal impairment, cardiovascular disease, diabetes, history of angioedema, history of suicidal ideation and behavior. Concurrent use of thiazolidine antidiabetics (e.g., Actos).

ACTION

Binds to calcium channel sites in CNS tissue, inhibiting excitatory neurotransmitter release. Exerts antinociceptive, anticonvulsant activity. May affect descending noradrenergic and serotonergic pain transmission pathways from the brainstem to spinal cord. **Therapeutic Effect:** Decreases symptoms of painful peripheral neuropathy; decreases frequency of partial seizures.

PHARMACOKINETICS

Well absorbed following PO administration. Excreted in urine unchanged. **Half-life:** 6 hrs.

⌛ LIFESPAN CONSIDERATIONS

Pregnancy/Lactation: Increased risk of fetal skeletal abnormalities. Unknown if distributed in breast milk.

Children: Safety and efficacy not established. **Elderly:** Age-related renal impairment may require dosage adjustment.

INTERACTIONS

DRUG: **Alcohol, CNS depressants (e.g., LORazepam, morphine, zolpidem)** may increase sedative effect. **HERBAL:** **Herbals with sedative properties (e.g., chamomile, kava kava, valerian)** may increase CNS depression. **FOOD:** None known. **LAB VALUES:** May increase CPK. May cause mild PR interval prolongation. May decrease platelet count.

AVAILABILITY (Rx)

Solution, Oral: 20 mg/mL.

Capsules: ***(Lyrica):*** 25 mg, 50 mg, 75 mg, 100 mg, 150 mg, 200 mg, 225 mg, 300 mg.

Tablet, Extended-Release: ***(Lyrica CR):*** 82.5 mg, 165 mg, 330 mg.

ADMINISTRATION/HANDLING

• Give without regard to food. • Administer whole; do not break, crush, or open capsule. • **Lyrica CR:** Give once daily in evening. • Discontinue pregabalin gradually over at least 1 wk. • Administer whole; do not break, cut, crush, or divide. Tablet cannot be chewed.

INDICATIONS/ROUTES/DOSAGE

Partial-Onset Seizures

PO: ADULTS, ELDERLY: Initially, 75 mg twice daily or 50 mg 3 times/day. May increase dose based on tolerability/effect. **Maximum:** 600 mg/day. **ADOLESCENTS, CHILDREN, 4 YRS AND OLDER WEIGHING 30 KG OR MORE:** Initially, 2.5 mg/kg/day in 2 or 3 divided doses. May increase wkly based on clinical response and tolerability. **Maximum:** 10 mg/kg/day (not to exceed 600 mg/day). **LESS THAN 30 KG:** Initially, 3.5 mg/kg/day in 2 or 3 divided doses. May increase wkly based on clinical response and tolerability. **Maximum:** 14 mg/kg/day. **CHILDREN YOUNGER THAN 4 YRS, INFANTS WEIGHING LESS THAN 30 KG:** Initially, 3.5 mg/kg/day in 3 divided doses. May increase wkly based on response and tolerability. **Maximum:** 14 mg/kg/day.

Neuropathic Pain (Diabetes-associated)

PO: ADULTS, ELDERLY: Initially, 25–75 mg/day once daily or in 2–3 divided doses. May increase within 1 wk based on response and tolerability. **Maximum:** 300–450 mg/day.

PO: ***(Lyrica CR):*** **ADULTS, ELDERLY:** Initially, 165 mg once daily. May increase to 330 mg/day within 1 wk. **Maximum:** 330 mg/day.

Postherpetic Neuralgia, Neuropathic Pain Associated With Spinal Cord Injury

PO: ADULTS, ELDERLY: Initially, 75 mg twice daily or 50 mg 3 times/day. May increase to 300 mg/day within 1 wk. May further increase to 600 mg/day after 2–4 wks. **Maximum:** 600 mg/day.

PO: ***(Lyrica CR):*** **ADULTS, ELDERLY:** Initially, 165 mg once daily. May increase to 330 mg/day within 1 wk. May further increase to 660 mg once daily after 2–4 wks. **Maximum:** 660 mg/day.

Fibromyalgia

PO: ADULTS, ELDERLY: ***(Immediate-Release):*** Initially, 75 mg twice daily. May increase to 150 mg twice daily within 1 wk. **Maximum:** 225 mg twice daily.

Dosage in Renal Impairment

Creatinine Clearance	Daily Dosage
30–60 mL/min	75–300 mg in 2–3 divided doses
15–29 mL/min	25–150 mg in 1 or 2 doses
Less than 15 mL/min	25–75 mg once daily

Dosage for Hemodialysis

◄ALERT► Take supplemental dose immediately following dialysis.

Daily Dosage	Supplemental Dosage
25 mg	Single dose of 25 mg or 50 mg
25–50 mg	Single dose of 50 mg or 75 mg
75 mg	Single dose of 100 mg or 150 mg

Dosage in Hepatic Impairment

No dose adjustment.

P

SIDE EFFECTS

Frequent (32%–12%): Dizziness, drowsiness, ataxia, peripheral edema. **Occasional (12%–5%):** Weight gain, blurred vision, diplopia, difficulty with concentration, attention, cognition; tremor, dry mouth, headache, constipation, asthenia. **Rare (4%–2%):** Abnormal gait, confusion, incoordination, twitching, flatulence, vomiting, edema, myopathy.

ADVERSE EFFECTS/TOXIC REACTIONS

Abrupt withdrawal increases risk of seizure frequency in pts with seizure disorders; withdraw gradually over a minimum of 1 wk. May increase risk of suicidal thoughts and behavior.

NURSING CONSIDERATIONS

BASELINE ASSESSMENT

Seizure: Review history of seizure disorder (type, onset, intensity, frequency, duration, LOC). **Pain:** Assess onset, type, location, and duration of pain. Question history of suicidal ideation and behavior.

INTERVENTION/EVALUATION

Assess for seizure activity. Assess for clinical improvement; record onset of relief of pain. Assess for peripheral edema. Question for changes in visual acuity. Monitor weight.

PATIENT/FAMILY TEACHING

• Do not abruptly stop taking drug; seizure frequency may be increased. • Avoid tasks that require alertness, motor skills until response to drug is established. • Avoid alcohol. • Seek immediate medical attention if thoughts of suicide, new-onset or worsening of anxiety, depression, or changes in mood occur.

primidone

prim-i-done
(Apo-Primidone ✱, Mysoline)
Do not confuse primidone with predniSONE or pyridoxine.

◆CLASSIFICATION

PHARMACOTHERAPEUTIC: Barbiturate. **CLINICAL:** Anticonvulsant.

USES

Management of psychomotor, generalized tonic-clonic (grand mal), and focal seizures. **OFF-LABEL:** Treatment of essential tremor (familial tremor).

PRECAUTIONS

Contraindications: Hypersensitivity to primidone, PHENobarbital; porphyria. **Cautions:** Renal/hepatic impairment, pulmonary insufficiency, elderly, debilitated, children, hypoadrenalism, pts at risk for suicidal thoughts/behavior, depression, history of drug abuse.

ACTION

Decreases neuron excitability. Raises seizure threshold. **Therapeutic Effect:** Reduces seizure activity.

PHARMACOKINETICS

Widely distributed. Protein binding: 99%. Metabolized in liver to PHENobarbital. Minimal excretion in urine. **Half-life:** 3–6 hrs. (PHENobarbital: 2–5 days.)

⌛ LIFESPAN CONSIDERATIONS

Pregnancy/Lactation: Crosses placenta; distributed in breast milk. **Children/Elderly:** May produce paradoxical excitement, restlessness.

INTERACTIONS

DRUG: **Alcohol, CNS depressants (e.g., LORazepam, morphine, zolpidem)** may increase CNS depression. **Valproic acid** increases concentration, risk of toxicity. **Strong CYP2C19 inducers (e.g., carBAMazepine, rifAMPin)** may decrease concentration/effect. **Strong CYP2C19 inhibitors (e.g., FLUoxetine, fluvoxaMINE)** may increase concentration/effect. May decrease effect of **dolutegravir, oral contraceptives, tenofovir, voriconazole, warfarin**. **HERBAL:** **Herbals with**

sedative properties (e.g., chamomile, kava kava, valerian) may increase CNS depression. FOOD: None known. LAB VALUES: May decrease serum bilirubin. **Therapeutic serum level:** 4–12 mcg/mL; **toxic serum level:** greater than 12 mcg/mL.

AVAILABILITY (Rx)

Tablets: 50 mg, 250 mg.

ADMINISTRATION/HANDLING

PO

- Give with food to minimize GI effects.

INDICATIONS/ROUTES/DOSAGE

Seizure Control

PO: ADULTS, ELDERLY, CHILDREN 8 YRS AND OLDER: Initially, 100–125 mg/day at bedtime for days 1–3. **Days 4–6:** 100–125 mg twice daily. **Days 7–9:** 100–125 mg 3 times/day. **Usual dose:** 750–1,500 mg/day in 3–4 divided doses. **Maximum:** 2 g/day. **CHILDREN YOUNGER THAN 8 YRS:** Initially, 50 mg/day at bedtime for days 1–3. **Days 4–6:** 50 mg twice daily. **Days 7–9:** 100 mg twice daily. **Usual dose:** 125–250 mg 3 times/day. **NEONATES:** 12–20 mg/kg/day in divided doses 2–4 times/day.

Dosage in Renal Impairment

Creatine Clearance	Interval
50 mL/min or greater	q12h
10–49 mL/min	q12–24h
Less than 10 mL/min	q24h
Hemodialysis (HD)	Administer dose post-HD

Dosage in Hepatic Impairment

No dose adjustment.

SIDE EFFECTS

Frequent: Ataxia, dizziness. **Occasional:** Anorexia, drowsiness, altered mental status, nausea, vomiting, paradoxical excitement. **Rare:** Rash.

ADVERSE EFFECTS/TOXIC REACTIONS

Abrupt withdrawal after prolonged therapy may produce effects ranging from markedly increased dreaming, nightmares, insomnia, tremor, diaphoresis, vomiting to hallucinations, delirium, seizures, status epilepticus. Skin eruptions may appear as hypersensitivity reaction. Blood dyscrasias, hepatic disease, hypocalcemia occur rarely. Overdose produces cold/clammy skin, hypothermia, severe CNS depression, followed by high fever, coma. May increase risk of suicidal thoughts and behavior.

NURSING CONSIDERATIONS

BASELINE ASSESSMENT

Review history of seizure disorder (intensity, frequency, duration, LOC). Observe frequently for recurrence of seizure activity. Initiate seizure precautions. Question history of suicidal ideation and behavior.

INTERVENTION/EVALUATION

Monitor for changes in behavior, depression, suicidal ideation. Monitor CBC, neurologic status (frequency, duration, severity of seizures). Monitor for **therapeutic serum level:** 4–12 mcg/mL; **toxic serum level:** more than 12 mcg/mL.

PATIENT/FAMILY TEACHING

- Do not abruptly discontinue medication after long-term use (may precipitate seizures). • Strict maintenance of drug therapy is essential for seizure control. • Avoid tasks that require alertness, motor skills until response to drug is established; drowsiness usually disappears during continued therapy. • Seek immediate medical attention if thoughts of suicide, new onset or worsening of anxiety, depression, or changes in mood occur.

propafenone

proe-**paf**-e-nown
(Apo-Propafenone ✦, Rythmol SR)

■ **BLACK BOX ALERT** ■ Mortality or nonfatal cardiac arrest rate (7.7% of pts) in asymptomatic

P

non–life-threatening ventricular arrhythmia pts with recent MI (more than 6 days but less than 2 yrs prior) reported.

◆CLASSIFICATION

PHARMACOTHERAPEUTIC: Class 1c antiarrhythmic. **CLINICAL:** Antiarrhythmic.

USES

Immediate-Release: Treatment of life-threatening ventricular arrhythmias (e.g., sustained ventricular tachycardias). To prolong time to recurrence of paroxysmal atrial fibrillation/flutter (PAF) or paroxysmal supraventricular tachycardia (PSVT) in pts with disabling symptoms and without structural heart disease. **Extended-Release:** Prolong the time to recurrence of atrial fibrillation/flutter or paroxysmal supraventricular tachycardia in pts with disabling symptoms without structural heart disease. **OFF-LABEL:** Treatment following cardioversion of recent-onset atrial fibrillation; supraventricular tachycardia in pts with Wolff-Parkinson-White syndrome.

P

PRECAUTIONS

Contraindications: Hypersensitivity to propafenone. Sinus bradycardia, bronchospastic disorders or severe obstructive pulmonary disease, cardiogenic shock, uncorrected electrolyte imbalance, sinoatrial, AV, intraventricular impulse generation or conduction disorders (e.g., sick sinus syndrome, AV block) without pacemaker, uncompensated HF, marked hypotension. **Cautions:** Renal/hepatic impairment, myasthenia gravis, pts at risk for QTc interval prolongation (congenital long QT syndrome, HF, medications that prolong QTc interval, hypokalemia, hypomagnesemia).

ACTION

Blocks fast inward sodium current. Slows the rate of increase of the action potential (prolongs conduction velocity, refractory period). **Therapeutic Effect:** Suppresses arrhythmias.

PHARMACOKINETICS

Nearly completely absorbed following PO administration. Protein binding: 85%–97%. Metabolized in liver. Primarily excreted in feces. **Half-life:** 2–10 hrs.

⌛ LIFESPAN CONSIDERATIONS

Pregnancy/Lactation: Crosses placenta, distributed in breast milk. **Children:** Safety and efficacy not established. **Elderly:** No age-related precautions noted.

INTERACTIONS

DRUG: **Amiodarone** may affect cardiac conduction, repolarization. May increase effects of **warfarin. CYP3A4 inhibitors (e.g., ketoconazole, erythromycin)** may increase concentration/toxicity. **Strong CYP2D6 inhibitors (e.g., buPROPion, FLUoxetine)** may increase concentration/effect. **QT interval–prolonging medications (e.g., amiodarone, azithromycin, ciprofloxacin, haloperidol, methadone, sotalol)** may increase risk of QTc interval prolongation. **HERBAL:** **St. John's wort** may decrease concentration/effect. **FOOD:** **Grapefruit products** may increase concentration. **LAB VALUES:** May cause ECG changes (e.g., QRS widening, PR interval prolongation), positive ANA titer.

AVAILABILITY (Rx)

Tablets: 150 mg, 225 mg, 300 mg.

Capsules, Extended-Release: 225 mg, 325 mg, 425 mg.

ADMINISTRATION/HANDLING

PO

• Give without regard to food. • Give whole; do not break, crush, divide, or open capsules.

INDICATIONS/ROUTES/DOSAGE

Ventricular Arrhythmias, PAT, PSVT

PO: ***(Immediate-Release):*** **ADULTS, ELDERLY:** Initially, 150 mg q8h. May increase at 3- to 4-day intervals to 225 mg q8h, then to 300 mg q8h. **Maximum:** 900 mg/day.

Atrial Fibrillation (Prevention of recurrence)
PO: ***(Immediate-Release):*** **ADULTS, ELDERLY:** Initially, 150 mg q8h. May increase at 3- to 4-day intervals to 225 mg q8h, then to 300 mg q8h. **Maximum:** 900 mg/day. ***(Extended-Release):*** **ADULTS, ELDERLY:** Initially, 225 mg q12h. May increase at 5-day intervals to 325 mg q12h. **Maximum:** 425 mg q12h.

Dosage in Renal Impairment
No dose adjustment.

Dosage in Hepatic Impairment
Use caution.

SIDE EFFECTS

Frequent (13%–7%): Dizziness, nausea, vomiting, altered taste, constipation. **Occasional (6%–3%):** Headache, dyspnea, blurred vision, dyspepsia. **Rare (less than 2%):** Rash, weakness, dry mouth, diarrhea, edema, hot flashes.

ADVERSE EFFECTS/TOXIC REACTIONS

May cause or worsen arrhythmias, HF. Overdose may produce hypotension, drowsiness, bradycardia, atrioventricular conduction disturbances.

NURSING CONSIDERATIONS

BASELINE ASSESSMENT

Correct electrolyte imbalance before administering medication. Obtain baseline ECG. Screen for cardiac contraindications.

INTERVENTION/EVALUATION

Assess pulse for quality, rhythm, rate. Monitor ECG for cardiac performance or changes, particularly widening of QRS complex, prolongation of PR interval. Question for visual disturbances, headache, GI upset. Monitor LFT. Monitor for therapeutic serum level (0.06–1 mcg/mL).

PATIENT/FAMILY TEACHING

• Compliance with therapy regimen is essential to control arrhythmias. • Altered taste sensation may occur. • Report headache, blurred vision. • Avoid tasks that require alertness, motor skills until response to drug is established. • Report chest pain, difficulty breathing, palpitations.

propofol

HIGH ALERT

proe-poe-fol
(Diprivan, Fresenius Propoven)
Do not confuse Diprivan with Diflucan or Ditropan, or propofol with fospropofol.

CLASSIFICATION

PHARMACOTHERAPEUTIC: Rapid-acting general anesthetic. **CLINICAL:** Sedative-hypnotic.

USES

Induction/maintenance of anesthesia. Continuous sedation in intubated and respiratory controlled adult pts in ICU. **OFF-LABEL:** Postop antiemetic, refractory status epilepticus.

PRECAUTIONS

Contraindications: Hypersensitivity to propofol, eggs, egg products, soybean or soy products. **Cautions:** Hemodynamically unstable pts, hypovolemia, severe cardiac/respiratory disease, elevated ICP, impaired cerebral circulation, preexisting pancreatitis, hyperlipidemia, seizure disorder, elderly, debilitated; peanut allergy.

ACTION

Causes CNS depression through agonist action of GABA receptors. **Therapeutic Effect:** Produces hypnosis rapidly.

PHARMACOKINETICS

Route	Onset	Peak	Duration
IV	40 sec	N/A	3–10 min

P

Rapidly, extensively distributed. Protein binding: 97%–99%. Metabolized in liver. Primarily excreted in urine. Unknown if removed by hemodialysis. Rapid awakening can occur 10–15 min after discontinuation. **Half-life:** 3–12 hrs.

LIFESPAN CONSIDERATIONS

Pregnancy/Lactation: Unknown if drug crosses placenta. Distributed in breast milk. Not recommended for obstetrics, breastfeeding mothers. **Children:** Safety and efficacy not established. FDA-approved for use in pts 2 mos and older. **Elderly:** No age-related precautions noted; lower dosages recommended.

INTERACTIONS

DRUG: **Alcohol, CNS depressants (e.g., LORazepam, morphine, zolpidem)** may increase CNS, respiratory depression, hypotensive effects. **Antihypertensive medications (e.g., amLODIPine, lisinopril, valsartan)** may increase hypotensive effects. HERBAL: **Herbals with sedative properties (e.g., chamomile, kava kava, valerian)** may increase CNS depression. **Herbals with hypotensive properties (e.g., garlic, ginger, gingko biloba)** may increase effect. FOOD: None known. LAB VALUES: May increase serum triglycerides.

AVAILABILITY (Rx)

Injection Emulsion: 10 mg/mL.

ADMINISTRATION/HANDLING

IV

◀ALERT▶ Do not give through same IV line with blood or plasma.

Reconstitution • May give undiluted, or dilute only with D_5W. • Do not dilute to concentration less than 2 mg/mL (4 mL D_5W to 1 mL propofol yields 2 mg/mL).

Rate of administration • Too-rapid IV administration may produce marked severe hypotension, respiratory depression, irregular muscular movements. • Observe for signs of extravasation (pain, discolored skin patches, white or blue color to peripheral IV site area, delayed onset of drug action).

Storage • Store at room temperature. • Discard unused portions. • Do not use if emulsion separates. • Shake well before using.

IV INCOMPATIBILITIES

Amikacin (Amikin), amphotericin B complex (Abelcet, AmBisome, Amphotec), bretylium (Bretylol), calcium chloride, ciprofloxacin (Cipro), diazePAM (Valium), digoxin (Lanoxin), DOXOrubicin (Adriamycin), gentamicin (Garamycin), methylPREDNISolone (SOLU-Medrol), minocycline (Minocin), phenytoin (Dilantin), tobramycin (Nebcin), verapamil (Isoptin).

IV COMPATIBILITIES

Acyclovir (Zovirax), bumetanide (Bumex), calcium gluconate, cefTAZidime (Fortaz), dexmedetomidine (Precedex), DOBUTamine (Dobutrex), DOPamine (Intropin), enalapril (Vasotec), fentaNYL, heparin, insulin, labetalol (Normodyne, Trandate), lidocaine, LORazepam (Ativan), magnesium, milrinone (Primacor), nitroglycerin, norepinephrine (Levophed), potassium chloride, vancomycin (Vancocin).

INDICATIONS/ROUTES/DOSAGE

Anesthesia

IV infusion: ADULTS, ELDERLY: Induction, 2–2.5 mg/kg (approximately 40 mg q10sec until onset of anesthesia). **Maintenance:** Initially, 100–200 mcg/kg/min or 6–12 mg/kg/hr for 10–15 min. Usual maintenance infusion: 50–100 mcg/kg/min or 3–6 mg/kg/hr. CHILDREN 3–16 YRS: Induction, 2.5–3.5 mg/kg over 20–30 sec, then infusion of 125–300 mcg/kg/min or 7.5–18 mg/kg/hr.

Sedation in ICU

IV infusion: ADULTS, ELDERLY: Initially, 5 mcg/kg/min (0.3 mg/kg/hr); increase by increments of 5–10 mcg/kg/min (0.3–

P

0.6 mg/kg/hr) q5–10 min until desired sedation level achieved. **Usual maintenance:** 5–50 mcg/kg/min (0.3–3 mg/kg/hr). Reduce dose after adequate sedation established, and adjust to response. Daily interruption with retitration (sedation vacation) recommended to minimize prolonged sedative effects.

Dosage in Renal/Hepatic Impairment
No dose adjustment.

SIDE EFFECTS

Frequent: Involuntary muscle movements, apnea (common during induction; often lasts longer than 60 sec), hypotension, nausea, vomiting, IV site burning/stinging. **Occasional:** Twitching, thrashing, headache, dizziness, bradycardia, hypertension, fever, abdominal cramps, paresthesia, coldness, cough, hiccups, facial flushing, green-tinted urine. **Rare:** Rash, dry mouth, agitation, confusion, myalgia, thrombophlebitis.

ADVERSE EFFECTS/TOXIC REACTIONS

Continuous infusion or repeated intermittent infusions of propofol may result in extreme drowsiness, respiratory depression, circulatory depression, delirium. Too-rapid IV administration may produce severe hypotension, respiratory depression, involuntary muscle movements. Pt may experience acute allergic reaction, characterized by abdominal pain, anxiety, restlessness, dyspnea, erythema, hypotension, pruritus, rhinitis, urticaria. May cause propofol infusion syndrome, a collection of metabolic disorders and organ system failures including metabolic acidosis, hyperkalemia, rhabdomyolysis, hepatomegaly; cardiac, renal failure.

NURSING CONSIDERATIONS

BASELINE ASSESSMENT

Resuscitative equipment, suction, O_2 must be available. Obtain vital signs before administration.

INTERVENTION/EVALUATION

Observe for signs of wakefulness, agitation. Monitor respiratory rate, B/P, heart rate, O_2 saturation, depth of sedation, serum lipid, triglycerides (if used longer than 24 hrs). May change urine color to green. If continuous high-dose infusions do not properly induce sedation, consider additional sedatives (e.g., opioids, hypnotics, benzodiazepines) to achieve desired response.

propranolol

HIGH ALERT

proe-**pran**-oh-lol
(Hemangeol, Inderal LA, Inderal XL, InnoPran XL)

BLACK BOX ALERT Severe angina exacerbation, MI, ventricular arrhythmias may occur in angina pts after abrupt discontinuation; must taper gradually over 1–2 wks.
Do not confuse Inderal LA with Adderall, Imdur, Isordil, or Toradol, or propranolol with Pravachol.

FIXED-COMBINATION(S)

Inderide: propranolol/hydroCHLOROthiazide (a diuretic): 40 mg/25 mg, 80 mg/25 mg. **Inderide LA:** propranolol/hydroCHLOROthiazide (a diuretic): 80 mg/50 mg, 120 mg/50 mg, 160 mg/50 mg.

CLASSIFICATION

PHARMACOTHERAPEUTIC: Nonselective beta-adrenergic blocker. **CLINICAL:** Antihypertensive, antianginal, antiarrhythmic, antimigraine.

USES

Treatment of angina pectoris, supraventricular arrhythmias, essential tremors, hypertension, ventricular tachycardia, symptomatic treatment of obstructive hypertrophic cardiomyopathy, treatment of proliferating infantile hemangioma requiring systemic therapy, migraine headache prophylaxis, pheochromocytoma,

P

prevention of MI. **Hemangeol:** Treatment of proliferating infantile hemangioma needing systemic therapy. **OFF-LABEL:** Treatment adjunct for anxiety, tremor due to Parkinson's disease, alcohol withdrawal, aggressive behavior, schizophrenia, antipsychotic-induced akathisia, variceal hemorrhage, acute panic.

PRECAUTIONS

Contraindications: Hypersensitivity to propranolol. Bronchial asthma, severe sinus bradycardia, cardiogenic shock, sick sinus syndrome, heart block greater than first-degree (unless pt has functional pacemaker), uncompensated HF. **Hemangeol (Additional):** Premature infants with corrected age younger than 5 wks, infants weighing less than 2.5 kg; history of bronchospasm, bradycardia (less than 80 beats/min), B/P less than 50/30 mm Hg, pheochromocytoma. **Cautions:** Diabetes, renal/hepatic impairment, Raynaud's disease, hyperthyroidism, myasthenia gravis, psychiatric disease, bronchospastic disease, elderly pts, history of severe anaphylaxis to allergens.

P

ACTION

Blocks $beta_1$-, $beta_2$-adrenergic receptors. **Therapeutic Effect:** Slows heart rate; decreases B/P, myocardial contractility, myocardial oxygen demand.

PHARMACOKINETICS

Route	Onset	Peak	Duration
PO	1–2 hrs	N/A	6 hrs

Widely distributed. Protein binding: 93%. Metabolized in liver. Primarily excreted in urine. Not removed by hemodialysis. **Half-life:** 4–6 hrs.

LIFESPAN CONSIDERATIONS

Pregnancy/Lactation: Crosses placenta. Distributed in breast milk. Avoid use during first trimester. May produce low-birth-weight infants, bradycardia, apnea, hypoglycemia, hypothermia during delivery. **Children:** No age-related precautions noted. **Elderly:** Age-related peripheral vascular disease may increase susceptibility to decreased peripheral circulation.

INTERACTIONS

DRUG: **Alpha$_2$ agonists (e.g., cloNIDine)** may increase AV-blocking effect. **Strong CYP3A4 inducers (e.g., carBAMazepine, phenytoin, rifAMPin)** may decrease concentration/effect. **Dronedarone, fingolimod, rivastigmine** may increase bradycardic effect. May increase vasoconstriction of **ergot derivatives (e.g., ergotamine)**. **HERBAL:** **Herbals with hypertensive properties (e.g., licorice, yohimbe) or hypotensive properties (e.g., garlic, ginger, ginkgo biloba)** may alter effects. **FOOD:** None known. **LAB VALUES:** May increase serum antinuclear antibody (ANA) titer, serum BUN, LDH, lipoprotein, alkaline phosphatase, potassium, uric acid, ALT, AST, triglycerides.

AVAILABILITY (Rx)

Injection Solution: 1 mg/mL. **Oral Solution:** 20 mg/5 mL, 40 mg/5 mL. **Oral Solution:** ***(Hemangeol):*** 4.28 mg/mL. **Tablets:** 10 mg, 20 mg, 40 mg, 60 mg, 80 mg.

Capsules, Extended-Release (24-HR): 60 mg, 80 mg, 120 mg, 160 mg.

ADMINISTRATION/HANDLING

IV

Reconstitution • Give undiluted for IV push. • For IV infusion, may dilute each 1 mg in 10 mL D_5W.

Rate of administration • Do not exceed 1 mg/min injection rate. • For IV infusion, give over 30 min.

Storage • Store at room temperature. • Once diluted, stable for 24 hrs at room temperature.

PO

• May crush scored tablets. • Do not break, crush, or open extended- or sustained-release capsules. • Give immediate-release tablets on empty stomach. • Give extended-release, sustained-release without regard to food.

IV INCOMPATIBILITIES

Amphotericin B complex (Abelcet, AmBisome, Amphotec).

IV COMPATIBILITIES

Alteplase (Activase), heparin, milrinone (Primacor), potassium chloride, propofol (Diprivan).

INDICATIONS/ROUTES/DOSAGE

Hypertension

PO: ADULTS, ELDERLY: *(Immediate-Release or Extended-Release):* Initially, 80 mg/day. May increase at greater than or equal to 1-wk intervals prn based on patient response. Usual dosage range: 80–160 mg/day.

Angina

PO: ADULTS, ELDERLY: *(Immediate-Release):* Initially, 80 mg/day. Increase dose at least 1 wk intervals as tolerated to desired effect. Range: 80–320 mg/day in 2–4 divided doses.

PO: *(Extended-Release [Inderal LA]):* Initially, 80 mg/day. Increase dose as tolerated to desired effect. Range: 80–320 mg/day.

Arrhythmia

IV: ADULTS, ELDERLY: 1 mg over 1 min. May repeat q2min up to maximum of 3 doses. **CHILDREN:** 0.01–0.15 mg/kg over 10 min. May repeat q6–8h. **Maximum:** Infants, 1 mg/dose; children, 3 mg/dose.

PO: ADULTS, ELDERLY: *(Immediate-Release):* 10–40 mg 3–4 times/day. **CHILDREN:** Initially, 0.5–1 mg/kg/day in divided doses q6–8h. May increase q3–5days. Usual dosage: 2–4 mg/kg/day. **Maximum:** 16 mg/kg/day or 60 mg/day.

Adjunct to Alpha-Blocking Agents to Treat Pheochromocytoma

PO: ADULTS, ELDERLY: *(Immediate-Release):* Initially, 10 mg q6h or 20 mg 3 times daily. Begin 3–4 days after initiation of an alpha-1 blocker and adjust to goal heart rate up to 120 mg/day in divided doses.

Migraine Headache

PO: ADULTS, ELDERLY: *(Immediate-Release or Extended-Release):* Initially, 40–80 mg/day. May increase gradually based on response and tolerability. Usual effective range: 40–160 mg/day. **CHILDREN 7 YRS AND OLDER:** *(Immediate-Release):* Initially, 10 mg daily. May increase at wkly intervals in 10 mg increments. Usual dose range: 10–20 mg 3 times/day.

Reduction of Cardiovascular Mortality, Reinfarction in Pts With Previous MI

PO: ADULTS, ELDERLY: *(Immediate-Release):* Initially, 60–120 mg/day in 2–3 divided doses. May increase dose based on heart rate and BP up to 240 mg/day.

Essential Tremor

PO: ADULTS, ELDERLY: *(Immediate-Release or Extended-Release):* Initially, 60–80 mg/day. May increase based on response and tolerability. Usual dosage range: 60–320 mg/day.

Infantile Hemangioma

Note: Separate doses by at least 9 hrs during or after feeding.

PO: INFANTS 5 WKS TO 5 MOS: Initially, 0.15 mL/kg (0.6 mg/kg) twice daily for 1 wk. Beginning with wk 2, increase to 0.3 mL/kg (1.1 mg/kg) twice daily. For wk 3, increase to maintenance dose of 0.4 mL/kg (1.7 mg/kg) twice daily. Maintain dose for 6 months. Readjust dose as weight increases.

Dosage in Renal/Hepatic Impairment

Use caution.

SIDE EFFECTS

Frequent: Diminished sexual function, drowsiness, difficulty sleeping, unusual fatigue/weakness. **Occasional:** Bradycardia, depression, sensation of coldness in extremities, diarrhea, constipation, anxiety, nasal congestion, nausea, vomiting. **Rare:** Altered taste, dry eyes, pruritus, paresthesia.

P

ADVERSE EFFECTS/TOXIC REACTIONS

Overdose may produce profound bradycardia, hypotension. Abrupt withdrawal may result in diaphoresis, palpitations, headache, tremulousness. May precipitate HF, MI in pts with cardiac disease, thyroid storm in pts with thyrotoxicosis, peripheral ischemia in pts with existing peripheral vascular disease. Hypoglycemia may occur in pts with previously controlled diabetes. **Antidote:** Glucagon (see Appendix J for dosage).

NURSING CONSIDERATIONS

BASELINE ASSESSMENT

Assess renal function, LFT. Assess B/P, heart rate, immediately before administering drug (if pulse is 60/min or less or systolic B/P is less than 90 mm Hg, withhold medication, contact physician). **Angina:** Record onset, quality, radiation, location, intensity, duration of anginal pain, precipitating factors (exertion, emotional stress).

INTERVENTION/EVALUATION

Assess pulse for quality, regularity, bradycardia. Monitor ECG for cardiac arrhythmias. Assess fingers for color, numbness (Raynaud's). Assess for evidence of HF (dyspnea [particularly on exertion or lying down], night cough, peripheral edema, distended neck veins). Monitor I&O (increase in weight, decrease in urinary output may indicate HF). Assess for rash, fatigue, behavioral changes. Therapeutic response time ranges from a few days to several wks. Measure B/P near end of dosing interval (determines if B/P is controlled throughout day).

PATIENT/FAMILY TEACHING

• Do not abruptly discontinue medication. • Compliance with therapy regimen is essential to control hypertension, arrhythmia, anginal pain. • To avoid hypotensive effect, slowly go from lying to standing. • Avoid tasks that require alertness, motor skills until response to drug is established. • Report excessively slow pulse rate (less than 50 beats/min), peripheral numbness, dizziness. • Do not use nasal decongestants, OTC cold preparations (stimulants) without physician approval. • Restrict salt, alcohol intake.

pyridostigmine

peer-id-oh-**stig**-meen
(Mestinon, Mestinon SR ✱, Regonol)
Do not confuse pyridostigmine with physostigmine, or Regonol with Reglan or Renagel.

◆CLASSIFICATION

PHARMACOTHERAPEUTIC: Anticholinesterase inhibitor. **CLINICAL:** Cholinergic muscle stimulant.

USES

Treatment of myasthenia gravis.

PRECAUTIONS

Contraindications: Hypersensitivity to pyridostigmine. Mechanical, intestinal or urinary obstruction. **Cautions:** Bronchial asthma, COPD, bradycardia, seizure disorder, hyperthyroidism, cardiac arrhythmias, peptic ulcer, renal impairment.

ACTION

Prevents destruction of acetylcholine by inhibiting the enzyme acetylcholinesterase, enhancing impulse transmission across neuromuscular junction. **Therapeutic Effect:** Produces miosis; increases intestinal, skeletal muscle tone; stimulates salivary, sweat gland secretions.

PHARMACOKINETICS

Poorly absorbed from GI tract. Metabolized in liver. Excreted primarily unchanged in urine. **Half-life:** 1–2 hrs.

⌛ LIFESPAN CONSIDERATIONS

Pregnancy/Lactation: Unknown if drug crosses placenta or is distributed in breast milk. **Children:** Safety and efficacy not established. **Elderly:** No age-related precautions noted.

INTERACTIONS

DRUG: None significant. **HERBAL:** None significant. **FOOD:** None known. **LAB VALUES:** None significant.

AVAILABILITY (Rx)

Injection Solution: ***(Regonol):*** 5 mg/mL. **Solution, Oral:** 60 mg/5 mL. **Tablets:** 30 mg, 60 mg.

Tablets: Extended-Release: 180 mg.

ADMINISTRATION/HANDLING

IV, IM

• Give large parenteral doses concurrently with 0.6–1.2 mg atropine sulfate IV to minimize side effects.

PO

• Give with food, milk. • Tablets may be crushed. Do not chew, crush extended-release tablets (may be broken). • Give larger dose at times of increased fatigue (e.g., for those with difficulty in chewing, 30–45 min before meals).

IV INCOMPATIBILITIES

Do not mix with any other medications.

INDICATIONS/ROUTES/DOSAGE

Note: Highly individualized dosing ranges.

Myasthenia Gravis

PO: ADULTS, ELDERLY: ***(Immediate-Release):*** Initially, 60 mg 3 times/day. Dosage increased at 48-hr intervals. **Maintenance:** 60 mg–1.5 g/day divided into 5–6 doses/day. (Usual dose: 600 mg/day.) **CHILDREN:** Initially, 1 mg/kg/dose q4–6h. **Maximum:** 7 mg/kg/24 hr divided into 5–6 doses. Usual dose: 600 mg/day.

PO: ***(Extended-Release):*** **ADULTS, ELDERLY:** 180–540 mg 1–2 times/day with at least a 6-hr interval between doses.

IV, IM: ADULTS, ELDERLY: 2 mg or 1/30th of oral dose q2–3h. **CHILDREN:** 0.05–0.15 mg/kg/dose. **Maximum single dose:** 10 mg.

Dosage in Renal/Hepatic Impairment

No dose adjustment.

SIDE EFFECTS

Frequent: Miosis, increased GI/skeletal muscle tone, bradycardia, constriction of bronchi/ureters, diaphoresis, increased salivation. **Occasional:** Headache, rash, temporary decrease in diastolic B/P with mild reflex tachycardia, short periods of atrial fibrillation (in hyperthyroid pts), marked drop in B/P (in hypertensive pts).

ADVERSE EFFECTS/TOXIC REACTIONS

Overdose may produce cholinergic crisis, manifested as increasingly severe descending muscle weakness (appears first in muscles involving chewing, swallowing, followed by muscle weakness of shoulder girdle, upper extremities), respiratory muscle paralysis, followed by pelvis girdle/leg muscle paralysis. Requires withdrawal of all cholinergic drugs and immediate use of 1–4 mg atropine sulfate IV for adults, 0.01 mg/kg for infants and children younger than 12 yrs.

NURSING CONSIDERATIONS

BASELINE ASSESSMENT

Larger doses should be given at time of greatest fatigue. Assess muscle strength before testing for diagnosis of myasthenia gravis and following drug administration. Avoid large doses in pts with megacolon, reduced GI motility.

INTERVENTION/EVALUATION

Have facial tissues readily available at pt's bedside. Monitor respirations closely during myasthenia gravis testing or if dosage is increased. Assess diligently for cholinergic reaction, bradycardia in myasthenic pt in crisis. Coordinate dosage time with periods of fatigue and increased/decreased muscle strength. Monitor for therapeutic response to

P

medication (increased muscle strength, decreased fatigue, improved chewing/swallowing functions).

PATIENT/FAMILY TEACHING

- Report nausea, vomiting, diarrhea, diaphoresis, profuse salivary secretions, palpitations, muscle weakness, severe abdominal pain, difficulty breathing.

P

QUEtiapine

TOP 100

kwet-**eye**-a-peen
(SEROquel, SEROquel XR)

BLACK BOX ALERT Increased risk of suicidal ideation and behavior in children, adolescents, young adults 18–24 yrs with major depressive disorder, other psychiatric disorders. Elderly with dementia-related psychosis are at increased risk for death.

Do not confuse QUEtiapine with OLANZapine, or SEROquel with SEROquel XR or SINEquan.

CLASSIFICATION

PHARMACOTHERAPEUTIC: Dibenzodiazepine derivative. **CLINICAL:** Second-generation (atypical) antipsychotic.

USES

Treatment of schizophrenia. Treatment of acute manic episodes associated with bipolar disorder (alone or in combination with lithium or valproate). Maintenance treatment of bipolar disorder as an adjunct to lithium or valproic acid. Treatment of acute depressive episodes associated with bipolar disorder. **Extended-Release Only:** Adjunctive treatment to antidepressants in major depressive disorder (MDD). **OFF-LABEL:** Delirium in critically ill pts, psychosis/agitation related to Alzheimer's dementia. Treatment of autism, treatment-resistant obsessive compulsive disorder.

PRECAUTIONS

Contraindications: Hypersensitivity to QUETiapine. **Cautions:** Renal/hepatic impairment, hyperlipidemia, pts at risk for aspiration pneumonia, cardiovascular disease (e.g., HF, history of MI), cerebrovascular disease, dehydration, hypovolemia, history of drug abuse/dependence, seizure disorder, hypothyroidism, pts at risk for suicide, Parkinson's disease, decreased GI motility, urinary retention, narrow-angle glaucoma, diabetes, visual problems, elderly, pts at risk for orthostatic hypotension. Avoid use in pts at risk for torsades de pointes (hypokalemia, hypomagnesemia, history of cardiac arrhythmias, congenital long QT syndrome, concurrent medications that prolong QT interval).

ACTION

Antagonizes DOPamine and serotonin (antipsychotic activity), histamine (somnolence), alpha$_1$-adrenergic (orthostatic hypotension) receptors. **Therapeutic Effect:** Diminishes symptoms associated with schizophrenia/bipolar disorders.

PHARMACOKINETICS

Rapidly absorbed. Protein binding: 83%. Widely distributed in tissues; CNS concentration exceeds plasma concentration. Metabolized in liver. Primarily excreted in urine. **Half-life:** 6 hrs.

LIFESPAN CONSIDERATIONS

Pregnancy/Lactation: Unknown if drug is distributed in breast milk. Not recommended for breastfeeding mothers. **Children:** Safety and efficacy not established in children less than 10 yrs of age (bipolar mania) or less than 13 yrs of age (schizophrenia). **Elderly:** No age-related precautions noted, but lower initial and target dosages may be necessary.

INTERACTIONS

DRUG: **QT interval–prolonging medications (e.g., amiodarone, azithromycin, ciprofloxacin, haloperidol, methadone, sotalol)** may increase risk of QTc interval prolongation. **Alcohol, CNS depressants (e.g., LORazepam, morphine, zolpidem)** may increase CNS depression. May increase hypotensive effects of **antihypertensives. Strong CYP3A4 inducers (e.g., carBAMazepine, phenytoin, rifAMPin)** may decrease concentration/effect. **Strong CYP3A4 inhibitors (e.g., clarithromycin, ketoconazole)** may increase concentration/effect. **Anticholinergic agents (e.g.,**

Q

aclidinium, ipratropium, tiotropium, umeclidinium) may increase anticholinergic effect. **HERBAL: Herbals with sedative properties (e.g., chamomile, kava kava, valerian)** may increase CNS depression. **St. John's wort** may decrease concentration/effect. **FOOD:** None known. **LAB VALUES:** May decrease total free thyroxine (T_4) serum levels. May increase serum cholesterol, triglycerides, ALT, AST, WBC, GGT. May produce false-positive pregnancy test result.

AVAILABILITY (Rx)

Tablets: 25 mg, 50 mg, 100 mg, 200 mg, 300 mg, 400 mg. **Tablets, Extended-Release:** 50 mg, 150 mg, 200 mg, 300 mg, 400 mg.

ADMINISTRATION/HANDLING

PO

• Give immediate-release tablets without regard to food. • Do not break, crush, dissolve, or divide extended-release tablets. • Extended-release tablets should be given without regard to food or with a light meal in evening.

Q

INDICATIONS/ROUTES/DOSAGE

• When restarting pts who have been off QUEtiapine for less than 1 wk, titration is not required and maintenance dose can be reinstituted. • When restarting pts who have been off QUEtiapine for longer than 1 wk, follow initial titration schedule. • When discontinuing, gradual tapering recommended to avoid withdrawal symptoms and minimize risk of relapse.

Schizophrenia

PO: ***(Immediate-Release):*** **ADULTS, ELDERLY:** Initially, 25 mg twice daily, then increase in 25–50-mg increments divided 2–3 times/day on the second and third days; may further increase up to target dose of 300–400 mg/day in 2–3 divided doses by the fourth day. Further adjustments of 25–50 mg twice daily may be made at intervals of 2 days or longer. **Maintenance:** 400-800 mg/day. **Maximum:** 800 mg/day. ***(Extended-Release):*** Initially, 300 mg/day. May increase in increments of up to 300 mg/day at intervals as short as 1 day. Range: 400–800 mg/day. **Maximum:** 800 mg/day. ***(Immediate-Release):*** **CHILDREN 13 YRS AND OLDER:** Initially, 25 mg twice daily on day 1, 50 mg twice daily on day 2, then increase by 100 mg/day to target dose of 400 mg twice daily on day 5. May further increase to 800 mg/day in increments of 100 mg or less daily. Range: 400–800 mg/day. **Maximum:** 800 mg. Total dose may be divided in 3 doses/day. ***(Extended-Release):*** Initially, 50 mg once daily on day 1, 100 mg on day 2, until 400 mg once daily is reached on day 5. Range: 400–800 mg/day. **Maximum:** 800 mg/day.

Mania in Bipolar Disorder

PO: ***(Immediate-Release):*** **ADULTS, ELDERLY:** Initially, 100-200 mg once daily at bedtime or in 2 divided doses on day 1. May increase in increments of 100 mg/day to 200 mg twice daily on day 4. May further increase in increments of 200 mg/day to 800 mg/day **Maximum:** 800 mg/day. ***(Extended-Release):*** Initially, 300 mg on day 1 in the evening; increase to 600 mg on day 2 . Adjust dose base on response/tolerability. **Maximum:** 800 mg/day. ***(Immediate-Release):*** **CHILDREN 10 YRS AND OLDER:** 25 mg twice daily on day 1, 50 mg twice daily on day 2, then 100 mg twice daily on day 3, 150 mg twice daily on day 4, then continue at target dose of 200 mg twice daily on day 5. Usual range: 200–300mg twice daily. **Maximum:** 600 mg/day. ***(Extended-Release):*** 50 mg on day 1; 100 mg on day 2; then increase by 100 mg/day until target dose of 400 mg once daily on day 5. Usual range: 400–600 mg once daily.

Depression in Bipolar Disorder

PO: ***(Immediate-Release):*** **ADULTS, ELDERLY:** Initially, 50 mg/day on day 1, increase to 100 mg/day on day 2, then increase by 50–100 mg/day up to target dose of 300 mg/day. ***(Extended-Release):*** Initially, 50 mg on day 1 in the evening, 100 mg on day 2, 200 mg on day 3, 300 mg on day 4 and thereafter.

Adjunctive Therapy in MDD

PO: ADULTS, ELDERLY: ***(Extended-Release):*** Initially, 50 mg on days 1 and 2; then 150 mg on days 3 and 4; then 150–300 mg/day thereafter.

Dosage in Hepatic Impairment

(Immediate-Release): Initially, 25 mg/day. Increase by 25–50 mg/day to effective dose. ***(Extended-Release):*** Initially, 50 mg/day, increase by 50 mg/day until effective dose.

Dosage in Renal Impairment

No dose adjustment.

SIDE EFFECTS

Frequent (19%–10%): Headache, drowsiness, dizziness. **Occasional (9%–3%):** Constipation, orthostatic hypotension, tachycardia, dry mouth, dyspepsia, rash, asthenia, abdominal pain, rhinitis. **Rare (2%):** Back pain, fever, weight gain.

ADVERSE EFFECTS/TOXIC REACTIONS

May increase risk of death in elderly pts with dementia-related psychosis. Most deaths appeared to be cardiovascular (e.g., HF, sudden death) or infectious (e.g., pneumonia) in nature. May increase risk of life-threatening neuroleptic malignant syndrome (NMS). Symptoms of NMS may include hyperpyrexia, muscle rigidity, altered mental status, autonomic instability (irregular pulse/blood pressure, tachycardia, diaphoresis, cardiac arrhythmias); elevated CPK, rhabdomyolysis, acute renal failure. Tardive dyskinesia (potentially irreversible, involuntary, dyskinetic movements) has occurred. Metabolic changes including hyperglycemia, ketoacidosis, hyperosmolar coma, diabetes, dyslipidemia may occur. Agranulocytosis, leukopenia, neutropenia was reported. Cognitive and motor impairment reported in 24% of pts. Other effects may include body temperature dysregulation, cataracts, dysphagia, dystonia, extrapyramidal symptoms, orthostatic hypotension, falls, syncope, seizures. Overdose may cause heart block, hypotension, hypokalemia, tachycardia.

NURSING CONSIDERATIONS

BASELINE ASSESSMENT

Obtain lipid profile, vital signs; CBC in pts with baseline leukopenia, neutropenia; pregnancy test in females of reproductive potential. Screen for active infection. Receive full medication history and screen for interactions. Question history as listed in Precautions. Assess risk of dysphagia, aspiration. Initiate fall precautions. Assess appearance, behavior, speech pattern, levels of interest. Offer emotional support.

INTERVENTION/EVALUATION

Monitor blood glucose in pts with diabetes; lipid profile after initiation and periodically thereafter. Monitor CBC, orthostatic vital signs frequently during the first mos of therapy. Monitor for hyperglycemia (blurred vision, confusion, excessive thirst, Kussmaul respirations, polyuria), infections (cough, fatigue, fever), body temperature dysregulation, dysphagia, dystonia, tardive dyskinesia, symptoms of NMS. Assess for therapeutic response (greater interest in surroundings, improved self-care, increased ability to concentrate, relaxed facial expression).

PATIENT/ FAMILY TEACHING

• Treatment may depress your immune system response and reduce your ability to fight infection. Report symptoms of infection such as body aches, chills, cough, fatigue, fever. Avoid those with active infection until response to drug is established. • Report symptoms of high blood sugar levels (e.g., blurred vision, excessive thirst/hunger, headache, frequent urination); nervous system changes (e.g., abnormal, involuntary movements (e.g., lip smacking, puckering, tongue protrusion or chewing, jaw movement, rapid blinking of the eye), difficulty swallowing, seizures, tremor; spasms of the neck, tongue, face). • Treatment may

Q

cause NMS (confusion, high fever, muscle rigidity, high or irregular B/P, heart arrhythmias), a life-threatening condition that can be confused with symptoms of severe infection. • Avoid tasks that require alertness, motor skills until response to drug is established. • Go slowly from lying to standing. • Do not take newly prescribed medications unless approved by prescriber who originally started treatment. • Avoid overheating, dehydration. • Seek immediate medical attention if thoughts of suicide, new onset or worsening of anxiety, depression, or changes in mood occur.

quinapril

kwin-a-pril
(Accupril)

BLACK BOX ALERT May cause fetal injury, mortality. Discontinue as soon as possible once pregnancy detected.

Do not confuse Accupril with Accolate, Accutane, Aciphex, or Monopril.

FIXED-COMBINATION(S)

Accuretic: quinapril/hydroCHLOROthiazide (a diuretic): 10 mg/12.5 mg, 20 mg/12.5 mg, 20 mg/25 mg.

CLASSIFICATION

PHARMACOTHERAPEUTIC: Angiotensin-converting enzyme (ACE) inhibitor. **CLINICAL:** Antihypertensive.

USES

Treatment of hypertension. Used alone or in combination with other antihypertensives. Adjunctive therapy in management of HF. **OFF-LABEL:** Treatment of pediatric hypertension.

PRECAUTIONS

Contraindications: Hypersensitivity to quinapril. History of angioedema from previous treatment with ACE inhibitors, concomitant use with aliskiren in pts with diabetes. Concomitant use with neprilysin inhibitor (e.g., sacubitril) or within 36 hrs of switching to or from neprilysin inhibitor. **Cautions:** Renal impairment, hypertrophic cardiomyopathy with outflow tract obstruction, major surgery, HF, hypovolemia, unstented bilateral renal artery stenosis, hyperkalemia, concurrent potassium supplements, severe aortic stenosis, ischemic heart disease, cerebrovascular disease.

ACTION

Suppresses renin-angiotensin-aldosterone system, preventing conversion of angiotensin I to angiotensin II, a potent vasoconstrictor. Lower angiotensin II causes an increase in plasma renin activity and decreased aldosterone secretion. **Therapeutic Effect:** Reduces peripheral arterial resistance, B/P.

PHARMACOKINETICS

Route	Onset	Peak	Duration
PO	1 hr	N/A	24 hrs

Widely distributed. Protein binding: 97%. Rapidly hydrolyzed to active metabolite. Primarily excreted in urine. Minimal removal by hemodialysis. **Half-life:** 1–2 hrs; metabolite, 3 hrs (increased in renal impairment).

LIFESPAN CONSIDERATIONS

Pregnancy/Lactation: Crosses placenta. Unknown if distributed in breast milk. May cause fetal, neonatal mortality or morbidity. **Children:** Safety and efficacy not established. **Elderly:** May be more sensitive to hypotensive effects.

INTERACTIONS

DRUG: **Aliskiren** may increase hyperkalemic effect. May increase potential for allergic reactions to **allopurinol.** **Angiotensin receptor blockers (e.g., losartan, valsartan)** may increase adverse effects. May increase adverse effects of **lithium, sacubitril.** **HERBAL:** **Herbals with hyper-**

tensive properties (e.g., licorice, yohimbe) or hypotensive properties (e.g., garlic, ginger, ginkgo biloba) may alter effects. **FOOD:** None known. **LAB VALUES:** May increase serum BUN, alkaline phosphatase, bilirubin, creatinine, potassium, ALT, AST. May decrease serum sodium. May cause positive antinuclear antibody (ANA) titer.

AVAILABILITY (Rx)

Tablets: 5 mg, 10 mg, 20 mg, 40 mg.

ADMINISTRATION/HANDLING

PO

• Give without regard to food. • Tablets may be crushed.

INDICATIONS/ROUTES/DOSAGE

Hypertension

PO: ADULTS: Initially, 10–20 mg/day. May adjust dosage at intervals of at least 2 wks or longer up to 80 mg/day in one or two divided doses. **ELDERLY:** Initially, 10 mg once daily. Titrate to optimal response.

Adjunct to Manage HF

PO: ADULTS, ELDERLY: Initially, 5 mg twice daily. Titrate at wkly intervals to 20–40 mg/day in 2 divided doses. Target dose: 20 mg twice daily.

Dosage in Renal Impairment

Hypertension

Creatinine Clearance	Initial Dose
More than 60 mL/min	10 mg
30–60 mL/min	5 mg
10–29 mL/min	2.5 mg

HF

Creatinine Clearance	Initial Dose
Greater than 30 mL/min	5 mg
10–30 mL/min	2.5 mg

Dosage in Hepatic Impairment

No dose adjustment.

SIDE EFFECTS

Frequent (7%–5%): Headache, dizziness. **Occasional (4%–2%):** Fatigue, vomiting, nausea, hypotension, chest pain, cough, syncope. **Rare (less than 2%):** Diarrhea, cough, dyspnea, rash, palpitations, impotence, insomnia, drowsiness, malaise.

ADVERSE EFFECTS/TOXIC REACTIONS

Excessive hypotension ("first-dose syncope") may occur in pts with HF, those who are severely salt/volume depleted. Angioedema, hyperkalemia occur rarely. Agranulocytosis, neutropenia may occur in pts with collagen vascular disease (scleroderma, systemic lupus erythematosus), renal impairment. Nephrotic syndrome may occur in pts with history of renal disease.

NURSING CONSIDERATIONS

BASELINE ASSESSMENT

Obtain renal function test. Obtain B/P immediately before each dose in addition to regular monitoring (be alert to fluctuations). In pts with prior renal disease, urine test for protein by dipstick method should be made with first urine of day before beginning therapy and periodically thereafter. In pts with renal impairment, autoimmune disease, or taking drugs that affect leukocytes or immune response, CBC, differential count should be performed before beginning therapy and q2wks for 3 mos, then periodically thereafter.

INTERVENTION/EVALUATION

Monitor B/P for hypotension; renal function, serum potassium, WBC. Assist with ambulation if dizziness occurs.

PATIENT/ FAMILY TEACHING

• Go slowly from lying to standing. • Full therapeutic effect may take 1–2 wks. • Report any sign of infection (sore throat, fever). • Skipping doses or voluntarily discontinuing drug may produce severe rebound hypertension. • Avoid tasks that require alertness, motor skills until response to drug is established. • Avoid alcohol.

Q

RABEprazole

TOP 100

ra-**bep**-ra-zole
(Aciphex, Aciphex Sprinkle, Pariet ✱)
Do not confuse Aciphex with Accupril or Aricept, or RABEprazole with ARIPiprazole, donepezil, lansoprazole, omeprazole, or raloxifene.

◆CLASSIFICATION

PHARMACOTHERAPEUTIC: Proton pump inhibitor. **CLINICAL:** Gastric acid inhibitor.

USES

Short-term treatment (4–8 wks), maintenance of erosive or ulcerative gastroesophageal reflux disease (GERD). Treatment of daytime/nighttime heartburn, other symptoms of GERD. Short-term treatment (4 wks or less) in healing, symptomatic relief of duodenal ulcers. Long-term treatment of pathologic hypersecretory conditions, including Zollinger-Ellison syndrome. Treatment of *H. pylori* (in combination with amoxicillin and clarithromycin). Sprinkle dose form approved for treatment of GERD in children 1–11 yrs. **OFF-LABEL:** Maintenance of healing and prevention of relapse of duodenal ulcers. Treatment of NSAID-induced ulcers.

PRECAUTIONS

Contraindications: Hypersensitivity to RABEprazole, other proton pump inhibitors (e.g., omeprazole). Concomitant use with rilpivirine-containing products. **Cautions:** Severe hepatic impairment, osteoporosis.

ACTION

Suppresses gastric acid secretion by inhibiting H^+/K^+–ATP pump. **Therapeutic Effect:** Increases gastric pH, reducing gastric acid production.

PHARMACOKINETICS

Rapidly absorbed after passing through stomach relatively intact as delayed-release tablet. Protein binding: 96%. Metabolized in liver. Excreted in urine (90%), feces. **Half-life:** 1–2 hrs (increased with hepatic impairment).

⌛ LIFESPAN CONSIDERATIONS

Pregnancy/Lactation: Unknown if drug crosses placenta or is distributed in breast milk. **Children:** Safety and efficacy not established. **Elderly:** No age-related precautions noted.

INTERACTIONS

DRUG: May decrease concentration/effects of **acalabrutinib, cefuroxime, erlotinib, neratinib, pazopanib. Strong CYP2C19 inducers (e.g., FLUoxetine), strong CYP3A4 inducers (e.g., carBAMazepine, phenytoin, rifAMPin)** may decrease concentration/effect. May decrease concentration of **ketoconazole, clopidogrel, atazanavir. HERBAL: St. John's wort** may decrease concentration/effects. **FOOD:** None known. **LAB VALUES:** May increase serum ALT, AST, thyroid-stimulating hormone (TSH).

AVAILABILITY (Rx)

Tablets, Delayed-Release: 20 mg. **Capsule, Sprinkle:** 5 mg, 10 mg.

ADMINISTRATION/HANDLING

PO

• May give without regard to food; best taken after breakfast. • Do not break, crush, dissolve, or divide tablet; give whole.

Sprinkle

• May give with antacid. • Administer 30 min before a meal. • Open capsule, sprinkle on soft food. Take within 15 min of preparation. • Do not chew, crush.

INDICATIONS/ROUTES/DOSAGE

GERD (Erosive or ulcerative)

PO: ADULTS, ELDERLY: 20 mg/day for 4–8 wks. If inadequate response, may repeat for additional 8 wks. **Maintenance:** 20 mg/day.

Short-Term Treatment of Symptomatic GERD
PO: ADULTS, ELDERLY, CHILDREN 12 YRS AND OLDER: 20 mg/day for 4 wks. If inadequate response, may repeat additional 4 wks. **CHILDREN, 1–11 YRS, WEIGHING 15 KG OR GREATER:** 10 mg once daily. **WEIGHING LESS THAN 15 KG:** 5 mg once daily; may increase to 10 mg once daily.

Duodenal Ulcer
PO: ADULTS, ELDERLY: 20 mg/day after morning meal for 4 wks.

Pathologic Hypersecretory Conditions
PO: ADULTS, ELDERLY: Initially, 60 mg once daily. May increase to 60 mg twice daily.

***H. pylori* Infection**
PO: ADULTS, ELDERLY: 20 mg twice daily for 10–14 days (given with various antibiotic regimens).

Dosage in Renal Impairment
No dose adjustment.

Dosage in Hepatic Impairment
Mild to moderate impairment: No dose adjustment. **Severe impairment:** Use caution.

SIDE EFFECTS

Rare (less than 2%): Headache, nausea, dizziness, rash, diarrhea, malaise.

ADVERSE EFFECTS/TOXIC REACTIONS

Hyperglycemia, hypokalemia, hyponatremia, hyperlipemia occur rarely. May increase risk of bone fractures, *C. difficile*-associated colitis, fundic gland polyps, interstitial nephritis, vitamin B_{12} deficiency.

NURSING CONSIDERATIONS

BASELINE ASSESSMENT

Question history of GI disease, ulcers, GERD.

INTERVENTION/EVALUATION

Evaluate for therapeutic response (relief of GI symptoms). Question if GI discomfort, nausea, diarrhea, headache occurs. Assess skin for evidence of rash. Observe for evidence of dizziness; utilize appropriate safety precautions.

PATIENT/FAMILY TEACHING

• Swallow tablets whole; do not break, chew, dissolve, or divide tablets. • Report headache.

raloxifene

TOP 100

ra-**lox**-i-feen
(Evista)

BLACK BOX ALERT Increases risk of deep vein thrombosis, pulmonary embolism. Women with coronary heart disease or pts at risk for coronary events are at increased risk for death due to stroke.
Do not confuse Evista with AVINza.

◆CLASSIFICATION

PHARMACOTHERAPEUTIC: Selective estrogen receptor modulator (SERM). **CLINICAL:** Osteoporosis preventive.

USES

Prevention/treatment of osteoporosis in postmenopausal women. Reduces risk of invasive breast cancer in postmenopausal women with osteoporosis and postmenopausal women at high risk for invasive breast cancer.

PRECAUTIONS

Contraindications: Hypersensitivity to raloxifene. Active or history of venous thromboembolic events, such as deep vein thrombosis (DVT), pulmonary embolism, retinal vein thrombosis; women who are or may become pregnant, breastfeeding. **Cautions:** Cardiovascular disease, renal/hepatic impairment, pts at risk for thrombosis (immobility, indwelling venous catheter/access device, morbid obesity, genetic hypercoagulable conditions),

R

unexplained uterine bleeding, elevated triglycerides in response to oral estrogen therapy.

ACTION

Selective estrogen receptor modulator (SERM) that binds to estrogen receptors, increasing bone mineral density. Blocks estrogen effects in breast/uterus. **Therapeutic Effect:** Reduces bone resorption, increases bone mineral density, reduces incidence of fractures.

PHARMACOKINETICS

Rapidly absorbed. Protein binding: 95%. Metabolized in liver. Excreted primarily in feces. Unknown if removed by hemodialysis. **Half-life:** 27.7–32.5 hrs.

⌛ LIFESPAN CONSIDERATIONS

Pregnancy/Lactation: Unknown if distributed in breast milk. Contraindicated in pregnancy, breastfeeding. **Children:** Not used in this pt population. **Elderly:** No age-related precautions noted.

INTERACTIONS

DRUG: **Bile acid sequestrants (e.g., cholestyramine)** may decrease absorption/effect. May decrease absorption of **levothyroxine.** **HERBAL:** None significant. **FOOD:** None known. **LAB VALUES:** May lower serum total cholesterol, LDL. May decrease platelet count, serum inorganic phosphate, albumin, calcium, protein.

AVAILABILITY (Rx)

Tablets: 60 mg.

ADMINISTRATION/HANDLING

PO

- Give without regard to food.

INDICATIONS/ROUTES/DOSAGE

Note: Discontinue at least 72 hrs prior to and during prolonged immobilization (may increase risk for DVT/PE).

Prophylaxis/Treatment of Osteoporosis, Breast Cancer Risk Reduction

PO: ADULTS, ELDERLY: 60 mg/day.

Dosage in Renal/Hepatic Impairment

No dose adjustment.

SIDE EFFECTS

Frequent (25%–10%): Hot flashes, flu-like symptoms, arthralgia, sinusitis. **Occasional (9%–5%):** Weight gain, nausea, myalgia, pharyngitis, cough, dyspepsia, leg cramps, rash, depression. **Rare (4%–3%):** Vaginitis, UTI, peripheral edema, flatulence, vomiting, fever, migraine, diaphoresis.

ADVERSE EFFECTS/TOXIC REACTIONS

Thromboembolic events (DVT, pulmonary embolism, superficial thrombophlebitis) may occur, esp. in pts with immobility. May increase risk of uterine bleeding, hypertriglyceridemia; death due to stroke.

NURSING CONSIDERATIONS

BASELINE ASSESSMENT

Obtain lipid panel. Question history of thrombosis (CVA, DVT, PE). Question for possibility of pregnancy. Drug should be discontinued 72 hrs before and during prolonged immobilization (postop recovery, prolonged bed rest). Therapy may be resumed only after pt is fully ambulatory.

INTERVENTION/EVALUATION

Monitor serum total cholesterol, total calcium, phosphate, total protein, albumin, bone mineral density, platelet count. Diligently monitor for CVA (aphasia, blindness, confusion, paresthesia, hemiparesis, syncope), DVT (arm/leg pain, swelling), pulmonary embolism (chest pain, dyspnea, hypoxia, tachycardia).

PATIENT/FAMILY TEACHING

• Avoid prolonged restriction of movement during travel (increased risk of venous thromboembolic events). • Take supplemental calcium, vitamin D if daily dietary intake is inadequate. • Engage in regular weight-bearing exercise. • Modify, discontinue habits of cigarette smoking, alcohol consumption. • Report symptoms of DVT (swelling, pain, hot feeling in the arms or legs), lung embolism (difficulty breathing, chest pain, rapid heart rate), stroke (blindness, confusion, difficulty speaking, one-sided weakness, passing out).

raltegravir

TOP 100

ral-**teg**-ra-veer
(Isentress, Isentress HD)

◆CLASSIFICATION

PHARMACOTHERAPEUTIC: Integrase inhibitor. **CLINICAL:** Antiretroviral (anti-HIV).

USES

Treatment of HIV-1 infection in adults and children and weighing at least 2 kg. Used in combination with at least two other antiretroviral agents. **OFF-LABEL:** Post-exposure prophylaxis for occupational exposure to HIV.

PRECAUTIONS

Contraindications: Hypersensitivity to raltegravir. **Cautions:** Elderly, pts at risk for creatine kinase (CK) elevations and/or skeletal muscle abnormalities.

ACTION

Inhibits activity of HIV-1 integrase, an enzyme that incorporates viral DNA into host cell. **Therapeutic Effect:** Prevents integration and replication of viral HIV-1.

PHARMACOKINETICS

Widely distributed. Protein binding: 83%. Metabolized in liver. Excreted in feces (51%), urine (32%). **Half-life:** 9 hrs.

LIFESPAN CONSIDERATIONS

Pregnancy/Lactation: May cross placenta. Breastfeeding not recommended. **Children:** Safety and efficacy not established in pts younger than 4 wks. **Elderly:** Age-related hepatic, renal, cardiac impairment requires strict monitoring.

INTERACTIONS

DRUG: Proton pump inhibitors (e.g., omeprazole, pantoprazole) may increase concentration. **Aluminum, magnesium salts, rifAMPin** may decrease levels/effect. **HERBAL:** None significant. **FOOD:** None known. **LAB VALUES:** May increase serum glucose, bilirubin, aminotransferase, alkaline phosphatase, amylase, lipase, creatine kinase. May decrease lymphocytes, neutrophils (ANC), Hgb, platelets.

AVAILABILITY (Rx)

Packet, Oral: 100 mg. **Tablets, Chewable:** 25 mg, 100 mg.

Tablets, Film-Coated: 400 mg, 600 mg.

ADMINISTRATION/HANDLING

PO

• Give without regard to food. • Do not break, crush, dissolve, or divide film-coated tablets. • Chewable tablets may be chewed or taken whole. • **Oral Packet:** Mix with 5 mL water to provide a concentration of 20 mg/mL. Once mixed, measure dose with oral syringe. Give within 30 min of mixing.

INDICATIONS/ROUTES/DOSAGE

HIV Infection

PO: ADULTS, ELDERLY, CHILDREN WEIGHING 40 KG OR MORE: Treatment naïve: 400 mg twice daily or 1,200 mg once daily. **Treatment experienced:** 400 mg twice daily. (Dosage increased to 800 mg twice daily when given with rifAMPin [treatment naïve or experienced]). **CHILDREN WEIGHING 25 KG OR MORE (WHO CAN SWALLOW A TABLET):** 400 mg twice daily. **CHILDREN 2–11 YRS WEIGHING 40 KG OR MORE (CHEWABLE TABLETS):** 300 mg twice daily. **WEIGHING 28–39 KG:** 200 mg twice daily. **WEIGHING 20–27 KG:** 150 mg twice daily. **WEIGHING 14–19 KG:** 100 mg twice daily. **WEIGHING 11–13 KG:** 75 mg twicedaily. **CHILDREN WEIGHING 14–19 KG (ORAL PACKET):** 100 mg twice daily. **WEIGHING 11–13 KG:** 80 mg twice daily.

WEIGHING 8–10 KG: 60 mg twice daily. **WEIGHING 6–7 KG:** 40 mg twice daily. **WEIGHING 4–5 KG:** 30 mg twice daily. **WEIGHING 3–4 KG:** 25 mg twice daily. **NEONATES (7 DAYS OR YOUNGER): 4 TO LESS THAN 5 KG:** 7 mg once daily. **3 TO LESS THAN 4 KG:** 5 mg once daily. **2 TO LESS THAN 3 KG:** 4 mg once daily. **(8–28 DAYS): 4 TO LESS THAN 5 KG:** 7 mg twice daily. **3 TO LESS THAN 4 KG:** 5 mg twice daily. **2 TO LESS THAN 3 KG:** 4 mg twice daily.

Dosage in Renal Impairment

Mild to severe impairment: No dose adjustment.

Dosage in Hepatic Impairment

Mild to moderate impairment: No dose adjustment. **Severe impairment:** Not recommended.

SIDE EFFECTS

Frequent (17%–10%): Diarrhea, nausea, headache. **Occasional (5%):** Fever. **Rare (2%–1%):** Vomiting, abdominal pain, fatigue, dizziness.

ADVERSE EFFECTS/TOXIC REACTIONS

Fatal cutaneous reactions including Stevens-Johnson syndrome, toxic epidermal necrolysis were reported. Hypersensitivity reactions including angioedema, eosinophilia, facial edema, malaise, rash, organ dysfunction, hepatic injury may occur. May induce immune reconstitution syndrome (inflammatory response to dormant opportunistic infections such as herpesvirus, *Mycobacterium avium*, cytomegalovirus, *Pneumocystis jiroveci* pneumonia, tuberculosis, or acceleration of autoimmune disorders such as Graves′ disease, polymyositis, Guillain-Barré). Chewable tablets (contain phenylalanine) may be harmful to pts with phenylketonuria. May increase risk of myopathy, rhabdomyolysis. Nephrolithiasis, renal failure reported in less than 2% of pts. May increase risk of suicidal ideation and behavior.

R

NURSING CONSIDERATIONS

BASELINE ASSESSMENT

Obtain CBC, BMP, CD4 count, viral load, HIV-1 RNA level; pregnancy test in females of reproductive potential. Question history of hepatic impairment, depression, suicidal ideation. Offer emotional support.

INTERVENTION/EVALUATION

Monitor CD4 count, viral load, HIV-1 RNA level for treatment effectiveness. Monitor renal function as clinically indicated. An increase in serum creatinine greater than 0.4 mg/dL from baseline may indicate renal impairment. Monitor LFT for hepatic injury (bruising, hematuria, jaundice, right upper abdominal pain, nausea, vomiting, weight loss). Obtain CK level if myopathy, rhabdomyolysis (joint/muscle pain, malaise) is suspected. Cough, dyspnea, fever, excess of band cells on CBC may indicate acute infection. (WBC count may be unreliable in pts with uncontrolled HIV infection.) Monitor for immune reconstitution syndrome. Assess skin for toxic skin reactions, rash. Screen for psychiatric symptoms, suicidal ideation and behavior.

PATIENT/FAMILY TEACHING

• Treatment does not cure HIV infection, nor does it reduce risk of transmission. Practice safe sex with barrier methods or abstinence. • Drug resistance can form if therapy is interrupted; do not run out of supply. • As immune system strengthens, it may respond to dormant infections hidden within the body. Report body aches, chills, cough, fever, night sweats, shortness of breath. • Report liver problems (abdominal pain, bruising, clay-colored stool, amber- or dark-colored urine, yellowing of the skin or eyes), kidney problems (decreased urine output, flank pain, darkened urine), toxic skin reactions (itching, peeling, rash, redness, swelling). • Do not breastfeed. • Seek immediate medical attention if thoughts of suicide, new onset or worsening of anxiety, depression, or changes in mood occur.

ramelteon

ra-**mel**-tee-on
(Rozerem)
Do not confuse ramelteon with Remeron, or Rozerem with Razadyne or Remeron.

◆CLASSIFICATION

PHARMACOTHERAPEUTIC: Melatonin receptor agonist. **CLINICAL:** Hypnotic.

USES

Treatment of insomnia in pts who experience difficulty with sleep onset.

PRECAUTIONS

Contraindications: Hypersensitivity to ramelteon. Concurrent fluvoxaMINE therapy, history of angioedema with previous ramelteon therapy. **Cautions:** Depression, other psychiatric conditions, alcohol consumption, other CNS depressants, moderate hepatic impairment, severe sleep apnea, COPD; concomitant strong CYP1A2 inhibitors (e.g., fluvoxaMINE).

ACTION

Selectively targets melatonin receptors thought to be involved in maintenance of circadian rhythm underlying normal sleep-wake cycle. **Therapeutic Effect:** Prevents insomnia characterized by difficulty with sleep onset.

PHARMACOKINETICS

Widely distributed. Protein binding: 82%. Metabolized in liver. Excreted in urine (84%), feces (4%). **Half-life:** 2–5 hrs.

⌛ LIFESPAN CONSIDERATIONS

Pregnancy/Lactation: Unknown if distributed in breast milk. Breastfeeding not recommended. **Children:** Safety and efficacy not established. **Elderly:** Age-related hepatic impairment may require dosage adjustment.

INTERACTIONS

DRUG: Fluconazole, ketoconazole may increase concentration/effect. **CNS depressants (e.g., alcohol, morphine, oxyCODONE, zolpidem)** may increase CNS depression. **Strong CYP3A4 inducers (e.g., carBAMazepine, rifAMPin)** may decrease concentration/effect. **FluvoxaMINE** may increase concentration/effect; increase risk of toxicity. **HERBAL: Herbals with sedative properties (e.g., chamomile, kava kava, valerian)** may increase CNS depression. **FOOD:** Onset of action may be reduced if taken with or immediately after a **high-fat meal. LAB VALUES:** May decrease serum cortisol.

AVAILABILITY (Rx)

Tablets, Film-Coated: ***(Rozerem):*** 8 mg.

ADMINISTRATION/HANDLING

PO

• Administer within 30 min before bedtime. • Do not give with, or immediately following, a high-fat meal. • Do not break, crush, dissolve, or divide tablet.

INDICATIONS/ROUTES/DOSAGE

Insomnia

PO: ADULTS, ELDERLY: 8 mg 30 min before bedtime. **Maximum:** 8 mg.

Dosage in Renal Impairment

No dose adjustment.

Dosage in Hepatic Impairment

Mild to moderate impairment: No dose adjustment. **Severe impairment:** Not recommended.

SIDE EFFECTS

Frequent (7%–5%): Headache, dizziness, drowsiness (expected effect). **Occasional (4%–3%):** Fatigue, nausea, exacerbated insomnia. **Rare (2%):** Diarrhea, myalgia, depression, altered taste, arthralgia.

ADVERSE EFFECTS/TOXIC REACTIONS

Severe hypersensitivity reactions including anaphylaxis, angioedema, dyspnea, throat constriction may occur. Angioedema involving larynx, glottis, tongue can be fatal. Worsening of insomnia may indicate underlying psychiatric illness. May cause amnesic events including cooking, sleepwalking, sexual activity, sleep-driving. May increase risk of suicidal ideation and behavior. May affect reproductive hormones in adults (decreased testosterone levels, increased prolactin levels), resulting in unexplained amenorrhea, galactorrhea, decreased libido, impaired fertility.

NURSING CONSIDERATIONS

BASELINE ASSESSMENT

Assess B/P, pulse, respirations. Raise bed rails, provide call light. Provide environment conducive to sleep (quiet environment, low/no lighting, TV off). Do not give unless a full night of sleep is planned.

INTERVENTION/EVALUATION

Assess sleep pattern of pt. Evaluate for therapeutic response: rapid induction of sleep onset, decrease in number of nocturnal awakenings.

PATIENT/FAMILY TEACHING

• Take within 30 min before going to bed; confine activities to those necessary to prepare for bed. • Avoid tasks that require alertness, motor skills until response to drug is established. • Therapy may need to be discontinued if cooking, driving, sleepwalking, sexual activity occurs without recollection. • Do not take unless a full night of sleep is planned. • Avoid alcohol. • Do not take medication with or immediately after a high-fat meal.

ramipril

ram-i-pril
(Altace)

■ **BLACK BOX ALERT** ■ May cause fetal injury, mortality. Discontinue as soon as possible once pregnancy is detected.
Do not confuse Altace with alteplase, Amaryl, or Artane, or ramipril with enalapril or Monopril.

◆CLASSIFICATION

PHARMACOTHERAPEUTIC: Angiotensin-converting enzyme (ACE) inhibitor. **CLINICAL:** Antihypertensive.

USES

Treatment of hypertension. Used alone or in combination with other antihypertensives. Treatment of HF following MI. Reduce risk of heart attack, stroke in pts 55 yrs and older at increased risk of developing major cardiovascular events. **OFF-LABEL:** HF. Delay progression of nephropathy, reduce risks of cardiovascular events in hypertensive pts with type 1 or type 2 diabetes.

PRECAUTIONS

Contraindications: Hypersensitivity to ramipril, other ACE inhibitors. History of ACE inhibitor–induced angioedema, concomitant use with aliskiren in pts with diabetes. Concomitant use or within 36 hrs of switching to or from a neprilysin inhibitor (e.g., sacubitril). **Cautions:** Renal impairment, elderly, collagen vascular disease, hyperkalemia, hypertrophic cardiomyopathy with outflow tract obstruction; unstented unilateral, bilateral renal artery stenosis; severe aortic stenosis; before, during, or immediately after major surgery; concomitant potassium supplements.

ACTION

Suppresses renin-angiotensin-aldosterone system. Blocks conversion of angiotensin I to angiotensin II, increases plasma renin activity, decreases aldosterone secretion. **Therapeutic Effect:** Reduces peripheral arterial resistance, decreasing B/P.

R

PHARMACOKINETICS

Route	Onset	Peak	Duration
PO	1–2 hrs	3–6 hrs	24 hrs

Widely distributed. Protein binding: 73%. Metabolized in liver. Primarily excreted in urine. Not removed by hemodialysis. **Half-life:** 5.1 hrs.

LIFESPAN CONSIDERATIONS

Pregnancy/Lactation: Crosses placenta. Distributed in breast milk. May cause fetal or neonatal mortality or morbidity. **Children:** Safety and efficacy not established. **Elderly:** May be more sensitive to hypotensive effects.

INTERACTIONS

DRUG: **Aliskiren** may increase hyperkalemic effect. May increase potential for allergic reactions to **allopurinol. Angiotensin receptor blockers (e.g., losartan, valsartan)** may increase adverse effects. May increase adverse effects of **lithium, sacubitril. HERBAL: Herbals with hypertensive properties (e.g., licorice, yohimbe) or hypotensive properties (e.g., garlic, ginger, ginkgo biloba)** may alter effects. **FOOD:** None known. **LAB VALUES:** May increase serum BUN, alkaline phosphatase, bilirubin, creatinine, potassium, ALT, AST. May decrease serum sodium. May cause positive antinuclear antibody (ANA) titer.

AVAILABILITY (Rx)

Capsules: 1.25 mg, 2.5 mg, 5 mg, 10 mg.

ADMINISTRATION/HANDLING

PO

• Give without regard to food. • May mix with water, apple juice/sauce.

INDICATIONS/ROUTES/DOSAGE

Hypertension

PO: ADULTS, ELDERLY: Initially, 2.5 mg/day. Titrate to desired effect after 2–4 wks up to 20 mg daily in 1 or 2 divided doses. **Pts with volume depletion:** Initially, 1.25 mg daily. Titrate to desired response.

HF Following MI

PO: ADULTS, ELDERLY: Initially, 1.25–2.5 mg twice daily. Continue for 1 wk, then titrate upward q3wks to target dose of 5 mg twice daily.

Risk Reduction for MI/Stroke

PO: ADULTS, ELDERLY: Initially, 2.5 mg/day for 7 days, then 5 mg/day for 21 days, then 10 mg/day as a single dose (or in divided doses in hypertensive or recent post-MI pts).

Dosage in Renal Impairment

CrCl equal to or less than 40 mL/min: 25% of normal dose.

Renal Failure and Hypertension

Initially, 1.25 mg/day titrated upward. **Maximum:** 5 mg/day. **Renal failure and HF:** Initially, 1.25 mg/day, titrated up to 2.5 mg twice daily.

Dosage in Hepatic Impairment

No dose adjustment. Discontinue for jaundice or marked elevation of hepatic enzymes.

SIDE EFFECTS

Frequent (12%–5%): Cough, headache. **Occasional (4%–2%):** Dizziness, fatigue, nausea, asthenia. **Rare (less than 2%):** Palpitations, insomnia, nervousness, malaise, abdominal pain, myalgia.

ADVERSE EFFECTS/TOXIC REACTIONS

Excessive hypotension ("first-dose syncope") may occur in pts with HF, severely salt or volume depleted. Angioedema, hyperkalemia occur rarely. Agranulocytosis, neutropenia may occur in pts with collagen vascular disease (scleroderma, systemic lupus erythematosus), renal impairment. Nephrotic syndrome may occur in pts with history of renal disease. May cause angioedema of the face, neck, throat, tongue. Cholestatic jaundice, fulminant hepatic necrosis may occur.

R

NURSING CONSIDERATIONS

BASELINE ASSESSMENT

Obtain B/P immediately before each dose, in addition to regular monitoring (be alert to fluctuations). Renal function tests should be performed before beginning therapy. Question history of hypersensitivity reaction, angioedema.

INTERVENTION/EVALUATION

In pts with prior renal disease, urine test for protein (by dipstick method) should be made with first urine of day before beginning therapy and periodically thereafter. In pts with renal impairment, autoimmune disease, or taking drugs that affect leukocytes or immune response, CBC, differential count should be performed before beginning therapy and q2wks for 3 mos periodically thereafter. Monitor B/P, renal function, serum potassium. Assess for cough (frequent effect). Assist with ambulation if dizziness occurs. Assess lung sounds for rales, wheezing in pts with HF. Monitor urinalysis for proteinuria. Monitor serum potassium in pts on concurrent diuretic therapy.

PATIENT/FAMILY TEACHING

• Do not discontinue medication without physician's approval. • Slowly go from lying to standing to minimize hypotensive effect. • Report palpitations, cough, chest pain. • Dizziness may occur in first few days. • Avoid alcohol. • Report swelling of the face, lips, or tongue.

ramucirumab

ra-mue-**sir**-ue-mab
(Cyramza)

■ **BLACK BOX ALERT** ■ May increase risk of severe, and sometimes fatal, hemorrhage, GI hemorrhage, and GI perforation. Permanently discontinue if severe bleeding occurs. May impair wound healing.

Do not confuse ramucirumab with ranibizumab.

◆CLASSIFICATION

PHARMACOTHERAPEUTIC: Vascular endothelial growth factor (VEGF) inhibitor. Monoclonal antibody. **CLINICAL:** Antineoplastic.

USES

As a single agent or in combination with PACLitaxel, for treatment of advanced or metastatic gastric or gastroesophageal junction adenocarcinoma with disease progression on or after prior fluoropyrimidine- or platinum-containing chemotherapy. In combination with DOCEtaxel, for treatment of metastatic non–small-cell lung cancer (NSCLC) with disease progression on or after platinum-based chemotherapy. In combination with FOLFIRI, for treatment of metastatic colorectal cancer with disease progression on or after therapy with bevacizumab, oxaliplatin, and a fluoropyrimidine. Treatment of advanced or relapsed/refractory hepatocellular carcinoma (as a single agent).

PRECAUTIONS

Contraindications: Hypersensitivity to ramucirumab. **Cautions:** History of arterial/venous thromboembolism (e.g., MI, cardiac arrest, CVA, cerebral ischemia), hepatic cirrhosis, electrolyte imbalance, hypertension, GI bleeding/perforation, chronic/unhealed wounds; baseline neutropenia, thrombocytopenia.

ACTION

Binds vascular endothelial growth factor (VEGF) receptor 2 and blocks binding of VEGF ligands, VEGF-A, VEGF-C, and VEGF-D. **Therapeutic Effect:** Inhibits/reduces tumor vascularity and growth.

PHARMACOKINETICS

Metabolism not specified. Elimination not specified.

LIFESPAN CONSIDERATIONS

Pregnancy/Lactation: May cause fetal harm. Females of reproductive potential should use effective contraception during treatment and up to 3 mos after discontinuation. Unknown if distributed in breast milk. **Children:** Safety and efficacy not established. **Elderly:** No age-related precautions noted.

INTERACTIONS

DRUG: May increase adverse effects/toxic reactions of **belimumab. HERBAL:** None significant. **FOOD:** None known. **LAB VALUES:** May increase urine protein. May decrease neutrophils, serum sodium.

AVAILABILITY (Rx)

Injection Solution: 100 mg/10 mL, 500 mg/50 mL.

ADMINISTRATION/HANDLING

IV

• Do not administer IV push or bolus. • Recommend premedication with IV histamine H_1 antagonist (e.g., diphenhydramine) prior to each infusion. Pts with prior Grade 1 or Grade 2 infusion reaction should also be premedicated with dexamethasone (or equivalent) and acetaminophen prior to each infusion. • Flush IV line with 0.9% NaCl upon infusion completion.

Reconstitution • Calculate dose, required solution volume, and number of vials needed using weight in kg. • Vials contain either 100 mg/10 mL or 500 mL/50 mL at concentration of 10 mg/mL. • Visually inspect for particulate matter. Discard if particulate matter or discoloration observed. • Using 250 mL 0.9% NaCl bag, withdraw and discard a volume equal to the total calculated volume of solution. • Slowly add required dose to diluent bag for final volume of 250 mL. Gently invert bag to mix; do not shake.

Rate of administration • Infuse over 60 min using 0.22-micron in-line filter via dedicated line.

Storage • Refrigerate vials in original carton until time of use. • Do not freeze. • Diluted solution may be refrigerated up to 24 hrs or stored at room temperature for up to 4 hrs. • Protect from light.

IV INCOMPATIBILITIES

Do not dilute in dextrose-containing fluids or infuse concomitantly with other electrolytes or medications.

INDICATIONS/ROUTES/DOSAGE

Gastric Cancer (Advanced or metastatic)

IV: ADULTS, ELDERLY: 8 mg/kg every 14 days, either as a single agent or in combination with wkly PACLitaxel. Continue until disease progression or unacceptable toxicity.

NSCLC

IV: ADULTS, ELDERLY: (Disease progression on or after platinum-based chemotherapy): 10 mg/kg on day 1 of a 21-day cycle in combination with DOCEtaxel. Continue until disease progression or unacceptable toxicity. **(First-line treatment):** 10 mg/kg once q2wks (in combination with erlotinib). Continue until disease progression or unacceptable toxicity.

Colorectal Cancer

IV: ADULTS, ELDERLY: 8 mg/kg q2wks, in combination with FOLFIRI (irinotecan, leucovorin, 5-fluorouracil). Continue until disease progression or unacceptable toxicity.

Hepatocellular Carcinoma

IV: ADULTS, ELDERLY: 8 mg/kg q2wks (as single agent). Continue until disease progression or unacceptable toxicity

Dose Modification

Based on Common Terminology Criteria for Adverse Events (CTCAE).

Infusion-related reaction: Reduce infusion rate by 50% for Grade 1 or Grade 2 reaction. Permanently discontinue for Grade 3 or Grade 4 reaction. **Severe hypertension:** Interrupt treatment until controlled with medical management. Permanently discontinue for severe hypertension that is not controlled

R

with antihypertensive therapy. **Proteinuria:** Interrupt treatment for urine protein level greater than or equal to 2 g/24 hrs. Restart treatment at reduced dose of 6 mg/kg every 14 days once urine protein level returns to less than 2 g/24 hrs. If level greater than or equal 2 g/24 hrs recurs, interrupt treatment and reduce dose to 5 mg/kg every 14 days once level returns to less than 2 g/24 hrs. Permanently discontinue for urine protein level greater than 3 g/24 hrs or in the setting of nephrotic syndrome. **Wound healing complications:** Interrupt treatment prior to scheduled surgery until wound is fully healed. **Arterial thromboembolic events, GI perforation, or Grade 3 or Grade 4 bleeding:** Permanently discontinue.

Dosage in Renal Impairment
No dose adjustment.

Dosage in Hepatic Impairment
Mild to moderate impairment: No dose adjustment. **Severe impairment:** Use caution.

SIDE EFFECTS

Occasional (16%–9%): Hypertension, diarrhea, headache. **Ramucirumab plus paclitaxel: Frequent (57%–20%):** Fatigue, diarrhea, peripheral edema, hypertension, stomatitis.

R

ADVERSE EFFECTS/TOXIC REACTIONS

Fatal hemorrhagic events including GI bleeding occurred in 3.4% of pts receiving single agent and in 4.3% of pts receiving combo therapy. GI perforations occurred in 0.7% of pts receiving single agent and in 1.2% of pts receiving combo therapy. Thromboembolic events including arterial thromboembolism, CVA, MI reported in 1.7% of pts. Severe hypertension occurred in 8% of pts receiving single agent and in 15% of pts receiving combo therapy despite medical management. Severe infusion-related reactions such as back pain/spasms, bronchospasm, chest pain, chills, dyspnea, flushing, hypotension, hypoxia, paresthesia, rigors/tremors, supraventricular tachycardia, wheezing occurred in 16% of pts. May cause ineffective wound healing or wound dehiscence requiring medical intervention. Reversible posterior leukoencephalopathy syndrome (RPLS) reported in less than 1% of pts. Proteinuria may indicate nephrotic syndrome. Clinical deterioration of hepatic cirrhosis, manifested by new-onset or worsening encephalopathy, ascites, or hepatorenal syndrome, was reported in pts receiving single agent. Other adverse reactions include epistaxis, intestinal obstruction, neutropenia, severe rash, thrombocytopenia. Immunogenicity (anti-ramucirumab antibodies) occurred in 6% of pts.

NURSING CONSIDERATIONS

BASELINE ASSESSMENT

Obtain CBC, BMP, vital signs; pregnancy test in females of reproductive potential. Question history of CVA, hepatic impairment/cirrhosis, hypertension, MI, prior hypersensitivity reaction. Offer emotional support.

INTERVENTION/EVALUATION

Monitor CBC, serum electrolytes, vital signs. Persistent diastolic hypertension may indicate hypertensive emergency. Obtain ECG for arrhythmia, chest pain, palpitation. Consider RPLS in pts with altered mental status, confusion, headache, seizure, visual disturbances. Screen for GI bleeding, GI perforation. Notify physician if any CTCAE toxicities occur (see Appendix M). Monitor for hypersensitivity reaction. Once infusion is completed, IV access must be flushed with NS.

PATIENT/FAMILY TEACHING

• Treatment may cause severe allergic reaction or infusion-related reaction. • Use effective contraception to avoid pregnancy. Do not breastfeed. • Neurologic changes, including altered mental status, headache, seizures, trouble speaking, may indicate high blood pressure crisis or life-threatening brain swelling. • Immediately report abdominal pain, GI bleeding, vomiting blood. • Therapy may cause severe blood-clotting events such as heart attack or stroke.

ranolazine

ra-**noe**-la-zeen
(Ranexa)
Do not confuse Ranexa with CeleXA.

CLASSIFICATION

PHARMACOTHERAPEUTIC: Cardiovascular agent. **CLINICAL:** Antianginal agent.

USES

Treatment of chronic angina.

PRECAUTIONS

Contraindications: Hypersensitivity to ranolazine. Hepatic cirrhosis, concurrent use of strong CYP3A inhibitors (e.g., rifAMPin, carBAMazepine) or CYP3A inducers (e.g., ketoconazole, itraconazole, fluconazole, clarithromycin, erythromycin). **Cautions:** Renal/hepatic impairment. Pts at risk for QTc interval prolongation (congenital long QT syndrome, HF, medications that prolong QTc interval, hypokalemia, hypomagnesemia).

ACTION

Inhibits inward current of sodium channel during cardiac repolarization, thereby reducing calcium influx. Decreased influx of calcium reduces ventricular tension, myocardial oxygen demand. Does not reduce heart rate, B/P. **Therapeutic Effect:** Exerts antianginal, anti-ischemic effects on cardiac tissue.

PHARMACOKINETICS

Absorption highly variable. Peak plasma concentration: 2–5 hrs. Rapidly, extensively metabolized in intestine, liver. Protein binding: 62%. Excreted in urine (75%), feces (25%). **Half-life:** 7 hrs.

LIFESPAN CONSIDERATIONS

Pregnancy/Lactation: Unknown if drug crosses placenta or is distributed in breast milk. **Children:** Safety and efficacy not established. **Elderly:** No age-related precautions noted.

INTERACTIONS

DRUG: See contraindications. **Strong CYP3A4 inducers (e.g., carBAMazepine, phenytoin, rifAMPin)** may decrease concentration/effect. **Calcium channel blockers (e.g., dilTIAZem, verapamil), strong CYP3A4 inhibitors (e.g., clarithromycin, ketoconazole)** may increase concentration/effect. May increase concentration/effect of **digoxin, simvastatin, tacrolimus. QT interval–prolonging medications (e.g., amiodarone, azithromycin, ciprofloxacin, haloperidol, methadone, sotalol)** may increase risk of QTc interval prolongation. **HERBAL: St. John's wort** may decrease concentration/effects. **FOOD: Grapefruit products** may increase plasma concentration, risk of QT prolongation. **LAB VALUES:** May slightly elevate serum BUN, creatinine.

AVAILABILITY (Rx)

Tablets, Extended-Release: 500 mg, 1,000 mg.

ADMINISTRATION/HANDLING

PO

• May give without regard to food. • Do not break, crush, dissolve, or divide extended-release tablets.

INDICATIONS/ROUTES/DOSAGE

Chronic Angina

PO: ADULTS, ELDERLY: Initially, 500 mg twice daily. May increase to 1,000 mg twice daily, based on clinical response. Dose should not exceed 500 mg twice daily when used concurrently with

R

moderate CYP3A inhibitors (e.g., fluconazole, dilTIAZem, verapamil).

Dosage in Renal/Hepatic Impairment
No dose adjustment (discontinue if acute renal failure develops). Contraindicated in pts with cirrhosis.

SIDE EFFECTS

Occasional (6%–4%): Dizziness, headache, constipation, nausea. **Rare (2%–1%):** Peripheral edema, abdominal pain, dry mouth, vomiting, tinnitus, vertigo, palpitations.

ADVERSE EFFECTS/TOXIC REACTIONS

Overdose manifested as confusion, diplopia, dizziness, paresthesia, syncope.

NURSING CONSIDERATIONS

BASELINE ASSESSMENT

Receive full medication history and screen for contraindications. Question history of hepatic impairment, long QT syndrome. Record onset, type (sharp, dull, squeezing), radiation, location, intensity, duration of anginal pain, precipitating factors (exertion, emotional stress). Obtain baseline ECG.

INTERVENTION/EVALUATION

Assist with ambulation if dizziness occurs. Give with food if nausea occurs. Assess for relief of anginal pain. Monitor ECG, pulse for irregularities.

PATIENT/FAMILY TEACHING

• Avoid grapefruit products. • Do not chew, crush, dissolve, or divide extended-release tablets. • Avoid tasks requiring alertness, motor skills until response to drug is established. • Treatment may affect the electrical properties of the heart; report palpitations, loss of consciousness.

rasagiline

ra-**sa**-ji-leen
(Azilect, Apo-Rasagiline ♣)

Do not confuse Azilect with Aricept.

◆CLASSIFICATION

PHARMACOTHERAPEUTIC: MAO type B inhibitor. **CLINICAL:** Antiparkinson agent.

USES

Treatment of signs/symptoms of Parkinson's disease as initial monotherapy or as adjunct therapy with or without levodopa.

PRECAUTIONS

Contraindications: Hypersensitivity to rasagiline. Concurrent use with methadone, traMADol, meperidine, MAOIs within 14 days of rasagiline, cyclobenzaprine, dextromethorphan, or St. John's wort. **Cautions:** Hepatic impairment (avoid use in moderate to severe impairment); cardiovascular, cerebrovascular disease, baseline hypotension. Avoid foods high in tyramine. Do not use within 5 wks of stopping FLUoxetine; do not start tricyclic, SSRI, or SNRI within 2 wks of stopping rasagiline. History of major psychotic disorder.

ACTION

Irreversibly and selectively inhibits monoamine oxidase type B, an enzyme that plays a major role in catabolism of DOPamine. Inhibition of DOPamine depletion reduces symptomatic motor deficits of Parkinson's disease. **Therapeutic Effect:** Reduces symptoms of Parkinson's disease; appears to delay disease progression.

PHARMACOKINETICS

Widely distributed. Protein binding: 88%–94%. Metabolized in liver. Excreted in urine (62%), feces (7%). **Half-life:** 1.3–3 hrs.

⌛ LIFESPAN CONSIDERATIONS

Pregnancy/Lactation: Unknown if distributed in breast milk. **Children:** Safety and efficacy not established. **Elderly:** No age-related precautions noted.

INTERACTIONS

DRUG: **Alcohol** may increase adverse effects. **Amphetamines, MAOIs (e.g., phenelzine, selegiline), sympathomimetics (e.g., DOPamine)** may cause hypertensive crisis. **Anorexiants (e.g., dexfenfluramine, fenfluramine, sibutramine), CNS stimulants (e.g., methylphenidate), cyclobenzaprine, dextromethorphan, meperidine, methadone, mirtazapine, serotonin or norepinephrine reuptake inhibitors (e.g., citalopram, sertraline, venlafaxine), tricyclic antidepressants (e.g., amitriptyline), venlafaxine** may cause serotonin syndrome. May increase risk of **atomoxetine, buPROPion** toxicity. **Levodopa** may cause hypertensive/hypotensive reaction. **HERBAL:** **Herbals with hypotensive properties (e.g., black cohosh, garlic)** may increase effect. **FOOD:** **Caffeine, foods/beverages containing tyramine** may result in hypertensive reaction, hypertensive crisis. **LAB VALUES:** May increase serum alkaline phosphatase, bilirubin, ALT, AST. May cause leukopenia.

AVAILABILITY (Rx)

Tablets: 0.5 mg, 1 mg.

ADMINISTRATION/HANDLING

PO

• Give without regard to food. • Avoid food, beverages containing tyramine (e.g., cheese, sour cream, yogurt, pickled herring, liver, figs, raisins, bananas, avocados, soy sauce, broad beans, yeast extracts, meat tenderizers, red wine, beer), excessive amounts of caffeine (e.g., coffee, tea).

INDICATIONS/ROUTES/DOSAGE

◀ALERT▶ When used in combination with levodopa, dosage reduction of levodopa should be considered.

Parkinson's Disease

PO: ADULTS, ELDERLY, MONOTHERAPY, ADJUNCTIVE THERAPY WITHOUT LEVODOPA: 1 mg once daily. **ADULTS, ELDERLY, ADJUNCTIVE THERAPY WITH LEVODOPA:** Initially, 0.5 mg once daily. If therapeutic response is not achieved, dose may be increased to 1 mg once daily. **ADJUNCTIVE THERAPY WITHOUT LEVODOPA:** 1 mg once daily.

Dose Modification

Concomitant use of CYP1A2 inhibitors, ciprofloxacin: 0.5 mg once daily.

Dosage in Hepatic Impairment

Mild impairment: 0.5 mg once daily. **Moderate to severe impairment:** Not recommended.

Dosage in Renal Impairment

No dose adjustment.

SIDE EFFECTS

Frequent (14%–12%): Headache, nausea. **Occasional (9%–5%):** Orthostatic hypotension, weight loss, dyspepsia, dry mouth, arthralgia, depression, hallucinations, constipation. **Rare (4%–2%):** Fever, vertigo, ecchymosis, rhinitis, neck pain, arthritis, paresthesia.

ADVERSE EFFECTS/TOXIC REACTIONS

Increase in dyskinesia (impaired voluntary movement), dystonia (impaired muscular tone) occurs in 18% of pts, angina occurs in 9%. Gastroenteritis, conjunctivitis occur rarely (3% of pts).

NURSING CONSIDERATIONS

BASELINE ASSESSMENT

Obtain LFT, B/P. Receive full medication history and screen for interactions. Question history of severe hepatic impairment, cardiovascular disease.

INTERVENTION/EVALUATION

Monitor B/P. Assess for clinical reversal of symptoms (improvement of tremor of head/hands at rest, mask-like facial expression, shuffling gait, muscular rigidity). If hallucinations or dyskinesia occurs, symptoms may be eliminated if levodopa dosage is reduced. Hallucinations generally are

R

accompanied by confusion and, to a lesser extent, insomnia.

PATIENT/FAMILY TEACHING

• Orthostatic hypotension may occur more frequently during initial therapy. • Avoid tasks that require alertness, motor skills until response to drug is established. • Hallucinations may occur (more so in the elderly with Parkinson's disease), typically within first 2 wks of therapy. • Avoid foods that contain tyramine (cheese, sour cream, beer, wine, pickled herring, liver, figs, raisins, bananas, avocados, soy sauce, yeast extracts, yogurt, papaya, broad beans, meat tenderizers), excessive amounts of caffeine (coffee, tea, chocolate), OTC preparations for hay fever, colds, weight reduction (may produce significant rise in B/P). • Do not take any newly prescribed medications unless approved by prescriber who originally started therapy.

rasburicase

ras-**bure**-i-kase
(Elitek, Fasturtec 🍁)

BLACK BOX ALERT Severe hypersensitivity reactions including anaphylaxis reported. May cause severe hemolysis in pts with glucose-6-phosphate dehydrogenase (G6PD) deficiency. Screen pts at high risk for G6PD (African or Mediterranean descent) prior to therapy. Methemoglobinemia has been reported. Blood samples left at room temperature may interfere with uric acid measurements. Must collect blood samples in prechilled tubes containing heparin and immediately immerse in ice water bath. Assay plasma samples within 4 hrs of collection. Elitek enzymatically degrades uric acid in blood samples left at room temperature.

◆CLASSIFICATION

PHARMACOTHERAPEUTIC: Urate-oxidase enzyme. **CLINICAL:** Antihyperuricemic.

USES

Initial management of uric acid levels in pts with leukemia, lymphoma, and solid tumor malignancies who are receiving chemotherapy expected to result in tumor lysis and subsequent elevation of plasma uric acid.

PRECAUTIONS

Contraindications: History of anaphylaxis or severe hypersensitivity to rasburicase. Prior rasburicase-associated drug reactions including hemolysis, methemoglobinemia. History of G6PD deficiency. **Cautions:** Pts at high risk for G6PD deficiency (e.g., African, Mediterranean, or Southeast Asian descent).

ACTION

A urate-oxidase enzyme that converts uric acid into allantoin (an inactive metabolite of uric acid). Does not inhibit formation of uric acid. **Therapeutic Effect:** Decreases uric acid levels.

PHARMACOKINETICS

Half-life: 16–23 hrs.

LIFESPAN CONSIDERATIONS

Pregnancy/Lactation: Unknown if distributed in breast milk. Unknown if crosses placenta. May cause fetal harm. **Children/Elderly:** No age-related precautions noted.

INTERACTIONS

DRUG: None significant. **HERBAL:** None significant. **FOOD:** None known. **LAB VALUES:** May increase serum bilirubin, ALT. May decrease serum phosphate.

AVAILABILITY (Rx)

Injection, Powder for Reconstitution: 1.5 mg/vial, 7.5 mg/vial.

ADMINISTRATION/HANDLING

IV

Reconstitution • Must use diluent provided in carton. • Reconstitute 1.5-mg vial with 1 mL of diluent or 7.5-mg vial with 5 mL of diluent to provide concentration of 1.5 mg/mL. • Gently swirl to mix. Do not shake. • Inspect for particulate matter or discoloration. • Inject calculated dose into appropriate volume of 0.9% NaCl to achieve a final volume of 50 mL.

Rate of administration • Infuse over 30 min. • Do not use filter during reconstitution or infusion.

Storage • Refrigerate solution until time of use. • Discard after 24 hrs following reconstitution.

IV INCOMPATIBILITIES

Do not mix with other IV medications.

INDICATIONS/ROUTES/DOSAGE

Note: Indicated only for a single course of treatment.

Management of Hyperuricemia

IV: ADULTS, ELDERLY, CHILDREN: (High risk): 0.2 mg/kg once daily (duration based on plasma uric acid levels). **(Intermediate risk):** 0.15 mg/kg (duration based on plasma uric acid levels). **(Low risk):** 0.1 mg/kg (duration based on clinical judgment).

Dosage in Renal/Hepatic Impairment

No dose adjustment.

SIDE EFFECTS

Frequent (50%–46%): Vomiting, fever. **Occasional (27%–13%):** Nausea, headache, abdominal pain, constipation, diarrhea, mucositis, rash.

ADVERSE EFFECTS/TOXIC REACTIONS

Hypersensitivity reactions occurred in 4.3% of pts including injection irritation, peripheral edema, urticaria, pruritus. Anaphylaxis, hemolysis, methemoglobinemia occurred in less than 1%. Pulmonary hemorrhage, respiratory failure, supraventricular arrhythmias, ischemic coronary artery disorders, sepsis, abdominal, gastrointestinal infections occurred in greater than 2% of pts. Anti-rasburicase antibodies reported.

NURSING CONSIDERATIONS

BASELINE ASSESSMENT

Obtain CBC, BMP, LFT, serum phosphate, uric acid level; pregnancy test in females of reproductive potential. Question for history of prior hypersensitivity reactions. Assess G6PD deficiency risk in potential candidates.

INTERVENTION/EVALUATION

Monitor CBC, BMP, LFT, serum phosphate. If hypersensitivity reaction occurs, stop infusion and immediately notify physician. Screen for clinical tumor lysis syndrome, hemolysis, methemoglobinemia. Follow strict procedure when collecting uric acid levels. Obtain ECG for chest pain/tightness, hyperkalemia, dyspnea. Assess skin for rash.

PATIENT/FAMILY TEACHING

- Report any allergic reaction, bronchospasm, chest pain or tightness, cough, difficulty breathing, dizziness, fainting, rash, or itching.

regorafenib

re-goe-**raf**-e-nib
(Stivarga)

BLACK BOX ALERT Severe, sometimes fatal, hepatotoxicity reported. Monitor hepatic function prior to and during treatment. Interrupt, reduce, or discontinue therapy if hepatotoxicity or hepatocellular necrosis occurs.

CLASSIFICATION

PHARMACOTHERAPEUTIC: Vascular endothelial growth factor (VEGF) inhibitor. Tyrosine kinase inhibitor. **CLINICAL:** Antineoplastic.

USES

Treatment of metastatic colorectal cancer in pts who have been previously treated

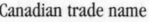

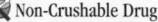

R

with fluoropyrimidine/oxaliplatin/irinotecan-based chemotherapy, anti-VEGF or anti-EGFR therapy. Locally advanced, unresectable, or metastatic GI stromal tumor previously treated with imatinib and SUNItinib. Treatment of hepatocellular carcinoma (HCC) previously treated with sorafenib.

PRECAUTIONS

Contraindications: Hypersensitivity to regorafenib. **Cautions:** Mild to moderate hepatic impairment (not recommended with severe hepatic impairment), hypertension (not recommended with severe or uncontrolled hypertension), recent surgical/dental procedures, chronic open wounds/ulcers, hemoptysis, concomitant warfarin therapy, cardiovascular disease, recent MI.

ACTION

Inhibits tyrosine kinase activity involved with tumor angiogenesis, oncogenesis, and maintenance of tumor microenvironment. **Therapeutic Effect:** Inhibits tumor cell growth and metastasis.

PHARMACOKINETICS

Widely distributed. Metabolized in liver. Protein binding: 99.5%. Peak plasma concentration: 4 hrs. Excreted in feces (71%), urine (19%). **Half-life:** 28 hrs (Range: 14–58 hrs).

R

LIFESPAN CONSIDERATIONS

Pregnancy/Lactation: Avoid pregnancy; may cause fetal harm. Females of reproductive potential must use effective contraception during treatment and for at least 2 mos after discontinuation. Breastfeeding not recommended during treatment and for at least 2 wks after discontinuation. **Children:** Safety and efficacy not established. **Elderly:** No age-related precautions noted.

INTERACTIONS

DRUG: Strong CYP3A4 inducers (e.g., carBAMazepine, phenytoin) may decrease concentration/effects. **Strong CYP3A4 inhibitors (e.g., clarithromycin, ketoconazole)** may increase concentration/effects. **HERBAL: St. John's wort** may decrease concentration/effects. **FOOD: Grapefruit products** may increase concentration/effects. **High-fat meal** may increase absorption/concentration. **LAB VALUES:** May decrease lymphocytes, neutrophils, platelets, serum calcium, phosphorus, potassium, sodium. May increase serum bilirubin, ALT, AST, lipase, amylase, INR, urine protein.

AVAILABILITY (Rx)

Tablets: 40 mg.

ADMINISTRATION/HANDLING

PO

• Take at same time each day with low-fat (less than 30%) breakfast. • Give whole; do not break, crush, dissolve, or divide tablet.

INDICATIONS/ROUTES/DOSAGE

Metastatic Colorectal Cancer, GI Stromal Tumor, Hepatocellular Carcinoma

PO: ADULTS/ELDERLY: 160 mg once daily for first 21 days of each 28-day cycle. Continue until disease progression or unacceptable toxicity.

Dosage Modification

Symptomatic Hypertension, Toxic Skin Reactions, Severe Side Effects (Grades 3–4)

PO: ADULTS/ELDERLY: Reduce dose to 120 mg once daily. If recovery does not occur within 7 days (despite dose reduction), interrupt treatment for minimum of 7 days and reassess. If recovery does not occur after interruption, reduce dose to 80 mg once daily. Discontinue for any of the following: intolerance of 80-mg dose; serum ALT or AST greater than 20 times upper limit of normal (ULN); serum ALT/AST greater than 3 times ULN and bilirubin greater than 2 times ULN; recurrent serum ALT/AST greater than 5 times ULN despite dose of 120 mg; recovery failure of Grade 3 or 4 side effects, toxic skin reaction.

Dosage in Renal Impairment
No dose adjustment.

Dosage in Hepatic Impairment
Mild to moderate impairment: No dose adjustment. **Severe impairment:** Not recommended.

SIDE EFFECTS

Frequent (64%–26%): Asthenia/fatigue, anorexia, diarrhea, mucositis, weight loss, hypertension, dysphonia, generalized pain, fever, rash. **Occasional (10%–5%):** Headache, alopecia, dysgeusia, musculoskeletal stiffness, dry mouth. **Rare (2% or less):** Tremor, gastric reflux.

ADVERSE EFFECTS/TOXIC REACTIONS

Myelosuppression (lymphopenia, neutropenia, thrombocytopenia) is an expected response to therapy. May cause GI perforation, GI fistula formation. Hemorrhaging of respiratory, GI, genitourinary tracts reported in 21% of pts. Hypertension (30% of pts) may lead to hypertensive crisis. May cause ineffective wound healing or wound dehiscence requiring medical intervention. Palmar-plantar erythrodysesthesia syndrome (PPES), a chemotherapy-induced skin condition that presents with redness, swelling, numbness, skin sloughing of hands, feet (45% of pts). Reversible posterior leukoencephalopathy syndrome (RPLS) reported in less than 1% of pts. May induce cardiac ischemia and/or MI. Severe, sometimes fatal, hepatotoxicity including hepatocellular necrosis reported in less than 1%. Infections including mucocutaneous and systemic infections, nasopharyngitis, pneumonia, UTI reported in 31% of pts (most likely due to neutropenia).

NURSING CONSIDERATIONS

BASELINE ASSESSMENT

Obtain CBC, BMP, LFT; pregnancy test in females of reproductive potential. Assess recent surgical/dental procedures. Obtain full medication history including herbal products. Question for history of hypertension, hepatic impairment, cardiovascular disease. Assess skin for open/unhealed wounds. Offer emotional support.

INTERVENTION/EVALUATION

Monitor B/P, CBC, serum electrolytes, urinalysis. Monitor LFT q2wks for 2 mos, then monthly; or every wk if elevated. Persistent diastolic hypertension may indicate hypertensive emergency. Obtain ECG for palpitation, chest pain, hypokalemia, hyperkalemia, hypocalcemia, bradycardia, ventricular arrhythmias. Reverse posterior leukoencephalopathy syndrome (RPLS) should be considered in pts with seizure, headache, visual disturbances, altered mental status, malignant hypertension. Assess hydration status. Encourage PO intake. Immediately report any hemorrhaging, bloody stools, hematuria, abdominal pain, hemoptysis (may indicate GI perforation/fistula formation).

PATIENT/FAMILY TEACHING

• Treatment may depress your immune system response and reduce your ability to fight infection. Report symptoms of infection such as body aches, chills, cough, fatigue, fever. Avoid those with active infection. • Report liver problems (abdominal pain, bruising, clay-colored stool, amber- or dark-colored urine, yellowing of the skin or eyes), symptoms of hemorrhagic stroke (confusion, difficulty speaking, one-sided weakness or paralysis, loss of vision, seizures). • Report neurologic changes including confusion, seizures, vision loss, high blood pressure crisis (may indicate RPLS). • Do not take herbal products. • Notify physician before any planned surgical/dental procedures. • Do not ingest grapefruit products. • Take with low-fat food only. • Use effective contraception to avoid pregnancy. Do not breastfeed. • Immediately report bleeding of any kind.

R

remdesivir

rem-**de**-si-vir
(Veklury)
Do not confuse remdesivir with oseltamivir, peramivir, or zanamivir.

◆Classification

PHARMACOTHERAPEUTIC: Nucleotide analog ribonucleic acid (RNA) polymerase inhibitor. **CLINICAL:** Antiviral.

USES

Treatment of coronavirus disease 2019 (COVID-19) in adults and pediatric pts (12 yrs and older and weighing at least 40 kg) who require hospitalization.

PRECAUTIONS

Contraindications: Hypersensitivity to remdesivir. **Cautions:** Renal impairment, hepatic disease. Avoid concomitant use of chloroquine phosphate, hydroxychloroquine.

ACTION

Inhibits SARS-CoV-2 RNA-dependent RNA polymerase, essential for viral replication. Distributes into cells and metabolizes into active nucleoside triphosphate metabolite, which competes for incorporation into RNA chains, resulting in chain termination. **Therapeutic Effect:** Inhibits viral replication of coronavirus associated with COVID-19.

PHARMACOKINETICS

Widely distributed. Primarily metabolized by enzymatic activity into active metabolite (minimal hepatic metabolism). Protein binding: 88%–94%. Peak plasma concentration: less than 1 hr. Excreted in urine (49%), feces (less than 1%). **Half-life:** 1 hr.

LIFESPAN CONSIDERATIONS

Pregnancy/Lactation: Unknown if distributed in breast milk. **Children:** Safety and efficacy not established in pts younger than 12 yrs or weighing less than 40 kg. **Elderly:** No age-related precautions noted.

INTERACTIONS

DRUG: **Chloroquine, hydroxychloroquine** may decrease antiviral/therapeutic effect. **Strong CYP3A4 inducers (e.g., carBAMazepine, phenytoin, rifAMPin)** may decrease concentration/effect. **HERBAL:** None significant. **FOOD:** None known. **LAB VALUES:** May increase serum ALT, AST, bilirubin, creatinine, glucose; prothrombin time. May decrease CrCl, estimated glomerular filtration rate (eGFR), Hgb, lymphocytes.

AVAILABILITY (Rx)

Injection, Powder for Reconstitution: 100 mg. **Injection Solution:** 100 mg/20 mL (5 mg/mL).

ADMINISTRATION/HANDLING

IV

Note: Must be prepared and administered in the healthcare setting by a healthcare provider.

Reconstitution/Preparation • Reconstitute lyophilized powder with 19 mL Sterile Water for injection. Discard vial if vacuum does not pull Sterile Water for Injection into vial. • Shake for 30 sec, then allow contents to settle for 2–3 min. Repeat until contents are completely dissolved (discard if not completely dissolved). • Reconstituted solution must be diluted in either 100 mL or 250 mL 0.9% NaCl infusion bag. Concentrated injection solution must be diluted in 250 mL 0.9% NaCl infusion bag only. • Visually inspect for particulate matter or discoloration. Solution should appear clear, colorless to slightly yellow. Do not use if solution is cloudy or discolored or if visible particles are observed. • Withdraw and discard a volume from the infusion bag that is equal to the required volume of dose (40 mL for loading dose; 20 mL for maintenance dose). • Transfer required volume of

dose to infusion bag. • Invert 20 times to mix. Do not shake.
Rate of administration • Infuse over 30–120 min based on tolerability.
Storage • Store unused vials containing lyophilized powder at controlled room temperature. Refrigerate unused vials containing concentrated injection solution or store at room temperature for up to 12 hrs. • May refrigerate diluted solution for up to 48 hrs or store at room temperature for up to 24 hrs. • Do not shake or freeze.

IV INCOMPATABILITIES

Do not mix or infuse with other medications or solutions.

INDICATIONS/ROUTES/DOSAGE

COVID-19 Infection

IV: ADULTS, CHILDREN 12 YRS AND OLDER WEIGHING AT LEAST 40 KG: 200 mg (as a single loading dose) on day 1, then 100 mg daily for 4 days or until hospital discharge. May continue for up to 10 days in pts without substantial clinical improvement at day 5. **Permanent discontinuation:** Discontinue in pts with hypersensitivity reactions, serum ALT greater than 10 times ULN, or serum ALT elevation associated with signs and symptoms of hepatic inflammation.

Dosage in Renal Impairment

eGFR 30 mL/min or greater: No dose adjustment. **eGFR less than 30 mL/min:** Not recommended.

Dosage in Hepatic Impairment.

Mild to severe impairment: Not specified; use caution.

SIDE EFFECTS

Rare (5% to less than 1%): Nausea, injection site erythema.

ADVERSE EFFECTS/TOXIC REACTIONS

Hypersensitivity reactions including anaphylaxis, angioedema, bradycardia, diaphoresis, dyspnea, fever, hypertension, hypotension, hypoxia, nausea, rash, shivering, tachycardia wheezing have occurred. Grade 1 or 2 transaminase elevations were reported. Seizure activity, acute kidney occur rarely.

NURSING CONSIDERATIONS

BASELINE ASSESSMENT

Obtain vital signs, renal function test (BUN, serum creatinine; CrCl, eGFR), LFT, prothrombin time. Confirm positive test for SARS-CoV-2. Question history of renal impairment, hepatic disease. Auscultate lung sounds. Assess for symptoms of COVID-19 (anosmia, cough, dysgeusia, dyspnea, fever, headache, muscle aches, respiratory failure, sepsis). Initiate isolation precautions.

INTERVENTION/EVALUATION

Monitor vital signs, eGFR, LFT, prothrombin time. Assess for hypersensitivity reactions, esp. during initial doses. Monitor I&Os. Assess for acute kidney injury, esp. in critically ill pts (decreased urinary output, edema, flank pain, seizures); hepatic injury (abdominal pain, encephalopathy, fatigue, jaundice, nausea, vomiting). Monitor for worsening of COVID-19–related symptoms.

PATIENT/FAMILY TEACHING

• Treatment is not a cure, but it may shorten recovery time and reduce symptoms associated with COVID-19. • Severe allergic reactions, including anaphylaxis, can occur. If allergic reaction occurs, seek immediate medical attention. • Report symptoms of liver inflammation (abdominal pain, confusion, nausea, vomiting, yellowing of skin or eyes); kidney inflammation (decreased urine output, flank pain, darkened urine).

reslizumab

res-li-**zoo**-mab
(Cinqair)

BLACK BOX ALERT
Anaphylaxis reported in less than 1% asthmatic pts, which usually occurred during or within 20 min of completion of infusion. Observe for appropriate period of time after administration.

Do not confuse reslizumab with certolizumab, daclizumab, eculizumab, efalizumab, mepolizumab, natalizumab, omalizumab, pembrolizumab, tocilizumab, or vedolizumab, or Cinqair with Cinryze, Cinolar, Cinobac, Sinemet, Singulair, or SINEquan.

◆CLASSIFICATION

PHARMACOTHERAPEUTIC: Interleukin-5 receptor antagonist. Monoclonal antibody. **CLINICAL:** Antiasthmatic.

USES

Add-on maintenance treatment of pts with severe asthma, aged 18 yrs and older, and with an eosinophil phenotype.

PRECAUTIONS

Contraindications: Hypersensitivity to reslizumab. **Cautions:** History of helminth (parasite) infection; long-term use of corticosteroids. Not indicated for treatment of other eosinophilic conditions; relief of acute bronchospasm, status asthmaticus, exercise-induced bronchospasm. History of anaphylaxis.

ACTION

Exact mechanism unknown. Inhibits signaling of interleukin-5 cytokine, reducing production and survival of eosinophils responsible for asthmatic inflammation and pathogenesis. **Therapeutic Effect:** Prevents inflammatory process. Decreases number of asthma exacerbations.

PHARMACOKINETICS

Widely distributed. Degraded into small peptides and amino acids via proteolytic enzymes. Peak plasma concentration: reached by end of infusion. Excretion not specified. **Half-life:** 24 days.

LIFESPAN CONSIDERATIONS

Pregnancy/Lactation: Unknown if distributed in breast milk. However, human immunoglobulin G (IgG) is present in breast milk and is known to cross placenta. **Children:** Safety and efficacy not established. **Elderly:** No age-related precautions noted.

INTERACTIONS

DRUG: None known. **HERBAL:** None significant. **FOOD:** None known. **LAB VALUES:** May increase creatine phosphokinase (CPK).

AVAILABILITY (Rx)

Injection Solution: 100 mg/10 mL (10 mg/mL).

ADMINISTRATION/HANDLING

IV

Preparation • Allow vial to warm to room temperature. • Visually inspect for particulate matter or discoloration. Solution should appear clear to slightly opalescent, colorless to pale yellow. • Proteinaceous particles may be present. • Air bubbles are expected and allowed. • Do not use if solution is cloudy or discolored or if foreign particles are observed. • Do not shake. • Withdraw proper dose volume from vial and dilute in 50 mL 0.9% NaCl bag. • Gently invert to mix. Do not shake (may cause foaming/precipitate formation). • Infuse via dedicated line. • After infusion is complete, flush IV line with 0.9% NaCl.

Rate of administration • Infuse over 20–50 min (depending on total volume of infusion), using an in-line, low protein-binding filter (pore size: 0.2 micron).

Storage • Refrigerate unused vials. • Do not freeze. • Diluted solution may be refrigerated or stored at room temperature for up to 16 hrs. • If refrigerated, allow diluted solution to warm to room temperature before use. • Protect from light.

IV INCOMPATIBILITIES

Do not mix or infuse with other medications.

INDICATIONS/ROUTES/DOSAGE

Asthma (Severe)

IV: ADULTS, ELDERLY: 3 mg/kg once q4wks.

Dosage in Renal/Hepatic Impairment

Not specified; use caution.

SIDE EFFECTS

Rare (3%–1%): Oropharyngeal pain, myalgia.

ADVERSE EFFECTS/TOXIC REACTIONS

Life-threatening anaphylaxis reported in less than 1% of pts. Hypersensitivity reactions including bronchospasm, dyspnea, hypoxia, rash, urticaria, vomiting usually occurred during infusion or within 20 min after completion. Less than 1% of pts reported at least one malignant neoplasm within 6 mos of initiation. Unknown if treatment will influence the immunologic response to helminth (parasite) infection. Immunogenicity (auto-reslizumab antibodies) reported in 5% of pts.

NURSING CONSIDERATIONS

BASELINE ASSESSMENT

Obtain serum CPK. Verify presence of eosinophil phenotype. Question history of hypersensitivity reaction. Therapy should be administered in a health care setting by medical professionals who are trained and prepared to readily manage anaphylaxis. Have anaphylactic medications (e.g., antihistamine, bronchodilator, corticosteroid, EPINEPHrine, H_2 receptor antagonist), intubation kit, supplemental oxygen readily available before initiation. Inhaled or systemic corticosteroids should not be suddenly discontinued upon initiation. Corticosteroids that are not gradually reduced may cause withdrawal symptoms or unmask conditions that were originally suppressed with corticosteroid therapy. Pts with preexisting helminth infection should be treated prior to initiation.

INTERVENTION/EVALUATION

Obtain serum CPK in pts complaining of myalgia. Diligently observe for hypersensitivity/anaphylactic reaction during infusion and directly after completion. If anaphylaxis occurs, discontinue infusion and provide immediate resuscitation support. Early detection is vital. Assess rate, depth, rhythm of respirations, oxygen saturation for therapeutic effectiveness. Assess lungs for wheezing, rales. Obtain pulmonary function test to assess disease improvement. Interrupt or discontinue therapy if helminth infection occurs, if worsening of asthma-related symptoms occurs (esp. in pts tapering off corticosteroids). Monitor for increased use of rescue inhalers; may indicate deterioration of asthma. Monitor for primary malignancies.

PATIENT/FAMILY TEACHING

• Treatment may cause life-threatening anaphylaxis. Immediately report allergic reactions such as difficulty breathing, hives, itching, low blood pressure, rash, swelling of the face or tongue, sudden coughing, vomiting, wheezing during infusion or immediately after infusion. • Therapy not indicated for relief of acute asthma or bronchospasm. • Have a rescue inhaler readily available. • Increased use of rescue inhalers may indicate worsening of asthma. • Seek medical attention if asthma symptoms worsen or remain uncontrolled. • Do not stop corticosteroid therapy unless directed by prescriber. • Treatment may increase risk of new cancers or alter the body's immune response to parasite infections.

ribavirin

rye-ba-**vye**-rin
(Virazole)

BLACK BOX ALERT
Significant teratogenic/embryocidal effects. Hemolytic anemia is significant toxicity, usually occurring within 1–2 wks. May worsen cardiac disease and lead to fatal or nonfatal MI. Inhalation may interfere with safe and effective assisted ventilation. Monotherapy not effective for chronic hepatitis C virus infection.

Do not confuse ribavirin with riboflavin, rifAMPin, or Robaxin.

FIXED-COMBINATION(S)

With interferon alfa-2b (**Rebetron**). Individually packaged.

◆CLASSIFICATION

PHARMACOTHERAPEUTIC: Synthetic nucleoside. **CLINICAL:** Antihepaciviral.

USES

Inhalation: Treatment of respiratory syncytial virus (RSV) infections (esp. in pts with underlying compromising conditions such as chronic lung disorders, congenital heart disease, recent transplant recipients). **Capsule/tablet/oral solution:** Treatment of chronic hepatitis C virus infection in pts with compensated hepatic disease in combination with other medications.

PRECAUTIONS

Contraindications: Hypersensitivity to ribavirin. **Inhalation:** Women who are pregnant or may become pregnant. **Oral formulations:** Hemoglobinopathies (e.g., sickle cell anemia), men whose female partner is pregnant, women of childbearing age who are pregnant or may become pregnant. Concomitant use of didanosine. **Ribasphere, Rebetol Only:** CrCl less than 50 mL/min. **Cautions: Inhalation:** Pts requiring assisted ventilation, COPD, asthma. **PO:** Baseline anemia, cardiac/pulmonary disease, elderly, renal impairment, history of sarcoidosis, psychiatric illness.

ACTION

Inhibits replication of viral RNA, DNA, influenza virus RNA polymerase activity; interferes with expression of messenger RNA. **Therapeutic Effect:** Inhibits viral protein synthesis.

PHARMACOKINETICS

Readily absorbed. Peak concentrations: **Inhalation:** At end of inhalation period. **Capsules:** 3 hrs. **Tablets:** 2 hrs. Protein binding: None. Metabolized in liver and intracellularly. Primarily excreted in urine. **Half-life: Inhalation:** 6.5–11 hrs. **Capsules:** 298 hr at steady state. **Tablets:** 120–170 hrs.

⌛ LIFESPAN CONSIDERATIONS

Pregnancy/Lactation: Contraindicated in pregnancy. Females and males with female partners of reproductive potential must use 2 forms of effective contraception during treatment and for at least 6 mos after discontinuation. Unknown if excreted in breast milk. **Children/Elderly:** No age-related precautions noted.

INTERACTIONS

DRUG: May increase the adverse effects of **didanosine. Zidovudine** may increase adverse effects. **HERBAL:** None significant. **FOOD:** None known. **LAB VALUES:** None significant.

AVAILABILITY (Rx)

Capsules: 200 mg. ***Powder for Solution, Nebulization: (Virazole):*** 6 g. **Solution, Oral:** 40 mg/mL. **Tablet:** 200 mg, 400 mg, 600 mg.

ADMINISTRATION/HANDLING

PO

• Capsules may be taken without regard to food. • Do not break, crush, or open capsules. • Use oral solution in children

5 yrs or younger, those 47 kg or less, or those unable to swallow. • Give capsules with food when combined with peginterferon alfa-2b. • Tablets should be given with food.

Inhalation

◀ALERT▶ May be given via nasal or oral inhalation.

• Solution appears clear, colorless; is stable for 24 hrs at room temperature. • Discard solution for nebulization after 24 hrs. • Discard if discolored or cloudy. • Add 50–100 mL Sterile Water for Injection or Inhalation to 6-g vial. • Transfer to a flask, serving as reservoir for aerosol generator. • Further dilute to final volume of 300 mL, giving solution concentration of 20 mg/mL. • Use only aerosol generator available from manufacturer of drug. • Do not give concomitantly with other drug solutions for nebulization. • Discard reservoir solution when fluid levels are low and at least q24h. • Only experienced personnel should administer drug.

INDICATIONS/ROUTES/DOSAGE

Note: Combination therapy with peginterferon alone is not recommended in HCV guidelines.

Chronic Hepatitis C Virus Infection

PO: ADULTS, ELDERLY WEIGHING MORE THAN 75 KG: 1,200 mg daily in 2 divided doses. **WEIGHING 74 KG OR LESS:** 1,000 mg daily in 2 divided doses. **LOW INITIAL DOSE:** 600 mg/day. May increase as tolerated.

Dosage in Renal Impairment

Capsules/Oral Solution

ADULTS: CrCl less than 50 mL/min: Contraindicated. **CHILDREN: Serum creatinine more than 2 mg/dL:** Discontinue treatment.

Ribasphere Tablets

ADULTS: CrCl less than 50 mL/min: Not recommended.

Dosage in Hepatic Impairment

Contraindicated.

Severe Lower Respiratory Tract Infection Caused by Respiratory Syncytial Virus (RSV)

Inhalation: CHILDREN, INFANTS: Use with Viratek small-particle aerosol generator at concentration of 20 mg/mL (6 g reconstituted with 300 mL Sterile Water for Injection) over 12–18 hrs/day for 3–7 days.

SIDE EFFECTS

Frequent (greater than 10%): Hemolytic anemia, dizziness, headache, fatigue, fever, insomnia, irritability, depression, emotional lability, impaired concentration, alopecia, rash, pruritus, nausea, anorexia, dyspepsia, vomiting, decreased hemoglobin, hemolysis, arthralgia, musculoskeletal pain, dyspnea, sinusitis, flu-like symptoms. **Occasional (10%–1%):** Nervousness, altered taste, weakness.

ADVERSE EFFECTS/ TOXIC REACTIONS

Cardiac arrest, apnea, ventilator dependence, bacterial pneumonia, pneumonia, pneumothorax occur rarely. If treatment exceeds 7 days, anemia may occur.

NURSING CONSIDERATIONS

BASELINE ASSESSMENT

Obtain sputum specimens before giving first dose or at least during first 24 hrs of therapy. Assess respiratory status for baseline. **PO:** Obtain CBC with differential, pretreatment and monthly pregnancy test for women of childbearing age.

INTERVENTION/EVALUATION

Monitor Hgb, Hct, platelets, LFT, I&O, fluid balance carefully. Check hematology reports for anemia due to reticulocytosis when therapy exceeds 7 days. For ventilator-assisted pts, watch for "rainout" in tubing and empty frequently; be alert to impaired ventilation/gas exchange due to drug precipitate. Assess skin for rash. Monitor B/P, respirations; assess lung sounds.

R

PATIENT/FAMILY TEACHING

• Report immediately any difficulty breathing, itching/swelling/redness of eyes, severe abdominal pain, bloody diarrhea, unusual bleeding/bruising. • Female pts should take measures to avoid pregnancy. • Male pts must use condoms during sexual activity.

ribociclib

rye-boe-**sye**-klib
(Kisqali)
Do not confuse ribociclib with palbociclib or riboflavin.

◆CLASSIFICATION

PHARMACOTHERAPEUTIC: Cyclin-dependent kinase inhibitor. **CLINICAL:** Antineoplastic.

USES

Used in combination with an aromatase inhibitor as initial endocrine-based therapy for treatment of postmenopausal women with hormone receptor (HR)–positive, human epidermal growth factor receptor 2 (HER2)–negative advanced or metastatic breast cancer. Treatment of HR-positive, HER2-negative advanced or metastatic breast cancer (in combination with fulvestrant) in pre-/perimenopausal or postmenopausal women as initial endocrine-based therapy.

PRECAUTIONS

Contraindications: Hypersensitivity to ribociclib. **Cautions:** Baseline cytopenias, hepatic impairment. Avoid concomitant use of strong CYP3A inhibitors, strong CYP3A inducers, QTc interval–prolonging medications. Avoid use in pts with or at risk for QTc prolongation (e.g., congenital long QT syndrome, hypokalemia, hypomagnesemia; uncontrolled, significant cardiac disease including MI, HF, unstable angina, bradyarrhythmias).

ACTION

Blocks retinoblastoma protein phosphorylation and prevents progression through cell cycle, resulting in arrest of G_1 phase. **Therapeutic Effect:** Inhibits tumor growth.

PHARMACOKINETICS

Widely distributed. Metabolized extensively in liver. Protein binding: 70%. Peak plasma concentration: 1–4 hrs. Excreted in feces (69%), urine (23%). **Half-life:** 30–55 hrs.

LIFESPAN CONSIDERATIONS

Pregnancy/Lactation: Indicated for postmenopausal women; however, may cause fetal harm/malformations when used during pregnancy. Females of reproductive potential should use effective contraception during treatment and for at least 3 wks after discontinuation. Unknown if distributed in breast milk. Breastfeeding not recommended during treatment and for at least 3 wks after discontinuation. **Children:** Safety and efficacy not established. **Elderly:** No age-related precautions noted.

INTERACTIONS

DRUG: Strong CYP3A inhibitors (e.g., clarithromycin, ketoconazole, ritonavir) may increase concentration/effect. **Strong CYP3A inducers (e.g., carBAMazepine, phenytoin, rifAMPin)** may decrease concentration/effect. **QT interval–prolonging medications (e.g., amiodarone, azithromycin, ceritinib, haloperidol, moxifloxacin)** may increase risk of QT interval prolongation, torsades de pointes. May increase concentration/effect of **aprepitant, bosutinib, budesonide, naloxegol, neratinib, olaparib, pimozide.** May decrease effect of **BCG vaccine.** May increase adverse effects/toxicity of **natalizumab, pimecrolimus, tacrolimus. HERBAL: Echinacea, St. John's wort** may decrease concentration/effect. **FOOD: Grapefruit products** may increase concentration/effect. **LAB VALUES:** May increase serum ALT, AST, bilirubin. May decrease ANC, Hgb, lymphocytes, leukocytes, neutrophils, platelets; serum potassium, phosphate.

AVAILABILITY (Rx)

Tablets: 200 mg. **Blister Pack:** (21 tablets, 42 tablets, 63 tablets).

ADMINISTRATION/HANDLING

PO

• Give without regard to food. Administer tablet whole; do not break, cut, or crush. • Do not give if tablet is cracked, broken, or not intact. • Tablets cannot be chewed. If a dose is missed or vomiting occurs after administration, do not give extra dose. Administer next dose at regularly scheduled time.

INDICATIONS/ROUTES/DOSAGE

Breast Cancer (Advanced or metastatic)

Note: A luteinizing hormone–releasing hormone (LHRH) agonist should be administered to premenopausal and perimenopausal women.

PO: ADULTS, ELDERLY: 600 mg once daily for 21 days, followed by 7 days off treatment of 28-day cycle. Use in combination with an aromatase inhibitor or fulvestrant. Continue until disease progression or unacceptable toxicity.

Dose Reduction Schedule

First reduction: 400 mg/day. **Second reduction:** 200 mg/day. **Unable to tolerate 200 mg/day:** Permanently discontinue.

Dose Modification

Based on Common Terminology Criteria for Adverse Events.

Hepatotoxicity

Note: Defined as hepatotoxicity without total bilirubin greater than 2 times upper limit of normal (ULN). If serum ALT, AST elevation greater than 3 times ULN with total bilirubin greater than 2 times ULN, permanently discontinue.

Grade 1 serum ALT, AST elevation (up to 3 times ULN): No dose adjustment. **Grade 2 serum ALT, AST elevation (greater than 3–5 times ULN) with baseline at less than Grade 2:** Withhold treatment until improved to baseline, then resume at same dose level. If baseline at less than Grade 2, do not withhold treatment. If Grade 2 serum ALT, AST elevation recurs, then resume at reduced dose level. **Grade 3 serum ALT, AST elevation (greater than 5–20 times ULN):** Withhold treatment until improved to baseline, then resume at reduced dose level. If Grade 3 serum ALT, AST elevation recurs, permanently discontinue. **Grade 4 serum ALT, AST elevation (greater than 20 times ULN):** Permanently discontinue.

Hematologic

Grade 1 or 2 neutropenia (ANC 1000 cells/mm³ to less than the lower limit of normal): No dose adjustment. **Grade 3 neutropenia (ANC 500 to less than 1000 cells/mm³:** Withhold treatment until recovery to Grade 2 or less, then resume at same dose level. If Grade 3 neutropenia recurs, withhold treatment until recovery to Grade 2 or less, then resume at reduced dose level. **Grade 3 febrile neutropenia:** Withhold treatment until recovery to Grade 2 or less, then resume at reduced dose level. **Grade 4 neutropenia (ANC less than 500 cells/mm³):** Withhold treatment until recovery to Grade 2 or less, then resume at reduced dose level.

QTc Interval Prolongation

QTc interval prolongation greater than 480 msec: Withhold treatment until resolved to less than 481 msec, then resume at same dose level. If QTc interval prolongation greater than 480 msec recurs, withhold treatment until resolved to less than 481 msec, then resume at reduced dose level. **QTc interval prolongation greater than 500 msec:** Withhold treatment if QTc interval prolongation greater than 500 msec on at least two separate ECGs (within same visit). If QTc interval prolongation resolves to less than 481 msec after withholding treatment, resume at reduced dose level. **QTc interval prolongation greater than 500 msec (or greater**

R

than 60 msec from baseline) with torsades de pointes, polymorphic ventricular tachycardia, unexplained syncope, symptoms of serious arrhythmia: Permanently discontinue.

Other Toxicities

Any other Grade 1 or 2 toxicities: No dose adjustment. **Any other Grade 3 toxicities:** Withhold treatment until resolved to Grade 1 or 0, then resume at same dose level. If Grade 3 toxicities recur, resume at reduced dose level. **Any other CTCAE Grade 4 toxicities:** Permanently discontinue.

Concomitant Use of Strong CYP3A Inhibitors

Reduce initial dose to 400 mg once daily if strong CYP3A inhibitor cannot be discontinued. If CYP3A inhibitor is discontinued, increase ribociclib dose (after at least 5 half-lives of CYP3A inhibitor have elapsed) to the dose used prior to initiating strong CYP3A inhibitor.

Dosage in Renal Impairment

Not specified; use caution.

Dosage in Hepatic Impairment

Mild impairment: No dose adjustment. **Moderate to severe impairment:** Reduce starting dose to 400 mg once daily.

SIDE EFFECTS

Frequent (52%–17%): Nausea, fatigue, diarrhea, alopecia, vomiting, constipation, headache, back pain, decreased appetite, rash. **Occasional (14%–11%):** Pruritus, pyrexia, insomnia, dyspnea, stomatitis, peripheral edema, abdominal pain.

ADVERSE EFFECTS/TOXIC REACTIONS

Myelosuppression (anemia, leukopenia, lymphopenia, neutropenia, thrombocytopenia) is an expected response to therapy, but more severe reactions, including febrile neutropenia, may be life-threatening. CTCAE Grade 3 or 4 neutropenia reported in 60% of pts. Severe hepatotoxicity reported in 10% of pts. QTc interval prolongation, infections including UTI may occur.

NURSING CONSIDERATIONS

BASELINE ASSESSMENT

Obtain ANC, CBC, BMP, LFT, vital signs, weight; pregnancy test in females of reproductive potential. Obtain ECG (note QTc interval). Initiate treatment only in pts with QTc interval less than 450 msec. Question history of cardiac disease, cardiac conduction disorders, hepatic impairment. Receive full medication history including herbal products and screen for interactions. Screen for risk of bleeding, QTc interval prolongation, active infection. Obtain dietary consult. Offer emotional support.

INTERVENTION/EVALUATION

Monitor ANC, CBC for myelosuppression; LFT for hepatotoxicity q2wks for the first 2 cycles, then prior to each subsequent cycle, then as clinically indicated. Monitor BMP, serum phosphate for electrolyte imbalance; consider correcting imbalances, esp. hypokalemia, hypomagnesemia (due to increased risk of cardiac arrhythmias, torsades de pointes). Obtain repeat ECG on day 14 of the first cycle and at the beginning of the second cycle, or more frequently if QTc interval prolongation occurs. Monitor daily pattern of bowel activity, stool consistency. Assess skin for rash, lesions. Monitor weight, I&O.

PATIENT/FAMILY TEACHING

• Treatment may depress your immune system and reduce your ability to fight infection. Report symptoms of infection such as body aches, burning with urination, chills, cough, fatigue, fever. Avoid those with active infection. • Report symptoms of bone marrow depression such as bruising, fatigue, fever, shortness of breath, weight loss;

bleeding easily, bloody urine or stool. • Do not take newly prescribed medications unless approved by the prescriber who originally started treatment. • Report liver problems such as bruising, confusion, amber or dark-colored urine; right upper abdominal pain, yellowing of the skin or eyes; heart arrhythmias (chest pain, difficulty breathing, palpitations, passing out). • Therapy indicated for postmenopausal women; however, birth defects may occur when used during pregnancy. Use effective contraception to avoid pregnancy. Do not breastfeed. • Do not ingest grapefruit products, Seville oranges, starfruit, pomegranate, herbal supplements. • Report planned surgical/dental procedures. • Immediately report bleeding of any kind.

rifAMPin

rif-**am**-pin
(Rifadin, Rofact ✱)
Do not confuse Rifadin with Rifater or Ritalin, or rifAMPin with ribavirin, rifabutin, Rifamate, rifapentine, rifAXIMin, or Ritalin.

FIXED-COMBINATION(S)

Rifamate: rifAMPin/isoniazid (an antitubercular): 300 mg/150 mg. **Rifater:** rifAMPin/isoniazid/pyrazinamide (an antitubercular): 120 mg/50 mg/300 mg.

◆CLASSIFICATION

PHARMACOTHERAPEUTIC: Rifamycin derivative. **CLINICAL:** Antitubercular.

USES

In combination with other antitubercular agents for initial treatment, retreatment of active tuberculosis. Eliminates meningococci from nasopharynx of asymptomatic carriers. **OFF-LABEL:** Prophylaxis of *H. influenzae* type B infection, *Legionella* pneumonia, serious infections caused by *Staphylococcus* spp. (in combination with other agents). Treatment of prosthetic joint infection.

PRECAUTIONS

Contraindications: Concomitant therapy with atazanavir, darunavir, fosamprenavir, saquinavir, ritonavir, tipranavir; hypersensitivity to rifAMPin, other rifamycins. **Cautions:** Hepatic impairment, active or treated alcoholism, porphyria. Concurrent medications associated with hepatotoxicity.

ACTION

Interferes with bacterial RNA synthesis by binding to DNA-dependent RNA polymerase, preventing attachment to DNA, thereby blocking RNA transcription. **Therapeutic Effect:** Bactericidal in susceptible microorganisms.

PHARMACOKINETICS

Widely distributed. Protein binding: 80%. Metabolized in liver. Primarily eliminated by biliary system. Not removed by hemodialysis. **Half-life:** 3–5 hrs (increased in hepatic impairment).

⌛ LIFESPAN CONSIDERATIONS

Pregnancy/Lactation: Crosses placenta. Distributed in breast milk. **Children/Elderly:** No age-related precautions noted.

INTERACTIONS

DRUG: May decrease concentration/effects of **atovaquone, dilTIAZem, disopyramide, edoxaban, esomeprazole, methadone, mycophenolate, omeprazole, oral anticoagulants (e.g., apixaban, warfarin), oral contraceptives, phenytoin, ranolazine, tacrolimus, tenofovir, zolpidem.** **HERBAL:** None significant. **FOOD:** **Food** decreases extent of absorption. **LAB VALUES:** May increase serum alkaline phosphatase, bilirubin, uric acid, ALT, AST.

AVAILABILITY (Rx)

Capsules: 150 mg, 300 mg. **Injection, Powder for Reconstitution:** 600 mg.

ADMINISTRATION/HANDLING

IV

Reconstitution • Reconstitute 600-mg vial with 10 mL Sterile Water for Injection to provide concentration of 60 mg/mL. • Withdraw desired dose and further dilute with 0.9% NaCl or D_5W to concentration not to exceed 6 mg/mL.

Rate of administration • For IV infusion only. Avoid IM, SQ administration. • Avoid extravasation (local irritation, inflammation). • Infuse over 30 min to 3 hrs.

Storage • Reconstituted vial is stable for 24 hrs. • Diluted solution is stable for 4 hrs in D_5W or 24 hrs in 0.9% NaCl.

PO

• Preferably give 1 hr before or 2 hrs following meals with 8 oz of water (may give with food to decrease GI upset; will delay absorption). • For pts unable to swallow capsules, contents may be mixed with applesauce, jelly. • Administer at least 1 hr before antacids, esp. those containing aluminum.

IV INCOMPATIBILITIES

DilTIAZem (Cardizem).

IV COMPATIBILITIES

D_5W if infused within 4 hrs (risk of precipitation beyond this time period).

INDICATIONS/ROUTES/DOSAGE

Tuberculosis

Note: A four-drug regimen (ethambutol, isoniazid, pyrazinamide, rifAMPin) is preferred for initial, empiric treatment.

PO, IV: ADULTS, ELDERLY: 10 mg/kg/day. **Maximum:** 600 mg/day. **CHILDREN:** 10–20 mg/kg/day usually as a single daily dose. **Maximum:** 600 mg/day.

Meningococcal Carrier

PO, IV: ADULTS, ELDERLY: 600 mg twice daily for 2 days. **PO only: CHILDREN 1 MO AND OLDER:** 10 mg/kg/dose q12h for 2 days. **Maximum:** 600 mg/dose. **CHILDREN YOUNGER THAN 1 MO:** 5 mg/kg/dose q12h for 2 days.

Dosage in Renal/Hepatic Impairment

No dose adjustment.

SIDE EFFECTS

Frequent: Red-orange or red-brown discoloration of urine, feces, saliva, skin, sputum, sweat, tears. **Occasional (5%–3%):** Hypersensitivity reaction (flushing, pruritus, rash). **Rare (2%–1%):** Diarrhea, dyspepsia, nausea, oral candida (sore mouth, tongue).

ADVERSE EFFECTS/TOXIC REACTIONS

Hepatotoxicity (risk is increased when rifAMPin is taken with isoniazid), hepatitis, blood dyscrasias, Stevens-Johnson syndrome, antibiotic-associated colitis occur rarely.

NURSING CONSIDERATIONS

BASELINE ASSESSMENT

Obtain CBC, renal function test, LFT. Screen for concomitant medications known to cause hepatotoxicity. Question for hypersensitivity to rifAMPin, rifamycins. Ensure collection of diagnostic specimens.

INTERVENTION/EVALUATION

Assess IV site at least hourly during infusion; restart at another site at the first sign of irritation or inflammation. Monitor LFT, assess for hepatitis: jaundice, anorexia, nausea, vomiting, fatigue, weakness (hold rifAMPin, inform physician at once). Report hypersensitivity reactions promptly: any type of skin eruption, pruritus, flu-like syndrome with high dosage. Monitor daily pattern of bowel activity, stool consistency (potential for antibiotic-associated colitis). Monitor CBC results for blood dyscrasias; be alert for infection (fever, sore throat), unusual bruising/bleeding, unusual fatigue/weakness.

PATIENT/FAMILY TEACHING

• Preferably take on empty stomach with 8 oz of water 1 hr before or 2 hrs after meal (with food if GI upset). • Avoid alcohol. • Do not take any other medications without consulting physician, including antacids; must take rifAMPin at least 1 hr before antacid. • Urine, feces, sputum, sweat, tears may become red-orange; soft contact lenses may be permanently stained. • Report any new symptom immediately such as yellow eyes/skin, fatigue, weakness, nausea/vomiting, sore throat, fever, flu, unusual bruising/bleeding. • If taking oral contraceptives, check with physician (reliability may be affected).

rifAXIMin

rif-**ax**-i-min
(Xifaxan, Zaxine ✦)
Do not confuse rifAXIMin with rifAMPin.

◆CLASSIFICATION

PHARMACOTHERAPEUTIC: Anti-infective. **CLINICAL:** Site-specific antibiotic.

USES

Treatment of traveler's diarrhea caused by noninvasive strains of *E. coli*. Reduction of risk for recurrence of overt hepatic encephalopathy. Treatment of irritable bowel syndrome with diarrhea (IBS-D) in adults. **OFF-LABEL:** Treatment of hepatic encephalopathy. Treatment of *C. difficile*–associated diarrhea.

PRECAUTIONS

Contraindications: Hypersensitivity to rifAXIMin, other rifamycin antibiotics. **Cautions:** Severe hepatic impairment.

ACTION

Inhibits bacterial RNA synthesis by binding to bacterial DNA-dependent RNA polymerase. **Therapeutic Effect:** Bactericidal.

PHARMACOKINETICS

Less than 0.4% absorbed after PO administration. Primarily excreted in feces. **Half-life:** 5.85 hrs.

⌛ LIFESPAN CONSIDERATIONS

Pregnancy/Lactation: Unknown if drug is distributed in breast milk. **Children:** Safety and efficacy not established in pts younger than 12 yrs for traveler's diarrhea; younger than 18 yrs for IBS-D. **Elderly:** No age-related precautions noted.

INTERACTIONS

DRUG: May decrease effect of **BCG (intravesical).** **HERBAL:** None significant. **FOOD:** None known. **LAB VALUES:** None significant.

AVAILABILITY (Rx)

Tablets: 200 mg, 550 mg.

ADMINISTRATION/HANDLING

PO

• Give without regard to food. • Do not break, crush, dissolve, or divide film-coated tablets.

INDICATIONS/ROUTES/DOSAGE

Traveler's Diarrhea

PO: ADULTS, ELDERLY, CHILDREN 12 YRS AND OLDER: 200 mg 3 times/day for 3 days.

Hepatic Encephalopathy

PO: ADULTS, ELDERLY: 550 mg 2 times/day or 400 mg 3 times/day.

IBS-D

PO: ADULTS, ELDERLY: 550 mg 3 times/day for 14 days. May repeat up to 2 times if symptoms recur.

Dosage in Renal/Hepatic Impairment

No dose adjustment.

SIDE EFFECTS

Occasional (11%–5%): Flatulence, headache, abdominal discomfort, rectal tenesmus, defecation urgency, nausea. **Rare (4%–2%):** Constipation, fever, vomiting.

R

ADVERSE EFFECTS/TOXIC REACTIONS

Hypersensitivity reaction, superinfection occur rarely.

NURSING CONSIDERATIONS

BASELINE ASSESSMENT

Check baseline hydration status: skin turgor, mucous membranes for dryness, urinary status. Assess stool frequency, consistency.

INTERVENTION/EVALUATION

Encourage adequate fluid intake. Assess bowel sounds for peristalsis. Monitor daily pattern of bowel activity, stool consistency. Assess for GI disturbances, blood in stool.

PATIENT/FAMILY TEACHING

• Report if diarrhea worsens or if blood occurs in stool, fever develops within 48 hrs.

rimegepant

ri-**me**-je-pant
(Nurtec ODT)
Do not confuse rimegepant with ubrogepant.

◆Classification

PHARMACOTHERAPEUTIC: Calcitonin gene–related peptide (CGRP) receptor antagonist. **CLINICAL:** Antimigraine.

USES

Treatment of migraines with or without aura in adults.

PRECAUTIONS

Contraindications: Hypersensitivity to rimegepant. **Cautions:** Not indicated for prevention of migraine.

ACTION

Exact mechanism of action unknown. Binds to and inhibits calcitonin gene–related peptide (CGRP) receptor. **Therapeutic Effect:** Relieves migraine headache.

PHARMACOKINETICS

Rapidly absorbed. Metabolized in liver. Protein binding: 96%. Peak plasma concentration: 1.5 hrs. Excreted in urine (51%), feces (42%). **Half-life:** 11 hrs.

⌛ LIFESPAN CONSIDERATIONS

Pregnancy/Lactation: Unknown if distributed in breast milk. **Children:** Safety and efficacy not established. **Elderly:** Safety and efficacy not established.

INTERACTIONS

DRUG: **Strong CYP3A4 inhibitors (e.g., clarithromycin, itraconazole, ketoconazole, ritonavir), moderate CYP3A inhibitors (e.g., dilTIAZem, fluconazole, verapamil), P-gp inhibitors (e.g., amiodarone, carvedilol, verapamil)** may increase concentration/effect. **Strong CYP3A4 inducers (e.g., carBAMazepine, phenytoin, rifAMPin), moderate CYP3A inducers (e.g., bosentan, nafcillin)** may decrease concentration/effect. **HERBAL:** None significant. **FOOD:** None known. **LAB VALUES:** None known.

AVAILABILITY (Rx)

Tablets, Orally Disintegrating: 75 mg.

ADMINISTRATION/HANDLING

Orally Disintegrating Tablets

• Do not remove from blister pack until needed. • Peel backing off; do not push tablet through blister pack. • Place tablet on or under tongue; allow to dissolve. Swallow with saliva.

INDICATIONS/ROUTES/DOSAGE

Migraine (with or without aura)

PO: ADULTS: 75 mg once prn. Do not exceed 75 mg in a 24-hr period.

Dose Modification

Concomitant Use of Strong/Moderate CYP3A4 Inhibitors: Avoid concomitant use of strong CYP3A4 inhibitors. Avoid second dose of rimegepant within 48 hrs of concomitant moderate CYP3A4 inhibitors.

Concomitant Use of Strong/Moderate CYP3A4 Inducers: Due to loss of efficacy, avoid concomitant use of strong or moderate CYP3A4 inducers.

Dosage in Renal Impairment

Mild to severe impairment: No dose adjustment.

Dosage in Hepatic Impairment

Mild to moderate impairment: No dose adjustment. **Severe impairment:** Avoid use.

SIDE EFFECTS

Rare (2%): Nausea.

ADVERSE EFFECTS/TOXIC REACTIONS

Hypersensitivity reactions including dyspnea, severe rash reported in less than 1% of pts.

NURSING CONSIDERATIONS

BASELINE ASSESSMENT

Question characteristics of migraine headaches (onset, location, duration, possible precipitating symptoms).

INTERVENTION/EVALUATION

Evaluate for relief of migraine headaches (photophobia, phonophobia, nausea, vomiting, pain, dizziness, fogginess). Monitor for hypersensitivity reactions.

PATIENT/FAMILY TEACHING

• Allergic reactions such as difficulty breathing, severe rash may occur. If allergic reaction occurs, seek immediate medical attention. • There is a high risk of interactions with other medications. Do not take newly prescribed medications unless approved by prescriber who originally started therapy.

ripretinib

ri-**pre**-tin-ib
(Qinlock)

Do not confuse ripretinib with avapritinib, ceritinib, imatinib, regorafenib, rucaparib, ruxolitinib, sunitinib.

◆Classification

PHARMACOTHERAPEUTIC: KIT inhibitor, PDGFR-alpha blocker. Tyrosine kinase inhibitor. **CLINICAL:** Antineoplastic.

USES

Treatment of adults with advanced gastrointestinal stromal tumor (GIST) who have received prior treatment with three or more kinase inhibitors (including imatinib).

PRECAUTIONS

Contraindications: Hypersensitivity to ripretinib. **Cautions:** Baseline hematologic cytopenias, hepatic impairment, dermatologic disease, cardiovascular disease, hypertension, HF; conditions predisposing to infection (e.g., diabetes, immunocompromised, open wounds); recent surgical incision, poorly healed wounds. Do not initiate in pts with uncontrolled hypertension.

ACTION

Inhibits KIT proto-oncogene receptor tyrosine kinase and platelet-derived growth factor receptor A (PDGFRA) kinase signaling, including wild-type, primary, secondary mutations of KIT and PDGFRA. **Therapeutic Effect:** Inhibits tumor growth.

PHARMACOKINETICS

Widely distributed. Metabolized in liver. Protein binding: greater than 99%. Steady state reached in 14 days. Excreted in feces (34%), urine (less than 1%). **Half-life:** 14.8.

R

LIFESPAN CONSIDERATIONS

Pregnancy/Lactation: Avoid pregnancy; may cause fetal harm. Females and males with female partners of reproductive potential must use effective contraception during treatment and for at least 7 days after discontinuation. Unknown if distributed in breast milk. Breastfeeding not recommended during treatment and for at least 7 days after discontinuation. **Males:** May impair fertility. **Children:** Safety and efficacy not established. **Elderly:** Safety and efficacy not established.

INTERACTIONS

DRUG: **Strong CYP3A4 inducers (e.g., carBAMazepine, phenytoin, rifAMPin)** may decrease concentration/effect. **Conivaptan, idelalisib** may increase serum concentration. **HERBAL:** None significant. **FOOD:** None known. **LAB VALUES:** May increase activated partial thromboplastin time (aPTT), INR; serum amylase, ALT, bilirubin, CPK, creatinine, lipase, triglycerides. May decrease serum phosphate, sodium; Hgb, neutrophils, RBCs.

AVAILABILITY (Rx)

Tablets: 50 mg.

ADMINISTRATION/HANDLING

PO

• Give without regard to food. • Administer tablets whole; do not break, crush, or divide. Tablet cannot be chewed. • If vomiting occurs after administration, give next dose at regularly scheduled time (do not give additional dose). • If a dose is missed, do not give if more than 8 hrs have passed since the missed scheduled dose.

INDICATIONS/ROUTES/DOSAGE

GI Stromal Tumor

PO: ADULTS: 150 mg once daily. Continue until disease progression or unacceptable toxicity.

Dose Reduction Schedule for Adverse Events.

First dose reduction: 100 mg once daily. **Unable to tolerate 100-mg dose:** Permanently discontinue.

Dose Modification

Based on Common Terminology Criteria for Adverse Events (CTCAE).

Arthralgia/Myalgia

Grade 2 arthralgia/myalgia: Withhold treatment until improved to grade 1 or baseline. If improved within 7 days, resume at same dose or consider reduced dose. Consider re-escalating if maintained at grade 1 or baseline for at least 28 days. If recurs, withhold treatment until improved to grade 1 or baseline, then resume at reduced dose regardless of the time symptoms improved.
Grade 3 arthralgia/myalgia: Withhold treatment for at least 7 days (or until improved to grade 1 or baseline), then resume at reduced dose. Consider re-escalating if maintained at grade 1 or baseline for at least 28 days.

Hypertension

Grade 3 hypertension: If symptomatic, withhold until symptoms resolve and B/P has improved. If B/P has improved to grade 1 or baseline, resume at same dose or consider reduced dose. If recurs, withhold treatment until symptoms resolve and B/P has improved, then resume at reduced dose.
Grade 4 hypertension: Permanently discontinue.

Left Ventricular Dysfunction

Grade 3 or 4 left ventricular dysfunction: Permanently discontinue.

Palmar-Plantar Erythrodysesthesia Syndrome (PPES)

Grade 2 PPES: Withhold treatment until improved to grade 1 or baseline. If improved within 7 days, resume at same dose or consider reduced dose. Consider re-escalating if maintained at grade 1 or baseline for at least 28 days. If recurs, withhold treatment until improved to grade 1 or baseline, then resume at reduced dose regardless of the time symptoms improved. **Grade 3 PPES:** Withhold treatment for at least 7 days (or until improved to grade 1 or baseline), then resume at reduced dose. Consider re-escalating if maintained at grade 1 or baseline for at least 28 days.

Other Toxicities

Other grade 3 or 4 toxicities: Withhold treatment up to a maximum of 28 days until improved to grade 1 or baseline, then resume at same dose or consider reduced dose. Consider re-escalating if maintained at grade 1 or baseline for at least 28 days. If recurs, permanently discontinue.

Dosage in Renal Impairment

Mild to moderate impairment: No dose adjustment. **Severe impairment:** Not specified; use caution.

Dosage in Hepatic Impairment

Mild impairment: No dose adjustment. **Moderate to severe impairment:** Not specified; use caution.

SIDE EFFECTS

Frequent (52%–19%): Alopecia, fatigue, nausea, abdominal pain, constipation, myalgia, diarrhea, decreased appetite, vomiting, headache, arthralgia, decreased weight. **Occasional (17%–7%):** Peripheral edema, muscle spasm, asthenia, dyspnea, dry skin, pruritus, stomatitis, agitation, hyperesthesia.

ADVERSE EFFECTS/TOXIC REACTIONS

Myelosuppression (anemia, neutropenia) is an expected response to therapy. PPES, a chemotherapy-induced skin condition that presents with redness, swelling, numbness, skin sloughing of the hands and feet, reported in 21% of pts. New primary malignancies including cutaneous squamous cell carcinoma, keratoacanthoma were reported. Grade 1–3 hypertension reported in 14% of pts. Cardiac dysfunction (cardiac failure, acute left ventricular failure, diastolic dysfunction, ventricular hypertrophy) reported in 2% of pts. Other cardiac events may include cardiac arrest, acute coronary syndrome, MI. Impaired wound healing may occur.

NURSING CONSIDERATIONS

BASELINE ASSESSMENT

Obtain CBC; B/P; pregnancy test in females of reproductive potential. Verify use of effective contraception. Question history of cardiovascular disease, hypertension, HF, dermatologic disease, hepatic impairment. Assess LVEF by echocardiogram. Conduct dermatologic exam; assess for open wounds, lesions, surgical incisions. Question for recent surgeries, invasive dental procedures. Screen for active infection. Receive full medication history and screen for interactions. Offer emotional support.

INTERVENTION/EVALUATION

Monitor CBC, B/P throughout therapy. Assess for drug toxicities if discontinuation or dose reduction of concomitant CYP3A inhibitor is unavoidable. Monitor for infection (cough, fatigue, fever). If serious infection, sepsis occurs, initiate appropriate antimicrobial therapy. Assess skin for dermal toxicities, PPES. Monitor skin for impaired wound healing, new skin lesions, rash, sloughing. Assess LVEF by echocardiogram at regular intervals. Monitor for symptoms of HF (dyspnea, edema, palpitations, syncope). Monitor daily pattern of bowel activity, stool consistency.

PATIENT/FAMILY TEACHING

• Treatment may depress your immune system response and reduce your ability to fight infection. Report symptoms of infection such as body aches, chills, cough, fatigue, fever. Avoid those with active infection. • Report symptoms of bone marrow depression such as

R

bruising, fatigue, fever, shortness of breath, weight loss; bleeding easily, bloody urine or stool. • Report liver problems (abdominal pain, bruising, clay-colored stool, dark or amber-colored urine, yellowing of the skin or eyes), toxic skin reactions (e.g., itching, peeling, rash, redness, swelling). • Treatment may reduce the heart's ability to pump effectively; expect routine echocardiograms. Report difficulty breathing, palpitations, swelling of extremities. • High blood pressure may occur; expect frequent blood pressure monitoring. • Notify physician before any planned surgeries/invasive dental procedures. • Use effective contraception to avoid pregnancy. Do not breastfeed. • Do not take newly prescribed medications unless approved by prescriber who originally started treatment. • Treatment may cause new cancers.

risankizumab-rzaa

ris-an-**kiz**-ue-mab-rzaa
(Skyrizi)
Do not confuse risankizumab with ixekizumab.

◆CLASSIFICATION

PHARMACOTHERAPEUTIC: Interleukin-23 antagonist. Monoclonal antibody. **CLINICAL:** Antipsoriatic agent.

USES

Treatment of moderate to severe plaque psoriasis in adults who are candidates for systemic therapy or phototherapy.

PRECAUTIONS

Contraindications: Hypersensitivity to risankizumab. **Cautions:** Conditions predisposing to infection (e.g., diabetes, immunocompromised pts, renal failure, open wounds), prior exposure to tuberculosis or use in pts who reside or travel to areas where TB is endemic. Avoid use during active infection. Concomitant use of live vaccines not recommended.

ACTION

Selectively binds to p19 subunit of interleukin-23 (IL-23) and inhibits interaction with IL-23 receptor. IL-23 is a cytokine that is involved in inflammatory and immune response. **Therapeutic Effect:** Alters biologic immune response; reduces inflammation of psoriatic lesions.

PHARMACOKINETICS

Widely distributed. Degraded into small peptides and amino acids via catabolic pathway. Peak plasma concentration: 3–14 days. Steady state reached in 16 wks. **Half-life:** 28 days.

⌛ LIFESPAN CONSIDERATIONS

Pregnancy/Lactation: Unknown if distributed in breast milk. However, human immunoglobulin G (IgG) is present in breast milk and is known to cross the placenta. **Children:** Safety and efficacy not established. **Elderly:** No age-related precautions noted.

INTERACTIONS

DRUG: May decrease therapeutic effects/increase adverse effects of **live vaccines. Belimumab, infliximab** may increase immunosuppressive effect. **HERBAL:** None significant. **FOOD:** None known. **LAB VALUES:** None known.

AVAILABILITY (Rx)

Injection Solution, Prefilled Syringe: 75 mg/0.83 mL.

ADMINISTRATION/HANDLING

SQ

Preparation • Remove prefilled syringe from refrigerator and allow solution to warm to room temperature (approx. 15–30 min) with needle cap intact. • Visually inspect for particulate matter or discoloration. Solution should appear clear to slightly opalescent, colorless to slightly yellow in color. Do not use if solution is cloudy or discolored or if visible particles are observed.

Administration • Insert needle subcutaneously into outer thigh or abdomen and inject solution. Injections to the outer arms may only be performed by a healthcare professional. • Do not inject into areas of active skin disease or injury such as sunburns, skin rashes, inflammation, skin infections, or active psoriasis. • Rotate injection sites. • Do not administer IV or intramuscularly. • If a dose is missed, administer as soon as possible, then give next dose at regularly scheduled time.

Storage • Refrigerate prefilled syringes in original carton until time of use. • Protect from light. • Do not shake. • Do not freeze or expose to heating sources.

INDICATIONS/ROUTES/DOSAGE

Plaque Psoriasis

SQ: ADULTS, ELDERLY: 150 mg (two 75-mg injections) at wk 0 and wk 4, then q12wks thereafter.

Dosage in Renal Impairment

Mild to severe impairment: Not specified; use caution.

Dosage in Hepatic Impairment

Mild to severe impairment: Not specified; use caution.

SIDE EFFECTS

Rare (4%–2%): Headache, tension headache, sinus headache, fatigue, asthenia, injection site reactions (bruising, erythema, extravasation, hematoma, hemorrhage, infection, inflammation, irritation, pain, pruritus, swelling, warmth).

ADVERSE EFFECTS/TOXIC REACTIONS

Upper respiratory tract infections (bacterial, viral, unspecified) including nasopharyngitis, pharyngitis, rhinitis, sinusitis, tonsillitis reported in 13% of pts. Tinea infections reported in 1% of pts. Serious infections including cellulitis, herpes zoster, osteomyelitis, sepsis occurred in less than 1% of pts. Immunogenicity (auto-risankizumab antibodies) reported in 24% of pts.

NURSING CONSIDERATIONS

BASELINE ASSESSMENT

Consider completion of age-appropriate immunizations prior to initiation. Pts should be evaluated for active tuberculosis and tested for latent infection prior to initiation and periodically during therapy. Induration of 5 mm or greater with tuberculin skin testing should be considered a positive test result when assessing if treatment for latent tuberculosis is necessary. Screen for active infection or chronic infections. Conduct dermatologic exam; record characteristics of psoriatic lesions. Assess pt's willingness to self-inject medication. Teach proper injection techniques.

INTERVENTION/EVALUATION

Assess skin for improvement of lesions. Monitor for symptoms of tuberculosis (cough, fatigue, hemoptysis, nocturnal sweating, weight loss), including those who tested negative for latent tuberculosis infection prior to initiating therapy. Interrupt or discontinue treatment if serious infection, opportunistic infection, or sepsis occurs.

PATIENT/FAMILY TEACHING

• Treatment may depress your immune system and reduce your ability to fight infection. Report symptoms of infection such as body aches, burning with urination, chills, cough, fatigue, fever; fungal infections. Avoid those with active infection. • Do not receive live vaccines. • Expect frequent tuberculosis screening. Report symptoms of tuberculosis such as cough, fatigue, night sweats, weight loss, or coughing up blood. • Report travel plans to possible endemic areas.

risedronate

ris-**ed**-roe-nate
(Actonel, Atelvia)
Do not confuse Actonel with Actos, or risedronate with alendronate.

FIXED-COMBINATION(S)

Actonel with Calcium: risedronate/calcium: 35 mg/6 × 500 mg.

◆CLASSIFICATION

PHARMACOTHERAPEUTIC: Bisphosphonate. **CLINICAL:** Calcium regulator.

USES

Actonel: Treatment of Paget's disease of bone. Treatment/prevention of osteoporosis in postmenopausal women, glucocorticoid-induced osteoporosis (daily dose 7.5 mg predniSONE or greater). Treatment of osteoporosis in men. **Atelvia:** Treatment of osteoporosis in postmenopausal women.

PRECAUTIONS

Contraindications: Hypersensitivity to risedronate, other bisphosphonates (e.g., alendronate); inability to stand or sit upright for at least 30 min; abnormalities of esophagus that delay esophageal emptying; hypocalcemia. **Cautions:** GI diseases (duodenitis, dysphagia, esophagitis, gastritis, ulcers [drug may exacerbate these conditions]), severe renal impairment (CrCl less than 30 mL/min).

ACTION

Inhibits bone resorption by action on osteoclasts or osteoclast precursors. **Therapeutic Effect: Osteoporosis:** Decreases bone resorption (indirectly increases bone mineral density). **Paget's Disease:** Inhibition of bone resorption causes a decrease (but more normal architecture) in bone formation.

PHARMACOKINETICS

Rapidly absorbed. Bioavailability decreased when administered with food. Protein binding: 24%. Not metabolized. Excreted unchanged in urine, feces. Not removed by hemodialysis. **Half-life:** 1.5 hrs (initial); 480 hrs (terminal).

LIFESPAN CONSIDERATIONS

Pregnancy/Lactation: Unknown if distributed in breast milk. **Children:** Not indicated for use in this pt population. **Elderly:** No age-related precautions noted.

INTERACTIONS

DRUG: Antacids containing aluminum, calcium, magnesium; vitamin D may decrease absorption (avoid administration within 30 min of **risedronate**). **Histamine H_2 receptor antagonists (e.g., famotidine, ranitidine), proton pump inhibitors (e.g., omeprazole, pantoprazole)** may decrease concentration/effect. **HERBAL:** None significant. **FOOD:** None known. **LAB VALUES:** None significant.

AVAILABILITY (Rx)

Tablets: ***(Actonel):*** 5 mg, 30 mg, 35 mg, 150 mg. **Tablets, Delayed-Release:** ***(Atelvia):*** 35 mg.

ADMINISTRATION/HANDLING

PO

Actonel: • Administer 30–60 min before any food, drink, other oral medications to avoid interference with absorption. • Give on empty stomach with full glass of plain water (not mineral water). • Pt must avoid lying down for at least 30 min after swallowing tablet (assists with delivery to stomach, reduces risk of esophageal irritation). • Give whole; do not break, crush, dissolve, or divide tablet. • **Atelvia:** Take in morning immediately following breakfast with at least 4 oz water. • Remain upright for 30 min after taking dose.

INDICATIONS/ROUTES/DOSAGE

Paget's Disease

PO: ***(Actonel):*** **ADULTS, ELDERLY:** 30 mg/day for 2 mos. Retreatment may occur after 2-mo post-treatment observation period.

Prophylaxis, Treatment of Postmenopausal Osteoporosis

PO: ***(Actonel):*** **ADULTS, ELDERLY:** 5 mg/day or 35 mg once wkly or 150 mg once monthly.

Treatment of Postmenopausal Osteoporosis

PO: ***(Atelvia):*** **ADULTS, ELDERLY:** 35 mg once wkly.

Treatment of Male Osteoporosis

PO: ***(Actonel):*** **ADULTS, ELDERLY:** 35 mg once wkly.

Treatment and Prevention of Glucocorticoid-Induced Osteoporosis

PO: ***(Actonel):*** **ADULTS, ELDERLY:** 5 mg/day.

Dosage in Renal Impairment

Not recommended with CrCl less than 30 mL/min.

Dosage in Hepatic Impairment

No dose adjustment.

SIDE EFFECTS

Frequent (30%): Arthralgia. **Occasional (12%–8%):** Rash, diarrhea, constipation, nausea, abdominal pain, dyspepsia, flu-like symptoms, peripheral edema. **Rare (5%–3%):** Bone pain, sinusitis, asthenia, dry eye, tinnitus.

ADVERSE EFFECTS/TOXIC REACTIONS

Overdose produces hypocalcemia, hypophosphatemia, significant GI disturbances, osteonecrosis of jaw.

NURSING CONSIDERATIONS

BASELINE ASSESSMENT

Assess symptoms of Paget's disease (bone pain, bone deformities). Hypocalcemia, vitamin D deficiency must be corrected before therapy begins. Obtain baseline laboratory studies, esp. serum electrolytes, renal function. Verify pt is able to stand or sit upright for at least 30 min.

INTERVENTION/EVALUATION

Check serum electrolytes (esp. calcium, ionized calcium, phosphorus, alkaline phosphatase levels). Monitor I&O, BUN, creatinine in pts with renal impairment.

PATIENT/FAMILY TEACHING

• Expected benefits occur only when medication is taken with full glass (6–8 oz) of plain water first thing in the morning and at least 30 min before first food, beverage, medication of the day. Any other beverage (mineral water, orange juice, coffee) significantly reduces absorption of medication. • Do not lie down for at least 30 min after taking medication (potentiates delivery to stomach, reduces risk of esophageal irritation). • Report swallowing difficulties, pain when swallowing, chest pain, new/worsening heartburn. • Consider weight-bearing exercises; modify behavioral factors (cigarette smoking, alcohol consumption). • Report jaw pain, incapacitating bone, joint, or muscle pain.

risperiDONE

ris-**per**-i-done
(Perseris, RisperDAL, RisperDAL Consta)

BLACK BOX ALERT Increased risk of mortality in elderly pts with dementia-related psychosis, mainly due to pneumonia, HF.

Do not confuse RisperDAL with Restoril.

◆CLASSIFICATION

PHARMACOTHERAPEUTIC: Benzisoxazole derivative. **CLINICAL:** Second-generation (atypical) antipsychotic. Antimanic agent.

USES

Oral: Treatment of schizophrenia, irritability/aggression associated with autistic disease in children. Treatment of acute mania associated with bipolar disorder (monotherapy in children and adults; in combination with lithium or valproate in adults). **IM:** Management of schizophrenia, maintenance treatment of bipolar 1 disorder (monotherapy or in combination with lithium or valproate in adults). **OFF-LABEL:** Tourette's syndrome. Posttraumatic stress syndrome. Major depressive disorder.

PRECAUTIONS

Contraindications: Hypersensitivity to risperiDONE. **Cautions:** Renal/hepatic impairment, seizure disorder, cardiac disease, recent MI, breast cancer or other prolactin-dependent tumors, Parkinson's disease, elderly; pts at risk for aspiration, orthostatic hypotension; diabetes, decreased GI motility, urinary retention, BPH, xerostomia, visual problems, pts exposed to temperature extremes, preexisting myelosuppression, narrow-angle glaucoma; history of suicidal ideation and behavior.

ACTION

May antagonize DOPamine, serotonin receptors in both CNS and periphery. **Therapeutic Effect:** Suppresses psychotic behavior.

PHARMACOKINETICS

Widely distributed. Protein binding: 90%. Metabolized in liver. Primarily excreted in urine. **Half-life:** 3–20 hrs; metabolite, 21–30 hrs (increased in elderly). **Injection:** 3–6 days.

LIFESPAN CONSIDERATIONS

Pregnancy/Lactation: Unknown if drug crosses placenta or is distributed in breast milk. Breastfeeding not recommended. **Children:** Safety and efficacy not established in children younger than 13 yrs for schizophrenia, 10 yrs for bipolar mania, and 5 yrs for autistic disorder. **Elderly:** More susceptible to postural hypotension. Age-related renal/hepatic impairment may require dosage adjustment.

INTERACTIONS

DRUG: Alcohol, CNS depressants (e.g., LORazepam, morphine, zolpidem) may increase CNS depression. **Strong CYP3A4 inducers (e.g., carBAMazepine, phenytoin, rifAMPin)** may decrease concentration/effect. **Anticholinergics (e.g., aclidinium, ipratropium, tiotropium, umeclidinium)** may increase anticholinergic effect. **HERBAL: Herbals with sedative properties (e.g., chamomile, kava kava, valerian)** may increase CNS depression. **FOOD:** None known. **LAB VALUES:** May increase serum prolactin, glucose, AST, ALT. May cause ECG changes.

AVAILABILITY (Rx)

Injection, Powder for Reconstitution: ***(RisperDAL Consta):*** 12.5 mg, 25 mg, 37.5 mg, 50 mg. **Oral Solution:** 1 mg/mL. **Syringe, Prefilled:** 90 mg, 120 mg. **Tablets:** 0.25 mg, 0.5 mg, 1 mg, 2 mg, 3 mg, 4 mg.

Tablets, Orally Disintegrating: 0.25 mg, 0.5 mg, 1 mg, 2 mg, 3 mg, 4 mg.

ADMINISTRATION/HANDLING

◀ALERT▶ Do not administer via IV route.

IM

Reconstitution • Use only diluent and needle supplied in dose pack. • Prepare suspension according to manufacturer's directions. • May be given up to 6 hrs after reconstitution, but immediate administration is recommended. • If 2 min pass between reconstitution and injection, shake upright vial vigorously back and forth to resuspend solution.

Rate of administration • Inject IM into upper outer quadrant of gluteus maximus or into deltoid muscle in upper arm.

Storage • Store at room temperature.

PO

• Give without regard to food. • May mix oral solution with water, coffee, orange juice, low-fat milk. Do not mix with cola, tea.

Orally Disintegrating Tablet

• Remove from blister pack immediately before administration. • Using gloves, place immediately on tongue. • Tablet dissolves in seconds. • Pt may swallow with or without liquid. • Do not split or chew.

SQ

Insert needle subcutaneously into abdomen only and inject solution. • Do not inject into areas of active skin disease or injury such as sunburns, skin rashes, inflammation, skin infections, or active psoriasis. • Rotate injection sites. • Do not rub injection site.

INDICATIONS/ROUTES/DOSAGE

Schizophrenia

PO: ADULTS: Initially, 1–2 mg/day as single or 2 divided doses. May increase gradually (1–2 mg/day at intervals of at least 24 hrs). Usual dosage range: 2–6 mg/day. **Usual maximum:** 6–8 mg/day. **ELDERLY:** Initially, 0.5 mg twice daily. May increase slowly at increments of no more than 0.5 mg twice daily. **CHILDREN 13–17 YRS:** Initially, 0.5 mg/day (as single daily dose). May increase by 0.5–1 mg/day at intervals of greater than 24 hrs to recommended dose of 3 mg/day. **IM: ADULTS, ELDERLY:** Initially, 25 mg q2wks. May increase based on response and tolerability in increments of 12.5–25 mg q4wks. **Maximum:** 50 mg q2wks. Dosage adjustments should not be made more frequently than every 4 wks.
SQ: ADULTS, ELDERLY: 90–120 mg once monthly.

Bipolar Mania

PO: ADULTS: Initially, 1–3 mg in 1 or 2 divided doses. May increase by 1 mg/day at 24-hr intervals. Usual dose: 4–6 mg/day. **ELDERLY:** Initially, 0.5 mg twice daily. Titrate slowly.
PO: CHILDREN 10–17 YRS: Initially, 0.5 mg/day. May increase by 0.5–1 mg/day at intervals of greater than 24 hrs to recommended dose of 2.5 mg/day. **IM: ADULTS, ELDERLY:** 25 mg q2wks. May increase dose in increments of 12.5 mg no sooner than 4 wks. **Maximum:** 50 mg q2wks.

Autism

CHILDREN 5 YRS AND OLDER WEIGHING MORE THAN 19 KG: Initially, 0.5 mg/day. May increase to 1 mg after 4 days. May further increase dose by 0.5 mg/day in greater than 2-wk intervals. Range: 0.5–3 mg/day. **CHILDREN 5 YRS AND OLDER WEIGHING 15–19 KG:** Initially, 0.25 mg/day. May increase to 0.5 mg/day after 4 days. May further increase dose by 0.25 mg/day in greater than 2-wk intervals. Range: 0.5–3 mg/day.

Dosage in Renal/Hepatic Impairment

Mild to moderate impairment: No dose adjustment. **Severe impairment:** Initial dosage for adults, elderly pts is 0.5 mg twice daily. Dosage is titrated slowly to desired effect.

SIDE EFFECTS

Frequent (26%–13%): Agitation, anxiety, insomnia, headache, constipation. **Occasional (10%–4%):** Dyspepsia, rhinitis, drowsiness, dizziness, nausea, vomiting, rash, abdominal pain, dry skin, tachycardia. **Rare (3%–2%):** Visual disturbances, fever, back pain, pharyngitis, cough, arthralgia, angina, aggressive behavior, orthostatic hypotension, breast swelling.

ADVERSE EFFECTS/TOXIC REACTIONS

Rare reactions include tardive dyskinesia (characterized by tongue protrusion, puffing of the cheeks, chewing or puckering of mouth), neuroleptic malignant syndrome (hyperpyrexia, muscle rigidity, altered mental status, irregular pulse or B/P, tachycardia, diaphoresis, cardiac arrhythmias, rhabdomyolysis, acute renal failure). Hyperglycemia, life-threatening events such as ketoacidosis and hyperosmolar coma, death have been reported.

NURSING CONSIDERATIONS

BASELINE ASSESSMENT

Renal function test, LFT should be performed before therapy begins. Assess behavior, appearance, emotional status, response to environment, speech pattern, thought content, baseline weight. Obtain fasting serum glucose, CBC. Question history of suicidal ideation and behavior.

R

INTERVENTION/EVALUATION

Monitor B/P, heart rate, weight, LFT, ECG. Monitor for fine tongue movement (may be first sign of tardive dyskinesia, which may be irreversible). Monitor for suicidal ideation. Assess for therapeutic response (greater interest in surroundings, improved self-care, increased ability to concentrate, relaxed facial expression). Monitor for potential neuroleptic malignant syndrome: fever, muscle rigidity, irregular B/P or pulse, altered mental status. Monitor fasting serum glucose periodically during therapy. Diligently screen for suicidal ideation and behavior; new onset or worsening of anxiety, depression, mood disorder.

PATIENT/FAMILY TEACHING

• Seek immediate medical attention if thoughts of suicide, new onset or worsening of anxiety, depression, or changes in mood occur. • Avoid tasks that may require alertness, motor skills until response to drug is established (may cause dizziness/drowsiness). • Avoid alcohol. • Go from lying to standing slowly. • Report trembling in fingers, altered gait, unusual muscular/skeletal movements, palpitations, severe dizziness/fainting, swelling/pain in breasts, visual changes, rash, difficulty breathing.

R

riTUXimab

TOP 100 HIGH ALERT

ri-**tux**-i-mab
(Rituxan, Rituxan Hycela, Ruxience, Truxima)

■ **BLACK BOX ALERT** ■ Profound, occasionally fatal infusion-related reactions reported during first 30–120 min of first infusion. Tumor lysis syndrome leading to acute renal failure may occur 12–24 hrs following first dose. Severe, sometimes fatal, mucocutaneous reactions resulting in progressive multifocal leukoencephalopathy (PML) and death reported. Test all pts for hepatitis B virus (HBV) infection prior to initiation. HBV reactivation may cause fulminant hepatitis, hepatic failure, and death.

Do not confuse Rituxan with Remicade, or riTUXimab with bevacizumab, inFLIXimab, brentuximab, obinutuzumab, ofatumumab, ramucirumab, ruxolitinib.

◆CLASSIFICATION

PHARMACOTHERAPEUTIC: Anti-CD20 monoclonal antibody. **CLINICAL:** Disease-modifying antirheumatic drug (DMARD), antineoplastic, immunosuppressant.

USES

RiTUXimab: Treatment of CD20-positive non-Hodgkin's lymphomas (NHL): relapsed or refractory, low-grade, or follicular B-cell NHL; follicular B-cell NHL (previously untreated); nonprogressive, low-grade B-cell NHL; diffuse large B-cell NHL, previously untreated. Treatment of CD20-positive chronic lymphocytic leukemia (CLL), in combination with fludarabine and cyclophosphamide (FC). Treatment of adults with moderate to severe active rheumatoid arthritis (RA), in combination with methotrexate, who have had an inadequate response to one or more TNF antagonists. Treatment of granulomatosis with polyangiitis (GPA) (Wegener's granulomatosis) and microscopic polyangiitis (MPA). Treatment of moderate to severe pemphigus vulgaris. **OFF-LABEL:** Treatment of autoimmune hemolytic anemia, chronic immune thrombocytopenic purpura (ITP), systemic autoimmune disease (other than rheumatoid arthritis), Burkitt's lymphoma, CNS lymphoma, Hodgkin's lymphoma. **Rituxan Hycela:** Treatment of adults with relapsed or refractory follicular lymphoma as a single agent; previously untreated follicular lymphoma, in combination with first-line chemotherapy and, in pts achieving a complete or partial response to rituximab in combination with chemotherapy, as a single agent; nonprogressing (including stable disease) follicular lymphoma as a single agent after first-line cyclophosphamide, vincristine and predniSONE chemotherapy. Treatment of adults with diffuse large B-cell lymphoma in adults (previous untreated) in combination with cyclophosphamide, doxorubicin, vincristine, predniSONE, or other anthracycline-based chemotherapy regimens. Treatment of CLL, in combination with fludarabine and cyclophosphamide (previously untreated and previously treated CLL). Limitations: Only indicated in pts who have had at least one full dose of intravenous rituximab. Not indicated for treatment of nonmalignant conditions.

PRECAUTIONS

Contraindications: Hypersensitivity to riTUXimab. **Cautions:** Baseline cytopenias, active infection, conditions predisposing to infection (e.g., diabetes, renal failure, immunocompromised pts, open wounds); pts at risk for tumor lysis syndrome (high tumor burden), cardiac disease, elderly, pulmonary disease, renal impairment, hepatitis B virus (HBV) infection, hepatitis C virus (HCV) infection; pts at risk for GI perforation (Crohn's disease, diverticulitis, GI tract malignancies, peptic ulcers, peritoneal malignancies). Avoid administration of live or live attenuated vaccines during treatment and after discontinuation until B cells are no longer depleted.

ACTION

Binds to CD20, the antigen found on surface of B lymphocytes. Activates B-cell cytotoxicity. B cells may also play a role in development/progression of RA. Hyaluronidase increases the absorption rate of rituximab by increasing permeability of SQ tissue. **Therapeutic Effect:** Produces cytotoxicity, reduces tumor size. Signs/symptoms of rheumatoid arthritis are reduced; structural damage delayed.

PHARMACOKINETICS

Rapidly depletes B cells. **Half-life:** 59.8 hrs after first infusion, 174 hrs after fourth infusion.

LIFESPAN CONSIDERATIONS

Pregnancy/Lactation: May cause fetal harm due to fetal B-cell depletion and lymphocytopenia in neonates. Unknown if distributed in breast milk. Females of reproductive potential should use effective contraception during treatment and for at least 12 mos after discontinuation. Breastfeeding not recommended during treatment and for at least 6 mos after discontinuation. **Children:** Safety and efficacy not established. **Elderly:** Increased risk of cardiac/pulmonary adverse reactions.

INTERACTIONS

DRUG: **Denosumab, pimecrolimus, tacrolimus** may increase risk of adverse effects. May increase toxic effects of **abatacept, belimumab, clozapine, leflunomide, natalizumab. Roflumilast** may increase immunosuppressive effect. May increase immunosuppressive effect of **fingolimod**. May decrease concentration/effect of **nivolumab, sipuleucel-T. Trastuzumab** may increase neutropenic effect. May decrease therapeutic effect; increase risk of adverse effect of **live vaccines.** **HERBAL:** **Echinacea** may decrease therapeutic effect. **FOOD:** None known. **LAB VALUES:** May increase serum creatinine, glucose; LDH. May decrease Hgb, Hct, leukocytes, lymphocytes, neutrophils, platelets, RBCs; B-cell counts, immunoglobulin concentrations. May diminish diagnostic effect of *Coccidioides immitis* skin test.

AVAILABILITY (Rx)

Injection Solution, IV: 10 mg/mL (10 mL, 50 mL). **Injection Solution, SQ:** ***(Rituxan Hycela):*** 1,400 mg/23,400 units, 1,600 mg/26,800 units.

ADMINISTRATION/HANDLING

IV

◀ALERT▶ Do not give by IV push or bolus. Must be administered by a health care professional who is experienced in management of severe infusion reactions.

R

Reconstitution • Dilute with 0.9% NaCl or D_5W to provide final concentration of 1–4 mg/mL in infusion bag.
Rate of administration • Initially infuse at rate of 50 mg/hr. If no hypersensitivity or infusion-related reaction, may increase infusion rate in 50 mg/hr increments q30min to maximum 400 mg/hr. • Subsequent infusion can be given at 100 mg/hr and increased by 100 mg/hr increments q30min to maximum 400 mg/hr.
Storage • Refrigerate vials. • Diluted solution is stable for 24 hrs if refrigerated or at room temperature.

SQ
Preparation • Visually inspect for particulate matter or discoloration. Solution should appear clear to opalescent, colorless to slightly yellow in color. Do not use if solution is cloudy, discolored, or if visible particles are observed.
Administration • For 1,400 mg/23,400 unit dose (11.7 mL), insert needle subcutaneously into abdomen and inject solution over 5 min. • For 1,600 mg/26,800 unit dose (13.4 mL), insert needle subcutaneously into abdomen and inject solution over 7 min. • Do not inject into areas of active skin disease or injury such as sunburns, skin rashes, inflammation, skin infections, or active psoriasis. • If administration is interrupted, continue administering at the same site (or at different site) but only in the SQ abdomen. • Do not administer IV or intramuscular. • Rotate injection sites.
Storage • Refrigerate unused vials until time of use. • Protect from light. • Do not freeze or expose to heating sources. • Once transferred to syringe, may refrigerate for up to 48 hrs or store at room temperature for up to 8 hrs.

IV INCOMPATIBILITIES

Do not mix with any other medications.

INDICATIONS/ROUTES/DOSAGE

NHL (Relapsed/refractory, low-grade or follicular CD20-positive B-cell)
IV: ADULTS: 375 mg/m^2 wkly for 4 or 8 doses.
SQ: ADULTS: 1,400 mg/23,400 units once wkly for 3 or 7 wks following full dose of IV rituximab at wk 1 (e.g., 4 or 8 wks total). **ADULTS (RETREATMENT):** 1,400 mg/23,400 units once wkly for 3 wks following full dose of IV rituximab at wk 1 (e.g., 4 wks total).

NHL (Diffuse large B-cell)
IV: ADULTS: 375 mg/m^2 on day 1 of each cycle up to 8 doses.
SQ: ADULTS: 1,400 mg/23,400 units on day 1 of cycles 2–8 of CHOP chemotherapy for up to 7 cycles following full dose of IV rituximab at day 1, cycle 1 of CHOP therapy.

NHL (Follicular, CD20-positive, B-cell, previously untreated)
IV: ADULTS: 375 mg/m^2 on day 1 of each cycle up to 8 doses. **Maintenance (single agent):** 375 mg/m^2 q8wks for 12 doses. **SQ: ADULTS:** 1,400 mg/23,400 units on day 1 of cycles 2–8 (q21 days), for up to 7 cycles following full dose of IV rituximab on day 1 of cycle 1 (e.g., up to 8 cycles total). In pts with partial or complete response, start maintenance therapy 8 wks after completion. Administer as single agent q8wks for 12 doses.

NHL (Nonprogressive, CD20-positive, B-cell following 6–8 cycles of cyclophosphamide, vinCRIStine, and prednisoLONE [CVP therapy])
IV: ADULTS: 375 mg/m^2 once wkly for 4 doses q6mos. **Maximum:** 16 doses. **SQ: ADULTS:** 1,400 mg/23,400 units once wkly for 3 wks (e.g., 4 wks total) at 6-mo intervals following completion of CVP therapy and a full dose of IV rituximab at wk 1. **Maximum:** 16 doses.

NHL (Combination with ibritumomab)
IV: ADULTS: 250 mg/m^2 day 1; repeat in 7–9 days with ibritumomab.

Rheumatoid Arthritis
IV: ADULTS: 1,000 mg every 2 wks times 2 doses in combination with methotrexate. May repeat course q24wks (if needed, no sooner than 16 wks).

CLL

IV: ADULTS, CHILDREN: (Induction): 375 mg/m² in first cycle (on day prior to fludarabine/cyclophosphamide) and 500 mg/m² on day 1 in cycles 2–6, administered every 28 days. **SQ: ADULTS:** 1,600 mg/26,800 units on day 1 of cycles 2–6 (q28 days) for a total of 5 cycles following full dose of IV rituximab on day 1 of cycle 1 (e.g., 6 cycles total).

GPA, MPA

IV: ***(Induction):*** **ADULTS, CHILDREN:** 375 mg/m² once wkly for 4 wks (in combination with methylPREDNISolone IV for 1–3 days, then daily predniSONE). ***(Follow-up therapy):*** **ADULTS:** 500 mg as 2 infusions separated by 2 wks, then 500 mg q6mos thereafter. **CHILDREN:** 250 mg/m2 q2wks for 2 doses, then 250 mg/m2 q6mos thereafter..

Pemphigus Vulgaris

IV: ADULTS, ELDERLY: 1,000 mg q2wks for 2 doses (in combination with a tapering course of glucocorticoids), then 500 mg at months 12 and 18 and q6mos thereafter.

Dosage in Renal/Hepatic Impairment

No dose adjustment.

SIDE EFFECTS

Note: Side effects may vary depending on dose and indicated treatment. **Frequent (53%–14%):** Fever, chills, asthenia, constipation, nausea, headache, paresthesia, night sweats, pyrexia, rash, pruritus, abdominal pain, alopecia. **Occasional (13%–5%):** Cough, pain, rhinitis, peripheral neuropathy, back pain, bone pain, diarrhea, vomiting, dizziness, myalgia, arthralgia, hypotension, insomnia, erythema, throat irritation, urticaria, muscle spasm, dyspnea, hypertension, chest pain, flushing, anxiety, peripheral edema.

ADVERSE EFFECTS/TOXIC REACTIONS

Myelosuppression (anemia, leukopenia, lymphopenia, neutropenia, thrombocytopenia) is an expected response to therapy. Severe infusion reactions including anaphylaxis, angioedema, ARDS, bronchospasm, hypotension, hypoxia, pulmonary infiltrates were reported. Cardiac events including cardiogenic shock, MI, ventricular fibrillation may occur, particularly in pts with history of preexisting cardiac conditions. Severe, and sometimes fatal, mucocutaneous reactions including paraneoplastic pemphigus, Stevens-Johnson syndrome, lichenoid dermatitis, vesiculobullous dermatitis, toxic epidermal necrolysis may occur. Progressive multifocal leukoencephalopathy (PML), an opportunistic viral infection of the brain caused by the JC virus, may result in progressive permanent disability and death. Infections including upper respiratory tract infection, pneumonia, pharyngitis, nasopharyngitis, bronchitis, UTI, sinusitis, conjunctivitis, influenza occurred in 15%–4% of pts. May cause HBV reactivation, resulting in fulminant hepatitis, hepatic failure, and death. Tumor lysis syndrome may present as acute renal failure, hypocalcemia, hyperuricemia, hyperphosphatemia. Fatal cases of bowel perforation/obstruction were reported.

NURSING CONSIDERATIONS

BASELINE ASSESSMENT

Obtain CBC; pregnancy test in females of reproductive potential; LFT in pts with history of HCV, HBV infection. Test all pts for hepatitis B virus infection. Initiate anti-HBV therapy if warranted. Recommend continuous ECG monitoring during initial infusions. Screen for active infection. Pretreatment with acetaminophen and diphenhydrAMINE before each infusion may prevent infusion-related effects. Confirm compliance of effective contraception. Conduct baseline dermatological exam and assess skin for open/unhealed wounds, lesions, moles. Receive full medication history and screen for interactions. Question history of cardiac disease, GI perforation, chronic infections, renal impairment. All pts planning

R

to receive SQ dose must complete at least one full intravenous dose. Recommend prophylactic treatment for *Pneumocystis jiroveci* (PCP) and herpes virus infection in pts with CLL during treatment and for up to 12 mos after discontinuation. Offer emotional support.

INTERVENTION/EVALUATION

Monitor CBC at regular intervals. Monitor serum calcium, phosphate, uric acid if tumor lysis syndrome is suspected (acute renal failure, electrolyte imbalance, cardiac arrhythmias, seizures). Monitor for infections of any kind. Monitor for an infusion-related reaction; generally occurs within 30 min–2 hrs of beginning first infusion. Slowing infusion resolves symptoms. If given SQ, monitor pt at least 15 min following administration. Pts who present with abdominal pain, fever, nausea, vomiting should be evaluated for bowel perforation/obstruction. Assess mouth for ulcerations; skin for cutaneous reactions. Closely monitor for exacerbation of hepatitis or HBV reactivation (amber- to orange-colored urine, fatigue, jaundice, nausea, vomiting). Due to risk of cardiovascular events, have emergency resuscitation equipment ready available. Offer antiemetic if nausea occurs, antidiarrheal if diarrhea occurs. Monitor daily pattern of bowel activity, stool consistency. Ensure adequate hydration, nutrition. Monitor weight, I&Os

PATIENT/FAMILY TEACHING

• Treatment may depress the immune system and reduce the ability to fight infection. Report symptoms of infection such as body aches, burning with urination, chills, cough, fatigue, fever. Avoid those with active infection. • Report symptoms of bone marrow depression such as bruising, fatigue, fever, shortness of breath, weight loss; bleeding easily, bloody urine or stool. • Therapy may cause tumor lysis syndrome (a condition caused by the rapid breakdown of cancer cells), which can cause kidney failure and can be fatal. Report decreased urination, amber-colored urine, confusion, difficulty breathing, fatigue, fever, muscle or joint pain, palpitations, seizures, vomiting. • Use effective contraception to avoid pregnancy. Do not breastfeed. • PML, an opportunistic viral infection of the brain, may cause progressive, permanent disabilities and death. Report symptoms of PML, brain hemorrhage such as confusion, memory loss, paralysis, trouble speaking, vision loss, seizures, weakness. • Immediately report symptoms of infusion reactions (difficulty breathing, itching, hives, palpitations, rash, swelling of the face or tongue); severe mucocutaneous reactions (blisters, peeling of skin, ulceration of the mouth); HBV reactivation (fatigue, yellowing of the skin or eyes); bowel obstruction or perforation (abdominal pain, fever, nausea, vomiting); cardiovascular events (chest pain, cold/clammy skin, difficulty breathing, fainting, irregular heartbeat, palpitations, sweating). • Do not take newly prescribed medications unless approved by the prescriber who originally started treatment.

rivaroxaban

TOP 100

rye-va-**rox**-a-ban
(Xarelto)

■ **BLACK BOX ALERT** ■ Epidural/spinal hematomas may occur in pts receiving neuraxial anesthesia or spinal puncture, resulting in long-term or permanent paralysis. Factors increasing risk of epidural/spinal hematoma include indwelling epidural catheters, concomitant drugs such as NSAIDs, platelet inhibitors, other anticoagulants; history of traumatic or repeated spinal or epidural punctures, history of spinal deformity or spinal surgery. Monitor for signs and symptoms of neurologic impairment. Consider benefits and risks before neuraxial intervention in anticoagulated pts or planned thromboprophylaxis. Increased risk of stroke may occur in pts with atrial fibrillation when discontinuing for reasons other than bleeding.

Do not confuse rivaroxaban with argatroban.

◆CLASSIFICATION

PHARMACOTHERAPEUTIC: Factor Xa inhibitor. Direct oral anticoagulant. **CLINICAL:** Anticoagulant.

USES

Prophylaxis of deep vein thrombosis (DVT) in pts undergoing knee or hip replacement surgery and in acutely ill medical pts. Prevents stroke/systemic embolism in pts with nonvalvular atrial fibrillation. Treatment of DVT/PE. Reduces risk of recurrent DVT/PE following 6 mos of treatment. In combination with aspirin, reduces risk of major CV events (e.g., MI, stroke) in pts with chronic coronary artery disease (CAD) or peripheral artery disease (PAD).

PRECAUTIONS

Contraindications: Hypersensitivity to rivaroxaban. Active major bleeding. **Cautions:** Renal/hepatic impairment, pts at increased risk of bleeding (e.g., thrombocytopenia, stroke, severe uncontrolled hypertension), elderly pts; avoid use with heparin, low molecular weight heparin (LMWH), aspirin, warfarin, NSAIDs. Pts with prosthetic heart valves or significant rheumatic heart disease.

ACTION

Selectively and reversibly blocks active site of factor Xa, a key factor in the intrinsic and extrinsic pathway of blood coagulation cascade. Inhibits platelet activation and fibrin clot formation. **Therapeutic Effect:** Inhibits blood coagulation.

PHARMACOKINETICS

Rapidly absorbed after PO administration. Peak plasma concentration: 2–4 hrs. Absorption dependent on site of drug release within GI tract. Avoid administration into small intestine due to reduced absorption. Protein binding: 92%–95%. Metabolized in liver. Excreted in urine (66%), feces (28%). **Half-life:** 5–9 hrs, 11–13 hrs (elderly pts).

⌛ LIFESPAN CONSIDERATIONS

Pregnancy/Lactation: Crosses placenta. Use during pregnancy should be avoided. Unknown if excreted in breast milk. **Children:** Safety and efficacy not established. **Elderly:** May be at increased risk for bleeding due to age-related renal impairment. Use caution.

INTERACTIONS

DRUG: **Strong CYP3A4 inhibitors (e.g., ketoconazole, clarithromycin, ritonavir)** may increase concentration, risk of bleeding. **Anticoagulants (e.g., heparin, warfarin), antiplatelets (e.g., aspirin, clopidogrel), NSAIDs (e.g., ibuprofen, ketorolac, naproxen)** may increase bleeding risk. **Apixaban, dabigatran, edoxaban** may increase anticoagulant effect. **HERBAL:** **Herbals with anticoagulant/antiplatelet properties (e.g., garlic, ginger, ginkgo biloba)** may increase risk of bleeding. **FOOD:** **Grapefruit products** may increase risk of bleeding. **LAB VALUES:** May decrease platelets. May increase serum ALT, AST, bilirubin.

AVAILABILITY (Rx)

Tablets: 2.5 mg, 10 mg, 15 mg, 20 mg.

ADMINISTRATION/HANDLING

PO

• Administer doses of 15 mg or greater with food; doses of 10 mg/day may be given without regard to food. • **DVT prophylaxis (knee, hip):** Give without regard to food. • **Nonvalvular atrial fibrillation:** Give with evening meal.

INDICATIONS/ROUTES/DOSAGE

Note: Avoid in pts with BMI greater than 40 kg/m^2 or weight greater than 120 kg due to lack of clinical data in this population.

DVT Prophylaxis, Knee Replacement

PO: ADULTS, ELDERLY: 10 mg daily for minimum 10–14 days up to 35 days. Initiate at least 6–10 hrs after surgery once hemostasis established. **CrCl less than 30 mL/min:** Avoid use.

R

DVT Prophylaxis, Hip Replacement
PO: ADULTS, ELDERLY: 10 mg daily for 10–14 days (minimum) up to 35 days. Initiate at least 6–10 hrs after surgery once hemostasis established. **CrCl less than 30 mL/min:** Avoid use.

DVT Prophylaxis, Acutely Ill
PO: ADULTS, ELDERLY: 10 mg once daily.

Nonvalvular Atrial Fibrillation
PO: ADULTS, ELDERLY: CrCl greater than 50 mL/min: 20 mg daily. **CrCl 15–50 mL/min:** 15 mg daily. **CrCl less than 15 mL/min:** Avoid use.

Treatment of DVT/PE
PO: ADULTS, ELDERLY: 15 mg twice daily for 3 wks, then 20 mg once daily.

Reduce Risk of DVT/PE (After 6 mos treatment)
PO: ADULTS, ELDERLY: 10 mg once daily up to 6–12 mos.

Reduce Risk of CV Events
PO: ADULTS, ELDERLY: 2.5 mg twice daily (in combination with aspirin [75–100 mg] once daily).

Dosage in Renal Impairment
CrCl less than 30 mL/min: Avoid use in DVT/PE, postoperative thromboprophylaxis. ***(Nonvalvular atrial fibrillation):*** **CrCl 15–50 mL/min:** 15 mg once daily with evening meal. **CrCl less than 15 mL/min:** Avoid use.

Dosage in Hepatic Impairment
Mild impairment: No dose adjustment. **Moderate to severe impairment:** Avoid use.

SIDE EFFECTS

Rare (3%–1%): Wound secretion/oozing, extremity pain, muscle spasm, syncope, pruritus.

ADVERSE EFFECTS/TOXIC REACTIONS

Increased risk of bleeding/hemorrhagic events including retroperitoneal hemorrhage, cerebral hemorrhage, subdural hematoma, epidural/spinal hematoma (esp. with epidural catheters, spinal trauma). Serious reactions including jaundice, cholestasis, cytolytic hepatitis, Stevens-Johnson syndrome, hypersensitivity reaction, anaphylaxis reported.

NURSING CONSIDERATIONS

BASELINE ASSESSMENT

Obtain ECG for pts with a history of atrial fibrillation. Question for history of bleeding disorders, recent surgery, spinal punctures, intracranial hemorrhage, bleeding ulcers, open wounds, anemia, renal/hepatic impairment. Receive full medication history including herbal products.

INTERVENTION/EVALUATION

Be alert for complaints of abdominal/back pain, headache, confusion, weakness, vision change (may indicate hemorrhage). Question for increased menstrual bleeding/discharge. Assess peripheral pulses; skin for ecchymosis, petechiae. Check for excessive bleeding from minor cuts, scratches. Assess urine output for hematuria. Immediately report suspected pregnancy.

PATIENT/FAMILY TEACHING

• Do not take/discontinue any medication except on advice of physician. • Avoid alcohol, aspirin, NSAIDs. • Consult physician before surgery, dental work. • Use electric razor, soft toothbrush to prevent bleeding. • Report any unusual bleeding/bruising, spinal/epidural hematomas (e.g., tingling, numbness, muscular weakness). • Report if pregnant or planning to become pregnant. • Avoid grapefruit products.

rivastigmine

riv-a-**stig**-meen
(Exelon)

◆ **CLASSIFICATION**

PHARMACOTHERAPEUTIC: Acetylcholinesterase inhibitor. **CLINICAL:** Anti-Alzheimer's dementia agent.

USES

Oral: Treatment of mild to moderate dementia of Alzheimer's or mild to moderate dementia of Parkinson's disease. **Transdermal:** Treatment of mild, moderate, or severe dementia of the Alzheimer type. Treatment of mild to moderate dementia associated with Parkinson's disease. **OFF-LABEL:** Lewy body dementia.

PRECAUTIONS

Contraindications: Hypersensitivity to rivastigmine, other carbamate derivatives (e.g., neostigmine), history of application site reactions with rivastigmine patch. **Cautions:** Peptic ulcer disease, concurrent use of NSAIDs, sick sinus syndrome, bradycardia or supraventricular conduction defects, urinary obstruction, seizure disorders, asthma, COPD, body weight less than 50 kg.

ACTION

Increases acetylcholine in CNS by reversibly inhibiting hydrolysis by cholinesterase. **Therapeutic Effect:** Slows progression of symptoms of Alzheimer's disease, dementia of Parkinson's disease.

PHARMACOKINETICS

Widely distributed. Penetrates blood-brain barrier. Metabolized via cholinesterase-mediated hydrolysis. Excreted in urine (97%), feces (0.4%). **Half-life:** 1 hr (oral); 8–16 hrs (transdermal patch).

LIFESPAN CONSIDERATIONS

Pregnancy/Lactation: Unknown if distributed in breast milk. **Children:** Not indicated in this pt population. **Elderly:** No age-related precautions noted.

INTERACTIONS

DRUG: May interfere with **anticholinergics (e.g., dicyclomine, glycopyrrolate, scopolamine)** effects. May increase the bradycardic effect of **beta blockers (e.g., atenolol, carvedilol, metoprolol)**. May increase the adverse effects of **metoclopramide.** **HERBAL:** None significant. **FOOD:** None known. **LAB VALUES:** None significant.

AVAILABILITY (Rx)

Transdermal Patch: 4.6 mg/24 hrs, 9.5 mg/24 hrs, 13.3 mg/24 hrs.

Capsules: 1.5 mg, 3 mg, 4.5 mg, 6 mg.

ADMINISTRATION/HANDLING

PO

• Give morning and evening doses with food. • Give capsule whole; do not break, cut, or open.

Transdermal Patch

• May apply the day following the last oral dose. • Apply to upper or lower back, upper arm, or chest. • Avoid reapplication to same spot of skin for 14 days. • Do not apply to red, irritated, or broken skin. • Avoid eye contact. • After removal, fold patch to press adhesive together and discard.

INDICATIONS/ROUTES/DOSAGE

Alzheimer's Dementia (Mild to moderate)

PO: ADULTS, ELDERLY: Initially, 1.5 mg twice daily. May increase at intervals of at least 2 wks to 3 mg twice daily, then 4.5 mg twice daily, and finally 6 mg twice daily. **Maximum:** 6 mg twice daily. **Transdermal:** Initially, 4.6 mg/24 hrs. May increase at intervals of at least 4 wks to 9.5 mg/24 hrs and then to 13.3 mg/24 hrs.

Alzheimer's Dementia (Severe)

Transdermal: ADULTS, ELDERLY: Initially, 4.6 mg/24 hrs. May increase at intervals of at least 4 wks to 9.5 mg/24 hrs and then to 13.3 mg/24 hrs.

Parkinson's Dementia

PO: ADULTS, ELDERLY: Initially, 1.5 mg twice daily. May increase at intervals of at least 4 wks to 3 mg twice daily, then

R

4.5 mg twice daily, and finally 6 mg twice daily. **Maximum:** 6 mg twice daily. **Transdermal:** Initially, 4.6 mg/24 hrs. May increase after 4 wks to 9.5 mg/24 hrs and then to 13.3 mg/24 hrs.

Dosage in Renal Impairment
No dose adjustment.

Dosage in Hepatic Impairment
Oral: No dose adjustment. **Transdermal: Maximum:** 4.6 mg/24 hrs.

SIDE EFFECTS

Frequent (47%–17%): Nausea, vomiting, dizziness, diarrhea, headache, anorexia. **Occasional (13%–6%):** Abdominal pain, insomnia, dyspepsia (heartburn, indigestion, epigastric pain), confusion, UTI, depression. **Rare (5%–3%):** Anxiety, drowsiness, constipation, malaise, hallucinations, tremor, flatulence, rhinitis, hypertension, flu-like symptoms, weight loss, syncope.

ADVERSE EFFECTS/TOXIC REACTIONS

Overdose can produce cholinergic crisis, characterized by severe nausea/vomiting, increased salivation, diaphoresis, bradycardia, hypotension, respiratory depression, seizures.

R

NURSING CONSIDERATIONS

BASELINE ASSESSMENT

Obtain vital signs. Assess history for peptic ulcer, urinary obstruction, asthma, COPD, cardiac disease. Assess cognitive, behavioral, functional deficits.

INTERVENTION/EVALUATION

Monitor for cholinergic reaction: GI discomfort/cramping, feeling of facial warmth, excessive salivation, diaphoresis, lacrimation, pallor, urinary urgency, dizziness. Monitor for nausea, diarrhea, headache, insomnia.

PATIENT/ FAMILY TEACHING

• Take with meals (at breakfast, dinner). • Swallow capsule whole. Do not break, chew, or divide capsules. • Report nausea, vomiting, diarrhea, diaphoresis, increased salivary secretions, severe abdominal pain, dizziness.

rizatriptan

rye-za-trip-tan
(Maxalt, Maxalt-MLT, Maxalt RPD 🍁)

◆CLASSIFICATION

PHARMACOTHERAPEUTIC: Serotonin 5-HT_1 receptor agonist. **CLINICAL:** Antimigraine.

USES

Treatment of acute migraine headache with or without aura.

PRECAUTIONS

Contraindications: Hypersensitivity to rizatriptan. Basilar or hemiplegic migraine, history of stroke or transient ischemic attack; severe cardiovascular disease, coronary artery vasospasm, peripheral vascular disease, ischemic bowel disease, uncontrolled hypertension, use within 24 hrs of ergotamine-containing preparations or another serotonin receptor agonist, MAOI use within 14 days. **Cautions:** Mild to moderate renal/hepatic impairment, end-stage renal disease requiring dialysis, elderly, cardiovascular risks (e.g., hypertension, diabetes, hypercholesterolemia).

ACTION

Binds selectively to serotonin 5-HT_1 receptors in cranial arteries producing vasoconstriction. **Therapeutic Effect:** Relieves migraine headache.

PHARMACOKINETICS

Widely distributed. Protein binding: 14%. Crosses blood-brain barrier. Metabolized by liver. Excreted primarily in urine (82%), feces (12%). **Half-life:** 2–3 hrs.

LIFESPAN CONSIDERATIONS

Pregnancy/Lactation: Unknown if drug is distributed in breast milk. **Children:** Safety and efficacy not established. **Elderly:** No age-related precautions noted.

INTERACTIONS

DRUG: **Ergot derivatives (e.g., ergotamine)** may increase vasoconstrictive effect. **Strong CYP3A4 inhibitors (e.g., clarithromycin, ketoconazole** may increase concentration/effect. **MAOIs (e.g., phenelzine, selegiline), propranolol** may dramatically increase concentration (avoid concurrent use). **HERBAL:** None significant. **FOOD:** **All foods** delay peak drug concentration by 1 hr. **LAB VALUES:** None significant.

AVAILABILITY (Rx)

Tablets ***(Maxalt)***: 5 mg, 10 mg. **Tablets, Orally Disintegrating:** ***(Maxalt-MLT)***: 5 mg, 10 mg.

ADMINISTRATION/HANDLING

PO

• Orally disintegrating tablet is packaged in individual aluminum pouch. • Open packet with dry hands. • Place tablet onto tongue, allow to dissolve, swallow with saliva. Administration with water is not necessary.

INDICATIONS/ROUTES/DOSAGE

Acute Migraine Headache

PO: ADULTS OLDER THAN 18 YRS, ELDERLY: 5–10 mg. If significant improvement is not attained, dose may be repeated after 2 hrs. **Maximum:** 30 mg/24 hrs. (Use 5 mg/dose in pts taking propranolol with maximum of 15 mg/24 hrs.) **CHILDREN 6–17 YRS WEIGHING 40 KG OR MORE:** 10 mg as single dose. (Maximum 5 mg as single dose with propranolol.) **WEIGHING LESS THAN 40 KG:** 5 mg as a single dose. (Not recommended if taking propranolol.)

Dosage in Renal/Hepatic Impairment

No dose adjustment.

SIDE EFFECTS

Frequent (9%–7%): Dizziness, drowsiness, paresthesia, fatigue. **Occasional (6%–3%):** Nausea, chest pressure, dry mouth. **Rare (2%):** Headache; neck, throat, jaw pressure; photosensitivity.

ADVERSE EFFECTS/TOXIC REACTIONS

Cardiac reactions (ischemia, coronary artery vasospasm, MI), noncardiac vasospasm-related reactions (hemorrhage, CVA) may occur, esp. in pts with hypertension, diabetes, strong family history of coronary artery disease, obesity, smokers, males older than 40 yrs, postmenopausal women.

NURSING CONSIDERATIONS

BASELINE ASSESSMENT

Question for history of peripheral vascular disease, renal/hepatic impairment. Question pt regarding onset, location, duration of migraine, possible precipitating symptoms.

INTERVENTION/EVALUATION

Monitor for evidence of dizziness. Evaluate for relief of migraine headaches (photophobia, phonophobia, nausea, vomiting, pain, dizziness, fogginess).

PATIENT/FAMILY TEACHING

• Take single dose as soon as symptoms of an actual migraine headache appear. • Medication is intended to relieve migraine, not to prevent or reduce number of attacks. • Avoid tasks that require alertness, motor skills until response to drug is established. • Report immediately if palpitations, pain/tightness in chest/throat, pain/weakness of extremities occurs. • Do not remove orally disintegrating tablet from blister pack until just before dosing.

rolapitant

roe-**la**-pi-tant
(Varubi)
Do not confuse rolapitant with aprepitant, fosaprepitant.

◆CLASSIFICATION

PHARMACOTHERAPEUTIC: Substance P/neurokinin (P/NK) receptor antagonist. **CLINICAL:** Antinausea, antiemetic.

USES

Prevention of delayed nausea and vomiting associated with initial and repeat courses of emetogenic cancer chemotherapy, including, but not limited to, highly emetogenic chemotherapy, in combination with other antiemetic agents.

PRECAUTIONS

Contraindications: Hypersensitivity to rolapitant. CYP2D6 substrates with a narrow therapeutic index (e.g., thioridazine). **Cautions:** Mild to moderate hepatic impairment, pts at risk for QT interval prolongation or ventricular arrhythmia (congenital long QT syndrome, medications that prolong QT interval, hypokalemia, hypomagnesemia). Not recommended in severe hepatic impairment.

R

ACTION

Selectively and competitively inhibits human substance P/NK_1 receptors. **Therapeutic Effect:** Decreases nausea and vomiting associated with chemotherapy.

PHARMACOKINETICS

Readily absorbed. Widely distributed. Metabolized in liver. Protein binding: greater than 99%. Peak plasma concentration: 4 hrs. Excreted in urine (14%), feces (73%). **Half-life:** 158 hrs.

⌛ LIFESPAN CONSIDERATIONS

Pregnancy/Lactation: Safety and efficacy not established during pregnancy. Unknown if distributed in breast milk. **Children:** Safety and efficacy not established. **Elderly:** No age-related precautions noted.

INTERACTIONS

DRUG: **Thioridazine** may increase risk of torsades de pointes, QT internal prolongation (contraindicated). **Strong CYP3A inducers (e.g., carBAMazepine, phenytoin, rifAMPin)** may decrease concentration/effect. May increase concentration/effect of **BCRP substrates (e.g., methotrexate, rosuvastatin), CYP2D6 substrates (e.g., pimozide), P-gp substrates (e.g., digoxin). QT interval–prolonging medications (e.g., amiodarone, azithromycin, ciprofloxacin, haloperidol, methadone, sotalol)** may increase risk of QTc interval prolongation. **HERBAL:** **St. John's wort** may decrease concentration/effect. **FOOD:** None significant. **LAB VALUES:** May decrease Hct, Hgb, neutrophils, RBC.

AVAILABILITY (Rx)

Emulsion, IV: 166.5 mg/92.5 ml. **Tablets:** 90 mg.

ADMINISTRATION/HANDLING

IV

Rate of administration • Infuse over 30 min. Do not dilute. • Solution is compatible with 0.9% NaCl, D5W or Lactated Ringers via Y-site.
Storage • Store at room temperature.

PO

• Administer approx. 1–2 hrs prior to chemotherapy. • Give without regard to food. Administer prior to initiation of each chemotherapy cycle at no less than 2-wk intervals.

INDICATIONS/ROUTES/DOSAGE

Chemotherapy-Associated Nausea/ Vomiting

PO: ADULTS, ELDERLY: 180 mg once on day 1 (in combination with dexamethasone and a 5-HT_3 receptor antagonist). Do not give rolapitant at intervals of less than 2 wks.

IV: ADULTS, ELDERLY: 166.5 mg given within 2 hrs prior to initiation of chemotherapy on day 1 (in combination with dexamethasone and a 5-HT_3 receptor antagonist).

Dosage in Renal Impairment

Mild to moderate impairment: No dose adjustment. **Severe impairment:** Not specified; use caution.

Dosage in Hepatic Impairment

Mild to moderate impairment: No dose adjustment. **Severe impairment:** Treatment not recommended.

SIDE EFFECTS

Occasional (9%–6%): Decreased appetite, hiccups, dizziness. **Rare (4%–3%):** Abdominal pain.

ADVERSE EFFECTS/TOXIC REACTIONS

Torsades de pointes, QT prolongation reported in pts taking thioridazine concomitantly; avoid use. Baseline electrolyte imbalance may increase risk of arrhythmias.

NURSING CONSIDERATIONS

BASELINE ASSESSMENT

Obtain CBC, BMP, serum magnesium. Question history of arrhythmias, hepatic impairment, congenital long QT syndrome. Receive medication history and screen for interactions. Assess hydration status. Obtain ECG in pts taking concomitant drugs that prolong QT interval.

INTERVENTION/EVALUATION

Periodically monitor CBC, BMP. Monitor hydration, nutritional status, I&O. Correct electrolyte imbalances prior to each dose. If CYP2D6 substrate medications cannot be withheld, diligently monitor for QT interval prolongation, ventricular arrhythmias. Assist with ambulation if dizziness occurs. Assess for anemia-related symptoms.

PATIENT/FAMILY TEACHING

• Therapy may alter effectiveness of other drugs. Do not take any newly prescribed medications unless approved by doctor who originally started treatment. • Report symptoms of arrhythmias such as chest pain, dizziness, fainting, fatigue, palpitations, shortness of breath. • Do not take herbal products or ingest grapefruit products. • Report persistent nausea, vomiting despite treatment.

romiDEPsin

roe-mi-**dep**-sin
(Istodax)

Do not confuse romiDEPsin with romiPLOStim.

CLASSIFICATION

PHARMACOTHERAPEUTIC: Histone deacetylase (HDAC) inhibitor. **CLINICAL:** Antineoplastic.

USES

Treatment of cutaneous T-cell lymphoma (CTCL) or peripheral T-cell lymphoma (PTCL).

PRECAUTIONS

Contraindications: Hypersensitivity to romiDEPsin. **Cautions:** Moderate or severe hepatic impairment, end-stage renal impairment, preexisting cardiac disease, pts at risk for QTc interval prolongation (congenital long QT syndrome, HF, medications that prolong QTc interval, hypokalemia, hypomagnesemia), conditions predisposing to infection (e.g., diabetes, immunocompromised pts, renal failure, open wounds), pts at risk for tumor lysis syndrome (high tumor burden), chronic viral infections (hepatitis B virus, herpesvirus). Avoid concomitant strong CYP3A4 inhibitors/inducers; caution with moderate CYP3A4 inhibitors or P-glycoprotein inhibitors.

ACTION

Catalyzes acetyl group removal from protein lysine residues, resulting in acetyl group accumulation, which alters chromatin structure and transcription

R

factor activation, terminating cell growth. **Therapeutic Effect:** Induces cell-cycle arrest, cell death.

PHARMACOKINETICS

Widely distributed. Metabolized in liver. Protein binding: 92%–94%. Excretion not specified. **Half-life:** 3 hrs.

⌛ LIFESPAN CONSIDERATIONS

Pregnancy/Lactation: Avoid pregnancy; may cause fetal harm. Females and males with female partners of reproductive potential must use effective contraception during treatment and for at least 1 mo after discontinuation. Consider nonhormonal contraception (condoms, intrauterine device). Breastfeeding not recommended during treatment and for at least 1 wk after discontinuation. May impair fertility in both females and males. **Children:** Safety and efficacy not established. **Elderly:** No age-related precautions noted.

INTERACTIONS

DRUG: Strong CYP3A4 inhibitors (e.g., clarithromycin, itraconazole, ritonavir) may increase concentration. **Strong CYP3A4 inducers (e.g., carBAMazepine, phenytoin, rifAMPin)** may decrease concentration. **QT interval–prolonging medications (e.g., amiodarone, azithromycin, ceritinib, haloperidol, moxifloxacin)** may increase risk of QT interval prolongation, cardiac arrhythmias. May increase adverse effects; decrease therapeutic effect of **vaccines (live). HERBAL: Echinacea** may decrease therapeutic effect. **FOOD: Grapefruit products** may increase concentration/effects. **LAB VALUES:** May decrease serum albumin, phosphate, potassium, sodium; Hgb, leukocytes, lymphocytes, platelets, neutrophils, RBCs. May increase serum ALT, AST, glucose, uric acid. May increase or decrease serum magnesium.

AVAILABILITY (Rx)

Injection, Powder for Reconstitution, 2-Vial Kit: 10 mg.

ADMINISTRATION/HANDLING

Reconstitution • Reconstitute with 2 mL of supplied diluent (80% propylene glycol, 20% dehydrated alcohol). • Swirl contents gently to dissolve powder. • Reconstituted solution provides 5 mg/mL. Further dilute in 500 mL 0.9% NaCl.

Rate of administration • Infuse over 4 hrs.

Storage • Reconstituted solution is stable for at least 24 hrs at room temperature. • Solution appears clear, colorless. Discard if precipitate is present or solution is discolored.

INDICATIONS/ROUTES/DOSAGE

CTCL, PTCL

IV: ADULTS, ELDERLY: 14 mg/m^2 administered over 4 hrs on days 1, 8, and 15 of a 28-day cycle. Repeat cycles every 28 days based on benefit and tolerability.

Dose Modification

Hematologic Toxicity

Grade 3 or 4 neutropenia or thrombocytopenia: Delay treatment until ANC 1,500 cells/mm^3 or more and/or platelets 75,000 cells/mm^3 or more (or baseline), then resume at 14 mg/m^2. **Grade 4 neutropenia or thrombocytopenia requiring platelet transfusion:** Delay treatment until recovered to Grade 1 or 0 (or baseline), then permanently reduce dose to 10 mg/m^2.

Nonhematologic Toxicity (Excluding alopecia)

Grade 2 or 3 toxicity: Delay treatment until recovered to Grade 1 or 0 (or baseline), then restart at 14 mg/m^2. **Grade 4, recurrent Grade 3 toxicity:** Delay treatment until recovered to Grade 1 or 0 (or baseline), then permanently reduce dose to 10 mg/m^2. **Recurrent Grade 3 or 4 toxicity (with dose reduction):** Permanently discontinue.

Dosage in Renal Impairment

No dose adjustment. Use caution in end-stage-renal disease.

Dosage in Hepatic Impairment
Mild impairment: No dose adjustment. **Moderate impairment:** Reduce starting dose to 7 mg/m². **Severe impairment:** Reduce starting dose to 5 mg/m².

SIDE EFFECTS

Frequent (57%–23%): Nausea, fatigue, vomiting, anorexia. **Occasional (20%–7%):** Diarrhea, fever, distorted sense of taste, constipation, hypotension, pruritus. **Rare (4%–2%):** Dermatitis, T-wave and ST-wave changes on ECG.

ADVERSE EFFECTS/TOXIC REACTIONS

Myelosuppression (anemia, lymphopenia, neutropenia, thrombocytopenia) is an expected response to therapy, but more severe reactions including febrile neutropenia may occur. Fatal infections including pneumonia, sepsis were reported. Increased risk of life-threatening infections are greater in pts treated with monoclonal antibodies directed at lymphocyte antigens and in pts with disease involvement of the bone marrow. Reactivation of hepatitis B virus, Epstein-Barr virus infection may occur. May cause cardiac conduction abnormalities (cardiac arrhythmias, T-wave, ST-segment changes, QT interval prolongation). Tumor lysis syndrome may present as acute renal failure, hypocalcemia, hyperuricemia, hyperphosphatemia.

NURSING CONSIDERATIONS

BASELINE ASSESSMENT

Obtain CBC, BMP, LFT; pregnancy test in females of reproductive potential. Confirm compliance of effective contraception. Screen for active infection. Question history of hepatic/renal impairment, cardiac disease. Receive full medication history and screen for interactions. Assess risk for QT interval prolongation, tumor lysis syndrome. Ensure adequate hydration. Offer emotional support.

INTERVENTION/EVALUATION

Monitor CBC, BMP, LFT. Monitor ECG for cardiac conduction abnormalities. Diligently monitor for infection (cough, fatigue, fever); reactivation of chronic viral infections. Monitor serum uric acid level if tumor lysis syndrome (acute renal failure, electrolyte imbalance, cardiac arrhythmias, seizures) is suspected.

PATIENT/FAMILY TEACHING

• Treatment may depress your immune system response and reduce your ability to fight infection. Report symptoms of infection such as body aches, chills, cough, fatigue, fever. Avoid those with active infection. • Report symptoms of bone marrow depression such as bruising, fatigue, fever, shortness of breath, weight loss; bleeding easily, bloody urine or stool. • Report palpitations, chest pain, shortness of breath, dizziness, fainting; may indicate arrhythmia. • Therapy may cause life-threatening tumor lysis syndrome (a condition caused by the rapid breakdown of cancer cells), which can cause kidney failure. Report decreased urination, amber-colored urine; confusion, difficulty breathing, fatigue, fever, muscle or joint pain, palpitations, seizures, vomiting. • Report liver problems (abdominal pain, bruising, clay-colored stool, amber- or dark-colored urine, yellowing of the skin or eyes), kidney problems (decreased urine output, flank pain, darkened urine). • Treatment may alter the electrical properties of the heart; report chest pain, difficulty breathing, palpitations. • Do not take newly prescribed medications unless approved by prescriber who originally started treatment. • Use effective contraception to avoid pregnancy. Do not breastfeed.

romosozumab-aqqg

roe-moe-**soz**-ue-mab
(Evenity)

BLACK BOX ALERT May increase risk of myocardial infarction (MI), cerebrovascular accident (CVA), cardiovascular death. Do not initiate in pts with recent (within 1 yr) MI, CVA. In pts with other cardiovascular risks, consider whether the benefits of treatment outweigh

R

the risks. Discontinue treatment in pts who develop MI, CVA.

Do not confuse romosozumab with atezolizumab, mepolizumab, pembrolizumab, trastuzumab, or vedolizumab, or Evenity with Emgality.

◆CLASSIFICATION

PHARMACOTHERAPEUTIC: Sclerostin inhibitor. Monoclonal antibody. **CLINICAL:** Osteoporosis agent.

USES

Treatment of postmenopausal women with osteoporosis at high risk for fracture, defined as history of osteoporotic fracture, multiple risk factors for fracture, or pts who have failed or intolerant to other osteoporosis therapy.

PRECAUTIONS

Contraindications: Hypersensitivity to romosozumab-aqqg. Hypocalcemia prior to initiation. **Cautions:** Severe renal impairment (eGFR 15–29 mL/min) or receiving dialysis; pts at risk for osteonecrosis of the jaw (cancer, radiotherapy, poor oral hygiene, preexisting dental disease or infection, anemia, coagulopathy, recent dental procedures, tooth extraction). History of MI, CVA, cardiovascular disease. Avoid use in pts with recent (within 1 yr) MI, CVA.

R

ACTION

Stimulates osteoblastic activity by inhibiting sclerostin, a regulatory factor in bone metabolism. **Therapeutic Effect:** Increases bone mass, improves bone structure and strength, decreases bone reabsorption.

PHARMACOKINETICS

Widely distributed. Degraded into small peptides and amino acids via catabolic pathway. Peak plasma concentration: 5 days. Steady state reached in 3 mos. **Half-life:** 12.8 days.

⌛ LIFESPAN CONSIDERATIONS

Pregnancy/Lactation: Not indicated in female pts of reproductive potential. **Children:** Safety and efficacy not established. **Elderly:** No age-related precautions noted.

INTERACTIONS

DRUG: None significant. **HERBAL:** None significant. **FOOD:** None known. **LAB VALUES:** May decrease calcium.

AVAILABILITY (Rx)

Injection Solution, Prefilled Syringe: 105 mg/1.17 mL.

ADMINISTRATION/HANDLING

SQ

Preparation • Remove prefilled syringe from refrigerator and allow solution to warm to room temperature (at least 30 min) with needle cap intact. • Visually inspect for particulate matter or discoloration. Solution should appear clear to opalescent, colorless to slightly yellow in color. Do not use if solution is cloudy or discolored or if visible particles are observed.

Administration • Insert needle subcutaneously into upper arm, outer thigh, or abdomen and inject solution. • Do not inject into areas of active skin disease or injury such as sunburns, skin rashes, inflammation, skin infections, or active psoriasis. • Rotate injection sites. • Do not administer IV or intramuscularly. • If a dose is missed, administer as soon as possible, then give next dose at the date of last dose.

Storage • Refrigerate prefilled syringes in original carton until time of use. • Protect from light. • Do not shake. • Do not freeze or expose to heating sources. • If not refrigerated, may store at room temperature (up to 77°F) for no more than 30 days. Discard of not used within 30 days.

INDICATIONS/ROUTES/DOSAGE

Postmenopausal Osteoporosis

SQ: ADULTS, ELDERLY: 210 mg (two 105-mg injections) once monthly for 12 mos.

Give with supplemental calcium and vitamin D.

Dosage in Renal Impairment

Mild to severe impairment: No dose adjustment.

Dosage in Hepatic Impairment

Mild to severe impairment: Not specified; use caution.

SIDE EFFECTS

Occasional (13%–6%): Arthralgia, headache. **Rare (4%–2%):** Injection site reactions (pain, erythema), muscle spasms, peripheral edema, asthenia, neck pain, insomnia, paresthesia.

ADVERSE EFFECTS/TOXIC REACTIONS

MI, CVA, cardiovascular death reported in less than 1% of pts. Hypocalcemia reported in less than 1% of pts. Pts with severe renal impairment (eGFR 15–29 mL/min) or receiving dialysis have an increased risk of hypocalcemia. Hypersensitivity reactions including angioedema, erythema multiforme, dermatitis, rash, urticaria may occur. Symptomatic hypocalcemia reported in 7% of pts. Osteonecrosis of the jaw may present as mandibular pain, jaw bone erosion, periodontal/gingival infection or ulceration, osteomyelitis, slow healing of the mouth after dental procedures. Pts with cancer, radiotherapy, poor oral hygiene, preexisting dental disease or infection, anemia, coagulopathy may be at increased risk of developing osteonecrosis of the jaw. Atypical subtrochanteric and diaphyseal femoral fractures may occur with little or no trauma. Immunogenicity (auto-romosozumab antibodies) reported in 18% of pts.

NURSING CONSIDERATIONS

BASELINE ASSESSMENT

Obtain serum calcium level. Hypocalcemia must be corrected prior to initiation. Calcium and vitamin D supplementation is recommended during treatment. Question history of MI, CVA, cardiovascular disease, renal impairment. Do not initiate in pts with recent (within 1 yr) MI, CVA. To assess the risk of osteonecrosis of the jaw, the prescriber should perform an oral examination prior to initiation. Question recent dental procedures or tooth extraction.

INTERVENTION/EVALUATION

Monitor serum calcium levels periodically, esp. in pts with severe renal impairment or receiving dialysis. Monitor for symptoms of CVA (aphasia, altered mental status, headache, hemiplegia, vision loss); MI (chest pain, dyspnea, syncope, diaphoresis, arm/jaw pain), osteonecrosis of the jaw (jaw pain/numbness, loosening of teeth, poor healing of the gums; hypocalcemia (muscle spasm, myalgia, paresthesia, seizures, QT interval prolongation, ventricular arrhythmias; Chvostek's sign, Trousseau's sign). A dull, aching thigh or groin pain should be evaluated for possible femoral fractures. Monitor for hypersensitivity reactions.

PATIENT/FAMILY TEACHING

• Report symptoms of heart attack (chest pain, difficulty breathing, jaw pain, nausea, pain that radiates to the arm or jaw, sweating), stroke (confusion, one-sided weakness, loss of consciousness, trouble speaking, vision loss); atypical leg fractures (dull, aching thigh or groin pain). • Treatment may cause low blood calcium levels; report difficulty swallowing, fatigue, muscle cramps, muscle weakness, palpations, paralysis, numbness, tingling, seizures. • Treatment may cause lack of blood supply to the jaw bone when the bone is exposed, which may lead to jaw necrosis. Report jaw pain or numbness, loosening of teeth, poor healing of the gums. Maintain proper oral hygiene. • Allergic reactions such as swelling of the face or tongue, rash, itching may occur.

rOPINIRole

roe-**pin**-i-role
(Requip XL)

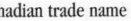

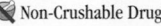

R

Do not confuse rOPINIRole with RisperDAL.

◆CLASSIFICATION

PHARMACOTHERAPEUTIC: DOPamine agonist. **CLINICAL:** Antiparkinson agent.

USES

Treatment of signs/symptoms of idiopathic Parkinson's disease. **Immediate-Release Only:** Treatment of moderate to severe primary restless legs syndrome (RLS).

PRECAUTIONS

Contraindications: Hypersensitivity to rOPINIRole. **Cautions:** History of orthostatic hypotension, cardiovascular or cerebrovascular disease, syncope, concurrent use of CNS depressants, preexisting dyskinesia, hepatic or severe renal dysfunction (end-stage renal disease [ESRD]), major psychotic disorder, elderly.

ACTION

Stimulates postsynaptic DOPamine receptors in caudate putamen in the brain. **Therapeutic Effect:** Relieves signs/symptoms of Parkinson's disease.

PHARMACOKINETICS

Widely distributed. Metabolized in liver. Protein binding: 40%. Steady state reached in 2 days. Excreted in urine. **Half-life:** 6 hrs.

R

LIFESPAN CONSIDERATIONS

Pregnancy/Lactation: Distributed in breast milk. Drug activity possible in breastfeeding infant. **Children:** Safety and efficacy not established. **Elderly:** No age-related precautions noted, but hallucinations may occur more frequently.

INTERACTIONS

DRUG: **Ciprofloxacin** may increase concentration/effect. **Alcohol, CNS depressants (e.g., LORazepam, morphine, zolpidem)** may increase CNS depressant effects. **Antipsychotic agents (e.g., haloperidol)** may decrease therapeutic effect. **HERBAL:** **Herbals with hypotensive properties (e.g., garlic, ginger, gingko biloba)** may increase hypotensive effect. **FOOD:** **All foods** delay peak plasma levels by 1 hr but do not affect drug absorption. **LAB VALUES:** May increase serum alkaline phosphatase.

AVAILABILITY (Rx)

Tablets: 0.25 mg, 0.5 mg, 1 mg, 2 mg, 3 mg, 4 mg, 5 mg.

Tablets, Extended-Release: 2 mg, 4 mg, 6 mg, 8 mg, 12 mg.

ADMINISTRATION/HANDLING

PO

- May give without regard to food.
- Do not break, crush, dissolve, or divide extended-release tablets.

INDICATIONS/ROUTES/DOSAGE

Parkinson's Disease

PO: ***(Immediate-Release):*** **ADULTS, ELDERLY:** Initially, 0.25 mg 3 times/day. Based on individual pt response, dosage should be titrated with wkly increments. **Wk 1:** 0.25 mg 3 times/day; total daily dose: 0.75 mg. **Wk 2:** 0.5 mg 3 times/day; total daily dose: 1.5 mg. **Wk 3:** 0.75 mg 3 times/day; total daily dose: 2.25 mg. **Wk 4:** 1 mg 3 times/day; total daily dose: 3 mg. **After wk 4:** May increase dose by 1.5 mg/day on wkly basis up to dose of 9 mg/day. May then further increase by 3 mg/day on wkly basis up to total dose of 24 mg/day (ESRD: 18 mg). ***(Extended-Release):*** Initially, 2 mg once daily for 1–2 wks. May increase by 2 mg/day at 1 wk or longer interval. **Maximum:** 24 mg/day. ESRD: 18 mg.

Discontinuation Taper

Gradually taper over 7 days as follows: Decrease frequency from 3 times/day to twice daily for 4 days, then decrease from twice daily to once daily for remaining 3 days.

Restless Legs Syndrome

PO: ***(Immediate-Release):*** **ADULTS, ELDERLY:** 0.25 mg once daily for days 1 and 2. May increase to 0.5 mg daily for days 3–7 and after 7 days to 1 mg daily. May further titrate upward in 0.5-mg increments q7days until reaching daily dose of 3 mg during wk 6. Daily dose may be increased to maximum of 4 mg beginning wk 7. Give all doses 1–3 hrs before bedtime. ESRD: 3 mg maximum.

Dosage in Renal/Hepatic Impairment

No dose adjustment. Use caution with severe renal impairment. Titrate cautiously in pts with hepatic impairment.

SIDE EFFECTS

Frequent (60%–40%): Nausea, dizziness, extreme drowsiness. **Occasional (12%–5%):** Syncope, vomiting, fatigue, viral infection, dyspepsia, diaphoresis, asthenia, orthostatic hypotension, abdominal discomfort, pharyngitis, abnormal vision, dry mouth, hypertension, hallucinations, confusion. **Rare (less than 4%):** Anorexia, peripheral edema, memory loss, rhinitis, sinusitis, palpitations, impotence.

ADVERSE EFFECTS/TOXIC REACTIONS

Dyskinesia, impulsive/compulsive behavior (pathologic gambling, hypersexuality, binge-eating) occur rarely.

NURSING CONSIDERATIONS

BASELINE ASSESSMENT

Parkinson's disease: Assess signs/symptoms (e.g., tremor, gait). **Restless legs syndrome:** Assess frequency of symptoms, sleep pattern.

INTERVENTION/EVALUATION

Assess for clinical improvement, clinical reversal of symptoms (improvement of tremors of head/hands at rest, mask-like facial expression, shuffling gait, muscular rigidity). Assist with ambulation if dizziness occurs. Monitor B/P, daytime alertness.

PATIENT/FAMILY TEACHING

• Drowsiness, dizziness may be an initial response. • Postural hypotension may occur more frequently during initial therapy. Slowly go from lying to standing. • Avoid tasks that require alertness, motor skills until response to drug is established. • If nausea occurs, take medication with food. • Hallucinations may occur, more so in the elderly than in younger pts with Parkinson's disease. • Report occurrence of falling asleep during activities of daily living, new or worsening symptoms, changes in B/P, fainting, unusual urges. • Avoid alcohol.

rosuvastatin

TOP 100

roe-**soo**-va-**sta**-tin
(Apo-Rosuvastatin ✦, Crestor, Ezallor Sprinkle)

Do not confuse rosuvastatin with atorvastatin, lovastatin, nystatin, pitavastatin, or simvastatin.

◆CLASSIFICATION

PHARMACOTHERAPEUTIC: HMG-CoA reductase inhibitor. **CLINICAL:** Antihyperlipidemic.

USES

Adjunct to diet therapy in pts with primary hyperlipidemia and mixed dyslipidemia; to decrease elevated total, LDL cholesterol, serum triglyceride levels; increases HDL. Adjunct to diet to slow progression of atherosclerosis in pts with elevated cholesterol. Treatment of primary dysbetalipoproteinemia, homozygous familial hypercholesterolemia (HoFH). Treatment of pts ages 10–17 yrs with heterozygous familial hypercholesterolemia (HeFH) to reduce elevated total cholesterol, LDL cholesterol, and apolipoprotein B. Primary prevention of cardiovascular disease (risk reduction of MI, stroke, arterial revascularization) without clinically evident CAD, but with multiple risk factors.

PRECAUTIONS

Contraindications: Hypersensitivity to rosuvastatin. Active hepatic disease, breastfeeding, pregnancy, unexplained, persistent elevations of hepatic enzymes. **Cautions:** Anticoagulant therapy, hepatic

R

impairment, substantial alcohol consumption, elective major surgery, renal impairment, acute renal failure, uncontrolled hypothyroidism, elderly.

ACTION

Interferes with cholesterol biosynthesis by inhibiting conversion of the enzyme HMG-CoA to mevalonate, a precursor to cholesterol. **Therapeutic Effect:** Decreases LDL, VLDL, plasma triglyceride levels; increases HDL concentration.

PHARMACOKINETICS

Protein binding: 88%. Minimal hepatic metabolism. Primarily excreted in feces. **Half-life:** 19 hrs (increased in severe renal dysfunction).

LIFESPAN CONSIDERATIONS

Pregnancy/Lactation: Contraindicated in pregnancy (suppression of cholesterol biosynthesis may cause fetal toxicity), lactation. Risk of serious adverse reactions in breastfeeding infants. **Children:** Safety and efficacy not established in children younger than 7 yrs. **Elderly:** No age-related precautions noted.

INTERACTIONS

DRUG: **Aluminum- and magnesium-containing antacids** may decrease concentration/effects. Increased risk of myopathy with **colchicine, cycloSPORINE, fenofibrate, fenofibrate derivatives, gemfibrozil, niacin.** May increase anticoagulant effect of **warfarin.** HERBAL: None significant. FOOD: **Red yeast rice** contains 2.4 mg **lovastatin** per 600 mg rice. LAB VALUES: May increase serum alkaline phosphatase, bilirubin, creatinine phosphokinase, glucose, transaminases. May produce hematuria, proteinuria.

AVAILABILITY (Rx)

Capsule, Sprinkle: 5 mg, 10 mg, 20 mg, 40 mg. **Tablets:** 5 mg, 10 mg, 20 mg, 40 mg.

ADMINISTRATION/HANDLING

PO

• Give without regard to food. May give at any time of day.

INDICATIONS/ROUTES/DOSAGE

Hyperlipidemia, Dyslipidemia, Atherosclerosis, Dysbetalipoproteinemia, Primary Prevention of Cardiovascular Disease

PO: ADULTS, ELDERLY: Usual starting dosage is 10–20 mg/day, with adjustments based on lipid levels; monitor q2–4wks until desired level is achieved. Lower starting dose of 5 mg is recommended in pts of Asian ancestry. **Maximum:** 40 mg/day. Range: 5–40 mg/day.

HoFH

PO: ADULTS, ELDERLY: Initially, 20 mg/day. **Range:** 5–40 mg/day. **Maximum:** 40 mg/day. **CHILDREN 7 YRS AND OLDER:** 20 mg once daily.

HeFH

PO: CHILDREN 10–17 YRS: Initially, 20 mg once daily. Range: 5–20 mg once daily. **Maximum:** 20 mg. **8–9 YRS:** 5–10 mg once daily. **Maximum:** 10 mg.

Concurrent CycloSPORINE Use

PO: ADULTS, ELDERLY: 5 mg/day maximum.

Concurrent Gemfibrozil, Atazanavir/Ritonavir, Lopinavir/Ritonavir or Simeprevir Therapy

PO: ADULTS, ELDERLY: Initially, 5 mg/day. 10 mg/day maximum.

Dosage in Renal Impairment (CrCl less than 30 mL/min)

PO: ADULTS, ELDERLY: 5 mg/day; do not exceed 10 mg/day.

Dosage in Hepatic Impairment

Contraindicated in active in liver disease.

SIDE EFFECTS

Generally well tolerated. Side effects are usually mild, transient. **Occasional (9%–3%):** Pharyngitis, headache, diarrhea, dyspepsia, nausea, depression. **Rare (less than 3%):** Myalgia, asthenia, back pain.

ADVERSE EFFECTS/TOXIC REACTIONS

Potential for ocular lens opacities. Hypersensitivity reaction, hepatitis, rhabdomyolysis occur rarely.

NURSING CONSIDERATIONS

BASELINE ASSESSMENT

Obtain lipid panel, LFT; pregnancy test in females of reproductive potential. Obtain dietary history, esp. fat consumption.

INTERVENTION/EVALUATION

Monitor serum cholesterol, HDL, LDL, triglycerides for therapeutic response. Lipid levels should be monitored within 2–4 wks of initiation of therapy or change in dosage. Monitor LFT at 12 wks following initiation of therapy, at any elevation of dose, and periodically (e.g., semiannually) thereafter. Monitor CPK if myopathy is suspected. Assess for headache, sore throat. Be alert for myalgia, weakness.

PATIENT/FAMILY TEACHING

• Use appropriate contraceptive measures. • Periodic lab tests are essential part of therapy. • Maintain appropriate diet (important part of treatment). • Report unexplained muscle pain, tenderness, weakness, esp. if associated with fever, malaise.

rucaparib

roo-**kap**-a-rib
(Rubraca)
Do not confuse rucaparib with neratinib, niraparib, olaparib.

◆CLASSIFICATION

PHARMACOTHERAPEUTIC: Poly (ADP-ribose) polymerase (PARP) inhibitor. **CLINICAL:** Antineoplastic.

USES

Treatment of deleterious germline and/or somatic BRCA mutation–associated (detected by FDA-approved test) advanced ovarian cancer in pts who have been treated with two or more lines of chemotherapy. Maintenance treatment of recurrent ovarian cancer in pts who are in complete or partial response to platinum-based chemotherapy. Treatment of deleterious BRCA mutation (germline and/or somatic)–associated metastatic castration-resistant prostate cancer in adults treated with androgen receptor–directed therapy and a taxane-based chemotherapy.

PRECAUTIONS

Contraindications: Hypersensitivity to rucaparib. **Cautions:** Baseline cytopenias, hepatic impairment.

ACTION

Inhibits poly (ADP-ribose) polymerase (PARP) enzymes (involved in DNA transcription, cell-cycle regulation, and DNA repair). By inhibiting PARP, may cause PARP DNA complexes resulting in DNA damage and cancer cellular death. **Therapeutic Effect:** Inhibits tumor cell growth and metastasis.

PHARMACOKINETICS

Widely distributed. Metabolized in liver. Protein binding: 70%. Peak plasma concentration: 1.9 hrs. Excretion not specified. **Half-life:** 17–19 hrs.

⌛ LIFESPAN CONSIDERATIONS

Pregnancy/Lactation: Avoid pregnancy; may cause fetal harm. Females of reproductive potential should use effective contraception during treatment and for at least 6 mos after discontinuation. Unknown if distributed in breast milk. Breastfeeding not recommended during treatment and for at least 2 wks after discontinuation. **Children:** Safety and efficacy not established. **Elderly:** No age-related precautions noted.

INTERACTIONS

DRUG: May decrease effect of **BCG vaccine.** May increase concentration/effect of **cilostazol, lomitapide, pimozide,**

R

rasagiline, tiZANidine. HERBAL: None significant. **FOOD:** None known. **LAB VALUES:** May increase serum ALT, AST, cholesterol, creatinine. May decrease ANC, Hgb, absolute lymphocyte count, platelets.

AVAILABILITY (Rx)

Tablets: 200 mg, 250 mg, 300 mg.

ADMINISTRATION/HANDLING

PO

• Give without regard to food. • If a dose is missed or vomiting occurs after administration, do not give extra dose. Administer next dose at regularly scheduled time.

INDICATIONS/ROUTES/DOSAGE

Note: Administer only to pts with deleterious germline and/or somatic BRCA mutation.

Ovarian Cancer (Advanced or maintenance of recurrent)

PO: ADULTS, ELDERLY: 600 mg twice daily about 12 hrs apart. Continue until disease progression or unacceptable toxicity.

Prostate Cancer

PO: ADULTS, ELDERLY: 600 mg twice daily. Continue until disease progression or unacceptable toxicity. Pts should also receive a gonadotropin-releasing hormone analog or have had bilateral orchiectomy.

Dose Reduction Schedule

Starting dose: 600 mg twice daily. **First dose reduction:** 500 mg twice daily. **Second dose reduction:** 400 mg twice daily. **Third dose reduction:** 300 mg twice daily.

Dose Modification

Adverse Events, Nonhematologic Toxicity

Either withhold treatment or reduce dosage per dose reduction schedule.

Hematologic Toxicity

Withhold treatment until improved to Grade 1 or 0 and investigate cause. If myelodysplastic syndrome or acute myeloid leukemia confirmed, permanently discontinue.

Dosage in Renal Impairment

Mild to moderate impairment: No dose adjustment. **Severe impairment, ESRD:** Not specified; use caution.

Dosage in Hepatic Impairment

Mild impairment: No dose adjustment. **Moderate to severe impairment:** Not specified; use caution.

SIDE EFFECTS

Frequent (77%–21%): Nausea, asthenia, fatigue, vomiting, constipation, dysgeusia, decreased appetite, diarrhea, abdominal pain, dyspnea. **Occasional (17%–9%):** Dizziness, rash, pyrexia, photosensitivity reaction, pruritus.

ADVERSE EFFECTS/TOXIC REACTIONS

Myelosuppression (anemia, lymphopenia, neutropenia, thrombocytopenia) is an expected response to therapy. Myelodysplastic syndrome/acute myeloid leukemia reported in less than 1% of pts. Infections including nasopharyngitis, pharyngitis, upper respiratory tract infection occurred in 43% of pts. Febrile neutropenia reported in less than 1% of pts. Palmar-plantar erythrodysesthesia syndrome (PPES), a chemotherapy-induced skin condition, that presents with redness, swelling, numbness, skin sloughing of the hands and feet, was reported in 2% of pts.

NURSING CONSIDERATIONS

BASELINE ASSESSMENT

Obtain CBC, vital signs, weight. Do not initiate therapy until hematologic toxicities have recovered from previous chemotherapy. Obtain pregnancy test in females of reproductive potential. Question plans of breastfeeding. Question history of hepatic/renal impairment, hypercholesterolemia. Screen for risk of bleeding, active infection. Offer emotional support.

INTERVENTION/EVALUATION

Monitor CBC monthly; creatinine periodically. For prolonged hematologic toxicities caused by other chemotherapies, monitor CBC wkly until recovery. If hematologic levels have not recovered to CTCAE Grade 1 or 0 after 4 wks, consider hematology consultation for further investigations including bone marrow analysis, blood sample for cytogenetics. Diligently monitor for infection (cough, fatigue, fever). Monitor for myelodysplastic syndrome, acute myeloid leukemia. Assess skin for rash, lesions, sloughing. Monitor for decreased urine output, renal dysfunction.

PATIENT/FAMILY TEACHING

• Treatment may depress your immune system response and reduce your ability to fight infection. Report symptoms of infection such as body aches, chills, cough, fatigue, fever. Avoid those with active infection. • Report bleeding or easy bruising, bloody urine or stool, frequent infections, fatigue, shortness of breath, weakness, weight loss; may indicate acute bone marrow depression or acute leukemia. • Use effective contraception to avoid pregnancy. Do not breastfeed. • Do not take herbal supplements. • Report planned surgical/dental procedures.

rufinamide

rue-**fin**-a-myde
(Banzel)

◆CLASSIFICATION

PHARMACOTHERAPEUTIC: Triazole derivative. **CLINICAL:** Anticonvulsant.

USES

Adjunctive therapy in treatment of seizures associated with Lennox-Gastaut syndrome in adults and children 1 yr and older.

PRECAUTIONS

Contraindications: Hypersensitivity to rufinamide. Familial short QT syndrome. **Cautions:** Concomitant use of QT interval-shortening drugs, depression, pts at high risk for suicide, mild to moderate hepatic impairment (not recommended in pts with severe hepatic impairment), concurrent use with hormonal contraceptives.

ACTION

Modulates activity of sodium channels. Prolongs inactive state of the sodium channel in cortical neurons, limits sustained repetitive firing of sodium-dependent action potential, inhibiting excitatory neurotransmitter release. **Therapeutic Effect:** Decreases frequency/severity of seizure activity.

PHARMACOKINETICS

Widely distributed. Protein binding: 34%. Extensively metabolized via hydrolysis. Excreted primarily in urine. **Half-life:** 6–10 hrs.

⌛ LIFESPAN CONSIDERATIONS

Pregnancy/Lactation: May produce fetal skeletal abnormalities. May be distributed in breast milk. **Children:** Safety and efficacy not established in pts younger than 4 yrs. **Elderly:** Age-related renal, hepatic, or cardiac impairment may require initiation of therapy at low end of dosing range.

INTERACTIONS

DRUG: May increase concentration/effect of **PHENobarbital, phenytoin.** May decrease concentration/effect of **carBAMazepine. Valproate** may increase concentration/effect. **Alcohol, CNS depressants (e.g., LORazepam, morphine, zolpidem)** may increase CNS depressant effect. **HERBAL:** None significant. **FOOD:** None known. **LAB VALUES:** May decrease WBCs.

AVAILABILITY (Rx)

Oral Suspension: 40 mg/mL. **Tablets, Film-Coated:** 200 mg, 400 mg.

ADMINISTRATION/HANDLING

PO

• Give with food. • Film-coated tablets may be cut or crushed for dosing

R

flexibility. • Shake oral suspension well before each dose; use bottle adapter and dosing syringes provided.

INDICATIONS/ROUTES/DOSAGE

Lennox-Gastaut Seizures

Note: Discontinue therapy gradually to minimize potential of increased seizure frequency (e.g., decrease by 25% q2days).
PO: ADULTS, ELDERLY: Initially, 400–800 mg/day, given in 2 equally divided doses. Dose should be increased by 400–800 mg/day every 2 days. **Maximum:** 3,200 mg/day, administered in 2 equally divided doses. CHILDREN 1 YR AND OLDER: Treatment should be initiated at a daily dose of 10 mg/kg/day, given in 2 equally divided doses. Increase by 10-mg/kg increments every other day to a target dose of 45 mg/kg/day or 3,200 mg/day, whichever is less, administered in 2 equally divided doses.

Dosage in Renal Impairment

No dose adjustment.

Dosage in Hepatic Impairment

Mild to moderate impairment: Use caution. **Severe impairment:** Not recommended.

SIDE EFFECTS

Children: Frequent (27%–11%): Headache, dizziness, fatigue, nausea, drowsiness, diplopia. Occasional (6%–4%): Tremor, nystagmus, blurred vision, vomiting. Rare (3%): Ataxia, upper abdominal pain, anxiety, constipation, dyspepsia, back pain, gait disturbance, vertigo. **Adults:** Frequent (17%–7%): Lethargy, vomiting, headache, fatigue, dizziness, nausea. Occasional (5%–4%): Influenza, nasopharyngitis, anorexia, rash, ataxia, diplopia. Rare (3%): Bronchitis, sinusitis, psychomotor hyperactivity, upper abdominal pain, aggression, ear infection, inattention, pruritus.

ADVERSE EFFECTS/TOXIC REACTIONS

Suicidal ideation or behavior occurs rarely, noted as early as 1 wk after initiation of therapy and persisting for at least 24 wks. Shortening of the QT interval (up to 20 msec), hypersensitivity reaction (rash, fever, urticaria) have been noted. Abrupt withdrawal may precipitate seizure, status epilepticus.

NURSING CONSIDERATIONS

BASELINE ASSESSMENT

Obtain ECG. Review history of seizure disorder (intensity, frequency, duration, level of consciousness). Initiate seizure precautions. Question history of suicidal ideation and behavior.

INTERVENTION/EVALUATION

Provide safety measures as needed. Observe frequently for recurrence of seizure activity. Assess for clinical improvement (decrease in intensity, frequency of seizures). Assist with ambulation if drowsiness, lethargy occur. Question for evidence of headache. Monitor for suicidal ideation and behavior.

PATIENT/FAMILY TEACHING

• Do not abruptly withdraw medication (may precipitate seizures). • Avoid tasks that require alertness, motor skills until response to drug is established. • Strict maintenance of drug therapy is essential for seizure control. • Avoid alcohol. • Use effective nonhormonal contraception to avoid pregnancy. • Seek immediate medical attention if thoughts of suicide, new onset or worsening of anxiety, depression, or changes in mood occur.

ruxolitinib

rux-oh-**li**-ti-nib
(Jakafi)

◆CLASSIFICATION

PHARMACOTHERAPEUTIC: Janus-associated tyrosine kinase inhibitor. **CLINICAL:** Antineoplastic.

USES

Treatment of intermediate or high-risk myelofibrosis, including primary myelofibrosis, post–polycythemia vera myelofibrosis, post–essential thrombocythemia myelofibrosis. Treatment of polycythemia vera. Treatment of steroid-refractory acute graft-versus-host disease (GVHD) in adults and children 12 yrs and older.

PRECAUTIONS

Contraindications: Hypersensitivity to ruxolitinib. **Cautions:** Conditions predisposing to infection (e.g., diabetes, renal failure, immunocompromised pts, open wounds), chronic opportunistic infections (e.g., herpesvirus infection, hepatitis B virus [HBV] infection, fungal infections), renal/hepatic impairment, concomitant use of strong CYP3A4 inhibitors, history of bradycardia, conduction disturbances, ischemic heart disease, HF.

ACTION

Inhibits Janus-associated kinases (JAKs) JAK1 and JAK2, which mediates the signaling of cytokines and growth factor important for hematopoiesis and immune function. In myelofibrosis and polycythemia vera JAK1/2 activity is dysregulated. **Therapeutic Effect:** Modulates the affected JAK1/2 activity.

PHARMACOKINETICS

Widely distributed. Protein binding: 97%. Metabolized in liver. Excreted in urine (74%), feces (22%). **Half-life:** 3–5 hrs.

LIFESPAN CONSIDERATIONS

Pregnancy/Lactation: Unknown if distributed in breast milk. Not recommended in nursing mothers. Must either discontinue drug or discontinue breastfeeding. **Children:** Safety and efficacy not established. **Elderly:** No age-related precautions noted.

INTERACTIONS

DRUG: Strong CYP3A4 inhibitors (e.g., clarithromycin, ketoconazole) may increase concentration/effect. May increase adverse effects; decrease therapeutic effect of **vaccines (live). HERBAL:** None known. **FOOD: Grapefruit products** may increase concentration. **LAB VALUES:** May decrease platelets, RBC, Hgb, Hct, WBC. May increase serum bilirubin, ALT, AST, cholesterol.

AVAILABILITY (Rx)

Tablets: 5 mg, 10 mg, 15 mg, 20 mg, 25 mg.

ADMINISTRATION/HANDLING

PO

- Give without regard to food.

Feeding Tube

- Suspend tablet in 40 mL water and stir for 10 min. • May administer suspension within 6 hrs after tablet has dispersed. • Flush with 75 mL water after administration.

INDICATIONS/ROUTES/DOSAGE

Myelofibrosis

PO: ADULTS: 20 mg twice daily if platelets greater than 200,000 cells/mm^3, or 15 mg twice daily if platelets 100,000–200,000 cells/mm^3, or 5 mg twice daily if platelets 50,000 to less than 100,000 cells/mm^3. Dose reduction based on platelet response. **Maximum:** 25 mg twice daily.

Polycythemia Vera

PO: ADULTS, ELDERLY: Initially, 10 mg bid. Doses titrated based on safety/efficacy.

GVHD

PO: ADULTS, ELDERLY, CHILDREN 12 YRS AND OLDER: Initially, 5 mg twice daily. May increase to 10 mg twice daily after at least 3 days (if ANC and platelets have not decreased by 50% or greater from baseline).

R

Dosage in Renal Impairment
Myelofibrosis

CrCl 15–59 mL/min	Platelets 100,000–150,000/mm^3	10 mg twice daily
CrCl 15–59 mL/min	Platelets 50,000 to less than 100,000/mm^3	5 mg once daily
CrCl 15–59 mL/min	Platelets less than 50,000/mm^3	Avoid use
End-stage renal disease (ESRD) on dialysis	Platelets 100,000–200,000/mm^3	15 mg after dialysis on days of dialysis
ESRD on dialysis	Platelets more than 200,000/mm^3	20 mg after dialysis on days of dialysis
ESRD not requiring dialysis		Avoid use

Polycythemia
CrCl 5–59 mL/min and any platelet count: 5 mg twice daily.
GVHD
CrCl 5–59 mL/min and any platelet count: 5 mg once daily. **ESRD on dialysis:** 5 mg once after dialysis. **ESRD not on dialysis:** Avoid use.

R

Dosage in Hepatic Impairment
Myelofibrosis

Hepatic impairment	Platelets 100,000–150,000/mm^3	10 mg twice daily
Hepatic impairment	Platelets 50,000 to less than 100,000/mm^3	5 mg once daily
Hepatic impairment	Platelets less than 50,000/mm^3	Avoid use

Polycythemia
Mild to severe and any platelet count: 5 mg twice daily.
GVHD
Stage 3 or 4 liver GVHD and any platelet count: 5 mg once daily.

SIDE EFFECTS

Frequent (23%–14%): Bruising, dizziness, vertigo, labyrinthitis, headache. **Occasional (9%–7%):** Weight gain, flatulence.

ADVERSE EFFECTS/TOXIC REACTIONS

May cause severe thrombocytopenia (70% of pts), anemia (96% of pts), neutropenia (18% of pts), which may improve with reduced dose or by temporarily withholding regimen. Anemic pts may require blood transfusions. Increased risk of developing opportunistic bacterial, mycobacterial, fungal, viral infections including herpes zoster, urinary tract infection, urosepsis, renal infection, pyuria. Increased risk of bleeding disorders including ecchymosis, hematoma, injection site hematoma, periorbital hematoma, petechiae, purpura.

NURSING CONSIDERATIONS

BASELINE ASSESSMENT

Obtain CBC, serum chemistries, renal function, LFT, urinalysis, cholesterol level. Assess recent vaccinations status. Receive full medication history including herbal products. Question for possibility of pregnancy, renal/hepatic impairment, HIV.

INTERVENTION/EVALUATION

Monitor CBC (every 2–4 wks until doses stabilized), serum chemistries, renal function, LFT, cholesterol. Obtain urinalysis with reflex culture for suspected UTI. Routinely assess vital signs, I&O, breath sounds, gait. Monitor temperature; be alert for fever, infectious process. Avoid IM injections, rectal temperatures, other traumas that induce bleeding. Assess skin for petechiae, hematoma, purpura.

PATIENT/FAMILY TEACHING

• Report any new bruising/bleeding, bloody stools or urine, fever, chills, rash, painful urination, suspected infection, fatigue, shortness of breath. • Do not breastfeed. • Avoid grapefruit products. • Open skin lesions, blisters may signal herpes infection. • Blood work will be routinely monitored; if on dialysis, take only following dialysis.

sacituzumab govitecan-hziy

sak-i-**tooz**-ue-mab **goe**-vi-**tee**-kan (Trodelvy)

■ BLACK BOX ALERT ■ Severe neutropenia may occur. Withhold treatment for absolute neutrophil count (ANC) less than 1,500 cells/mm³ or febrile neutropenia. Initiate antimicrobial therapy in pts with febrile neutropenia. Consider granulocyte colony-stimulating factor prophylaxis. Severe diarrhea may occur. If not contraindicated, administer atropine for early diarrhea of any severity. For onset of late diarrhea, evaluate for infectious processes.

Do not confuse sacituzumab govitecan with fam-trastuzumab deruxtecan, sarilumab, secukinumab.

◆CLASSIFICATION

PHARMACOTHERAPEUTIC: Anti-Trop-2, antibody drug conjugate, topoisomerase I inhibitor. Monoclonal antibody. **CLINICAL:** Antineoplastic.

USES

Treatment of adults with metastatic triple-negative breast cancer (mTNBC) who have received two or more prior therapies for metastatic disease.

PRECAUTIONS

Contraindications: Hypersensitivity to sacituzumab govitecan-hziy. **Cautions:** Baseline hematologic cytopenias, hepatic impairment, dehydration; conditions predisposing to infection (e.g., diabetes, renal failure, immunocompromised pts, open wounds), chronic opportunistic infections (e.g., herpesvirus infection, fungal infections). Do not substitute with other drugs containing irinotecan or its active metabolites. Pts who are homozygous for the UGT1A1*28 allele are at increased risk for neutropenia.

ACTION

An antibody drug conjugate consisting of a humanized antitrophoblast cell-surface antigen 2 (Trop-2) monoclonal antibody coupled to the topoisomerase I inhibitor SN-38. Trop-2 is overexpressed and is associated with cancer cell growth. Binds to Trop-2 and is internalized; SN-38 is release in tumors. **Therapeutic Effect:** Causes DNA damage, apoptosis, and cell death.

PHARMACOKINETICS

Widely distributed. Metabolized by UGT1A1 enzymes. Excretion not specified. **Half-life:** 16 hrs, (SN-38): 18 hrs.

LIFESPAN CONSIDERATIONS

Pregnancy/Lactation: Avoid pregnancy; may cause fetal harm. Females of reproductive potential should use effective contraception during treatment and for at least 6 mos after discontinuation. Unknown if distributed in breast milk. Breastfeeding not recommended during treatment and for at least 1 mo after discontinuation. May impair fertility. **Males:** Males with female partners of reproductive potential should use effective contraception during treatment and for at least 3 mos after discontinuation. **Children:** Safety and efficacy not established. **Elderly:** Safety and efficacy not established.

INTERACTIONS

DRUG: **UGT1A1 inhibitors (e.g., atazanavir, ketoconazole)** may increase adverse effects. **UGT1A1 inducers (e.g., carBAMazepine, phenytoin, ritonavir)** decrease concentration/effect. May decrease therapeutic effect of **BCG (intravesical), vaccines (live). Irinotecan, pimecrolimus, tacrolimus (topical)** may enhance the adverse/toxic effects. **HERBAL:** **Echinacea** may decrease therapeutic effect. **FOOD:** None known. **LAB VALUES:** May increase activated partial thromboplastin time (aPTT), serum alkaline phosphatase,

S

AST, ALT, magnesium. May decrease serum albumin, calcium, magnesium, potassium, phosphate, sodium; Hgb, leukocytes, neutrophils, platelets, RBCs. May increase or decrease serum glucose. May diminish diagnostic effect of *Coccidioides immitis* skin test.

AVAILABILITY (Rx)

Injection, Powder for Reconstitution: 180 mg.

ADMINISTRATION/HANDLING

IV

Premedication • Give antipyretic, H1 and H2 blocker, antiemetic (either two- or three-drug combination) prior to each infusion. May give a corticosteroid in pts with prior infusion reaction.

Reconstitution • Must be prepared by personal trained in aseptic manipulations and admixing of cytotoxic drugs. • Calculate the number of vials needed for reconstitution based on weight in kg at the beginning of each treatment cycle (or more frequently if body weight has changed by more than 10%). • Allow vial to warm to room temperature. • Reconstitute each vial with 20 mL of 0.9% NaCl to a final concentration of 10 mg/mL. • Swirl vial gently for up to 15 min until powder is completely dissolved. Do not shake or agitate. • Visually inspect for particulate matter or discoloration. Solution should appear clear and yellow in color. Do not use if solution is cloudy, discolored, or if visible particles are observed. • Dilute in an infusion bag containing 0.9% NaCl to a final concentration of 1.1–3.4 mg/mL (do not exceed 500 mL). Infusion bag must be made of polypropylene to minimize foaming.

Infusion Guidelines • Do not administer as IV push or bolus. • Flush IV line with 20 mL of 0.9% NaCl after infusion is complete.

Rate of administration • **First Infusion:** Infuse over 3 hrs. • **Subsequent Infusions:** Infuse over 1–2 hrs if previously tolerated. May slow or interrupt infusion if infusion reactions occur.

Storage • Refrigerate unused vials in original carton. • May refrigerate diluted solution for up to 4 hrs. After refrigeration, diluted solution must be infused within 4 hrs (includes infusion time). • Protect from light. • Do not shake, agitate, or freeze.

IV INCOMPATABILITIES

Do not mix or infuse with other solutions or medications.

INDICATIONS/ROUTES/DOSAGE

Note: Withhold dose on day 1 of any cycle for ANC less than 1,500/mm^3; withhold on day 8 of any cycle for ANC less than 1,000/mm^3.

Breast Cancer (triple-negative)

IV Infusion: ADULTS: 10 mg/kg on days 1 and 8 of 21-day cycle. Continue until disease progression or unacceptable toxicity. **Maximum:** 10 mg/kg/dose.

Dose Modification

Based on Common Terminology Criteria for Adverse Events (CTCAE).

Note: Do not re-escalate if a dose reduction is made.

Neutropenia

Grade 3 febrile neutropenia; grade 4 neutropenia for 7 days or greater; grade 3 or 4 neutropenia that delays dosing by 2 or 3 wks for recovery to less than or equal to grade 1: For first occurrence, reduce dose by 25% and give granulocyte colony-stimulating factor. For second occurrence, reduce dose by 50%. For third occurrence, permanently discontinue. **Grade 3 or 4 neutropenia that delays dosing beyond 3 wks for recovery to less than or equal to grade 1:** Permanently discontinue. Severe Non-Neutropenic Toxicity. **Grade 4 nonhematologic toxicity of any duration;**

S

any grade 3 or 4 treatment-induced nausea, vomiting, diarrhea (not controlled by antiemetics/antidiarrheal agents); other grade 3 or 4 nonhematologic toxicity lasting greater than 48 hrs (despite medical management); grade 3 or 4 nonneutropenic toxicity that delays dosing by 2 or 3 wks for recovery to less than or equal to grade 1: For first occurrence, reduce dose by 25%. For second occurrence, reduce dose by 50%. For third occurrence, permanently discontinue. **Grade 3 or 4 nonneutropenia hematologic toxicity that does not improve to less than or equal grade 1 within 3 wks:** Permanently discontinue.

Dosage in Renal Impairment

Mild impairment: No dose adjustment. **Moderate to severe impairment:** Not specified; use caution.

Dosage in Hepatic Impairment

Mild to severe impairment: Not specified; use caution.

SIDE EFFECTS

Frequent (69–21%): Nausea, diarrhea, fatigue, vomiting, alopecia, constipation, rash, skin irritation/exfoliation, decreased appetite, abdominal pain/distension, headache, back pain, cough, dizziness, dyspnea. **Occasional (19%–11%):** Edema, pruritus, arthralgia, dry skin, mucositis, stomatitis, esophagitis, mucosal inflammation, pyrexia, insomnia, dehydration, dysgeusia, extremity pain.

ADVERSE EFFECTS/TOXIC REACTIONS

Myelosuppression (anemia, leukopenia, neutropenia, thrombocytopenia) is an expected response to therapy, but more severe reactions including severe neutropenia, febrile neutropenia may be life-threatening. Pts with uridine diphosphate-glucuronosyl transferase 1A1 (UGT1A1)*28 allele are at an increased risk of neutropenia, other adverse reactions. Diarrhea occurred in 63% of pts. Grade 3 or 4 diarrhea reported in 9% of pts. Life-threatening hypersensitivity reactions, including anaphylaxis, may occur. Grade 3 or 4 nausea and vomiting was reported. Pleural effusion reported in 2% of pts. Infections including bronchitis, influenza, pneumonia, respiratory syncytial virus infection, upper respiratory tract infection, UTI, viral infection were reported. Neuropathies including hypoesthesia, gait disturbance, muscular weakness, paresthesia, peripheral motor/sensorimotor neuropathy reported in 24% of pts. Immunogenicity (auto-sacituzumab govitecan-hziy antibodies) reported in 2% of pts.

NURSING CONSIDERATIONS

BASELINE ASSESSMENT

Obtain ANC, CBC, LFT; pregnancy test in females of reproductive potential. Confirm compliance of effective contraception. Confirm triple-negative breast cancer status. Obtain weight in kilograms. Verify status of UGT1A1*28 allele. Question occurrence of infusion reactions prior to each dose. Question history of hepatic impairment. Screen for active infection. Assess usual bowel movement patterns, stool characteristics. Assess and correct hydration status prior to each dose. Receive full medication history and screen for interactions. Offer emotional support.

INTERVENTION/EVALUATION

Monitor ANC, CBC for myelosuppression. Monitor for severe neutropenia, febrile neutropenia (esp. in pts with reduced UGT1A1 activity); infections (cough, fatigue, fever). If serious infection occurs, initiate appropriate antimicrobial therapy. Monitor for hypersensitivity reactions, infusion reactions during infusion and for at least 30 min after completion. If infusion-related reaction occurs, interrupt infusion and

S

manage symptoms. Permanently discontinue if life-threatening infusion reaction, hypersensitivity reaction occurs. Diarrhea must be treated promptly. If diarrhea occurs, evaluate for infectious processes. If negative for infectious processes, recommend loperamide (antidiarrheal agent) 4 mg initially, then 2 mg with every episode of diarrhea up to a maximum of 16 mg/day. Discontinue antidiarrheal agent 12 hrs after diarrhea subsides. May give atropine for subsequent treatments in pts who exhibit excessive cholinergic response (e.g., abdominal cramping, diarrhea, salivation). Adequate fluid and electrolyte resuscitation should be considered. Offer antiemetics if nausea or vomiting occurs. Monitor I&Os, hydration status. Monitor for neuropathies.

PATIENT/FAMILY TEACHING

• Treatment may depress your immune system response and reduce your ability to fight infection. Report symptoms of infection such as body aches, chills, cough, fatigue, fever. Avoid those with active infection. • Report symptoms of bone marrow depression (e.g., bruising, fatigue, fever, shortness of breath, weight loss; bleeding easily, bloody urine or stool). • Severe allergic reactions, including anaphylaxis, can occur. If allergic reaction occurs, seek immediate medical attention. • Severe diarrhea may cause dehydration, electrolyte imbalance. Drink plenty of fluids. Report diarrhea that does not improve with medical management. Maintain proper hydration and nutrition. • Use effective contraception to avoid pregnancy. Do not breastfeed. • Nausea and vomiting is a common side effect. • Report nervous system changes (gait disturbance, pain, numbness, trouble walking); UTI (fever, urinary frequency, burning during urination, foul-smelling urine). • Do not take newly prescribed medications unless approved by the prescriber who originally started treatment.

S

sacubitril-valsartan

sak-**ue**-bi-tril
(Entresto)

■ BLACK BOX ALERT ■ May cause fetal harm, mortality. Discontinue as soon as pregnancy detected.

◆CLASSIFICATION

PHARMACOTHERAPEUTIC: Combination of sacubitril, a neprilysin inhibitor, and valsartan, an angiotensin II receptor blocker. **CLINICAL:** Reduces risk of complications in HF.

USES

To reduce the risk of cardiovascular death and hospitalization in pts with chronic HF (NYHA class II-IV) and reduced ejection fraction. Treatment of symptomatic HF with systemic left ventricular systolic dysfunction in pediatric pts 1 yr and older.

PRECAUTIONS

Contraindications: Hypersensitivity to sacubitril or valsartan; history of angioedema related to angiotensin-converting enzyme (ACE) inhibitor or angiotensin receptor blockers (ARB); concomitant use or within 36 hrs of ACE inhibitors; concomitant use of aliskiren in pts with diabetes. **Cautions:** Baseline anemia, dehydration, hypovolemia, sodium depletion; concomitant use of potassium-sparing diuretics or potassium supplements; hepatic/renal impairment; unstented bilateral/unilateral renal artery stenosis; significant aortic/mitral stenosis. Pts with orthostatic hypotension.

ACTION

Sacubitril inhibits neprilysin, increasing peptide levels that are degraded by neprilysin (e.g., natriuretic peptides). Valsartan directly antagonizes angiotensin II receptors; blocks vasoconstrictor, aldosterone secreting effects of angiotensin II, inhibiting binding of angiotensin II to AT_1 receptors. **Therapeutic Effect:** Decreases risk of mortality in pts with chronic HF; produces vasodilation; decreases peripheral resistance; decreases B/P.

PHARMACOKINETICS

Widely distributed. Sacubitril is converted by esterases; not significantly metabolized after conversion. Valsartan is minimally metabolized in liver. Protein binding (both): 94%–97%. Peak plasma concentration: sacubitril: 30 min, valsartan: 1.5 hrs. Steady-state concentration: 3 days. Excretion: sacubitril: urine (52%–68%), feces (37%–48%); valsartan: feces (86%), urine (13%). **Half-life:** sacubitril: 1.4 hrs; valsartan: 9.9 hrs.

LIFESPAN CONSIDERATIONS

Pregnancy/Lactation: Avoid pregnancy; may cause fetal harm/mortality. Unknown if distributed in breast milk. Breastfeeding not recommended. **Children:** Safety and efficacy not established. **Elderly:** No age-related precautions noted.

INTERACTIONS

DRUG: **ACE inhibitors (e.g., enalapril, ramipril)** may increase risk of angioedema (contraindicated). **Potassium-sparing diuretics (e.g., spironolactone)** may increase risk of hyperkalemia. **NSAIDs (e.g., ibuprofen, naproxen)** may worsen renal function. May increase concentration/effect of **lithium**. **HERBAL:** **Herbals with hypertensive properties (e.g., licorice, yohimbe) or hypotensive properties (e.g., garlic, ginger, ginkgo biloba)** may alter effects. **FOOD:** None known. **LAB VALUES:** May increase serum BUN, creatinine, potassium. May decrease Hct, Hgb.

AVAILABILITY (Rx)

Fixed-Dose Combination Tablets: ***(Sacubitril/valsartan):*** 24 mg/26 mg, 49 mg/51 mg, 97 mg/103 mg.

ADMINISTRATION/HANDLING

PO

- Give without regard to food.

INDICATIONS/ROUTES/DOSAGE

HF

Note: Allow a 36-hr washout period when switching from or to an ACE inhibitor. After initial dose, may double dose as tolerated q2–4wks to target dose of 97 mg/103 mg.
PO: ADULTS, ELDERLY: (Previously taking high dose of ACE inhibitor [greater than 10 mg enalapril or equivalent] or ARB [greater than 160 mg valsartan or equivalent]): Initially, 49 mg/51 mg twice daily. **CHILDREN WEIGHING MORE THAN 50 KG:** Initially, 49 mg/51 mg twice daily. **40–50 KG:** Initially, 24 mg/26 mg twice daily. **LESS THAN 40 KG:** Initially, 1.6 mg/kg/dose twice daily. (Previously taking low dose of ACE inhibitor [10 mg or less of enalapril or equivalent] or ARB): 24 mg/26 mg twice daily. (Not currently taking an ACE inhibitor or ARB): 24 mg/26 mg twice daily. **CHILDREN, ADOLESCENTS WEIGHING MORE THAN 50 KG:** Initially, 24 mg/26 mg twice daily. **WEIGHING 50 KG OR LESS:** Initially, 0.8 mg/kg/dose twice daily.

Dosage in Renal Impairment

Mild to moderate impairment: No dose adjustment. **Severe impairment:** Initially, 24 mg/26 mg twice daily. **Maintenance:** May double each dose every 2–4 wks up to 97 mg/103 mg twice daily based on tolerability.

Dosage in Hepatic Impairment

Mild impairment: No dose adjustment. **Moderate impairment:** Initially, 24 mg/26 mg twice daily. **Maintenance:** May double each dose every 2–4 wks up to 97 mg/103 mg twice daily based on tolerability. **Severe impairment:** Treatment not recommended.

SIDE EFFECTS

Occasional (9%): Cough, dizziness.

ADVERSE EFFECTS/TOXIC REACTIONS

Angioedema (less than 1% of pts), hypotension (18% of pts), orthostatic

S

hypotension (2% of pts), impairment/decrease in renal function due to inhibition of renin-angiotensin-aldosterone system (5% of pts), elevation of serum creatinine greater than 50% from baseline (1.4% of pts), renal impairment including oliguria, azotemia, acute renal failure (5% of pts), hyperkalemia (12% of pts), serum potassium elevation greater than 5.5 mEq/L (4% of pts) have occurred.

NURSING CONSIDERATIONS

BASELINE ASSESSMENT

Obtain baseline BMP; CBC in pts with baseline anemia. Obtain B/P, heart rate immediately before each dose, in addition to regular monitoring (be alert for fluctuations). Assess hydration status. Correct hydration/sodium depletion prior to initiation. Receive medication history and screen for interactions, esp. concomitant use of aliskiren, ACE inhibitors, ARBs, potassium-sparing diuretics, potassium supplements. Verify negative pregnancy status. Question history of hepatic/renal impairment, renal artery stenosis; angioedema, hypersensitivity reaction.

INTERVENTION/EVALUATION

Monitor BMP, esp. serum BUN, creatinine, potassium. Monitor for hyperkalemia, hypotension. If hypotension occurs, place pt in supine position, feet slightly elevated; consider interrupting treatment or altering dose of diuretic, antihypertensive drugs and screen for dehydration/serum sodium depletion. If pt positive for dehydration, be cautious with PO/IV administration. Overhydration may exacerbate HF. Assist with ambulation if dizziness occurs. Monitor for hypersensitivity reaction, including angioedema. If angioedema occurs, interrupt treatment and institute therapy to protect airway patency.

PATIENT/FAMILY TEACHING

• Be cautious of fluid intake. Overhydration may lead to worsening of HF, while underhydration may lead to low blood pressure. • Report urine changes such as darkened urine, decreased output. • Immediately report allergic reactions such as difficulty breathing, itching, rash, tongue swelling; symptoms of high potassium levels such as extreme fatigue, muscle weakness, palpitations; suspected pregnancy. • Do not breastfeed. • Diuretics (water pills) may increase risk of low pressure or low potassium levels.

salmeterol

TOP 100

sal-**met**-er-all
(Serevent Diskus)

■ BLACK BOX ALERT ■ Long-acting beta$_2$-adrenergic agonists may increase risk of asthma-related deaths and asthma-related hospitalizations in pediatric and adolescent pts. Use only as adjuvant therapy in pts who are currently receiving but not adequately controlled on long-term asthma control medication.

Do not confuse salmeterol with Solu-Medrol, or Serevent with Atrovent, Combivent, Serentil, or Sinemet.

FIXED-COMBINATION(S)

Advair Diskus: salmeterol/fluticasone (a corticosteroid): 50 mcg/100 mcg, 50 mcg/250 mcg, 50 mcg/500 mcg. **Advair HFA:** salmeterol/fluticasone (a corticosteroid): 21 mcg/45 mcg, 21 mcg/115 mcg, 21 mcg/230 mcg.

◆CLASSIFICATION

PHARMACOTHERAPEUTIC: Beta$_2$-adrenergic agonist (long-acting). **CLINICAL:** Bronchodilator.

USES

Prevention of exercise-induced bronchospasm, bronchospasm; maintenance treatment of asthma and prevention of bronchospasm in pts with reversible obstructive airway disease, including those with symptoms of nocturnal asthma. Long-term maintenance treatment of bronchospasm associated with COPD (including emphysema and chronic bronchitis).

PRECAUTIONS

Contraindications: Hypersensitivity to salmeterol. Treatment of status asthmaticus, acute episodes of asthma or COPD. Use as monotherapy in treatment of asthma without concomitant long-term asthma control medication (e.g., inhaled corticosteroids). **Cautions:** Not for acute symptoms; may cause paradoxical bronchospasm, severe asthma. Cardiovascular disorders (coronary insufficiency, arrhythmias, hypertension), seizure disorders, diabetes, hyperthyroidism, hepatic impairment, hypokalemia.

ACTION

Stimulates $beta_2$-adrenergic receptors in lungs, resulting in relaxation of bronchial smooth muscle. **Therapeutic Effect:** Relieves bronchospasm, reducing airway resistance.

PHARMACOKINETICS

Route	Onset	Peak	Duration
Inhalation (asthma)	30–45 min	2–4 hrs	12 hrs
Inhalation (COPD)	2 hrs	3.25–4.75 hrs	12 hrs

Low systemic absorption; acts primarily in lungs. Protein binding: 95%. Metabolized in liver. Excreted in urine (25%), feces (60%). **Half-life:** 5.5 hrs.

LIFESPAN CONSIDERATIONS

Pregnancy/Lactation: Unknown if distributed in breast milk. **Children:** No age-related precautions in pts older than 4 yrs. **Elderly:** Lower dosages may be needed (may be more susceptible to tachycardia, tremors).

INTERACTIONS

DRUG: **Beta blockers (e.g., carvedilol, metoprolol)** may reduce effect; may produce bronchospasm. **Strong CYP3A4 inhibitors (e.g., clarithromycin, ketoconazole, ritonavir), MAOIs (e.g., phenelzine, selegiline), tricyclic antidepressants (e.g., amitriptyline, doxepin)** may increase concentration/effects (wait 14 days after stopping MAOIs, tricyclic antidepressants before starting salmeterol). **HERBAL:** None significant. **FOOD:** None known. **LAB VALUES:** May decrease serum potassium. May increase serum glucose.

AVAILABILITY (Rx)

Aerosol Powder Breath Activated, Inhalation: 50 mcg/inhalation.

ADMINISTRATION/HANDLING

Inhalation

• Do not shake or prime. Before inhaling the dose, breath out fully (do not exhale into Diskus device). Activate and use only in level horizontal position. • Inhale quickly and deeply through Diskus. • Hold breath as long as possible before exhaling slowly. • Do not use a spacer or wash mouthpiece.

INDICATIONS/ROUTES/DOSAGE

Maintenance and Prevention Therapy for Asthma, Bronchospasm

Inhalation: ADULTS, ELDERLY, CHILDREN 4 YRS AND OLDER: 1 inhalation (50 mcg) q12h (used in combination with inhaled corticosteroids not as monotherapy).

Prevention of Exercise-Induced Bronchospasm

Inhalation: ADULTS, ELDERLY, CHILDREN 4 YRS AND OLDER: 1 inhalation at least 30 min before exercise. Additional doses should not be given for 12 hrs. Do not administer if already giving salmeterol twice daily.

Maintenance Therapy for COPD

Inhalation: ADULTS, ELDERLY: 1 inhalation (50 mcg) q12h.

Dosage in Renal/Hepatic Impairment

No dose adjustment.

SIDE EFFECTS

Frequent (28%): Headache. **Occasional (7%–3%):** Cough, tremor, dizziness, vertigo, throat dryness/irritation, pharyngitis. **Rare (less than 3%):** Palpitations, tachycardia, nausea, heartburn, GI distress, diarrhea.

S

ADVERSE EFFECTS/TOXIC REACTIONS

May prolong QT interval (can precipitate ventricular arrhythmias). Hypokalemia, hyperglycemia may occur.

NURSING CONSIDERATIONS

BASELINE ASSESSMENT

Question history of cardiac disease, hepatic impairment, seizure disorder. Screen for concomitant medications known to prolong QT interval. Assess lung sounds, vital signs.

INTERVENTION/EVALUATION

Monitor rate, depth, rhythm, type of respiration; quality/rate of pulse, B/P. Assess lungs for wheezing, rales, rhonchi. Periodically evaluate serum potassium levels.

PATIENT/FAMILY TEACHING

• Not for relief of acute episodes. • Keep canister at room temperature (cold decreases effects). • Do not stop medication or exceed recommended dosage. • Report chest pain, dizziness. • Wait at least 1 full min before second inhalation. • Administer dose 30–60 min before exercise when used to prevent exercise-induced bronchospasm. • Avoid excessive use of caffeine derivatives (coffee, tea, colas, chocolate).

S

sargramostim

sar-**gra**-moe-stim
(Leukine)
Do not confuse Leukine with leucovorin or Leukeran.

◆CLASSIFICATION

PHARMACOTHERAPEUTIC: Colony-stimulating factor. **CLINICAL:** Hematopoietic agent.

USES

Acute myelogenous leukemia (AML: following induction chemotherapy): Shortens time to neutrophil recovery; reduces incidence of severe infections. **Bone marrow transplant (allogeneic or autologous):** For graft failure, engraftment delay. **Myeloid reconstitution** following allogeneic or autologous bone marrow transplant. **Peripheral stem cell transplant (allogeneic or autologous):** Mobilizes hematopoietic progenitor cells. **Hematopoietic radiation injury syndrome (acute):** Treatment to increase survival due to acute exposure to myelosuppressive radiation doses. **OFF-LABEL:** Primary prophylaxis of neutropenia.

PRECAUTIONS

Contraindications: Hypersensitivity to sargramostim. Concurrent (24 hrs preceding or following) myelosuppressive chemotherapy or radiation, pts with excessive leukemic myeloid blasts in bone marrow or peripheral blood (greater than 10%), known hypersensitivity to yeast-derived products. **Cautions:** Preexisting HF, fluid retention, cardiovascular disease, pulmonary disease (hypoxia, pulmonary infiltrates), renal/hepatic impairment.

ACTION

Stimulates proliferation/differentiation and functional activity of eosinophils, monocytes, neutrophils, and macrophages. **Therapeutic Effect:** Assists bone marrow in making new WBCs, increases their chemotactic, antifungal, antiparasitic activity. Increases cytoneoplastic cells, activates neutrophils to inhibit tumor cell growth.

PHARMACOKINETICS

Route	Onset	Peak	Duration
IV (increase WBCs)	7–14 days	N/A	1 wk

Detected in serum within 5 min after SQ administration. **Peak serum levels:** 1–3 hrs. **Half-life: IV:** 1 hr; **SQ:** 3 hrs.

⌛ LIFESPAN CONSIDERATIONS

Pregnancy/Lactation: Unknown if drug crosses placenta or is distributed in breast milk. **Children:** Safety and efficacy not established. **Elderly:** No age-related precautions noted.

INTERACTIONS

DRUG: May increase adverse effects of **tisagenlecleucel, vaccines (live).** May decrease therapeutic effect of **vaccines (live). Corticosteroids (e.g., dexamethasone, predniSONE)** may increase myeloproliferative effect. **HERBAL:** None significant. **FOOD:** None known. **LAB VALUES:** May increase serum ALT, AST, bilirubin, creatinine. May decrease serum albumin.

AVAILABILITY (Rx)

Injection, Powder for Reconstitution: 250 mcg.

ADMINISTRATION/HANDLING

SQ

May be given without further dilution.

IV

Reconstitution • To 250-mcg vial, add 1 mL Sterile Water for Injection (preservative free) or Bacteriostatic Water for Injection. Direct diluent to side of vial, gently swirl contents to avoid foaming; do not shake or vigorously agitate. • After reconstitution, further dilute in 25–50 mL 0.9% NaCl to a concentration of 10 mcg/mL or greater. If final concentration less than 10 mcg/mL, 1 mg of human albumin per 1 mL of 0.9% NaCl should be added to provide a final albumin concentration of 0.1% (e.g., 1 mL 5% albumin per 50 mL 0.9% NaCl).

◀ALERT▶ Albumin is added before addition of sargramostim (prevents drug adsorption to components of drug delivery system).

Rate of administration • Give each single dose over 30 min, 2 hr, 6 hr, or continuous infusion.

Storage • Refrigerate powder, reconstituted solution, diluted solution for injection. • Do not shake. • Reconstituted solutions are clear, colorless. • Use within 6 hrs; discard unused portions. • Use 1 dose per vial; do not reenter vial.

IV INCOMPATIBILITIES

Amphotericin B complex (Abelcet, AmBisome, Amphotec), ondansetron (Zofran).

IV COMPATIBILITIES

Dexamethasone (Decadron), diphenhydrAMINE (Benadryl), famotidine (Pepcid), granisetron (Kytril), heparin, metoclopramide (Reglan), promethazine (Phenergan).

INDICATIONS/ROUTES/DOSAGE

Neutrophil Recovery Following Chemotherapy in AML

IV infusion: ADULTS 55 YRS OR OLDER: 250 mcg/m^2/day (as 4-hr infusion) starting approximately 4 days following completion of induction chemotherapy (if day 10 bone marrow is hypoplastic with less than 5% blasts). Continue until ANC is greater than 1,500 cells/mm^3 for 3 consecutive days or a maximum of 42 days. If WBC greater than 50,000 cells/mm^3 and/or ANC greater that 20,000 cells/mm^3, interrupt treatment or reduce dose by 50%.

Myeloid Recovery Following Bone Marrow Transplant (BMT)

IV infusion: ADULTS, ELDERLY: Usual parenteral dosage: 250 mcg/m^2/day (as 2-hr infusion). Begin 2–4 hrs after autologous bone marrow infusion and not less than 24 hrs after last dose of chemotherapy or last radiation treatment, when post marrow infusion ANC is less than 500 cells/mm^3. Continue until ANC greater than 1,500 cells/mm^3 for 3 consecutive days. If WBC greater than 50,000 cells/mm^3 and/or ANC greater that 20,000 cells/mm^3, interrupt treatment or reduce dose by 50%. Discontinue if blast cells appear or underlying disease progresses.

Bone Marrow Transplant Failure, Engraftment Delay

IV infusion: ADULTS, ELDERLY: 250 mcg/m^2/day for 14 days. Infuse over 2 hrs. May repeat after 7 days off therapy if engraftment has not occurred. A third course with 500 mcg/m^2/day for 14 days may be tried if engraftment still has not occurred.

Stem Cell Transplant, Mobilization

IV, SQ: ADULTS: 250 mcg/m²/day IV (as 24-hr infusion) or SQ once daily. Continue same dose throughout peripheral blood progenitor cell collection. If WBC greater than 50,000 cells/mm³, reduce dose by 50%.

Stem Cell Transplant, Post-transplant

IV, SQ: ADULTS, ELDERLY: 250 mcg/m²/day IV (as 24-hr infusion) or SQ once daily beginning immediately following infusion of progenitor cells. Continue until ANC greater than 1,500 cells/mm³ for 3 consecutive days.

Hematopoietic Radiation Injury Syndrome (Acute)

SQ: ADULTS, ELDERLY WEIGHING MORE THAN 40 KG: 7 mcg/kg once daily. Begin treatment as soon as possible after suspected or confirmed exposure to radiation doses greater than 2 (gray) Gy. Do not delay if CBC not available. Continue until ANC remains greater than 1,000/cells mm³ for 3 consecutive CBCs (obtain q3days) or ANC exceeds 10,000/cells mm³ after radiation-induced nadir.

Dosage in Renal/Hepatic Impairment

No dose adjustment.

SIDE EFFECTS

Frequent: GI disturbances (nausea, diarrhea, vomiting, stomatitis, anorexia, abdominal pain), arthralgia or myalgia, headache, malaise, rash, pruritus. **Occasional:** Peripheral edema, weight gain, dyspnea, asthenia, fever, leukocytosis, capillary leak syndrome (fluid retention, irritation at local injection site, peripheral edema). **Rare:** Tachycardia, arrhythmias, thrombophlebitis.

ADVERSE EFFECTS/TOXIC REACTIONS

Pleural/pericardial effusion occurs rarely after infusion.

NURSING CONSIDERATIONS

BASELINE ASSESSMENT

Obtain CBC, BMP, LFT, vital signs. Question history of cardiac/pulmonary disease, renal/hepatic impairment.

INTERVENTION/EVALUATION

Monitor CBC with differential, serum renal/hepatic function, pulmonary function, vital signs, weight. Monitor for supraventricular arrhythmias during administration (particularly in pts with history of cardiac arrhythmias). Assess closely for dyspnea during and immediately following infusion (particularly in pts with history of lung disease). If dyspnea occurs during infusion, cut infusion rate by half. If dyspnea continues, stop infusion immediately. If neutrophil count exceeds 20,000 cells/mm³ or platelet count exceeds 500,000 cells/mm³, reduce dose by half, based on clinical condition of pt. Blood counts return to normal or baseline 3–7 days after discontinuation of therapy.

PATIENT/FAMILY TEACHING

• Report difficulty breathing, esp. during or immediately after infusion. • May increase risk of cardiac arrhythmias; report dizziness, fainting, palpitations. • Treatment may cause edema, fluid collection in the lungs or around the heart.

sarilumab

sar-**il**-ue-mab
(Kevzara)

BLACK BOX ALERT

Tuberculosis (TB), invasive fungal infections, other opportunistic infections leading to hospitalization and death were reported. Avoid use in pts with active infection. Withhold treatment until serious infection is controlled. Test for TB prior to and during treatment, regardless of initial result; if positive, start treatment for TB prior to initiation.

Do not confuse sarilumab with adalimumab, avelumab, belimumab, brodalumab, dupilumab, ipilimumab, nivolumab, or panitumumab.

◆CLASSIFICATION

PHARMACOTHERAPEUTIC: Interleukin-6 receptor antagonist. Monoclonal antibody. **CLINICAL:** Antirheumatic, disease modifying.

USES

Treatment of adults with moderately to severely active rheumatoid arthritis who have had an inadequate response or intolerance to one or more DMARDs. May use as monotherapy or in combination with nonbiologic DMARDs (do not use in combination with biologic DMARDs).

PRECAUTIONS

Contraindications: Hypersensitivity to sarilumab. **Cautions:** Hyperlipidemia, hypertriglyceridemia, active hepatic disease or hepatic impairment; recent travel or residence in endemic TB or mycosis areas; history of chronic opportunistic infections (esp. bacterial, invasive fungal, mycobacterial, protozoal, viral, TB); conditions predisposing to infection (e.g., diabetes, immunocompromised pts, renal failure, open wounds); history of HIV, herpes zoster, hepatitis B virus (HBV) infection, malignancies; baseline neutropenia, thrombocytopenia; pts at risk for GI perforation (Crohn's disease, diverticulitis, GI tract malignancies, peptic ulcers, peritoneal malignancies). Not recommended in pts with active infection, concomitant use of biological DMARDs; baseline ANC less than 2000 cells/mm^3, platelet count less than 150,000 cells/mm^3, serum ALT, AST above 1.5 times upper limit of normal (ULN).

ACTION

Binds to interleukin-6 (IL-6) receptor, inhibiting signaling of IL-6, a cytokine involved in inflammatory and immune responses. **Therapeutic Effect:** Reduces inflammation of RA.

PHARMACOKINETICS

Widely distributed. Peak plasma concentration: 2–4 days. Excretion (200 mg dose): linear, nonsaturable proteolytic pathway. (150 mg dose): Nonlinear, saturable target medicated pathway. **Half-life:** Concentration dependent: 200 mg q2wks (up to 10 days); 150 mg q2wks (up to 8 days).

LIFESPAN CONSIDERATIONS

Pregnancy/Lactation: Crosses the placental barrier, esp. during the third trimester. Unknown if distributed in breast milk; however, maternal immunoglobulin G (IgG) is present in breast milk. **Children:** Safety and efficacy not established. **Elderly:** Use caution (increased incidence of infections).

INTERACTIONS

DRUG: May decrease therapeutic effect of **BCG (intravesical), vaccines (live)**. May increase adverse effects of **belimumab, natalizumab, vaccines (live)**. **HERBAL:** **Echinacea** may decrease therapeutic effect. **FOOD:** None known. **LAB VALUES:** May increase serum ALT, AST, cholesterol, LDL, HDL, triglycerides. May decrease leukocytes, neutrophils, platelets.

AVAILABILITY (Rx)

Injection Solution: 150 mg/1.14 mL, 200 mg/1.14 mL.

ADMINISTRATION/HANDLING

SQ

Preparation • Remove prefilled syringe from refrigerator and allow solution to warm to room temperature (approx. 30 min). • Visually inspect for particulate matter or discoloration. Solution should appear clear, colorless to slightly yellow in color. Do not use if solution is cloudy, discolored, or visible particles are observed.

Administration • Insert needle subcutaneously into upper arms, outer thigh, or abdomen and inject solution. • Do not inject into areas of active skin disease or injury such as sunburns, skin rashes, inflammation, skin infections, or active psoriasis. • Do not administer IV or intramuscularly. • Rotate injection sites.

S

Storage • Refrigerate in original carton until time of use. • Protect from light. • May store at room temperature for up to 14 days. Once warmed to room temperature, do not place back into refrigerator. • Do not freeze or expose to heating sources. • Do not shake.

INDICATIONS/ROUTES/DOSAGE

Note: Do not initiate if ANC is less than 2,000 cells/mm^3; platelets less than 150,000 cells/mm^3; or serum ALT or AST greater than 1.5 times ULN.

Rheumatoid Arthritis

SQ: ADULTS, ELDERLY: 200 mg once q2wks.

Dose Modification

Neutropenia

ANC greater than 1000 cells/mm^3: No dose adjustment. **ANC 500–1000 cells/mm^3:** Withhold treatment until ANC greater than 1000 cells/mm^3, then resume at 150 mg once q2wks. May increase to 200 mg once q2wks as clinically indicated. **ANC less than 500 cells/mm^3:** Permanently discontinue.

Hepatotoxicity

Serum ALT elevation up to 3 times ULN: Consider modifying dose of concomitant DMARDs. **Serum ALT elevation greater than 3–5 times ULN:** Withhold treatment until serum ALT less than 3 times ULN, then resume at 150 mg once q2wks. May increase to 200 mg once q2wks as clinically indicated. **Serum ALT elevation greater than 5 times ULN:** Permanently discontinue.

Serious Infection

Withhold treatment until serious infection is controlled, then resume as clinically indicated.

Thrombocytopenia

Platelet count 50,000–100,000 cells/mm^3: Withhold treatment until platelet count greater than 100,000 cells/mm^3, then resume at 150 mg once q2wks. May increase to 200 mg once q2wks as clinically indicated. **Platelet count less than 50,000 cells/mm^3:** Permanently discontinue if confirmed by repeat testing.

Dosage in Renal Impairment

Mild to moderate impairment: No dose adjustment. **Severe impairment:** Not specified; use caution.

Dosage in Hepatic Impairment

Not specified; use caution.

SIDE EFFECTS

Rare (4%–2%): Injection site reactions (pain, erythema, pruritus).

ADVERSE EFFECTS/TOXIC REACTIONS

Serious, sometimes fatal, infections including aspergillosis, candidiasis, cellulitis, *Cryptococcus*, histoplasmosis, pneumonia, sepsis, tuberculosis; bacterial, mycobacterial, invasive fungal, opportunistic, viral infections were reported. Nasopharyngitis, upper respiratory tract infections, urinary tract infections occurred in 2–4% of pts. Neutropenia may increase risk of serious infection. GI perforation may occur, esp. in pts with history of diverticulitis or concomitant use of NSAIDs, corticosteroids. May increase risk for new malignancies. Hypersensitivity reactions including rash, urticaria reported in less than 1% of pts. May increase risk of HBV reactivation, which may result in fulminant hepatitis, hepatic failure, death. Immunogenicity (auto-sarilumab antibodies) was reported.

NURSING CONSIDERATIONS

BASELINE ASSESSMENT

Obtain CBC, LFT, lipid panel. Assess onset, location, duration of pain, inflammation. Inspect appearance of affected joints for immobility, deformities. Pts should be evaluated for active tuberculosis and tested for latent infection prior to initiation and periodically during therapy. Induration of 5 mm or greater with tuberculin skin testing should be considered a positive test result when assessing if treatment for latent tuberculosis is necessary. Question history of

S

chronic infections, opportunistic infections, herpes infection. Screen for active infection. Assess skin for open wounds. Question history of active hepatic disease, GI perforation, malignancies, HIV, HBV, hypersensitivity reactions. Receive full medication history and screen for interactions. Assess pt's willingness to self-inject medication.

INTERVENTION/EVALUATION

Assess for therapeutic response: relief of pain, stiffness, swelling; increased joint mobility; reduced joint tenderness; improved grip strength. Monitor neutrophil count, platelet count, LFT 4–6 wks after initiation, then q3mos thereafter. Monitor lipid panel 4–6 wks after initiation, then q6mos thereafter. Monitor for symptoms of tuberculosis, including those who tested negative for latent tuberculosis infection prior to initiating therapy. Interrupt or discontinue treatment if serious infection, opportunistic infection, or sepsis occurs and initiate appropriate antimicrobial therapy. Closely monitor for HBV reactivation.

PATIENT/FAMILY TEACHING

• Treatment may depress your immune system and reduce your ability to fight infection. Report symptoms of infection such as body aches, burning with urination, chills, cough, fatigue, fever. Avoid those with active infection. • Do not receive live vaccines. • Expect frequent tuberculosis screening. Report travel plans to possible endemic areas. • A health care provider will show you how to properly prepare and inject medication. You must demonstrate correct preparation and injection techniques before using medication at home. • Report allergic reactions such as itching, hives, rash. • Immediately report severe or persistent abdominal pain, bloody stool, fever; may indicate rupture in GI tract. • Treatment may cause reactivation of HBV, new cancers. • Therapy may decrease platelet count, which may increase risk of bleeding. • Report liver problems such as bruising, confusion, amber or dark-colored urine; right upper abdominal pain; yellowing of the skin or eyes.

sAXagliptin

sax-a-**glip**-tin
(Onglyza)
Do not confuse SAXagliptin with SITagliptin or SUMAtriptan.

FIXED-COMBINATION(S)

Kombiglyze XR: SAXagliptin/metFORMIN (an antidiabetic): 2.5 mg/1,000 mg, 5 mg/500 mg, 5 mg/1,000 mg.

◆CLASSIFICATION

PHARMACOTHERAPEUTIC: DDP-4 inhibitor (gliptins). **CLINICAL:** Antidiabetic agent.

USES

Adjunctive treatment to diet and exercise to improve glycemic control in pts with type 2 diabetes as monotherapy or in combination with other antidiabetic agents.

PRECAUTIONS

Contraindications: Hypersensitivity to SAXagliptin. Type 1 diabetes, ketoacidosis. **Cautions:** Concurrent use of other glucose-lowering agents, moderate to severe renal impairment, end-stage renal disease requiring hemodialysis, concurrent use of strong CYP3A4 inhibitors (e.g., clarithromycin); history of pancreatitis.

ACTION

Slows the inactivation of incretin hormones by inhibiting DDP-4 enzyme. Incretin hormones increase insulin synthesis/release from pancreas and decrease glucagon secretion. **Therapeutic Effect:** Regulates glucose homeostasis.

PHARMACOKINETICS

Widely distributed. Metabolized in liver. Peak plasma concentration: 2 hrs. Excreted in urine (75%), feces (22%).

S

Half-life: 2.5 hrs; metabolite, 3.1 hrs.

LIFESPAN CONSIDERATIONS

Pregnancy/Lactation: Unknown if distributed in breast milk. **Children:** Safety and efficacy not established. **Elderly:** Age-related renal impairment may require dosage adjustment.

INTERACTIONS

DRUG: May increase hypoglycemic effects of **insulin, sulfonylureas (e.g., glipiZIDE, glyBURIDE). Strong CYP3A4 inhibitors (e.g., clarithromycin, ketoconazole)** may increase concentration/effect. **CYP3A4 inducers (e.g., carBAMazepine, phenytoin, rifAMPin)** may decrease concentration/effect. **HERBAL: Herbals with hypoglycemic properties (e.g., fenugreek)** may increase effect. **FOOD: Grapefruit products** may increase concentration/effect. **LAB VALUES:** May slightly decrease WBCs, lymphocytes. May increase serum creatinine.

AVAILABILITY (Rx)

Tablets, Film-Coated: 2.5 mg, 5 mg.

ADMINISTRATION/HANDLING

PO

- May give without regard to food.
- Do not break, crush, dissolve, or divide film-coated tablets.

INDICATIONS/ROUTES/DOSAGE

Type 2 Diabetes

PO: ADULTS, ELDERLY: 2.5 or 5 mg once daily. **Concurrent strong CYP3A4 inhibitors (e.g., ketoconazole):** 2.5 mg once daily. **Hemodialysis:** Give dose after dialysis.

Dosage in Renal Impairment

Mild impairment: No dose adjustment. **Moderate to severe impairment: CrCl less than 50 mL/min:** 2.5 mg once daily.

Dosage in Hepatic Impairment

No dose adjustment.

SIDE EFFECTS

Occasional (7%): Headache. **Rare (3%–1%):** Peripheral edema, sinusitis, abdominal pain, gastroenteritis, vomiting, rash.

ADVERSE EFFECTS/TOXIC REACTIONS

May cause HF, esp. in pts with cardiovascular disease. Concomitant use of hypoglycemic agents may increase risk of hypoglycemia. Pancreatitis reported in less than 1%. Hypersensitivity reactions including anaphylaxis, angioedema (tongue/lip swelling), exfoliative skin conditions. Other reactions include bullous pemphigoid, severe/disabling arthralgia. Infections including upper respiratory tract infection (8% of pts), UTI (7% of pts) may occur.

NURSING CONSIDERATIONS

BASELINE ASSESSMENT

Obtain blood glucose, hemoglobin A1c, renal function. Assess pt's understanding of diabetes management, routine home glucose monitoring. Receive full medication history and screen for interactions. Question history renal impairment, cardiovascular disease, pancreatitis.

INTERVENTION/EVALUATION

Monitor blood glucose, hemoglobin A1c level, renal function. Assess for hypoglycemia (diaphoresis, tremors, dizziness, anxiety, headache, tachycardia, perioral numbness, hunger, diplopia, difficulty concentrating), hyperglycemia (polyuria, polyphagia, polydipsia, nausea, vomiting, fatigue, Kussmaul breathing), hypersensitivity reactions. Concomitant use of beta blockers (e.g., carvedilol, metoprolol) may mask symptoms of hypoglycemia. Screen for glucose-altering conditions: fever, increased activity or stress, surgical procedures. Obtain dietary consult for nutritional education. Severe abdominal pain, nausea may indicate pancreatitis.

PATIENT/FAMILY TEACHING

- Diabetes mellitus requires lifelong control. Diet and exercise are principal

S

parts of treatment; do not skip or delay meals. Test blood sugar regularly. Monitor daily calorie intake. • When taking combination drug therapy or when glucose conditions are altered (excessive alcohol ingestion, insufficient carbohydrate intake, hormone deficiencies, critical illness), have a low blood sugar treatment available (e.g., glucagon, oral dextrose). • Persistent, severe abdominal pain that radiates to the back (with or without vomiting) may indicate acute pancreatitis. • Report joint pain; allergic reactions of any kind.

scopolamine

skoe-**pol**-a-meen
(Trans-Derm Scop, Buscopan ✱)

FIXED-COMBINATION(S)

Donnatal: scopolamine/atropine (anticholinergic)/hyoscyamine (anticholinergic)/PHENobarbital (sedative): 0.0065 mg/0.0194 mg/0.1037 mg/16.2 mg.

◆CLASSIFICATION

PHARMACOTHERAPEUTIC: Anticholinergic. **CLINICAL:** Antinausea, antiemetic.

USES

Prevention of motion sickness, postop nausea/vomiting. **OFF-LABEL:** Breakthrough treatment of nausea/vomiting associated with chemotherapy.

PRECAUTIONS

Contraindications: Hypersensitivity to scopolamine. Narrow-angle glaucoma. **Cautions:** Hepatic/renal impairment, cardiac disease (hypertension, HF), seizure disorder, psychoses, coronary artery disease, prostatic hyperplasia, urinary retention, reflux esophagitis, ulcerative colitis, hyperthyroidism, GI obstruction, hiatal hernia, elderly.

ACTION

Competitively inhibits action of acetylcholine in smooth muscle, secretory glands, and CNS. **Therapeutic Effect:** Prevents motion-induced nausea/vomiting.

⌛ LIFESPAN CONSIDERATIONS

Pregnancy/Lactation: Crosses placenta; unknown if distributed in breast milk. **Children:** May be more susceptible to adverse effects. **Elderly:** Dizziness, hallucinations, confusion may require dosage adjustment. Use caution.

INTERACTIONS

Transdermal: DRUG: None significant. **HERBAL:** None significant. **FOOD: Grapefruit products** may increase concentration/effect. **LAB VALUES:** May interfere with gastric secretion test.

AVAILABILITY (Rx)

Transdermal System: ***(Trans-Derm Scop):*** 1.5 mg.

ADMINISTRATION/HANDLING

Transdermal

• Apply patch to hairless area behind one ear. • If dislodged or on for more than 72 hrs, replace with fresh patch. • Do not cut/trim. • Limit contact with water.

INDICATIONS/ROUTES/DOSAGE

Prevention of Motion Sickness

Transdermal: ADULTS: One system at least 4 hrs prior to exposure and q72h as needed.

Postop Nausea/Vomiting

Transdermal: ADULTS, ELDERLY: 1 system no sooner than 1 hr before surgery and removed 24 hrs after surgery.

Dosage in Renal/Hepatic Impairment

No dose adjustment.

SIDE EFFECTS

Frequent (greater than 15%): Dry mouth, drowsiness, blurred vision. **Rare (5%–1%):** Dizziness, restlessness, hallucinations, confusion, difficulty urinating, rash.

ADVERSE EFFECTS/TOXIC REACTIONS

None known.

NURSING CONSIDERATIONS

BASELINE ASSESSMENT

Assess for use of CNS depressants, anticholinergics. Question medical history as listed in Precautions.

INTERVENTION/EVALUATION

Monitor for dehydration. Observe for improvement of symptoms.

PATIENT/FAMILY TEACHING

• Avoid tasks requiring alertness, motor skills until response to drug is established (may cause drowsiness, disorientation, confusion). • Use only 1 patch at a time; do not cut. • Wash hands after administration.

secukinumab

sek-ue-**kin**-ue-mab
(Cosentyx, Cosentyx Sensor Pen)
Do not confuse secukinumab with canakinumab, ranibizumab, trastuzumab, ustekinumab

◆CLASSIFICATION

PHARMACOTHERAPEUTIC: Monoclonal antibody. Human interleukin-17A antagonist. **CLINICAL:** Antipsoriasis agent.

USES

Treatment of moderate to severe plaque psoriasis in adult pts who are candidates for systemic therapy or phototherapy, active psoriatic arthritis (PsA), active ankylosing spondylitis (AS). Treatment of active nonradiographic axial spondyloarthritis in adults with objective signs of inflammation.

PRECAUTIONS

Contraindications: Hypersensitivity to secukinumab. **Cautions:** Elderly, active Crohn's disease, HIV infection, concomitant use of immunosuppressants; conditions predisposing to infections (e.g., diabetes, renal failure, immunocompromised pts, open wounds); hypersensitivity to latex (injector pen/prefilled syringe), preexisting or recent-onset CNS demyelinating disorders (e.g., multiple sclerosis, polyneuropathy); exposure to tuberculosis. Administration of live vaccines not recommended.

ACTION

Selectively binds to the interleukin-17A (IL-17A) cytokine, inhibiting its interaction with the IL-17 receptor. IL-17A is involved in inflammatory and immune responses. **Therapeutic Effect:** Inhibits release of proinflammatory cytokines.

PHARMACOKINETICS

Widely distributed. Degraded into small peptides and amino acids via catabolic pathway. Peak plasma concentration: 6 days. Steady state reached in 24 wks. Excretion not defined. **Half-life:** 22–31 days.

⌛ LIFESPAN CONSIDERATIONS

Pregnancy/Lactation: Unknown if distributed in breast milk. **Children:** Safety and efficacy not established. **Elderly:** No age-related precautions noted.

INTERACTIONS

DRUG: May decrease efficacy/immune response of **live vaccines;** may increase risk of toxic effects of **live vaccines. HERBAL: Echinacea** may decrease the therapeutic effect. **FOOD:** None known. **LAB VALUES:** None significant.

AVAILABILITY (Rx)

Injector Pen: 150 mg/mL solution. **Prefilled Syringe:** 150 mg/mL solution.

ADMINISTRATION/HANDLING

SQ

• Follow instructions for preparation according to manufacturer guidelines.

Administration • Insert needle subcutaneously into upper arms, outer thigh, or abdomen and inject solution. • Do not inject into areas of active skin disease or injury such as sunburns, skin rashes, inflammation, skin infections, or active psoriasis. • Rotate injection sites.

Storage • Refrigerate until time of use. • Allow injector pen/prefilled syringe/vial to warm to room temperature before use (15–30 min). Do not freeze.

INDICATIONS/ROUTES/DOSAGE

Plaque Psoriasis

SQ: ADULTS, ELDERLY: 300 mg every wk for 5 doses, then 300 mg q4wks. (Some pts may only require 150 mg.)

PsA, AS, Axial Spondyloarthritis (Nonradiographic)

Note: With coexistent plaque psoriasis, use dose for plaque psoriasis.

SQ: ADULTS, ELDERLY: Initially, 150 mg at wks 0, 1, 2, 3, and 4, then q4wks or 150 mg q4wks. For active PsA, may consider dose of 300 mg.

Dosage in Renal/Hepatic Impairment

Not studied; use caution.

SIDE EFFECTS

Rare (4%–1%): Diarrhea, urticaria, rhinorrhea.

ADVERSE EFFECTS/TOXIC REACTIONS

May increase risk tuberculosis. Infections including nasopharyngitis (11% of pts), upper respiratory tract infection (2.5% of pts), mucocutaneous infection with *Candida* (1.2% of pts), rhinitis, pharyngitis, oral herpes (1% of pts) have occurred. May cause exacerbation of Crohn's disease. Hypersensitivity reactions including anaphylaxis were reported. Immunogenicity (auto-secukinumab antibodies) occurred in less than 1% of pts.

NURSING CONSIDERATIONS

BASELINE ASSESSMENT

Pts should be evaluated for active tuberculosis and tested for latent infection prior to initiating treatment and periodically during therapy. Induration of 5 mm or greater with tuberculin skin testing should be considered a positive test result when assessing if treatment for latent tuberculosis is necessary. Antifungal therapy should be considered for those who reside or travel to regions where mycoses are endemic. Do not initiate therapy during active infection. Question history of active Crohn's disease, hepatitis B or C virus infection, HIV infection, demyelinating disorders, cardiovascular disease; concomitant use of immunosuppressive agents.

INTERVENTION/EVALUATION

Monitor skin for disease improvement. Monitor for symptoms of tuberculosis, including those who tested negative for latent tuberculosis infection prior to initiating therapy. Interrupt or discontinue treatment if serious infection, opportunistic infection, or sepsis occurs. Monitor for hypersensitivity reaction.

PATIENT/FAMILY TEACHING

• Treatment may depress your immune system response and reduce your ability to fight infection. Report symptoms of infection such as body aches, chills, cough, fatigue, fever. Avoid those with active infection. • Do not receive live vaccines. • Expect frequent tuberculosis screening. • Report travel plans to possible endemic areas. • Injector pen/prefilled syringe should not be used by pts with latex allergy. • Immediately report itching, hives, rash, swelling of the face or tongue; may indicate allergic reaction. • Treatment may cause worsening of Crohn's disease.

S

selegiline

se-**le**-ji-leen
(Emsam, Zelapar)

■ BLACK BOX ALERT ■ Antidepressants increase risk of suicidal thoughts and behavior in pediatrics and young adults. Monitor closely for changes in behavior, suicidal ideation.

Do not confuse Eldepryl with Elavil or enalapril, selegiline with Salagen, sertraline, or Stelazine, or Zelapar with Zaleplon, Zemplar, or ZyPREXA.

◆CLASSIFICATION

PHARMACOTHERAPEUTIC: MAOI type B. **CLINICAL:** Antiparkinson agent, antidepressant.

USES

Oral: Adjunct to levodopa/carbidopa in treatment of Parkinson's disease. **Transdermal:** Treatment of major depressive disorder (MDD). **OFF-LABEL:** Treatment of ADHD, early Parkinson's disease.

PRECAUTIONS

Contraindications: Hypersensitivity to selegiline. Concurrent use of meperidine. **Orally Disintegrating Tablet (additional):** Concurrent use of cyclobenzaprine, dextromethorphan, methadone, St. John's wort, traMADol, oral selegiline, other MAOIs within 14 days of selegiline. **Transdermal (additional):** Pheochromocytoma; concurrent use of buPROPion, SSRIs (e.g., FLUoxetine), SNRIs (e.g., DULoxetine), tricyclic antidepressants, busPIRone, traMADol, methadone, dextromethorphan, St. John's wort, mirtazapine, cyclobenzaprine, oral selegiline, other MAOIs, carBAMazepine, OXcarbazepine, sympathomimetics (e.g., amphetamines, cold products containing vasoconstrictors). Elective surgery requiring general anesthesia, local anesthesia containing sympathomimetics; foods high in tyramine content. **Cautions:** Renal/hepatic impairment, depression, elderly pts, major psychiatric disorder; pts at high risk of suicide; pts at high risk of hypotension (cerebrovascular disease, cardiovascular disease, hypovolemia).

ACTION

May increase dopaminergic activity by interfering with dopamine reuptake at the synapse. **Therapeutic Effect:** Relieves signs/symptoms of Parkinson's disease (tremor, akinesia, posture/equilibrium disorders, rigidity). Improves mood with MDD.

PHARMACOKINETICS

Route	Onset	Peak	Duration
PO	1 hr	—	24–72 hrs

Rapidly absorbed from GI tract. Crosses blood-brain barrier. Protein binding: 90%. Metabolized in liver. Primarily excreted in urine. **Half-life: PO:** 10 hrs. **Transdermal:** 18–25 hrs.

⌛ LIFESPAN CONSIDERATIONS

Pregnancy/Lactation: Unknown if drug crosses placenta or is distributed in breast milk. **Children:** Safety and efficacy not established. **Elderly:** No age-related precautions noted.

INTERACTIONS

DRUG: **FLUoxetine, fluvoxaMINE, meperidine, PARoxetine, sertraline, venlafaxine** may cause mania, serotonin syndrome (altered mental status, restlessness, diaphoresis, diarrhea, fever). **Tricyclic antidepressants (e.g., amitriptyline, doxepin)** may cause diaphoresis, hypertension, syncope, altered mental status, hyperpyrexia, seizures, tremors (wait 14 days between stopping selegiline and starting tricyclic antidepressants). **Alcohol** may increase adverse effects. **HERBAL:** **Herbals with hypotensive properties (e.g., garlic, ginger, ginkgo biloba)** may increase hypotensive effect. **FOOD:** **Tyramine-rich**

foods may produce hypertensive reactions. **LAB VALUES:** None significant.

AVAILABILITY (Rx)

Capsules: 5 mg. **Tablets:** 5 mg. **Tablets, Orally Disintegrating:** ***(Zelapar):*** 1.25 mg. **Transdermal:** ***(Emsam):*** 6 mg/24 hrs, 9 mg/24 hrs, 12 mg/24 hrs.

ADMINISTRATION/HANDLING

PO

• Give without regard to food. • Avoid tyramine-containing foods, large quantities of caffeine-containing beverages.

PO (Orally Disintegrating Tablets)

• Give in morning before breakfast and without liquid. • Peel off backing with dry hands (do not push tablets through foil). • Immediately place on top of tongue, allow to disintegrate. • Avoid food, liquids for 5 min before and after taking selegiline.

Transdermal

• Apply to dry, intact skin on upper torso or thigh, outer surface of upper arm. • Avoid exposure to external heat source. • Normal exposure to water unlikely to affect adhesion. • If patch becomes loose, press back into place. If patch falls off again, apply a new patch; follow same dose schedule. • Rotate application sites.

INDICATIONS/ROUTES/DOSAGE

Adjunctive Treatment of Parkinson's Disease

PO: ADULTS: ***(Capsule, Tablet):*** 5 mg at breakfast and lunch, given concomitantly with each dose of carbidopa and levodopa. **ELDERLY:** Initially, 5 mg in the morning. May increase up to 10 mg/day. **ADULTS, ELDERLY:** ***(Orally Disintegrating Tablet):*** Initially, 1.25 mg daily for at least 6 wks. May increase to maximum of 2.5 mg/day.

Major Depressive Disorder

Transdermal: ADULTS: Initially, 6 mg/24 hrs. May increase in 3 mg/24 hrs increments at minimum of 2 wks. **Maximum:** 12 mg/24 hrs. **ELDERLY:** **Maximum:** 6 mg/24 hrs.

Dosage in Renal/Hepatic Impairment

Orally disintegrating tablet: Not recommended in severe impairment. **Oral:** Use caution. **Transdermal:** No dose adjustment.

SIDE EFFECTS

Frequent (10%–4%): Nausea, dizziness, light-headedness, syncope, abdominal discomfort. **Occasional (3%–2%):** Confusion, hallucinations, dry mouth, vivid dreams, dyskinesia. **Rare (1%):** Headache, myalgia, anxiety, diarrhea, insomnia.

ADVERSE EFFECTS/TOXIC REACTIONS

Symptoms of overdose may vary from CNS depression (sedation, apnea, cardiovascular collapse, death) to severe paradoxical reactions (hallucinations, tremor, seizures). Impaired motor coordination, (loss of balance, blepharospasm, facial grimaces, feeling of heaviness in lower extremities), depression, nightmares, delusions, overstimulation, sleep disturbance, anger, hallucinations, confusion may occur.

NURSING CONSIDERATIONS

BASELINE ASSESSMENT

Receive full medication history and screen for contraindications/interactions. Question medical history as listed in Precautions. Assess current state of mental health.

INTERVENTION/EVALUATION

Be alert to neurologic effects (headache, lethargy, mental confusion, agitation). Monitor for evidence of dyskinesia (difficulty with movement). Assess for clinical reversal of symptoms (improvement of tremors of head/hands at rest, mask-like facial expression, shuffling gait, muscular rigidity). Monitor for unusual behavior, worsening depression, suicidal ideation, especially at initiation of therapy or with changes in dosage.

S

PATIENT/FAMILY TEACHING

• Tolerance to dizziness, light-headedness develops during therapy. • Avoid tasks that require alertness, motor skills until response to drug is established. • Dry mouth, drowsiness, dizziness may be an expected response to drug. • Avoid alcohol. • Report worsening depression, unusual behavior, thoughts of suicide. • Avoid tyramine-rich foods. • Do not take newly prescribed medications unless approved by prescriber who originally started treatment. • Do not take herbal supplements.

selinexor

sel-i-**nex**-or
(Xpovio)
Do not confuse selinexor with Effexor or selegiline. Xpovio with Xeloda, Xgeva, Xtandi.

◆CLASSIFICATION

PHARMACOTHERAPEUTIC: Nuclear export inhibitor. **CLINICAL:** Antineoplastic.

USES

Treatment of adults with relapsed or refractory multiple myeloma (in combination with dexamethasone) who have received at least four prior therapies and whose disease is refractory to at least two proteasome inhibitors, at least two immunomodulatory agents, and an anti-CD38 monoclonal antibody. Treatment of adults with relapsed or refractory diffuse large B-cell lymphoma (DLBCL), not otherwise specified, including DLBCL arising from follicular lymphoma, after at least two lines of systemic therapy.

PRECAUTIONS

Contraindications: Hypersensitivity to selinexor. **Cautions:** Baseline cytopenias, hepatic impairment, optic disorders, uncorrected hyponatremia, fall risk, elderly, conditions predisposing to infection (e.g., diabetes, renal failure, immunocompromised pts, open wounds), chronic opportunistic infections (e.g., herpesvirus infection, fungal infections), pts at risk for bleeding (e.g., history of intracranial/GI/GU bleeding, coagulation disorders, recent trauma, concomitant use of anticoagulants, NSAIDs, antiplatelets).

ACTION

Reversibly inhibits nuclear export of tumor suppressor proteins, growth regulators, messenger RNA of oncogenic proteins by blocking protein exportin 1 (XPO1), leading to blockage of exportin 1. **Therapeutic Effect:** Reduces oncogenic proteins, causes cell cycle arrest and cancer cell apoptosis.

PHARMACOKINETICS

Widely distributed. Metabolized in liver. Protein binding: 95%. Peak plasma concentration: 4 hrs. Excretion not specified. **Half-life:** 6–8 hrs.

⌛ LIFESPAN CONSIDERATIONS

Pregnancy/Lactation: Avoid pregnancy; may cause fetal harm. Females and males with female partners of reproductive potential must use effective contraception during treatment and for at least 1 wk after discontinuation. Unknown if distributed in breast milk. Breastfeeding not recommended during treatment and for at least 1 wk after discontinuation. May impair fertility in females. **Children:** Safety and efficacy not established. **Elderly:** May have increased risk of serious or fatal adverse reactions.

INTERACTIONS

DRUG: May decrease therapeutic effect of **BCG (Intravesical), vaccines (live). Pimecrolimus, tacrolimus (topical)** may enhance the adverse/toxic effects. May increase adverse effects of **natalizumab. HERBAL: Echinacea** may decrease therapeutic effect. **FOOD:**

None known. **LAB VALUES:** May increase serum ALT, AST, bilirubin, creatine kinase, glucose, creatinine. May decrease serum albumin, calcium, sodium, magnesium, phosphate; absolute neutrophil count (ANC), Hgb, Hct, leukocytes, lymphocytes, neutrophils, platelets, RBCs. May increase or decrease serum potassium.

AVAILABILITY (Rx)

Tablets: 20 mg.

ADMINISTRATION/HANDLING

PO

• Give without regard to food. • Administer tablets whole with water; do not break, crush, or divide. Tablets cannot be chewed. • If a dose is missed or vomiting occurs after administration, give next dose at regularly scheduled time (do not give additional dose).

INDICATIONS/ROUTES/DOSAGE

Multiple Myeloma (relapsed or refractory)

PO: ADULTS: 80 mg on days 1 and 3 of each wk (in combination with dexamethasone 20 mg on day 1 and 3 each wk). Continue until disease progression or unacceptable toxicity.

DLBCL (relapsed or refractory)

PO: ADULTS: 60 mg on days 1 and 3 of each wk. Continue until disease progression or unacceptable toxicity.

Dose Reduction Schedule

(Multiple myeloma): First dose reduction: 100 mg once wkly. **Second dose reduction:** 80 once wkly. **Third dose reduction:** 60 mg once wkly. **Unable to tolerate 60-mg dose:** Permanently discontinue.

(DLBCL): First dose reduction: 40 mg on day 1 and 3 each of wk (80 mg total). **Second dose reduction:** 60 once wkly. **Third dose reduction:** 40 mg once wkly. **Unable to tolerate 40-mg dose:** Permanently discontinue.

Dose Modification

Based on Common Terminology Criteria for Adverse Events (CTCAE).

Anemia

(Multiple myeloma/DLBCL): Hgb less than 8 mg/dL: Reduce one dose level. **Life-threatening anemia:** Withhold treatment until Hgb improves to 8 g/dL, then resume at reduced dose level.

Neutropenia

(Multiple myeloma): ANC 500–1,000 cells/mm³ *without* fever: Reduce one dose level. **ANC less than 500 cells/mm³ or febrile neutropenia:** Withhold treatment until ANC improves to 1,000 cells/mm³, then resume at reduced dose level.

(DLBCL): ANC 500–1,000 cells/mm³ *without* fever: For first occurrence, withhold treatment until ANC improves to 1,000 cells/mm³, then resume at same dose. If recurs, reduce one dose level. **ANC less than 500 cells/mm³ or febrile neutropenia:** Withhold treatment until ANC improves to 1,000 cells/mm³, then resume at reduced dose level.

Thrombocytopenia

(Multiple myeloma): Platelet count 25,000–74,999 cells/mm³: Reduce one dose level. **Platelet count 25,000–74,999 cells/mm³ *with* bleeding:** Withhold treatment until bleeding resolves, then resume at reduced dose level. **Platelet count less than 25,000 cells/mm³:** Withhold treatment until platelet count improves to 50,000 cells/mm³, then resume at one reduced dose level.

(DLBCL): Platelet count 50,000–74,999 cells/mm³: Interrupt one dose, then resume at same dose. **Platelet count 25,000–49,999 cells/mm3 *without* bleeding:** For first occurrence, withhold treatment until platelet count improves to greater than or equal to 50,000 cells/mm³, then resume at reduced dose level. **Platelet count 25,000–49,999 cells/mm³ *with* bleeding:** Withhold treatment until bleeding resolves and platelet count improves to 50,000 cells/mm³, then resume at reduced dose level. **Platelet count less than 25,000 cells/mm³:** Withhold treatment until platelet count improves to 50,000 cells/mm³, then resume at reduced dose level.

S

Diarrhea

Grade 2 diarrhea: For first occurrence, maintain dose. If recurs, reduce one dose level. **Grade 3 or 4 diarrhea:** Withhold treatment until improved to grade 2 or less, then resume at reduced dose level.

Fatigue

Grade 2 fatigue (lasting longer than 7 days); grade 3 fatigue: Withhold treatment until improved to grade 1 or baseline, then resume at reduced dose level.

Hyponatremia

Serum sodium level 130 mmol/L or less: Withhold treatment until improved to greater than 130 mmol/L, then resume at reduced dose level.

Nausea/Vomiting

Grade 1 or 2 nausea/vomiting: Maintain dose. **Grade 3 nausea; grade 3 or 4 vomiting:** Withhold treatment until improved to grade 2 or less, then resume at one reduced dose level.

Ocular Toxicity

Grade 2 ocular toxicity (excluding cataract): Withhold treatment until improved to grade 1 or baseline, then resume at one reduced dose level. **Grade 3 or 4 ocular toxicity:** Permanently discontinue. **Grade 2 (or higher) cataract:** Reduce one dose level.

Weight Loss/Anorexia

Weight loss of 10% to less than 20%; anorexia associated with significant weight loss or malnutrition: Withhold treatment until improved to more than 90% of baseline weight, then resume at one reduced dose level.

Other Nonhematologic Toxicity

Any other grade 3 or 4 toxicity: Withhold treatment until improved to grade 2 or lower, then resume at one reduced dose level.

Dosage in Renal Impairment

Mild to severe impairment: No dose adjustment. **ESRD, dialysis:** Not specified; use caution.

Dosage in Hepatic Impairment

Mild impairment: No dose adjustment. **Moderate to severe impairment:** Not specified; use caution.

SIDE EFFECTS

Note: Frequency and occurrence of side effects may vary based on indicated treatment. **Frequent (73–24%):** Fatigue, asthenia, nausea, decreased appetite, decreased weight, diarrhea, vomiting, constipation, dyspnea. **Occasional (17%–10%):** Edema, cough, pyrexia, musculoskeletal pain, dizziness, insomnia, dehydration, dysgeusia, ageusia, vision blurred, reduced visual acuity, hypotension. headache, abdominal pain, peripheral neuropathy.

ADVERSE EFFECTS/TOXIC REACTIONS

Note: Frequency and occurrence of adverse reactions may vary based on indicated treatment.

Myelosuppression (anemia, leukopenia, lymphopenia, neutropenia, thrombocytopenia) is an expected response to therapy, but more severe reactions including febrile neutropenia, hemorrhagic thrombocytopenia may occur. Hemorrhagic events (corneal bleeding epistaxis, GI/rectal bleeding, hematoma, hematuria, subdural hematoma) reported in 10% of pts. GI toxicities (anorexia, diarrhea, nausea, vomiting, weight loss) reported in 80% of pts. Life-threatening hyponatremia reported in 39%–62% of pts. Serious and fatal infections (adenovirus, bronchitis, bronchiolitis, herpesvirus infection, pharyngitis, nasopharyngitis, parainfluenza, pneumonia, respiratory syncytial virus infection, rhinitis, rhinovirus, sepsis, UTI) were reported. Life-threatening neurologic toxicities (amnesia, decreased level of consciousness, confusion, delirium, hallucinations) reported in 30% of pts. Falls reported in 8% of pts. Cardiac failure, cataracts reported in 3% of pts.

S

NURSING CONSIDERATIONS

BASELINE ASSESSMENT

Obtain ANC, CBC, BMP, body weight; pregnancy test in females of reproductive potential. Confirm compliance of effective contraception. Administer prophylactic antiemetic prior to each dose. Question history of hepatic impairment, herpesvirus infection, chronic opportunistic infections, optic disorders. Assess nutritional/hydration status. Obtain dietary consultation. Assess risk for bleeding. Screen for active infection. Initiate fall precautions. Assess usual bowel movement patterns, stool characteristics. Offer emotional support.

INTERVENTION/EVALUATION

Monitor ANC, CBC, BMP, body weight frequently during the first 3 mos of treatment, then as indicated. Diligently monitor for infections (cough, fever, fatigue), esp. respiratory tract infections, herpesvirus infection, sepsis. If serious infection or sepsis occurs, initiate appropriate antimicrobial therapy. Assess for symptoms of hyponatremia (coma, confusion, headache, lethargy, nausea, seizures, vomiting). Administer RBC transfusion per clinical guidelines if anemia occurs. Administer platelet transfusion per clinical guidelines if bleeding occurs in pts with thrombocytopenia. Consider growth colony-stimulating factor in pts with neutropenia. Withhold treatment 24 hrs before and 72 hrs after cataract surgery. Assess proper hydration/nutritional intake, I&Os. Offer antiemetics if nausea/vomiting occurs; antidiarrheal agent if diarrhea occurs. Monitor daily pattern of bowel activity, stool consistency. Monitor for neurologic toxicities (confusion, hallucinations, lethargy). Assess for visual changes at each office visit. If change of vision occurs, consider referral to ophthalmologist. Monitor for GI/genitourinary bleeding, bloody stool; symptoms of intracranial bleeding (aphasia, blindness, confusion, facial droop, hemiplegia, seizures).

PATIENT/FAMILY TEACHING

• Treatment may depress your immune system and reduce your ability to fight infection. Report symptoms of infection such as body aches, burning with urination, chills, cough, fatigue, fever. Avoid those with active infection. • Report symptoms of bone marrow depression (e.g., bruising, fatigue, fever, shortness of breath, weight loss; bleeding easily, bloody urine or stool). • Report liver problems (abdominal pain, bruising, clay-colored stool, dark or amber-colored urine, yellowing of the skin or eyes), nervous system changes (confusion, delirium, difficulty speaking, dizziness, hallucinations, pain, paralysis, numbness), change of vision, fatigue, weight loss, bleeding of any kind. • Diarrhea, nausea, vomiting are common side effects that may cause dehydration, electrolyte imbalance, malnutrition. Drink plenty of fluids. Maintain proper caloric and nutritional intake. • Use effective contraception to avoid pregnancy. Do not breastfeed. • Avoid tasks that require alertness, motor skills until response to drug is established.

selpercatinib

sel-per-**ka**-tih-nib
(Retevmo)
Do not confuse selpercatinib with selinexor, selumetinib, or tucatinib.

CLASSIFICATION

PHARMACOTHERAPEUTIC: RET kinase inhibitor, tyrosine kinase inhibitor. **CLINICAL:** Antineoplastic.

USES

Treatment of adults with metastatic RET fusion-positive non–small cell lung cancer (NSCLC). Treatment of adults and pediatric pts 12 yrs and older with

S

advanced or metastatic RET-mutant medullary thyroid cancer (MTC) who require systemic therapy; or advanced, metastatic RET fusion-positive thyroid cancer who require systemic therapy and who are radioactive iodine refractory (if radioactive iodine is appropriate).

PRECAUTIONS

Contraindications: Hypersensitivity to selpercatinib. **Cautions:** Baseline cytopenias, hepatic impairment, hypertension, conditions predisposing to infection (e.g., diabetes, immunocompromised pts, renal failure, open wounds); pts at risk for QTc interval prolongation, cardiac arrhythmias (congenital long QT syndrome, HF, QT interval–prolonging medications, hypokalemia, hypomagnesemia); pts at risk for bleeding (e.g., history of intracranial/GI/GU bleeding, coagulation disorders, recent trauma, concomitant use of anticoagulants, NSAIDs, antiplatelets). Do not initiate in pts with uncontrolled hypertension.

ACTION

Inhibits wild-type RET, multiple mutated RET fusion proteins, vascular endothelial growth factor (VEGFR) 1 and VEGFR3 receptors, and fibroblast growth factor receptor (FGFR). Mutations in RET can result in activated RET fusion proteins, which can act as oncogenic drivers, promoting tumor cell line proliferation. **Therapeutic Effect:** Exhibits antitumor activity in cells with activation of RET proteins.

S

PHARMACOKINETICS

Widely distributed. Metabolized in liver. Protein binding: 97%. Peak plasma concentration: 2 hrs. Excreted in feces (69%), urine (24%). **Half-life:** 32 hrs.

LIFESPAN CONSIDERATIONS

Pregnancy/Lactation: Avoid pregnancy; may cause fetal harm. Females and males with female partners of reproductive potential must use effective contraception during treatment and for at least 1 wk after discontinuation. Unknown if distributed in breast milk. Breastfeeding not recommended during treatment and for at least 1 wk after discontinuation. May impair fertility in both females and males. **Children:** Safety and efficacy not established in pts younger than 12 yrs. **Elderly:** No age-related precautions noted.

INTERACTIONS

DRUG: **Strong CYP3A4 inhibitors (e.g., clarithromycin, ketoconazole, ritonavir), moderate CYP3A4 inhibitors (e.g., erythromycin, dilTIAZem, fluconazole)** may increase concentration/effect. **Strong CYP3A4 inducers (e.g., carBAMazepine, phenytoin, rifAMPin), moderate CYP3A4 inducers (e.g., bosentan, nafcillin)** may decrease concentration/effect. **Histamine-2 receptor antagonists (e.g., famotidine); antacids containing magnesium, calcium, aluminum, bicarbonate; proton pump inhibitors (e.g., omeprazole, pantoprazole)** may reduce concentration/effect. **QT interval–prolonging medications (e.g., amiodarone, azithromycin, entrectinib, haloperidol, methadone, quetiapine, ribociclib)** may increase risk of QTc interval prolongation, cardiac arrhythmias. **HERBAL:** None significant. **FOOD:** **Grapefruit products** may increase concentration/effect. **LAB VALUES:** May increase serum alkaline phosphatase, ALT, AST, bilirubin, cholesterol (total), potassium. May decrease serum albumin, calcium, creatinine, magnesium, sodium; leukocytes, platelets. May increase or decrease serum glucose.

AVAILABILITY (Rx)

Capsules: 40 mg, 80 mg.

ADMINISTRATION/HANDLING

PO.

• If concomitant use of proton pump inhibitor (e.g., pantoprazole) is unavoidable, give selpercatinib with food; otherwise, may give without regard to food. •

Give 2 hrs before or 10 hrs after histamine-2 receptor antagonist (e.g., famotidine). • Give 2 hrs before or 2 hrs after locally acting antacid (e.g., magnesium-, calcium-, aluminum-, bicarbonate-containing antacids). • Administer capsules whole; do not break, cut, or open. • Capsules cannot be chewed. • Do not give a missed dose within 6 hrs of next dose. • If vomiting occurs after administration, give next dose at regularly scheduled time (do not give additional dose).

INDICATIONS/ROUTES/DOSAGE

NSCLC (Metastatic RET fusion-positive), MTC (Advanced or metastatic RET-mutant), Thyroid Cancer (Advanced, metastatic RET fusion-positive)

PO: ADULTS, CHILDREN 12 YRS AND OLDER: (LESS THAN 50KG): 120 mg twice daily. **(50 KG OR GREATER):** 160 mg twice daily. Continue until disease progression or unacceptable toxicity.

Dose Reduction Schedule

Dose Reduction for Adverse Reactions	Weighing less than 50 kg	Weighing 50 kg or greater
First reduction	80 mg twice daily	120 mg twice daily
Second reduction	40 mg twice daily	80 mg twice daily
Third reduction	40 mg once daily	40 mg twice daily
Permanently discontinue in pts unable to tolerate 3 dose reductions.		

Dose Modification

Based on Common Terminology Criteria for Adverse Events (CTCAE).

Hepatotoxicity

Grade 3 or 4 hepatotoxicity: Withhold treatment and monitor serum ALT/AST wkly until improved to grade 1 or baseline, then resume at a reduced dose by 2 dose levels. Continue to monitor serum ALT/AST wkly until 4 wks after reaching the dose prior to grade 3 or 4 hepatotoxicity, then increase dose by 1 dose level (after at least 2 wks without recurrence), then increase to dose taken prior to grade 3 or 4 hepatotoxicity (after at least 4 wks without recurrence).

Hemorrhagic Events

Grade 3 or 4 hemorrhage: Withhold treatment until improved to grade 1 or 0. **Severe or life-threatening hemorrhage:** Permanently discontinue

Hypersensitivity Reactions

Any grade hypersensitivity reaction: Withhold treatment until resolved with corticosteroids, then resume at a reduced dose by 3 dose levels (while continuing corticosteroids). May increase dose by 1 dose level each wk until reaching the dose prior to hypersensitivity reaction, then taper corticosteroids.

Hypertension

Grade 3 hypertension (despite optimal hypertensive therapy): Withhold treatment until adequately controlled, then resume at reduced dose level. **Grade 4 hypertension:** Permanently discontinue.

QT Interval Prolongation

Grade 3 QT interval prolongation: Withhold treatment until improved to grade 1 or 0 (or baseline), then resume at reduced dose level. **Grade 4 QT interval prolongation:** Permanently discontinue.

Other Toxicities

Any grade 3 or 4 toxicities: Withhold treatment until improved to grade 1 or 0, then resume at reduced dose level.

Concomitant Use of CYP3A Inhibitor: LESS THAN 50KG: Moderate CYP3A inhibitor: Reduce dose to 80 mg twice daily. **Strong CYP3A inhibitor:** Reduce dose to 40 mg twice daily. **50 KG OR GREATER:** Moderate CYP3A inhibitor: Reduce dose to 120 mg twice daily. **Strong CYP3A inhibitor:** Reduce dose to 80 mg twice daily.

Dosage in Renal Impairment

Mild to moderate impairment: No dose adjustment. **Severe impairment:** Not specified; use caution.

S

Dosage in Hepatic Impairment
Mild to moderate impairment: No dose adjustment. **Severe impairment:** Reduce dose to 80 mg twice daily.

SIDE EFFECTS

Frequent (39%–23%): Dry mouth, diarrhea, hypertension, fatigue, asthenia, malaise, edema (eye, eyelid, face, localized, lymph, peripheral, scrotal), rash, constipation, nausea, headache, abdominal pain. **Occasional (18%–16%):** Cough, dyspnea, vomiting.

ADVERSE EFFECTS/TOXIC REACTIONS

Leukopenia, thrombocytopenia is an expected response to therapy. Serious hepatotoxicity reported in 3% of pts. Serum ALT/AST elevation reported in 45% and 51% of pts, respectively. Grade 3 hypertension (17% of pts), grade 4 hypertension (less than 1% of pts) has occurred. Concentration-dependent QT interval prolongation may occur, increasing risk of cardiac arrhythmias. Life-threatening hemorrhagic events (intraabdominal, GI, facial, genitourinary, intracranial, pulmonary, rectal, vaginal hemorrhage), ecchymosis, epistaxis, hematoma, hemoptysis, tracheal site hemorrhage may occur. Symptoms of hypersensitivity reactions including arthralgia, fever, myalgia, rash may occur with concurrent thrombocytopenia, transaminitis. May cause impaired wound healing.

S

NURSING CONSIDERATIONS

BASELINE ASSESSMENT

Obtain CBC, serum electrolytes, LFT, TSH, ECG, B/P; pregnancy test in females of reproductive potential. Confirm compliance of effective contraception. Verify presence of a RET gene fusion (NSCLC, thyroid cancer) or specific RET gene mutation (MTC) in tumor specimens or plasma. Withhold treatment at least 7 days prior to elective surgery. Do not administer for at least 2 wks after major surgery. Assess skin for open wounds, surgical incisions. Question history of hypertension, hepatic impairment, recent surgery. Assess risk for bleeding. Screen for active infection. Receive full medication history and screen for interactions.

INTERVENTION/EVALUATION

Monitor CBC, serum electrolytes, LFT, TSH, ECG periodically; LFT q2wks for the first 3 mos, then monthly thereafter (or wkly in pts with hepatotoxicity); B/P after 1 wk, then at least monthly thereafter. Manage hypersensitivity reactions with corticosteroids therapy. Assess for toxicities if concomitant use of CYP3A4 inhibitor is unavoidable. If concomitant use QT interval–prolonging medications is unavoidable, monitor ECG for QT interval prolongation, cardiac arrhythmias. Assess wounds/incisions for adequate healing following any surgery. Monitor daily pattern of bowel activity, stool consistency, I&Os. Monitor for bleeding of any kind; symptoms of intracranial bleeding (aphasia, blindness, confusion, facial droop, hemiplegia, seizures).

PATIENT/FAMILY TEACHING

• Treatment may depress your immune system and reduce your ability to fight infection. Report symptoms of infection such as body aches, burning with urination, chills, cough, fatigue, fever. Avoid those with active infection. • Report liver problems (abdominal pain, bruising, clay-colored stool, dark or amber-colored urine, yellowing of the skin or eyes), allergic reactions (rash, fever, muscle or joint pain), hemorrhagic stroke (confusion, difficulty speaking, one-sided weakness or paralysis, loss of vision), bleeding of any kind. • Use effective contraception to avoid pregnancy. Do not breastfeed. • Treatment may cause or worsen high blood pressure. • There is a high risk of interactions with other medications. Do not take newly prescribed medications unless approved by prescriber who originally started treatment. Do not ingest grapefruit products or herbal supplements. Avoid use of acid-reducing medications. • Treatment may affect the electrical conduction of the heart, which may lead to arrhythmias; report chest pain, dizziness, fainting, palpitations. • Notify physician before any planned surgeries/dental procedures.

semaglutide

sem-a-**gloo**-tide
(Ozempic, Rybelsus)

■ BLACK BOX ALERT ■ Thyroid C-cell tumors have occurred in rodent studies with glucagon-like peptide-1 (GLP-1) receptor agonists; unknown if relevant in humans. Contraindicated in pts with a personal/family history of medullary thyroid carcinoma or in pts with multiple endocrine neoplasia syndrome type 2.

Do not confuse semaglutide with albiglutide, dulaglutide, liraglutide, or teduglutide.

◆CLASSIFICATION

PHARMACOTHERAPEUTIC: Glucagon-like peptide-1 (GLP-1) receptor agonist. **CLINICAL:** Antidiabetic.

USES

Adjunct to diet and exercise to improve glycemic control in adults with type 2 diabetes mellitus. Risk reduction of major cardiovascular (CV) events in adults with type 2 diabetes mellitus and established cardiovascular disease.

PRECAUTIONS

Contraindications: Hypersensitivity to semaglutide. Personal/family history of medullary thyroid carcinoma (MTC). Pts with multiple endocrine neoplasia syndrome type 2 (MEN2). **Cautions:** Mild to moderate gastroparesis, renal impairment. History of pancreatitis. Not recommended in pts with severe GI disease, diabetic ketoacidosis, type 1 diabetes mellitus, or pancreatitis, or for use as first-line treatment regimen.

ACTION

Agonist of human glucagon-like peptide-1 (GLP-1). Increases glucose-dependent insulin secretion. Decreases inappropriate glucagon secretion. Slows gastric emptying. **Therapeutic Effect:** Augments glucose-dependent insulin secretion.

PHARMACOKINETICS

Widely distributed. Metabolized by proteolytic enzymes via protein degradation into small peptides, amino acids. Protein binding: greater than 99%. Peak plasma concentration: 1–3 days. Steady state reached in 4–5 wks. Excreted in urine (3% unchanged), feces. **Half-life:** 7 days.

⌛ LIFESPAN CONSIDERATIONS

Pregnancy/Lactation: Unknown if distributed in breast milk. Due to extended clearance period, recommend discontinuation of therapy at least 2 mos before planned pregnancy. **Children:** Safety and efficacy not established. **Elderly:** No age-related precautions noted.

INTERACTIONS

DRUG: May increase hypoglycemic effect of **insulins, sulfonylureas (e.g., glipiZIDE, glyBURIDE).** **HERBAL: Herbals with hypoglycemic properties (e.g., fenugreek)** may increase effect. **FOOD:** None known. **LAB VALUES:** Expected to decrease serum glucose, Hgb A1c. May increase serum amylase, lipase.

AVAILABILITY (Rx)

Injection Solution, Prefilled Injector Pen: 1 mg/dose or 0.25 mg or 0.5 mg per dose (2 mg/1.5 mL). **Tablets:** 3 mg, 7 mg, 14 mg.

ADMINISTRATION/HANDLING

PO

• Administer on an empty stomach, at least 30 min before the first food intake, beverage, or other oral medications of the day. • Take with 4 oz of plain water only. Eat 30–60 min after dose. • Administer whole; do not break, cut, or crush. Tablets cannot be chewed.

SQ

Guidelines • Administer any time of the day, without regard to food, on the same day of each wk. May change administration day if the time between two doses is at least 2 days. • If dose is missed, administer within 5 days of missed dose. If more than 5 days pass after missed dose, wait until next regularly scheduled dose.

Preparation • Visually inspect for particulate matter or discoloration. Solution should appear clear, colorless, and free of particles. Do not use if solution is cloudy, discolored, or visible particles are observed.

Administration • Insert needle subcutaneously into abdomen, outer thigh, or upper arm, and inject solution. • Do not inject into areas of active skin disease or injury such as sunburns, skin rashes, inflammation, skin infections, or active psoriasis. • Do not administer IV or intramuscular. • Rotate injection sites.

Storage • Refrigerate unused injector pens. • Once used, may refrigerate or store at room temperature for up to 56 days. • Do not freeze. • Protect from sunlight.

S

INDICATIONS/ROUTES/DOSAGE

Type 2 Diabetes Mellitus, Risk Reduction of Major CV Events

SQ: ADULTS, ELDERLY: Initially, 0.25 mg once wkly for 4 wks, then increase to 0.5 mg once wkly for at least 4 wks. If glycemic response is inadequate, may further increase to a maximum of 1 mg once wkly.

PO: ADULTS, ELDERLY: Initially, 3 mg once daily for 30 days, then increase to 7 mg once daily for at least 30 days. May further increase to 14 mg once daily. **Note:** The 3 mg dose is intended only for therapy initiation.

Dosage in Renal/Hepatic Impairment

Mild to severe impairment: No dose adjustment.

SIDE EFFECTS

Occasional (15%–5%): Nausea, vomiting, diarrhea, abdominal pain, constipation. **Rare (less than 1%):** Injection site reactions (pain, erythema), fatigue, dysgeusia, dizziness.

ADVERSE EFFECTS/TOXIC REACTIONS

May increase risk of acute renal failure or worsening of chronic renal impairment (esp. with dehydration), severe gastroparesis, pancreatitis, thyroid C-cell tumors. Hypersensitivity reactions including anaphylaxis, angioedema were reported. May increase risk of hypoglycemia when used with other hypoglycemic agents, insulin. Diabetic retinopathy complications reported in 1% of pts. Worsening of diabetic retinopathy has been associated with rapid improvement of glucose control. Cholelithiasis reported in 2% of pts. Immunogenicity (anti-semaglutide antibody formation) reported in 1% of pts.

NURSING CONSIDERATIONS

BASELINE ASSESSMENT

Obtain glucose level, Hgb A1c. Obtain BUN, serum creatinine, eGFR, CrCl in pts with renal impairment. Question history of medullary thyroid carcinoma, multiple endocrine neoplasia syndrome type 2, hypersensitivity reaction, pancreatitis. Screen for use of other hypoglycemic agents, insulin. Assess pt's understanding of diabetes management, routine home glucose monitoring. Assess hydration status. Obtain dietary consult for nutritional education. Assess pt's willingness to self-inject medication.

INTERVENTION/EVALUATION

Monitor capillary blood glucose levels, Hgb A1c; renal function in pts with renal impairment reporting severe GI symptoms such as diarrhea, gastroparesis, vomiting. Monitor for hypersensitivity reaction. Screen for thyroid tumors (dysphagia, dyspnea, persistent hoarseness, neck mass). If tumor is suspected, consider endocrinologist consultation. Assess for hypoglycemia (anxiety, confusion, diaphoresis, diplopia, dizziness, headache, hunger, perioral numbness, tachycardia, tremors), hyperglycemia (confusion, fatigue, Kussmaul breathing, nausea, polyuria, vomiting). Screen for glucose-altering conditions: fever, stress, surgical procedures, trauma. Monitor for pancreatitis (severe, steady abdominal pain often radiating to the back [with or without vomiting]). Encourage fluid intake. Monitor I&Os.

PATIENT/FAMILY TEACHING

• A health care provider will show you how to properly prepare and inject medication. You must demonstrate correct preparation and injection techniques before using medication at home. • Diabetes mellitus requires lifelong control. Diet and exercise are principal parts of treatment; do not skip or delay meals. • Test blood sugar regularly. • Monitor daily calorie intake. • When taking additional medications to lower blood sugar or when glucose demands are altered (excessive alcohol ingestion, insufficient carbohydrate intake, hormone deficiencies, critical illness), have low blood sugar treatment available (glucagon, oral dextrose). • Therapy may increase risk of thyroid cancer; report lumps or swelling of the neck, hoarseness, shortness of breath, trouble swallowing. • Persistent, severe abdominal pain that radiates to the back (with or without vomiting) may indicate acute pancreatitis. • Report allergic reactions of any kind, esp. difficulty breathing, itching, rash, swelling of the face or throat. • Kidney injury or kidney failure may occur; report decreased urine output, amber-colored urine, flank pain.

sertraline

ser-tra-leen
(Zoloft)

BLACK BOX ALERT Increased risk of suicidal ideation and behavior in children, adolescents, young adults 18–24 yrs with major depressive disorder, other psychiatric disorders.

Do not confuse sertraline with cetirizine, selegiline, Serentil, or Serevent, or Zoloft with Zocor.

CLASSIFICATION

PHARMACOTHERAPEUTIC: Selective serotonin reuptake inhibitor. **CLINICAL:** Antidepressant, anxiolytic, obsessive-compulsive disorder adjunct.

USES

Treatment of major depressive disorders, panic disorder, obsessive-compulsive disorder (OCD), posttraumatic stress disorder (PTSD), premenstrual dysphoric disorder (PMDD), social anxiety disorder. **OFF-LABEL:** Eating disorders, bulimia nervosa, generalized anxiety disorder (GAD).

PRECAUTIONS

Contraindications: Hypersensitivity to sertraline. MAOI use within 14 days (concurrently or within 14 days of stopping an MAOI or sertraline). Concurrent use of oral concentrate (contains alcohol) with disulfiram. Concurrent use with pimozide; initiation in pts treated with linezolid or methylene blue. **Cautions:** Seizure disorder, hepatic impairment, pts at risk for uric acid nephropathy, elderly, pts in third trimester of pregnancy, pts at high risk for suicide, family history of bipolar disorder or mania, pts with risk factors for QT prolongation (e.g., hypokalemia, hypomagnesemia), alcoholism. Pts in whom weight loss is undesirable.

S

ACTION

Blocks reuptake of the neurotransmitter serotonin at CNS neuronal presynaptic membranes, increasing availability at postsynaptic receptor sites. **Therapeutic Effect:** Relieves depression, reduces obsessive-compulsive behavior, decreases anxiety.

PHARMACOKINETICS

Widely distributed. Protein binding: 98%. Metabolized in liver. Excreted in urine (45%), feces (45%). Not removed by hemodialysis. **Half-life:** 26 hrs.

LIFESPAN CONSIDERATIONS

Pregnancy/Lactation: Unknown if drug crosses placenta or is distributed in breast milk. **Children:** Children and adolescents are at increased risk for suicidal ideation and behavior or worsening of depression, esp. during the first few mos of therapy. **Elderly:** No age-related precautions noted, but lower initial dosages recommended.

INTERACTIONS

DRUG: **Alcohol, disulfiram** may increase adverse effects. **Anticoagulants (e.g., heparin, rivaroxaban, warfarin), antiplatelets (e.g., aspirin, clopidogrel), NSAIDs (e.g., diclofenac, meloxicam, naproxen)** may increase risk of bleeding. **MAOIs (e.g., phenelzine, selegiline)** may cause neuroleptic malignant syndrome, serotonin syndrome. **Serotonergic drugs (e.g., busPIRone, carBAMazepine, fentaNYL, linezolid, lithium, SNRIs [e.g., DULoxetine, venlafaxine])** may cause serotonin syndrome. May increase concentration, toxicity of **tricyclic antidepressants (e.g., amitriptyline, doxepin).** HERBAL: **Glucosamine, herbals with anticoagulant/antiplatelet properties (e.g., garlic, ginger, ginkgo biloba, ginseng)** may increase concentration/effect. FOOD: **Grapefruit products** may increase concentration/effect. LAB VALUES: May increase total serum cholesterol, triglycerides, ALT, AST. May decrease serum uric acid.

AVAILABILITY (Rx)

Oral Concentrate: 20 mg/mL. **Tablets:** 25 mg, 50 mg, 100 mg.

ADMINISTRATION/HANDLING

PO

• Give with food, milk if GI distress occurs. • Oral concentrate must be diluted before administration. Mix with 4 oz water, ginger ale, lemon/lime soda, or orange juice *only*. Give immediately after mixing.

INDICATIONS/ROUTES/DOSAGE

Depression

PO: ADULTS: Initially, 50 mg/day. May increase by 25–50 mg/day at 7-day intervals up to 300 mg/day. **ELDERLY:** Initially, 25 mg/day. May increase by 25–50 mg/day at 7-day intervals up to 300 mg/day.

Obsessive-Compulsive Disorder (OCD)

PO: ADULTS, CHILDREN 13–17 YRS: Initially, 50 mg/day with morning or evening meal. May increase by 25–50 mg/day at 7-day intervals up to 200 mg/day. **ELDERLY, CHILDREN 6–12 YRS:** Initially, 25 mg/day. May increase by 25–50 mg/day at 7-day intervals. **Maximum:** 200 mg/day.

Panic Disorder

PO: ADULTS, ELDERLY: Initially, 25 mg once daily for 3–7 days. May increase to 50 mg/day. May further increase dose based on response and tolerability in increments of 25–50 mg at intervals of at least 1 wk. **Maximum:** 200 mg/day.

Posttraumatic Stress Disorder (PTSD), Social Anxiety Disorder (SAD)

PO: ADULTS, ELDERLY: Initially, 25–50 mg/day. May increase by 25–50 mg/day at 7-day intervals. Range: 50–200 mg/day. **Maximum:** 200 mg/day.

Premenstrual Dysphoric Disorder (PMDD)

PO: ADULTS: (Continuous daily dosing): Initially, 25 mg once daily. Over first month, increase to 50 mg once daily. In subsequent menstrual cycles, an increase up to 200 mg/day may be necessary. **(Luteal phase dosing):** Initially, 25 mg once daily during luteal phase. Over first month, increase to 50 mg once daily. In subsequent menstrual cycles, an increase up to 150 mg/day may be necessary.

Dosage in Renal Impairment
No dose adjustment.

Dosage in Hepatic Impairment
Use caution.

SIDE EFFECTS

Frequent (26%–12%): Headache, nausea, diarrhea, insomnia, drowsiness, dizziness, fatigue, rash, dry mouth. **Occasional (6%–4%):** Anxiety, nervousness, agitation, tremor, dyspepsia, diaphoresis, vomiting, constipation, sexual dysfunction, visual disturbances, altered taste. **Rare (less than 3%):** Flatulence, urinary frequency, paresthesia, hot flashes, chills.

ADVERSE EFFECTS/TOXIC REACTIONS

Serotonin syndrome (seizures, arrhythmias, high fever), neuroleptic malignant syndrome (muscle rigidity, cognitive changes), suicidal ideation have occurred.

NURSING CONSIDERATIONS

BASELINE ASSESSMENT

Assess appearance, behavior, speech patterns, level of interest, mood. For pts on long-term therapy, CBC, renal function, LFT should be performed periodically. Question history of suicidal ideation and behavior.

INTERVENTION/EVALUATION

Assess mental status for depression, suicidal ideation (esp. at beginning of therapy or change in dosage), anxiety, social function, panic attack. Monitor daily pattern of bowel activity, stool consistency. Assist with ambulation if dizziness occurs.

PATIENT/FAMILY TEACHING

• Report headache, fatigue, tremor, sexual dysfunction. • Avoid tasks that require alertness, motor skills until response to drug is established (may cause dizziness, drowsiness). • Take with food if nausea occurs. • Avoid alcohol. • Do not take OTC medications without consulting physician. • Seek immediate medical attention if thoughts of suicide, new onset or worsening of anxiety, depression, or changes in mood occur.

sevelamer

TOP 100

se-**vel**-a-mer
(Renagel, Renvela)
Do not confuse Renagel with Reglan, Regonol, or Renvela, or sevelamer with Savella.

◆ CLASSIFICATION

PHARMACOTHERAPEUTIC: Polymeric phosphate binder. **CLINICAL:** Electrolyte modifier, antihyperphosphatemia agent.

USES

Control of serum phosphorus in pts with chronic renal disease on hemodialysis.

PRECAUTIONS

Contraindications: Hypersensitivity to sevelamer. Bowel obstruction. **Cautions:** Dysphagia, severe GI tract motility disorders, major GI tract surgery.

ACTION

Binds with phosphate within the intestinal lumen without altering calcium, aluminum, or bicarbonate concentration. **Therapeutic Effect:** Inhibits phosphate absorption. Decreases serum phosphate concentration.

PHARMACOKINETICS

Not absorbed systemically. Unknown if removed by hemodialysis.

⌛ LIFESPAN CONSIDERATIONS

Pregnancy/Lactation: Not distributed in breast milk. **Children:** Safety and efficacy not established. **Elderly:** No age-related precautions noted.

INTERACTIONS

DRUG: May decrease concentration/effect of **fluoroquinolones (e.g., levoFLOXacin), levothyroxine, mycophenolate.** **HERBAL:** None significant. **FOOD:** May cause reduced absorption of **vitamins D, E, K, folic acid.** **LAB VALUES:** Expected to decrease serum phosphate.

AVAILABILITY (Rx)

Powder for Oral Suspension: ***(Renvela):*** 0.8 g/pack, 2.4 g/pack.

Tablets: 800 mg.

ADMINISTRATION/HANDLING

PO

• Give with meals. • Space other medication by at least 1 hr before or 3 hrs after sevelamer. • Give tablets whole; do not break, crush, dissolve, or divide. • **Oral Suspension:** Mix 0.8 g with 30 mL water (2.4 g with 60 mL water). Stir vigorously to suspend (does not dissolve) just prior to drinking.

INDICATIONS/ROUTES/DOSAGE

Hyperphosphatemia

PO: ADULTS, ELDERLY: 800–1,600 mg with each meal, depending on severity of hyperphosphatemia (5.5–7.4 mg/dL: 800 mg 3 times/day; 7.5–8.9 mg/dL: 1,200–1,600 mg 3 times/day; 9 mg/dL or greater: 1,600 mg 3 times/day). **Maintenance:** Based on serum phosphorus concentrations. Goal range: 3.5–5.5 mg/dL.

Serum Phosphorus Concentration	Dosage
Greater than 5.5 mg/dL	Increase by 400–800 mg per meal at 2-wk intervals
3.5–5.5 mg/dL	Maintain current dosage
Less than 3.5 mg/dL	Decrease by 400–800 mg per meal

Dosage in Renal/Hepatic Impairment

No dose adjustment.

SIDE EFFECTS

Frequent (20%–11%): Infection, pain, hypotension, diarrhea, dyspepsia, nausea, vomiting. **Occasional (10%–1%):** Headache, constipation, hypertension, increased cough.

ADVERSE EFFECTS/TOXIC REACTIONS

Thrombosis occurs rarely.

NURSING CONSIDERATIONS

BASELINE ASSESSMENT

Obtain serum calcium, phosphate. Question history of bowel obstruction, GI motility disorders.

INTERVENTION/EVALUATION

Monitor serum phosphate, calcium.

PATIENT/FAMILY TEACHING

• Take with meals, swallow tablets whole; do not chew, crush, dissolve, or divide tablets. • Report persistent headache, nausea, vomiting, diarrhea, hypotension.

simvastatin

TOP 100

sim-va-sta-tin

(FloLipid, Zocor)

Do not confuse simvastatin with atorvastatin, lovastatin, nystatin, pitavastatin, or pravastatin, or Zocor with Cozaar, Lipitor, Zoloft, or ZyrTEC.

FIXED-COMBINATION(S)

Juvisync: simvastatin/SITagliptin (an antidiabetic agent): 10 mg/100 mg, 20 mg/100 mg, 40 mg/100 mg. **Simcor:** simvastatin/niacin (an antilipemic agent): 20 mg/500 mg, 40 mg/500 mg, 20 mg/750 mg, 20 mg/1000 mg, 40 mg/1000 mg. **Vytorin:** simvastatin/ezetimibe (a cholesterol absorption inhibitor): 10 mg/10 mg, 20 mg/10 mg, 40 mg/10 mg, 80 mg/10 mg.

◆CLASSIFICATION

PHARMACOTHERAPEUTIC: Hydroxymethylglutaryl-CoA (HMG-CoA) reductase inhibitor. **CLINICAL:** Antihyperlipidemic.

USES

Secondary prevention of cardiovascular events in pts with hypercholesterolemia and coronary heart disease (CHD) or at high risk for CHD. Treatment of hyperlipidemias to reduce elevations in total serum cholesterol, LDL-C, apolipoprotein B, triglycerides, VLDL-C and increase HDL-C. Treatment of homozygous familial hypercholesterolemia (HoFH). Treatment of heterozygous familial hypercholesterolemia (HeFH) in adolescents (10–17 yrs, females more than 1 yr postmenarche).

PRECAUTIONS

Contraindications: Hypersensitivity to simvastatin. Active hepatic disease or unexplained, persistent elevations of hepatic transaminases, pregnancy, breastfeeding, concurrent use of strong CYP3A4 inhibitors (e.g., clarithromycin, cycloSPORINE, gemfibrozil). **Cautions:** Hepatic disease, diabetes, severe renal impairment, substantial alcohol consumption. Withholding or discontinuing simvastatin may be necessary when pt is at risk for renal failure secondary to rhabdomyolysis. Concomitant use of other medications associated with myopathy.

ACTION

Interferes with cholesterol biosynthesis by inhibiting conversion of the enzyme HMG-CoA to mevalonate. **Therapeutic Effect:** Decreases LDL, cholesterol, VLDL, triglyceride levels; increase in HDL concentration.

PHARMACOKINETICS

Well absorbed from GI tract. Protein binding: 95%. Metabolized in liver. Excreted in feces (60%), urine (13%). Unknown if removed by hemodialysis.

Route	Onset	Peak	Duration
PO (to reduce cholesterol)	3 days	14 days	N/A

LIFESPAN CONSIDERATIONS

Pregnancy/Lactation: Contraindicated in pregnancy (suppression of cholesterol biosynthesis may cause fetal toxicity), lactation. Risk of serious adverse reactions in breastfeeding infants. **Children:** Safety and efficacy not established in children less than 10 yrs of age or in premenarchal girls. **Elderly:** No age-related precautions noted.

INTERACTIONS

DRUG: **CycloSPORINE, Strong CYP3A4 inhibitors (e.g., clarithromycin, ketoconazole), amiodarone, calcium channel blockers (e.g., dilTIAZem, verapamil), colchicine, fibrates, gemfibrozil, niacin, ranolazine** may increase risk of acute renal failure, rhabdomyolysis. **Strong CYP3A4 inducers (e.g., carBAMazepine, phenytoin, rifAMPin)** may decrease concentration/effect. **HERBAL:** **St. John's wort** may decrease concentration/effect. **FOOD:** **Grapefruit products** may increase concentration, toxicity. **Red yeast rice** contains 2.4 mg **lovastatin** per 600 mg rice. **LAB VALUES:** May increase serum creatine kinase (CK), transaminase.

AVAILABILITY (Rx)

Oral Suspension: 20 mg/5 mL, 40 mg/5 mL. **Tablets:** 5 mg, 10 mg, 20 mg, 40 mg, 80 mg.

ADMINISTRATION/HANDLING

PO

• Give without regard to food. • Administer in evening for maximum efficacy. Shake suspension well for 20 sec before administering.

INDICATIONS/ROUTES/DOSAGE

Note: Limit 80-mg dose to pts taking simvastatin longer than 12 mos without evidence of myopathy.

S

Prevention of Cardiovascular Events
PO: ADULTS, ELDERLY: Initially, 10–20 mg once daily. Range: 5–40 mg/day.

Hyperlipidemias
PO: ADULTS, ELDERLY: Initially, 10–20 mg once daily. **Pts with CHD or CHD risk equivalents:** Initially, 40 mg/day. **Range:** 5–40 mg/day.

Homozygous Familial Hypercholesterolemia (HoFH)
PO: ADULTS, ELDERLY: 40 mg once daily in evening.

Heterozygous Familial Hypercholesterolemia (HeFH)
PO: CHILDREN 10–17 YRS: 10 mg once daily in evening. May increase to 20 mg once daily after 6 wks. May further increase to 40 mg once daily after additional 6 wks. **Maximum dose:** 40 mg/day.

Dosing Adjustment With Medications
(CycloSPORINE, gemfibrozil): Do not exceed 10 mg/day. ***(Amiodarone, amLODIPine, ranolazine):*** Do not exceed 20 mg/day. ***(DilTIAZem, dronedarone, verapamil):*** Do not exceed 10 mg/day. ***(Lomitapide):*** Reduce simvastatin dose by 50% when initiating lomitapide. Do not exceed 20 mg/day.

Dosage in Renal Impairment
CrCl less than 30 mL/min: Initially, 5 mg/day.

S

Dosage in Hepatic Impairment
Contraindicated with active hepatic disease.

SIDE EFFECTS

Generally well tolerated. Side effects are usually mild and transient. **Occasional (3%–2%):** Headache, abdominal pain/cramps, constipation, upper respiratory tract infection. **Rare (less than 2%):** Diarrhea, flatulence, asthenia, nausea/vomiting, depression.

ADVERSE EFFECTS/TOXIC REACTIONS

May cause ocular lens opacities. Hypersensitivity reaction, hepatitis occur rarely. Myopathy (muscle pain, tenderness, weakness with elevated serum creatine kinase [CK], sometimes taking the form of rhabdomyolysis) has occurred.

NURSING CONSIDERATIONS

BASELINE ASSESSMENT

Obtain lipid panel, LFT; urine pregnancy test in females of reproductive potential.

INTERVENTION/EVALUATION

Monitor serum cholesterol, triglyceride lab results for therapeutic response. Monitor LFT. Assess for headache, myopathy.

PATIENT/FAMILY TEACHING

• Use appropriate contraceptive measures. • Periodic lab tests are essential part of therapy. • Maintain appropriate diet. Avoid grapefruit products. • Report unexplained muscle pain, tenderness, weakness.

siponimod

si-**pon**-i-mod
(Mayzent)
Do not confuse siponimod with fingolimod or ozanimod.

◆CLASSIFICATION

PHARMACOTHERAPEUTIC: Sphingosine-1-phosphate receptor modulator. **CLINICAL:** Multiple sclerosis agent.

USES

Treatment of relapsing forms of multiple sclerosis (MS), including clinically isolated syndrome, relapsing-remitting disease, and active secondary progressive disease, in adults.

PRECAUTIONS

Contraindications: Hypersensitivity to siponimod. Pts with CYP2C9*3/*3 genotype. Recent (within 6 mos) MI, unstable angina, CVA, TIA, decompensated HF requiring hospitalization, NYHA class III/IV HF, sick sinus syndrome, Mobitz type II second- or third-degree AV block (unless pt has functioning pacemaker). **Cautions:** Conditions predisposing to infection (e.g., diabetes, immunocompromised pts, renal failure, open wounds), baseline sinus bradycardia, severe hepatic impairment, hypertension, altered pulmonary function, pts at risk for developing AV block (congenital heart disease, ischemic heart disease, HF), pts at risk for macular edema (e.g., diabetes, history of uveitis); history of syncope, thromboembolic events (CVA, pulmonary embolism, MI [more than 6 mos prior]). Concomitant use of antiarrhythmics, beta blockers, calcium channel blockers, immunosuppressants, immune modulators, antineoplastics, QT interval–prolonging medications. Not recommended in pts with severe active infection; history of cardiac arrest, cerebrovascular disease, uncontrolled hypertension, or severe, untreated sleep apnea unless approved by a cardiologist.

ACTION

Blocks capacity of lymphocytes to move out from lymph nodes, reducing the number of lymphocytes available to the CNS. **Therapeutic Effect:** May involve reduction of lymphocyte migration into the CNS, reducing inflammation.

PHARMACOKINETICS

Widely distributed. Metabolized in liver. Protein binding: 68%. Peak plasma concentration: 4 hrs. Steady state reached in 6 days. Excreted primarily in feces. **Half-life:** 30 hrs.

⌛ LIFESPAN CONSIDERATIONS

Pregnancy/Lactation: Avoid pregnancy; may cause fetal harm. Females of reproductive potential should use effective contraception during treatment and up to 10 days after discontinuation. Unknown if distributed in breast milk. **Children:** Safety and efficacy not established. **Elderly:** Age-related hepatic impairment may increase risk of adverse effects/hepatic injury.

INTERACTIONS

DRUG: **Beta blockers (e.g., carvedilol, metoprolol), bretylium, calcium channel blockers (e.g., dilTIAZem, verapamil), ceritinib, digoxin, lacosamide** may increase risk of AV block, bradycardia. May increase QT interval–prolonging effect of **amiodarone, azithromycin, haloperidol.** May decrease therapeutic effect of **BCG (intravesical), live vaccines.** May increase toxic effect of **live vaccines. Fluconazole** may increase concentration/effect. **RifAMPin** may decrease concentration/effect. May increase toxic effects of **denosumab, leflunomide, natalizumab, tacrolimus.** May decrease therapeutic effect of **nivolumab, sipuleucel-T, tertomotide.** May increase immunosuppressive effect of **tofacitinib, other immunosuppressants.** **HERBAL:** **Echinacea** may decrease therapeutic effect. **FOOD:** None known. **LAB VALUES:** May increase serum ALT, AST, bilirubin, GGT. Expected to cause a dose-dependent reduction in peripheral lymphocyte count to 20%–30% of baseline values.

AVAILABILITY (Rx)

Tablets: 0.25 mg, 2 mg.

ADMINISTRATION/HANDLING

PO

• Give without regard to meals. • Starter pack should be used in pts who titrate to 2 mg maintenance dose. Do not use starter pack in pts who titrate to 1 mg maintenance dose. • If one dose titration is missed for more than 24 hrs, reinitiate treatment starting with day 1 of titration regimen. • If treatment is interrupted for more than 4 consecutive days after initial titration is completed, reinitiate treatment starting with day 1 of titration regimen.

INDICATIONS/ROUTES/DOSAGE

Multiple Sclerosis (Relapsing)

PO: ADULTS, ELDERLY: (Pts with CYP2C9 genotypes *1/*1, *1/*2, or *2/*2):

S

0.25 mg on day 1, then 0.25 mg on day 2, then 0.5 mg on day 3, then 0.75 mg on day 4, then 1.25 mg on day 5. **Maintenance:** 2 mg once daily starting on day 6. **(Pts with CYP2C9 genotypes *1/*3 or *2/*3):** 0.25 mg on day 1, then 0.25 mg on day 2, then 0.5 mg on day 3, then 0.75 mg on day 4. **Maintenance:** 1 mg once daily starting on day 5.

Dosage in Renal Impairment

Mild to severe impairment: No dose adjustment.

Dosage in Hepatic Impairment

Mild to moderate impairment: No dose adjustment. **Severe impairment:** Use caution.

SIDE EFFECTS

Occasional (15%–6%): Headache, hypertension, peripheral edema, nausea, dizziness, diarrhea, extremity pain.

ADVERSE EFFECTS/TOXIC REACTIONS

Life-threatening infections (bronchitis, sinusitis, upper respiratory tract infection, fungal skin infection) reported in 3% of pts. Fatal cases of cryptococcal meningitis, disseminated cryptococcal infections were reported. Herpes zoster infections reported in 5% of pts. Reactivation of herpes viral infection may cause varicella zoster meningitis. Progressive multifocal leukoencephalopathy (PML), an opportunistic viral infection of the brain caused by the JC virus, may result in progressive permanent disability and death. Posterior reversible encephalopathy syndrome, a dysfunction of the brain that may evolve into an ischemic CVA or cerebral hemorrhage, may occur. Macular edema reported in 2% of pts. Pts with diabetes or history of uveitis are at an increased risk for developing macular edema. Bradycardia reported in 4% of pts. AV conduction delays reported in 5% of pts. Dose-dependent reductions of pulmonary function (absolute forced expiratory volume over 1 sec) reported in 3% of pts. Hepatic injury (transaminitis) reported in 10% of pts. Seizures reported in 2% of pts. Falls reported in 11% of pts. Rebound or severe exacerbation of disease may occur after discontinuation. May increase risk of hypertension, new malignancies. Fatal thromboembolic events including CVA, pulmonary embolism, MI reported in 3% of pts.

NURSING CONSIDERATIONS

BASELINE ASSESSMENT

Obtain CBC, LFT, ECG. Test all pts for CYP2C9 variants to determine CYP2C9 genotype. Assess baseline symptoms of MS (e.g., bladder/bowel dysfunction, cognitive impairment, depression, dysphagia, fatigue, gait disorder, numbness/tingling, pain, seizures, spasticity, tremors, weakness). Consultation with a cardiologist is advised in pts with QT interval prolongation greater than 500 msec; arrhythmias requiring treatment with Class Ia or Class III antiarrhythmic; ischemic heart disease, HF, history of cardiac arrest, recent MI; history of Mobitz type II second- or third-degree AV block, sick sinus syndrome, sinoatrial heart block. First-dose monitoring is recommended in pts with preexisting cardiac conditions (baseline sinus bradycardia, first- or second-degree [Mobitz type I], history of MI [more than 6 mos prior], HF) in a medical setting that can adequately treat symptomatic bradycardia. Pts without a documented history of vaccination against varicella zoster or a confirmed history of varicella infection (chickenpox) should be tested for antibodies prior to initiation. A full vaccination course for varicella in antibody-negative pts is recommended prior to initiation. Perform baseline ophthalmologic evaluation of the fundus (including the macula) prior to initiation. Receive full medication history and screen for interaction (esp. immunosuppressants; drugs known to bradycardia, AV conduction delay). Question history as listed in Precautions. Screen for active infection.

INTERVENTION/EVALUATION

At initial treatment (within first 4–6 hrs after dose), therapy reduces heart rate,

S

AV conduction. In pts with preexisting cardiac conditions, monitor for symptomatic bradycardia for at least 6 hrs after first dose with hourly pulse, B/P, and then obtain ECG at the end of day 1. If heart rate is less than 45 beats/min, QTc interval is 500 msec or greater, or new-onset second-degree (or higher) AV block is present after 6 hrs of first dose, continue monitoring until resolved. If intervention is required, continue heart monitoring overnight and repeat 6-hr monitoring after second dose. Conduct ophthalmic examination with any change of vision. Pts with altered mental status, seizures, visual disturbances, unilateral weakness should be evaluated for cryptococcal meningitis, varicella zoster meningitis, posterior reversible encephalopathy syndrome, PML. Persistent immunosuppressive effects may occur for up to 3–4 wks after discontinuation. Closely monitor for adverse effects if other immunosuppressants are initiated within the first 3–4 wks after discontinuation. Monitor B/P for hypertension. Monitor for systemic or local infections, herpetic infections; symptoms of new malignancies. Conduct neurologic assessment. Assess for symptoms improvement of MS. Monitor for symptoms of MI (chest pain, diaphoresis, left arm/jaw pain, increased serum troponin, ST segment elevation), CVA (aphasia, altered mental status, facial droop, hemiplegia, vision loss), pulmonary embolism (chest pain, dyspnea, tachycardia).

PATIENT/FAMILY TEACHING

• Treatment may depress your immune system and reduce your ability to fight infection. Report symptoms of infection such as body aches, burning with urination, chills, cough, fatigue, fever. Avoid those with active infection. • Any change of vision will require an immediate eye examination. • PML, an opportunistic viral infection of the brain, may cause progressive, permanent disabilities or death. Report symptoms of PML such as confusion, memory loss, paralysis, trouble speaking, vision loss, seizures, weakness. • Treatment may worsen high blood pressure or cause new cancers. • Report liver problems (abdominal pain, bruising, clay-colored stool, amber or dark colored urine, yellowing of the skin or eyes), lung problems (reduced lung function, shortness of breath), heart arrhythmias (chest pain, dizziness, fainting, palpitations, slow or rapid heart rate, irregular heart rate). • Posterior reversible encephalopathy syndrome, a dysfunction of the brain that may cause a stroke or bleeding in the brain, may occur. • Treatment may cause life-threatening blood clots; report symptoms of heart attack (chest pain, difficulty breathing, jaw pain, nausea, pain that radiates to the left arm, sweating), lung embolism (difficulty breathing, chest pain, rapid heart rate), stroke (confusion, difficulty speaking, one-sided weakness or paralysis, loss of vision). • Use effective contraception to avoid pregnancy. Do not breastfeed. • Due to high risk of interactions, do not take newly prescribed medications unless approved by the provider who originally started treatment. • Do not receive live vaccines for at least 4 wks after last dose. • Severe worsening of MS symptoms may occur after stopping treatment.

sirolimus

sir-**oh**-li-mus
(Rapamune)

BLACK BOX ALERT Increased susceptibility to infection and potential for development of lymphoma may result from immunosuppression. Not recommended for liver or lung transplant pts. Use only by physicians experienced in immunosuppressive therapy and management of transplant pts.

Do not confuse Rapamune with Rapaflo, or sirolimus with everolimus, pimecrolimus, tacrolimus, or temsirolimus.

CLASSIFICATION

PHARMACOTHERAPEUTIC: mTOR kinase inhibitor. **CLINICAL:** Immunosuppressant.

USES

Prophylaxis of organ rejection in pts receiving renal transplant (in combination with cycloSPORINE and corticosteroids). Treatment of lymphangioleiomyomatosis. **OFF-LABEL:** Prophylaxis of organ rejection in heart transplant recipients. Prevention of acute graft-vs-host disease in allogeneic stem cell transplantation. Treatment of refractory acute or chronic graft-vs-host disease. Rescue agent for acute and chronic organ rejection.

PRECAUTIONS

Contraindications: Hypersensitivity to sirolimus. **Cautions:** Cardiovascular disease (HF, hypertension); pulmonary disease, hepatic impairment, renal impairment, hyperlipidemia, perioperative period due to increased chance of surgical complications from impaired wound and tissue healing. Concurrent use with medications that may alter renal function.

ACTION

Inhibits T-lymphocyte activation and proliferation in response to antigenic and cytokine stimulation, and inhibits antibody production. **Therapeutic Effect:** Inhibits acute rejection of allografts and prolongs graft survival.

PHARMACOKINETICS

Widely distributed. Protein binding: 92%. Extensively metabolized in liver. Primarily excreted in feces (91%). **Half-life:** 57–63 hrs.

LIFESPAN CONSIDERATIONS

Pregnancy/Lactation: Unknown if crosses placenta or is distributed in breast milk. **Children:** Safety and efficacy not established in pts younger than 13 yrs. **Elderly:** No age-related precautions noted.

INTERACTIONS

DRUG: **CYP3A4 inducers (e.g., carBAMazepine, rifabutin, rifAMPin)** may decrease concentration/effect. **CYP3A4 inhibitors (e.g., clarithromycin, erythromycin, itraconazole, verapamil)** may increase concentration, toxicity. May increase concentration/effect of **cycloSPORINE** (take sirolimus 4 hrs after cycloSPORINE for renal transplant). May decrease the therapeutic effect; increase adverse effects of **vaccines (live)**. **HERBAL:** **St. John's wort** may decrease concentration/effect. **Echinacea** may decrease the therapeutic effect. **FOOD:** **Grapefruit products** may increase risk of myelotoxicity, nephrotoxicity. **LAB VALUES:** May increase serum ALT, AST, alkaline phosphatase, LDH, BUN, creatine phosphate, cholesterol, triglycerides, creatinine. May alter WBC, serum glucose, calcium. May decrease Hgb, Hct.

AVAILABILITY (Rx)

Oral Solution: 1 mg/mL.

Tablets: 0.5 mg, 1 mg, 2 mg.

ADMINISTRATION/HANDLING

• Doses should be taken 4 hrs after cycloSPORINE. • Take consistently with or without food. • Do not break, crush, dissolve, or divide tablets. • Mix oral solution with only water or orange juice, stir vigorously, drink immediately.

INDICATIONS/ROUTES/DOSAGE

ALERT Tablets and oral solution are not bioequivalent. (However, clinical equivalence shown at 2 mg dose.)

Prevention of Organ Transplant Rejection (Low to moderate risk)

PO: ADULTS, CHILDREN 13 YRS AND OLDER WEIGHING MORE THAN 40 KG: Loading dose: 6 mg on day 1. **Maintenance:** 2 mg/day. **ADULTS, CHILDREN 13 YRS AND OLDER WEIGHING LESS THAN 40 KG:** Loading dose: 3 mg/m^2 on day 1. **Maintenance:** 1 mg/m^2/day.

Prevention of Organ Transplant Rejection (High risk)
PO: ADULTS: Loading dose: Up to 15 mg on day 1. **Maintenance:** 5 mg/day. Obtain trough between 5–7 days. Continue therapy for 1 yr following transplantation. Further adjustments based on clinical status.

Lymphangioleiomyomatosis
PO: ADULTS, ELDERLY: Initially, 2 mg/day with dosage adjustment to maintain concentration between 5–15 ng/mL. Obtain serum trough level after 10–20 days. Once maintenance dose is adjusted, further adjustments should be made at 7- to 14-day intervals. Once a stable dose is attained, serum trough levels should be assessed at least q3mos.

Dosage in Renal Impairment
No dose adjustment.

Dosage in Hepatic Impairment
Loading dose: No change. **Maintenance dose: Mild to moderate impairment:** Reduce dose by 33%. **Severe impairment:** Reduce dose by 50%.

SIDE EFFECTS

Occasional: Hypercholesterolemia, hyperlipidemia, hypertension, rash. **High doses (5 mg/day):** Anemia, arthralgia, diarrhea, hypokalemia, peripheral edema, thrombocytopenia.

ADVERSE EFFECTS/TOXIC REACTIONS

Hepatotoxicity occurs rarely. Skin carcinoma (including basal cell, squamous cell, melanoma) has been observed.

NURSING CONSIDERATIONS

BASELINE ASSESSMENT

Obtain LFT; pregnancy test in females of reproductive potential. Question for medication usage (esp. cycloSPORINE, dilTIAZem, ketoconazole, rifAMPin). Determine if pt has chickenpox, herpes zoster, malignancy, infection.

INTERVENTION/EVALUATION

Monitor renal function, LFT periodically. Monitor serum cholesterol, triglycerides, platelets; Hgb. Obtain trough concentration 10–20 days after dose. Once maintenance dose is adjusted, make further adjustments at intervals of 7–14 days. Once stable dose is attained, assess trough concentration at least q3mos.

PATIENT/FAMILY TEACHING

• Avoid those with colds, other infections. • Avoid grapefruit products. • Avoid exposure to sunlight, artificial light sources. • Strict monitoring is essential in identifying, preventing symptoms of organ rejection. • Do not chew, crush, dissolve, or divide tablets.

SITagliptin

TOP 100 HIGH ALERT

sit-a-**glip**-tin
(Januvia)
Do not confuse Januvia with Enjuvia, Jantoven, or Janumet, or SITagliptin with SAXagliptin or SUMAtriptan.

FIXED-COMBINATION(S)

Janumet, Janumet XR: SITagliptin/metFORMIN (an antidiabetic): 50 mg/500 mg, 50 mg/1,000 mg.

◆CLASSIFICATION

PHARMACOTHERAPEUTIC: DPP-4 inhibitors (gliptins). **CLINICAL:** Antidiabetic agent.

USES

Adjunctive treatment to diet, exercise to improve glycemic control in pts with type 2 diabetes as monotherapy or in combination with other antidiabetic agents.

PRECAUTIONS

Contraindications: Hypersensitivity to SITagliptin. **Cautions:** Type 1 diabetes, diabetic ketoacidosis, renal impairment, end-stage renal disease, history of

S

pancreatitis, angioedema with other DPP-4 inhibitors. Concurrent use of other glucose-lowering agents may increase risk of hypoglycemia.

ACTION

Inhibits DPP-4 enzyme, causing prolonged active incretin levels. Incretin regulates glucose homeostasis. **Therapeutic Effect:** Regulates glucose homeostasis. Increases synthesis and release of insulin from pancreatic cells; lowers glucagon secretion from pancreas, decreases hepatic glucose production.

PHARMACOKINETICS

Route	Onset	Peak	Duration
PO	N/A	1–4 hrs	24 hrs

Rapidly absorbed. Protein binding: 38%. Excreted in urine (87%), feces (13%). **Half-life:** 12 hrs.

LIFESPAN CONSIDERATIONS

Pregnancy/Lactation: Unknown if distributed in breast milk. **Children:** Safety and efficacy not established. **Elderly:** No age-related precautions noted.

INTERACTIONS

DRUG: May enhance hypoglycemic effect of **insulin, sulfonylureas (e.g., glipiZIDE, glyBURIDE).** **HERBAL:** None significant. **FOOD:** None known. **LAB VALUES:** May slightly increase WBCs, particularly neutrophil count. May increase serum creatinine.

AVAILABILITY (Rx)

Tablets, Film-Coated: 25 mg, 50 mg, 100 mg.

ADMINISTRATION/HANDLING

PO

• May give without regard to food. • Do not break, crush, dissolve, or divide film-coated tablets.

INDICATIONS/ROUTES/DOSAGE

Type 2 Diabetes

PO: ADULTS OVER 18 YRS, ELDERLY: 100 mg once daily.

Dosage in Renal Impairment

CrCl 30 mL/min to less than 50 mL/min: 50 mg once daily. **CrCl less than 30 mL/min, ESRD, dialysis:** 25 mg once daily.

Dosage in Hepatic Impairment

No dose adjustment.

SIDE EFFECTS

Occasional (5% and greater): Headache, nasopharyngitis. **Rare (3%–1%):** Diarrhea, abdominal pain, nausea.

ADVERSE EFFECTS/TOXIC REACTIONS

Hypersensitivity reactions including angioedema, Stevens-Johnson syndrome reported. Acute pancreatitis occurs rarely.

NURSING CONSIDERATIONS

BASELINE ASSESSMENT

Obtain renal function test, serum glucose; Hgb A1c. Assess pt's understanding of diabetes management, routine home glucose monitoring. Obtain dietary consult for nutritional education. Question history of renal impairment, type 1 diabetes, ketoacidosis, pancreatitis. Receive full medication history and screen for interactions.

INTERVENTION/EVALUATION

Monitor blood glucose, hemoglobin A1c level, renal function. Assess for hypoglycemia (diaphoresis, tremors, dizziness, anxiety, headache, tachycardia, perioral numbness, hunger, diplopia, difficulty concentrating), hyperglycemia (polyuria, polyphagia, polydipsia, nausea, vomiting, fatigue, Kussmaul breathing), hypersensitivity reaction. Concomitant use of beta blockers (e.g., carvedilol, metoprolol) may mask symptoms of hypoglycemia. Screen for glucose-altering conditions: fever, increased activity or stress, surgical procedures. Dietary consult for nutritional education. Severe abdominal pain, nausea may indicate pancreatitis.

PATIENT/FAMILY TEACHING

• Diabetes mellitus requires lifelong control. Diet and exercise is a principal part of treatment; do not skip or delay meals. Test blood sugar regularly. Monitor daily calorie intake. • When taking combination drug therapy or when glucose conditions are altered (excessive alcohol ingestion, insufficient carbohydrate intake, hormone deficiencies, critical illness), have a low blood sugar treatment available (e.g., glucagon, oral dextrose). • Persistent, severe abdominal pain that radiates to the back (with or without vomiting) may indicate acute pancreatitis. • Report joint pain; allergic reactions of any kind.

sodium bicarbonate

soe-dee-um bye-**kar**-boe-nate
(Neut)

◆CLASSIFICATION

PHARMACOTHERAPEUTIC: Alkalinizing agent. **CLINICAL:** Antacid, electrolyte supplement, urinary/systemic alkalinizer.

USES

Management of metabolic acidosis, gastric hyperacidity. Alkalinization agent for urine; hyperkalemia treatment; management of overdose of tricyclic antidepressants and aspirin. **OFF-LABEL:** Prevention of contrast-induced nephropathy.

PRECAUTIONS

Contraindications: Hypersensitivity to sodium bicarbonate. Hypernatremia, alkalosis, unknown abdominal pain, hypocalcemia, severe pulmonary edema. **Cautions:** HF, edematous states, renal insufficiency, cirrhosis.

ACTION

Dissociates to provide bicarbonate ion. **Therapeutic Effect:** Neutralizes hydrogen ion concentration, raises blood, urinary pH.

PHARMACOKINETICS

Route	Onset	Peak	Duration
PO	15 min	N/A	1–3 hrs
IV	Immediate	N/A	8–10 min

Well absorbed following PO administration, sodium bicarbonate dissociates to sodium and bicarbonate ions. With increased hydrogen ion concentrations, bicarbonate ions combine with hydrogen ions to form carbonic acid, which then dissociates to CO_2, which is excreted by the lungs. Plasma concentration regulated by kidney (ability to form, excrete bicarbonate).

LIFESPAN CONSIDERATIONS

Pregnancy/Lactation: May produce hypernatremia, increase tendon reflexes in neonate or fetus whose mother is administered chronically high doses. May be distributed in breast milk. **Children:** No age-related precautions noted. Do not use as antacid in pts younger than 6 yrs. **Elderly:** Age-related renal impairment may require dosage adjustment.

INTERACTIONS

DRUG: May increase concentration, toxicity of **quiNIDine, quiNINE.** May decrease effects of **lithium. HERBAL:** None significant. **FOOD: Milk, other dairy products** may result in milk-alkali syndrome. **LAB VALUES:** May increase serum, urinary pH.

AVAILABILITY (Rx)

Injection Solution (Rx): 0.5 mEq/mL (4.2%), 1 mEq/mL (8.4%). **Tablets (OTC):** 325 mg, 650 mg.

ADMINISTRATION/HANDLING

IV

◀ALERT▶ For direct IV administration in neonates or infants, use 0.5 mEq/mL concentration.

Reconstitution • May give undiluted.

Rate of administration • For IV push, give up to 1 mEq/kg over 1–3 min for cardiac arrest. • For IV infusion, do not exceed rate of infusion of 1 mEq/kg/hr. • For children younger than 2 yrs, premature infants, neonates, administer by slow infusion, up to 10 mEq/min.

Storage • Store at room temperature.

PO

• Give 1–3 hrs after meals.

IV INCOMPATIBILITIES

Amiodarone (Cordarone), ascorbic acid, calcium chloride, dilTIAZem (Cardizem), DOBUTamine (Dobutrex), DOPamine (Intropin), HYDROmorphone (Dilaudid), magnesium sulfate, midazolam (Versed), norepinephrine (Levophed), ondansetron (Zofran).

IV COMPATIBILITIES

Dexmedetomidine (Precedex), furosemide (Lasix), heparin, insulin, lidocaine, mannitol, milrinone (Primacor), morphine, phenylephrine (Neo-Synephrine), potassium chloride, propofol (Diprivan), vancomycin (Vancocin).

INDICATIONS/ROUTES/DOSAGE

◀ALERT▶ May give by IV push, IV infusion, or orally. Dose individualized based on severity of acidosis, laboratory values, pt age, weight, clinical conditions. Do not fully correct bicarbonate deficit during the first 24 hrs (may cause metabolic alkalosis).

Cardiac Arrest

◀ALERT▶ Routine use not recommended.

IV: ADULTS, ELDERLY: Initially, 1 mEq/kg. May repeat based on arterial blood gases. **CHILDREN, INFANTS:** Initially, 0.5–1 mEq/kg. May repeat based on arterial blood gases.

Metabolic Acidosis (Mild to moderate)

IV: ADULTS, ELDERLY, CHILDREN: 2–5 mEq/kg over 4–8 hrs. May repeat based on acid-base status.

Prevention of Contrast-Induced Nephropathy

IV infusion: ADULTS, ELDERLY: 154 mEq/L sodium bicarbonate in D_5W solution: 3 mL/kg/hr 1 hr immediately before contrast injection, then 1 mL/kg/hr during contrast exposure and for 6 hrs after procedure.

Metabolic Acidosis (Associated with chronic renal failure)

PO: ADULTS, ELDERLY: Initially, 15.4–23.1 mEq/day in divided doses. Titrate to normal serum bicarbonate level of 23–29 mEq/L.

Renal Tubular Acidosis (Distal)

PO: ADULTS, ELDERLY: 0.5–2 mEq/kg/day in 4–6 divided doses. **CHILDREN:** 2–3 mEq/kg/day in divided doses.

Renal Tubular Acidosis (Proximal)

PO: ADULTS, ELDERLY, CHILDREN: 5–10 mEq/kg/day in divided doses. Maintenance dose to maintain serum bicarbonate in normal range.

Urine Alkalinization

PO: ADULTS, ELDERLY: Initially, 4 g, then 1–2 g q4h. **Maximum:** 16 g/day (8 g/day in adults older than 60 yrs).

Antacid

PO: ADULTS, ELDERLY: 300 mg–2 g 1–4 times/day.

Hyperkalemia

IV: ADULTS, ELDERLY: 50 mEq over 5 min.

SIDE EFFECTS

Frequent: Abdominal distention, flatulence, belching.

ADVERSE EFFECTS/TOXIC REACTIONS

Excessive, chronic use may produce metabolic alkalosis (irritability, twitching, paresthesia, cyanosis, slow or shallow respirations, headache, thirst, nausea). Fluid overload results in headache, weakness, blurred vision, behavioral changes, incoordination, muscle twitching, elevated B/P, bradycardia, tachypnea, wheezing, coughing, distended neck veins. Extravasation may occur at the IV site, resulting in tissue necrosis, ulceration.

NURSING CONSIDERATIONS

BASELINE ASSESSMENT

Assess for symptoms of acidosis, alkalosis. Do not give PO medication within 1 hr of antacids.

INTERVENTION/EVALUATION

Monitor serum, urinary pH, CO_2 level, serum electrolytes, plasma bicarbonate levels. Monitor for metabolic alkalosis, fluid overload. Assess for clinical improvement of metabolic acidosis (relief from hyperventilation, weakness, disorientation). Monitor serum phosphate, calcium, uric acid levels. Assess for relief of gastric distress.

sodium chloride HIGH ALERT

so-dee-um **klor**-ide
(Muro 128, Nasal Moist, Ocean, SalineX)

◆CLASSIFICATION

PHARMACOTHERAPEUTIC: Electrolyte supplement. **CLINICAL:** Electrolyte, isotonic volume expander, ophthalmic adjunct.

USES

Parenteral: Source of hydration; prevention/treatment of sodium, chloride deficiencies (hypertonic for severe deficiencies). Prevention of muscle cramps, heat prostration occurring with excessive perspiration. **Nasal:** Restores moisture, relieves dry, inflamed nasal membranes. **Ophthalmic:** Therapy in reduction of corneal edema, diagnostic aid in ophthalmoscopic exam.

PRECAUTIONS

Contraindications: Hypersensitivity to sodium chloride. Fluid retention, hypernatremia, hypertonic uterus. **Cautions:** HF, renal impairment, cirrhosis, hypertension, edema. Do not use sodium chloride preserved with benzyl alcohol in neonates.

ACTION

Sodium is a major cation of extracellular fluid. **Therapeutic Effect:** Controls water distribution, fluid and electrolyte balance, osmotic pressure of body fluids; maintains acid-base balance.

PHARMACOKINETICS

Widely distributed. Primarily excreted in urine and, to a lesser degree, in sweat, tears, saliva.

LIFESPAN CONSIDERATIONS

Pregnancy/Lactation: No precautions noted. **Children/Elderly:** No age-related precautions noted.

INTERACTIONS

DRUG: May decrease effect of **lithium**. May enhance adverse/toxic effects of **tolvaptan.** **HERBAL:** None significant. **FOOD:** None known. **LAB VALUES:** None significant.

AVAILABILITY (Rx)

Injection Concentrate (Rx): 23.4% (4 mEq/mL). **Injection Solution (Rx):** 0.45%, 0.9%, 3%. **Irrigation (Rx):** 0.45%, 0.9%. **Nasal Gel (OTC):** ***(Nasal Moist):*** 0.65%. **Nasal Solution (OTC):** ***(SalineX):*** 0.4% ***(Nasal Moist, Ocean):*** 0.65%. **Ophthalmic Ointment (OTC):** ***(Muro 128):*** 5%. **Ophthalmic Solution (OTC):** ***(Muro 128):*** 2%, 5%.

Tablets (OTC): 1 g.

ADMINISTRATION/HANDLING

IV

• Hypertonic solutions (3% or 5%) are administered via large vein; avoid infiltration; do not exceed 100 mL/hr. • Vials containing 2.5–4 mEq/mL (concentrated NaCl) must be diluted with D_5W or $D_{10}W$ before administration.

PO

• Do not crush/break enteric-coated or extended-release tablets. • Administer with full glass of water.

Nasal

• Instruct pt to begin inhaling slowly just before releasing medication into nose.

• Instruct pt to inhale slowly, then release air gently through mouth. • Continue technique for 20–30 sec.

Ophthalmic

• Place gloved finger on lower eyelid and pull out until pocket is formed between eye and lower lid. • Place prescribed number of drops (or ¼–½ inch of ointment) into pocket. • Instruct pt to close eye gently for 1–2 min so that medication will not be squeezed out of sac. • When lower lid is released, have pt keep eye open without blinking for at least 30 sec for solution; for ointment, have pt close eye, roll eyeball around to distribute medication. • When using drops, apply gentle finger pressure to lacrimal sac at inner canthus for 1 min to minimize systemic absorption.

INDICATIONS/ROUTES/DOSAGE

◀ALERT▶ Dosage based on age, weight, clinical condition; fluid, electrolyte, acid-base balance status.

Usual Parenteral Dosage

IV: ADULTS, ELDERLY, CHILDREN: Determined by laboratory determinations (mEq). Dosage varies widely based on clinical conditions.

Usual Oral Dosage

PO: ADULTS, ELDERLY: 1–2 g 3 times/day.

Usual Nasal Dosage

Intranasal: ADULTS, ELDERLY, CHILDREN: 2–3 sprays as needed.

Usual Ophthalmic Dosage

Ophthalmic solution: ADULTS, ELDERLY: Apply 1–2 drops q3–4h.

Ophthalmic ointment: ADULTS, ELDERLY: Apply once daily or as directed.

SIDE EFFECTS

Frequent: Facial flushing. **Occasional:** Fever; irritation, phlebitis, extravasation at injection site. **Ophthalmic:** Temporary burning, irritation.

ADVERSE EFFECTS/TOXIC REACTIONS

Too-rapid administration may produce peripheral edema, HF, pulmonary edema. Excessive dosage may produce hypokalemia, hypervolemia, hypernatremia.

NURSING CONSIDERATIONS

BASELINE ASSESSMENT

Obtain serum electrolytes, B/P. Assess fluid balance (I&O, daily weight, lung sounds, edema).

INTERVENTION/EVALUATION

Monitor serum electrolytes, acid-base balance, B/P. Monitor fluid balance (I&O, daily weight, lung sounds, edema), IV site for extravasation. Hypernatremia associated with edema, weight gain, elevated B/P; hyponatremia associated with muscle cramps, nausea, vomiting, dry mucous membranes.

PATIENT/FAMILY TEACHING

• Temporary burning, irritation may occur upon instillation of eye medication. • Discontinue eye medication and report if severe pain, headache, rapid change in vision (peripheral, direct), sudden appearance of floating spots, acute redness of eyes, pain on exposure to light, double vision occurs.

sofosbuvir/ velpatasvir

soe-**fos**-bue-vir/vel-**pat**-as-vir
(Epclusa)

Do not confuse sofosbuvir with boceprevir, dasabuvir, fosamprenavir, or simeprevir, or velpatasvir with daclatasvir, grazoprevir, or paritaprevir.

◆CLASSIFICATION

PHARMACOTHERAPEUTIC: Nucleotide analog NS5B polymerase inhibitor, NS5A inhibitor. **CLINICAL:** Antiviral.

USES

Treatment of chronic hepatitis C virus (HCV) genotype 1, 2, 3, 4, 5, or 6 infection in adults and pediatric pts 6 yrs and older or weighing at least 17 kg without cirrhosis, or with compensated cirrhosis, or in combination with ribavirin in pts with decompensated cirrhosis.

PRECAUTIONS

Contraindications: Hypersensitivity to sofosbuvir, velpatasvir. If given with ribavirin, contraindications to ribavirin apply. **Cautions:** Anemia (when used with ribavirin), renal impairment, end-stage renal disease requiring hemodialysis, hepatic disease unrelated to HCV infection, HIV infection. Concomitant use of amiodarone (with or without beta blockers) in pts with underlying cardiac disease. Concomitant use of P-glycoprotein inducers, moderate CYP2B6 inducers, strong CYP2C8 inducers, moderate or strong CYP3A4 inducers not recommended.

ACTION

Sofosbuvir inhibits the HCV NS5B RNA-dependent RNA polymerase. Velpatasvir inhibits the VCV NS5A protein. **Therapeutic Effect:** Inhibits viral replication of HCV.

PHARMACOKINETICS

Widely distributed. Metabolized in liver. Protein binding: sofosbuvir: 61%–68%; velpatasvir: greater than 99.5%. Peak plasma concentration: sofosbuvir: 0.5–1 hr; velpatasvir: 3 hrs. Excretion: sofosbuvir: urine (80%), feces (14%); velpatasvir: feces (94%), urine (0.4%). **Half-life:** sofosbuvir: 0.5 hr; velpatasvir: 15 hrs.

LIFESPAN CONSIDERATIONS

Pregnancy/Lactation: When used with ribavirin, therapy is contraindicated in pregnant women and in men whose female partners are pregnant. Females and males with female partners of reproductive potential must use effective contraception for at least 6 mos following discontinuation (if therapy includes ribavirin). Unknown if distributed in breast milk. **Children:** Safety and efficacy not established. **Elderly:** No age-related precautions noted.

INTERACTIONS

DRUG: Moderate or strong inducers of CYP2B6, CYP2C8, CYP3A4, P-glycoprotein (e.g., carBAMazepine, phenytoin, OXcarbazepine, rifampicin) may decrease concentration/effect of sofosbuvir/velpatasvir. **Amiodarone (with or without beta blockers [e.g., carvedilol, metoprolol])** may significantly increase risk of symptomatic bradycardia. **Proton pump inhibitors (e.g., omeprazole, pantoprazole)** may decrease concentration/effect. **HERBAL:** None significant. **FOOD:** None known. **LAB VALUES:** May increase serum bilirubin (indirect), creatine phosphokinase (CPK), lipase.

AVAILABILITY (Rx)

Tablets, Fixed-Dose: sofosbuvir 400 mg/velpatasvir 100 mg, sofosbuvir 200 mg/velpatasvir 50 mg.

ADMINISTRATION/HANDLING

PO

- Give without regard to food.

INDICATIONS/ROUTES/DOSAGE

Hepatitis C Virus Infection

PO: ADULTS, ELDERLY: 400 mg/100 mg once daily. **CHILDREN 6 YRS AND OLDER (WEIGHING AT LEAST 17 KG): 30 KG OR GREATER:** 400 mg/100 mg once daily. **17–29 KG:** 200 mg/50 mg once daily.

Treatment Regimen and Duration

Pts without cirrhosis or pts with compensated cirrhosis (Child-Pugh A): 400 mg/100 mg once daily for 12 wks. **Pts with decompensated cirrhosis (Child-Pugh B or C):** 1 tablet once daily with ribavirin for 12 wks.

Dosage in Renal Impairment

Mild to moderate impairment: CrCl greater than or equal to 30 mL/min: No dose adjustment. **Severe impairment: CrCl less than 30 mL/min,**

S

end-stage renal disease: Not specified; use caution.

Dosage in Hepatic Impairment
Mild to severe impairment: No dose adjustment.

SIDE EFFECTS

Frequent (22%–15%): Headache, fatigue. **Occasional (9%–5%):** Nausea, asthenia, insomnia, irritability. **Rare (2%):** Rash.

ADVERSE EFFECTS/TOXIC REACTIONS

Symptomatic bradycardia requiring pacemaker intervention was reported in pts taking amiodarone and sofosbuvir, in combination with daclatasvir or simeprevir. Cardiac arrest was reported in a pt taking amiodarone in combination with sofosbuvir and ledipasvir. Bradycardia usually occurred within hrs to days, but may occur up 2 wks after initiation (when used with amiodarone). Pts with underlying cardiac disease or advanced hepatic disease or taking concomitant beta blockers are at an increased risk for bradycardia when used concomitantly with amiodarone. Depression reported in 1% of pts.

NURSING CONSIDERATIONS

BASELINE ASSESSMENT

Obtain CBC (when used with ribavirin), renal function test, LFT, HCV-RNA level; serum lipase, CPK; pregnancy test in female pts of reproductive potential. Confirm hepatitis C virus genotype. Question history of renal impairment, hepatic disease unrelated to HCV infection; HIV infection or use of antiretroviral therapy. Receive full medication history, and screen for interactions (esp. concomitant use of amiodarone).

INTERVENTION/EVALUATION

Monitor serum lipase, CPK. Periodically monitor HCV-RNA level for treatment effectiveness. If unable to discontinue amiodarone, recommend inpatient cardiac monitoring for at least 48 hrs, followed by outpatient or self-monitoring of HR for at least 2 wks after initiation. Cardiac monitoring is also recommended in pts who discontinue amiodarone just prior to initiation. Reinforce birth control compliance and obtain monthly pregnancy tests in female pts of reproductive potential taking concomitant ribavirin. Encourage nutritional intake.

PATIENT/FAMILY TEACHING

- Pts who take amiodarone during therapy may require inpatient and outpatient cardiac monitoring (and in some cases, pacemaker implantation) due to an increased risk of slow heartbeats or cardiac arrest. If amiodarone cannot be interrupted or discontinued, immediately report symptoms of slow heartbeat such as chest pain, confusion, dizziness, fainting, light-headedness, memory problems, palpitations, weakness. • Treatment may be used in combination with ribavirin. Inform pt of contraindications/adverse effects of ribavirin therapy. Use effective contraception to avoid pregnancy. Do not breastfeed. • Do not take newly prescribed medications unless approved by prescriber who originally started treatment. • Do not take herbal products. • Avoid alcohol. • Maintain proper nutritional intake.

solifenacin

TOP 100

sol-i-**fen**-a-sin
(VESIcare, VESIcare LS)

CLASSIFICATION

PHARMACOTHERAPEUTIC: Anticholinergic agent, muscarinic receptor antagonist. **CLINICAL:** Urinary antispasmodic.

USES

Treatment of overactive bladder with symptoms of urinary frequency, urgency, or urge incontinence. Treatment of neurogenic detrusor overactivity (NDO) in children 2 yrs and older.

PRECAUTIONS

Contraindications: Hypersensitivity to solifenacin. Gastric retention, uncontrolled narrow-angle glaucoma, urinary retention. **Cautions:** Bladder outflow obstruction, GI obstructive disorders, decreased GI motility, controlled narrow-angle glaucoma, renal/hepatic impairment, pts at risk for QTc interval prolongation (congenital long QT syndrome, HF, medications that prolong QTc interval, hypokalemia, hypomagnesemia), hot weather and/or exercise.

ACTION

Inhibits muscarinic receptors. **Therapeutic Effect:** Decreases urinary bladder contractions, increases residual urine volume, decreases detrusor muscle pressure.

PHARMACOKINETICS

Well absorbed. Protein binding: 98%. Metabolized in liver. Excreted in urine (69%), feces (23%). **Half-life:** 40–68 hrs.

LIFESPAN CONSIDERATIONS

Pregnancy/Lactation: Unknown if drug crosses placenta or is distributed in breast milk. **Children:** Safety and efficacy not established. **Elderly:** No age-related precautions noted.

INTERACTIONS

DRUG: CYP3A4 inhibitors (e.g., ketoconazole, erythromycin, azole antifungals, clarithromycin) may increase concentration/effect. **Aclidinium, ipratropium, tiotropium, umeclidinium** may increase anticholinergic effect. **Strong CYP3A4 inducers (e.g., carBAMazepine, phenytoin, rifAMPin)** may decrease concentration/effect. **QT interval–prolonging medications (e.g., amiodarone, azithromycin, ciprofloxacin, haloperidol, methadone, sotalol)** may increase risk of QTc interval prolongation. **HERBAL: St. John's wort** may decrease concentration/effect. **FOOD: Grapefruit products** may increase concentration/effect. **LAB VALUES:** None known.

AVAILABILITY (Rx)

Oral Suspension: 5 mg/5 mL.
Tablets: 5 mg, 10 mg.

ADMINISTRATION/HANDLING

PO

- Give without regard to food. Swallow tablets whole, with liquids.

INDICATIONS/ROUTES/DOSAGE

Overactive Bladder

PO: ADULTS, ELDERLY: 5 mg/day; if tolerated, may increase to 10 mg/day.

NDO

PO: CHILDREN (WEIGHING MORE THAN 60 KG): 5 mg once daily. **Maximum:** 10 mg. **(46–60 KG):** 4 mg once daily. **Maximum:** 8 mg. **(31–45 KG):** 3 mg once daily. **Maximum:** 6 mg. **(16–30 KG):** 3 mg once daily. **Maximum:** 5 mg. **(9–15 KG):** 2 mg once daily. **Maximum:** 4 mg.

Dose Modification

Concomitant Use of Strong CYP3A4 Inhibitors

Maximum: 5 mg/day.

Dosage in Renal/Hepatic Impairment

Severe renal impairment (CrCl less than 30 mL/min) or moderate hepatic impairment: Maximum dosage is 5 mg/day. Not recommended in severe hepatic impairment.

SIDE EFFECTS

Frequent (28%–13%): Dry mouth, constipation. **Occasional (5%–3%):** Blurred vision, UTI, dyspepsia, nausea. **Rare (2%–1%):** Dizziness, dry eyes, fatigue, depression, edema, hypertension, epigastric pain, vomiting, urinary retention.

ADVERSE EFFECTS/TOXIC REACTIONS

Angioneurotic edema, GI obstruction occur rarely. Overdose can result in severe anticholinergic effects.

NURSING CONSIDERATIONS

BASELINE ASSESSMENT

Assess symptoms of overactive bladder before beginning the drug. Question medical

S

history as listed in Precautions. Screen for concomitant medications known to prolong QT interval. Obtain baseline ECG.

INTERVENTION/EVALUATION

Monitor I&O, anticholinergic effects, creatinine clearance. Assess for decrease in symptoms. Obtain bladder scan if urinary retention is suspected.

PATIENT/FAMILY TEACHING

• Avoid tasks requiring alertness, motor skills until response to drug is established. • Anticholinergic side effects include constipation, urinary retention, blurred vision, heat prostration in hot environment. • Use caution during exercise, exposure to heat.

somatropin

soe-ma-**troe**-pin
(Genotropin, Genotropin Miniquick, Humatrope, Norditropin FlexPro, Nutropin, Nutropin AQ NuSpin, Omnitrope, Saizen, Serostim, Zomacton, Zorbtive)
Do not confuse somatropin with SUMAtriptan.

◆CLASSIFICATION

PHARMACOTHERAPEUTIC: Polypeptide hormone. **CLINICAL:** Growth hormone.

USES

Adults: Growth deficiency due to pituitary disease, hypothalamic disease, surgery, radiation, or trauma. **Serostim:** AIDS-related wasting or cachexia. **Zorbtive:** Short bowel syndrome. **Children:** Long-term treatment of growth failure due to lack of or inadequate endogenous growth hormone secretion; chronic renal insufficiency; short stature, Turner's syndrome, Prader-Willi syndrome, or homeobox gene deficiency; idiopathic short stature. **OFF-LABEL:** Treatment of pediatric HIV pts with wasting/cachexia; HIV adipose redistribution syndrome.

PRECAUTIONS

Contraindications: Hypersensitivity to growth hormone. Pts with Prader-Willi syndrome with growth hormone deficiency who are severely obese or have severe respiratory impairment, Prader-Willi syndrome without growth hormone deficiency, children with closed epiphyses, acute critical illness due to complications after open heart or abdominal surgery, multiple accidental trauma, acute respiratory failure, active neoplasia, diabetic retinopathy. Active malignancy, progression of active growing intracranial lesion or tumor. **Cautions:** Diabetes, elderly.

ACTION

Stimulates cartilaginous growth areas of long bones; increases number, size of skeletal muscle cells; influences size of organs; increases RBC mass by stimulating erythropoietin. Influences metabolism of carbohydrates (decreases insulin sensitivity), fats (mobilizes fatty acids), minerals (retains phosphorus, sodium, potassium by promotion of cell growth), proteins (increases protein synthesis). **Therapeutic Effect:** Stimulates growth.

PHARMACOKINETICS

Well absorbed after SQ, IM administration. Localized primarily in kidneys, liver. **Half-life: IV:** 20–30 min; **SQ, IM:** 3–5 hrs.

⌛ LIFESPAN CONSIDERATIONS

Pregnancy/Lactation: Unknown if drug is distributed in breast milk. **Children/Elderly:** No age-related precautions noted.

INTERACTIONS

DRUG: **Corticosteroids (e.g., hydrocortisone, predniSONE)** may inhibit growth response. **Oral estrogens** may decrease response to somatropin. **HERBAL:** None significant. **FOOD:** None known. **LAB VALUES:** May increase serum alkaline phosphatase, inorganic phosphorus, parathyroid hormone. May decrease glucose tolerance. May slightly decrease thyroid function.

AVAILABILITY (Rx)

Injection, Powder for Reconstitution: ***(Genotropin):*** 5 mg, 12 mg. ***(Genotropin Miniquick):*** 0.2 mg, 0.4 mg, 0.6 mg, 0.8 mg, 1 mg, 1.2 mg, 1.4 mg, 1.6 mg, 1.8 mg, 2 mg. ***(Humatrope):*** 5 mg, 6 mg, 12 mg, 24 mg. ***(Omnitrope):*** 5.8 mg. ***(Saizen):*** 5 mg, 8.8 mg. ***(Serostim):*** 4 mg, 5 mg, 6 mg. **(Zomacton):** 5 mg, 10 mg. ***(Zorbtive):*** 8.8 mg. **Injection Solution:** ***(Omnitrope):*** 5 mg/1.5 mL, 10 mg/1.5 mL. ***(Norditropin FlexPro Pen):*** 5 mg/1.5 mL, 10 mg/1.5 mL, 15 mg/1.5 mL, 30 mg/3 mL. ***(Nutropin AQ NuSpin):*** 5 mg/2 mL, 10 mg/2 mL, 20 mg/2 mL.

ADMINISTRATION/HANDLING

◀ALERT▶ Neonate: Benzyl alcohol as a preservative has been associated with fatal toxicity (gasping syndrome) in premature infants. Reconstitute with Sterile Water for Injection only. Use only 1 dose per vial. Discard unused portion.

Reconstitution • Genotropin, Genotropin Miniquick: Reconstitute with diluent provided. **Humatrope:** Reconstitute with 1.5–5 mL diluent provided, swirl gently, do not shake. **Humatrope Cartridge:** Dilute with solution provided with cartridge only. **Nutropin:** Reconstitute each 5 mg with 1.5–5 mL diluent, swirl gently, do not shake. **Omnitrope:** Reconstitute with diluents provided, swirl gently, do not shake. **Saizen:** 5 mg: Reconstitute with 1–3 mL diluent provided, swirl gently, do not shake. 8.8 mg: Reconstitute with 2–3 mL diluent provided, swirl gently, do not shake. **Serostim:** Reconstitute with Sterile Water for Injection. **Zorbtive:** Reconstitute with 1–2 mL Bacteriostatic Water for Injection.

Storage • Long-term: Refrigerate all products except Zorbtive. Once reconstituted, Humatrope, Nutropin, Saizen, Zorbtive stable for 14 days, Genotropin for 21 days, Humatrope Cartridge for 28 days. **Genotropin Miniquick:** Refrigerate, use within 24 hrs.

INDICATIONS/ROUTES/DOSAGE

Growth Hormone Deficiency

SQ: ***(Genotropin, Omnitrope):*** **ADULTS:** 0.04 mg/kg wkly divided into 6–7 equal doses/wk. May increase at 4- to 8-wk intervals to maximum of 0.08 mg/kg/wk. **CHILDREN:** 0.16–0.24 mg/kg wkly divided into equal daily doses.

SQ: ***(Humatrope):*** **ADULTS:** 0.006 mg/kg once daily. May increase to maximum of 0.0125 mg/kg/day. **CHILDREN:** 0.18–0.3 mg/kg wkly divided into alternate-day doses or 6 doses/wk.

SQ: ***(Norditropin):*** **ADULTS:** 0.004 mg/kg/day. May increase after 6 wks up to 0.016 mg/kg/day. **CHILDREN:** 0.024–0.034 mg/kg/dose 6–7 days/wk.

SQ: ***(Nutropin, Nutropin AQ):*** **ADULTS:** 0.006 mg/kg once daily. May increase to maximum of 0.025 mg/kg/day (younger than 35 yrs) or 0.0125/kg/day (35 yrs and older). **CHILDREN:** 0.3–0.7 mg/kg wkly divided into equal daily doses.

SQ: ***(Saizen):*** **ADULTS:** 0.005 mg/kg/day. May increase up to 0.01 mg/kg/day after 4 wks. **CHILDREN:** 0.18 mg/kg/wk divided into equal daily doses or 0.06 mg/kg 3 times/wk or as 0.03 mg/kg administered 6 days/wk.

Noonan Syndrome

SQ: ***(Norditropin):*** Up to 0.066 mg/kg/day.

Chronic Renal Insufficiency

SQ: ***(Nutropin, Nutropin AQ):*** **CHILDREN:** 0.35 mg/kg wkly divided into equal daily doses. Continue until the time of renal transplantation.

Idiopathic Short Stature

SQ: ***(Genotropin, Omnitrope):*** 0.47 mg/kg wkly divided into equal doses 6–7 times/wk. ***(Humatrope):*** 0.37 mg wkly divided into equal doses 6–7 times/wk. ***(Nutropin, Nutropin AQ):*** Up to 0.3 mg/kg wkly divided into daily doses.

Turner's Syndrome

SQ: ***(Humatrope, Nutropin, Nutropin AQ):*** **CHILDREN:** 0.375 mg/kg wkly divided into equal doses 3–7 times/wk.

S

(Genotropin, Omnitrope): 0.33 mg/kg wkly divided into 6–7 doses.

AIDS-Related Wasting

SQ: *(Serostim):* **ADULTS WEIGHING MORE THAN 55 KG:** 6 mg once daily at bedtime. **ADULTS WEIGHING 45–55 KG:** 5 mg once daily at bedtime. **ADULTS WEIGHING 35–44 KG:** 4 mg once daily at bedtime. **ADULTS WEIGHING LESS THAN 35 KG:** 0.1 mg/kg once daily at bedtime.

Prader-Willi Syndrome

SQ: *(Genotropin, Omnitrope):* 0.24 mg/kg wkly divided into equal doses 6–7 times/wk.

Short Bowel Syndrome

SQ: *(Zorbtive):* **ADULTS:** 0.1 mg/kg/day. **Maximum:** 8 mg/day.

Dosage in Renal/Hepatic Impairment

No dose adjustment.

SIDE EFFECTS

Frequent: Otitis media, other ear disorders (with Turner's syndrome). **Occasional:** Carpal tunnel syndrome, gynecomastia, myalgia, peripheral edema, fatigue, asthenia. **Rare:** Rash, pruritus, visual changes, headache, nausea, vomiting, injection site pain/swelling, abdominal pain, hip/knee pain.

ADVERSE EFFECTS/TOXIC REACTIONS

May cause fluid retention, glucose tolerance, lipoatrophy. Intracranial hypertension may manifest as change, of vision, headache, papilledema, nausea, vomiting. May increase risk of malignancy progression. Rapid growth may cause slipped capital femoral epiphyses. Hypersensitivity reactions including angioedema, anaphylaxis were reported.

NURSING CONSIDERATIONS

BASELINE ASSESSMENT

Obtain baseline lab chemistries, thyroid function, serum glucose, height, weight. Obtain full medical history (drug has multiple contraindications).

INTERVENTION/EVALUATION

Monitor bone growth, growth rate in relation to pt's age. Monitor serum calcium, glucose, phosphorus levels; renal, parathyroid, thyroid function. Observe for decreased muscle wasting in AIDS pts.

PATIENT/FAMILY TEACHING

• Follow correct procedure to reconstitute drug for administration and for safe handling/disposal of needles. • Regular follow-up with physician is important part of therapy. • Report development of severe headache, visual changes, pain in hip/knee, limping.

sonidegib

soe-ni-**deg**-ib
(Odomzo)

■ BLACK BOX ALERT ■ May cause embryo-fetal death/severe malformations when given during pregnancy. Verify pregnancy status before initiation. Female patients of reproductive potential must use effective contraception during treatment and for at least 20 mos after discontinuation. Due to the potential risk of exposure through semen, male patients must use condoms during sexual activity (even after a vasectomy) during treatment and for at least 8 mos after discontinuation.

Do not confuse sonidegib with vismodegib.

◆ CLASSIFICATION

PHARMACOTHERAPEUTIC: Hedgehog pathway inhibitor. **CLINICAL:** Antineoplastic.

USES

Treatment of adult pts with locally advanced basal cell carcinoma that has recurred following surgery or radiation therapy, or those who are not candidates for surgery or radiation.

PRECAUTIONS

Contraindications: Hypersensitivity to sonidegib. **Cautions:** Renal/hepatic impairment. Avoid concomitant use of strong or moderate CYP3A inhibitors, strong or moderate CYP3A inducers.

ACTION

Basal cell cancer is associated with mutation in Hedgehog pathway components, which can activate the pathway, causing nonrestrictive proliferation of skin basal cells. Binds to and inhibits smoothened homologue (SMO), the protein involved in Hedgehog signal transduction. **Therapeutic Effect:** Inhibits tumor cell growth and survival.

PHARMACOKINETICS

Poorly absorbed after PO administration (less than 10%). Metabolized in liver. Protein binding: greater than 97%. Peak plasma concentration: 2–4 hrs. Steady state reached in 4 mos. Excreted in feces (70%), urine (30%). **Half-life:** 28 days.

⌛ LIFESPAN CONSIDERATIONS

Pregnancy/Lactation: Avoid use; may cause fetal harm. Females of reproductive potential must use effective contraception during treatment and up to 20 mos after discontinuation. May impair fertility. **Males:** Males must use condoms during sexual activity (even after a vasectomy) during treatment and up to 8 mos after discontinuation. **Children:** Safety and efficacy not established. **Elderly:** May have increased risk of severe musculoskeletal adverse events (e.g., muscle spasms, myopathy).

INTERACTIONS

DRUG: **Strong CYP3A inhibitors (e.g., clarithromycin, ketoconazole), moderate CYP3A inhibitors (e.g., atazanavir, fluconazole)** may increase concentration/effect. **Strong CYP3A inducers (e.g., carBAMazepine, phenytoin, rifAMPin)** may decrease concentration/effect. **HERBAL:** None significant. **FOOD:** **High-fat meals** may increase absorption/concentration. **LAB VALUES:** May increase serum ALT/AST, amylase, creatinine, CK, glucose, lipase. May decrease Hct, Hgb, lymphocytes.

AVAILABILITY (Rx)

Capsules: 200 mg.

ADMINISTRATION/HANDLING

PO

- Give on an empty stomach at least 1 hr before or 2 hrs after a meal.

INDICATIONS/ROUTES/DOSAGE

Basal Cell Carcinoma

PO: ADULTS, ELDERLY: 200 mg once daily. Continue until disease progression or unacceptable toxicity.

Dose Modification

Interrupt therapy for severe or intolerable musculoskeletal adverse reactions; first occurrence of serum CK level 2.5–10 times upper limit of normal (ULN); recurrent serum CK level 2.5–5 times ULN. Once resolved, resume at 200 mg once daily.

Discontinuation

Permanently discontinue for serum CK level greater than 2.5 times ULN with worsening renal function; serum CK level greater than 10 times ULN; recurrent serum CK level greater than 5 times ULN; recurrent severe or intolerable musculoskeletal adverse reactions.

Dosage in Renal Impairment

No dose adjustment.

Dosage in Hepatic Impairment

Mild impairment: No dose adjustment. **Moderate to severe impairment:** Not studied; use caution.

SIDE EFFECTS

Frequent (54%–23%): Muscle spasm, alopecia, dysgeusia, fatigue, nausea, diarrhea, musculoskeletal pain, decreased appetite. **Occasional (19%–10%):** Myalgia, abdominal pain, headache, generalized pain, vomiting, pruritus.

S

ADVERSE EFFECTS/TOXIC REACTIONS

Musculoskeletal events occurred in 68% of pts. Common Terminology Criteria for Adverse Events (CTCAE) Grade 3 or 4 musculoskeletal events (9% of pts) may require administration of muscle relaxants, analgesics/narcotics, magnesium supplementation, IV hydration. Serum CK level elevations usually occur before musculoskeletal pain or spasms. Increased serum CK levels reported in 61% of pts. The median onset of serum CK elevation was approx. 12 wks. May increase risk of rhabdomyolysis. Amenorrhea lasting longer than 18 mos has occurred.

NURSING CONSIDERATIONS

BASELINE ASSESSMENT

Obtain CBC, BMP, LFT; pregnancy test in females of reproductive potential. Receive medication history and screen for interactions. Assess hydration status. Offer emotional support.

INTERVENTION/EVALUATION

Monitor renal function, serum CK levels periodically and with any musculoskeletal adverse events. If musculoskeletal adverse reactions occur with serum CK levels greater than 2.5 times ULN, obtain serum CK level at least wkly until resolution. Monitor urine color, output. Serum CK level elevation or worsening of renal function may indicate rhabdomyolysis. Monitor pregnancy status during therapy.

PATIENT/FAMILY TEACHING

• Treatment may cause severe muscle damage, which may cause kidney damage. • Report dark-colored urine or decreased urine output despite hydration. • Immediately report musculoskeletal symptoms such as muscle pain/spasms/tenderness/weakness. • Do not donate blood or blood products during treatment and up to 20 mos after discontinuation. • Use effective contraception to avoid pregnancy. Do not breastfeed. • Take on empty stomach at least 1 hr before or 2 hrs after a meal.

SORAfenib

soe-**raf**-e-nib
(NexAVAR)
Do not confuse NexAVAR with NexIUM, or SORAfenib with imatinib or SUNItinib.

◆CLASSIFICATION

PHARMACOTHERAPEUTIC: Vascular endothelial growth factor (VEGF) inhibitor. Tyrosine kinase inhibitor. **CLINICAL:** Antineoplastic.

USES

Treatment of advanced renal cell carcinoma (RCC), unresectable hepatocellular carcinoma (HCC), locally recurrent or metastatic progressive differentiated thyroid carcinoma (DTC) refractive to radioactive iodine treatment. **OFF-LABEL:** Recurrent or metastatic angiosarcoma, resistant gastrointestinal stromal tumor.

PRECAUTIONS

Contraindications: Hypersensitivity to SORAfenib. Use in combination with CARBOplatin and PACLitaxel in pts with squamous cell lung cancer. **Cautions:** Uncontrolled hypertension, pulmonary disease, pts at risk for GI perforation (e.g., Crohn's disease, diverticulitis, GI tract malignancies, peptic ulcers, peritoneal malignancies), pts at risk for QTc interval prolongation (congenital long QT syndrome, HF, medications that prolong QTc interval, hypokalemia, hypomagnesemia), pts at risk for bleeding (e.g., history of intracranial/GI/genitourinary bleeding, coagulation disorders, recent trauma, concomitant use of anticoagulants, antiplatelets); unstable coronary artery disease, recent MI, HF, concurrent use with strong CYP3A4 inducers.

ACTION

Inhibits tumor cell proliferation by inhibiting intracellular Raf kinases and cell surface kinase receptors. **Therapeutic Effect:** Inhibits tumor growth and survival.

PHARMACOKINETICS

Metabolized in liver. Protein binding: 99.5%. Excreted in feces (77%), urine (19%). **Half-life:** 25–48 hrs.

LIFESPAN CONSIDERATIONS

Pregnancy/Lactation: Avoid use; may cause fetal harm. Females of reproductive potential should use effective contraception during treatment and for at least 6 mos after discontinuation. Breastfeeding not recommended during treatment and for at least 2 wks after discontinuation. **Males:** Males with female partners of reproductive potential should use effective contraception during treatment and for at least 3 mos after discontinuation. May impair fertility. **Children:** Safety and efficacy not established. **Elderly:** No age-related precautions noted.

INTERACTIONS

DRUG: **Strong CYP3A4 inducers (e.g., carBAMazepine, PHENobarbital, rifAMPin)** may decrease concentration/effect. **QT interval–prolonging medications (e.g., amiodarone, azithromycin, ceritinib, haloperidol, moxifloxacin)** may increase risk of QT interval prolongation, cardiac arrhythmias. May increase adverse effects of **carboplatin**. May increase anticoagulant effect of **warfarin**. HERBAL: **Echinacea** may decrease the therapeutic effect. **St. John's wort** may decrease concentration/effect. FOOD: **High-fat meals** decrease effectiveness. LAB VALUES: May increase serum lipase, amylase, bilirubin, alkaline phosphatase, transaminases. May decrease serum phosphorus, lymphocytes, WBCs, Hgb, Hct.

AVAILABILITY (Rx)

Tablets: *(NexAVAR):* 200 mg.

ADMINISTRATION/HANDLING

PO

• Give 1 hr before or 2 hrs after meal (high-fat meal reduces effectiveness). • Swallow tablet whole; do not break, crush, dissolve, or divide tablet.

INDICATIONS/ROUTES/DOSAGE

Renal Cell Carcinoma, Hepatocellular Carcinoma, Thyroid Carcinoma

PO: ADULTS, ELDERLY: 400 mg (2 tablets) twice daily without food. Continue until disease progression or unacceptable toxicity.

Dose Reduction Schedule

HCC/RCC: First dose reduction: 400 mg once daily. **Second dose reduction:** 200 mg once daily or 400 mg every other day.

DTC: First dose reduction: 400 mg once in the morning and 200 mg once at night (12 hrs apart). **Second dose reduction:** 200 mg twice daily. **Third dose reduction:** 200 mg once daily

Dose Modification

Based on Common Terminology Criteria for Adverse Events.

Cardiac Toxicity

Grade 3 congestive HF: Withhold treatment until improved to Grade 1 or 0, then resume at reduced dose level. Permanently discontinue for Grade 3 congestive HF that does not improve within 30 days; Grade 4 congestive HF; Grade 2 or greater cardiac ischemia/infarction.

Dermatologic Toxicity

Note: If improved to Grade 1 or 0 from Grade 2 or 3 toxicity for at least 28 days, may increase dose by one dose level.

HCC/RCC: Grade 2 toxicity: (First occurrence): Continue same dose and start topical therapy. **(Not improved within 7 days; second or third occurrence):** Withhold treatment until improved to Grade 1 or 0, then resume at reduced dose level. **(Fourth occurrence):** Permanently discontinue. **Grade 3 toxicity: (First or second occurrence):** Withhold treatment until improved to Grade 1 or 0, then resume at reduced dose level. **(Third occurrence):** Permanently discontinue.

DTC: Grade 2 toxicity: (First occurrence): Reduce dose to 600 mg once daily. **(Not improved within 7 days; second or third occurrence):** Withhold treatment until improved to Grade 1, then reduce dose by one dose level (for

S

second occurrence) or by two dose levels (for third occurrence). **(Fourth occurrence):** Permanently discontinue. **Grade 3 toxicity: (First occurrence):** Withhold treatment until improved to Grade 1, then resume at reduced dose level. **(Second occurrence):** Withhold treatment until improved to Grade 1, then reduce dose by two dose levels. **(Third occurrence):** Permanently discontinue.

Hypertension

Grade 2 (symptomatic/persistent) hypertension; Grade 2 symptomatic increase greater than 20 mm Hg (diastolic); B/P greater than 140/90 mm Hg if previously within normal limits; Grade 3 hypertension: Withhold treatment until symptoms resolve and diastolic B/P is less than 90 mm Hg, then resume at reduced dose level. May further reduce if needed. **Grade 4 hypertension; more than 2 dose reductions are required:** Permanently discontinue.

Nonhematologic Toxicity

Any Grade 2 toxicity: Reduce dose by one dose level. **Any Grade 3 toxicity: (First occurrence):** Withhold treatment until Grade 2 or less, then resume at reduced dose level. **(Not improved within 7 days; second or third occurrence):** Withhold treatment until Grade 2 or less, then reduce dose by two dose levels. **(Fourth occurrence):** Withhold treatment until Grade 2 or less, then reduce dose by two dose levels for HCC and RCC, or 3 dose levels for DTC.

QT Interval Prolongation

QT interval greater than 500 msec; increase of 60 msec or greater from baseline: Withhold treatment and correct electrolyte abnormalities. May restart based on clinical judgment.

Permanent Discontinuation

Grade 2 or greater hemorrhage requiring medical intervention; any grade GI perforation; Grade 3 or 4 serum ALT elevation; serum ALT/ALT elevation greater than 3 times ULN with serum bilirubin 2 times ULN.

Dosage in Renal Impairment

Mild to severe impairment (not requiring dialysis): No dose adjustment.

Dosage in Hepatic Impairment

Mild to moderate impairment: No dose adjustment. **Severe impairment:** Not specified.

SIDE EFFECTS

Frequent (43%–16%): Diarrhea, rash, fatigue, exfoliative dermatitis, alopecia, nausea, pruritus, hypertension, anorexia, vomiting. **Occasional (15%–10%):** Constipation, minor bleeding, dyspnea, sensory neuropathy, cough, abdominal pain, dry skin, weight loss, joint pain, headache. **Rare (9%–1%):** Acne, flushing, stomatitis, mucositis, dyspepsia, arthralgia, myalgia, hoarseness.

ADVERSE EFFECTS/TOXIC REACTIONS

Myelosuppression (anemia, leukopenia, neutropenia, thrombocytopenia) is an expected response to the therapy. Cardiac ischemia/MI reported in 3% of pts. Fatal hemorrhage (esophageal hemorrhage, bleeding from any site) was reported. Life-threatening cutaneous toxicities including Stevens-Johnson syndrome, toxic epidermal necrolysis, hand-foot skin reactions may occur. GI perforation reported in less than 1% of pts. May impair healing of wounds. An increased risk of mortality was reported in pts receiving other chemotherapeutic agents. May cause QT interval prolongation, thyroid-stimulating hormone (TSH) suppression, hepatotoxicity, neuropathy, intracranial hemorrhage, interstitial lung disease, pneumonitis, thrombotic microangiopathy, osteonecrosis of the jaw; arterial aneurysms, dissections, rupture.

NURSING CONSIDERATIONS

BASELINE ASSESSMENT

Obtain CBC, BMP, LFT, TSH, B/P; pregnancy test in females of reproductive potential. Screen for active infection. Question history as listed in Precautions. Receive full medication history and screen for interac-

S

tions. Conduct dermatologic exam. Assess for poorly healed wounds/recent surgical wounds. Assess risk for QT interval prolongation. Offer emotional support.

INTERVENTION/EVALUATION

Monitor CBC, serum electrolytes, ECG; TSH (if applicable), LFT for hepatic injury (abdominal pain, jaundice, nausea, transaminitis, vomiting). Monitor B/P frequently. Diligently assess skin for cutaneous toxicities, impaired wound healing. Monitor for cardiac ischemia/infarction (chest pain, diaphoresis, left arm or jaw pain, ST segment elevation, serum troponin elevation), GI perforation (abdominal pain, fever, nausea, vomiting), infection (cough, fatigue, fever); neuropathy (gait disturbance, fine motor control difficulties, numbness); hypersensitivity reactions (anaphylaxis, urticaria), bleeding of any kind.

PATIENT/FAMILY TEACHING

• Treatment may depress your immune system response and reduce your ability to fight infection. Report symptoms of infection such as body aches, chills, cough, fatigue, fever. Avoid those with active infection. • Report symptoms of bone marrow depression (e.g., bruising, fatigue, fever, shortness of breath, weight loss; bleeding easily, bloody urine or stool). • Report symptoms of lung inflammation (excessive coughing, difficulty breathing, chest pain); liver problems (abdominal pain, bruising, clay-colored stool, dark or amber- colored urine, yellowing of the skin or eyes), toxic skin reactions (rash, redness, sloughing, swelling). • Life-threatening cardiac events may occur; report symptoms of heart attack (chest pain, difficulty breathing, jaw pain, nausea, pain that radiates to the arm or jaw, sweating). • Treatment may affect the heart's ability to pump blood or alter the electrical conduction of the heart, which may lead to HF, cardiac arrhythmias; report chest pain, difficulty breathing, dizziness, swelling of extremities, fainting, palpitations. • Bleeding of any kind can be life-threatening • Use effective contraception to avoid pregnancy. Do not breastfeed. • Do not take newly prescribed medications unless approved by prescriber who originally started treatment. • Treatment may worsen high blood pressure. • Immediately report severe or persistent abdominal pain, bloody stool, fever, vomiting blood; may indicate rupture in GI tract.

sotalol

HIGH ALERT

soe-ta-lol
(Betapace, Betapace AF, Sorine, Sotylize)

BLACK BOX ALERT Initiation, titration to occur in a hospital setting with continuous ECG to monitor potential onset of life-threatening arrhythmias. Calculate CrCl prior to dosing. Adjust dose based on CrCl. Betapace should not be substituted for Betapace AF.

Do not confuse Betapace with Betapace AF, or sotalol with Stadol or Sudafed.

CLASSIFICATION

PHARMACOTHERAPEUTIC: Nonselective beta-adrenergic blocking agent. **CLINICAL:** Antiarrhythmic Class II, Class III.

USES

Treatment of documented, life-threatening ventricular arrhythmias. Maintain normal sinus rhythm in pts with symptomatic atrial fibrillation/flutter. **OFF-LABEL:** Fetal tachycardia, treatment of atrial fibrillation with hypertrophic cardiomyopathy.

PRECAUTIONS

Contraindications: Hypersensitivity to sotalol. Cardiogenic shock, congenital or acquired long QT syndrome, second- or third-degree heart block (unless functioning pacemaker is present), sinus bradycardia, uncontrolled HF, bronchial asthma or related bronchospastic conditions. **Betapace, Betapace AF, Sotylize (additional):** Baseline QT interval

S

greater than 450 msec, bronchospastic conditions, CrCl less than 40 mL/min, serum potassium less than 4 mEq/L, sick sinus syndrome. **Cautions:** Pts with history of ventricular tachycardia, ventricular fibrillation, cardiomegaly, compensated HF, diabetes mellitus, QT interval prolongation, concurrent medications that prolong QT interval, hypokalemia, hypomagnesemia, renal impairment, within first 2 wks post MI, peripheral vascular disease, Raynaud's syndrome, myasthenia gravis, psychiatric disease, bronchospastic disease. Concurrent use of digoxin, verapamil, dilTIAZem, history of severe anaphylaxis to allergens.

ACTION

Class II effects: Increases sinus cycle length, AV nodal refractoriness; decreases AV nodal conduction; slows heart rate. **Class III effects:** Prolongs atrial/ventricular action potentials, inducing effective refractory prolongation of atrial/ventricular muscle and atrial/ventricular accessory pathways. **Therapeutic Effect:** Produces antiarrhythmic activity.

PHARMACOKINETICS

Route	Onset	Peak	Duration
PO	1–2 hrs	2.5–4 hrs	8–16 hrs

Widely distributed. Primarily excreted unchanged in urine. Removed by hemodialysis. **Half-life:** 12 hrs (increased in elderly, renal impairment).

S

⌛ LIFESPAN CONSIDERATIONS

Pregnancy/Lactation: Crosses placenta. Distributed in breast milk. **Children:** Safety and efficacy not established. **Elderly:** Age-related peripheral vascular disease may increase susceptibility to decreased peripheral circulation. Age-related renal impairment may require dosage adjustment.

INTERACTIONS

DRUG: **Calcium channel blockers (e.g., dilTIAZem, verapamil)** may increase effect on AV conduction, B/P. May mask symptoms of hypoglycemia, prolong hypoglycemic effects of **insulin, oral hypoglycemics (e.g., glipiZIDE, metFORMIN). QT-prolonging medications (e.g., amiodarone, ciprofloxacin, haloperidol, ondansetron)** may increase risk of prolonged QT interval. **HERBAL:** **Herbals with hypotensive properties (e.g., garlic, ginger, ginkgo biloba)** may alter effects. **FOOD:** None known. **LAB VALUES:** May increase serum BUN, glucose, alkaline phosphatase, LDH, lipoprotein, ALT, AST, triglycerides, potassium, uric acid.

AVAILABILITY (Rx)

Solution, Intravenous: 150 mg/10 mL. **Solution, Oral:** 5 mg/mL. **Tablets:** 80 mg, 120 mg, 160 mg, 240 mg.

ADMINISTRATION/HANDLING

PO

• Give without regard to food. • Give at same time each day.

INDICATIONS/ROUTES/DOSAGE

Note: Baseline QTc interval and CrCl must be determined before initiation.

Ventricular Arrhythmias

PO: ADULTS, ELDERLY: Initially, 80 mg twice daily. May increase in 80 mg/day increments at 3-day intervals. Range: 160–320 mg/day in 2 divided doses. **Maximum:** 640 mg/day in life-threatening refractive arrhythmias.

IV: Initially, 75 mg infused over 5 hrs twice daily. Range: 75–150 mg twice daily. **Maximum:** 300 mg twice daily.

Atrial Fibrillation, Atrial Flutter

PO: ADULTS, ELDERLY: Initially, 80 mg twice daily. May increase to 120–160 mg twice daily.

IV: Initially, 75 mg infused over 5 hrs twice daily. Usual dose: 112.5 mg twice daily. **Maximum:** 150 mg twice daily.

Usual Dosage for Children

PO: Initially, 90 mg/m^2/day in 3 divided doses. May incrementally increase up to a maximum of 180 mg/m^2/day not to exceed maximum adult dose of 320 mg/day.

Dosage in Renal Impairment
Dosage interval is modified based on creatinine clearance.

Atrial Fibrillation/Flutter

Creatinine Clearance	Dosage
Greater than 60 mL/min	12 hrs
40–60 mL/min	24 hrs
Less than 40 mL/min	Contraindicated

Ventricular Arrhythmias

Creatinine Clearance	Dosage
Greater than 60 mL/min	12 hrs
30–60 mL/min	24 hrs
10–29 mL/min	q36–48h

Dosage in Hepatic Impairment
No dose adjustment.

SIDE EFFECTS

Frequent: Diminished sexual function, drowsiness, insomnia, asthenia. **Occasional:** Depression, cold hands/feet, diarrhea, constipation, anxiety, nasal congestion, nausea, vomiting. **Rare:** Altered taste, dry eyes, pruritus, paresthesia of fingers, toes, scalp.

ADVERSE EFFECTS/TOXIC REACTIONS

Bradycardia, HF, hypotension, bronchospasm, hypoglycemia, prolonged QT interval, torsades de pointes, ventricular tachycardia, premature ventricular complexes may occur.

NURSING CONSIDERATIONS

BASELINE ASSESSMENT

Baseline QTc interval and CrCl must be determined prior to initiation. Pt must be on continuous cardiac monitoring upon initiation of therapy. Do not administer without consulting physician if pulse is 60 beats/min or less. Question medical history as listed in Precautions.

INTERVENTION/EVALUATION

Diligently monitor for arrhythmias. Assess B/P for hypotension, pulse for bradycardia. Assess for HF: dyspnea, peripheral edema, jugular vein distention, increased weight, rales in lungs, decreased urinary output.

PATIENT/FAMILY TEACHING

• Do not discontinue, change dose without physician approval. • Avoid tasks requiring alertness, motor skills until response to drug is established (may cause drowsiness). • Periodic lab tests, ECGs are essential part of therapy. • Report rapid heartbeat, chest pain, swelling of ankles/legs, difficulty breathing.

spironolactone

spir-**on**-oh-**lak**-tone
(Aldactone, CaroSpir)

BLACK BOX ALERT Has been shown to produce tumors in chronic toxicity animal studies.
Do not confuse Aldactone with Aldactazide.

FIXED-COMBINATION(S)

Aldactazide: spironolactone/hydro-CHLOROthiazide (a thiazide diuretic): 25 mg/25 mg, 50 mg/50 mg.

CLASSIFICATION

PHARMACOTHERAPEUTIC: Aldosterone receptor antagonist. **CLINICAL:** Potassium-sparing diuretic, antihypertensive.

USES

Ascites due to cirrhosis: Management of edema in cirrhotic pts when edema is unresponsive to fluid and sodium restriction. Heart failure (NYHA class III–IV and reduced ejection fraction) to increase survival, manage edema, and to reduce need for hospitalization for HF. Management of hypertension (unresponsive to other therapies). Treatment of primary hyperaldosteronism. **OFF-LABEL:** Treatment of edema, hypertension in children, female acne, female hirsutism. Ascites due to cirrhosis.

PRECAUTIONS

Contraindications: Hypersensitivity to spironolactone. Hyperkalemia, Addison's disease, concomitant use with eplerenone. **Cautions:** Dehydration, hyponatremia, concurrent use of supplemental potassium, elderly. Mild renal impairment, declining renal function, ACE inhibitors or angiotensin receptor blockers.

ACTION

Interferes with sodium reabsorption by competitively inhibiting action of aldosterone in distal tubule, promoting sodium and water excretion, increasing potassium retention. May decrease effect of aldosterone on arteriolar smooth muscle. **Therapeutic Effect:** Produces diuresis, lowers B/P.

PHARMACOKINETICS

Widely distributed. Protein binding: 91%–98%. Metabolized in liver to active metabolite. Primarily excreted in urine. Unknown if removed by hemodialysis. **Half-life:** 78–84 min.

LIFESPAN CONSIDERATIONS

Pregnancy/Lactation: Active metabolite excreted in breast milk. Breastfeeding not recommended. **Children:** No age-related precautions noted. **Elderly:** May be more susceptible to developing hyperkalemia. Age-related renal impairment may require dosage adjustment.

INTERACTIONS

S

DRUG: **ACE inhibitors (e.g., captopril, lisinopril), angiotensin receptor blockers (e.g., valsartan), eplerenone, potassium-containing medications, potassium supplements** may increase risk of hyperkalemia. May decrease therapeutic effect of **digoxin. NSAIDs (e.g., ibuprofen, ketorolac, naproxen)** may decrease antihypertensive effect. **HERBAL:** **Herbals with hypertensive properties (e.g., licorice, yohimbe) or hypotensive properties (e.g., garlic, ginger, ginkgo biloba)** may alter effects. **FOOD:** **Food** increases absorption. **LAB VALUES:** May increase urinary calcium excretion, serum BUN, glucose, creatinine, magnesium, potassium, uric acid. May decrease serum sodium.

AVAILABILITY (Rx)

Oral Suspension: 25 mg/5 mL.
Tablets: 25 mg, 50 mg, 100 mg.

ADMINISTRATION/HANDLING

PO

• Take with food to reduce GI irritation and increase absorption. **Suspension:** • Shake well. • May give with or without food (give consistently with respect to food).

INDICATIONS/ROUTES/DOSAGE

Ascites (due to cirrhosis)

PO: ADULTS, ELDERLY: ***(Tablet):*** Initially, 100 mg/day as single dose. May titrate q3–5 days based on response and tolerability. **Maximum dose:** 400 mg once daily.

Hypertension

PO: ADULTS, ELDERLY: ***(Tablet):*** Initially, 12.5–25 mg once daily. May titrate q2wks as needed. **Maximum:** 100 mg. ***(Suspension):*** 20–75 mg daily in 1 or 2 divided doses. May titrate q2wks based on response and tolerability.

Primary Aldosteronism

PO: ADULTS, ELDERLY: Initially, 12.5–25 mg once daily. Gradually titrate to the lowest effective dose. **Maximum dose:** 400 mg/day.

HF

PO: ADULTS, ELDERLY: ***(Tablet):*** Initially, 12.5–25 mg/day. May double the dose q4wks if serum potassium remains less than 5 mEq/L and renal function remains stable. **Maximum:** 50 mg/day. in 1 or 2 divided doses. ***(Suspension):*** Initially, 10–20 mg once daily. May titrate to 37.5 mg once daily if serum potassium remains less than 5 mEq/L and renal function remains stable.

Dosage in Renal Impairment

CrCl 50 mL/min or greater: Initially, 12.5–25 mg once daily. **Maintenance:** 25 mg once or twice daily. **CrCl 30–49 mL/min:** Initially, 12.5 mg once daily or every other day. **Maintenance:** 12.5–25 mg once daily. **CrCl less than 30 mL/min:** Not recommended.

Dosage in Hepatic Impairment
No dose adjustment.

SIDE EFFECTS

Frequent: Hyperkalemia (in pts with renal insufficiency, those taking potassium supplements), dehydration, hyponatremia, lethargy. **Occasional:** Nausea, vomiting, anorexia, abdominal cramps, diarrhea, headache, ataxia, drowsiness, confusion, fever. **Male:** Gynecomastia, impotence, decreased libido. **Female:** Menstrual irregularities (amenorrhea, postmenopausal bleeding), breast tenderness. **Rare:** Rash, urticaria, hirsutism.

ADVERSE EFFECTS/TOXIC REACTIONS

Severe hyperkalemia may produce arrhythmias, bradycardia, ECG changes (tented T waves, widening QRS complex, ST segment depression). May proceed to cardiac standstill, ventricular fibrillation. Cirrhosis pts at risk for hepatic decompensation if dehydration, hyponatremia occurs. Pts with primary aldosteronism may experience rapid weight loss, severe fatigue during high-dose therapy.

NURSING CONSIDERATIONS

BASELINE ASSESSMENT

Obtain serum electrolytes, renal function test, weight; B/P. Assess hydration status.

INTERVENTION/EVALUATION

Monitor serum electrolyte values, esp. for increased potassium, BUN, creatinine. Monitor B/P. Monitor for hyponatremia: mental confusion, thirst, cold/clammy skin, drowsiness, dry mouth. Monitor for hyperkalemia: colic, diarrhea, muscle twitching followed by weakness/paralysis, arrhythmias. Obtain daily weight. Note changes in edema, skin turgor.

PATIENT/FAMILY TEACHING

• Expect increase in volume, frequency of urination. • Therapeutic effect takes several days to begin and can last for several days when drug is discontinued. • Report irregular or slow pulse, symptoms of electrolyte imbalance (see previous Intervention/Evaluation). • Avoid foods high in potassium, such as whole grains (cereals), legumes, meat, bananas, apricots, orange juice, potatoes (white, sweet), raisins. • Avoid alcohol.

sulfamethoxazole-trimethoprim

sul-fa-meth-**ox**-a-zole-trye-**meth**-oh-prim
(Bactrim, Bactrim DS, Sulfatrim)
Do not confuse Bactrim with bacitracin or Bactroban.

FIXED-COMBINATION(S)

Bactrim, Septra: sulfamethoxazole/trimethoprim: 5:1 ratio remains constant in all dosage forms (e.g., 400 mg/80 mg).

◆CLASSIFICATION

PHARMACOTHERAPEUTIC: Sulfonamide derivative. **CLINICAL:** Antibiotic.

USES

Treatment of susceptible infections due to *S. pneumoniae, H. influenzae, E. coli, Klebsiella* spp., *Enterobacter* spp., *M. morganii, P. mirabilis, P. vulgaris, S. flexneri, Pneumocystis jiroveci,* including acute or complicated and recurrent or chronic UTI, *Pneumocystis jiroveci* pneumonia (PCP), shigellosis, enteritis, otitis media, chronic bronchitis, traveler's diarrhea. Prophylaxis of PCP. Acute exacerbation of COPD. **OFF-LABEL:** Chronic prostatitis, prophylaxis for UTI, MRSA infections, prosthetic joint infection.

PRECAUTIONS

Contraindications: Hypersensitivity to any sulfa medication, trimethoprim. History

S

of drug-induced immune thrombocytopenia with sulfonamides or trimethoprim, infants younger than 4 wks, megaloblastic anemia due to folate deficiency, severe hepatic/renal impairment. Concomitant administration of dofetilide. **Cautions:** Pts with G6PD deficiency, hepatic/renal/thyroid impairment, porphyria, asthma, elderly, concurrent anticonvulsant therapy.

ACTION

Sulfamethizole: Interferes with bacterial folic acid synthesis and growth. **Trimethoprim:** Inhibits dihydrofolic acid reduction. **Therapeutic Effect:** Bactericidal in susceptible microorganisms.

PHARMACOKINETICS

Widely distributed. Protein binding: 45%–60%. Metabolized in liver. Excreted in urine. Minimally removed by hemodialysis. **Half-life:** sulfamethoxazole, 6–12 hrs; trimethoprim, 6–17 hrs (increased in renal impairment).

LIFESPAN CONSIDERATIONS

Pregnancy/Lactation: Contraindicated during pregnancy at term and during lactation. Readily crosses placenta. Distributed in breast milk. May produce kernicterus in newborn. **Children:** Contraindicated in pts younger than 2 mos; may increase risk of kernicterus in newborn. **Elderly:** Increased risk for severe skin reaction, myelosuppression, decreased platelet count.

S

INTERACTIONS

DRUG: May increase concentration/effects of **phenytoin, digoxin, oral hypoglycemics (e.g., glipiZIDE, metFORMIN), warfarin.** May increase adverse effects of **methotrexate. Strong CYP3A4 inducers (e.g., carBAMazepine, phenytoin, rifAMPin)** may decrease concentration/effect. Trimethoprim may increase concentration/effect of **dofetilide. Leucovorin** may increase adverse effects of trimethoprim. **HERBAL: St. John's wort** may decrease concentration/effect. **Herbals with hypoglycemic properties (e.g., fenugreek)** may increase concentration/effect. **FOOD:** None known. **LAB VALUES:** May increase serum BUN, creatinine, ALT, AST, bilirubin.

AVAILABILITY (Rx)

◀ALERT▶ All dosage forms have same 5:1 ratio of sulfamethoxazole (SMZ) to trimethoprim (TMP).

Injection Solution: SMZ 80 mg and TMP 16 mg per mL. **Oral Suspension:** SMZ 200 mg and TMP 40 mg per 5 mL. **Tablets:** ***(Bactrim):*** SMZ 400 mg and TMP 80 mg. **Tablets, Double Strength:** ***(Bactrim DS):*** SMZ 800 mg and TMP 160 mg.

ADMINISTRATION/HANDLING

IV

Reconstitution • Dilute each 5 mL with 75–125 mL D_5W. • Do not mix with other drugs or solutions.

Rate of administration • Infuse over 60–90 min. Must avoid bolus or rapid infusion. • Do not give IM.

Storage • IV infusion (piggyback) stable for 2 hrs (5 mL/75 mL D_5W), 4 hrs (5 mL/100 mL D_5W), 6 hrs (5 mL/125 mL D_5W). • Discard if cloudy or precipitate forms.

PO

• Administer without regard to food. • Give with at least 8 oz water.

IV INCOMPATIBILITIES

Fluconazole (Diflucan), foscarnet (Foscavir), midazolam (Versed), vinorelbine (Navelbine).

IV COMPATIBILITIES

Dexmedetomidine (Precedex), dilTIAZem (Cardizem), heparin, HYDROmorphone (Dilaudid), LORazepam (Ativan), magnesium sulfate, morphine, niCARdipine (Cardene).

INDICATIONS/ROUTES/DOSAGE

Usual Adult/Elderly Dosage Range

PO: 1–2 double-strength tablets q12–24h. **IV:** 8–20 mg/kg/day as trimethoprim in divided doses q6–12h.

Usual Dosage Range for Infants 2 Mos and Older, Children, Adolescents

PO/IV: 6–12 mg TMP/kg/day in divided doses q12h. **Maximum single dose:** 160 mg TMP.

Dosage in Renal Impairment

Creatinine Clearance	Dosage
15–30 mL/min	50% of usual dosage
Less than 15 mL/min	Not recommended
HD	2.5–10 mg/kg trimethoprim q24h (or 5–20 mg/kg 3 times/wk) (give after HD)
CRRT	2.5–7.5 mg/kg trimethoprim q12h

Dosage in Hepatic Impairment

No dose adjustment.

SIDE EFFECTS

Frequent: Anorexia, nausea, vomiting, rash (generally 7–14 days after therapy begins), urticaria. **Occasional:** Diarrhea, abdominal pain, pain/irritation at IV infusion site. **Rare:** Headache, vertigo, insomnia, seizures, hallucinations, depression.

ADVERSE EFFECTS/TOXIC REACTIONS

Rash, fever, sore throat, pallor, purpura, cough, shortness of breath may be early signs of serious adverse effects. Fatalities are rare but have occurred in sulfonamide therapy following Stevens-Johnson syndrome, toxic epidermal necrolysis, fulminant hepatic necrosis, agranulocytosis, aplastic anemia, other blood dyscrasias. Myelosuppression, decreased platelet count, severe dermatologic reactions may occur, esp. in the elderly.

NURSING CONSIDERATIONS

BASELINE ASSESSMENT

Obtain history for hypersensitivity to trimethoprim or any sulfonamide, sulfite sensitivity, bronchial asthma. Determine serum renal, hepatic, hematologic baselines.

INTERVENTION/EVALUATION

Monitor daily pattern of bowel activity, stool consistency. Assess skin for rash, pallor, purpura. Check IV site, flow rate. Monitor renal, hepatic, hematology function. Assess I&O. Check for CNS symptoms (headache, vertigo, insomnia, hallucinations). Monitor for cough, shortness of breath. Assess for overt bleeding, ecchymosis, edema.

PATIENT/FAMILY TEACHING

• Continue medication for full length of therapy. • Take oral doses with 8 oz water and drink several extra glasses of water daily. • Report immediately any new symptoms, esp. rash, other skin changes, bleeding/bruising, fever, sore throat, diarrhea. • Avoid prolonged exposure to UV, direct sunlight.

sulfaSALAzine

sul-fa-**sal**-a-zeen

(Apo-SulfaSALAzine ✦, Azulfidine, Azulfidine EN-tabs, Salazopyrin ✦)

Do not confuse Azulfidine with Augmentin or azaTHIOprine, or sulfaSALAzine with sulfADIAZINE or sulfiSOXAZOLE.

◆CLASSIFICATION

PHARMACOTHERAPEUTIC: 5-Aminosalicylic acid derivative. **CLINICAL:** Anti-inflammatory.

USES

Treatment of mild to moderate ulcerative colitis, adjunctive therapy in severe ulcerative colitis, rheumatoid arthritis (RA), juvenile rheumatoid arthritis. **OFF-LABEL:** Treatment of ankylosing spondylitis, Crohn's disease, psoriasis, psoriatic arthritis.

PRECAUTIONS

Contraindications: Hypersensitivity to sulfaSALAzine, sulfa, salicylates; porphyria; GI or GU obstruction. **Cautions:** Severe

S

allergies, bronchial asthma, impaired hepatic/renal function, G6PD deficiency, blood dyscrasias, history of recurring or chronic infections.

ACTION

Modulates local mediators of inflammatory response. Inhibits tumor necrosis factor (TNF). **Therapeutic Effect:** Decreases inflammatory response, interferes with GI secretion. Effect appears topical rather than systemic.

PHARMACOKINETICS

Poorly absorbed from GI tract. Cleaved, absorbed in colon by intestinal bacteria, forming sulfapyridine and mesalamine (5-ASA). Widely distributed. Metabolized via colonic intestinal flora. Primarily excreted in urine. **Half-life:** 5.7–10 hrs.

LIFESPAN CONSIDERATIONS

Pregnancy/Lactation: May produce infertility, oligospermia in men while taking medication. Readily crosses placenta; if given near term, may produce jaundice, hemolytic anemia, kernicterus in newborn. Distributed in breast milk. Pt should not breastfeed premature infant or those with hyperbilirubinemia or G6PD deficiency. **Children:** No age-related precautions noted in pts older than 2 yrs. **Elderly:** No age-related precautions noted.

S

INTERACTIONS

DRUG: None significant. **HERBAL:** None significant. **FOOD:** Impairs folate absorption. **LAB VALUES:** None significant.

AVAILABILITY (Rx)

Tablets: ***(Azulfidine):*** 500 mg.

Tablets, Delayed-Release: ***(Azulfidine EN-tabs):*** 500 mg.

ADMINISTRATION/HANDLING

PO

• Space doses evenly (intervals not to exceed 8 hrs). • Administer after meals or with food. • Swallow enteric-coated tablets whole; do not break, crush, dissolve, or divide. • Give with 8 oz of water; encourage several glasses of water between meals.

INDICATIONS/ROUTES/DOSAGE

Ulcerative Colitis

PO: ADULTS, ELDERLY: ***(Immediate-Release, Delayed-Release):*** Initially, 3–4 g/day in divided doses q8h. May initiate at 1–2 g/day to reduce GI intolerance. **Maximum:** 6 g/day. **Maintenance:** 2 g/day in divided doses at intervals less than or equal to q8h. **CHILDREN 6 YRS AND OLDER:** Initially, 40–70 mg/kg/day in 3–6 divided doses. **Maximum initial dose:** 4 g/day. **Maintenance:** 30–70 mg/kg/day in 3–6 divided doses. **Maximum daily dose:** 4 g/day.

Rheumatoid Arthritis (RA)

PO: ***(Delayed-Release Tablets):*** **ADULTS, ELDERLY:** Initially, 0.5 g once daily or 1 g/day in 2 divided doses for 1 wk. Increase by 0.5 g/wk, up to 2 g/day in 2 divided doses. **Maximum:** 3 g/day (if response to 2 g/day is inadequate after 12 wks of treatment).

Juvenile Rheumatoid Arthritis (JRA)

PO: ***(Delayed-Release Tablets):*** **CHILDREN 6–16 YRS:** Initially, 10 mg/kg/day. May increase by 10 mg/kg/day at wkly intervals. Range: 30–50 mg/kg/day. **Maximum:** 2 g/day.

Dosage in Renal/Hepatic Impairment

Use caution.

SIDE EFFECTS

Frequent (33%): Anorexia, nausea, vomiting, headache, oligospermia (generally reversed by withdrawal of drug). **Occasional (3%):** Hypersensitivity reaction (rash, urticaria, pruritus, fever, anemia). **Rare (less than 1%):** Tinnitus, hypoglycemia, diuresis, photosensitivity.

ADVERSE EFFECTS/TOXIC REACTIONS

Anaphylaxis, Stevens-Johnson syndrome, hematologic toxicity (leukopenia, agranulocytosis), hepatotoxicity, nephrotoxicity occur rarely.

NURSING CONSIDERATIONS

BASELINE ASSESSMENT

Obtain CBC, LFT. Question history of prior hypersensitivity reactions.

INTERVENTION/EVALUATION

Monitor I&O, urinalysis, renal function tests; ensure adequate hydration (minimum output 1,500 mL/24 hrs) to prevent nephrotoxicity. Assess skin for rash (discontinue drug, notify physician at first sign). Monitor daily pattern of bowel activity, stool consistency. (Dosage increase may be needed if diarrhea continues, recurs.) Monitor CBC closely; assess for and report immediately any hematologic effects (bleeding, ecchymoses, fever, pharyngitis, pallor, weakness, purpura). Monitor LFT; observe for jaundice.

PATIENT/FAMILY TEACHING

• May cause orange-yellow discoloration of urine, skin. • Take after or with food with 8 oz of water; drink several glasses of water between meals. • Continue for full length of treatment; may be necessary to take drug even after symptoms relieved. • Routinely monitor blood levels. • Inform dentist, surgeon of sulfaSALAzine therapy. • Avoid exposure to sun, ultraviolet light until photosensitivity determined (may last for mos after last dose).

SUMAtriptan

soo-ma-**trip**-tan
(Imitrex, Onzetra, Sumavel DosePro, Tosymra, Xsail, Zembrace SymTouch)
Do not confuse SUMAtriptan with SAXagliptin, SITagliptin, somatropin, or ZOLMitriptan.

FIXED-COMBINATION(S)

Treximet: SUMAtriptan/naproxen (an NSAID): 85 mg/500 mg, 10 mg/60 mg.

◆CLASSIFICATION

PHARMACOTHERAPEUTIC: Serotonin 5-HT_1 receptor agonist. **CLINICAL:** Antimigraine.

USES

PO, SQ, Intranasal, Transdermal: Acute treatment of migraine headache with or without aura. **SQ: (Excluding Zembrace)** Treatment of cluster headaches.

PRECAUTIONS

Contraindications: Hypersensitivity to SUMAtriptan. Management of hemiplegic or basilar migraine, peripheral vascular disease, CVA, ischemic heart disease (including angina pectoris, history of MI, silent ischemia, Prinzmetal's angina), severe hepatic impairment, transient ischemic attack, uncontrolled hypertension, MAOI use within 14 days, use within 24 hrs of ergotamine preparations or another 5-HT_1 agonist. **Cautions:** Mild to moderate hepatic impairment, seizure disorder, hypertension, elderly.

ACTION

Binds selectively to serotonin 5-HT_1 receptors in cranial arteries, producing vasoconstrictive effect on cranial blood vessels. **Therapeutic Effect:** Relieves migraine headache.

PHARMACOKINETICS

Route	Onset	Peak	Duration
Nasal	15 min	N/A	24–48 hrs
PO	30 min	2 hrs	24–48 hrs
SQ	10 min	1 hr	24–48 hrs

Widely distributed. Metabolized in liver. Protein binding: 10%–21%. Excreted in urine. **Half-life:** 2 hrs.

⌛ LIFESPAN CONSIDERATIONS

Pregnancy/Lactation: Unknown if distributed in breast milk. **Children:** Safety and efficacy not established. **Elderly:** No age-related precautions noted.

S

INTERACTIONS

DRUG: **Ergotamine-containing medications** may produce vasospastic reaction. **MAOIs (e.g., phenelzine, selegiline)** may increase concentration, half-life. **SSRIs (e.g., escitalopram, PARoxetine, sertraline)** and **SNRIs (e.g., DULoxetine, venlafaxine)** may increase risk of serotonin syndrome. **HERBAL:** None significant. **FOOD:** None known. **LAB VALUES:** None significant.

AVAILABILITY (Rx)

Injection, Prefilled Autoinjector: 4 mg/0.5 mL, 6 mg/0.5 mL. ***(Zembrace SymTouch):*** 3-mg prefilled syringe. **Injection Solution:** 6 mg/0.5 mL. ***(Sumavel DosePro):*** 4 mg/0.5 mL, 6 mg/0.5 mL. **Nasal Powder:** ***(Onzetra, Xsail):*** **Capsules:** 11 mg (to be used with Xsail breath powdered nasal device). **Nasal Spray:** ***(Imitrex Nasal):*** 5 mg/actuation, 20 mg/actuation. ***(Tosymra):*** 10 mg/actuation. **Tablets:** ***(Imitrex):*** 25 mg, 50 mg, 100 mg.

ADMINISTRATION/HANDLING

SQ

• Follow manufacturer's instructions for autoinjection device use. • Administer needleless (Sumavel DosePro) only to abdomen or thigh.

PO

• Swallow tablets whole. Do not break, crush, dissolve, or divide. • Take with full glass of water.

Nasal

• Unit contains only one spray—do not test before use. • Instruct pt to gently blow nose to clear nasal passages. • With head upright, close one nostril with index finger, breathe out gently through mouth. • Have pt insert nozzle into open nostril about one-half inch, close mouth and, while taking a breath through nose, release spray dosage by firmly pressing plunger. • Instruct pt to remove nozzle from nose and gently breathe in through nose and out through mouth for 10–20 sec; do not breathe in deeply.

INDICATIONS/ROUTES/DOSAGE

Acute Migraine Headache

PO: ADULTS, ELDERLY: 50–100 mg. Dose may be repeated after at least 2 hrs. **Maximum:** 100 mg/single dose; 200 mg/24 hrs.

SQ: ADULTS, ELDERLY: Initially, up to 6 mg. **Maximum:** Up to two 6-mg injections/24 hrs (separated by at least 1 hr). ***(Zembrace SymTouch):*** 3-mg single dose. **Maximum:** 12 mg/24 hrs. Separate dose by at least 1 hr.

Intranasal: ADULTS, ELDERLY: ***(Spray):*** Initially, 5 mg, 10 mg, or 20 mg once in one nostril. May repeat once after at least 2 hrs. **Maximum:** 40 mg/24h. ***(Tosymra):*** Initially, 10 mg once in one nostril. If initial dose was partially effective or headache recurs, may repeat dose once after at least 1 hr. **Maximum:** 30 mg/4 hrs. ***(Nasal Powder):*** Initially, a single dose of 22 mg (11 mg in each nostril). May repeat once after at least 2 hrs. **Maximum:** 44 mg/24 hrs separated by at least 2 hrs.

Cluster Headaches

SQ: ADULTS, ELDERLY: Initially, 6 mg. May repeat after 1 hr. **Maximum:** 6 mg/dose; two 6-mg doses/24 hrs.

Dosage in Renal Impairment

No dose adjustment.

Dosage in Hepatic Impairment

Mild to moderate impairment: Maximum PO dose: 50 mg. **Severe impairment:** Contraindicated.

SIDE EFFECTS

Frequent: PO (10%–5%): Tingling, nasal discomfort. **SQ (greater than 10%):** Injection site reactions, tingling, warm/hot sensation, dizziness, vertigo. **Nasal (greater than 10%):** Altered taste, nausea, vomiting. **Occasional: PO (5%–1%):** Flushing, asthenia, visual disturbances. **SQ (10%–2%):** Burning sensation, numbness, chest discomfort, drowsiness, asthenia. **Nasal (5%–1%):** Nasopharyngeal discomfort, dizziness. **Rare: PO (less than 1%):** Agitation, eye irritation, dysuria. **SQ (less than

2%): Anxiety, fatigue, diaphoresis, muscle cramps, myalgia. **Nasal (less than 1%):** Burning sensation.

ADVERSE EFFECTS/TOXIC REACTIONS

Excessive dosage may produce tremors, redness of extremities, reduced respirations, cyanosis, seizures, paralysis. Serious arrhythmias occur rarely, esp. in pts with hypertension, obesity, smokers, diabetes, strong family history of coronary artery disease. Serotonin syndrome may occur (agitation, confusion, hallucinations, hyperreflexia, myoclonus, shivering, tachycardia).

NURSING CONSIDERATIONS

BASELINE ASSESSMENT

Receive full medical history, medication history and screen for contraindications. Obtain pregnancy test in female pts of reproductive potential. Question regarding onset, location, duration of migraine, possible precipitating symptoms.

INTERVENTION/EVALUATION

Evaluate for relief of migraine headache and resulting photophobia, phonophobia (sound sensitivity), nausea, vomiting.

PATIENT/FAMILY TEACHING

• Follow proper technique for loading of autoinjector, injection technique, discarding of syringe. • Do not use more than 2 injections during any 24-hr period and allow at least 1 hr between injections. • Report immediately if wheezing, palpitations, skin rash, facial swelling, pain/tightness in chest/throat occur.

SUNItinib

HIGH ALERT

soo-**nit**-in-ib
(Sutent)

■ BLACK BOX ALERT ■ Hepatotoxicity may be severe and/or result in fatal liver failure.

Do not confuse SUNItinib with imatinib or SORAfenib.

CLASSIFICATION

PHARMACOTHERAPEUTIC: Vascular endothelial growth factor (VEGF) inhibitor. Tyrosine kinase inhibitor. **CLINICAL:** Antineoplastic.

USES

Treatment of GI stromal tumor (GIST) after disease progression while on or demonstrating intolerance to imatinib. Treatment of advanced renal cell carcinoma (RCC). Adjuvant treatment of adults at high risk of recurrent RCC following nephrectomy. Treatment of pancreatic neuroendocrine tumor (PNET). **OFF-LABEL:** Non-GI stromal tumor, soft tissue sarcomas, advanced thyroid cancer.

PRECAUTIONS

Contraindications: Hypersensitivity to SUNItinib. **Cautions:** Cardiac dysfunction, bradycardia, electrolyte imbalance, bleeding tendencies, hypertension, history of prolonged QT interval, medications that prolong QT interval, hypokalemia, hypomagnesemia, concurrent use of strong CYP3A4 inducers or inhibitors, HF, renal/hepatic impairment, pregnancy.

ACTION

Inhibitory action against multiple receptor tyrosine kinases including growth factor receptors, vascular endothelial growth factors, colony-stimulating factor receptors, glial cell-line neurotrophic factor receptors. **Therapeutic Effect:** Prevents tumor cell growth, produces tumor regression, inhibits metastasis.

PHARMACOKINETICS

Metabolized in liver. Protein binding: 95%. Excreted in feces (61%), urine (16%). **Half-life:** 40–60 hrs.

LIFESPAN CONSIDERATIONS

Pregnancy/Lactation: Has potential for embryotoxic, teratogenic effects. Breastfeeding not recommended. **Children:** Safety and efficacy not established. **Elderly:** No age-related precautions noted.

S

INTERACTIONS

DRUG: **Strong CYP3A4 inhibitors (e.g., clarithromycin, itraconazole, ketoconazole, voriconazole)** may increase concentration, toxicity. **Strong CYP3A4 inducers (e.g., carBAMazepine, PHENobarbital, phenytoin, rifAMPin)** may decrease concentration/effects. **QT interval–prolonging medications (e.g., amiodarone, haloperidol, moxifloxacin)** may increase risk of QT interval prolongation, cardiac arrhythmias. May increase adverse effects of **bevacizumab**. May increase adverse effects; decrease therapeutic effect of **vaccines (live)**. HERBAL: **St. John's wort** may decrease concentration. **Herbals with hypoglycemic properties (e.g., fenugreek)** may increase hypoglycemic effect. **Echinacea** may decrease therapeutic effect. FOOD: **Grapefruit products** may increase concentration/effect. LAB VALUES: May increase serum alkaline phosphatase, bilirubin, amylase, lipase, creatinine, ALT, AST. May alter serum potassium, sodium, uric acid. May produce thrombocytopenia, neutropenia. May decrease serum phosphate, thyroid function levels.

AVAILABILITY (Rx)

Capsules: 12.5 mg, 25 mg, 37.5 mg, 50 mg.

ADMINISTRATION/HANDLING

S

PO

• Give without regard to food. Avoid grapefruit products.

INDICATIONS/ROUTES/DOSAGE

GI Stromal Tumor, Renal Cell Carcinoma, RCC (Adjuvant treatment)

PO: ADULTS, ELDERLY: 50 mg once daily for 4 wks, followed by 2 wks off in 6-wk cycle.

Pancreatic Neuroendocrine Tumor

PO: ADULTS, ELDERLY: 37.5 mg once daily continuously without a scheduled off-treatment period. **Maximum:** 50 mg/day.

Dose Modification

PO: ADULTS, ELDERLY: Dosage increase or reduction in 12.5-mg increments is recommended based on safety and tolerability.

Concomitant Use of Strong CYP3A4 Inhibitors

Consider a dose reduction to a minimum of 37.5 mg/day (GIST, RCC) or 25 mg/day (PNET).

Concomitant Use of CYP3A4 Inducers

Consider a dose increase (monitor carefully for toxicity) to maximum of 87.5 mg/day (GIST, RCC) or 62.5 mg (PNET).

Dosage in Renal Impairment

No initial dose adjustment; subsequent adjustment may be needed.

Dosage in Hepatic Impairment

No dose adjustment initially; Grade 3 or 4 hepatotoxicity during treatment: withhold/discontinue if hepatotoxicity does not resolve.

SIDE EFFECTS

Stromal tumor: Common (42%–30%): Fatigue, diarrhea, anorexia, abdominal pain, nausea, hyperpigmentation. Frequent (29%–18%): Mucositis/stomatitis, vomiting, asthenia, altered taste, constipation, fever. Occasional (15%–8%): Hypertension, rash, myalgia, headache, arthralgia, back pain, dyspnea, cough. **Renal carcinoma:** Common (74%–43%): Fatigue, diarrhea, nausea, mucositis/stomatitis, dyspepsia, altered taste. Frequent (38%–20%): Rash, vomiting, constipation, hyperpigmentation, anorexia, arthralgia, dyspnea, hypertension, headache, abdominal pain. Occasional (18%–11%): Limb pain, peripheral/periorbital edema, dry skin, hair color change, myalgia, cough, back pain, dizziness, fever, tongue pain, flatulence, alopecia, dehydration.

ADVERSE EFFECTS/TOXIC REACTIONS

Palmar-plantar erythrodysesthesia syndrome (PPES) occurs occasionally (14%), manifested as blistering/rash/peeling of skin on palms of hands, soles of feet. Bleeding, decrease in left ventricular ejection fraction, deep vein thrombosis (DVT), pancreatitis, neutropenia, seizures occur rarely.

NURSING CONSIDERATIONS

BASELINE ASSESSMENT

Question possibility of pregnancy. Obtain baseline CBC, BMP, LFT before beginning therapy and prior to each treatment. Obtain baseline ECG, thyroid function tests. Question medical history as listed in Precautions.

INTERVENTION/EVALUATION

Assess eye area, lower extremities for early evidence of fluid retention. Offer antiemetics to control nausea, vomiting. Monitor daily pattern of bowel activity, stool consistency. Monitor CBC for evidence of neutropenia, thrombocytopenia; assess LFT for hepatotoxicity. Monitor for PPES. Monitor B/P.

PATIENT/FAMILY TEACHING

• Treatment may depress your immune system response and reduce your ability to fight infection. Report symptoms of infection such as body aches, chills, cough, fatigue, fever. Avoid those with active infection. • Avoid pregnancy; use effective contraceptive measures. • Promptly report fever, unusual bruising/bleeding from any site.

S

tacrolimus

ta-**kroe-li**-mus
(Astagraf XL, Envarsus XR, Prograf, Protopic)

BLACK BOX ALERT Increased susceptibility to infection and potential for development of lymphoma. Extended-release associated with increased mortality in female liver transplant recipients. Topical form associated with rare cases of malignancy. Topical form should be used only for short-term and intermittent treatment. Not recommended in children younger than 2 yrs. Use only 0.03% ointment for children 2–15 yrs of age. Administer under supervision of physician experienced in immunosuppressive therapy.

Do not confuse Protopic with Protonix, or tacrolimus with everolimus, pimecrolimus, sirolimus, or temsirolimus.

◆CLASSIFICATION

PHARMACOTHERAPEUTIC: Calcineurin inhibitor. **CLINICAL:** Immunosuppressant.

USES

PO, Injection: Prevention of organ rejection in pts receiving allogeneic liver, kidney, heart transplant. Should be used concurrently with adrenal corticosteroids. In heart and kidney transplant pts, should be used in conjunction with azaTHIOprine or mycophenolate. **Topical:** Moderate to severe atopic dermatitis in immunocompetent pts. **OFF-LABEL:** Prevention of organ rejection in lung, small bowel recipients; prevention and treatment of graft-vs-host disease in allogeneic hematopoietic stem cell transplantation.

PRECAUTIONS

Contraindications: Hypersensitivity to tacrolimus. **Cautions:** Hypersensitivity to HCO-60 polyoxyl 60 hydrogenated castor oil (used in solution for injection). Renal/hepatic impairment cardiac disease; history of chronic, opportunistic infections, concurrent use with other nephrotoxic drugs (e.g., cycloSPORINE), concurrent use of strong CYP3A4 inhibitors or inducers. Avoid use of potassium-sparing diuretics, ACE inhibitors, potassium-based salt substitutes. Pts at risk for pure red cell aplasia (e.g., concurrent use of mycophenolate); pts at risk for QTc interval prolongation (congenital long QT syndrome, HF, medications that prolong QTc interval, hypokalemia, hypomagnesemia). **Topical:** Exposure to sunlight.

ACTION

Inhibits T-lymphocyte activation by binding to intracellular protein FKBP-12, forming a complex with calcineurin-dependent proteins, inhibiting calcineurin phosphatase activity. **Therapeutic Effect:** Suppresses immunological-mediated inflammatory response; prevents organ transplant rejection.

PHARMACOKINETICS

Variably absorbed after PO administration (food reduces absorption). Protein binding: 99%. Metabolized in liver. Primarily excreted in feces. Not removed by hemodialysis. **Half-life:** 21–61 hrs.

⌛ LIFESPAN CONSIDERATIONS

Pregnancy/Lactation: Crosses placenta. Hyperkalemia, renal dysfunction noted in neonates. Distributed in breast milk. Breastfeeding not recommended. **Children:** May require higher dosages (decreased bioavailability, increased clearance). May make post-transplant lymphoproliferative disorder more common, esp. in pts younger than 3 yrs. **Elderly:** Age-related renal impairment may require dosage adjustment.

INTERACTIONS

DRUG: **Aluminium-containing antacids** may increase concentration. **Strong CYP3A4 inhibitors (e.g., clarithromycin, ketoconazole, ritonavir), calcium channel blockers (e.g., dilTIAZem, verapamil)** may increase concentration/effect. **Strong CYP3A4 inducers**

(e.g., carBAMazepine, phenytoin, rifAMPin) may decrease concentration/effect. **CycloSPORINE, foscarnet may** increase nephrotoxic effect. May decrease therapeutic effect; increase adverse effect of **vaccines (live). Enzalutamide** may decrease concentration/effect. **Eplerenone, potassium-sparing diuretics (e.g., spironolactone)** may increase hyperkalemic effect. **QT interval–prolonging medications (e.g., amiodarone, azithromycin, ciprofloxacin, haloperidol, methadone, sotalol)** may increase risk of QTc interval prolongation. **HERBAL: Echinacea** may decrease therapeutic effect. **St. John's wort** may decrease concentration/effect. **FOOD: Food** decreases rate/extent of absorption. **Grapefruit products** may increase concentration, toxicity (potential for nephrotoxicity). **LAB VALUES:** May increase serum ALT, AST, amylase, bilirubin, BUN, cholesterol, creatinine, potassium, glucose, triglycerides. May decrease serum magnesium; Hgb, Hct, platelets. May alter leukocytes.

AVAILABILITY (Rx)

Capsules: ***(Prograf):*** 0.5 mg, 1 mg, 5 mg. **Injection Solution:** ***(Prograf):*** 5 mg/mL. **Ointment:** ***(Protopic):*** 0.03%, 0.1%. **Packet, Oral:** 0.2 mg, 2 mg.

Capsules, Extended-Release: ***(Astagraf XL):*** 0.5 mg, 1 mg, 5 mg. **Tablets, Extended-Release:** ***(Envarsus XR):*** 0.75 mg, 1 mg, 4 mg.

ADMINISTRATION/HANDLING

IV

Reconstitution • Dilute with appropriate amount (250–1,000 mL, depending on desired dose) 0.9% NaCl or D_5W to provide concentration between 0.004 and 0.02 mg/mL.

Rate of administration • Give as continuous IV infusion. • Continuously monitor pt for anaphylaxis for at least 30 min after start of infusion. • Stop infusion immediately at first sign of hypersensitivity reaction.

Storage • Store diluted infusion solution in glass or polyethylene containers and discard after 24 hrs. • Do not store in PVC container (decreased stability, potential for extraction).

PO

• Avoid grapefruit products. • **Immediate-Release:** Administer without regard to food. Be consistent with timing of administration. • **Extended-Release:** Administer at least 1 hr before or 2 hrs after a meal. Do not crush, cut, dissolve, or divide; swallow whole. • **Granules for Oral Suspension:** Mix with 15–30 mL of water (do not sprinkle on food). Give immediately after mixing. Add additional 15–30 mL of water to rinse cup and ensure all medication is taken.

Topical

• For external use only. • Do not cover with occlusive dressing. • Rub gently, completely onto clean, dry skin.

IV INCOMPATIBILITIES

Acyclovir.

IV COMPATIBILITIES

Calcium gluconate, dexamethasone (Decadron), diphenhydrAMINE (Benadryl), DOBUTamine (Dobutrex), DOPamine (Intropin), furosemide (Lasix), heparin, HYDROmorphone (Dilaudid), insulin, leucovorin, LORazepam (Ativan), morphine, nitroglycerin, potassium chloride.

INDICATIONS/ROUTES/DOSAGE

Note: Give initial postoperative dose no sooner than 6 hrs after liver or heart transplant and within 24 hrs of kidney transplant.

Prevention of Liver Transplant Rejection

PO: ADULTS, ELDERLY: ***(Immediate-Release):*** 0.1–0.15 mg/kg/day in 2 divided doses 12 hrs apart (in combination with corticosteroids). Titrate to target trough concentration. **CHILDREN:** 0.15–0.2 mg/kg/day in 2 divided doses 12 hrs apart. Titrate to target trough concentration.

IV: ADULTS, ELDERLY, CHILDREN: 0.03–0.05 mg/kg/day as continuous infusion.

Prevention of Kidney Transplant Rejection

PO: ADULTS, ELDERLY: ***(Immediate-Release):*** 0.2 mg/kg/day (in combination with azaTHIOprine) in 2 divided doses 12 hrs apart or 0.1 mg/kg/day (in combination with mycophenolate) in 2 divided doses 12 hrs apart. Titrate to target trough concentration. **CHILDREN:** 0.2–0.3 mg/kg/day divided q12h. ***(Extended-Release [Astagraf XL]): (With Basiliximab Induction):*** (Prior to or within 48 hrs of transplant completion): 0.15–0.2 mg/kg once daily (in combination with corticosteroids and mycophenolate). Titrate to target trough concentration. **CHILDREN 4 YRS AND OLDER:** 0.3 mg/kg once daily. ***(Without Basiliximab Induction):*** Preoperative dose: 0.1 mg/kg (administer within 12 hrs prior to reperfusion). Post-operative dosing: 0.2 mg/kg once daily (in combination with corticosteroids and mycophenolate). Give at least 4 hrs after pre-operative dose and within 12 hrs of reperfusion. Titrate to target trough concentration. ***(Extended-Release [Envarsus XL]):*** 0.14 mg/kg/day.

IV: ADULTS, ELDERLY: Initially, 0.03–0.05 mg/kg/day as continuous infusion.

Prevention of Heart Transplant Rejection

Note: Recommended in combination with azaTHIOprine or mycophenolate. May also use with an mTOR kinase inhibitor (e.g., sirolimus).

PO: ADULTS, ELDERLY: Initially, 0.075 mg/kg/day in 2 divided doses 12 hrs apart. Titrate to target trough concentration.

IV: ADULTS, ELDERLY: Initially, 0.01 mg/kg/day as continuous infusion.

Atopic Dermatitis

Topical: ADULTS, ELDERLY, CHILDREN 15 YRS AND OLDER: Apply 0.03% or 0.1% ointment to affected area twice daily. **CHILDREN 2–15 YRS:** Use 0.03% ointment twice daily. Continue treatment for 1 wk after symptoms have resolved. If no improvement within 6 wks, re-examine to confirm diagnosis.

SIDE EFFECTS

Frequent (greater than 30%): Headache, tremor, insomnia, paresthesia, diarrhea, nausea, constipation, vomiting, abdominal pain, hypertension. **Occasional (29%–10%):** Rash, pruritus, anorexia, asthenia, peripheral edema, photosensitivity.

ADVERSE EFFECTS/TOXIC REACTIONS

Hypersensitivity reactions, including anaphylaxis, were reported. Cardiac toxicities including myocardial hypertrophy, QT interval prolongation, torsades de pointes, MI, pericardial effusion, SVT, ventricular arrhythmias, may occur. May increase risk of new-onset diabetes after transplantation. May cause acute renal failure, GI perforation, hepatotoxicity, hyperkalemia, hypertension, myelosuppression (anemia, leukopenia, neutropenia, thrombocytopenia), new malignancies, pure red cell aplasia, thrombotic microangiopathy. Fatal infections including bacterial, fungal, protozoal, opportunistic, viral infections (including cytomegalovirus) were reported. Progressive multifocal leukoencephalopathy (PML), an opportunistic viral infection of the brain caused by the JC virus, may result in progressive permanent disability and death. Nephrotoxicity may occur with high doses. Neurotoxicities (e.g., confusion, depression, encephalopathy, myasthenia, myoclonus, neuralgia, neuropathy, paralysis, seizures) were reported.

NURSING CONSIDERATIONS

BASELINE ASSESSMENT

Obtain CBC, BMP, LFT; ECG; pregnancy test in females of reproductive potential. Question history of hepatic/renal impairment, cardiac disease, chronic opportunistic infections. Screen for active infection. Receive full medication history and screen for interaction (esp. use of other immunosuppressants). Have aqueous solution of EPINEPHrine 1:1,000, O_2 available at bedside before beginning IV infusion.

INTERVENTION/EVALUATION

CBC should be performed wkly during first mo of therapy, twice monthly during second and third mos of treatment, then monthly throughout the first yr. Monitor BUN, serum creatinine, CrCL, eGFR pts with renal impairment. Monitor LFT periodically. Assess continuously for first 30 min following start of infusion and at frequent intervals thereafter. Monitor I&O closely. Monitor for infections (cough, fatigue fever), neurotoxicities, psychiatric symptoms. Monitor for cardiac ischemia/infarction (chest pain, diaphoresis, left arm or jaw pain, ST segment elevation, serum troponin elevation), GI perforation (abdominal pain, fever, nausea, vomiting), infection (cough, fatigue, fever); neuropathy (gait disturbance, fine motor control difficulties, numbness); hypersensitivity reactions (anaphylaxis, urticaria), bleeding of any kind.

PATIENT/FAMILY TEACHING

• Treatment may depress your immune system and reduce your ability to fight infection. Report symptoms of infection such as body aches, burning with urination, chills, cough, fatigue, fever. Avoid those with active infection. • Report lung problems (excessive coughing, difficulty breathing, chest pain); liver problems (abdominal pain, bruising, clay-colored stool, dark or amber-colored urine, yellowing of the skin or eyes), kidney problems (decreased urine output, flank pain, darkened urine), skin toxicities (rash, peeling); symptoms of heart attack (chest pain, difficulty breathing, jaw pain, nausea, pain that radiates to the left arm, sweating); bleeding of any kind. • Allergic reactions, including anaphylaxis, may occur. • Treatment may alter the electrical conduction of the heart, which may lead to cardiac arrhythmias; report chest pain, difficulty breathing, dizziness, swelling of extremities, fainting, palpitations. • Use effective contraception to avoid pregnancy. Do not breastfeed. • Do not take newly prescribed medications unless approved by prescriber who originally started treatment. • Treatment may worsen high B/P. • Avoid exposure to sun, artificial light (may cause photosensitivity reaction). • Do not take within 2 hrs of taking antacids. • Do not ingest grapefruit products.

talazoparib

tal-a-**zoe**-pa-rib
(Talzenna)
Do not confuse talazoparib with niraparib, olaparib, or rucaparib, or Talzenna with Senna.

◆CLASSIFICATION

PHARMACOTHERAPEUTIC: Poly (ADP-ribose) polymerase (PARP) inhibitor. **CLINICAL:** Antineoplastic.

USES

Treatment of adults with deleterious or suspected deleterious germline BRCA-mutation *(gBRCAm)* HER2-negative locally advanced or metastatic breast cancer.

PRECAUTIONS

Contraindications: Hypersensitivity to talazoparib. **Cautions:** Baseline cytopenias, renal/hepatic impairment, conditions predisposing to infection (e.g., diabetes, renal failure, immunocompromised pts, open wounds); concomitant use of P-gp inhibitors. Do not initiate in pts who have not recovered from hematological toxicities related to prior chemotherapy.

T

ACTION

Inhibits poly (ADP-ribose) polymerase (PARP) enzymatic activity. PARP enzymes are involved in DNA transcription, cell cycle regulation and DNA repair. Inhibition causes cell death due to DNA damage. **Therapeutic Effect:** Inhibits tumor cell growth and survival.

PHARMACOKINETICS

Widely distributed. Metabolized by oxidation, dehydrogenation, and conjugation (with minimal hepatic metabolism). Protein binding: 74%. Peak plasma concentration: 1–2 hrs. Excreted in urine (69%), feces (20%). **Half-life:** 90 (±58) hrs.

LIFESPAN CONSIDERATIONS

Pregnancy/Lactation: Avoid pregnancy; may cause fetal harm. Females of reproductive potential must use effective contraception during treatment and for at least 7 mos after discontinuation. Unknown if distributed in breast milk. Breastfeeding not recommended during treatment and for at least 1 mo after discontinuation. **Males:** Males with female partners of reproductive potential must use effective contraception during treatment and for at least 4 mos after discontinuation. May impair fertility. **Children:** Safety and efficacy not established. **Elderly:** No age-related precautions noted.

INTERACTIONS

DRUG: **Certain P-gp inhibitors (e.g., amiodarone, carvedilol, clarithromycin, itraconazole, verapamil)** may significantly increase concentration/effect. **Cladribine** may increase myelosuppression. **HERBAL:** None significant. **FOOD:** None known. **LAB VALUES:** May increase serum alkaline phosphatase, ALT, AST, glucose. May decrease Hgb, leukocytes, neutrophils, lymphocytes, platelets; serum calcium.

T

AVAILABILITY (Rx)

Capsules: 0.25 mg, 1 mg.

ADMINISTRATION/HANDLING

PO

• Give without regard to meals. • Administer capsules whole; do not break, cut, or open. Capsules cannot be chewed. • If a dose is missed or vomiting occurs after administration, do not give extra dose. Administer next dose at regularly scheduled time.

INDICATIONS/ROUTES/DOSAGE

Note: Administer only to pts with germline BRCA mutation.

Breast Cancer

PO: ADULTS, ELDERLY: 1 mg once daily. Continue until disease progression or unacceptable toxicity.

Dose Reduction Schedule

First reduction: 0.75 mg once daily. **Second reduction:** 0.5 mg once daily. **Third reduction:** 0.25 mg once daily. **Unable to tolerate 0.25 mg dose:** Permanently discontinue.

Dose Modification

Based on Common Terminology Criteria for Adverse Events (CTCAE).

Hematologic Toxicity

Hemoglobin less than 8 g/dL: Withhold treatment until improved to 9 g/dL (or greater), then resume at next reduced dose.

Platelet count less than 50,000 cells/mm3: Withhold treatment until improved to 75,000 cells/mm3 (or greater), then resume at next reduced dose. **Neutrophil count less than 1,000 cells/mm3:** Withhold treatment until improved to 1,500 cells/mm3 (or greater), then resume at next reduced dose.

Nonhematologic Toxicity

Any Grade 3 or 4 adverse reaction: Withhold treatment until improved to Grade 1 or 0, then consider resuming at a reduced dose or discontinue.

Concomitant Use of P-gp Inhibitors

Reduce dose to 0.75 mg once daily. If P-gp inhibitor is discontinued for 3–5 half-lives, resume talazoparib dose to the dose used prior to starting P-gp inhibitor.

Dosage in Renal Impairment

Mild impairment: No dose adjustment. **Moderate impairment (CrCl 30–59 mL/min):** Reduce dose to 0.75 mg once daily. **Severe impairment:** Not specified; use caution.

Dosage in Hepatic Impairment

Mild impairment: No dose adjustment. **Moderate to severe impairment:** Not specified; use caution.

SIDE EFFECTS

Frequent (62%–21%): Fatigue, asthenia, nausea, headache, vomiting, alopecia, diarrhea, decreased appetite.

ADVERSE EFFECTS/TOXIC REACTIONS

Myelosuppression (anemia, leukopenia, neutropenia, thrombocytopenia) is an expected response to therapy. Grade 3 (or higher) anemia, neutropenia, thrombocytopenia reported in 39%–15% of pts. Acute myeloid leukemia, myelodysplastic syndrome was reported in pts who received prior chemotherapy with platinum agents and/or DNA-damaging agents.

NURSING CONSIDERATIONS

BASELINE ASSESSMENT

Obtain CBC; pregnancy test in females of reproductive potential. Obtain renal function test (BUN, serum creatinine, CrCl, eGFR) in pts with renal impairment; LFT in pts with hepatic impairment. Question history of hepatic/renal impairment, prior treatment with other chemotherapeutic agents. Receive full medication history and screen for interactions (esp. P-gp inhibitors). Screen for active infection. Do not initiate in pts who have not recovered from hematological toxicities related to prior chemotherapy. Offer emotional support.

INTERVENTION/EVALUATION

Monitor CBC monthly. If hematologic toxicities occur, monitor CBC wkly until blood counts recover. If blood counts do not recover, consider hematology consultation for further investigations such as bone marrow analysis and blood sample for cytogenetics. Monitor for acute myeloid leukemia, myelodysplastic syndrome (bleeding, bruising easily; fatigue, frequent infections, pyrexia, hematuria, melena, weakness, weight loss; cytopenias, increased requirements for blood transfusion). If acute myeloid leukemia or myelodysplastic syndrome occurs, discontinue treatment. If concomitant use of P-gp inhibitor is unavoidable, monitor for adverse reactions/drug toxicities. Diligently screen for infections (cough, fatigue, fever). Monitor daily pattern of bowel activity, stool consistency. Encourage nutritional intake.

PATIENT/FAMILY TEACHING

• Treatment may depress your immune system and reduce your ability to fight infection. Report symptoms of infection such as body aches, burning with urination, chills, cough, fatigue, fever. Avoid those with active infection. • Treatment may cause severe bone marrow depression or new-onset myeloid leukemia; report bruising, fatigue, fever, frequent infections, shortness of breath, weight loss; bleeding easily, blood in urine or stool. • Use effective contraception to avoid pregnancy. Do not breastfeed. • Report liver problems (abdominal pain, bruising, clay-colored stool, amber- or dark-colored urine, yellowing of the skin or eyes). • Do not take newly prescribed medications unless approved by prescriber who originally started treatment.

tamoxifen

HIGH ALERT

ta-**MOKS**-i-fen
(Nolvadex-D ✦, Soltamox)

■ BLACK BOX ALERT ■ Serious, possibly life-threatening CVA, pulmonary emboli, uterine malignancy (endometrial adenocarcinoma, uterine sarcoma) have occurred.

Do not confuse tamoxifen with pentoxifylline, tamsulosin, or temazepam.

CLASSIFICATION

PHARMACOTHERAPEUTIC: Selective estrogen receptor modulator (SERM). Estrogen receptor antagonist. **CLINICAL:** Antineoplastic.

T

USES

Adjunct treatment in advanced breast cancer after primary treatment with surgery and radiation, reduction of risk of breast cancer in women at high risk, reduction of risk of invasive breast cancer in women with ductal carcinoma in situ (DCIS), metastatic breast cancer in women and men. **OFF-LABEL:** Ovarian cancer (advanced and/or recurrent), treatment of endometrial cancer; risk reduction of breast cancer in women with Paget's disease of the breast.

PRECAUTIONS

Contraindications: Hypersensitivity to tamoxifen. Concomitant warfarin therapy when used in treatment of breast cancer in high-risk women, history of deep vein thrombosis (DVT) or pulmonary embolism (in high-risk women for breast cancer and in women with DCIS). **Cautions:** Thrombocytopenia, pregnancy, history of thromboembolic events, hyperlipidemia, concomitant use of strong CYP2D6 inhibitors and/or moderate CYP2D6 inhibitors.

ACTION

Competitively binds to estrogen receptors on tumor, producing a complex. **Therapeutic Effect:** Inhibits DNA synthesis and estrogen effects. Slows tumor growth.

PHARMACOKINETICS

Well absorbed from GI tract. Metabolized in liver. Primarily excreted in feces. **Half-life:** 7 days.

T

LIFESPAN CONSIDERATIONS

Pregnancy/Lactation: If possible, avoid use during pregnancy, esp. first trimester. May cause fetal harm. Unknown if distributed in breast milk. Breastfeeding not recommended. Nonhormonal contraceptives recommended during therapy and for at least 2 mos after discontinuation. **Children:** Safe and effective in girls 2–10 yrs with McCune-Albright syndrome, precocious puberty. **Elderly:** No age-related precautions noted.

INTERACTIONS

DRUG: **Strong CYP3A4 inducers (e.g., carBAMazepine, phenytoin, rifAMPin)** may decrease concentration/effect. **Strong CYP3A4 inhibitors (e.g., clarithromycin, ketoconazole)** may increase concentration/effect. May increase anticoagulant effect of **warfarin.** May decrease effect of **anastrozole. Moderate/strong CYP2D6 inhibitors (e.g., FLUoxetine, sertraline)** may decrease efficacy and increase risk of breast cancer. **HERBAL:** **St. John's wort** may decrease concentration/effect. **FOOD:** None known. **LAB VALUES:** May increase serum cholesterol, calcium, triglycerides, AST, ALT.

AVAILABILITY (Rx)

Solution, Oral: ***(Soltamox):*** 10 mg/5 mL. **Tablets:** 10 mg, 20 mg.

ADMINISTRATION/HANDLING

PO

• Give without regard to food. • Use supplied dosing cup for oral solution.

INDICATIONS/ROUTES/DOSAGE

Metastatic Breast Cancer (Males and females)

PO: ADULTS, ELDERLY: 20–40 mg/day. Give doses greater than 20 mg/day in 2 divided doses. **Premenopausal:** Tamoxifen may be given (with ovarian suppression) in pts with no prior endocrine therapy or prior treatment with ovarian suppression and an AI. **Postmenopausal:** Tamoxifen may be given in pts with no prior endocrine therapy or prior endocrine therapy with an AI.

Breast Cancer Treatment

PO: ADJUVANT THERAPY (FEMALES), PREMENOPAUSAL WOMEN: 20 mg once daily for 5 yrs. May continue for total of 10 yrs if premenopausal or perimenopausal after 5 yrs. If postmenopausal after 5 yrs, may continue for total of 10 yrs or switch to an AI up to total of 10 yrs of endocrine therapy. **POSTMENOPAUSAL WOMEN:** Total duration of 10 yrs, or tamoxifen for an initial duration of 5 yrs, followed by an AI for up to 5 yrs (for total duration of 10 yrs) or tamoxifen for 2–3 yrs, followed by an AI for up to 5 yrs (for a total duration of 7–8 yrs) or an AI for 5 yrs.

Ductal Carcinoma in Situ (DCIS)

PO: ADULTS, ELDERLY: 20 mg once daily for 5 yrs.

Breast Cancer Risk Reduction

PO: ADULTS, ELDERLY: 20 mg once daily for 5 yrs.

Dosage in Renal/Hepatic Impairment

No dose adjustment.

SIDE EFFECTS

Frequent: Women (greater than 10%): Hot flashes, nausea, vomiting. **Occasional:** Headache, nausea, vomiting, rash, bone pain, confusion, weakness, drowsiness. **Women (9%–1%):** Changes in menstruation, genital itching, vaginal discharge, endometrial hyperplasia, polyps. **Men:** Impotence, decreased libido.

ADVERSE EFFECTS/TOXIC REACTIONS

Retinopathy, corneal opacity, decreased visual acuity noted in pts receiving extremely high dosages (240–320 mg/day) for longer than 17 mos.

NURSING CONSIDERATIONS

BASELINE ASSESSMENT

Obtain CBC, serum calcium, estrogen receptor assay prior to therapy. Obtain baseline breast and gynecologic exams, mammogram results. Question history of thrombosis (DVT, PE).

INTERVENTION/EVALUATION

Obtain CBC, serum calcium periodically. Monitor for increased bone pain; ensure adequate pain relief. Monitor I&O, weight. Monitor for symptoms of DVT (leg or arm pain/swelling), PE (chest pain, dyspnea, tachycardia). Assess for hypercalcemia (increased urinary volume, excessive thirst, nausea, vomiting, constipation, hypotonicity of muscles, deep bone/flank pain, renal stones).

PATIENT/FAMILY TEACHING

• Report vaginal bleeding/discharge/itching, leg cramps, weight gain, shortness of breath, weakness. • May initially experience increase in bone, tumor pain (appears to indicate good tumor response). • Report persistent nausea, vomiting. • Report symptoms of DVT (e.g., swelling, pain, hot feeling in the arms or legs; discoloration of extremity), lung embolism (e.g., difficulty breathing, chest pain, rapid heart rate). • Nonhormonal contraceptives are recommended during treatment.

tamsulosin

tam-**soo**-loe-sin
(Flomax, Flomax CR✱)

Do not confuse Flomax with Flonase, Flovent, Foltx, Fosamax, or Volmax, or tamsulosin with tamoxifen or terazosin.

FIXED-COMBINATION(S)

Jalyn: tamsulosin/dutasteride (an androgen hormone inhibitor): 0.4 mg/0.5 mg.

◆CLASSIFICATION

PHARMACOTHERAPEUTIC: Alpha$_1$-adrenergic blocker. **CLINICAL:** Benign prostatic hyperplasia agent.

USES

Treatment of symptoms of benign prostatic hyperplasia (BPH). **OFF-LABEL:** Treatment of bladder outlet obstruction or dysfunction. To facilitate expulsion of ureteral stones (distal).

PRECAUTIONS

Contraindications: Hypersensitivity to tamsulosin. **Cautions:** Concurrent use

T

of phosphodiesterase (PDE5) inhibitors (e.g., sildenafil, tadalafil, vardenafil), baseline orthostatic hypotension.

ACTION

Antagonist of alpha receptors in prostate. **Therapeutic Effect:** Relaxes smooth muscle in bladder neck and prostate; improves urinary flow, symptoms of prostatic hyperplasia.

PHARMACOKINETICS

Widely distributed. Protein binding: 94%–99%. Metabolized in liver. Primarily excreted in urine. Unknown if removed by hemodialysis. **Half-life:** 9–13 hrs.

LIFESPAN CONSIDERATIONS

Pregnancy/Lactation: Not indicated for use in women. **Children:** Not indicated in this pt population. **Elderly:** No age-related precautions noted.

INTERACTIONS

DRUG: **Other alpha-adrenergic blocking agents (e.g., doxazosin, prazosin, terazosin)** may increase alpha-blockade effects. **Sildenafil, tadalafil, vardenafil** may cause symptomatic hypotension. **Strong CYP3A4 inhibitors (e.g., clarithromycin, ketoconazole, ritonavir)** may increase concentration/effect. **Strong CYP3A4 inducers (e.g., carBAMazepine, phenytoin, rifAMPin)** may decrease concentration/effect. **HERBAL:** **Herbals with hypotensive properties (e.g., garlic, ginger, ginkgo biloba)** may alter effects. **St. John's wort** may decrease concentration/effect. **FOOD:** **Grapefruit products** may increase risk for orthostatic hypotension. **LAB VALUES:** None known.

AVAILABILITY (Rx)

Capsules: 0.4 mg.

ADMINISTRATION/HANDLING

PO

- Give at same time each day, 30 min after the same meal. • Do not break, crush, or open capsule.

INDICATIONS/ROUTES/DOSAGE

Benign Prostatic Hyperplasia (BPH)

PO: ADULTS: 0.4 mg once daily, approximately 30 min after same meal each day. May increase dosage to 0.8 mg if inadequate response in 2–4 wks. If therapy discontinued or interrupted for several days, restart at 0.4 mg once daily.

Dosage in Renal/Hepatic Impairment

No dose adjustment.

SIDE EFFECTS

Frequent (9%–7%): Dizziness, drowsiness. **Occasional (5%–3%):** Headache, anxiety, insomnia, orthostatic hypotension. **Rare (less than 2%):** Nasal congestion, pharyngitis, rhinitis, nausea, vertigo, impotence.

ADVERSE EFFECTS/TOXIC REACTIONS

First-dose syncope (hypotension with sudden loss of consciousness) may occur within 30–90 min after initial dose. May be preceded by tachycardia (pulse rate of 120–160 beats/min).

NURSING CONSIDERATIONS

BASELINE ASSESSMENT

Obtain vital signs. Assess history of prostatic hyperplasia (difficulty initiating urine stream, dribbling, sense of urgency, leaking). Question for sensitivity to tamsulosin, or use of other alpha-adrenergic blocking agents.

INTERVENTION/EVALUATION

Assist with ambulation if dizziness occurs. Monitor renal function, I&O, weight changes, peripheral edema, B/P. Monitor for first-dose syncope.

PATIENT/FAMILY TEACHING

- Take at same time each day, 30 min after the same meal. • Go from lying to standing slowly. • Avoid tasks that require alertness, motor skills until response to drug is established. • Avoid grapefruit products.

T

tapentadol

ta-**pen**-ta-dol
(Nucynta, Nucynta ER, Nucynta IR ✦)

BLACK BOX ALERT

Exposes pt to risks of opioid addiction, abuse, misuse. Serious, life-threatening respiratory depression may occur. Accidental ingestion can result in a fatal overdose. May cause neonatal opioid withdrawal syndrome. Avoid alcohol while taking tapentadol ER. Benzodiazepines, CNS depressants may cause profound sedation, respiratory depression, coma, or death. **Do not confuse tapentadol with traMADol.**

◆CLASSIFICATION

PHARMACOTHERAPEUTIC: Centrally acting opioid (Schedule II). **CLINICAL:** Analgesic.

USES

Nucynta: Relief of moderate to severe acute pain in adults 18 yrs and older. **Nucynta ER:** Management of moderate to severe chronic or neuropathic pain associated with diabetic peripheral neuropathy when around-the-clock analgesic is needed for extended period.

PRECAUTIONS

Contraindications: Hypersensitivity to tapentadol. Severe respiratory depression, acute or severe bronchial asthma, hypercapnia in uncontrolled settings, known or suspected paralytic ileus, concurrent use or ingestion within 14 days of MAOI use. **Cautions:** Respiratory disease or respiratory compromise (e.g., hypoxia, hypercapnia, or decreased respiratory reserve), asthma, COPD, severe obesity, sleep apnea syndrome, CNS depression; history of drug abuse and misuse, drug-seeking behavior, dependency; head injury, intracranial lesions, pancreatic or biliary disease, renal or hepatic impairment, seizure disorder; baseline hypotension, adrenal insufficiency, elderly, debilitated, cachexia; concomitant use with serotonergic agents.

ACTION

Binds to mu-opioid receptors in the central nervous system, causing inhibition of ascending pain pathways; increases norepinephrine by inhibiting its reabsorption into nerve cells. **Therapeutic Effect:** Produces analgesia. Reduces level of pain perception.

PHARMACOKINETICS

Widely distributed. Metabolized in liver. Protein binding: 20%. Excreted in urine (99%). **Half-life:** 4 hrs (immediate-release); 5–6 hrs (extended-release).

LIFESPAN CONSIDERATIONS

Pregnancy/Lactation: Unknown if drug crosses placenta or is distributed in breast milk. **Children:** Not recommended for use in this pt population. **Elderly:** Age-related renal impairment may increase risk of side effects.

INTERACTIONS

DRUG: **Alcohol, CNS depressants (e.g., LORazepam, morphine, zolpidem)** may increase CNS depression, respiratory depression. **MAOIs (e.g., phenelzine, selegiline), SSRIs (e.g., FLUoxetine)** may increase risk of serotonin syndrome. **HERBAL:** **Herbals with sedative properties (e.g., chamomile, kava kava, valerian)** may increase CNS depression. **FOOD:** None known. **LAB VALUES:** None significant.

AVAILABILITY (Rx)

Tablets: 50 mg, 75 mg, 100 mg.

Tablets, Extended-Release: 50 mg, 100 mg, 150 mg, 200 mg, 250 mg.

ADMINISTRATION/HANDLING

PO

• Give without regard to food. • Tablets may be crushed. • Give extended-release tablets whole; do not break, crush, dissolve, or divide.

INDICATIONS/ROUTES/DOSAGE

Note: Not recommended in severe renal or hepatic impairment.

Pain Control

PO: ADULTS, ELDERLY: ***(Nucynta):*** 50–100 mg q4–6h as needed (may administer an additional dose 1h or longer after initial dose). **Maximum:** 600 mg/day (700 mg on day 1). ***(Nucynta ER):*** Initially, 50 mg twice daily (12 hrs apart). May increase by 50 mg twice daily q3days to effective dose. Range: 100–250 mg twice daily. **Maximum:** 500 mg/day.

Conversion to Extended-Release

Conversion from other oral opioids: Initially, 50 mg q12h. ***(Immediate-Release Tapentadol):*** Use same total daily dose but divide into 2 equal doses given twice daily. **Maximum:** 500 mg daily.

Neuropathic Pain Associated With Diabetic Peripheral Neuropathy

PO: ADULTS, ELDERLY: ***(Extended-Release):*** Initially, 50 mg q12h. Titrate in increments of 50 mg no more frequently than twice daily q3days. Range: 100–250 mg q12h.

Dosage in Renal Impairment

CrCl 30 mL/min or greater: No adjustment. **CrCl less than 30 mL/min:** Not recommended.

Dosage in Hepatic Impairment

(Immediate-Release): Moderate impairment: 50 mg q8h. **Maximum:** 3 doses/24 hrs. ***(Extended-Release):*** Initially, 50 mg/day. **Maximum:** 100 mg/day.

SIDE EFFECTS

Frequent (greater than 10%): Nausea, dizziness, vomiting, sleepiness, headache.

ADVERSE EFFECTS/TOXIC REACTIONS

Respiratory depression, serotonin syndrome have been reported.

NURSING CONSIDERATIONS

BASELINE ASSESSMENT

Assess onset, type, location, and duration of pain. Obtain vital signs. If respirations are 12/min or lower, withhold medication, contact physician. Question medical history as listed in Precautions. Assess for potential of abuse/misuse (e.g., drug-seeking behavior, mental health conditions, history of substance abuse).

INTERVENTION/EVALUATION

Monitor for decreased respirations or B/P. Initiate deep breathing and coughing exercises, particularly in pts with impaired pulmonary function. Assess for clinical improvement and record onset of pain relief. Screen for drug abuse and misuse, drug-seeking behavior.

PATIENT/FAMILY TEACHING

• Avoid tasks that require alertness, motor skills until response to drug is established. • Avoid alcohol, CNS depressants. • Report nausea, vomiting, shortness of breath, difficulty breathing. • Chronic use may increase risk of opioid dependency, addiction.

telavancin

tel-a-**van**-sin
(Vibativ)

BLACK BOX ALERT Pts with preexisting renal impairment (CrCl less than 50 mL/min) who are treated for hospital-acquired pneumonia may have increased mortality risk when compared to vancomycin. May cause new or worsening renal impairment. May cause fetal harm (low birth weight, limb malformations). Women of childbearing potential should have pregnancy test before treatment; avoid use during pregnancy unless benefit to pt outweighs fetal risk.

Do not confuse telavancin with dalbavancin or oritavancin; or Vibativ with Vibra-Tabs or vigabatrin.

◆ CLASSIFICATION

PHARMACOTHERAPEUTIC: Lipoglycopeptide antibacterial. **CLINICAL:** Antibiotic.

USES

Treatment of complicated skin, soft tissue infections (cSSSI) caused by gram-positive microorganisms, including methicillin-susceptible or methicillin-resistant *S. aureus*, vancomycin-susceptible *Enterococcus*. Treatment of hospital-acquired and ventilator-associated bacterial pneumonia (HABP/VABP) caused by susceptible isolates of *S. aureus*.

PRECAUTIONS

Contraindications: Prior hypersensitivity reactions to telavancin. Concomitant use of IV unfractionated heparin. **Cautions:** Renal impairment (CrCl 50 mL/min or less), concomitant use of other nephrotoxic medications (e.g., NSAIDs, ACE inhibitors, aminoglycosides). Avoid use in pts with history of congenital QT syndrome, known prolongation of QT interval, uncompensated HF, severe left ventricular hypertrophy, or receiving treatment with other drugs known to prolong QT interval, hypokalemia, hypomagnesemia; known vancomycin hypersensitivity.

ACTION

Inhibits bacterial cell wall synthesis by blocking polymerization and cross-linking of peptidoglycan. Disrupts membrane potential and changes cell wall permeability. **Therapeutic Effect:** Bactericidal. Antibiotic.

PHARMACOKINETICS

Not metabolized in liver; pathway unspecified. Protein binding: 90%. Primarily excreted unchanged in urine. Not removed by hemodialysis. **Half-life:** 8–9 hrs.

LIFESPAN CONSIDERATIONS

Pregnancy/Lactation: May cause fetal harm at regular dosage. Unknown if distributed in breast milk. **Children:** Safety and efficacy not established. **Elderly:** Age-related renal impairment may increase risk of nephrotoxicity; dosage adjustment recommended.

INTERACTIONS

DRUG: **QT interval–prolonging medications (e.g., amiodarone, azithromycin, ciprofloxacin, haloperidol, methadone, sotalol)** may increase risk of QTc interval prolongation, cardiac arrhythmias. May decrease therapeutic effect of **heparin.** **HERBAL:** None significant. **FOOD:** None known. **LAB VALUES:** May alter serum potassium. May increase serum bilirubin, ALT, AST, BUN, creatinine; PT, aPTT, INR. May decrease Hgb, Hct, WBC count.

AVAILABILITY (Rx)

Injection, Powder for Reconstitution: 750 mg.

ADMINISTRATION/HANDLING

IV

◄ALERT► Give by intermittent IV infusion (piggyback). Do not give by IV push (may result in hypotension).

Reconstitution • Reconstitute with 45 mL Sterile Water for Injection, D_5W, or 0.9% NaCl to provide concentration of 15 mg/mL (total volume approximately 50 mL). • Prior to administration, further dilute with D_5W or 0.9% NaCl to final concentration of 0.6–8 mg/mL. • Do not shake.

Rate of administration • Infuse over at least 60 min. Flush line with D_5W or 0.9% NaCl before and after administration.

Storage • Discard if particulate is present. • Diluted solution is stable for 4 hrs at room temperature or 72 hrs if refrigerated in vial or infusion bag.

IV INCOMPATIBILITIES

Amphotericin, colistimethate, levoFLOXacin (Levaquin), micafungin (Mycomine).

IV COMPATIBILITIES

Azithromycin, caspofungin, cefepime, cefTAZidime, cefTRIAXone, ciprofloxa-

T

cin, doripenem, doxycycline, gentamicin, ertapenem, fluconazole, meropenem, tobramycin, pantoprazole, piperacillin-tazobactam, tigecycline.

INDICATIONS/ROUTES/DOSAGE

Usual Parenteral Dosage

IV infusion: ADULTS, ELDERLY: 10 mg/kg once every 24 hrs for 7–14 days (cSSSI); 7–21 days (HABP/VABP). Duration based on severity, infection site, and clinical progress of pt.

Dosage in Renal Impairment

Creatinine Clearance	Dosage
50 mL/min or greater	10 mg/kg every 24 hrs
30–49 mL/min	7.5 mg/kg every 24 hrs
10–29 mL/min	10 mg/kg every 48 hrs
Less than 10 mL/min	No dose adjustment (not studied)

Dosage in Hepatic Impairment

No dose adjustment (unless concomitant renal impairment).

SIDE EFFECTS

Frequent (33%–27%): Altered taste, nausea. **Occasional (14%–6%):** Vomiting, foamy urine, diarrhea, dizziness, pruritus. **Rare (4%–2%):** Rigors, rash, infusion site pain, anorexia, infusion site erythema.

T

ADVERSE EFFECTS/TOXIC REACTIONS

Nephrotoxicity (acute kidney injury, acute tubular necrosis, renal failure), diarrhea due to *C. difficile* may occur. "Red-man syndrome" (characterized by erythema on face, neck, upper torso), tachycardia, hypotension, myalgia, angioedema may occur from too-rapid rate of infusion. May cause QT interval prolongation.

NURSING CONSIDERATIONS

BASELINE ASSESSMENT

Obtain pregnancy test in females of reproductive potential. Obtain baseline serum BUN, creatinine, creatinine clearance prior to initiating therapy, every 48–72 hrs, and after treatment is completed. Obtain culture and sensitivity tests before giving first dose (therapy may begin before results are known). Question history of renal impairment, long QT interval syndrome, HF.

INTERVENTION/EVALUATION

Monitor renal function tests, I&O. Assess skin for rash. Avoid rapid infusion ("red-man syndrome"). Monitor daily pattern of bowel activity, stool consistency. Obtain *C. difficile* PCR test if diarrhea occurs. Monitor ECG for QT interval prolongation, cardiac arrhythmias.

PATIENT/FAMILY TEACHING

• Use effective contraception during treatment. • Report rash, signs/symptoms of nephrotoxicity, diarrhea. • Report chest pain, irregular heart rhythm, palpitations, passing out.

telmisartan

tel-mi-**sar**-tan

(Apo-Telmisartan 🍁, Micardis)

BLACK BOX ALERT May cause fetal injury, mortality. Discontinue as soon as possible once pregnancy is detected.

FIXED-COMBINATION(S)

Micardis HCT: telmisartan/hydroCHLOROthiazide (a diuretic): 40 mg/12.5 mg, 80 mg/12.5 mg. **Twynsta:** telmisartan/amLODIPine (a calcium channel blocker): 40 mg/5 mg, 40 mg/10 mg, 80 mg/5 mg, 80 mg/10 mg.

◆CLASSIFICATION

PHARMACOTHERAPEUTIC: Angiotensin II receptor antagonist. **CLINICAL:** Antihypertensive.

USES

Treatment of hypertension alone or in combination with other antihypertensives. Reduces cardiovascular risk in pts 55 yrs of age and older unable to take ACE inhibitors and at high risk of major cardiovascular event (e.g., MI, stroke).

PRECAUTIONS

Contraindications: Hypersensitivity to telmisartan. Concurrent use with aliskiren in pts with diabetes. **Cautions:** Hypovolemia, hyperkalemia, hepatic/renal impairment, renal artery stenosis (unilateral, bilateral), biliary obstructive disease, significant aortic/mitral stenosis. Concurrent use with ramipril not recommended. Avoid potassium supplements.

ACTION

Blocks vasoconstrictor and aldosterone-secreting effects of angiotensin II, inhibiting binding of angiotensin II to AT_1 receptors. **Therapeutic Effect:** Causes vasodilation, decreases peripheral resistance, decreases B/P.

PHARMACOKINETICS

Widely distributed. Protein binding: greater than 99%. Metabolized in liver. Excreted in feces. **Half-life:** 24 hrs.

LIFESPAN CONSIDERATIONS

Pregnancy/Lactation: May cause fetal harm. Unknown if distributed in breast milk. **Children:** Safety and efficacy not established. **Elderly:** No age-related precautions noted.

INTERACTIONS

DRUG: NSAIDs (e.g., diclofenac, meloxicam, naproxen) may increase adverse effects. May increase **lithium** concentration, risk of toxicity. **Aliskiren** may increase hyperkalemic effect. May increase adverse effect/toxicity of **ACE inhibitors (e.g., benazepril, lisinopril, ramipril). HERBAL: Herbals with hypertensive properties (e.g., licorice, yohimbe) or hypotensive properties (e.g., garlic, ginger, ginkgo biloba)** may alter effects. **FOOD:** None known. **LAB VALUES:** May increase serum BUN, creatinine, uric acid, cholesterol. May decrease Hgb, Hct.

AVAILABILITY (Rx)

Tablets: 20 mg, 40 mg, 80 mg.

ADMINISTRATION/HANDLING

PO

- Give without regard to food.

INDICATIONS/ROUTES/DOSAGE

Hypertension

PO: ADULTS, ELDERLY: Initially, 20–40 mg once daily. Titrate based on pt's response up to 80 mg once daily.

Cardiovascular Risk Reduction

PO: ADULTS, ELDERLY: 80 mg once daily.

Dosage in Renal Impairment

No dose adjustment.

Dosage in Hepatic Impairment

Use with caution.

SIDE EFFECTS

Occasional (7%–3%): Upper respiratory tract infection, sinusitis, back/leg pain, diarrhea. **Rare (1%):** Dizziness, headache, fatigue, nausea, heartburn, myalgia, cough, peripheral edema.

ADVERSE EFFECTS/TOXIC REACTIONS

Overdosage may manifest as hypotension, tachycardia; bradycardia occurs less often.

NURSING CONSIDERATIONS

BASELINE ASSESSMENT

Obtain renal function test. Obtain B/P, heart rate immediately before each dose, in addition to regular monitoring (be alert to fluctuations). Assess medication history (esp. diuretics). Question for history of hepatic/renal impairment, renal artery stenosis.

INTERVENTION/EVALUATION

Monitor B/P, pulse, serum electrolytes, renal function.

T

PATIENT/FAMILY TEACHING

Report symptoms of low blood pressure (pale, clammy skin; dizziness, fainting, weakness). • Maintain proper hydration. • Avoid pregnancy. • Immediately report suspected pregnancy. • Avoid excessive exertion during hot weather (risk of dehydration, hypotension).

temozolomide

HIGH ALERT

tem-oh-**zoe**-loe-myde
(Temodal ✱, Temodar)
Do not confuse Temodar with Tambocor.

◆CLASSIFICATION

PHARMACOTHERAPEUTIC: Imidazotetrazine derivative, alkylating agent. **CLINICAL:** Antineoplastic.

USES

Treatment of adults with refractory anaplastic astrocytoma, newly diagnosed glioblastoma multiforme (concomitantly with radiotherapy, then as maintenance therapy). **OFF-LABEL:** Malignant glioma, metastatic melanoma, metastatic CNS lesions, cutaneous T-cell lymphomas, advanced neuroendocrine tumors, soft tissue sarcoma, pediatric neuroblastoma. Ewing's sarcoma (recurrent or progressive).

PRECAUTIONS

Contraindications: Hypersensitivity to temozolomide, dacarbazine. **Cautions:** Baseline cytopenias, severe hepatic/renal impairment, pulmonary disease, seizure disorder, hypothyroidism, conditions predisposing to infection (e.g., diabetes, immunocompromised pts, renal failure, open wounds); history of chronic opportunistic infections (bacterial, fungal, protozoal, viral).

ACTION

Produces cytotoxic effect through alkylation of DNA, causing DNA double strand breaks and apoptosis. **Therapeutic Effect:** Inhibits DNA replication, causing cell death.

PHARMACOKINETICS

Widely distributed. Penetrates blood-brain barrier. Metabolized via hydrolysis. Protein binding: 15%. Peak plasma concentration: 1 hr. Excreted in urine (38%), feces (less than 1%). **Half-life:** 1.6–1.8 hrs.

⧗ LIFESPAN CONSIDERATIONS

Pregnancy/Lactation: Avoid pregnancy; may cause fetal harm. Females of reproductive potential must use effective contraception during treatment and for at least 6 mos after discontinuation. Breastfeeding not recommended during treatment and for at least 1 wk after discontinuation. **Males:** Males with female partners of reproductive potential must use effective contraception and must not donate sperm during treatment and for at least 3 mos after discontinuation. May impair fertility. **Children:** Safety and efficacy not established. **Elderly:** Pts older than 70 yrs may experience higher risk of developing Grade 4 neutropenia, thrombocytopenia.

INTERACTIONS

DRUG: **Valproic acid** may increase adverse effects. **Bone marrow depressants (e.g., cladribine)** may increase myelosuppression. **Live virus vaccines** may potentiate virus replication, increase vaccine side effects, decrease pt's antibody response to vaccine. **HERBAL:** **Echinacea** may decrease effects. **FOOD:** **All foods** decrease rate, extent of drug absorption. **LAB VALUES:** May decrease Hgb, neutrophils, platelets, WBC count, lymphocytes.

AVAILABILITY (Rx)

Capsules: 5 mg, 20 mg, 100 mg, 140 mg, 180 mg, 250 mg. **Injection, Powder for Reconstitution:** 100 mg.

ADMINISTRATION/HANDLING

IV

• Reconstitute each 100-mg vial with 41 mL Sterile Water for Injection to provide concentration of 2.5 mg/mL. • Swirl gently; do not shake. • Do NOT further dilute. • Infuse over 90 min. • Stable for 14 hrs (includes infusion time).

PO

• High-fat food reduces absorption; increases risk of nausea, vomiting. • For best results, administer at bedtime. • Give capsule whole with water. Do not break, open, or crush capsules.

INDICATIONS/ROUTES/DOSAGE

Anaplastic Astrocytoma (Refractory)

IV infusion, PO: ADULTS, ELDERLY: Initially, 150 mg/m²/day for 5 consecutive days of 28-day treatment cycle. Subsequent doses of 100–200 mg/m²/day based on platelet count, absolute neutrophil count (ANC) during previous cycle. **Maintenance:** 200 mg/m²/day for 5 days q4wks if ANC greater than 1,500 cells/mm³ and platelets more than 100,000 cells/mm³. Continue until disease progression is observed. Minimum: 100 mg/m²/day for 5 days q4wks.

Glioblastoma Multiforme

Note: ***Pneumocystis carinii*** pneumonia (PCP) prophylaxis required during concomitant phase and continue in pts who develop lymphocytopenia until recovery to Grade 1 or less. **IV infusion, PO: ADULTS, ELDERLY: Concomitant phase:** 75 mg/m² daily for 42 days (with focal radiotherapy) if ANC 1,500 cells/mm³ or greater, platelet count 100,000 cells/mm³ or greater, and nonhematologic toxicity Grade 1 or less. **Maintenance phase: (begin 4 wks after concomitant phase completion): (Cycle 1):** 150 mg/m² once daily for 5 days followed by 23 days without treatment. **(Cycles 2–6):** May increase to 200 mg/m² once daily for 5 days followed by 23 days without treatment if ANC greater than 1,500 cells/mm³, platelets greater than 100,000 cells/mm³, and nonhematologic toxicity with previous cycle is Grade 2 or less (exclude alopecia, nausea, vomiting).

Dosage in Renal/Hepatic Impairment

Mild to moderate impairment: No dose adjustment. **Severe impairment:** Not specified; use caution.

SIDE EFFECTS

Frequent (53%–33%): Nausea, vomiting, headache, fatigue, constipation. **Occasional (16%–5%):** Diarrhea, asthenia, pyrexia, dizziness, peripheral edema, coordination abnormality, amnesia, insomnia, anorexia, abdominal pain, back pain, paresthesia, somnolence, paresis, urinary incontinence, ataxia, rash, pruritus, dysphagia, anxiety, abnormal gait, increased urination, breast pain, confusion, weight increase, myalgia, diplopia, vision changes.

ADVERSE EFFECTS/TOXIC REACTIONS

Myelosuppression (anemia, leukopenia, pancytopenia) is an expected response to therapy, but fatal outcomes were reported. Elderly pts and women showing higher incidence of developing severe myelosuppression. Usually occurs within first few cycles; is not cumulative. Nadir occurs in approximately 26–28 days, with recovery within 14 days of nadir. Prolonged pancytopenia may result in aplastic anemia, which can be fatal. May increase occurrence of *Pneumocystis carinii* pneumonia, myelodysplastic syndrome including myeloid leukemia, or secondary malignancies. Fatal infections including bacterial, fungal, protozoal, viral (new or chronic) infections may occur. Upper respiratory tract infections, pharyngitis, sinusitis reported in 6%–8% of pts. Convulsion reported in 23% of pts. Adrenal hypercorticism reported in 8% of pts. Skin toxicities including Stevens-Johnson syndrome, toxic epidermal necrolysis may occur. Fatal hepatotoxicity, hyperbilirubinemia, cholestasis,

T

hepatitis may occur. May cause *Pneumocystis carinii* pneumonia, myelodysplastic syndrome (including myeloid leukemia), secondary malignancies, interstitial lung disease, pneumonitis, alveolitis, pulmonary fibrosis, diabetes insipidus.

NURSING CONSIDERATIONS

BASELINE ASSESSMENT

Obtain CBC, LFT; pregnancy test in females of reproductive potential. ANC must be greater than 1500 cells/mm^3 and platelet count greater than 100,000 cells/mm^3. Question history of seizure disorder, pulmonary disease. Screen for active infection, dormant opportunistic infections. Offer emotional support.

INTERVENTION/EVALUATION

Obtain CBC on day 22 (21 days after first dose) or within 48 hrs of that day, and wkly, until ANC is greater than 1,500 cells/mm^3 and platelet count is greater than 100,000 cells/mm^3. Monitor LFT for hepatic injury (abdominal pain, jaundice, nausea, transaminitis, vomiting). Assess skin for cutaneous toxicities. Monitor for infection (cough, fatigue, fever), myelodysplastic syndrome (bone pain, decreased appetite, fatigue, fever; unusual bruising, bleeding). Consider ABG, radiologic test if ILD/pneumonitis (excessive cough, dyspnea, fever, hypoxia) is suspected. Consider treatment with corticosteroids if ILD/pneumonitis is confirmed.

PATIENT/FAMILY TEACHING

• Treatment may depress your immune system response and reduce your ability to fight infection. Report symptoms of infection such as body aches, chills, cough, fatigue, fever. Avoid those with active infection. • Report symptoms of bone marrow depression (e.g., bruising, fatigue, fever, shortness of breath, weight loss; bleeding easily, bloody urine or stool). • Report symptoms of lung inflammation (excessive coughing, difficulty breathing, chest pain); liver problems (abdominal pain, bruising, clay-colored stool, dark or amber-colored urine, yellowing of the skin or eyes), toxic skin reactions (rash, redness, sloughing, swelling). • Use effective contraception to avoid pregnancy. Do not breastfeed. • Maintain proper hydration and nutrition. • Do not take newly prescribed medications unless approved by prescriber who originally started treatment. • Secondary cancers may occur.

temsirolimus

HIGH ALERT

tem-sir-**oh**-li-mus
(Torisel)
Do not confuse temsirolimus with everolimus, sirolimus, or tacrolimus.

◆CLASSIFICATION

PHARMACOTHERAPEUTIC: mTOR kinase inhibitor. **CLINICAL:** Antineoplastic.

USES

Treatment of advanced renal cell carcinoma.

PRECAUTIONS

Contraindications: Hypersensitivity to temsirolimus. Moderate to severe hepatic impairment; serum bilirubin greater than 1.5 times upper limit of normal (ULN). **Cautions:** Hypersensitivity to sirolimus, hepatic/renal impairment, baseline cytopenias, pulmonary disease, conditions predisposing to infection (e.g., diabetes, renal failure, immunocompromised pts, open wounds), pts at risk for GI perforation (e.g., Crohn's disease, diverticulitis, GI tract malignancies, peptic ulcers, peritoneal malignancies), thrombosis (immobility, indwelling venous catheter/access device, morbid obesity, genetic hypercoagulable conditions); history of chronic opportunistic infections (esp. bacterial, invasive fungal, mycobacterial, protozoal, viral, TB); poorly healed wounds/recent incisions, diabetes, hyperlipidemia. Concurrent use with other medication that may cause angioedema (e.g., ACE inhibitors).

ACTION

Binds to FKBP12, an intracellular protein–forming complex that inhibits mTOR signaling, arresting the cell cycle at G1 phase in tumor cells. **Therapeutic Effect:** Inhibits tumor cell growth, produces tumor regression.

PHARMACOKINETICS

Metabolized in liver. Excreted in feces (78%), urine (5%). **Half-life:** 17 hrs.

LIFESPAN CONSIDERATIONS

Pregnancy/Lactation: Avoid pregnancy; may cause fetal harm. Females and males with female partners of reproductive potential must use effective contraception during treatment and for at least 3 mos after discontinuation. Breastfeeding not recommended during treatment and for at least 3 wks after discontinuation. May impair fertility in both females and males. **Children:** Safety and efficacy not established. **Elderly:** May have increased risk of adverse reactions.

INTERACTIONS

DRUG: **CYP3A4 inhibitors (e.g., clarithromycin, ketoconazole, ritonavir)** may increase concentration/effect. **CYP3A4 inducers (e.g., carBAMazepine, phenytoin, rifAMPin)** may decrease concentration/effect. May decrease therapeutic effect; increase adverse effects of **vaccines (live)**. **HERBAL:** **St. John's wort** may decrease concentration/effect. **Echinacea** may decrease therapeutic effect. **FOOD:** **Grapefruit products** may increase plasma concentration/effect. **LAB VALUES:** May increase serum alkaline phosphatase, AST, bilirubin, creatinine, glucose, cholesterol, triglycerides. May decrease Hgb, leukocytes, lymphocytes, neutrophils, platelets; serum phosphorus, potassium.

AVAILABILITY (Rx)

Injection Solution Kit: 25 mg/mL supplied with 1.8-mL diluent vial.

ADMINISTRATION/HANDLING

IV

Reconstitution • Inject 1.8 mL of diluent into vial. • The vial contains an overfill of 0.2 mL (30 mg/1.2 mL). • Due to the overfill, the drug concentration of resulting solution will be 10 mg/mL. • A total volume of 3 mL will be obtained, including the overfill. • Mix well by inverting the vial. Allow sufficient time for air bubbles to subside. • Dilute in 250 mL 0.9% NaCl. • Invert bag to mix; avoid excessive shaking (may cause foaming).

Rate of administration • Administer through an in-line filter not greater than 5 microns; infuse over 30–60 min. • Infusion should be completed within 6 hrs (includes preparation time).

Storage • Refrigerate kit. • Reconstituted solution appears clear to slightly turbid, colorless to yellow, and free from visible particulates. • The 10 mg/mL drug solution/diluent mixture is stable for up to 24 hrs at room temperature. • Solutions diluted for infusion (in 250 mL 0.9% NaCl) must be infused within 6 hrs of preparation.

IV INCOMPATIBILITIES

Both acids and bases degrade solution; combinations of temsirolimus with agents capable of modifying solution pH should be avoided.

INDICATIONS/ROUTES/DOSAGE

◀ALERT▶ Pretreat with IV diphenhydrAMINE 25–50 mg, 30 min before infusion.

Renal Cancer

IV: ADULTS/ELDERLY: 25 mg once wkly. Treatment should continue until disease progresses or unacceptable toxicity occurs.

Dose Modification

Concomitant CYP3A4 inhibitors: Consider dose of 12.5 mg/wk.

T

Concomitant CYP3A4 inducers: Consider dose of 50 mg/wk.

Dosage in Renal Impairment
No dose adjustment.

Dosage in Hepatic Impairment
Mild impairment: Reduce dose to 15 mg/wk. **Moderate to severe impairment:** Contraindicated.

SIDE EFFECTS

Common (51%–32%): Asthenia, rash, mucositis, nausea, edema (facial edema, peripheral edema), anorexia. **Frequent (28%–20%):** Generalized pain, dyspnea, diarrhea, cough, fever, abdominal pain, constipation, back pain, impaired taste. **Occasional (19%–8%):** Weight loss, vomiting, pruritus, chest pain, headache, nail disorder, insomnia, nosebleed, dry skin, acne, chills, myalgia.

ADVERSE EFFECTS/TOXIC REACTIONS

Hypersensitivity reactions including apnea, chest pain, dyspnea, flushing, hypotension, anaphylaxis may occur. May cause acute renal failure, deep vein thrombosis (DVT), GI perforation, hepatotoxicity, hyperglycemia/glucose intolerance, hyperlipidemia, proteinuria, nephrotic syndrome; fatal interstitial lung disease, pneumonitis. May impair healing of wounds. May increase risk of intracranial hemorrhage in pts with CNS tumors or receiving anticoagulation therapy.

T

NURSING CONSIDERATIONS

BASELINE ASSESSMENT

Obtain CBC, BMP, LFT; pregnancy test in females of reproductive potential. Screen for active infection. Question history of hepatic/renal impairment, latent chronic infections, thromboembolism. Receive full medication history and screen for interactions. Assess risk of bleeding. Assess skin for poorly healed wounds/recent surgery. Offer emotional support.

INTERVENTION/EVALUATION

Monitor CBC for myelosuppression, LFT for hepatic injury (abdominal pain, jaundice, nausea, transaminitis, vomiting); blood glucose for hyperglycemia (fatigue, Kussmaul respirations, polyphagia, polyuria, polydipsia, nausea, vomiting); lipid panel. Obtain urine protein periodically; proteinuria may indicate nephrotic syndrome. Monitor for infections (cough, fatigue, fever). Monitor daily pattern of bowel activity, stool consistency. Consider ABG, radiologic test if ILD/pneumonitis (excessive cough, dyspnea, fever, hypoxia) is suspected. Consider treatment with corticosteroids if ILD/pneumonitis is confirmed. Assess skin for impaired wound healing. Monitor for symptoms of DVT (leg or arm pain/swelling, redness), GI perforation (abdominal pain, fever, nausea, vomiting), hypersensitivity reactions (anaphylaxis, urticaria), bleeding of any kind. Assess oral cavity for stomatitis.

PATIENT/FAMILY TEACHING

• Treatment may depress your immune system response and reduce your ability to fight infection. Report symptoms of infection such as body aches, chills, cough, fatigue, fever. Avoid those with active infection. • Report symptoms of bone marrow depression (e.g., bruising, fatigue, fever, shortness of breath, weight loss; bleeding easily, bloody urine or stool). • Treatment may cause reactivation of chronic viral infections, new cancers. • Report symptoms of DVT (swelling, pain, hot feeling in the arms or legs; discoloration of extremity), lung inflammation (excessive coughing, difficulty breathing, chest pain); liver problems (abdominal pain, bruising, clay-colored stool, dark or amber-colored urine, yellowing of the skin or eyes), high blood sugar (fatigue, Kussmaul respirations, polyphagia, polyuria, polydipsia, nausea, vomiting), bleeding of any kind. • Immediately report severe or persistent abdominal pain, bloody stool, fever; may indicate rupture in GI tract. • Use effective contraception to avoid pregnancy. Do not breastfeed.

teriflunomide

ter-i-**floo**-noe-myde
(Aubagio)

■ BLACK BOX ALERT ■ May result in major birth defects. Pregnancy must be excluded before initiating therapy and must be avoided during treatment or prior to completion of an accelerated elimination procedure. Severe hepatic injury may occur. Do not initiate in pts with acute/chronic liver disease or serum ALT greater than 2 times upper limit of normal.

Do not confuse teriflunomide with leflunomide.

◆CLASSIFICATION

PHARMACOTHERAPEUTIC: Pyrimidine synthesis inhibitor, immunomodulatory agent. **CLINICAL:** Multiple sclerosis agent.

USES

Treatment of relapsing forms of multiple sclerosis, including clinically isolated syndrome, relapsing-remitting disease, and active secondary progressive disease.

PRECAUTIONS

Contraindications: Hypersensitivity to teriflunomide, leflunomide. Pregnant women or women of childbearing potential who are not using reliable contraception, severe hepatic impairment, concurrent use of leflunomide. **Cautions:** Baseline cytopenias, diabetes, pts older than 60 yrs, pulmonary disease, mild to moderate hepatic disease; conditions predisposing to infection (e.g., diabetes, renal failure, immunocompromised pts, open wounds); history of chronic opportunistic infections (esp. fungal/viral infections, TB); concomitant use of nephrotoxic medications. Not recommended in pts with severe immunodeficiency, bone marrow disease; severe, active infection. Do not initiate in pts with active or chronic infections until resolved.

ACTION

Inhibits pyrimidine synthesis, exhibiting anti-inflammatory and antiproliferative properties. **Therapeutic Effect:** May reduce number of activated lymphocytes in the CNS. May slow progression of multiple sclerosis.

PHARMACOKINETICS

Widely distributed. Peak concentration: 1–4 hrs. Protein binding: greater than 99%. Metabolized by hydrolysis. Excreted in urine (23%), feces (38%). **Half-life:** 18–19 days.

⌛ LIFESPAN CONSIDERATIONS

Pregnancy/Lactation: Avoid pregnancy; may cause fetal harm. Females and males with female partners of reproductive potential must use effective contraception during treatment and until plasma drug concentrations are at least 0.02 mg/L following accelerated elimination procedure. Breastfeeding not recommended. **Children:** Safety and efficacy not established. **Elderly:** No age-related precautions noted.

INTERACTIONS

DRUG: May increase concentration/effects of **CYP2C8 substrates (e.g., repaglinide, PACLitaxel, rosuvastatin, topotecan).** May decrease concentration/effects of **warfarin, CYP1A2 substrates (e.g., DULoxetine, tiZANidine).** May decrease therapeutic effect; increase adverse effects of **vaccines (live). HERBAL: Echinacea** may decrease therapeutic effect. **FOOD:** None known. **LAB VALUES:** May increase serum potassium, ALT, AST, alkaline phosphatase, bilirubin. May decrease WBCs, neutrophil count.

AVAILABILITY (Rx)

Tablets: 7 mg, 14 mg.

ADMINISTRATION/HANDLING

PO

- Give without regard to food.

INDICATIONS/ROUTES/DOSAGE

Multiple Sclerosis

PO: ADULTS, ELDERLY: 7 mg or 14 mg once daily.

Adjustment of Toxicity

ALT elevation greater than 3 times ULN: Discontinue teriflunomide and initiate drug elimination procedures: cholestyramine 8 g q8h for 11 days (if not tolerated, may decrease to 4 g q8h) or activated charcoal 50 g q12h for 11 days. **Note:** The 11 days do not need to be consecutive unless plasma concentration needs to be lowered rapidly.

Dosage in Renal Impairment

No dose adjustment.

Dosage in Hepatic Impairment

Mild to moderate impairment: No dose adjustment. **Severe impairment:** Contraindicated.

SIDE EFFECTS

Frequent (19%–6%): Headache, diarrhea, nausea, alopecia, paresthesia, upper abdominal pain. **Occasional (4%–3%):** Hypertension, oral herpes, anxiety, hypertension, toothache, musculoskeletal pain. **Rare (2%–1%):** Seasonal allergy, sciatica, burning sensation, carpal tunnel syndrome, blurred vision, acne, pruritus, myalgia, abdominal distention, conjunctivitis.

ADVERSE EFFECTS/TOXIC REACTIONS

Myelosuppression (lymphopenia, neutropenia, thrombocytopenia) was reported. Severe hepatic injury, hepatotoxicity may occur. Infections, opportunistic infections including aspergillosis, influenza, *Klebsiella* pneumonia, *Pneumocystis jiroveci* pneumonia, TB were reported (mainly occurring in pts taking concomitant immunosuppressive therapy). May increase risk of malignancies, proliferative disorders. Hypersensitivity reactions including angioedema, dyspnea, urticaria, and anaphylaxis may occur. May cause acute renal failure, peripheral neuropathy, hypertension, interstitial lung disease, pneumonitis, sudden cardiac death. Skin toxicities including Steven-Johnson syndrome, toxic epidermal necrolysis may occur.

NURSING CONSIDERATIONS

BASELINE ASSESSMENT

Obtain CBC, LFT; pregnancy test in females of reproductive potential. Assess baseline symptoms of MS (e.g., bladder/bowel dysfunction, cognitive impairment, depression, dysphagia, fatigue, gait disorder, numbness/tingling, pain, seizures, spasticity, tremors, weakness). Screen for active infection. Question history of hepatic/renal impairment, pulmonary disease, neuropathy; chronic, opportunistic infections. Evaluate for active TB and test for latent infection prior to and during treatment. Induration of 5 mm or greater with purified protein derivative (PPD) is considered a positive result when assessing for latent TB. Consider treatment with antimycobacterial therapy in pts with latent TB.

INTERVENTION/EVALUATION

Monitor CBC for myelosuppression; LFT for hepatic injury (abdominal pain, jaundice, nausea, transaminitis, vomiting) at least monthly for 6 mos. Conduct neurologic assessment. Assess for symptomatic improvement of MS. Monitor for neuropathy. Consider ABG, radiologic test if ILD/pneumonitis (excessive cough, dyspnea, fever, hypoxia) is suspected. Consider treatment with corticosteroids if ILD/pneumonitis is confirmed. Monitor for TB regardless of baseline PPD. Diligently monitor for acute infection (cough, fatigue, fever), opportunistic infections; reactivation of chronic infections. Monitor B/P for hypertension. Assess skin for cutaneous toxicities. Due to extended drug clearance (elimination may take up to 2 yrs), an accelerated elimination program may be needed (e.g., cholestyramine 8 g q8h for 11 days; activated charcoal 50 g q12h for 11 days).

PATIENT/FAMILY TEACHING

• Treatment may depress your immune system and reduce your ability to fight infection. Report symptoms of infection such as body aches, burning with urination, chills, cough, fatigue, fever. Avoid those with active infection. • Report symptoms of bone marrow depression (e.g., bruising, fatigue, fever, shortness of breath, weight loss; bleeding easily, bloody urine or stool). • Expect routine tuberculosis screening. Report any travel plans to possible endemic areas. • Do not receive live vaccines. • Report liver problems (abdominal pain, bruising, clay-colored stool, dark or amber-colored urine, yellowing of the skin or eyes), kidney problems (decreased urine output, flank pain, darkened urine); skin toxicities (rash, peeling, sloughing), nervous system pain/weakness/tingling. • Allergic reactions such as difficulty breathing, hives, rash, swelling of the face or tongue, can happen at any time. If allergic reaction occurs, seek immediate medical attention. • Treatment may worsen high blood pressure or cause new cancers. • Severe worsening of MS symptoms may occur after stopping treatment. • Use effective contraception to avoid pregnancy. Do not breastfeed.

teriparatide

ter-i-**par**-a-tide
(Forteo)

BLACK BOX ALERT Increased risk of osteosarcoma; risk dependent on dose and duration.

◆ CLASSIFICATION

PHARMACOTHERAPEUTIC: Parathyroid hormone analog. **CLINICAL:** Osteoporosis agent.

USES

Treatment of postmenopausal women with osteoporosis who are at increased risk for fractures. Treatment of men with primary or hypogonadal osteoporosis who are at high risk for fractures. High-risk pts include those with a history of osteoporotic fractures, who have failed previous osteoporosis therapy, or were intolerant of previous osteoporosis therapy. Treatment of glucocorticoid-induced osteoporosis in men and women.

PRECAUTIONS

Contraindications: Hypersensitivity to teriparatide. **Cautions:** Conditions that increase risk of osteosarcoma (e.g., Paget's disease, unexplained elevations of alkaline phosphatase level, children or young adults with open epiphyses, prior skeletal radiation therapy, implant therapy), hypercalcemia, hypercalcemic disorders (e.g., hyperparathyroidism), bone metastases, history of skeletal malignancies, metabolic bone diseases other than osteoporosis, cardiac disease, renal/hepatic impairment, pts at risk for orthostasis, active or recent urolithiasis.

ACTION

Stimulates osteoblast function. Increases calcium absorption from GI tract/renal tubular reabsorption. **Therapeutic Effect:** Increases bone mineral density, bone mass/strength, reduces osteoporosis-related fractures.

PHARMACOKINETICS

Widely distributed. Metabolized in liver. Excreted in urine. **Half-life:** 1 hr.

⌛ LIFESPAN CONSIDERATIONS

Pregnancy/Lactation: Unknown if drug crosses placenta or is distributed

T

in breast milk. **Children:** Safety and efficacy not established. **Elderly:** No age-related precautions noted.

INTERACTIONS

DRUG: None significant. **HERBAL:** None significant. **FOOD:** None known. **LAB VALUES:** May increase serum calcium (transient), uric acid.

AVAILABILITY (Rx)

Injection Solution: 600 mcg/2.4 mL (injector pen containing 28 daily doses of 20 mcg).

ADMINISTRATION/HANDLING

SQ

- Refrigerate, but minimize time out of refrigerator. Do not freeze; discard if frozen. • Administer into thigh, abdominal wall.

INDICATIONS/ROUTES/DOSAGE

Osteoporosis

SQ: ADULTS, ELDERLY: 20 mcg once daily into thigh, abdominal wall. Continue for up to 2 yrs (lifetime duration).

Dosage in Renal/Hepatic Impairment

No dose adjustment.

SIDE EFFECTS

Occasional: Leg cramps, nausea, dizziness, headache, orthostatic hypotension, tachycardia.

ADVERSE EFFECTS/TOXIC REACTIONS

Angina pectoris has been reported.

NURSING CONSIDERATIONS

BASELINE ASSESSMENT

Obtain serum calcium, phosphate, PTH, bone mineral density. Question medical history as listed in Precautions.

INTERVENTION/EVALUATION

Monitor bone mineral density, serum calcium, phosphate, PTH. Observe for symptoms of hypercalcemia (anxiety, bradycardia, facial twitching; muscle cramps, spasm, weakness; seizures). Monitor B/P for hypotension, pulse for tachycardia.

PATIENT/FAMILY TEACHING

- Go from lying to standing slowly.
- Report persistent symptoms of hypercalcemia (nausea, vomiting, constipation, lethargy, asthenia).

testosterone

TOP 100 HIGH ALERT

tes-**tos**-te-rone

(Androderm, AndroGel Pump, Aveed, Depo-Testosterone, Fortesta, Jatenzo, Natesto, Striant, Testim, Testopel, Vogelxo)

BLACK BOX ALERT Virilization in children and women may occur following secondary exposure to testosterone topical gel and solution. Aveed: Serious pulmonary oil microembolism reaction and anaphylaxis reported during or immediately after administration.

Do not confuse testosterone with testolactone.

◆CLASSIFICATION

PHARMACOTHERAPEUTIC: Androgen. **CLINICAL:** Sex hormone.

USES

Androgen replacement therapy in treatment of delayed male puberty, male hypogonadism (congenital or acquired), inoperable female breast cancer pts who are 1–5 yrs postmenopausal.

PRECAUTIONS

Contraindications: Hypersensitivity to testosterone. Breastfeeding, pregnant or who may become pregnant, prostate (known or suspected) or breast cancer in males. **Depo-Testosterone (additional):** Severe cardiac/hepatic/renal disease. **Cautions:** Renal/hepatic/cardiac dysfunction, pts with history of MI or CAD; conditions influenced by edema (e.g., seizure disorder, migraines).

ACTION

Principal endogenous androgen promoting growth, development of male sex organs, maintains secondary sex characteristics in androgen-deficient males. **Therapeutic Effect:** Relieves androgen deficiency.

PHARMACOKINETICS

Well absorbed after IM administration. Protein binding: 98%. Metabolized in liver. Primarily excreted in urine. Unknown if removed by hemodialysis. **Half-life:** 10–100 min.

LIFESPAN CONSIDERATIONS

Pregnancy/Lactation: Contraindicated in pregnant women, women who may become pregnant, or during lactation. **Children:** Safety and efficacy not established; use with caution. **Elderly:** May increase risk of hyperplasia, stimulate growth of occult prostate carcinoma.

INTERACTIONS

DRUG: May increase hepatotoxic effect of **cycloSPORINE**. May increase the anticoagulant effect of **warfarin**. **HERBAL:** None significant. **FOOD:** None known. **LAB VALUES:** May increase Hgb, Hct, LDL, serum alkaline phosphatase, bilirubin, calcium, potassium, sodium, AST. May decrease HDL.

AVAILABILITY (Rx)

Capsule: *(Jatenzo):* 158 mg, 198 mg, 237 mg. **Gel, Topical:** *(AndroGel, Testim):* 1%, 1.62%. *(Vogelxo):* 50-mg packet or tube, 12.5 mg/actuation metered dose pump. *(Fortesta):* 10 mg/actuation. **Injection:** *(Cypionate [Depo-Testosterone]):* 100 mg/mL, 200 mg/mL. *(Enanthate [Delatestryl]):* 200 mg/mL. *(Aveed [Undecanoate]):* 750 mg/3 mL. **Mucoadhesive, for Buccal Application:** *(Striant):* 30 mg. **Nasal Gel:** *(Natesto):* 5.5 mg/actuation. **Pellet for SQ Implantation:** *(Testopel):* 75 mg. **Solution, Metered Dose Pump:** *(Axiron):* 30 mg/activation. **Transdermal System Patch:** *(Androderm):* 2 mg/day or 4 mg/day.

ADMINISTRATION/HANDLING

IM

• Give deep in gluteal muscle. • Do not give IV. • Warming or shaking redissolves crystals that may form in long-acting preparations. • Wet needle of syringe may cause solution to become cloudy; this does not affect potency.

PO

• Give with meals. • Administer capsule whole; do not break, cut, or crush. Capsule cannot be chewed.

Buccal

• *(Striant):* Apply to gum area (above incisor tooth). • Hold firmly in place for 30 sec to ensure adhesion. Instruct pt to not chew or swallow. • Not affected by food, toothbrushing, gum, chewing, alcoholic beverages. • Remove before placing new system.

Transdermal

• *(Androderm):* Apply to clean, dry area on skin on back, abdomen, upper arms, thighs. • Do not use tape to secure. Avoid bathing, swimming for at least 3 hrs after each application. • Do not apply to bony prominences (e.g., shoulder) or oily, damaged, irritated skin. Do not apply to scrotum. • Rotate application site with 7-day interval to same site.

Transdermal Gel

• *(AndroGel, Testim, Vogelxo):* Apply (morning preferred) to clean, dry, intact skin of shoulder, upper arms. (AndroGel 1% may also be applied to abdomen.) • Upon opening packet(s), squeeze entire contents into palm of hand, immediately apply to application site. • Allow to dry. • Do not apply to genitals. • *(Fortesta):* Apply to skin of front and inner thighs.

Topical Solution

• *(Axiron):* Apply using applicator to axilla at same time each morning. • Avoid washing site for 2 hrs after application.

T

INDICATIONS/ROUTES/DOSAGE

Male Hypogonadism (Primary or hypogonadotropic)

IM: ADULTS: *(Cypionate or Enanthate):* 75–100 mg/wk or 150–200 mg q2wks. *(Undecanoate):* 750 mg at initiation, 4 wks and q10 wks thereafter. **CHILDREN 12 YRS AND OLDER:** *(Cypionate or Enanthate):* Initiation of pubertal growth: 25–75 mg q3–4wks, gradually titrate q6–9mos to 100–150 mg. Duration: 3–4yrs. **Maintenance virilizing dose:** 200–250 mg q3–4wks. May convert to other testosterone replacement dosages once expected adult height and adequate virilization achieved.

PO: *(Capsules):* 237 mg twice daily in morning and evening. Range: 158–396 mg twice daily.

SQ: *(Pellets):* **ADULTS, CHILDREN 12 YRS AND OLDER:** 150–450 mg q3–6mos. *(Enanthate):* **ADULTS, ELDERLY:** 75 mg once wkly. Range: 50–100 mg once wkly.

Topical gel: *(Fortesta):* 40 mg once daily in morning. Range: 10–70 mg. **Maximum:** 70 mg. *(Vogelxo):* 50 mg once daily (one tube or one packet or 4 pump actuations).

Topical solution: *(Axiron):* **ADULTS, ELDERLY:** 60 mg once daily (1 pump activation of 30 mg to each axilla). Range: 30–120 mg.

Transdermal patch: *(Androderm):* **ADULTS, ELDERLY:** Start therapy with 4 mg/day patch applied at night. Apply patch to abdomen, back, thighs, upper arms. Dose adjustment based on testosterone levels. Range: 2–6 mg/day.

Transdermal gel: ADULTS, ELDERLY: *(AndroGel 1%):* Initial dose of 5 g delivers 50 mg testosterone and is applied once daily to abdomen, shoulders, upper arms. May increase to 7.5 g (75 mg testosterone), then to 10 g (100 mg testosterone), if necessary. *(AndroGel 1.62%):* Initial dose of 40.5 mg applied once daily in the morning to shoulder and upper arms. May increase to 81 mg. Further adjustments based on testosterone levels.

Transdermal gel: *(Testim, Vogelxo):* **ADULTS, ELDERLY:** Initial dose of 5 g delivers 50 mg testosterone and is applied once daily to the shoulders, upper arms. May increase to 10 g (100 mg testosterone).

Buccal: *(Striant):* **ADULTS, ELDERLY:** 30 mg q12h.

Nasal gel: *(Natesto):* **ADULTS ELDERLY:** 11 mg (2 actuations, 1 per each nostril) 3 times/day (6–8 hrs apart).

Delayed Male Puberty

IM: *(Enanthate):* **ADOLESCENTS:** 50–200 mg q2–4wks for limited duration (4–6 months).

SQ: *(Pellets):* **ADULTS:** 150–450 mg q3–6mos.

Breast Carcinoma

IM: *(Ethanate):* **ADULTS:** 200–400 mg q2–4wks.

Dosage in Renal/Hepatic Impairment

Use caution.

SIDE EFFECTS

Frequent: Gynecomastia, acne. **Females:** Hirsutism, amenorrhea, other menstrual irregularities; deepening of voice; clitoral enlargement (may not be reversible when drug is discontinued). **Occasional:** Edema, nausea, insomnia, oligospermia, priapism, male-pattern baldness, bladder irritability, hypercalcemia (in immobilized pts, those with breast cancer), hypercholesterolemia, inflammation/pain at IM injection site. **Transdermal:** Pruritus, erythema, skin irritation. **Rare:** Polycythemia (with high dosage), hypersensitivity.

ADVERSE EFFECTS/TOXIC REACTIONS

Peliosis hepatitis (presence of blood-filled cysts in parenchyma of liver), hepatic neoplasms, hepatocellular carcinoma have been associated with prolonged high-dose therapy. Anaphylactic reactions occur rarely. Venous thromboembolism (e.g., DVT, PE) reported.

NURSING CONSIDERATIONS

BASELINE ASSESSMENT

Obtain CBC, BMP, LFT, lipid panel; weight, B/P. Wrist X-rays may be ordered to determine bone maturation in children. Question history of hepatic/renal impairment, seizure disorder, thromboembolism (CVA, MI, pulmonary embolism).

INTERVENTION/EVALUATION

Weigh daily, report wkly gain of more than 5 lb; evaluate for edema. Monitor B/P. Assess serum electrolytes, cholesterol, Hgb, Hct (periodically for high dosage), LFT, radiologic exam of wrist, hand (when using in prepubertal children). With breast cancer or immobility, check for hypercalcemia (anxiety, bradycardia, facial twitching; muscle cramps, spasm, weakness; seizures). Ensure adequate intake of protein, calories. Assess for virilization. Monitor sleep patterns. Monitor for CVA (aphasia, confusion, paresthesia, hemiparesis, seizures), MI (chest pain, diaphoresis, left arm/jaw pain, increased serum troponin, ST segment elevation), pulmonary embolism (chest pain, dyspnea, hypoxia, tachycardia).

PATIENT/FAMILY TEACHING

• Do not take any other medication without consulting physician. • Maintain diet high in protein, calories. • Weigh daily; report 5 lb/wk gain. • Report nausea, vomiting, acne, pedal edema. • **Females:** Promptly report menstrual irregularities, hoarseness, deepening of voice. • **Males:** Report frequent erections, difficulty urinating, gynecomastia. • Treatment may cause arterial or venous blood clots; report symptoms of heart attack (chest pain, difficulty breathing, jaw pain, nausea, pain that radiates to the left arm, sweating), stroke (blindness, confusion, one-sided weakness, loss of consciousness, trouble speaking, seizures); DVT (swelling, pain, hot feeling in the arms or legs), lung embolism (difficulty breathing, chest pain, rapid heart rate).

tiaGABine

tye-a-ga-been
(Gabitril)
Do not confuse tiaGABine with tiZANidine.

◆CLASSIFICATION

PHARMACOTHERAPEUTIC: Selective GABA reuptake inhibitor. **CLINICAL:** Anticonvulsant.

USES

Adjunctive therapy for treatment of partial seizures in adults and children 12 yrs or older.

PRECAUTIONS

Contraindications: Hypersensitivity to tiaGABine. **Cautions:** Hepatic impairment. Pts at risk for suicidal behavior/thoughts.

ACTION

Enhances activity of gamma-aminobutyric acid (GABA), the major inhibitory neurotransmitter in the CNS. **Therapeutic Effect:** Inhibits seizure activity.

PHARMACOKINETICS

Widely distributed. Protein binding: 96%. Metabolized in liver. Primarily excreted in feces. **Half-life:** 2–5 hrs.

LIFESPAN CONSIDERATIONS

Pregnancy/Lactation: May cause fetal harm. Distributed in breast milk. **Children:** Safety and efficacy not established in pts younger than 12 yrs. **Elderly:** Age-related hepatic impairment may require dosage adjustment.

INTERACTIONS

DRUG: CNS depressants (e.g., alcohol, morphine, oxyCODONE, zolpidem) may increase CNS depression. **Strong CYP3A4 inducers (e.g., carBAMazepine, phenytoin, rifAMPin)** may decrease concentration/effect. **Strong CYP3A4 inhibitors**

T

(e.g., clarithromycin, ketoconazole) may increase concentration/effect. HERBAL: **Herbals with sedative properties (e.g., chamomile, kava kava, valerian)** may increase CNS depression. **St. John's wort** may decrease concentration/effect. FOOD: None known. LAB VALUES: None significant.

AVAILABILITY (Rx)

Tablets: 2 mg, 4 mg, 12 mg, 16 mg.

ADMINISTRATION/HANDLING

- Give with food.

INDICATIONS/ROUTES/DOSAGE

Note: Pts not taking enzyme-inducing antiepileptic drugs (AEDs): Lower doses required and slower titration may be needed. Do not use a loading dose, rapid titration, and/or increase in large-dose increments.

Partial Seizures

PO: ADULTS, ELDERLY: **Pts receiving enzyme-inducing AED regimens:** Initially, 4 mg once daily. May increase by 4–8 mg/day at wkly intervals. **Maintenance:** 32–56 mg/day in 2–4 divided doses. CHILDREN 12–18 YRS: **Pts receiving enzyme-inducing AED regimens:** Initially, 4 mg once daily for 1 wk. May increase by 4 mg in 2 divided doses for 1 wk, then may increase by 4–8 mg at wkly intervals thereafter. **Maximum:** 32 mg/day in 2–4 divided doses.

T

Dosage in Renal Impairment

No dose adjustment.

Dosage in Hepatic Impairment

Use caution.

SIDE EFFECTS

Frequent (34%–20%): Dizziness, asthenia (loss of strength, energy), drowsiness, nervousness, confusion, headache, infection, tremor. Occasional: Nausea, diarrhea, abdominal pain, impaired concentration.

ADVERSE EFFECTS/TOXIC REACTIONS

Overdose characterized by agitation, confusion, hostility, weakness. Full recovery occurs within 24 hrs of discontinuation. Depression, suicidal ideation.

NURSING CONSIDERATIONS

BASELINE ASSESSMENT

Review history of seizure disorder (intensity, frequency, duration, level of consciousness). Observe frequently for recurrence of seizure activity. Initiate seizure precautions.

INTERVENTION/EVALUATION

For pts on long-term therapy, serum hepatic/renal function tests, CBC should be performed periodically. Assist with ambulation if dizziness occurs. Assess for clinical improvement (decrease in intensity, frequency of seizures). Monitor for depression, unusual behavior, suicidal ideation or thoughts.

PATIENT/FAMILY TEACHING

• Go from lying to standing slowly. • Avoid tasks that require alertness, motor skills until response to drug is established. • Avoid alcohol. • Report worsening seizure activity, thoughts of suicide, increased depression.

ticagrelor

tye-**ka**-grel-or
(Brilinta)

■ BLACK BOX ALERT ■ May cause significant, sometimes fatal bleeding. Do not use with active bleeding or history of intracranial bleeding. Do not initiate in pts planning urgent coronary artery bypass graft (CABG) surgery. Discontinue at least 5 days prior to any surgery. Suspect bleeding in any pt who is hypotensive and has had recent percutaneous coronary intervention (PCI), CABG, or other surgical procedures. If possible, manage bleeding without discontinuing therapy to decrease risk of cardiovascular events. Aspirin maintenance doses greater than 100 mg/day may reduce effectiveness and should be strictly avoided.

◆**CLASSIFICATION**

PHARMACOTHERAPEUTIC: $P2Y_{12}$ platelet aggregation inhibitor. **CLINICAL:** Antiplatelet.

USES

Reduce rate of cardiovascular death, MI, stroke in pts with acute coronary syndrome (ACS) or history of MI. Reduce rate of stent thrombosis in pts who have been stented for treatment of ACS. Reduce risk of first MI or stroke in pts with coronary artery disease (CAD) at high risk for such events.

PRECAUTIONS

Contraindications: Hypersensitivity to ticagrelor. History of intracranial hemorrhage, active pathologic bleeding, severe hepatic impairment. **Cautions:** Moderate hepatic impairment, renal impairment, history of hyperuricemia or gouty arthritis. Pts at increased risk of bradycardia, concurrent use of strong CYP3A4 inhibitors or inducers, elderly. (Recommend holding dose 5 days before planned surgery if applicable.) Pts with risk factors for bleeding (e.g., trauma, peptic ulcer disease).

ACTION

Reversibly inhibits platelet $P2Y_{12}$ ADP receptor to prevent signal transduction and platelet activation. **Therapeutic Effect:** Reduces platelet aggregation.

PHARMACOKINETICS

Readily absorbed after PO administration. Protein binding: 99%. Metabolized in liver. Primarily excreted in feces (58%), urine (26%). **Half-life:** 7–9 hrs.

LIFESPAN CONSIDERATIONS

Pregnancy/Lactation: Unknown if distributed in breast milk. **Children:** Safety and efficacy not established. **Elderly:** No age-related precautions noted.

INTERACTIONS

DRUG: **Aspirin** greater than 100 mg/day may decrease effect. **CYP3A4 inhibitors (e.g., clarithromycin, ketoconazole)** may increase concentration/effect. **Strong CYP3A4 inducers (e.g., carBAMazepine, phenytoin, rifAMPin)** may decrease concentration/effect. **Anticoagulants (e.g., warfarin), antiplatelets (e.g., aspirin, clopidogrel), NSAIDs (e.g., ibuprofen, ketorolac, naproxen)** may increase risk of bleeding. May increase adverse effects of **apixaban, dabigatran, edoxaban**. May increase concentration/effect of **digoxin, simvastatin, lovastatin.** **HERBAL:** **St. John's wort** may decrease concentration/effect. **Herbals with anticoagulant/antiplatelet properties (e.g., garlic, ginger, ginkgo biloba), glucosamine** may increase risk of bleeding. **FOOD:** **Grapefruit products** may increase potential for bleeding. **LAB VALUES:** May increase serum uric acid, creatinine.

AVAILABILITY (Rx)

Tablets: 60 mg, 90 mg.

ADMINISTRATION/HANDLING

PO

• Give without regard to food. • May be crushed, mixed with water, and drunk immediately (refill glass with water, stir and drink contents).

INDICATIONS/ROUTES/DOSAGE

Acute Coronary Syndrome

PO: ADULTS: Initially, 180 mg once, then 90 mg twice daily. (begin 12h after initial loading dose). Give with aspirin 325 mg once (loading dose), then maintain with aspirin 75–100 mg daily. Continue for up to 12 mos, then decrease dose to 60 mg twice daily.

CAD (With high risk for cardiovascular events, primary prevention)

PO: ADULTS, ELDERLY: 60 mg twice daily (in combination with aspirin). Continue indefinitely.

Dosage in Renal Impairment

No dose adjustment.

T

Dosage in Hepatic Impairment
Mild impairment: No dose adjustment. **Moderate impairment:** Use caution. **Severe impairment:** Avoid use.

SIDE EFFECTS

Occasional (13%–7%): Dyspnea, headache. **Rare (5%–3%):** Cough, dizziness, nausea, diarrhea, back pain, fatigue.

ADVERSE EFFECTS/TOXIC REACTIONS

Life-threatening events including intracranial bleeding, epistaxis, intrapericardial bleeding with cardiac tamponade, hypovolemic shock requiring vasopressive support or blood transfusion was reported. Pts with history of sick sinus syndrome, second- or third-degree AV block, bradycardic syncope have increased risk of bradycardia. May cause atrial fibrillation, hypotension, hypertension. Gynecomastia reported in less than 1% of men.

NURSING CONSIDERATIONS

BASELINE ASSESSMENT

Obtain CBC, BMP, LFT. Question for history of bleeding, stomach ulcers, colon polyps, head trauma, cardiac arrhythmias, unstable angina, recent MI, hepatic impairment, hypertension, stroke, pulmonary disease. Receive full medication history including herbal products.

INTERVENTION/EVALUATION

Routinely screen for bleeding. Assess skin for bruising, hematoma. Monitor renal function, uric acid, digoxin levels if applicable. Report hematuria, epistaxis, coffee-ground emesis, black/tarry stools.

PATIENT/FAMILY TEACHING

• It may take longer to stop bleeding during therapy. • Do not vigorously blow nose. • Use soft toothbrush, electric razor to decrease risk of bleeding. • Immediately report bloody stool, urine, or nosebleeds. • Report all newly prescribed medications. • Inform physician of any planned dental procedures or surgeries.

T

tigecycline

tye-gee-**sye**-kleen
(Tygacil)

■ **BLACK BOX ALERT** ■ An increase in all-cause mortality observed in Phase 3 and 4 clinical trials. Use is reserved when alternate treatment is not appropriate.

◆CLASSIFICATION

PHARMACOTHERAPEUTIC: Glycylcycline. **CLINICAL:** Antibiotic.

USES

Treatment of susceptible infections due to *E. coli, E. faecalis, S. aureus, S. agalactiae, S. anginosus* group (includes *S. anginosus, S. intermedius, S. constellatus), S. pyogenes, B. fragilis, Citrobacter freundii, E. cloacae, K. oxytoca, K. pneumoniae, B. thetaiotaomicron, B. uniformis, B. vulgatus, C. perfringens, Peptostreptococcus micros* including complicated skin/skin structure infections, complicated intra-abdominal infections, community-acquired bacterial pneumonia.

PRECAUTIONS

Contraindications: Hypersensitivity to tigecycline. **Cautions:** Hypersensitivity to tetracyclines, pregnancy, hepatic impairment, monotherapy for pts with intestinal perforation. Do not use for diabetic foot infections, healthcare (hospital)-acquired pneumonia, or ventilator-associated pneumonia.

ACTION

Inhibits protein synthesis by binding to ribosomal receptor sites of bacterial cell wall. **Therapeutic Effect:** Bacteriostatic effect.

PHARMACOKINETICS

Widely distributed. Metabolized in liver. Protein binding: 71%–89%. Excreted in feces (59%), urine (33%). **Half-life:** Single dose: 27 hrs; following multiple doses: 42 hrs.

LIFESPAN CONSIDERATIONS

Pregnancy/Lactation: May cause fetal harm. May be distributed in breast milk. Permanent discoloration of the teeth (brown-gray) may occur if used during tooth development. **Children:** Safety and efficacy not established in pts younger than 8 yrs. Use is reserved for when no effective alternative is available. **Elderly:** No age-related precautions noted.

INTERACTIONS

DRUG: May increase concentration/ effect of **warfarin.** **HERBAL:** None significant. **FOOD:** None known. **LAB VALUES:** May increase serum alkaline phosphatase, amylase, BUN, bilirubin, glucose, LDH, ALT, AST. May decrease serum potassium; Hgb, leukocytes, platelets.

AVAILABILITY (Rx)

Injection, Powder for Reconstitution: ***(Tygacil):*** 50-mg vial.

ADMINISTRATION/HANDLING

IV

Reconstitution • Reconstitute with 5.3 mL 0.9% NaCl or D_5W to a concentration of 10 mg/mL. Dilute in 100 mL 0.9% NaCl or D_5W.

Rate of administration • Infuse over 30–60 min. Flush IV line after infusion is complete.

Storage • Refrigerate diluted solution for up to 24 hrs or store at room temperature for up to 6 hrs. • Reconstituted solution appears yellow to red-orange. • Discard if solution is discolored (green, black) or precipitate forms.

IV INCOMPATIBILITIES

Amphotericin B, methylPREDNISolone, voriconazole.

IV COMPATIBILITIES

Amikacin, azithromycin, aztreonam, cefepime, cefTAZidime, ciprofloxacin, doripenem, ertapenem, fluconazole, gentamicin, linezolid, piperacillin-tazobactam, potassium chloride, telavancin, tobramycin, vancomycin.

INDICATIONS/ROUTES/DOSAGE

Systemic Infections

IV: ADULTS OVER 18 YRS, ELDERLY: Initially, 100 mg, followed by 50 mg q12h for 5–14 days. **CHILDREN 12 YRS AND OLDER:** 50 mg q12h. **CHILDREN 8–11 YRS:** 1.2–2 mg/kg q12h. **Maximum:** 50 mg/dose.

Dosage in Renal Impairment

No dose adjustment.

Dosage in Hepatic Impairment

Mild to moderate impairment: No dose adjustment. **Severe impairment: IV: ADULTS OVER 18 YRS, ELDERLY:** Initially, 100 mg, followed by 25 mg q12h.

SIDE EFFECTS

Frequent (29%–13%): Nausea, vomiting, diarrhea. **Occasional (7%–4%):** Headache, hypertension, dizziness, increased cough, delayed healing. **Rare (3%–2%):** Peripheral edema, pruritus, constipation, dyspepsia, asthenia (loss of strength, energy), hypotension, phlebitis, insomnia, rash, diaphoresis.

ADVERSE EFFECTS/TOXIC REACTIONS

Dyspnea, abscess, pseudomembranous colitis (abdominal cramps, severe watery diarrhea, fever) ranging from mild to life-threatening may result from altered bacterial balance in GI tract.

NURSING CONSIDERATIONS

BASELINE ASSESSMENT

Obtain CBC, LFT. Question for history of allergies, esp. tetracyclines.

INTERVENTION/EVALUATION

Monitor daily pattern of bowel activity, stool consistency. Be alert for superinfection: fever, anal/genital pruritus, oral mucosal changes (ulceration, pain, erythema).

PATIENT/FAMILY TEACHING

- Report diarrhea, rash, mouth soreness, other new symptoms.

tildrakizumab-asmn

til-dra-**kiz**-ue-mab-asmn
(Ilumya)
Do not confuse tildrakizumab-asmn with atezolizumab, benralizumab, certolizumab, daclizumab, eculizumab, efalizumab, mepolizumab, tositumomab, or trastuzumab.

◆CLASSIFICATION

PHARMACOTHERAPEUTIC: Interleukin-23 antagonist. Monoclonal antibody. **CLINICAL:** Antipsoriatic agent.

USES

Treatment of moderate to severe plaque psoriasis in adults who are candidates for systemic therapy or phototherapy.

PRECAUTIONS

Contraindications: Hypersensitivity to tildrakizumab-asmn. **Cautions:** Conditions predisposing to infection (e.g., diabetes, immunocompromised pts, renal failure, open wounds), prior exposure to tuberculosis. Concomitant use of live vaccines not recommended.

T

ACTION

Selectively binds to p19 subunit of interleukin-23 (IL-23) and inhibits interaction with IL-23 receptor. IL-23 is a cytokine that is involved in inflammatory and immune response. **Therapeutic Effect:** Alters biologic immune response; reduces inflammation.

PHARMACOKINETICS

Widely distributed. Degraded into small peptides and amino acids via catabolic pathway. Peak plasma concentration: 6 days. Steady state reached in 16 wks. **Half-life:** 23 days.

⌛ LIFESPAN CONSIDERATIONS

Pregnancy/Lactation: Unknown if distributed in breast milk. However, human immunoglobulin G (IgG) is present in breast milk and is known to cross the placenta. **Children:** Safety and efficacy not established. **Elderly:** No age-related precautions noted.

INTERACTIONS

DRUG: May decrease therapeutic effect of **live vaccines.** May increase risk of adverse effects/toxic reactions of **belimumab, live vaccines. HERBAL:** None significant. **FOOD:** None known. **LAB VALUES:** None known.

AVAILABILITY (Rx)

Injection Solution, Prefilled Syringe: 100 mg/mL.

ADMINISTRATION/HANDLING

SQ

Preparation • Remove prefilled syringe from refrigerator and allow solution to warm to room temperature (approx. 30 min). • Visually inspect for particulate matter or discoloration. Solution should appear clear to slightly opalescent, colorless to slightly yellow in color. Do not use if solution is cloudy, discolored, or if visible particles are observed. • If present, air bubbles do not need to be removed before administration.

Administration • Insert needle subcutaneously into upper arm, outer thigh, or abdomen and inject solution. • Do not inject into areas of active skin disease or injury such as sunburns, skin rashes, inflammation, skin infections, or active psoriasis. • Do not administer IV or intramuscular. • Rotate injection sites.

Storage • Refrigerate prefilled syringes in original carton until time of use. • Protect from light. • May store at room temperature for up to 30 days. Once warmed to room temperature, do not place back into refrigerator. • Do not freeze or expose to heating sources. • Do not shake.

INDICATIONS/ROUTES/DOSAGE

Plaque Psoriasis

SQ: ADULTS, ELDERLY: 100 mg at wk 0 and wk 4, then q12wks thereafter.

Dosage in Renal /Hepatic Impairment

Not specified; use caution.

SIDE EFFECTS

Rare (3%–2%): Injection site reactions (bruising, edema, erythema, hematoma, hemorrhage, inflammation, pain, pruritus, swelling, urticaria), diarrhea.

ADVERSE EFFECTS/TOXIC REACTIONS

Hypersensitivity reactions including angioedema, urticaria may occur. Upper respiratory tract infections reported in 14% of pts. Infections reported in 23% of pts. May increase risk of serious infections. Immunogenicity (auto-tildrakizumab-asmn antibodies) occurred in 7% of pts.

NURSING CONSIDERATIONS

BASELINE ASSESSMENT

Consider completion of immunizations before initiation. Pts should be evaluated for active tuberculosis and tested for latent infection before initiation and periodically during therapy. Induration of 5 mm or greater with tuberculin skin testing should be considered a positive test result when assessing if treatment for latent tuberculosis is necessary. Screen for active infection. Question history of chronic infections, hypersensitivity reactions. Conduct dermatologic exam; record characteristics of psoriatic lesions.

INTERVENTION/EVALUATION

Assess skin for improvement of lesions. Monitor for symptoms of tuberculosis, including those who tested negative for latent tuberculosis infection before initiating therapy. Interrupt or discontinue treatment if serious infection, opportunistic infection, or sepsis occurs. Monitor for hypersensitivity reaction, angioedema.

PATIENT/FAMILY TEACHING

• Treatment may depress your immune system and reduce your ability to fight infection. Report symptoms of infection such as body aches, burning with urination, chills, cough, fatigue, fever. Avoid those with active infection. • Do not receive live vaccines. • Expect frequent tuberculosis screening. • Report travel plans to possible endemic areas. • Report allergic reactions such as itching, swelling of the face or tongue.

tiotropium

TOP 100

tye-oh-**trope**-ee-yum
(Spiriva HandiHaler, Spiriva Respimat)

Do not confuse Spiriva with Inspra, or tiotropium with ipratropium.

FIXED-COMBINATION(S)

Stiolto Respimat: tiotropium/olodaterol (a bronchodilator): 2.5 mcg/ 2.5 mcg.

◆CLASSIFICATION

PHARMACOTHERAPEUTIC: Anticholinergic (long-acting). **CLINICAL:** Bronchodilator.

USES

Long-term maintenance treatment of bronchospasm associated with COPD, including chronic bronchitis, emphysema, and for reducing COPD exacerbations. **Spiriva Respimat only:** Maintenance treatment of asthma in pts 6 yrs and older.

PRECAUTIONS

Contraindications: Hypersensitivity to tiotropium. History of hypersensitivity

T

to ipratropium. **Cautions:** Narrow-angle glaucoma, prostatic hypertrophy, bladder neck obstruction, moderate to severe renal impairment, history of hypersensitivity to atropine, myasthenia gravis.

ACTION

Competitively and reversibly inhibits action of acetylcholine at muscarinic receptors in bronchial smooth muscle. **Therapeutic Effect:** Causes bronchodilation.

PHARMACOKINETICS

Binds extensively to tissue. Protein binding: 72%. Metabolized by oxidation. Excreted in urine. **Half-life:** 5–6 days.

LIFESPAN CONSIDERATIONS

Pregnancy/Lactation: Unknown if distributed in breast milk. **Children:** Safety and efficacy not established. **Elderly:** Higher frequency of dry mouth, constipation, UTI noted with increasing age.

INTERACTIONS

DRUG: Concurrent administration with **anticholinergics (e.g., aclidinium, umeclidinium, ipratropium)** may increase adverse effects. **HERBAL:** None significant. **FOOD:** None known. **LAB VALUES:** None significant.

AVAILABILITY (Rx)

Inhalation Spray: ***(Spiriva Respimat):*** 1.25 mcg/actuation, 2.5 mcg/actuation. **Powder for Inhalation:** ***(Spiriva):*** 18 mcg/capsule (in blister packs).

ADMINISTRATION/HANDLING

Inhalation

• ***(Spiriva):*** Open dustcap of HandiHaler by pulling it upward, then open mouthpiece. • Place capsule in center chamber and firmly close mouthpiece until a click is heard, leaving the dustcap open. • Hold HandiHaler device with mouthpiece upward, press piercing button completely in once, and release. • Instruct pt to breathe out completely before breathing in slowly and deeply but at rate sufficient to hear the capsule vibrate. • Have pt hold breath as long as it is comfortable until exhaling slowly. • Instruct pt to repeat once again to ensure full dose is received. • ***(Spiriva Respimat):*** Refer to manufacturer's pt instructions.

Storage • Store at room temperature. Do not expose capsules to extreme temperature, moisture. • Do not store capsules in HandiHaler device. • Use immediately once foil is peeled back or removed.

INDICATIONS/ROUTES/DOSAGE

COPD (Maintenance treatment, reduction of COPD exacerbations)

Inhalation: ADULTS, ELDERLY: ***(Spiriva):*** 18 mcg (1 capsule)/day via HandiHaler inhalation device. ***(Spiriva Respimat [2.5 mcg/actuation]):*** 2 inhalations (2.5 mcg/inhalation) once daily.

Asthma

Inhalation: ADULTS, ELDERLY, CHILDREN 6 YRS AND OLDER: ***(Spiriva Respimat [1.25 mcg/actuation]):*** 2 inhalations of 1.25 mcg once daily. Maximum benefit may take up to 4–8 wks.

Dosage in Renal Impairment

CrCl 60 mL/min or less: Use caution in moderate to severe impairment.

Dosage in Hepatic Impairment

No dose adjustment.

SIDE EFFECTS

Frequent (16%–6%): Dry mouth, sinusitis, pharyngitis, dyspepsia, UTI, rhinitis. **Occasional (5%–4%):** Abdominal pain, peripheral edema, constipation, epistaxis, vomiting, myalgia, rash, oral candidiasis.

ADVERSE EFFECTS/TOXIC REACTIONS

Angina pectoris, depression, flu-like symptoms, glaucoma, increased intraocular pressure occur rarely.

NURSING CONSIDERATIONS

BASELINE ASSESSMENT

Question history of glaucoma, bladder outlet obstruction, renal impairment, myasthenia gravis. Auscultate lung sounds.

INTERVENTION/EVALUATION

Monitor rate, depth, rhythm, type of respiration; quality, rate of pulse. Assess lung sounds for rhonchi, wheezing, rales. Monitor ABGs. Observe for clavicular retractions, hand tremor. Evaluate for clinical improvement (quieter, slower respirations, relaxed facial expression, cessation of clavicular retractions).

PATIENT/FAMILY TEACHING

• Increase fluid intake (decreases lung secretion viscosity). • Do not use more than 1 capsule for inhalation in a 24-h period. • Rinsing mouth with water immediately after inhalation may prevent mouth/throat dryness, thrush. • Avoid excessive use of caffeine derivatives (chocolate, coffee, tea, cola, cocoa). • Report eye pain/discomfort, blurred vision, visual halos.

tipiracil/trifluridine

trye-**flure**-i-deen/tye-**pir**-a-sil
(Lonsurf)

Do not confuse trifluridine with floxuridine, or tipiracil with tipifarnib or Pipracil.

◆CLASSIFICATION

PHARMACOTHERAPEUTIC: Antimetabolite/thymidine phosphorylase inhibitor. **CLINICAL:** Antineoplastic.

USES

Treatment of pts with metastatic colorectal cancer who have been previously treated with fluoropyrimidine-, oxaliplatin-, and irinotecan-based chemotherapy, an anti–vascular endothelial growth factor (VEGF) biological therapy, and if RAS wild-type, an anti–epidermal growth factor (EGFR) therapy. Treatment of metastatic gastric or gastroesophageal junction adenocarcinoma previously treated with a fluoropyrimidine, a platinum, and either a taxane or irinotecan.

PRECAUTIONS

Contraindications: Hypersensitivity to trifluridine or tipiracil. **Cautions:** Baseline cytopenias, conditions predisposing to infection (e.g., diabetes, renal failure, immunocompromised pts, open wounds), pts at risk for tumor lysis syndrome (high tumor burden, dehydration), history of pulmonary embolism; pregnancy, moderate to severe hepatic impairment.

ACTION

Trifluridine (active cytotoxic component) interferes with DNA synthesis and cell proliferation of cancer cells. Tipiracil increases exposure of trifluridine by inhibiting metabolism via thymidine phosphorylase. **Therapeutic Effect:** Inhibits tumor cell growth and metastasis.

PHARMACOKINETICS

Widely distributed. Metabolized by thymidine phosphorylase (not metabolized in liver). Protein binding: trifluridine: 96%; tipiracil: 8%. Peak plasma concentration: 2 hrs. Excreted primarily in urine (50%). **Half-life:** trifluridine: 1.4 hrs (2.1 hrs at steady state); tipiracil: 2.1 hrs (2.4 hrs at steady state).

⌛ LIFESPAN CONSIDERATIONS

Pregnancy/Lactation: Avoid pregnancy; may cause fetal harm. Females and males with females partners of reproductive potential must use effective contraception during treatment and for at least 3 mo after discontinuation. Breastfeeding not recommended during treatment and for at least 1 day after discontinuation. **Children:** Safety and efficacy not established. **Elderly:** May have increased risk of neutropenia, thrombocytopenia.

T

INTERACTIONS

DRUG: May decrease therapeutic effect; increase adverse effects of **vaccines (live)**. **HERBAL:** **Echinacea** may decrease therapeutic effect. **FOOD:** None known. **LAB VALUES:** May decrease Hct, Hgb, platelets, neutrophils, RBC, WBC.

AVAILABILITY (Rx)

Fixed-Dose Combination Tablets: ***(Trifluridine/Tipiracil):*** 15 mg/6.14 mg, 20 mg/8.19 mg.

ADMINISTRATION/HANDLING

PO

• Give within 1 hr of completion of morning and evening meals. Do not give on empty stomach.

INDICATIONS/ROUTES/DOSAGE

Note: Do not initiate the cycle until ANC is 1,500 cells/mm^3 or greater; febrile neutropenia is resolved; platelet count is 75,000 cells/mm^3 or greater; Grade 3 or 4 nonhematologic toxicity is resolved to Grade 1 or 0.

Colorectal, Gastric Cancer

PO: ADULTS, ELDERLY: (Dose based on trifluridine component) 35 mg/m^2 (rounded to nearest 5-mg increment) twice daily on days 1–5 and days 8–12 of 28-day cycle. Continue until disease progression or unacceptable toxicity. **Maximum:** 80 mg/dose (based on trifluridine component).

Dose Modification

Based on Common Terminology Criteria for Adverse Events (CTCAE).

Hematologic/Nonhematologic Toxicity

Interrupt treatment for ANC less than 500 cells/mm^3; febrile neutropenia; platelet count less than 50,000 cells/mm^3; Grade 3 or 4 nonhematologic toxicity. Do not restart until ANC is 1,500 cells/mm^3 or greater; febrile neutropenia is resolved; platelet count is 75,000 cells/mm^3 or greater; Grade 3 or 4 nonhematologic toxicity is resolved to Grade 1 or 0 (except Grade 3 nausea and/or vomiting controlled by antiemetic therapy; Grade 3 diarrhea responsive to antidiarrheal medication). Once resolved, resume at decreased incremental dose of 5 mg/m^2 from previous dose. A maximum of 3 dose reductions is allowed to dosage minimum of 20 mg/m^2 twice daily. Do not increase dose after it has been reduced.

Dosage in Renal Impairment

Mild to moderate impairment: No dose adjustment. **Severe impairment:** Reduce dose to 20 mg/m^2 twice daily on days 1–5 and days 8–12 of a 28-day cycle. May further reduce dose to 15 mg/m^2 twice daily if unable to tolerate 20 mg/m^2 dose. Permanently discontinue if unable to tolerate 15 mg/m^2 dose.

Dosage in Hepatic Impairment

Mild impairment: No dose adjustment. **Moderate to severe impairment:** Avoid use.

SIDE EFFECTS

Frequent (52%–19%): Asthenia, fatigue, nausea, diarrhea, decreased appetite, vomiting, abdominal pain, pyrexia. **Occasional (8%–7%):** Stomatitis, dysgeusia, alopecia.

ADVERSE EFFECTS/TOXIC REACTIONS

Severe and/or life-threatening myelosuppression including anemia (77% of pts), Grade 3 anemia (18% of pts), neutropenia (67% of pts), Grade 3 or 4 neutropenia (27% and 11% of pts), thrombocytopenia (42% of pts), Grade 3 or 4 thrombocytopenia (5% and 1% of pts), febrile neutropenia (3.8% of pts) may occur. Infections including nasopharyngitis, UTI reported in 2%–4% of pts. Pulmonary embolism occurred in 2% of pts. Interstitial lung disease occurs rarely.

NURSING CONSIDERATIONS

BASELINE ASSESSMENT

CBC; pregnancy test in females of reproductive potential. Screen for active infection, history of pulmonary embolism. Assess hydration status. Question pt's usual stool characteristics (color, frequency, consistency).

INTERVENTION/EVALUATION

Follow proper handling and disposal procedures for cytotoxic drugs. Monitor ANC, CBC on day 15 of each cycle. If any Grade 3 or 4 hematologic toxicity occurs, repeat ANC, CBC more frequently. If chest pain, dyspnea, tachycardia occurs, provide supplemental O_2 and obtain radiologic testing to rule out pulmonary embolism. Diligently monitor for infection (cough, fatigue, fever). Monitor daily stool pattern, consistency. Encourage PO intake. Monitor for bleeding if thrombocytopenia occurs.

PATIENT/FAMILY TEACHING

• Treatment may depress your immune system response and reduce your ability to fight infection. Report symptoms of infection such as body aches, chills, cough, fatigue, fever. Avoid those with active infection. • Report symptoms of bone marrow depression (e.g., bruising, fatigue, fever, shortness of breath, weight loss; bleeding easily, bloody urine or stool). • Use effective contraception to avoid pregnancy. Do not breastfeed. • Immediately report chest pain, difficult breathing, fast heart rate, rapid breathing; may indicate life-threatening blood clot in the lungs. • Drink plenty of fluids. • Report diarrhea, nausea, vomiting that is not controlled by antinausea, antidiarrheal medication. • Report bleeding of any kind.

tisagenlecleucel

tis-a-jen-lek-loo-sel
(Kymriah)

BLACK BOX ALERT Life-threatening cytokine release syndrome (CRS) was reported. Do not administer in pts with inflammatory disorders or severe active infection. Treat CRS with tocilizumab and corticosteroids. Life-threatening neurologic toxicities may occur. Monitor for neurological events after treatment.

Do not confuse tisagenlecleucel with sipuleucel-T or Kymriah with Kynamro.

◆CLASSIFICATION

PHARMACOTHERAPEUTIC: Anti-CD19. Chimeric antigen receptor (CAR) T-cell immunotherapy. **CLINICAL:** Antineoplastic.

USES

Treatment of B-cell precursor acute lymphoblastic leukemia (ALL) that is refractory or in second or later relapse in pts up to 25 yrs of age. Treatment of adults with relapsed or refractory large B-cell lymphoma after two or more lines of systemic therapy including diffuse large B-cell lymphoma (DLBCL) not otherwise specified, high-grade B-cell lymphoma and DLBCL arising from follicular lymphoma. Limitations: Not indicated for treatment of primary central nervous system lymphoma.

PRECAUTIONS

Contraindications: Hypersensitivity to tisagenlecleucel. **Cautions:** Baseline cytopenias, elderly, cardiac/pulmonary disease, conditions predisposing to infection (e.g., diabetes, renal failure, immunocompromised pts, open wounds); history of venous thromboembolism (DVT, PE); pts at risk for acute thrombosis (immobility, indwelling venous catheter/access device, morbid obesity, underlying atherosclerosis, genetic hypercoagulable conditions); history of HIV infection, hepatitis B or C virus infection; pts at risk for tumor lysis syndrome (high tumor burden). Not recommended during active infection or in pts with inflammatory disorders. Avoid administration of live vaccines during treatment and after discontinuation until B cells are no longer depleted.

T

ACTION

A CD-19–directed genetically modified autologous T-cell immunotherapy that reprograms T cells with a transgene encoding a chimeric antigen receptor, which identifies and eliminates CD19-expressing malignant and normal cells. CAR recognizes CD19 and is fused to CD137 (enhances expansion and persistence of tisagenlecleucel) and CD3 zeta (a critical component for initiating T-cell activation and antitumor activity). **Therapeutic Effect:** Causes antitumor activity by initiating activation of T cells.

PHARMACOKINETICS

Highly distributed into bone marrow. Peak plasma concentration: approx. 10 days. **Half-life:** 17 days (ALL); 45 days (DCBC).

LIFESPAN CONSIDERATIONS

Pregnancy/Lactation: May cause fetal harm due to fetal B-cell depletion and neonatal lymphocytopenia. Unknown if distributed in breast milk. **Children:** Safety and efficacy has been established. **Elderly:** Safety and efficacy not established.

INTERACTIONS

DRUG: **Systemic corticosteroids (e.g., dexamethasone, prednisone)** may decrease therapeutic effect; may increase risk of infection. May decrease therapeutic effect of **vaccines.** May increase adverse/toxic effects of **live vaccines. Granulocyte colony-stimulating factors, sargramostim** may increase adverse/toxic effects of tisagenlecleucel. **HERBAL:** None significant. **FOOD:** None known. **LAB VALUES:** May increase serum ALT, AST, bilirubin. May decrease serum potassium, phosphorus, sodium; B-cell counts, fibrinogen, immunoglobulin concentrations, leukocytes, lymphocytes, neutrophils, platelets. May prolong aPTT.

AVAILABILITY (Rx)

Patient-Specific Autologous Infusion: 0.2–5 × 10^6 CAR-positive viable T cells/kg, 0.1–2.5 × 10^8 CAR-positive viable T cells, 0.6–6 × 10^8 CAR-positive viable T cells.

ADMINISTRATION/HANDLING

◀ALERT▶ Premedicate with acetaminophen and diphenhydramine (or another H1 antihistamine) approx. 30–60 min before infusion. Do not use a leukocyte-depleting filter during infusion. Infusion bags contain human cells genetically modified with a lentivirus. Follow biosafety handling and safety guidelines.

IV

Preparation • Verify the number of infusion bags needed for dose (up to 3 cryopreserved patient-specific infusion bags may be required to complete a single dose). • Verify dose with Certificate of Conformance (CoC) and Certificate of Analysis (CoA). • Thawing time must be coordinated with infusion time. If more than 1 bag is needed for dose, recommend thawing 1 bag at a time (allows verification that the previous bag was administered safely). • Match pt identity with infusion bag identifiers. • Visually inspect for cracks or breaks. Do not infuse if cracks or breaks are present. • Prime infusion tubing with 0.9% NaCl. • **Thawing:** Place infusion bag inside a second sterile bag to safeguard infusion bag from leaks and to protect ports from contamination. • Thaw 1 bag at a time using either a water bath at 37°C or dry thawing method. • Continue to thaw until no ice is visible on infusion bag. Then remove bag from thawing device. • Visually inspect for clumps. Gently mix if clumps are present (small clumps should disperse). • Do not infuse if bag is leaking, damaged, or if clumps do not disperse after gentle mixing. • Do not spin down, wash, or resuspend contents.

Rate of administration • Infuse at 10–20 mL/min (adjust as needed for small children who require smaller volumes) until all contents are infused. • Upon completion, rinse infusion bag with 10–30 mL of 0.9% NaCl (while maintaining a closed system) to ensure that as many cells as possible are administered.

Storage • Infusion bags are frozen until time of use. • Thawed infusion bags that have reached room temperature must be infused within 30 min. • Do not store thawed infusion bags at 37°C.

INDICATIONS/ROUTES/DOSAGE

Note: Single-dose infusion(s) contains specimen of chimeric antigen receptor (CAR)–positive viable T cells. Dose is based on weight at the time of leukapheresis.

ALL (Relapsed/refractory)

Note: Give 2–14 days following lymphodepleting chemotherapy with fludarabine and cyclophosphamide.

IV: ADULTS YOUNGER THAN 25 YRS, CHILDREN WEIGHING 50 KG OR LESS: 0.2–5 $\times 10^6$ CAR-positive viable T cells/kg. **WEIGHING 50 KG OR MORE:** 0.1–2.5 $\times 10^8$ CAR-positive viable T cells.

DLBCL (Relapsed/refractory)

Note: Give 2–11 days following lymphodepleting chemotherapy with fludarabine and cyclophosphamide.

IV: ADULTS: 0.6–6 $\times 10^8$ CAR-positive viable T cells.

Dosage in Renal /Hepatic Impairment

Not specified; use caution.

SIDE EFFECTS

Frequent (40%–18%): Pyrexia, decreased appetite, headache, migraine, tachycardia, nausea, diarrhea, vomiting, fatigue, malaise, cough, edema (generalized, peripheral), delirium, agitation, hallucination, irritability, restlessness, generalized pain, constipation. **Occasional (16%–6%):** Abdominal pain, rash (maculopapular, papular, pruritic), myalgia, arthralgia, anxiety, tachypnea, chills, fluid overload, back pain, sleep disorder, insomnia, nightmares, nasal congestion, tremor, dizziness, oropharyngeal pain. **Rare (3%–1%):** Speech disorder (dysarthria, aphasia), visual impairment, motor dysfunction, muscle spasm.

ADVERSE EFFECTS/TOXIC REACTIONS

Myelosuppression (anemia leukopenia, lymphopenia, neutropenia, thrombocytopenia) is an expected response to therapy, but more severe reactions including bone marrow depression, febrile neutropenia may be life-threatening. Prolonged cytopenias may occur for several wks following lymphodepleting chemotherapy. Life-threatening CRS reported in up to 79% of pts. Symptoms of CRS may include asthenia, hypotension, nausea, pyrexia; elevated ALT/AST, bilirubin; disseminated intravascular coagulation (DIC), capillary leak syndrome, hemophagocytic lymphohistiocytosis/macrophage activation syndrome (HLH/MAS). Infusion reactions may be clinically indistinguishable from CRS. Life-threatening neurological toxicities including altered mental status, balance disorders, confusion, disorientation, encephalopathy, seizures, speech disorders, syncope occurred in up to 72% of pts. Cardiac events including cardiac failure, cardiac arrest may occur, esp. in pts with history of cardiac disease. Life-threatening opportunistic infections, bacterial/viral/fungal infections, sepsis were reported. Other life-threatening or fatal events may include abdominal compartment syndrome, acute kidney injury, ARDS, graft-versus-host disease, multiple organ dysfunction syndrome, respiratory distress/failure, seizures, thrombosis (DVT, PE, venous thrombosis). May cause HBV reactivation, resulting in fulminant hepatitis, hepatic failure, or death. Tumor lysis syndrome may present as acute renal failure, hypocalcemia, hyperuricemia, hyperphosphatemia. Hypogammaglobulinemia, agammaglobulinemia (IgG) (related to B-cell aplasia) reported in 43% of pts. May increase risk of new malignancies. Hypersensitivity reactions

T

including anaphylaxis may occur. Immunogenicity (anti-mCAR19 antibodies) occurred in 5% of pts.

NURSING CONSIDERATIONS

BASELINE ASSESSMENT

Obtain CBC, BMP, LFT, vital signs; pregnancy test in females of reproductive potential. Test all pts for hepatitis B or C virus infection, HIV infection before cell collection. Withhold infusion if any of the following are present: active graft-versus-host disease, unresolved adverse effect from previous chemotherapies (e.g., cardiac reactions, hypotension, pulmonary reactions); severe, uncontrolled infection; worsening of leukemia burden following lymphodepleting chemotherapy. Ensure that tocilizumab, emergency resuscitative equipment are readily available before initiation and following completion. Question history of cardiac disease, pulmonary disease, chronic infections, renal impairment, thrombosis. Question for recent administration of vaccines, live vaccines. Offer emotional support.

INTERVENTION/EVALUATION

Monitor ANC, CBC, BMP, LFT, vital signs as clinically indicated; immunoglobulin levels after treatment (and in newborns of treated mothers). Manage hypogammaglobulinemia as clinically appropriate. Obtain serum calcium, phosphate, uric acid if tumor lysis syndrome is suspected. Diligently monitor for CRS. Recommend observation 2–3 times/wk during the first wk at a health care facility. Follow manufacturer's guidelines regarding management of CRS (e.g., administration of IV fluids, vasopressors, tocilizumab). Monitor for infections of any kind. Due to risk of cardiovascular events, have emergency resuscitation equipment readily available. Conduct routine neurological assessments. Monitor for symptoms of DVT (leg or arm pain/swelling), PE (chest pain, dyspnea, tachycardia). Monitor for bleeding events, renal toxicity (anuria, hypertension, generalized edema, flank pain), secondary malignancies, recurrence of cancer, HBV reactivation (amber to orange-colored urine, fatigue, jaundice, nausea, vomiting), neurological toxicities. Monitor weight, I&Os; daily pattern of bowel activity, stool consistency. Ensure adequate hydration, nutrition.

PATIENT/FAMILY TEACHING

• Treatment may depress your immune system and reduce your ability to fight infection. Report symptoms of infection such as body aches, burning with urination, chills, cough, fatigue, fever. Avoid those with active infection. • Report symptoms of bone marrow depression such as bruising, fatigue, fever, shortness of breath, weight loss, bleeding easily, bloody urine or stool. • CRS, a life-threatening condition caused by immune activation, may occur; report difficulty breathing, headache, fever, low blood pressure, rash, rapid heart rate. Stay within the proximity of a health care facility for at least 4 wks after infusion. • Therapy may cause tumor lysis syndrome (a condition caused by the rapid breakdown of cancer cells), which can cause kidney failure and can be fatal. Report decreased urination, amber-colored urine, confusion, difficulty breathing, fatigue, fever, muscle or joint pain, palpitations, seizures, vomiting. • Effective contraception may be required based on treatment with other medications. • Report cardiovascular events (e.g., difficulty breathing, fainting, irregular heartbeats, palpitations, sweating). • Report bleeding of any kind. • If applicable, vaccinations should be up-to-date at least 6 wks before starting treatment. Do not receive live vaccines. • Report symptoms of DVT (e.g., swelling, pain, hot feeling in the arms or legs; discoloration of extremity), lung embolism (e.g., difficulty breathing, chest pain, rapid heart rate). • Report liver problems such as bruising, confusion, dark or amber-colored urine, right upper abdominal pain, or yellowing of the skin or eyes; kidney problems such as de-

T

creased urine output, dark-colored urine; allergic reactions such as difficulty breathing, hives, low blood pressure, rash, swelling of the face or tongue. • Treatment may cause reactivation of chronic viral infections, new cancers.

tiZANidine

tye-**zan**-i-deen
(Zanaflex)
Do not confuse tiZANidine with tiaGABine.

CLASSIFICATION

PHARMACOTHERAPEUTIC: Alpha$_2$-adrenergic agonist. **CLINICAL:** Antispastic.

USES

Acute and intermittent management of muscle spasticity (spasms, stiffness, rigidity), spasticity associated with multiple sclerosis or spinal cord injury.

PRECAUTIONS

Contraindications: Hypersensitivity to tiZANidine. Concurrent use with strong CYP1A2 inhibitors (e.g., ciprofloxacin, fluvoxamine). **Cautions:** Renal/hepatic disease, pts at risk for severe hypotensive effects, cardiac disease, psychiatric disorders, elderly.

ACTION

Increases presynaptic inhibition of spinal motor neurons mediated by alpha$_2$-adrenergic agonists, reducing facilitation to postsynaptic motor neurons. **Therapeutic Effect:** Reduces muscle spasticity.

PHARMACOKINETICS

Metabolized in liver. Primarily excreted in urine. **Half-life:** 2 hrs.

INTERACTIONS

DRUG: **Alcohol, other CNS depressants (e.g., LORazepam, morphine, zolpidem)** may increase CNS depressant effects. **Strong CYP1A2 inhibitors (e.g., ciprofloxacin, fluvoxaMINE)** may increase concentration/adverse effects (contraindicated). **HERBAL:** **Herbals with hypotensive properties (e.g., garlic, ginger, ginkgo biloba)** may alter effects. **Herbals with sedative properties (e.g., chamomile, kava kava, valerian)** may increase CNS depression. **FOOD:** None known. **LAB VALUES:** May increase serum alkaline phosphatase, ALT, AST.

AVAILABILITY (Rx)

Capsules: 2 mg, 4 mg, 6 mg. **Tablets:** 2 mg, 4 mg.

ADMINISTRATION/HANDLING

PO

• Capsules may be opened and sprinkled on food. • May give without regard to food. • Administration should be consistent and not switched between giving with or without food.

INDICATIONS/ROUTES/DOSAGE

Muscle Spasticity

PO: ADULTS, ELDERLY: Initially, 2 mg once daily at bedtime. May increase by 2–4 mg at intervals of 1–4 days. **Maximum:** 36 mg/day in 3–4 divided doses. **Discontinuation of therapy:** Gradually taper dose by 2–4 mg daily.

Dosage in Renal Impairment

May require dose reduction/less frequent dosing. **CrCl less than 25 mL/min:** Reduce dose by 50%. If higher doses needed, increase dose instead of frequency.

Dosage in Hepatic Impairment

Avoid use if possible. If used, monitor for adverse effects (e.g., hypotension).

SIDE EFFECTS

Frequent (49%–41%): Dry mouth, drowsiness, asthenia. **Occasional (16%–4%):** Dizziness, UTI, constipation. **Rare**

T

(3%): Nervousness, amblyopia, pharyngitis, rhinitis, vomiting, urinary frequency.

ADVERSE EFFECTS/TOXIC REACTIONS

Hypotension may be associated with bradycardia, orthostatic hypotension, and, rarely, syncope. Risk of hypotension increases as dosage increases; hypotension is noted within 1 hr after administration. May cause visual hallucinations.

NURSING CONSIDERATIONS

BASELINE ASSESSMENT

Obtain LFT. Record onset, type, location, duration of muscular spasm. Check for immobility, stiffness, swelling.

INTERVENTION/EVALUATION

Assist with ambulation at all times. For those on long-term therapy, serum hepatic/renal function tests should be performed periodically. Evaluate for therapeutic response (decreased intensity of skeletal muscle pain/tenderness, improved mobility, decrease in spasticity). Go from lying to standing slowly.

PATIENT/FAMILY TEACHING

• Avoid tasks that require alertness, motor skills until response to drug is established. • Avoid sudden changes in posture. • May cause hypotension, sedation, impaired coordination. • Avoid alcohol.

T

tobramycin

toe-bra-**mye**-sin
(TOBI, Tobrex)

BLACK BOX ALERT May cause neurotoxicity, nephrotoxicity, ototoxicity. Ototoxicity usually is irreversible. Increased risk of neuromuscular blockade, including respiratory paralysis, particularly when given after anesthesia or muscle relaxants. May cause fetal harm.

Do not confuse tobramycin with vancomycin, or Tobrex with TobraDex.

FIXED-COMBINATION(S)

TobraDex: tobramycin/dexamethasone (a steroid): 0.3%/0.1% per mL or per g. **Zylet:** tobramycin/loteprednol: 0.3%/0.5%.

◆CLASSIFICATION

PHARMACOTHERAPEUTIC: Aminoglycoside. **CLINICAL:** Antibiotic.

USES

Treatment of susceptible infections due to *P. aeruginosa,* other gram-negative organisms including skin/skin structure, bone, joint, respiratory tract infections; postop, burn, intra-abdominal infections; complicated UTI; septicemia; meningitis. **Ophthalmic:** Superficial eye infections: blepharitis, conjunctivitis, keratitis, corneal ulcers. **Inhalation:** Bronchopulmonary infections *(Pseudomonas aeruginosa)* in pts with cystic fibrosis.

PRECAUTIONS

Contraindications: Hypersensitivity to tobramycin, other aminoglycosides (cross-sensitivity) and their components. **Cautions:** Renal impairment, auditory or vestibular impairment, conditions that depress neuromuscular transmission, Parkinson's disease, myasthenia gravis, hypocalcemia, pregnancy, elderly.

ACTION

Irreversibly binds to protein on bacterial ribosomes. **Therapeutic Effect:** Interferes with protein synthesis of susceptible microorganisms.

PHARMACOKINETICS

Widely distributed. Protein binding: less than 30%. Excreted in urine. Removed by hemodialysis. **Half-life:** 2–4 hrs (increased in renal impairment, neonates; decreased in cystic fibrosis, febrile, or burn pts).

LIFESPAN CONSIDERATIONS

Pregnancy/Lactation: Readily crosses placenta; distributed in breast milk. May cause fetal nephrotoxicity. Ophthalmic form should not be used in breastfeeding mothers and only when specifically indicated in pregnancy. **Children:** Immature renal function in neonates, premature infants may increase risk of toxicity. **Elderly:** Age-related renal impairment may increase risk of toxicity; dosage adjustment recommended.

INTERACTIONS

DRUG: May decrease therapeutic effect of **BCG (intravesical), vaccine (live). Foscarnet, mannitol** may increase nephrotoxic effect. **Penicillin** may decrease concentration/effect. **HERBAL:** None significant. **FOOD:** None known. **LAB VALUES:** May increase serum BUN, bilirubin, creatinine, alkaline phosphatase, LDH, ALT, AST. May decrease serum calcium, magnesium, potassium, sodium. Therapeutic peak serum level: 5–20 mcg/mL; therapeutic trough serum level: 0.5–2 mcg/mL. Toxic peak serum level: greater than 20 mcg/mL; toxic trough serum level: greater than 2 mcg/mL.

AVAILABILITY (Rx)

Infusion, Premix: 60 mg/50 mL, 80 mg/100 mL. **Inhalation Powder:** ***(TOBI Podhaler):*** 28 mg in a capsule. **Injection, Powder for Reconstitution:** 1.2 g. **Injection Solution:** 10 mg/mL, 40 mg/mL. **Ointment, Ophthalmic:** ***(Tobrex):*** 0.3%. **Solution, Nebulization:** ***(TOBI):*** 60 mg/mL. **Solution, Ophthalmic:** ***(Tobrex):*** 0.3%.

ADMINISTRATION/HANDLING

◀ALERT▶ Coordinate peak and trough lab draws with administration times.

IV

Reconstitution • Dilute with 50–100 mL D_5W or 0.9% NaCl. Amount of diluent for infants, children depends on individual need.

Rate of administration • Infuse over 30–60 min.

Storage • Store vials at room temperature. • Solutions may be discolored by light or air (does not affect potency). • Refrigerate diluted solution for up to 96 hrs or store at room temperature for up to 24 hrs.

IM

• To minimize discomfort, give deep IM slowly. • Less painful if injected into gluteus maximus rather than lateral aspect of thigh.

Inhalation

• Refrigerate. • May store at room temperature up to 28 days after removing from refrigerator. • Do not use if cloudy or contains particulates. • **Podhaler:** Capsules must not be swallowed. • Doses should be as close as possible to 12 hrs apart and not less than 6 hrs apart. • Use Podhaler device supplied.

Ophthalmic

• Place gloved finger on lower eyelid, pull out until pocket is formed between eye and lower lid. • Place correct number of drops (1/4–1/2 inch ointment) into pocket. • **Solution:** Apply digital pressure to lacrimal sac for 1–2 min (minimizes drainage into nose/throat, reducing risk of systemic effects). • **Ointment:** Instruct pt to close eye for 1–2 min, rolling eyeball (increases contact area of drug to eye). • Remove excess solution/ointment around eye.

IV INCOMPATIBILITIES

Amphotericin B complex (Abelcet, AmBisome, Amphotec), heparin, indomethacin (Indocin), piperacillin-tazobactam (Zosyn), propofol (Diprivan), sargramostim (Leukine, Prokine).

IV COMPATIBILITIES

Amiodarone (Cordarone), calcium gluconate, cefepime, ceftaroline, cefTAZidime, dexmedetomidine (Precedex), dilTIAZem (Cardizem), furosemide (Lasix), HYDROmorphone (Dilaudid), insulin, linezolid (Zyvox), magnesium sulfate, midazolam (Versed), morphine, niCARdipine (Cardene), tigecycline (Tygacil).

INDICATIONS/ROUTES/DOSAGE

◀ALERT▶ Space parenteral doses evenly around the clock. Dosage based on ideal body weight. Peak, trough levels determined periodically to maintain desired serum concentrations (minimizes risk of toxicity). Recommended peak level: 4–10 mcg/mL; trough level: 0.5–2 mcg/mL.

Usual Parenteral Dosage

IV: ADULTS, ELDERLY: 3–7.5 mg/kg/day in 3 divided doses. Once-daily dosing: 4–7 mg/kg every 24 hrs. **CHILDREN, ADOLESCENTS:** 6–7.5 mg/kg/day divided q6–8h. **NEONATES LESS THAN 1 KG (14 DAYS OR YOUNGER):** 5 mg/kg/dose q48h; **(15–28 DAYS):** 5 mg/kg/dose q36h. **1–2 KG (7 DAYS OR YOUNGER):** 5 mg/kg/dose q48h; **(8–28 DAYS):** 5 mg/kg/dose q36h. **GREATER THAN 2 KG (7 DAYS OR YOUNGER):** 4 mg/kg q24h; **(8–28 DAYS):** 4–5 mg/kg q24h.

Usual Ophthalmic Dosage

Ophthalmic ointment: ADULTS, ELDERLY, CHILDREN 2 MOS AND OLDER: Apply 1/2 inch to conjunctiva q8–12h (q3–4h for severe infections).

Ophthalmic solution: ADULTS, ELDERLY, CHILDREN 2 MOS AND OLDER: 1–2 drops in affected eye q4h (2 drops/hr for severe infections).

Usual Inhalation Dosage (Cystic fibrosis)

Inhalation high dose: ADULTS, CHILDREN 6 YRS AND OLDER: 300 mg q12h 28 days on, 28 days off. ***(Tobi Podhaler):*** Four 28-mg capsules twice daily for 28 days followed by 28 days off.

Dosage in Renal Impairment

After loading dose of 1–2 mg/kg, maintenance dose and frequency are based on serum creatinine levels, creatinine clearance.

Creatinine Clearance	Dosing Interval
41–60 mL/min	q12h
21–40 mL/min	q24h
10–20 mL/min	q48h
Less than 10 mL/min	q72h
Hemodialysis	Loading dose 2–3 mg/kg then 1–2 mg/kg q48–72h
Continuous renal replacement therapy	Loading dose 2–3 mg/kg then 1–2.5 mg/kg q24–48h

Dosage in Hepatic Impairment

No dose adjustment.

SIDE EFFECTS

Occasional: IM: Pain, induration. **IV:** Phlebitis, thrombophlebitis. **Topical:** Hypersensitivity reaction (fever, pruritus, rash, urticaria). **Ophthalmic:** Tearing, itching, redness, eyelid swelling. **Rare:** Hypotension, nausea, vomiting.

ADVERSE EFFECTS/TOXIC REACTIONS

Nephrotoxicity (acute kidney injury, acute tubular necrosis, renal failure) may occur. Irreversible ototoxicity (dizziness, ringing/roaring in ears, hearing loss), neurotoxicity (headache, dizziness, lethargy, tremor, visual disturbances) occur occasionally. Risk increases with higher dosages or prolonged therapy or if solution is applied directly to mucosa. Superinfections, particularly fungal infections, may result from bacterial imbalance with any administration route. Anaphylaxis may occur.

NURSING CONSIDERATIONS

BASELINE ASSESSMENT

Dehydration must be treated before beginning parenteral therapy. Question for history of allergies, esp. aminoglycosides, sulfite (and parabens for topical, ophthalmic routes). Establish baseline hearing acuity. Obtain baseline lab tests, esp. renal function.

INTERVENTION/EVALUATION

Monitor I&O (maintain hydration), urinalysis, renal function. Monitor results of peak/trough blood tests. **Therapeutic serum level:** peak: 5–20 mcg/mL; trough: 0.5–2 mcg/mL. **Toxic serum level:** peak: greater than 20 mcg/mL; trough: greater than 2 mcg/mL. Be alert to ototoxic, neurotoxic symptoms. Evaluate IV site for phlebitis (heat, pain, red streaking over vein). Assess for rash. Monitor for superinfection, particularly anal/genital pruritus, changes of oral mucosa, diarrhea. When treating pts with neuromuscular disorders, assess respiratory response carefully. **Ophthalmic:** Assess for redness, swelling, itching, tearing.

PATIENT/FAMILY TEACHING

• Report any hearing, visual, balance, urinary problems, even after therapy is completed. • **Ophthalmic:** Blurred vision, tearing may occur briefly after application. • Report persistent tearing, redness, irritation.

tocilizumab

toe-si-**liz**-oo-mab
(Actemra)

BLACK BOX ALERT Tuberculosis, serious invasive fungal infections, other opportunistic infections have occurred. Test for tuberculosis prior to and during treatment, regardless of initial result. Consider treatment of latent TB prior to initiation.

CLASSIFICATION

PHARMACOTHERAPEUTIC: Interleukin (IL)-6 receptor inhibitor. **CLINICAL:** Antirheumatic, disease-modifying agent.

USES

Treatment of moderate to severe rheumatoid arthritis in adults who had inadequate response to disease-modifying antirheumatic drugs (DMARDs). Treatment of active systemic juvenile idiopathic arthritis (SJIA) in pts 2 yrs of age and older. Treatment of active polyarticular juvenile idiopathic arthritis (PJIA) in pts 2 yrs and older. Treatment of adults and children 2 yrs of age and older with chimeric antigen receptor (CAR) T-cell–induced severe or life-threatening cytokine release syndrome. Treatment of giant cell arteritis in adults.

PRECAUTIONS

Contraindications: Hypersensitivity to tocilizumab. **Cautions:** Preexisting or recent-onset demyelinating disorders (e.g., multiple sclerosis), elderly, recent travel or residence in TB- or mycosis-endemic areas; history of chronic opportunistic infections (esp. bacterial, invasive fungal, mycobacterial, protozoal, viral, TB); history of HIV, herpes zoster, hepatitis B or C virus infection; conditions predisposing to infection (e.g., diabetes, renal failure, immunocompromised pts, open wounds), pts at risk for GI perforation (e.g., Crohn's disease, diverticulitis, GI tract malignancies, peptic ulcers, peritoneal malignancies). Do not initiate in pts with active infection; platelet count 100,000 cells/mm^3 or less, ANC less than 2,000 cells/mm^3; serum ALT, AST greater than 1.5 times ULN.

ACTION

Binds to IL-6 receptors, inhibiting signals of proinflammatory cytokines. **Therapeutic Effect:** Inhibits/slows structural joint damage, improves physical function.

PHARMACOKINETICS

Distributed in steady state of plasma and tissue compartments. Undergoes biphasic elimination from circulation. **Half-life:** 11–13 days.

LIFESPAN CONSIDERATIONS

Pregnancy/Lactation: Unknown if distributed in breast milk; however, immunoglobulin G (IgG) is present in breast milk and is known to cross the placenta. **Children:** Safety and efficacy not established in conditions other than SJIA, severe or life-threatening CAR T-cell–induced cytokine release syndrome. **Elderly:** Cautious use due to increased risk of serious infections, malignancy.

INTERACTIONS

DRUG: May increase adverse effects of **abatacept, belimumab, natali-**

T

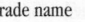

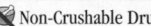

zumab, tofacitinib, vaccines (live). May decrease therapeutic effect of **vaccines (live). Baricitinib** may increase adverse effects. May increase immunosuppressive effect of **anti-TNF agents (e.g., adalimumab, etanercept, infliximab). HERBAL: Echinacea** may alter levels/effects. **FOOD:** None known. **LAB VALUES:** May increase serum ALT, AST, lipids. May decrease platelets, neutrophils.

AVAILABILITY (Rx)

Injection Solution: 20 mg/mL (80 mg/4 mL, 200 mg/10 mL, 400 mg/20 mL). **Syringe for SQ Administration:** 162 mg/0.9 mL. **Syringe Auto-injector:** 162 mg/0.9 mL.

ADMINISTRATION/HANDLING

◀ALERT▶ Do not infuse IV push or bolus.

IV

Reconstitution • Dilute in 100 mL 0.9% NaCl (50 mL 0.9% NaCl for SJIA pts weighing less than 30 kg). • Prior to mixing, withdraw and discard volume of NaCl equal to volume of patient-dosed solution. • Invert bag to avoid foaming. • Inject solution and dilute for mixture that equals 50 mL or 100 mL in NaCl bag.

Rate of administration • Infuse over 1 hr.

Storage • Refrigerate vials; do not freeze. • Diluted solutions may be stored for 24 hrs at room temperature or refrigerated. • Protect from light until time of use. • Solution appears colorless. Discard solution if it appears cloudy, discolored, or contains particulate.

INDICATIONS/ROUTES/DOSAGE

Note: Do not infuse concomitantly in same IV line with other drugs. Do not begin if ANC less than 2,000 cells/mm^3, platelets less than 100,000 cells/mm^3, or ALT or AST more than 1.5 times ULN.

Moderate to Severely Active Rheumatoid Arthritis

IV: ADULTS, ELDERLY: 4 mg/kg every 4 wks initially. May increase to 8 mg/kg every 4 wks. **Maximum:** 800 mg per dose. **SQ: ADULTS, ELDERLY WEIGHING 100 KG OR GREATER:** 162 mg/wk. **WEIGHING LESS THAN 100 KG:** 162 mg every other wk. May increase to every wk based on clinical response.

Cytokine Release Syndrome

IV: ADULTS, CHILDREN WEIGHING 30 KG OR GREATER: 8 mg/kg. **PTS WEIGHING LESS THAN 30 KG:** 12 mg/kg. If no clinical improvement, 3 additional doses may be given with an interval of at least 8 hrs. **Maximum:** 800 mg/dose.

Giant Cell Arteritis

SQ: ADULTS, ELDERLY: 162 mg once every wk (in combination with tapering course of glucocorticoid). May be given alone following discontinuation of glucocorticoid.

Dosage Modification

Hepatic enzyme levels greater than ULN.

Lab Value	Recommendation
1–3 times ULN	Dose modify concomitant DMARDs or reduce dose to 4 mg/kg until ALT, AST normalized
Greater than 3–5 times ULN	Interrupt treatment until ALT, AST less than 3 times ULN, then follow guidelines for 1–3 times ULN
Greater than 5 times ULN	Discontinue treatment

SJIA

IV: CHILDREN WEIGHING 30 KG OR MORE: 8 mg/kg q2wks. **CHILDREN WEIGHING LESS THAN 30 KG:** 12 mg/kg q2wks.

SQ: CHILDREN WEIGHING 30 KG OR MORE: 162 mg once every wk. **CHILDREN WEIGHING LESS THAN 30 KG:** 162 mg q2wks.

PJIA

IV: CHILDREN WEIGHING 30 KG OR MORE: 8 mg/kg q4wks. **CHILDREN WEIGHING LESS THAN 30 KG:** 10 mg/kg q4wks.

SQ: WEIGHING 30 KG OR MORE: 162 mg q2wks. **WEIGHING LESS THAN 30 KG:** 162 mg q3wks.

Dosage in Renal Impairment

Mild impairment: No dose adjustment. **Moderate to severe impairment:** Use caution (not studied).

Dosage in Hepatic Impairment

Not recommended.

SIDE EFFECTS

Occasional (8%–6%): Upper respiratory tract infection, nasopharyngitis, headache, hypertension. **Rare (5%–3%):** Infusion reaction, dizziness, bronchitis, rash, oral ulceration.

ADVERSE EFFECTS/TOXIC REACTIONS

Neutropenia may increase risk of infections. Fatal infections (bacterial arthritis, cellulitis, herpes zoster, pneumonia, UTI, gastroenteritis, diverticulitis), opportunistic infections (aspergillosis, candidiasis, cryptococcus, pneumocystosis, TB) were reported. Serious hepatotoxicity may lead to liver transplantation or death. Hypersensitivity reactions (anaphylaxis, erythema, rash, urticaria) may occur. Demyelinating disorders (multiple sclerosis, chronic inflammatory demyelinating polyneuropathy) may occur. May increase risk of GI perforation, new malignancies. Other reactions may include Stevens-Johnson syndrome, pancreatitis.

NURSING CONSIDERATIONS

BASELINE ASSESSMENT

Obtain CBC, BMP, LFT, lipid panel; pregnancy test in females of reproductive potential. Assess onset, location, duration of pain, inflammation. Inspect appearance of affected joints for immobility, deformities. Evaluate for active TB and test for latent infection prior to and during treatment. An induration of 5 mm or greater with purified protein derivative (PPD) is considered a positive result when assessing for latent TB. Consider treatment with antimycobacterial therapy in pts with latent TB. Screen for active infection; history of chronic, opportunistic infections. Question history of hepatic impairment, malignancies; prior hypersensitivity reactions. Screen for concomitant use of other immunosuppressants.

INTERVENTION/EVALUATION

Monitor neutrophil, platelet count 4–8 wks after initiation, then q3mos thereafter. Monitor LFT for hepatic injury (abdominal pain, jaundice, nausea, transaminitis, vomiting) q4–8 wks for 6 mos after initiation, then q3mos thereafter. Obtain lipid panel 4–8 wks after initiation. Monitor for TB infection regardless of baseline PPD. Consider discontinuation if serious infection, opportunistic infection, sepsis occurs. Monitor for hypersensitivity reactions, demyelinating disorders, new malignancies. Report abdominal pain, GI hemorrhage, melena, hematemesis (may indicate GI perforation). Assess skin for cutaneous toxicities. Assess for therapeutic response: relief of pain, stiffness, swelling; increased joint mobility; reduced joint tenderness; improved grip strength.

PATIENT/FAMILY TEACHING

• Treatment may depress your immune system response and reduce your ability to fight infection. Report symptoms of infection such as body aches, chills, cough, fatigue, fever. Avoid those with active infection. • Expect routine tuberculosis screening. Report any travel plans to possible endemic areas. • Do not receive live vaccines. • Report liver problems (abdominal pain, bruising, clay-colored stool, dark or amber-colored urine, yellowing of the skin or eyes), skin reactions (rash, redness, swelling). • Immediately report severe or persistent abdominal pain, bloody stool, fever, vomiting blood; may indicate rupture in GI tract. • Treatment may cause reactivation of chronic viral infections; new cancers; demyelinating disorders such as MS. • Immediately report

T

allergic reactions of any kind. • Other immunosuppressant drugs may increase risk of infection, bleeding.

tofacitinib

toe-fa-**sye**-ti-nib
(Xeljanz, Xeljanz XR)

■ BLACK BOX ALERT ■ Increased risk for developing bacterial, viral, invasive fungal, other opportunistic infections including tuberculosis, cryptococcosis, pneumocystosis that may lead to hospitalization or death; infections often occurred in combination with other immunosuppressants (methotrexate, corticosteroids). Closely monitor for development of infection. Test for latent tuberculosis prior to treatment and during treatment, regardless of initial result. Treatment for latent TB should be initiated before use. Malignancies including lymphoma, nonmelanoma skin cancer reported. Increased rate of Epstein-Barr virus–associated post-transplant lymphoproliferative disorder observed in renal transplant pts who are treated with tofacitinib and other immunosuppressive therapy drugs.

Do not confuse tofacitinib with tipifarnib or Xeljanz with Xeloda.

◆CLASSIFICATION

PHARMACOTHERAPEUTIC: Janus-associated kinase (JAK) inhibitor. **CLINICAL:** Antirheumatic, disease-modifying.

T

USES

Treatment of adult pts with moderate to severe active rheumatoid arthritis with previous inadequate response or intolerance to methotrexate. May be used as monotherapy or in combination with methotrexate or other nonbiologic disease-modifying antirheumatic drugs (DMARDs). Treatment of active psoriatic arthritis (PsA) in pts who have had inadequate response to methotrexate, other DMARDs. Treatment of moderate to severe active ulcerative colitis (UC) in adults who have had an inadequate response or intolerance to tumor necrosis factor blockers. Treatment of active polyarticular course juvenile idiopathic arthritis (pcJIA) in pts 2 yrs and older. Do not use in combination with other biologic DMARDs or with potent immunosuppressants (e.g., azaTHIOprine, cycloSPORINE).

PRECAUTIONS

Contraindications: Hypersensitivity to tofacitinib. **Cautions:** Baseline cytopenias, hepatic/renal impairment, elderly, pulmonary disease, hyperlipidemia, pts who resided in or traveled to endemic areas; cardiac conduction abnormalities, HF; Asian ancestry, conditions predisposing to infection (e.g., diabetes, renal failure, immunocompromised pts, open wounds), pts at risk for GI perforation (e.g., Crohn's disease, diverticulitis, GI tract malignancies, peptic ulcers, peritoneal malignancies), history of chronic opportunistic infections (esp. bacterial, invasive fungal, mycobacterial, protozoal, viral infections including TB); thrombosis (arterial thrombosis, DVT, pulmonary embolism).

ACTION

Inhibits JAK enzymes, which are intracellular enzymes involved in stimulating hematopoiesis and immune cell functioning through a signaling pathway. **Therapeutic Effect:** Reduces inflammation, tenderness, swelling of joints; slows or prevents progressive joint destruction in rheumatoid arthritis (RA). Prevents cytokine or growth factor gene expression, reducing circulating natural killer cells and increasing B cells.

PHARMACOKINETICS

Widely distributed. Metabolized in liver. Protein binding: 40%. Peak plasma concentration: 30–60 min (instant-release); 4 hrs (extended-release). Steady state reached in 24–48 hrs. Excreted primarily in urine. **Half-life:** 3 hrs (instant-release); 6–8 hrs (extended-release).

LIFESPAN CONSIDERATIONS

Pregnancy/Lactation: Females of reproductive potential should use effective contraception during treatment. Breastfeeding not recommended during treatment and for at least 18 hrs after discontinuation. **Children:** Safety and efficacy not established in pts younger than 2 yrs. **Elderly:** Increased risk for serious infections, malignancy.

INTERACTIONS

DRUG: **Immunosuppressants (e.g., azaTHIOprine, cycloSPORINE)** may increase risk for added immunosuppression, infection. **Strong CYP3A4 inhibitors (e.g., clarithromycin, ketoconazole, ritonavir)** may increase concentration/effect. **Strong CYP3A4 inducers (e.g., carBAMazepine, phenytoin, rifAMPin)** may decrease concentration/effect. May increase adverse effects; decrease therapeutic effect of **vaccines (live)**. **HERBAL:** **St. John's wort** may decrease concentration/effect. **Echinacea** may decrease the therapeutic effect. **FOOD:** None known. **LAB VALUES:** May increase ALT, AST, bilirubin, lipids, creatinine. May decrease Hgb, neutrophils, lymphocytes.

AVAILABILITY (Rx)

Tablets, Film-Coated: *(Xeljanz):* 5 mg, 10 mg. *(Xeljanz XR):* 11 mg, 22 mg. **Oral Solution:** 1 mg/mL.

ADMINISTRATION/HANDLING

PO

• Give without regard to food. • Do not cut, split, crush, or chew XR tablet.

INDICATIONS/ROUTES/DOSAGE

◀ALERT▶ Do not initiate treatment in pts with baseline active infection (systemic/localized), severe hepatic impairment, lymphocytes less than 500 cells/mm³, ANC less than 1,000 cells/mm³, Hgb less than 9 g/dL.

Rheumatoid Arthritis (Monotherapy or with nonbiologic DMARD)

PO: ADULTS/ELDERLY: *(Xeljanz):* 5 mg twice daily. *(Xeljanz XR):* 11 mg once daily.

PsA (With nonbiologic DMARD)

PO: ADULTS/ELDERLY: *(Xeljanz):* 5 mg twice daily. *(Xeljanz XR):* 11 mg once daily.

UC

PO: ADULTS/ELDERLY: *(Xeljanz):* Induction: 10 mg twice daily for 8 wks. May transition to maintenance dose or continue 10 mg twice daily for additional 8 wks. Discontinue if 10 mg twice daily is ineffective after 4 mos. **Maintenance:** 5 mg twice daily. May increase to 10 mg twice daily for shortest duration. Use lowest effective dose to maintain response. *(Xeljanz XR):* **Induction:** 22 mg once daily for at least 8 wks. May continue for maximum of 16 wks or transition to maintenance dose. Discontinue if 22 mg once daily dose is ineffective after 16 wks. **Maintenance:** 11 mg once daily. May increase to 22 mg once daily for shortest duration. Use lowest effective dose to maintain response.

pcJIA

PO: CHILDREN 2 YRS AND OLDER WEIGHING 10–19 KG: 3.2 mg (3.2 mL oral solution) twice daily. **20–39 KG:** 4 mg (4 mL oral solution) twice daily. **40 KG OR GREATER:** 5 mg (one 5-mg tablet or 5 mL oral solution) twice daily.

Dose Modification for RA/Psoriatic Arthritis

Hematologic Toxicity

ANC 500–1,000 cells/mm³: Withhold treatment until ANC is 1,000 cells/mm³, then resume previous dose based on response and tolerability. **ANC or lymphocyte count less than 500 cells/mm³:** Permanently discontinue. **Hgb less than 8 g/dL or a decrease of more than 2 g/dL:** Withhold treatment until Hgb level normalizes.

Concomitant Use of Strong/Moderate CYP3A4 Inhibitor, Strong CYPC19 Inhibitor

Reduce dose to 5 mg once daily (if taking 5 mg twice daily or 11 mg once daily).

Dose Modification for UC

Hematologic Toxicity

ANC 500–1,000 cells/mm³: *(Instant-Release):* Reduce dose to 5 mg twice daily

T

(if taking 10 mg twice daily) or withhold treatment (if taking 5 mg twice daily) until ANC is greater than 1,000 cells/mm³, then resume previous dose based on response and tolerability. ***(Extended-Release):*** Reduce dose to 11 mg once daily (if taking 22 mg once daily) or withhold treatment (if taking 11 mg once daily) until ANC is greater than 1000 cells/mm³, then resume previous dose based on response and tolerability. **ANC or lymphocyte count less than 500 cells/mm³:** Permanently discontinue. **Hgb less than 8 g/dL or a decrease of more than 2 g/dL:** Withhold treatment until Hgb level normalizes.

Concomitant Use of Strong/Moderate CYP3A4 Inhibitor, Strong CYPC19 Inhibitor

(Instant-Release): Reduce dose to 5 mg twice daily (if taking 10 mg twice daily) or 5 mg once daily (if taking 5 mg twice daily). ***(Extended-Release):*** Reduce dose to 11 mg once daily (if taking 22 mg once daily) or 5 mg once daily (if taking 11 mg once daily).

Dose Modification for pcJIA

Hematologic Toxicity

ANC 500–1,000 cells/mm³: Withhold treatment until ANC is greater than 1,000 cells/mm³. **ANC or lymphocyte count less than 500 cells/mm³:** Permanently discontinue. **Hgb less than 8 g/dL or a decrease of more than 2 g/dL:** Withhold treatment until Hgb level normalizes.

Concomitant Use of Strong/Moderate CYP3A4 Inhibitor, Strong CYPC19 Inhibitor

Reduce dose to 3.2 mg once daily (if taking 3.2 mg twice daily), or 4 mg once daily (if taking 4 mg twice daily), or 5 mg once daily (if taking 5 mg twice daily).

Dosage in Renal Impairment

Mild impairment: No dose adjustment. **Moderate to severe impairment: (RA/Psoriatic arthritis):** Reduce dose to 5 mg once daily (if 5 mg twice daily or 11 mg once daily). **(UC):** ***(Instant-Release):*** If taking 10 mg twice daily, reduce to 5 mg twice daily. If taking 5 mg twice daily, reduce to 5 mg once daily. ***(Extended-Release):*** Reduce dose to 11 mg once daily (if taking 22 mg once daily) or 5 mg once daily (if taking 11 mg once daily). **(pcJIA):** Reduce dose to 3.2 mg once daily (if taking 3.2 mg twice daily), or 4 mg once daily (if taking 4 mg twice daily), or 5 mg once daily (if taking 5 mg twice daily).

Dosage in Hepatic Impairment

Mild impairment: No dose adjustment. **Moderate impairment: (RA/Psoriatic arthritis):** Reduce dose to 5 mg once daily (if 5 mg twice daily or 11 mg once daily). **(UC):** ***(Instant-Release):*** If taking 10 mg twice daily, reduce to 5 mg twice daily. If taking 5 mg twice daily, reduce to 5 mg once daily. ***(Extended-Release):*** Reduce dose to 11 mg once daily (if taking 22 mg once daily) or 5 mg once daily (if taking 11 mg once daily). **(pcJIA):** Reduce dose to 3.2 mg once daily (if taking 3.2 mg twice daily), or 4 mg once daily (if taking 4 mg twice daily), or 5 mg once daily (if taking 5 mg twice daily). **Severe impairment:** Not recommended.

SIDE EFFECTS

Rare (4%–2%): Upper respiratory tract infection, diarrhea, nasopharyngitis, headache, hypertension.

ADVERSE EFFECTS/TOXIC REACTIONS

Neutropenia, lymphopenia may increase risk for infection. Serious infections may include aspergillosis, BK virus, cellulitis, coccidioidomycosis, cryptococcus, cytomegalovirus, esophageal candidiasis, histoplasmosis, invasive fungal infections, listeriosis, pneumocystosis, pneumonia, tuberculosis, UTI, sepsis. May cause viral reactivation of herpes zoster infection. May increase risk of GI perforation, lymphoma, new malignancies (breast, lung, pancreatic, prostate cancer; melanoma, nonmelanoma skin cancer). Pts older than 50 yrs with at least one cardiovascular risk factors are at increased risk of sudden cardiac death if taking higher dose. Thrombotic events (arterial thrombosis, DVT, pulmonary embolism) have occurred. Hypersensitivity reactions (angioedema, urticaria) were reported. Hepatotoxicity reported in 1% of pts. Fatal interstitial lung disease may occur.

NURSING CONSIDERATIONS

BASELINE ASSESSMENT

Obtain CBC, BMP, LFT, lipid panel; pregnancy test in females of reproductive potential. Assess onset, location, duration of pain, inflammation. Inspect appearance of affected joints for immobility, deformities in pts with RA. Assess usual bowel movement patterns, stool characteristics in pts with UC. Evaluate for active TB and test for latent infection prior to and during treatment. An induration of 5 mm or greater with purified protein derivative (PPD) is considered a positive result when assessing for latent TB. Consider treatment with antimycobacterial therapy in pts with latent TB. Screen for active infection; history of chronic, opportunistic infections. Question history of hepatic/renal impairment, pulmonary disease, cardiovascular risk, thrombosis, malignancies; prior hypersensitivity reactions. Receive full medication history and screen for interactions.

INTERVENTION/EVALUATION

Monitor neutrophil, platelet count 4–8 wks after initiation, then q3mos thereafter. Monitor LFT for hepatic injury (abdominal pain, jaundice, nausea, transaminitis, vomiting) q4–8 wks for 6 mos after initiation, then q3mos thereafter. Obtain lipid panel 4–8 wks after initiation. Monitor for TB infection regardless of baseline PPD. Consider discontinuation if serious infection, opportunistic infection, sepsis occurs. Monitor for hypersensitivity reactions, new malignancies; symptoms of arterial thrombosis, DVT (leg or arm pain/swelling); PE (chest pain, dyspnea, tachycardia). Report abdominal pain, GI hemorrhage, melena, hematemesis (may indicate GI perforation). Monitor daily pattern of bowel activity, stool consistency. Consider ABG, radiologic test if ILD/pneumonitis (excessive cough, dyspnea, fever, hypoxia) is suspected. Consider treatment with corticosteroids if ILD/pneumonitis is confirmed. Assess for therapeutic response (arthritis): relief of pain, stiffness, swelling; increased joint mobility, improved grip strength; (UC): decreased abdominal pain, cramping, diarrhea; increased appetite, weight gain.

PATIENT/FAMILY TEACHING

• Treatment may depress your immune system response and reduce your ability to fight infection. Report symptoms of infection such as body aches, chills, cough, fatigue, fever. Avoid those with active infection. • Expect routine tuberculosis screening. Report any travel plans to possible endemic areas. • Do not receive live vaccines. • Report liver problems (abdominal pain, bruising, clay-colored stool, dark or amber-colored urine, yellowing of the skin or eyes), symptoms of lung inflammation (excessive coughing, difficulty breathing, chest pain); DVT (swelling, pain, hot feeling in the arms or legs; discoloration of extremity), lung embolism (difficulty breathing, chest pain, rapid heart rate). • Immediately report severe or persistent abdominal pain, bloody stool, fever, vomiting blood; may indicate rupture in GI tract. • Treatment may cause reactivation of chronic viral infections, new cancers. • Immediately report allergic reactions of any kind. • Avoid pregnancy. Do not breastfeed.

T

tolterodine

tol-**ter**-oh-deen
(Detrol, Detrol LA)
Do not confuse Detrol with Ditropan, or tolterodine with fesoterodine.

CLASSIFICATION

PHARMACOTHERAPEUTIC: Antimuscarinic agent. **CLINICAL:** Antispasmodic.

USES

Treatment of overactive bladder in pts with symptoms of urinary frequency, urgency, or urge incontinence.

PRECAUTIONS

Contraindications: Hypersensitivity to tolterodine or fesoterodine. Gastric retention, uncontrolled narrow-angle glaucoma, urinary retention. **Cautions:** Renal impairment, bladder outflow obstruction (risk of urinary retention), GI motility disorders (e.g., pyloric stenosis [risk of gastric retention]), treated narrow-angle glaucoma, myasthenia gravis, pts risk for QTc interval prolongation (congenital long QT syndrome, HF, medications that prolong QTc interval, hypokalemia, hypomagnesemia), hepatic impairment, elderly.

ACTION

Antagonist of muscarinic receptors mediating urinary bladder contraction. Increases residual urine volume, reduces detrusor muscle pressure. **Therapeutic Effect:** Decreases urinary frequency, urgency.

PHARMACOKINETICS

Widely distributed. Protein binding: 96%. Metabolized in liver. Primarily excreted in urine. **Half-life:** Immediate-release: 2–10 hrs. Extended-release: 7–18 hrs.

T

LIFESPAN CONSIDERATIONS

Pregnancy/Lactation: Unknown if drug is distributed in breast milk. Breastfeeding not recommended. **Children:** Safety and efficacy not established. **Elderly:** No age-related precautions noted.

INTERACTIONS

DRUG: **Strong CYP3A4 inhibitors (e.g., clarithromycin, ketoconazole, ritonavir)** may increase concentration/effect. **Strong CYP3A4 inducers (e.g., carBAMazepine, phenytoin, rifAMPin)** may decrease concentration/effect. **Anticholinergics (e.g., aclidinium, ipratropium, tiotropium, umeclidinium)** may increase anticholinergic effect. **Strong CYP2D6 inhibitors (e.g., FLUoxetine, PARoxetine)** may inhibit drug metabolism. **QT interval–prolonging medications (e.g., amiodarone, azithromycin, ciprofloxacin, haloperidol, methadone, sotalol)** may increase risk of QTc interval prolongation. **HERBAL:** **St. John's wort** may decrease concentration/effects. **FOOD:** None known. **LAB VALUES:** None known.

AVAILABILITY (Rx)

Tablets: 1 mg, 2 mg.

Capsules, Extended-Release: 2 mg, 4 mg.

ADMINISTRATION/HANDLING

PO

• May give without regard to food. • Give extended-release capsules whole; do not break, crush, or open.

INDICATIONS/ROUTES/DOSAGE

Overactive Bladder

PO: ADULTS, ELDERLY: ***(Immediate-Release):*** 1–2 mg twice daily. **With CYP3A4 inhibitors:** 1 mg twice daily. ***(Extended-Release):*** 2–4 mg once daily. **With CYP3A4 inhibitors:** 2 mg once daily.

Dosage in Renal/Hepatic Impairment

Mild to moderate impairment: ***(Immediate-Release):*** 1 mg twice daily. Use caution. ***(Extended-Release):*** 2 mg once daily. Use caution. **Severe impairment:** Not recommended.

SIDE EFFECTS

Frequent (40%): Dry mouth. **Occasional (11%–4%):** Headache, dizziness, fatigue, constipation, dyspepsia, upper respiratory tract infection, UTI, dry eyes, abnormal vision (accommodation problems), nausea, diarrhea. **Rare (3%):** Drowsiness, chest/back pain, arthralgia, rash, weight gain, dry skin.

ADVERSE EFFECTS/TOXIC REACTIONS

Hypersensitivity reactions (angioedema, airway obstruction, dyspnea, hypotension) resulting in hospitalization were reported. May cause gastric retention in pts with gastric motility disorders. Overdose can result in severe anticholinergic effects, including abdominal cramps, facial warmth, excessive salivation/lacrimation, diaphoresis, pallor, urinary urgency, blurred vision, prolonged QT interval.

NURSING CONSIDERATIONS

BASELINE ASSESSMENT

Assess degree of overactive bladder (urinary urgency, frequency, incontinence). Question history as listed in Precautions.

INTERVENTION/EVALUATION

Assist with ambulation if dizziness occurs. Question for visual changes. Monitor incontinence, postvoid residuals. Monitor ECG in pts at risk for QT interval prolongation.

PATIENT/FAMILY TEACHING

• May cause blurred vision, dry eyes/mouth, constipation. • Report any confusion, altered mental status. • Avoid tasks that require alertness, motor skills until response to drug is established.

topiramate

toe-**peer**-a-mate
(Qudexy XR, Topamax, Topamax Sprinkle, Trokendi XR)
Do not confuse Topamax or topiramate with TEGretol, TEGretol XR, or Toprol XL.

◆CLASSIFICATION

PHARMACOTHERAPEUTIC: Miscellaneous agent. **CLINICAL:** Anticonvulsant.

USES

Monotherapy for treatment of partial-onset or primary generalized tonic-clonic seizures in pts 2 yrs and older (immediate-release, Qudexy XR) or 6 yrs and older (Trokendi XR). Adjunctive therapy for partial-onset, primary generalized tonic-clonic seizures or seizures associated with Lennox-Gastaut syndrome in pts 2 yrs and older (immediate-release, Qudexy XR) or 6 yrs and older (Trokendi XR). Prevention of migraine headache in pts 12 yrs and older. **OFF-LABEL:** Neuropathic pain, diabetic neuropathy, prophylaxis of cluster headaches, infantile spasms.

PRECAUTIONS

Contraindications: Hypersensitivity to topiramate. **Extended-Release: Trokendi XR:** Recent alcohol use (within 6 hrs prior to or after). **Qudexy XR:** Pts with metabolic acidosis who are taking metFORMIN. **Cautions:** Hepatic/renal impairment, elderly, respiratory impairment, strenuous exercise, heat exposure, concomitant use anticholinergic agents; history of congenital metabolism dysfunction, decreased mitochondrial activity; suicidal ideation and behavior.

ACTION

Blocks neuronal sodium channels, enhances GABA activity; antagonizes glutamate receptors and weakly inhibits carbonic anhydrase. **Therapeutic Effect:** Decreases seizure activity.

PHARMACOKINETICS

Widely distributed. Protein binding: 15%–41%. Metabolized in liver. Primarily excreted unchanged in urine. Removed by hemodialysis. **Half-life:** 21 hrs.

⌛ LIFESPAN CONSIDERATIONS

Pregnancy/Lactation: Unknown if distributed in breast milk. **Children:** Safety and efficacy not established in pts younger than 2 yrs. **Elderly:** Age-related renal impairment may require dosage adjustment.

T

INTERACTIONS

DRUG: **Alcohol, CNS depressants (e.g., LORazepam, morphine, zolpidem)** may increase CNS depression. **Strong CYP3A4 inducers (e.g., carBAMazepine, phenytoin, rifAMPin)** may decrease concentration/effect. **Carbonic anhydrase inhibitors** may increase risk of kidney stone formation and severity of metabolic acidosis. May decrease therapeutic effect of **oral contraceptives. Salicylates (e.g., aspirin), thiazide diuretics (e.g., hydrochlorothiazide)** may increase concentration/effect. **HERBAL:** **Herbals with sedative properties (e.g., chamomile, kava kava, valerian)** may increase CNS depression. **FOOD:** None known. **LAB VALUES:** May reduce serum bicarbonate, increase ALT, AST.

AVAILABILITY (Rx)

Capsules (Sprinkle): 15 mg, 25 mg.
Tablets: ***(Topamax):*** 25 mg, 50 mg, 100 mg, 200 mg.

Capsules, Extended-Release: ***(Trokendi XR):*** 25 mg, 50 mg, 100 mg, 200 mg. ***(Qudexy XR):*** 25 mg, 50 mg, 100 mg, 150 mg, 200 mg.

ADMINISTRATION/HANDLING

PO

• Do not break, crush, dissolve, or divide tablets (bitter taste). • Give without regard to food. • Sprinkle capsules may either be swallowed whole or contents sprinkled on teaspoonful of soft food and swallowed immediately; do not chew. • ***(Trokendi XR):*** Give whole. Do not sprinkle on food, chew, or crush. ***(Qudexy XR):*** Swallow whole; may open and sprinkle on spoonful of soft food.

INDICATIONS/ROUTES/DOSAGE

Note: Do not abruptly discontinue; taper gradually to prevent rebound effects.

Adjunctive Treatment of Partial-Onset Seizures, Lennox-Gastaut Syndrome (LGS), Tonic-Clonic Seizures

PO: ADULTS, ELDERLY, CHILDREN 17 YRS AND OLDER: ***(Immediate-Release):*** Initially, 25 mg once or twice daily for 1 wk. May increase by 25–50 mg/day at wkly intervals. Usual maintenance dose: 100–200 mg twice daily (partial-onset) or 200 mg 2 times/day (primary tonic-clonic). **Maximum:** 400 mg/day. **CHILDREN 2–16 YRS:** Initially, 1–3 mg/kg/day to maximum of 25 mg at night for 1 wk. May increase by 1–3 mg/kg/day at wkly intervals given in 2 divided doses. **Maintenance:** 5–9 mg/kg/day in 2 divided doses. **ADULTS, ELDERLY:** ***(Extended-Release):*** Initially, 25–50 mg/day. Increase by 25–50 mg/day at wkly intervals, up to 400 mg/day. **CHILDREN 2 YRS AND OLDER:** Initially, 25 mg (based on range of 1–3 mg/kg) once daily at bedtime for 1 wk. Increase dose by 1–3 mg/kg at 1–2 wk intervals up to 5–9 mg/kg once daily.

Monotherapy With Partial-Onset, Tonic-Clonic Seizures

PO: ADULTS, ELDERLY, CHILDREN 10 YRS AND OLDER: ***(Immediate-Release):*** Initially, 25 mg twice daily. May increase at wkly intervals up to 400 mg/day according to the following schedule: Wk 1, 25 mg twice daily. Wk 2, 50 mg twice daily. Wk 3, 75 mg twice daily. Wk 4, 100 mg twice daily. Wk 5, 150 mg twice daily. Wk 6, 200 mg twice daily. **CHILDREN 2–9 YRS:** Initially, 25 mg once daily. Then 25 mg 2 times/day Wk 2; then increase by 25–50 mg/day at wkly intervals up to minimum dose. (See table below.) **ADULTS, ELDERLY, CHILDREN 10 YRS OR OLDER:** ***(Extended-Release): (Qudexy XR, Trokendi XR):*** Initially, 50 mg once daily for 1 wk. Increase by 50 mg/day at wkly intervals for first 4 wks, then by 100 mg/day for Wks 5 and 6, up to 400 mg/day.

Wgt.	Minimum	Maximum
11 kg or less	150 mg/day in 2 divided doses	250 mg/day in 2 divided doses
12–22 kg	200 mg/day in 2 divided doses	300 mg/day in 2 divided doses
23–31 kg	200 mg/day in 2 divided doses	350 mg/day in 2 divided doses

Wgt.	Minimum	Maximum
32–38 kg	250 mg/day in 2 divided doses	350 mg/day in 2 divided doses
39 kg or greater	250 mg/day in 2 divided doses	400 mg/day in 2 divided doses

Migraine Prevention

PO: ADULTS, ELDERLY, CHILDREN 12 YRS AND OLDER: Initially, 25 mg/day. May increase by 25–50 mg/day at 7-day intervals up to a total daily dose of 100 mg/day in 2 divided doses.

Dosage in Renal Impairment

Reduce dose by 50% and titrate more slowly in pts who have CrCl less than 70 mL/min.

Dosage in Hepatic Impairment

Use caution.

SIDE EFFECTS

Frequent (30%–10%): Drowsiness, dizziness, ataxia, nervousness, nystagmus, diplopia, paresthesia, nausea, tremor. **Occasional (9%–3%):** Confusion, breast pain, dysmenorrhea, dyspepsia, depression, asthenia, pharyngitis, weight loss, anorexia, rash, musculoskeletal pain, abdominal pain, difficulty with coordination, sinusitis, agitation, flu-like symptoms. **Rare (3%–2%):** Mood disturbances (e.g., irritability, depression), dry mouth, aggressive behavior, impaired heat regulation.

ADVERSE EFFECTS/TOXIC REACTIONS

Psychomotor slowing, impaired concentration, language problems (esp. word-finding difficulties), memory disturbances occur occasionally. Metabolic acidosis, suicidal ideation occur rarely.

NURSING CONSIDERATIONS

BASELINE ASSESSMENT

Seizures: Review history of seizure disorder (intensity, frequency, duration, level of consciousness). Initiate seizure precautions. Provide quiet, dark environment. Question history of suicidal ideation and behavior; congenital metabolism dysfunction. **Migraine:** Assess pain location, duration, intensity. Assess renal function.

INTERVENTION/EVALUATION

Monitor renal function tests, LFT. Observe frequently for recurrence of seizure activity. Assess for clinical improvement (decrease in intensity/frequency of seizures). Diligently screen for suicidal ideation and behavior; new onset or worsening of anxiety, depression, mood disorder.

PATIENT/FAMILY TEACHING

• Avoid tasks that require alertness, motor skills until response to drug is established (may cause dizziness, drowsiness, impaired concentration). • Drowsiness usually diminishes with continued therapy. • Avoid use of alcohol, other CNS depressants. • Do not abruptly discontinue drug (may precipitate seizures). • Strict maintenance of drug therapy is essential for seizure control. • Maintain adequate fluid intake (decreases risk of renal stone formation). • Report blurred vision, eye pain. • Report suicidal ideation, depression, unusual behavior. • Use caution with activities that may increase core temperature (exposure to extreme heat, dehydration). • Oral contraceptives may become ineffective. Use other contraceptive measures to avoid pregnancy.

T

topotecan

HIGH ALERT

toe-poe-**tee**-kan
(Hycamtin)

■ BLACK BOX ALERT ■ Severe myelosuppression may occur. Do not administer first cycle in pts with neutrophil count less than 1,500 cells/mm^3 and platelet count less than 100,000 cells/mm^3.

Do not confuse Hycamtin with Hycomine, Mycamine, or topotecan with irinotecan.

◆CLASSIFICATION

PHARMACOTHERAPEUTIC: Topoisomerase inhibitor. **CLINICAL:** Antineoplastic.

USES

Treatment of metastatic ovarian cancer, relapsed or refractory small-cell lung cancer, recurrent or resistant cervical cancer (in combination with CISplatin). **OFF-LABEL:** Treatment of central nervous system lesions/lymphoma, Ewing's sarcoma, rhabdomyosarcoma, neuroblastoma, acute myeloid leukemia.

PRECAUTIONS

Contraindications: Hypersensitivity to topotecan. Baseline neutrophil count less than 1,500 cells/mm^3 and platelet count less than 100,000 cells/mm^3, severe myelosuppression. **Cautions:** Mild myelosuppression, renal impairment, pulmonary disease, elderly, conditions predisposing to infection (e.g., diabetes, renal failure, immunocompromised pts, open wounds).

ACTION

Interacts with topoisomerase I, an enzyme that relieves torsional strain in DNA by inducing reversible single-strand breaks. Prevents religation of DNA strand, resulting in damage to double-strand DNA, cell death. Acts at S phase of cell cycle. **Therapeutic Effect:** Produces cytotoxic effect.

PHARMACOKINETICS

Widely distributed. Metabolized via enzymatic hydrolysis. Protein binding: 35%. Excreted in urine (51%), feces (18%). **Half-life:** 2–3 hrs (increased in renal impairment).

LIFESPAN CONSIDERATIONS

Pregnancy/Lactation: Avoid pregnancy; may cause fetal harm. Females of reproductive potential must use effective contraception during treatment and for at least 6 mos after discontinuation. Breastfeeding not recommended during treatment and for at least 1 wk after discontinuation. May impair fertility in both females and males. **Males:** Males with female partners of reproductive potential must use effective contraception during treatment and for at least 3 mos after discontinuation. **Children:** Safety and efficacy not established. **Elderly:** Age-related renal impairment may require dosage adjustment.

INTERACTIONS

DRUG: **Live virus vaccines** may potentiate virus replication, increase vaccine side effects, decrease pt's antibody response to vaccine. **Other bone marrow depressants (e.g., cladribine)** may increase risk of myelosuppression. **BCRP/ABCG2 inhibitors (e.g., omeprazole, verapamil), P-glycoprotein/ABCB1 inhibitors (e.g., amLODIPine, digoxin)** may increase concentration/effect. **HERBAL:** **Echinacea** may decrease therapeutic effect. **FOOD:** None known. **LAB VALUES:** May increase serum ALT, AST, bilirubin. May decrease Hgb, leukocytes, neutrophils, platelets, RBCs.

AVAILABILITY (Rx)

Injection, Powder for Reconstitution: 4 mg (single-dose vial). **Injection Solution:** 1 mg/mL (4 mL).

Capsules: 0.25 mg, 1 mg.

ADMINISTRATION/HANDLING

◄ALERT► Due to cytotoxic properties, handle with extreme care during preparation/administration.

PO

• Give without regard to food. • Administer whole; do not break, crush, dissolve, or divide capsule. • Do not give replacement dose if vomiting occurs.

IV

Reconstitution • Calculate the number of vials needed for reconstitution based on body surface area. • Swirl vial gently until powder is completely dissolved. Do not shake or agitate. • Visually inspect for particulate matter or discoloration. Solution should appear light yellow to greenish in color. Dilute in 50–100 mL 0.9% NaCl or D_5W.

Rate of administration • Infuse over 30 min.

Storage • Store unused vials in original carton at room temperature. • May store diluted solution at controlled room temperature for no more than 24 hrs. • Protect from light.

IV INCOMPATIBILITIES

Dexamethasone (Decadron), 5-fluorouracil, mitoMYcin (Mutamycin).

IV COMPATIBILITIES

CARBOplatin (Paraplatin), CISplatin (Platinol AQ), cyclophosphamide (Cytoxan), DOXOrubicin (Adriamycin), etoposide (VePesid), gemcitabine (Gemzar), granisetron (Kytril), ondansetron (Zofran), PACLitaxel (Taxol), palonosetron (Aloxi), vinCRIStine (Oncovin).

INDICATIONS/ROUTES/DOSAGE

◀ALERT▶ Do not give if baseline neutrophil count is less than 1,500 cells/mm^3 and platelet count is less than 100,000 cells/mm^3. For retreatment, neutrophils should be greater than 1,000 cells/mm^3, platelets greater than 100,000 cells/mm^3, and Hgb 9 g/dL or greater.

Ovarian Carcinoma

IV: ADULTS, ELDERLY: 1.5 mg/m^2/day for 5 consecutive days, beginning on day 1 of 21-day course. Continue until disease progression or unacceptable toxicity. **Neutrophils less than 500 cells/mm^3 or platelets less than 25,000 cells/mm^3:** Reduce dose to 1.25 mg/m^2/day for subsequent cycles.

Small-Cell Lung Cancer

PO: ADULTS, ELDERLY: 2.3 mg/m^2/day for 5 days; repeat q21days (dose rounded to nearest 0.25 mg). **Severe neutropenia or prolonged neutropenia, platelets less than 25,000 cells/mm^3, recovery from Grade 3 or 4 diarrhea:** Reduce dose by 0.4 mg/m^2/day for subsequent cycles.

IV: ADULTS, ELDERLY: 1.5 mg/m^2/day for 5 consecutive days q21days. **Neutrophils less than 500 cells/mm^3 or platelets less than 25,000 cells/mm^3:** Reduce dose to 1.25 mg/m^2/day for subsequent cycles.

Cervical Cancer

IV: ADULTS, ELDERLY: 0.75 mg/m^2/day for 3 days (followed by CISplatin 50 mg/m^2 on day 1 only). Repeat q21days (baseline neutrophil count greater than 1,500 cells/mm^3 and platelet count greater than 100,000 cells/mm^3). **Severe febrile neutropenia (neutrophils less than 1,000 cells/mm^3 with temperature of 38°C) or platelet count less than 25,000 cells/mm^3:** Reduce dose to 0.6 mg/m^2/day for subsequent cycles. If necessary, further decrease dose to 0.45 mg/m^2/day. Continue for a maximum of 6 cycles (in nonresponders) or until disease progression or unacceptable toxicity.

Dosage in Renal Impairment

IV: No dosage adjustment in pts with mild renal impairment (CrCl 40–60 mL/min). **CrCl 20–29 mL/min:** 0.75 mg/m^2.

PO: CrCl 30–49 mL/min: 1.5 mg/m^2/day. May increase by 0.4 mg/m^2/day following first cycle if no GI/hematologic toxicities occur. **CrCl less than 30 mL/min:** Decrease dose to 0.6 mg/m^2/day. May increase by 0.4 mg/m^2/day following first cycle if no GI/hematologic toxicities occur.

Dosage in Hepatic Impairment

No dose adjustment.

SIDE EFFECTS

Frequent (77%–21%): Nausea, vomiting, diarrhea, total alopecia, headache, dyspnea. **Occasional (9%–3%):** Paresthesia, constipation, abdominal pain. **Rare:** Anorexia, malaise, arthralgia, asthenia, myalgia.

T

ADVERSE EFFECTS/TOXIC REACTIONS

Myelosuppression (anemia, neutropenia, thrombocytopenia) is an expected response to therapy, but more severe reactions including Grade 4 neutropenia, thrombocytopenia, Grade 3 or 4 anemia, febrile neutropenia, neutropenic enterocolitis may occur. Life-threatening sepsis reported. Fatal interstitial lung disease, pneumonitis was reported. May cause severe extravasation and tissue injury. Hypersensitivity reactions including anaphylaxis, angioedema may occur.

NURSING CONSIDERATIONS

BASELINE ASSESSMENT

Obtain CBC (prior to each dose), LFT; pregnancy test in females of reproductive potential. Assess LVEF by echocardiogram. Question history pulmonary disease, renal impairment. Screen for active infection. Consider premedication with antiemetic at least 30 min before each dose. Due to high risk of extravasation and tissue injury with infusion, ensure patency of IV catheter. Assess hydration status. Offer emotional support.

INTERVENTION/EVALUATION

Monitor CBC for myelosuppression, LFT for hepatic injury (abdominal pain, jaundice, nausea, transaminitis, vomiting), renal function test in pts with renal impairment. Monitor for severe neutropenia, febrile neutropenia, infections (cough, fatigue, fever); thrombocytopenia-associated bleeding. Monitor daily pattern of bowel activity, stool consistency. Consider ABG, radiologic test if ILD/pneumonitis (excessive cough, dyspnea, fever, hypoxia) is suspected. Consider treatment with corticosteroids if ILD/pneumonitis is confirmed. Monitor for hypersensitivity reactions (anaphylaxis, angioedema).

PATIENT/FAMILY TEACHING

• Treatment may depress your immune system response and reduce your ability to fight infection. Report symptoms of infection such as body aches, chills, cough, fatigue, fever. Avoid those with active infection. • Report symptoms of bone marrow depression (e.g., bruising, fatigue, fever, shortness of breath, weight loss; bleeding easily, bloody urine or stool). • Seek immediate medical attention if severe allergic reactions (anaphylaxis, difficulty breathing; swelling of the face, tongue, throat) occur. • Report symptoms of lung inflammation (excessive coughing, difficulty breathing, chest pain); liver problems (abdominal pain, bruising, clay-colored stool, dark or amber-colored urine, yellowing of the skin or eyes). • Maintain proper hydration and nutrition. • Use effective contraception to avoid pregnancy. Do not breastfeed.

torsemide

tore-se-myde
Do not confuse torsemide with furosemide.

CLASSIFICATION

PHARMACOTHERAPEUTIC: Loop diuretic. **CLINICAL:** Antihypertensive, diuretic.

USES

Treatment of hypertension either alone or in combination with other antihypertensives. (Not recommended for initial treatment of hypertension.) Edema associated with HF, hepatic/renal impairment.

PRECAUTIONS

Contraindications: Hypersensitivity to torsemide or any sulfonylurea. Anuria, hepatic coma. **Cautions:** Pts with cirrhosis, hypotension, hypokalemia.

ACTION

Enhances excretion of sodium, chloride, potassium, water at ascending limb of loop of Henle and distal renal tubules. Reduces plasma, extracellular fluid volume. **Therapeutic Effect:** Produces diuresis, relieves edema; lowers B/P.

PHARMACOKINETICS

Route	Onset	Peak	Duration
PO (diuresis)	30–60 min	1–2 hrs	6–8 hrs

Widely distributed. Protein binding: 97%–99%. Metabolized in liver. Primarily excreted in urine. Not removed by hemodialysis. **Half-life:** 2–4 hrs.

LIFESPAN CONSIDERATIONS

Pregnancy/Lactation: Unknown if drug is distributed in breast milk. **Children:** Safety and efficacy not established. **Elderly:** No age-related precautions noted.

INTERACTIONS

DRUG: **NSAIDs (e.g., diclofenac, meloxicam, naproxen), aspirin** may increase risk of renal toxicity. May increase risk of **digoxin** toxicity associated with torsemide-induced hypokalemia. May increase risk of **lithium** toxicity. **Bile acid sequestrants (e.g., cholestyramine), sucralfate** may decrease absorption. May increase hyponatremic effect of **desmopressin**. May increase concentration/effect of **foscarnet**. **HERBAL:** **Herbals with hypertensive properties (e.g., licorice, yohimbe) or hypotensive properties (e.g., garlic, ginger, ginkgo biloba)** may alter effects. **Licorice** may increase hypokalemic effect. **FOOD:** None known. **LAB VALUES:** May increase serum BUN, creatinine, uric acid. May decrease serum calcium, chloride, magnesium, potassium, sodium.

AVAILABILITY (Rx)

Tablets: 5 mg, 10 mg, 20 mg, 100 mg.

ADMINISTRATION/HANDLING

PO

- Give without regard to food. Give with food to avoid GI upset, preferably with breakfast (prevents nocturia).

INDICATIONS/ROUTES/DOSAGE

Hypertension

PO: ADULTS, ELDERLY: Initially, 2.5–5 mg/day. May increase to 10 mg/day if no response in 4–6 wks. **Range:** 5–10 mg/day.

Edema Associated With HF

PO: ADULTS, ELDERLY: Initially, 10–20 mg/day. May increase by approximately doubling dose until desired therapeutic effect is attained. **Maximum:** 200 mg.

Edema Associated With Chronic Renal Failure

PO: ADULTS, ELDERLY: Initially, 20 mg/day. May increase by approximately doubling dose until desired therapeutic effect is attained. **Maximum:** 200 mg/day.

Edema Associated With Hepatic Cirrhosis

PO: ADULTS, ELDERLY: Initially, 5–10 mg once daily. May increase gradually by doubling dose until the desired diuretic response is achieved. **Maximum single dose:** 40 mg.

Dosage in Renal/Hepatic Impairment

No dose adjustment.

SIDE EFFECTS

Frequent (10%–4%): Headache, dizziness, rhinitis. **Occasional (3%–1%):** Asthenia, insomnia, nervousness, diarrhea, constipation, nausea, dyspepsia, edema, ECG changes, pharyngitis, cough, arthralgia, myalgia. **Rare (less than 1%):** Syncope, hypotension, arrhythmias.

ADVERSE EFFECTS/TOXIC REACTIONS

Ototoxicity may occur with too-rapid IV administration or with high doses; must be given slowly. Overdose produces acute, profound water loss, volume/electrolyte depletion, dehydration, decreased blood volume, circulatory collapse.

NURSING CONSIDERATIONS

BASELINE ASSESSMENT

Obtain renal function test, serum electrolyte levels, esp. potassium. Obtain weight,

T

B/P. Assess for peripheral edema. Assess lungs for crackles, signs of HF.

INTERVENTION/EVALUATION

Monitor B/P, renal function, serum electrolytes (esp. potassium), I&O, weight. Monitor for ototoxicity. Auscultate lungs for crackles. Check for signs of edema, particularly of dependent areas. Although less potassium is lost with torsemide than with furosemide, assess for signs of hypokalemia (change of muscle strength, tremor, muscle cramps, altered mental status, cardiac arrhythmias).

PATIENT/FAMILY TEACHING

• Take medication in morning to prevent excessive urination at night. • Expect increased urinary volume, frequency. • Report palpitations, muscle weakness, cramps, nausea, dizziness. • Do not take other medications (including OTC drugs) without consulting physician. • Eat foods high in potassium such as whole grains (cereals), legumes, meat, bananas, apricots, orange juice, potatoes (white, sweet), raisins.

trabectedin

tra-**bek**-te-din
(Yondelis)

◆CLASSIFICATION

PHARMACOTHERAPEUTIC: Alkylating agent. **CLINICAL:** Antineoplastic.

USES

Treatment of unresectable or metastatic soft tissue sarcoma (liposarcoma or leiomyosarcoma) in pts who have received a prior anthracycline-containing regimen.

PRECAUTIONS

Contraindications: Hypersensitivity reaction, anaphylactic reaction to trabectedin. **Cautions:** Baseline cytopenias, hepatic impairment, cirrhosis, renal impairment; history of DVT, pulmonary embolism; recent MI, cardiomyopathy, HF. Concomitant use of strong CYP3A inducers, strong CYP3A inhibitors not recommended.

ACTION

Binds to guanine residues in the minor groove of DNA, leading to cell cycle disruption and cellular death. Blocks cell cycle at G_2/M phase. **Therapeutic Effect:** Inhibits tumor cell growth and metastasis.

PHARMACOKINETICS

Widely distributed. Metabolized in liver. Protein binding: 97%. Excreted in feces (58%), urine (6%). Hemodialysis not expected to enhance elimination. **Half-life:** 175 hrs.

⌛ LIFESPAN CONSIDERATIONS

Pregnancy/Lactation: Avoid pregnancy; may cause fetal harm/malformations. Females of reproductive potential should use effective contraception during treatment and for at least 2 mos after discontinuation. Breastfeeding not recommended. **Males:** Males with female partners of reproductive potential should use effective contraception during treatment and up to 5 mos after discontinuation. May impair fertility in both females and males. **Children:** Safety and efficacy not established. **Elderly:** Safety and efficacy not established.

INTERACTIONS

DRUG: **Strong CYP3A4 inducers (e.g., carBAMazepine, phenytoin, rifAMPin)** may decrease concentration/effect. **Strong CYP3A4 inhibitors (e.g., clarithromycin, ketoconazole, ritonavir)** may increase concentration/effect. **Alcohol** may increase hepatotoxic effect. May decrease therapeutic effect; increase adverse effects of **vaccines (live)**. **HERBAL:** **Echinacea** may decrease therapeutic effect. **FOOD:** None known. **LAB VALUES:** May decrease Hgb, Hct, platelets, neutrophils, RBCs; serum albumin, phosphate. May increase serum alkaline phosphatase, ALT, AST, bilirubin, CPK, creatinine. May reduce diagnostic effect of *Coccidioides immitis* skin test.

AVAILABILITY (Rx)

Powder for Reconstitution: 1 mg.

ADMINISTRATION/HANDLING

IV

Reconstitution • Contents are hazardous; use cytotoxic precautions during handling and disposal. • Reconstitute with 20 mL Sterile Water for Injection for final concentration of 0.05 mg/mL. • Shake until fully dissolved. • Visually inspect solution for particulate matter or discoloration. Solution should appear clear, colorless to pale brownish-yellow in color. Discard if solution is discolored or particles are observed. • Dilute in 500 mL 0.9% NaCl or D_5W. • See manufacturer guidelines for materials/containers that are compatible with diluted solution.

Infusion guidelines • Premedicate with dexamethasone 20 mg IV (or appropriate corticosteroid) 30 min prior to each infusion. • Infuse diluted solution immediately after reconstitution. • Use an in-line, 0.2-micron polyethersulfone filter. • Infuse via dedicated central venous line using an infusion pump.

Rate of administration • Infuse over 24 hrs.

Storage • Refrigerate unused vials. • Diluted solution must be administered within 30 hrs of reconstitution.

IV INCOMPATIBILITIES

Do not mix or infuse with other medications.

INDICATIONS/ROUTES/DOSAGE

Liposarcoma, Leiomyosarcoma

IV infusion: ADULTS, ELDERLY: 1.5 mg/m^2 once q3wks until disease progression or unacceptable toxicity.

Dosage in Renal Impairment

CrCl greater than or equal to 30 mL/min or greater: No dose adjustment. **CrCl less than 30 mL/min or end-stage renal disease:** Not specified; use caution.

Dosage in Hepatic Impairment

Mild impairment: No dose adjustment. **Moderate impairment:** 0.9 mg/m^2 once q3wks. **Severe impairment:** Not recommended.

Dose Reduction for Normal Hepatic Function or Mild Hepatic Impairment

Initial dose: 1.5 mg/m^2 once q3wks. **First dose reduction:** 1.2 mg/m^2 once q3wks. **Second dose reduction:** 1 mg/m^2 once q3wks.

Dose Reduction for Moderate Hepatic Impairment

Initial dose: 0.9 mg/m^2 once q3wks. **First dose reduction:** 0.6 mg/m^2 once q3wks. **Second dose reduction:** 0.3 mg/m^2 once q3wks.

Dose Modification

Hepatotoxicity

Serum ALT/AST greater than 2.5 times upper limit of normal (ULN): Delay next dose for up to 3 wks.

Serum alkaline phosphatase greater than 2.5 times ULN; serum ALT/AST greater than 5 times ULN; total serum bilirubin greater than ULN: Delay next dose for up to 3 wks, then resume at reduced dose level.

Hematologic Toxicity

Absolute neutrophil count (ANC) less than 1,500 cells/mm³: Delay next dose for up to 3 wks. **ANC less than 1,000 cells/mm³ with fever or infection; ANC less than 500 cells/mm³ lasting more than 5 days:** Delay next dose for up to 3 wks, then resume at reduced dose level. **Platelet count less than 100,000 cells/mm³:** Delay next dose for up to 3 wks. **Platelet count less than 25,000 cells/mm³:** Delay next dose for up to 3 wks, then resume at reduced dose level.

Nonhematologic Toxicity

CPK greater than 2.5 times ULN: Delay next dose for up to 3 wks. **CPK greater**

T

than 5 times ULN: Delay next dose for up to 3 wks, then resume at reduced dose level.
Decreased LVEF less than lower limit of normal or clinical evidence of cardiomyopathy: Delay next dose for up to 3 wks. **Decreased LVEF with an absolute decrease of 10% or more from baseline and less than lower limit of normal, or clinical evidence of cardiomyopathy:** Delay next dose for up to 3 wks, then resume at reduced dose level.
Any other Grade 3 or 4 reaction: Delay next dose for up to 3 wks, then resume at reduced dose level.

Permanent Discontinuation

Permanently discontinue for persistent adverse effects requiring a delay of treatment for more than 3 wks; continued adverse effects after reducing dose to 1 mg/m^2 in pts with normal hepatic function, or 0.3 mg/m^2 in pts with preexisting moderate hepatic impairment; severe hepatic dysfunction with bilirubin 2 times ULN, and ALT/AST 3 times ULN, and alkaline phosphatase less than 2 times ULN in prior treatment cycle in pts with baseline normal hepatic function; exacerbation of hepatic dysfunction in pts with preexisting moderate hepatic impairment.

SIDE EFFECTS

Frequent (75%–25%): Nausea, fatigue, asthenia, malaise, vomiting, decreased appetite, constipation, diarrhea, peripheral edema, dyspnea, headache. **Occasional (15%–11%):** Insomnia, arthralgia, myalgia, paresthesia.

T

ADVERSE EFFECTS/TOXIC REACTIONS

Myelosuppression (anemia, neutropenia, thrombocytopenia) is an expected response to therapy, but more severe reactions including Grade 3 or 4 neutropenia, febrile neutropenia, fatal sepsis may occur. Fatal rhabdomyolysis, muscular toxicity may result in renal failure. CPK elevation occurred in 32% of pts; Grade 3 or 4 CPK elevation occurred in 6% of pts. Hepatotoxicity, including hepatic failure, may occur. LFT elevation occurred in 70%–90% of pts. Cardiomyopathy including decreased ejection fraction, diastolic dysfunction, HF, right ventricular dysfunction reported in 6% of pts; Grade 3 or 4 cardiomyopathy reported in 4% of pts. Drug extravasation may result in tissue necrosis requiring debridement. Other adverse effects may include phlebitis (15% of pts), pulmonary embolism (less than 10% of pts), hypersensitivity reaction.

NURSING CONSIDERATIONS

BASELINE ASSESSMENT

Obtain ANC, CBC, CPK, BMP, LFT; vital signs prior to each dose and periodically thereafter. Obtain LVEF by echocardiogram. Verify placement of central venous line. Receive full medication history. Assess nutritional status. Question history of DVT, pulmonary embolism, cardiac disease, recent MI; renal/hepatic impairment; prior hypersensitivity reaction. Screen for active infection. Offer emotional support.

INTERVENTION/EVALUATION

Monitor ANC, CBC for myelosuppression; CPK, serum creatinine for rhabdomyolysis, renal failure; LFT for hepatotoxicity; BMP for electrolyte imbalance (esp. in pts with diarrhea, vomiting, malnutrition); vital signs. Assess LVEF by echocardiogram at 2- to 3-mo intervals (or more frequently in pts with cardiomyopathy). Diligently screen for infections (cough, fatigue fever), sepsis. Monitor for DVT (leg or arm pain/swelling), rhabdomyolysis (decreased urinary output, amber-colored urine, fatigue, muscle pain/weakness), pulmonary embolism (sudden chest pain, dyspnea, hypoxia, tachycardia), HF (dyspnea, fatigue, palpitations, edema, exercise intolerance); hypersensitivity reaction; side effects of dexamethasone (e.g., hyperglycemia, weight loss, decreased appetite). Monitor I&O. Monitor daily pattern of bowel activity, stool consistency.

PATIENT/FAMILY TEACHING

• Treatment may depress your immune system and reduce your ability to fight infection. Report symptoms of infection such as body aches, chills, cough, fatigue, fever. Avoid those with active infection. • Life-threatening events, such as HF (shortness of breath, fast or slow heart rate, palpitations, swelling of the ankles or legs), liver injury or failure (abdominal pain, easy bruising, clay-colored stools, dark-amber urine, fatigue, loss of appetite, yellowing of skin or eyes), muscle toxicity (muscle pain/weakness, kidney failure), blood clots in lungs (difficulty breathing, fast heart rate, chest pain), may occur. • Use effective contraception to avoid pregnancy. Do not breastfeed. • Avoid grapefruit products, herbal supplements. • Do not receive live vaccines.

traMADol

tram a dol
(Apo-TraMADol ✤, ConZip, Ultram)

■ **BLACK BOX ALERT** ■ May cause opioid addiction, abuse, misuse. Serious, life-threatening respiratory depression may occur. Extended-release tablets must be swallowed whole. Crushing, chewing, or dissolving of ER tablets can result in a fatal overdose. May cause neonatal opioid withdrawal syndrome. Concomitant use of alcohol, benzodiazepines, CNS depressants may cause profound sedation, respiratory depression, coma, or death. Use with any CYP3A4 inhibitor may result in increased concentration/effect, which may cause potentially fatal respiratory depression.

Do not confuse traMADol with tapentadol, Toradol, or Trandate, or Ultram with Ultracet.

FIXED-COMBINATION(S)

Ultracet: traMADol/acetaminophen (a non-narcotic analgesic): 37.5 mg/325 mg.

◆CLASSIFICATION

PHARMACOTHERAPEUTIC: Centrally acting synthetic opioid. **CLINICAL:** Analgesic.

USES

Immediate-Release: Management of moderate to moderately severe pain. **Extended-Release:** Around-the-clock management of moderate to moderately severe pain for extended period.

PRECAUTIONS

Contraindications: Hypersensitivity to traMADol, opioids. Pediatric pts under 12 yrs of age; postop management in pts under 18 yrs following tonsillectomy and/or adenoidectomy; severe respiratory depression; acute bronchial asthma in absence of appropriate monitoring; GI obstruction (paralytic ileus [known or suspected]). Concomitant use with or within 14 days following MAOI therapy. **Cautions:** CNS depression, anoxia, advanced hepatic cirrhosis, respiratory depression, elevated ICP, seizure disorder, hepatic/renal impairment, treatment of acute abdominal conditions, opioid-dependent pts, head injury, myxedema, hypothyroidism, hypoadrenalism, pregnancy. Avoid use in pts who are suicidal or addiction prone, emotionally disturbed, depressed, heavy alcohol users, elderly, debilitated.

ACTION

Binds to mu-opioid receptors in CNS, inhibiting ascending pain pathway. Inhibits reuptake of norepinephrine, serotonin, inhibiting descending pain pathways. **Therapeutic Effect:** Reduces pain.

PHARMACOKINETICS

Route	Onset	Peak	Duration
PO	Less than 1 hr	2–3 hrs	9 hrs

Widely distributed. Protein binding: 20%. Metabolized in liver (reduced in pts with advanced cirrhosis). Primarily excreted in urine. **Half-life:** 6–7 hrs (increased in renal/hepatic failure).

T

LIFESPAN CONSIDERATIONS

Pregnancy/Lactation: Crosses placenta. Distributed in breast milk. **Children:** Safety and efficacy not established in children younger than 17 yrs. **Elderly:** Age-related renal impairment may require dosage adjustment.

INTERACTIONS

DRUG: **Alcohol, CNS depressants (e.g., LORazepam, morphine, zolpidem)** may increase CNS depression. **Strong CYP3A4 inhibitors (e.g., clarithromycin, ketoconazole, ritonavir)** may increase concentration/effect. May increase CNS depressant effect; decrease therapeutic effect of **carBAMazepine**. **CarBAMazepine** may decrease concentration/effect. **Strong CYP2D6 inhibitors (e.g., FLUoxetine, PARoxetine)** may decrease therapeutic effect. **Linezolid, MAOIs (e.g., phenelzine, selegiline), ondansetron, SNRIs (e.g., DULoxetine, venlafaxine), SSRIs (e.g., escitalopram, PARoxetine, sertraline)** may increase risk of serotonin syndrome, seizure activity. HERBAL: **Herbals with sedative properties (e.g., chamomile, kava kava, valerian)** may increase CNS depression. **St. John's wort** may decrease concentration/effect. FOOD: None known. LAB VALUES: May increase serum creatinine, ALT, AST, urine protein. May decrease Hgb.

T

AVAILABILITY (Rx)

Tablets, Immediate-Release: 50 mg. **Suspension, Oral:** ***(Synapryn FusePaq):*** 10 mg/mL.

Capsules, Extended-Release: 100 mg, 150 mg, 200 mg, 300 mg. **Tablets, Extended-Release:** 100 mg, 200 mg, 300 mg.

ADMINISTRATION/HANDLING

PO

• Give without regard to food but consistently with or without meals. • ***(Extended-Release):*** Administer whole; do not break, crush, dissolve, or divide.

INDICATIONS/ROUTES/DOSAGE

Moderate to Moderately Severe Pain

PO: ***(Immediate-Release):*** **ADULTS, ELDERLY, CHILDREN 17 YRS AND OLDER:** 50 mg q4–6h as needed. May increase to 50–100 mg q4–6h as needed. **Maximum:** 400 mg/day for pts 75 yrs and younger; 300 mg/day for pts older than 75 yrs.

PO: ***(Extended-Release):*** **ADULTS, ELDERLY, CHILDREN 18 YRS AND OLDER:** Initially, 100 mg once daily. Titrate q5days. **Maximum:** 300 mg once daily.

Dosage in Renal Impairment

(Immediate-Release): For pts with CrCl less than 30 mL/min, increase dosing interval to q12h. **Maximum:** 200 mg/day. Do not use extended-release.

Dosage in Hepatic Impairment

(Immediate-Release): Cirrhosis: Dosage is decreased to 50 mg q12h. Do not use extended-release with severe hepatic impairment.

SIDE EFFECTS

Frequent (25%–15%): Dizziness, vertigo, nausea, constipation, headache, drowsiness. **Occasional (10%–5%):** Vomiting, pruritus, CNS stimulation (e.g., nervousness, anxiety, agitation, tremor, euphoria, mood swings, hallucinations), asthenia, diaphoresis, dyspepsia, dry mouth, diarrhea. **Rare (less than 5%):** Malaise, vasodilation, anorexia, flatulence, rash, blurred vision, urinary retention/frequency, menopausal symptoms.

ADVERSE EFFECTS/TOXIC REACTIONS

May cause seizure activity at usual dosages. Serotonin syndrome (altered mental status, autonomic instability, clonus, diaphoresis, hyperthermia, hyperreflexia, tremor) was reported. Hypersensitivity reactions (anaphylaxis, angioedema, bronchospasm), toxic skin reactions (Stevens Johnson syndrome, toxic epidermal necrolysis), severe hypotension, respiratory depression, secondary hypogonadism, thyroid dysfunction, psychosis may occur. May increase risk of suicidal ideation and behavior.

NURSING CONSIDERATIONS

BASELINE ASSESSMENT

Assess onset, type, location, duration of pain. Receive full medication history (esp. serotonergic agents, CNS depressants). Question history as listed in Precautions. Assess risk of drug abuse and misuse.

INTERVENTION/EVALUATION

Monitor heart rate, B/P. Assist with ambulation if dizziness, vertigo occurs. Palpate bladder for urinary retention. Diligently screen for suicidal ideation and behavior; new onset or worsening of anxiety, depression, mood disorder. Screen for drug abuse and misuse, drug-seeking behavior. Monitor for seizure activity; symptoms of serotonin syndrome. Assess for clinical improvement, record onset of relief of pain. Monitor closely for misuse or abuse.

PATIENT/FAMILY TEACHING

• May cause physical dependence. • Pts with history of drug abuse are at increased risk for misuse or abuse. Take medication only as prescribed. • Avoid alcohol, other narcotics, sedatives. • Avoid tasks requiring alertness, motor skills until response to drug is established. • Report severe confusion, excessive sweating, difficulty breathing, excessive sedation, seizures, muscle weakness, tremors, chest pain, palpitations.

trametinib

tra-**me**-ti-nib
(Mekinist)
Do not confuse trametinib with imatinib or tipifarnib.

◆CLASSIFICATION

PHARMACOTHERAPEUTIC: MEK inhibitor. **CLINICAL:** Antineoplastic.

USES

Used as a single agent or in combination with dabrafenib for treatment of unresectable or metastatic melanoma with BRAF V600E or V600L mutations, as detected by FDA-approved test. Single-agent regimen is not indicated in pts who have received prior BRAF-inhibitor therapy. Adjuvant treatment of melanoma in combination with dabrafenib in pts with BRAF V600E or BRAF V600K mutations and lymph node involvement, following complete resection. Treatment of locally advanced or metastatic anaplastic thyroid cancer (in combination with dabrafenib). Treatment of metastatic non–small-cell lung cancer (NSCLC) in pts with BRAF V600E mutation in combination with dabrafenib.

PRECAUTIONS

Contraindications: Hypersensitivity to trametinib. **Cautions:** Baseline cytopenias, cardiac disease (cardiomyopathy), diabetes, ocular disease, hepatic impairment, history of thromboembolic events (CVA, DVT, MI, pulmonary embolism [PE], pts at risk for GI perforation (e.g., Crohn's disease, diverticulitis, GI tract malignancies, peptic ulcers, peritoneal malignancies), interstitial lung disease (sarcoidosis, pulmonary fibrosis); conditions predisposing to infection (e.g., diabetes, immunocompromised pts, renal failure, open wounds).

ACTION

Inhibits mitogen-activated extracellular kinase (MEK). MEK is a downstream effector of protein kinase Braf (BRAF). **Therapeutic Effect:** Inhibits cell proliferation and causes cell cycle arrest.

PHARMACOKINETICS

Widely distributed. Protein binding: 97.4%. Peak plasma concentration: 1.5 hrs. Metabolized in liver. Excreted in feces (80%), urine (20%). **Half-life:** 3.9–4.8 days.

LIFESPAN CONSIDERATIONS

Pregnancy/Lactation: Avoid pregnancy; may cause fetal harm. Females and males with female partners of reproductive potential must use effective contraception during treatment and for at least 4 mos after discontinuation. Breastfeeding not recommended during treatment and for at least 4 mos after discontinuation. May impair fertility in females. **Children:** Safety and efficacy not established. **Elderly:** May have increased risk of adverse effects, skin lesions, primary malignancies. **Males:** May decrease sperm count.

INTERACTIONS

DRUG: None significant. **HERBAL:** None known. **FOOD: High-fat meals** may decrease absorption/effect. **LAB VALUES: Single regimen:** May increase serum alkaline phosphatase, ALT, AST. May decrease serum albumin; Hgb, Hct. **Combination regimen:** May increase serum alkaline phosphatase, ALT, AST, bilirubin, calcium, creatinine, glucose, GGT, potassium. May decrease Hgb, Hct, leukocytes, lymphocytes, neutrophils, platelets; serum albumin, calcium, magnesium, phosphorus, potassium, sodium.

AVAILABILITY (Rx)

Tablets: 0.5 mg, 2 mg.

ADMINISTRATION/HANDLING

PO

- Administer at least 1 hr before or 2 hrs after meal.

INDICATIONS/ROUTES/DOSAGE

T

Melanoma (Metastatic or unresectable)

PO: ADULTS/ELDERLY: 2 mg once daily (either as a single agent or in combination with dabrafenib). Continue until disease progression or unacceptable toxicity.

Melanoma (Adjuvant treatment)

PO: ADULTS, ELDERLY: 2 mg once daily (in combination with dabrafenib). Continue for up to 1 yr in absence of disease progression or unacceptable toxicity.

Thyroid Cancer

PO: ADULTS, ELDERLY: 2 mg once daily (in combination with dabrafenib). Continue until disease progression or unacceptable toxicity.

NSCLC (Metastatic)

PO: ADULTS, ELDERLY: 2 mg once daily in combination with dabrafenib. Continue until disease progression or unacceptable toxicity.

Dose Reduction Schedule

Trametinib regimen: FIRST DOSE REDUCTION: 1.5 mg once daily. **SECOND DOSE REDUCTION:** 1 mg once daily. Discontinue if unable to tolerate 1-mg dose. **Dabrafenib combination regimen: FIRST DOSE REDUCTION:** 100 mg twice daily. **SECOND DOSE REDUCTION:** 75 mg twice daily. **THIRD DOSE REDUCTION:** 50 mg twice daily. Discontinue if unable to tolerate 50-mg dose.

Dose Modification

Based on Common Terminology Criteria for Adverse Events.

Cardiotoxicity

Asymptomatic decrease of left ventricular ejection fraction (LVEF) greater than 10% from baseline: Withhold trametinib up to 4 wks. If LVEF improved, resume at lower dose level. Discontinue if not improved. Do not modify dabrafenib dose. **Symptomatic HF or decrease of LVEF greater than 20% from baseline:** Discontinue trametinib. Withhold dabrafenib until improved, then resume at lower dose level.

Cutaneous Toxicity

Intolerable Grade 2 skin toxicity; Grade 3 or 4 skin toxicity: Withhold both regimens for up to 3 wks. If improved, resume both at lower dose level. Discontinue both regimens if not improved.

Febrile Events

Fever of 101.3°F–104°F (38.5°C–40°C): Do not modify trametinib dose. Withhold dabrafenib until fever resolved, then resume at either same dose or lower dose level. **Fever greater than 104°F (40°C) or complicated fever (dehydration, hypotension, renal failure):** Withhold trametinib until resolved, then resume at either same dose or lower dose level. Withhold dabrafenib until resolved, then resume at either lower dose level or discontinue.

New Primary Malignancies

Cutaneous: No changes required for either regimen. **Noncutaneous:** Do not change trametinib dose. Discontinue dabrafenib in pts who develop RAS mutation-positive malignancies.

Nonspecific Adverse Reactions

Other intolerable Grade 2 reactions; any other Grade 3 reactions: Withhold both regimens until resolved to Grade 0–1, then resume at lower dose level. Discontinue both regimens if not improved. **First occurrence of any other Grade 4 reaction:** Withhold both regimens until resolved to Grade 0–1, then resume at lower dose level or discontinue.

Ocular Toxicity

Grade 2 or 3 retinal pigment epithelial detachment: Withhold trametinib up to 3 wks. If improved to Grade 0–1, resume at lower dose level. Discontinue if not improved. Do not modify dabrafenib. **Retinal vein occlusion:** Discontinue trametinib. Do not modify dabrafenib. **Uveitis or iritis:** Do not modify trametinib. Withhold dabrafenib for up to 6 wks. If improved to Grade 0–1, then resume at same dose level. Discontinue if not improved.

Pulmonary Toxicity

Interstitial lung disease: Discontinue trametinib. Do not modify dabrafenib.

Venous Thromboembolism

Uncomplicated DVT/PE: Withhold trametinib for up to 3 wks. If improved to Grade 0–1, then resume at lower dose level. Discontinue if not improved. Do not modify dabrafenib. **Life-threatening PE:** Discontinue both regimens.

Dosage in Renal/Hepatic Impairment

No dose adjustment.

SIDE EFFECTS

Single Regimen

Frequent (57%–32%): Rash, diarrhea, lymphedema, peripheral edema. **Occasional (19%–10%):** Dermatitis acneiform, hypertension, stomatitis, mouth ulceration, mucosal ulceration, abdominal pain, dry skin, pruritus, paronychia, folliculitis, cellulitis, dizziness, dysgeusia, blurred vision, dry eye.

Combination Regimen

Frequent (71%–40%): Pyrexia, chills, fatigue, rash, nausea, vomiting. **Occasional (36%–11%):** Diarrhea, abdominal pain, peripheral edema, headache, cough, arthralgia, night sweats, myalgia, constipation, decreased appetite, back pain, dry skin, insomnia, dermatitis acneiform, dizziness, muscle spasm, extremity pain, actinic keratosis, erythema, oral/throat pain, pruritus, dry mouth, dehydration.

ADVERSE EFFECTS/TOXIC REACTIONS

Primary malignancies (basal or squamous cell carcinoma, keratoacanthoma, pancreatic adenocarcinoma, glioblastoma) were reported. DVT, PE reported in 9% of pts. May increase cell proliferation of wild-type BRAF melanoma or new malignant melanomas. Serious, sometimes fatal intracranial or GI bleeding occurred in 5% of pts. Other hemorrhagic events may include conjunctival/gingival/rectal/hemorrhoidal/vaginal bleeding, epistaxis, melena. Cardiomyopathy, HF, decreased LVEF reported in 7%–9% of pts. Ocular toxicities such as retinal vein occlusion, retinal detachment, vision loss, glaucoma, uveitis, iritis were reported. Cough, dyspnea, hypoxia, pleural effusion, infiltrates may indicate interstitial lung disease. Serious febrile reactions may lead to renal failure, severe dehydration, hypotension, rigors. Skin toxicities including palmar-plantar erythrodysesthesia syndrome (PPES), papilloma have occurred. Hyperglycemia reported in 2%–5% of pts. Other adverse effects may include hypertension, rhabdomyolysis, QT interval prolongation.

NURSING CONSIDERATIONS

BASELINE ASSESSMENT

Obtain CBC, BMP, LFT, ECG, vital signs; pregnancy test in females of reproductive

T

potential. Verify BRAF V600E status. Obtain LVEF by echocardiogram. Assess skin for moles, lesions. Receive full medication history and screen for interactions. Screen for active infection. Question history as listed in Precautions. Offer emotional support.

INTERVENTION/EVALUATION

Monitor CBC for myelosuppression, LFT for hepatic injury (abdominal pain, jaundice, nausea, transaminitis, vomiting), ECG. Monitor for severe neutropenia, febrile neutropenia, infections (cough, fatigue, fever); symptoms of hyperglycemia (dehydration, confusion, extreme thirst, sweet-smelling breath, Kussmaul respirations, nausea); GI perforation (abdominal pain, fever, hematemesis). Assess skin for new lesion, toxicities q2mos. Assess LVEF for cardiomyopathy (dyspnea, edema, palpitations) by echocardiogram 1 mo after initiation, then q2–3mos thereafter. Obtain ophthalmologic exam for change of vision, eye irritation. Consider ABG, radiologic test if ILD/pneumonitis (excessive cough, dyspnea, fever, hypoxia) is suspected. Consider treatment with corticosteroids if ILD/pneumonitis is confirmed. Monitor for ocular toxicities; symptoms of DVT (leg or arm pain/swelling), intracranial hemorrhage (aphasia, altered mental status, facial droop, hemiplegia, vision loss), PE (chest pain, dyspnea, tachycardia). Bleeding of any kind can be life threatening and must be treated promptly.

PATIENT/FAMILY TEACHING

• Treatment may depress your immune system response and reduce your ability to fight infection. Report symptoms of infection such as body aches, chills, cough, fatigue, fever. Avoid those with active infection. • Report symptoms of bone marrow depression (e.g., bruising, fatigue, fever, shortness of breath, weight loss; bleeding easily, bloody urine or stool). • Report liver problems (abdominal pain, bruising, clay-colored stool, dark or amber-colored urine, yellowing of the skin or eyes), eye toxicities (eye redness, irritation; change of vision), heart problems (swelling of extremities, palpitations), symptoms of lung inflammation (excessive coughing, difficulty breathing, chest pain), DVT (swelling, pain, hot feeling in the arms or legs; discoloration of extremity), lung embolism (difficulty breathing, chest pain, rapid heart rate), high blood sugar levels (confusion, frequent urination, hunger, thirst). • Treatment may reduce the heart's ability to pump effectively; expect routine echocardiograms. • Use effective contraception to avoid pregnancy. Do not breastfeed. • New cancers may occur. • Immediately report severe or persistent abdominal pain, bloody stool, fever, vomiting blood; may indicate rupture in GI tract. • Bleeding may be life-threatening; report GI bleeding, symptoms of hemorrhagic stroke (confusion, one-sided weakness or paralysis, difficulty speaking).

trastuzumab

TOP 100 HIGH ALERT

tras-**too**-zoo-mab
(Herceptin)

■ BLACK BOX ALERT ■ Subclinical and clinical HF (manifested as CHF, decreased left ventricular ejection fraction) may occur, esp. in pts receiving concomitant anthracycline therapy. Fatal infusion reactions and pulmonary toxicities may occur. Monitor for anaphylaxis, angioedema, interstitial pneumonitis, acute respiratory distress syndrome. Exposure during pregnancy may cause fetal harm and neonatal death.

Do not confuse trastuzumab with ado-trastuzumab, fam-trastuzumab (or biosimilars).

◆CLASSIFICATION

PHARMACOTHERAPEUTIC: HER2 receptor antagonist. Monoclonal antibody. **CLINICAL:** Antineoplastic.

USES

Treatment of HER2-overexpressing breast cancer (adjuvant), metastatic breast cancer, metastatic gastric or gastroesophageal junction adenocarcinoma (in pts without prior treatment). **OFF-LABEL:** Treatment of HER2-positive metastatic breast cancer in pts who have not received prior anti-HER2 therapy or in pts whose cancer has progressed on prior trastuzumab therapy (in combination with lapatinib).

PRECAUTIONS

Contraindications: Hypersensitivity to trastuzumab. **Cautions:** Baseline cytopenias, cardiac disease (cardiomyopathy, HF), pts at risk for interstitial lung disease (sarcoidosis, pulmonary fibrosis), tumor lysis syndrome (high tumor burden, dehydration); conditions predisposing to infection (e.g., diabetes, immunocompromised pts, renal failure, open wounds).

ACTION

Binds to extracellular domain of human epidermal growth factor receptor 2 (HER2) protein, inhibiting proliferation of tumor cells that overexpresss HER2 protein. **Therapeutic Effect:** Inhibits tumor cell growth and survival; mediates antibody-dependent cellular cytotoxicity.

PHARMACOKINETICS

Half-life: 11–23 days.

LIFESPAN CONSIDERATIONS

Pregnancy/Lactation: Females of reproductive potential should use effective contraception during treatment and for at least 7 mos after discontinuation. Unknown if distributed in breast milk. Breastfeeding not recommended. **Children:** Safety and efficacy not established. **Elderly:** Age-related cardiac dysfunction may require dosage adjustment.

INTERACTIONS

DRUG: May increase levels/toxicity of **belimumab.** May decrease concentration/effect of **paclitaxel (conventional).** **HERBAL:** None significant. **FOOD:** None known. **LAB VALUES:** None significant.

AVAILABILITY (Rx)

Injection, Powder for Reconstitution: 150 mg, 420 mg.

ADMINISTRATION/HANDLING

IV

Reconstitution • Reconstitute 420-mg vial with 20 mL Bacteriostatic Water for Injection (150-mg vial with 7.4 mL Sterile Water for Injection) to yield concentration of 21 mg/mL. • Gently swirl vial to mix. Do not shake. • If foaming appears, allow vial to stand for up to 5 min. • Visually inspect for particulate matter or discoloration. Solution should appear clear to slightly opalescent, colorless to pale yellow. Do not use if cloudy or discolored or if visible particles are observed. • Dilute in 250 mL 0.9% NaCl (do not dilute in D_5W). • Gently invert bag to mix.

Rate of administration • Do not give IV push or bolus. • Infuse loading dose (4 mg/kg) over 90 min. Infuse maintenance infusion (2 mg/kg) over 30–90 min.

Storage • Refrigerate unused vials. • May refrigerate diluted solution for up to 24 hrs. • Do not freeze.

IV INCOMPATIBILITIES

Do not mix with D_5W or any other medications.

INDICATIONS/ROUTES/DOSAGE

Note: Do not substitute with ado-trastuzumab emtansine.

Breast Cancer (Adjuvant)

IV: ADULTS, ELDERLY: (With concurrent PACLitaxel or DOCEtaxel): Initially, 4 mg/kg (loading dose), then 2 mg/kg wkly for 12 wks, followed 1 wk later (when concurrent chemotherapy completed) by 6 mg/kg q3wks for total therapy duration of 52 wks. **(With DOCEtaxel/CARBOplatin):** Initially, 4 mg/kg (loading dose), then 2 mg/kg wkly for a total of 18 wks, followed 1 wk later (when concurrent chemotherapy completed) by 6 mg/kg q3wks for total therapy duration of 52 wks. **(Following**

T

multimodality chemotherapy): Initially, 8 mg/kg (loading dose), then 6 mg/kg q3wks for total of 52 wks.

Breast Cancer (Metastatic)
IV: ADULTS, ELDERLY: (Either as single agent or in combination with PACLitaxel): Initially, 4 mg/kg (loading dose), then 2 mg/kg wkly until disease progression.

Gastric Cancer
IV: ADULTS, ELDERLY: (In combination with CISplatin and either capecitabine or fluorouracil for 6 cycles, then as monotherapy): Initially, 8 mg/kg (loading dose), then 6 mg/kg q3wks until disease progression.

Dosage Adjustment in Cardiotoxicity
Left ventricular ejection fraction (LVEF) 16% or greater decrease from baseline WNL (within normal limits) or LVEF below normal limits and 10% or greater decrease from baseline: Hold treatment for 4 wks. Repeat LVEF q4wks. Resume therapy if LVEF returns to normal limits in 4–8 wks and remains at 15% or less decrease from baseline.

Dosage in Renal/Hepatic Impairment
No dose adjustment.

SIDE EFFECTS

Frequent (47%–18%): Generalized pain, asthenia, fever, nausea, chills, headache, cough, diarrhea, abdominal pain, dyspnea, rash. **Occasional (14%–6%):** Anorexia, insomnia, dizziness, peripheral edema, paresthesia, edema, nausea, vomiting, bone pain, arthralgia, accidental injury. **Rare (5%–1%):** Tachycardia, acne, peripheral neuritis, neuropathy.

ADVERSE EFFECTS/TOXIC REACTIONS

Myelosuppression (anemia, neutropenia, thrombocytopenia) is an expected response to therapy, but more severe reactions including febrile neutropenia may occur. May cause decrease in LVEF, cardiac arrhythmias, hypertension, HF, cardiomyopathy, cardiac death. Infusion reactions (asthenia, chills, fever, hypotension, nausea, vomiting, rash) have occurred, but more severe reactions including anaphylaxis, angioedema, hypoxia, severe hypotension can be fatal. Pulmonary toxicities (acute respiratory distress syndrome, dyspnea, interstitial pneumonitis, pulmonary infiltrates), infections (influenza, pharyngitis, rhinitis, sinusitis) were reported. Tumor lysis syndrome may present as acute renal failure, hypocalcemia, hyperuricemia, hyperphosphatemia.

NURSING CONSIDERATIONS

BASELINE ASSESSMENT

Obtain CBC, ECG; pregnancy test in females of reproductive potential. Assess LVEF by echocardiogram. Screen for active infection. Question for history of cardiac/pulmonary disease, infusion reactions. Offer emotional support.

INTERVENTION/EVALUATION

Monitor CBC for myelosuppression. Monitor for severe neutropenia, febrile neutropenia, infections (cough, fatigue, fever). Monitor serum uric acid level if tumor lysis syndrome (acute renal failure, electrolyte imbalance, cardiac arrhythmias, seizures) is suspected. Assess LVEF for cardiomyopathy (dyspnea, edema, palpitations) by echocardiogram q3mos (monthly if treatment is withheld for severe cardiomyopathy), then q6mos for 2 yrs after discontinuation. Diligently monitor infusion reactions. Have resuscitative equipment available if infusion reactions occur. Consider ABG, radiologic test if ILD/pneumonitis (excessive cough, dyspnea, fever, hypoxia) is suspected. Consider treatment with corticosteroids if ILD/pneumonitis is confirmed.

PATIENT/FAMILY TEACHING

- Treatment may depress your immune system response and reduce your ability to fight infection. Report symptoms of infection such as body aches, chills,

T

cough, fatigue, fever. Avoid those with active infection. • Report symptoms of bone marrow depression (e.g., bruising, fatigue, fever, shortness of breath, weight loss; bleeding easily, bloody urine or stool). • Treatment may reduce the heart's ability to pump effectively; expect routine echocardiograms. • Report heart problems (difficulty breathing, swelling of extremities, palpitations), kidney problems (decreased urine output, flank pain, darkened urine); symptoms of lung inflammation (excessive coughing, difficulty breathing, chest pain). • Use effective contraception to avoid pregnancy. Do not breastfeed. • Life-threatening infusion reactions may occur. Immediately report difficulty breathing, dizziness, rash; swelling of face, tongue, throat.

trastuzumab/ hyaluronidase

tras-**tu**-zoo-mab **hye**-al-ure-**on**-i-dase
(Herceptin Hylecta)

BLACK BOX ALERT May cause cardiac failure, esp. in pts with anthracycline-containing chemotherapy regimens. Monitor left ventricular function prior to initiation and during treatment. Serious and fatal cases of interstitial lung disease (ILD), pneumonitis were reported. Symptoms usually occurred during or within 24 hrs of administration. Permanently discontinue if anaphylaxis, ILD, acute respiratory distress syndrome occurs. Treatment may cause fetal harm. Recommend effective contraception.

Do not confuse trastuzumab/ hyaluronidase with ado-trastuzumab emtansine, daratumumab/hyaluronidase, fam-trastuzumab deruxtecan, pertuzumab, trastuzumab (or biosimilars), or rituximab/ hyaluronidase.

CLASSIFICATION

PHARMACOTHERAPEUTIC: Human epidermal growth factor receptor 2 (HER2) antagonist; monoclonal antibody. **CLINICAL:** Antineoplastic.

USES

Adjuvant treatment of adults with HER2-overexpressing node-positive or node-negative (estrogen receptor [ER]/progesterone receptor [PR]–negative or with one high-risk feature) breast cancer: as part of a treatment regimen consisting of doxorubicin, cyclophosphamide, and either paclitaxel or docetaxel; as part of a treatment regimen with docetaxel and carboplatin; as a single agent following multimodal anthracycline-based therapy. Treatment of adults as first-line therapy for HER2-overexpressing metastatic breast cancer (in combination with paclitaxel); as a single agent for HER2-overexpressing breast cancer in pts who have received one or more chemotherapy regimens for metastatic disease.

PRECAUTIONS

Contraindications: Hypersensitivity to trastuzumab/hyaluronidase, trastuzumab-containing regimens. **Cautions:** Baseline cytopenias, active infection, pulmonary disorders (e.g., COPD, emphysema, pulmonary fibrosis), cardiovascular disease, HF, conditions predisposing to infection (e.g., diabetes, renal failure, immunocompromised pts, open wounds). Do not substitute with ado-trastuzumab or intravenous trastuzumab.

ACTION

Binds to extracellular domain of HER2 protein, inhibiting proliferation of HER2-overexpressing tumor cells. Mediates antibody-dependent cellular toxicity. Hyaluronidase increases dispersion and absorption of SQ injected medications by increasing permeability. **Therapeutic Effect:** Inhibits proliferation of cells overexpressing HER2 protein.

T

PHARMACOKINETICS

Widely distributed. Peak plasma concentration: 3 days. Eliminated by parallel and nonlinear saturable target mediated clearance. **Half-life:** Not specified.

LIFESPAN CONSIDERATIONS

Pregnancy/Lactation: Avoid pregnancy; may cause fetal harm. Females of reproductive potential should use effective contraception during treatment and for at least 7 mos after discontinuation. Breastfeeding not recommended during treatment and for at least 7 mos after discontinuation. **Children:** Safety and efficacy not established. **Elderly:** May have increased risk of cardiac dysfunction.

INTERACTIONS

DRUG: May increase cardiotoxic effects of **anthracyclines (e.g., daunorubicin, doxorubicin, epirubicin).** **HERBAL:** None significant. **FOOD:** None known. **LAB VALUES:** May decrease Hgb, neutrophils, RBCs.

AVAILABILITY (Rx)

Injection Solution: trastuzumab 600 mg/hyaluronidase 10,000 units (120 mg/2,000 units/mL).

ADMINISTRATION/HANDLING

Subcutaneous

Preparation • Visually inspect for particulate matter or discoloration. Solution should appear clear to opalescent, colorless to yellow in color. Do not use if solution is cloudy or discolored or visible particles are observed. • Withdraw contents from vial into syringe. • To avoid clogging, immediately attach a hypodermic needle or subcutaneous infusion set to syringe.

Administration • Insert needle subcutaneously into left or right thigh (only), approx. 2.5 cm from previous injection sites. • Do not inject into areas of active skin disease or injury such as sunburns, skin rashes, inflammation, skin infections, or active psoriasis. • Rotate injection sites. • Do not administer IV or intramuscularly. • If a dose is missed, administer as soon as possible and adjustment schedule to maintain dosing intervals.

Rate of administration • Inject over 2–5 min.

Storage • Refrigerate vials in original carton until time of use. • Protect from light. • Do not shake or freeze. • After vial is removed from refrigerator, use within 4 hrs. • May store syringe containing solution at room temperature for up to 4 hrs or refrigerate for up to 24 hrs.

INDICATIONS/ROUTES/DOSAGE

Breast Cancer (HER2-positive) (adjuvant)

SQ: ADULTS: 600 mg/10,000 units q3wks (21-day cycle) for 52 wks or until disease recurrence. Extending treatment beyond 1 yr is not recommended.

Breast Cancer (HER2-positive, metastatic)

SQ: ADULTS: 600 mg/10,000 units q3wks (21-day cycle). Continue until disease progression or unacceptable toxicity.

Dose Modification

Cardiac Toxicity

Withhold treatment for 4 wks for an absolute decrease in left ventricular ejection fraction (LVEF) that is greater than or equal to 16% from baseline; absolute decrease in LVEF below institutional limits of normal and greater than or equal to 10% from baseline. May resume if LVEF returns to normal limits and the absolute decrease from baseline is greater than or equal to 15% within 4–8 wks. Permanently discontinue if left ventricular dysfunction persists longer than 8 wks or treatment is withheld on more than three occasions for cardiac toxicity.

Dosage in Renal Impairment

Mild to severe impairment: Not specified; use caution.

Dosage in Hepatic Impairment

Mild to severe impairment: Not specified; use caution.

SIDE EFFECTS

Frequent (33%–17%): Fatigue, diarrhea, arthralgia, injection site reactions (e.g., bruising, pain, dermatitis, discoloration, discomfort, erythema, fibrosis, hematoma, hemorrhage, induration, irritation, nodule, rash, ulcer), rash, myalgia. **Occasional (15%–6%):** Nausea, peripheral neuropathy, headache, flushing, edema, cough, extremity pain, pyrexia, nail disorder, abdominal pain, alopecia, erythema, constipation, hypertension, stomatitis, dyspnea, back pain, generalized pain, vomiting, insomnia, mucosal inflammation, pruritus, dizziness, paresthesia, nasal inflammation/discomfort.

ADVERSE EFFECTS/TOXIC REACTIONS

Myelosuppression (anemia, neutropenia) is an expected response to therapy. Cardiomyopathy reported in 5% of pts. Other cardiac disorders may include tachycardia, palpitations, congestive HF. Pulmonary toxicities (acute respiratory distress syndrome, dyspnea, hypoxia, ILD, noncardiogenic pulmonary edema, pneumonitis, pleural effusions, pulmonary fibrosis, pulmonary infiltrates, pulmonary insufficiency) were reported. Infections (upper respiratory tract infections, UTI, viral infections) were reported. Epistaxis reported in 6% of pts. Hypersensitivity reactions, including anaphylaxis, may occur. Immunogenicity (auto-trastuzumab antibodies) reported in 10% of pts.

NURSING CONSIDERATIONS

BASELINE ASSESSMENT

Obtain CBC; pregnancy test in females of reproductive potential. Confirm compliance of effective contraception. Verify presence of HER2 protein overexpression or HER2 gene amplification in tumor specimen. Assess LVEF by echocardiogram. Question history of cardiovascular disease, HF, hypersensitivity reactions, pulmonary disease. Screen for active infection. Offer emotional support.

INTERVENTION/EVALUATION

Monitor CBC periodically. Consider ABG, radiologic test if ILD/pneumonitis (excessive cough, dyspnea, fever, hypoxia) is suspected. Consider treatment with corticosteroids if ILD/pneumonitis is confirmed. Auscultate lung sounds. Monitor for symptoms of HF (chest pain, dyspnea, palpitations, swelling of extremities). Assess LVEF by echocardiogram q3mos. If treatment withheld due to change in LVEF, monitor LVEF at 4-wk intervals. If treatment is used as adjuvant therapy, assess LVEF q6mos for at least 2 yrs upon completion. Monitor for infections (cough, fatigue, fever). If serious infection occurs, initiate appropriate antimicrobial therapy. Monitor daily pattern of bowel activity, stool consistency. Offer antiemetic if nausea/vomiting occurs. Monitor for hypersensitivity reactions.

PATIENT/FAMILY TEACHING

• Treatment may depress your immune system response and reduce your ability to fight infection. Report symptoms of infection such as body aches, chills, cough, fatigue, fever. Avoid those with active infection. • Report symptoms of bone marrow depression (e.g., bruising, fatigue, fever, shortness of breath, weight loss; bleeding easily, bloody urine or stool). • Report symptoms of lung inflammation (excessive coughing, difficulty breathing, chest pain); heart failure (e.g., chest pain, difficulty breathing, palpitations, swelling of extremities); UTI (fever, urinary frequency, burning during urination, foul-smelling urine). • Treatment may reduce the heart's ability to pump effectively; expect routine echocardiograms. • Use effective contraception to avoid pregnancy. Do not breastfeed. • Nausea/vomiting is a common side effect. • Maintain proper hydration and nutrition. • Severe allergic re-

T

actions, including anaphylaxis, can occur. If allergic reaction occurs, seek immediate medical attention.

traZODone

traz-o-done
(Apo-TraZODone ✱)

■ BLACK BOX ALERT ■ Increased risk of suicidal ideation and behavior in children, adolescents, young adults 18–24 yrs with major depressive disorder, other psychiatric disorders. **Do not confuse traZODone with traMADol or ziprasidone.**

◆CLASSIFICATION

PHARMACOTHERAPEUTIC: Serotonin reuptake inhibitor/antagonist. **CLINICAL:** Antidepressant.

USES

Treatment of major depressive disorder (MDD). **OFF-LABEL:** Insomnia.

PRECAUTIONS

Contraindications: Hypersensitivity to traZODone. Use of MAOIs (concurrently or within 14 days of discontinuing traZODone or MAOI); initiation in pt receiving linezolid or IV methylene blue. **Cautions:** Cardiac disease, cardiac conduction disorders, seizure disorder, elderly, hepatic/renal impairment, cerebrovascular disease; history of suicidal ideation and behavior, conditions predisposing to priapism (e.g., sickle cell disease), concomitant use of antihypertensives.

T

ACTION

Blocks reuptake of serotonin at neuronal presynaptic membranes, increasing its availability at postsynaptic receptor sites. **Therapeutic Effect:** Relieves depression.

PHARMACOKINETICS

Widely distributed. Protein binding: 85%–95%. Metabolized in liver. Primarily excreted in urine. **Half-life:** 5–9 hrs (increased in elderly).

⌛ LIFESPAN CONSIDERATIONS

Pregnancy/Lactation: Crosses placenta; minimally distributed in breast milk. **Children:** Safety and efficacy not established in pts younger than 6 yrs. **Elderly:** More likely to experience sedative, hypotensive effects; lower dosage recommended.

INTERACTIONS

DRUG: **Strong CYP3A4 inhibitors (e.g., clarithromycin, ketoconazole)** may increase concentration/effect. May increase concentration/effect of **phenytoin. Strong CYP3A4 inducers (e.g., carBAMazepine, rifAMPin)** may decrease concentration/effect. May increase QT interval-prolonging effect of **clarithromycin. Linezolid, venlafaxine** may increase serotonergic effect. **MAOIs (e.g., phenelzine, selegiline)** may increase adverse effects. **HERBAL: St. John's wort** may decrease concentration/effect. **FOOD:** None known. **LAB VALUES:** May decrease neutrophils, WBCs.

AVAILABILITY (Rx)

Tablets: 50 mg, 100 mg, 150 mg, 300 mg.

ADMINISTRATION/HANDLING

PO

• Give shortly after snack, meal (reduces risk of dizziness). • Tablets may be crushed.

INDICATIONS/ROUTES/DOSAGE

◀ALERT▶ Therapeutic effect may take up to 6 wks to occur.

Depression

PO: ADULTS: Initially, 50 mg twice daily. May increase in increments of 50 mg/day q3–7 days up to 75–150 mg twice daily. May further increase by 50–100 mg/day q2–4 wks. Usual dosage range: 200 to 400 mg/day. **Maximum:** 600 mg/day. **ELDERLY:** Initially, 25–50 mg at bedtime.

May increase by 25–50 mg every 3–7 days. Range: 75–150 mg/day.

Dosage in Renal/Hepatic Impairment
Use caution.

SIDE EFFECTS

Frequent (9%–3%): Drowsiness, dry mouth, light-headedness, dizziness, headache, blurred vision, nausea, vomiting. **Occasional (3%–1%):** Nervousness, fatigue, constipation, myalgia/arthralgia, mild hypotension. **Rare:** Photosensitivity reaction.

ADVERSE EFFECTS/TOXIC REACTIONS

Priapism, altered libido, retrograde ejaculation, impotence occur rarely. Appears to be less cardiotoxic than other antidepressants, although arrhythmias may occur in pts with preexisting cardiac disease.

NURSING CONSIDERATIONS

BASELINE ASSESSMENT

Assess mental status, mood, behavior. For pts on long-term therapy, serum hepatic/renal function tests, blood counts should be performed periodically. Question history as listed in Precautions.

INTERVENTION/EVALUATION

Monitor for suicidal ideation (esp. at beginning of therapy or dosage change). Assess appearance, behavior, speech pattern, level of interest, mood. Assist with ambulation if dizziness, light-headedness occurs.

PATIENT/FAMILY TEACHING

• Immediately discontinue medication, consult physician if priapism occurs. • **Immediate-Release:** May take after meal, snack. • **Extended-Release:** Take on empty stomach. • May take at bedtime if drowsiness occurs. • Change positions slowly to avoid hypotensive effect. • Avoid tasks that require alertness, motor skills until response to drug is established. • Photosensitivity to sun may occur. • Report visual disturbances, worsening depression, suicidal ideation, unusual changes in behavior. • Do not abruptly discontinue medication. • Avoid alcohol.

trospium

tro-spee-um
(Trosec ✱)

◆CLASSIFICATION

PHARMACOTHERAPEUTIC: Anticholinergic. **CLINICAL:** Antispasmodic.

USES

Treatment of overactive bladder with symptoms of urge urinary incontinence, urgency, urinary frequency.

PRECAUTIONS

Contraindications: Hypersensitivity to trospium. Pts with or at increased risk of gastric retention, uncontrolled narrow-angle glaucoma, urinary retention. **Cautions:** Decreased GI motility, renal/hepatic impairment, obstructive GI disorders, ulcerative colitis, intestinal atony, myasthenia gravis, controlled narrow-angle glaucoma, bladder flow obstruction, Alzheimer's disease, hot weather/exercise, elderly.

ACTION

Antagonizes effect of acetylcholine on muscarinic receptors, producing parasympatholytic action. **Therapeutic Effect:** Reduces smooth muscle tone in bladder.

PHARMACOKINETICS

Minimally absorbed after PO administration. Protein binding: 50%–85%. Distributed in plasma. Excreted in feces (82%), urine (6%). **Half-life:** 20 hrs.

⌛ LIFESPAN CONSIDERATIONS

Pregnancy/Lactation: Unknown if drug crosses placenta or is distributed in breast milk. **Children:** Safety and efficacy not established. **Elderly:** Higher

T

incidence of dry mouth, constipation, dyspepsia, UTI, urinary retention in pts 75 yrs and older.

INTERACTIONS

DRUG: **Alcohol** may increase CNS depression. **Anticholinergics (e.g., aclidinium, ipratropium, tiotropium, umeclidinium)** may increase anticholinergic effect. **HERBAL:** None significant. **FOOD:** **High-fat meals** may reduce absorption. **LAB VALUES:** None significant.

AVAILABILITY (Rx)

Tablets: 20 mg. **Capsules, Extended-Release:** 60 mg.

ADMINISTRATION/HANDLING

PO

• Give at least 1 hr before meals or on an empty stomach. • Do not break, crush, dissolve, or divide tablets or extended-release capsules; administer whole. • Administer tablets at bedtime, capsules in morning with full glass of water, 1 hr before eating.

INDICATIONS/ROUTES/DOSAGE

Overactive Bladder

PO: ADULTS: ***(Immediate-Release):*** 20 mg twice daily. **ELDERLY 75 YRS AND OLDER:** 20 mg once daily. **ADULTS, ELDERLY:** ***(Extended-Release):*** 60 mg once daily in the morning.

Dosage in Renal Impairment

CrCl less than 30 mL/min: Immediate-release dose is reduced to 20 mg once daily at bedtime. Extended-release not recommended.

Dosage in Hepatic Impairment

Mild impairment: No dose adjustment. **Moderate to severe impairment:** Use with caution.

SIDE EFFECTS

Frequent (20%): Dry mouth. **Occasional (10%–4%):** Constipation, headache. **Rare (less than 2%):** Fatigue, upper abdominal pain, dyspepsia (heartburn, indigestion, epigastric pain), flatulence, dry eyes, urinary retention.

ADVERSE EFFECTS/TOXIC REACTIONS

Overdose may result in severe anticholinergic effects, characterized by nervousness, restlessness, nausea, vomiting, confusion, diaphoresis, facial flushing, hypertension, hypotension, respiratory depression, irritability, lacrimation. Supraventricular tachycardia and hallucinations occur rarely.

NURSING CONSIDERATIONS

BASELINE ASSESSMENT

Assess for dysuria, urinary urgency, frequency, incontinence.

INTERVENTION/EVALUATION

Monitor for symptomatic relief. Monitor I&O; palpate bladder for retention. Monitor daily pattern of bowel activity, stool consistency.

PATIENT/FAMILY TEACHING

• Report nausea, vomiting, diaphoresis, increased salivary secretions, palpitations, severe abdominal pain. • Swallow tablets, extended-release capsules whole. • Take 1 hr before meals.

tucatinib

too-**ka**-ti-nib
(Tukysa)

Do not confuse tucatinib with afatinib, dasatinib, lapatinib, neratinib, talazoparib, tofacitinib, or trametinib.

◆Classification

PHARMACOTHERAPEUTIC: Human epidermal growth factor receptor 2 (HER2) antagonist, tyrosine kinase inhibitor. **CLINICAL:** Antineoplastic.

USES

Treatment of adults with advanced unresectable or metastatic HER2-positive breast cancer (in combination with trastuzumab and capecitabine), including pts with or without brain metastases, who have received one or more prior anti-HER2-based regimens in the metastatic setting.

PRECAUTIONS

Contraindications: Hypersensitivity to tucatinib. **Cautions:** Baseline anemia, hepatic/renal impairment, dehydration, conditions predisposing to infection (e.g., diabetes, renal failure, immunocompromised pts, open wounds); concomitant use of CYP3A substrates, P-glycoprotein substrates, moderate CYP2C8 inhibitors. Avoid concomitant use of strong CYP2C8 inhibitors.

ACTION

Highly selective for HER2 kinase domain. Inhibits HER2 phosphorylation, causing downstream inhibition of MAPK and AKT signaling and cell proliferation. **Therapeutic Effect:** Shows antitumor activity in HER2-expressing tumor cells and inhibits the growth of HER2-expressing tumors.

PHARMACOKINETICS

Widely distributed. Metabolized in liver. Protein binding: 97%. Peak plasma concentration: 2 hrs. Excreted in feces (86%), urine (4%). **Half-life:** 8.5 hrs.

LIFESPAN CONSIDERATIONS

Pregnancy/Lactation: Avoid pregnancy; may cause fetal harm. Females and males with female partners of reproductive potential must use effective contraception during treatment and for at least 1 wk after discontinuation. Unknown if distributed in breast milk. Breastfeeding not recommended during treatment and for at least 1 wk after discontinuation. May impair fertility. **Children:** Safety and efficacy not established. **Elderly:** May have increased risk of adverse effects/toxic reactions.

INTERACTIONS

DRUG: Strong CYP2C8 inhibitors (e.g., gemfibrozil, clopidogrel), moderate CYP2C8 inhibitors (e.g., irbesartan, efavirenz) may increase concentration/effect. **Strong CYP3A4 inducers (e.g., carBAMazepine, phenytoin), moderate CYP2C8 inducers (e.g., rifAMPin)** may decrease concentration/effect. May increase concentration/effect of **acalabrutinib, axitinib, bosutinib, cyclosporine, irinotecan, ranolazine, simvastatin, tamsulosin, topotecan, trazodone.** **HERBAL:** None significant. **FOOD:** None known. **LAB VALUES:** May increase serum alkaline phosphatase, ALT, AST, bilirubin, creatinine. May decrease serum magnesium, phosphate, potassium, sodium; Hgb.

AVAILABILITY (Rx)

Tablets: 50 mg, 150 mg.

ADMINISTRATION/HANDLING

PO

• Give without regard to food. Administer tablet whole; do not break, cut, or crush. • Do not give if tablet is cracked, broken, or not intact. • Tablets cannot be chewed. • If a dose is missed or vomiting occurs after administration, give next dose at regularly scheduled time (do not give additional dose).

T

INDICATIONS/ROUTES/DOSAGE

Breast Cancer (HER2-positive, unresectable or metastatic)

PO: ADULTS: 300 mg twice daily (in combination with trastuzumab and capecitabine). Continue until disease progression or unacceptable toxicity.

Dose Reduction Schedule

First dose reduction: 250 mg twice daily. **Second dose reduction:** 200 mg twice daily. **Third dose reduction:** 150 mg twice daily. **Unable to tolerate 150-mg dose:** Permanently discontinue.

Dose Modification

Based on Common Terminology Criteria for Adverse Events (CTCAE).

Diarrhea

Grade 3 diarrhea *without* antidiarrheal therapy: Start antidiarrheal therapy. Withhold treatment until improved to Grade 1 or 0, then resume at same dose. **Grade 3 diarrhea *with* antidiarrheal therapy:** Start or intensify antidiarrheal therapy. Withhold treatment until improved to Grade 1 or 0, then resume at reduced dose level. **Grade 4 diarrhea:** Permanently discontinue.

Hepatotoxicity (During treatment)

Grade 2 serum bilirubin elevation: Withhold treatment until improved to Grade 1 or 0, then resume at same dose. **Grade 3 serum ALT/AST or bilirubin elevation:** Withhold treatment until improved to Grade 1 or 0, then resume at reduced dose level. **Grade 4 serum ALT/AST or bilirubin elevation:** Permanently discontinue. Serum ALT/AST elevation greater than 3 times ULN *with* serum bilirubin elevation 2 times ULN: Permanently discontinue.

Other Toxicities

Any other Grade 3 toxicities: Withhold treatment until improved to Grade 1 or 0, then resume at reduced dose level. **Any other Grade 4 toxicities:** Permanently discontinue.

Concomitant Use of Strong CYP2C8 Inhibitor

If strong CYP2C8 inhibitor cannot be discontinued, reduce dose to 100 mg twice daily. If strong CYP2C8 inhibitor is discontinued for 3 eliminated half-lives, may resume dose prior to starting CYP2C8 inhibitor.

Dosage in Renal Impairment

Mild to moderate impairment: No dose adjustment. **Severe impairment:** Not recommended.

Dosage in Hepatic Impairment

Mild to moderate impairment: No dose adjustment. **Severe impairment:** Reduce dose to 200 mg twice daily.

SIDE EFFECTS

Note: Frequency and occurrence of side effects may vary based on combination regimen. **Frequent (80%–20%):** Diarrhea, nausea, vomiting, stomatitis, oropharyngeal pain/discomfort, oral ulceration/blistering, decreased appetite, rash. **Occasional (15%–13%):** Arthralgia, decreased weight, peripheral neuropathy.

ADVERSE EFFECTS/TOXIC REACTIONS

Anemia is an expected response to therapy. Life-threatening diarrhea may cause dehydration, electrolyte imbalance, hypotension, acute kidney injury, and death. Median onset of diarrhea was 12 days. Severe hepatotoxicity may occur. Palmar-plantar erythrodysesthesia syndrome (PPES), a chemotherapy-induced skin condition that presents with redness, swelling, numbness, skin sloughing of the hands and feet, reported in 63% of pts. Epistaxis reported in 12% of pts.

NURSING CONSIDERATIONS

BASELINE ASSESSMENT.

Obtain CBC, BMP, LFT; pregnancy test in females of reproductive potential. Confirm compliance of effective contraception. Confirm HER2-positive status. Question history of hepatic/renal impairment. Assess usual bowel movement patterns, stool characteristics. Assess and correct hydration status prior to initiation. Receive full medication history and screen for interactions. Offer emotional support.

INTERVENTION/EVALUATION.

Monitor LFT q3wks (or more frequently in pts with hepatotoxicity). Monitor CBC, renal function, electrolytes periodically. An increase of serum creatinine greater than 0.4 mg/dL from baseline may indicate renal impairment. Diarrhea must be treated promptly. If diarrhea occurs, initiate antidiarrheal therapy and evaluate for other causes (infectious processes). Consider IV hydration if severe dehydra-

T

tion occurs. Replete electrolytes as clinically indicated. Assess skin for dermal toxicities, PPES. Monitor for toxicities if discontinuation or dose reduction if concomitant strong or moderate CYP2C8 inhibitors, P-glycoprotein substrates, CYP3A substrates is unavoidable.

PATIENT/FAMILY TEACHING.

• Diarrhea, nausea, vomiting is a common side effect. • Diarrhea may cause dehydration, electrolyte imbalance, low blood pressure, kidney injury, and may be life threatening. Drink plenty of fluids. Report diarrhea or dehydration that does not improve with medical management. • Report toxic skin reactions (itching, peeling, rash, redness, swelling); liver problems (abdominal pain, bruising, clay-colored stool, dark or amber-colored urine, yellowing of the skin or eyes), kidney problems (decreased urine output, flank pain, darkened urine). • There is a high risk of interactions with other medications. Do not take newly prescribed medications unless approved by prescriber who originally started therapy. • Avoid herbal supplements (esp. St. John's wort). • Use effective contraception to avoid pregnancy. Do not breastfeed.

ubrogepant

ue-**broe**-je-pant
(Ubrelvy)
Do not confuse ubrogepant with atogepant or rimegepant.

◆Classification

PHARMACOTHERAPEUTIC: Calcitonin gene–related peptide (CGRP) receptor antagonist. **CLINICAL:** Antimigraine.

USES

Treatment of migraines with or without aura in adults.

PRECAUTIONS

Contraindications: Hypersensitivity to ubrogepant. Concomitant use of strong CYP3A4 inhibitors. **Cautions:** Hepatic/renal impairment. Not indicated for prevention of migraine. Avoid concomitant use of strong CYP3A4 inducers.

ACTION

Exact mechanism of action unknown. Binds to and inhibits calcitonin gene–related peptide (CGRP) receptor. **Therapeutic Effect:** Relieves migraine headache.

PHARMACOKINETICS

Rapidly absorbed. Metabolized in liver. Protein binding: 87%. Peak plasma concentration: 1.5 hrs. Excreted in feces (42%), urine (6%). **Half-life:** 5–7 hrs.

U

⧗ LIFESPAN CONSIDERATIONS

Pregnancy/Lactation: May cause fetal harm. Unknown if distributed in breast milk. **Children:** Safety and efficacy not established. **Elderly:** No age-related precautions noted.

INTERACTIONS

DRUG: Strong CYP3A4 inhibitors (e.g., clarithromycin, ketoconazole, ritonavir), moderate CYP3A inhibitors (e.g., cyclosporine, fluconazole, verapamil), P-gp inhibitors (e.g., amiodarone, carvedilol, clarithromycin, itraconazole, verapamil) may increase concentration/effect. **Strong CYP3A4 inducers (e.g., carBAMazepine, phenytoin, rifAMPin), moderate CYP3A inducers (e.g., bosentan, nafcillin)** may decrease concentration/effect. **HERBAL: St. John's wort** may decrease concentration/effect. **FOOD:** None known. **LAB VALUES:** None known.

AVAILABILITY (Rx)

Tablets: 50 mg, 100 mg.

ADMINISTRATION/HANDLING

PO

- Give without regard to food.

INDICATIONS/ROUTES/DOSAGE

Migraine (with or without aura)

PO: ADULTS: 50 mg or 100 mg as needed. May repeat dose at least 2 hrs after initial dose. Do not exceed 200 mg in a 24-hr period.

Dose Modification

Concomitant Drug	Initial Dose	Second Dose (if needed)
Moderate CYP3A4 inhibitors	50 mg	Avoid within 24 hrs
Weak CYP3A4 inhibitors	50 mg	50 mg
BCRP and/or P-gp only inhibitors	50 mg	50 mg
Strong CYP3A4 inducers	Avoid Use	Avoid use
Weak or moderate CYP3A4 inducers	100 mg	100 mg

Dosage in Renal Impairment

Mild to moderate impairment: No dose adjustment. **Severe impairment (CrCl 15–29 mL/min):** Initially, 50 mg. May repeat 50 mg dose at least 2 hrs after initial dose. **ESRD (CrCl less than 15 mL/min):** Avoid use.

Dosage in Hepatic Impairment

Mild to moderate impairment: No dose adjustment. **Severe impairment:** Initially, 50 mg. May repeat 50 mg dose at least 2 hrs after initial dose.

SIDE EFFECTS

Rare (2%–1%): Nausea, somnolence, dry mouth.

ADVERSE EFFECTS/TOXIC REACTIONS

None known.

NURSING CONSIDERATIONS

BASELINE ASSESSMENT

Question characteristics of migraine headaches (onset, location, duration, possible precipitating symptoms). Receive full medication history and screen for interactions. Question history of hepatic/renal impairment.

INTERVENTION/EVALUATION

Evaluate for relief of migraine headaches (photophobia, phonophobia, nausea, vomiting, pain, dizziness, fogginess).

PATIENT/FAMILY TEACHING

• There is a high risk of interactions with other medications. Do not take newly prescribed medications unless approved by prescriber who originally started therapy. Do not take herbal products (esp. St. John's wort) or ingest grapefruit products. • Avoid tasks that require alertness, motor skills until response to drug is established.

umeclidinium

ue-**mek**-li-**din**-ee-um
(Incruse Ellipta)
Do not confuse umeclidinium with aclidinium or clidinium.

FIXED-COMBINATION(S)

Anoro Ellipta: umeclidinium/vilanterol (bronchodilator): 62.5 mcg/25 mcg. **Trelegy Ellipta:** umeclidium/fluticasone (corticosteroid)/vilanterol (bronchodilator): 62.5 mcg/100 mcg/25 mcg.

◆CLASSIFICATION

PHARMACOTHERAPEUTIC: Anticholinergic. **CLINICAL:** Bronchodilator (long-acting).

USES

Long-term, once-daily maintenance treatment of airflow obstruction in pts with COPD including chronic bronchitis and/or emphysema.

PRECAUTIONS

Contraindications: Hypersensitivity to umeclidinium. Severe hypersensitivity to milk proteins or any drug components. **Cautions:** Bladder neck obstruction, myasthenia gravis, narrow-angle glaucoma, prostatic hypertrophy, urinary retention. Not recommended in pts with acutely deteriorating COPD requiring emergent relief of acute symptoms.

ACTION

Inhibits muscarinic M_3 receptor in lungs, resulting in relaxation of bronchial smooth muscle. **Therapeutic Effect:** Relieves bronchospasm, reduces airway resistance, improves bronchodilation.

PHARMACOKINETICS

Rapidly absorbed following inhalation. Primarily metabolized by enzyme cytochrome P4502D6. Protein binding: 89%. Peak concentration: 5–15 min. Steady state reached within 14 days. **Half-life:** 11 hrs.

LIFESPAN CONSIDERATIONS

Pregnancy/Lactation: Unknown if distributed in breast milk. Must either discontinue drug or discontinue breastfeeding.

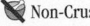

Children: Not indicated in this pt population. **Elderly:** No age-related precautions noted.

INTERACTIONS

DRUG: **Anticholinergics (e.g., aclidinium, ipratropium, tiotropium)** may increase anticholinergic effect. **HERBAL:** None significant. **FOOD:** None known. **LAB VALUES:** None known.

AVAILABILITY (Rx)

Inhalation Powder: 62.5 mcg/capsule (in blister packs containing 7 or 30 doses).

ADMINISTRATION/HANDLING

Inhalation

Administration • Follow instructions for preparation according to manufacturer guidelines. • Do not shake or prime. Prior to inhaling dose, exhale fully (do not exhale into inhaler). Close lips tightly around inhaler and inhale (rapidly, steadily, and deeply). Do not breathe through nose or block air vent with fingers. • Remove mouthpiece and hold breath for 3–4 sec, then breathe out slowly and gently. Do not close container until medication has been inhaled. • Close lid cover.

Storage • Store at room temperature up to 6 wks after opening tray. • Do not refrigerate or freeze. • Protect from sunlight and moisture. • Discard after counter reaches 0. • Do not reuse inhaler.

INDICATIONS/ROUTES/DOSAGE

COPD

Inhalation: ADULTS, ELDERLY: One inhalation (62.5 mcg) once daily, at same time each day. **Maximum:** 1 inhalation/24 hrs.

Dose Modification

Deterioration of COPD: Discontinue treatment. Initiate short-acting bronchodilators and supportive pulmonary therapy.

Dosage in Renal Impairment

No dose adjustment.

Dosage in Hepatic Impairment

Mild to moderate impairment: No dose adjustment. **Severe impairment:** Use caution.

SIDE EFFECTS

Occasional (8%–5%): Nasopharyngitis, upper respiratory tract infection. **Rare (3%–1%):** Cough, arthralgia, viral respiratory tract infection, pharyngitis, myalgia, abdominal pain, toothache, tachycardia.

ADVERSE EFFECTS/TOXIC REACTIONS

Life-threatening asthma-related events, bronchospasm, worsening of COPD-related symptoms have been reported. Hypersensitivity reactions may occur (esp. in pts with undiagnosed severe milk protein allergy or allergy to products containing lactose). Worsening of narrow-angle glaucoma (eye pain, blurry vision, visual halos, colored images in association with red eyes from conjunctival congestion and corneal edema) may occur. May cause worsening of urinary retention, esp. in pts with prostatic hypertrophy or bladder neck obstruction.

NURSING CONSIDERATIONS

BASELINE ASSESSMENT

Obtain O_2 saturation, vital signs; pulmonary function test, if applicable. Assess respiratory rate, depth, rhythm. Assess lung sounds for wheezing. Screen for concomitant use of anticholinergic medications. Question history of asthma, BPH, bladder neck obstruction, glaucoma. Teach proper inhaler priming and administration techniques. Conduct ophthalmologic exam in pts with narrow-angle glaucoma.

INTERVENTION/EVALUATION

Routinely monitor O_2 saturation, vital signs. Auscultate lung sounds and monitor for symptom improvement. Recommend discontinuation of short-acting beta$_2$-agonists while on long-term therapy. Monitor for COPD deterioration, narrow-angle glaucoma, urinary retention/obstruction. Monitor for increased use of rescue inhaler; may indicate worsening of respiratory status.

PATIENT/FAMILY TEACHING

• Report fever, productive cough, body aches, paradoxical bronchospasm, difficulty breathing; may indicate lung infection, worsening of COPD. • Therapy not intended for acute COPD symptom relief, and extra doses are not advised. • Report symptoms of acute narrow-angle glaucoma, urinary retention, bladder distention. • Refill prescription when counter on left of inhaler reaches red area of scale. • Follow manufacturer guidelines for proper use of inhaler. • Drink plenty of fluids (decreases lung secretion viscosity). • Rinse mouth with water after inhalation to decrease mouth/throat irritation.

upadacitinib

TOP 100

ue-**pad**-a-**sye**-ti-nib
(Rinvoq)

BLACK BOX ALERT Increased risk for developing bacterial, invasive fungal, viral, other opportunistic infections (including tuberculosis, herpes zoster, cryptococcosis, pneumocystosis), which may lead to hospitalization or death. Infections often occurred in combination with other immunosuppressants (methotrexate, other disease-modifying antirheumatic drugs). Closely monitor for infections. Test for latent tuberculosis prior to initiation and during treatment, regardless of initial result. Latent TB should be treated prior to initiation. Lymphomas, other malignancies were reported. Thromboembolic events, including deep vein thrombosis (DVT), pulmonary embolism (PE), arterial thrombosis, have occurred.

Do not confuse upadacitinib with baricitinib or tofacitinib.

◆CLASSIFICATION

PHARMACOTHERAPEUTIC: Janus kinase (JAK) inhibitor. **CLINICAL:** Disease-modifying antirheumatic drug (DMARD).

USES

Treatment of adults with moderately to severely active rheumatoid arthritis who have had an inadequate response or intolerance to methotrexate.

PRECAUTIONS

Contraindications: Hypersensitivity to upadacitinib. **Cautions:** Baseline cytopenias, hepatic/renal impairment, elderly, uncontrolled hyperlipidemia; history of arterial or venous thrombosis (CVA, DVT, MI, PE); pts at risk for thrombosis (immobility, indwelling venous catheter/access device, morbid obesity, underlying atherosclerosis, genetic hypercoagulable conditions), recent travel or residence in TB- or mycosis-endemic areas; history of chronic opportunistic infections (bacterial, invasive fungal, mycobacterial, protozoal, viral, TB); infections including HIV, herpes zoster, hepatitis B or C virus; conditions predisposing to infection (e.g., diabetes, renal failure, immunocompromised pts, open wounds), pts at risk for GI perforation (e.g., Crohn's disease, diverticulitis, GI tract or abdominal malignancies, GI ulcers). Use of live, attenuated vaccines is not recommended.

ACTION

Inhibits JAK enzymes, which are intracellular enzymes involved in stimulating hematopoiesis and immune cell function via signaling pathway. **Therapeutic Effect:** Reduces inflammation, tenderness, swelling of joints; slows or prevents progressive joint destruction in rheumatoid arthritis (RA).

PHARMACOKINETICS

Rapidly absorbed and widely distributed. Metabolized in liver. Protein

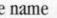

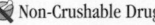

U

binding: 52%. Peak plasma concentration: 2–4 hrs. Excreted in feces (38%), urine (24%). **Half-life:** 8–14 hrs.

LIFESPAN CONSIDERATIONS

Pregnancy/Lactation: Avoid pregnancy; may cause fetal harm. Females of reproductive potential must use effective contraception during treatment and for at least 4 wks after discontinuation. Unknown if distributed in breast milk. Breastfeeding not recommended during treatment and for at least 6 days after discontinuation. **Children:** Safety and efficacy not established. **Elderly:** No age-related precautions noted.

INTERACTIONS

DRUG: May diminish therapeutic effect of **vaccines, BCG (intravesical).** May increase adverse/toxic effects of **natalizumab, live vaccines. Strong CYP3A4 inhibitors (e.g., clarithromycin, ketoconazole, ritonavir)** may increase concentration/effect. **Strong CYP3A4 inducers (e.g., rifAMPin, phenytoin, carBAMazepine, phenobarbital)** may decrease concentration/effect. **HERBAL: Echinacea** may decrease therapeutic effect. **FOOD:** None known. **LAB VALUES:** May increase serum ALT, AST, creatine phosphokinase, low-density lipoprotein (LDL), high-density lipoprotein (HDL), total cholesterol. May decrease absolute lymphocyte count, absolute neutrophil count (ANC), Hgb.

AVAILABILITY (Rx)

Tablets, Extended-Release: 15 mg.

ADMINISTRATION/HANDLING

PO

• Give without regard to food. • Administer tablet whole; do not break, cut, or crush. • Tablets cannot be chewed.

INDICATIONS/ROUTES/DOSAGE

ALERT Do not initiate in pts with severe, active infection (systemic/localized), absolute lymphocyte count less than 500 cells/mm³, ANC less than 1,000 cells/mm³, Hgb less than 8 g/dL; severe hepatic impairment. Do not use in combination with other JAK inhibitors, biologic DMARDs, strong immunosuppressants (e.g., azathioprine, cycloSPORINE).

Rheumatoid Arthritis

PO: ADULTS: 15 mg once daily.

Dose Modification

Hematologic Toxicity

Hgb less than 8 g/dL: Withhold treatment until Hgb is greater than or equal to 8 gm/dL, then resume treatment. **Absolute lymphocyte count (ALC) less than 500 cells/mm³:** Withhold treatment until ALC is greater than or equal to 500 cells/mm³, then resume treatment. **ANC less than 1000 cells/mm³:** Withhold treatment until ANC is greater than or equal to 1,000 cells/mm³, then resume treatment.

Hepatotoxicity

Withhold treatment until hepatotoxicity is resolved, then resume if clinically indicated.

Serious Infection

Withhold treatment until serious infection is resolved, then resume if clinically indicated.

Dosage in Renal Impairment

Mild to severe impairment: No dose adjustment.

Dosage in Hepatic Impairment

Mild to moderate impairment: No dose adjustment. **Severe impairment:** Not recommended.

SIDE EFFECTS

Rare (4%–1%): Nausea, cough, pyrexia.

ADVERSE EFFECTS/TOXIC REACTIONS

Neutropenia, lymphopenia may increase risk of infection. Serious and sometimes fatal infections (bacterial, mycobacterial, invasive fungal, viral, other opportunistic infections) may occur. Serious infections may include cellulitis, cryptococcosis, esophageal candidiasis, herpes zoster, pneumonia, pneumocystosis, TB. Upper respiratory tract infections (laryngitis, nasopharyngitis, pharyngitis, pharyngotonsillitis, rhinitis, sinusitis, tonsillitis, viral infection) reported in 14% of pts. May cause viral reactivation of hepatitis B virus, herpes zoster. New nonmelanoma skin malignancies, lymphomas were reported. Thromboembolic events including DVT, pulmonary embolism, arterial thrombosis have occurred. May increase risk of GI perforation.

NURSING CONSIDERATIONS

BASELINE ASSESSMENT.

Obtain CBC, LFT, lipid panel; pregnancy test in females of reproductive potential. Confirm compliance of effective contraception. Evaluate for active TB and test for latent TB infection. An induration of 5 mm or greater with purified protein derivative (PPD) is considered a positive result when assessing for latent TB. Consider treatment with antimycobacterial therapy in pts with latent TB. Screen for active infection. Question history of arterial/venous thrombosis, hepatic/renal impairment; chronic infections including HIV, hepatitis B or C virus, herpes zoster. Assess risk of GI perforation. Receive full medication history and screen for interactions. Recommend up-to-date vaccinations (non-live, attenuated), including prophylactic zoster vaccination, prior to initiation. Assess onset, location, duration of pain, inflammation. Inspect appearance of affected joints for immobility, deformities.

INTERVENTION/EVALUATION

Monitor CBC, LFT periodically; lipid panel 12 wks after initiation and as indicated thereafter. Monitor for TB regardless of baseline PPD. Diligently monitor for infections (cough, fatigue, fever). If severe acute infection, opportunistic infection occurs, withhold treatment and initiate appropriate antimicrobial therapy. Monitor for symptoms of GI perforation (abdominal pain, fever, melena, hematemesis); DVT (leg or arm pain/swelling), CVA (aphasia, altered mental status, hemiplegia, vision loss, seizures); MI (arm/jaw pain, chest pain, diaphoresis, dyspnea), PE (chest pain, dyspnea, tachycardia), hepatotoxicity (bruising, jaundice, right upper abdominal pain, nausea, vomiting, weight loss), viral infection reactivation. Assess for therapeutic response: relief of pain, stiffness, swelling; increased joint mobility; reduced joint tenderness; improved grip strength.

PATIENT/FAMILY TEACHING

• Treatment may depress your immune system response and reduce your ability to fight infection. Report symptoms of infection such as body aches, chills, cough, fatigue, fever. Avoid those with active infection. • Expect routine tuberculosis screening. Report any travel plans to possible endemic areas. • Do not receive live vaccines. • Report liver problems (abdominal pain, bruising, clay-colored stool, dark or amber-colored urine, yellowing of the skin or eyes); symptoms of DVT (swelling, pain, hot feeling in the arms or legs; discoloration of extremity). • Life-threatening arterial blood clots may occur; report symptoms of heart attack (chest pain, difficulty breathing, jaw pain, nausea, pain that radiates to the arm, sweating), lung embolism (difficulty breathing, chest pain, rapid heart rate), stroke (confusion, difficulty speaking, one-sided weakness or paralysis, loss of vision). • Report severe or persistent abdominal pain, bloody stool, fever, vomiting; may indicate rupture in GI tract. • Treatment may cause reactivation of chronic infections, new cancers. • Use effective contraception to avoid pregnancy. Do not breastfeed.

U

ustekinumab

TOP 100

yoo-ste-**kin**-ue-mab
(Stelara)
Do not confuse Stelara with Aldara, or ustekinumab with inFLIXimab or riTUXimab.

◆CLASSIFICATION

PHARMACOTHERAPEUTIC: Interleukin-12, interleukin-23 inhibitor, monoclonal antibody. **CLINICAL:** Antipsoriasis agent.

USES

Treatment of adults, adolescents 6 yrs or older with moderate to severe plaque psoriasis who are candidates for systemic therapy or phototherapy. Treatment of adults with active psoriatic arthritis alone or in combination with methotrexate. Treatment of adults with moderate to severe active Crohn's disease. Treatment of adults with moderate to severe active ulcerative colitis.

PRECAUTIONS

Contraindications: Hypersensitivity to ustekinumab. **Cautions:** Prior malignancies (esp. skin cancer), pts who resided or traveled to endemic areas; conditions predisposing to infection (e.g., diabetes, renal failure, immunocompromised pts, open wounds), history of chronic opportunistic infections (esp. bacterial, invasive fungal, mycobacterial, protozoal, viral infections including herpes zoster, TB). Avoid use of live vaccines.

ACTION

Binds to and interferes with proinflammatory cytokines, interleukin-12, and interleukin-23, reducing these proinflammatory signalers. **Therapeutic Effect:** Shows clinical improvement of psoriasis, psoriatric arthritis.

PHARMACOKINETICS

Widely distributed. Degraded into small peptides and amino acids via catabolic pathways. Steady state reached in 28 wks. **Half-life:** 10–126 days.

⌛ LIFESPAN CONSIDERATIONS

Pregnancy/Lactation: Unknown if distributed in breast milk. **Children:** Safety and efficacy not established in pts younger than 6 yrs. **Elderly:** May have increased risk of infections.

INTERACTIONS

DRUG: May increase immunosuppressive effect of **inFLIXimab.** May decrease therapeutic effect; increase adverse effects of **vaccines (live), BCG (intravesical).** **HERBAL:** **Echinacea** may decrease therapeutic effect. **FOOD:** None known. **LAB VALUES:** May increase lymphocyte count.

AVAILABILITY (Rx)

Injection Solution, Intravenous: 130 mg/26 mL. **Injection Solution, SQ (Prefilled Syringes):** 45 mg/0.5 mL, 90 mg/mL.

ADMINISTRATION/HANDLING

IV

Reconstitution • Calculate the number of vials needed for dose based on pt's weight. • Withdraw and discard a volume from 250-mL 0.9% NaCl infusion bag equal to the volume of vials needed for dose. • Withdraw calculated dose from vial or vials and add to infusion bag to equal a final volume of 250 mL. • Visually inspect for particulate matter or discoloration. Do not use if solution is cloudy, discolored, or if visible particles are observed.

Rate of administration • Infuse over at least 60 min. Use an in-line, low-protein-binding filter (0.2 microns).

Storage • Refrigerate unused vials in original carton until time of use. • Protect from light. • Keep vials upright. • Diluted solution may be stored at room temperature for up to 4 hrs.

SQ

Preparation • Visually inspect for particulate matter or discoloration. Solution should appear clear and colorless to slightly yellow in color. • Solution may contain a few small translucent or white particles.

Administration • Insert needle subcutaneously into upper arm, outer thigh, or abdomen and inject solution. • Do not inject into areas of active skin disease or injury such as sunburns, skin rashes, inflammation, skin infections, or active psoriasis. • Do not administer IV or intramuscular. • Rotate injection sites.

Storage • Refrigerate prefilled syringes in original carton until time of use. • Protect from light. • Do not freeze or expose to heating sources. • Do not shake.

INDICATIONS/ROUTES/DOSAGE

Plaque Psoriasis

SQ: ADULTS, ELDERLY WEIGHING 100 KG OR LESS: Initially, 45 mg, then 45 mg 4 wks later, followed by 45 mg every 12 wks. **WEIGHING MORE THAN 100 KG:** Initially, 90 mg, then 90 mg 4 wks later, followed by 90 mg every 12 wks. **Note:** 45 mg also efficacious; however, 90 mg is recommended due to greater efficacy. **CHILDREN 6 YRS AND OLDER WEIGHING MORE THAN 100 KG:** Initially, 90 mg, repeat in 4 wks, then q12 wks. **WEIGHING 61–100 KG:** Initially, 45 mg, repeat in 4 wks, then q12 wks. **WEIGHING 60 KG OR LESS:** Initially, 0.75 mg/kg, repeat in 4 wks, then q12 wks.

Psoriatic Arthritis

SQ: ADULTS, ELDERLY: Initially, 45 mg repeated in 4 wks followed by 45 mg q12wks. **PTS WITH COEXISTENT MODERATE TO SEVERE PLAQUE PSORIASIS WEIGHING MORE THAN 100 KG:** Initially, 90 mg repeated in 4 wks, then 90 mg q12wks.

Crohn's Disease

IV infusion: ADULTS, ELDERLY: Initially, (as a single dose) 520 mg (greater than 85 kg); 390 mg (56–85 kg); 260 mg (up to 54 kg).

SQ: Maintenance: 90 mg q8wks beginning 8 wks following the IV induction dose.

Ulcerative Colitis

IV: ADULTS, ELDERLY WEIGHING MORE THAN 85 KG: Induction: 520 mg as single dose. **WEIGHING 56–85 KG:** 390 mg as single dose. **WEIGHING LESS THAN 55 KG:** 260 mg as single dose.

SQ: Maintenance: 90 mg q8wks (starting 8 wks after IV induction dose).

Dosage in Renal/Hepatic Impairment

No dose adjustment.

SIDE EFFECTS

Occasional (8%–4%): Nasopharyngitis, upper respiratory tract infection, headache. **Rare (3%–1%):** Fatigue, diarrhea, back pain, dizziness, pruritus, injection site erythema, myalgia, depression.

ADVERSE EFFECTS/TOXIC REACTIONS

May increase risk of acute infections; reactivation of latent infections. Serious invasive and opportunistic bacterial, mycobacterial, fungal, viral infections (anal abscess, appendicitis, cellulitis, cholecystitis, diverticulitis, gastroenteritis, listeria meningitis, listeriosis, ophthalmic herpes zoster, osteomyelitis, pneumonia, sepsis, TB, UTI, viral infections) requiring hospitalization were reported. May increase risk of new malignancies. Hypersensitivity reactions including angioedema, anaphylaxis were reported. Reversible posterior leukoencephalopathy syndrome (RPLS) may present as aphasia, altered mental status, paralysis, vision loss, weakness. Noninfectious pneumonias (interstitial/eosinophilic/cryptogenic-organizing pneumonia) were reported. Immunogenicity (auto-ustekinumab antibodies) reported in 12% of pts. Pts genetically deficient in IL-12/IL-23 are at an increased risk of disseminated infections from mycobacteria (non-tuberculosis, environmental mycobacterial), salmonella, BCG vaccines.

U

NURSING CONSIDERATIONS

BASELINE ASSESSMENT

Obtain pregnancy test in females of reproductive potential. Conduct dermatological exam; record characteristics of psoriatic lesions. Assess degree of abdominal pain, cramping; usual bowel movement patterns, stool characteristics in pts with UC. Evaluate for active TB and test for latent infection. An induration of 5 mm or greater with purified protein derivative (PPD) is considered a positive result when assessing for latent TB. Screen for active infection; history of chronic, opportunistic infections. Question history of prior malignancies. Consider completion of age-appropriate immunizations prior to initiation. BCG vaccines should not be given 1 yr prior to initiation or 1 yr after discontinuation.

INTERVENTION/EVALUATION

Obtain CBC if infection is suspected. Monitor for symptoms of TB (cough, fatigue, hemoptysis, nocturnal sweating, weight loss), including those who tested negative for latent TB infection. Monitor for infections (abdominal pain, cough, fatigue, fever). Interrupt or discontinue treatment if serious infection, opportunistic infection, or sepsis occurs. RPLS should be considered in pts with altered mental status, confusion, headache, seizures, visual disturbances. Assess skin for improvement of lesions in pts with psoriasis; decreased abdominal pain, cramping, diarrhea; increased appetite, weight gain in pts with UC.

PATIENT/FAMILY TEACHING

• Treatment may depress your immune system and reduce your ability to fight infection. Report symptoms of infection such as body aches, burning with urination, chills, cough, fatigue, fever; fungal infections. Avoid those with active infection. • Report travel plans to possible endemic areas. • Do not receive live vaccines, BCG vaccines. • Expect frequent TB screening. • Dormant or chronic viral, invasive fungal infections may become reactivated. • Nervous system changes including altered mental status, seizures, headache, blurry vision, high blood pressure, trouble speaking, one-sided weakness may indicate life-threatening brain dysfunction/swelling. • Treatment may cause new cancers. • Life-threatening allergic reactions (anaphylaxis, swelling of face, tongue, throat) must be reported immediately, regardless of the time the dose was administered.

valACYclovir

val-a-**sye**-kloe-veer
(Valtrex)
Do not confuse valACYclovir with acyclovir or valGANciclovir, or Valtrex with Keflex or Valcyte.

◆CLASSIFICATION

PHARMACOTHERAPEUTIC: Nucleoside analogue DNA polymerase inhibitor. **CLINICAL:** Antiviral.

USES

Treatment of herpes zoster (shingles) in immunocompetent pts. Treatment of initial and recurrent genital herpes in immunocompetent adults. Prevention of recurrent genital herpes and reduction of transmission of genital herpes in immunocompetent pts. Suppression of genital herpes in HIV-infected pts. Treatment of herpes labialis (cold sores). Treatment of chickenpox in immunocompetent children. **OFF-LABEL:** Prophylaxis and treatment of cancer-related HSV, VZV.

PRECAUTIONS

Contraindications: Hypersensitivity to acyclovir, valACYclovir. **Cautions:** Renal impairment, concurrent use of nephrotoxic agents, elderly pts.

ACTION

Converted to acyclovir by intestinal/hepatic metabolism. Competes for viral DNA polymerase; inhibits incorporation into viral DNA. **Therapeutic Effect:** Inhibits DNA synthesis and viral replication.

PHARMACOKINETICS

Widely distributed to tissues, body fluids (including CSF). Protein binding: 13%–18%. Rapidly converted by hydrolysis to active compound acyclovir. Primarily excreted in urine. Removed by hemodialysis. **Half-life: Acyclovir:** 2.5–3.3 hrs (increased in renal impairment).

⌛ LIFESPAN CONSIDERATIONS

Pregnancy/Lactation: May cross placenta. May be distributed in breast milk. **Children:** Safety and efficacy not established in children younger than 2 yrs (chickenpox); younger than 12 yrs (cold sores). **Elderly:** Age-related renal impairment may require dosage adjustment.

INTERACTIONS

DRUG: **Nephrotoxic medications (e.g., foscarnet, gentamicin)** may increase risk of nephrotoxicity, renal impairment. May increase concentration/effect of **tiZANidine**. **HERBAL:** None significant. **FOOD:** None known. **LAB VALUES:** None significant.

AVAILABILITY (Rx)

Tablets: 500 mg, 1,000 mg.

ADMINISTRATION/HANDLING

PO

• Give without regard to food. • If GI upset occurs, give with meals.

INDICATIONS/ROUTES/DOSAGE

Herpes Zoster (shingles)

PO: ADULTS, ELDERLY: (Immunocompetent): 1 g 3 times/day for 7 days. **(Immunocompromised):** 1 g 3 times/day for 7–14 days.

Herpes Simplex (Cold sores)

PO: ADULTS, ELDERLY: (Immunocompetent [Primary]): 2 g twice daily for 1 day (separate by 12 hrs). **(Suppressive):** 500 mg or 1 g once daily. **(Immunocompetent [Primary]):** 1 g 2 times/day for 5–10 days. **(Suppressive):** 500 mg twice daily.

Initial Episode of Genital Herpes

PO: ADULTS, ELDERLY: (Immunocompetent): 1 g twice daily for 7–10 days. **(Immunocompromised):** 1 g 2 times/day for 5–10 days.

Recurrent Episodes of Genital Herpes

PO: ADULTS, ELDERLY: (Immunocompetent): 500 mg twice daily for 3 days or 1 g twice daily for 5 days. **(Immunocompromised):** 1 g 2 times/day for 5–10 days.

V

Suppressive Therapy of Genital Herpes

PO: ADULTS, ELDERLY: **(Immunocompetent):** 500 mg twice daily or 1 g once daily (500 mg once daily in pts with 9 or fewer recurrences/yr). **(Immunocompromised):** 500 mg 2 times/day.

Chickenpox

PO: CHILDREN 2–17 YRS: **(Immunocompetent):** 20 mg/kg/dose 3 times/day for 5 days. **Maximum:** 1 g 3 times/day.

Dosage in Renal Impairment

Dosage and frequency are modified based on creatinine clearance. **HD:** Give dose postdialysis.

Cold Sores/Herpes Zoster

Creatinine Clearance	Herpes Zoster	Cold Sores
30–49 mL/min	1 g q12h	1 g q12h × 2 doses
10–29 mL/min	1 g q24h	500 mg q12h × 2 doses
Less than 10 mL/min	500 mg q24h	500 mg as single dose

Genital Herpes

Creatinine Clearance	Initial Episode	Recurrent Episode	Suppressive Therapy
10–29 mL/min	1 g q24h	500 mg q24h	500 mg q24–48h
Less than 10 mL/min	500 mg q24h	500 mg q24h	500 mg q24–48h

Dosage in Hepatic Impairment

No dose adjustment.

SIDE EFFECTS

Frequent: **Herpes zoster (17%–10%):** Nausea, headache. **Genital herpes (17%):** Headache. Occasional: **Herpes zoster (7%–3%):** Vomiting, diarrhea, constipation (50 yrs and older), asthenia, dizziness (50 yrs and older). **Genital herpes (8%–3%):** Nausea, diarrhea, dizziness. Rare: **Herpes zoster (3%–1%):** Abdominal pain, anorexia. **Genital herpes (3%–1%):** Asthenia, abdominal pain.

ADVERSE EFFECTS/TOXIC REACTIONS

Neutropenia, thrombocytopenia, renal failure occur rarely.

NURSING CONSIDERATIONS

BASELINE ASSESSMENT

Tissue cultures for herpes zoster, herpes simplex should be obtained before giving first dose (therapy may proceed before results are known). Assess medical history, esp. HIV infection, bone marrow or renal transplantation, renal/hepatic impairment. Assess characteristics, frequency of lesions.

INTERVENTION/EVALUATION

Monitor CBC, LFT, renal function, urinalysis. Evaluate cutaneous lesions. Provide analgesics, comfort measures for herpes zoster (esp. exhausting to elderly). Encourage fluids.

PATIENT/FAMILY TEACHING

• Drink adequate fluids. • Do not touch lesions with fingers to avoid spreading infection to new site. • **Genital herpes:** Continue therapy for full length of treatment. • Space doses evenly. • Avoid sexual intercourse during duration of lesions to prevent infecting partner. • ValACYclovir does not cure herpes. • Report if lesions recur or do not improve. • Pap smears should be done at least annually due to increased risk of cervical cancer in women with genital herpes. • Initiate treatment at first sign of recurrent episode of genital herpes or herpes zoster (early treatment within first 24–48 hrs is imperative for therapeutic results).

V

valGANciclovir

val-gan-**sye**-kloe-veer
(Apo-ValGANciclovir ✦, Valcyte)

■ **BLACK BOX ALERT** ■ May adversely affect spermatogenesis, fertility. Risk for granulocytopenia, anemia, thrombocytopenia.

Do not confuse Valcyte with Valium or Valtrex, or valGANciclovir with valACYclovir.

◆CLASSIFICATION

PHARMACOTHERAPEUTIC: Synthetic nucleoside. **CLINICAL:** Antiviral.

USES

Adults: Treatment of cytomegalovirus (CMV) retinitis in AIDS. Prevention of CMV disease in high-risk renal, cardiac, renal-pancreas transplant pts. **Children:** Prevention of CMV disease in high-risk renal (4 mos to 16 yrs) and cardiac transplant pts (1 mo to 16 yrs).

PRECAUTIONS

Contraindications: Hypersensitivity to valGANciclovir, ganciclovir. **Cautions:** Use extreme caution in children due to long-term carcinogenicity, reproductive toxicity. Renal impairment, concurrent nephrotoxic medications, preexisting bone marrow suppression or cytopenias, baseline cytopenias, elderly (at greater risk for renal impairment).

ACTION

Inhibits binding of deoxyguanosine triphosphate to DNA polymerase. **Therapeutic Effect:** Inhibits viral DNA synthesis.

PHARMACOKINETICS

Widely distributed including CSF, ocular tissue. Slowly metabolized intracellularly. Primarily excreted in urine. Removed by hemodialysis. **Half-life: Ganciclovir:** 4 hrs (increased in renal impairment).

LIFESPAN CONSIDERATIONS

Pregnancy/Lactation: Avoid pregnancy; may cause fetal harm. Females of reproductive potential should use effective contraception during treatment. Breastfeeding not recommended during treatment and for at least 3 days after discontinuation. May impair fertility in both females and males. **Children:** Safety and efficacy not established in pts younger than 1 month. **Elderly:** Age-related renal impairment may require dosage adjustment.

INTERACTIONS

DRUG: Bone marrow depressants may increase myelosuppression. May increase concentration/effect of **didanosine, mycophenolate. Probenecid** may decrease renal clearance, increase concentration. May increase nephrotoxic effect of **amphotericin**, **cycloSPORINE**. May increase adverse effects of **zidovudine**. **Zidovudine (AZT)** may increase risk of hematologic toxicity. **HERBAL:** None significant. **FOOD:** None known. **LAB VALUES:** May decrease creatinine clearance, platelet count, neutrophils, Hgb, Hct. May increase serum creatinine.

AVAILABILITY (Rx)

Powder for Oral Solution: 50 mg/mL (100 mL).

Tablets: 450 mg.

ADMINISTRATION/HANDLING

PO

• Take with meals. • Do not break, crush, dissolve, or divide tablets; give whole (potential carcinogen). • Avoid contact with skin. • Wash skin with soap, water if contact occurs. • Store oral suspension in refrigerator. Discard after 49 days.

INDICATIONS/ROUTES/DOSAGE

Note: Do not use if absolute neutrophil count (ANC) less than 500 cells/mm^3, platelets less than 25,000 cells/mm^3, or Hgb less than 8 g/dL.

Cytomegalovirus (CMV) Retinitis (AIDS-related)

PO: ADULTS: Induction: 900 mg (two 450-mg tablets) twice daily for 14–21 days. **Maintenance:** 900 mg once daily.

Prevention of CMV After Transplant

PO: ADULTS, ELDERLY: 900 mg once daily (duration dependent on type of transplant, donor, and recipient serostatus). **CHILDREN 1 MO–16 YRS:** Once daily based on body surface area (BSA) and CrCl using formula: (Dose = 7 × BSA × CrCl). **Maximum:** 900 mg/day.

Dosage in Renal Impairment

Dosage and frequency are modified based on creatinine clearance.

Creatinine Clearance	Induction Dosage	Maintenance Dosage
60 mL/min or higher	900 mg twice daily	900 mg once daily
40–59 mL/min	450 mg twice daily	450 mg once daily
25–39 mL/min	450 mg once daily	450 mg every 2 days
10–24 mL/min	450 mg every 2 days	450 mg twice wkly

Dosage in Hepatic Impairment

No dose adjustment.

SIDE EFFECTS

Frequent (16%–9%): Diarrhea, neutropenia, headache. **Occasional (8%–3%):** Nausea. **Rare (less than 3%):** Insomnia, paresthesia, vomiting, abdominal pain, fever.

ADVERSE EFFECTS/TOXIC REACTIONS

Hematologic toxicity, including severe neutropenia (most common), anemia, thrombocytopenia, leukopenia, aplastic anemia, pancytopenia, bone marrow suppression may occur. Retinal detachment occurs rarely. Overdose may result in renal toxicity.

NURSING CONSIDERATIONS

BASELINE ASSESSMENT

Obtain CBC, renal function test; pregnancy test in females of reproductive potential. Receive full medication history and screen for interactions.

INTERVENTION/EVALUATION

Monitor CBC for myelosuppression. Obtain ophthalmic exam q4–6wks during treatment. Monitor for change of vision (may indicate retinal detachment). Ensure adequate hydration (minimum of 1,500 mL/24 hrs). Monitor I&Os.

PATIENT/FAMILY TEACHING

• Treatment may depress your immune system response and reduce your ability to fight infection. Report symptoms of infection such as body aches, chills, cough, fatigue, fever. Avoid those with active infection. • Report symptoms of bone marrow depression (e.g., bruising, fatigue, fever, shortness of breath, weight loss; bleeding easily, bloody urine or stool). • Therapy only provides viral suppression and is not a cure. • Expect frequent eye exams if being treated for CMV retinitis. Report change of vision. • Use effective contraception to avoid pregnancy. Do not breastfeed.

valproic acid

val-**pro**-ick **as**-id

(Apo-Divalproex ✱, Depakote, Depakote ER, Depakote Sprinkle)

■ **BLACK BOX ALERT** ■ Embryo, fetal neural tube defects (spina bifida) have occurred. Life-threatening pancreatitis, complete hepatic failure have occurred.

Do not confuse Depakene with Depakote.

◆CLASSIFICATION

PHARMACOTHERAPEUTIC: Histone deacetylase inhibitor. **CLINICAL:** Anticonvulsant, antimanic, antimigraine.

V

USES

Monotherapy/adjunctive therapy of complex partial seizures, simple and complex absence seizures. Adjunctive therapy of multiple seizures including absence seizures. **Additional uses for Depakote, Depakote ER:** Treatment of manic episodes with bipolar disorder, prophylaxis of migraine headaches. **OFF-LABEL:** Refractory status epilepticus, diabetic neuropathy. Mood stabilizer for behaviors in dementia.

PRECAUTIONS

Contraindications: Hypersensitivity to valproic acid. Active hepatic disease, urea cycle disorders, known mitochondrial disorders caused by mutation in mitochondrial DNA polymerase gamma (POLG). Children under 2 yrs of age suspected of having POLG-related disorder. Migraine prevention in pregnant women. **Cautions:** Children younger than 2 yrs. Hepatic impairment, pts at risk for hepatotoxicity (e.g., cirrhosis, concomitant use of hepatotoxic medications), pts at high risk for suicide (e.g., history of ideation and behavior; depression), elderly, therapy requiring multiple anticonvulsants; congenital metabolic disorders, severe seizure disorders (accompanied by mental retardation), organic brain disease.

ACTION

Directly increases concentration of inhibitory neurotransmitter gamma-aminobutyric acid (GABA). **Therapeutic Effect:** Decreases seizure activity, stabilizes mood, prevents migraine headache.

PHARMACOKINETICS

Widely distributed. Protein binding: 80%–90%. Metabolized in liver. Primarily excreted in urine. Not removed by hemodialysis. **Half-life:** 9–16 hrs (may be increased in hepatic impairment, elderly pts, children younger than 18 mos).

LIFESPAN CONSIDERATIONS

Pregnancy/Lactation: Drug crosses placenta; is distributed in breast milk. **Children:** Increased risk of hepatotoxicity in pts younger than 2 yrs. **Elderly:** May have increase incidence of insomnia.

INTERACTIONS

DRUG: **Cholestyramine, rifAMPin** may decrease concentration/effect. May increase adverse effects of **lamoTRIgine, LORazepam**. **HERBAL:** None significant. **FOOD:** None known. **LAB VALUES:** May increase serum LDH, bilirubin, ALT, AST. May cause false interpretation of urine ketone test. **Therapeutic serum level:** 50–100 mcg/mL; **toxic serum level:** greater than 100 mcg/mL.

AVAILABILITY (Rx)

Capsules: 250 mg. **Capsules, Sprinkle:** ***(Depakote Sprinkle):*** 125 mg. **Injection Solution:** 100 mg/mL. **Oral Solution:** 250 mg/5 mL.

Tablets, Delayed-Release: ***(Depakote):*** 125 mg, 250 mg, 500 mg. **Tablets, Extended-Release:** ***(Depakote ER):*** 250 mg, 500 mg.

ADMINISTRATION/HANDLING

IV

Reconstitution • Dilute each single dose with at least 50 mL D_5W, 0.9% NaCl, or lactated Ringer's.

Rate of administration • Infuse over 60 min at rate of 20 mg/min or less. • Alternatively, single doses of up to 45 mg/kg given over 5–10 min (1.5–6 mg/kg/min).

Storage • Store vials at room temperature. • Diluted solutions stable for 24 hrs. • Discard unused portion.

PO

• Give without regard to food. Do not mix oral solution with carbonated beverages (may cause mouth/throat irritation). • May sprinkle capsule (Depakote Sprinkle) contents on applesauce and give immediately (do not chew sprinkle beads). • Give delayed-release/extended-release tablets whole. Do not crush, break, open delayed-release capsule (Stavzor). • Regular-release and delayed-release formulations usually given in 2–4 divided doses/day. Extended-release formulation (Depakote ER) usually given once daily.

IV COMPATIBILITIES

Cefepime, cefTAZidime.

INDICATIONS/ROUTES/DOSAGE

Seizures

PO: ADULTS, ELDERLY, CHILDREN 10 YRS AND OLDER: Initially, 10–15 mg/kg/day. May increase by 5–10 mg/kg/day at wkly intervals up to 60 mg/kg/day. **Usual adult dosage:** 1,000–2,500 mg/day.

IV: ADULTS, ELDERLY, CHILDREN: Same daily dose divided q6h.

Manic Episodes

PO: ADULTS, ELDERLY: Initially, 500–750 mg/day. May increase by 250–500 mg q1–3days to reach desired clinical effect and therapeutic serum concentration. **Maximum:** 60 mg/kg/day.

Prevention of Migraine Headaches

PO: ***(Extended-Release [Depakote ER]):*** **ADULTS, ELDERLY:** Initially, 500 mg once daily. May increase up to 1,000 mg once daily.

PO: ***(Delayed-Release [Depakote]):*** **ADULTS, ELDERLY, CHILDREN 16 YRS AND OLDER:** Initially, 250 mg twice daily. May increase up to 1,000 mg/day in 2 divided doses.

Dosage in Renal Impairment

No dose adjustment.

Dosage in Hepatic Impairment

Mild to moderate impairment: Not recommended. **Severe impairment:** Contraindicated.

SIDE EFFECTS

Frequent: Epilepsy: Abdominal pain, irregular menses, diarrhea, transient alopecia, indigestion, nausea, vomiting, tremors, fluctuations in body weight. **Mania (22%–19%):** Nausea, drowsiness. **Occasional: Epilepsy:** Constipation, dizziness, drowsiness, headache, skin rash, unusual excitement, restlessness. **Mania (12%–6%):** Asthenia, abdominal pain, dyspepsia, rash. **Rare: Epilepsy:** Mood changes, diplopia, nystagmus, spots before eyes, unusual bleeding/bruising.

ADVERSE EFFECTS/TOXIC REACTIONS

Thrombocytopenia-associated bleeding, hyperammonemia, hypothermia were reported. Fatal hepatic failure may occur (particularly within the first 6 mos of treatment) and may be preceded by anorexia, facial edema, lethargy malaise, weakness, vomiting. Life-threatening pancreatitis may occur, which may include hemorrhage with rapid deterioration from initial symptoms to death. May increase risk of suicidal ideation and behavior. Drug reaction with eosinophilia and systemic symptoms (DRESS), also known as multiorgan hypersensitivity, has been reported. DRESS may present with facial swelling, eosinophilia, fever, lymphadenopathy, rash, which may be associated with other organ systems, such as hepatitis, hematologic abnormalities, myocarditis, nephritis.

NURSING CONSIDERATIONS

BASELINE ASSESSMENT

Obtain CBC, LFT. Question history of suicidal ideation and behavior. **Anticonvulsant:** Review history of seizure disorder (intensity, frequency, duration, level of consciousness). Initiate safety measures, quiet dark environment. **Antimanic:** Assess behavior, appearance, emotional status, response to environment, speech pattern, thought content. **Antimigraine:** Question characteristics of migraine headaches (onset, location, duration, possible precipitating symptoms).

INTERVENTION/EVALUATION

Monitor CBC, LFT, serum ammonia. Monitor for symptoms of DRESS. Diligently assess for suicidal ideation and behavior; new onset or worsening of anxiety, depression, mood disorder. **Anticonvulsant:** Observe frequently for recurrence of seizure activity. Assess skin for ecchymoses, petechiae. Monitor for clinical improvement (decrease in intensity/frequency of seizures). **Antimanic:** Assess for therapeutic response (interest in surroundings, increased ability to concentrate, relaxed facial expression). **Antimigraine:** Evaluate for relief of migraine headache and resulting photophobia, phonophobia, nausea, vomiting. **Therapeutic serum level:** 50–100 mcg/mL; **toxic serum level:** greater than 100 mcg/mL.

PATIENT/ FAMILY TEACHING

• Do not abruptly discontinue medication after long-term use (may precipitate seizures). • Strict maintenance of drug therapy is essential for seizure control. • Avoid tasks that require alertness, motor skills until response to drug is established. • Drowsiness usually disappears during continued therapy. • Avoid alcohol. • Report liver problems such as nausea, vomiting, lethargy, altered mental status, weakness, loss of appetite, abdominal pain, yellowing of skin, unusual bruising/bleeding. • Seek immediate medical attention if thoughts of suicide, new onset or worsening of anxiety, depression, or changes in mood occur.

valsartan

val-**sar**-tan
(Apo-Valsartan ✱, Diovan)

■ BLACK BOX ALERT ■ May cause fetal injury, mortality. Discontinue as soon as possible once pregnancy is detected.

Do not confuse Diovan with Zyban, or valsartan with losartan or Valstar.

FIXED-COMBINATION(S)

Diovan HCT: valsartan/hydroCHLOROthiazide (a diuretic): 80 mg/12.5 mg, 160 mg/12.5 mg, 160 mg/25 mg, 320 mg/12.5 mg, 320 mg/25 mg. **Byvalson:** valsartan/nebivolol (a beta blocker): 80 mg/5 mg. **Exforge:** valsartan/amLODIPine (a calcium channel blocker): 160 mg/5 mg, 160 mg/10 mg, 320 mg/5 mg, 320 mg/10 mg. **Exforge HCT:** valsartan/amLODIPine (a calcium channel blocker)/hydroCHLOROthiazide (a diuretic): 160 mg/5 mg/12.5 mg, 160 mg/5 mg/25 mg, 160 mg/10 mg/12.5 mg, 160 mg/10 mg/25 mg, 320 mg/10 mg/25 mg. **Valturna:** valsartan/aliskiren (a direct renin inhibitor): 160 mg/150 mg, 320 mg/300 mg.

◆CLASSIFICATION

PHARMACOTHERAPEUTIC: Angiotensin II receptor antagonist. **CLINICAL:** Antihypertensive.

V

USES

Treatment of hypertension alone or in combination with other antihypertensives. Treatment of HF (NYHA Class II–IV). Reduce mortality in high-risk pts (left ventricular failure/dysfunction) following MI.

PRECAUTIONS

Contraindications: Hypersensitivity to valsartan. Concomitant use with aliskiren in pts with diabetes. **Cautions:** Concurrent use of potassium-sparing diuretics or potassium supplements, mild to severe hepatic impairment, unstented bilateral/unilateral renal artery stenosis, renal impairment, significant aortic/mitral stenosis, elderly.

ACTION

Directly antagonizes angiotensin II receptors. Blocks vasoconstrictor, aldosterone-secreting effects of angiotensin II, inhibiting binding of angiotensin II to AT_1 receptors. **Therapeutic Effect:** Produces vasodilation, decreases peripheral resistance, decreases B/P.

PHARMACOKINETICS

Widely distributed. Food decreases peak plasma concentration. Protein binding: 95%. Metabolized in liver. Excreted in feces (83%), urine (13%). Unknown if removed by hemodialysis. **Half-life:** 6 hrs.

LIFESPAN CONSIDERATIONS

Pregnancy/Lactation: May cause fetal harm. Unknown if distributed in breast milk. **Children:** Safety and efficacy not established. **Elderly:** No age-related precautions noted.

V

INTERACTIONS

DRUG: **Potassium-sparing drugs (e.g., spironolactone, triamterene), potassium supplements** may increase serum potassium. **Aliskiren** may increase hyperkalemic effect. May increase adverse/toxicity of **ACE inhibitors (e.g., benazepril, lisinopril)**. **HERBAL:** **Herbals with hypertensive properties (e.g., licorice, yohimbe) or hypotensive properties (e.g., garlic, ginger, ginkgo biloba)** may alter effects. **FOOD:** None known. **LAB VALUES:** May increase serum bilirubin, ALT, AST, BUN, creatinine, potassium. May decrease Hgb, Hct, WBC.

AVAILABILITY (Rx)

Tablets: 40 mg, 80 mg, 160 mg, 320 mg.

ADMINISTRATION/HANDLING

PO

- Give without regard to food.

INDICATIONS/ROUTES/DOSAGE

Hypertension

PO: ADULTS, ELDERLY: Initially, 80–160 mg/day in pts who are not volume depleted. Titrate based on response. **Maximum:** 320 mg/day. **CHILDREN 6–16 YRS:** Initially, 1.3 mg/kg once daily (**Maximum:** 40 mg). May increase up to 2.7 mg/kg once daily (**Maximum:** 160 mg/day).

HF

PO: ADULTS, ELDERLY: Initially, 20–40 mg twice daily. Titrate to 80 mg twice daily. May increase up to 160 mg twice daily. **Maximum:** 320 mg/day.

Post-MI, Left Ventricular Dysfunction

PO: ADULTS, ELDERLY: May initiate 12 hrs or longer following MI. Initially, 20 mg twice daily. May increase within 7 days to 40 mg twice daily. May further increase up to target dose of 160 mg twice daily.

Dosage in Renal Impairment

CrCl greater than 30 mL/min: No dose adjustment. **CrCl 30 mL/min or less: ADULTS:** Safety/efficacy not established. **CHILDREN 6–16 YRS:** Not recommended.

Dosage in Hepatic Impairment

No dose adjustment.

SIDE EFFECTS

Rare (2%–1%): Insomnia, fatigue, heartburn, abdominal pain, dizziness, headache, diarrhea, nausea, vomiting, arthralgia, edema.

ADVERSE EFFECTS/TOXIC REACTIONS

Overdosage may manifest as hypotension, tachycardia. Bradycardia occurs less often. Viral infection, upper respiratory tract infection (cough, pharyngitis, sinusitis, rhinitis) occur rarely.

NURSING CONSIDERATIONS

BASELINE ASSESSMENT

Obtain renal function test; pregnancy in females of reproductive potential. Obtain B/P, heart rate immediately before each dose, in addition to regular monitoring (be alert to fluctuations). Assess medication history (esp. diuretic). Question for history of hepatic/renal impairment, renal artery stenosis, severe HF.

INTERVENTION/EVALUATION

Maintain hydration (offer fluids frequently). Assess for evidence of upper respiratory infection. Monitor serum electrolytes, renal function, B/P, pulse. Observe for symptoms of hypotension.

PATIENT/ FAMILY TEACHING

• Use effective contraception to avoid pregnancy. • Report heart problems (difficulty breathing, palpitations, swelling of extremities), symptoms of low blood pressure (cold, clammy skin; dizziness, fast heart rate, sweating), kidney problems (decreased urine output, flank pain, darkened urine).

vancomycin

van-koe-**mye**-sin
(Vancocin)
Do not confuse vancomycin with clindamycin, gentamicin, tobramycin, or Vibramycin.

◆CLASSIFICATION

PHARMACOTHERAPEUTIC: Tricyclic glycopeptide antibiotic. **CLINICAL:** Antibiotic.

USES

Systemic: Treatment of infections caused by staphylococcal, streptococcal spp. bacteria. **PO:** Treatment of *C. difficile*–associated diarrhea and treatment of enterocolitis caused by *S. aureus* (including MRSA). **OFF-LABEL:** Treatment of infections caused by gram-positive organisms in pts with serious allergies to beta-lactam antibiotics; treatment of beta-lactam–resistant gram-positive infections. Surgical prophylaxis, treatment of prosthetic joint infection.

PRECAUTIONS

Contraindications: Hypersensitivity to vancomycin. **Cautions:** Renal impairment, elderly, dehydration, pts at risk for extravasation (e.g., peripheral IV catheters, midline catheters, elderly, poor peripheral vasculature), concomitant use of other ototoxic, nephrotoxic medications.

ACTION

Binds to bacterial cell walls, altering cell membrane permeability, inhibiting RNA synthesis. **Therapeutic Effect:** Bactericidal.

PHARMACOKINETICS

PO: Poorly absorbed from GI tract. Primarily excreted in feces. **Parenteral:** Widely distributed (except CSF). Protein binding: 10%–50%. Primarily excreted unchanged in urine. Not removed by hemodialysis. **Half-life:** 4–11 hrs (increased in renal impairment).

⌛ LIFESPAN CONSIDERATIONS

Pregnancy/Lactation: Drug crosses placenta, distributed in breast milk following IV administration. **Children:** Close monitoring of serum levels recommended in premature neonates, young infants. **Elderly:** Age-related renal impairment may increase risk of ototoxicity, nephrotoxicity; dosage adjustment recommended.

INTERACTIONS

DRUG: May increase concentration/effects of **aminoglycosides (e.g., amikacin, gentamicin)**. **Bile acid sequestrants (e.g., cholestyramine)** may decrease therapeutic effect (oral vancomycin). **HERBAL:** None significant. **FOOD:** None known. **LAB VALUES:** May increase BUN. **Therapeutic peak serum level:** (Not routinely obtained) 20–40 mcg/mL; **therapeutic trough serum level:** 10–20 mcg/mL. **Toxic peak serum level:** greater than 40 mcg/mL; **toxic trough serum level:** greater than 20 mcg/mL.

AVAILABILITY (Rx)

Capsules: 125 mg, 250 mg. **Infusion, *Premix:*** 500 mg/100 mL, 750 mg/150 mL, 1 g/200 mL. **Injection, Powder for Reconstitution:** 500 mg, 750 mg, 1 g. **Oral Solution:** 25 mg/mL, 50 mg/mL.

ADMINISTRATION/HANDLING

IV

◀ALERT▶ Give by intermittent IV infusion (piggyback) or continuous IV infusion. Do not give IV push (may result in exaggerated hypotension or red man syndrome). Due to high risk of extravasation, consider infusion via central venous catheter.

Reconstitution • For intermittent IV infusion (piggyback), reconstitute each 500-mg vial with 10 mL Sterile Water for Injection (20 mL for 1-g vial) to provide concentration of 50 mg/mL. • Further dilute with D_5W or 0.9% NaCl to final concentration not to exceed 5 mg/mL.

Rate of administration • Administer over 60 min or longer (30 min for each 500 mg recommended). • Monitor B/P closely during IV infusion.

Storage • Reconstituted vials are stable for 14 days at room temperature or if refrigerated. • Diluted solutions are stable for 14 days if refrigerated or 7 days at room temperature. • Discard if precipitate forms.

PO

• May give with food. • Powder for injection may be reconstituted and diluted for oral administration.

IV INCOMPATIBILITIES

Albumin, amphotericin B complex (Abelcet, AmBisome, Amphotec), aztreonam (Azactam), ceFAZolin (Ancef), cefotaxime (Claforan), cefOXitin (Mefoxin), cefTAZidime (Fortaz), cefTRIAXone (Rocephin), cefuroxime (Zinacef), foscarnet (Foscavir), heparin, nafcillin (Nafcil), piperacillin, and tazobactam (Zosyn).

IV COMPATIBILITIES

Amiodarone (Cordarone), calcium gluconate, dexmedetomidine (Precedex), dilTIAZem (Cardizem), HYDROmorphone (Dilaudid), insulin, LORazepam (Ativan), magnesium sulfate, midazolam (Versed), morphine, niCARdipine (Cardene), potassium chloride, propofol (Diprivan).

INDICATIONS/ROUTES/DOSAGE

Note: Initial IV dosing in nonobese pts is based on actual body weight. Subsequent dosing is adjusted based on serum trough concentrations and renal function. Pt-specific dosing may be necessary to determine dose and interval (e.g., morbid obesity, critical illness, unstable renal function).

Usual Parenteral Dosage

IV: ADULTS, ELDERLY: 15–20 mg/kg/dose (rounded to nearest 250 mg) q8–12h. Dosage requires adjustment in renal impairment. **Usual Maximum Dose:** 2 g. **ADOLESCENTS, CHILDREN, INFANTS:** 45–60 mg/kg/day divided q6–8h. Dose- and frequency-based serum concentrations. **NEONATES:** Loading dose of 20 mg/kg; then, 10–20 mg/kg/dose q12–48h.

Staphylococcal Enterocolitis, Antibiotic–Associated Pseudomembranous Colitis Caused by *Clostridium Difficile*

PO: ADULTS, ELDERLY: 125–500 mg 4 times/day for 10–14 days. **CHILDREN:** 40 mg/kg/day in 3–4 divided doses for 7–10 days. **Maximum:** 2 g/day.

Dosage in Renal Impairment
After loading dose, subsequent dosages and frequency are modified based on creatinine clearance, severity of infection, and serum concentration of drug.

Dosage in Hepatic Impairment
No dose adjustment.

SIDE EFFECTS

Frequent: PO: Bitter/unpleasant taste, nausea, vomiting, mouth irritation (with oral solution). **Rare: Parenteral:** Phlebitis, thrombophlebitis, pain at peripheral IV site, dizziness, vertigo, tinnitus, chills, fever, rash, necrosis with extravasation. **PO:** Rash.

ADVERSE EFFECTS/TOXIC REACTIONS

Nephrotoxicity (acute kidney injury, acute tubular necrosis, renal failure), ototoxicity (temporary or permanent hearing loss) may occur. Too-rapid infusion may cause red man syndrome, a common adverse reaction characterized by pruritus, urticaria, erythema, angioedema, tachycardia, hypotension, myalgia, maculopapular rash (usually appears on face, neck, upper torso). Cardiovascular toxicity (cardiac depression, arrest) occurs rarely. Onset usually occurs within 30 min of start of infusion, resolves within hrs following infusion. May result from too-rapid rate of infusion. Extravasation may cause tissue necrosis. Infusions via peripheral IV or midline access may cause thrombophlebitis.

NURSING CONSIDERATIONS

BASELINE ASSESSMENT

Avoid other ototoxic, nephrotoxic medications if possible. Obtain culture, sensitivity test before giving first dose (therapy may begin before results are known). Consider placement of central venous line/PICC line.

INTERVENTION/EVALUATION

Monitor serum renal function tests, I&O. Assess skin for rash. Check hearing acuity, balance. Monitor B/P carefully during infusion. Monitor for red man syndrome. Evaluate IV site for phlebitis (heat, pain, red streaking over vein). Obtain vancomycin peak/trough level as ordered by physician or pharmacist. **Therapeutic serum level: peak:** 20–40 mcg/mL; **trough:** 10–20 mcg/mL. **Toxic serum level: peak:** greater than 40 mcg/mL; **trough:** greater than 20 mcg/mL.

PATIENT/ FAMILY TEACHING

• Continue therapy for full length of treatment. • Doses should be evenly spaced. • Report ringing in ears, hearing loss, changes in urinary frequency or consistency. • Lab tests are important part of total therapy.

vandetanib

van-**det**-a-nib
(Caprelsa)

■ **BLACK BOX ALERT** ■ Can prolong QT interval (torsades de pointes and sudden cardiac death reported). Do not use in pts with hypokalemia, hypocalcemia, hypomagnesemia, congenital long QT syndrome. Electrolyte imbalances must be corrected prior to initiating therapy. If medication that prolongs QT interval is needed, more frequent ECG monitoring is recommended. ECGs should be obtained during wks 2–4 and wks 8–12 after starting therapy and 3 mos thereafter. Any dose reduction or interruption related to QT prolongation greater than 2 wks must have frequent ECG monitoring as noted above. Only certified prescribers and pharmacies with a restricted distribution program are able to prescribe and dispense.

◆CLASSIFICATION

PHARMACOTHERAPEUTIC: Epidermal growth factor receptor (EGFR) inhibitor. Vascular endothelial growth factor (VEGF) inhibitor. Tyrosine kinase inhibitor. **CLINICAL:** Antineoplastic.

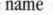

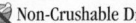

V

USES

Treatment of symptomatic or progressive medullary thyroid cancer in pts with unresectable locally advanced or metastatic disease.

PRECAUTIONS

Contraindications: Hypersensitivity to vandetanib. Congenital long QT syndrome. **Cautions:** Baseline cytopenias, pts at risk for QTc interval prolongation (congenital long QT syndrome, HF, medications that prolong QTc interval, hypokalemia, hypomagnesemia), hypothyroidism, cerebrovascular disease, moderate to severe renal/hepatic impairment, hypertension, uncompensated HF, history of torsades de pointes.

ACTION

Inhibits tyrosine kinases including epidermal growth factor (EGF) and vascular endothelial growth factor (VEGF). Blocks intracellular signaling, angiogenesis, and cellular proliferation. **Therapeutic Effect:** Inhibits thyroid tumor cell growth and survival.

PHARMACOKINETICS

Widely distributed. Peak concentration: 4–10 hrs. Metabolized in liver. Protein binding: 90%. Excreted in feces (44%), urine (25%). **Half-life:** 19 days.

LIFESPAN CONSIDERATIONS

Pregnancy/Lactation: Avoid pregnancy; may cause fetal harm. Females of reproductive potential must use effective contraception during treatment and for at least 4 mos after treatment. Unknown if distributed in breast milk. **Children:** Safety and efficacy not established. **Elderly:** No age-related precautions noted.

INTERACTIONS

DRUG: **QT interval–prolonging medications (e.g., amiodarone, azithromycin, ciprofloxacin, haloperidol, methadone, sotalol)** may increase risk of QTc interval prolongation. **Strong CYP3A4 inducers (e.g., carBAMazepine, phenytoin, rifAMPin)** may decrease concentration/effect. **HERBAL:** **St. John's wort** may decrease concentration/effect. **FOOD:** **Grapefruit products** may increase risk of torsades de pointes, myelotoxicity. **LAB VALUES:** May decrease WBC, Hgb, neutrophils. May increase serum bilirubin, ALT, AST, creatinine; urine protein. May alter serum calcium, glucose, magnesium, potassium.

AVAILABILITY (Rx)

Tablets: 100 mg, 300 mg.

ADMINISTRATION/HANDLING

PO

• Give without regard to food. • Do not crush. • May disperse in 2 oz of noncarbonated water and stir for 10 min until tablet is evenly dispersed (will not completely dissolve). Administer dispersion immediately. Rinse residue in glass with 4 oz water and administer. Can be given via feeding tube. • Direct contact of crushed tablets with skin or mucous membranes should be strictly avoided. If contact occurs, wash thoroughly.

Storage • Contact pharmacy to properly discard out-of-date tablets.

INDICATIONS/ROUTES/DOSAGE

Thyroid Cancer

Note: Do not begin unless QT_c interval is less than 450 msec. Maintain serum calcium and magnesium within normal limits. Maintain serum potassium at least 4 mEq/L or greater.

PO: ADULTS, ELDERLY: 300 mg once daily. Continue until disease progression or unacceptable toxicity.

Dosage Adjustment for QT Prolongation or Toxicity

Interrupt therapy until resolved or improved, then restart at 100–200 mg once daily.

Dosage in Renal Impairment

CrCl less than 50 mL/min: 200 mg once daily. Closely monitor QT interval.

Dosage in Hepatic Impairment

Mild impairment: No dose adjustment. **Moderate to severe impairment:** Not recommended.

SIDE EFFECTS

Frequent (57%–21%): Diarrhea/colitis, rash, dermatitis acneiform/acne, nausea, headache, fatigue, anorexia, abdominal pain. **Occasional (15%–10%):** Dry skin, vomiting, asthenia, photosensitivity, insomnia, nasopharyngitis, dyspepsia, cough, pruritus, weight decrease, depression.

ADVERSE EFFECTS/TOXIC REACTIONS

Prolonged QT interval resulting in torsades de pointes, ventricular arrhythmias, sudden cardiac death have been reported. Frequent diarrhea may result in electrolyte imbalances. Severe skin reactions, including Stevens-Johnson syndrome, have been reported. Interstitial lung disease (ILD) or pneumonitis reported (may result in respiratory-related death). Consider ILD in pts with hypoxia, pleural effusion, cough, dyspnea. Ischemic cerebrovascular events have been reported. Life threatening events including hypertensive crisis, reversible posterior leukoencephalopathy syndrome (RPLS) have been noted. Adverse reactions resulting in death included respiratory failure/arrest, aspiration pneumonia, cardiac failure, sepsis, GI bleeding.

NURSING CONSIDERATIONS

BASELINE ASSESSMENT

Obtain CBC with differential, serum chemistries, magnesium, ionized calcium, TSH, UA, ECG, vital signs. Obtain negative urine pregnancy before therapy. Question for history of congenital long QT syndrome, HF, arrhythmias, hepatic/renal impairment, seizures, CVA, hemorrhagic events, HTN. Obtain full medication history including contraception. Perform full head-to-toe exam including visual acuity, thorough skin assessment.

INTERVENTION/EVALUATION

Monitor CBC, serum electrolytes. Obtain ECG during wks 2–4, wks 8–12, then every 3 mos thereafter. Obtain ECG for palpitations, chest pain, hypokalemia, hyperkalemia, hypocalcemia, bradycardia, ventricular arrhythmias, syncope. Report any respiratory changes including dyspnea, cough (may indicate ILD). Reversible posterior leukoencephalopathy syndrome should be considered in pts with seizures, headache, visual disturbances, confusion, altered mental status. Ophthalmologic exams including slit lamp recommended in pts with visual disturbances.

PATIENT/FAMILY TEACHING

• Blood levels, ECGs will be routinely monitored. • Use effective contraception to avoid pregnancy. • Changes in mental status, seizures, headache, blurry vision, trouble speaking, one-sided weakness may indicate stroke, high blood pressure crisis, or life-threatening brain swelling. Immediately report any newly prescribed medications. • Do not take herbal products. • Limit exposure to sunlight. • Report any yellowing of skin or eyes, abdominal pain, bruising, black/tarry stools, dark urine, decreased urine output, skin changes. • Report palpitations, chest pain, shortness of breath, dizziness, fainting (may indicate arrhythmia).

varenicline

var-**en**-i-kleen
(Champix ✤, Chantix)

BLACK BOX ALERT Risk of psychiatric symptoms and suicidal behavior. Agitation, hostility, depressed mood have been reported.

◆CLASSIFICATION

PHARMACOTHERAPEUTIC: Selective partial nicotine agonist. **CLINICAL:** Smoking deterrent.

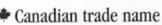

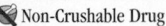

V

USES

Aid to smoking-cessation treatment.

PRECAUTIONS

Contraindications: Hypersensitivity to varenicline. **Cautions:** Renal impairment, history of suicidal ideation or preexisting psychiatric illness, bipolar disorder, depression, schizophrenia, pts at risk for seizures (e.g., head trauma, seizure disorder).

ACTION

Prevents nicotine stimulation of mesolimbic dopamine system associated with nicotine addiction. **Therapeutic Effect:** Decreases desire to smoke.

PHARMACOKINETICS

Widely distributed. Absorption unaffected by food, time-of-day dosing. Peak plasma concentration: 3–4 hrs. Steady state reached within 4 days. Protein binding: 20%. Minimal metabolism. Removed by hemodialysis. Primarily excreted unchanged in urine. **Half-life:** 24 hrs.

⌛ LIFESPAN CONSIDERATIONS

Pregnancy/Lactation: Unknown if distributed in breast milk. **Children:** Not recommended. **Elderly:** Age-related renal impairment may require dosage adjustment.

INTERACTIONS

DRUG: Histamine H_2 receptor antagonists (e.g., famotidine, ranitidine) may increase concentration/effect. May increase concentration/effect of **nicotine** **HERBAL:** None significant. **FOOD:** None known. **LAB VALUES:** None significant.

AVAILABILITY (Rx)

Tablets, Film-Coated: 0.5 mg, 1 mg.

ADMINISTRATION/HANDLING

• Give after meal and with full glass of water. • Do not break, crush, dissolve, or divide film-coated tablets.

INDICATIONS/ROUTES/DOSAGE

◀ALERT▶ Therapy should start 1 wk before stopping smoking.

Smoking Deterrent

PO: ADULTS, ELDERLY: Days 1–3: 0.5 mg once daily. **Days 4–7:** 0.5 mg twice daily. **Day 8–end of treatment:** 1 mg twice daily. Therapy should last for total of 12 wks. Pts who have successfully stopped smoking at the end of 12 wks should continue with an additional 12 wks of treatment to increase likelihood of long-term abstinence.

Dosage in Renal Impairment

CrCl less than 30 mL/min: 0.5 mg once daily. **Maximum:** 0.5 mg twice daily.

End-stage renal disease, undergoing hemodialysis: Maximum: 0.5 mg once daily.

Dosage in Hepatic Impairment

No dose adjustment.

SIDE EFFECTS

Frequent (30%–13%): Nausea, insomnia, headache, abnormal dreams. **Occasional (8%–5%):** Constipation, abdominal discomfort, fatigue, dry mouth, flatulence, altered taste, dyspepsia, vomiting, anxiety, depression, irritability. **Rare (3%–1%):** Drowsiness, rash, increased appetite, lethargy, nightmares, gastroesophageal reflux disease, rhinorrhea, agitation, mood swings.

ADVERSE EFFECTS/TOXIC REACTIONS

Abrupt withdrawal may cause irritability, sleep disturbances in 3% of pts. Hypertension, angina pectoris, arrhythmia, bradycardia, coronary artery disease, gingivitis, anemia, lymphadenopathy occur rarely. May cause bizarre behavior, suicidal ideation.

NURSING CONSIDERATIONS

BASELINE ASSESSMENT

Screen, evaluate for coronary heart disease (history of MI, angina pectoris), cardiac arrhythmias, suicidal ideation. Assess smoking pack/yr history.

INTERVENTION/EVALUATION

Discontinue use if cardiovascular symptoms occur or worsen. Monitor for psychiatric symptoms (changes in behavior, mood, level of interest, appearance). Assess for cravings, noncompliance with cessation.

PATIENT/FAMILY TEACHING

• Initiate treatment 1 wk before quit-smoking date. • Take with food and with full glass of water. • With twice-daily dosing, take 1 tablet in morning, 1 in evening. • Report persistent nausea, insomnia. • Seek immediate medical attention if thoughts of suicide, new onset or worsening of anxiety, depression, or changes in mood occur.

vasopressin

vay-soe-**pres**-in
(Pressyn ✦, Pressyn AR ✦, Vasostrict)
Do not confuse Pitressin with Pitocin.

◆CLASSIFICATION

PHARMACOTHERAPEUTIC: Posterior pituitary hormone. **CLINICAL:** Vasopressor, antidiuretic hormone analogue.

USES

Vasoconstriction: To increase blood pressure in adults with vasodilatory shock who remain hypotensive despite fluids and catecholamines. **OFF-LABEL:** Adjunct in treatment of acute massive GI hemorrhage or esophageal varices.

PRECAUTIONS

Contraindications: Hypersensitivity to vasopressin. **Cautions:** Seizure disorder, migraine, asthma, vascular disease, renal/cardiac disease, goiter (with cardiac complications), arteriosclerosis, nephritis, elderly.

ACTION

Stimulates a family of arginine vasopressin (AVP) receptors. **Therapeutic Effect:** Increases systemic vascular resistance and mean arterial BP; increases water permeability at renal tubules, causing a decreased urine volume and increased osmolality; causes smooth muscle contraction in GI tract.

PHARMACOKINETICS

Route	Onset	Peak	Duration
IV	N/A	N/A	0.5–1 hr
IM, SQ	1–2 hrs	N/A	2–8 hrs

Widely distributed. Metabolized in liver, kidney. Primarily excreted in urine. **Half-life:** 10–20 min.

LIFESPAN CONSIDERATIONS

Pregnancy/Lactation: Caution in giving to breastfeeding women. **Children/Elderly:** Caution due to risk of water intoxication/hyponatremia.

INTERACTIONS

DRUG: None significant. **HERBAL:** None significant. **FOOD:** None known. **LAB VALUES:** None significant.

AVAILABILITY (Rx)

Injection Solution: 20 units/mL.

ADMINISTRATION/HANDLING

IV

Reconstitution • Dilute in D_5W or 0.9% NaCl to concentration of 0.1–1 unit/mL (usual concentration: 100 units/500 mL D_5W).
Rate of administration • Give as IV infusion.
Storage • Store at room temperature.

IM, SQ

• Give with 1–2 glasses of water to reduce side effects.

IV INCOMPATIBILITIES

Furosemide (Lasix), phenytoin (Dilantin).

V

IV COMPATIBILITIES

Amiodarone, argatroban, dilTIAZem (Cardizem), DOBUTamine (Dobutrex), DOPamine (Intropin), heparin, insulin, milrinone (Primacor), nitroglycerin, norepinephrine (Levophed), pantoprazole (Protonix), phenylephrine (Neo-Synephrine).

INDICATIONS/ROUTES/DOSAGE

Vasodilatory Shock

IV infusion: ADULTS, ELDERLY: Initially, 0.03 units/min. Titrate by 0.005 units/min at 10–15-min intervals. **Maximum:** 0.1 units/min.

Dosage in Renal/Hepatic Impairment

No dose adjustment.

SIDE EFFECTS

Frequent: Pain at injection site (with vasopressin tannate). **Occasional:** Abdominal cramps, nausea, vomiting, diarrhea, dizziness, diaphoresis, pale skin, circumoral pallor, tremors, headache, eructation, flatulence. **Rare:** Chest pain, confusion, allergic reaction (rash, urticaria, pruritus, wheezing, difficulty breathing, facial/peripheral edema), sterile abscess (with vasopressin tannate).

ADVERSE EFFECTS/TOXIC REACTIONS

Anaphylaxis, MI, water intoxication have occurred. Elderly, very young are at higher risk for water intoxication. May increase risk of ischemia (cardiac, mesenteric, limb, skin). Extravasation may cause tissue necrosis.

V

NURSING CONSIDERATIONS

BASELINE ASSESSMENT

Establish baselines for weight, B/P, pulse, serum electrolytes, urine specific gravity.

INTERVENTION/EVALUATION

Monitor I&O closely, restrict intake as necessary to prevent water intoxication. Weigh daily if indicated. Check B/P, pulse frequently. Monitor serum electrolytes, urine specific gravity. Evaluate injection site for erythema, pain, abscess. Report side effects to physician for dose reduction. Be alert for early signs of water intoxication (drowsiness, listlessness, headache, seizures). Observe for evidence of GI bleeding. Withhold medication, report immediately any chest pain, allergic symptoms.

PATIENT/FAMILY TEACHING

• Promptly report headache, chest pain, shortness of breath, other symptoms. • Stress importance of I&O. • Avoid alcohol. • Report confusion, seizure activity.

vedolizumab

ve-doe-**liz**-ue-mab
(Entyvio)
Do not confuse vedolizumab with certolizumab, eculizumab, natalizumab, omalizumab, tocilizumab.

◆CLASSIFICATION

PHARMACOTHERAPEUTIC: Selective adhesion molecule inhibitor. Monoclonal antibody. **CLINICAL:** GI agent.

USES

Treatment of adult pts with moderately to severely active ulcerative colitis (UC) who have had an inadequate response with, lost response to, or were intolerant to a tumor necrosis factor (TNF) blocker or immunomodulator; or had an inadequate response with, were intolerant to, or demonstrated dependence on corticosteroids. Treatment of adult pts with moderately to severely active Crohn's disease (CD) who have had an inadequate response with, lost response to, or were intolerant to a TNF blocker or immunomodulator; or had an inadequate response with, were intolerant to, or demonstrated dependence on corticosteroids.

PRECAUTIONS

Contraindications: Hypersensitivity to vedolizumab. **Cautions:** Hepatic impairment, pts who resided or traveled to endemic areas; conditions predisposing to infection (e.g., diabetes, renal failure, immunocompromised pts, open wounds), history of chronic opportunistic infections (esp. bacterial, invasive fungal, mycobacterial, protozoal, viral infections including herpes zoster, TB), prior malignancies. Preexisting or recent-onset CNS demyelinating disorders including multiple sclerosis.

ACTION

Binds to T-lymphocyte integrin receptors and blocks the interaction with mucosal addressin cell adhesion molecule-1 (MAdCAM-1). Inhibits migration and homing of memory T-lymphocytes into inflamed GI tissue. **Therapeutic Effect:** Reduces chronic inflammation of colon.

PHARMACOKINETICS

Metabolism not specified. Excretion not specified. **Half-life:** 25 days.

LIFESPAN CONSIDERATIONS

Pregnancy/Lactation: Unknown if distributed in breast milk. Use caution when administering to nursing women. **Children:** Safety and efficacy not established. **Elderly:** No age-related precautions noted.

INTERACTIONS

DRUG: **Anti-TNF agents (e.g., adalimumab, certolizumab, etanercept, infliximab)** may increase adverse effects. May decrease the therapeutic effect; increase adverse effects of **vaccines (live)**. **HERBAL:** **Echinacea** may decrease the therapeutic effect. **FOOD:** None known. **LAB VALUES:** May increase serum ALT, AST, bilirubin.

AVAILABILITY (Rx)

Lyophilized Powder for Injection: 300 mg.

ADMINISTRATION/HANDLING

IV

Infusion guidelines • Do not administer IV push or bolus. • Reconstitute with Sterile Water for Injection and subsequently dilute with 0.9% NaCl only. • After infusion completed, flush IV line with 30 mL of 0.9% NaCl.

Reconstitution • Reconstitute with 4.8 mL Sterile Water for Injection. Direct stream toward glass wall to avoid excessive foaming. • Gently swirl contents for at least 15 sec until completely dissolved. • Do not shake or agitate. • Allow solution to sit at room temperature for up to 20 min to allow remaining foam to settle and powder to dissolve. If not fully dissolved after 20 min, allow additional 10 min for dissolution. Do not use if product is not dissolved within 30 min. • Visually inspect for particulate matter and discoloration. Do not use if discolored or if particulate matter is observed. • Prior to withdrawing solution, invert vial 3 times to ensure mixing. • Withdraw 5 mL and further dilute in 250 mL 0.9% NaCl bag. • Infuse immediately.

Rate of administration • Infuse over 30 min.

Storage • Reconstituted solution should appear clear to opalescent, colorless to light brownish yellow and free of particles. • May refrigerate diluted solution for up to 4 hrs.

INDICATIONS/ROUTES/DOSAGE

Ulcerative Colitis and Crohn's Disease

IV: ADULTS, ELDERLY: 300 mg once at wk 0, wk 2, and wk 6, then every 8 wks thereafter. Discontinue in pts who do not show evidence of therapeutic benefit by wk 14.

Dosage in Renal Impairment

Use caution.

V

Dosage in Hepatic Impairment

Use caution. Discontinue for jaundice or signs/symptoms of hepatic injury.

SIDE EFFECTS

Occasional (13%–4%): Nasopharyngitis, headache, arthralgia, nausea, pyrexia, upper respiratory tract infection, fatigue, cough, bronchitis, influenza, back pain. **Rare (3%):** Rash, pruritus, sinusitis, oropharyngeal pain, extremity pain.

ADVERSE EFFECTS/TOXIC REACTIONS

Infusion-related reactions, including anaphylaxis, characterized by bronchospasm, dyspnea, flushing, hypotension, laryngeal edema, nausea, pyrexia, tachycardia, wheezing, vomiting, reported in less than 1% of pts. May increase risk of severe infections such as anal abscess, cytomegaloviral colitis, giardiasis, *Listeria* meningitis, *Salmonella* sepsis, TB, UTI, which may lead to fatal sepsis. PML (weakness, paralysis, vision loss, aphasia, cognition impairment) has occurred rarely; however, immunocompromised pts are at increased risk for development. Hepatotoxicity with serum ALT, AST greater than 3 times upper limit of normal reported in less than 2% of pts. Malignancies including B-cell lymphoma, breast cancer, colon cancer, lung cancer of primary neuroendocrine carcinoma, lung neoplasm, malignant hepatic neoplasm, melanoma, renal cancer, squamous cell carcinoma, transitional cell carcinoma occur rarely. Immunogenicity (anti-vedolizumab antibodies) occurred in 4%–13% of pts.

V

NURSING CONSIDERATIONS

BASELINE ASSESSMENT

Obtain CBC, LFT; pregnancy test in females of reproductive potential. Screen for active infection; history of chronic, opportunistic infections. Question history of prior malignancies. Consider completion of age-appropriate immunizations prior to initiation. Evaluate for active TB and test for latent infection prior to and during treatment. An induration of 5 mm or greater with tuberculin skin test should be considered a positive result when assessing for latent TB. Antifungal therapy should be considered for those who reside in or travel to regions where mycoses are endemic. Have supplemental oxygen, anaphylaxis kit readily available. Assess degree of abdominal pain, cramping; usual bowel movement patterns, stool characteristics.

INTERVENTION/EVALUATION

Monitor LFT. Obtain CBC if infection is suspected. Monitor for symptoms of TB (cough, fatigue, hemoptysis, nocturnal sweating, weight loss), including those who tested negative for latent TB infection. Monitor for infections (abdominal pain, cough, fatigue, fever). Interrupt or discontinue treatment if serious infection, opportunistic infection, or sepsis occurs. Monitor for hypersensitivity reaction. Infusion-related reactions generally occur within 2 hrs after infusion. Consider administration of antihistamine, antipyretic, and/or corticosteroid if mild to moderate hypersensitivity reaction occurs. If anaphylaxis occurs, provide immediate resuscitation support. Monitor for new onset or worsening of neurologic symptoms, esp. in pts with CNS disorders; may indicate PML.

PATIENT/FAMILY TEACHING

• Treatment may depress your immune system and reduce your ability to fight infection. Report symptoms of infection such as body aches, burning with urination, chills, cough, fatigue, fever; fungal infections. Avoid those with active infection. • Report travel plans to possible endemic areas. • Do not receive live vaccines. • Expect frequent TB screening. • Dormant or chronic viral, invasive fungal infections may become reactivated. • Treatment may cause new cancers. • Infusion may cause severe allergic reactions such as face/tongue swelling, hives, itching, low blood pressure, trouble breathing, or, in some cases, anaphylaxis. • Do not breastfeed. • Abdominal pain, bruising, clay-colored stools, dark-amber urine, fatigue, loss of appetite, yellowing of skin or eyes may indicate liver problem. • Paralysis, vision changes, impaired speech, altered mental status may indicate life-threatening neurologic event called progressive multifocal leukoencephalopathy (PML).

vemurafenib

vem-ue-**raf**-e-nib
(Zelboraf)

CLASSIFICATION

PHARMACOTHERAPEUTIC: BRAF kinase inhibitor. **CLINICAL:** Antineoplastic.

USES

Treatment of unresectable or metastatic melanoma with a BRAF V600E mutation as detected by FDA-approved test. Treatment of Erdheim-Chester disease (ECD) in pts with a BRAF V600E mutation.

PRECAUTIONS

Contraindications: Hypersensitivity to vemurafenib. **Cautions:** Hepatic impairment, pts at risk for QTc interval prolongation (congenital long QT syndrome, HF, medications that prolong QTc interval, hypokalemia, hypomagnesemia), elderly, prior radiation therapy.

ACTION

Inhibits kinase activity of certain mutated forms of BRAF. **Therapeutic Effect:** Blocks tumor cell proliferation in melanoma with the mutation.

PHARMACOKINETICS

Widely distributed. Protein binding: 99%. Minimally metabolized in liver. Primarily excreted in feces (94%). **Half-life:** 57 hrs. Range: 30–120 hrs.

LIFESPAN CONSIDERATIONS

Pregnancy/Lactation: Avoid pregnancy; may cause fetal harm. Females of reproductive potential must use effective contraception during treatment and for at least 2 mos after discontinuation. Unknown if distributed in breast milk. **Children:** Safety and efficacy not established. **Elderly:** May have increased risk of adverse reactions, side effects.

INTERACTIONS

DRUG: **Strong CYP3A4 inhibitors (e.g., clarithromycin, ketoconazole)** may increase concentration/effect. **Strong CYP3A4 inducers (e.g., carBAMazepine, phenytoin, rifAMPin)** may decrease concentration/effect. May increase concentration/effect of **digoxin. QT interval–prolonging medications (e.g., amiodarone, azithromycin, ciprofloxacin, haloperidol, methadone, sotalol)** may increase risk of QTc interval prolongation. May increase bleeding effect with **warfarin.** **HERBAL:** **St. John's wort** may decrease concentration/effect. **FOOD:** None known. **LAB VALUES:** May increase serum alkaline phosphatase, ALT, AST, gamma-glutamyl transferase (GGT), bilirubin.

AVAILABILITY (Rx)

Film-Coated Tablets: 240 mg.

ADMINISTRATION/HANDLING

PO

• Give without regard to food in the morning and evening, approx. 12 hrs apart with a full glass of water. • Administer tablets whole; do not break, crush, divide, or dissolve.

INDICATIONS/ROUTES/DOSAGE

Note: Management of adverse drug reactions may require dose reduction, treatment interruption, or discontinuation.

ECD, Melanoma

PO: ADULTS, ELDERLY: 960 mg twice daily (in morning and evening about 12

V

hrs apart). Continue until disease progression or unacceptable toxicity.

Dosage Modification

Based on Common Terminology Criteria for Adverse Events (CTCAE). **Grade 1 or Grade 2 (tolerable) toxicity:** No dose adjustment. **Grade 2 (intolerable) or Grade 3 toxicity: First occurrence:** Interrupt treatment until toxicity returns to Grade 0 or 1, then resume at 720 mg twice daily. **Second occurrence:** Interrupt treatment, then resume at 480 mg twice daily. **Third occurrence:** Discontinue. **Grade 4 toxicity: First occurrence:** Interrupt treatment, then resume at 480 mg twice daily. **Second occurrence:** Discontinue.

Dosage in Renal/Hepatic Impairment

Mild to moderate impairment: No dose adjustment. **Severe impairment:** Use with caution.

SIDE EFFECTS

Frequent (53%–33%): Arthralgia, alopecia, fatigue, rash, nausea. **Occasional (28%–11%):** Diarrhea, hyperkeratosis, headache, pruritus, pyrexia, dry skin, extremity pain, anorexia, vomiting, peripheral edema, erythema, dysgeusia, myalgia, constipation, asthenia. **Rare (8%–5%):** Maculopapular rash, actinic keratosis, musculoskeletal pain, back pain, cough, papular rash.

ADVERSE EFFECTS/TOXIC REACTIONS

Cutaneous squamous cell carcinoma (cuSCC) and keratoacanthomas reported in 24% of pts. Pts at increased risk of cuSCC include elderly pts, pts with prior skin cancer, chronic sun exposure. Hypersensitivity reactions including erythema, hypotension, anaphylaxis reported. Mild to severe photosensitivity was reported. Serious dermatologic reactions include Stevens-Johnson syndrome, toxic epidermal necrolysis. Ophthalmologic reactions including uveitis reported. Hepatotoxicity may lead to discontinuation.

NURSING CONSIDERATIONS

BASELINE ASSESSMENT

Obtain serum chemistries, renal function test, serum magnesium, ionized calcium, ECG, PT/INR if taking warfarin. Confirm presence of BRAF V600E mutation. Review history for previous radiation therapy. Assess skin for moles, lesions, papilloma, and perform full dermatologic exam. Obtain baseline ophthalmologic exam, visual acuity. Assess medication history for QT-prolonging drugs. Obtain negative urine pregnancy before initiating treatment. Offer emotional support.

INTERVENTION/EVALUATION

Monitor ECG 15 days after initiation, then monthly for first 3 mos, then q3mos thereafter. Routinely assess skin during treatment and for 6 mos after discontinuation. Immediately report any new skin lesions. Obtain ECG for palpitations, chest pain, hypokalemia, hyperkalemia, hypocalcemia, bradycardia, ventricular arrhythmias, syncope. Monitor PT/INR while pt is on warfarin. Pruritus, difficulty breathing, erythema, hypotension may indicate anaphylaxis.

PATIENT/FAMILY TEACHING

• Treatment may cause new cancers. • Use effective contraception to avoid pregnancy. • Avoid sunlight exposure. • Report any skin changes, including new warts, sores, reddish bumps that bleed or do not heal, change in mole size or color. • Report yellowing of skin or eyes, abdominal pain, bruising, black/tarry stools, dark urine, decreased urine output, skin changes. • Report palpitations, chest pain, shortness of breath, dizziness, fainting (may indicate arrhythmia).

venetoclax

ven-**et**-oh-klax
(Venclexta)
Do not confuse venetoclax or Venclexta with Venelex.

◆ **CLASSIFICATION**

PHARMACOTHERAPEUTIC: B-cell lymphoma 2 (BCL-2) inhibitor. **CLINICAL:** Antineoplastic.

USES

Monotherapy or in combination with rituximab for treatment of pts with chronic lymphocytic leukemia (CLL) or small lymphocytic leukemia (SLL) with or without 17p deletion who have received at least one prior therapy. Treatment of newly diagnosed acute myeloid leukemia (AML) (in combination with azacitidine, decitabine, or low-dose cytarabine) in pts 75 yrs of age or older, or with comorbidities precluding use of intensive induction chemotherapy.

PRECAUTIONS

Contraindications: Hypersensitivity to venetoclax. Concomitant use of strong CYP3A inhibitors at initiation and during ramp-up phase. **Cautions:** Baseline cytopenias, concomitant use of moderate CYP3A inhibitors, P-gp inhibitors; conditions predisposing to infection (e.g., diabetes, renal failure, immunocompromised pts, open wounds), hepatic/renal impairment, electrolyte imbalance; history of gout; pts at high risk for tumor lysis syndrome (high tumor burden).

ACTION

Binds to and selectively inhibits B-cell lymphoma-2 protein and displaces proapoptotic proteins, restoring process of apoptosis. **Therapeutic Effect:** Inhibits tumor cell growth and metastasis.

PHARMACOKINETICS

Widely distributed. Metabolized in liver. Protein binding: highly bound (unspecified). Peak plasma concentration: 5–8 hrs. Excreted in feces (greater than 99%). **Half-life:** 26 hrs.

LIFESPAN CONSIDERATIONS

Pregnancy/Lactation: Avoid pregnancy; may cause fetal harm/malformations. Females and males with female partners of reproductive potential should use effective contraception during treatment and for at least 30 days after discontinuation. Unknown if distributed in breast milk. Breastfeeding not recommended. May impair fertility in males. **Children:** Safety and efficacy not established. **Elderly:** No age-related precautions noted.

INTERACTIONS

DRUG: **Strong CYP3A inhibitors (e.g., clarithromycin, ketoconazole), moderate CYP3A inhibitors (e.g., dilTIAZem, fluconazole, verapamil), P-gp inhibitors (e.g., cycloSPORINE, ranolazine, ticagrelor)** may increase concentration/effect. **Strong CYP3A inducers (e.g., carBAMazepine, phenytoin, rifAMPin)** may decrease concentration/effect. May increase concentration/effect of **digoxin**. May decrease the therapeutic effect; increase adverse effects of **vaccines (live)**. **HERBAL:** **Bitter orange** may increase concentration/effect. **FOOD:** **Grapefruit products, Seville oranges, starfruit** may increase concentration/effect. Low-fat meals, high-fat meals increase exposure/concentration. **LAB VALUES:** May decrease Hgb, Hct, neutrophils, platelets, RBCs; serum calcium, potassium. Tumor lysis syndrome may result in elevated serum phosphate, potassium, uric acid.

AVAILABILITY (Rx)

Tablets: 10 mg, 50 mg, 100 mg.

ADMINISTRATION/HANDLING

PO

• Give with food and water at same time each day. • Administer tablets whole; do not cut, crush, or divide. • If a dose is missed by no more than 8 hrs, administer as soon as possible. If dose is missed by more than 8 hrs or if vomiting occurs after dosing, skip dose and administer the next dose on schedule.

INDICATIONS/ROUTES/DOSAGE

CLL

PO: ADULTS, ELDERLY: Week 1: 20 mg once daily for 7 days. **Week 2:** 50 mg once daily for 7 days. **Week 3:** 100 mg once daily for 7 days. **Week 4:** 200 mg once daily for 7 days. **Week 5 and thereafter:** 400 mg once daily. Continue until disease progression or unacceptable toxicity. **In combination with rituximab: Week 5 and thereafter:** 400 mg once daily. Continue until disease progression or unacceptable toxicity for up to 24 mos from day 1 (cycle 1) of rituximab. Begin rituximab after receiving venetoclax at 400 mg once daily for 7 days. **In combination with obinutuzumab**: Obinutuzumab begins on day 1 of cycle 1. Begin venetoclax on day 22 of cycle 1 (based on 5-wk ramp-up schedule). Ramp-up is completed at end of cycle 2. **Cycle 3 (day 1 and beyond):** 400 mg once daily until end of cycle 12. Each cycle is 28 days.

AML

PO: ADULTS 75 YRS OR OLDER: Day 1: 100 mg once daily. **Day 2:** 200 mg once daily. **Day 3:** 400 mg once daily. **In combination with azaCITIDine or decitabine: Day 4 and beyond:** 400 mg once daily. Continue until disease progression or unacceptable toxicity. **In combination with low-dose cytarabine: Day 4 and beyond:** 600 mg once daily. Continue until disease progression or unacceptable toxicity.

Dose Modification

Based on Common Terminology Criteria for Adverse Events (CTCAE). For pts with dose interruption greater than 1 wk during 5-wk ramp-up phase or greater than 2 wks at 400 mg daily dose, reassess risk of tumor lysis syndrome to determine if reinitiation with a reduced dose is needed. Consider discontinuation in pts who require reduced dosage of less than 100 mg for more than 2 wks.

Dose Reduction Schedule

Note: During ramp-up phase, continue reduced dose for 1 wk before increasing dose. **Dose interruption at 400 mg:** Resume at 300 mg. **Dose interruption at 300 mg:** Resume at 200 mg. **Dose interruption at 200 mg:** Resume at 100 mg. **Dose interruption at 100 mg:** Resume at 50 mg. **Dose interruption at 50 mg:** Resume at 20 mg. **Dose interruption at 20 mg:** Resume at 10 mg.

Tumor Lysis Syndrome

Any occurrence of blood chemistry abnormalities: Withhold next dose, then resume at same dose if resolved within 24–48 hrs of last dose. If not resolved within 48 hrs, resume at reduced dose.

Any event of tumor lysis syndrome: Resume at reduced dose once resolved.

Grade 3 or 4 Nonhematologic Toxicity

First occurrence: Withhold treatment until resolved to Grade 1 or baseline, then resume at same dose. **Second and subsequent occurrences:** Withhold treatment until resolved, then follow dose reduction schedule (or reduce dose at prescriber's discretion).

Hematologic Toxicity

First occurrence of Grade 3 or 4 neutropenia with infection or fever; Grade 4 hematologic toxicity (except lymphopenia): Withhold treatment until resolved to Grade 1 or baseline, then resume at same dose. **Second and subsequent occurrences:** Withhold treatment until resolved, then follow dose reduction schedule (or reduce dose at prescriber's discretion).

Concomitant Use CYP3A Inhibitors, P-gp Inhibitors

Strong CYP3A inhibitors: Avoid inhibitor or reduce venetoclax dose by at least 75%. **Moderate CYP3A inhibitors or P-gp Inhibitors:** Avoid inhibitor or reduce venetoclax dose by at least 50%.

Dosage in Renal/Hepatic Impairment

Mild to moderate impairment: No dose adjustment. **Severe impairment:** Not specified; use caution.

SIDE EFFECTS

Frequent (35%–14%): Diarrhea, nausea, fatigue, pyrexia, vomiting, headache, constipation. **Occasional (13%–10%):** Cough, peripheral edema, back pain.

ADVERSE EFFECTS/TOXIC REACTIONS

Myelosuppression (anemia, neutropenia, thrombocytopenia) is an expected response to therapy. Grade 3 or 4 neutropenia reported in 41% of pts. Pts with high tumor burden, renal impairment, concomitant use of strong or moderate CYP3A inhibitors, P-gp inhibitors may experience life-threatening tumor lysis syndrome, which mainly occurs during the 5-wk ramp-up phase and as early as 6–8 hrs after dose (hospitalization may be necessary). Tumor lysis syndrome may cause renal failure requiring emergent dialysis. Other reactions may include upper respiratory tract infection, pneumonia, autoimmune hemolytic anemia.

NURSING CONSIDERATIONS

BASELINE ASSESSMENT

Obtain ANC, CBC, BMP, renal function test; serum phosphate, calcium; vital signs prior to initiation and periodically thereafter. Obtain pregnancy test in female pts of reproductive potential. Question history of hepatic/renal impairment, gout. Assess all pts for high risk of tumor lysis syndrome and provide adequate hydration and antihyperuricemics (according to manufacturer guidelines) prior to first dose. Conduct tumor burden assessments including blood chemistries, radiologic testing (e.g., CT scan). Correct electrolyte imbalances prior to initiation. Receive full medication history (esp. CYP3A inhibitors, P-gp inhibitors, drugs with narrow therapeutic index). Screen for active infection. Offer emotional support.

INTERVENTION/EVALUATION

Monitor ANC, CBC for myelosuppression. Diligently monitor for tumor lysis syndrome (acute renal failure, electrolyte imbalance, cardiac arrhythmias, seizures). Monitor for infection and provide appropriate antimicrobial therapy if indicated. To reduce risk of neutropenia-associated infection, consider administration of granulocyte-colony stimulating factor (e.g., filgrastim). Monitor for toxicities if discontinuation of CYP3A inhibitors, P-gp inhibitors is unavoidable. Monitor I&O. Assess hydration status.

PATIENT/FAMILY TEACHING

• Treatment may depress your immune system and reduce your ability to fight infection. Report symptoms of infection such as body aches, chills, cough, fatigue, fever. Avoid those with active infection. • Therapy may cause tumor lysis syndrome (a condition caused by the rapid breakdown of cancer cells), which can cause kidney failure and may lead to death. Report decreased urination, amber-colored urine, confusion, difficulty breathing, fatigue, fever, muscle or joint pain, palpitations, seizures, vomiting. • Drink at least 6–8 glasses of water every day. • Use effective contraception to avoid pregnancy. Do not breastfeed. • Avoid grapefruit products, herbal supplements. • Do not take newly prescribed medications unless approved by prescriber who originally started therapy. • Do not receive live vaccines.

venlafaxine

ven-la-**fax**-een
(Effexor XR)

BLACK BOX ALERT Increased risk of suicidal ideation and behavior in children, adolescents, young adults 18–24 yrs with major depressive disorder, other psychiatric disorders.

CLASSIFICATION

PHARMACOTHERAPEUTIC: Serotonin-norepinephrine reuptake inhibitor (SNRI). **CLINICAL:** Antidepressant.

USES

Treatment of depression. Treatment of generalized anxiety disorder (GAD), social anxiety disorder (SAD). Treatment of panic disorder, with or without agoraphobia. **OFF-LABEL:** Treatment of attention-deficit hyperactivity disorder (ADHD), obsessive-compulsive disorder (OCD), hot flashes, diabetic neuropathy, posttraumatic stress disorder (PTSD).

PRECAUTIONS

Contraindications: Hypersensitivity to venlafaxine. Use of MAOIs intended to treat psychiatric disorders concurrently or within 14 days of discontinuing MAOI. Initiation of MAOI to treat psychiatric disorder within 7 days of discontinuing venlafaxine, initiation in pts receiving linezolid or IV methylene blue. **Cautions:** Seizure disorder, renal/hepatic impairment, pts at high risk for suicide, recent MI, mania, volume-depleted pts, narrow-angle glaucoma, HF, hyperthyroidism, abnormal platelet function, elderly.

ACTION

Potentiates CNS neurotransmitter activity by inhibiting reuptake of serotonin, norepinephrine, and, to lesser degree, DOPamine. **Therapeutic Effect:** Relieves depression.

PHARMACOKINETICS

Widely distributed. Protein binding: 25%–30%. Metabolized in liver. Primarily excreted in urine. Not removed by hemodialysis. **Half-life:** 3–7 hrs; metabolite, 9–13 hrs (increased in hepatic/renal impairment).

LIFESPAN CONSIDERATIONS

Pregnancy/Lactation: Unknown if distributed in breast milk. **Children:** Children, adolescents are at increased risk for suicidal ideation and behavior, worsening depression, esp. during first few mos of therapy. **Elderly:** Use caution.

INTERACTIONS

DRUG: **Strong CYP3A4 inhibitors (e.g., clarithromycin, ketoconazole, ritonavir)** may increase concentration/effect. **MAOIs (e.g., phenelzine, selegiline)** may cause neuroleptic malignant syndrome, autonomic instability (including rapid fluctuations of vital signs), extreme agitation, hyperthermia, altered mental status, myoclonus, rigidity, coma. **Strong CYP3A4 inducers (e.g., carBAMazepine, phenytoin, rifAMPin)** may decrease concentration/effect. May increase risk of bleeding with **NSAIDs (e.g., diclofenac, meloxicam, naproxen), aspirin, warfarin.** **HERBAL:** **St. John's wort** may decrease concentration/effect. **Herbals with anticoagulant/antiplatelet properties (e.g., garlic, ginger, ginkgo biloba), glucosamine** may increase risk of bleeding. **FOOD:** **Grapefruit products** may increase concentration/effect. **LAB VALUES:** May increase serum cholesterol CPK, LDH, prolactin, GGT.

AVAILABILITY (Rx)

Tablets: 25 mg, 37.5 mg, 50 mg, 75 mg, 100 mg.

Capsules, Extended-Release: ***(Effexor XR):*** 37.5 mg, 75 mg, 150 mg. **Tablets, Extended-Release:** 37.5 mg, 75 mg, 150 mg, 225 mg.

ADMINISTRATION/HANDLING

PO

• Give with food. • Scored tablet may be crushed. • Do not break, crush, dissolve, or divide extended-release tablets. • May open capsule, sprinkle on applesauce. Give immediately without chewing and follow with full glass of water.

INDICATIONS/ROUTES/DOSAGE

Depression

PO: ***(Immediate-Release):*** **ADULTS, ELDERLY:** Initially, 37.5–75 mg/day in 2–3 divided doses with food. May increase up to 75 mg/day at intervals of 4 days or longer. Usual dose: 75–375 mg/day. **Maximum:** 375 mg/day in 3 divided doses.

PO: ***(Extended-Release):*** **ADULTS, ELDERLY:** Initially, 37.5–75 mg/day as single dose with food. May increase by 75 mg/day at intervals of 4 days or longer. Usual dose: 75–225 mg once daily. **Maximum:** 225 mg/day.

Generalized Anxiety Disorder (GAD)

PO: ***(Extended-Release):*** **ADULTS, ELDERLY:** Initially, 37.5–75 mg/day (pts initiated at 37.5 mg once daily may increase to 75 mg once daily after 4–7 days). May increase by 75 mg/day at 4-day intervals up to 225 mg/day.

Panic Disorder

PO: ***(Extended-Release):*** **ADULTS, ELDERLY:** Initially, 37.5 mg/day. May increase to 75 mg after 7 days followed by increases of 75 mg/day at 7-day intervals up to 225 mg/day.

Social Anxiety Disorder (SAD)

PO: ***(Extended-Release):*** **ADULTS, ELDERLY:** 75 mg once daily.

Dosage in Renal/Hepatic Impairment

Consider decreasing venlafaxine dosage by 50% in pts with moderate hepatic impairment, 25% in pts with mild to moderate renal impairment, 50% in pts on dialysis (withhold dose until completion of dialysis). When discontinuing therapy, taper dosage slowly over 2 wks.

SIDE EFFECTS

Frequent (greater than 20%): Nausea, drowsiness, headache, dry mouth. **Occasional (20%–10%):** Dizziness, insomnia, constipation, diaphoresis, nervousness, asthenia, ejaculatory disturbance, anorexia. **Rare (less than 10%):** Anxiety, blurred vision, diarrhea, vomiting, tremor, abnormal dreams, impotence.

ADVERSE EFFECTS/TOXIC REACTIONS

Sustained increase in diastolic B/P of 10–15 mm Hg occurs occasionally. Serotonin syndrome (agitation, confusion, hallucinations, hyperreflexia), neuroleptic malignant syndrome (muscular rigidity, fever, cognitive changes), suicidal ideation have occurred.

NURSING CONSIDERATIONS

BASELINE ASSESSMENT

Obtain weight, B/P. Assess appearance, behavior, speech pattern, level of interest, mood. Assess risk of suicide.

INTERVENTION/EVALUATION

Monitor signs/symptoms of depression, B/P, weight. Assess sleep pattern for evidence of insomnia. Check during waking hours for drowsiness, dizziness, anxiety; provide assistance as necessary. Assess appearance, behavior, speech pattern, level of interest, mood for therapeutic response. Monitor for suicidal ideation (esp. at initiation of therapy or changes in dosage).

PATIENT/ FAMILY TEACHING

• Take with food to minimize GI distress • Do not increase, decrease, suddenly stop medication. • Avoid tasks that require alertness, motor skills until response to drug is established. • Report if breastfeeding, pregnant, or planning to become pregnant. • Avoid alcohol. • Seek immediate medical attention if thoughts of suicide, new onset or worsening of anxiety, depression, or changes in mood occur.

verapamil

ver-**ap**-a-mil
(Calan SR, Verelan, Verelan PM, Isoptin SR ✱)
Do not confuse Verelan with Voltaren.

FIXED-COMBINATION(S)

Tarka: verapamil/trandolapril (an ACE inhibitor): 240 mg/1 mg, 180 mg/2 mg, 240 mg/2 mg, 240 mg/4 mg.

V

◆ CLASSIFICATION

PHARMACOTHERAPEUTIC: Calcium channel blocker (nondihydropyridine). **CLINICAL:** Antihypertensive, antianginal, antiarrhythmic (class IV).

USES

Parenteral: Management of supraventricular tachyarrhythmias (SVT, rapid conversion to sinus rhythm), temporary control of rapid ventricular rate in atrial flutter/fibrillation. **PO:** Treatment of angina at rest (e.g., vasospastic angina, unstable angina, chronic stable angina). Control of ventricular rate at rest and during stress in chronic atrial flutter and/or fibrillation. Management of hypertension. Prophylaxis of repetitive paroxysmal supraventricular tachycardia (PSVT).

PRECAUTIONS

Contraindications: Hypersensitivity to verapamil. Atrial fibrillation/flutter in presence of accessory bypass tract (e.g., Wolff-Parkinson-White, Lown-Ganong-Levine syndromes), severe left ventricular dysfunction, cardiogenic shock, second- or third-degree heart block (except with pacemaker), hypotension (SBP less than 90 mm Hg), sick sinus syndrome (except with pacemaker). **IV:** Current use of IV beta-blocking agents, ventricular tachycardia. **Cautions:** Renal/hepatic impairment, concomitant use of beta blockers and/or digoxin, myasthenia gravis, elderly, hypertrophic cardiomyopathy. Avoid use in HF.

ACTION

Inhibits calcium ion entry across cardiac, vascular smooth-muscle cell membranes, dilating coronary arteries, peripheral arteries, arterioles. **Therapeutic Effect:** Decreases heart rate, myocardial contractility; slows SA, AV conduction. Decreases total peripheral vascular resistance by vasodilation.

PHARMACOKINETICS

Widely distributed. Protein binding: 90% (60% in neonates). Metabolized in liver. Primarily excreted in urine. Not removed by hemodialysis. **Half-life: Single dose:** 2–8 hrs; **multiple doses:** 4.5–12 hrs.

LIFESPAN CONSIDERATIONS

Pregnancy/Lactation: Drug crosses placenta; distributed in breast milk. Breastfeeding not recommended. **Children:** No age-related precautions noted. **Elderly:** Age-related renal impairment may require dosage adjustment.

INTERACTIONS

DRUG: May increase hypotensive effect of **beta blockers (e.g., carvedilol, metoprolol)**. May increase concentration/effects of **statins (e.g., atorvastatin, simvastatin), dofetilide. Strong CYP3A4 inhibitors (e.g., clarithromycin, ketoconazole)** may increase concentration/effect. May increase concentration of **cycloSPORINE, carBAMazepine. Strong CYP3A4 inducers (e.g., carBAMazepine, phenytoin, rifAMPin)** may decrease concentration/effect. **HERBAL: St. John's wort** may decrease concentration/effect. **Herbals with hypertensive properties (e.g., licorice, yohimbe) or hypotensive properties (e.g., garlic, ginger, ginkgo biloba)** may alter effects. **FOOD: Grapefruit products** may increase concentration/effect. **LAB VALUES:** ECG may show prolonged PR interval. **Therapeutic serum level:** 0.08–0.3 mcg/mL; **toxic serum level:** N/A.

AVAILABILITY (Rx)

Injection Solution: 2.5 mg/mL. **Tablets:** 40 mg, 80 mg, 120 mg.

Capsules, Extended-Release: 100 mg, 120 mg, 180 mg, 200 mg, 240 mg, 300 mg, 360 mg. **Tablets, Extended-Release:** 120 mg, 180 mg, 240 mg.

ADMINISTRATION/HANDLING

IV

Reconstitution • May give undiluted.
Rate of administration • Administer IV push over 2 min for adults, children; give over 3 min for elderly. • Continuous ECG monitoring during IV injection is required for children, recommended for adults. • Monitor ECG for rapid ventricular rate, extreme bradycardia, heart block, asystole, prolongation of PR interval. Notify physician of any significant changes. • Monitor B/P q5–10min. • Pt should remain recumbent for at least 1 hr after IV administration.
Storage • Store vials at room temperature.

PO

• Do not give with grapefruit products. • Do not crush or cut extended-release tablets, capsules. Give extended-release tablets with food. • Sustained-release capsules may be opened and sprinkled on applesauce, then swallowed immediately (do not chew).

IV INCOMPATIBILITIES

Albumin, amphotericin B complex (Abelcet, AmBisome, Amphotec), nafcillin (Nafcil), propofol (Diprivan), sodium bicarbonate.

IV COMPATIBILITIES

Amiodarone (Cordarone), calcium chloride, calcium gluconate, dexamethasone (Decadron), digoxin (Lanoxin), DOBUTamine (Dobutrex), DOPamine (Intropin), furosemide (Lasix), heparin, HYDROmorphone (Dilaudid), lidocaine, magnesium sulfate, metoclopramide (Reglan), milrinone (Primacor), morphine, multivitamins, nitroglycerin, norepinephrine (Levophed), potassium chloride, potassium phosphate, procainamide (Pronestyl), propranolol (Inderal).

INDICATIONS/ROUTES/DOSAGE

Supraventricular Tachyarrhythmias (SVT)

IV: ADULTS, ELDERLY: Initially, 5 to 10 mg (0.075 to 0.15 mg/kg) over 2 min. Repeat dose: 10 mg (0.15 mg/kg) 30 min after initial dose. **CHILDREN:** Initially, 0.1 to 0.3 mg/kg (2 to 5 mg) over 2 min. Repeat dose: 0.1 to 0.3 mg/kg 30 min after the initial dose. **PO: ADULTS, ELDERLY: (Prophylaxis):** 240–480 mg/day in 3–4 divided doses. **Maximum:** 480 mg/day.

Angina, Unstable Angina, Chronic Stable Angina

PO: ***(Immediate-Release):*** **ADULTS, ELDERLY:** 80–160 mg 3 times daily.

Atrial Fibrillation (Rate control)

IV: ADULTS, ELDERLY: Initially, 0.075–0.15 mg/kg (usual: 5–10 mg) over 2 min. May repeat with 10 mg after 15–30 min.
PO: ***(Immediate-Release):*** 240–480 mg/day in 3–4 divided doses.

Hypertension

PO: ***(Immediate-Release):*** **ADULTS, ELDERLY:** Initially, 40–120 mg 3 times/day. Range: 240 – 480 mg/day in divided doses.
PO: ***(Extended-Release [Calan SR]):*** **ADULTS, ELDERLY:** Initially, 120–180 mg once daily. May increase at wkly intervals to 240 mg once daily, then 180 mg twice daily. **Maximum:** 240 mg twice daily.
PO: ***(Extended-Release [Verelan]):*** **ADULTS, ELDERLY:** Initially, 120–240 mg once daily. May increase dose at wkly intervals to 180 mg/day, then 240 mg/day, then 360 mg/day, then 480 mg/day maximum.
PO: ***(Extended-Release [Verelan PM]):*** **ADULTS, ELDERLY:** Initially, 100–200 mg once daily at bedtime. May increase dose at wkly intervals to 300 mg once daily, then 400 mg once daily maximum.

Chronic Atrial Fibrillation (Rate control), SVT

PO: ***(Immediate-Release):*** **ADULTS, ELDERLY:** 240–480 mg/day in 3–4 divided doses. Usual range: 120–360 mg/day.

Dosage for Renal Impairment

CrCl less than 10 mL/min: Dose reduction (50%–75%) of normal dose recommended.

Dosage in Hepatic Impairment

Dose reduction (20%–50%) of normal dose recommended.

V

SIDE EFFECTS

Frequent (7%): Constipation. **Occasional (4%–2%):** Dizziness, light-headedness, headache, asthenia, nausea, peripheral edema, hypotension. **Rare (less than 1%):** Bradycardia, dermatitis, rash.

ADVERSE EFFECTS/TOXIC REACTIONS

Rapid ventricular rate in atrial flutter/fibrillation, marked hypotension, extreme bradycardia, HF, asystole, second- or third-degree AV block occur rarely.

NURSING CONSIDERATIONS

BASELINE ASSESSMENT

Obtain ECG, B/P, heart rate. Record onset, type (sharp, dull, squeezing), radiation, location, intensity, duration of anginal pain, precipitating factors (exertion, emotional stress).

INTERVENTION/EVALUATION

Assess pulse for quality, rate, rhythm. Monitor B/P. Monitor ECG for cardiac changes, particularly prolongation of PR interval. Assist with ambulation if dizziness occurs. Assess for peripheral edema. For those taking oral form, monitor daily pattern of bowel activity, stool consistency. **Therapeutic serum level:** 0.08–0.3 mcg/mL; **toxic serum level:** N/A.

PATIENT/FAMILY TEACHING

• Do not abruptly discontinue medication. • Compliance with therapy regimen is essential to control anginal pain. • Go from lying to standing slowly. • Avoid tasks that require alertness, motor skills until response to drug is established. • Limit caffeine. • Avoid or limit alcohol. • Report continued, persistent angina pain, irregular heartbeats, shortness of breath, swelling, dizziness, constipation, nausea, hypotension. • Avoid grapefruit products.

vilazodone

vil-**az**-oh-done
(Viibryd)

■ BLACK BOX ALERT ■ Increased risk of suicidal ideation and behavior in children, adolescents, and young adults 18–24 yrs of age with major depressive disorder, other psychiatric disorders.

◆CLASSIFICATION

PHARMACOTHERAPEUTIC: Selective serotonin reuptake inhibitor. **CLINICAL:** Antidepressant.

USES

Treatment of major depressive disorder.

PRECAUTIONS

Contraindications: Hypersensitivity to vilazodone. Use of MAOIs intended to treat psychiatric disorders (with or within 14 days of stopping vilazodone or MAOI), starting vilazodone in pts receiving linezolid or methylene blue. **Cautions:** Seizure disorder, pts at risk for suicide (history of ideation and behavior; depression), hepatic impairment, elderly.

ACTION

Enhances serotonergic activity in CNS by selectively inhibiting reuptake of serotonin. **Therapeutic Effect:** Relieves depression.

PHARMACOKINETICS

Widely distributed. Peak concentration: 4–5 hrs. Protein binding: 96%–99%. Metabolized in liver. **Half-life:** 25 hrs.

⌛ LIFESPAN CONSIDERATIONS

Pregnancy/Lactation: Unknown if drug crosses placenta or is excreted in breast milk. **Children:** Safety and efficacy not established. **Elderly:** No age-related precautions noted.

INTERACTIONS

DRUG: **Alcohol** may increase adverse effects. **Aspirin, NSAIDs (e.g., diclofenac, meloxicam, naproxen), warfarin** may increase risk of bleeding. **Strong CYP3A4 inhibitors (e.g., clarithromycin, ketoconazole)** may

V

increase concentration. **BusPIRone, lithium, MAOIs (e.g., phenelzine, selegiline) naratriptan, SNRIs (e.g., venlafaxine), SSRIs (e.g., sertraline), traMADol, tryptophan** may increase risk of serotonin syndrome. **HERBAL:** **Herbals with anticoagulant/antiplatelet properties (e.g., garlic, ginger, ginkgo biloba), glucosamine** may increase risk of bleeding. **St. John's wort** may decrease concentration/effect. **FOOD:** None known. **LAB VALUES:** None significant.

AVAILABILITY (Rx)

Tablets: 10 mg, 20 mg, 40 mg.

ADMINISTRATION/HANDLING

PO

- Give with food (administration without food can result in inadequate drug concentration, may diminish effectiveness).

INDICATIONS/ROUTES/DOSAGE

Depression

PO: **ADULTS, ELDERLY:** Initially, 10 mg once daily for 7 days, followed by 20 mg once daily. May increase to 40 mg once daily after a minimum of 7 days. **Note:** When discontinuing treatment, reduce dose gradually. From 40 mg/day: taper to 20 mg/day for 4 days, then 10 mg/day for 3 days. From 20 mg/day: taper to 10 mg/day for 7 days.

Concomitant Moderate/Strong CYP3A4 Inhibitors

PO: **ADULTS, ELDERLY:** 20 mg/day.

Concomitant Strong CYP3A4 Inducers

May increase dose to 80 mg/day when used concomitantly for more than 14 days.

Dosage in Renal/Hepatic Impairment

No dose adjustment.

SIDE EFFECTS

Frequent (28%–23%): Diarrhea, nausea. **Occasional (9%–3%):** Dizziness, dry mouth, insomnia, vomiting, decreased libido, abnormal dreams, fatigue, sweating. **Rare (2%):** Dyspepsia, flatulence, paresthesia, restlessness, arthralgia, abnormal orgasm, delayed ejaculation, increased appetite, palpitations, tremor.

ADVERSE EFFECTS/TOXIC REACTIONS

Serotonin syndrome (agitation, confusion, hallucinations, hyperreflexia), neuroleptic malignant syndrome (fever, muscular rigidity, cognitive changes).

NURSING CONSIDERATIONS

BASELINE ASSESSMENT

Assess behavior, appearance, emotional status, response to environment, speech pattern, thought content, risk of suicide.

INTERVENTION/EVALUATION

Monitor B/P, heart rate, weight. Monitor for suicidal ideation (esp. at initiation of therapy or changes in dosage). Assess for therapeutic response (greater interest in surroundings, improved self-care, increased ability to concentrate, relaxed facial expression).

PATIENT/FAMILY TEACHING

- Avoid tasks that may require alertness, motor skills until response to drug is established (may cause dizziness). • Slowly go from lying to standing. • Take with food. • Do not suddenly stop taking medication; withdraw gradually. • Seek immediate medical attention if thoughts of suicide, new onset or worsening of anxiety, depression, or changes in mood occur. • Avoid alcohol.

V

vinBLAStine HIGH ALERT

vin-**blas**-teen

BLACK BOX ALERT Must be administered by personnel trained in administration/handling of chemotherapeutic agents. For IV use only. Fatal if given intrathecally (ascending paralysis, death). Vesicant; avoid extravasation.

Do not confuse vinBLAStine with vinCRIStine or vinorelbine.

CLASSIFICATION

PHARMACOTHERAPEUTIC: Antimicrotubular. Vinca alkaloid. **CLINICAL:** Antineoplastic.

USES

Treatment of Hodgkin's lymphoma, non-Hodgkin's lymphoma, Langerhans cell histiocytosis, advanced testicular carcinoma, Kaposi's sarcoma, Letterer-Siwe disease. **OFF-LABEL:** Treatment of bladder, ovarian cancer; non–small-cell lung cancer; soft tissue sarcoma, melanoma.

PRECAUTIONS

Contraindications: Hypersensitivity to vinBLAStine. Bacterial infection, significant granulocytopenia (unless as a result of condition being treated). **Cautions:** Hepatic impairment, cardiovascular disease (e.g., cardiomyopathy, hypertension), pulmonary disease, baseline cytopenias, conditions predisposing to infection (e.g., diabetes, renal failure, immunocompromised pts, open wounds); history of thrombosis (CVA, MI); pts at risk for extravasation (e.g., peripheral IV catheters, elderly, poor peripheral vasculature), recent exposure to radiation therapy, chemotherapy.

ACTION

Binds to tubulin, inhibiting microtubule formation; may interfere with nucleic acid, protein synthesis. **Therapeutic Effect:** Inhibits cell division by disrupting mitotic spindle.

PHARMACOKINETICS

Does not cross blood-brain barrier. Protein binding: 99%. Metabolized in liver. Excreted in urine (14%), feces (10%). **Half-life:** 24.8 hrs.

LIFESPAN CONSIDERATIONS

Pregnancy/Lactation: Avoid pregnancy; may cause fetal harm. Females of reproductive potential must use effective contraception during treatment and for at least 6 mos after discontinuation. Breastfeeding not recommended during treatment and for at least 1 wk after discontinuation. May impair fertility. **Males:** Males with female partners of reproductive potential must use effective contraception during treatment and for at least 3 mos after discontinuation. **Children/Elderly:** No age-related precautions noted.

INTERACTIONS

DRUG: **Strong CYP3A4 inhibitors (e.g., clarithromycin, ketoconazole, ritonavir), moderate CYP3A inhibitors (e.g., dilTIAZem, fluconazole, verapamil)** may increase concentration/effect. **Strong CYP3A4 inducers (e.g., carBAMazepine, phenytoin, rifAMPin), moderate CYP3A inducers (e.g., bosentan, nafcillin)** may decrease concentration/effect. May decrease therapeutic effect of **BCG (intravesical). Bone marrow depressants (e.g., cladribine)** may increase myelosuppression. **Live virus vaccines** may potentiate virus replication, increase vaccine side effects, decrease pt's antibody response to vaccine. **HERBAL:** **St. John's wort** may decrease concentration. **Echinacea** may decrease the therapeutic effect. **FOOD:** None known. **LAB VALUES:** May increase serum uric acid.

AVAILABILITY (Rx)

Injection Solution: 1 mg/mL.

ADMINISTRATION/HANDLING

◄ALERT► May be carcinogenic, mutagenic, teratogenic. Handle with extreme care during preparation and administration. Give by IV injection. Leakage from IV site into surrounding tissue may produce extreme irritation. Avoid eye contact with solution (severe eye irritation, possible corneal ulceration may result).

If eye contact occurs, immediately irrigate eye with water.

IV

Note: In order to prevent inadvertent intrathecal administration, dispense as a piggyback (not a syringe).

Reconstitution • Using 1 mg/mL solution, further dilute in 25–50 mL D_5W or 0.9% NaCl.

Rate of administration • Infuse over 5–15 min. Prolonged administration time and/or increased volume may increase risk of vein irritation and extravasation.

Storage • Refrigerate unopened vials. • Solution appears clear, colorless. • Following dilution, solution is stable for up to 21 days if protected from light (consult manufacturer prescribing information). • Discard if solution is discolored or precipitate forms.

IV INCOMPATIBILITIES

Furosemide (Lasix).

IV COMPATIBILITIES

Allopurinol (Aloprim), CISplatin (Platinol AQ), cyclophosphamide (Cytoxan), DOXOrubicin (Adriamycin), etoposide (VePesid), 5-fluorouracil, gemcitabine (Gemzar), granisetron (Kytril), heparin, leucovorin, methotrexate, ondansetron (Zofran), PACLitaxel (Taxol), vinorelbine (Navelbine).

INDICATIONS/ROUTES/DOSAGE

◄ALERT► Dosage individualized based on clinical response, tolerance to adverse effects. When used in combination therapy, consult specific protocols for optimum dosage, sequence of drug administration.

Usual Dosage

IV: ADULTS, ELDERLY: Initially, 3.7 mg/m² (adjust dose q7days based on WBC response) up to 5.5 mg/m² (second wk), 7.4 mg/m² (third wk), 9.25 mg/m² (fourth wk), and 11.1 mg/m² (fifth wk). **Maximum:** 18.5 mg/m². **CHILDREN:** 3–6 mg/m² q7–14days. **Maximum:** 12.5 mg/m²/wk.

Dosage in Renal Impairment

No dose adjustment.

Dosage in Hepatic Impairment

Direct serum bilirubin concentration 1.5–3 mg/dL: Reduce dose by 50%. **Greater than 3 mg/dL:** Avoid use.

SIDE EFFECTS

Frequent: Nausea, vomiting, alopecia. **Occasional:** Constipation, diarrhea, rectal bleeding, headache, paresthesia (occur 4–6 hrs after administration, persist for 2–10 hrs), malaise, asthenia, dizziness, pain at tumor site, jaw/face pain, depression, dry mouth. **Rare:** Dermatitis, stomatitis, phototoxicity, hyperuricemia.

ADVERSE EFFECTS/TOXIC REACTIONS

Hematologic toxicity manifested most commonly as leukopenia, less frequently as anemia. WBC reaches its nadir 4–10 days after initial therapy, recovers within 7–14 days (high dosage may require 21-day recovery period). Thrombocytopenia is usually mild and transient, with recovery occurring in a few days. Hepatic insufficiency may increase risk of toxicity. Acute shortness of breath, bronchospasm may occur, particularly when administered concurrently with mitoMYcin. Extravasation may cause severe tissue necrosis. Neurotoxicity (seizures, severe CNS damage), cardiovascular toxicities (angina pectoris, cardiomyopathy, CVA, hypertension, limb ischemia, MI, Raynaud's phenomenon), GI toxicities (hemorrhagic enterocolitis, GI bleeding, intestinal obstruction, paralytic ileus, toxic megacolon) may occur.

NURSING CONSIDERATIONS

BASELINE ASSESSMENT

Obtain CBC, LFT; pregnancy test in females of reproductive potential. Screen for active infection. Question history of cardiac/pulmonary disease, hepatic impairment. Assess patency of IV access. Offer emotional support.

INTERVENTION/EVALUATION

Monitor CBC for myelosuppression, LFT for hepatic injury (abdominal pain, jaundice, nausea, transaminitis, vomiting). Monitor for infections (cough, fatigue, fever), neurotoxicities (seizures, CNS effects), stomatitis, pulmonary toxicities (bronchospasm, dyspnea); symptoms of CVA (aphasia, altered mental status, facial droop, hemiplegia, vision loss); MI (chest pain, diaphoresis, left arm/jaw pain, increased serum troponin, ST segment elevation). Extravasation may result in cellulitis, phlebitis. Large amount of extravasation may result in tissue sloughing. If extravasation occurs, give local injection of hyaluronidase, apply warm compresses.

PATIENT/FAMILY TEACHING

• Treatment may depress your immune system response and reduce your ability to fight infection. Report symptoms of infection such as body aches, chills, cough, fatigue, fever. Avoid those with active infection. • Report symptoms of bone marrow depression (e.g., bruising, fatigue, fever, shortness of breath, weight loss; bleeding easily, bloody urine or stool). • Avoid pregnancy. Do not breastfeed. • Treatment may reduce the heart's ability to pump effectively. • Report heart problems (difficulty breathing, swelling of extremities, palpitations), liver problems (abdominal pain, bruising, clay-colored stool, dark or amber-colored urine, yellowing of the skin or eyes), skin reactions (rash, redness, swelling), seizures. • Life-threatening cardiovascular events may occur; report symptoms of heart attack (chest pain, difficulty breathing, jaw pain, nausea, pain that radiates to the arm or jaw, sweating), stroke (confusion, one-sided weakness or paralysis, difficulty speaking).

vinCRIStine

HIGH ALERT

vin-**cris**-teen
(Marqibo)

BLACK BOX ALERT Must be administered by personnel trained in administration/handling of chemotherapeutic agents. For IV use only. Fatal if given intrathecally (ascending paralysis, death). Vesicant; avoid extravasation. Marqibo and Vincasar are not interchangeable.

Do not confuse vinCRIStine with vinBLAStine.

CLASSIFICATION

PHARMACOTHERAPEUTIC: Antimicrotubular. Vinca alkaloid. **CLINICAL:** Antineoplastic.

USES

Treatment of acute lymphocytic leukemia (ALL), Hodgkin's lymphoma, advanced non-Hodgkin's lymphomas, neuroblastoma, rhabdomyosarcoma, Wilms tumor. **Marqibo:** Relapsed Philadelphia chromosome negative (Ph^-) ALL in adults whose disease has progressed after 2 or more antileukemic therapies. **OFF-LABEL:** Treatment of multiple myeloma, chronic lymphocytic leukemia (CLL), brain tumors, small-cell lung cancer, ovarian germ cell tumors, Ewing's sarcoma, gestational trophoblastic tumors, retinoblastoma.

PRECAUTIONS

Contraindications: Hypersensitivity to vinCRIStine. Demyelinating form of Charcot-Marie-Tooth syndrome. Intrathecal administration. **Cautions:** Hepatic impairment, elderly, preexisting neuromuscular disorders, conditions predisposing to infection (e.g., diabetes, renal failure, immunocompromised pts, open wounds); pts at risk for extravasation (e.g., peripheral IV catheters, elderly, poor peripheral vasculature), recent exposure to radiation therapy, chemotherapy; pts at risk for tumor lysis syndrome (high tumor burden, dehydration); history of GI obstruction.

ACTION

Binds to tubulin, inhibiting microtubule formation; may interfere with nucleic

V

acid/protein synthesis. **Therapeutic Effect:** Inhibits cell division by disrupting mitotic spindle.

PHARMACOKINETICS

Does not cross blood-brain barrier. Protein binding: 75%. Metabolized in liver. Primarily excreted in feces by biliary system. **Half-life:** 24 hrs. **Marqibo:** 45 hrs.

LIFESPAN CONSIDERATIONS

Pregnancy/Lactation: If possible, avoid use during pregnancy, esp. first trimester. May cause fetal harm. Breastfeeding not recommended. **Children:** No age-related precautions noted. **Elderly:** More susceptible to neurotoxic effects.

INTERACTIONS

DRUG: **Strong CYP3A4 inhibitors (e.g., clarithromycin, ketoconazole, ritonavir), moderate CYP3A inhibitors (e.g., dilTIAZem, fluconazole, verapamil)** may increase concentration/effect. **Strong CYP3A4 inducers (e.g., carBAMazepine, phenytoin, rifAMPin), moderate CYP3A inducers (e.g., bosentan, nafcillin)** may decrease concentration/effect. May decrease therapeutic effect of **BCG (intravesical). Live virus vaccines** may potentiate virus replication, increase vaccine side effects, decrease pt's antibody response to vaccine. **HERBAL:** **St. John's wort** may decrease concentration/effect. **Echinacea** may decrease the therapeutic effect. **FOOD:** None known. **LAB VALUES:** May increase serum uric acid.

AVAILABILITY (Rx)

Injection Solution: 1 mg/mL. **Injection Suspension:** ***(Marqibo):*** 5 mg/31 mL.

ADMINISTRATION/HANDLING

Note: In order to prevent inadvertent intrathecal administration, dispense as a piggyback. (not a syringe).

IV

◀ALERT▶ May be carcinogenic, mutagenic, teratogenic. Handle with extreme care during preparation and administration. Use extreme caution in calculating, administering vinCRIStine. Overdose may result in serious or fatal outcome.

Injection Solution

Reconstitution • Dilute in 25–50 mL D_5W or 0.9% NaCl.

Rate of administration • Administer as 5–10 min infusion (preferred). • Do not infuse into extremity with impaired, potentially impaired circulation caused by compression or invading neoplasm, phlebitis, varicosity.

Storage • Refrigerate unopened vials. • Solution appears clear, colorless. • Discard if solution is discolored or precipitate forms. • Diluted solutions are stable for 7 days refrigerated or 2 days at room temperature.

Injection Suspension

• Calculate dose of vinCRIStine and remove volume equal to volume of intended solution from 100 mL 0.9% NaCl or D_5W infusion bag. Inject vinCRIStine into infusion bag (total volume: 100 mL).

Rate of administration • Administer over 60 min.

Storage • Must be administered within 12 hrs of preparation.

IV INCOMPATIBILITIES

Furosemide (Lasix), IDArubicin (Idamycin).

IV COMPATIBILITIES

Allopurinol (Aloprim), CISplatin (Platinol AQ), cyclophosphamide (Cytoxan), cytarabine (Ara-C, Cytosar), DOXOrubicin (Adriamycin), etoposide (VePesid), 5-fluorouracil, gemcitabine (Gemzar), granisetron (Kytril), leucovorin, methotrexate, ondansetron (Zofran), PACLitaxel (Taxol), vinorelbine (Navelbine).

INDICATIONS/ROUTES/DOSAGE

Note: Dosing may be capped at 2 mg/dose. Dosing and frequency may vary by

V

protocol and/or treatment phase. Dispense in mini bag (not syringe).

Usual Dosage Injection Solution

IV: ADULTS, ELDERLY: 1.4 mg/m^2, frequency may vary based on protocol. **CHILDREN WEIGHING MORE THAN 10 KG:** 1.5–2 mg/m^2, frequency may vary based on protocol. **CHILDREN WEIGHING LESS THAN 10 KG:** 0.05 mg/kg once wkly. **Maximum:** 2 mg.

Dosage in Renal Impairment

No dose adjustment.

Dosage in Hepatic Impairment

Bilirubin	Dosage
Bilirubin greater than 3 mg/dL	50% of normal

ALL Injection Suspension

IV: ADULTS, ELDERLY: 2.25 mg/m^2 q7days. Infuse over 1 hr.

Dosage in Renal/Hepatic Impairment

No dose adjustment.

SIDE EFFECTS

Expected: Peripheral neuropathy (occurs in nearly every pt; first clinical sign is depression of Achilles tendon reflex). **Frequent:** Peripheral paresthesia, alopecia, constipation/obstipation (upper colon impaction with empty rectum), abdominal cramps, headache, jaw pain, hoarseness, diplopia, ptosis/drooping of eyelid, urinary tract disturbances. **Occasional:** Nausea, vomiting, diarrhea, abdominal distention, stomatitis, fever.

ADVERSE EFFECTS/TOXIC REACTIONS

Myelosuppression (anemia, neutropenia, thrombocytopenia) is an expected response to therapy, but more severe reactions, including febrile neutropenia, may occur. Acute dyspnea, bronchospasm may occur, esp. when administered concurrently with mitoMYcin. Prolonged or high-dose therapy may produce foot/wrist drop, difficulty walking, slapping gait, ataxia, muscle wasting. Extravasation may cause severe tissue necrosis. Tumor lysis syndrome may present as acute renal failure, hypocalcemia, hyperuricemia, hyperphosphatemia. Paralytic ileus, bowel obstruction, colonic pseudo-obstruction may occur. Hepatotoxicity reported in 6%–11% of pts. Infections including pneumonia, sepsis, Staphylococcal bacteremia may occur. Cardiac arrest reported in 5% of pts.

NURSING CONSIDERATIONS

BASELINE ASSESSMENT

Obtain CBC, LFT; pregnancy test in females of reproductive potential. Screen for active infection. Question history of hepatic impairment, neuromuscular disease. Assess risk of tumor lysis syndrome. Assess patency of IV access. Offer emotional support.

INTERVENTION/EVALUATION

Monitor CBC for myelosuppression; LFT for hepatic injury (abdominal pain, jaundice, nausea, transaminitis, vomiting). Monitor for infections (cough, fatigue, fever), sepsis, neurotoxicities, pulmonary toxicities (bronchospasm, dyspnea). Monitor serum uric acid level if tumor lysis syndrome (acute renal failure, electrolyte imbalance, cardiac arrhythmias, seizures) is suspected. Monitor for GI obstruction (abdominal pain, fever, nausea, vomiting). Extravasation produces stinging, burning, edema at injection site. Terminate injection immediately, locally inject hyaluronidase, apply heat (disperses drug, minimizes discomfort, cellulitis).

PATIENT/FAMILY TEACHING

• Immediately report any pain/burning at injection site during administration. • Treatment may depress your immune system response and reduce your ability to fight infection. Report symptoms of infection such as body aches,

V

chills, cough, fatigue, fever. Avoid those with active infection. • Report symptoms of bone marrow depression (e.g., bruising, fatigue, fever, shortness of breath, weight loss; bleeding easily, bloody urine or stool). • Use effective contraception to avoid pregnancy. Do not breastfeed. • Report liver problems (abdominal pain, bruising, clay-colored stool, dark or amber-colored urine, yellowing of the skin or eyes), skin reactions (rash, redness, swelling). • Life-threatening tumor lysis syndrome (a condition caused by the rapid breakdown of cancer cells), which can cause kidney failure, may occur. Report decreased urination, amber-colored urine; confusion, difficulty breathing, fatigue, fever, muscle or joint pain, palpitations, seizures, vomiting. • Report abdominal pain, fever, nausea, vomiting; may indicate GI obstruction.

vinorelbine HIGH ALERT

vin-oh-**rel**-been
(Navelbine)

BLACK BOX ALERT Must be administered by personnel trained in administration/handling of chemotherapeutic agents. Severe myelosuppression, resulting in serious infections, shock, death, may occur.

Do not confuse vinorelbine with vinBLAStine or vinCRIStine.

◆CLASSIFICATION

PHARMACOTHERAPEUTIC: Antimicrotubular. Vinca alkaloid. **CLINICAL:** Antineoplastic.

USES

Single agent or in combination with CISplatin for treatment of unresectable, advanced or metastatic, non–small-cell lung cancer (NSCLC). **OFF-LABEL:** Treatment of metastatic breast cancer, cervical carcinoma, ovarian carcinoma, malignant pleural mesothelioma, soft tissue sarcoma, small-cell lung cancer.

PRECAUTIONS

Contraindications: Hypersensitivity to vinorelbine. **Cautions:** Compromised marrow reserve due to prior chemotherapy/radiation therapy; hepatic impairment, neuropathy, pulmonary impairment.

ACTION

Binds to tubulin, inhibiting microtubule formation; may interfere with nucleic acid protein synthesis. **Therapeutic Effect:** Prevents cellular division by disrupting formation of mitotic spindle.

PHARMACOKINETICS

Widely distributed. Protein binding: 80%–90%. Metabolized in liver. Primarily excreted in feces by biliary system. **Half-life:** 28–43 hrs.

LIFESPAN CONSIDERATIONS

Pregnancy/Lactation: Avoid pregnancy; may cause fetal harm. Females of reproductive potential must use effective contraception during treatment and for at least 1 mo after discontinuation. Breastfeeding not recommended during treatment and for at least 9 days after discontinuation. May impair fertility in both females and males. **Males:** Males with female partners of reproductive potential must use effective contraception during treatment and for at least 3 mos after discontinuation. **Children:** Safety and efficacy not established. **Elderly:** No age-related precautions noted.

INTERACTIONS

DRUG: **CISplatin** may increase risk of granulocytopenia. **Live virus vaccines** may potentiate virus replication, increase vaccine side effects, decrease pt's antibody response to vaccine. **Strong CYP3A4 inhibitors (e.g., clarithromycin, ketoconazole)** may increase concentration/effects. **HERBAL:** **St. John's wort** may decrease concentration. **Echinacea** may decrease the therapeutic effect. **FOOD:** None known. **LAB VALUES:** May increase serum bilirubin, alkaline phosphatase, ALT, AST.

V

AVAILABILITY (Rx)

Injection Solution: 10 mg/mL (5-mL vials).

ADMINISTRATION/HANDLING

IV

◀ALERT▶ IV needle, catheter must be correctly positioned before administration. Leakage into surrounding tissue produces extreme irritation, local tissue necrosis, thrombophlebitis. Handle drug with extreme care during administration; wear protective clothing per protocol. If solution comes in contact with skin/mucosa, immediately wash thoroughly with soap, water.

Reconstitution • Must be diluted and administered via syringe or IV bag.

Syringe Dilution

• Dilute calculated vinorelbine dose with D_5W or 0.9% NaCl to concentration of 1.5–3 mg/mL.

IV Bag Dilution

• Dilute calculated vinorelbine dose with D_5W, 0.45% or 0.9% NaCl, 5% dextrose and 0.45% NaCl, Ringer's or lactated Ringer's to concentration of 0.5–2 mg/mL.

Rate of administration • Administer diluted vinorelbine over 6–10 min into side port of free-flowing IV closest to IV bag followed by flushing with 75–125 mL of one of the solutions. • If extravasation occurs, stop injection immediately; give remaining portion of dose into another vein.

Storage • Refrigerate unopened vials. • Protect from light. • Unopened vials are stable at room temperature for 72 hrs. • Do not administer if particulate has formed. • Diluted vinorelbine may be used for up to 24 hrs under normal room light when stored in polypropylene syringes or polyvinyl chloride bags at room temperature.

IV INCOMPATIBILITIES

Acyclovir (Zovirax), allopurinol (Aloprim), amphotericin B (Fungizone), amphotericin B complex (Abelcet, AmBisome, Amphotec), ampicillin (Omnipen), ceFAZolin (Ancef), cefTRIAXone (Rocephin), cefuroxime (Zinacef), 5-fluorouracil (5-FU), furosemide (Lasix), ganciclovir (Cytovene), methylPREDNISolone (SOLU-Medrol), sodium bicarbonate.

IV COMPATIBILITIES

Calcium gluconate, CARBOplatin (Paraplatin), CISplatin (Platinol AQ), cyclophosphamide (Cytoxan), cytarabine (ARA-C, Cytosar), dacarbazine (DTIC), DAUNOrubicin (Cerubidine), dexamethasone (Decadron), diphenhydrAMINE (Benadryl), DOXOrubicin (Adriamycin), etoposide (VePesid), gemcitabine (Gemzar), granisetron (Kytril), HYDROmorphone (Dilaudid), IDArubicin (Idamycin), methotrexate, morphine, ondansetron (Zofran), vinBLAStine (Velban), vinCRIStine (Oncovin).

INDICATIONS/ROUTES/DOSAGE

◀ALERT▶ Dosage adjustments should be based on granulocyte count obtained on the day of treatment, as follows:

Granulocyte Count (cells/mm³) on Day of Treatment	Dosage
1,500 or higher	100% of starting dose
1,000–1,499	50% of starting dose
Less than 1,000	Do not administer

NSCLC Monotherapy

IV injection: ADULTS, ELDERLY: 30 mg/m² q7days.

NSCLC Combination Therapy With CISplatin

IV injection: ADULTS, ELDERLY: 25–30 mg/m² q7days.

Dosage in Renal Impairment

No dose adjustment. **HD:** Decrease dose to 20 mg/m²/wk given post-HD or on non-HD days.

Dosage in Hepatic Impairment

Serum Bilirubin	Dosage
2 mg/dL or less	100% of dose

Serum Bilirubin	Dosage
2.1–3 mg/dL	50% of dose
Greater than 3 mg/dL	25% of dose

SIDE EFFECTS

Frequent (35%–12%): Asthenia, nausea, constipation, erythema, pain, vein discoloration at injection site, fatigue, peripheral neuropathy manifested as paresthesia, hyperesthesia, diarrhea, alopecia. **Occasional (10%–5%):** Phlebitis, dyspnea, loss of deep tendon reflexes. **Rare:** Chest pain, jaw pain, myalgia, arthralgia, rash.

ADVERSE EFFECTS/TOXIC REACTIONS

Myelosuppression (anemia, leukopenia, neutropenia, thrombocytopenia) is an expected response to therapy. Hemorrhagic cystitis, syndrome of inappropriate antidiuretic hormone reported in less than 1% of pts. Acute shortness of breath, severe bronchospasm occur infrequently, particularly in pts with preexisting pulmonary dysfunction. Hepatic toxicity may occur.

NURSING CONSIDERATIONS

BASELINE ASSESSMENT

Obtain CBC prior to each dose. Granulocyte count should be at least 1,000 cells/mm^3 before vinorelbine administration. Granulocyte nadirs occur 7–10 days following dosing. Do not give hematologic growth factors within 24 hrs before administration of chemotherapy or earlier than 24 hrs following cytotoxic chemotherapy. Advise women of childbearing potential to avoid pregnancy during drug therapy. Offer emotional support.

INTERVENTION/EVALUATION

Diligently monitor injection site for swelling, redness, pain. Monitor CBC for myelosuppression during and following therapy (infection [fever, sore throat, signs of local infection], unusual bleeding/bruising, anemia [excessive fatigue, weakness]). Monitor pts developing severe granulocytopenia for evidence of infection, fever. Crackers, dry toast, sips of cola may help relieve nausea. Monitor daily pattern of bowel activity, stool consistency. Question for tingling, burning, numbness of hands/feet (peripheral neuropathy). Pt complaint of "walking on glass" is sign of hyperesthesia.

PATIENT/FAMILY TEACHING

- Treatment may depress your immune system response and reduce your ability to fight infection. Report symptoms of infection such as body aches, chills, cough, fatigue, fever. Avoid those with active infection.
- Report symptoms of bone marrow depression (e.g., bruising, fatigue, fever, shortness of breath, weight loss; bleeding easily, bloody urine or stool).
- Use effective contraception to avoid pregnancy. Do not breastfeed.
- Report liver problems (abdominal pain, bruising, clay-colored stool, dark or amber-colored urine, yellowing of the skin or eyes), skin reactions (rash, redness, swelling).
- Report new or worsening signs of neuropathy.

vismodegib

vis-moe-**deg**-ib
(Erivedge)

BLACK BOX ALERT May result in embryo-fetal death or severe birth defects including missing digits, midline defects, irreversible malformations due to embryotoxic and teratogenic properties. Verify pregnancy status prior to initiation. Advise use of effective contraception in female pts. Advise male pts of potential exposure risk through seminal fluid.

CLASSIFICATION

PHARMACOTHERAPEUTIC: Hedgehog pathway inhibitor. **CLINICAL:** Antineoplastic.

V

USES

Treatment of adults with metastatic basal cell carcinoma, locally advanced basal cell carcinoma with recurrence after surgery, or pts who are not candidates for surgery or radiation.

PRECAUTIONS

◀ALERT▶ Do not donate blood products for at least 7 mos after discontinuation.

Contraindications: Hypersensitivity to vismodegib. **Cautions:** Hepatic impairment.

ACTION

An inhibitor of Hedgehog pathway, binding to and inhibiting smoothened, a transmembrane protein involved in Hedgehog signal transduction. **Therapeutic Effect:** Inhibits tumor cell growth and survival.

PHARMACOKINETICS

Metabolized in liver. Protein binding: 99%. Excreted in feces (82%), urine (4%). **Half-life:** 4 days (daily dosing), 12 days (single dose).

LIFESPAN CONSIDERATIONS

Pregnancy/Lactation: Avoid pregnancy; may cause fetal harm. Females of reproductive potential must use effective contraception during treatment and for at least 24 mos after discontinuation. Breastfeeding not recommended during treatment and for at least 24 mos after discontinuation. May impair fertility. **Males:** Males with female partners of reproductive potential must use effective contraception during treatment and for at least 3 mos after discontinuation. **Children:** Safety and efficacy not established. **Elderly:** Safety and efficacy not established.

INTERACTIONS

DRUG: None significant. **HERBAL:** None significant. **FOOD:** None known. **LAB VALUES:** May decrease potassium, sodium, GFR. May increase serum BUN, creatinine.

AVAILABILITY (Rx)

Capsules: 150 mg.

ADMINISTRATION/HANDLING

PO

• Give without regard to food. • Give whole. Do not break, crush, or open capsule.

INDICATIONS/ROUTES/DOSAGE

Advanced or Metastatic Basal Cell Carcinoma

PO: ADULTS/ELDERLY: 150 mg once daily. Continue until disease progression or unacceptable toxicity.

Dosage in Renal/Hepatic Impairment

No dose adjustment.

SIDE EFFECTS

Frequent (71%–40%): Muscle spasm, alopecia, dysgeusia, weight loss, fatigue. **Occasional (30%–11%):** Nausea, amenorrhea, diarrhea, anorexia, constipation, vomiting, arthralgia, loss of taste.

ADVERSE EFFECTS/TOXIC REACTIONS

Severe cutaneous reactions including Stevens-Johnson syndrome, toxic epidermal necrolysis. Drug reaction with eosinophilia and systemic symptoms (DRESS), also known as multiorgan hypersensitivity, has been reported. DRESS may present with facial swelling, eosinophilia, fever, lymphadenopathy, rash, which may be associated with other organ systems, such as hepatitis, hematologic abnormalities, myocarditis, nephritis.

NURSING CONSIDERATIONS

BASELINE ASSESSMENT

Obtain pregnancy test in females of reproductive potential. Question history of hepatic impairment. Offer emotional support.

V

INTERVENTION/EVALUATION

Monitor for cutaneous toxicities; symptoms of DRESS.

PATIENT/FAMILY TEACHING

• Use effective contraception to avoid pregnancy. Do not breastfeed. • Do not donate blood for at least 2 yrs. • Toxic skin reactions (necrosis, redness, sloughing) may occur. • Severe multiorgan hypersensitivity reaction (DRESS) may cause life-threatening organ dysfunction; report chest pain, decreased urinary output, facial swelling, fever, rash, swelling of lymph nodes.

vitamin D (vitamin D analogues)

calcitriol

kal-si-**trye**-ole
(Calcijex ✱, Rocaltrol, Vectical)

doxercalciferol

dox-er-kal-**sif**-e-role
(Hectorol)

ergocalciferol

er-goe-kal-**sif**-e-role
(Drisdol)

paricalcitol

par-i-**kal**-si-tol
(Zemplar)

◆CLASSIFICATION

PHARMACOTHERAPEUTIC: Fat-soluble vitamin. **CLINICAL:** Vitamin D analogue.

USES

Calcitriol: Manage hypocalcemia in pts on chronic renal dialysis, secondary hypoparathyroidism in chronic kidney disease (CKD), manage hypocalcemia in hypoparathyroidism. **(Topical):** Treatment of mild to moderate plaque psoriasis. **Doxercalciferol:** Treatment of secondary hyperparathyroidism in CKD. **Ergocalciferol:** Treatment of refractory rickets, hypophosphatemia, hypoparathyroidism, dietary supplement. **Paricalcitol: (Intravenous):** Treatment/prevention of secondary hyperparathyroidism associated with stage 5 CKD. **(PO):** Treatment/prevention of secondary hyperparathyroidism associated with stage 3 and 4 CKD and stage 5 CKD pts on hemodialysis or peritoneal dialysis. **OFF-LABEL: Calcitriol:** Vitamin D–dependent rickets. **Ergocalciferol:** Prevention/treatment of vitamin D deficiency in pts with CKD, osteoporosis prevention.

PRECAUTIONS

Contraindications: Hypersensitivity to cholecalciferol, ergocalciferol. Vitamin D toxicity, hypercalcemia. **Cautions:** Pts with malabsorption syndrome. Concurrent use with digoxin.

ACTION

Calcitriol: Stimulates calcium transport in intestines, resorption in bones, and tubular reabsorption in kidney; suppresses parathyroid hormone (PTH) secretion/synthesis. **Doxercalciferol:** Regulates blood calcium levels, stimulates bone growth, suppresses PTH secretion/synthesis. **Ergocalciferol:** Promotes active absorption of calcium and phosphorus, increasing serum levels to allow bone mineralization; mobilizes calcium and phosphate from bone, increases reabsorption of calcium and phosphate by renal tubules. **Paricalcitol:** Suppresses PTH secretion/synthesis.

V

Therapeutic Effect: Essential for absorption, utilization of calcium, phosphate, control of PTH levels.

PHARMACOKINETICS

Calcitriol: Rapidly absorbed. Protein binding: 99.9%. Metabolized to active metabolite (ergocalciferol). Excreted in feces (49%), urine (16%). **Half-life:** 5–8 hrs. **Doxercalciferol:** Metabolized in liver. **Half-life:** 32–37 hrs. **Ergocalciferol:** Metabolized in liver. **Paricalcitol:** Readily absorbed. Protein binding: 99.8%. Metabolized in liver. Primarily excreted in feces. **Half-life:** 5–7 hrs.

LIFESPAN CONSIDERATIONS

Pregnancy/Lactation: Unknown if drug crosses placenta. Infant risk cannot be excluded. **Children/Elderly:** No age-related precautions noted.

INTERACTIONS

DRUG: **Calcium-containing products, concurrent vitamin D (or derivatives)** may increase risk of hypercalcemia. May increase **digoxin** toxicity due to hypercalcemia (may cause arrhythmias). May increase concentration/effect of **aluminum hydroxide, sucralfate. Bile acid sequestrants (e.g., cholestyramine)** may decrease absorption. **HERBAL:** None significant. **FOOD:** None known. **LAB VALUES:** May increase serum cholesterol, calcium, magnesium, phosphate, ALT, AST, BUN, creatinine.

AVAILABILITY (Rx)

Calcitriol

Capsules, Softgel: ***(Rocaltrol):*** 0.25 mcg, 0.5 mcg. **Injection Solution:** 1 mcg/mL. **Oral Solution:** ***(Rocaltrol):*** 1 mcg/mL.

Doxercalciferol

Capsules, Softgel: ***(Hectorol):*** 0.5 mcg, 1 mcg, 2.5 mcg. **Injection Solution:** ***(Hectorol):*** 2 mcg/mL.

Ergocalciferol

Capsules: ***(Drisdol):*** 50,000 units (1.25 mg). **Liquid, Oral:** ***(Drisdol):*** 8,000 units/mL (200 mcg/mL). **Tablets:** 400 units.

Paricalcitol

Capsules, Gelatin: ***(Zemplar):*** 1 mcg, 2 mcg, 4 mcg. **Injection Solution:** ***(Zemplar):*** 2 mcg/mL.

ADMINISTRATION/HANDLING

Calcitriol

PO

• May take without regard to food.

IV

• May give as IV bolus at end of dialysis.

Doxercalciferol

PO

• May take without regard to food.

IV

• May give as IV bolus via catheter at end of dialysis.

Ergocalciferol

PO

• May take without regard to food.

Paricalcitol

PO

• May take without regard to food. • For 3 times/wk dosing, give no more frequently than every other day.

IV

• Give bolus anytime during dialysis. • Do not give more frequently than every other day.

INDICATIONS/ROUTES/DOSAGE

Calcitriol

Hypocalcemia on Chronic Renal Dialysis

PO: ADULTS, ELDERLY: ***(Rocaltrol):*** Initially, 0.25 mcg/day or every other day. May increase by 0.25 mcg/day at 4- to 8-wk intervals. **Range:** 0.5–1 mcg/day.

IV: ADULTS, ELDERLY: 1–2 mcg 3 times/wk. Adjust dose at 2- to 4-wk intervals. Range: 0.5–4 mcg 3 times/wk.

Hypocalcemia in Hypoparathyroidism

PO: ADULTS, CHILDREN 6 YRS AND OLDER: ***(Rocaltrol):*** Initially, 0.25 mcg/day. May increase at 2- to 4-wk intervals. Range: 0.5–2 mcg/day. **CHILDREN 1–5 YRS:** 0.25–0.75 mcg once daily.

Secondary Hyperparathyroidism Associated With Moderate to Severe CKD Not on Dialysis

PO: ADULTS, ELDERLY, CHILDREN 3 YRS AND OLDER: ***(Rocaltrol):*** Initially, 0.25 mcg/day. May increase to 0.5 mcg/day. **CHILDREN YOUNGER THAN 3 YRS:** Initially, 0.01–0.015 mcg/kg/day.

Doxercalciferol

Secondary Hyperparathyroidism (Dialysis)

PO: ADULTS, ELDERLY: Initial dose (intact parathyroid hormone [iPTH] greater than 400 pg/mL): 10 mcg 3 times/wk at dialysis. Dose titrated to lower iPTH to 150–300 pg/mL, with dosage adjustments made at 8-wk intervals. **Maximum:** 20 mcg 3 times/wk.

IV: ADULTS, ELDERLY: Initial dose (iPTH greater than 400 pg/mL): 4 mcg 3 times/wk after dialysis, given as bolus dose. Dose titrated to lower iPTH to 150–300 pg/mL, with dosage adjustments made at 8-wk intervals. **Maximum:** 18 mcg/wk.

Secondary Hyperparathyroidism (Predialysis)

PO: ADULTS, ELDERLY: Initially, 1 mcg/day. Titrate dose to lower iPTH to 35–70 pg/mL for stage 3 CKD and 70–110 pg/mL for stage 4 CKD. **Maximum:** 3.5 mcg/day.

Ergocalciferol (Dietary supplement)

PO: ADULTS, ELDERLY, CHILDREN: 10 mcg (400 units)/day. **NEONATES:** 10–20 mcg (400–800 units)/day.

Hypoparathyroidism

PO: ADULTS, ELDERLY: 625 mcg–5 mg (25,000–200,000 units)/day (with calcium supplements). **CHILDREN:** 1.25–5 mg (50,000–200,000 units)/day (with calcium supplements).

Plaque Psoriasis

Topical: ADULTS, ELDERLY: Apply to affected area twice daily.

Paricalcitol

Secondary Hyperparathyroidism in Stage 5 CKD

IV: ADULTS, ELDERLY, CHILDREN 5 YRS AND OLDER: Initially, 0.04–0.1 mcg/kg given as bolus dose no more frequently than every other day at any time during dialysis. May increase by 2–4 mcg every 2–4 wks. Dose is based on serum iPTH levels.

Secondary Hyperparathyroidism in Stages 3 and 4 CKD

Note: Initial dose based on baseline serum iPTH levels. Dose adjusted q2wks based on iPTH levels relative to baseline.

PO: ADULTS, ELDERLY: (iPTH 500 PG/ML OR LESS): 1 mcg/day or 2 mcg 3 times/wk. **(iPTH GREATER THAN 500 PG/ML):** 2 mcg/day or 4 mcg 3 times/wk.

Dosage in Renal/Hepatic Impairment

No dose adjustment.

SIDE EFFECTS

Frequencies not defined. **Calcitriol:** Cardiac arrhythmias, headache, pruritus, hypercalcemia, polydipsia, abdominal pain, metallic taste, nausea, vomiting, myalgia, soft tissue calcification. **Doxercalciferol:** Edema, pruritus, nausea, vomiting, headache, dizziness, dyspnea, malaise, hypercalcemia. **Ergocalciferol:** Hypercalcemia, hypervitaminosis D, decreased renal function, soft tissue calcification, bone demineralization, nausea, constipation, weight loss. **Paricalcitol:** Edema, nausea, vomiting, hypercalcemia.

ADVERSE EFFECTS/TOXIC REACTIONS

Early signs of overdose manifested as weakness, headache, drowsiness, nausea, vomiting, dry mouth, constipation, muscle/bone pain, metallic taste. Later signs of overdose evidenced by polyuria, polydipsia, anorexia, weight loss, noctu-

V

ria, photophobia, rhinorrhea, pruritus, disorientation, hallucinations, hyperthermia, hypertension, cardiac dysrhythmias.

NURSING CONSIDERATIONS

BASELINE ASSESSMENT

Obtain serum calcium, phosphate, PTH.

INTERVENTION/EVALUATION

Monitor serum calcium, phosphate, PTH. (therapeutic calcium level: 9–10 mg/dL). Estimate daily dietary calcium intake. Encourage adequate fluid intake. Monitor for signs/symptoms of vitamin D intoxication.

PATIENT/FAMILY TEACHING

• Adequate calcium intake should be maintained. • Dietary phosphorus may need to be restricted (foods high in phosphorus include beans, dairy products, nuts, peas, whole-grain products). • Oral formulations may cause hypersensitivity reactions. Avoid excessive doses. • Report signs/symptoms of hypercalcemia (headache, weakness, drowsiness, nausea, vomiting, dry mouth, constipation, metallic taste, muscle or bone pain). • Maintain adequate hydration. • Avoid changes in diet or supplemental calcium intake (unless directed by health care professional). • Avoid magnesium-containing antacids in pts with renal failure.

V

voriconazole

vor-i-**kon**-a-zole
(Vfend, Apo-Voriconazole ✱)

Do not confuse voriconazole with fluconazole or Vfend with Venofer or Vimpat.

◆CLASSIFICATION

PHARMACOTHERAPEUTIC: Azole derivative. **CLINICAL:** Antifungal.

USES

Treatment of invasive aspergillosis, esophageal candidiasis. Treatment of serious fungal infections caused by *Scedosporium apiospermum, Fusarium* spp. Treatment of candidemia in nonneutropenic pts. Treatment of disseminated *Candida* infections of skin and abdomen, kidney, bladder wall, and wounds. **OFF-LABEL:** Empiric treatment of fungal meningitis or osteoarticular infections, coccidioidomycosis in HIV pts, fungal endophthalmitis, infection prophylaxis of graft-vs-host disease or pts with allogeneic hematopoietic stem cell transplant.

PRECAUTIONS

Contraindications: Hypersensitivity to voriconazole. Concurrent administration of barbiturates (long acting), carBAMazepine, efavirenz (400 mg/day or greater), ergot alkaloids, pimozide, quiNIDine (may cause prolonged QT interval, torsades de pointes), rifabutin, rifAMPin, ritonavir (800 mg/day or greater), sirolimus, St. John's wort. **Cautions:** Severe renal/hepatic impairment, hypersensitivity to other azole antifungal agents. Pts at risk for acute pancreatitis, pts with fructose intolerance, glucose-galactose malabsorption; concomitant nephrotoxic medications; pts at risk for QTc interval prolongation (congenital long QT syndrome, HF, medications that prolong QTc interval, hypokalemia, hypomagnesemia).

ACTION

Interferes with fungal cytochrome P450 activity, decreasing ergosterol synthesis, inhibiting fungal cell membrane formation. **Therapeutic Effect:** Damages fungal cell wall membrane.

PHARMACOKINETICS

Widely distributed. Protein binding: 58%. Metabolized in liver. Primarily excreted as metabolite in urine. **Half-life:** Variable, dose dependent.

LIFESPAN CONSIDERATIONS

Pregnancy/Lactation: May cause fetal harm. **Children:** Safety and efficacy not established in pts younger than 12 yrs. **Elderly:** No age-related precautions noted.

INTERACTIONS

DRUG: May increase concentration, risk of toxicity of **calcium channel blockers (e.g., dilTIAZem, verapamil), cycloSPORINE, ergot alkaloids, HMG-CoA reductase inhibitors (e.g., lovastatin), methadone, sirolimus, tacrolimus, warfarin. CarBAMazepine, rifabutin, rifAMPin** may decrease concentration/effect. **QT interval–prolonging medications (e.g., amiodarone, azithromycin, ciprofloxacin, haloperidol, methadone, sotalol)** may increase risk of QTc interval prolongation. **HERBAL: St. John's wort** may significantly decrease concentration. **FOOD:** None known. **LAB VALUES:** May increase serum alkaline phosphatase, ALT, AST, bilirubin, creatinine. May decrease potassium.

AVAILABILITY (Rx)

Injection, Powder for Reconstitution: 200 mg. **Powder for Oral Suspension:** 200 mg/5 mL. **Tablets:** 50 mg, 200 mg.

ADMINISTRATION/HANDLING

IV

Reconstitution • Reconstitute 200-mg vial with 19 mL Sterile Water for Injection to provide concentration of 10 mg/mL. Dilute in 0.9% NaCl or D_5W to provide concentration of 0.5–5 mg/mL.

Rate of administration • Infuse over 1–2 hrs at a rate not to exceed 3 mg/kg/hr. • Do not infuse concomitantly into same line with other drug infusions. • Do not infuse concomitantly even in separate lines with concentrated electrolyte solutions or blood products.

Storage • Store powder for injection at room temperature. • Use reconstituted solution immediately. • Do not use after 24 hrs when refrigerated.

PO

• Give 1 hr before or 1 hr after a meal.
• Do not mix oral suspension with any other medication or flavoring agent.
• Shake suspension for about 10 sec before use.

IV INCOMPATIBILITIES

Tigecycline (Tygacil).

IV COMPATIBILITIES

Anidulafungin, caspofungin, ceftaroline, doripenem.

INDICATIONS/ROUTES/DOSAGE

Invasive Aspergillosis

IV: ADULTS, ELDERLY, ADOLESCENTS 15 YRS AND OLDER: Initially, 6 mg/kg q12h for 2 doses, then 4 mg/kg q12h. **CHILDREN 12–14 YRS WEIGHING 50 KG OR MORE:** 6 mg/kg q12h for 2 doses, then 4 mg/kg q12h. **WEIGHING LESS THAN 50 KG:** 9 mg/kg q12h for 2 doses, then 8 mg/kg q12h. **CHILDREN 2–11 YRS:** 9 mg/kg q12h for 2 doses, then 8 mg/kg q12h.

PO: ADULTS, ELDERLY, ADOLESCENTS 15 YRS AND OLDER: 200–300 mg q12h or 3–4 mg/kg q12h. **CHILDREN 12–14 YRS WEIGHING 50 KG OR MORE:** 200–300 mg q12h. **WEIGHING LESS THAN 50 KG:** 9 mg/kg q12h. **Maximum:** 350 mg/dose. **CHILDREN 2–11 YRS:** 9 mg/kg q12h. **Maximum:** 350 mg/dose.

Candidemia, Other Deep Tissue *Candida* Infections

IV: ADULTS, ELDERLY, ADOLESCENTS 15 YRS AND OLDER: Initially, 400 mg (6 mg/kg) q12h for 2 doses, then 200 mg (3 mg/kg) IV or PO q12h. **CHILDREN 12–14 YRS WEIGHING 50 KG OR MORE:** 400 mg (6 mg/kg) q12h for 2 doses, then 4 mg/kg q12h. **WEIGHING LESS THAN 50 KG:** 9 mg/kg q12h for 2 doses, then 8 mg/kg q12h. **CHILDREN 2–11 YRS:** 9 mg/kg q12h for 2 doses, then 8 mg/kg q12h.

PO: ADULTS, ELDERLY, ADOLESCENTS 15 YRS AND OLDER: See IV. **CHILDREN 12–14 YRS WEIGHING 50 KG OR MORE:** 200 mg (3 mg/kg) q12h. **WEIGHING LESS THAN 50**

V

KG: 9 mg/kg q12h. **Maximum:** 350 mg/dose. **CHILDREN 2–11 YRS:** 9 mg/kg q12h. **Maximum:** 350 mg/dose.

Esophageal Candidiasis

PO: ADULTS, ELDERLY, ADOLESCENTS 15 YRS AND OLDER WEIGHING 40 KG OR MORE: 200 mg q12h. **Maximum:** 600 mg daily. **WEIGHING LESS THAN 40 KG:** 100 mg q12h. **Maximum:** 300 mg daily. **CHILDREN 12–14 YRS WEIGHING 50 KG OR GREATER:** 200 mg q12h. **WEIGHING LESS THAN 50 KG:** 9 mg/kg q12h. **Maximum:** 350 mg/dose. **CHILDREN 2–11 YRS:** 9 mg/kg q12h. **Maximum:** 350 mg/dose.

Scedosporiosis, Fusariosis

IV: ADULTS, EDLERLY: Initially, 6 mg/kg q12h for 2 doses, then 4 mg/kg q12h for at least 7 days. **PO: WEIGHING 40 KG OR MORE:** 200 mg q12h. **WEIGHING LESS THAN 40 KG:** 100 mg q12h.

Dosage in Pts Receiving Phenytoin

IV: Increase maintenance dose to 5 mg/kg q12h.

PO: Increase 200 mg q12h to 400 mg q12h (pts weighing 40 kg or more) or 100 mg q12h to 200 mg q12h (pts weighing less than 40 kg).

Dosage in Pts Receiving Efavirenz

Increase dose to 400 mg q12h and reduce efavirenz to 300 mg/day.

Dosage in Renal Impairment

No dose adjustment. IV dosing not recommended in pts with CrCl 50 mL/min or less.

Dosage in Hepatic Impairment

Mild to moderate impairment: Reduce maintenance dose by 50%. **Severe impairment:** Use only if benefits outweigh risks. Monitor closely for toxicity.

SIDE EFFECTS

Frequent (20%–6%): Abnormal vision, fever, nausea, rash, vomiting. **Occasional (5%–2%):** Headache, chills, hallucinations, photophobia, tachycardia, hypertension.

ADVERSE EFFECTS/TOXIC REACTIONS

Hepatotoxicity (jaundice, hepatitis, hepatic failure), acute renal failure have occurred in severely ill pts.

NURSING CONSIDERATIONS

BASELINE ASSESSMENT

Obtain BMP, LFT; ECG. Correct electrolyte deficiencies prior to initiating treatment. Receive full medication history and screen for interactions. Question medical history as listed in Precautions.

INTERVENTION/EVALUATION

Monitor serum renal function, LFT. Monitor visual function (visual acuity, visual field, color perception) for drug therapy lasting longer than 28 days.

PATIENT/FAMILY TEACHING

• Take at least 1 hr before or 1 hr after a meal. • Avoid grapefruit products. • Report visual changes (blurred vision, photophobia, yellowing of skin/eyes). • Avoid performing hazardous tasks if changes in vision occur. • Avoid direct sunlight. • Women of childbearing potential should use effective contraception.

vorinostat

vor-**in**-o-stat
(Zolinza)

Do not confuse vorinostat with Votrient.

◆CLASSIFICATION

PHARMACOTHERAPEUTIC: Histone deacetylase (HDAC) inhibitor. **CLINICAL:** Antineoplastic.

USES

Treatment of cutaneous manifestations in pts with cutaneous T-cell lymphoma (CTCL) with progressive, persistent, or

V

recurrent disease, on or following two systemic therapies.

PRECAUTIONS

Contraindications: Hypersensitivity to vorinostat. **Cautions:** Diabetes, history of thrombosis events (DVT, PE); pts at risk for thrombosis (immobility, indwelling venous catheter/access device, morbid obesity, underlying atherosclerosis, genetic hypercoagulable conditions); pts at risk for QTc interval prolongation (congenital long QT syndrome, HF, medications that prolong QTc interval, hypokalemia, hypomagnesemia); pts at risk for bleeding (e.g., history of intracranial, GI, genitourinary bleeding; coagulation disorders, recent trauma, concomitant use of anticoagulants, antiplatelets). Use caution during perioperative period in pts requiring bowel surgery.

ACTION

Inhibits activity of histone deacetylase enzymes that catalyze removal of acetyl groups from protein lysine residues, causing accumulation of acetylated histones. **Therapeutic Effect:** Terminates cell growth, causes apoptosis.

PHARMACOKINETICS

Protein binding: 71%. Metabolized to inactive metabolites. Excreted in urine. **Half-life:** 2 hrs.

LIFESPAN CONSIDERATIONS

Pregnancy/Lactation: May cause fetal harm. Unknown if distributed in breast milk. **Children:** Safety and efficacy not established. **Elderly:** No age-related precautions noted.

INTERACTIONS

DRUG: May increase effect of **warfarin. Valproic acid** increases risk of GI bleeding, thrombocytopenia. **QT interval–prolonging medications (e.g., amiodarone, azithromycin, ciprofloxacin, haloperidol, methadone, sotalol)** may increase risk of QTc interval prolongation. **HERBAL:** None significant. **FOOD:** None known. **LAB VALUES:** May decrease serum calcium, potassium, sodium, phosphate, platelet count. May increase serum glucose, creatinine; urine protein.

AVAILABILITY (Rx)

Capsules: 100 mg.

ADMINISTRATION/HANDLING

PO

- Do not break, crush, dissolve, or divide capsules. • Give with food. • Maintain adequate hydration during treatment.

INDICATIONS/ROUTES/DOSAGE

Cutaneous T-Cell Lymphoma (CTCL)

PO: ADULTS, ELDERLY: 400 mg once daily with food. Continue until disease progression or unacceptable toxicity.

Dose Modification

Intolerance or toxicity: Reduce dose to 300 mg once daily. **Unable to tolerate daily dose:** May further reduce to 300 mg once daily for 5 consecutive days per wk (5 out of 7 days).

Dosage in Renal Impairment

Use caution.

Dosage in Hepatic Impairment

Mild to moderate impairment: 300 mg once daily. **Severe impairment:** 100–200 mg once daily.

SIDE EFFECTS

Frequent (50%–24%): Fatigue, diarrhea, nausea, altered taste, anorexia. **Occasional (21%–11%):** Weight decrease, muscle spasms, alopecia, dry mouth, chills, vomiting, constipation, dizziness, peripheral edema, headache, pruritus, cough, fever.

ADVERSE EFFECTS/TOXIC REACTIONS

Thrombocytopenia occurs in 25% of pts, anemia in 15%. Pulmonary embolism occurs in 4% of pts. Deep vein thrombosis (DVT) occurs rarely.

NURSING CONSIDERATIONS

BASELINE ASSESSMENT

Obtain CBC, BMP; PT/INR in pts taking concomitant warfarin; pregnancy test in females of reproductive potential. Screen for active infection. Question history of thrombosis (DVT, PE). Receive full medication history and screen for interactions.

INTERVENTION/EVALUATION

Monitor CBC, serum electrolytes q2wks for 2 mos, then monthly. Replace electrolyte as indicated to prevent cardiac arrhythmias. Monitor for symptoms of DVT (leg or arm pain/swelling), PE (chest pain, dyspnea, tachycardia). Bleeding of any kind can be life-threatening and must be treated promptly. Encourage fluid intake, approximately 2 L/day input. Assess for evidence of dehydration. Provide antiemetics to control nausea/vomiting. Monitor daily pattern of bowel activity, stool consistency.

PATIENT/FAMILY TEACHING

• Drink at least 2 L/day of fluids to prevent dehydration. • Treatment may cause life-threatening blood clots; report symptoms of DVT (swelling, pain, hot feeling in the arms or legs; discoloration of extremity), lung embolism (difficulty breathing, chest pain, rapid heart rate). • Use effective contraception to avoid pregnancy. Do not breastfeed. • Treatment may increase risk of bleeding. Report bleeding of any kind.

V

vortioxetine

vor-tye-**ox**-e-teen
(Trintellix)

■ **BLACK BOX ALERT** ■ Antidepressants have an increased risk of suicidal ideation and behavior in children, adolescents, and young adults. Monitor closely for worsening or emergence of suicidal thoughts and behaviors.

Do not confuse vortioxetine with FLUoxetine, PARoxetine, or venlafaxine.

◆ CLASSIFICATION

PHARMACOTHERAPEUTIC: Selective serotonin reuptake inhibitor (SSRI). **CLINICAL:** Antidepressant.

USES

Treatment of major depressive disorder.

PRECAUTIONS

Contraindications: Hypersensitivity to vortioxetine. Use of monoamine oxidase inhibitors (MAOIs) intended to treat psychiatric disorders concurrently or within 21 days of stopping vortioxetine; do not use vortioxetine within 14 days of stopping an MAOI. Initiation of vortioxetine in pts receiving linezolid or intravenous methylene blue. **Cautions:** Dehydration, hepatic impairment, elderly, pts at risk for bleeding (e.g., history of intracranial/GI/genitourinary bleeding, coagulation disorders, recent trauma, concomitant use of anticoagulants, antiplatelets); history of suicidal ideation and behavior; family history of bipolar disorder, mania, hypomania.

ACTION

Blocks reuptake of neurotransmitter serotonin at CNS presynaptic membranes, increasing availability at postsynaptic receptor sites. **Therapeutic Effect:** Relieves depression.

PHARMACOKINETICS

Widely distributed. Metabolized in liver. Protein binding: 98%. Peak plasma concentration: 7–11 hrs. Steady state reached within 2 wks. Excreted in urine (59%), feces (26%). **Half-life:** 66 hrs.

⌛ LIFESPAN CONSIDERATIONS

Pregnancy/Lactation: May cause fetal harm when administered in third trimester. Unknown if distributed in breast milk. Exposed neonates are at increased risk of apnea, cyanosis, prolonged hospitalization, pulmonary hypertension, seizures, serotonin syndrome. **Children:** Safety and efficacy not established in pediatric population. **Elderly:** May have increased risk of dehydration, hyponatremia.

INTERACTIONS

DRUG: **Strong CYP3A4 inducers (e.g., carBAMazepine, phenytoin, rifAMPin)** may decrease concentration/effects. **Strong CYP2D6 inhibitors (e.g., buPROPion, FLUoxetine, PARoxetine)** may increase concentration/effect. **MAOIs (e.g., phenelzine, selegiline)** contraindicated; may cause malignant hyperthermia, hypertensive crisis, hyperreflexia, seizures, serotonin syndrome. **Alcohol** may increase adverse effects. **Serotonergic drugs (e.g., busPIRone, linezolid, lithium, traMADol)** may increase risk of serotonin syndrome. **Anticoagulants, antiplatelets, NSAIDs** may increase risk of bleeding. HERBAL: **St. John's wort** may decrease concentration/effect. **Herbals with anticoagulant/antiplatelet properties (e.g., garlic, ginger, ginkgo biloba), glucosamine** may increase risk of bleeding. FOOD: None known. LAB VALUES: May decrease serum sodium.

AVAILABILITY (Rx)

Tablets: 5 mg, 10 mg, 20 mg.

ADMINISTRATION/HANDLING

PO

- Give without regard to food. May administer with milk or food if GI upset occurs.

INDICATIONS/ROUTES/DOSAGE

Major Depressive Disorder

PO: ADULTS/ELDERLY: Initially, 10 mg once daily. May increase to 20 mg as tolerated. **Maintenance:** 5–20 mg once daily.

Dose Modification

Concomitant use of strong CYP2D6 inhibitors: Reduce dose by half of intended therapy. **Maximum:** 10 mg once daily. **Concomitant use of strong CYP inducers:** If coadministered for more than 14 days, consider increasing vortioxetine dose. **Maximum:** Do not exceed more than 3 times original dose. **CYP2D6 poor metabolizers: Maximum:** 10 mg once daily.

Discontinuation

Gradually taper dose to minimize incidence of withdrawal symptoms and to allow detection of re-emerging symptoms.

Dosage in Renal Impairment

No dose adjustment.

Dosage in Hepatic Impairment

Mild to moderate impairment: No dose adjustment. **Severe impairment:** Not recommended.

SIDE EFFECTS

Frequent (32%–22%): Nausea, sexual dysfunction. **Occasional (10%–3%):** Diarrhea, dizziness, dry mouth, constipation, vomiting, flatulence, abnormal dreams, pruritus.

ADVERSE EFFECTS/TOXIC REACTIONS

Life-threatening serotonin syndrome may include mental status changes (agitation, hallucinations, delirium, coma), autonomic instability (tachycardia, labile blood pressure, dizziness, sweating, flushing, hyperthermia), neuromuscular symptoms (tremor, rigidity, myoclonus [localized muscle twitching], hyperactive reflexes, incoordination), seizures, GI symptoms (nausea, vomiting, diarrhea). May increase risk of bleeding events such as ecchymosis, hematoma, epistaxis (nosebleed), petechiae. Mania/hypomania may indicate baseline bipolar disorder. Syndrome of inappropriate antidiuretic hormone (SIADH), also known as water intoxication or dilutional hyponatremia, may induce seizures, coma, or death. Angioedema, dyspnea, rash may indicate allergic reaction. May increase risk of suicidal ideation and behavior once treatment is therapeutic. May alter sexual

V

drive, ease of arousal, ease of reaching orgasm, or cause erectile dysfunction in men or decreased lubrication in women.

NURSING CONSIDERATIONS

BASELINE ASSESSMENT

Obtain serum electrolytes. Note serum sodium level. Assess appearance, behavior, speech pattern, level of interest, mood. Assess risk for bleeding. Receive full medication history including herbal products.

INTERVENTION/EVALUATION

Monitor serum sodium levels. Screen for signs of SIADH (confusion, seizures). Diligently screen for suicidal ideation and behavior; new onset or worsening of anxiety, depression, mood disorder. Assess for improvement of depression (improved emotion, self-image, interest in activities; decreased agitation, loneliness, self-harm). Monitor for symptoms of serotonin syndrome, mania/hypomania. Monitor for allergic reactions.

PATIENT/FAMILY TEACHING

• Report neurologic changes: confusion, excessive talking, hallucinations, headache, hyperactivity, insomnia, racing thoughts, seizure-like activity, tremors; sexual dysfunction; fever; or any type of allergic reaction. • Avoid tasks that require alertness, motor skills until response to drug is established (may cause dizziness, drowsiness). • Seek immediate medical attention if thoughts of suicide, new onset or worsening of anxiety, depression, or changes in mood occur. • Report bleeding, bruising. • Severe allergic reaction may occur; report rash; swelling of the face, tongue, throat.

V

warfarin

TOP 100 HIGH ALERT

war-far-in

(Coumadin, Jantoven)

BLACK BOX ALERT May cause major or fatal bleeding. Risk factors include history of GI bleeding, hypertension, cerebrovascular disease, heart disease, malignancy, trauma, anemia, renal insufficiency, age 65 yrs and older, high anticoagulation factor (INR greater than 4). Consider cardiac/hepatic function, age, nutritional status, concurrent medications, risk of bleeding when dosing warfarin. Genetic variations have been identified as factors associated with dosage and bleeding risk. Genotyping tests are available. **Do not confuse Coumadin with Kemadrin, or Jantoven with Janumet or Januvia.**

CLASSIFICATION

PHARMACOTHERAPEUTIC: Vitamin K antagonist. **CLINICAL:** Anticoagulant.

USES

Prophylaxis, treatment of thromboembolic disorders and embolic complications arising from atrial fibrillation or valve replacement. Risk reduction of systemic embolism following MI (e.g., recurrent MI, stroke). **OFF-LABEL:** Adjunct treatment in transient ischemic attacks.

PRECAUTIONS

Contraindications: Hypersensitivity to warfarin. Hemorrhagic tendencies (e.g., cerebral aneurysms, bleeding from GI tract), recent or potential surgery of eye or CNS, neurosurgical procedures, open wounds, severe uncontrolled or malignant hypertension, spinal puncture procedures, uncontrolled bleeding, ulcers, unreliable or noncompliant pts, unsupervised pts, blood dyscrasias, pericarditis or pericardial effusion, pregnancy (except in women with mechanical heart valves at high risk for thromboembolism), bacterial endocarditis, threatened abortion. Major regional lumbar block anesthesia or traumatic surgery, eclampsia/preeclampsia. **Cautions:** Active tuberculosis, acute infection, diabetes, heparin-induced thrombocytopenia and deep vein thrombosis, pts at risk for hemorrhage, moderate to severe renal impairment, moderate to severe hypertension, thyroid disease, polycythemia vera, vasculitis, open wound, menstruating and postpartum women, indwelling catheters, trauma, prolonged dietary deficiencies, disruption of GI normal flora, history of peptic ulcer disease, protein C deficiency, elderly.

ACTION

Interferes with hepatic synthesis of vitamin K–dependent clotting factors, resulting in depletion of coagulation factors II, VII, IX, X. **Therapeutic Effect:** Prevents further extension of formed existing clot; prevents new clot formation, secondary thromboembolic complications.

PHARMACOKINETICS

Route	Onset	Peak	Duration
PO	1.5–3 days	5–7 days	2–5 days

Widely distributed. Protein binding: 99%. Metabolized in liver. Primarily excreted in urine. Not removed by hemodialysis. **Half-life:** 20–60 hrs.

LIFESPAN CONSIDERATIONS

Pregnancy/Lactation: Contraindicated in pregnancy (fetal, neonatal hemorrhage, intrauterine death). Crosses placenta; is not distributed in breast milk. **Children:** More susceptible to effect. **Elderly:** Increased risk of hemorrhage; lower dosage recommended.

INTERACTIONS

DRUG: **Amiodarone, azole antifungals (e.g., fluconazole), cimetidine, disulfiram, sulfamethoxazole-trimethoprim, levothyroxine, metroNIDAZOLE, NSAIDs (e.g., diclofenac, meloxicam, naproxen), omeprazole, platelet aggregation inhibitors (e.g., clopidogrel), salicylates (e.g.,**

W

aspirin), thrombolytic agents (e.g., alteplase), thyroid hormones (e.g., levothyroxine), may increase effect. **Strong CYP3A inducers (e.g., carBAMazepine, phenytoin, rifAMPin), nafcillin, oral contraceptives, sucralfate, vitamin K** may decrease effects. **HERBAL: Herbals with anticoagulant/antiplatelet properties (e.g., garlic, ginger, ginkgo biloba), fenugreek, glucosamine** may increase risk of bleeding. **FOOD: Foods rich in vitamin K (e.g., spinach, brussels sprouts, meat)** may decrease effect. **Cranberry juice** may increase effect. **LAB VALUES:** None known.

AVAILABILITY (Rx)

Tablets: ***(Coumadin, Jantoven):*** 1 mg, 2 mg, 2.5 mg, 3 mg, 4 mg, 5 mg, 6 mg, 7.5 mg, 10 mg.

ADMINISTRATION/HANDLING

PO

• Give without regard to food. Give with food if GI upset occurs. • Give at same time each day.

INDICATIONS/ROUTES/DOSAGE

◀ALERT▶ Initial dosing must be individualized with use of recommended institutional protocols. Response is influenced by numerous factors (e.g., age, organ function, genetic variations).

Anticoagulant

PO: ADULTS, ELDERLY: Initially, 2–5 mg once daily (for most pts). **Maintenance:** 2–10 mg once daily. Once INR is therapeutic and stable, subsequent dosage may be guided by use of a maintenance dosing nomogram. INR should be checked wkly when out of range and approximately q4wks when stable and therapeutic.

Dosage in Renal/Hepatic Impairment

No dose adjustment. Closely monitor INR.

SIDE EFFECTS

Occasional: GI distress (nausea, anorexia, abdominal cramps, diarrhea). **Rare:** Hypersensitivity reaction (dermatitis, urticaria), esp. in those sensitive to aspirin.

ADVERSE EFFECTS/TOXIC REACTIONS

Bleeding complications ranging from local ecchymoses to major hemorrhage (intracranial hemorrhage, GI/GU/nasal/oral/rectal bleeding) may occur. Hepatotoxicity, blood dyscrasias, necrosis, vasculitis, local thrombosis occur rarely. **Antidote:** Vitamin K. Amount based on INR, significance of bleeding. Range: 2.5–10 mg given orally or slow IV infusion (see Appendix J for dosage).

NURSING CONSIDERATIONS

BASELINE ASSESSMENT

Obtain CBC, PT/INR before administration and daily following therapy initiation. Obtain genotyping prior to initiating therapy if available. Screen for major active bleeding. Question recent history of bleeding, recent trauma, surgical procedures, epidural anesthesia.

INTERVENTION/EVALUATION

When stabilized, follow with INR determination q4–6wks. Assess CBC for anemia; urine/stool for occult blood. Monitor for hypotension; complaints of abdominal/back pain, severe headache, confusion, seizures, hemiparesis, aphasia (may be sign of hemorrhage). Question for increase in amount of menstrual discharge. Assess for ecchymoses, petechiae. Check for excessive bleeding from minor cuts, scratches.

PATIENT/FAMILY TEACHING

• Blood levels will be monitored routinely. • Do not take, discontinue any other medication except on advice of physician. • Avoid alcohol, aspirin, drastic dietary changes. • Consult with physician before surgery, dental work. • Urine may become red-orange. • Falls, subtle injuries, esp. head or abdominal trauma, can be life-threatening. • Report bleeding, bruising, red or brown urine, black stools. • Use electric razor, soft toothbrush to prevent bleeding. • Report coffee-ground vomitus, blood-tinged mucus from cough. • Seek immediate medical attention for stroke-like symptoms (confusion, difficulty speaking, headache, one-sided weakness); bloody stool or urine.

zanamivir

zan-**am**-i-veer
(Relenza Diskhaler)

◆CLASSIFICATION

PHARMACOTHERAPEUTIC: Neuraminidase inhibitor. **CLINICAL:** Antiviral, anti-influenza.

USES

Treatment of uncomplicated acute illness due to influenza virus A and B in adults, children 7 yrs and older who have been symptomatic for less than 2 days. Prevention of influenza A and B in adults and children 5 yrs and older.

PRECAUTIONS

Contraindications: Hypersensitivity to zanamivir. **Cautions:** Not recommended in respiratory disease (e.g., COPD, asthma).

ACTION

Inhibits influenza virus enzyme neuraminidase, essential for viral replication. **Therapeutic Effect:** Prevents viral release from infected cells.

PHARMACOKINETICS

Widely distributed. Protein binding: less than 10%. Not metabolized. Excreted unchanged in urine. **Half-life:** 2.5–5.1 hrs.

⌛ LIFESPAN CONSIDERATIONS

Pregnancy/Lactation: Unknown if drug crosses placenta or is distributed in breast milk. **Children:** Safety and efficacy not established in pts younger than 7 yrs (treatment) or younger than 5 yrs (prevention). **Elderly:** No age-related precautions noted.

INTERACTIONS

DRUG: May decrease levels/effect of **influenza virus vaccine. HERBAL:** None significant. **FOOD:** None known. **LAB VALUES:** None significant.

AVAILABILITY (Rx)

Powder for Inhalation: 5 mg/blister.

ADMINISTRATION/HANDLING

Inhalation

• Instruct pt to use Diskhaler device provided, exhale completely; then, holding mouthpiece 1 inch away from lips, inhale and hold breath as long as possible before exhaling. • Rinse mouth with water immediately after inhalation (prevents mouth/throat dryness). • Store at room temperature.

INDICATIONS/ROUTES/DOSAGE

Treatment of Influenza Virus

Inhalation: ADULTS, ELDERLY, CHILDREN 7 YRS AND OLDER: 2 inhalations (one 5-mg blister per inhalation for total dose of 10 mg) twice daily (approximately 12 hrs apart) for 5 days.

Prevention of Influenza Virus

Inhalation: ADULTS, ELDERLY, CHILDREN 5 YRS AND OLDER: 2 inhalations (10 mg) once daily for duration of exposure period (7 days for household exposure, 28 days for community exposure).

Dosage in Renal/Hepatic Impairment

No dose adjustment.

SIDE EFFECTS

Occasional (3%–2%): Diarrhea, sinusitis, nausea, bronchitis, cough, dizziness, headache. **Rare (less than 1.5%):** Malaise, fatigue, fever, abdominal pain, myalgia, arthralgia, urticaria.

ADVERSE EFFECTS/TOXIC REACTIONS

May cause neutropenia. Bronchospasm may occur in those with history of COPD, bronchial asthma. Neuropsychiatric events (e.g., confusion, seizures, hallucinations) have been reported.

Z

NURSING CONSIDERATIONS

BASELINE ASSESSMENT

Pts requiring an inhaled bronchodilator at same time as zanamivir should use the bronchodilator before zanamivir administration.

INTERVENTION/EVALUATION

Provide assistance if dizziness occurs. Monitor daily pattern of bowel activity, stool consistency.

PATIENT/FAMILY TEACHING

• Follow manufacturer guidelines for use of delivery device. • Avoid contact with those who are at high risk for influenza. • Continue treatment for full 5-day course. • In pts with respiratory disease, an inhaled bronchodilator should be readily available.

zanubrutinib

zan-ue-**broo**-ti-nib
(Brukinsa)
Do not confuse zanubrutinib with acalabrutinib or ibrutinib; Brukinsa with Imbruvica.

CLASSIFICATION

PHARMACOTHERAPEUTIC: Bruton tyrosine kinase (BTK) inhibitor. **CLINICAL:** Antineoplastic.

USES

Treatment of adults with relapsed or refractory mantle cell lymphoma (MCL) who have received at least one prior therapy.

PRECAUTIONS

Contraindications: Hypersensitivity to zanubrutinib. **Cautions:** Baseline cytopenias, hepatic/renal impairment, conditions predisposing to infection (e.g., diabetes, renal failure, immunocompromised pts, open wounds), chronic opportunistic infections (e.g., herpesvirus infection, hepatitis B virus [HBV] infection, fungal infections), pts at risk for bleeding (e.g., history of intracranial/GI/genitourinary bleeding, coagulation disorders, recent trauma, concomitant use of anticoagulants, antiplatelets); history of atrial fibrillation, atrial flutter, cardiac disease. Avoid concomitant use of strong or moderate CYP3A4 inducers.

ACTION

Highly selective BTK inhibitor that forms a covalent bond with a cysteine residue in the BTK active site, inhibiting activity of BKT. BKT is a signaling molecule of pathways necessary for B-cell proliferation. **Therapeutic Effect:** Inhibits malignant B-cell proliferation and reduces tumor growth.

PHARMACOKINETICS

Rapidly absorbed and widely distributed. Metabolized in liver. Protein binding: 94%. Peak plasma concentration: 2 hrs. Excreted in feces (87%), urine (8%). **Half-life:** 2–4 hrs.

LIFESPAN CONSIDERATIONS

Pregnancy/Lactation: Avoid pregnancy; may cause fetal harm. Females of reproductive potential and males with female partners of reproductive potential must use effective contraception during treatment and for at least 1 wk after discontinuation. Unknown if distributed in breast milk. Breastfeeding not recommended during treatment and for at least 2 wks after discontinuation. **Children:** Safety and efficacy not established. **Elderly:** No age-related precautions noted.

INTERACTIONS

DRUG: May enhance effect/adverse effects of **anticoagulants (e.g., heparin, warfarin), antiplatelets (e.g., aspirin, clopidogrel)**, increasing risk of bleeding. **Strong CYP3A4 inhibitors (e.g., clarithromycin, ketoconazole, ritonavir), moderate CYP3A inhibitors (e.g., erythromycin, ciprofloxacin, dilTIAZem, fluconazole, verapamil)** may increase concentration/effect. **Strong**

Z

CYP3A4 inducers (e.g., rifAMPin, phenytoin, carBAMazepine, phenobarbital), moderate CYP3A inducers (e.g., bosentan, nafcillin) may decrease concentration/effect. May decrease effects of **BCG (intravesical), vaccines (live).** May increase toxic effects **of natalizumab, live vaccines. Pimecrolimus, tacrolimus** may increase adverse/toxic effect. **HERBAL: Echinacea** may decrease therapeutic effect. **FOOD:** None known. **LAB VALUES:** May increase serum ALT, bilirubin, uric acid. May decrease Hgb, leukocytes, lymphocytes, platelets, neutrophils, RBCs.

AVAILABILITY (Rx)

Capsules: 80 mg.

ADMINISTRATION/HANDLING

PO

• Give without regard to food. • Administer capsule whole; do not break, cut, or open. • If a dose is missed, administer as soon as possible on same day, then follow usual dosing schedule the following day.

INDICATIONS/ROUTES/DOSAGE

MCL

PO: ADULTS, ELDERLY: 160 mg twice daily or 320 mg once daily. Continue until disease progression or unacceptable toxicity.

Dose Modification

Based on Common Terminology Criteria for Adverse Events (CTCAE). **Grade 3 or 4 nonhematologic toxicity; Grade 3 thrombocytopenia *with* bleeding; Grade 4 thrombocytopenia (lasting more than 10 days); Grade 3 febrile neutropenia; Grade 4 neutropenia lasting more than 7 days: (First occurrence):** Withhold treatment until improved to Grade 1 or 0 (or baseline), then resume at 160 mg twice daily or 320 mg once daily. **(Second occurrence):** Withhold treatment until improved to Grade 1 or 0 (or baseline), then resume at 80 mg twice daily or 160 mg once daily. **(Third occurrence):** Withhold treatment until improved to Grade 1 or 0 (or baseline), then resume at 80 mg once daily. **(Fourth occurrence):** Permanently discontinue.

Concomitant Use of CYP3A Inhibitors/Inducers

Strong CYP3A inhibitors: Reduce dose to 80 mg once daily. **Moderate CYP3A inhibitors:** Reduce dose to 80 mg twice daily. **Strong or moderate CYP3A inhibitors:** Avoid concomitant use.

Dosage in Renal Impairment

Mild to moderate impairment: No dose adjustment. **Severe impairment, hemodialysis:** Monitor for adverse reactions/toxic effects.

Dosage in Hepatic Impairment

Mild to moderate impairment: No dose adjustment. **Severe impairment:** Reduce dose to 80 mg twice daily.

SIDE EFFECTS

Frequent (36%–23%): Rash, diarrhea. **Occasional (14%–12%):** Bruising, musculoskeletal pain, myalgia, back pain, arthralgia, constipation, cough, hypertension. **Rare (4%):** Headache.

ADVERSE EFFECTS/TOXIC REACTIONS

Myelosuppression (anemia, leukopenia, lymphopenia, neutropenia, thrombocytopenia) is an expected response to therapy, but more severe reactions including febrile neutropenia, hemorrhagic thrombocytopenia may occur. Life-threatening hemorrhagic events including intracranial hemorrhage, GI bleeding, hematuria, hemothorax occurred in 2% of pts. Petechiae, purpura reported in 50% of pts. Life-threatening bacterial, invasive fungal, viral, other opportunistic infections; pneumonia may occur. Grade 3 infections reported in 23% of pts. Reactivation of HBV infection was reported. UTI reported in 11% of pts. New primary malignancies including basal cell carcinoma, squamous cell carcinoma (6% of pts), nonskin carcinomas (9% of pts) have occurred. Atrial fibrillation/atrial flutter reported in 2% of pts.

NURSING CONSIDERATIONS

BASELINE ASSESSMENT

Obtain CBC; PT/INR (if on anticoagulation therapy); pregnancy test in female of reproductive potential. Confirm compliance of effective contraception. Assess risk for bleeding. Question history of atrial fibrillation, atrial flutter, cardiac disease; intracranial/GI/genitourinary bleeding, coagulation disorders, recent trauma; previous skin cancers. Assess usual bowel movement patterns, stool characteristics. Receive full medication history and screen for interactions. Screen for active infection. Consider prophylactic treatment of herpes simplex virus, *pneumocystis jirovecii* pneumonia, other infections. Offer emotional support.

INTERVENTION/EVALUATION

Monitor CBC periodically for cytopenias. Diligently monitor for infections (cough, fever, fatigue), esp. respiratory tract infections, herpesvirus infection, opportunistic infections, sepsis. If serious infection or sepsis occurs, initiate appropriate antimicrobial therapy. Monitor for HBV reactivation, new malignancies (skin and nonskin). Obtain ECG if chest pain, dyspnea, palpitations occur. Monitor for hemorrhagic events including intracranial hemorrhage (altered mental status, aphasia, blindness, hemiparesis, unequal pupils, seizures), GI bleeding (hematemesis, melena, rectal bleeding), genitourinary bleeding (hematuria), epistaxis. Monitor daily pattern of bowel activity, stool consistency. Monitor for drug toxicities if discontinuation or dose reduction of concomitant CYP3A inhibitor is unavoidable.

PATIENT/FAMILY TEACHING

• Treatment may depress your immune system and reduce your ability to fight infection. Report symptoms of infection such as body aches, burning with urination, chills, cough, fatigue, fever. Avoid those with active infection. • Report symptoms of bone marrow depression such as bruising, fatigue, fever, shortness of breath, weight loss; bleeding easily, bloody urine or stool. • Treatment may cause new cancers; reactivation of HBV. • Report liver problems (abdominal pain, bruising, clay-colored stool, dark or amber-colored urine, yellowing of the skin or eyes), heart arrhythmias (chest pain, dizziness, fainting, palpitations, slow or rapid heart rate, irregular heart rate); symptoms of hemorrhagic stroke (confusion, difficulty speaking, one-sided weakness or paralysis, loss of vision, seizures). • Immediately report bleeding of any kind. • Use effective contraception to avoid pregnancy. Do not breastfeed. • There is a high risk of interactions with other medications. Do not take newly prescribed medications unless approved by prescriber who originally started therapy. • Avoid grapefruit products, herbal supplements (esp. St. John's wort).

zidovudine

zye-**doe**-vue-deen
(Retrovir)

BLACK BOX ALERT Neutropenia, severe anemia may occur. Lactic acidosis, severe hepatomegaly with steatosis (fatty liver), including fatalities, have occurred. Symptomatic myopathy, myositis associated with prolonged use.

Do not confuse Retrovir with acyclovir or ritonavir.

FIXED-COMBINATION(S)

Combivir: zidovudine/lamiVUDine (an antiviral): 300 mg/150 mg. **Trizivir:** zidovudine/lamiVUDine/abacavir (an antiviral): 300 mg/150 mg/300 mg.

CLASSIFICATION

PHARMACOTHERAPEUTIC: Nucleoside reverse transcriptase inhibitors. **CLINICAL:** Antiretroviral.

Z

USES

Treatment of HIV infection in combination with at least two other antiretroviral agents. Prevention of maternal/fetal HIV transmission. **OFF-LABEL:** Prophylaxis in health care workers at risk for acquiring HIV after occupational exposure (part of multidrug regimen).

PRECAUTIONS

Contraindications: Potentially life-threatening allergic reactions to zidovudine or its components. **Cautions:** Bone marrow compromise, renal/hepatic impairment. Combination with interferon with or without ribavirin in HIV/hepatitis C virus (HCV) coinfection.

ACTION

Interferes with viral RNA-dependent DNA polymerase, an enzyme necessary for viral HIV replication. **Therapeutic Effect:** Slows HIV replication, reducing progression of HIV infection.

PHARMACOKINETICS

Widely distributed. Protein binding: 25%–38%. Metabolized in liver. Crosses blood-brain barrier and is widely distributed, including to CSF. Primarily excreted in urine. **Half-life:** 0.5–3 hrs (increased in renal impairment).

LIFESPAN CONSIDERATIONS

Pregnancy/Lactation: Unknown if drug crosses placenta or is distributed in breast milk. Unknown if fetal harm or effects on fertility can occur. **Children:** No age-related precautions noted. **Elderly:** Information not available.

Z

INTERACTIONS

DRUG: May decrease therapeutic effect of **cladribine, DOXOrubicin, ganciclovir, interferons, valganciclovir.** **HERBAL:** None significant. **FOOD:** None known. **LAB VALUES:** May increase mean corpuscular volume (MCV).

AVAILABILITY (Rx)

Capsules: 100 mg. **Injection Solution:** ***(Retrovir):*** 10 mg/mL. **Syrup:** 50 mg/5 mL. **Tablets:** 300 mg.

ADMINISTRATION/HANDLING

IV

Reconstitution • Dilute in D_5W to provide concentration no greater than 4 mg/mL.

Rate of administration • Infuse over 1 hr. May infuse over 30 min in neonates.

Storage • Refrigerate diluted solution for up to 24 hrs or store at room temperature for up to 8 hrs. • Do not use if solution is discolored or precipitate forms.

PO

• Keep capsules in cool, dry place. Protect from light. • Give without regard to food. • Space doses evenly around the clock. • Pt should maintain an upright position when given medication to prevent esophageal ulceration.

IV COMPATIBILITIES

Dexamethasone (Decadron), DOBUTamine (Dobutrex), DOPamine (Intropin), heparin, LORazepam (Ativan), morphine, potassium chloride.

INDICATIONS/ROUTES/DOSAGE

HIV Infection

PO: ADULTS, ELDERLY: 300 mg q12h. **CHILDREN 4 WKS TO 18 YRS WEIGHING 30 KG OR MORE:** 300 mg q12h. **WEIGHING 9–29 KG:** 9 mg/kg q12h. **WEIGHING 4–8 KG:** 12 mg/kg q12h. **PREMATURE NEONATES, GA 35 WKS OR MORE:** 4 mg/kg q12h, increase to 12 mg/kg q12h after 4 wks of age. **GA 30–34 WKS:** 2 mg/kg q12h for 2 wks, then 3 mg/kg q12h, then 12 mg/kg q12h after 6–8 wks. **GA LESS THAN 30 WKS:** 2 mg/kg q12h, then 3 mg/kg q12h at 4 wks of age, then 12 mg/kg q12h after 8–10 wks of age.

IV: ADULTS, ELDERLY, CHILDREN OLDER THAN 12 YRS: 1 mg/kg/dose q4h around the clock. **CHILDREN 12 YRS AND YOUNGER, FULL-TERM NEONATES:** 3 mg/kg/dose q12h. **OLDER THAN 4 WKS:** Increase to 9 mg/kg/dose q12h. **PREMATURE NEONATES:** 1.5–2.3 mg/kg/dose q12h based on gestation at birth. **6–10 WKS:** Increase to 9 mg/kg/dose q12h.

Prevention of Maternal/Fetal HIV Transmission

Note: Zidovudine should be given IV near delivery regardless of antepartum regimen or mode of delivery in women with HIV RNA level greater than 1,000 copies/mL (or unknown status). Other antiretrovirals should be continued orally. Zidovudine IV is not required in pts receiving HIV therapy with HIV RNA level less than 1,000 copies/mL near delivery.

IV: DURING LABOR AND DELIVERY: 2 mg/kg loading dose, then IV infusion of 1 mg/kg/hr until delivery. For scheduled cesarean section, begin IV zidovudine 3 hrs before surgery. **NEONATAL:** Begin 6–12 hrs after birth and continue for first 6 wks of life. Use IV route only until oral therapy can be administered.

PO: FULL-TERM INFANTS: 4 mg/kg/dose q12h (IV: 3 mg/kg/dose q12h). **INFANTS 30–34 WKS' GESTATION:** 2 mg/kg/dose q12h; increase to 3 mg/kg/dose at 2 wks of age (IV: 1.5 mg/kg/dose q12h; increase to 2.3 mg/kg/dose q12h at 2 wks of age). **INFANTS LESS THAN 30 WKS' GESTATION:** 2 mg/kg/dose q12h. (IV: 1.5 mg/kg/dose q12h.)

Dosage in Renal Impairment

ADULTS, ELDERLY: CrCl less than 15 mL/min, including hemodialysis or peritoneal dialysis: PO: 100 mg q8h or 300 mg once daily. **IV:** 1 mg/kg q6–8hr. **INFANTS OLDER THAN 6 WKS, CHILDREN, ADOLESCENTS: GFR 10 mL/min/1.73m^2 or greater:** No adjustment. **GFR less than 10 mL/min/1.73m^2:** Administer 50% of dose q8h.

Dosage in Hepatic Impairment

No dose adjustment.

SIDE EFFECTS

Expected (46%–42%): Nausea, headache. **Frequent (20%–16%):** Abdominal pain, asthenia, rash, fever, acne. **Occasional (12%–8%):** Diarrhea, anorexia, malaise, myalgia, drowsiness. **Rare (6%–5%):** Dizziness, paresthesia, vomiting, insomnia, dyspnea, altered taste.

ADVERSE EFFECTS/TOXIC REACTIONS

Anemia (occurring most commonly after 4–6 wks of therapy), granulocytopenia may occur in pts with pretherapy low baselines. Neurotoxicity (ataxia, fatigue, lethargy, nystagmus, seizures) may occur.

NURSING CONSIDERATIONS

BASELINE ASSESSMENT

Obtain CBC, CD4 cell count, HIV RNA plasma level, viral load. Obtain specimens for viral diagnostic tests before starting therapy (therapy may begin before results are obtained).

INTERVENTION/EVALUATION

Monitor CBC, CD4 cell count, HIV RNA plasma levels. Monitor for bleeding. Assess for headache, dizziness. Monitor daily pattern of bowel activity, stool consistency. Evaluate skin for acne, rash. Monitor for opportunistic infections (fever, chills, cough, myalgia). Monitor I&O, serum renal function, LFT.

PATIENT/FAMILY TEACHING

• Treatment is not a cure for HIV infection, nor does it reduce risk of transmission to others. • Do not take any medications without physician's approval. • Bleeding from gums, nose, rectum may occur and should be reported to physician immediately. • Dental work should be done before therapy or after blood counts return to normal (often wks after therapy has stopped). • Inform physician if muscle weakness, difficulty breathing, headache, inability to sleep, unusual bleeding, rash, signs of infection occur.

ziprasidone

zi-**pras**-i-done
(Geodon, Zeldox ✦)

■ BLACK BOX ALERT ■ Increased risk of mortality in elderly pts with dementia-related psychosis, mainly due to pneumonia, HF.

Do not confuse ziprasidone with traZODone.

◆ CLASSIFICATION

PHARMACOTHERAPEUTIC: Second-generation (atypical) antipsychotic. **CLINICAL:** Antipsychotic.

USES

Treatment of schizophrenia, acute agitation in pts with schizophrenia. Treatment of acute mania or mixed episodes associated with bipolar disorder with or without psychosis. Maintenance treatment of bipolar disorder as adjunct to lithium or valproic acid. **OFF-LABEL:** Major depressive disorder (adjunct to antidepressants).

PRECAUTIONS

Contraindications: Hypersensitivity to ziprasidone. Conditions associated with risk of prolonged QT interval, congenital long QT syndrome, concurrent use of other QT-prolongation medications (e.g., amiodarone, moxifloxacin, tacrolimus, thioridazine). Uncompensated HF. Recent MI. **Cautions:** Pts with bradycardia, hypokalemia, hypomagnesemia may be at greater risk for torsades de pointes. History of MI or unstable heart disease, seizure disorder, cardiac arrhythmias, disorders in which CNS depression is a feature; pts at risk for aspiration pneumonia, hypotension, suicide; elderly, diabetes, hepatic impairment, Parkinson's disease, pts with breast cancer or other prolactin-dependent tumors.

ACTION

Exact mechanism unknown. Antagonizes alpha-adrenergic, DOPamine, histamine, serotonin receptors; inhibits reuptake of serotonin, norepinephrine. **Therapeutic Effect:** Diminishes symptoms of schizophrenia, depression.

PHARMACOKINETICS

Widely distributed. Food increases bioavailability. Protein binding: 99%. Metabolized in liver. Excreted in feces. Not removed by hemodialysis. **Half-life: PO:** 7 hrs; **IM:** 2–5 hrs.

⌛ LIFESPAN CONSIDERATIONS

Pregnancy/Lactation: Unknown if drug crosses placenta or is distributed in breast milk. **Children:** Safety and efficacy not established. **Elderly:** No age-related precautions noted. Use caution.

INTERACTIONS

DRUG: Alcohol, CNS depressants (e.g., LORazepam, morphine, zolpidem) may increase CNS depression. **CarBAMazepine** may decrease concentration. **QT interval–prolonging medications (e.g., amiodarone, azithromycin, ciprofloxacin, haloperidol, methadone, sotalol)** may increase risk of QTc interval prolongation. **HERBAL: Herbals with sedative properties (e.g., chamomile, kava kava, valerian)** may increase CNS depression. **FOOD: All foods** enhance bioavailability. **LAB VALUES:** May prolong QT interval. May increase serum glucose, prolactin levels.

AVAILABILITY (Rx)

Capsules: 20 mg, 40 mg, 60 mg, 80 mg. **Injection, Powder for Reconstitution:** 20 mg.

Z

ADMINISTRATION/HANDLING

IM

• Store vials at room temperature; protect from light. • Reconstitute each vial with 1.2 mL Sterile Water for Injection to provide concentration of 20 mg/mL. • Reconstituted solution stable for 24 hrs at room temperature or 7 days if refrigerated.

PO

• Give with food containing at least 500 calories (increases bioavailability).

INDICATIONS/ROUTES/DOSAGE

◀ALERT▶ Dosage greater than 80 mg twice daily is not recommended in most pts. **To discontinue therapy:** Gradually discontinue to avoid withdrawal symptoms, minimize risk of relapses.

Schizophrenia

PO: ADULTS, ELDERLY: Initially, 20 mg twice daily with food. Titrate at intervals of no less than 2 days based on response and tolerability. **Maintenance:** 40 80 mg twice daily.

Acute Agitation (Schizophrenia)

IM: ADULTS, ELDERLY: 10 mg q2h or 20 mg q4h. **Maximum:** 40 mg/day. Switch to oral therapy as soon as possible.

Bipolar Disorder (Acute and maintenance as adjunct to lithium or valproate)

PO: ADULTS, ELDERLY (Acute): Initially, 40 mg twice daily. May increase to 60–80 mg twice daily on second day of treatment. **Maintenance:** 40–80 mg twice daily.

Dosage in Renal Impairment

Oral: No dose adjustment. **IM:** Use caution.

Dosage in Hepatic Impairment

Use caution.

SIDE EFFECTS

Frequent (30%–16%): Headache, drowsiness, dizziness. **Occasional:** Rash, orthostatic hypotension, weight gain, restlessness, constipation, dyspepsia. **Rare:** Hyperglycemia, priapism.

ADVERSE EFFECTS/TOXIC REACTIONS

Prolongation of QT interval (as seen on ECG) may produce torsades de pointes, a form of ventricular tachycardia.

NURSING CONSIDERATIONS

BASELINE ASSESSMENT

Obtain serum magnesium, potassium; ECG to assess risk for QT interval prolongation. Assess pt's behavior, appearance, emotional status, response to environment, speech pattern, thought content.

INTERVENTION/EVALUATION

Assess for therapeutic response (greater interest in surroundings, improved self-care, increased ability to concentrate, relaxed facial expression). Monitor weight.

PATIENT/FAMILY TEACHING

• Avoid tasks that require alertness, motor skills until response to drug is established. • Avoid alcohol. • Report chest pain, shortness of breathing, irregular heartbeats, fainting, palpitations.

ziv-aflibercept

ziv-a-**flib**-er-sept
(Zaltrap)

■ BLACK BOX ALERT ■ Severe, and sometimes fatal, hemorrhagic events including GI hemorrhage were reported in pts receiving concomitant FOLFIRI therapy. Do not initiate in pts with severe hemorrhage. Fatal GI perforation may occur. Discontinue treatment in pts with impaired wound healing. Withhold treatment for at least 4 wks prior to elective surgery. Do not resume treatment for at least 4 wks after major surgery until wound is fully healed.

Z

Do not confuse ziv-aflibercept with abatacept, Aricept, or etanercept.

◆CLASSIFICATION

PHARMACOTHERAPEUTIC: Vascular endothelial growth factor (VEGF) inhibitor. **CLINICAL:** Antineoplastic.

USES

Treatment of metastatic colorectal cancer (mCRC) (in combination with 5-fluorouracil, leucovorin, irinotecan [FOLFIRI]) in pts resistant to or has progressed following an oxaliplatin-containing regimen.

PRECAUTIONS

Contraindications: Hypersensitivity to ziv-aflibercept. **Cautions:** Baseline cytopenias, conditions predisposing to infection (e.g., diabetes, renal failure, immunocompromised pts, open wounds), pts at risk for bleeding (e.g., history of intracranial/GI/GU bleeding, coagulation disorders, recent trauma; concomitant use of anticoagulants, antiplatelet medication, NSAIDs), hypertension, elderly, history of arterial/venous thrombosis (e.g., CVA, DVT, MI, pulmonary embolism), GI perforation or hemorrhage.

ACTION

A recombinant fusion protein, comprising portions of binding domains of vascular endothelial growth factor (VEGF) receptors. Acts as a decoy receptor that prevents VEGF receptor binding/activation. **Therapeutic Effect:** Produces anti-angiogenesis/tumor regression.

PHARMACOKINETICS

Half-life: 6 days (range: 4–7 days).

LIFESPAN CONSIDERATIONS

Pregnancy/Lactation: Avoid pregnancy; may cause fetal harm. Females of reproductive potential and males should use effective contraception during therapy and for at least 3 mos after discontinuation. Unknown if distributed in breast milk. **Children:** Safety and efficacy not established. **Elderly:** May have increased risk of side effects, esp. diarrhea, dehydration, dizziness, weakness, weight loss.

INTERACTIONS

DRUG: May decrease therapeutic effect of **BCG (intravesical). Anticoagulants (e.g., heparin, warfarin), antiplatelets (e.g., aspirin, clopidogrel), NSAIDS (e.g., diclofenac, meloxicam, naproxen), thrombolytic therapy (e.g., alteplase)** may increase risk of bleeding in pts with treatment-induced thrombocytopenia. **Cladribine** may increase myelosuppressive effect. **HERBAL:** None significant. **FOOD:** None known. **LAB VALUES:** May increase serum ALT, AST, serum creatinine; urine protein. May decrease leukocytes, neutrophils, platelets.

AVAILABILITY (Rx)

Injection Solution: 100 mg/4 mL (25mg/mL), 200 mg/8mL (25 mg/mL).

ADMINISTRATION/HANDLING

IV

Preparation • Visually inspect for particulate matter or discoloration. Solution should appear clear, colorless to pale yellow in color. Discard if solution is cloudy, discolored, or if visible particles are observed. • Withdraw proper dose from vial and dilute in 0.9% NaCl or D_5W to a final concentration of 0.6–8 mg/mL. Use polyvinyl chloride (PVC) infusion bags containing bis (2-ethylhexyl) phthalate (DEHP) or polyolefin. • Mix by gentle inversion. • Do not shake or agitate. • Discard unused portions.

Rate of administration • Infuse over 60 min via dedicated IV line using an in-line 0.2-micron polyethersulfone filter and an infusion set made of one of the following: polypropylene, polyethylene-lined PVC, polyurethane, DEHP-free PVC-containing trioctyl-trimellitate (TOTM), PVC containing DEHP. • Do not use in-line filters made of polyvinylidene fluoride

(PVDF) or nylon. • Do not administer as IV push or bolus.
Storage • Refrigerate unused vials. • Do not shake. • Protect from light. • May refrigerate diluted solution for up to 24 hrs or at controlled room temperature for up to 8 hrs.

IV INCOMPATIBILITIES

Do not infuse with other medications or solutions.

INDICATIONS/ROUTES/DOSAGE

Note: Delay treatment until ANC 1,500 cells/mm^3 or greater.

Metastatic Colorectal Cancer

IV: ADULTS, ELDERLY: 4 mg/kg (based on actual body weight) q2wks (in combination with 5-fluorouracil, leucovorin, and irinotecan). Continue until disease progression or unacceptable toxicity.

Dose Modification

Hypertension (Treatment-Induced)

Severe hypertension, recurrent hypertension: Withhold treatment until hypertension is controlled, then permanently reduce to 2 mg/kg q2wks.

Proteinuria

Urine protein greater than or equal to 2 g/24 hrs: Withhold treatment until urine protein less than 2 g/24 hrs, then resume at previous dose. **Recurrent urine protein greater than 2 g/24 hrs:** Withhold treatment until urine protein less than 2 g/24 hrs, then resume with a permanent reduction to 2 mg/kg q2wks.

Permanent Discontinuation

Permanently discontinue if severe hemorrhage, GI perforation, impaired wound healing, fistula formation, hypertensive crisis, arterial thromboembolism, nephrotic syndrome, thrombotic microangiopathy, reversible posterior leukoencephalopathy occurs.

Dosage in Renal/Hepatic Impairment

No dose adjustment.

SIDE EFFECTS

Frequent (57%–24%): Diarrhea, fatigue, stomatitis, abdominal pain, decreased appetite. **Occasional (13%–9%):** Asthenia, dyspnea, headache. **Rare (3%–2%):** Skin hyperpigmentation, dystonia, oropharyngeal pain, dehydration, rhinorrhea, hemorrhoids, proctalgia.

ADVERSE EFFECTS/TOXIC REACTIONS

Leukopenia, neutropenia, thrombocytopenia are expected responses to therapy, but more severe reactions including bone marrow depression, febrile neutropenia may be life-threatening. Severe, sometimes fatal, hemorrhagic events including intracranial/GI/GU/nasal/postprocedural hemorrhage may occur. GI perforations occurred in less than 1% of pts. May cause impaired wound healing or wound dehiscence requiring medical intervention, GI or non-GI fistula formation, severe hypertension, severe proteinuria, nephrotic syndrome, severe diarrhea, dehydration. Arterial thromboembolism including CVA, MI, TIA reported in up to 3% of pts. Reversible posterior leukoencephalopathy syndrome (RPLS) may present as aphasia, altered mental status, paralysis, vision loss, weakness. UTI reported in 6% of pts. Palmar-plantar erythrodysesthesia syndrome (PPES), a chemotherapy-induced skin condition that presents with redness, swelling, numbness, skin sloughing of the hands and feet, reported in 4% of pts. Immunogenicity (auto-ziv-aflibercept antibodies) occurred in up to 3% of pts.

NURSING CONSIDERATIONS

BASELINE ASSESSMENT

Obtain CBC, BUN, serum creatinine, LFT; urine protein; vital signs. Obtain pregnancy test in females of reproductive potential. Question for recent surgeries, dental procedures. Question history of thromboembolism (CVA, DVT, MI, pulmonary embolism), hypertension, hemorrhagic events. Screen for active infection. Screen for home medications that may increase risk of hemorrhage. Assess skin for open wounds, lesions,

Z

surgical incisions. Obtain dietary consult. Assess hydration status. Offer emotional support.

INTERVENTION/EVALUATION

Monitor ANC, CBC for myelosuppression prior to each cycle; renal function test, LFT, urine protein periodically. Monitor B/P at least q2wks. Persistent diastolic hypertension may indicate hypertensive crisis. If urine dipstick proteinuria is greater than or equal to 2+, obtain 24-hr urine protein test. Withhold treatment for at least 4 wks prior to elective surgery or for at least 4 wks after major surgery and until wound is fully healed. Due to high risk for arterial occlusions, be vigilant when screening for CVA (aphasia, confusion, paresthesia, hemiparesis, seizures), MI (chest pain, diaphoresis, left arm/jaw pain, increased serum troponin, ST segment elevation). RPLS should be considered in pts with altered mental status, confusion, headache, seizures, visual disturbances. Report abdominal pain, fever, hemoptysis, melena (may indicate GI perforation/fistula formation). Monitor skin for impaired wound healing, new skin lesions, rash, sloughing. Monitor for decreased urine output, renal dysfunction, nephrotic syndrome. Encourage fluid intake. Monitor daily pattern of bowel activity, stool consistency.

PATIENT/FAMILY TEACHING

• Life-threatening blood clots of the arteries and veins have occurred; report symptoms of heart attack (chest pain, difficulty breathing, jaw pain, nausea, pain that radiates to the left arm, sweating), stroke (blindness, confusion, one-sided weakness, loss of consciousness, trouble speaking, seizures), DVT (swelling, pain, hot feeling in the arms or legs), lung embolism (difficulty breathing, chest pain, rapid heart rate). Report liver problems (abdominal pain, bruising, clay-colored stool, amber or dark-colored urine, yellowing of the skin or eyes); skin changes (sloughing, rash, poor healing of wounds). • Life-threatening bleeding may occur; report bloody stool or urine, rectal bleeding, nosebleeds, vomiting up blood. • Treatment may depress your immune system response and reduce your ability to fight infection. Report symptoms of infection such as body aches, chills, cough, fatigue, fever. Avoid those with active infection. • Avoid pregnancy; treatment may cause birth defects. Females and males of childbearing potential should use effective contraception during treatment and for at least 3 mos after last dose. • Nervous system changes, including altered mental status, seizures, headache, blurry vision, high blood pressure, trouble speaking, one-sided weakness, may indicate stroke, high blood pressure crisis, life-threatening brain dysfunction/swelling. • Notify physician before any planned surgeries/dental procedures. • Severe diarrhea may lead to dehydration; drink plenty of fluids.

zoledronic acid

zoe-le-**dron**-ik **as**-id
(Aclasta🍁, Reclast)
Do not confuse Zometa with Zofran or Zoladex.

◆CLASSIFICATION

PHARMACOTHERAPEUTIC: Bisphosphonate. **CLINICAL:** Calcium regulator, bone resorption inhibitor.

USES

Zometa: Treatment of hypercalcemia of malignancy, bone metastases from solid tumors. Treatment of multiple myeloma osteolytic lesions. **Reclast:** Treatment and prevention of postmenopausal osteoporosis, glucocorticoid-induced osteoporosis, treatment of Paget's disease. Treatment of osteoporosis in men to increase bone mass. **OFF-LABEL:** Prevention of bone loss associated with aromatase inhibitor therapy in postmenopausal

Z

women with breast cancer or androgen deprivation therapy in men with prostate cancer. Post–renal transplant bone loss.

PRECAUTIONS

Contraindications: Hypersensitivity to zoledronic acid, other bisphosphonates (e.g., alendronate, risedronate). **Reclast only:** CrCl less than 35 mL/min, acute renal impairment, hypocalcemia. **Cautions:** Elderly. **Oncology indications:** History of aspirin-sensitive asthma, mild to moderate renal impairment. **Non-oncology indications:** Pts with disturbances of calcium and mineral metabolism (e.g., hypoparathyroidism, malabsorption syndrome).

ACTION

Inhibits bone resorption by action on osteoclasts. Inhibits osteoclast activity/skeletal calcium release induced by tumors; inhibits osteoclast-mediated resorption. **Therapeutic Effect: Tumor:** Increases urinary calcium, phosphorus excretion; decreases serum calcium, phosphorus levels. **Osteoporosis:** Reduces bone turnover.

LIFESPAN CONSIDERATIONS

Pregnancy/Lactation: Unknown if drug crosses placenta or is distributed in breast milk. Recommend discontinuation of therapy as early as possible prior to a planned pregnancy. **Children:** Safety and efficacy not established. **Elderly:** Age-related renal impairment may require dosage adjustment.

INTERACTIONS

DRUG: **Aminoglycosides (e.g., amikacin, gentamicin), calcitonin** may increase hypocalcemic effect. **NSAIDs (e.g., diclofenac, meloxicam, naproxen)** may increase adverse effects. **Proton pump inhibitors (e.g., lansoprazole, pantoprazole)** may decrease therapeutic effect. **HERBAL:** None significant. **FOOD:** None known. **LAB VALUES:** May decrease serum magnesium, calcium, phosphate.

AVAILABILITY (Rx)

Injection Solution: 4 mg/5 mL vial, 4 mg/100 mL single-use ready-to-use bottle. 5 mg diluted in 100 mL ready-to-infuse solution.

ADMINISTRATION/HANDLING

◀ALERT▶ Pt should be adequately rehydrated before administration of zoledronic acid.

IV (Zometa)

Reconstitution • Dilute in 100 mL 0.9% NaCl or D_5W.

Rate of administration • Infuse over at least 15 min.

Storage • Store unused vials at room temperature. • Infusion of solution must be completed within 24 hrs.

IV (Reclast)

• Infuse over at least 15 min. • Follow infusion with a 10-mL 0.9% NaCl flush of IV line.

IV INCOMPATIBILITIES

Do not mix with other medications.

INDICATIONS/ROUTES/DOSAGE

Hypercalcemia Malignancy (Zometa)

IV: ADULTS, ELDERLY: 4 mg infused over at least 15 min. Retreatment may be considered, but at least 7 days should elapse to allow for full response to initial dose.

Multiple Myeloma, Osteolytic Lesions, Bone Metastases From Solid Tumors (Zometa)

IV: ADULTS, ELDERLY: 4 mg q3–4wks.

Paget's Disease (Reclast)

IV: ADULTS, ELDERLY: 5 mg as a single dose. Data about retreatment not available (seldom required within 5 yrs).

Osteoporosis Treatment (Reclast)

IV: ADULTS, ELDERLY: 5 mg once yearly. Consider discontinuing after 3–5 yrs in pts with low risk of fractures.

Z

Treatment/Prevention of Glucocorticoid-Induced Osteoporosis (Reclast)
IV: ADULTS, ELDERLY: 5 mg once yearly.

Prevention of Postmenopausal Osteoporosis (Reclast)
IV: ADULTS, ELDERLY: 5 mg once q2yrs.

Dosage in Renal Impairment
***(Reclast):* CrCl less than 35 mL/min:** Contraindicated.
(Zometa): Multiple myeloma, metastatic bone lesions of solid tumors.

Creatinine Clearance	Dosage
50–60 mL/min	3.5 mg
40–49 mL/min	3.3 mg
30–39 mL/min	3 mg
Less than 30 mL/min	Not recommended

(Zometa): Hypercalcemia of malignancy. **Mild to moderate impairment:** No adjustment. **Severe impairment: (SCr greater than 4.5 mg/dL):** Use caution only after considering risk versus benefit.

Dosage in Hepatic Impairment
No dose adjustment.

SIDE EFFECTS

Frequent (44%–26%): Fever, nausea, vomiting, constipation. **Occasional (15%–10%):** Hypotension, anxiety, insomnia, flu-like symptoms (fever, chills, bone pain, myalgia, arthralgia). **Rare:** Conjunctivitis.

ADVERSE EFFECTS/TOXIC REACTIONS

Renal toxicity may occur if IV infusion is administered in less than 15 min.

Z

NURSING CONSIDERATIONS

BASELINE ASSESSMENT

Obtain renal function test; serum calcium, phosphate. Assess hydration status (adequate hydration is essential to reduce renal injury). Obtain dental exam for pts at risk for osteonecrosis.

INTERVENTION/EVALUATION

Monitor renal function; serum calcium, phosphate. Assess vertebral bone mass (document stabilization, improvement). Assess for fever. Monitor food intake, daily pattern of bowel activity, stool consistency. Check I&O, serum BUN, creatinine in pts with renal impairment.

ZOLMitriptan

zole-mi-**trip**-tan
(Zomig, Zomig Rapimelt ❋, Zomig-ZMT)
Do not confuse ZOLMitriptan with almotriptan, rizatriptan or SUMAtriptan.

◆ CLASSIFICATION

PHARMACOTHERAPEUTIC: Serotonin 5-HT_1 receptor agonist. **CLINICAL:** Antimigraine.

USES

Oral: Treatment of acute migraine attack with or without aura in adults. **Nasal:** Treatment of acute migraine with or without aura in adults and children 12 yrs and older. **OFF-LABEL:** Short-term prevention of menstrual migraines.

PRECAUTIONS

Contraindications: Hypersensitivity to ZOLMitriptan. Arrhythmias associated with conduction disorders (e.g., Wolff-Parkinson-White syndrome), basilar or hemiplegic migraine, coronary artery disease, ischemic heart disease (including angina pectoris, history of MI, silent ischemia, Prinzmetal's angina), uncontrolled hypertension, use within 24 hrs of ergotamine-containing preparations or another serotonin receptor agonist, MAOI used within 14 days. **Additional for nasal spray:** Cerebrovascular syndromes (e.g., stroke), peripheral vascular disease. **Cautions:** Hepatic impairment, cardiovascular risks (e.g., hypertension, hypercholesterolemia, smoking, obesity, diabetes), elderly.

ACTION

Binds selectively to serotonin receptors, producing vasoconstrictive effect and reducing inflammation on cranial blood vessels. **Therapeutic Effect:** Relieves migraine headache.

PHARMACOKINETICS

Widely distributed. Protein binding: 25%. Metabolized in liver. Excreted in urine (60%), feces (30%). **Half-life:** 2.8–3.7 hrs.

LIFESPAN CONSIDERATIONS

Pregnancy/Lactation: Unknown if drug is distributed in breast milk. **Children:** Safety and efficacy not established in pts younger than 12 yrs. **Elderly:** No age-related precautions noted.

INTERACTIONS

DRUG: **Ergot derivatives (e.g., ergotamine)** may increase vasoconstrictive effect. **MAOIs (e.g., phenelzine, selegiline)** may increase concentration/effect. **HERBAL:** None significant. **FOOD:** None known. **LAB VALUES:** None significant.

AVAILABILITY (Rx)

Nasal Spray: ***(Zomig):*** 2.5 mg, 5 mg. **Tablets:** 2.5 mg, 5 mg.

Tablets, Orally Disintegrating ***(Zomig-ZMT):*** 2.5 mg, 5 mg.

ADMINISTRATION/HANDLING

PO

• Give without regard to food. Tablets may be broken.

Orally Disintegrating Tablet (ODT)

• Give whole; do not break, crush, cut. • Place on pt's tongue; allow to dissolve. • Not necessary to administer with liquid.

Nasal

• Instruct pt to clear nasal passages as much as possible before use. • With head upright, pt should close one nostril with index finger, breathe out gently through mouth. • Instruct pt to insert nozzle into open nostril about one-half inch, close mouth, and while taking a breath through nose, release spray dosage by firmly pressing plunger. • Have pt remove nozzle from nose, gently breathe in through nose and out through mouth for 15–20 sec. Tell pt to avoid breathing in deeply.

INDICATIONS/ROUTES/DOSAGE

Acute Migraine Attack

PO: ADULTS, ELDERLY, CHILDREN OLDER THAN 18 YRS: Initially, 1.25–2.5 mg (**Maximum:** 5 mg). If headache returns, may repeat dose after 2 hrs. **Maximum:** 10 mg/24 hrs.

Orally disintegrating tablet: ADULTS, ELDERLY: Initially, 2.5 mg (**maximum:** 5 mg) at onset of migraine headache. If headache returns, may repeat dose after 2 hrs. **Maximum:** 10 mg/24 hrs.

Intranasal: ADULTS, ELDERLY, CHILDREN 12 YRS AND OLDER: Initially, 2.5 mg (**Maximum:** 5 mg). If headache returns, may repeat dose after 2 hrs. **Maximum:** 10 mg/24 hrs.

Dosage in Renal Impairment

No dose adjustment.

Dosage in Hepatic Impairment

Nasal/ODT: Mild impairment: No dose adjustment. **Moderate to severe impairment:** Not recommended. **Tablet: Mild:** No dose adjustment. **Moderate to severe impairment:** Initially, 1.25 mg. **Maximum daily dose:** 5 mg in severe impairment.

SIDE EFFECTS

Frequent (8%–6%): PO: Dizziness, paresthesia, neck/throat/jaw pressure, drowsiness. **Nasal:** Altered taste, paresthesia.

Z

Occasional (5%–3%): PO: Warm/hot sensation, asthenia, chest pressure. **Nasal:** Nausea, drowsiness, nasal discomfort, dizziness, asthenia, dry mouth. **Rare (2%–1%):** Diaphoresis, myalgia.

ADVERSE EFFECTS/TOXIC REACTIONS

Cardiac events (ischemia, coronary artery vasospasm, MI), noncardiac vasospasm-related reactions (hemorrhage, stroke) occur rarely, particularly in pts with hypertension, diabetes, strong family history of coronary artery disease; pts who are obese; smokers; males older than 40 yrs; postmenopausal women.

NURSING CONSIDERATIONS

BASELINE ASSESSMENT

Question for history of peripheral vascular disease, coronary artery disease, renal/hepatic impairment, MAOI use. Question characteristics of migraine headaches (onset, location, duration, possible precipitating symptoms).

INTERVENTION/EVALUATION

Monitor for evidence of dizziness. Monitor B/P, esp. in pts with hepatic impairment. Evaluate for relief of migraine headaches (photophobia, phonophobia, nausea, vomiting, pain, dizziness, fogginess).

PATIENT/FAMILY TEACHING

• Take single dose as soon as symptoms of actual migraine attack appear. • Medication is intended to relieve migraine, not to prevent or reduce number of attacks. • Avoid tasks that require alertness, motor skills until response to drug is established. • Report chest pain; palpitations; tightness in throat; edema of face, lips, eyes; rash; easy bruising; blood in urine or stool; pain or numbness in arms or legs.

zolpidem

zole-**pi**-dem
(Ambien, Ambien CR, Edluar, Intermezzo, Sublinox ♣, Zolpimist)
Do not confuse Ambien with Abilify, Ativan, or zolpidem with LORazepam, zaleplon, or Zyloprim.

◆CLASSIFICATION

PHARMACOTHERAPEUTIC: Hypnotic, miscellaneous (Schedule IV). **CLINICAL:** Sedative-hypnotic.

USES

Ambien, Edluar, Zolpimist: Short-term treatment of insomnia (with difficulty of sleep onset). **Ambien CR:** Treatment of insomnia (with difficulty of sleep onset and/or sleep maintenance). **Intermezzo:** Treatment of insomnia characterized by middle-of-the-night awakening followed by difficulty returning to sleep in pts with 4 or more hrs of sleep time remaining.

PRECAUTIONS

Contraindications: Hypersensitivity to zolpidem. **Cautions:** Hepatic impairment, obstructive sleep apnea, debilitated, elderly, respiratory disease (e.g., COPD, emphysema), myasthenia gravis, depressive disorders; history of drug abuse and misuse.

ACTION

Enhances action of inhibitory neurotransmitter gamma-aminobutyric acid (GABA). Increases chloride conduction, neuronal hyperpolarization; inhibits action potential and decreases neuronal excitability. **Therapeutic Effect:** Induces sleep with fewer nightly awakenings, improves sleep quality.

PHARMACOKINETICS

Route	Onset	Peak	Duration
PO	30 min	N/A	6–8 hrs

Widely distributed. Protein binding: 92%. Metabolized in liver; excreted in urine. Not removed by hemodialysis. **Half-life:** 1.4–4.5 hrs (increased in hepatic impairment).

LIFESPAN CONSIDERATIONS

Pregnancy/Lactation: Drug crosses placenta and is distributed in breast milk. **Children:** Safety and efficacy not established. **Elderly:** More likely to experience falls or confusion; decreased initial doses recommended. Age-related hepatic impairment may require dosage adjustment.

INTERACTIONS

DRUG: **Alcohol, CNS depressants (e.g., gabapentin, LORazepam, morphine)** may increase CNS depression. **Strong CYP3A4 inducers (e.g., carBAMazepine, phenytoin, rifAMPin)** may decrease concentration/effect. **Strong CYP3A4 inhibitors (e.g., clarithromycin, ketoconazole)** may increase concentration/effect. HERBAL: **Herbals with sedative properties (e.g., chamomile, kava kava, valerian)** may increase CNS depression. **St. John's wort** may decrease concentration/effect. FOOD: None known. LAB VALUES: None significant.

AVAILABILITY (Rx)

Oral Solution: *(Zolpimist):* 5 mg/actuation. **Tablets:** 5 mg, 10 mg. **Tablets, Sublingual** *(Edluar):* 5 mg, 10 mg. *(Intermezzo):* 1.75 mg, 3.5 mg.

Tablets, Extended-Release: 6.25 mg, 12.5 mg.

ADMINISTRATION/HANDLING

PO

• For faster sleep onset, do not give with or immediately after a meal. • Give extended-release tablets whole; do not break, crush, dissolve, or divide. • Edluar sublingual tablets to be placed under tongue and allowed to disintegrate. Do not give with water or allow pt to swallow tablet. • Spray Zolpimist directly into mouth over tongue.

INDICATIONS/ROUTES/DOSAGE

Note: Dosage adjustment is recommended for female pts.

Insomnia

PO, spray, sublingual: *(Edluar, Zolpimist):* ADULTS: 5–10 mg (males), 5 mg (females) immediately before bedtime. ELDERLY, DEBILITATED: 5 mg immediately before bedtime. *(Intermezzo):* ADULTS, ELDERLY: 3.5 mg (males), 1.75 mg (females), taken once in middle of night with 4 or more hrs of expected sleep yet to come.

PO: *(Extended-Release):* ADULTS: 6.25–12.5 mg (males), 6.25 mg (females) immediately before bedtime. ELDERLY, DEBILITATED: 6.25 mg immediately before bedtime.

Dosage in Renal Impairment

No dose adjustment; use caution.

Dosage in Hepatic Impairment

Mild to moderate impairment: *(Immediate-Release Tablet, Spray, Sublingual Tablet):* 5 mg. *(Extended-Release Tablet):* 6.25 mg. *(Intermezzo):* 1.75 mg. **Severe impairment:** Avoid use.

SIDE EFFECTS

Occasional (7%): Headache, change in appetite. **Rare (less than 2%):** Dizziness, nausea, diarrhea, muscle pain, sleepwalking.

ADVERSE EFFECTS/TOXIC REACTIONS

Overdose may produce severe ataxia (clumsiness, unsteadiness), bradycardia, diplopia, severe drowsiness, nausea, vomiting, difficulty breathing, unconsciousness. Abrupt withdrawal following long-term use may produce weakness, facial flushing, diaphoresis, vomiting,

Z

tremor. Drug tolerance/dependence may occur with prolonged use of high dosages. May cause amnesic events that include cooking, sleepwalking, sexual activity, driving.

NURSING CONSIDERATIONS

BASELINE ASSESSMENT

Assess vital signs, mental status, sleep patterns. Raise bed rails, provide call light. Provide environment conducive to sleep (back rub, quiet environment, low lighting). Do not give unless a full night of sleep is planned.

INTERVENTION/EVALUATION

Monitor sleep pattern. Evaluate for therapeutic response to insomnia: decrease in number of nocturnal awakenings, increase in length of sleep. Monitor daytime alertness, respiratory rate, behavior profile.

PATIENT/FAMILY TEACHING

• Do not abruptly discontinue medication after long-term use. • Avoid alcohol and tasks that require alertness, motor skills until response to drug is established. • Tolerance, dependence may occur with prolonged use of high dosages. • Do not break, chew, crush, dissolve, or divide extended-release tablets; swallow whole. • Therapy may need to be discontinued if cooking, driving, sleepwalking occurs without recollection. • Do not take unless a full 8 hrs of sleep is planned.

zonisamide

zoe-**nis**-a-mide
(Zonegran)
Do not confuse Zonegran with SINEquan, or zonisamide with lacosamide.

◆CLASSIFICATION

PHARMACOTHERAPEUTIC: Anticonvulsant, miscellaneous. **CLINICAL:** Anticonvulsant.

USES

Adjunctive therapy in treatment of partial seizures in adults, children older than 16 yrs with epilepsy. **OFF-LABEL:** Bipolar disorder.

PRECAUTIONS

Contraindications: Hypersensitivity to zonisamide. Allergy to sulfonamides. **Cautions:** Renal/hepatic impairment, metabolic acidosis (e.g., severe respiratory disease); history of suicidal ideation and behavior.

ACTION

Exact mechanism unknown. May stabilize neuronal membranes, suppress neuronal hypersynchronization by blocking sodium, calcium channels. **Therapeutic Effect:** Reduces seizure activity.

PHARMACOKINETICS

Widely distributed. Metabolized in liver. Extensively bound to RBCs. Protein binding: 40%. Primarily excreted in urine. **Half-life:** 63 hrs (plasma), 105 hrs (RBCs).

⌛ LIFESPAN CONSIDERATIONS

Pregnancy/Lactation: Crosses placenta. Unknown if distributed in breast milk. **Children:** Safety and efficacy not established in pts younger than 16 yrs. **Elderly:** No age-related precautions noted, but lower dosages recommended.

INTERACTIONS

DRUG: **Alcohol, CNS depressants (e.g., LORazepam, morphine, zolpidem)** may increase sedative effect. **Strong CYP3A4 inducers (e.g., carBAMazepine, phenytoin, rifAMPin)** may increase metabolism, decrease effect. **HERBAL:** **Herbals with sedative properties (e.g., chamomile, kava kava, valerian)** may increase CNS depression. **St. Johns wort** may decrease concentration/effect. **FOOD:** None known. **LAB VALUES:** May increase serum BUN, creatinine.

AVAILABILITY (Rx)

Capsules: 25 mg, 50 mg, 100 mg.

ADMINISTRATION/HANDLING

PO

• Give without regard to food. • Give capsules whole; do not break, cut, or crush. • Do not give to pts allergic to sulfonamides.

INDICATIONS/ROUTES/DOSAGE

Note: Do not use if CrCl is less than 50 mL/min. Discontinue gradually to minimize the potential of increased seizure activity and withdrawal symptoms.

Partial Seizures

PO: ADULTS, ELDERLY, CHILDREN OLDER THAN 16 YRS: Initially, 100 mg/day. May increase to 200 mg/day after 2 wks. Further increases to 300 mg/day and 400 mg/day can be made with minimum of 2 wks between adjustments. **Range:** 100–600 mg/day.

Dosage in Renal Impairment

Not recommended with CrCl less than 50 mL/min.

Dosage in Hepatic Impairment

Use with caution.

SIDE EFFECTS

Frequent (17%–9%): Drowsiness, dizziness, anorexia, headache, agitation, irritability, nausea. **Occasional (8%–5%):** Fatigue, ataxia, confusion, depression, impaired memory/concentration, insomnia, abdominal pain, diplopia, diarrhea, speech difficulty. **Rare (4%–3%):** Paresthesia, nystagmus, anxiety, rash, dyspepsia, weight loss.

ADVERSE EFFECTS/TOXIC REACTIONS

Overdose characterized by bradycardia, hypotension, respiratory depression, coma. Leukopenia, anemia, thrombocytopenia occur rarely.

NURSING CONSIDERATIONS

BASELINE ASSESSMENT

Review history of seizure disorder (intensity, frequency, duration, level of consciousness). Initiate seizure precautions. CBC, LFT should be performed before therapy begins and periodically during therapy.

INTERVENTION/EVALUATION

Observe frequently for recurrence of seizure activity. Assess for clinical improvement (decrease in intensity, frequency of seizures). Assist with ambulation if dizziness occurs.

PATIENT/FAMILY TEACHING

• Strict maintenance of drug therapy is essential for seizure control. • Avoid tasks that require alertness, motor skills until response to drug is established. • Avoid alcohol. • Report if rash, back/abdominal pain, blood in urine, fever, sore throat, ulcers in mouth, easy bruising occur. • Seek immediate medical attention if thoughts of suicide, new onset or worsening of anxiety, depression, or changes in mood occur.

Z

Appendix A

CALCULATION OF DOSES

Frequently, dosages ordered do not correspond exactly to what is available and must be calculated.

RATIO/PROPORTION:

A pt is to receive 65 mg of a medication. It is available as 80 mg/2 mL. What volume (mL) needs to be administered to the patient?

STEP 1: Set up ratio.

$$\frac{80\text{ mg}}{2\text{ mL}} = \frac{65\text{ mg}}{\text{x (mL)}}$$

STEP 2: Cross multiply and divide each side by the number with x to determine volume to be administered.

$$80\text{ mg} \times (\text{x})\text{ mL} = 65\text{ mg} \times 2\text{ mL}$$
$$80\text{ x} = 130$$
$$\text{x} = \frac{130}{80} = 1.625\text{ mL}$$

CALCULATIONS IN MICROGRAMS PER KILOGRAM PER MINUTE (mcg/kg/min):

A 63-year-old pt (weight 165 lb) is to receive medication A at a rate of 8 mcg/kg/min. Given a solution containing medication A in a concentration of 500 mg/250 mL, at what rate (mL/hr) would you infuse this medication?

STEP 1: Convert to same units. In this problem, the dose is expressed in mcg/kg; therefore, convert weight to kg (2.2 lb = 1 kg) and drug concentration to mcg/mL (1 mg = 1,000 mcg).

165 lb divided by 2.2 = 75 kg

$$\frac{500\text{ mg}}{250\text{ mL}} = \frac{2\text{ mg}}{\text{mL}} = \frac{2{,}000\text{ mcg}}{\text{mL}}$$

STEP 2: Number of mcg/hr.

(75 kg) × 8 mcg/kg/min = 600 mcg/min or 36,000 mcg/hr

STEP 3: Number of mL/hr.

36,000 mcg/hr divided by 2,000 mcg/mL = 18 mL/hr

Appendix B

CONTROLLED DRUGS (UNITED STATES)

Schedule I: Medications having no legal medical use. These substances may be used for research purposes with proper registration (e.g., heroin, LSD).

Schedule II: Medications having a legitimate medical use but are characterized by a very high abuse potential and/or potential for severe physical and psychic dependency. Emergency telephone orders for limited quantities of these drugs are authorized, but the prescriber must provide a written, signed prescription order (e.g., morphine, amphetamines, HYDROcodone, oxyCODONE).

Schedule III: Medications having significant abuse potential (less than Schedule II). Telephone orders are permitted (e.g., codeine in combination with other substances such as butalbital).

Schedule IV: Medications having a low abuse potential. Telephone orders are permitted (e.g., benzodiazepines, traMADol, zolpidem).

Schedule V: Medications having the lowest abuse potential of the controlled substances. Some Schedule V products may be available without a prescription (e.g., certain cough preparations containing limited amounts of an opiate).

Appendix C

WOUND CARE

A wound is any process that disrupts the normal structure and function of tissues. Wounds can be closed (e.g., bruise, sprain) or open (e.g., abrasion, surgical wound). The most common chronic wounds are nonhealing surgical wounds, pressure ulcers, diabetic foot ulcers, and venous ulcers.

TYPES OF OPEN WOUNDS

Superficial	Damage only to the epithelium; heals rapidly via regeneration of epithelial cells.
Partial thickness	Involves the dermal layer and is associated with blood vessel damage.
Full thickness	Involves subcutaneous fat and deeper layers (e.g., muscle, bone). Requires the longest time to heal. Connective tissue needs to regenerate; contraction occurs during the healing process.

WOUND HEALING

Wound healing is a complex process resulting in restored cell structure and tissue layers after an injury. When skin is damaged, it begins to heal from the bottom layer up and from the outside inward. Wound healing involves cellular, physiologic, biochemical, and molecular processes. They are interdependent and overlapping. An acute wound usually heals within several wks, whereas chronic wounds take 6 wks or longer to heal. Additionally, other factors can delay the healing process. These include trauma/edema, infection, necrosis, lack of oxygen delivery to the tissues, advanced age, obesity, chronic diseases (e.g., diabetes, anemia), vascular insufficiency, immobility, pressure necrosis, and immunodeficiency.

Wound healing can be divided into three phases: inflammation, proliferation, and maturation.

Inflammation	Occurs within seconds of the injury and can last up to 3 days. Associated with redness, heat, swelling, and pain. Immediate vasoconstriction of damaged blood vessels, and coagulation limiting blood loss occurs. Following vasoconstriction, histamine and other chemical mediators are released from damaged cells, causing vasodilation and release of growth factors essential for wound healing (e.g., increased capillary permeability and release of exudate).
Proliferation	Granulation tissue composed of macrophages, fibroblasts, immature collagen, blood vessels, and ground substance is formed. Fibroblasts stimulate production of collagen and elastin, increasing the strength of the wound and stimulating growth of new blood vessels. As granulation fills the wound site, the edges of the wound pull together, decreasing the surface of the wound.

	Epithelialization then occurs: Epithelial cells migrate from the wound edge, covering the wound and resulting in scar formation. This phase usually lasts 2 to 3 wks.
Maturation	Collagen fibers cross link and reorganize, increasing the strength of scar. This process can take anywhere from 3 wks to 2 yrs.

WOUND DRESSINGS

Dressings play a major role in wound management. They protect the wound, keeping it moist, and thus promote healing (only diabetic, dry, gangrenous toes require a moisture-free environment for effective healing).

Hydrocolloid, hydrogel, film, and foam dressing can handle large amounts of exudate and promote auto-debridement. Alginate and collagen-based dressings promote granulation of tissue. Silver and iodine dressings are used to avoid infections, which may delay wound healing.

WOUND CARE PRODUCTS

Description	General Uses	Comments
Alginate dressings: Spun fibers of brown seaweed that act as ion exchange mechanisms to absorb serous fluid or exudate, forming a gel-like covering that conforms to the shape of the wound. Facilitate autolytic débridement and maintain a moist wound environment. **Products:** Algicell, Carra Sorb. Available as ropes, pads.	Abrasions/lacerations/skin tears Arterial/venous ulcers Deep and tunneling wounds Diabetic ulcers Pressure ulcers Second-degree burns Odorous wounds Contaminated and infected wounds	Good for moderately to heavily exudative wounds and hemorrhagic wounds Can be left in place until soaked with exudate Requires a secondary dressing (e.g., transparent film, foam, hydrocolloids) Do not moisten prior to use Nonadhesive, nonocclusive Contraindicated in third-degree burns; not recommended for dry or minimally exudative wounds
Collagenase ointment: Sterile enzymatic débriding ointment that possesses the ability to digest collagen in necrotic tissue. **Products:** Santyl.	Débriding chronic dermal ulcers and severely burned areas	Can be used for infected wounds Gauze is used as a secondary dressing Discontinue when granulation tissue is present Optimal pH for enzymatic action is 6–8 Avoid acidic agents for cleansing; avoid detergents and agents containing heavy metal (e.g., mercury or silver), which may adversely affect enzymatic activity

Continued

Description	General Uses	Comments
Trypsin, castor oil, Peru balsam: Trypsin is a mild débriding agent that helps shed damaged skin cells. **Castor oil** acts as a lubricant to protect tissue. **Peru balsam** increases blood flow to a wound area, reduces wound odor. **Products:** Granulex, Xenaderm. Available as gel, ointment, spray.	Promotes healing/ treatment of decubitus ulcers, varicose ulcer, and dehiscent wounds	Can be used for infected wounds Avoid concurrent use of silver-containing products (may reduce efficacy) Promotes healing and relieves pain caused by bed sores and other skin ulcers
Hydrophilic polyurethane foam: Also called open cell foam dressings. Sheets of foamed solutions of polymers containing variably sized open cells that can hold wound exudate away from wound bed. Maintains moist wound environment. **Products:** Curafoam, Lyofoam. Available as sheets in a wide variety of formulations.	Moderate to heavy exudative wounds with or without a clean granular wound bed Diabetic ulcers, pressure ulcers, venous stasis ulcers Draining surgical incisions Superficial burns Tube and drain sites	Contraindicated for use in third-degree burns Not recommended for wounds with little to no exudate or when tunneling is present Good for cavitating wounds Highly absorbent, semiocclusive dressing Usual dressing change is up to 3 times/wk Can be worn during bathing
Hydrocolloids: Formulations of elastomeric, adhesive, and gelling agents; the most common absorbent ingredient is carboxymethylcellulose. Most hydrocolloids are backed with a semiocclusive film layer. The wound side of the dressing is adhesive, adhering to a moist surface as well as to dry skin but not to the moist wound bed. As wound fluid is absorbed, the hydrocolloid forms a viscous gel in the wound bed, enhancing a moist wound environment. **Products:** Hydrocol, Tegasorb. Available as dressings, granules, patches, paste.	Minimal to moderate exudate in partial and full thickness wounds Cuts and abrasions First- and second-degree burns Pressure ulcers Stasis ulcers	Not for wounds producing heavy exudate, infected wounds, dry eschar-covered wounds May provide pain relief Good for chronic wounds that are epithelializing Can be left in place for up to 7 days Contraindicated for third-degree burns Can shower while wearing

Description	General Uses	Comments
Hydrogels: Glycerin- or water-based dressings designed to hydrate the wound. May absorb small amounts of exudate. **Products:** Curacel, Duo Derm, Intra Site. Available as gel, sheets, gauze.	Partial and full thickness wounds Dry to minimal exudate Cuts and abrasions First- and second-degree burns Pressure ulcers Stasis ulcers	Not for wounds producing moderate to heavy exudate Not for infected wounds May provide pain relief Good for wounds that are debriding Good for keeping a dry wound moist Can be left in place for 1–3 days
Iodine compounds: Cadexomer iodine: Iodine is complexed with a polymeric cadexomer starch vehicle, forming a topical gel or paste. The cadexomer moiety absorbs exudate and debris and releases iodine for antimicrobial activity. **Products:** Iodosorb, iodoflex. Available as gel, dressing, ointment, powder.	Chronic nonhealing, exuding wounds including pressure or leg ulcers and exuding, infected wounds	Requires use of a secondary dressing Contraindicated in pts with iodine sensitivity, Hashimoto's thyroiditis, nontoxic nodular goiter, children Dressing to be changed when it turns white, indicating that the iodine has been depleted Do not use on dry necrotic tissue
Silver compounds Silver sulfadiazine cream: Silver possesses bactericidal properties. Has been shown to reduce bacterial density, vascular margination, migration of inflammatory cells. Enhances rate of re-epithelialization. **Products:** Silvadene, SSD, Thermazene.	Prevent infection in second- and third-degree burns Prevent or treat infection in chronic wounds	May have cytotoxic effects that could delay wound healing Allergic reactions may occur Use should be limited to a 2- to 4-wk period Bacteria may become resistant with prolonged use Avoid use with collagenase- or trypsin-containing debriding agents
Transparent film dressings: Polyurethane sheets coated on one side with an adhesive that is inactivated by moisture and will not adhere to a moist surface such as the wound bed. Have no absorbent capacity and are impermeable to fluids and bacteria but are semipermeable to oxygen and water vapor. **Products:** Bioclusive, CarraFilm, Tegaderm HP. Available in a variety of sizes and features.	Prophylaxis on high-risk intact skin Superficial wounds with minimal or no exudate Wounds on elbows, heels, or flat surfaces; covering of blisters; and retention of primary dressing	Prevents wound desiccation and contamination by bacteria Contraindicated in third-degree burns Promotes autolysis of necrotic tissue in the wound; maintains moist environment Avoid in arterial ulcers and infected wounds requiring frequent monitoring Do not use as primary dressing on wounds with depth or tunneling May provide pain relief Usually changed up to 3 times/wk

Continued

Description	General Uses	Comments
Becaplermin gel: Recombinant formulation of platelet-derived growth factor that promotes cell mitogenesis and proliferation of cells involved in wound repair. Enhances formation of granulation tissue. **Products:** Regranex.	Diabetic foot ulcers that extend into subcutaneous tissue or beyond and have an adequate blood supply	Usually applied daily Adequate blood supply and absence of necrotic tissue are needed for efficacy Repeated use (3 or more tubes) may increase risk of cancer-related death Use cautiously in pts with known malignancy

Appendix D

DRUGS OF ABUSE

Substance	Brand/ Street Names	Administered	Effects of Intoxication	Potential Health Consequences
Amphetamine	*Adderall, Dexedrine;* bennies, black beauties, hearts, speed, truck drivers, uppers	Injection, smoked, snorted	Increased heart rate, blood pressure, body temperature, metabolism; increased energy, mental alertness; tremors; reduced appetite; irritability; anxiety; panic; violent behavior; psychosis	Weight loss, insomnia, cardiac or cardiovascular complications, stroke, seizures, addiction, tremor, irritability
Barbiturates	*Nembutal, Seconal, Phenobarbital;* barbs, reds, phennies, yellows, yellow jackets	Injection, oral	Reduction of pain and anxiety; feeling of well-being; lowered inhibitions; slowed pulse/breathing; lowered blood pressure; poor concentration; sedation, drowsiness	Confusion, fatigue; impaired coordination, memory, judgment; respiratory depression or arrest; addiction; depression; unusual excitement; fever; irritability; slurred speech; dizziness
Benzodiazepines	*Ativan, Librium, Valium, Xanax;* candy, downers, tranks, Xannies, Xannie bars	Oral	Reduction of pain and anxiety; feeling of well-being; lowered inhibitions; slowed pulse/breathing; lowered blood pressure; poor concentration; sedation, drowsiness	Confusion, fatigue; impaired coordination, memory, judgment; respiratory depression or arrest; addiction; dizziness

Continued

Substance	*Brand/* Street Names	Administered	Effects of Intoxication	Potential Health Consequences
Bupropion	*Wellbutrin;* poor man's cocaine	Oral	Increased heart rate, B/P, and temperature; mental alertness; feel euphoric, exhilarated, energetic	Seizures, tachycardia, arrhythmias, loss of consciousness
Cocaine	Blow, bump, candy, coke, crack, rock, snow, toot	Injection, smoked, snorted	Increased heart rate, blood pressure, body temperature, metabolism; increased energy, mental alertness; tremors; reduced appetite; irritability; anxiety; panic; violent behavior; psychosis	Weight loss, insomnia, cardiac or cardiovascular complications, stroke, seizures, addiction, nasal damage from snorting, rapid or irregular heartbeat, headaches, malnutrition
Codeine	*Fiorinal with codeine, Tylenol with codeine;* Captain Cody, schoolboy, loads, pancakes and syrup	Injection, oral	Pain relief, euphoria, drowsiness	Respiratory depression and arrest, nausea, confusion, constipation, sedation, unconsciousness, coma, tolerance, addiction
Dextromethorphan	Found in some cough and cold medications; poor man's PCP, velvet, Robo, Triple C	Oral	Impaired motor function, feeling of being separated from one's body and environment; euphoria; slurred speech; confusion; dizziness; distorted visual perceptions	

Substance	*Brand/* Street Names	Administered	Effects of Intoxication	Potential Health Conse-quences
Flunitraze-pam	*Rohypnol;* forget-me pill, Mexican Valium, roofies, roofinol, rope, rophies	Oral, snorted	Sedation, mus-cle relaxation, confusion, memory loss, dizziness, impaired coor-dination, reduced pain/ anxiety, feeling of well-being	Addiction; confusion, fatigue, memory loss, respiratory depression
Gabapentin	*Neurontin, Lyrica, Lycia;* gabbie	Oral	Self-treatment of alcohol, cocaine, or opioid craving; euphoria, relaxation	Diarrhea, double vision, drowsiness, lethargic, slurred speech
GHB	Georgia home boy, grievous bodily harm, liquid ecstasy, goop, liquid X	Oral	Drowsiness, nausea, head-ache, disorien-tation, loss of coordination, memory loss	Uncon-sciousness, seizures, coma, confu-sion, nausea, vomiting, headache
Heroin	Smack, brown sugar, dope, junk, white horse, China white	Injection, smoked, snorted	Euphoria, drowsiness, impaired coor-dination, dizzi-ness, confusion, nausea, seda-tion, feeling of heaviness in the body, slowed breathing	Constipation, confusion, sedation, respiratory depression, coma, addic-tion
Hydroco-done	*Vicodin, Lortab;* vike, watson-387	Oral	Pain relief, euphoria, drowsiness	Respiratory depression and arrest, nausea, confusion, constipation, sedation, uncon-sciousness, coma, tolerance, addiction

Continued

Substance	*Brand/* Street Names	Administered	Effects of Intoxication	Potential Health Consequences
Inhalants	Solvents (paint thinner, glues), nitrites (laughing gas, snappers, poppers)	Inhaled through nose or mouth	Stimulation, loss of inhibition, headache, nausea or vomiting, slurred speech, loss of motor coordination, wheezing	Cramps, muscle weakness, depression, memory impairment, damage to cardiovascular and nervous systems, unconsciousness, sudden death
Ketamine	*Ketalar;* cat Valium, Special K, kit kat, vitamin K	Injection, snorted, smoked	Increased heart rate and blood pressure, impaired motor function, feelings of being separated from one's body and environment; at high doses: delirium, depression, respiratory depression or arrest; death	Memory loss, numbness, nausea/vomiting, anxiety, tremors, respiratory depression
Loperamide	*Imodium;* poor man's methadone	Oral	Reducing symptoms of opioid withdrawal	CNS depression, intestinal blockage
LSD	Acid, cubes, microdot, yellow sunshine, blotter, bloomers	Oral, absorbed through mouth tissues	Altered states of perception and feeling; hallucinations; nausea; increased body temperature, heart rate, blood pressure; loss of appetite; sweating; sleeplessness; numbness; dizziness; weakness; tremors; impulsive behavior; rapid shifts in emotion	Flashbacks, hallucinogen persisting perception disorder

Substance	*Brand/* Street Names	Administered	Effects of Intoxication	Potential Health Consequences
Marijuana	Blunt, ganja, grass, joint, Mary Jane, pot, reefer, sinsemilla, skunk, weed	Oral, smoked	Euphoria, relaxation, slowed reaction time, impaired balance and coordination, increased heart rate and appetite, impaired learning and memory, anxiety, panic attacks, psychosis	Cough, impaired memory and learning, anxiety, panic attacks, frequent respiratory infections, possible mental health decline, addiction
MDMA	Ecstasy, Adam, clarity, Eve, lover's speed, peace, Molly	Injection, oral, snorted	Mild hallucinogenic effects, increased tactile sensitivity, empathic feelings, lowered inhibition, anxiety, chills, sweating, teeth clenching, muscle cramping	Reduced appetite, irregular heartbeat, heart failure, impaired memory, hyperthermia, addiction
Mescaline	Buttons, cactus, peyote	Oral, smoked	Altered states of perception and feeling; hallucinations; nausea; increased body temperature, heart rate, blood pressure; loss of appetite; sweating; sleeplessness; numbness; dizziness; weakness; tremors; impulsive behavior; rapid shifts in emotion	Loss of appetite, nausea, weakness, chronic mental disorders

Continued

Substance	*Brand/* Street Names	Administered	Effects of Intoxication	Potential Health Consequences
Methamphetamine	*Desoxyn*; meth, ice, crank, crystal, go fast, speed	Oral, injection, smoked, snorted	Increased heart rate, blood pressure, body temperature, metabolism; increased energy, mental alertness; tremors; reduced appetite; irritability; anxiety; panic; violent behavior; psychosis	Weight loss, insomnia, cardiac or cardiovascular complications, stroke, seizures, addiction, severe dental problems, behavior/memory loss, impaired memory and learning, tolerance, addiction
Methylphenidate	*Ritalin*; JIF, MPH, Skippy, smart drug, vitamin R	Injection, oral, snorted	Increase or decrease in blood pressure; psychotic episodes	Digestive problems, loss of appetite, weight loss, reduced appetite, rapid irregular heartbeat, heart failure, seizures, stroke
Morphine	*Roxanol, Duramorph;* M, Miss Emma, monkey, white stuff	Injection, oral, smoked	Pain relief, euphoria, drowsiness	Respiratory depression and arrest, nausea, confusion, constipation, sedation, unconsciousness, coma, tolerance, addiction
Oxycodone	*OxyContin, Percodan;* oxycotton, oxycet, hillbilly heroin, killers, OCs	Injection, oral	Pain relief, euphoria, drowsiness	Respiratory depression and arrest, nausea, confusion, constipation, sedation, unconsciousness, coma, tolerance, addiction

Substance	*Brand/* Street Names	Administered	Effects of Intoxication	Potential Health Consequences
PCP	*Phencyclidine;* angel dust, boat, hog, love boat, peace pill	Injection, oral, smoked	Impaired motor function, feelings of being separated from one's body and environment, analgesia, psychosis, aggression, violence, slurred speech, loss of coordination, hallucinations	Memory loss, loss of appetite, panic, aggression, violence
Psilocybin	Magic mushrooms, purple passion, shrooms	Oral	Altered states of perception and feeling, hallucinations, nausea, nervousness, paranoia, panic	Chronic mental disorders
Quetiapine	*Seroquel;* baby heroin, Suzie-Q, Q-ball	Oral	Reduced anxiety, sedation	Arrhythmias, coma, death (with overdose)

Appendix E

EQUIANALGESIC DOSING

Guidelines for equianalgesic dosing of commonly used analgesics are presented in the following table. The dosages are approximate to 10 mg of morphine intramuscularly. These guidelines are for the management of acute pain in the opioid-naïve pt. Dosages may vary for the opioid-tolerant pt and for the management of chronic pain. Dosing adjustments for renal or hepatic insufficiency may also be necessary. Clinical response is the criterion that must be applied for each pt with titration to desired response.

Name	Equianalgesic Oral Dose	Equianalgesic Parenteral Dose (IV, IM, SQ)
Codeine	200 mg	100–130 mg
FentaNYL	Not available	0.1 mg (100 mcg)
HYDROcodone	30–45 mg	Not available
HYDROmorphone (Dilaudid)	7.5–8 mg	1.5–2 mg
HYDROmorphone (Dilaudid) (Controlled-Release)	7.5 mg	N/A
Meperidine (Demerol)	300 mg	75 mg
Methadone (Dolophine)	10–20 mg	10 mg
Morphine	30 mg	10 mg
OxyCODONE (OxyContin)	20–30 mg	Not available
OxyMORphone	10 mg	1 mg
OxyMORphone (Extended-Release)	10 mg	N/A

Appendix F

HERBALS: COMMON NATURAL MEDICINES

The use of herbal therapies is increasing in the United States. Because of the rise in the use of herbal therapy, the following is presented to provide some basic information on some of the more popular herbs. Please note this is not an all-inclusive list, which is beyond the scope of this handbook.

Name	Uses	Comments
Aloe vera	Orally: osteoarthritis, inflammatory bowel diseases (e.g., ulcerative colitis), fever, itching, inflammation. Topically: burns, wound healing, psoriasis, sunburn, frostbite, cold sores.	Well tolerated. Orally can cause abdominal pain, cramps; topically can cause burning, itching, contact dermatitis. May lower blood glucose levels and have additive effects with antidiabetic medications.
Bilberry	Orally: improve visual acuity (e.g., night vision, cataracts), atherosclerosis, chronic fatigue syndrome, venous insufficiency, varicose veins, hemorrhoids. Topically: mild inflammation of mouth and throat mucous membranes.	Can inhibit platelet aggregation, increase risk of bleeding when combined with antiplatelet or anticoagulant medications (e.g., aspirin, clopidogrel, enoxaparin, warfarin). May lower blood glucose.
Bitter orange	Orally: appetite stimulant, dyspepsia. Topically: inflammation of the eyelid, conjunctiva, retina.	May cause hypertension, cardiovascular toxicity. May increase concentration/ effects of midazolam; concurrent use with MAOIs may increase blood pressure (avoid use); combination with caffeine can increase blood pressure, heart rate.
Black cohosh	Orally: symptoms of menopause, premenstrual syndrome (PMS), dysmenorrhea, dyspepsia, inducing labor in pregnant women, anxiety, fever, cough, cardiovascular disease, cognitive function, infertility, osteoarthritis, osteoporosis, rheumatoid arthritis. Topically: acne, mole, and wart removal; improve skin appearance.	Can cause GI upset, rash, headache, dizziness, increased weight, cramping, breast tenderness, vaginal spotting/ bleeding. May decrease effects of cisplatin; may increase risk of hepatic damage with hepatotoxic medications.

Continued

Name	Uses	Comments
Capsicum (cayenne pepper)	Orally: dyspepsia, flatulence, diarrhea, cramps, toothache, hyperlipidemia. Topically: pain of shingles, osteoarthritis, rheumatoid arthritis, postherpetic neuralgia, diabetic neuralgia, trigeminal neuralgia.	Orally can cause upper abdominal discomfort (e.g., gas, bloating, nausea, diarrhea, belching); topically can cause burning, stinging, erythema. May increase effects/adverse effects of antiplatelet medications.
Chamomile	Prepared as a tea and used as a mild sedative, relaxant, and sleeping aid; used for indigestion, itching, and inflammation.	Large amounts may cause vomiting.
Chasteberry	Orally: menstrual irregularities (e.g., dysmenorrhea, amenorrhea, metrorrhagia).	Can cause GI upset, headache, diarrhea, nausea, itching, urticaria, rash, insomnia, increased weight, irregular menstrual bleeding. Can interfere with efficacy of oral contraceptives, hormone replacement therapy.
Clove (clove oil)	Orally: dyspepsia, expectorant, diarrhea, halitosis, flatulence, nausea, vomiting. Topically: toothache, mouth and throat inflammation.	Topically can cause tissue irritation, allergic dermatitis.
Co-enzyme Q-10	Heart failure, angina, diabetes, hypertension.	Can cause GI side effects (e.g., nausea, vomiting, diarrhea, appetite suppression, heartburn, epigastric discomfort). Can decrease blood pressure and have an additive effect with antihypertensive medications; may reduce anticoagulant effects of warfarin.
Cranberry	Prevention/treatment of urinary tract infections, neurogenic bladder, urinary deodorizer in incontinence, kidney stones, prevention of urinary catheter blockage.	Usually well tolerated. Large amounts can cause GI upset, diarrhea, nausea, vomiting. Greater than 1,000 mL daily can increase risk of uric acid, kidney stone formation.
DHEA	Slow or reverse aging, weight loss, metabolic syndrome, increase immune and cognitive function.	At high dose can cause acne, hirsutism, hair loss, voice deepening, insulin resistance, altered menstrual pattern. May interfere with antiestrogen effects of anastrozole, letrozole, or other aromatase inhibitors; may overcome estrogen receptor antagonist activity of tamoxifen in estrogen receptor positive cancer cells.

Name	Uses	Comments
Dong quai	Dysmenorrhea, premenstrual syndrome, menopausal symptoms.	May cause photosensitivity and photodermatitis. May increase effect/risk of bleeding with antiplatelet and anticoagulant medications (e.g., aspirin, warfarin).
Echinacea	Treat/prevent common cold, influenza, other upper respiratory tract infections.	Usually well tolerated. Can cause GI effects (e.g., nausea, abdominal pain, diarrhea, vomiting). Stimulates immune function—may exacerbate autoimmune diseases (e.g., multiple sclerosis, rheumatoid arthritis, systemic lupus erythematosus).
Eucalyptus	Orally: infections, fever, dyspepsia, expectorant for coughs. Topically: inflammation of respiratory tract mucous membranes, rheumatoid arthritis, nasal stuffiness.	Orally: GI effects (e.g., nausea, vomiting, diarrhea). Topically (prolonged exposure/large amounts): agitation, drowsiness, muscle weakness, ataxia.
Evening primrose oil	Premenstrual syndrome (PMS), endometriosis, symptoms of menopause (e.g., hot flashes).	May increase risk of bruising/bleeding with antiplatelet/anticoagulant medications (e.g., aspirin, clopidogrel, enoxaparin, warfarin).
Feverfew	Orally: fever, headaches, prevention of migraines, menstrual irregularities. Topically: toothaches, antiseptic.	Orally: GI effects (e.g., heartburn, nausea, diarrhea, constipation, abdominal pain, bloating, flatulence). Topically: contact dermatitis. May have additive effects, increase risk of bleeding with antiplatelet medications.
Fish oil	Hyperlipidemia, hypertriglyceridemia, hypertension, stroke, depression, rheumatoid arthritis, osteoporosis, psoriasis, Crohn's disease.	Can cause a fishy aftertaste, halitosis, heartburn, dyspepsia, nausea, loose stools, rash. May have additive effect with antihypertensive medication.
Garlic	Hypertension, hyperlipidemia, age-related vascular changes, atherosclerosis, chronic fatigue syndrome, menstrual disorders, coronary heart disease, peripheral arterial disease.	Dose-related effects including breath/body odor, mouth and GI burning/irritation, heartburn, flatulence, nausea, vomiting, diarrhea. May increase effects of antiplatelets (e.g., aspirin, clopidogrel, enoxaparin), anticoagulants (e.g., warfarin); may decrease effects of oral contraceptives, cyclosporine, protease inhibitors, and non-nucleoside reverse transcriptase inhibitors (NNRTIs).

Continued

Name	Uses	Comments
Ginger	Motion sickness, morning sickness, dyspepsia, rheumatoid arthritis, osteoarthritis, loss of appetite, migraine headache, diarrhea, flatulence, irritable bowel syndrome, dysmenorrhea.	Usually well tolerated. At high doses of 5 g/day may cause abdominal discomfort, heartburn, diarrhea, irritant effect in mouth and throat. May increase risk of bleeding with antiplatelet medications and anticoagulants (e.g., aspirin, clopidogrel, enoxaparin, warfarin).
Ginkgo	Dementia (including Alzheimer's), vascular dementia, mixed dementia.	Mild GI upset, headache, dizziness, constipation, palpitations, allergic skin reactions. Large doses can cause diarrhea, nausea, vomiting, weakness. Decreases platelet aggregation; may increase risk of bleeding with antiplatelet and anticoagulants (e.g., aspirin, clopidogrel, enoxaparin, warfarin).
Ginseng	Increases resistance to environmental stress, improves well-being, boosts energy, diuretic.	May cause insomnia, vaginal bleeding, headache, hypertension, hypotension, decreased appetite, edema. May decrease effectiveness of warfarin.
Glucosamine	Osteoarthritis, glaucoma, temporomandibular joint arthritis.	May cause mild GI effects (e.g., nausea, heartburn, diarrhea, constipation). May increase risk of bleeding with anticoagulants (e.g., warfarin).
Gotu kola	Reduce fatigue, anxiety, depression, improve memory and intelligence.	May cause GI upset, nausea, drowsiness. May cause additive sedative effects/side effects with CNS depressants (e.g., clonazePAM, LORazepam, zolpidem).
Grapefruit	Hyperlipidemia, atherosclerosis, weight loss and obesity.	May increase concentrations/effects of benzodiazepines, calcium channel blockers, carBAMazepine, carvedilol, clomiPRAMINE, cycloSPORINE, estrogens, lovastatin, simvastatin, atorvastatin.
Green tea	Improves cognitive performance and mental alertness.	Can cause nausea, vomiting, abdominal bloating, dyspepsia, flatulence, diarrhea. Higher doses can cause dizziness, insomnia, fatigue, agitation. May increase effects of amphetamines, caffeine.

Name	Uses	Comments
Hawthorn	Congestive HF, coronary heart disease, angina, arrhythmias.	Generally well tolerated. Can cause vertigo, dizziness, nausea, GI complaints, fatigue, sweating, rash.
Kava kava	Anxiety disorders, stress, attention-deficit hyperactivity disorder (ADHD), insomnia, restlessness.	GI upset, headache, dizziness, drowsiness, enlarged pupils and disturbances of oculomotor equilibrium and accommodation, dry mouth, allergic skin reactions. May increase drowsiness, motor reflex depression with alcohol, benzodiazepines, other CNS depressants.
L-carnitine	Treatment of primary L-carnitine deficiency, acute myocardial infarction, supplement to total parenteral nutrition, L-carnitine deficiency in those requiring hemodialysis.	Can cause nausea, vomiting, abdominal cramps, heartburn, gastritis, diarrhea, body odor, seizures.
Licorice	Gastric and duodenal ulcers, sore throat, bronchitis, dyspepsia, cough, osteoarthritis, chronic gastritis, menopausal symptoms, osteoporosis, bacterial/viral infections.	Excessive ingestion can cause pseudohyperaldosteronism with sodium and water retention, hypokalemia, alkalosis. May lead to hypertension, edema, arrhythmias. May reduce effect of antihypertensive medication therapy, warfarin.
Melatonin	Jet lag, insomnia, shift-work disorder.	Can cause daytime drowsiness, headache, dizziness. May increase effect of antiplatelets, anticoagulants (e.g., aspirin, clopidogrel, enoxaparin, warfarin). May cause additive sedation with CNS depressants (e.g., alcohol, benzodiazepines).
Milk thistle	Liver disorders, chronic inflammatory liver disease, hepatic cirrhosis, chronic hepatitis.	Usually well tolerated. Can cause nausea, diarrhea, dyspepsia, flatulence, abdominal bloating, anorexia.
Nettle	Urinary disorders associated with benign prostatic hyperplasia (e.g., nocturia, frequency, dysuria, urinary retention).	Generally well tolerated. May cause GI complaints, sweating, allergic skin reactions. May decrease effects of warfarin.
Peppermint	Common cold, cough, inflammation of mouth and pharynx, sinusitis, fever, cramps of upper GI tract, dyspepsia, flatulence, irritable bowel syndrome (IBS), fever, tension headache.	Can cause heartburn, nausea, vomiting, allergic reactions including flushing and headache. May increase concentration/effects of cyclosporine.

Continued

Name	Uses	Comments
Red yeast	Maintain desirable cholesterol levels in healthy people; reduce cholesterol in hyperlipidemia; indigestion; diarrhea; improve blood circulation.	Can cause abdominal discomfort, heartburn, flatulence, dizziness. May increase cyclosporine concentration.
SAMe	Depression, anxiety, heart disease, fibromyalgia, osteoarthritis, tendonitis, dementia, Alzheimer's disease, Parkinson's disease.	Higher doses can cause flatulence, nausea, vomiting, diarrhea, constipation, headache, mild insomnia, anorexia, sweating, dizziness, nervousness. May have additive adverse effects with MAOIs including hypertension, hyperthermia, agitation, confusion, coma. May have additive serotonergic effects and serotonin syndrome-like effects (e.g., agitation, tremors, tachycardia, diarrhea, hyperreflexia, shivering, diaphoresis) with antidepressants.
Saw palmetto	Symptoms of benign prostatic hyperplasia (BPH).	Can cause dizziness, headache, GI complaints (e.g., nausea, vomiting, constipation, diarrhea). May increase effect of antiplatelets, anticoagulants (e.g., aspirin, clopidogrel, enoxaparin, warfarin). May interfere with contraceptives.
St. John's wort	Depression, anxiety, heart palpitations; mood disturbances associated with menopause, ADHD, obsessive-compulsive disorder (OCD), seasonal affective disorder (SAD), premenstrual syndrome (PMS), social phobia.	Usually well tolerated. Can cause insomnia, vivid dreams, restlessness, agitation, irritability, GI discomfort, diarrhea, fatigue, dry mouth, dizziness, headache. May decrease effect of alprazolam, amitriptyline, oral contraceptives, cyclosporine, imatinib, irinotecan, NNRTIs, phenytoin, protease inhibitors, tacrolimus, warfarin. May cause additive serotonergic effects with antidepressants, paroxetine, sertraline, tramadol.
Turmeric	Osteoarthritis, rheumatoid arthritis, dyspepsia, abdominal pain, Crohn's disease, ulcerative colitis, diarrhea, flatulence, loss of appetite, hepatitis, *H. pylori,* peptic ulcers, irritable bowel syndrome.	Usually well tolerated. Can cause dyspepsia, diarrhea, distention, GERD, nausea, vomiting. May increase risk of bleeding with antiplatelets/anticoagulants. May increase risk of hypoglycemia with antidiabetic drugs.

Name	Uses	Comments
Valerian	Insomnia, anxiety-associated restlessness, sleeping disorders.	Can cause headache, excitability, insomnia, gastric discomfort, dry mouth, vivid dreams, morning drowsiness. May have additive sedative effects with alcohol, benzodiazepines, other CNS depressants.
Yohimbe	Aphrodisiac, impotence, exhaustion, angina, hypertension, diabetic neuropathy, postural hypotension.	Can cause excitation, tremors, insomnia, anxiety, hypertension, tachycardia, dizziness, irritability, headache, fluid retention, rash, nausea, vomiting. High doses can cause respiratory depression. May have additive effects with MAOIs. Tyramine-containing foods increase risk of hypertensive crisis.

Appendix G

LIFESPAN, CULTURAL ASPECTS, AND PHARMACOGENOMICS OF DRUG THERAPY

LIFESPAN

Drug therapy is unique to pts of different ages. Age-specific competencies involve understanding the development and health needs of the various age groups. Pregnant pts, children, and elderly people represent different age groups with important considerations during drug therapy.

CHILDREN

In pediatric drug therapy, drug administration is guided by the age of the child, weight, level of growth and development, and height. The dosage ordered is to be given either by kilogram of body weight or by square meter of body surface area, which is based on the height and weight of the child. Many dosages based on these calculations must be individualized based on pediatric response.

If the oral route of administration is used, often syrup or chewable tablets are given. Additionally, sometimes medication is added to liquid or mixed with foods. Remember to never force a child to take oral medications because choking or emotional trauma may ensue.

If an intramuscular injection is ordered, the vastus lateralis muscle in the midlateral thigh is used because the gluteus maximus is not developed until walking occurs and the deltoid muscle is too small. For intravenous medications, administer very slowly in children. If given too quickly, high serum drug levels will occur with the potential for toxicity.

PREGNANCY

Women of childbearing years should be asked about the possibility of pregnancy before any drug therapy is initiated. Advise a woman who is either planning a pregnancy or believes she may be pregnant to inform her physician immediately. During pregnancy, medications given to the mother pass to the fetus via the placenta. Teratogenic (fetal abnormalities) effects may occur. Breastfeeding while the mother is taking certain medications may not be recommended due to the potential for adverse effects on the newborn.

The choice of drug ordered for pregnant women is based on the stage of pregnancy because the fetal organs develop during the first trimester. Cautious use of drugs in women of reproductive age who are sexually active and who are not using contraceptives is essential to prevent the potential for teratogenic or embryotoxic effects.

ELDERLY

Elderly people are more likely to experience an adverse drug reaction owing to physiologic changes (e.g., visual, hearing, mobility changes, chronic diseases) and cognitive changes (short-term memory loss or alteration in the thought process) that may lead to multiple medication dosing. In chronic disease states such as hypertension, glaucoma, asthma, or arthritis, the daily ingestion of multiple medications increases the potential for adverse reactions and toxic effects.

Decreased renal or hepatic function may lower the metabolism of medications in the liver and reduce excretion of medications, thus prolonging the half-life of the drug and the potential for toxicity. Dosages in elderly people should initially be smaller than for the general adult population and then slowly titrated based on pt response and therapeutic effect of the medication.

CULTURE

The term *ethnopharmacology* was first used to describe the study of medicinal plants used by indigenous cultures. More recently, it is being used as a reference to the action and effects of drugs in people from diverse racial, ethnic, and cultural backgrounds. Although there are insufficient data from investigations involving people from diverse backgrounds that would provide reliable information on ethnic-specific responses to all medications, there is growing evidence that modifications in dosages are needed for some members of racial and ethnic groups. There are wide variations in the perception of side effects by pts from diverse cultural backgrounds. These differences may be related to metabolic differences that result in higher or lower levels of the drug, individual differences in the amount of body fat, or cultural differences in the way individuals perceive the meaning of side effects and toxicity. Nurses and other healthcare providers need to be aware that variations can occur with side effects, adverse reactions, and toxicity so that pts from diverse cultural backgrounds can be monitored.

Some cultural differences in response to medications include the following:

African Americans: Generally, African Americans are less responsive to beta blockers (e.g., propranolol [Inderal]) and angiotensin-converting enzyme (ACE) inhibitors (e.g., enalapril [Vasotec]).

Asian Americans: On average, Asian Americans have a lower percentage of body fat, so dosage adjustments must be made for fat-soluble vitamins and other drugs (e.g., vitamin K used to reverse the anticoagulant effect of warfarin).

Hispanic Americans: Hispanic Americans may require lower dosages and may experience a higher incidence of side effects with tricyclic antidepressants (e.g., amitriptyline).

Native Americans: Alaskan Eskimos may suffer prolonged muscle paralysis with the use of succinylcholine when administered during surgery.

There has been a desire to exert more responsibility over one's health and, as a result, a resurgence of self-care practices. These practices are often influenced by folk remedies and the use of medicinal plants. In the United States, there are several major ethnic population subgroups (white, black, Hispanic, Asian, and Native Americans). Each of these ethnic groups has a wide range of practices that influence beliefs and interventions related to health and illness. At any given time, in any group, treatment may consist of the use of traditional herbal therapy, a combination of ritual and prayer with medicinal plants, customary dietary and environmental practices, or the use of Western medical practices.

AFRICAN AMERICANS

Many African Americans carry the traditional health beliefs of their African heritage. Health denotes harmony with nature of the body, mind, and spirit, whereas illness is seen as disharmony that results from natural causes or divine punishment. Common practices to the art of healing include treatments with herbals and rituals known empirically to restore health. Specific forms of healing include using home remedies, obtaining medical advice from a physician, and seeking spiritual healing.

Examples of healing practices include the use of hot baths and warm compresses for rheumatism, the use of herbal teas for respiratory illnesses, and the use of kitchen condiments in folk remedies. Lemon, vinegar, honey, saltpeter, alum, salt, baking soda, and Epsom salt are common kitchen ingredients used. Goldenrod, peppermint, sassafras, parsley, yarrow, and rabbit tobacco are a few of the herbals used.

HISPANIC AMERICANS

The use of folk healers, medicinal herbs, magic, and religious rituals and ceremonies are included in the rich and varied customs of Hispanic Americans. This ethnic group believes that God is responsible for allowing health or illness to occur. Wellness may be viewed as good luck, a reward for good behavior, or a blessing from God. Praying, using herbals and spices, wearing religious objects such as medals, and maintaining a balance in diet and physical activity are methods considered appropriate in preventing evil or poor health.

Hispanic ethnopharmacology is more complementary to Western medical practices. After the illness is identified, appropriate treatment may consist of home remedies (e.g., use of vegetables and herbs), use of over-the-counter patent medicines, and use of physician-prescribed medications.

ASIAN AMERICANS

For Asian Americans, harmony with nature is essential for physical and spiritual well-being. Universal balance depends on harmony among the elemental forces: fire, water, wood, earth, and metal. Regulating these universal elements are two forces that maintain physical and spiritual harmony in the body: the *yin* and the *yang*. Practices shared by most Asian cultures include meditation, special nutritional programs, herbology, and martial arts.

Therapeutic options available to traditional Chinese physicians include prescribing herbs, meditation, exercise, nutritional changes, and acupuncture.

NATIVE AMERICANS

The theme of total harmony with nature is fundamental to traditional Native American beliefs about health. It is dependent on maintaining a state of equilibrium among the physical body, the mind, and the environment. Health practices reflect this holistic approach. The method of healing is determined traditionally by the medicine man, who diagnoses the ailment and recommends the appropriate intervention.

Treatment may include heat, herbs, sweat baths, massage, exercise, diet changes, and other interventions performed in a curing ceremony.

EUROPEAN AMERICANS

Europeans often use home treatments as the front-line interventions. Traditional remedies practiced are based on the magical or empirically validated experience of ancestors. These cures are often practiced in combination with religious rituals or spiritual ceremonies.

Household products, herbal teas, and patent medicines are familiar preparations used in home treatments (e.g., saltwater gargle for sore throat).

PHARMACOGENOMICS

Traditionally, medications are prescribed using a "one size fits all" philosophy. In general, the genetic makeup is similar in all humans, regardless of race or sex. However, people inherit variations in their genes, which can affect the way a person responds to a medication. A genetic variation may make a medication stay in the body longer, causing serious side effects, or a variation may make the medication less potent.

For example, two people taking the same cancer medication may have very different responses. One may have severe, life-threatening side effects, whereas the second may have few, if any, side effects. The drug may shrink a tumor in one person but not in another.

Pharmacogenomics examines how a person's genetic makeup affects response to medications. Although widespread application still lies in the future, pharmacogenomics has the potential to personalize medical therapies. Physicians eventually will be able to prescribe medications based on an individual's genotype, thereby maximizing effectiveness and minimizing side effects.

Pharmacogenomics is an expanding field that explores the effect of interindividual genetic differences on pharmacokinetics, pharmacodynamics, drug efficiency, and safety of drug treatments. Pharmacogenomic biomarkers (proteins) can provide predictive tools for improving drug response and reducing adverse drug reactions. These biomarkers mainly originate from genes encoding drug-metabolizing enzymes, drug transporters, drug targets, and human leukocyte antigens. Currently, more than 100 drugs contain pharmacogenomic information in the package labeling. The goal is to develop personalized genetic-based strategies that will optimize therapeutic outcomes.

Personalized treatments are especially warranted when prescribing medications with a narrow therapeutic index or when toxicity can be life-threatening. Antineoplastics, anticoagulants, and anti-HIV therapies are often administered at maximum tolerated doses. This approach can result in toxicity and/or produce a poor response to therapy. Severe adverse drug reactions are one of the most common reasons for hospital admissions. Genetic testing for drug responses is expected to decrease hospitalizations by as much as 30%.

Carbamazepine (Tegretol) has been linked to dose-dependent side effects and life-threatening adverse effects. It is metabolized by enzymes encoded by the CYP3A4 gene to its active metabolite. An association has been found between the HLA-B*1502 allele and risk of Stevens-Johnson syndrome/toxic epidermal necrolysis, particularly in Asians. Before initiating carbamazepine treatment in high-risk patients, genetic testing for the HLA-B*1502 allele is recommended by the Food and Drug Administration (FDA).

Tumor cells carry the same genetic polymorphisms of normal cells. However, malignant cells are genetically unstable and can produce genetic changes that can alter disposition of active drug at the tumor site. Genetic analysis of tumors can help predict therapeutic benefit (or lack thereof) of targeted biologics such as **trastuzumab (Herceptin)** for ERBB2 *(HER2)*-amplified breast cancers or **erlotinib (Tarceva)** for epidermal growth factor receptor (EGFR)-overexpressing lung cancers.

Genetic mutations in tumors can also predict resistance to treatment, as noted in colorectal cancers, where activating mutations in *KRAS* are known to be a predictive marker for resistance to the EGFR-specific monoclonal antibodies **cetuximab (Erbitux)** and **panitumumab (Vectibix).**

By utilizing the information provided by pharmacogenomic testing, drug therapy is changing to a more individualized approach. Anticipated benefits of pharmacogenomics include creation of better vaccines, safer medications targeted to specific diseases, and more appropriate dosing of medications at the onset of therapy. Ultimately, we may see a decrease in healthcare costs due to more efficient clinical trials, reduced adverse drug reactions, and less time needed to find effective therapy for patients.

Appendix H

NORMAL LABORATORY VALUES

HEMATOLOGY/COAGULATION

Test	Normal Range
Activated partial thromboplastin time (aPTT)	25–35 sec
Erythrocyte count (RBC count)	M: 4.5–5.5 million cells/mm^3 F: 4.0–4.9 million cells/mm^3
Hematocrit (HCT, Hct)	M: 41%–50% F: 36%–44%
Hemoglobin (Hb, Hgb)	M: 13.5–16.5 g/dL F: 12.0–15.0 g/dL
Leukocyte count (WBC count)	4.5–10.0 thousand cells/mm^3
Leukocyte differential count	
Basophils	0%–0.75%
Eosinophils	1%–3%
Lymphocytes	25%–33%
Monocytes	3%–7%
Neutrophils—bands	3%–5%
Neutrophils—segmented	54%–62%
Mean corpuscular hemoglobin (MCH)	26–34 pg/cell
Mean corpuscular hemoglobin concentration (MCHC)	31%–37% Hb/cell
Mean corpuscular volume (MCV)	80–100 fL
Partial thromboplastin time (PTT)	60–85 sec
Platelet count (thrombocyte count)	100–450 thousand/mm^3
Prothrombin time (PT)	11–13.5 sec
RBC count (see Erythrocyte count)	

CLINICAL CHEMISTRY (SERUM PLASMA, URINE)

Test	Normal Range
Alanine aminotransferase (ALT)	8–36 units/L 8–78 units/L (children 0–2 mos)
Albumin	3.2–5 g/dL
Alkaline phosphatase	33–131 (adults 25–60 yrs) 51–153 (adults older than 60 yrs)
Amylase	30–110 units/L
Aspartate aminotransferase (AST)	5–35 units/L
Bilirubin (direct)	0–0.3 mg/dL
Bilirubin (total)	0.1–1.2 mg/dL
BUN	7–20 mg/dL

Test	Normal Range
Calcium, ionized	2.24–2.46 mEq/L
Calcium (total)	8.6–10.3 mg/dL
Carbon dioxide (CO_2) total	23–30 mEq/L
Chloride	95–108 mEq/L
Cholesterol (total) HDL cholesterol LDL cholesterol	Less than 200 mg/dL 40–60 mg/dL Less than 160 mg/dL
Creatinine	0.5–1.4 mg/dL
Creatinine clearance	M: 80–125 mL/min/1.73 m^2 F: 75–115 mL/min/1.73 m^2
Creatine kinase (CK) isoenzymes CK-BB CK-MB (cardiac) CK-MM (muscle)	0% 0%–3.9% 96%–100%
Creatine phosphokinase (CPK)	8–150 units/L
Ferritin	13–300 ng/mL
Glucose (preprandial)	Less than 115 mg/dL
Glucose (fasting)	60–110 mg/dL
Glucose (nonfasting, 2 hrs postprandial)	Less than 120 mg/dL
Hemoglobin A1c	Less than 8 mg/dL
Iron	66–150 mcg/dL
Iron-binding capacity, total (TIBC)	250–420 mcg/dL
Lactate dehydrogenase (LDH)	56–194 units/L
Lipase	23–208 units/L
Magnesium	1.6–2.5 mg/dL
Osmolality	289–308 mOsm/kg
Oxygen saturation	90–95 (arterial) 40–70 (venous)
pH	7.35–7.45 (arterial) 7.32–7.42 (venous)
Phosphorus, inorganic	2.8–4.2 mg/dL
Potassium	3.5–5.2 mEq/L
Protein (total)	6.5–7.9 g/dL
Sodium	134–149 mEq/L
Thyroid-stimulating hormone (TSH)	0.7–6.4 milliunits/L (adults 20 yrs or younger) 0.4–4.2 milliunits/L (adults 21–54 yrs) 0.5–8.9 milliunits/L (adults 55–87 yrs)
Transferrin	Greater than 200 mg/dL
Triglycerides (TG)	45–155 mg/dL
Urea nitrogen	7–20 mg/dL
Uric acid	M: 2–8 mg/dL F: 2–7.5 mg/dL

Appendix I

DRUG INTERACTIONS

OVERVIEW

A drug interaction is a situation in which a substance (e.g., another drug, food, or herbal) can affect the activity of a drug when administered together. This action can be synergistic (drug effect is increased) or antagonistic (drug effect is decreased). Drugs that increase the concentration of another drug can lead to an increase in side effects or even a drug overdose. Drugs that decrease the concentration of another drug may decrease the therapeutic effect.

Factors that may contribute to drug interactions include:

- Old age: Liver metabolism, renal function, nerve transmission decrease with age. Also a sensory decrease increases the chance of errors in drug administration.
- Polypharmacy: As the number of medications taken increases, the potential that some of them will interact is more likely.
- Genetic factors: Genes synthesize enzymes that metabolize drugs. Some races have genotypic variations that may decrease or increase the activity of these enzymes. This is seen in variations in the isozymes of cytochrome P450.
- Hepatic or renal diseases: Blood concentrations of drugs that are metabolized in the liver and/or eliminated by the kidneys may be altered if these organs are not functioning correctly.

Drug interactions may be the result of various processes. These processes may include alterations in the pharmacokinetics of the drug such as in the absorption, distribution, metabolism, and excretion or the result of pharmacodynamics properties of the drug (e.g., coadministration of a receptor antagonist and an agonist for the same receptor).

PHARMACOKINETIC INTERACTIONS

Modifying the effect of a drug may be caused by differences in absorption, distribution, metabolization, or excretion of one or both of the drugs compared with the expected behavior of each drug when taken individually.

ABSORPTION

Changes in motility: Some drugs such as the prokinetic agents increase the speed that a substance passes through the intestines. If a drug is present in the digestive tract's absorption zone for less time, its blood concentration will decrease. The opposite will occur with drugs that decrease intestinal motility.

Certain drugs require an acid stomach pH for absorption while others require the basic pH of the intestines. Modification in the pH could change this absorption. In the case of antacids, an increase in pH can alter the absorption of other drugs.

Drug solubility—Food: Absorption of some drugs can be reduced if administered together with food (e.g., warfarin and avocado).

Formation of nonabsorbable complexes:

- Chelation: The presence of di- or trivalent cations can cause the chelation of certain drugs, making them harder to absorb (e.g., tetracyclines or fluoroquinolones and dairy products).

- Binding with proteins: Some drugs (e.g., sucralfate) bind to proteins and for this reason, sucralfate is contraindicated in enteral feeding.
- Drugs that are retained in the intestinal lumen can form large complexes that impede their absorption. This can occur with cholestyramine if associated with drugs such as digoxin or warfarin.

Action on the P-glycoprotein of the enterocytes appears to be one of the mechanisms promoted by consumption of grapefruit juice in increasing the bioavailability of various drugs.

DISTRIBUTION

The main interaction mechanism is competition for plasma protein transport. The drug that arrives first binds with the plasma protein, leaving the second drug dissolved in plasma, which modifies its concentration (e.g., displacement of bilirubin from albumin binding site by ceftriaxone increases the risk of kernicterus in neonates).

METABOLISM

Most drugs are eliminated from the body, at least in part, by being changed chemically to a less lipid-soluble product (i.e., metabolized) and thus more likely to be excreted from the body via the kidney or bile. Drugs may go through two different metabolic processes: phase 1 and phase 2 metabolism.

In phase 1 metabolism, hepatic microsomal enzymes found in the endothelium of liver cells metabolize drugs via hydrolysis and oxidation and reduction reactions. These chemical reactions make the drug more water soluble. In phase 2 metabolism, large water-soluble substances (e.g., glucuronic acid, sulfate) are attached to the drug, forming inactive, or significantly less active, water-soluble metabolites. Phase 2 processes include glucuronidation, sulfation, conjugation, acetylation, and methylation.

Virtually any of the phase 1 and phase 2 enzymes can be inhibited, and some of these enzymes can be induced by drugs. Inhibiting the activity of metabolic enzymes results in increased concentrations of the drug (substrate), whereas inducing metabolic enzymes results in decreased concentrations of the drug (substrate).

The term "cytochrome P450" (CYP enzymes) refers to a family of more than 100 enzymes in the human body that modulate various physiologic functions. First identified in the 1950s, the CYP enzyme system contains two large subgroups: steroidogenic and xenobiotic enzymes. Only the xenobiotic group is involved in the metabolism of drugs. The xenobiotic group includes four major enzyme families: CYP1, CYP2, CYP3, and CYP4. The primary role of these families is the metabolism of drugs. These families are further subdivided into subfamilies designated by a capital letter and given a specific enzyme number (1, 2, 3, etc.) according to the similarity in amino acid sequence it shares with other enzymes (e.g., CYP1A2).

The key CYP450 enzymes include CYP1A2, CYP2C9, CYP2C19, CYP2D6, and CYP3A4 and may be responsible for metabolism of 75% of all drugs, with the CYP3A subfamily responsible for nearly half of this activity.

The CYP enzymes are found in the endoplasmic reticulum of cells in a variety of human tissue but are primarily concentrated in the liver and intestine. CYP enzymes can be both inhibited and induced, leading to increased or decreased serum concentration of the drug (along with its effects).

The following tables of CYP substrates, inhibitors, and inducers provide a perspective on drugs that are affected by, or affect, cytochrome P450 (CYP) enzymes.

CYP substrate includes drugs reported to be metabolized, at least in part, by one or more CYP enzymes. **CYP inhibitor** includes drugs reported to inhibit one or more CYP enzymes. **CYP inducer** contains drugs reported to induce one or more CYP enzymes.

P450 ENZYMES: SUBSTRATES, INHIBITORS, INDUCERS
CYP1A2 ENZYME

CYP1A2 SUBSTRATES	CYP1A2 INHIBITORS	CYP1A2 INDUCERS
Clozapine (Clozaril)	Cimetidine (Tagamet)	Barbiturates
Mirtazapine (Remeron)	Ciprofloxacin (Cipro)	Carbamazepine (Tegretol)
Olanzapine (Zyprexa)	Fluvoxamine	Rifampin (Rifadin)
Ramelteon (Rozerem)		Smoking
Ropinirole (Requip)		
Tizanidine (Zanaflex)		

- CYP1A2 enzyme is increasingly involved in drug interactions.
- More potent inhibitors include cimetidine, ciprofloxacin, and fluvoxamine.
- Smoking is the most important inducer, but rifampin and barbiturates also can increase enzyme activity.
- Example of reaction: Tizanidine plasma concentrations increased more than 30-fold when the inhibitor fluvoxamine was given concurrently.

CYP2C9 ENZYME

CYP2C9 SUBSTRATES	CYP2C9 INHIBITORS	CYP2C9 INDUCERS
Candesartan (Atacand)	Amiodarone (Cordarone)	Barbiturates
Celecoxib (Celebrex)	Clopidogrel (Plavix)	Carbamazepine (Tegretol)
Diclofenac (Voltaren)	Fluconazole (Diflucan)	Rifampin (Rifadin)
Glipizide (Glucotrol)	Metronidazole (Flagyl)	St. John's wort
Glyburide (DiaBeta)	Sulfamethoxazole	
Ibuprofen (Advil, Motrin)	Valproic acid (Depakote)	
Irbesartan (Avapro)		
Meloxicam (Mobic)		
Warfarin (Coumadin)		

- More potent inhibitors include amiodarone, metronidazole, and sulfamethoxazole.
- All of the inducers can substantially increase enzyme activity.
- Both warfarin and oral hypoglycemics are of serious concern with regard to drug interactions. Substrates warranting attention include warfarin and oral hypoglycemics.

CYP2C19 ENZYME

CYP2C19 SUBSTRATES	CYP2C19 INHIBITORS	CYP2C19 INDUCERS
Citalopram (Celexa)	Cimetidine (Tagamet)	Barbiturates
Diazepam (Valium)	Clopidogrel (Plavix)	Carbamazepine (Tegretol)
Escitalopram (Lexapro)	Esomeprazole (Nexium)	Rifampin (Rifadin)
Omeprazole (Prilosec)	Fluconazole (Diflucan)	St. John's wort
Pantoprazole (Protonix)	Fluvoxamine	
Sertraline (Zoloft)	Modafinil (Provigil)	

- Inhibition by itself does not frequently cause adverse effects compared with other CYP enzymes because many of the substrates do not have serious toxicity.
- Inhibition or induction of the enzyme nonetheless may result in an adverse drug interaction.
- Racial background is important in the likelihood of being deficient in this enzyme (e.g., 3%–5% of Caucasians and 12%–23% of Asians are poor metabolizers of this enzyme).

CYP2D6 ENZYME

CYP2D6 SUBSTRATES	CYP2D6 INHIBITORS	CYP2D6 INDUCERS
Amitriptyline (Elavil)	Amiodarone (Cordarone)	See comment below
Duloxetine (Cymbalta)	Bupropion (Wellbutrin)	
Fluoxetine (Prozac)	Fluoxetine (Prozac)	
Metoclopramide (Reglan)	Paroxetine (Paxil)	
Metoprolol (Lopressor)		
Paroxetine (Paxil)		
Risperidone (Risperdal)		
Tamoxifen (Nolvadex)		
Tolterodine (Detrol)		
Tramadol (Ultram)		
Venlafaxine (Effexor)		

- Potent inhibitors include fluoxetine and paroxetine.
- Evidence suggests that this enzyme is not very susceptible to enzyme induction.
- Genetics, rather than drug therapy, account for most ultra-rapid metabolizers (e.g., Greeks, Portuguese, Saudis, and Ethiopians have high enzyme activity).

CYP3A4 ENZYME

CYP3A4 SUBSTRATES	CYP3A4 INHIBITORS	CYP3A4 INDUCERS
Alfuzosin (Uroxatral)	Amiodarone (Cordarone)	Carbamazepine (Tegretol)
Alprazolam (Xanax)	Clarithromycin (Biaxin)	Efavirenz (Sustiva)
Budesonide (Entocort EC)	Diltiazem (Cardizem)	Phenobarbital
Carbamazepine (Tegretol)	Fluconazole (Diflucan)	Rifampin (Rifadin)
Cyclosporine (Neoral)	Fluoxetine (Prozac)	St. John's wort
Fluticasone (Flovent)	Itraconazole (Sporanox)	
Lovastatin (Mevacor)	Ketoconazole (Nizoral)	
Sildenafil (Viagra)	Verapamil (Calan, Isoptin)	
Simvastatin (Zocor)		

- This enzyme metabolizes about half of all medications on the market.
- Drug toxicity of CYP3A4 substrates due to inhibition of CYP3A4 is relatively common.
- This enzyme is very sensitive to induction, tending to lower plasma concentrations of substrates, resulting in reduced efficacy of the substrate.
- Most potent inhibitors include clarithromycin, itraconazole, and ketoconazole.

- Rifampin is a potent inducer and may reduce serum concentrations of substrates by as much as 90%.

EXCRETION

RENAL EXCRETION

Only the free fraction of a drug that is dissolved in the blood is removed via the kidneys. Drugs that are tightly bound to proteins are not available for renal excretion, as long as they are not metabolized when they may be excreted as metabolites. Creatinine clearance is used as a measure of kidney function.

BILE EXCRETION

Bile excretion always involves energy in active transport across the epithelium of the bile duct against a concentration gradient. Bile excretion of drugs mainly occurs when their molecular weight is greater than 300 and contain both polar and lipophilic groups. Glucuronidation of the drug in the kidney will also enhance bile excretion.

PHARMACODYNAMIC INTERACTIONS

PHARMACOLOGIC RECEPTORS

- **Pure agonists:** Drugs bind to the main locus of the receptor, causing a similar effect to that of the main drug. For example, fentanyl and midazolam can lead to increased sedation, or vancomycin and an aminoglycoside can lead to increased potential for nephrotoxicity.
- **Partial agonists:** Drugs bind to one of the receptor's secondary loci, having the same effect to that of the main drug but with lower intensity.
- **Antagonists:** Drugs bind directly to the receptor's main locus but their effect is opposite to that of the main drug. For example, an opioid and naloxone cause a decreased effect of the opioid, reversal of sedation, respiratory depression, and hypotension.

SIGNAL TRANSDUCTION MECHANISMS

These are processes that commence after the interaction of the drug with the receptor. For example, hypoglycemia produces a release of catecholamines, which triggers compensation mechanisms that increase blood glucose levels. For example, if a patient is taking both insulin (which reduces glucose) and also a beta blocker for heart disease, the beta blocker will block the catecholamine receptors. This will block the reaction triggered by the catecholamines if hypoglycemia occurs, with an increased risk of a serious reaction.

Appendix J

ANTIDOTE/REVERSAL AGENTS

Agent	Antidote/ Reversal Agents	Dosage
Acetaminophen	Acetylcysteine (Acetadote, Mucomyst)	PO: ADULTS, CHILDREN: Loading dose: 140 mg/kg, then 70 mg/kg q4h for a total of 18 doses. Total dose delivered: 1,330 mg/kg. IV: ADULTS, CHILDREN: Loading dose: 150 mg/kg over 60 min, then 50 mg/kg over 4 hrs, then 100 mg/kg over 16 hrs. Total dose delivered: 300 mg/kg.
Anticholinergic agents (e.g., atropine)	Physostigmine	IM/IV/SQ: ADULTS: Initially, 0.5–2 mg, then repeat q20min until response occurs or adverse effects occur. Repeat 1–4 mg q30–60min as life-threatening symptoms recur. IV: CHILDREN (Reserve for life-threatening situation only): 0.01–0.03 mg/kg/dose. May repeat after 15–20 min to maximum total dose of 2 mg, or until response occurs or adverse cholinergic effects occur.
Apixaban (Eliquis)	Kcentra Prothrombin Complex concentrate (Factors II, VII, IX, X, Protein C, Protein S)	Dose based on pre-dose INR, expressed in units of factor IX activity. (Give with Vitamin K) **INR 2 to <4**: 25 units/kg. **Maximum:** 2,500 units. **INR 4–6**: 35 units/kg. **Maximum:** 3,500 units. **INR >6**: 50 units/kg. **Maximum:** 5,000 units.
Apixaban (Eliquis)/ rivaroxaban (Xarelto)	Andexanet alfa (Andexxa)	Apixaban (5 mg or less)/rivaroxaban (10 mg or less): 4 mg IV bolus, then 4 mg/min for up to 120 min. Apixaban (more than 5 mg)/rivaroxaban (more than 10 mg): 800 mg IV bolus, then 8 mg/min for up to 120 min.
Arsenic	Dimercaprol (BAL in oil)	Mild Poisoning IM: ADULTS, CHILDREN: 2.5 mg/kg/dose q6h for 2 days, then q12h for 1 day, then once daily for 10 days. Severe Poisoning IM: ADULTS, CHILDREN: 3 mg/kg/dose q4h for 2 days, then q6h for 1 day, then q12h for 10 days.
Benzodiazepines (e.g., midazolam)	Flumazenil (Romazicon)	IV: ADULTS: 0.2 mg over 30 sec. May give 0.3-mg dose after 30 sec if desired LOC not obtained. Additional doses of 0.5 mg can be given over 30 sec at 1-min intervals up to cumulative dose of 3 mg. CHILDREN: 0.01 mg/kg (**maximum:** 0.2 mg) with repeat doses of 0.01 mg/kg (**maximum:** 0.2 mg) given every minute to maximum total cumulative dose of 1 mg.
Beta blockers (e.g., propranolol)	Glucagon	IV: ADULTS: 5–10 mg over 1 min, followed by infusion of 1–10 mg/hr.

Continued

Agent	Antidote/ Reversal Agents	Dosage
Calcium channel blockers (e.g., verapamil)	Glucagon	IV: ADULTS: 5–10 mg over 1 min, followed by infusion of 1–10 mg/hr.
Carbamate pesticides	Atropine	IV: ADULTS: Initially, 1–5 mg doubled q5min until signs of muscarinic excess abate. IV INFUSION: ADULTS: 0.5–1 mg/hr. IM: ADULTS (Mild symptoms): 2 mg. If severe symptoms develop after first dose, 2 additional doses should be repeated in 10 min. (Severe symptoms): Immediately administer three 2-mg doses. IV: CHILDREN: 0.02–0.05 mg/kg q10–20min until atropine effect observed, then q1–4h for at least 24 hrs. IM: 0.5–2 mg/dose based on weight (0.5 mg: 15–40 lb, 1 mg: 41–90 lb, 2 mg: greater than 90 lb). (Mild symptoms): 1 injection. (Severe symptoms): 2 additional injections given in rapid succession 10 min after receiving first injection.
Dabigatran (Pradaxa)	Idarucizumab (Praxbind)	IV: 5 g (give as 2 separate 2.5 g doses no more than 15 minutes apart).
Digoxin (Lanoxin)	Digoxin immune FAB (Digibind)	**ADULTS** Unknown amount of ingestion: 800 mg IV infusion if acute ingestion, 240 mg IV infusion if chronic ingestion. **Dosing for Ingestion of Single Large Dose** Dose (in no. of vials) = (Total digitalis body load in mg)/(0.5 mg of digitalis bound per vial). Total digitalis body load in mg = (No. of tablets/capsules ingested) × (mg strength of tablet/capsule) × (bioavailability of tablet/capsule). Digoxin tablets and elixir are 80% bioavailable. Digoxin capsules and injection are 100% bioavailable. **Dosing Based on Serum Level** Digoxin: Dose (in no. of vials) = (Serum digoxin level in ng/mL) × (weight in kg)/(100). Digitoxin: Dose (in no. of vials) = (Serum digitoxin level in ng/mL) × (weight in kg)/(1,000). **CHILDREN** **Dosing for Ingestion of Single Large Dose** Dose (in no. of vials) = (Total digitalis body load in mg)/(0.5 mg of digitalis bound per vial). Total digitalis body load in mg = (No. of tablets/capsules ingested) × (mg strength of tablet/capsule) × (bioavailability of tablet/capsule). Digoxin tablets and elixir are 80% bioavailable. Digoxin capsules and injection are 100% bioavailable. WEIGHING 20 kg or less: Dilution of reconstituted vial to 1 mg/mL may be desirable for doses of 3 mg or less. Dose (in no. of mg) = Dose (in no. of vials) × 38 mg/vial. Dose (in no. of vials) = (Serum digoxin level in ng/mL) × (weight in kg)/(100).

Agent	Antidote/ Reversal Agents	Dosage
Edoxaban (Savaysa)	See apixaban (Eliquis)	See apixaban (Eliquis)
Ethylene glycol	Fomepizole (Antizol)	IV: ADULTS, CHILDREN: Loading dose 15 mg/kg, then 10 mg/kg q12h for 4 doses, then 15 mg/kg q12h thereafter until ethylene glycol levels reduced to less than 20 mg/dL and patient is asymptomatic with normal pH.
Extravasation vasoconstrictive agents (e.g., dopamine)	Phentolamine (Regitine)	ADULTS, CHILDREN: Infiltrate area with small amount of solution made by diluting 5–10 mg in 10 mL 0.9% NaCl within 12 hrs of extravasation. In general, do not exceed 0.1–0.2 mg/kg (5 mg total).
Heparin	Protamine	IV: ADULTS, CHILDREN: Dosage is determined by most recent dosage of heparin or low molecular weight heparin (LMWH): 1 mg protamine neutralizes 90–115 units of heparin and 1 mg (100 units) of LMWH. **Maximum:** 50 mg.
Hyperkalemia	Sodium polystyrene sulfonate (Kayexalate, SPS)	PO: ADULTS, ELDERLY: 15 g 1–4 times/day. CHILDREN: 1g/kg q6h.
Hypoglycemia	Glucagon	IM/IV/SQ: ADULTS, ELDERLY, CHILDREN: 1 mg, may repeat in 15 min as needed. If pt fails to respond, IV dextrose must be given.
Iron	Deferoxamine (Desferal)	Acute IM: ADULTS: Initially, 1,000 mg, then 500 mg q4h for 2 doses. Additional doses of 0.5 g q4–12h. **Maximum:** 6 g/24 hrs. CHILDREN 3 YRS AND OLDER: 90 mg/kg/dose q8h (not to exceed 1 g/dose). **Maximum:** 6 g/24 hrs. IV: ADULTS, CHILDREN: 15 mg/kg/hr. **Maximum:** 6 g/24 hrs. Chronic IM: ADULTS: 500–1,000 mg/day. IV: ADULTS, CHILDREN: 15 mg/kg/hr. **Maximum:** 12 g/24 hrs.
Isoniazid	Pyridoxine (vitamin B_6)	IV: ADULTS, CHILDREN: Total dose of pyridoxine equal to amount of isoniazid ingested as first dose of 1–4 g IV, then 1 g IM q30min until total dose completed. If not known, give 5 g at rate of 1 g/min. May repeat q5–10min.

Continued

Agent	Antidote/ Reversal Agents	Dosage
Lead	Calcium EDTA	Symptomatic Treat for 3–5 days; give in conjunction with dimercaprol. IM: ADULTS, CHILDREN: 167 mg/m^2 q4h. IV: ADULTS, CHILDREN: 1 g/m^2 as 8- to 24-hr infusion or divided q12h. Lead Encephalopathy Treat for 5 days; give concurrently with dimercaprol. IM: ADULTS, CHILDREN: 250 mg/m^2 q4h. IV: ADULTS, CHILDREN: 50 mg/kg/day as 24-hr continuous infusion.
Lead	Dimercaprol (BAL in oil)	Mild IM: ADULTS, CHILDREN: Loading dose 4 mg/kg, then 3 mg/kg/dose q4h for 2–7 days. Begin calcium EDTA with second dose. Severe and Lead Encephalopathy IM: ADULTS, CHILDREN: 4 mg/kg/dose q4h for 3–5 days. Begin calcium EDTA with second dose.
Lead	Succimer (Chemet)	PO: ADULTS, CHILDREN: 10 mg/kg/dose q8h for 5 days, then q12h for 14 days. **Maximum:** 500 mg/dose. Note: For children younger than 5 yrs, dose based on mg/m^2.
Methanol	Fomepizole (Antizol)	IV: ADULTS, CHILDREN: Loading dose 15 mg/kg, then 10 mg/kg q12h for 4 doses, then 15 mg/kg q12h thereafter until ethylene glycol levels reduced to less than 20 mg/dL and patient is asymptomatic with normal pH.
Opioids (e.g., morphine)	Naloxone (Narcan)	IV/IM/SQ: ADULTS: 0.4–2 mg/dose. May repeat every 2–3 min as needed. Therapy may need to be reassessed if no response is seen after cumulative dose of 10 mg. CHILDREN (5 YRS OR OLDER or WEIGHING 20 KG OR GREATER): 2 mg/dose IV/IM/SQ. May repeat every 2–3 min as needed. Therapy may need to be reassessed if no response is seen after cumulative dose of 10 mg. CHILDREN (WEIGHING LESS THAN 20 KG): 0.1 mg/kg/dose. May repeat every 2–3 min as needed.

Agent	Antidote/ Reversal Agents	Dosage
Organophosphate pesticides	Atropine	IV: ADULTS: Initially, 1–5 mg doubled q5min until signs of muscarinic excess abate. IV INFUSION: ADULTS: 0.5–1 mg/hr. IM: ADULTS (Mild symptoms): 2 mg. If severe symptoms develop after first dose, 2 additional doses should be repeated in 10 min. (Severe symptoms): Immediately administer three 2-mg doses. IV: CHILDREN: 0.02–0.05 mg/kg q10–20min until atropine effect observed, then q1–4h for at least 24 hrs. IM: 0.5–2 mg/dose based on weight (0.5 mg: 15–40 lb, 1 mg: 41–90 lb, 2 mg: greater than 90 lb). (Mild symptoms): 1 injection. (Severe symptoms): 2 additional injections given in rapid succession 10 min after receiving first injection.
Organophosphate pesticides	Pralidoxime (Protopam)	IM/IV: ADULTS: 1–2 g. Repeat in 1–2 hrs if muscle weakness has not been relieved, then at 10- to 12-hr intervals if cholinergic signs recur. CHILDREN: 20–50 mg/kg/dose. Repeat in 1–2 hrs if muscle weakness is not relieved, then at 10- to 12-hr intervals if cholinergic signs recur.
Rivaroxaban (Xarelto)	See apixaban (Eliquis)	See apixaban (Eliquis)
Warfarin (Coumadin)	Phytonadione (vitamin K)	PO/IV/SQ: ADULTS: 2.5–10 mg/dose. May repeat in 12–48 hrs if given PO, 6–8 hrs if given by IV or SQ route. CHILDREN: 0.5–5 mg depending on need for further anticoagulation, severity of bleeding.

Appendix K

PREVENTING MEDICATION ERRORS AND IMPROVING MEDICATION SAFETY

Medication safety is a high priority for the healthcare professional. Prevention of medication errors and improved safety for the pt are important, esp. in today's healthcare environment when today's pt is older and sometimes sicker and the drug therapy regimen can be more sophisticated and complex.

A medication error is defined by the National Coordinating Council for Medication Error Reporting and Prevention (NCC MERP) as "any preventable event that may cause or lead to inappropriate medication use or pt harm while the medication is in the control of the health care professional, pt, or consumer."

Most medication errors occur as a result of multiple, compounding events as opposed to a single act by a single individual.

Use of the wrong medication, strength, or dose; confusion over sound-alike or look-alike drugs; administration of medications by the wrong route; miscalculations (esp. when used in pediatric pts or when administering medications intravenously); and errors in prescribing and transcription all can contribute to compromising the safety of the pt. The potential for adverse events and medication errors is definitely a reality and is potentially tragic and costly in both human and economic terms.

Healthcare professionals must take the initiative to create and implement procedures to prevent medication errors from occurring and implement methods to reduce medication errors. The first priority in preventing medication errors is to establish a multidisciplinary team to improve medication use. The goal for this team would be to assess medication safety and implement changes that would make it difficult or impossible for mistakes to occur. Some important criteria in making improved medication safety successful include the following:

- Promote a nonpunitive approach to reducing medication errors.
- Increase the detection and the reporting of medication errors, near misses, and potentially hazardous situations that may result in medication errors.
- Determine root causes of medication errors.
- Educate about the causes of medication errors and ways to prevent these errors.
- Make recommendations to allow organization-wide, system-based changes to prevent medication errors.
- Learn from errors that occur in other organizations and take measures to prevent similar errors.

Some common causes and ways to prevent medication errors and improve safety include the following:

Handwriting: Poor handwriting can make it difficult to distinguish between two medications with similar names. Also, many drug names sound similar, esp. when the names are spoken over the telephone, poorly enunciated, or mispronounced.

- Take time to write legibly.
- Keep phone or verbal orders to a minimum to prevent misinterpretation.

- Repeat back orders taken over the telephone.
- When ordering a new or rarely used medication, print the name.
- Always specify the drug strength, even if only one strength exists.
- Express dosages for oral liquids only in metric weights or volumes (e.g., mg or mL), not by teaspoon or tablespoon.
- Print generic and brand names of look-alike or sound-alike medications.

Zeros and decimal points: Hastily written orders can present problems even if the name of the medication is clear.

- Never leave a decimal point "naked." Place a zero before a decimal point when the number is less than a whole unit (e.g., use 0.25 mg or 250 mcg, **not** .25 mg).
- Never have a trailing zero following a decimal point (e.g., use 2 mg, **not** 2.0 mg).

Abbreviations: Errors can occur because of a failure to standardize abbreviations. Establishing a list of abbreviations that should never be used is recommended.

- Never abbreviate unit as "U"; spell out "unit."
- Do not abbreviate "once daily" as OD or QD or "every other day" as QOD; spell it out.
- Do not use D/C, as this may be misinterpreted as either discharge or discontinue.
- Do not abbreviate drug names; spell out the generic and/or brand names.

Ambiguous or incomplete orders: These types of orders can cause confusion or misinterpretation of the writer's intention. Examples include situations when the route of administration, dose, or dosage form has not been specified.

- Do not use slash marks—they may be read as the number one (1).
- When reviewing an unusual order, verify the order with the person writing the order to prevent any misunderstanding.
- Read over orders after writing.
- Encourage that the drug's indication for use be provided on medication orders.
- Provide complete medication orders—do not use "resume preop" or "continue previous meds."
- Provide the age and, when appropriate, the weight of the pt.

High-alert medications: Medications in this category have an increased risk of causing significant pt harm when used in error. Mistakes with these medications may or may not be more common but may be more devastating to the pt if an error occurs. A list of high-alert medications can be obtained from the Institute for Safe Medication Practices (ISMP) at www.ismp.org.

Technology available today that can be used to address and help solve potential medication problems or errors includes the following:

- Electronic prescribing systems—This refers to computerized prescriber order entry systems. Within these systems is the capability to incorporate medication safety alerts (e.g., maximum dose alerts, allergy screening). Additionally, these systems should be integrated or interfaced with pharmacy and laboratory systems to provide drug-drug and drug-disease interactions alerts and include clinical order screening capability.
- Bar codes—These systems are designed to use bar-code scanning devices to validate identity of pts, verify medications administered, document administration, and provide safety alerts.

- "Smart" infusion pumps—These pumps allow users to enter drug infusion protocols into a drug library along with predefined dosage limits. If a dosage is outside the limits established, an alarm is sounded and drug delivery is halted, informing the clinician that the dose is outside the recommended range.
- Automated dispensing systems; point-of-use dispensing system—These systems should be integrated with information systems, esp. pharmacy systems.
- Pharmacy order entry system—This should be fully integrated with an electronic prescribing system with the capability of producing medication safety alerts. Additionally, the system should generate a computerized medication administration record (MAR), which would be used by the nursing staff while administering medications.

Medication reconciliation: Medication errors generally occur at transition points in the pt's care (admission, transfer from one level of care to another [e.g., critical care to general care area], and discharge). Incomplete documentation can account for up to 60% of potential medication errors. Therefore, it becomes necessary to accurately and completely reconcile medication across the continuum of care. This includes the name, dosage, frequency, and route of medication administration.

Medication reconciliation programs are a process of identifying the most accurate list of all medications a pt is taking and using this list to provide correct medications anywhere within the healthcare system. The focus is on not only compiling a list but using the list to reduce medication errors and provide quality pt care.

Additional Strategies to Reduce Medication Errors

The ISMP, Food and Drug Administration (FDA), and other agencies have identified high-risk areas associated with medication errors. They include the following:

At-risk population: At-risk populations primarily include pediatric and geriatric pts. For both, this risk is due to altered pharmacokinetic parameters with little published information regarding medication use in these groups. Additionally, in the pediatric population, the risk is due to the need for calculating doses based on age and weight, lack of available dosage forms, and concentrations for smaller children.

In a USP report, more than one-third of medication errors reaching the pt occurred in pts 65 yrs of age and older. Almost 40% of people 60 yrs and older take at least five medications. More than 50% of fatal hospital medication errors involve seniors. In the senior population, age-related physiologic changes (e.g., decreased renal function, reduced muscle mass) increase the risk for adverse events.

Avoid abbreviations and nomenclature: The confusion caused by abbreviations has prompted the ISMP to develop a list of abbreviations that should be avoided (see back cover of handbook).

Recognize prescription look-alike and sound-alike medications: The ISMP has developed an extensive list of confused drug names (see www.jointcommission.org). See individual monographs for **DO NOT CONFUSE** information.

Focus on high-alert medications: High-alert medications are medications that bear a heightened risk of causing significant pt harm if incorrectly used. High-alert medications in the handbook have a colored background for the entire monograph.

Look for duplicate therapies and interactions: Drug interactions and duplicate therapies can increase risk of adverse reactions. Refer to individual monographs for significant interaction information (drug, herbal, food).

Report errors to improve process: This action plays an important role in preventing further errors. The intent is to identify system failures that can be altered to prevent further errors.

Appendix L

PARENTERAL FLUID ADMINISTRATION

Replacing fluids in the body is based on body fluid needs. Water comprises approximately 60% of the adult body. Approximately 40% is intracellular fluid and 20% is extracellular fluid, of which 15% is interstitial (tissues) and 5% is intravascular. The walls separating these compartments are porous, allowing water to move freely between them. Small particles such as sodium and chloride can pass through the walls, but larger molecules such as proteins and starches usually are unable to pass through the walls.

Hydrostatic and osmotic pressures are forces that move water and regulate the body's water. Intravenous fluid manipulates these two pressures. Hydrostatic pressure reflects the weight and volume of water. The greater the volume, the higher the blood pressure.

Effects of Osmotic Pressure: *Osmosis* is the diffusion of water across a semipermeable membrane from an area of high concentration to an area of low concentration (water moves into the compartment of higher concentration of particles, or solute). This is similar to the action of a sponge soaking up water. This pull is referred to as *osmotic pressure.* It is the number of particles in each compartment that keeps water where it is supposed to be. By administering fluids with more (or fewer) particles than blood plasma, fluid is pulled into the compartment where it is needed the most.

How do we know where the water is needed? To assess water balance, measure the *osmolality* of blood plasma (number of particles [osmoles] in a kilogram of fluid). *Osmolarity* is the number of particles in a liter of fluid. Normal serum osmolality is approximately 300 milliosmoles (mOsm) per liter.

Crystalloids are made of substances that form crystals (e.g., sodium chloride) and are small, so easy movement between compartments is possible. Crystalloids are categorized by their tonicity (a synonym for osmolality). An isotonic solution has the same number of particles (osmolality) as plasma and will not promote a shift of fluids into or out of cells. Examples of isotonic crystalloid solutions are 0.9% sodium chloride and lactated Ringer's solution. Dextrose 5% in water is another isotonic crystalloid. However, it is quickly metabolized, and the fluid quickly becomes hypotonic. Hypotonic solutions (e.g., D_5W, 0.45% sodium chloride) are a good source of free water, causing a shift out of the vascular bed and into cells by way of osmosis. Hypotonic solutions are given to correct cellular dehydration and hypernatremia. Hypertonic solutions have more particles than body water and pull water back into the circulation, which can shrink cells.

SODIUM CHLORIDE

USES

- Extracellular fluid replacement when chloride loss is greater than or equal to sodium loss
- Treatment of metabolic alkalosis in the presence of fluid loss; chloride ions cause a compensatory decrease of bicarbonate ions
- Sodium depletion, extracellular fluid volume deficit with sodium deficit
- Initiation and termination of blood transfusion, preventing hemolysis of RBCs (occurs with Dextrose in Water solutions)

SIDE EFFECTS/ABNORMALITIES

- Hypernatremia
- **Acidosis:** 0.9% sodium chloride contains one-third more chloride ions than is present in extracellular fluid; excess chloride ions cause loss of bicarbonate, resulting in acidosis
- **Hypokalemia:** Increased potassium excretion at the same time extracellular fluid is increasing, which further decreases potassium concentration in extracellular fluid
- Circulatory overload

DEXTROSE (GLUCOSE)

EFFECTS

- Provides calories for essential energy
- Improves hepatic function because it is converted into glycogen
- Spares body protein, preventing unnecessary breakdown of protein tissue
- Prevents ketosis
- Stored in the liver as glycogen, causing a shift of potassium from extracellular to intracellular fluid compartment

USES

- Dehydration
- Hyponatremia
- Hyperkalemia
- Vehicle of drug delivery and nutrition

Note: Once infused, dextrose is rapidly metabolized to water and carbon dioxide, becoming hypotonic rather than isotonic.

SIDE EFFECTS/ABNORMALITIES

- Dehydration: Osmotic diuresis occurs if dextrose is given faster than the pt's ability to metabolize it
- Hypokalemia (see Effects)
- Hyperinsulinism due to rapid infusion of hypertonic solution
- Water intoxication due to an imbalance based on increase in extracellular fluid volume from water alone

SELECTED PARENTERAL FLUIDS

Solution	Comments
Dextrose 5% in Water (D_5W)	Supplies approximately 170 cal/L and free water to aid in renal excretion of solutes Avoid excessive volumes in pts with increased antidiuretic hormone activity or to replace fluids in hypovolemic pts
0.9% Sodium chloride (0.9% NaCl)	Isotonic fluid commonly used to expand extracellular fluid in presence of hypovolemia Can be used to treat mild metabolic alkalosis

Solution	Comments
0.45% Sodium chloride (0.45% NaCl)	Hypotonic solution that provides sodium, chloride, and free water; sodium and chloride allow kidneys to select and retain needed amounts Free water is desirable as aid to kidneys in elimination of solutes
3% Sodium chloride	Used only to treat severe hyponatremia
Lactated Ringer's solution	Isotonic solution that contains sodium, potassium, calcium, and chloride in approximately the same concentrations as found in plasma Used to treat hypovolemia, burns, and fluid loss as bile or diarrhea

Appendix M

COMMON TERMINOLOGY CRITERIA FOR ADVERSE EVENTS (CTCAE)

The Common Terminology Criteria for Adverse Events (CTCAE) is descriptive terminology used for reporting an adverse event (AE) in a concise and standardized manner. It is supported by the U.S. Department of Health and Human Services, National Institutes of Health, and National Cancer Institute. An AE term is a unique representation of a specific event that can be used for medical documentation and scientific analyses. Along with cancer medications, other drugs may use the CTCAE system for dose and treatment modifications.

CTCAE terms are grouped by system organ classes, such as *Blood/Lymphatic, GI, Nervous, Renal,* and *Respiratory* disorders. Within each system organ class, AEs are listed and accompanied by a brief description. A grading scale is then provided for each AE term, and each grade refers to a specific severity.

The CTCAE grading scale displays grades 1–5 with particular descriptions and/or recommendations. The severity for each AE is based on the following generalized guidelines: **Grade 1**: Asymptomatic or mild symptoms; clinical or diagnostic observations only; intervention not indicated. **Grade 2**: Moderate; minimal, local, or noninvasive intervention indicated; limiting age-appropriate instrumental activity of daily living (ADL). **Grade 3**: Severe or medically significant but not immediately life-threatening; hospitalization or prolonged hospitalization indicated; disabling; limiting self-care ADL. **Grade 4**: Life-threatening consequences; urgent intervention indicated. **Grade 5**: Death related to AE.

CTCAE EXAMPLES

Adverse Event	Grade				
	1	2	3	4	5
Blood/ Lymphatic **Anemia**	Hgb < lower limit of normal–10 g/dL	Hgb 8–10 g/dL	Hgb <8 g/dL; transfusion indicated	Life-threatening consequences Urgent intervention indicated	Death
Gastrointestinal **Diarrhea**	Increase of <4 stools/day over baseline Mild ostomy output	Increase of 4–6 stools/day over baseline Moderate ostomy output	Increase of 7 stools/day over baseline Severe ostomy output Hospitalization required	Life-threatening consequences Urgent intervention indicated	Death
General **Fever**	38–39°C (100.4–102.2°F)	>39–40°C (102.3–104°F)	>40°C (>104° F) for less than 24 hrs	>40°C (>104°F) for more than 24 hrs	Death

Adverse Event	Grade 1	2	3	4	5
Infections **UTI**	N/A	Localized; local intervention indicated (topical, antifungal, antiviral)	IV antibiotic, antifungal, antiviral intervention indicated. Radiologic or surgical intervention indicated	Life-threatening consequences Urgent intervention indicated	Death
Investigations **Lipase increased**	>ULN–1.5 times ULN	>1.5–2 times ULN	>2–5 times ULN	>5 times ULN	N/A
Metabolism/ Nutrition **Hyperkalemia**	>ULN–5.5 mmol/L	>5.5–6 mmol/L	>6–7 mmol/L	>7 mmol/L; life-threatening consequences	Death

ULN, Upper limit of normal.

Index

COMMONLY USED ABBREVIATIONS

ABG(s)—arterial blood gas(es)
ACE—angiotensin-converting enzyme
ADHD—attention-deficit hyperactivity disorder
AIDS—acquired immunodeficiency syndrome
ALT—alanine aminotransferase, serum
ANC—absolute neutrophil count
aPTT—activated partial thromboplastin time
AST—aspartate aminotransferase, serum
AV—atrioventricular
bid—twice per day
BMP—basic metabolic panel
B/P—blood pressure
BSA—body surface area
BUN—blood urea nitrogen
CBC—complete blood count
CrCl—creatinine clearance
CNS—central nervous system
CO—cardiac output
COPD—chronic obstructive pulmonary disease
CPK—creatine phosphokinase
CSF—cerebrospinal fluid
CT—computed tomography
CVA—cerebrovascular accident
D_5W—dextrose 5% in water
dL—deciliter
DNA—deoxyribonucleic acid
DVT—deep vein thrombosis
ECG—electrocardiogram
EEG—electroencephalogram
esp.—especially
g—gram
GGT—gamma glutamyl transpeptidase
GI—gastrointestinal
GU—genitourinary
H_2—histamine
Hct—hematocrit
HDL—high-density lipoprotein
HF—heart failure
Hgb—hemoglobin
HIV—human immunodeficiency virus
HMG-CoA—3-hydroxy-3-methylglutaryl-coenzyme A (HMG-CoA) reductase inhibitors (statins)
hr/hrs—hour/hours
HTN—hypertension
I&O—intake and output
ICP—intracranial pressure
IgA—immunoglobulin A
IM—intramuscular
IOP—intraocular pressure
IV—intravenous
K—potassium
kg—kilogram
LDH—lactate dehydrogenase
LDL—low-density lipoprotein
LFT—liver function test
LOC—level of consciousness
MAC—*Mycobacterium avium* complex
MAOI—monoamine oxidase inhibitor
mcg—microgram
mEq—milliequivalent
mg—milligram
MI—myocardial infarction
min—minute(s)
mo/mos—month/months
N/A—not applicable
Na—sodium
NaCl—sodium chloride
NG—nasogastric
NSAID(s)—nonsteroidal anti-inflammatory drug(s)
OD—right eye
OS—left eye
OTC—over the counter
OU—both eyes
PCP—Pneumocystis jiroveci pneumonia
PO—orally, by mouth
prn—as needed
PSA—prostate-specific antigen
pt/pts—patient/patients
PT—prothrombin time
PTCA—percutaneous transluminal coronary angiography
q—every
RBC—red blood cell count
REM—rapid eye movement
RNA—ribonucleic acid
SA—sinoatrial node
subQ—subcutaneous
sec—second(s)
SSRI—selective serotonin reuptake inhibitor
tbsp—tablespoon
tid—three times daily
TNF—tumor necrosis factor
tsp—teaspoon
UTI—urinary tract infection
VLDL—very-low-density lipoprotein
WBC—white blood cell count
wk/wks—week/weeks
yr/yrs—year/years

IV Compatibilities

The IV compatibility table provides data when 2 or more medications are given in a Y-site of administration. The data in this table largely represent physical incompatibilities (e.g., haze, precipitate, change in color). Therapeutic incompatibilities have not been included, so when using the table, professional judgement should be exercised.

C Physically compatible via Y-site administration.
I Physically incompatible.
N Information on compatibility not available or conflicting

	Dextrose 5%	Sodium Chloride	Acyclovir	Amikacin	Amiodarone	Anidulafungin	Argatroban	Azithromycin	Aztreonam	Bivalirudin	Bumetanide	Calcium Gluconate	Cefazolin	Cefepime	Ceftaroline Fosamil	Ceftriaxone	Ciprofloxacin	Clindamycin	Daptomycin	Dexamethasone	Dexmedetomidine	Diltiazem	Diphenhydramine	Dobutamine	Dopamine	Enalapril	Epinephrine	Eptifibatide	Esmolol	Famotidine	Fluconazole	Furosemide	Gentamicin	Granisetron	Heparin	Hydrocortisone	Hydromorphone	Imipenem	Insulin	Labetalol	Levofloxacin	Linezolid	Lorazepam	Magnesium	Mannitol	Meropenem	Methylprednisolone	Metoclopramide	Metronidazole	Midazolam	Morphine	Nicardipine	Nitroglycerin	Nitroprusside	Norepinephrine	Octreotide	Ondansetron	Pantoprazole	Phenylephrine	Piperacillin/Tazobactam	Potassium Chloride	Propofol	Sodium Bicarbonate	Tigecycline	Tobramycin	Vancomycin	Vasopressin
Heparin	C	C	C	I	I	C	N	N	C	C	N	C	C	C	C	C	I	C	C	C	C	C	C	C	C	C	C	N	C	C	C	C	I	C	—	C	C	N	C	C	I	C	C	C	N	C	C	C	C	C	C	I	C	C	C	N	C	I	N	C	C	C	C	C	I	I	C
Hydrocortisone	C	C	C	C	N	C	C	N	C	C	N	C	N	N	C	N	I	C	N	C	N	C	N	N	C	C	C	N	C	C	N	C	N	C	C	—	N	N	N	N	N	C	C	C	N	N	N	N	N	I	C	C	N	N	C	N	C	N	N	C	N	C	C	N	N	N	N
Hydromorphone	C	C	C	C	N	N	N	N	C	C	N	N	I	N	C	N	N	C	N	C	C	C	C	C	C	N	C	N	N	C	N	C	C	C	C	N	—	N	N	C	N	C	C	C	N	N	N	N	C	C	C	C	C	N	C	N	C	I	N	C	N	C	N	N	C	C	N
Imipenem	C	C	C	N	I	C	N	I	C	N	N	N	N	N	N	N	N	N	N	N	N	C	C	N	N	N	N	N	N	C	I	N	N	C	N	N	N	—	C	N	N	C	I	N	N	N	N	N	N	I	N	N	N	N	N	N	C	N	N	N	N	C	I	C	N	N	C
Insulin	N	C	N	N	C	N	N	N	C	N	N	N	C	C	C	N	N	N	N	N	N	N	N	C	I	N	N	N	C	C	N	N	C	N	C	N	N	C	—	I	C	N	N	C	N	C	N	N	N	N	C	N	C	N	N	N	N	C	N	N	N	C	C	N	C	C	C
Labetalol	C	C	N	C	C	N	N	N	N	C	N	C	C	N	I	I	N	C	N	N	C	C	N	C	C	C	C	N	C	C	N	I	C	N	C	N	C	N	I	—	N	C	C	C	N	N	N	N	C	C	C	C	C	C	C	N	N	N	N	N	C	C	N	N	C	C	N
Levofloxacin	C	C	I	C	N	C	N	I	N	C	N	N	N	N	C	N	N	C	C	C	C	N	N	C	C	N	C	N	N	N	N	I	C	N	I	N	C	N	I	N	—	C	C	C	N	N	N	N	N	N	C	N	I	I	N	N	N	N	C	N	C	N	C	N	N	C	N
Linezolid	C	C	C	C	N	C	N	N	C	N	N	C	C	N	N	C	C	C	N	C	C	N	C	C	C	C	N	N	C	C	N	C	C	C	C	C	C	C	N	C	C	—	C	C	C	C	C	N	C	C	C	C	C	N	N	N	C	N	N	C	C	N	C	C	C	C	C
Lorazepam	N	C	C	C	C	N	N	N	I	C	C	N	N	N	C	N	C	N	N	C	C	C	N	C	C	N	C	N	N	C	C	C	C	C	C	C	C	C	N	C	C	C	—	N	N	N	N	N	C	C	C	C	C	N	C	N	I	N	N	C	C	C	N	N	N	C	N
Magnesium	C	C	C	C	I	N	N	N	C	C	N	C	C	N	C	N	I	C	N	N	C	N	N	C	N	C	N	N	C	C	N	N	C	C	C	C	C	N	C	C	C	C	N	—	N	N	N	N	C	N	C	C	N	C	N	N	C	N	N	C	C	C	N	N	C	C	N
Mannitol	—	—	N	C	N	N	N	N	C	C	N	N	N	N	C	N	N	N	N	N	N	N	N	N	N	N	N	N	N	N	N	C	N	N	N	N	N	N	N	N	N	C	N	N	—	N	N	N	N	N	N	N	N	N	N	N	N	I	N	N	C	C	N	N	N	N	N
Meropenem	N	C	I	N	N	C	N	N	N	N	N	C	N	N	N	N	N	N	N	C	N	N	C	N	N	C	N	N	N	N	C	C	C	N	C	N	N	N	C	N	N	C	N	N	N	—	N	C	N	N	C	N	N	N	C	N	I	N	N	N	C	N	N	N	N	C	C
Methylprednisolone	C	C	C	N	C	C	N	N	C	C	N	I	N	C	C	N	I	C	N	N	C	I	N	N	C	C	N	N	N	C	N	N	N	C	C	N	N	N	N	N	N	C	N	N	N	N	—	N	C	C	C	C	N	N	N	N	I	I	N	C	I	I	C	I	N	N	N
Metoclopramide	C	C	C	N	N	N	N	N	C	C	N	I	N	N	C	N	C	C	N	C	C	C	C	N	N	N	N	N	N	C	C	I	N	C	C	N	N	N	N	N	N	N	N	N	N	C	N	—	N	C	C	N	N	N	N	N	C	N	N	C	N	N	N	C	N	N	N
Metronidazole	—	—	C	N	N	C	N	N	I	C	N	N	C	C	C	N	C	N	N	N	C	C	N	N	C	C	N	N	C	N	C	N	N	C	C	N	C	N	N	C	N	C	C	C	N	N	C	N	—	C	C	C	N	N	N	N	N	N	N	C	N	N	N	N	N	N	C
Midazolam	C	C	N	C	C	C	C	N	N	C	I	C	C	I	C	N	C	C	N	I	C	C	C	C	C	N	C	N	N	C	C	C	C	N	C	I	C	I	N	C	N	C	C	N	N	N	C	C	N	—	C	C	C	C	C	N	N	I	N	N	C	C	I	N	C	C	N
Morphine	C	C	C	C	C	C	C	I	C	C	C	N	C	C	C	C	N	C	N	C	C	C	C	C	C	C	C	N	C	C	C	C	C	C	C	C	C	N	C	C	C	C	C	C	N	C	C	C	C	C	—	C	C	C	C	N	C	C	N	C	C	C	C	N	C	C	N
Nicardipine	C	C	N	C	N	N	N	N	C	N	N	C	C	I	N	N	N	C	N	N	N	C	N	C	C	C	C	N	C	C	N	I	C	N	I	C	C	N	N	C	N	C	C	C	N	N	C	N	C	C	C	—	C	C	C	N	N	N	N	N	C	N	N	N	C	C	N
Nitroglycerin	C	C	N	N	C	N	C	N	N	C	N	N	N	N	N	N	N	N	N	N	C	C	N	C	C	C	C	N	C	C	C	I	N	N	C	N	C	N	C	C	I	C	C	N	N	N	N	N	N	C	C	C	—	C	C	N	N	C	N	N	N	C	N	N	N	N	C
Nitroprusside	C	C	N	N	I	N	C	N	N	C	N	N	N	N	N	N	N	N	N	N	C	C	N	C	C	C	C	N	C	C	N	C	N	N	C	N	N	N	N	C	I	N	N	C	N	N	N	N	N	C	C	C	C	—	C	N	N	N	N	N	N	C	N	N	N	N	N
Norepinephrine	C	C	N	C	C	C	C	N	N	C	N	C	N	N	C	N	C	N	N	N	C	C	N	C	C	N	C	N	C	C	N	C	N	N	C	C	C	N	N	C	N	N	C	N	N	C	N	N	N	C	C	C	C	C	—	N	N	C	N	N	C	C	N	N	N	N	C
Octreotide	C	C	N	N	N	N	N	N	N	N	N	N	N	N	N	N	N	N	N	N	N	N	N	N	N	N	N	N	N	N	N	N	N	N	N	N	N	N	N	N	N	N	N	N	N	N	N	N	N	N	N	N	N	N	N	—	N	I	N	N	N	N	N	N	N	N	N
Ondansetron	C	C	I	C	N	N	N	C	C	N	N	N	C	N	C	N	N	C	N	C	C	N	C	N	C	N	N	N	N	C	C	C	C	N	C	C	C	C	N	N	N	C	I	C	N	I	I	C	N	N	C	N	N	N	N	N	—	N	N	C	C	N	I	N	N	C	N
Pantoprazole	C	C	N	I	I	C	N	N	I	N	N	I	C	N	C	C	I	N	N	I	N	N	I	I	C	N	I	N	I	N	I	C	N	N	I	N	I	N	C	N	N	N	N	N	I	N	I	N	N	I	C	N	C	N	C	I	N	—	N	N	C	N	N	N	N	I	C
Phenylephrine	C	C	N	N	C	C	C	N	N	C	N	N	N	N	N	N	N	N	N	N	C	N	N	N	N	N	N	N	N	C	N	I	N	N	N	N	N	N	N	N	C	N	N	N	N	N	N	N	N	N	N	N	N	N	N	N	N	N	—	N	N	N	N	N	N	N	C
Piperacillin/Tazobactam	C	C	I	N	I	C	N	I	C	C	C	C	N	N	N	N	N	C	N	C	C	N	C	I	C	C	N	N	N	I	C	C	N	C	C	C	C	N	N	N	N	C	C	C	N	N	C	C	C	N	C	N	N	N	C	N	C	N	N	—	C	N	C	C	I	I	C
Potassium Chloride	C	C	C	C	C	C	N	I	C	C	N	C	N	C	C	N	C	C	N	C	C	C	C	C	C	C	N	N	C	C	C	C	C	N	C	N	N	N	N	C	C	C	C	C	C	C	I	N	N	C	C	C	N	C	C	N	C	C	N	C	—	C	C	C	N	N	N
Propofol	C	C	C	I	N	N	N	N	C	N	C	C	C	I	C	C	N	C	N	C	C	N	C	C	C	C	C	N	C	C	C	C	I	N	C	C	C	C	C	C	N	N	C	C	C	N	I	N	N	C	C	N	C	C	C	N	N	N	C	N	C	—	C	N	I	C	N
Sodium Bicarbonate	C	C	C	C	I	I	N	N	C	C	N	C	N	N	C	C	I	C	N	C	C	I	N	N	N	N	I	N	C	C	N	C	N	C	C	C	N	I	C	N	C	C	N	N	N	N	C	N	N	I	C	N	N	N	N	N	I	N	N	C	C	C	—	N	N	C	C
Tigecycline	C	C	N	C	N	N	N	C	N	N	N	N	N	I	N	C	C	N	N	N	N	N	N	C	C	N	C	N	N	N	C	N	C	N	C	N	N	C	N	N	N	C	N	N	N	N	I	C	N	N	N	N	N	N	N	N	N	N	N	C	C	N	N	—	C	C	N
Tobramycin	C	C	C	N	C	C	N	I	C	C	N	C	N	I	C	N	C	C	N	N	C	C	N	N	N	N	N	N	C	N	C	C	N	C	I	N	C	N	C	C	N	C	N	C	N	N	N	N	N	C	C	C	N	N	N	N	N	N	N	I	N	I	N	C	—	N	N
Vancomycin	C	C	C	C	C	C	N	N	C	I	N	C	I	C	N	I	N	N	N	N	C	C	N	N	N	C	N	N	C	C	C	N	N	C	I	N	C	N	C	C	C	C	C	C	N	C	N	N	N	C	C	C	N	N	N	N	C	I	N	I	N	C	C	C	N	—	N
Vasopressin	—	C	N	N	C	N	C	N	N	N	N	N	N	N	C	N	C	N	N	N	N	C	N	C	C	N	C	N	N	N	C	I	C	N	C	N	N	C	C	N	N	C	N	N	N	C	N	N	C	N	N	N	C	N	C	N	N	C	C	C	N	N	C	N	N	N	—

IV Compatibilities

The IV compatibility table provides data when 2 or more medications are given in a Y-site of administration. The data in this table largely represent physical incompatibilities (e.g., haze, precipitate, change in color). Therapeutic incompatibilities have not been included, so when using the table, professional judgement should be exercised.

C Physically compatible via Y-site administration.
I Physically incompatible.
N Information on compatibility not available or conflicting

	Dextrose 5%	Sodium Chloride	Acyclovir	Amikacin	Amiodarone	Anidulafungin	Argatroban	Azithromycin	Aztreonam	Bivalirudin	Bumetanide	Calcium Gluconate	Cefazolin	Cefepime	Ceftaroline Fosamil	Ceftriaxone	Ciprofloxacin	Clindamycin	Daptomycin	Dexamethasone	Dexmedetomidine	Diltiazem	Diphenhydramine	Dobutamine	Dopamine	Enalapril	Epinephrine	Eptifibatide	Esmolol	Famotidine	Fluconazole	Furosemide	Gentamicin	Granisetron	Heparin	Hydrocortisone	Hydromorphone	Imipenem	Insulin	Labetalol	Levofloxacin	Linezolid	Lorazepam	Magnesium	Mannitol	Meropenem	Methylprednisolone	Metoclopramide	Metronidazole	Midazolam	Morphine	Nicardipine	Nitroglycerin	Nitroprusside	Norepinephrine	Octreotide	Ondansetron	Pantoprazole	Phenylephrine	Piperacillin/Tazobactam	Potassium Chloride	Propofol	Sodium Bicarbonate	Tigecycline	Tobramycin	Vancomycin	Vasopressin
Acyclovir	C	C	—	C	N	C	N	N	I	N	N	N	C	N	C	C	N	C	N	C	N	I	C	I	I	N	N	N	N	C	C	N	C	C	C	C	C	C	N	N	I	C	C	C	N	I	C	C	C	N	C	N	N	N	N	N	I	N	N	I	C	C	C	N	C	C	N
Amikacin	C	C	C	—	C	C	N	I	C	C	N	C	C	C	C	C	C	C	C	C	C	C	C	N	N	C	C	N	C	N	C	C	N	C	I	C	C	N	N	C	C	C	C	C	C	N	N	N	N	C	C	C	N	N	C	N	C	I	N	N	C	I	C	C	N	C	N
Amiodarone	C	C	N	C	—	N	I	N	N	N	N	C	I	N	C	C	C	C	N	N	C	N	N	C	C	N	C	C	C	C	C	C	C	N	I	N	N	I	C	C	N	N	C	I	N	N	C	N	N	C	C	N	C	I	C	N	N	I	C	I	C	N	I	N	C	C	C
Anidulafungin	C	C	C	C	N	—	N	N	N	N	N	N	C	C	N	C	C	C	N	C	N	N	N	C	C	N	C	N	N	C	C	C	C	N	C	C	N	C	N	N	C	C	N	N	N	C	C	N	C	C	C	N	N	N	C	N	N	C	C	C	C	N	I	N	C	C	N
Argatroban	C	C	N	N	I	N	—	N	N	N	N	N	N	N	N	N	N	N	N	N	N	C	C	C	C	N	N	C	N	N	N	C	N	N	N	C	N	N	N	N	N	N	N	N	N	N	N	N	N	C	C	N	C	C	C	N	N	N	C	N	N	N	N	N	N	N	C
Azithromycin	C	C	N	I	N	N	N	—	I	C	N	N	N	N	C	I	I	I	N	N	C	N	N	N	N	N	N	N	N	I	N	I	I	N	N	N	N	I	N	N	I	N	N	N	N	N	N	N	N	N	I	N	N	N	N	N	C	N	N	I	I	N	N	C	I	N	N
Aztreonam	C	C	I	C	N	N	N	N	—	C	C	N	C	N	N	C	C	C	C	C	C	C	C	C	C	C	N	N	N	C	C	C	C	C	C	C	C	C	C	N	N	C	I	C	C	N	C	C	I	N	C	C	N	N	N	N	C	I	N	C	C	C	C	N	C	C	N
Bivalirudin	C	C	N	C	I	N	N	C	C	—	C	C	C	C	N	C	C	C	N	C	N	C	C	C	C	C	C	C	C	C	C	C	C	N	C	C	C	N	N	C	C	N	C	C	C	N	C	C	C	C	C	N	C	C	C	N	N	N	C	C	C	N	C	N	C	I	N
Bumetanide	C	C	N	N	N	N	N	N	C	C	—	N	N	N	C	N	N	N	N	N	C	C	N	I	N	N	N	N	N	N	N	C	N	C	N	N	N	N	N	N	N	N	C	N	N	N	N	N	N	I	C	N	N	N	N	N	N	N	N	C	I	N	N	N	N	N	N
Calcium Gluconate	C	C	N	C	C	N	N	N	C	C	N	—	C	N	C	I	C	N	N	N	C	N	N	C	N	C	C	N	N	C	I	C	N	C	C	C	N	N	N	C	N	C	N	C	N	C	I	I	N	C	N	C	N	N	C	N	N	I	N	C	C	C	C	N	C	C	N
Cefazolin	C	C	C	C	I	C	N	N	C	C	N	C	—	N	N	N	N	C	N	N	C	C	N	N	N	C	N	N	C	C	C	N	I	C	C	N	I	N	C	C	N	C	N	C	N	N	N	N	C	C	C	C	N	N	N	N	C	C	N	N	N	C	N	N	N	I	N
Cefepime	C	C	N	C	N	C	N	N	N	C	N	N	N	—	N	N	N	C	N	N	C	N	N	I	C	N	N	N	N	N	C	C	C	C	C	N	N	N	C	N	N	N	N	N	N	N	C	N	C	I	C	I	N	N	N	N	N	N	N	N	C	I	N	I	I	C	N
Ceftaroline Fosamil	C	C	C	C	C	N	N	C	N	N	C	C	N	N	—	N	C	N	N	C	N	C	C	I	C	C	N	N	N	C	C	C	C	C	C	C	C	N	C	I	C	N	C	C	C	N	C	C	C	C	C	N	N	N	C	N	C	C	N	N	C	C	C	N	C	N	C
Ceftriaxone	C	C	C	C	C	C	N	I	C	C	N	I	N	N	N	—	N	I	C	N	C	C	N	N	N	N	N	N	N	C	I	N	N	C	C	N	N	N	N	I	N	C	N	N	N	N	N	N	N	N	C	N	N	N	N	N	N	C	N	N	N	C	C	C	N	I	C
Ciprofloxacin	C	C	N	C	C	C	N	I	C	C	N	C	N	N	C	N	—	I	N	I	C	C	C	C	C	N	N	N	N	N	N	I	C	C	I	I	N	N	N	N	N	C	C	I	N	N	I	C	C	C	N	N	N	N	C	N	N	I	N	N	C	N	I	C	C	N	C
Clevidipine	C	C	N	N	N	N	N	N	N	N	N	N	N	N	N	N	N	N	N	N	N	N	N	N	N	N	N	N	N	N	N	N	N	N	N	N	N	N	N	N	N	N	N	N	N	N	N	N	N	N	N	N	N	N	N	N	N	N	N	N	N	N	N	N	N	N	N
Clindamycin	C	C	C	C	C	C	N	I	C	C	N	N	C	C	C	I	I	—	N	N	C	C	N	N	N	C	N	N	C	N	I	N	C	C	C	C	C	N	N	C	C	C	N	C	N	N	C	C	N	C	C	C	N	N	N	N	C	N	N	C	C	C	C	N	C	N	N
Daptomycin	I	C	N	C	N	N	N	N	C	N	N	N	N	N	N	C	N	N	—	N	N	N	N	N	C	N	N	N	N	N	C	N	C	N	C	N	N	N	N	N	C	N	N	N	N	N	N	N	N	N	N	N	N	N	N	N	N	N	N	N	N	N	N	N	N	N	N
Dexamethasone	C	C	C	C	N	C	N	N	C	C	N	N	N	N	C	N	I	N	N	—	C	N	I	N	N	N	N	N	N	C	C	N	N	C	C	C	C	N	N	N	C	C	C	N	N	C	N	C	N	I	C	N	N	N	N	N	C	N	C	C	C	C	C	N	N	N	N
Dexmedetomidine	C	C	N	C	C	N	N	C	C	N	C	C	C	C	N	C	C	C	N	C	—	C	C	C	C	N	C	N	C	C	C	C	C	C	C	N	C	N	N	C	C	C	C	C	N	N	C	C	C	C	C	N	C	C	C	N	C	N	C	C	C	C	C	N	C	C	N
Diltiazem	C	C	I	C	N	N	C	N	C	C	C	N	C	N	C	C	C	C	N	N	C	—	N	C	N	N	C	N	C	N	C	I	C	N	C	C	C	C	N	C	N	N	C	N	N	N	I	C	C	C	C	C	C	C	C	N	N	N	N	N	C	N	I	N	C	C	C
Diphenhydramine	C	C	C	C	N	N	C	N	C	C	N	N	N	N	C	N	C	N	N	I	C	N	—	N	N	N	N	N	N	C	C	N	N	C	C	N	C	C	N	N	N	C	N	N	N	C	N	C	N	C	C	N	N	N	N	N	C	I	N	C	C	C	N	N	N	N	N
Dobutamine	C	C	I	N	C	C	C	N	C	C	I	C	N	C	I	N	C	N	N	N	C	C	N	—	C	C	C	N	N	C	C	I	N	C	C	N	C	N	C	C	C	C	C	C	N	N	N	N	N	C	C	C	C	C	C	N	N	I	N	I	C	C	N	C	N	N	C
Dopamine	C	C	I	N	C	C	C	N	C	C	N	N	N	C	C	N	C	N	C	N	C	C	N	C	—	C	C	N	C	C	C	I	N	C	C	C	C	N	I	C	C	C	C	N	N	N	C	N	C	C	C	C	C	C	C	N	C	C	N	C	C	C	N	C	N	N	C
Enalapril	C	C	N	C	N	N	N	N	C	C	N	C	C	N	C	N	N	C	N	N	C	N	N	C	C	—	N	N	C	C	N	N	C	C	C	C	N	N	N	C	N	C	N	C	N	C	C	N	C	N	C	C	C	C	N	N	N	N	N	C	C	C	N	N	N	C	N
Epinephrine	C	C	N	C	C	C	N	N	N	C	N	C	N	N	N	N	N	N	N	N	C	C	N	C	C	N	—	N	N	N	N	C	N	N	C	C	C	N	N	C	C	N	C	N	N	N	N	N	N	C	C	C	C	C	C	N	N	I	N	N	N	C	I	C	N	N	C
Eptifibatide	C	C	N	N	C	N	C	N	N	C	N	N	N	N	N	N	N	N	N	N	N	N	N	N	N	N	N	—	N	N	N	N	N	N	N	N	N	N	N	N	N	N	N	N	N	N	N	N	N	N	N	N	N	N	N	N	N	N	N	N	N	N	N	N	N	N	N
Esmolol	C	C	N	C	C	N	N	N	N	C	N	N	C	N	N	N	N	C	N	N	C	C	N	N	C	C	N	N	—	C	N	I	C	N	C	C	N	N	C	C	N	C	N	C	N	N	N	N	C	N	C	C	C	C	C	N	N	I	N	N	C	C	C	N	C	C	N
Famotidine	C	C	C	N	C	C	N	I	C	C	N	C	C	N	C	C	N	N	N	C	C	N	C	C	C	C	N	N	C	—	C	C	C	C	C	C	C	C	C	C	N	C	C	C	N	N	C	C	N	C	C	C	C	C	C	N	N	N	C	I	C	C	C	N	N	C	N
Fluconazole	C	C	C	C	C	C	N	N	C	C	N	I	C	C	C	I	N	I	C	C	C	C	C	C	C	N	N	N	N	C	—	I	C	C	C	N	N	I	N	N	N	N	C	N	N	C	N	C	C	C	C	N	C	N	N	N	C	I	N	C	C	C	N	C	C	C	C
Furosemide	C	C	N	C	C	C	C	I	C	C	C	C	N	C	C	N	I	N	N	N	C	I	N	I	I	N	C	N	I	C	I	—	I	C	C	C	C	N	N	I	I	C	C	N	C	C	N	I	N	C	C	I	I	C	C	N	C	C	I	C	C	C	C	N	C	N	I
Gentamicin	C	C	C	N	C	C	N	I	C	C	N	N	I	C	C	N	C	C	C	N	C	C	N	N	N	C	N	N	C	C	C	I	—	C	I	N	C	N	C	C	C	C	C	C	N	C	N	N	N	C	C	C	N	N	N	N	C	N	N	N	C	I	N	C	N	N	C
Granisetron	C	C	C	C	N	N	N	N	C	N	C	C	C	C	C	C	C	C	N	C	C	N	C	C	C	C	N	N	N	C	C	C	C	—	C	C	C	C	N	N	N	C	C	C	N	N	C	C	C	N	C	N	N	N	N	N	N	N	N	C	N	N	C	N	C	N	N